GEORGE WASHINGTON UNIVERSITY
PAUL HIMMELFARB HEALTH SCIENCES LIBRARY
2300 EYE STREET, N. W.
WASHINGTON, D. C. 20037

DISCARDED

AF327162

GEORGE WASHINGTON UNIVERSITY
PAUL HIMMELFARB HEALTH SCIENCES LIBRARY
2300 EYE STREET, N. W.
WASHINGTON, D. C. 20037

Musculoskeletal Disorders of the

Lower Extremities

Musculoskeletal Disorders of the Lower Extremities

Lawrence M. Oloff, D.P.M.

Vice President and Dean for Academic Affairs
Professor, Department of Surgery
Co-Director, Special Problems Clinic
California College of Podiatric Medicine
San Francisco, California

Clinical Assistant Professor
Podiatric Section
Division of Orthopedic Surgery
Department of Functional Restoration
Stanford University Medical Center
Palo Alto, California

Private Practice
Sports Orthopedic and Rehabilitation
Menlo Park, California

W.B. SAUNDERS COMPANY
A Division of Harcourt Brace & Company
Philadelphia   London   Toronto   Montreal   Sydney   Tokyo

W.B. SAUNDERS COMPANY
A Division of
Harcourt Brace & Company

The Curtis Center
Independence Square West
Philadelphia, Pennsylvania 19106

Library of Congress Cataloging-in-Publication Data

Musculoskeletal disorders of the lower extremities / [edited by]
Lawrence M. Oloff.

    p.   cm.

ISBN 0–7216–3716–7

1. Extremities, Lower—Diseases.   2. Musculoskeletal system—
    Diseases.   I. Oloff, Lawrence M.

[DNLM: 1. Musculoskeletal Diseases. 2. Leg. WE 850 M985 1994]

RC951.M87 1994

617.5′8—dc20

DNLM/DLC   93-7250

Musculoskeletal Disorders of the Lower Extremities   ISBN 0–7216–3716–7

Copyright © 1994 by W.B. Saunders Company

All rights reserved. No part of this publication may be reproduced or transmitted in any form or by any means, electronic or mechanical, including photocopy, recording, or any information storage and retrieval system, without permission in writing from the publisher.

Printed in the United States of America.

Last digit is the print number: 9   8   7   6   5   4   3   2   1

RC
51
187
994

Contributors

Todd S. Anhalt, M.D.
Clinical Associate Professor of Dermatology; Deputy Chief, Dermatology Services, Stanford University Medical Center, Stanford; Chief of Dermatology Clinics, Palo Alto Veterans Administration Medical Center, Palo Alto, California
Cutaneous Signs of Systemic Disease

Richard Berenter, D.P.M.
Associate Professor, California College of Podiatric Medicine, San Francisco, California
Biomechanics of Musculoskeletal Diseases

Ann Gabrielle Bergman, M.D.
Assistant Professor of Radiology, Stanford University; Assistant Professor of Radiology and Chief, Musculoskeletal Imaging Section, Radiology Department, Stanford University Medical Center, Stanford, California
Imaging of Musculoskeletal Tumors

Allan Bernstein, D.P.M.
Director of Podiatric Education, Western Medical Center, Santa Ana/Anaheim; Clinical Professor of Podiatric Surgery, California College of Podiatric Medicine; Chief, Department of Podiatric Surgery, West Medical Center, Santa Ana, California
Radiographic Evaluations of Bone and Joint Infections

Richard T. Bouché, D.P.M.
Member, Residency Training Committee, Fifth Avenue Medical Center; Attending Staff, Virginia Mason Sports Medicine Center and Virginia Mason Hospital, Seattle, Washington
Athletic Injuries
Compartment Syndromes

Albert Burns, D.P.M.
Chairman and Professor, Department of Podiatric Surgery, California College of Podiatric Medicine; Chief of Podiatric Surgery, Pacific Coast Hospital, San Francisco, California
Forefoot Implant Arthroplasty

Walter A. Carpenter, Ph.D., M.D.
Assistant Professor of Radiology, Emory University School of Medicine; Radiologist, Emory University Hospital, Atlanta, Georgia
Radiologic Manifestations of Arthritides Involving the Foot

Paul D. Dayton, D.P.M.
Clinical Assistant Professor, California College of Podiatric Medicine, San Francisco; Staff, Department of Surgery, Santa Teresa Community Hospital, San Jose, California
Compartment Syndromes

Michael S. Downey, D.P.M.
Chairman and Associate Professor, Department of Surgery, Pennsylvania College of Podiatric Medicine; Chairman, Division of Podiatric Surgery, Presbyterian Medical Center of Philadelphia, Philadelphia, Pennsylvania; Faculty, The Podiatry Institute, Tucker, Georgia
Surgical Treatment of Peripheral Nerve Entrapment Syndromes

Charles A. Eiser, D.P.M.
Clinical Assistant Professor, Division of Orthopedic Surgery, Stanford University School of Medicine, Palo Alto; California College of Podiatric Medicine, San Francisco; and Dr. William Scholl College of Podiatric Medicine, Chicago; Chief, Podiatric Section and Residency Director, Department of Veterans Affairs Medical Center, Livermore; Asso-

ciate Residency Director, Department of Veterans Affairs Medical Center, Palo Alto, California
Connective Tissue Diseases

Flair David Goldman, D.P.M.

Associate Clinical Professor, Department of Basic Medical Science, California College of Podiatric Medicine, San Francisco; Chief, Division of Podiatric Surgery, Department of Orthopedic Surgery, Kaiser Hospital, Santa Clara, California
Afflictions of Nerves and Muscles

Jeffrey Lee Halbrecht, M.D.

Director of Sports Medicine, California College of Podiatric Medicine; Assistant Clinical Professor, Graduate Department of Physical Therapy, University of California, San Francisco, School of Medicine; Medical Director, Women's Pro Ski Tour; Attending Physician, California Pacific Medical Center, Mt. Zion Hospital, and Pacific Coast Hospital, San Francisco, California
The Kinetic Chain: Back, Hip, and Knee Dysfunction in Relation to the Foot

Carolyn K. Harvey, D.P.M.

Associate Professor, Department of Podiatric Medicine, California College of Podiatric Medicine; Staff Member and Service Chief of Podiatric Medicine, Pacific Coast Hospital; San Francisco, California
HIV Infection and AIDS

Geoffrey Heard, D.P.M.

Visiting Professor, California College of Podiatric Medicine, San Francisco, California
Bone and Cartilage: Physiology and Repair

Vincent J. Hetherington, D.P.M.

Academic Dean and Professor, Department of Surgery, Ohio College of Podiatric Medicine, Cleveland, Ohio
Biomaterials: Soft Tissue and Bone Reaction to Implants

Juerg Hodler, M.D.

Assistant Professor, University of Zurich; Chief, Musculoskeletal Radiology Section, Balgrist Clinic, Zurich, Switzerland
Cross-Sectional Imaging

Douglas J. Ichikawa, D.P.M.

Active Staff and Member, Residency Training Committee, Fifth Avenue Hospital; Active Staff, Virginia Mason Hospital, Seattle, Washington
Athletic Injuries

Stephen Jackson, M.D.

Staff, Department of Anesthesiology, Good Samaritan Hospital, San Jose, California
Anesthesia Considerations

Richard M. Jay, D.P.M.

Director of Pediatrics and Professor of Foot and Ankle Orthopaedics, Pennsylvania College of Podiatric Medicine; Director of Foot and Ankle Surgical Residency Programs, The Graduate Hospital, Philadelphia, Pennsylvania
Congenital Deformities

William M. Jenkin, D.P.M.

Professor, Department of Surgery, and Co-Director, Special Problems Clinic, California College of Podiatric Medicine, San Francisco; Active Staff, Pacific Coast Hospital; Courtesy Staff, California Pacific Medical Center and Marin General Hospital, Stanford, California
Central Metatarsophalangeal Joint Arthrosis: Evaluation and Surgical Management

Warren S. Joseph, D.P.M.

Associate Professor of Medicine and Chief, Infectious Diseases, Pennsylvania College of Podiatric Medicine, Philadelphia, Pennsylvania
Septic Arthritis

Thomas J. Kaschak, D.P.M.

Clinical Assistant Professor, Department of Functional Restoration, Stanford University Medical Center, Palo Alto; Vice Chairman, Department of Surgery, Podiatric Section, San Jose Medical Center, San Jose, California
The Inflammatory Reaction
Laboratory Testing in Arthritic Disease
Pharmacologic Management of Inflammatory Joint Disease

Daniel K. Kosai, D.P.M.

Assistant Professor, Department of Biomechanics, California College of Podiatric Medicine, San Francisco; Staff, Doctor's Hospital of Pinole and Brookside Hospital, San Pablo, California
Biomechanics of Musculoskeletal Diseases

Barbara M. Kriz, Ph.D.

Professor of Anatomy and Chair, Department of Basic Sciences, California College of Podiatric Medicine, San Francisco, California
Articular Anatomy and Histology

Wilfred Laine, D.P.M.

Clinical Professor, Division of Orthopaedics, Stanford University School of Medicine, Palo Alto; Clinical Associate Professor, California College of Podiatric Medicine, San Francisco; Chief, Podiatric Section, Stanford University Medical Center; Chief, Podiatric Section, Surgical Service, Department of Veterans Affairs Medical Center, Palo Alto; Surgical Staff, Stanford University Hospital, Palo Alto, California
Seronegative Spondyloarthropathies

George Lampe, M.D.

Assistant Clinical Professor, Department of Anesthesiology, University of California, San Francisco; Staff Anesthesiologist, Good Samaritan Hospital, San Jose, California
Anesthesia Considerations

Christopher J. Lamy, D.P.M.

Staff, Southwest Washington Medical Center; Attending Staff, Good Samaritan Hospital and Medical Center and Emanuel Hospital and Medical Center; Private Practice, Vancouver, Washington
Septic Arthritis

Richard O. Lundeen, D.P.M.

Director, Residency Training, and Director, Regional Foot and Ankle Center, Midwest Medical Center, Indianapolis, Indiana
Role of Arthroscopy in the Treatment of Arthritic Ankle Disorders

Kieran T. Mahan, M.S., D.P.M.

Vice President for Academic Affairs and Dean; Professor, Department of Surgery, Pennsylvania College of Podiatric Medicine; Staff, Presbyterian Medical Center, Philadelphia, Pennsylvania
Joint Preservation Techniques in Hallux Limitus/Rigidus Repair

James L. McGuire, M.D.

Associate Dean for Graduate Medical Education and Clinical Affairs and Associate Professor of Medicine, Stanford University School of Medicine; Chief of Staff, Stanford University Hospital, Palo Alto, California
Seronegative Spondyloarthropathies

Jack L. Morris, D.P.M.

Professor and Chairman, Department of Biomechanics, California College of Podiatric Medicine; Staff, Pacific Coast Hospital, San Francisco, California
Biomechanics of Musculoskeletal Diseases

David Mullens, D.P.M.

Clinical Associate Professor, Department of Functional Restoration, Stanford University School of Medicine; Attending Surgeon, Stanford University Hospital; Private Practice, Palo Alto, California
Vascular Manifestations of Articular Disease

Brad L. Naylor, D.P.M.

Clinical Assistant Professor, Section of Podiatric Surgery, Division of Functional Restoration, Stanford University Hospital/Clinics; Clinical Associate Professor of Podiatric Medicine, California College of Podiatric Medicine, San Francisco; Chief of Podiatric Surgery, St. Luke's Hospital; Active Staff, Davies Medical Center, Pacific Coast Hospital, Stanford University Hospital, Stanford, and Veterans Administration Medical Center, Palo Alto, California
Contrast Radiography

Jon Nordgaard, D.P.M., P.T.

Private Practice, Santa Cruz Medical Clinic, Santa Cruz, California
Rehabilitation of the Arthritic Patient

Robert G. O'Keefe, D.P.M.

Senior Attending Medical Staff, Columbus Hospital of Chicago; Attending Medical Staff, Lutheran General Hospital; Consultant, Lutheran General Medical Group, Park Ridge, Illinois
Surgical Management of Soft Tissue Tumors

Lawrence M. Oloff, D.P.M.

Vice President and Dean for Academic Affairs, Professor, Department of Surgery, and Co-Director, Special Problems Clinic, California College of Podiatric Medicine, San Francisco; Clinical Assistant Professor, Department of Functional Restoration, Stanford University Medical Center, Palo Alto; Private Practice, Sports Orthopedic and Rehabilitation, Menlo Park; Podiatric Consultant, Varsity Teams, Stanford University, Stanford, and the San Francisco 49ers, San Francisco, California
Tendon Dysfunction

Jeffrey C. Page, D.P.M.

Associate Dean for Clinical Affairs and Associate Professor, Departments of Podiatric Medicine and Surgery, California College of Podiatric Medicine, San Francisco, California
Avascular Necrosis of Bone

Steven J. Palladino, D.P.M.

Professor, Department of Podiatric Surgery, California College of Podiatric Medicine, San Francisco; Attending Staff, Department of Orthopedics, Kaiser Permanente Medical Center, Santa Rosa, California
The Diabetic Foot
Post-Traumatic Painful Ankle

Divyang Patel, D.P.M.

Visiting Fellow, Califorina College of Podiatric Medicine, San Francisco, California
Crystalline Deposition Disease

Irving Pikscher, D.P.M.

Academic Director, Podiatric Surgical Residency, Edgewater Medical Center; Staff, Little Company of Mary Hospital, Evergreen Park, and Edgewater Medical Center, Chicago; Academic Director of Podiatric Surgical Residency Program, Suburban Hospital, Hinsdale, Illinois
Forefoot Arthroplasty

Donald Resnick, M.D.

Professor of Radiology, University of California, San Diego; Chief of Radiology, Department of Veterans Affairs Medical Center, San Diego, California
Radiologic Manifestations of Arthritides Involving the Foot

Jon R. Risser, D.P.M.

Co-Residency Director, Kaiser Hospital, Santa Clara, California
Afflictions of Nerves and Muscles

Richard D. Roth, D.P.M.

Adjunct Faculty, New York College of Podiatric Medicine, New York City, New York; Active Staff and Trustee, Palm Beach–Martin County Medical Center, Jupiter; Active Staff, Palm Beach Gardens Medical Center, Palm Beach Gardens
Rheumatoid Arthritis
Glucocorticoids: Use in the Management of Rheumatic Disorders

David J. Sartoris, M.D.

Associate Professor of Radiology, University of California, San Diego, School of Medicine; Chief, Quantitative Bone Densitometry, University of California, San Diego, Medical Center, San Diego, California
Cross-Sectional Imaging

John M. Schuberth, D.P.M.

Attending Staff, Department of Orthopedic Surgery, Kaiser Foundation Hospital, San Francisco, California
Fusions in the Arthritic Patient
Tendon Transfers

Mark E. Schweitzer, M.D.

Assistant Professor of Radiology, Jefferson Medical College; Staff, Thomas Jefferson University Hospital, Philadelphia, Pennsylvania
Cross-Sectional Imaging

Joyce M. Senick, D.P.M.

Staff, Leonard Hospital, Albany, and Private Practice, Malta, New York
Biomaterials: Soft Tissue and Bone Reaction to Implants

Donald Silcox, M.D.

Professor of Clinical Medicine, Division of Rheumatology, Stanford University Medical School; Staff, Stanford University Hospital, Palo Alto, and Department of Internal Medicine, Good Samaritan Hospital, San Jose, California
Anesthesia Considerations

James Stavosky, D.P.M.

Chairman and Associate Professor, Department of Podiatric Medicine, California College of Podiatric Medicine, San Francisco, California
Crystalline Deposition Disease

Mark G. Stein, M.B.B.Ch., B.Sc.

Assistant Clinical Professor of Radiology, University of California, Irvine; Staff Radiologist, Western Medical Center, Santa Ana, California
Radiographic Evaluations of Bone and Joint Infections

John J. Stienstra, D.P.M.

Attending Podiatrist, The Permanente Medical Group, Union City, California
Septic Arthritis

Richard G. Stiles, M.D.
Assistant Professor of Radiology, Emory University School of Medicine; Radiologist, Emory University Hospital, Atlanta, Georgia
Radiologic Manifestations of Arthritides Involving the Foot

Gideon Strich, M.D.
Assistant Clinical Professor, Department of Radiologic Sciences, University of California, Irvine; Staff Radiologist, Western Medical Center and West Coast Radiology Center, Santa Ana, California
Radiographic Evaluations of Bone and Joint Infections

Katrina Sullivan, D.P.M.
Auxiliary Faculty, Department of Medicine, University of Washington; Staff Podiatrist, Sports Medicine Clinic; Director, Foot Clinic and Pioneer Square Clinic; Staff, University of Washington Medical Center, Seattle, Washington
Athletic Injuries

Marley M. Taylor, D.P.M.
Clinical Instructor, Division of Orthopedic Surgery, Stanford University School of Medicine; Clinical Assistant Professor, California College of Podiatric Medicine, San Francisco; Dr. William Scholl College of Podiatric Medicine, Chicago; Associate Residency Director, Department of Veterans Affairs Medical Center, Livermore; Faculty Consultant, Division of Orthopedic Surgery, Stanford University School of Medicine, and Department of Veterans Affairs Medical Center, Palo Alto, California
Connective Tissue Diseases

John V. Vanore, D.P.M.
Staff, Trinity Hospital, Humana Hospital—Michael Reese, and Doctors Hospital of Hyde Park; Private Practice, Chicago, Illinois
Forefoot Arthroplasty
First Metatarsophalangeal Joint Arthrodesis

Craig Wargon, D.P.M.
Co-Residency Director and Staff Podiatrist, Kaiser Hospital, Santa Clara, California
Afflictions of Nerves and Muscles

Michael S. Weingarten, M.D.
Clinical Associate Professor of Surgery, University of Pennsylvania; Chief, Division of Vascular Surgery, The Graduate Hospital, Philadelphia, Pennsylvania
Advances in Wound Healing

Pamela K. Westfahl, Ph.D.
Associate Professor, Department of Basic Sciences, California College of Podiatric Medicine, San Francisco, California
Physiology of Pain

Bernard R. Wilcosky, Jr., M.D.
Chairman, Department of Anesthesiology, and Associate Medical Director, Sequoia Pain Treatment Clinic, Sequoia Hospital District, Redwood City, California
Medical Management of Chronic Pain

Bennett G. Zier, M.D.
Chairman and Professor of General Medicine, California College of Podiatric Medicine; Associate Clinical Professor, Internal Medicine, University of California, San Francisco; Chief of Medicine, Pacific Coast Hospital; Attending Staff, University of California, San Francisco/Mt. Zion Medical Center, San Francisco, California
Perioperative Considerations

Acknowledgments

I want to express my sincere appreciation to all the contributors, who gave countless hours of their time in the preparation of this text. I also thank the families of the contributors for letting me borrow from their already limited time.

In this same vein, I offer my deepest thanks to my family. This book is dedicated to them: To my wife Linda, for her unending love and support, and for her keeping the home together when projects such as this prevented me from doing my part. To my children Nicole, Dana, and Jacqueline, who always seem to make do with all too little time.

To my parents, whose love, support, and guidance instilled in me the desire to strive for the very best. It is with the deepest regrets that my father was not alive for this project, for my chosen profession was realized through his vision.

I would also like to thank Larry McGrew, Rosanne Hallowell, Lisette Bralow, and others at W. B. Saunders, whose efforts ultimately resulted in the completion of this text. And thanks to Tanya Chandler and Kristin Greene for their administrative assistance.

I am also appreciative of the encouragement that I received from the educational community at the California College of Podiatric Medicine and from my colleagues at Sports Orthopedic and Rehabilitation.

LAWRENCE M. OLOFF

Preface

Foot specialists need to concern themselves with the multitude of systemic diseases that manifest in the lower extremities, as well as those conditions that are peculiar to the foot and ankle. This first edition of *Musculoskeletal Disorders of the Lower Extremities* was created with this thought in mind. As a result, the authorship comprises a variety of specialists, each of whom lends expertise in the treatment of conditions of the foot and ankle. The intent was to provide a vast array of information, yet to do so in a logical progression, and to focus on the information that would most likely interest the clinician. This textbook was compiled with all these purposes in mind.

The textbook is divided into several sections. The emphasis is on bone and joint pathology, and the clinician is the target audience. The Basic Science section in itself exemplifies this approach and sets the tone for much of the book. Building blocks are laid in the Basic Science section, such as with the chapter entitled *The Inflammatory Reaction,* whereby a later chapter on the *Pharmacologic Management of Inflammatory Joint Disease* may be better appreciated. Traditional subject matter is discussed as with most standard texts, but the information is tipped towards a clinician's perspective, such as in the chapter on *Bone and Cartilage: Physiology and Repair.* Perhaps somewhat unconventional subjects such as biomechanics and implant reaction are dealt with in the initial section as well. This reflects a growing trend to define basic sciences in a more practical sense.

Later sections attempt to consolidate information that is usually only retrieved by referring to several textbooks. The presentation of topics such as the inflammatory arthritides emphasizes information that the evolving foot and ankle specialist will need to know or refer to on occasion. Present times and predictive future medical needs are reflected in the chapter on *HIV Infection and AIDS.* Chapters in the section on Radiologic Evaluation emphasize the practical application of the modern age of diagnostic radiology. Chapters in the section on Surgical Management focus in synopsis form on the common techniques performed on the patient with musculoskeletal disorders. Finally, a section on Chronic Pain Syndromes illustrates the trend to greater emphasis on these disorders.

It is hoped that this textbook fulfills its practical intents. It is unlikely that this textbook will gather dust on a shelf. This work should prove to be a valuable resource to podiatric medical and surgical specialists on a practical, day-to-day basis. It is also intended for other clinicians actively involved in the management of foot and ankle disorders.

LAWRENCE M. OLOFF

Contents

SECTION ONE

Basic Science, 1

CHAPTER 1
Articular Anatomy and Histology, 1
Barbara M. Kriz, Ph.D.

CHAPTER 2
Bone and Cartilage: Physiology and Repair, 15
Geoffrey Heard, D.P.M.

CHAPTER 3
The Inflammatory Reaction, 34
Thomas J. Kaschak, D.P.M.

CHAPTER 4
Advances in Wound Healing, 52
Michael S. Weingarten, M.D.

CHAPTER 5
Biomechanics, 65

PART I
Biomechanics of Musculoskeletal Diseases, 65
Jack L. Morris, D.P.M., Richard Berenter, D.P.M., and Daniel K. Kosai, D.P.M.

PART II
The Kinetic Chain: Back, Hip, and Knee Dysfunction in Relation to the
Foot, 83
Jeffrey Lee Halbrecht, M.D.

CHAPTER 6
Biomaterials: Soft Tissue and Bone Reaction to Implants, 91
Vincent J. Hetherington, D.P.M., and Joyce M. Senick, D.P.M.

SECTION TWO

Clinical Features of Articular Disease, 103

CHAPTER 7
Rheumatoid Arthritis, 103
Richard D. Roth, D.P.M.

CHAPTER 8
Seronegative Spondyloarthropathies,   132
James L. McGuire, M.D., and Wilfred Laine, D.P.M.

CHAPTER 9
Crystalline Deposition Disease,   141
Divyang Patel, D.P.M., and James Stavosky, D.P.M.

CHAPTER 10
Connective Tissue Diseases,   152
Charles A. Eiser, D.P.M., and Marley M. Taylor, D.P.M.

CHAPTER 11
Cutaneous Signs of Systemic Disease,   169
Todd S. Anhalt, M.D.

CHAPTER 12
Vascular Manifestations of Articular Disease,   201
David Mullens, D.P.M.

CHAPTER 13
Septic Arthritis,   207
John J. Stienstra, D.P.M., Christopher J. Lamy, D.P.M., and Warren S. Joseph, D.P.M.

CHAPTER 14
Laboratory Testing in Arthritic Disease,   220
Thomas J. Kaschak, D.P.M.

CHAPTER 15
Athletic Injuries,   234
Richard T. Bouché, D.P.M., Katrina Sullivan, D.P.M., and Douglas J. Ichikawa, D.P.M.

SECTION THREE

Musculoskeletal Manifestations of Specific Systemic Diseases,   261

CHAPTER 16
The Diabetic Foot,   261
Steven J. Palladino, D.P.M.

CHAPTER 17
Afflictions of Nerves and Muscles,   284
Craig Wargon, D.P.M., Jon R. Risser, D.P.M., and Flair David Goldman, D.P.M.

CHAPTER 18
HIV Infection and AIDS,   300
Carolyn K. Harvey, D.P.M.

SECTION FOUR

Radiologic Evaluation,   307

CHAPTER 19
Radiologic Manifestations of Arthritides Involving the Foot,   307
Richard G. Stiles, M.D., Walter A. Carpenter, Ph.D., M.D., and
Donald Resnick, M.D.

CHAPTER 20
Imaging of Musculoskeletal Tumors,   322
Ann Gabrielle Bergman, M.D.

CHAPTER 21
Radiographic Evaluations of Bone and Joint Infections,   340
Allan Bernstein, D.P.M., Gideon Strich, M.D., and
Mark G. Stein, M.B.B.Ch., B.Sc.

CHAPTER 22
Contrast Radiography,   365
Brad L. Naylor, D.P.M.

CHAPTER 23
Cross-Sectional Imaging,   377
Mark E. Schweitzer, M.D., Juerg Hodler, M.D., and David J. Sartoris, M.D.

SECTION FIVE

Medical Management,   397

CHAPTER 24
Pharmacologic Management of Inflammatory Joint Disease,   397
Thomas J. Kaschak, D.P.M.

CHAPTER 25
Glucocorticoids: Use in the Management of Rheumatic Disorders,   437
Richard D. Roth, D.P.M.

CHAPTER 26
Rehabilitation of the Arthritic Patient,   449
Jon Nordgaard, D.P.M., P.T.

SECTION SIX

Surgical Management,   457

CHAPTER 27
Perioperative Considerations,   457
Bennett G. Zier, M.D.

CHAPTER 28
Anesthesia Considerations,   464
Stephen Jackson, M.D., George Lampe, M.D., and Donald Silcox, M.D.

CHAPTER 29
Central Metatarsophalangeal Joint Arthrosis: Evaluation and Surgical
Management,   481
William M. Jenkin, D.P.M.

CHAPTER 30
Forefoot Arthroplasty,   496
John V. Vanore, D.P.M., and Irving Pikscher, D.P.M.

CHAPTER 31
Forefoot Implant Arthroplasty,   516
Albert Burns, D.P.M.

CHAPTER 32
Joint Preservation Techniques in Hallux Limitus/Rigidus Repair,   529
Kieran T. Mahan, M.S., D.P.M.

CHAPTER 33
First Metatarsophalangeal Joint Arthrodesis,   545
John V. Vanore, D.P.M.

CHAPTER 34
Fusions in the Arthritic Patient,   559
John M. Schuberth, D.P.M.

CHAPTER 35
Tendon Dysfunction,   577
Lawrence M. Oloff, D.P.M.

CHAPTER 36
Tendon Transfers,   588
John M. Schuberth, D.P.M.

CHAPTER 37
Role of Arthroscopy in the Treatment of Arthritic Ankle Disorders,   612
Richard O. Lundeen, D.P.M.

CHAPTER 38
Surgical Management of Soft Tissue Tumors,   626
Robert G. O'Keefe, D.P.M.

CHAPTER 39
Avascular Necrosis of Bone,   639
Jeffrey C. Page, D.P.M.

CHAPTER 40
Congenital Deformities,   652
Richard M. Jay, D.P.M.

SECTION SEVEN

Chronic Pain Syndromes,   673

CHAPTER 41
Physiology of Pain,   673
Pamela K. Westfahl, Ph.D.

CHAPTER 42
Medical Management of Chronic Pain,   678
Bernard R. Wilcosky, Jr., M.D.

CHAPTER 43
Surgical Treatment of Peripheral Nerve Entrapment Syndromes,   685
Michael S. Downey, D.P.M.

CHAPTER 44
Post-Traumatic Painful Ankle,   718
Steven J. Palladino, D.P.M.

CHAPTER 45
Compartment Syndromes,   726
Paul D. Dayton, D.P.M., and Richard T. Bouché, D.P.M.

INDEX,   737

Basic Science

CHAPTER 1

Articular Anatomy and Histology

Barbara M. Kriz, Ph.D.

A structural or anatomic classification of joints typically results in three major categories, according to the predominant tissue or design holding the articulating elements together; that is, joints are called *fibrous, cartilaginous,* or *synovial.*

CLASSIFICATION

Fibrous Joints

Fibrous joints are solid.[1–6] The principal material binding the articulating elements together is fibrous connective tissue, although other tissue types may also be present. Fiber density, length, and specific arrangement vary considerably according to the location of the joint and its functional requirements. Three groups of fibrous joints are traditionally described: *sutures, gomphoses,* and *syndesmoses.*

Sutures exist only in the skull where, in the adult, bones are held together closely by short, dense connective tissue fibers forming so-called sutural ligaments. These fibers are considerably longer in the fontanelles of fetal and infant skulls, where they are gradually replaced by bone.

Gomphoses are restricted to the maxillae and mandible and refer to the attachment of the peglike teeth in the alveolar sockets. Again, a short ligament of fibrous tissue forms the connection.

All other joints in which the articulating elements of the skeleton are held together primarily by fibrous connective tissue are classified as syndesmoses. This is a controversial classification, in that all ligaments may be said to fulfill this description; yet, in only a few areas is the ligament truly the only or principal connecting structure. True syndesmoses include the interosseous membranes of the forearm and leg and the interosseous ligament of the distal tibiofibular joint.

Fibrous joints are generally regarded as allowing for little or no movement; however, it is more accurate to state that a range of movement exists within this class. Neither the su-tures in the adult nor the gomphoses allow significant movement. Syndesmoses are characterized by connective tissue fibers of greater length; interosseous membranes, for example, consist of sheets of parallel, obliquely oriented fibers, whose purpose is to allow considerable movement between bones of the forearm during supination and pronation or between bones of the leg during dorsiflexion and plantarflexion of the ankle joint. In summary, the amount of movement possible at a fibrous joint varies directly with the length of the fibers.

The permanence of fibrous joints is also variable. For example, sutures frequently become ossified and, therefore, obliterated in middle to old age. Any joint that is replaced completely by bone is then called a *synostosis.* Although this process does not usually occur with other normal fibrous joints, it is observed in the lower extremity in the case of some syndesmotic tarsal coalitions.[7] Movement, already restricted by a fibrous coalition, is lost once the synostosis is formed.

Cartilaginous Joints

Cartilaginous joints,[1–6] like fibrous joints, are solid. The principal tissue intervening between the articulating parts of the skeleton is cartilage. Two structural types of cartilage, hyaline cartilage and fibrocartilage, form the basis for subcategories, which are sometimes referred to as the *primary* and *secondary cartilaginous joints*, but more commonly are known as *synchondroses* and *symphyses*, respectively.

In a synchondrosis, bones are connected by hyaline cartilage. By far the most numerous of the synchondroses are in the epiphyseal discs between areas of developing bone; thus, most synchondroses are temporary and function as areas that allow growth of the developing skeleton. When ossification is complete, the synchondroses of these epiphyseal areas are fully replaced by bone and, therefore, become synostoses. A few synchondroses remain as permanent parts of the skeleton; included in this group are the first sternocostal joints and several cranial synchondroses. In the lower extremity there are occurrences of synchondrotic tarsal coalitions that may or may not become ossified.[7]

Synchondroses allow very little movement. Epiphyseal discs are deformable but are not primarily for movement. The synchondroses of the rib cage contribute to the ability of this area to expand with respiration. This movement is exceedingly important in its totality but is fairly limited at individual joints.

In a symphysis, the surfaces of the two articulating bones are generally covered with a layer of hyaline cartilage; however, the principal intervening structure is a fibrocartilaginous disc. Intervertebral discs constitute the majority of symphyses. These discs consist of an outer fibrous region, the annulus fibrosus, and an inner gelatinous mucopolysaccharide region, the nucleus pulposus. This arrangement confers both toughness and deformability on the disc and allows for significant movement between vertebrae. Other symphyses include the manubriosternal joint and the pubic symphysis.

Symphyses are sometimes referred to as the *slightly movable joints* or *amphiarthroses* to signify that they allow more movement than do fibrous joints. In fact, a considerable range of movement exists within this group. The manubriosternal joint allows much less movement than does an intervertebral disc, although the hinging of the manubrium on the body of the sternum in this location is significant for rib cage expansion. Movement at the pubic symphysis is generally slight, but it becomes particularly important to allow expansion of the female pelvic cavity during childbirth.

Most symphyses are permanent; however, those of the sacrum and coccyx degenerate, with subsequent fusion between adjacent vertebral bodies as part of the normal development of these bones. In middle to old age, the manubriosternal disc also frequently degenerates, and the two parts of the sternum fuse wholly or partially.

Synovial Joints

Synovial joints are cavitated; that is, the two skeletal elements are held together by a sleeve or capsule of connective tissue that encloses a cavity and several other specialized tissues.[1–6] This is the principal joint type found in the limbs. Synovial joints are the most mobile of joints; however, even within this class, mobility varies tremendously. Subcategories are based on the specific shape or architecture of the joint surfaces involved (e.g., planar, saddle, and ball-and-socket) and on the types of movements allowed (e.g., flexion and extension; medial and lateral rotation).

All synovial joints have five basic structural features: a fibrous *capsule* that encloses a joint *cavity*, a specialized *articular cartilage* covering the articular surfaces, and *synovial membrane* lining the inner surface of the capsule and secreting a unique lubricating *synovial fluid.* Some synovial joints have one or more additional intra-articular structures; included among such structures are discs, menisci, labra, fat pads, tendons, and ligaments (Fig. 1–1).[8]

By far the majority of synovial joints develop as and remain synovial throughout the life of the individual. Nevertheless, even synovial joints may be temporary. For example, with advancing age, the cavity of the sacroiliac joint may become completely infiltrated by fibrocartilage. It may even

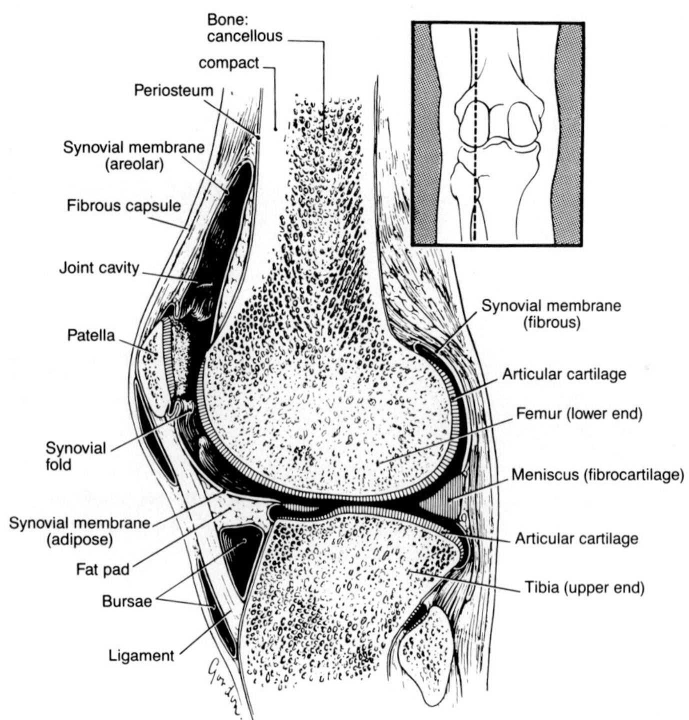

FIGURE 1–1. Sagittal section of a human knee joint. In addition to all the basic components of a synovial joint, the knee joint contains several intra-articular structures, including menisci, a fat pad, tendons, and ligaments. (From Cormack DH: Ham's Histology, 9th ed. Philadelphia, JB Lippincott, 1987, p 325.)

become fully ossified; that is, it may be converted to a synostosis.

EMBRYOLOGY OF JOINTS

Skeletal elements and joints, as well as many other tissues, are derived from the multipotential primitive connective tissue known as *mesenchyme.*[1, 6] This material, at first loosely organized, condenses in the developing skeleton and undergoes an orderly process of chondrification and ossification. Simultaneously, at the site of future joints, the so-called *interzonal* mesenchyme develops in accordance with the requirements of the site. Where fibrous joints will be located, fibrous connective tissue of the appropriate density and fiber length is formed. At the site of future synchondroses and symphyses, hyaline cartilage and fibrocartilage are, respectively, the predominant tissue types deposited. Where synovial joints will be located, the peripheral part of the interzonal mesenchyme at first condenses at the site of the future joint capsule. The enclosed mesenchyme then subdivides further into distinct zones that give rise to all the remaining parts of the joint, including the articular cartilage, synovial membrane, intracapsular structures (e.g., discs, menisci, ligaments), and the joint cavity. The last forms by the merging of small spaces in the central and most loosely organized region of the interzonal mesenchyme.

In view of the common tissue of origin for all of the joint categories, it is not surprising that considerable overlap exists between them under normal circumstances. Examples include the presence in many so-called fibrous joints of substantial cartilaginous areas, the cavitation of certain sym-

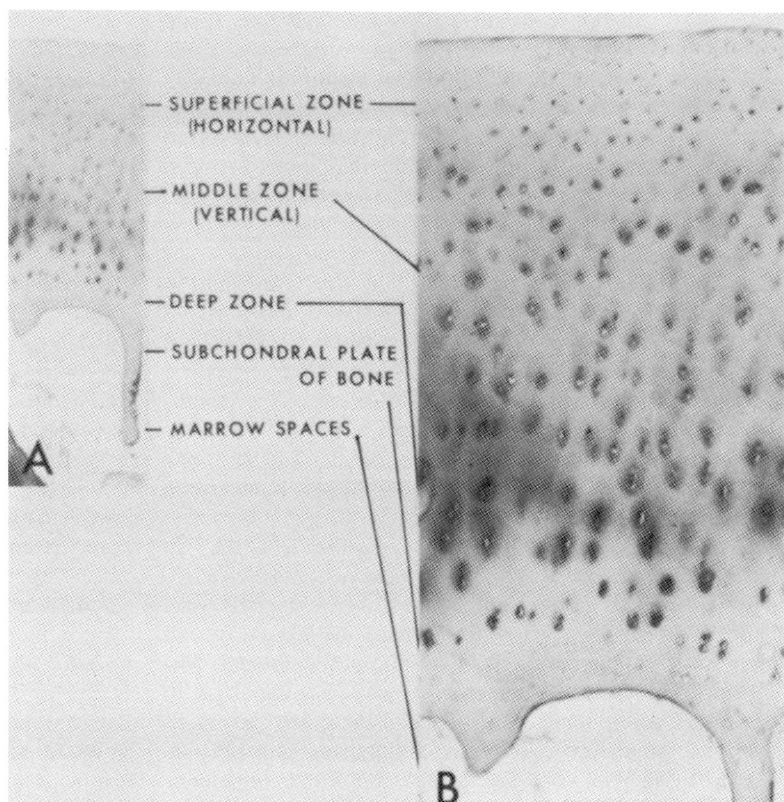

FIGURE 1–2. Low-power (*A*) and high-power (*B*) photomicrographs of human articular cartilage. In this preparation, three zones are identified: superficial, middle, and deep. The middle zone includes both the transitional and radial zones described by some authors. (From Salter RB: Textbook of Disorders and Injuries of the Musculoskeletal System, 2nd ed, p 18. © 1983, the Williams & Wilkins Co., Baltimore.)

physes, and common age-related changes in the structure of certain joints, including conversion of many joints to synostoses. Under abnormal circumstances, this basic potential for overlap may be magnified.

COMPONENTS OF SYNOVIAL JOINTS

Because synovial joints are the most numerous and the most important for the mobility of the skeleton, the remainder of this chapter focuses especially on this joint category. In particular, the histology of each of the structures found in synovial joints is detailed.

Articular Cartilage

In most synovial joints the ends of articulating bones are covered with a specialized type of hyaline cartilage. There are a few exceptions. In the zygapophyseal joints of the vertebral column, in the acromioclavicular, sternoclavicular, and temporomandibular joints, and in the glenoid fossa of the shoulder and the acetabulum of the hip joint, the articular cartilage contains a significant amount of fibrocartilage. All articular cartilages, however, are similar in that they are without perichondrium, blood vessels, lymphatics, or nerves. Young articular cartilage has a translucent, bluish-white appearance; with age, it becomes increasingly opaque and slightly yellow. Physical properties of articular cartilage include toughness and resilience, which allow it to support and transmit high loads, withstand shearing forces, and absorb shock. Some elasticity is lost with age. The surface of articular cartilage, as lubricated by synovial fluid, provides for an extremely low coefficient of friction during movement. This is due mainly to the unique structure of this tissue.[1, 6]

In most synovial joints, the hyaline cartilage contains within it a characteristic arrangement of collagen fibrils. In early morphologic studies by Benninghoff[9] it was suggested that these fibrils are organized as a network of arches, which have come to be known as Benninghoff arcades. An arcade arrangement is consistent with the observation that there is a high density of these collagen fibrils near the articular surface, where they are arranged parallel or tangential to the surface. In contrast, fibrils deeper in the tissue are sparser and oriented nearly perpendicular to the surface. This arrangement has long been more presumed than proven, because individual fibrils cannot readily be traced from end to end in sectioned material. However, in recent work using cryofractured articular cartilage viewed by scanning electron microscopy, it is reported that entire bundles of fibrils originating deep in the cartilage can indeed be traced to the surface where they arch and flatten together.[10]

The collagen fibrils are embedded in a matrix that is nearly three fourths water by weight and is rich in proteoglycans, especially chondroitin sulfates bound to protein.[4, 8, 11] Chondrocytes are interspersed in this matrix and are variously described as existing in either three or four layers, or zones, that overlie the mature subchondral bone (Fig. 1–2).[4] The cells in zone I, nearest the surface, are relatively small and elongated and lie parallel to the surface, as do the collagen fibrils in this area. This may be called the *tangential, superficial,* or *gliding zone.* Beneath this lies zone II, the *transitional* or *intermediate zone,* in which chondrocytes have a more typical oval or round appearance and are dispersed randomly throughout the collagen fibrils and matrix. Zone III, sometimes called the *deep* or *radial zone,* is the largest layer. In this zone cells are enlarged and arranged in groups or columns. (Sometimes zones II and III are combined, as in

Figure 1–2.) Finally, in the deepest or *calcified zone* (zone IV), matrix is impregnated with calcium salt crystals. Cells are sparse, and many appear to be degenerate. The arcades of collagen fibrils of the other three zones are embedded and attached in this calcified zone, which, in turn, is anchored to the subchondral bone by means of interdigitations between the two layers. In some histologic preparations, a thin basophilic line called the *tidemark* is observed in the most superficial part of the calcified cartilage zone.[6, 11]

The basic elements of articular cartilage—cells and matrix, with the latter consisting of ground substance and fibrils— show gradations of change from one zone to another; as a result, each zone has distinct combinations of characteristics. Some studies suggest that certain zones merit further subdivision according to ultrastructural and histochemical criteria.[12, 13] The following is a description of each of the aforementioned elements, taking into account the major interzonal modifications.

Cartilage cells, or chondrocytes, appear most ''active'' in the middle zones (zones II and III), because organelles associated with matrix component synthesis are especially well developed here (Fig. 1–3).[11, 12, 14] These include the rough endoplasmic reticulum and Golgi system of membranes. Mitochondria are also more numerous as well as being larger in these zones. Additionally, the surface of these cells has more plasma membrane projections. By comparison, cells of zone I appear to be relatively quiescent.[11, 12, 14] Other organelles and inclusions are not obviously distributed according to zone. For example, lipid droplets are occasionally observed in chondrocytes, regardless of zone. Micropinocytotic vesicles are few in some cells and numerous in others. Glycogen is also abundant in some cells. Lysosomes and microtubules are relatively infrequent, whereas intracytoplasmic filaments are abundant. Occasionally, cells with cilia are observed; the function of these is uncertain. Some of these intracellular components (e.g., glycogen, lysosomes, and filaments) become more numerous with age, in response to experimentally induced injury or to intra-articular injection of a variety of materials, and in diseases such as osteoarthritis, hemarthrosis, and chondromalacia.[11]

Collagen fibrils in the most superficial part of zone I are densely packed, such that both ground substance and cells are relatively sparse in this area. In one study[12] the collagen fibrils were measured as having a diameter of about 32 nm and a periodicity of 64 nm, which is typical of type II collagen. (Periodicity is 67 nm when measured by x-ray diffraction; however, in ultrastructural studies some shrinkage due to fixation is to be expected.) The collagen fibers in the superficial part of zone I occur both singly and in bundles of 30 fibrils or more. Deeper in zone I, collagen fiber bundles are smaller with greater intervening space. In addition, smaller collagenous elements are also seen in zone I. It has been reported that there is a concentration of 4-nm filaments in the immediate pericellular area, with 12-nm fibrils increasing in number at a greater distance from the cell, and typical 32-nm fibrils prominent at a still greater distance from the cell.[15] In zone II, fibrous elements of all sizes are fewer and spaced more widely, with correspondingly more intervening ground substance. Collagen fibrils most often are single rather than in bundles, are randomly oriented, and have typical 64-nm periodicity but have a larger diameter than in zone I (ranging from 30 to 60 nm). Zone III is similar, except that the diameter of the collagen fibrils ranges widely from 40 to 80 nm.[12] It has been reported that the fibrils in this zone form a meshwork around the chondrocytes that may serve a protective function. The increased diameter of fibrils in zones II

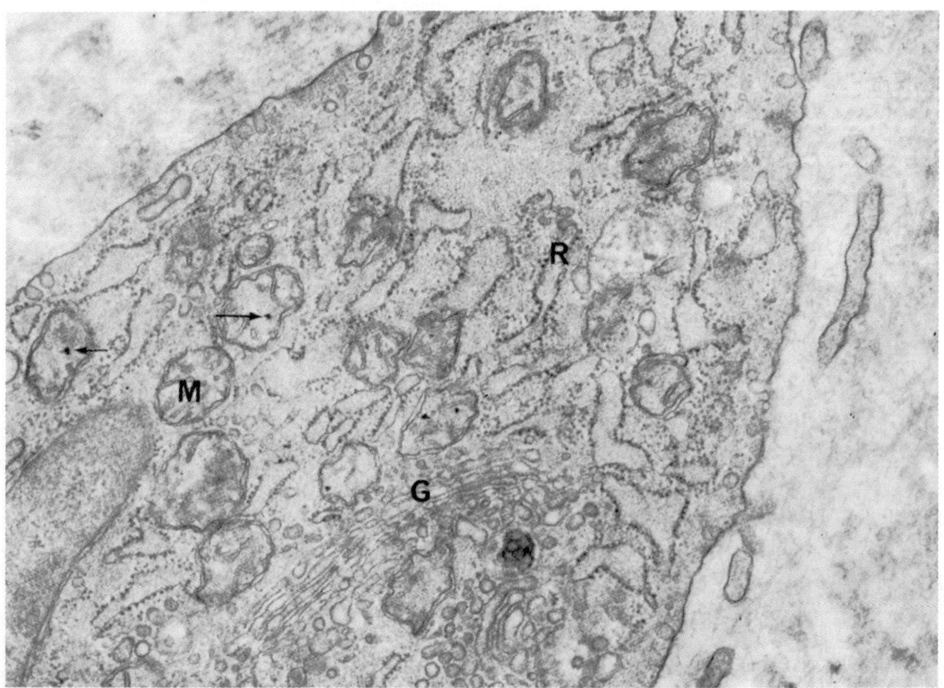

FIGURE 1–3. Electron micrograph of a typical chondrocyte from zone II articular cartilage of a rabbit aged 5 months. The cell contains abundant rough endoplasmic reticulum (R) and mitochondria (M), and the Golgi apparatus (G) is well developed. *Arrows* indicate dense bodies common in the mitochondria of these cells. ×40,000. (From Ghadially FN and Roy S: Ultrastructure of Synovial Joints in Health and Disease. London, Butterworth-Heinemann Ltd., 1969, p 39.)

and III is due to collagen cross-linking. Increased fibril diameter also occurs with age and in certain pathologic conditions. Very thick fibrils have been observed, for example, in osteoarthritic cartilage.[11]

The ground substance or interfibrillary matrix is a gel containing approximately 75% tissue fluid by wet weight, plus glycosaminoglycans, noncollagenic proteins, and glycoproteins. Chondroitin-4-sulfate and chondroitin-6-sulfate are the predominant glycosaminoglycans; these plus keratan sulfate and some dermatan sulfate are attached covalently to noncollagenic proteins to form proteoglycans.[8, 16] Hyaluronic acid is also present. Histochemical staining confirms that the interfibrillary matrix is more abundant in deeper zones than it is in zone I, where the fibrillary matrix predominates. Some studies suggest that the chondroitin sulfates are especially concentrated in pericellular areas. Aggregates of proteoglycans forming particles of 30 to 70 nm in diameter have been noted to have a similar distribution. Keratan sulfate, on the other hand, is found in matrix farther away from the chondrocytes.[11]

Lipid granules or lipid-containing vesicles are also found within the ground substance of the matrix, especially in deep zones. Lipid accumulates with age and injury and probably represents debris from necrotic cells and cell surface processes that have been shed. Calcium salts are deposited in the lipid granules of arthritic cartilage.[11]

Calcium salt crystals are, of course, also deposited in the matrix of zone IV, with the amount increasing with age. In zone IV of mature articular cartilage, chondrocytes are embedded and effectively isolated in a calcified matrix, although each cell has a narrow pericellular zone of uncalcified matrix.[11]

Between zones III and IV is the tidemark, originally noted as a distinctly basophilic layer in routine histologic preparations. More recent and intensive study suggests that the tidemark has a distinct substructure and probably represents an area of delicate balance, with cells on one side (zone III) producing factors that inhibit calcification and cells on the other side (zone IV) producing factors that promote calcification.[17] When articular cartilage from patients with osteoarthritis is examined, the tidemark is structurally disrupted or even destroyed, with resultant advance of mineralization into the upper hyaline cartilage zones.[18]

A thin, brightly appearing layer at the free surface of articular cartilage was first identified by phase-contrast microscopy and termed the *lamina splendens*.[19] It was thought to be a zone of pure hyaline. This area has been the subject of intense debate and is thought by many to be a "halo" artifact of the microscopic method employed. More recent ultrastructural studies do identify a 3-μm layer at the surface of zone I that is acellular but rich in apparently randomly oriented fine fibers and filaments.[12] Still more recent studies, employing polarized light microscopy and interference microscopy that should eliminate the problems associated with the phase-contrast approach, also report a distinct surface lamina.[13] Others believe that the lamina is merely an electron-dense coating of variable thickness, deposited on the articular surface and consisting of synovial fluid containing lipid-rich cellular debris and fine filaments.[1, 11]

Articular cartilage varies in thickness both from one joint to another and within a given joint. It apparently is thickest where the load is greatest. One study of femoral heads, for example, demonstrated a range of articular cartilage thickness from 0.4 to 3.5 mm, with the thickest cartilage occurring lateral to the fovea capitis, where the load is greatest, and thickness decreasing more gradually lateral to compared with medial to the fovea. Closer examination of this variation revealed that the calcified layer (zone IV) also varied in thickness and in a pattern that correlated closely with that of the full thickness of cartilage.[20]

Adult articular cartilage receives its nourishment by diffusion of the synovial fluid in the joint. There is debate as to whether capillary loops in the subchondral bone also feed the deeper layers of cartilage. Although this is likely in young cartilage prior to full development of the calcified zone, it appears that a mature calcified zone forms a considerable barrier to encroachment of vessels. A recent scanning electron microscope study of lower extremity joints in humans and other species showed almost all vessels in the subchondral area surrounded by lamellar bone. Rarely were vascular channels seen in direct contact with uncalcified articular cartilage, and never were they seen above the tidemark. Thus, subchondral vessels do not appear to be a normal source of nutrition for adult articular cartilage.[21]

Articular cartilage has a limited capacity for repair or regeneration. The mitotic index is low, even in young cartilage. Experimentally produced wounds in articular cartilage heal slowly and incompletely and, although the first cartilage to be deposited may be hyaline in type, fibrous tissue often eventually predominates in such sites.[11]

Joint Capsule

The capsules of synovial joints are sleeves of dense, fibrous connective tissue that enclose the joint cavity. These fibers are generally longitudinally oriented with respect to the joint, although interlacing of fibers occurs. The joint capsule blends with the periosteum of the articulating bones; anchoring to the bone is by typical Sharpey's fibers. This attachment usually occurs quite near the margin of the articular cartilage, although the distance from that margin varies considerably, and in some joints there is a substantial amount of intra-articular bone surface. The joint capsule is penetrated by vessels and nerves serving it and the synovial membrane that lines it. Gaps may be found in the capsule, through which outpocketings of synovial membrane protrude and form bursae.[1, 3, 8]

Most joint capsules are relatively thin where reinforcement is not required or would be a hindrance to movement. Local thickenings, on the other hand, occur where limitation of excessive movement is necessary. These thickenings of the capsule are often termed *capsular ligaments*; they are fully a part of the capsule and are distinct from so-called *accessory ligaments* that may be either *extracapsular* or *intracapsular*. Such accessory ligaments are, nevertheless, often immediately adjacent to the capsule and, particularly in the case of the extracapsular ligaments, frequently blend directly with it.[1, 3]

Synovial Membrane

Synovial membrane is not a classic membrane but rather is a complex, multilayered structure that primarily lines the internal surface of the fibrous joint capsule. It also invests or lines certain other components of the joint, as will be discussed. Synovial membrane produces some components of the synovial fluid and maintains the health of the joint by continuously processing this fluid to remove waste materials.

Synovial membrane consists of an inner lining, or *intima,* that faces the joint cavity and a loosely organized, vascular connective tissue region, or *subintima,* that blends with the joint capsule (Fig. 1–4).[1, 8] On gross examination the intimal layer appears translucent and smooth, and subintimal vessels and fat are visible through it. The membrane is reflected off the deep surface of the joint capsule onto the intra-articular bone, where it blends with the periosteum (see Fig. 1–1).[8] Synovial membrane never extends onto the articular cartilage surface but stops short of its margins. In joints with capsules that attach a considerable distance from the articular cartilage margin, there is likewise considerable intra-articular periosteum lined by synovial membrane. In such joints, of which the knee is a good example, the reflection of synovial membrane onto periosteum creates synovial membrane–lined recesses in the joint cavity. These are normally collapsed, potential spaces, but particulate material, cells, and other material may accumulate there. Furthermore, these may be early sites of erosion and other pathologic changes. These recesses are also frequent sites of small synovial protrusions, or villi. Such protrusions are normal structures that are thought to provide some flexibility for the membrane as the joint moves through its entire permitted range. They also increase the surface area of the membrane, potentially adding

to both its secretory and absorptive capability, as well as increasing the ability of the membrane to move fluid throughout the joint cavity. Villi may hypertrophy, become hypervascular, or show other changes in diseased joints.[22]

In addition to capsule and periosteum, some other intra-articular structures are typically invested in synovial membrane. For example, ligaments and tendons that are within the line of capsular attachment are usually lined by synovial membrane. This means that the subintimal side of the membrane blends with these structures and the intimal ''secreting'' surface faces the joint cavity. Thus, intracapsular ligaments and tendons are lined with membrane but are not bathed with fluid.[1] Other intra-articular structures, such as discs and menisci, are generally regarded as being unlined by membrane, although one study of menisci in rabbit knee joints reports the presence of synovial lining.[23] Unlined structures, just like the articular cartilage, are bathed directly in synovial fluid.

The nature of the tissue that is lined by the synovial membrane provided the basis for an early classification scheme that is still in use. Synovial membrane may be described as *fibrous, adipose,* or *areolar* in type, with gradations among these three also noted (see Fig. 1–4).[8, 24] These various types do not reflect substantial differences in the lining cells but rather variations in the subintimal zone. Fibrous synovial membrane lines dense connective tissue structures such as intra-articular tendons and ligaments and tends to have a relatively thin subintima. Adipose synovial membrane typically overlies fat pads and also contains substantial adipose tissue within its subintima. Areolar synovial tissue is the predominant category and is characterized by a loosely organized subintima. It is located where the membrane is thrown into folds or villi and where it reflects off the capsule onto the periosteum, creating the recesses noted previously. A single joint may have one or more of these types of synovial membrane, according to the area studied.[22]

The lining cell layer varies from about one to three cells in thickness, with fibrous synovial membrane having the thinnest lining and adipose synovial membrane typically having the thickest.[24] The lining is loosely organized; individual cells have long cytoplasmic processes that intertwine with one another extensively (Fig. 1–5).[25] Gaps between cells are common, such that intercellular spaces are continuous with the synovial joint cavity. These spaces contain both fibrillar and amorphous material. Collagen periodicity is observed on fibers of deeper layers, but banding is less apparent nearer the joint cavity. No basal lamina is apparent except as associated with the blood vessels in the subintima. Junctions between cells have not been identified in human synovial membrane, although they have been observed in other species.[1]

Electron microscopy reveals lining cells of two types, referred to as type A (Fig. 1–6) and type B (Fig. 1–7).[14, 26, 27] Type A cells are more abundant in humans and resemble macrophages. They are characterized by a well-developed Golgi apparatus and many vacuoles 0.4 to 1.5 μm in diameter and containing dense material. These cells also contain numerous vesicles indicative of active pinocytosis, as well as many mitochondria, filopodia or surface ruffles, and intracellular filaments 5 to 15 nm in diameter. Type A cells have a poorly developed, rough endoplasmic reticulum. In contrast, type B cells, which are more abundant in animals other than humans, resemble fibroblasts. They have a large amount of

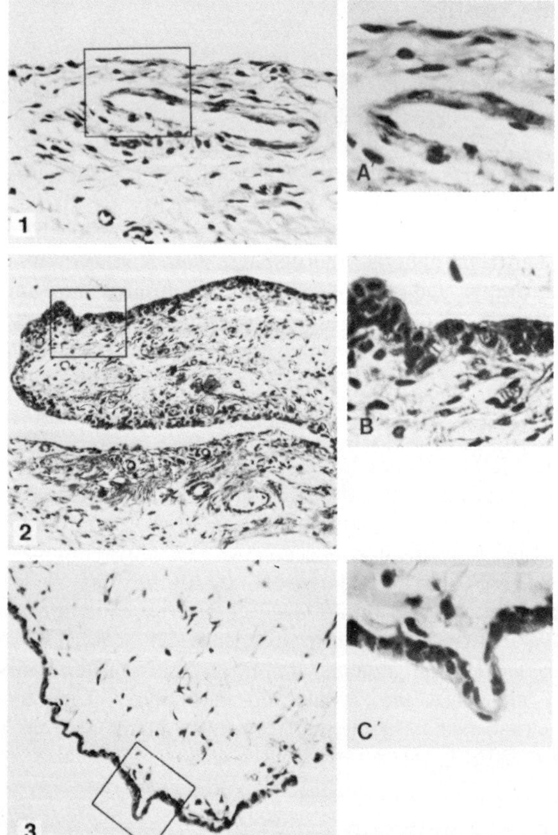

FIGURE 1–4. Light micrographs (low-power and high-power views) of the three types of synovial membrane: fibrous (*1* and *A'*), areolar (*2* and *B'*), and adipose (*3* and *C'*). In each, a lining, or intimal layer, faces the joint cavity and a vascular subintimal layer lies just beneath. (From Cormack DH: Ham's Histology, 9th ed. Philadelphia, JB Lippincott, 1987, p 334.)

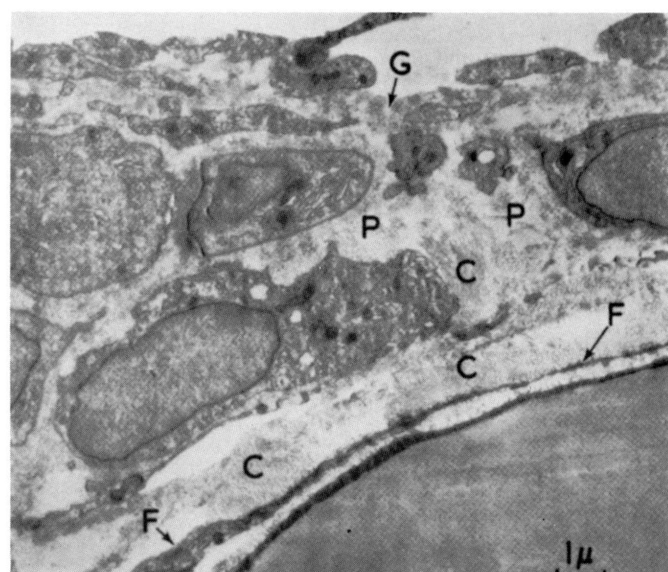

FIGURE 1–5. Low-power electron micrograph of synovial lining (intima) from the knee joint of a rabbit. The superficial cell layer is discontinuous; that is, large, intercellular spaces are in direct communication with the synovial cavity. Cells have long, intertwining cytoplasmic processes. A basement membrane is absent. F, fibrocytes; C, banded collagen; P, aperiodic fibers; G, granular material. ×9000. (From Ghadially FN and Roy S: Ultrastructure of rabbit synovial membrane. Ann Rheum Dis 25:318, 1966.)

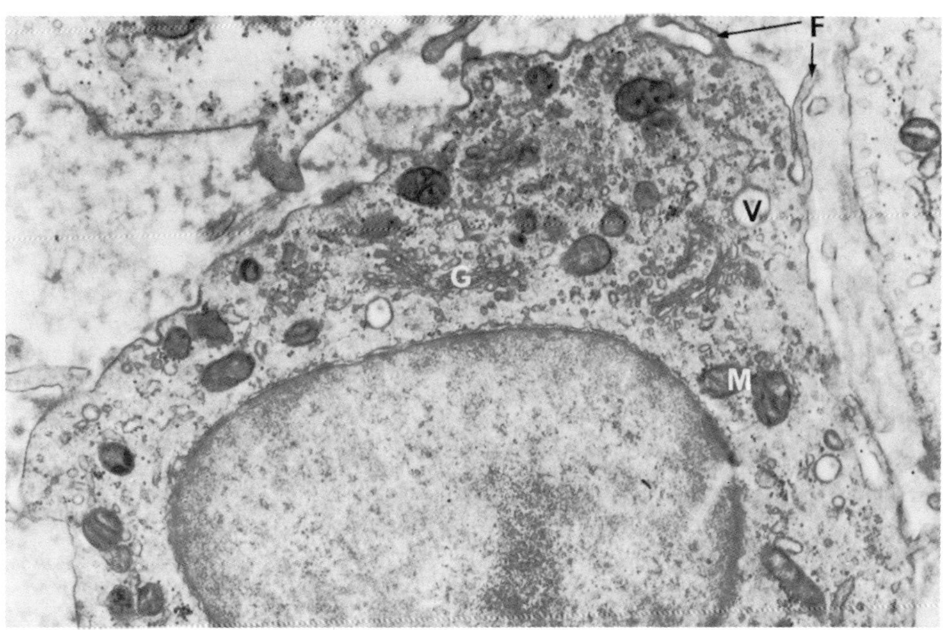

FIGURE 1–6. Electron micrograph of a type A cell from human synovial membrane. The cell resembles a macrophage and contains extensive Golgi membranes (G), many vacuoles (V), mitochondria (M), and filopodia (F). Rough endoplasmic reticulum is scanty. ×25,000. (From Ghadially FN and Roy S: Ultrastructure of Synovial Joints in Health and Disease. London, Butterworth-Heinemann Ltd., 1969, p 9.)

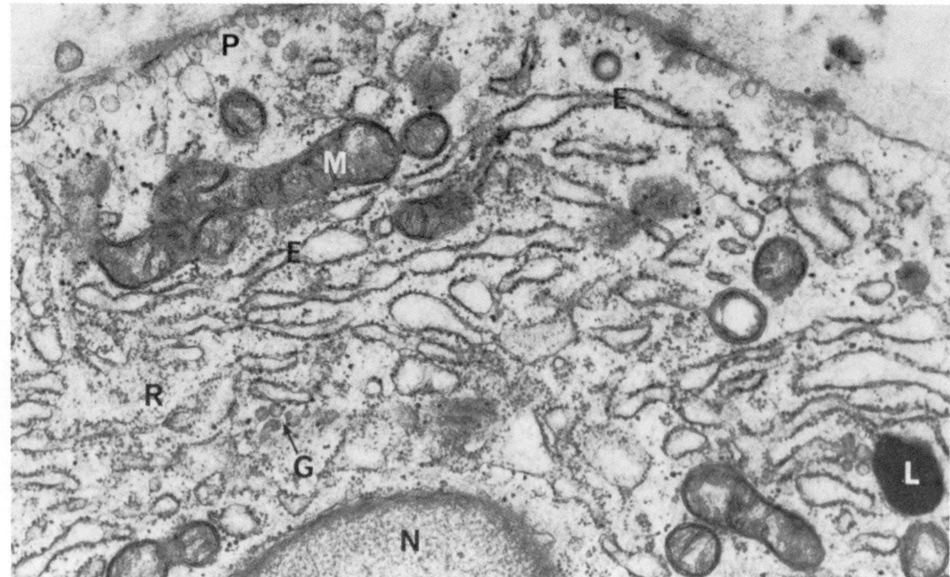

FIGURE 1–7. Electron micrograph of a type B cell from human synovial membrane. This cell type appears to be more actively involved in protein synthesis, because it is richly endowed with rough endoplasmic reticulum (E). Other organelles shown include ribosomes (R), Golgi vesicles (G), nucleus (N), mitochondria (M), micropinocytotic vesicles (P), and lysosome (L). ×41,500. (From Ghadially FN and Roy S: Ultrastructure of Synovial Joints in Health and Disease. London, Butterworth-Heinemann Ltd., 1969, p 11.)

rough endoplasmic reticulum and fewer vacuoles, vesicles, and mitochondria. For years there has been discussion of whether the two cell types truly have separate origins or whether they simply represent two different functional states of the same cell type. Recent evidence suggests that the type B cell is derived locally and replaced via cell turnover within the synovial membrane, whereas at least some of the type A cells are recruited from the bone marrow.[26] Thus, current belief favors the theory that the two cell types are indeed distinct.

The synovial subintima is a region of varying thickness and composition, depending on whether it is of the fibrous, areolar, or adipose type. It primarily consists of either loose areolar or denser fibrous connective tissue and also commonly contains elastic fibers, which presumably prevent unwanted redundancy in the synovial membrane during joint motion.[6] Subintima is typically a richly vascularized region of the synovial membrane. Adipose and areolar types of membrane have particularly large concentrations of capillaries.[24] These vessels are located throughout the subintima and characteristically form loops or networks that course immediately adjacent to the intimal cell layer. Most of the capillaries appear to be of the fenestrated type, which is consistent with a tissue actively involved in exchange of water and small molecules.[3, 22] Several cell types are commonly observed in the subintima. These include fibroblasts, adipocytes, macrophages, and mast cells. The latter are concentrated around blood vessels, but their precise function there is not known.[22]

Lymphatic vessels are found in the synovial subintima; however, they are less numerous and situated farther from the intima than are blood capillaries. They appear structurally similar to lymphatics elsewhere in the body and probably perform similar functions, such as the return of excess fluid, serum proteins and other macromolecules, and certain cells to the blood circulation. These lymphatics drain into larger lymphatic vessels located in the joint capsule and periosteum. Lymphatic vessels in the subintima appear to decrease in number with age, which raises interesting questions about

their potential role in the aging process as it relates to various joint diseases.[22]

There are few nerves in synovial membrane. Most appear to be associated with blood vessels in the deeper parts of the subintima and are probably vasomotor in nature.

Several functions can be attributed to the synovial membrane. Because of its flexibility and many folds and villi, it accommodates the necessary range of motion at each individual joint and also serves to circulate synovial fluid to all parts of the enclosed joint cavity. The synovial membrane is directly involved in the exchange of fluid and small molecules between the blood and the synovial fluid within the joint cavity. This is critical for the supply of nutrients to the articular cartilage, which is itself avascular. Conversely, the membrane participates in fluid uptake and in the removal of waste products from the synovial fluid. Depending on their size, these materials may be removed via the blood or the lymphatic circulation. Type A intimal lining cells are active in both pinocytosis and phagocytosis and, once they have ingested material, probably migrate to the deeper parts of the subintima where they can convey the larger waste products to the lymphatic system.[1] Some lining cells are known to express class II major histocompatibility complex antigens, suggesting that they may present these to T lymphocytes, thus initiating an immune response.[26] Synovial intimal cells and, in particular, type B cells are well equipped for synthesis and secretion, and a wide variety of products have been attributed to these cells. Among them are collagen, fibronectin, proteoglycans of the extracellular matrix, lysosomal enzymes, and complement proteins. Some glycosaminoglycans are probably synthesized by the intimal cells, but it is uncertain whether hyaluronic acid is one of these or whether this product is present in the cells as a result of pinocytosis from the synovial fluid. Hyaluronic acid may, at least in part, also be synthesized by fibroblasts or other cells in the subintima. Finally, type B cells are thought to be involved in the secretion of lubricin, a glycoprotein that aids in lubrication of the articular cartilage.[1, 6, 22, 27]

Type A synovial lining cells are strongly implicated in the

pathogenesis of rheumatoid arthritis. Their numbers increase markedly in early stages of this disease, apparently owing to increased recruitment from the bone marrow rather than by mitosis of local cells. Progressive digestion of articular cartilage matrix closely follows the synovial lining cell hyperplasia. This may be due to a direct release of lytic enzymes by the synovial cells or to an indirect effect of cytokines such as interleukin-1 which, in turn, induce autolytic processes in cells of the articular cartilage.[26]

Synovial Fluid

Synovial fluid has two principal functions. First, it provides nutrition for the articular cartilage and, if they are present, for intra-articular discs and menisci. Second, it lubricates the joint surfaces, thus both protecting them and increasing the efficiency of their action. To fulfill these functions, the properties of the fluid must be maintained within strict limits.

The synovial fluid of healthy joints at rest is a clear, colorless to pale yellow liquid of slightly alkaline pH. It contains few cells (according to one study, an average of 60 cells/ml), and these include monocytes, lymphocytes, macrophages, polymorphonuclear leukocytes, and sloughed synovial intimal cells.[1] A small amount of fibrous and particulate material, including some broken cells, is typically also found and probably represents normal wear and tear. The amount of synovial fluid is normally very small; even a large joint such as the knee has no more than 0.5 ml of synovial fluid. It has unique physical properties, being both highly viscous and elastic, resembling the egg white from which it received its name. Viscosity increases as dilution, pH, temperature, or shear rate (i.e., movement) decreases. Elasticity changes similarly, except that it decreases with decreased shear rate.[1, 6]

Synovial fluid is an ultrafiltrate of blood, containing approximately one third of the amount of protein found in blood plasma plus added protein produced by cells of the synovial membrane. Proteins from the blood include primarily albumin, but also enzymes such as alkaline phosphatase, complement proteins, and other larger proteins present in only small quantities. The loosely organized synovial membrane, with its numerous surface projections and capillaries in close proximity to the surface, is ideally constructed for transport of these blood-derived components to the joint cavity.

Some of the protein of synovial fluid is covalently bound to the glycosaminoglycan hyaluronic acid to form a material called mucin. The hyaluronic acid of mucin is highly polymerized and is thought to be the basis of the viscous and elastic properties of synovial fluid. The source of mucin has not been clearly identified; articular cartilage, subintimal mast cells and fibroblasts, and type A and type B cells of the synovial intima have all been proposed as potential sources. Various histochemical techniques have shown that glycosaminoglycans are present in type A intimal cells; however, it is very possible that hyaluronic acid is produced by one of the other suggested sources as well.[1]

The hyaluronic acid of mucin is thought to function by retaining water in the joint cavity during movement. Thus, the fluid is prevented or retarded from escaping through the intercellular spaces of the synovial membrane and into the

lymphatic vessels of the subintima as joint movement and compression occur. In this way the articular surfaces are protected by the retained fluid cushion present between them.[28] This function, however, does not fulfill the need for actual lubrication of the joint surfaces. Hyaluronic acid has been shown to be ineffective as a lubricant of articular cartilage.[1]

Many different theories of articular cartilage lubrication have been proposed. Some are variations on a general theme of fluid film lubrication operating according to hydrodynamic principles. Other theories invoke an active ingredient in the synovial fluid that acts as a boundary lubricant. A glycoprotein termed *lubricin*, which is thought to be a product of type B synovial intimal cells, has been identified and associated with this function. Most recently, the boundary lubrication theory has been further advanced with the proposal that phospholipids in oligolamellar form, much like natural membranes, provide the lubricating properties of synovial fluid.[29] According to this theory, phospholipid ''sheets'' arranged parallel to the joint surfaces slide against one another with minimal friction. Electron microscopic evidence for such oligolamellar structures has been reported from a study of the stifle joints of sheep.[29] In this study, lamellar bodies of varying stages of maturation were found close to, or within, invaginations of the articular surfaces. This suggests that the articular cartilage may be the source of the phospholipid material, in which case the function of lubricin remains in question. On the other hand, it has also been proposed that lubricin may be involved in the transport of the phospholipid to the articular surface. Synovial joint lubrication clearly promises to continue as an active area of research.

Discs and Menisci

In addition to the obligatory components that all synovial joints possess, several joints contain intra-articular structures. Discs and menisci are examples of such structures. They differ from one another mainly in that a disc is a circular structure that may completely subdivide a joint cavity so that it is, in reality, two joints in series, whereas a meniscus is usually a crescent-shaped structure that only partially subdivides the joint. Complete discs are found in the sternoclavicular joint and in the radiocarpal joint. Discs in the acromioclavicular and temporomandibular joints may be partial or complete. Menisci are located in the tibiofemoral portion of the knee joint. In all cases, the structures are attached peripherally to the fibrous joint capsule. Blood vessels and nerves penetrate for a variable distance from this peripheral attachment, but typically most of the disc or meniscus is avascular. Little is known of the types or distribution of nerves and nerve endings in these structures. Some are undoubtedly autonomic fibers associated with the vessels; however, other fibers enter the discs or menisci independently.[1, 2, 6, 30]

Discs and menisci are usually described as being composed of fibrocartilage and containing few cells; in reality, however, the composition varies considerably from one species to another, from one joint to another, and at different ages within the same location. For example, the disc of the human sternoclavicular joint is quite cellular and is composed of dense fibrous tissue until the third decade, when cartilage first appears. The disc of the temporomandibular joint may contain little or no cartilage but does contain considerable elastic tissue.[30] The menisci of the human knee joint are predominantly composed of fibrous connective tissue with only a few elastic fibers, whereas knee menisci from other species may contain much cartilage or even bone.[31] All discs and menisci appear to be subject to loss of cellularity, thinning, and other degenerative changes with age; discs frequently become perforated centrally, and menisci may develop clefts or frayed edges.[1, 30]

Discs and menisci, according to nearly all descriptions, are unlined by synovial membrane. One contradictory report suggests that menisci of the knee joints of rabbits are lined by synovial membrane[23]; however, ultrastructural evidence is lacking. As mentioned earlier, the cellularity of such intra-articular structures is highly variable. Some discs or menisci may have a discontinuous layer of cells at the surface, but these cells could also be fibroblasts or chondrocytes, distinct from synovial intimal cells.[30]

A variety of functions have been proposed for intra-articular discs and menisci. Because they are found where bone congruity is poor, one of their major functions is undoubtedly to improve congruity and, therefore, stability between articular surfaces. Other likely roles include shock absorption; facilitation of certain movements and, in particular, combinations of movements; limitation of other movements; protection of articular surfaces; distribution of weight over a large surface; and improved lubrication by facilitation of synovial fluid circulation throughout the joint.[1, 6, 30] There is an apparent physiologic basis for conserving the structures, at least in certain locations, as evidenced by the observation that, subsequent to surgical removal, menisci of the knee joint may regenerate near-perfect duplicates.[8]

Labra

Another type of intra-articular structure is the labrum. In humans, labra are found only in the glenohumeral and hip joints. They are circumferential structures, attached to the rim of the glenoid and acetabular sockets. Labra are distinct from articular cartilage; they consist of fibrocartilage and are triangular in cross-section, with their bases attached to the articular margins and their free apical surfaces lined by synovial membrane.

Like discs and menisci, labra serve to improve fit and, therefore, stability of the joints in which they are located; in this instance, they do so by deepening the glenoid and acetabular surfaces of the scapula and os coxae, respectively. The flexible nature of this fibrocartilaginous lip is also presumed to facilitate adjustment of the socket shape to the irregular convex head of the humerus or femur during all phases and extremes of movement at these joints. Other proposed functions include protecting the articular margins during extremes of movement and providing assistance in spreading synovial fluid throughout the joint.[1, 30]

Fat Pads

Localized accumulations of fat are found in several synovial joints, although only those in the hip joint (acetabular fat pad) and knee joint (infrapatellar fat pad) are named. All of the fat pads are similar in that they have a lobulated organization, with lobules separated by fibrous connective tissue septa; some septa contain considerable elastic tissue as well. These septa serve to distribute a rich blood supply derived from the general vascular anastomosis of the joint. Lymphatics are few; on the other hand, nerve endings, especially pain receptors, are abundant in fat pads. Fat pads are lined by synovial membrane.

Suggested functions for fat pads include protection of other intra-articular structures (e.g., ligament of the head of the femur) and serving as cushions or space-fillers, thus contributing to smoother, more efficient movement throughout the entire available range. Lubrication of joint surfaces may also be facilitated indirectly by the filling of excess space with fat pads.[6, 30]

Intra-Articular Folds

With the description of synovial membrane it was noted that the surface of this tissue frequently possesses small villi, especially in the recesses of joint cavities. Larger folds are also common. They range from very large, named synovial membrane–lined structures, such as the alar folds and ligamentum mucosum of the knee joint,[6, 30] to a variety of small, unnamed, yet constant structures that surround or intervene between articular surfaces. Although it has been presumed that these are all variations on a theme, namely, synovial membrane modification, they are included here as a separate, catch-all category of intra-articular structures because, in fact, the histologic nature of many of these structures remains to be established. That all these structures are indeed lined by synovial membrane remains to be shown. Furthermore, some may contain fibrocartilage and, therefore, be more properly classified as menisci or even labra, one or the other of which many of these structures resemble. Indeed, the term *meniscoid* has been applied to structures observed routinely in the zygapophyseal joints between lumbar vertebrae.[32] Studies in progress are focused on determining the histologic nature of a meniscus-like structure in the calcaneocuboid joint (Hollander JD and Kriz BM, Unpublished data). That such structures are extremely common in normal joints of both upper and lower extremities was reported more than 60 years ago; however, as was noted then, they are likely to be overlooked owing to their small size and the likelihood of being destroyed upon incision of the joint.[33] One can only speculate that the functions of these folds are similar to those of the other intra-articular structures that have been described to date. It has even been suggested that the larger, classically described discs, menisci, and labra merely represent enlargements or modifications of these simple intra-articular folds found in numerous other joints.[30]

PERIARTICULAR STRUCTURES

All of the structures described in the previous section either are constant components of joints or structures that, when present, are always intra-articular. There are still other categories of structures that, although they exist independently of joints in various locations, may also be associated with joints as either intra-articular or extra-articular features. Because these may also be implicated in joint disorders, they are discussed briefly here.

Bursae

Bursae are enclosed, self-contained, flattened sacs, typically with a synovial lining. They facilitate movement of musculoskeletal tissues over one another and thus are located between pairs of structures (e.g., between ligament and tendon, two ligaments, two tendons, or skin and bone). Bursae are classified as either deep or superficial (subcutaneous). Deep bursae, such as the iliopsoas bursa or the deep retrocalcaneal bursa, develop along with joints and by a similar series of steps during the embryonic period. Superficial bursae, such as the olecranon and prepatellar bursae, appear after birth; it is hypothesized that they develop in response to the stimulus of applied pressure.[34]

Histologic and ultrastructural studies suggest that the synovial lining of both deep and superficial bursae is similar and resembles the synovial membrane of joints.[34] On the other hand, fluid taken from deep bursae has been found to contain a much higher content of hyaluronic acid and to be more similar to joint fluid than is fluid sampled from superficial bursae.[35] Although it is well known that fluid from inflamed superficial bursae has a low viscosity, such sampling studies suggest that this alone may not indicate pathologic change. Histologic observations further suggest that movement of the loose areolar connective tissue that surrounds many superficial bursae may be as important as secreted fluid in accounting for their ability to reduce friction between apposing structures.[35]

Bursae located near joints frequently establish communication with them. Such communications increase with age; for example, communication between the gastrocnemius-semimembranosus bursa and the knee joint is reported to be essentially absent before 10 years of age but to be present in approximately 50% of knees by 50 years of age.[34] Adventitious bursae also may appear in response to abnormal pressure exerted (e.g., by a deformity such as a hallux valgus, by an atypical bone prominence or exostosis, or by an internal fixation device).[6]

Tendons

Tendons are located at the ends of many muscles and are the means by which these muscles are attached to bone or other skeletal elements. Tendons are characterized by great tensile strength, flexibility, and resistance to compression. These qualities are conferred by a highly ordered arrangement of predominantly type I collagen fibrils aligned longitudinally and embedded in a matrix that is mostly water and proteoglycan. The tendon is surrounded by an areolar covering called *epitendineum*, which conveys neurovascular elements. Branches of these vessels and nerves are further distributed via a connective tissue *endotendineum* that surrounds individual fascicles of collagen fibrils within the tendon.[4, 6, 34]

At the myotendineal junction, the collagen fibrils of the tendon are embedded in invaginations of the muscle cell membrane. At the bone attachment, or *enthesis*, four distinct histologic zones have been identified (Fig. 1–8).[36] They are, from tendon toward bone, respectively: zone 1, typical tendinous collagen structure (i.e., fibers oriented longitudinally, with interspersed fibroblasts); zone 2, unmineralized fibrocartilage, with chondrocytes arranged in pairs or rows and lying in lacunae between collagen fibrils; zone 3, mineralized fibrocartilage, with crystals clearly evident between collagen fibrils; and zone 4, bone, with mineralized fibrocartilage no longer distinguishable from the collagen of bone matrix.[36] This mechanism, by which the collagen fibrils of tendon

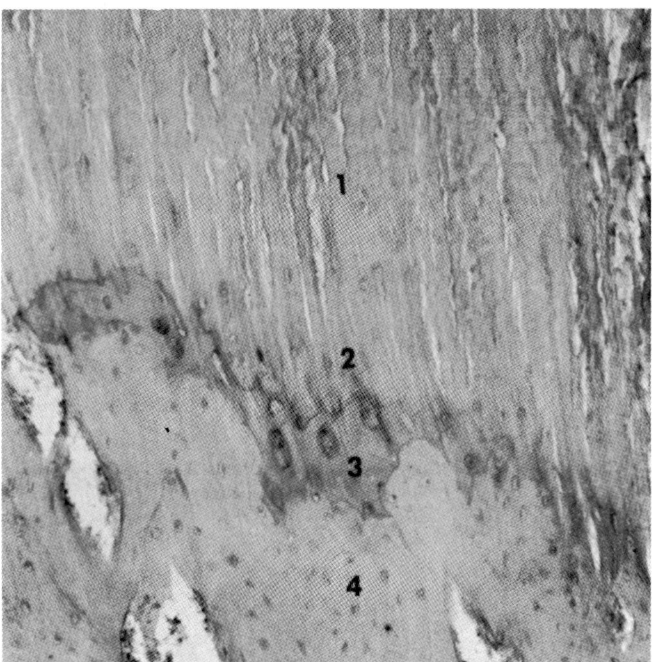

FIGURE 1–8. Light micrograph of the insertion of the quadriceps femoris tendon, by way of the patellar ligament, into the tibia. Four zones are visible: (1) tendon, (2) unmineralized fibrocartilage, (3) mineralized fibrocartilage, and (4) lamellar bone. (From Cooper JJ and Misol S: Tendon and ligament insertion. J Bone Joint Surg 52A:1, 1970.)

actually penetrate and blend with the bone substance, is also referred to as attachment by *Sharpey's fibers*. This type of arrangement is extremely strong. In a traction injury, it is not likely that a tendon would be extracted from the bone to which it is attached; rather, the tendon would more likely tear or avulse a bone fragment.[4]

Age-related changes in the relative proportions of collagen and matrix, as well as in the size of collagen fibrils, have been described. A peak size of collagen fibril diameter correlating with a peak in tensile strength is achieved at maturity but declines in senescent animals.[34] The proportion of elastic fibers, on the other hand, increases with age. Similar changes in collagen biochemistry and in relative proportions of tendon components, resulting in decreased tensile strength, may well be associated with the variety of conditions in which tendon weakening and rupture are observed. To list only a few, these include rheumatoid arthritis, systemic lupus erythematosus, hyperparathyroidism, and renal failure. Prolonged treatment with corticosteroids also may result in tendon weakening.[34]

Tendon Sheaths

At potential sites of friction, such as where tendons pass close to each other or to other structures, they are often enveloped in synovial sheaths. The osseofibrous tunnels created by retinacula of the wrist and ankle are examples of such locations. These sheaths develop at the same time as the joints, associated tendons, and deep bursae. In fact, synovial tendon sheaths embryologically are regarded as examples of deep bursae.[6, 34]

The synovial tendon sheath resembles a closed tube of synovial membrane into which the tendon is invaginated

(Fig. 1–9).[37] Thus one layer of membrane, the visceral layer, lies in close approximation to the tendon, whereas a second or parietal layer lies slightly outside the first and separated from it by a thin layer of fluid. The two layers are continuous by means of a *mesotendon* that carries vessels and nerves to the tendon. The mesotendon may be complete or discontinuous, in which case the smaller strands are termed *vincula*. The synovial tendon sheath, in turn, is surrounded and protected by a fibrous connective tissue sheath. Because the synovial sheath consists of a secretory layer similar to that of the synovial membrane of joints, the effect is to promote the ability of the tendon to glide smoothly in relation to surrounding structures. The secreted fluid may also contribute to the nutrition of the associated region of tendon.[4, 6, 34, 36]

Ligaments

Ligaments are dense bands of connective tissue that connect skeletal elements to each other, either creating (as in the case of syndesmoses) or supporting joints. They are attached in such a manner as to allow desired movement and to limit undesired movement at the joint spanned. Ligaments may be classified by composition, embryologic derivation, or location, the last being perhaps the most practical method. According to one system of classification by location, ligaments may be intracapsular, capsular (i.e., inseparable from the capsule), or extracapsular.[1, 3]

Structurally, ligaments closely resemble tendons in that they consist predominantly of type I collagen and their attachment to bone comprises the same four histologic zones. They are nourished by the same system of arteries that supplies the capsule and other tissues of the joint (see later). They are also affected similarly to tendons by a wide array of inflammatory and degenerative processes.[6, 34]

Where ligaments and tendons are intracapsular, they both typically have synovial membrane reflected off their surface. As a result, they are not bathed directly in synovial fluid, although they both may still have indirect benefit of lubrication. For example, evaginations of synovial membrane intervene between the cruciate ligaments of the knee and promote their gliding against one another. Similarly, the popliteus tendon lies on, and its movement is facilitated by, the subpopliteal recess of the knee joint.[1]

Retinacula

The classic retinacula are bands of thickened, transversely or obliquely oriented deep fascia that are attached at each end to bony prominences and thus create osseofibrous tunnels through which tendons and neurovascular structures pass into the foot and hand.[1] In many retinacula, fascial septa further compartmentalize the tunnel, and tendons passing through the compartments are enclosed in synovial tendon sheaths to reduce friction. The retinacula serve to protect all the structures that pass deep to them and also hold the tendons in close apposition to the bones. The latter increases the efficiency of the tendons by preventing their bowing out of position on muscle contraction.

The term *retinaculum* is also applied elsewhere to indicate connective tissue that is thickened to add support to a region. The patellar retinacula are thickened fascial expansions arising from the vastus medialis and vastus lateralis muscles and extending to either side of the knee joint, where they blend with ligaments and other supporting structures. The retinacula of the hip joint capsule are thickenings within this structure that protect and carry the major blood vessels of the head and neck of the femur.

Sesamoid Bones

Sesamoid bones are wholly or partially osseous structures that are generally quite small and are found embedded within tendons, either separately or in association with joint capsules.[1, 6] In the lower extremity, examples of the first type of sesamoid bone include those of the tibialis anterior, tibialis posterior, and peroneus longus. These bones are located within the tendons either near the point of insertion or where the tendon is abruptly and sharply angled in its passage. The point of contact actually resembles a joint, in that the apposed surfaces are covered with cartilage, and the area is typically enclosed by a small synovial bursa. Examples of the second type of sesamoid bone include the patella (by far the largest bone of this type), the tibial and fibular sesamoids of the first metatarsophalangeal joint, and the variable sesamoids of other joints in the toes. In all these examples the sesamoid bones are embedded within a complex of structures that includes the joint capsule, inserting tendons, and associated ligaments. Sesamoid bones are thought to protect from wear or excessive friction those structures within which they are found. They are also thought to change the direction of pull of tendons, presumably to improve their efficiency. Of common concern from a clinical standpoint are inflammation, varying degrees of displacement, frank dislocation, and fracture of sesamoid bones.

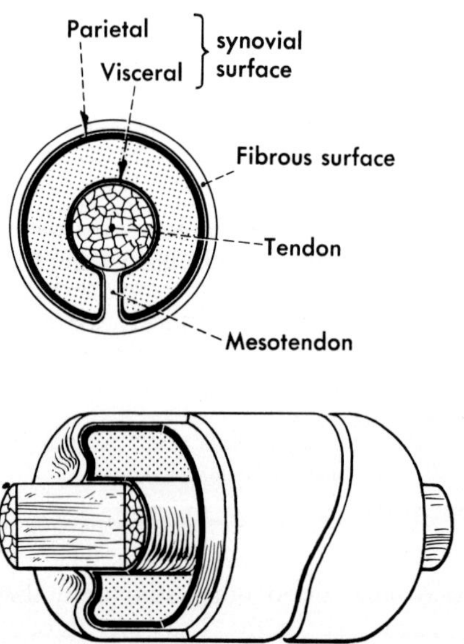

FIGURE 1–9. Diagram of a synovial tendon sheath. The upper view is a cross-section, the lower view shows the tendon sheath from the side, with a gap indicating that a segment has been removed. In this lower view, layers have been cut away at various levels so that the interior of the sheath can be seen. The space in which synovial fluid would be located is indicated with stippling. (From Hollinshead WH and Jenkins DB: Functional Anatomy of the Limbs and Back, 5th ed. Philadelphia, WB Saunders, 1981, p 32.)

BLOOD SUPPLY, LYMPHATIC DRAINAGE, AND INNERVATION OF JOINTS

Synovial joints typically receive a generous blood supply, delivered by branches from all major arteries passing near the articulation. Extensive anastomoses between the terminal branches of these arteries occur in tissues surrounding the joint as well as within the capsule and synovial membrane. In the extremities, anastomoses ensure that the blood supply to the joint and more distal parts of the limb is maintained in the event of interruption of blood flow through a major artery. Such a circumstance may be normal and temporary, such as that related to the motion of the joint, or may be due to a progressive and pathologic obstruction.

Many of the details of the arterial supply of joints were first described in 1743 by William Hunter. He observed that arteries piercing the joint capsule divide numerous times and form a network between the capsule and the synovial membrane; this network surrounds the joint at the point of capsular attachment to bone. Hunter termed this arrangement the *circulus articuli vasculosus*. From this circular network, branches arise to supply all parts of the joint except the articular cartilage, which is avascular. Branches to the joint capsule and associated tendons and ligaments usually run longitudinally between fascicles of connective tissue fibers and anastomose at intervals by transversely arranged branches. This has been described as a "ladder-like" pattern.[30, 38] Nevertheless, some regions of tendons are relatively hypovascular, even under normal circumstances. Examples include the middle third of the tendocalcaneus and of the patellar tendon, and it has been suggested that spontaneous rupture of these structures may be related to ischemia.[36]

At the attachments of the capsule, superficial vessels anastomose with periosteal vessels, whereas deeper vessels either terminate in capillary loops or enter the bone and anastomose with epiphyseal arteries. On the other hand, few vessels actually enter the bone at the entheses of intracapsular tendons and ligaments, which in part explains the slowness of the repair process in these structures.[38]

The synovial membrane of joints is particularly well supplied with blood and may, if it is thick and areolar in type, possess a series of as many as three layers of arterial plexuses. The first or outermost of these consists of larger arterial branches in direct communication with those of the capsule and the circulus articuli vasculosus. From this plexus, branches feed an intermediate subintimal plexus of finer vessels from which, in turn, a third and innermost plexus of precapillary arterioles is formed. The last supplies a dense meshwork of capillaries that lies immediately beneath the intimal layer of synovial cells. At the margins of the articular cartilage, capillaries of this part of the synovial membrane terminate as a series of loops oriented toward the synovial cavity.[30, 38]

The richness of the blood supply to areolar synovial membrane coupled with its extreme proximity to the joint cavity explains both the rapidity of fluid exchange across the membrane and the frequency with which even minor trauma or articular disease results in hemarthrosis. Thinner types of synovial membrane and regions of membrane subject to greater mechanical forces are less well vascularized.[38]

Intra-articular discs and menisci receive arterial branches from a peripheral plexus, located where these structures are attached to the joint capsule. The branches penetrate for a short distance into the disc or meniscus, where they terminate in capillary loops. Most of the structure is avascular, receiving its nutrition from the synovial fluid. The proportion of avascular tissue increases with age, which may account for the gradual degeneration that is commonly observed in discs and menisci.[30, 38]

The veins of articular tissues essentially follow the pattern of the arteries; they are extremely numerous and have abundant anastomoses. In the synovial membrane, one vein usually accompanies each artery of the outer plexuses, whereas two veins accompany each artery in the innermost plexus. Arteriovenous anastomoses are also common within the synovial membrane and other articular tissues. Although their precise function is unknown, it is presumed that they act as shunts for redirecting blood flow to areas of greatest need.[30, 38]

As previously discussed, the lymphatic system of the synovial membrane is involved in the absorption of certain components of the synovial fluid and, thus, in the maintenance of a healthy joint. There is a single plexus of lymphatic vessels in the synovial membrane, and it is located in the subintima. From this plexus branches terminating as blind-ending sacs extend toward the intimal surface but do not approach it as closely as do the blood capillaries of that layer. The lymphatics of the synovial membrane and those of the capsule are drained by larger vessels that accompany major blood vessels and pass to the regional deep lymph nodes.[30]

Most joints are innervated from several different sources. First, there are one or more primary, independent, articular branches from adjacent peripheral nerves. These often travel along fascial planes in neurovascular bundles with major blood vessels. Second, most joints receive accessory articular innervation from branches of nerves concerned primarily with the supply of muscles that act on or pass near to the joint. Finally, some joints receive fine articular branches that arise from cutaneous nerves supplying overlying skin. Because of the multiplicity of nerve sources, the indirect routes taken by some branches, and the microscopic size of many articular nerves, it is extremely difficult to completely denervate a joint.[30, 39]

All joints that have been studied appear similar in the general pattern of nerve distribution and in the variety of encapsulated and free nerve endings present. Joint capsules and ligaments are highly innervated tissues, with those regions most subject to compression or deformation being particularly heavily supplied with proprioceptors providing feedback to the central nervous system. On the other hand, synovial membrane, intra-articular discs, and menisci are relatively less well supplied with nerves. Functionally, the different types of sensory receptors fall within four major groups.[30, 39, 40] The first includes mechanoreceptors of the Ruffini type that are stimulated by changes in the position or tension of the joint capsule as it passes through its range of motion. The second group includes mechanoreceptors of the pacinian type. These receptors are also found in capsules as well as in other articular tissues, such as ligaments and tendons. They are rapidly adapting receptors that respond to acceleration, speed of movement, and vibration. The third category of nerve ending is essentially a Golgi type of tendon organ and is located in ligaments. This type of receptor responds to high tensions such as those applied at the extremes of joint position. The fourth group consists of nociceptors, free nerve endings that function as pain receptors responding to extremes of tension or to critical levels of certain chemicals that are released, for example, by ischemic or inflamed tissues. Such substances include, among others, lactic acid, histamine, and potassium ions. The joint capsule and associated ligaments are richly supplied with free nerve endings and are the major source of joint pain. Early experimental studies of knee joints in human volunteers showed that the synovial membrane, on the other hand, is relatively insensitive to pain.[41]

Finally, there are many small, unmyelinated fibers terminating on vessel walls and located throughout the capsule and associated tissues, including the synovial membrane. These are presumed to be sympathetic and vasomotor in function.

References

1. Williams PL, Warwick R, Dyson M, et al: Gray's Anatomy, 37th (British) ed. London, Churchill Livingstone, 1989, pp 460–485.
2. Leeson TS, Leeson CR, and Paparo AA: Text/Atlas of Histology. Philadelphia, WB Saunders, 1988, pp 189–194.
3. Jee WSS. The skeletal tissues. *In* Weiss T (ed): Histology: Cell and Tissue Biology. New York, Elsevier Biomedical, 1983, pp 247–254.
4. Salter RB: Textbook of Disorders and Injuries of the Musculoskeletal System, 2nd ed. Baltimore, Williams & Wilkins, 1983, pp 14–24.
5. Junqueira LC, Carneiro J, and Long JA: Basic Histology. Los Altos, Lange Medical Publications, 1986, pp 161–165.
6. Resnick D and Niwayama G: Diagnosis of Bone and Joint Disorders, Vol 2. Philadelphia, WB Saunders, 1988, pp 615–645.
7. Jacobs AM, Sollecito V, Oloff L, et al: Tarsal coalitions: An instructional review. J Foot Surg 20:214–221, 1981.
8. Cormack DH: Ham's Histology, 9th ed. Philadelphia, JB Lippincott, 1987, pp 324–338.
9. Benninghoff A: Form und bau der gelenkknorpel in ihren beziehungen zur funktion. II: Der aufbau des gelenk-knorpels in seinen beziehungen zur funktion. Z Zellforsch U Mikroskop Anat (Berlin) 2:783–862, 1925.
10. Clark JM: The organisation of collagen fibrils in the superficial zones of articular cartilage. J Anat 171:117–130, 1990.
11. Ghadially FN: Structure and function of articular cartilage. Clin Rheum Dis 7:3–28, 1981.
12. Weiss C, Rosenberg L, and Helfet AJ: An ultrastructural study of normal young adult human articular cartilage. J Bone Joint Surg 50A:663–674, 1968.
13. Dunham J, Shackleton DR, Billingham MEJ, et al: A reappraisal of the structure of normal canine articular cartilage. J Anat 157:89–99, 1988.
14. Ghadially FN and Roy S: Ultrastructure of Synovial Joints in Health and Disease. London, Butterworth, 1969, pp 1–59.
15. Lane JM and Weiss C: Review of articular cartilage collagen research. Arthritis Rheum 18:553–562, 1975.
16. Malemud CJ and Moskowitz RW: Physiology of articular cartilage. Clin Rheum Dis 7:29–55, 1981.
17. Oettmeier R, Abendroth K, and Oettmeier S: I. Analyses of the tidemark on human femoral heads. Acta Morphol Hung 37:155–168, 1989.
18. Oettmeier R, Abendroth K, and Oettmeier S: II. Tidemark changes in osteoarthritis—a histological and histomorphometric study in non-decalcified preparations. Acta Morphol Hung 37:169–180, 1989.
19. MacConaill MA: The movements of bones and joints: IV. The mechanical structure of articulating cartilage. J Bone Joint Surg 33B:251–257, 1951.
20. Muller-Gerbl M, Schulte E, and Putz R: The thickness of the calcified layer of articular cartilage: A function of the load supported? J Anat 154:103–111, 1987.
21. Clark JM: The structure of vascular channels in the subchondral plate. J Anat 171:105–115, 1990.
22. Hasselbacher P: Structure of the synovial membrane. Clin Rheum Dis 7:57–69, 1981.
23. Hu S, Zeng T, and Zuo R: Evidence that the meniscus is covered by synovial membrane. Can J Sport Sci 14:197–199, 1989.
24. Castor CW: The microscopic structure of normal human synovial tissue. Arthritis Rheum 3:140–151, 1960.
25. Ghadially FN and Roy S: Ultrastructure of rabbit synovial membrane. Ann Rheum Dis 25:318–326, 1966.
26. Henderson B: The synovial lining cell and synovitis. Scand J Rheumatol Suppl 76:33–38, 1988.
27. Barland P, Novikoff AB, and Hamerman D: Electron microscopy of the human synovial membrane. J Cell Biol 14:207–220, 1962.
28. Edwards JCW: Viewpoint: The synovial lining—a movable feast. Br J Rheumatol 28:534–536, 1989.
29. Hills BA: Oligolamellar nature of the articular surface. J Rheumatol 17:349–356, 1990.
30. Barnett CH, Davies DV, and MacConaill MA: Synovial Joints: Their Structure and Mechanics. Springfield, Charles C. Thomas, 1961, pp 54–73.
31. LeMinor JM: Comparative morphology of the lateral meniscus of the knee in primates. J Anat 170:161–171, 1990.
32. Engel R and Bogduk N: The menisci of the lumbar zygapophyseal joints. J Anat 135:795–809, 1982.
33. Grant JCB: Intraarticular synovial folds. Br J Surg 18:636–640, 1931.
34. Canoso JJ: Bursae, tendons, and ligaments. Clin Rheum Dis 7:189–221, 1981.
35. Canoso JJ, Stack MT, and Brandt KD: Hyaluronic acid content of deep and subcutaneous bursae of man. Ann Rheum Dis 42:171–175, 1983.
36. Cooper RR and Misol S: Tendon and ligament insertion. J Bone Joint Surg 52A:1–20, 1970.
37. Hollinshead WH and Jenkins DB: Functional Anatomy of the Limbs and Back. Philadelphia, WB Saunders, 1981, p 32.
38. Liew M and Dick WC: The anatomy and physiology of blood flow in a diarthrodial joint. Clin Rheum Dis 7:131–148, 1981.
39. Wyke B: The neurology of joints: A review of general principles. Clin Rheum Dis 7:223–239, 1981.
40. Zimny ML: Mechanoreceptors in articular tissues. Am J Anat 182:16–32, 1988.
41. Kellgren JH and Samuel EP: The sensitivity and innervation of the articular capsule. J Bone Joint Surg 32B:84–92, 1950.

CHAPTER 2

Bone and Cartilage: Physiology and Repair

Geoffrey Heard, D.P.M.

Bone and cartilage are similar in that they are specialized connective tissues that share a common mesenchymal origin and they consist of cells embedded in an intercellular matrix permeated by a system of collagenous fibers. However, bone and cartilage are quite dissimilar in other features such as degree of vascularity and patterns of growth. In addition, bone is dynamic and undergoes constant remodeling via resorption of old bone and production of new bone, whereas cartilage is relatively static and incapable of the same degree of remodeling as bone. These differences between bone and cartilage have profound consequences as far as their respective abilities to adapt to new stresses and repair themselves after injury.

BONE

Development

Bone formation is usually described as occurring in one of two distinct manners: endochondral or membranous. This distinction is based on whether bone is formed de novo from mesenchymal tissue or by osseous replacement of a cartilage model. An understanding of the differences between these two processes is helpful when discussing bone healing, but it should be emphasized that both patterns of bone formation are basically alike. The formation of bone is always the end result of bone-forming cells called *osteoblasts* functioning in a vascular environment to produce an organic matrix that will become calcified.

Endochondral Ossification

All the bones of the lower extremity develop by endochondral ossification. In this type of bone formation, the construction of bone via osteoblasts is preceded by a hyaline cartilage model that is gradually supplanted by bone. Initially, there is a condensation of mesenchyme, with cartilaginous cells forming a model of the future bone and secreting an extracellular matrix. The cells at the periphery of the cartilaginous bone model form a connective tissue sheath that surrounds the cartilage model, the perichondrium. At a certain stage of development that is specific for each bone, a primary ossification center develops. In long bones the primary ossification is always in the shaft or *diaphysis*. The cartilage cells in this

ossification center become enlarged, their borders calcify, and the cells die.

Because cartilage is avascular, it is totally dependent on blood vessels on its periphery to provide nutrients.[1] As these blood vessels infiltrate the perichondrium, they carry with them osteoprogenitor cells that turn into bone-forming osteoblast cells. These cells then lay down osteoid, the intercellular matrix of bone, and the matrix starts to calcify. This process results in the formation of a bony collar around the periphery of the cartilage model and the conversion of the perichondrium into periosteum. As diffusion of nutrients to the center of the cartilaginous shaft decreases, more cartilage cells start to die. Blood vessels then grow into the spaces left by the dead cartilage cells, bringing with them osteoblasts that will eventually replace the dying cartilage cells with bone cells.[2]

At both ends of the diaphysis are areas of spongy bone called the *metaphyses.* Beyond the metaphyses are the *epiphyses,* which are cartilaginous early in life. At specific times after birth, secondary centers of ossification form in the epiphyses that are similar to the primary centers in the diaphysis. As bone formation at the primary ossification center in the diaphysis starts to advance toward the epiphyses, the secondary centers of ossification begin formation of bone that advances toward the diaphysis. Eventually, all the cartilage is replaced by bone except for a single area of cartilage. This area of cartilage is referred to as the *physis,* or *growth plate.* Most bones have two growth plates, but the metatarsals and phalanges have only one.

Bone is capable only of appositional growth, that is, circumferential growth like that exhibited by the growth rings of trees. Cartilage, on the other hand, is capable of appositional and interstitial growth. Interstitial growth allows for longitudinal increases in bone length, and interstitial growth at the growth plate is solely responsible for the postfetal growth in bone length.

The growth plate has an orderly structure, and the cartilage cells, or chondrocytes, are arranged in a characteristic columnar pattern. Differences in the morphology of these chondrocytes allow for the division of the growth plate into distinctive zones. Cartilage cells on the epiphyseal side of the growth plate undergo interstitial growth via mitotic division, whereas the cartilage cells on the diaphyseal side of the growth plate are replaced by bone. The process occurring at the growth plate can be likened to a race, with the cartilage cells constantly increasing their numbers via mitotic division in an attempt to avoid being overtaken by bone-forming cells. Once the bone-forming cells overtake the cartilage cells, the growth plate closes and longitudinal bone growth ceases.

Various nomenclature has been used to describe the zones of the growth plate, and the number of zones delineated by investigators differs, but they all describe essentially the same process. The zone closest to the epiphysis is the *resting, or germinal, zone,* which contains the cells that initiate interstitial growth. These cells undergo mitosis, and the newly formed cells displace the older cells, which line up in longitudinal columns. As the older cells advance, they pass into the next layer, the *zone of proliferating cells.* The cells in this zone are actively involved in cellular division and the production of cartilage intercellular substance. The next layer contains large cells that are no longer undergoing mitotic division and is termed the *transitional zone.* The cells in the transitional zone continue their migration while hypertrophying to as much as five times their normal size, eventually forming the *zone of hypertrophy* (Fig. 2–1).[3]

Chondrocytes starting out in the germinal and proliferating zones are in close contact with the epiphyseal vessels. As these cells move away from the epiphyseal vessels that they rely on for their metabolic needs, they enlarge, become vacuolated, and eventually die. While this process is occurring, the extracellular matrix between the chondrocytes becomes mineralized in a process still not well understood. Multiple capillary loops from the metaphyseal vessels enter from the diaphyseal side of the growth plate in fingerlike projections, carrying with them multinuclear cells that resorb the dead chondrocytes and primitive cells that differentiate into osteoblasts. These osteoblasts lay down a thin layer of bone matrix on the remains of the calcified cartilage. This matrix starts to mineralize while new matrix is laid down appositionally. As the bone grows out in length and width via interstitial and appositional growth, respectively, bone is resorbed at an equal rate from the center of the bone. Were this resorption not to occur, adult bone would be solid throughout instead of possessing a medullary cavity in the middle of the diaphysis.[4]

Because the bone formation occurring at the ossification centers and at the growth plate involves the replacement of cartilage by bone, both processes have been termed *endochondral ossification.* The bone repair seen in most fractures also involves the gradual replacement of a cartilage precursor by bone and is commonly referred to as *endochondral bone repair.* This terminology has caused some confusion when used to describe the events occurring during this type of bone repair and has led to the belief by some that these events are similar to those at the growth plate. However, during fracture repair there is no formation of an orderly structure like a growth plate and no continued proliferation of cartilage cells on one side and ossification on the other. If such conditions did exist, all fractures would heal lengthened. Increased bone length after fracture repair can occur in children, but this is probably a result of increased blood supply, electronegativity, or both, at the growth plate and not any increase in length occurring at the fracture site itself.

Because endochondral bone repair has been likened to the healing by secondary intention seen in soft tissue, it is also referred to as *secondary bone healing.* This is an unfortunate choice of terms. Unlike soft tissue healing, where the gap is filled by granulation tissue with subsequent healing by scar tissue, in most cases of fracture repair the granulation tissue is eventually replaced by bone and not scar tissue. Furthermore, the term *secondary* can imply ''less frequent'' or ''inferior,'' when in reality this is the most common mechanism of fracture repair and achieves stability sooner than so-called primary healing (discussed later).

Membranous Ossification

Membranous ossification is seen in flat bones, such as the skull and the clavicle, and occurs via direct differentiation of mesenchymal cells into osteoblasts. This type of bone formation without an intermediate cartilage stage is similar to the other type of fracture repair, which is often referred to as *primary bone healing* owing to its similarity to soft tissue healing by primary intention. The term *primary bone healing* may give the impression that this process is the more normal and desirable method. In actuality, this type of fracture repair occurs only in a minority of cases, such as when there is

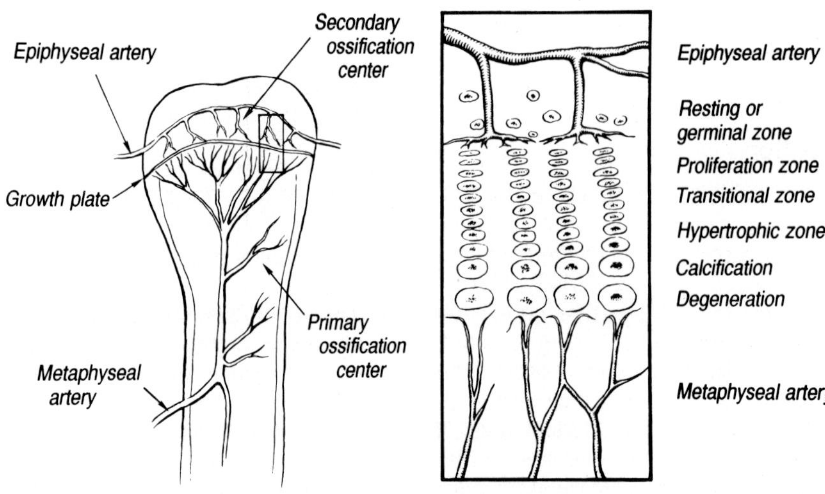

FIGURE 2–1. Zones of the growth plate.

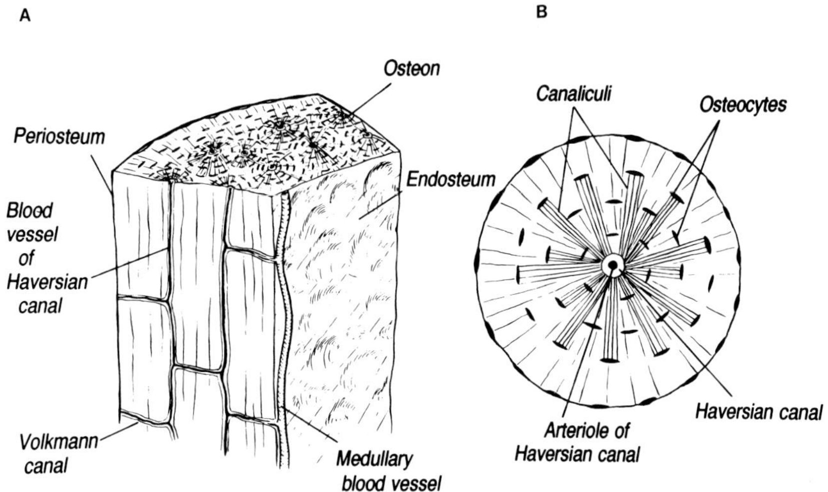

FIGURE 2–2. *A,* Structure of cortical (compact) bone. *B,* Structure of osteon.

little or no movement between the fracture ends and the blood supply is largely undamaged, or in those cases when rigid fixation is employed to repair the fracture.

Composition and Structure

Cell Types. There are three distinct groups of bone cells that have been clearly identified. Research continues into the origins and mechanisms of these cells and the possibility that other cells may play key roles in bone formation and remodeling. However, this section focuses primarily on the three most recognized cell types and what is currently known about them.

The osteoblasts, as stated earlier, are responsible for laying down osteoid, which will eventually become calcified to form bone. As osteoblasts lay down osteoid around them, they eventually become entrapped in their own matrix. When this occurs, they become osteocytes.

Osteocytes are the principal cells of mature bone, and they lie within lacunae. The exact role of osteocytes is still a source of controversy, but there is little evidence to support earlier suggestions that osteocytes serve a dual role in bone formation and resorption.

Osteoclasts are multinucleated cells whose function is bone resorption. These cells are located in Howship's lacunae found on the edges of bone surfaces where bone resorption is occurring.

Woven Versus Lamellar Bone. The bone formed during embryonic development, active growth in children, or the initial repair of fractures is referred to as *woven, fibrous,* or *immature bone.* Woven bone derives its name from the random, intertwining appearance of coarse bundles of collagen fibers.

Lamellar or mature bone replaces woven bone and is the bone seen in the normal adult skeleton. Lamellar bone derives its name from the sheetlike arrangement of mineralized bone matrix, referred to as *lamellae.*

Typical lamellar bone is approximately 8% water and 92% solid material. The solid portion of bone can be divided into an organic matrix, known as *osteoid,* and an inorganic com-ponent. Approximately 98% of the osteoid consists of type I collagen fibers that are embedded in the ground substance that constitutes the other 2% of the matrix. The ground substance comprises glycosaminoglycans (GAGs) and proteoglycans. GAGs are repeating disaccharide units with a net negative charge due to attached carboxyl and sulfate groups, and proteoglycans consist of multiple GAGs attached to a core protein. The inorganic phase of bone is composed primarily of hydroxyapatite and, to a lesser degree, calcium carbonate.[5]

The collagen fibers are aligned parallel to the tensile and compressive stresses the bone is subjected to, and the needle-shaped hydroxyapatite crystals are oriented parallel to the collagen fibers.

Cortical Versus Cancellous Bone. The morphology of mature bone is either cortical or cancellous. Cortical bone is hard and compact, and the basic unit is the osteon. Each osteon consists of a centrally located haversian canal through which one or more blood vessels run. The haversian canal is surrounded by concentric lamellae, each with a lacuna containing an osteocyte. Cytoplasmic processes extend from the osteocyte through canaliculi, enabling the osteocyte to communicate with the vessels in the haversian canal.[6] Another series of canals, Volkmann's canals, traverse from the periosteum of the outer cortex to the medullary cavity in the center of the bone. Each of these canals contains a blood vessel and communicates with the vessels in the haversian canals of the osteons it traverses (Fig. 2–2).

Cancellous bone, also known as *spongy* or *trabecular bone,* comprises a network of partitions or columns called *trabeculae* that enclose marrow-containing cavities. The trabeculae are oriented along lines of stress to maximize their weightbearing potential. Cancellous bone is different from cortical bone in that it has no haversian canals and is much more porous. The difference in porosity between cancellous and cortical bone has an effect on how revascularization and healing occur and is discussed further in the section on bone grafts.

The shaft, or diaphysis, of mature long bone consists of a tube of cortical bone that surrounds the medullary cavity, a largely hollow center containing fatty and hematopoietic marrow. The lining of the marrow cavity is known as the *endosteum*, and located within the endosteum are undifferentiated mesenchymal cells that will serve as the source of osteoblasts for fracture repair. These cells are also called *fibroblasts*, or *osteoprogenitor, cells.* The term *osteoprogenitor* has been used to distinguish them from osteoblasts, which have lost the capability of cellular division.[7]

The expanded ends, or metaphyses, of mature long bone are composed of cancellous bone surrounded by cortical bone. The cortical bone at the ends of bone is thinner than that in the shaft. With the exception of the ends where there is hyaline cartilage, the entire external surface of long bones is covered by a fibrous sheet called the *periosteum* (Fig. 2–3). The outside layer of the periosteum is fibrous and appears to be purely supportive in function. The innermost layer of the periosteum is the cambium layer; like the endosteum, it contains osteogenic cells. Because of the presence of these cells, every attempt should be made to preserve the periosteum when any bone work is performed, although the endosteum ultimately plays the most critical role in bone healing.

Blood Supply

The blood vessels providing circulation to long bones have been classified by Rhinelander into three groups, according to function rather than anatomic location.[8, 9]

The first group is the afferent vascular system, which consists of arteries and arterioles carrying blood and nutrients to the bone. This is the system of most concern to clinicians and is the only one discussed in detail. The second group is the efferent vascular system, which consists of veins and venules carrying blood and waste products away from the bone. The third system, the intermediate vascular system of compact bone, serves the purpose of the capillary network seen in soft tissues. This is not a true capillary system, however, because nutrients do not diffuse directly into the tissues being supplied but cross the cortex in canaliculi. These canaliculi enclose the bone tissue fluid in a compartment separate from that of the interstitial fluid surrounding

soft tissue blood vessels.[10] In addition, the size of these vessels is determined by the bony canals they travel through and does not vary under different conditions.

Normal blood flow through the diaphyseal cortex of long bone is mainly centrifugal, that is, from the medulla out to the periosteum. This blood flow pattern is primarily the result of a higher intravascular pressure in the medulla than in the periosteal area.[8, 11]

Adult long bone has three main afferent blood supplies: the principal nutrient artery, the metaphyseal-epiphyseal arteries, and the periosteal network of arterioles (Fig. 2–4). The principal nutrient artery (or arteries) penetrates the cortex through a foramen and enters directly into the medullary cavity. Once in the medulla, it divides into the ascending and descending medullary arteries that provide the main blood supply to the diaphysis.

The metaphyseal-epiphyseal arteries are numerous and penetrate the cortex at both metaphyses. These vessels anastomose at each end of the medulla with the medullary arteries to supply the spongy medulla. Under normal circumstances these vessels contribute minimally to the medullary circulation. However, when the principal artery is damaged owing to surgery or fracture, these vessels can become the sole blood supply to the medullary cavity.

The periosteal network of arterioles supplies only the outer one third to one fourth of the cortical bone. Rhinelander demonstrated that even when the medullary arterial supply was obliterated by an intramedullary nail, the periosteal network was still able to supply only the outer cortex.[8]

Both the principal nutrient artery and the periosteal network of arterioles enter the cortex only at the site of major fascial attachments, whereas the metaphyseal-epiphyseal arteries enter at all sides of the proximal and distal metaphyses. Because of this, all attempts should be made to minimize soft tissue dissection of bone at major fascial attachments.

During repair of a fracture or osteotomy, all three components of the afferent vascular system become transiently enhanced locally. In addition, the injured soft tissues adjacent to the fracture-osteotomy furnish an extraosseous blood supply to healing bone.[9, 12]

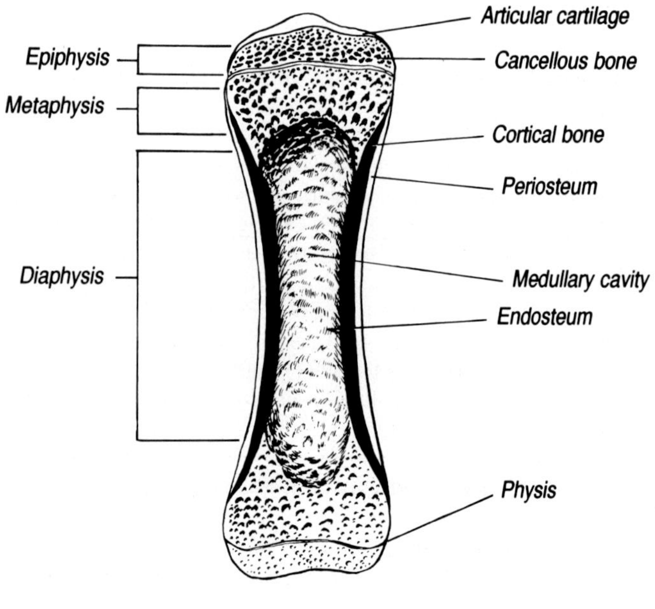

FIGURE 2–3. Structure of typical long bone. In mature long bone, the physis is absent.

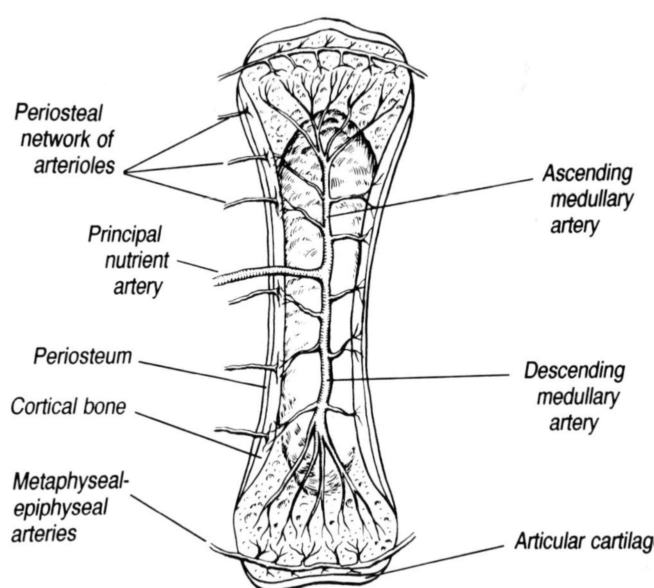

FIGURE 2–4. Diagrammatic representation of the blood supply to mature long bone.

Electrical Properties of Bone

Two different types of electrical potentials have been described as occurring in bone: stress-generated potentials and steady-state bioelectrical potentials. Stress-generated potentials are not dependent on cell viability and are found even in dead bone, whereas steady-state potentials are found only in viable bone.

Stress-Generated Potentials. Stress-generated potentials were first described in the 1950s by Fukada and Yasuda, who discovered that bone generated electrical signals when external forces were applied.[13] When nonuniform forces were applied to bone, those regions under tension exhibited positive potentials, whereas those regions under compression exhibited negative potentials.

It was hypothesized that these findings might offer a mechanism to explain Wolff's law of bone formation in areas of compression and bone resorption in areas of tension. If the application of physical forces to bone produced electrical potentials, it was postulated that these potentials might mediate the cellular response leading to remodeling. This hypothesis was strengthened by microelectrode studies that showed haversian canals in osteons under tension become more positive, and haversian canals in osteons under compression become more negative.[14]

Much of the early research on bone's endogenous electrical properties attempted to determine whether the source of these stress-generated potentials was due to piezoelectrical or electrokinetic effects.

Piezoelectricity is a generic term used to describe the generation of an electrical current by certain materials when they are stressed. The collagen portion of bone appears to account for the piezoelectrical properties of bone, with the mineral phase contributing little if anything.[15]

Electrokinetics involves the nonuniform spatial distribution of charges near the interface between a solid surface and an ion-containing fluid. All the parameters required for electrokinetic potentials exist in bone, and it has been hypothesized that this potential, also known as a *streaming potential,* could be generated by bone fluid flowing through canaliculi and haversian canals. These same streaming potentials have been shown to exist in cartilage under oscillatory compression.[16]

It is now believed that both piezoelectricity and streaming potentials are responsible for stress-generated potentials. The degree to which each contributes varies with differing conditions.

Steady-State Potentials. A different type of potential was reported by Friedenberg and Brighton, who recorded electrical potentials from bone in the absence of any external forces.[17] In a normal bone these steady-state potentials were electronegative in the metaphyseal regions and approached isopolarity in the diaphyseal regions. Actively growing regions of bone, such as the epiphyseal plate, exhibit electronegativity. In fractured bone the entire shaft becomes electronegative, with the fracture site and metaphyseal regions becoming relatively even more electronegative. Once the fracture is repaired, the potentials return to those seen in normal bone.

Fracture Healing

Any discussion of bone healing should begin with the understanding that most of the research on fracture repair has been carried out with animals. Although there are undoubtedly many similarities between the findings in certain animals and in humans, there are also some dissimilarities. For example, the size and volume of bones and cortices differ according to the size of the animal, but cell and fiber size stay fairly constant. Therefore, the relative length that cell and tissue types have to travel to effect repair differs. Animals also have different metabolic rates than humans, especially smaller animals such as rats and rabbits, which are commonly used in bone-healing studies.

Another factor often overlooked when reviewing the literature on osseous repair is that in some studies the bone was fractured, whereas in others an osteotomy was performed. Obviously, an osteotomy carried out under surgical conditions is going to be less damaging and disruptive to the soft and osseous tissues than a traumatic fracture.

Secondary Repair. The normal fracture repair process

seen in nonrigidly fixated fractures has been studied extensively. Numerous investigators have divided this sequence into different numbers of stages with various names, but all describe basically the same progression. Although well-defined steps are helpful in providing rough guidelines on which to base clinical decisions, it is important for the clinician to avoid thinking of stages in fracture healing as separate and distinct entities that occur within rigidly fixed time frames. Each stage is dependent on the stage that preceded it, and there is some overlap of these stages because more than one stage is usually present when fracture sites are explored surgically. In addition, fractures of different bones, and even fractures in the same bone but at different levels, may heal at significantly different rates. Individual variations may also occur owing to considerations such as the age of the patient and systemic factors.

Stages of Repair. The *inflammatory phase* begins immediately after the injury and consists of formation of a hematoma from disrupted blood vessels of the bone and surrounding soft tissues. The size of the hematoma is a function of the amount of bone and soft tissue damaged. Necrosis of the bone ends and clotting of blood vessels lead to vasodilatation, and the infiltration of plasma exudates brings with it the hallmark inflammatory cells such as mast cells, macrophages, and polymorphonuclear neutrophils (PMNs) as well as lysosomal enzymes. This stage correlates clinically with the development of pain and swelling, with the pain causing the patient to splint the injured area and the edema serving to partially immobilize the fractured bone. This usually lasts 3 or 4 days, with decrease in the pain and swelling marking the end of this phase.

The *reparative,* or *proliferative, phase* begins as capillaries and pluripotential mesenchymal cells begin to invade the fibrin scaffold provided by the hematoma and replace it with granulation tissue. In undisplaced fractures this process is dominated by the endosteum, whereas in displaced fractures the periosteal tissues dominate initially but are eventually replaced by the endosteal tissues. Within a few days callus formation begins as islands of cartilage and osteoid cells form in the granulation tissue. The osteogenic cells adjacent to the fracture site beneath the proliferating periosteum form bone directly via membranous ossification. This forms the base of the callus that will ultimately span the fracture site and has been likened to the towers of a suspension bridge by Urist and Johnson (Fig. 2–5).[18] Within 7 to 10 days, chondrocytes further away from the bone ends in a relatively avas-

cular environment proliferate and fabricate the matrix that ultimately spans the fracture gap, encompassing the bone ends and stabilizing the fracture fragments. This cartilage is gradually resorbed and replaced by bone via endochondral ossification. Although this type of fracture healing is referred to as *endochondral ossification,* it actually has components of membranous and endochondral ossification, with the former occurring first and the latter occurring subsequently and predominating the repair process.

The *remodeling phase,* the final stage, occurs once the fracture has been satisfactorily bridged. This phase is characterized by osteoclastic resorption of immature woven bone and its replacement with lamellar bone oriented according to lines of stress, reconstruction of the medullary canal, and restoration of the bone's preinjury diameter. This process appears to be governed by Wolff's law of bone formation at sites of compression and bone resorption at sites of tension. This phase can be quite prolonged and may continue for years, depending on the degree of the angulation and comminution of the fracture, the bone involved, and the age and condition of the patient.

Although the sequence of events seen during fracture healing is fairly well known, the underlying biochemical and physical effectors responsible for these events are not. Most research into bone healing currently is directed at identifying these substances and understanding their mechanisms of action. A more detailed understanding of these effectors of fracture healing is afforded by examining them within the framework of Heppenstall's classification, which divides fracture repair into a series of six stages,[6] as follows: (1) impact, (2) induction, (3) inflammation, (4) soft callus, (5) hard callus, and finally (6) remodeling. The first three stages are subdivisions of the inflammatory stage described earlier. The soft and hard callus stages are subdivisions of the proliferative stage.

Impact. The impact stage begins when more energy is applied to the bone than it can absorb without breaking and ends when the bone is fractured and the energy dissipated.

Induction. The events occurring in the induction stage have been at the vanguard of bone research during the last 20 years. At the impact stage, the local tissues contain few osteoblasts and no chondroblasts. Homeostatic regulation of bone volume is maintained through a continual balance of resorption of old bone and formation of new bone, so there are bone-forming cells active at the impact stage. However, these cells are active only to the extent that is necessary to

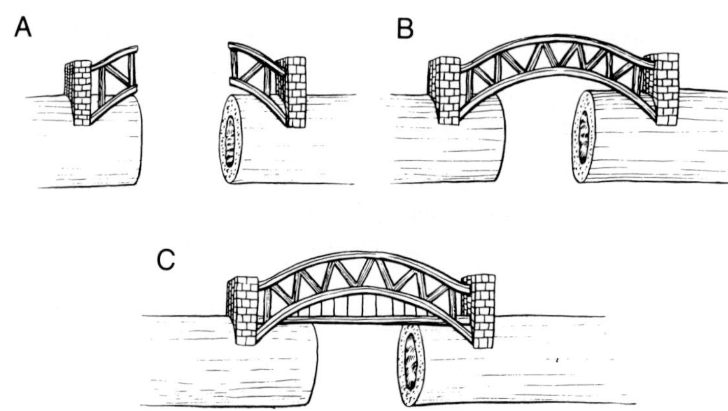

FIGURE 2–5. Urist and Johnson's analogy of long bone fracture repair with construction of an arched bridge. *A,* The towers represent initial periosteal bone formation. *B,* The arch represents continued subperiosteal trabeculation that spans the fracture ends and stabilizes the fracture. *C,* Once the fracture is stabilized, compact bone (represented by the roadway) bridges the fracture ends, replacing the fibrocartilaginous callus.

replace bone lost to normal resorption. The number of bone-forming cells and their activity level are not capable of producing the large amounts of bone needed to repair a fracture. It has been estimated that if a femoral shaft fracture were to depend solely on preexisting osteoblasts, between 200 and 1000 years would be required for healing.[19] To meet the demands required for fracture healing, two critical phenomena need to occur. First, all of the osteoblasts available need to be stimulated. Modulation is the method by which these cells are activated to begin the repair process. Even with modulation of the entire pool of available differentiated bone-forming cells, termed *determined osteogenic precursor cells* (DOPCs) by Friedenstein,[20] there are still not enough DOPCs in the fracture area to complete bone repair. Therefore, the second event that needs to occur is the recruitment of osteoprogenitor cells to the repair site. This second pool of cells consists of pluripotential fibroblast cells present in the marrow and surrounding soft tissue that are undifferentiated at the time of fracture. These cells acquire the ability to form bone in the presence of an inducing agent and have been termed *inducible osteogenic precursor cells* (IOPCs) by Friedenstein.[20] Induction is the process by which these cells differentiate and become bone-forming cells.

Although severe metabolic bone diseases such as scurvy, osteomalacia, osteoporosis, and Paget's disease suppress the normal repair process on a systemic level, most biologic causes of nonunions are local in nature. It is becoming increasingly clear that the local factors most responsible for noniatrogenic complications in bone healing are due to abnormalities in modulation and induction.[19]

It has been theorized for some time that the hypoxic, acidic environment following fracture-induced disruption of the blood supply may play a crucial role in modulation and induction.[6] Studies on chick embryonic tibial mesenchymal cells have shown that when these cells are subjected to low oxygen tensions and compression, they are transformed into cartilage-producing chondroblasts. When these cells are exposed to higher oxygen tensions and compression, they are transformed into bone-producing osteoblasts.[21] The list of possible modulators and inductors that have been identified over the last 20 years has grown to include a plethora of substances that include growth factors, mitogens, and chemotactic and differentiating agents.[22–24]

One of the more studied and earliest recognized inductors is bone morphogenetic protein (BMP). In 1965 Urist discovered that the implantation of demineralized bone matrix into the muscles of rodents induced ectopic bone formation.[25] Urist's initial findings have been corroborated by many subsequent investigators, and the ability of demineralized bone to induce bone formation was ascribed to a soluble, diffusible low-molecular-weight protein. This protein was given the name *bone morphogenetic protein* by Urist, although at the time it was not certain whether the effects of BMP were due to a single molecule or aggregates of molecules. In the 1980s when it was found that noncollagenous proteins (NCPs) induced bone formation, research emphasis shifted from looking at demineralized matrix to isolating BMP and associated NCPs from the bone matrix.

In 1984 Urist and colleagues were able to obtain purified BMP from bovine bone,[26] and since then several BMPs have been isolated from bone in sufficient quantity and quality to furnish amino acid sequencing. Wozney and associates were able to use oligonucleotide probes derived from the amino acid sequences of tryptic fragments of three BMP peptides to isolate complementary deoxyribonucleic acid (cDNA) clones, allowing for the expression of three recombinant human proteins.[27] These proteins have been named BMP-1, BMP-2A, and BMP-3 (also known as *osteogenin*). BMP-1 appears to be a novel regulatory protein, whereas BMP-2A and BMP-3 are new members of the transforming growth factor-β supergene family. Presently, seven proteins, BMP1–7, have been isolated and sequenced.

The current belief is that during fracture, transplantation, or even normal bone turnover, BMP is released from an aggregate of NCPs. There are also other growth factors found in bone matrix that seem to be released in the same manner as BMP and most likely play significant roles in induction, growth, and differentiation by exerting paracrine or autocrine effects. Among these are transforming growth factor-β, epidermal growth factor, insulin-like growth factors I and II, platelet-derived growth factor, and fibroblast growth factors (acidic and basic). Not all of these factors have been definitively shown to have chondrogenic or osteogenic activity in vivo, but it appears that the process of bone repair involves the interaction of many factors. Because these factors act in concert, with both concentration and time variables affecting the overall process, determining the effect of a single factor is difficult if not impossible.

Inflammation. Heppenstall's third stage is inflammation. The major events occurring during this stage (i.e., the influx of PMNs, neutrophils, mast cells, and macrophages) will be discussed in detail in Chapter 3. Because of its associated swelling and pain, clinicians often consider the inflammatory stage as nothing more than an unavoidable annoyance to both patient and clinician that must be tolerated while waiting for the important ensuing stages of repair to commence. In reality, the inflammatory phase is an important stage of repair, because the events commencing in this period are crucial to the progression of bone repair. For example, mast cells and certain types of leukocytes are first seen during the inflammatory stage. The exact role of these supporting cells is still subject to debate, but they undoubtedly serve an important role because they remain present long after the inflammatory phase passes.

Prostaglandins are released in large concentrations during the inflammatory phase, and their role in bone repair has been the focus of considerable research. Prostaglandins have been shown to have bone resorption effects similar to parathyroid hormone, and it has been proposed that prostaglandins may be responsible for the vascular changes and increase in osteogenic cells seen after bone fractures.

As discussed in greater detail later, a certain amount of motion appears to maximize the conditions that regulate fracture repair. In vitro studies have demonstrated that the application of mechanical forces to bone cells results in rapid increases in prostaglandin E_2 (PGE_2) production. Coinciding with this was an increase in cyclic adenosine monophosphate (cAMP) production and subsequent DNA synthesis. When PGE_2 was added to the cells, the effect on cAMP production was analogous to that seen with the application of mechanical forces. When these cells were pretreated with indomethacin (a prostaglandin inhibitor), application of mechanical forces failed to stimulate DNA synthesis.[28] These findings suggest that prostaglandins may mediate mechanogenic osteogenesis by acting on bone receptor mechanisms that, in turn, stimulate cAMP and DNA synthesis. It has been shown that PGE$_2$ accelerates the healing of bone in an in vivo dog model, whereas high doses of indomethacin were shown to decrease osteogenesis and increase fibrogenesis in a rat model of fracture healing.[29, 30] These results illustrate the double-edged sword that nonsteroidal antiinflammatory drug use may pose and argue for their judicious use in humans. Although such drugs may decrease the pain and swelling associated with the inflammatory stage, they may also impede the normal course of events required for uneventful bone healing.

Soft Callus. During this stage there is active proliferation of osteoblasts in the cambium layer of the periosteum and chondroblasts in the fracture gap. The endosteal blood supply begins to reestablish itself throughout this period, but owing to the profuse increases in cellularity, there is still a relative hypoxia. Clinically, this period is characterized by increased stability and decreased pain and swelling at the fracture site.

Heppenstall describes the formation of both an external and internal callus. The external callus is actually the result of two different mechanisms, as elaborated by McKibbin, who described three types of callus that appear during fracture repair: the primary callus response, the bridging external callus, and the late medullary callus.[7] The primary callus response and bridging callus formation can be considered as separate but interrelated phases that together constitute the external callus as defined by Heppenstall. McKibbin's late medullary callus is synonymous with Heppenstall's internal callus.

The first, or primary, callus begins within a week after the impact stage and is found in all fractures, irrespective of fixation. This is the callus described earlier that forms from the DPOCs beneath the intact periosteum and manufactures bone directly via membranous ossification. This response seems to be almost independent of environmental or hormonal circumstances, is short lived, and ceases if contact is not made with another fragment. Consequently, its ability to bridge gaps is limited.

If the gap existing between fracture fragments is too large for the primary callus to bridge, the next callus seen is the bridging external callus. Many of the events precipitated via induction come to fruition during formation of the bridging external callus. The bridging external callus is the callus characteristically seen in radiographs of nonfixated diaphyseal fractures; it seems to originate from the IOPCs in the neovascular and surrounding soft tissues. It appears that this response is governed by humoral induction as well as mechanical factors, because the magnitude of its response is directly proportional to the amount of motion at the fracture site. The greater the amount of motion at the fracture site, the larger the callus, whereas rigid immobilization inhibits callus formation. These mechanical effects are most likely mediated by bioelectrical phenomena that are still not well understood, because it is during this period that the entire shaft of the fractured bone becomes electronegative, and the fracture site and metaphyseal regions become even more electronegative. Once the fracture is repaired, the potentials return to those seen in normal bone. The primary purpose of the bridging external callus is believed to be stabilization of the fracture ends. This would provide a stable platform for osteoprogenitor cells to lay down bone and prevent disruption of fragile new vessels entering the fracture site from the medullary cavity.

The third type of callus described by McKibbin is the late medullary callus. It arises principally from the medullary cavity and is a prolonged process that may continue for months. The amount of cartilage found in this callus is much less than that found in the first two calluses. Mechanical stability appears to promote a later stage of medullary callus that replaces fibrous tissue with woven bone, probably to enable new osteons to pass across small gaps. Because of the larger amounts of endosteal bone surface and greater vascularity present in cancellous bone, this is the type of callus response that predominates in the healing of cancellous bone. This is also the principal form of fracture healing occurring in plate-fixated fractures with imperfect apposition of bone ends.

Hard Callus. During this stage the cartilaginous callus is transformed to woven bone via endochondral ossification. In addition to the osteoblasts laying down new bone, the osteoclasts are still actively removing the remaining necrotic bone. The vascular supply increases as the endosteal blood supply continues to reestablish itself, but the conditions remain hypoxic owing to cellular proliferation and activity. This stage begins at 3 or 4 weeks and persists until the fracture ends are solidly bridged with new bone.

Remodeling. As described earlier, this last stage of fracture repair involves the resorption of immature woven bone by osteoclasts and its replacement with lamellar bone by osteoblasts. During this period the medullary canal is reconstructed, the external callus is resorbed, and the bone returns to its prefracture dimensions. This process appears to be governed by Wolff's law of bone resorption at sites of tension and bone formation at sites of compression, with the new bone oriented along lines of compressive and tensile forces. This phase can last from several months to years, depending on the degree of the angulation and comminution of the fracture, the bone involved, and the age and condition of the patient.

Primary Healing. In those rare instances when a stable fracture site and close apposition of the bone ends occur naturally, or when rigid internal fixation is employed to attain these objectives in a fracture or osteotomy, bone repair proceeds without the formation of an external callus and without an intermediary cartilaginous stage. Primary healing was first observed radiographically in plated fractures by Danis in 1949, who described this manner of union as *soudure autogene,* or autogenous weld.[31] Schenk and Willenegger were the first to describe the underlying histologic events observed in a dog radius, and their findings have been confirmed by others using different bones and different animal models.[32]

In primary healing of bone, fracture-induced disruption of the local vascular supply results in the death of the osteons close to the fracture site, but the dead ends of the bone are not resorbed. Instead, the dead ends are recanalized by osteoclasts that form spearheads at the ends of the haversian canals in viable bone close to the fracture site. These spearheads (often referred to as *cutting cones*) advance across the fracture site, producing enlarged haversian canals that slowly cross the fracture site. As the cutting cones traverse across the fracture site, blood vessels and osteoblasts follow, laying down new bone to bridge the fracture site. In those areas where the bone ends are not in intimate contact, the gaps are filled by bone arising from the endosteum of the haversian system. This bone then serves as a bridge to allow new haversian systems to traverse the gap.

Schenk and Willeneger used tetracycline labeling in a dog

model to calculate the rate of primary bone repair. Osteoblastic tunneling did not commence for 3 weeks, and the cutting cones advanced at a rate of only 50 to 80 μm/day.[32] This translates to 1 mm in 12 to 20 days and is a relatively slow rate of fracture healing. These calculations were made on osteotomies performed with fine saw cuts under ideal conditions and likely do not accurately depict those conditions seen in all osteotomies or fractures.

CLINICAL APPLICATIONS

Debate on Rigid Fixation

One of the questions about fracture healing that remains unanswered, and is of particular importance to the clinician dealing with the lower extremity, is what constitutes the ideal mechanical environment. The goals of fracture repair are to restore as close to normal those conditions that were present before the injury. This is not limited to restoration of the original shape of the bone but also must take into account the condition of any associated joints and soft tissue. Rigid internal fixation was developed in an attempt to achieve all these goals.

Although there are distinct advantages to internal fixation of fractures, including avoidance of external immobilizers, earlier mobilization of the limb, and maintenance of length and correction, it is not necessarily better than secondary healing. There are some well-documented disadvantages of internal fixation, and debate continues on what conditions, if any, internal fixation should be used.

As noted earlier, even under ideal conditions bone repair by primary healing is a slow process. The question of how advantageous it is to promote bone healing without formation of an external callus then arises, because formation of external callus is the quickest manner to bridge a fracture gap. In those instances when there is a gap between the fracture ends, primary healing takes even longer. The extra dissection necessary for adequate surgical exposure to place drill holes and position the plate can cause additional vascular compromise, which can slow down the repair process even further. Application of a plate to the bone can temporarily decrease the efflux of blood via the efferent vascular system. Because the normal centrifugal blood flow is due to higher pressure in the medulla than the periosteum, any increase in the periosteal pressure by blockage of the efferent system can suppress the influx of blood from the medulla.

Plating of a fracture can also impede the rate of bone healing in other ways. There is substantial experimental and clinical evidence to suggest that a certain amount of mechanical loading serves as a stimulus to promote bone healing. Too much motion can prevent bone healing, but rigid immoblization can retard it. Plating of a fracture also shields it from the mechanical stresses that would normally pass through a repaired bone and strengthen it. The plate must be removed to allow the underlying bone to regain its prefracture strength. This plate should not be removed before 12 to 18 months, and even then there is the real possibility of refracture until the bone completely remodels. Attempts to overcome the problems posed by absolute rigidity yet retain the benefits of some stability have led to preliminary studies of alternative biomaterials. Among those materials being examined are carbon fiber–reinforced methyl methacrylate polymers and biodegradable polymers. The latter have been used successfully in the treatment of ankle fractures and have the added advantage of dissolving with time, avoiding the necessity for a second surgery to remove them.[33]

Bone Grafts

Bone grafts have been employed for more than 300 years, and approximately 1 million bone grafts are performed in the United States annually.[34] They are used in a variety of situations, including the treatment of delayed unions and nonunions, pseudarthroses, replacement of osseous defects left after trauma, infection or tumors, arthrodesis of joints, and reconstruction of congenital defects or deficits.

The terminology used when describing bone grafting is often confusing. The current term for tissue transplanted from one part of the body to another is *autograft.* The adjective used to describe this type of tissue is *autogeneic,* but the older terms *autogenous* and *autologous* are sometimes still found in the literature. The new term for tissue transplanted between members of the same species is *allograft,* replacing the older term *homograft.* The newer adjective to describe this tissue is *allogeneic,* replacing the old adjective *homogenous.* Urist recommends that the term *allograft* be restricted to living tissue, and when nonviable bone prepared by chemical agents, irradiation, freezing, or freeze-drying is transplanted, the term *alloimplant* be used.[35] This terminology has not been universally accepted as evidenced by the term *freeze-dried allograft.*

The term *syngraft* or *isograft* is used to describe tissue transplanted between genetically identical members of the same species (such as twins or an inbred strain), and *syngeneic* and *isogeneic* are the respective adjectives. *Xenograft* describes tissue transplanted between members of different species, and the corresponding adjective is *xenogeneic.* Syngrafts and xenografts are rarely used clinically and are mentioned only for completeness.

There are three mechanisms by which bone grafts effect osseous repair: osteogenesis, osteoinduction, and osteoconduction.[36] Some bone grafts exhibit all of these properties to varying degrees, whereas others exhibit only one or two. Knowledge of these differences enables the clinician to determine which type of graft is most appropriate for a given situation.

Osteogenesis is the formation of new bone by living cells in the graft and is seen only in autogeneic bone. Vascularized grafts (discussed later) have greater osteogenic capability than nonvascularized grafts. Few osteocytes and osteoblasts in nonvascularized grafts survive transplantation, but preosteoblasts, preosteoclasts, and osteoclasts on the surface of the graft do survive.[37, 38] The exact percentage of cells remaining viable after transplantation is unknown, but more cells survive in nonvascularized autogeneic cancellous grafts than nonvascularized autogeneic cortical grafts.

Osteoinduction is the ability some substances have to transform pluripotent stem cells in recipient bone and soft tissue into bone-forming cells. A number of polypeptide growth factors are believed to possess osteoinductive potential, most notably BMP.[39, 40]

Osteoconduction is the process whereby a material provides a nonviable scaffold for the ingrowth of blood vessels and osteoprogenitor cells from the recipient site. Axhausen referred to this process as *schleichender ersatz,* which has been translated to ''creeping substitution.''[41] Although this is a passive characteristic of bone grafts, as opposed to the active processes of osteogenesis and osteoinduction, it serves an equally important purpose. For newly formed bone produced at the graft site to be functional, it must be properly oriented and unite with the host bone. Osteoconduction occurs on viable biologic materials such as autogenous bone; on nonviable biologic materials such as frozen or freeze-dried, demineralized, or deproteinized allogeneic bone; and on nonbiologic materials such as ceramics or titanium and cobalt-chrome alloys.

The end result of any bone graft is a function of many variables, including the rate and extent of remodeling the graft undergoes and the loading demands placed on the graft. However, the most important determinant in the ultimate outcome of a bone graft is the degree and speed with which revascularization takes place. Grafts classified by this criteria can be placed broadly into three main categories, with special subsets within each category. These categories are vascularized autografts, nonvascularized autografts, and alloimplants.

Vascularized Autografts. Vascularized autografts can be either free or pedicled. By reestablishing the blood supply in a free graft via microsurgical reanastomosis or maintaining it via a pedicled graft, vascularized grafts show accelerated healing and repair compared with nonvascularized grafts. It is often stated that vascularized bone grafts heal similarly to a fracture, and although this is true to a large degree, the analogy is not exact. When a vascularized graft is placed in the lower extremity, a significant amount of remodeling must occur throughout the graft to accommodate the new stress patterns being passed through the bone from weightbearing.

Free Vascularized Grafts. Free vascularized grafts are more commonly used in the lower extremity than are pedicled grafts. In nonvascularized bone grafts the only cells that survive are restricted to the periphery of the graft, and these cells rely on diffusion of nutrients from the recipient site for their survival. Free vascularized autografts solve this problem by removing a section of bone along with its nutrient artery and veins and reanastomosing them at the recipient site using microsurgical techniques.

The first successful case of a free vascularized bone graft was reported in 1973 by McCullough and Fredrickson, who transplanted a rib to restore a mandibular defect.[42] The first reported use of a free vascularized autograft to treat a bony defect in the lower extremity was reported by Taylor and colleagues in 1975.[43]

The most commonly used donor sites are the rib, the fibula, and the iliac crest. Because of its size, shape, and composition, the rib is not suitable for use in the lower extremity and is usually used for mandibular defects. The fibula and iliac crest, however, are useful in lower extremity reconstruction.

As much as 20 cm of the proximal end of the fibula can be used as a graft, as long as the distal quarter is left intact to ensure stability of the ankle joint. Because of its length and cortical structure, the fibula is ideally suited for bridging long defects that require strength. The vascular supply to the fibula is consistent and comprises the relatively large peroneal artery. The fibula thus offers distinct technical advantages.

The nutrient vessels to the iliac crest are the deep circumflex iliac vessels. The iliac crest is a good source for cancellous bone and can provide more volume of bone than the fibula.

Pedicled Vascular Grafts. Pedicled grafts maintain blood supply to the transplanted bone not by microsurgical reanastomosis but by preservation of muscles attached to the bone that supply it with blood. Because the bone is on a pedicle, there are restrictions on how far the grafts can be moved that limit their use. The two most common clinical applications of these grafts in the lower extremity are the transfer of the posterior portion of the greater trochanter on the quadratus lumborum muscle for nonunions of the femoral neck[44] and the transfer of the fibula on the peroneal muscles for defects in the tibia.[45]

Theoretically, the ability to maintain circulation in transplanted bone makes vascularized autografts ideal. Clinically, vascularized bone grafts are particularly well suited for specific instances such as avascular necrosis and filling defects larger than 6 to 8 cm. However, there are limitations and drawbacks to their use. The surgery is a lengthy procedure that is technically demanding. Furthermore, these grafts are not structurally adequate for all uses, and it may take longer than a year for these grafts to hypertrophy to the size necessary to handle functional loading. The fracture rate in fibular grafts can approach 30%.

Nonvascularized Autografts. Fresh autogeneic nonvascularized bone grafts are the most commonly used grafts and the standard with which other grafts are compared. There are three types of grafts: cancellous, cortical, and corticocancellous. Each of these exhibits unique characteristics that determine the application for which they are best suited. In general, there is an inverse relationship between the stability of a graft and its osteogenic capability and rate of revascularization. Cancellous grafts possess good osteogenic, osteoconductive, and osteoinductive properties and are rapidly revascularized but offer little stability. Cortical grafts offer good stability but have less osteogenic and osteoinductive properties and revascularize at a much slower rate.

The healing of all nonvascularized bone grafts can be thought of as occurring in four stages: (1) an inflammatory response, (2) revascularization, (3) new bone formation, and (4) remodeling. The inflammatory response is similar between autogeneic cancellous and cortical grafts and is comparable with that seen in fracture repair.[37] This response occurs within minutes to hours and consists of the classic inflammatory cells such as PMNs, plasma cells, and leukocytes. During this period osteoclasts begin resorption of the graft, and the necrotic tissue is removed by macrophages.

The effects of structural differences between autogeneic cancellous and cortical grafts first begin to manifest themselves during osteoclastic resorption. These differences continue through the revascularization, new bone formation, and remodeling stages. These differences significantly affect the rate of revascularization, the degree of creeping substitution, and the extent of remodeling that occur in the two different types of grafts.[46]

The greater porosity and surface area of cancellous grafts compared with cortical grafts allow for increased osteoclast and macrophage access. Once the bone is degraded by osteoclasts and the necrotic tissue is removed by macrophages, the spaces evacuated are ready for revascularization. All nonvascularized autografts and alloimplants revascularize via the ingrowth of capillary buds from the host bed, but vessels from the host bed appear to be capable of revascularizing a cancellous autograft via reanastomosis. As a result of these factors, revascularization of cancellous autografts can begin sooner, sometimes within days, and to a fuller degree than with cortical grafts. Revascularization of the cancellous graft can be completed within 2 weeks, and as this occurs, primitive mesenchymal cells lining the trabeculae differentiate into osteoblasts and begin depositing seams of osteoid along the dead trabeculae of the bone graft.[47] Osteogenesis is additionally enhanced in cancellous grafts because larger numbers of preosteoblasts survive transplantation than in cortical grafts. The reason is that preosteoblasts in cancellous bone are not sequestered deep in the cortical matrix, and nutrients from the host bed can diffuse to them more easily. Moreover, cancellous grafts possess greater osteoinductive properties than cortical grafts because the increased surface area of cancellous bone also allows for greater diffusion of osteoinductive proteins. Because cancellous autografts are able to begin repair with bone formation and bone resorption occurring concomitantly, they exhibit initial strengthening.

Cortical grafts, on the other hand, show initial weakening, because they must undergo considerable resorption before revascularization and new bone formation can begin. New vessels from the host are unable to penetrate the dense cortical matrix and must enter the graft through existing haversian and Volkmann's canals on the periphery of the graft. For this to occur, osteoclastic resorption of these canals must first take place. The resultant increase in graft porosity leads to a decrease in the mechanical strength of the graft. This is significant because the strength of a graft appears to be related to the degree of porosity and not the completeness of repair, that is, the percentage of new and necrotic bone. Using a dog model, Enneking and coworkers showed that this increased porosity greatly weakened cortical bone grafts from 6 weeks to 6 months, and it was nearly a year before the strength of the transplant appeared normal.[48] In an attempt to accelerate the rate of repair with cortical autogeneic bone grafts, Burchardt and associates drilled holes in the graft.[49] Although this did not appear to decrease the strength of the graft, neither did it appear to accelerate the repair process. Drilling, however, did seem to lead to early formation of biologic pegs that may enhance the graft union to host bone.[49]

One last major difference between cancellous and cortical grafts is the amount of remodeling that eventually occurs. In cancellous grafts, all the necrotic bone is eventually resorbed and replaced by new bone. In cortical bone, certain areas of the graft become entrapped, because appositional new bone formation occurs before all the necrotic bone has been resorbed. This new bone essentially walls off the necrotic bone from osteoclastic resorption, and the end result is a mixture of viable new bone and necrotic old bone.

Corticocancellous grafts are a sort of hybrid that offer the stability of cortical grafts and the osteogenic, osteoinductive, and revascularization advantages of cancellous bone. When a corticocancellous graft is used, optimal incorporation is achieved by placing the cancellous portion next to the most vascular area in the recipient bed, usually the surrounding soft tissues.

By recognizing a few basic surgical principles, the clinician can optimize the osteogenic potential of nonvascularized autografts. Because the surviving cells in a graft are susceptible to the effects of both ischemia and the outside environment until they are placed at the host site, the time between harvesting and implantation should be kept to a minimum. During this period the graft should be kept moist and at physiologic temperatures, preferably in blood-soaked sponges. Finally, as mentioned earlier, the surviving cells in a graft are on the surface. Because these cells depend on receiving nutrients via diffusion from the vascular supply at the host site, it is best to keep the grafts as thin as possible and place them in the most vascular environment the host site can offer.

No discussion of nonvascularized autografts would be complete without mentioning the newest addition to the clinician's armamentarium: percutaneous bone marrow injection. The osteogenic properties of bone marrow have been known for some time, and bone marrow transplants have been used for decades to replace cancerous marrow destroyed by radiation and chemotherapy. Salama and Weissman first reported the use of autogeneic bone marrow–xenograft bone composites in 1978.[50] In 1986 Connolly and Shindell documented the first use of percutaneous marrow injection to treat an infected nonunion of the tibia,[51] and Connolly and colleagues also reported the ability to increase the osteogenic capability of bone marrow by differential centrifugation in animal studies.[52] Although the results thus far are preliminary and more studies need to be performed, marrow injection appears to be as effective as open autologous grafting with fewer disadvantages.[53]

Allografts and Alloimplants. Autografts are ideal in terms of osteogenesis, osteoinduction, osteoconduction, and immunologic compatibility. However, there are certain difficulties associated with their use. Among these problems are those risks posed by a second surgical site, including dehiscence, infection, and hematoma. In addition, there are also complications unique to bone graft harvesting such as donor site pain, limited amounts of bone available to fill large defects, and fatigue fractures. Because of these drawbacks, allografts are occasionally employed.

Because of the immune response, as well as the possibility of transmission of disease, fresh allogeneic bone is no longer used clinically. Two methods that sterilize allogeneic bone and reduce its antigenicity are freezing and freeze-drying. Although these two treatments markedly decrease the immunogenicity of allogeneic bone, they do not completely eradicate it. Freeze-dried bone, sometimes referred to as *lyophilized bone,* has the advantage of being less antigenic than frozen bone, and it can be stored easier and for much longer periods. With both frozen and freeze-dried bone, cortical bone appears to be less antigenic than cancellous bone.

Because freezing and freeze-drying destroy all living bone cells, these allogeneic grafts are therefore more properly referred to as *alloimplants.* Because alloimplants consist of nonviable bone and provide merely the form and matrix of bone tissue, they serve almost exclusively an osteoconductive function.

Alloimplants exhibit the same four-step repair process as autografts, but there are differences that are probably the result of their residual antigenicity.[54, 55] The inflammatory phase is prolonged and of a greater magnitude than with autografts, and revascularization is also slowed down. Consequently, incorporation is slower and less complete.

Chemosterilized, Allogeneic, Autolyzed, Antigen-Extracted Bone. Normal frozen or freeze-dried bone loses its BMP owing to enzymatic autolysis. Urist developed a method of preparing cortical allogeneic bone that reduces antigenicity even further than freezing or freeze-drying and preserves BMP activity.[56] Allogeneic, autolyzed, antigen-extracted (AAA) bone has greater osteoinductive capability, is incorporated more rapidly than other types of allogeneic bone, and can serve as a substitute for autogeneic bone. However, AAA bone lacks mechanical stability and is not practical in those situations in which graft strength is important. Urist has used AAA bone in arthrodesis of the knee and ankle.[57]

Demineralized Bone Matrix. Urist also reported the clinical usage of the osteoinductive capability of acid demineralized bone matrix (DBM) in 1968.[58] The osteoinductive, antigenic, and strength characteristics of DBM are similar to those of AAA. DBM can be easily molded into different shapes and has been used in the repair of craniofacial defects.[59, 60]

Nonunions

In spite of continuing advances in surgical techniques and increasing knowledge about bone healing, approximately 5% of all long bone fractures will go on to nonunion, resulting in 100,000 nonunions each year in the United States. The number of delayed unions each year is even greater. These are significant numbers, especially considering the potential difficulties one may encounter in dealing with these complications.

When presented with the possibility of a nonunion, two immediate questions face the clinician. The first question is determining what constitutes a normal repair period. The rate at which a fracture heals depends on many factors, such as the bone involved, the location of the fracture on the bone, the severity of the fracture, the method used to repair the fracture, the weightbearing status, the damage to surrounding soft tissue, the blood supply, the age of the patient, and patient compliance. Despite all these variables, most fractures either unite or show progressive signs of healing via serial radiographs at 4 to 6 months.[61] If a fracture has failed to heal in this period, it is generally considered a delayed union. If after 6 to 8 months there appears to be complete cessation of the repair process and there is no bridging of the fracture gap, or bridging by fibrous or fibrocartilaginous tissue, most authors consider this a nonunion.[62] Although these parameters provide the clinician with helpful time frames, a better definition of nonunion would be when a fracture fails to unite within the normal period exhibited for similar fractures.

Once a nonunion is diagnosed, the second question facing the clinician is determining its cause. No single treatment is universally successful, and to choose the most appropriate and effective treatment, it is necessary to attempt to resolve those factors responsible for the nonunion. No issue in orthopedics has elicited more discussion and controversy than the causes of nonunion. Attempts to classify the causes of nonunions as systemic versus local factors (and combinations of the two) may be more complex than once thought, as further discussed later. A more appropriate and useful division may be to classify the major causes of nonunions as technical failures, biologic failures, and combinations of the two.[63]

Technical Failures. The causes of technical failure have been well documented and include distraction, poor reduction, soft tissue interposition, failure to débride an infection, extensive soft tissue and vascular compromise, and excessive motion at the fracture site.

In an attempt to classify nonunions as either viable (i.e., capable of biologic reaction) or nonviable (i.e., incapable of biologic reaction), Weber and Cech compared standard radiographs with strontium radioisotope studies.[64] They then divided viable nonunions into three different classes based on the degree of callus present. The hypertrophic type of nonunion exhibits proliferative callus and is also known as "elephant foot." This most commonly occurs from inadequate fixation or premature weightbearing. The slightly hypertrophic type is a milder form and is also called the "horse hoof" callus. This is usually the result of loosening or breakage of a fixation plate. The third category of viable nonunion, the oligotrophic type, is often the result of incomplete fracture reduction or major displacement of the fracture followed by distraction. These exhibit no callus radiographically, appear inactive, and may be hard to differentiate from nonunions. However, bone scans and serial radiographs reveal that the bone ends are vascular and therefore biologically capable.

Because by definition the viable nonunions listed earlier show biologic activity, and most result from technical failures, these cannot be called true or complete biologic failures. There may be some biologic problem occurring concomitantly with the technical failure, but the predominant cause is technical.

Biologic Failures. During the last 20 years, as we have come to a fuller appreciation of the complexities of fracture repair, it has become apparent that the biologic causes of nonunion are equally complex. It is only logical that until all of the processes and variables involved in normal bone repair have been defined, our understanding of the myriad of possible ways bone repair can malfunction will be incomplete. Even if identification of all the processes and variables of normal bone repair is accomplished, there remains the even more daunting task of developing animal models to mimic specific malfunctions. For this reason the causes of biologic failure are much more difficult to identify than technical failures.

There are biologic causes of nonunions that are purely local in nature as well as those that are purely systemic. However, it may be more difficult than once believed to clearly delineate the cause of most biologic failures as one versus another. There is some ongoing degree of interaction between local and systemic factors.[37] Once normal fracture healing starts, there is almost a cascade effect where the completion of one stage initiates the start of the next. However, this cascade is neither necessarily automatic nor self-perpetuating. Any stage of bone repair can fail, irrespective of the other stages, raising the possibility that new systemic cofactors are constantly being recruited into local pathways.

Purely systemic causes of nonunion are rare. Among the conditions that predispose toward delayed healing or nonunions are osteomalacia, iron deficiency anemia, lack of vitamins C and D, primary hyperparathyroidism, and hypothyroidism. Medications can also exert systemic effects that can affect bone healing. Cortisone in large doses has been shown to suppress bone healing,[65] and although not a cause of nonunion, it may be a predisposing factor. The effects of anticoagulants, however, are not so clear cut. Stinchfield and coworkers asserted that anticoagulants impeded fracture healing,[66] but these claims were not substantiated by Flatmark.[67] As mentioned earlier in the discussion on fracture repair, indomethacin may hamper normal bone repair and predispose toward delayed unions or nonunions.

Another systemic factor often mentioned as a contributor to nonunions is age. The identification of this factor followed from the observation that nonunions are relatively rare in juveniles. This has often been attributed to the thicker periosteum found in children and, therefore, greater potential for osteogenesis. This may be a component cause of the decreased incidence of nonunion seen in children, but other factors that probably contribute have also been identified. Urist and associates demonstrated a decrease in the amount of BMP present in adults as they age,[68] and the findings of Strates and coworkers suggest that formation of new bone from demineralized bone matrix and marrow is reduced with aging.[69]

Before our current understanding of the intricacies of bone repair, it was believed that the primary cause of "local" bone repair failure lay with the osteoblasts. With elucidation of some of the events occurring during modulation and induction, this belief has changed. If there are no osseous pathologic changes prior to a fracture, there is no reason to believe that the existing osteoblasts are defective. These osteoblasts appear capable of handling the everyday task of replacing resorbed bone with new bone and maintaining an equilibrium between bone lost and bone gained. As stated earlier in discussing fracture healing, few osteoblasts are present at the time of fracture. Because they do not control their time or rate of reproduction, osteoblasts are dependent on modulation and induction to provide the stimuli to perform these functions. Therefore, it is currently believed that most biologic failures in bone repair are due to defects in the mediator mechanisms and not the osteoblasts themselves.[63]

It is fortunate that although our understanding of the biologic causes of nonunions is vague, our ability to recognize them and therefore attempt to treat them accordingly is somewhat less obtuse. Weber and Cech's classification of viable nonunions was described in the earlier section on technical failures.[64] Examination of their classification of nonviable nonunions, although not foolproof, does offer a starting point for reasonable treatment. The Weber-Cech classification divides nonviable nonunions into four different types.

Dystrophic nonunions are characterized by the presence of an intermediate fragment that has healed to only one of the major fragments. As a consequence, the intermediate fragment has a patent blood supply only on one of its sides, and the other nonvascularized side is unable to bridge the gap with the second major fragment.

The *necrotic type* of nonunion is most commonly the result of a comminuted fracture. These types can be difficult to diagnose with plain radiographs because the gap (or gaps) between the fragments is not always visible, and a callus is absent. Serial radiographs can often help as the fragment (or fragments) die and become more radiopaque than the surrounding bone.

The *defect type* of nonunion is distinguished by a gap present as the result of bone loss. The bone loss can be a result of sequestration following the initial injury or overzealous surgical débridement.

The fourth category of nonviable nonunion, the *atrophic type,* is typically the end result of one of the three nonviable types listed earlier.

Although it is often stated that the four nonviable nonunions could be due to a lack of blood supply, this line of thinking can be an oversimplification and misleading. An otherwise healthy patient may have a good blood supply to the limb involved. Lack of blood to the nonunion site may be due to failures in the mechanisms of revascularization and angiogenesis and not any preexisting circulatory deficiency.

Rationale for Treatment of Nonunions

Technical Failures. Most cases of technical failure have a fairly good prognosis once the cause is recognized and treated accordingly. If there is no hardware distracting or maintaining the fracture gap, thereby necessitating surgical removal, and the fracture ends are in good alignment, further immobilization may be all that is required.

The use of immobilization to heal fractures has been employed since fractures were first recognized clinically. Although the rationale that immobilization heals most fractures is based on the observation that many fractures heal if their ends are stabilized, its universal application to all cases of nonunion can be disastrous. The classic criterion for immobilization would be the delayed union or nonunion exhibiting profuse callus formation. This may be present without internal fixation or with internal fixation as long as the fixation is not maintaining the fracture gap. Further immobilization of an atrophic nonunion, or one in which the internal fixation is preventing osseous union, is ill advised.

In those instances where further immobilization is attempted, it may be carried out in conjunction with electrical stimulation. As described later, there are noninvasive and invasive methods of applying electrical stimulation. If nonsurgical methods, such as casting, are indicated in the initial treatment of a nonunion and the addition of electrical stimulation is being comtemplated, it must be realized that noninvasive units are not applicable in all situations. Specific contraindications include the treatment of a pseudarthrosis and osseous gaps greater than one half the diameter of the bone involved.

The first reported case of electrical stimulation used to heal a fracture was reported more than 150 years ago. Various reports of the use of electricity to cure nonunions appeared in the literature during the next 20 years, but it eventually fell into disuse. Interest was regenerated in the 1950s with the findings of Fukada and Yasuda, described earlier in the section on the endogenous electrical properties of bone.[13] Yasuda expanded his investigations to include the effect of exogenous electrical potentials on bone. By implanting electrodes and continuously applying a 1-μA electrical current for 3 weeks to the femur of a live rabbit, he found greater bone formation at the cathode than the anode.[70] The exact mechanisms of electrical stimulation are not clearly understood and are the subject of many current investigations. A review of the latest experimental findings and current theories is beyond the scope of this chapter, but the different types of systems presently available are briefly outlined.

Noninvasive methods of stimulation include inductive and capacitive coupling. Inductive coupling, also known as *pulsed electromagnetic field* (PEMF), uses the placement of a coil or pair of coils to generate a time-varying magnetic field. This magnetic field in turn produces voltage gradients and local current flow. The main disadvantage of this system is the need for patient compliance because the unit must be plugged into the wall to recharge the battery, the average recommended period of each daily treatment is 10 hours, and the placement of the coil (or coils) is more critical than with capacitive coupling electrodes.

With capacitive coupling, electrodes are placed on the skin at opposite sides of the nonunion. As alternating current is passed between the electrodes, an internal time-varying field potential creates voltage gradients and local current flow. The main disadvantage is the possibility of skin irritation at the electrode sites.

A semi-invasive method of electrical stimulation uses a Teflon-coated cathode resembling a Kirschner wire that is placed percutaneously at the fracture site. The anode is a pad that is placed on the skin, and the power supply can be embedded in the cast. The advantages of this system are that it does not require an open surgical procedure, and removal is easily accomplished. The disadvantages of this system are that it requires patient compliance, shifting and displacement of the wires is a possibility as are possible pin tract infections, and the anode must be replaced frequently. In addition, as with the two noninvasive methods discussed earlier, contraindications to its use are synovial pseudarthrosis and a nonunion gap wider than one half the diameter of the bone.

If surgical treatment of a nonunion is necessary (e.g., to remove hardware, realign bone, débride an infection, or treat a pseudarthrosis), there is one completely invasive method of electrical stimulation that entails implanting a cathode at the nonunion site and placing the anode somewhere away from the bone to prevent resorption. In the lower extremity this is most commonly accomplished by placing the anode, as well as the generator, in the calf muscle. The advantage of this system is that it requires no patient compliance. The major disadvantage is that it requires a second surgery to retrieve the system once bone healing is accomplished.

Biologic Failures. Unlike nonunions that are primarily or entirely technical in nature and often respond well to conservative measures once the problem is recognized and corrected, nonunions due to biologic failure usually require more drastic treatment. Because these nonunions lack osteogenic potential by their nature, bone grafts are commonly employed. When the use of cancellous bone grafts is desirable owing to their superior osteogenic qualities, concomitant rigid fixation is often necessary to provide the structural strength missing from the graft.

CARTILAGE

As stated at the beginning of this chapter, cartilage is similar to bone in that it is a specialized connective tissue consisting of cells embedded in an extracellular matrix that is permeated by collagenous fibers. However, there are major differences between bone and cartilage.

Chondrocytes are different from osteoblasts in that they produce type II collagen, not type I, and they are unique in their ability to synthesize greater amounts of specific proteoglycans and collagen than almost any other type of cell.

Cartilage is also dissimilar from bone in that it lacks nerves and blood or lymphatic vessels. Because of the low oxygen consumption of cartilage, it is sometimes stated that the metabolic rate of chondrocytes is also low. This belief is likely due in part to the fact that articular cartilage consists of relatively small numbers of cells distributed throughout an abundant extracellular matrix. In reality, the metabolic activity of individual chondrocytes approaches that of other tissue cells.

Classification and Structure

Cartilage is usually classified as either hyaline, yellow elastic, or white fibrous. Articular cartilage can be either hyaline or white fibrous, depending on the mode of development of the bone on which it lies. Those bones that undergo endochondral ossification have hyaline cartilage, and those that undergo membranous ossification have predominantly white fibrocartilage. This white fibrocartilage is found in

intervertebral discs, the temporomandibular joint, the pubis symphysis, and the acromioclavicular and sternoclavicular joints. Hyaline articular cartilage is discussed because it is the predominant articular cartilage found in the lower extremity.

Normal articular cartilage has a specific structure that enables it to withstand the unique demands placed on it, and an understanding of the complexity of normal articular cartilage is necessary to determine the appropriateness of any tissue that replaces it.

There still exists some uncertainty about the exact structure of hyaline articular cartilage, but most authors have divided it into three or four layers. These layers, or zones, are based on variations in the distribution of cells and matrix constituents (Fig. 2–6).[71]

Zone I, the superficial or tangential layer, is composed mainly of thin, tightly packed collagen fibers that run parallel to the articular surface. The cells in this layer are small and elongated and also lie parallel to the articular surface. Weiss and colleagues further divided this layer into a superficial zone IS and a deeper zone ID, called the *cellular zone.*[72] The collagen bundles run parallel to the articular surface in zones IS and ID, but the fibers are grouped into smaller bundles in zone ID, and there is greater ground substance between the fibers than in zone IS. In addition, the cells are usually larger and less elongated in zone ID than zone IS.

MacConaill observed a thin, bright line at the cartilage surface in untreated specimens examined by phase-contrast microscopy.[73] This layer, thought to be devoid of collagen fibers and to consist solely of hyaline, was termed the *lamina splendens.* Since it was first described, the existence of the lamina splendens has been a source of controversy. Aspden and Hukins claimed that the bright line is an artifact, or "halo," produced by phase-contrast microscopy.[74] Others using transmission electron microscopy have noted an extremely fine filamentous and particulate electron-dense material lying on top of the collagen fibrils, but they ascribe this to a combination of precipitated synovial fluid and lipid debris from the cartilage matrix. Dunham and coworkers recently demonstrated the presence of a lamina splendens using both polarized light microscopy and interference microscopy, neither of which produces a halo.[75]

Zone II is the transitional zone and contains larger and more rounded cells embedded in a proteoglycan matrix and collagen fibers oriented obliquely to the surface.

Zone III is the radial zone and contains cells similar in size to those found in zone II and oriented in columns perpendicular to the joint surface. The cells in zones II and III are actively involved in protein synthesis.

Zone IV is the calcified zone and interdigitates with the subchondral bone to firmly join cartilage and subchondral bone together. The cells in zone IV display the characteristics of cell death.

Between zones III and IV is a region referred to as the *tidemark.*[76] This area, which stains blue with hematoxylin-eosin stain in preparations of decalcified material, is the level at which almost all transverse fractures occur.[77]

Some investigators have described the arrangement of collagen fibers as if there was no interrelationship between the fibers in zone I and those found in zones II and III. Benninghoff, however, suggested that the collagen fibers in zone I did not constitute an independent layer resting on a random network of noncontiguous fibers in the lower zones but that

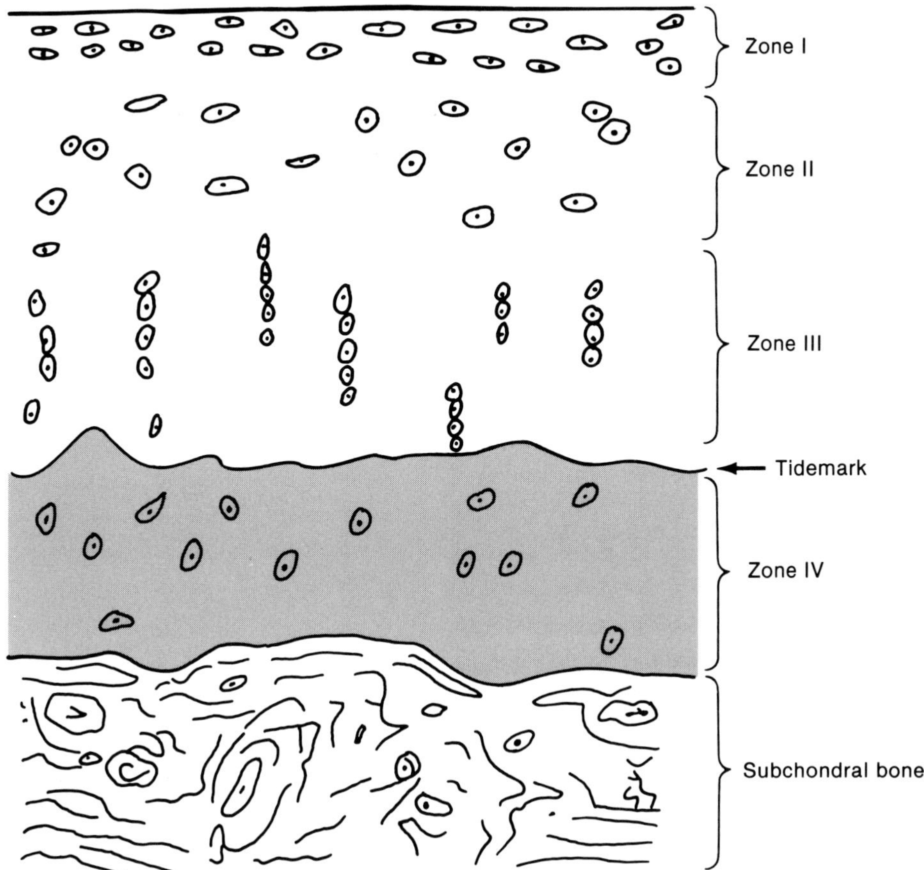

FIGURE 2–6. Zones of articular cartilage.

collagen fibers anchored in zone IV formed arcades as they approached the articular surface.[78] It was proposed that these fibers ran vertically toward the surface through zone III, turned oblique in zone II, and finally ran horizontal to the articular surface in zone I. The essential features of Benninghoff's model have recently been verified by Clark, who used scanning electron microscopy to trace fibers from zone III to zone I, where they flattened out to run parallel to the articular surface.[79] This orientation of collagen fibers at the surface of the joint provides resistance to shearing forces and surface wear, whereas the orientation in the deeper layers serves to resist compressive loading and allow for resilience.

The extracellular matrix of hyaline articular cartilage is manufactured by the chondrocytes and consists of matrix proteins, type II collagen, and proteoglycans. Proteoglycans (discussed earlier in the section on bone) are found throughout connective tissue. However, the proteoglycans found in cartilage are unique. Proteoglycans can exist as monomers, but those in hyaline cartilage are able to attach to hyaluronic acid via link proteins to form huge multimolecular aggregates. A single hyaluronic acid chain can bind as much as 250 times its weight in proteoglycans (Fig. 2–7).

GAGs carry negatively charged carboxyl and sulfate groups that are in close proximity. These like charges repel each other, causing the proteoglycans to spread out over a large area. It has been proposed that the large size of the proteoglycan aggregates may serve to immobilize them within the collagen network, increase their resilience to compressive forces, and make them more resistant to proteinases

than monomers would be. Fibrocartilage is inferior to hyaline cartilage owing to the presence of large amounts of dermatan sulfate, which is smaller than the other GAGs and does not bind to hyaluronic acid to form huge aggregates.

The structural framework for cartilage is provided by the collagen, which accounts for approximately 50% of the dry weight of cartilage. The proteoglycan aggregates expand until they are constrained by the collagen fibers that surround them. The elastic properties of the proteoglycan aggregates combined with the tensile forces of the collagen fibers imbue hyaline cartilage with its unique viscoelastic characteristics. When cartilage is compressed and water squeezed out, the negative charges on the proteoglycans repel each other and resist compression of the cartilage, allowing water back into the matrix. The volume of the cartilage then increases until the collagen fibers stop further increases.

The water content of articular cartilage approaches 80%, and the flow of synovial fluid in and out of matrix is critical because it appears to be the predominant, if not sole, manner in which nutrients are delivered to the cartilage.[80, 81] Lack of synovial fluid flow has been proposed as the cause of cartilage damage after long-term immobilization of joints. The presence of capillaries that appear to cross from subchondral bone into cartilage has spawned a debate about whether blood-borne nutrients may also supply the deeper layers of cartilage. These vessels may serve an important role in nourishment during growth, but scanning electron microscopic findings seem to corroborate earlier tracer studies that cast doubt on this function in adults.[82]

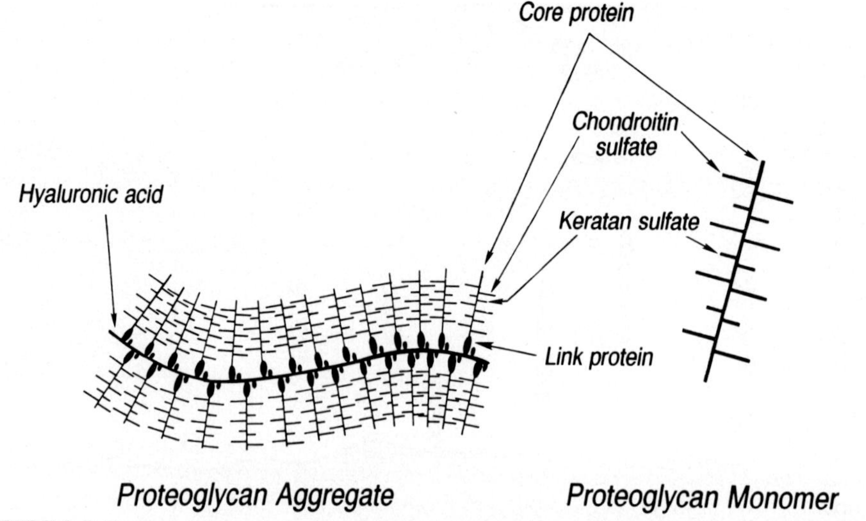

FIGURE 2–7. Diagrammatic representation of proteoglycan aggregate and proteoglycan monomer subunit.

Cartilage Repair

The repair of cartilage defects has proved to be a perplexing problem for years. Most of the studies that have examined cartilage repair after penetrating injuries have been conducted on rabbits and horses. As with animal studies of bone repair, caution must be exercised when attempts are made to extrapolate these findings to humans. In addition to the normal caveats, one must be cognizant of elements specific to cartilage studies when attempting to determine the applicability of animal models to humans, and even when comparing different studies involving the same species.

The degree to which cartilage can respond to injury is governed primarily by whether the injury is confined to the cartilage or extends into the subchondral bone.[83–87] However, other factors may affect the repair process to a lesser degree. The size of the defect must be considered, both in terms of its absolute size and its percentage of the total joint surface. The location of the defect in the joint is a factor. Lesions in an area of heavy weightbearing, such as the middle of the medial or lateral femoral condyle, may be expected to heal differently than lesions in areas of lessened weightbearing, such as the intercondylar groove. Another factor to be considered is the postoperative course. Whether the animal was immobilized, was allowed full or partial-weightbearing, underwent continuous passive motion, or any combination of these variables has to be considered. The length of any treatment, or treatments, as well as the length of follow-up must be regarded. Numerous studies have shown a change in the composition of the repair tissue over time. When dissimilar joints are compared, it should be recognized that contrasts between the biomechanics of each joint will result in different stresses and strains placed on the cartilage. Finally, the age of the animal must also be considered, because cartilage in skeletally immature animals may be capable of greater repair than that in older animals.

The normal repair of tissue usually consists of three phases. These three phases were described earlier in the section on bone healing, but a brief review will aid the discussion of cartilage repair. The initial stage is the inflammatory, or exudative, stage that starts with cellular necrosis and a transient vasoconstriction of the blood vessels in the area followed by a vasodilatation that brings white and red blood cells and an influx of undifferentiated cells. The second, or proliferative, stage is when fibroblasts proliferate and synthesize collagen to form a scar. The third stage is the remodeling, or maturation, phase and consists of intermolecular cross-linking of the collagen. Ultimately, either fibrous scar tissue is left, as is the case in skin, or there is regeneration of tissue identical to that present before the injury, such as described earlier for bone.

When an injury or laceration occurs on the articular surface and remains superficial to the subchondral bone, there is a cellular response. The chondrocytes near the partial-thickness defect proliferate, forming small clusters of new cells, and synthesize new proteoglycans.[86, 87] However, neither the quantities of cells or proteoglycans necessary to fill the defect are manufactured, nor are those cells and proteoglycans capable of migrating to fill the defect, because they are constrained by the extracellular matrix. In addition, the extent of this response is severely curtailed owing to the absence of a vascular supply to provide the components necessary for an inflammatory response. Without an inflammatory response, there can be no influx of fibroblasts to proliferate and therefore no real proliferative phase.

Although partial-thickness defects do not heal, somewhat surprisingly, they usually do not progress and rarely show any significant degree of collapse, fragmentation, or fibrillation.[77] Most of the human and animal evidence suggests that superficial injuries to cartilage do not progress further in a joint that is otherwise normal and stable. It is difficult, if not impossible, to create an animal model of progressive joint degeneration simply by making incisions in the surface of a normal joint.[86] For example, most animal knee models of osteoarthritis require the severing of a collateral and cruciate ligament in addition to intentional iatrogenic damage to the cartilage.

Unlike partial-thickness defects that show no real capability of repair, defects that extend into the subchondral bone are capable of repair. Most full-thickness defects show similar reparative patterns, but the amount and type of repair as well as time frames differ somewhat according to the size of the defect and the species of animal involved.

Once subchondral bone is violated, cells from the vascular

network in the subchondral bone that are capable of taking part in a classic inflammatory response gain access to the defect site. A fibrin clot then forms that fills the defect. This clot is then invaded by, and replaced with, undifferentiated cells resembling fibroblasts. Within 1 or 2 weeks these fibroblasts differentiate into cells resembling chondrocytes. Between 1 and 2 months after injury, the repair tissue appears similar to hyaline cartilage[88] and the matrix stains heavily with safranin O, indicating the presence of proteoglycans. However, at 3 or 4 weeks, most collagen present is type I, not type II.[89] By 8 weeks the type of collagen present is either all type II[90, 91] or predominantly type II but with significant amounts of type I collagen.[89] The type I collagen persists in significant amounts even after 1 year.

At first the repair tissue appears to be satisfactory, but as early as 6 months and no later than 1 year the cartilage becomes more fibrous and shows fibrillations and degenerative lesions.[92] The amount of safranin O staining and the hexosamine content of the repair tissue both decrease, indicating a loss of proteoglycan.[89] In addition to the presence of type I collagen and decrease in proteoglycan content, the repair tissue does not usually exhibit the classic zones found in hyaline cartilage. These findings all suggest that full-thickness defects of articular cartilage undergo repair that is satisfactory in the early stages (2 to 6 months), but that with time, the repair tissue degenerates into an inferior fibrocartilage-type tissue.

The question is then raised as to the cause of the inferior quality of the repair cartilage. Both the type of collagen found and the apparent loss of proteoglycans with time offer some clues. Connective tissues such as tendon and ligament that usually synthesize and secrete type I collagen also synthesize and secrete dermatan sulfate–containing proteoglycans. Dermatan sulfate–containing proteoglycans are much smaller and have inferior elastic properties compared with the cartilage-specific proteoglycans discussed earlier. This has led to the hypothesis that the repair tissue has dermatan sulfate in place of the chondroitin and keratin sulfates normally found in articular cartilage, thus accounting for the decreased capacity of the reparative tissue to withstand long-term stresses.[87]

Another possible explanation is offered by Furukawa and associates, who suggest that the increasing fibrous texture of the repair tissue seen with time may be due to a loss of proteoglycans rather than a change in the type of collagen.[89]

Methods of Repairing Cartilage

The pain and disability that can result from damage to the articular surfaces of synovial joints have spurred clinicians to attempt to develop methods of restoring these joints to as normal function as possible. None of the methods presently used is totally satisfactory.

Mitchell and Shepard[92] demonstrated that large areas of damaged articular cartilage can be repaired by drilling multiple small holes into the subchondral bone, eliciting the response described earlier. This method has been employed in the lower extremity to treat osteochondritis dissecans and degenerative metatarsophalangeal joints, but the results are unpredictable. In addition, although this method may produce an improved or pain-free joint in the short term, its long-term efficacy is questionable. When débriding any damaged carti-

lage before drilling, it appears as if the best results are obtained by keeping the margins of any articular defect perpendicular to the joint surface. Rudd and colleagues[93] demonstrated that beveling the edges of full-thickness articular defects in puppies resulted in further damage, whereas keeping the defects perpendicular did not. This would seem to coincide with the findings of Calandruccio and Gilmar, who noticed the flow of ground substance from cartilage adjacent to the site of injury into the defect.[83] This phenomenon, which they termed *matrix flow,* was observed only in partial-thickness defects with nearly vertical walls.

If subchondral drilling is performed, early joint motion appears to optimize the quality of repair. DePalma and co-workers showed that full-thickness defects healed more quickly and produced more repair tissue in weightbearing than non-weightbearing areas.[84] Salter and associates also demonstrated that continuous passive motion hastened the repair process and produced repair tissue that more closely resembled hyaline cartilage.[94]

One of the newer methods that shows great promise is the grafting of perichondrium taken from the rib.[95] This technique has been used clinically in a variety of joints and has proved to be successful.[96–99] The tissue formed has the same viscoelastic properties as hyaline cartilage, and after 1 year the histologic and biochemical characteristics are similar to those of normal articular cartilage.[100, 101]

In an attempt to determine the origin of the hyaline cartilage produced by the graft, Zarnett and Salter transplanted grafts from male rabbits into 15 female rabbits.[102] In 33% of the rabbits, all of the regenerated tissue contained Y chromosomes only, indicating that the new cartilage was derived exclusively from the progenitor cells of the graft. The karyotypes of the other 67% of the rabbits were mosaics, indicating the new cartilage was derived from both the graft and the pluripotential mesenchymal cells in the subchondral bone. Further evidence that elements in the subchondral bone may take part in the repair process was offered by Billings and colleagues.[103] They showed that DBM mixed with perichondrium produced higher quality repair tissue than DBM alone or perichondrium and an autogenous bone plug. This suggests, not surprisingly, that bone matrix contains factors that may govern cartilage as well as bone growth and differentiation.

References

1. Ham AW: Histology, 8th ed. Philadelphia, JB Lippincott, 1979.
2. Jotereau FV and LeDouarin NW: The developmental relationship between osteocytes and osteoclasts: A study using the quail-chick nuclear marker in endochondral ossification. Dev Biol 63:253, 1978.
3. Salter RS: Normal structure and function of musculoskeletal tissues. *In* Textbook of Disorders and Injuries of the Musculoskeletal System, 2nd ed. Baltimore, Williams & Wilkins, 1983.
4. Lacroix P: The internal remodeling of bone. *In* Bourne GH (ed): The Biochemistry and Physiology of Bone, Vol 3, 2nd ed. New York, Academic Press, 1971, pp 35–64.
5. Loutit JF and Nisbet NW: Resorption of bone. Lancet 2:26, 1979.
6. Heppenstall RB: Fracture Treatment and Healing. Philadelphia, WB Saunders, 1980.
7. McKibbin B: The biology of fracture healing in long bones. J Bone Joint Surg [Br] 60:150, 1978.
8. Rhinelander FW: Circulation in bone. *In* Bourne GH (ed): The Biochemistry and Physiology of Bone, Vol 2, 2nd ed. New York, Academic Press, 1972.
9. Rhinelander FW: Tibial blood supply in relation to fracture healing. Clin Orthop 105:34, 1974.
10. Hughes MS, Davies R, Kahn R, et al: Fluid space in bone. Clin Orthop 134:332, 1978.
11. Brookes M: The Blood Supply of Bone. London, Butterworth, 1971.

12. Gothman L: Vascular reactions in experimental fractures. Acta Chir Scand Suppl 284:1–34, 1961.
13. Fukada E and Yasuda I: On the piezoelectric effect of bone. J Physical Soc Jpn 10:1158, 1957.
14. Pollack SR, Korostoff E, Starkebaum W, et al: Microelectrode studies of stress-generated potentials in bone. *In* Brighton CT, Black J, and Pollack SR (eds): Electrical Properties of Bone and Cartilage. New York, Grune and Stratton, 1979, pp 69–81.
15. Marino A, Becker R, and Soderholm S: Origin of the piezoelectric effect in bone. Calcif Tissue Res 8:327, 1971.
16. Lee RC, Frank EH, Grodzinsky AJ, et al: Oscillatory compressional behavior of articular cartilage and its associated electromechanical properties. J Biomech Eng 103:280, 1981.
17. Friedenberg ZB and Brighton CT: Bioelectric potentials in bone. J Bone Joint Surg 48A:915, 1966.
18. Urist MR and Johnson RW Jr: IV Calcification and ossification: The healing of fractures in man under clinical conditions. J Bone Joint Surg 25:375, 1943.
19. Frost HM: The biology of fracture healing: An overview for clinicians: I. Clin Orthop 248:283, 1989.
20. Friedenstein AJ: Determined and inducible osteogenic precursor cells. *In* Ciba Foundation Symposium II: Hard Tissue Growth, Repair and Remineralization. Amsterdam, Associated Science Publishers, 1973, pp 169–185.
21. Peacock EE Jr and Van Winkle W: Wound Repair. Philadelphia, WB Saunders, 1976.
22. Mohan S and Baylink DJ: Bone growth factors. Clin Orthop 263:30, 1991.
23. Wozney JM: Bone morphogenetic protein. Prog Growth Factor Res 1:267, 1989.
24. Bonewald LF and Mundy GR: Role of transforming growth factor-beta in bone remodeling. Clin Orthop 250:261, 1990.
25. Urist MR: Bone formation by autoinduction. Science 150:893, 1965.
26. Urist MR, Huo YK, Brownell AG, et al: Purification of bovine bone morphogenetic protein by hydroxyapatite chromotography. Proc Natl Acad Sci USA 81:371, 1984.
27. Wozney JM, Rosen V, Celeste AJ, et al: Novel regulators of bone formation: Molecular clones and activities. Science 242:1528, 1988.
28. Somjen D, Binderman I, Berger E, et al: Bone remodeling induced by physical stress is prostaglandin E_2 mediated. Biochem Biophys Acta 627:91, 1980.
29. Elves MW, Bayley F, and Raylance PJ: The effect of indomethacin upon experimental fractures in the rat. Acta Orthop Scand 53:35, 1982.
30. Ro J, Sudmann E, and Marton PF: Effect of indomethacin on fracture healing in rats. Acta Orthop Scand 47:588, 1976.
31. Danis R: Theorie et pratique de l'osteosynthese. Paris, Masson et Cie, 1949.
32. Schenk P and Willeneger H: Morphological findings in primary fracture healing. Symp Biol Hung 7:75, 1967.
33. Bostman O, Vainionpaa S, Hirvensalo et al: Biodegradable internal fixation for malleolar fractures. J Bone Joint Surg [Br] 69:615, 1987.
34. Friedlander GE: Bone grafts. *In* Orthopaedic Knowledge Update Park Ridge, IL, American Academy of Orthopaedic Surgeons, January 3, 1990.
35. Urist MR: Bone transplants and implants. *In* Urist MR (ed): Fundamental and Clinical Bone Physiology. Philadelphia, JB Lippincott, 1980, p 331.
36. Bassett CAL and Ruedi-Lindesker A: Bibliography of bone transplantation. Transplantation 2:688, 1964.
37. Burchardt H: The biology of bone graft repair. Clin Orthop 174:28, 1983.
38. Burwell RC: Studies on the transplantation of bone: VII. The fresh composite homo-autograft of cancellous bone: An analysis of factors leading to osteogenesis in marrow transplants and in marrow containing bone grafts. J Bone Joint Surg 46B:110, 1964.
39. Urist MR, Silverman BF, Buring K, et al: The bone induction principle. Clin Orthop 53:243, 1967.
40. Reddi AM, Weintraoub S, and Muthukumaran N: Biologic principles of bone induction. Bone Graft 18:207, 1987.
41. Axhausen G: Ueber den histologischen vorgang bei der transplantation von gelenkenden. Arch Klin Chir 99:1, 1912.
42. McCullough DW and Fredrickson JM: Neovascularized rib grafts to reconstruct mandibular defects. Can J Otolaryngol 2:96, 1973.
43. Taylor GI, Miller GDH, and Ham FJ: The free vascularized bone graft. Plast Reconstr Surg 55:533, 1975.
44. Meyers M: The role of posterior bone grafts (muscle-pedicle) in femoral neck fractures. Clin Orthop 152:143, 1980.
45. Chacha PB: Vascularized pedicular bone grafts. Int Orthop 8:117, 1984.
46. Burchardt H: Biology of bone transplantation. Orthop Clin North Am 18:187, 1987.
47. Ray RD: Vascularization of bone grafts and implants. Clin Orthop 87:43, 1972.
48. Enneking WF, Burchardt H, Puhl JJ, et al: Physical and biological aspects of repair in dog cortical bone transplants. J Bone Joint Surg 51A:232, 1975.
49. Burchardt H, Glowczewskie FP, and Enneking WF: Allogenic segmental fibular transplants in azathioprine-immunosuppressed dogs. J Bone Joint Surg 59A:881, 1977.
50. Salama R and Weissman SL: The clinical use of combined xenografts of bone and autologous red marrow: A preliminary report. J Bone Joint Surg 60B:111, 1978.
51. Connolly JF and Shindell R: Percuataneous marrow injection for an ununited tibia. Neb Med J 4:105, 1986.
52. Connolly JF, Guse R, Lippiello L, et al: Development of an osteogenic bone marrow preparation. J Bone Joint Surg 71A:684, 1989.
53. Connolly J, Guse R, Tiedeman J, et al: Autologous marrow injection as a substitute for operative grafting of tibial nonunions. Clin Orthop 266:259, 1990.
54. Bos GD, Goldberg VM, Powell AE, et al: The effect of histocompatibility matching on canine frozen bone allografts. J Bone Joint Surg 65A:89, 1983.
55. Stevenson S, Hohn RB, and Templeton JW: Effects of tissue antigen matching on the healing of fresh cancellous bone allografts in dogs. Am J Vet Res 44:202, 1983.
56. Urist MR: Bone transplants and implants. *In* Urist MR (ed): Fundamental and Clinical Bone Physiology. Philadelphia, JB Lippincott, 1980, p 331.
57. Urist MR: Chemosterilized antigen-extracted surface-demineralized autolysed allogeneic (AAA) bone for arthrodesis. *In* Friedlander GE, Mankin HJ, and Sell KW (eds): Osteochondral Allografts. Boston, Little, Brown, 1983, p 193.
58. Urist MR: Surface decalcified allogeneic bone (SDAB) implants. Clin Orthop 56:37, 1968.
59. Glowacki J and Mulliken JB: Demineralized bone implants. Clin Plast Surg 12:233, 1985.
60. Mulliken JB, Kaban LB, and Glowacki J: Induced osteogenesis: The biologic principle and clinical applications. J Surg Res 37:487, 1984.
61. Muller ME, Allgower M, Schneider R, et al: Manual of Internal Fixation Techniques Recommended by the AO Group. New York, Springer-Verlag, 1979.
62. Boyd HB: Causes and treatment of non-union of the shafts of the long bones with a review of 741 patients. *In* Instructional Course Lectures, American Academy of Orthopaedic Surgeons, Vol. 17. St. Louis, CV Mosby, 1960, p 165.
63. Frost HM: The biology of fracture healing: An overview for clinicians: II. Clin Orthop 248:294, 1989.
64. Weber BG and Cech O: Pseudoarthrosis. Bern, Hans Huber, 1976.
65. Sissons HA and Hadfield GJ: The influence of cortisone on the repair of experimental fractures in the rabbit. Br J Surg 38:172, 1951.
66. Stinchfield FE, Sankaran B, and Samilson R: Effect of anticoagulant therapy on bone repair. J Bone Joint Surg 38A:270, 1956.
67. Flatmark AL: Fracture union in the presence of delayed blood coagualtion: A clinico-experimental investigation. Acta Chir Scand Suppl 344, 1964.
68. Urist MR, Hudak RT, Huo YK, et al: Osteoporosis: A bone morphogenetic protein autoimmune disease. *In* Dixon A and Sarnat BG (eds): Second International Conference on Bone Growth, January 3–5, 1985. New York, AR Liss, 1985, pp 77–96.
69. Strates BS, Stock A, and Connolly JF: Skeletal repair in the aged: A preliminary study in rabbits. Am J Med Sci 296:266, 1988.
70. Yasuda I: Fundamental aspects of fracture treatment. J Kyoto Med Soc 4:395, 1952.
71. Williams PL, Warwick R, Dyson M, et al: Gray's Anatomy, 37th ed. London, Churchill Livingstone, 1989, pp 460–485.
72. Weiss C, Rosenberg L, and Helfet AJ: An ultrastructural study of normal young adult human articular cartilage. J Bone Joint Surg 50A4:663, 1968.
73. MacConaill MA: The movements of bones and joints: IV. The mechanical structure of articulating cartilage. J Bone Joint Surg 33B:251, 1951.
74. Aspden RM and Hukins DWL: The lamina splendens of articular cartilage is an artefact of phase-contrast microscopy. Proc Roy Soc Lond [Biol] 206:109, 1979.
75. Dunham J, Shackleton DR, Billingham MEJ, et al: A reappraisal of the structure of normal canine articular cartilage. J Anat 157:89, 1988.
76. Fawns HT and Landells JW: Histochemical studies of rheumatic conditions: I. Observation of the fine structures of the matrix of normal bone and cartilage. Ann Rheum Dis 12:105, 1953.
77. Landells JW: The reactions of injured human articular cartilage. J Bone Joint Surg 39B3:548, 1957.
78. Benninghoff A: Form und bau der gelenkknorpel in ihren beziehungen zur funkton: II. Der aufbau des gelen-knorpels in seinen beziehungen sur funktion. Z Zellforsch U Mikroskop Anat 2:783, 1925.
79. Clark JM: The organisation of collagen fibrils in the superficial zones of articular cartilage. J Anat 171:117, 1990.
80. Miles JS and Eichelberger L: Biochemical studies of human cartilage during the aging process. J Am Geriatr Soc 12:1, 1964.
81. Linn FC and Sokoloff L: Movement and composition of interstitial fluid of cartilage. Arthritis Rheum 8:481, 1965.
82. Clark JM: The structure of vascular channels in the subchondral plate. J Anat 171:105, 1990.
83. Calandruccio RA and Gilmar WS: Proliferation, regeneration and repair of articular cartilage of immature animals. J Bone Joint Surg 44A:431, 1962.
84. DePalma AF, McKeever CD, and Subin DK: Process of repair of articular cartilage demonstrated by histology and autoradiography with tritiated thymidine. Clin Orthop 48:229, 1966.
85. Meachim GF and Roberts C: Repair of the joint surface from subarticular tissue in the rabbit knee. J Anat 109:317, 1971.
86. Coutts RD, Buckwalter JA, Johnson LL, et al: Symposium: The diagnosis and treatment of injuries involving the articular cartilage. Contemp Orthop 19:401, 1989.
87. Buckwalter J, Rosenberg L, Coutts R, et al: Articular cartilage: Injury and repair. *In* Woo SL and Buckwalter JA (eds): Repair of the Musculoskeletal Soft Tissues. Park Ridge, IL, American Academy of Orthopaedic Surgeons, 1988, pp 465–482.
88. Koide S, Shapiro F, and Glimcher MJ: Nature and source of repair tissue in articular cartilage defects: A histological study. Trans Orthop Res Soc 4:160, 1979.
89. Furukawa T, Eyre DR, Koide S, et al: Biochemical studies on repair cartilage resurfacing experimental defects in the rabbit knee. J Bone Joint Surg 62A1:79, 1980.
90. Cheung HS, Cottrell WH, Stephenson K, et al: In vitro biosynthesis in healing and normal rabbit articular tissue. J Bone Joint Surg 60A8:1076, 1978.
91. Cheung HS, Lynch KL, and Brewer BJ: In vitro synthesis of tissue specific type II collagen by healing cartilage. Arthritis Rheum 23:211, 1980.

92. Mitchell N and Shepard N: The resurfacing of adult rabbit articular cartilage by multiple perforations through the subchondral bone. J Bone Joint Surg 58A2:230, 1976.

93. Rudd RG, Visco DM, Kincaid SA, et al: The effects of beveling the margins of articular cartilage defects in immature dogs. Vet Surg 16:378, 1987.

94. Salter RB, Simmonds DF, Malcolm BW, et al: The biological effect of continuous passive motion on the healing of full-thickness defects in articular cartilage. J Bone Joint Surg 62A8:1232, 1980.

95. Skoog T and Johansson SH: The formation of articular cartilage from free perichondrial grafts. Plast Reconstr Surg 57:1, 1976.

96. Tajima S, Aoyagi F, and Maruyama Y: Free perichondrial grafting in the treatment of temporomandibular joint ankylosis. Plast Reconstr Surg 61:876, 1978.

97. Pastacaldi P and Engkvist O: Perichondrial wrist arthroplasty in rheumatoid patients. Hand 11:184, 1979.

98. Sully L, Jackson IT, and Sommerlad BC: Perichondrial grafting in rheumatoid metacarpophalangeal joints. Hand 12:137, 1980.

99. Jackson IT, Sully L, Tanner NSB, et al: An interpositional elastomeric cap for metacarpophalangeal joint perichondrioplasty in rheumatoid arthritis. Hand 13:58, 1981.

100. Woo SL, Kwan MK, and Lee TQ: Perichondrial autograft for articular cartilage. Acta Orthop Scand 58:510, 1987.

101. Amiel D, Coutts RD, Harwood Fl, et al: The chondrogenesis of rib perichondrial grafts for repair of full-thickness articular defects in a rabbit model: A one-year postoperative assessment. Connect Tissue Res 18:27, 1988.

102. Zarnett R and Salter RB: Periosteal neochondrogenesis for biologically resurfacing joints: Its cellular origin. Can J Surg 32:171, 1989.

103. Billings E, von Schroeder HP, Mai MT, et al: Cartilage resurfacing of the rabbit knee. Acta Orthop Scand 61:201, 1990.

CHAPTER 3

The Inflammatory Reaction

Thomas J. Kaschak, D.P.M.

Inflammation is the normal body's response to injury or invasion by a foreign element. When controlled, inflammation leads to repair of damaged tissue or the elimination of infective agents. Uncontrolled, it can produce tissue damage and disease. An impaired or absent inflammatory response to an appropriate stimulus defines the immunocompromised host.

Four cardinal signs characterize inflammation: heat *(calor)*, redness *(rubor)*, swelling *(tumor)*, and pain *(dolor)*, which altogether can lead to loss of function of the affected part *(functio laesa)*. Warmth and redness result from the dilatation of arterioles, venules, and capillaries and from the increase in blood flow. Exudation of vascular fluids causes tissues to swell. Humoral elements are produced that promote pain, thus impeding function.[1]

Acute inflammation is the body's initial protective response to invasion or injury. It lasts several minutes to several days and is characterized clinically by the appearance of the four cardinal signs described earlier. When the inflammation is severe, local tissue destruction may occur, as seen in abscess formation. If the inciting agent or event persists, *chronic inflammation* can develop. This form of inflammation is of longer duration and generally follows the acute reaction, but it may develop from the outset in particular cases.[2] Tissue proliferation is the hallmark of a chronic inflammatory response. Overlapping features of both forms may be found in any inflammatory reaction.[2, 3]

The inflammatory process occurs through a complicated interaction of cellular and chemical elements. Most of these elements are transported by the vascular system to the damaged or invaded site, where their actions help restore tissue integrity. Local tissues contribute to these defensive and restorative processes as well. Cellular and humoral factors participate through an elaborate series of signals that augment, propagate, and ultimately terminate the reaction.

Many diseases have as their hallmark acute or chronic inflammatory reactions. This is especially true of the arthritides. Gouty arthritis can serve as the prototype for an acute response. In this disorder, a readily identifiable antigen, monosodium urate crystals, stimulates the cascade of events recognized as acute inflammation. The affected joint becomes red, hot, swollen, and painful, and function of the limb becomes hindered. The humoral and cellular elements continue their offensive until the antigen is neutralized or its activity is suppressed by pharmacologic agents. Repeated attacks can result in joint changes more characteristic of chronic inflammation.

Rheumatoid arthritis represents the clinical prototype for chronic inflammation. In this disorder, an antigenic stimulus leads to a protracted, smoldering immunologic response. Symptoms can pursue a slow, progressive course ranging from an uncomfortable morning stiffness to pain and severe joint deformity. Tissue proliferation is characteristic as invading pannus destroys the structural and functional integrity of the joint. The chronic inflammation of rheumatoid arthritis can be punctuated by episodes of acute inflammatory flares. The inciting antigenic agent for rheumatoid arthritis has not been clearly elucidated.

The role that each humoral and cellular element plays in inflammation and joint disease must be identified and evaluated so that effective therapeutic agents can be developed. The cascade of events that occurs with inflammation has been the focus of much study, and many targets for the pharmacologic control of these processes have been identified. The magnitude and complexity of these interactions, however, present serious obstacles to treatment, because not only would the harmful effects of inflammation be suppressed but also would those processes essential to good health.

HUMORAL FACTORS OF INFLAMMATION

Immunoglobulins, complement, prostaglandins, leukotrienes, thromboxanes, cytokines, and many other soluble elements interact with one another and with immunologically active cells to restore the integrity of infected or damaged tissue. Some of the best known products of inflammation are the prostaglandins. This family of molecules has been a prime target for inflammatory joint disease (IJD) therapy. More recently, the role of leukotrienes in inflammation has been appreciated, and these alternate products of the arachidonic acid cascade may prove important in the genesis and control of the arthritic disease process.[4] The prostaglandins and leukotrienes are members of a group of biologically active compounds called *eicosanoids*. This group also includes prostacyclin, thromboxanes, and lipoxins.[5]

The Arachidonic Acid Cascade

Arachidonic acid is a normal constituent of cells. This phospholipid must be released from its membrane-bound position before it can be converted to biologically active, immunologically important mediators. The release is brought about through the action of a class of enzymes called *phospholipases.* These enzymes are activated by several tissue-specific or organ-specific stimulants such as the neurotransmitter norepinepherine, by hormones such as angiotensin II, or even by mechanical disruption of the cell.[6] Phospholipase A_2 hydrolyzes an ester group on the phospholipid component, thus releasing arachidonic acid, a process effectively inhibited by corticosteroids.[2, 7] The freed arachidonic acid substrate can then be converted to its inflammatory mediators by the action of one of two important enzymes: cyclooxygenase and lipoxygenase.

The Cyclooxygenase Pathway. After its release from the cell membrane, cyclooxygenase catalyzes the addition of molecular oxygen to the arachidonic acid molecule to form the cyclic endoperoxide prostaglandin G_2 (PGG_2) (Fig. 3–1). A hydroperoxidase then reduces the PGG_2 molecule with release of a highly reactive singlet oxygen free radical, creating another cyclic endoperoxide, PGH_2. Cell-specific metabolism of PGH_2 produces the biologically active prostanoid linked most specifically to the function of that particular type of cell.[2, 7–9] For instance, the enzyme thromboxane synthetase catalyzes the production of thromboxane A_2 (TXA_2) in platelets, whereas prostacyclin synthetase converts PGH_2 to prostacyclin (PGI_2) in endothelial cells.[8, 10, 11] PGD_2 is produced in mast cells, through the action of endoperoxide-D isomerase, and in stomach, kidney, intestine, and possibly microvascular endothelium. PGH_2 is converted to PGE_2 by the catalytic enzyme endoperoxide-E isomerase.[8, 11] Finally, in human erythrocytes and placenta, PGH_2 is reduced by endoperoxide reductase to $PGF_{2\alpha}$.[11]

The activities of these end products are varied and sometimes antagonistic. TXA_2 stimulates platelet activation, thus causing irreversible platelet aggregation. It also promotes the contraction of vascular and bronchial smooth muscle. Actions are restricted to the local microenvironment because TXA_2 is rapidly hydrolyzed (half-life of 30 seconds) to the inactive end product TXB_2. Prostacyclin, on the other hand, is a potent platelet inhibitor and vasodilator. Together, these two prostanoids serve to modulate vascular tone and patency.[8, 12, 13]

PGD_2 has been found to inhibit platelet aggregation, but not to the same extent as prostacyclin. It is a potent dilator of systemic resistance vessels, but it causes constriction of pulmonary arterioles and bronchioles.[8] In the kidney, PGD_2 produces a large increase in renal blood flow, with redistribution of flow from cortical to juxtaglomerular nephrons.[14]

Along with prostacyclin, PGE_2 is a potent mediator of the vascular phase of inflammation. Both act synergistically with vasoactive amines and kinins to increase vascular permeability. They also contribute at least partially to the joint erosions found in IJD by stimulating bone osteoclast activity.[2, 15]

Except in high concentrations, PGE_2 does not seem to cause pain directly. Instead, PGE_2 acts to potentiate the noxious effects of other chemical mediators of pain, such as bradykinin and histamine.[2, 16] PGE_2 was found to produce fever when injected into the cerebral ventricles or directly into the anterior hypothalamus.[17] In low concentrations, PGE_2 potentiates adenosine diphosphate–induced platelet aggregation, whereas in higher concentrations, platelet inhibition is observed. Thus, PGE_2 exerts a biphasic effect on platelet cell activity.[17] PGE_2 inhibits T cell suppressor function, thus enhancing immunoglobulin synthesis, while exerting anti-inflammatory activity through its ability to suppress B cell growth and differentiation.[2]

The Lipoxygenase Pathway. The products of the lipoxygenase pathway constitute an important group of proinflammatory elements whose primary actions promote modulation of microvascular permeability, smooth muscle tone, and inflammatory and immune cell function.[4] These elements are the products of leukocytes, including polymorphonuclear leukocytes, mast cells, monocytes, macrophages, eosinophils, and basophils. Platelets also are able to synthesize an important lipoxygenase product from cell membrane precursors.[2, 18, 19]

The enzyme 5-lipoxygenase catalyzes the stereospecific addition of molecular oxygen to the membrane-released arachidonic acid. The position of the carbon atom to which oxygen is inserted determines the chemical name of the product. The insertion of the oxygen atom serves as the ''energy currency'' of the product, affecting the molecule's spectrum of biologic activity.[5]

The first product of this reaction, 5-hydroperoxyeicosatetraenoic acid (5-HPETE), undergoes spontaneous or peroxidase-catalyzed degradation to the end product 5-hydroxyeicosatetraenoic acid (5-HETE). Alternatively, the 5-lipoxygenase enzyme can catalyze the conversion of 5-HPETE to the epoxide leukotriene A_4 (LTA_4). LTA_4 may then be converted to LTB_4 by the action of LTA_4 epoxide hydrolase, or, LTC_4 synthetase can effect the conjugation of LTA_4 with reduced glutathione to produce LTC_4. Subsequent metabolism of LTC_4 by γ-glutamyl transpeptidases and dipeptidases can occur within the cell membrane, in secreted cell granules, or in plasma containing these enzymes.[4] This activity successively generates the biologically active products LTD_4, LTE_4, and LTF_4.[2, 4, 5, 19] As with the products of

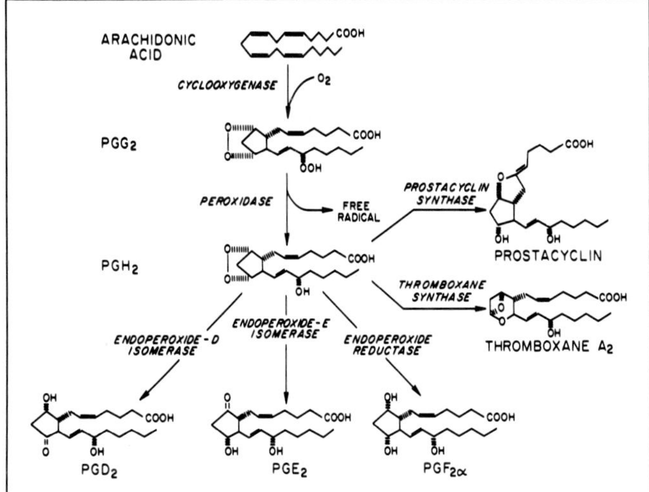

FIGURE 3–1. Metabolism of arachidonic acid by cyclooxygenase-initiated pathways. The subscript for each prostaglandin (e.g., PGE_2) designates the number of double bonds. In the platelet, catalysis of the conversion of PGH_2 to thromboxane A_2 also yields 12-hydroxy-5,8,10-hepatodecatrienoic acid and malodialdehyde. In addition to acting as a substrate for the cyclooxygenase, arachidonic acid undergoes catalysis by a number of other enzymes, including lipoxygenases and isozymes of cytochrome P-450. (From Oates JA, Fitzgerald GA, Branch RA, et al: Clinical implications of prostaglandin and thromboxane A_2 formation: I. Reprinted with permission from *The New England Journal of Medicine*, 319:689–698, 1988.)

cyclooxygenase, the products of 5-lipoxygenase have a varied effect on tissues and organs owing to differences in end site sensitivity to these products.[4]

The various types of leukotrienes are synthesized preferentially by each of the white blood cell types. LTB_4 is primarily a product of neutrophils, whereas LTB_4 and LTC_4 are products of monocytes and macrophages. Basophils, eosinophils, and certain mast cells mostly produce LTC_4. Endothelial cells appear to have the capacity to convert the precursor LTA_4 to the active product LTC_4.[4, 19] Finally, platelets can convert arachidonic acid from membrane phospholipids to the unstable 12-HPETE through the action of 12-lipoxygenase. This compound is then reduced to 12-HETE, a chemotactic factor for neutrophils, monocytes, and eosinophils.[20]

The activities of the 5-lipoxygenase pathway products are quite varied, especially in their relation to IJD. In this respect, LTB_4 plays a most prominent role.

LTB_4 is highly chemotactic for neutrophils and summons eosinophils and monocytes to the inflammatory theater of action. Essentially, this product induces an increase in both directed and random inflammatory cell movement, a process termed *chemokinesis*.[4] LTB_4 also promotes adherence of neutrophils to endothelial cells, particularly in the venule walls of injured tissues.

Reactions involving LTB_4 can result in the production of toxic superoxide ions (O_2^-). In concert with the vasodilatory prostaglandins PGI_2 and PGE_2, LTB_4 promotes leakage of plasma from vessels into the surrounding tissue. Its effects in IJD are noted most prominently in rheumatoid arthritis, ankylosing spondylitis, and gout.[4, 5, 21, 22]

A curious substance was discovered in the late 1930s by Feldberg and Kellaway while experimenting with dog lung tissue that had been perfused with cobra snake venom. These investigators noted a slow onset of contraction of guinea pig jejunum exposed to a substance produced by the lung tissue.[23] The active principal recovered was later termed *slow-reacting substance of anaphylaxis* (SRS-A), and further studies led to the suspicion that it was the mediator of the symptoms of asthma.[4] It is now believed that LTC_4, LTD_4, and LTE_4 are responsible for the action of SRS-A, with LTD_4 playing a major role.[22]

LTC_4, LTD_4, LTE_4, and LTF_4 are classified as *sulfidopeptide leukotrienes*, describing the sulfidopeptide conjugates with glutathione.[4] Their role in human disease is most noted in allergic and respiratory disorders. LTC_4, LTD_4, and LTE_4 are two to three times more potent than histamine in promoting bronchoconstriction and contraction of isolated airway smooth muscle. LTC_4 and LTD_4 induce the production of mucus by bronchial tissues, and they have been shown to suppress bronchial ciliary function. The well-recognized wheal-and-flare response of human skin after trauma or allergen exposure is mediated either directly by LTB_4, LTD_4, and LTE_4 or through their stimulated release of other endogenous mediators.[4, 5, 22]

Arachidonic acid also serves as a substrate for the enzyme 15-lipoxygenase in the production of 15-HPETE. Further metabolism of 15-HPETE yields several eicosanoids important to inflammation. The first of these, 8,15, diHETE, is comparable in chemotactic activity to LTB_4. The second product, 15-HETE, is weakly chemotactic and stimulates mast cells and their release of histamine.[24] It may also play a role as an inhibitor of the enzyme PGI_2 synthetase.[25]

Another group of biologically active compounds occurs through further metabolism of 15-HPETE. These compounds, designated lipoxin A (LxA) and lipoxin B (LxB), are primarily the products of human leukocytes. LxA and LxB have been found to inhibit natural killer (NK) cell activity. LxA can stimulate the release of superoxide anions, elastase, and hydrolytic lysosomal enzyme from polymorphonuclear neutrophils (PMNs). It can also cause arteriolar dilatation, bronchial smooth muscle contraction, and enzyme protein kinase C activation and possibly stimulate leukocyte chemotaxis without causing aggregation.[2, 26]

Cytokines

Cytokines are a group of protein growth factors produced and released by cells that affect the functional properties of other cells of the same organism (Fig. 3–2).[2, 27] The group includes interleukins, interferon, tumor necrosis factor, granulocyte macrophage colony-stimulating factor (GM-CSF), lymphotoxins, chemotactic factors, and other polypeptide growth factors. These proteins are produced only during the first few days after insult, and they contribute to inflammation and disease in a variety of ways. For the most part, they are responsible for most of the noxious effects associated with sepsis and acute generalized inflammatory diseases.

The properties of the individual cytokines function in concert, with the effects of each cytokine dependent on the presence or absence of the other factors. The interactions and effects may be synergistic, additive, or antagonistic.[28]

Interleukin-1. The biologic activities of human interleukin-1 (IL-1) occur through the action of two distinct proteins: IL-1α and IL-1β. These proteins share about 26% amino acid homology and bind to the same target cell receptor, causing similar biologic actions.[27] Monocytes and macrophages produce IL-1 in response to stimulation by immune complexes, bacterial endotoxins, C5a (a complement cleav-

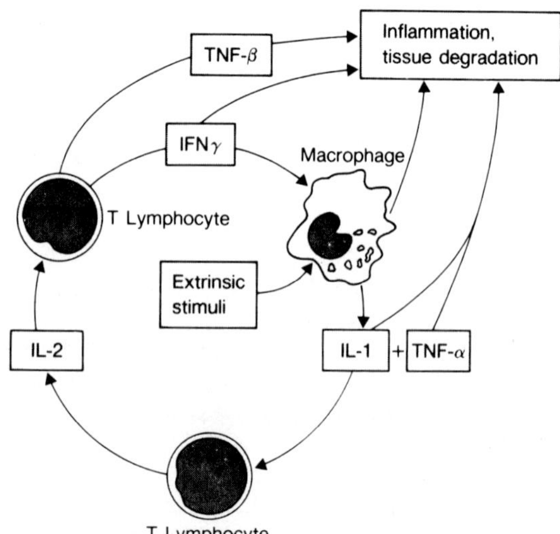

FIGURE 3–2. Cytokine network involved in inflammation. Topical stimulation by an extrinsic stimulus (e.g., lipopolysaccharide) leads to local release of various cytokines, including interleukin-1 (IL-1), tumor necrosis factor (TNF [α and β]), and interferon-γ (IFN-γ). Through their effects on vascular endothelia, IL-1 and TNF promote inflammation, vascular damage, and coagulation. IFN-γ synergizes with these cytokines by enhancing their production and action. (From Heremans H and Billiau A: The potential role of interferons and interferon antagonists in inflammatory disease. Drugs 38:957–972, 1989.)

age product), and other cytokines, including tumor necrosis factor-α (TNF-α), interferon-γ (IFN-γ), and macrophage colony-stimulating factor (M-CSF).[29] Endothelial cells, large granular lymphocytes (NK cells), keratinocytes, endothelial cells, and other cell types have the capacity to secrete IL-1.[29, 30] Receptors for this cytokine are found on many cells, including leukocytes, hematopoietic cells, smooth muscle cells, endothelial cells, fibroblasts, chondrocytes, hepatocytes, epidermal cells, and pituitary cells.[29, 31]

IL-I secreted at immunologically active sites appears to play a substantial role in the development and maintenance of chronic inflammation. It mediates accessory cell activity of macrophages important to the activation of T and B cells. It is highly chemotactic for both lymphocytes and neutrophils[32] and has been implicated as a cause of some of the systemic symptoms associated with inflammatory diseases.

On a cellular level, IL-1 stimulates immunocompetent cell activity. It promotes the proliferation of both T and B cell lines and induces the NK cell response. IL-1 stimulates prostaglandin production by synoviocytes and fibroblasts and the production and release of PGI_2, PGE_2, and platelet-activating factor from endothelial cells. IL-1 has been observed to directly increase the transcription of types I, III, and IV collagen leading to tissue fibrosis, and it is thought to provoke pannus production in the rheumatoid joint.[26, 28, 30, 33] Chondrocyte production of cartilage-degrading enzymes is increased by IL-1, and proteoglycan biosynthesis is diminished in its presence.[34]

In rheumatoid arthritis, osteoarthritis, and other IJDs, collagen degradation becomes an important factor in the loss of bone and joint structures. The enzyme collagenase helps initiate collagen breakdown at these sites. Hyperplastic synovial tissues found in rheumatoid arthritis serve as an abundant source of this protein. The IL-1 present in arthritic joint fluid may provide the stimulus for collagenase production. IL-1 elevates the levels of messenger ribonucleic acid (mRNA) encoding the enzyme in human synovial cell cultures.[35] Thus, by increasing the production of collagenase by joint tissue cells, IL-1 contributes significantly to the degradation of joint structures. In addition, the breakdown products of bone—collagen, hydroxyapatite, and bone particles themselves—stimulate adherent monocytes or peripheral blood mononuclear cells to increase IL-1 release, conceivably initiating this destructive cycle.[36]

Systemically, IL-1 has been implicated in the acute-phase responses associated with chronic arthropathy. It promotes the synthesis and release of acute-phase reactants from the liver, including C-reactive protein, amyloid A, and serum proteins.[37] Its action induces symptoms including fever and malaise, and at higher levels, IL-1 can cause hypotension and a shocklike state. A diminished ability to produce this agent in the elderly probably accounts for the lower incidence of fever during an acute-phase response such as that occurring with sepsis.[37] Important to animal species' survival, IL-1 has been found to cause a reduction in appetite and to inhibit potentially dangerous food-seeking behavior. It can bring about the desire to sleep, conserving energy and metabolic needs at a time when the organism requires rest for healing and repair.[38]

Interleukin-2. IL-2 is a cytokine produced exclusively by T cells.[29, 39] As with other cytokines, the actions of IL-2 are mediated when it becomes bound to specific cell membrane receptors. Unlike the receptors for other cell growth factors, however, those for IL-2 are not expressed on the surface of resting target cells. Instead, antigenic stimulation of the cell is required before receptor expression can occur.

The proliferation of T cell lines through the influence of IL-2 provides an interesting example of immune response regulation whereby factors produced during an immune response ultimately serve to regulate the progression of the response. Unstimulated T cells remain in the resting, or G_0, phase of the cell cycle. On simultaneous exposure to antigen and the macrophage-derived growth factor IL-1, the T lymphocyte is stimulated to produce and secrete IL-2. Concurrently, a subpopulation of T lymphocytes is incited to produce the IL-2 receptor.[40]

The process begins when antigen, in the presence of IL-1, activates the cell, moving it from the G_0 phase of the cell cycle into the G_1 phase. The G_1 phase is characterized by the production and accumulation of structural RNA, mRNA, and proteins in preparation for chromosomal replication. In this phase, the T cell accumulates and expresses IL-2 receptor (IL-2R) on its cell surface. Some IL-2R is released as a soluble protein and can be detected in synovial fluid and serum.[41] Further progression of the cell through the cell cycle then depends on binding of IL-2 to IL-2R. When this occurs, the cell enters the S, or synthesis, phase, during which deoxyribonucleic acid (DNA) synthesis and replication occur.[42] Proliferation and differentiation of the cell line then proceeds.

In addition to activating T lymphocytes, IL-2 triggers resting B lymphocytes that have been exposed to antigen to proliferate and differentiate into immunoglobulin M (IgM)-secreting cells.[43] Because there are no selective effects on particular B cell lines, it has been suggested that other antibody isotypes can be produced in addition to IgM, specifically, IgG_1, IgG_2, IgA, and IgE.[29] Other cytokines may then amplify the antibody production promoted by IL-2.

IL-2 helps keep the reticuloendothelial system active. Macrophages are activated by this growth factor, which is responsible for enhancing the function of NK cells.[29]

Interleukin-3. Produced mainly by T lymphocytes, IL-3 appears to stimulate mast cells and the production of IgG by B cells.[37] It is a hematopoietin that promotes the replication of pluripotent stem cells and participates in the regulation of neutrophils and monocytes, erythroid progenitor cells, and megakaryocytes.[44]

Interleukin-4. T lymphocytes and mast cells are the major sources of IL-4. This cytokine functions to promote T cell proliferation and enhance IL-2 production and responsiveness. It plays a central role in regulating the function of B cells and enhances the production of IgG isotype 1 (IgG_1) and IgE. Some studies suggest, however, that in humans, IL-4 may function to limit, rather than facilitate, antibody formation. It can also act as a co-stimulatory growth factor for mast cells and hematopoietic precursor cells.[29] IL-4 has also been found to inhibit the release of TNF.[37]

Interleukin-5. T cell–derived IL-5 induces mucosal leukocytes to produce IgA, a factor important for protection against pathogen invasion.[37]

Interleukin-6. Activated T cells and IL-1–stimulated monocytes and fibroblasts serve as the primary sources of IL-6. Smooth muscle and endothelial cells can also produce this growth factor.[29] IL-6 is made during the early stages of infection, stimulating the liver to produce the acute-phase reactants of inflammation.[37] IL-6 does not appear to have any effect on resting B cells that lack an IL-6 receptor, but it does play a major role in the maturation and differentiation of these cells into immunoglobulin-secreting cells. It appears to enhance the generation of immunoglobulin by B cells in the presence of IL-2, but alone, IL-6 has minimal capacity to activate the B cells.[29]

Interleukin-7. IL-7 is produced by the thymus gland and appears to stimulate the growth of lymphoid tissue.[37]

Interleukin-10. IL-10 has been found to be a potent inhibitor of TNF. This property offers a potential role in the treatment of acquired immunodeficiency syndrome (AIDS). TNF is known to stimulate the propagation of the HIV particle. IL-10 can potentially be used to suppress the endogenous production of this growth factor in the hope of controlling TNF-stimulated proliferation of the virus.[37]

Tumor Necrosis Factor. TNF was named when it was observed to cause necrosis in certain tumor masses.[45] It has since been revealed that TNF is identical to a substance called *cachectin,* a mediator of hemodynamic shock and cachexia in certain diseases.

Monocytes and macrophages are the primary sources of TNF, but lymphocytes, endothelial cells, and keratinocytes can also produce this polypeptide.[33] Many of the biologic properties attributed to IL-1 have also been observed with TNF. Like IL-1, TNF has been shown to stimulate synviocyte production of PGE_2, hyaluronic acid, and collagenase, but with less vigor. However, TNF and IL-1 can act synergistically to stimulate the synthesis and release of these compounds.[46] Unlike IL-1, TNF does not seem to facilitate T and B cell activity.[29]

TNF is produced in response to microbial invasion or as a consequence of tissue injury. The bacterial endotoxin lipopolysaccharide (LPS) appears to potently stimulate TNF synthesis and release, and in the case of gram-negative sepsis, high levels of TNF have been associated with an increased rate of mortality. TNF, along with IL-1, has the dubious reputation of causing corporal wasting.[30] The importance of this cytokine's influence in disease is supported by studies that have shown an improved rate of survival for septic patients who were treated with antibodies to TNF.[37]

The site of tissue production of TNF was found to influence the metabolic effects of this cytokine. When produced in the brain, TNF induces anorexia and a metabolic state reminiscent of acute protein-calorie starvation. In peripheral tissues, it initiates the gradual development of cachexia with anemia and loss of protein and lipid tissue.[47] Its most dramatic effect is on endothelial cells, for which even low concentrations of TNF will cause death.

Interferon. The IFNs make up a family of protein molecules composed of three members: IFN-α, IFN-β, and IFN-γ. Early studies showed that cells infected with a viral agent produced and released a protein substance that appeared to render other cells resistant to further viral spread. This substance came to be known as *interferon* for its ability to interfere with viral replication.

For experimental use, mixtures of these proteins have generally been prepared. Mixtures of IFN-α and IFN-β are commonly referred to as *type 1 IFN,* whereas IFN-γ has been named *type 2,* or immune, *IFN.*[48] Conventional terminology dictates the use of IFN-α, IFN-β, or IFN-γ when referring to these substances.

The macrophage appears to be the major source of IFN-α

and IFN-β, whereas IFN-γ is produced mainly by activated T lymphocytes and NK cells.[29, 49, 50] These cells produce IFNs in response to viral infection and on stimulation by nonviral agents, including protozoa and bacteria and their subcellular components, such as LPS.[49]

The IFNs function to activate macrophages and stimulate the release of a multitude of inflammatory factors by these cells. They promote T lymphocyte recruitment during immunologic reactions, and they participate in the regulation of IgE antibody secretion and production. IFNs are also known to induce the expression of major histocompatibility complex (MHC) antigens, which are important to the pathogenesis of rheumatoid arthritis, and to foster the production of acute-phase proteins.[48]

IFN-γ is the IFN type most frequently cited in scientific literature relating to inflammation and arthritis. This protein appears to advance autoimmune-mediated activity and may contribute to allograft rejection. IFN-γ activates macrophages and enhances their ability to produce reactive oxygen molecules. Exposure of T lymphocytes and NK cells to IFN-γ increases their capacity to differentiate into cytotoxic effector cells. Production of IL-1 and TNF by their source cells is augmented in the presence of IFN-γ. The antiviral effects of IFN-γ are less pronounced than those of IFN-α or IFN-β, but IFN-γ appears to offer more protection against parasitic and other intracellular pathogens.[29]

IFN-γ, or perhaps an atypical form of IFN-α, has been reported as present in the sera of some patients with certain autoimmune disorders, including rheumatoid arthritis and insulin-dependent diabetes mellitus. It is postulated that circulating IFNs may be the cause of some of the pathologic changes associated with autoimmune disorders. IFN-γ may play a pivotal role in the onset of autoimmune disease by virtue of its ability to induce class II MHC expression in situ, leading to enhanced presentation of tissue-specific antigens to autoreactive lymphocytes.[48] In rheumatoid and osteoarthritic joints, IFN-γ stimulates synovial cell proliferation, but it appears to inhibit the bone resorption stimulated by IL-1 and TNF, and to inhibit cartilage degradation promoted by TNF.[51]

Different activities have been attributed to the IFNs, depending on their site of production. For instance, when IFN-γ is produced near a focus of inflammation, it appears to act as a proinflammatory cytokine, but when present in the general circulation, all three IFNs function as antiinflammatory hormones.[48] The temporal occurrence of the IFNs, their concentration, and the presence of other cytokines and factors associated with inflammation all contribute to the overall effect these agents have on the inflammatory response.

Granulocyte Macrophage Colony-Stimulating Factor. GM-CSF is one of several myeloid growth factors that tightly regulate the production of blood and immune response cells from bone marrow precursor cells. It is produced mainly by activated T lymphocytes, endothelial cells, and some fibroblast cells in response to specific inducers. These inducers include TNF, IL-1, and endotoxins. Receptors for this colony-stimulating factor (CSF) have been identified on mature neutrophils, monocytes, and eosinophils.[44]

When sensitized T lymphocytes encounter antigen, a set of events follows, recognized as the cell-mediated immune response. The T cell becomes activated during this interaction with antigen, causing it to produce the glycoprotein GM-

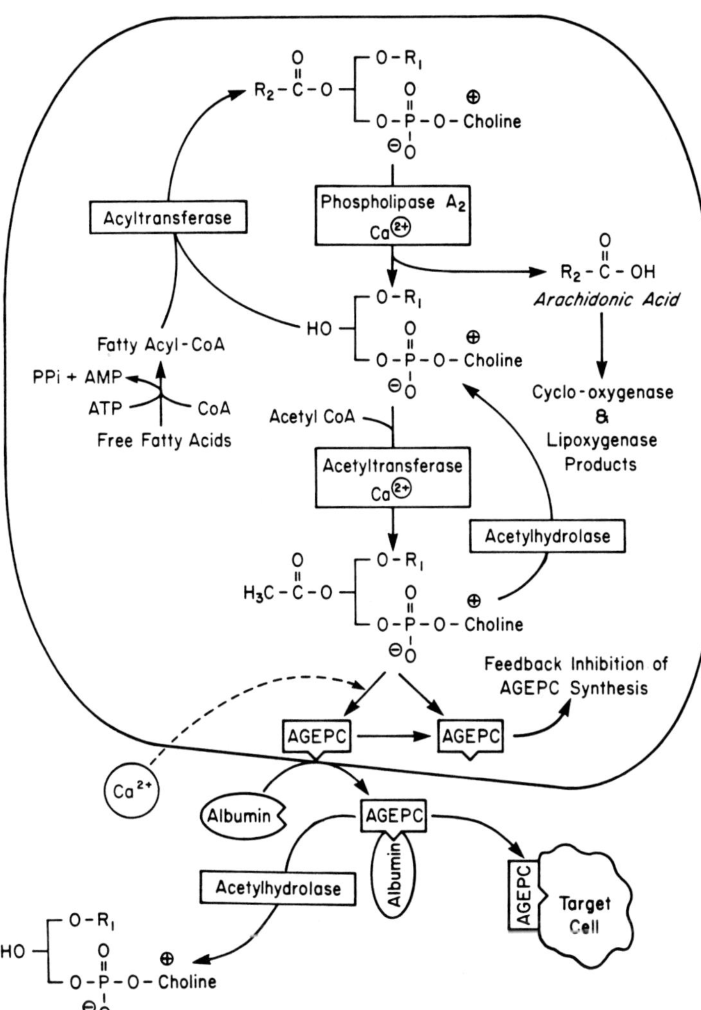

FIGURE 3–3. Proposed biosynthetic pathway for AGEPC (platelet-activating factor [PAF]). The deacylation-reacetylation pathway is the principal route of PAF biosynthesis by stimulated inflammatory cells. Activation of phospholipase A₂ hydrolyzes the long-chain fatty acyl group (predominantly arachidonic acid) at the two position of PAF precursors, followed by reacetylation of this position by acetyltransferase. The mechanisms for PAF release are currently unknown but may be coupled to sustained PAF synthesis. Degradation of PAF occurs via deacetylation of PAF by acetylhydrolase. (From Pinckard RN, Ludwig JC, and McManus LM: Platelet activating factors. *In* Gallin JI, Goldstein IM, and Snyderman R [eds]: Inflammation: Basic Principles and Clinical Correlates. New York, Raven Press, 1988, pp 139–167.)

CSF and other lymphokines. GM-CSF then stimulates the production of immune effector cells and local proliferation of mononuclear phagocytes. It also arouses the chemotactic urges of granulocytes, eosinophils, and mononuclear phagocytes, summoning these cells to the site of inflammation.[44]

A notable effect of GM-CSF on neutrophils is its ability to prime these cells for enhanced oxidative metabolism, resulting in a pronounced increase in superoxide production. It boosts neutrophil cytotoxicity and enhances their ability to phagocytize opsonized bacteria. GM-CSF induces eosinophils to augment their production of LTC₄ and effects macrophage tumoricidal activity.[44]

Macrophage Colony-Stimulating Factor. Produced by many types of tissue cells, M-CSF is a macrophage-specific growth factor. It stimulates the proliferation of macrophages and activates the tumoricidal activity of these cells. Macrophages exposed to M-CSF are stimulated to produce and release PGE, TNF, and IL-1.[44]

Granulocyte Colony-Stimulating Factor. The cellular sources of granulocyte colony-stimulating factor (G-CSF) have not yet been clearly identified. This growth factor appears to be neutrophil specific, stimulating the growth of pure neutrophil colonies. G-CSF induces increased oxidative metabolism of these cells, and it augments neutrophil antibody–dependent cell-mediated cytotoxicity.[44]

Platelet-Activating Factor

Platelet-activating factor (PAF) is a product of cell membrane phospholipids, and it appears to be the only phospholipid possessing strong biologic activity.[52] This autocoid does not exist as a stored product; rather, it is synthesized de novo by a variety of immunologically stimulated cell types. Cellular sources of PAF include neutrophils, monocytes, macrophages, NK cells, eosinophils, basophils, mast cells, vascular endothelial cells, platelets, and other cell types.[52, 53]

Pools of long-chain fatty acyl precursor residues are first acted on by phospholipase A₂, which yields a lysophospholipid product. This product is next acetylated by a specific acetyltransferase, forming the biologically active molecule, 1-*O*-alkyl-2-acetyl-*sn*-glycero-3-phosphocholine, or simply, PAF (Fig. 3–3). The reaction can also generate arachidonic acid, ostensibly from the same precursor molecule. A second pathway for PAF production has been identified that uses choline phosphotransferase as the catalytic enzyme for production of PAF from a different substrate molecule.[53]

The initiation of PAF synthesis depends on endogenous stores of intracellular calcium ion (Ca²⁺), whereas extracellular Ca²⁺ is required to sustain the synthesis and release of the molecule. The presence of albumin is also required to preserve the synthesis and release of the autocoid.[53]

The actions of PAF are initiated when the molecule binds

with specific target cell membrane receptors. It induces a wide range of biologic activities in addition to platelet activation and aggregation implied by its name. PAF promotes chemotaxis, aggregation, and granule secretion of neutrophils and monocytes; it causes contraction of smooth muscle in lung parenchyma and the intestine; and it induces microvascular permeability by causing contraction of endothelial cells in postcapillary venules.[52, 53] It is conceivable that the arachidonic acid produced during the synthesis of PAF feeds the cyclooxygenase and lipoxygenase pathways, thus further contributing to the inflammatory reaction.

The Complement Cascade and Active Complement Fragments

The complement system is composed of 11 proteins designated by the letter C followed by a signature number. The first of these is an assembly of several subunits identified as C1q, C1r, and C1s. These subunits require the presence of a calcium ion to hold the assembly together.

The complement system provides the host with a critical defensive barrier against foreign cells. Antibody recognizes and combines with the invading cell or molecule (antigen), thereby establishing a binding site for the C1q complement subunit. What follows is a complex series of reactions culminating in the formation of ion-permeable and water-permeable pores that cause the doomed cell to lyse. The system effectively prevents the development and spread of infection when its action is restricted to invading foreign cells, but disruption of the system can occur, allowing the host's cells to be targeted by the complement barrage. This self-destruction is recognized as allergy or hypersensitivity.

The complement cascade can follow either of two pathways. The classic pathway is initiated when complement becomes activated by the antigen-antibody complex (Fig. 3–4). The other, perhaps more primitive, pathway is a less specific means of immunologic defense (Fig. 3–5). It requires the presence of certain serum enzymes that work together with complement proteins to promote defense and inflammation. These serum proteins are known as the *properdin system,* and it was this protein system that contributed the name *properdin pathway* to the immunologic cascade.[54]

The C3 complement subunit is the preeminent protein in the properdin pathway system because it participates in every step. The pathway is activated by certain particulate polysaccharides, fungi, bacteria, viruses, certain mammalian cells, and aggregates of immunoglobulins.[55]

Many of the proteins and protein products of the complement cascade exhibit inherent biologic activity important to inflammation and disease. The C3a, C4a, and C5a fragments are active anaphylatoxins, forcing the release of histamine from mast cells and basophils, inducing contraction of smooth muscle, and promoting increased permeability of small blood vessels. In this respect, C5a appears to be the most potent of the three, whereas C4a possesses the least activity. The C5a fragment acts as a chemotactic agent for PMNs, monocytes, and macrophages.[18, 56, 57]

Vasoactive Amines

Histamine and 5-hydroxytryptamine (5-HT), or serotonin, are important mediators of vasodilatation and vascular permeability during the immediate phase of inflammation.[58] Of these two amines, it is histamine that proves to be more important in human disease.[59]

Histamine is stored preformed in granules of mast cells and basophils, and it is also present in platelets. It is liberated by physical events, such as trauma and exposure to temperature extremes; by the immunologic reaction of IgE binding to mast cell receptors; through the influence of the complement fragments C5a and C3a; and by certain low-molecular-weight mast cell degranulators and neutrophil-derived cationic proteins.[59, 60] IL-1, adenosine triphosphate, and the neurohormone substance P also have the capacity to cause mast cell degranulation and release of the vasoactive amine.[61]

Both histamine and 5-HT occur in platelets, and their release is stimulated during platelet aggregation or activation. Certain factors produced by IgE-activated basophils and mast cells also induce the release of these amines from platelets.[59]

The physiologic actions of histamine are mediated through its binding to either of two distinct receptors. These receptors, denoted as H_1 and H_2, are present on many immunologic and organ tissue cells. They are defined pharmacologically by the ability of their respective agonists and antagonists to cause tissue stimulation.[61]

In humans, stimulation of H_1 receptors produces contraction of smooth muscle, increased vascular permeability, pruritus, and generation of certain prostaglandins. An H_1-mediated decrease in atrioventricular conduction time in part leads to the tachycardia produced by histamine. Activation of airway vagal afferent nerves also occurs through H_1 stimulation. Diphenhydramine and chlorpheniramine are two of the classic antagonists to H_1-mediated histamine activity.[61]

The effects of H_2 stimulation are noted primarily in the pulmonary and gastrointestinal systems. These effects include the stimulation of gastric acid secretion, esophageal contraction, bronchial dilatation, and airway mucus production. H_2 antagonists include cimetidine and ranitidine.[61]

Stimulation of both H_1 and H_2 receptors produces multiple systemic effects, including headache, tachycardia, hypotension, and flushing.[61]

The Kinin System

Bradykinin is a vasoactive peptide that potently increases vascular permeability. This protein can cause smooth muscle contraction, blood vessel dilatation, and pain. The effects of bradykinin are potentiated by PGE_2.[59]

The cascade that leads to the production of bradykinin begins with the activation of factor XII (Hageman factor) of the clotting system through contact with surface-active agents, many of which are present in synovial fluid. Chondroitin sulfate, microcrystals, and components of the articular cartilage itself may all activate factor XII, as can endotoxins, basement membrane material, collagen, and certain other factors.[59, 62]

Activation of factor XII creates the enzyme designated *prekallikrein activator,* or factor XIIA, which cleaves the single-chain, gamma globulin glycoprotein, prekallikrein. Limited proteolytic digestion of this glycoprotein produces the enzyme kallikrein. Kallikrein can then react with any of three different plasma substrates important to the coagulation, kinin, or fibrinolytic system.[62]

High-molecular-weight kininogen, a plasma glycoprotein

precursor, is cleaved by kallikrein to produce the active product bradykinin. Bradykinin's activity is short lived because it is rapidly inactivated by two proteases: kininase I and kininase II. Kininase I is the same enzyme responsible for the inactivation of complement factors C3a, C4a, and C5a, whereas kininase II appears identical to angiotensin-converting enzyme (Fig. 3–6).[62]

Kallikrein is an important activator of factor XII. By causing factor XII activation, kallikrein can greatly amplify the kinin-generating system. The enzyme may also possess chemotactic activity.[52, 60]

Kallikrein may be important in the pathogenesis of IJD. The enzyme can convert collagenase in rheumatoid synovial fluid to active collagen, resulting in the proliferation of fibrous tissue and impaired joint function.[62]

The Clotting System

Factor XII activation is the initial step in the clotting cascade that ultimately leads to the production of the protein fibrin (Fig. 3–7). The clotting cascade can follow either of two pathways: extrinsic or intrinsic. The extrinsic pathway is initiated by tissue trauma, whereas the intrinsic pathway begins in the blood. Both pathways pursue complicated courses to produce the enzyme prothrombin activator.

Prothrombin activator splits prothrombin to form another enzyme, thrombin. Thrombin catalyzes the reaction that generates fibrin from its precursor molecule, fibrinogen. Fibrin is a monomer chain with the capacity to polymerize with other chains, forming a fibrin reticulum that traps blood cells, platelets, and plasma. The clot thus formed prevents loss of blood from the injured vessel. Calcium ions are necessary in all of these reactions, except during the first two steps of the intrinsic pathway.[63]

During the clotting cascade, fibrinopeptides are formed that may be important to inflammation. These fibrinopeptides are thought to possess chemotactic activity for neutrophils, and they have been shown to induce increased vascular permeability.[52, 63]

Plasminogen-activating factor, a product of vascular endothelium and certain other tissues, cleaves the protein plasminogen to generate the protease plasmin. Plasmin has many functions in addition to its role in lysing fibrin clots and controlling extensive, prolonged blood coagulation. The enzyme can activate clotting factor XII; it can cleave the C3 component of the complement system; and it can induce the formation of fibrin-split products, which have been shown to increase vascular permeability.[63]

Activated Oxygen

The body's primary defense against invading organisms is provided by the group of cells called *phagocytes*. These cells are charged with the responsibility of contacting, engulfing, and finally killing the offenders. Reactive oxygen species are used as lethal agents by the phagocytes to ensure a kill of an engulfed organism. Properly stimulated, immune cells produce these toxic oxygen species, which occasionally escape the confines of the cell and are released to the surrounding environment. The host tissues are then submitted to the same toxic effects normally exerted on an invader.

Molecular oxygen occurs as a pair of atoms covalently bonded, electrically neutral, and stable. But unlike most stable molecules, molecular oxygen contains two unpaired electrons in its orbitals. Partial reduction of the molecule creates oxygen free radicals and other reactive species. These toxic intermediates include the superoxide anion ($O^-\cdot_2$), hydrogen peroxide (H_2O_2), and the hydroxyl radical ($OH\cdot$). Singlet oxygen ($^1O_2$) can also be produced, and it can occur in either of two forms: Δ singlet oxygen ($^{1\Delta}O_2$) with paired electrons sharing the same orbital while the other orbital remains empty, and Σ singlet oxygen ($^{1\Sigma}O_2$), in which two electrons of opposite spins occupy different orbitals (Fig. 3–8).[64]

These reactive oxygen species are important contributors to tissue damage during inflammation and disease. They act as potent oxidizing or reducing agents—reacting with lipids, proteins, and other tissue components—thereby disrupting the tissue's integrity and biologic function. Certain of the antirheumatic pharmaceuticals function in part to scavenge these toxic species.

CELLULAR FACTORS OF INFLAMMATION

The cellular defense system comprises several types of specialized white blood cells working to eliminate infectious agents and damaged tissue from the body's internal environment. This system includes neutrophils, monocytes, macrophages, T and B lymphocytes, eosinophils, basophils, mast cells, platelets, fibroblasts, and a variety of other specialized cells. They function primarily to rid the tissues of foreign agents and to effect repair of tissues damaged in the exchange. They are also important in returning wounded tissues to proper order.

The activities of immune-rendering cells vary in time and manner. Their appearance at the site of inflammation follows a specific order where each defender arrives in sequence. These cells are called to order by various chemical attractants, including immune complexes, complement, and factors discussed earlier. Changes in the local environment (e.g., prostaglandin-induced vasodilatation) increase circulation and delivery of these cellular elements to the front lines.

Neutrophils. PMNs arise from blast cells in bone marrow and emerge as segmented end cells after undergoing approximately five cell divisions. Once released to the circulation, these cells circulate for about 10 hours before entering tissues or marginating in the postcapillary venules. Their life span is probably no more than 2 days. Although their ultimate fate is still speculated, it is thought that most senescent cells are removed by the spleen.[65, 66]

PMNs are the first cells to gather at the site of inflammation. They function primarily as a first line of defense by phagocytosing and killing invading bacteria.

Neutrophils help determine the continued course of an inflammatory reaction. They contain two types of granules—azurophil and specific—that provide factors important to this function. Azurophil granules contain microbicidal enzymes, neutral proteinases, acid hydrolases, and other agents, all of which help eliminate the inflammatory stimulant, establish an inflammatory environment, or chemotactically attract monocytes. Specific granules also contain agents functional to inflammation and defense, including lysozyme, collagenase, plasminogen activator, and others.[60, 65, 67]

Monocytes and Macrophages. Mononuclear phagocytes have been regarded as the body's scavenger cells.[60] Mono-

Text continued on page 46

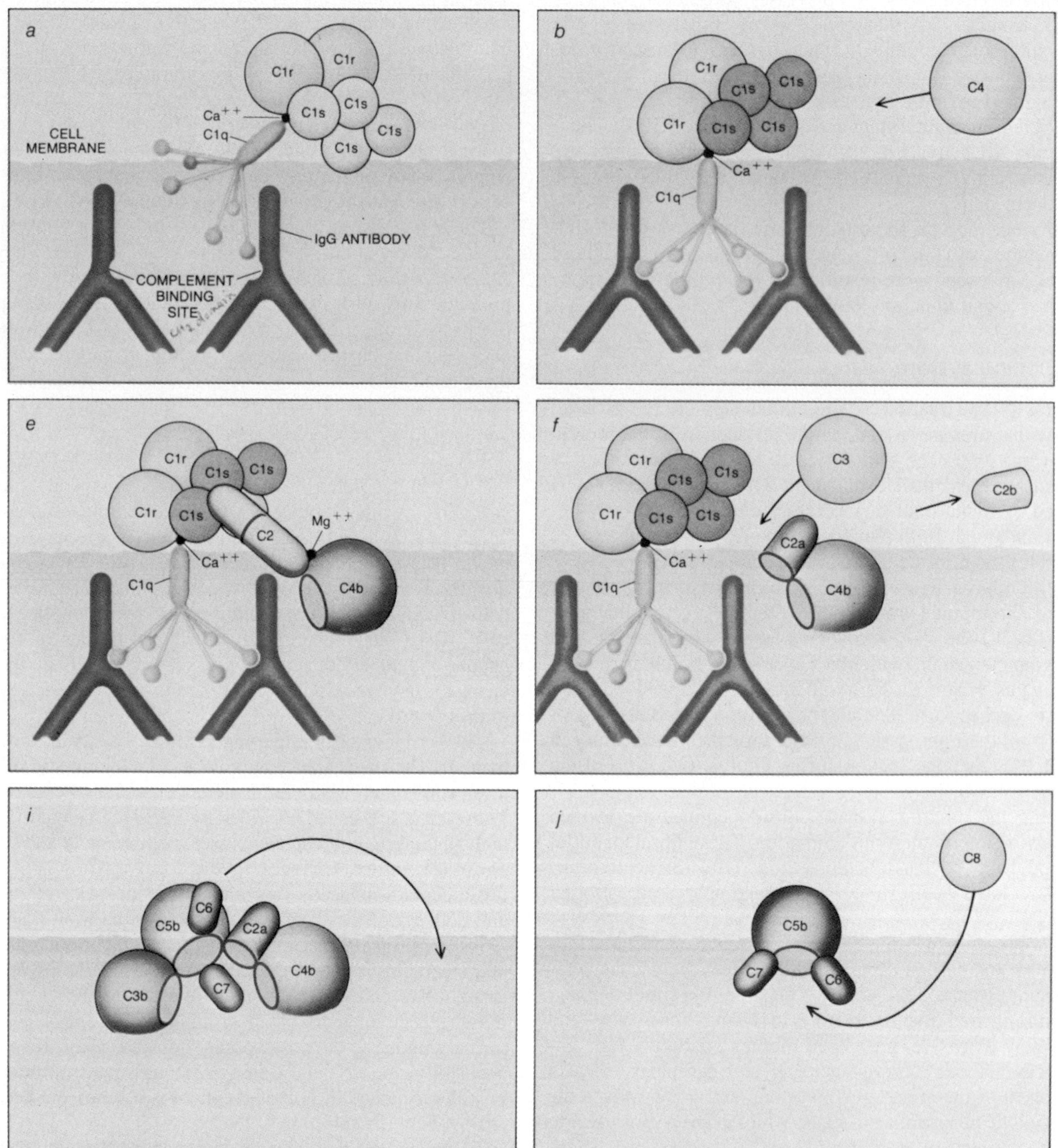

FIGURE 3–4. Complement cascade: the classic pathway. Foreign cells are recognized by antibodies, which bind to antigenic sites on the cell's surface. When two immunoglobulin G (IgG) antibodies are bound to adjacent sites, they can activate complement factor C1, which is inactive until it binds to the antibodies. C1 consists of three subunits, C1q, C1s, and C1r, held together by a calcium ion. The C1q subunit is able to bind to the complement-binding sites on antibodies *(a)*. When it is bound, the C1 complex becomes enzymatically active and will activate complement protein C4 that comes in contact with a C1s subunit *(b and c)*. C4 breaks into two parts, C4a and C4b, and the latter binds to the cell surface nearby *(d)*. When C2 comes in contact with the activated C1s *(e)*, it also is split. The C2a fragment combines with C4b to form an enzyme, which splits C3 *(f)*. The C3b fragment binds to the surface *(g)*. If it is near enough to the C4b,2a enzyme, together they bind C5 *(h)*. C6 and C7 bind to C5b *(i)*. The C5b,6,7 complex then binds to the cell surface at a new site *(j)*. C8 joins the C5b,6,7 complex. The components assemble themselves in such a way that a small hole is formed in the membrane through which a few ions can pass *(k)*. The addition of C9 greatly enlarges the hole and speeds up the flow of water and ions into the cell *(l)*, causing it to swell and burst. The C3a and C5a fragments produced also play a role in immune and allergic reactions; they cause the release of histamine from cells. (From Mayer MM: The complement system. *In* Burnet FM [ed]: Immunology: Readings from Scientific American. San Francisco, WH Freeman, 1975. © Scientific American Inc., George V. Kelvin.)

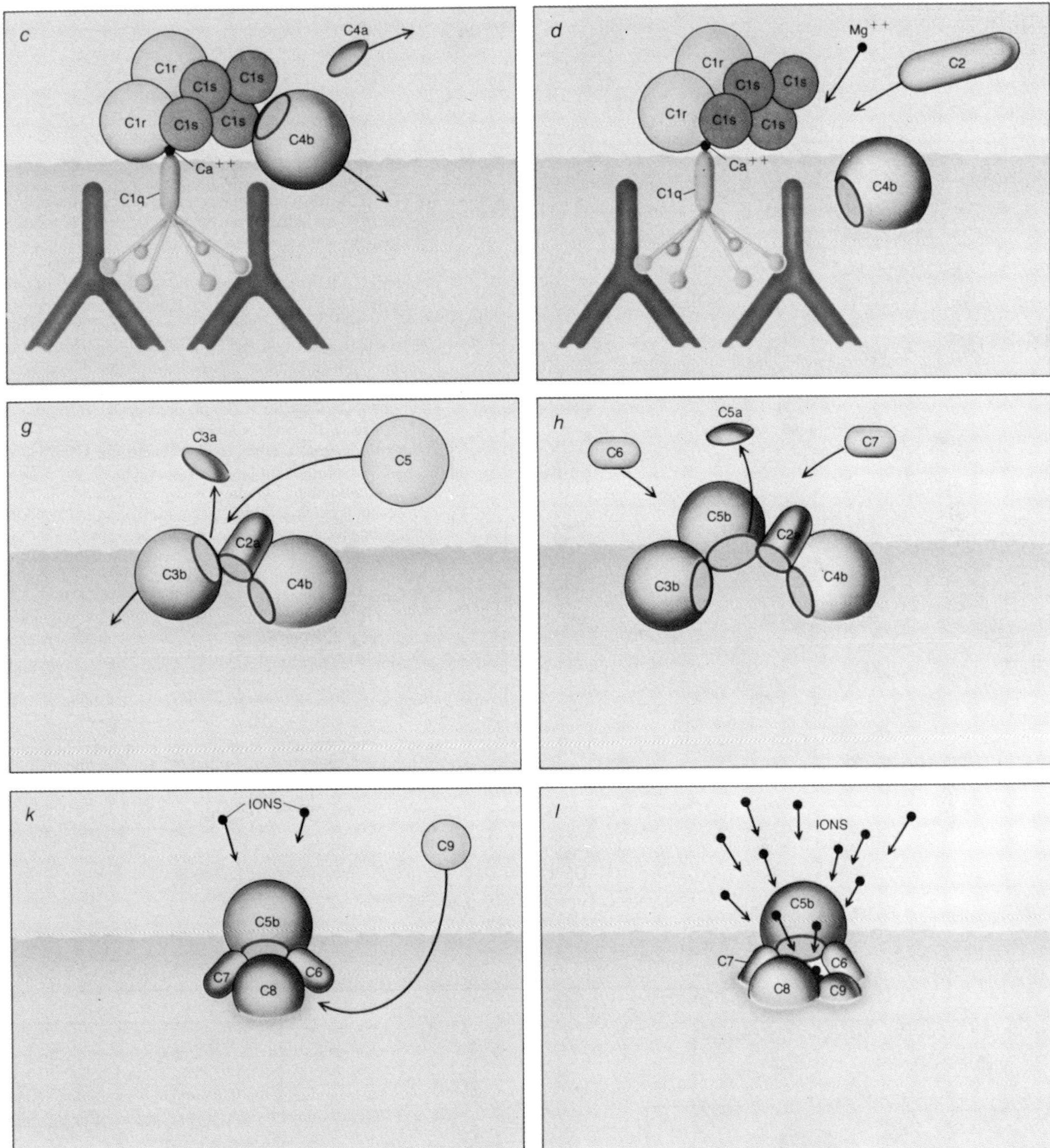

FIGURE 3–4 *Continued*

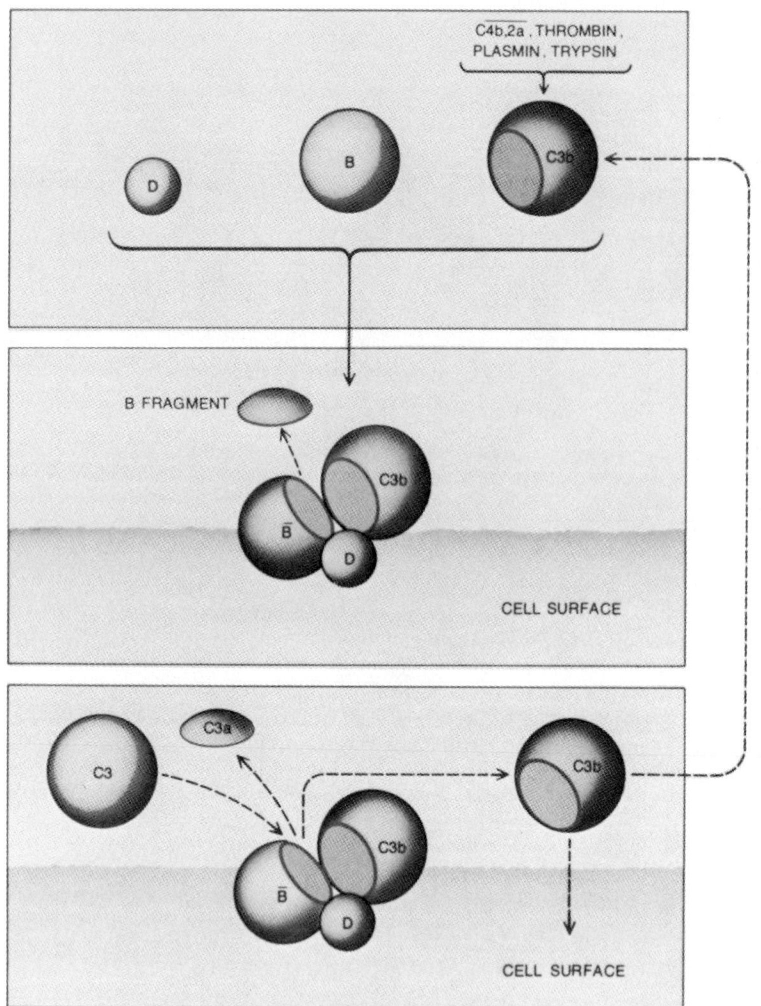

FIGURE 3–5. Complement cascade: the properdin pathway. The term *properdin* refers to a system of factors in blood serum that act together with complement in several immunologic processes. The properdin pathway is activated by microbial cells or by bacteria. Little is known about the properdin enzymes, but three subunits—factor B, factor D, and the complement fragment C3b—have been identified *(top panel).* Other subunits have been indicated in studies but have not yet been implicated definitively. Factor D activates factor B by cleavage *(middle panel),* and the activated fragment is designated *B̄.* The other B fragment goes into the fluid phase. C3b also plays a role, but its precise function is not known. Possible sources of the C3b that helps initiate the properdin system are the complement enzyme C4b,2a or plasmin, trypsin, or thrombin in blood serum. Factor B, factor D, and C3b become assembled on the surface of a microbial cell into a properdin system enzyme that corresponds in function to the complement enzyme C4b,2a, that is, they split C3 into C3a and C3b *(bottom panel).* C5 also is cleaved *(not shown),* but there are indications that the properdin system enzyme that is involved differs slightly from the enzyme that cleaves C3, possibly with respect to an unidentified subunit. The C3b that is generated may bind to the microbial cell surface, where it promotes phagocytosis (the engulfing of the cell by white blood cells). Or the C3b may join and yield another properdin enzyme complex, thus setting up a positive feedback process. Reactions after cleavage of C3 and C5 may follow the same sequence as found in the classic pathway, but details are not known. (From Mayer MM: The complement system. *In* Burnet FM [ed]: Immunology: Readings from Scientific American. San Francisco, WH Freeman, 1975. © Scientific American Inc., George V. Kelvin.)

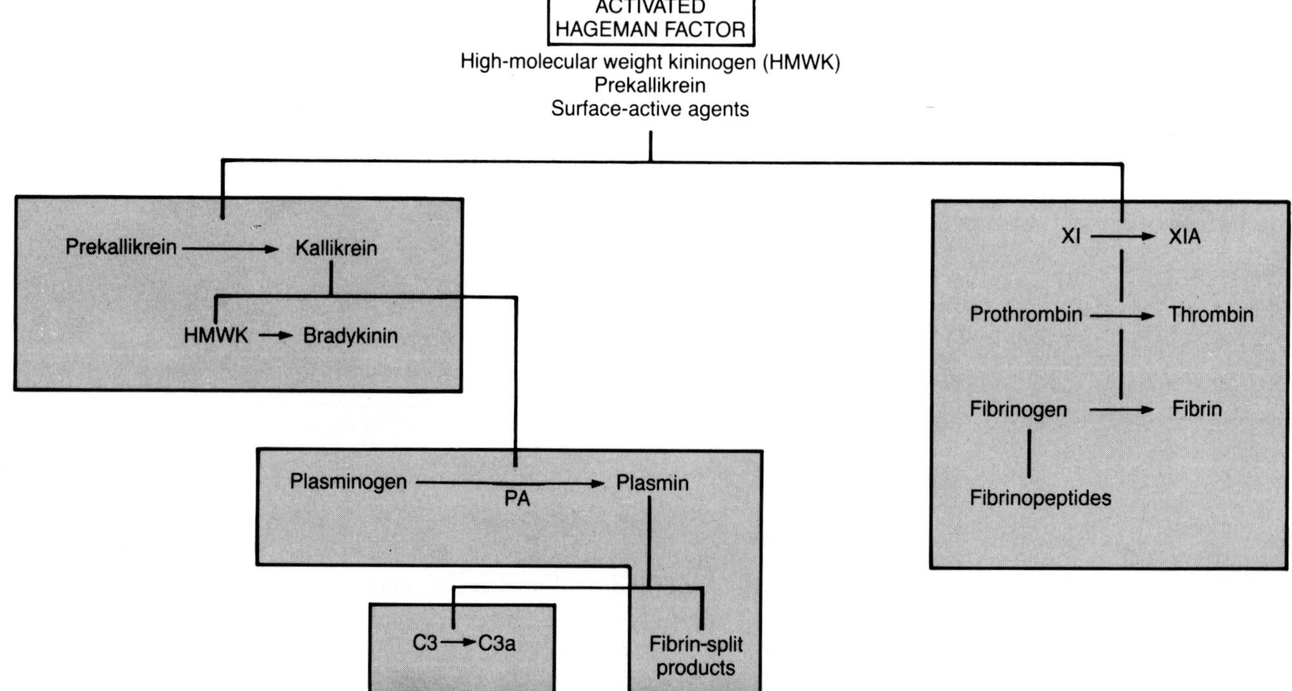

FIGURE 3–6. Generation of bradykinin: plasma mediator systems triggered by activation of Hageman factor. PA, plasminogen activator. (From Robbins SL, Cotran RS, and Kumar V: Robbins Pathologic Basis of Disease, 4th ed. Philadelphia, WB Saunders, 1989, p 55.)

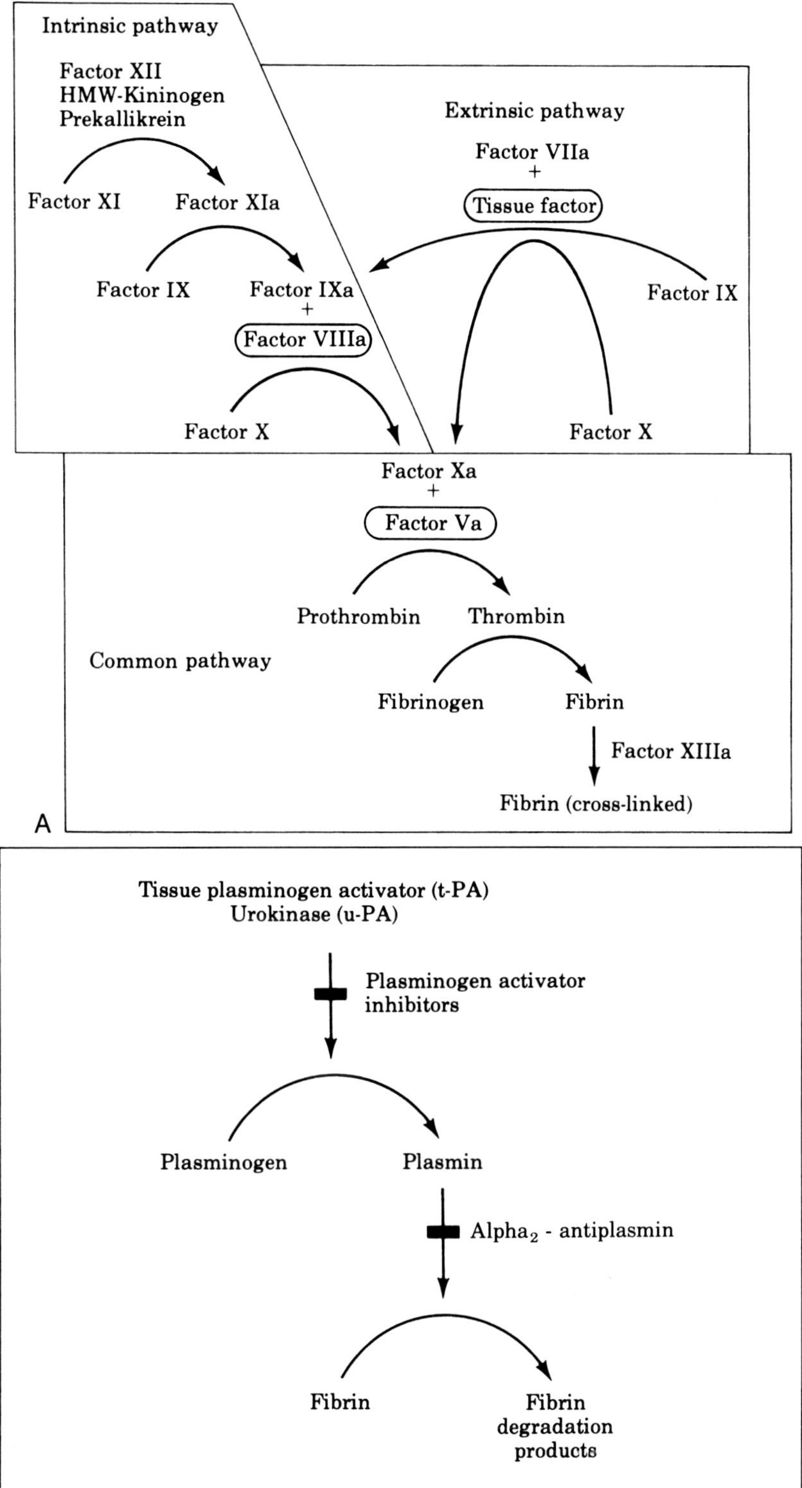

FIGURE 3–7. *A,* Blood coagulation cascade. Plasma zymogens are sequentially converted to active proteases as depicted by the arrows. Nonenzymatic protein cofactors *(ovals)* are required at several stages of the cascade. Factors IX, X, and prothrombin are activated on phospholipid surfaces. Thrombin cleaves fibrinogen, yielding fibrin monomers that polymerize to form a clot. (HMW, high molecular weight.) *B,* Fibrinolysis. The protease plasmin is generated enzymatically from fibrin-bound plasminogen by tissue plasminogen activator, or independent of fibrin by urokinase. The bacterial cofactor streptokinase forms a nonenzymatic complex with plasminogen, resulting in the conversion of additional plasminogen to plasmin. Plasmin degrades fibrin clots, generating fibrin degradation products. Plasminogen activation and fibrin degradation are inhibited by plasminogen activator inhibitors and alpha₂-antiplasmin, respectively. (Reprinted with permission from Lentz SR: Disorders of hemostasis. *In* Manual of Medical Therapeutics, 27th ed. Boston, Little, Brown and Company, 1992, pp 324–325.)

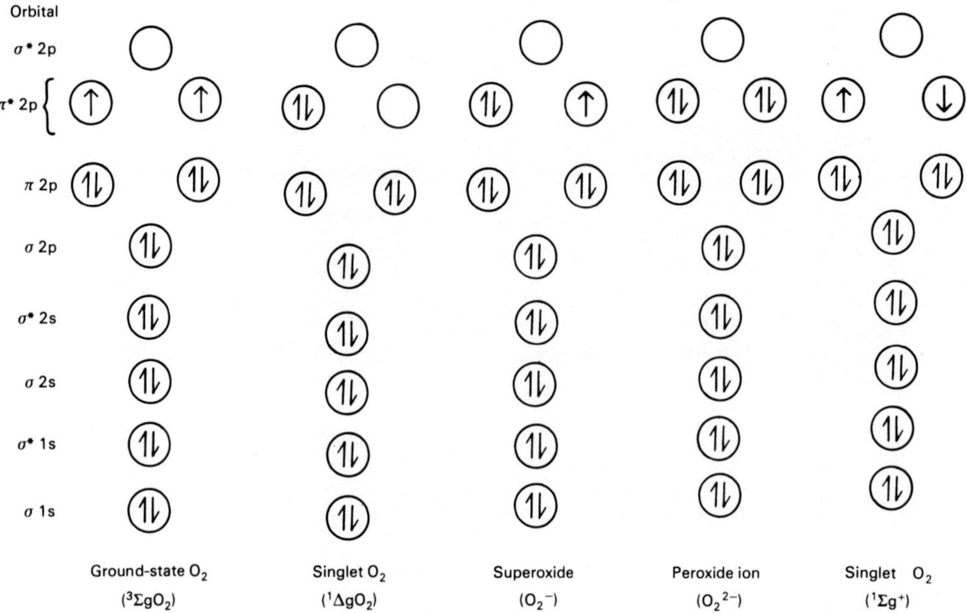

FIGURE 3–8. Electronic structure of several oxygen species. (From Halliwell B and Gutteridge JMC: Oxygen toxicity, oxygen radicals, transition metals and disease. Biochem J 219:1–14, 1984.)

cytes evolve from precursor cells in the bone marrow. Newly formed cells are present for less than a day in the marrow before emigrating to the circulation, where they spend about 32 hours before entering the tissues. During inflammation, the cell cycle time of promonocytes is shortened, substantially increasing the number of circulating monocytes.[68]

Monocytes are recognized by their indented nucleus, ruffled cytoplasmic membrane, and many pinocytotic vesicles. They are avid phagocytes, ingesting foreign particles and debris from injured cells and taking in proteins leaked from killed or damaged tissues. Neutrophils that have taken their complement of particles and debris are also fair game for monocytes.[60]

Under normal steady-state conditions, monocytes migrate to tissues and body cavities where they can then further differentiate into macrophages. A small percentage of new macrophages may also arise from dividing macrophages already located in the tissues.[67] Macrophage numbers increase during inflammation because of continued influx and differentiation of monocytes and a rise in cellular divisions of the existing local cells.[60, 67]

Macrophages become activated through their interaction with immune-sensitized T lymphocytes or through direct contact with bacterial products and other chemicals. Activation causes the cells to enlarge, increase their metabolism, and refine their ability to engulf and neutralize antigen. The cells are also prompted to release chemotactic and permeability factors, factors to aid healing, and proteins important in defense.[60]

Macrophages play an important role in projecting the immune reaction. The cells have receptors on their surface for the Fc fragment of immunoglobulin and for the complement protein C3b. When a macrophage engages antigen, the antigen is engulfed and processed and reduced to simple peptides. These peptides are then expressed on the cell's surface in conjunction with MHC determinants before being presented to T lymphocytes for further immunologic processing.[68]

Macrophages can inflict considerable damage on inflamed tissues through the action of the many toxic products secreted by the cell in the name of host protection. Hydrolytic enzymes, proteases such as collagenase, and activated forms of oxygen all can promote substantial injury to local tissues. The macrophages themselves can attack and destroy host cells should they sport antibodies recognized by the macrophage as foreign.[69, 70]

T and B Lymphocytes (T and B cells). T lymphocytes are antigen-specific, thymus-derived cells that function as effector cells for cell-mediated immune reactions. Several phenotypically discrete populations of T cells occur that display surface molecules correspondent with their functional heterogeneity. These surface molecules have been designated as *differentiation clusters* (CD); they have roles important in transmembrane signaling and antigen recognition. They include types CD2, CD3, CD4, and CD8.[71, 72]

Surface molecules of types CD2 and CD3 appear to function in transmitting signals across the cell membrane. The CD4 molecule may function as an adhesive necessary for T cell activation depending on antigen presentation in conjunction with class II MHC gene products. Cells of this type function as helper cells for B cell differentiation and as effector cells in delayed-type hypersensitivity reactions. The CD4 molecule also serves as the receptor for the human T cell lymphotropic virus III. By comparison, the CD8 molecule serves a similar role for activation of T cells dependent on antigen presentation in conjunction with class I MHC gene products. These cells function predominantly to kill cells infected by viruses.[71]

T cells are not activated by antigen encounters. Instead, the antigen must be presented to the cell in association with the MHC by a macrophage. Alternatively, an infected cell—as in the case of a viral infection—may express antigen on its surface in conjunction with the MHC, activating the T cell when contacted. Among other things, activation causes the T cell to produce cytokines, including IL-2, which expands that population of cells activated by antigen.[71]

Two major functions are defined for T cells: effector (cellular immune) and regulatory. Effector functions include delayed hypersensitivity reactions, resistance against infectious agents, tissue rejection reactions, and activity against certain tumors. Regulatory functions include the T cell's role in facilitating or suppressing immune reactions. Those designated as T helper cells assist other T and B cells to optimally respond to antigen, whereas T suppressor cells help suppress and control the immune reaction.[60]

B cells are produced by fetal liver and adult bone marrow tissue. They function as the effector arm of the humoral immune response. Initially, the B cell displays on its surface molecules of IgM that function as antigen receptors. If the cell encounters antigen at this stage, however, it becomes inactivated. Only later, when the cell expresses IgD as well, will antigenic encounter lead to further B cell differentiation. So stimulated, the B cell will then go on to express one of the several classes or subclasses of immunoglobulins (IgG, IgA, IgD, and IgM), before differentiating into a plasma cell capable of secreting antigen-specific immunoglobulin of the same class.[60, 71]

Activation and differentiation of the B cell line proceed with T cell cooperation. When the B cell reacts with antigen, it is stimulated to produce and express on its surface, receptors for specific growth factors. T cells stimulated by the same antigen release B cell growth factor, which causes the B cell line to proliferate. The T cell also releases B cell differentiation factors, provoking the B cell to differentiate into an immunoglobulin-secreting plasma cell.[71]

Mast Cells and Basophils. Mast cells and basophils are both derived from bone marrow precursor cells. They have within their cytoplasm large granules containing histamine and other mediators that stain dark blue with basic dyes. Receptors on the surface of these cells avidly bind the Fc portion of IgE. Stimulation of these receptors causes the release of histamine and other factors important to inflammation. Mast cells and basophils play a role critical to immediate hypersensitivity reactions.[73]

Basophils mature in the bone marrow before entering the general circulation. Here, they circulate for about 2 weeks before dying. Mast cells, on the other hand, enter into the tissues and probably maintain the capacity to proliferate. They are usually located adjacent to blood vessels and beneath epithelial surfaces.[73]

Eosinophils. Eosinophils are derived from bone marrow precursors and are identified by their acidophilic cytoplasmic granules that stain red or pink. These granules contain abundant peroxidase and lysosomal enzymes. Cationic proteins produced by the cell can cause membrane damage to infecting organisms by producing transmembrane pores.[65]

Eosinophils are found in the circulating blood and body tissues, particularly in the gastrointestinal tract. Their presence in the blood lasts about 2 days, whereas their life span in tissues may be as long as 2 weeks. The cells increase in number during allergic reactions and with parasitic infection. Tissue and blood eosinopenia occurs during inflammation and acute stress, but its relevance is unknown.[65]

Platelets. Thrombocytes, or platelets, are anuclear cell fragments that function primarily to initiate hemostasis.[74] They are derived from giant cells in the bone marrow called *megakaryocytes*.[75] Fragments of cytoplasm from these large cells break off and enter the circulation as platelets. In addi-

tion to their primary role in hemostasis, platelets are also important participants in the inflammatory response.

Platelets flow through normal blood vessels without incident. When a platelet encounters injured vascular endothelium (particularly arterial), it adheres via glycoprotein surface receptors to exposed von Willebrand factor in the vascular subendothelium. This activates the cell, causing it to flatten, spread, and develop numerous filapodia. Other changes in the platelet's surface cause activation of coagulation factors resulting in the production of fibrin, the entrapment of erythrocytes, and the formation of a hemostatic plug. Arachidonic acid is released from membrane phospholipids, and TXA_2 and 12-HETE are produced. These products promote further platelet aggregation and vasoconstriction. Histamine and serotonin (5-HT), also present in platelets, help occlude the hemorrhaging vessel by causing contraction of vascular smooth muscle cells.[75] In veins, where stasis is likely, platelets play a lesser role in initiating the coagulation process.[74]

Platelets play many roles during inflammation. They can activate and regulate the complement cascades, alter vascular permeability, and bind to microorganisms. Many of the factors produced by activated platelets are chemotactic for monocytes and PMNs. These factors include platelet-derived growth factor (PDGF), 12-HETE, and PAF. Platelets also help increase the monocyte's ability to adhere to surfaces. TXA_2, the main eicosanoid product released from platelets, enhances the adhesiveness of PMNs.[74]

Platelet activity is influenced by the many mediators released during inflammation and repair. Acute-phase reactants such as fibrinogen and derivatives of C-reactive protein increase platelet aggregation. Immune complexes stimulate platelet aggregation, but platelets that have adsorbed IgG to their surfaces may be susceptible to the same protective mechanisms facing invading microorganisms. Spent platelets are removed from the circulation by the spleen.[74]

Many inflammatory mediators, such as IL-1, TNF, and bacterial LPS, can alter the vascular endothelium, secondarily activating the platelets by contact with the thrombogenic surfaces. This process leads to local thrombosis, which is characteristic of inflammatory reactions.[74]

Endothelial Cells. Endothelial cells line all blood vessels and allow smooth flow of cells and fluid through the conduits. They are attached to the vessels by a basement membrane containing collagen, glycosaminoglycans, elastin, and other substances.[76]

The subendothelium becomes exposed when endothelial cells are stimulated to contract or when they are removed by trauma. The exposure of this layer to platelets causes their adherence to the subendothelium and their subsequent degranulation. The platelet-clotting cascade is thus initiated.[77]

Endothelial cells help regulate coagulation in a number of ways. They actively produce and secrete von Willebrand factor and other factors important to the initiation and advancement of the clotting cascade. On the other hand, these cells produce anticoagulant factors such as antithrombin III, protein C, and protease nexin. Both antithrombin III and protease nexin inhibit thrombin, whereas protein C appears to inactivate clotting factors Va and VIIIa. They produce and secrete antiplatelet factors, including prostacyclin, a potent vasodilator and platelet inhibitor. Endothelial cells produce two forms of plasminogen activator—urokinase and tissue plasminogen activator—both active in dissolving clots, but they also produce an inhibitor of plasminogen activator, suggesting a regulatory role.[77]

Half of the body's PMNs are included in the marginal pool, those cells that adhere to the endothelial lining of the blood vessels. Monocytes and lymphocytes are also capable of endothelial cell adherence, especially when the endothelium is stimulated by IL-1, TNF, or endotoxin. Once these cells become adherent to the endothelium, they move about the surface and can then migrate into the tissues via intercellular junctions. The endothelial cells release factors chemotactic for PMNs, including LTB$_4$.[77]

Fibroblasts. Fibroblasts are the most common cells found in connective tissue.[78] They are important during morphogenesis, directing structure formation and placement in the developing organism. In the adult, fibroblasts help maintain the structural integrity of the tissues. They are crucial to the repair of tissues that have sustained injury through trauma or infection. The activity of fibroblasts is probably not autonomous; rather, they are modulated by other connective tissue and immune cells.[79]

Fibroblasts and other connective tissue cells are responsible for producing the various matrix constituents of connective tissue. These products include the collagens; proteoglycans; glycoproteins, including fibronectin; and other components. Fibroblasts also produce matrix-degrading enzymes, including collagenase, elastase, proteoglycanases, glycosaminoglycanases, and glycoproteinases.[79] These enzymes are necessary for reducing the components of damaged connective tissue before new tissue can be constructed.

T cells stimulated by antigen produce the protein lymphocyte-derived chemotactic factor-F (LDCF-F), a chemotactic factor for fibroblasts. LTB$_4$ from leukocytes and PDGF and transforming growth factor-β (TGF-β) from platelets are also potent chemoattractants for fibroblasts. A C5-derived product from the complement protein, as well as three matrix components (collagen, fibronectin, and elastin), can also summon fibroblasts to areas of damage and repair.[79]

Fibroblast growth is regulated by "competence" and "progression" factors. The competence factors prepare the cells for growth, whereas progression factors stimulate DNA synthesis of the competent cells. PDGF is one of several competence factors; epidermal growth factor and TGF-β are examples of progression factors.[79]

Natural Killer Cells. NK cells have been described as large granular lymphocytes that demonstrate appreciable cytotoxic activity. They are nonphagocytic, nonadherent cells that lack surface immunoglobulins. These cells may impart a genetic resistance to viral and certain intracellular bacterial infections and may possess activity responsible for rejection of hematopoietic allografts.[80, 81]

Synovial Cells. Inflammation is the primary pathologic process that promotes the destruction of joint structures in arthritis. The invasion of synovium over the cartilage surface is a major cause of such destruction.

Normally a few cells thick, the synovium in arthritis is induced to proliferate into a structure many times thicker and more active. Unlike malignancy, the invasive synovial tissue is heterogenous, composed of endothelial cells, synovial cells, lymphocytes and plasma cells, mast cells, multinucleate cells, and rare PMNs. There are many factors contained in the fluid bathing the synovium that stimulate its growth, including synovial fibroblast-activating factor, PDGF, IL-1,

and other chemotactic agents previously discussed. Some inhibiting factors may be present as well.[82]

ACUTE INFLAMMATION

An acute inflammatory reaction generally occurs after the body experiences the insult of trauma or infection. Initially, there is an inconsistent, transient, local vasoconstriction lasting only several seconds, followed by vasodilatation and an increase in blood flow. The augmented blood flow and volume produce the characteristic warmth and redness typical of this reaction. Hydrostatic pressure increases, and a low-protein transudate may be forced into the extravascular space. Local release of the humoral factors PGE$_2$, PGI$_2$, LTE$_4$, PAF, and others further stimulates vasodilatation and increases vascular permeability, particularly in the postcapillary venules.[81, 83]

In mild, superficial inflammatory reactions, a low-protein serous fluid escapes into the local dermal tissues, causing blistering of the skin. In most acute reactions, increased vascular permeability allows protein-rich fluid to enter the extravascular tissues, increasing blood viscosity and causing rouleau formation of the red blood cells and margination of the white blood cells. The now protein-laden interstitium develops an increased osmotic pressure and produces a net outflow of fluid into the intercellular space. The edema of inflammation is now established.

Marginated leukocytes emigrate from the blood vessels between widening endothelial gaps, through the basement membrane, and into the perivascular tissues. PMNs are the primary immunologic cells present at the site of inflammation, attracted by LTB$_4$, 12-HETE, and other chemotactic factors. Neutrophils, which predominate at the site of inflammation during the first 6 to 24 hours, release chemotactic factors for monocytes that replace the PMNs in 24 to 48 hours. In suppurative or purulent acute inflammatory reactions, large amounts of pus may form. Masses of PMNs aggregate at the site, and coagulation of the pus can develop. Such reactions occur in acute appendicitis or may be more localized, as in tissue abscess formation.

Neutrophils are activated in response to an inflammatory stimulus through the process of stimulus-response coupling. Seconds after engaging a stimulant, the cell transforms into one capable of secreting factors that can cause significant tissue injury. Chemoattractants, leukotrienes, and immune complexes are all efficient stimulants capable of engaging neutrophil surface receptors and activating the stimulus-response cascade. Binding of these ligands causes phospholipase C to hydrolyze the membrane constituent phosphatidylinositol 4,5 bisphosphate, a process regulated by a guanosine triphosphate–binding protein (G protein). This results in the production of the "twin signals" inositol 1,4,5 triphosphate (IP$_3$) and *sn*-1,2-diacylglycerol (DG), which synergistically activate the cell. The water-soluble IP$_3$ enters the cytoplasm and activates receptors on the endoplasmic reticulum or calcium-containing organelles, causing the release of intracellular calcium. This action precedes the release of neutrophil lysosomal enzymes, cell aggregation, and assembly of the superoxide anion system at the plasmalemma. DG remains associated with the plasma membrane, where it activates the enzyme protein kinase C, which then catalyzes the phosphor-

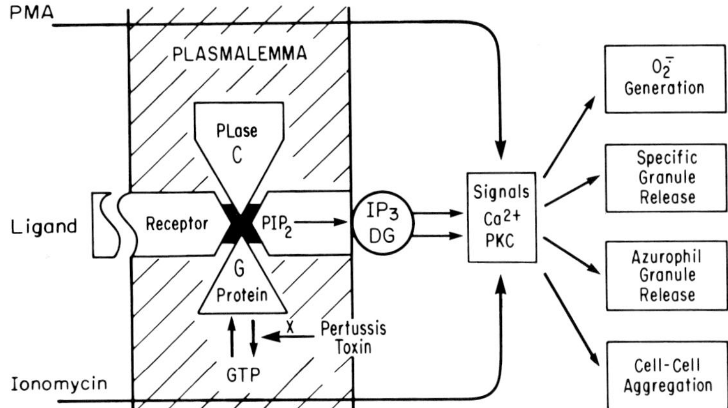

FIGURE 3–9. Stimulus-response coupling in the neutrophil. X represents the insertion into the lipid bilayer and the potential uncoupling of protein–protein interactions by nonsteroidal antiinflammatory drugs (NSAIDs). PMA, phorbol myristate acetate; PLase C, phospholipase C; PIP$_2$, phosphatidylinositol 4,5-bisphosphate; IP$_3$, inositol 1,4,5-triphosphate; DG, *sn*-1,2-diacylglycerol; PKC, protein kinase C; GTP, guanosine trisphosphate. (From Abramson SB and Weissmann G: The mechanisms of action of nonsteroidal anti-inflammatory drugs. Arthritis Rheum 32:1–9, 1989.)

ylation of those proteins responsible for regulating cell activation (Fig. 3–9).[84]

CHRONIC INFLAMMATION

Tissue proliferation is the hallmark of a chronic inflammatory reaction (manifested as erosive pannus formation in diseases such as rheumatoid arthritis), and control of this proliferation is central to the control of the disease process.[85]

There are three ways in which chronic inflammation can develop. First, bouts of acute inflammation followed by resolution generally lead to local tissue damage and scarring. Repeated damaging events promote a continuous effort at repair, thus establishing the chronic reaction. Second, chronic inflammation may arise as a result of a persistent inciting stimulant or through impairment of the healing process. Third, chronic inflammation may develop as a result of a low-grade, mild response to an antigenic stimulus that continues to smolder, causing tissue proliferation and destruction of normal anatomic structure. Such a state develops from persistent infection or prolonged exposure to toxic substances, or through autoimmune stimulation. The pathologic changes in rheumatoid arthritis may be typical of this last mechanism.[81, 85, 86]

The cells most important to chronic inflammation include macrophages, lymphocytes, plasma cells, and proliferating fibroblasts. Monocytes appear about 48 hours into developing inflammation and transform into larger macrophages that persist throughout the remainder of the reaction. IL-1 mediates the accessory cell activity of the macrophages. They are believed to play a central role in the processing of antigen and its presentation to lymphocytes. In chronic inflammation with granuloma formation, both cell types may transform into epithelioid cells, or they may form multinucleate giant cells by fusion of young, newly arrived cells with older, elicited cells.[67, 81] T lymphocytes are important in the cell-mediated arm of inflammation, whereas B lymphocytes and plasma cells play a major role in the humoral response and the production of antibody.

Lymphocytes play an important role in the pathogenesis of rheumatoid arthritis. Increased lymphocyte activity has been found in synovial fluid taken from rheumatoid patients as compared with their peripheral blood leukocytes. These activated cells are present early in the disease process, supporting the contention that they are indeed very early participants in the pathogenesis of rheumatoid arthritis. Further

support for the role of lymphocytes is found in studies that demonstrate the effects of thoracic duct drainage and total lymphoid irradiation for intractable rheumatoid arthritis.[87–89] These reports show that lymphocyte removal or suppression of their activity can lead to a marked diminution of joint inflammation. Certain lymphocyte subpopulations play a more prominent role than others in synovial inflammation.[89, 90]

The significance of mast cells in chronic inflammation has been greatly overlooked. Several lines of evidence suggest that mast cell numbers may be governed by immunologic events. Mast cells are a prominent feature in both extraosseous pannus and intraosseous invasive tissue. This raises the question of a possible role in the pathogenesis of rheumatoid arthritis. In synovium from patients with rheumatoid arthritis, the mast cells found in the tissue are positively correlated with the intensity of the lymphocyte infiltration. Mast cells here generate chemotactic factors for leukocyte subpopulations in obvious relevance to the pathogenesis of acute and chronic inflammation.[91–93] An increase in the number of mast cells occurs in the early stages of disease activity, whereas a decrease occurs as the lesion matures. Flare followed by relative quiescence is typical of IJDs, suggesting that mast cell concentration in tissues may serve as an indirect measure of the stage of the inflammatory response.[92]

Fibronectin, a high-molecular-weight glycoprotein, has been recognized for its actions in chronic systemic inflammatory disease. Made in large quantities by both type A (macrophage like) and type B (fibroblast like) synovial cells, its biologic activities include the enhancement of phagocytosis, chemotaxis, cell adhesion, and binding to both fibrinogen and collagen. Its concentration in synovial fluids is elevated during rheumatic joint disorders owing to local synthesis.[94, 95]

Deposits of fibrinlike material are common at sites of chronic inflammatory activity. It has been recognized that fibrinolysis is inhibited in these areas. Low fibrinolytic activity in chronically inflamed tissues may be a result of this inhibition, causing persistence of fibrinlike deposits in rheumatoid joints.[96]

References

1. Gallin JI, Goldstein IM, and Snyderman R (eds): Inflammation: Basic Principles and Clinical Correlates. New York, Raven Press, 1988, p 1.
2. Schumacher HR, Klippel JH, and Robinson DR (eds): Mediators of inflammation. *In* Primer on the Rheumatic Diseases, 9th ed. Atlanta, Arthritis Foundation, 1988, pp 24–30.

3. Zvaifler NJ: Overview of etiology and pathogenesis. *In* Utsinger PD, Zvaisler N, and Ehrlich GE (eds): Rheumatoid Arthritis: Etiology, Diagnosis, and Management. Philadelphia, JB Lippincott, 1985, pp 154–156.

4. Newcombe DS: Leukotrienes: Regulation of biosynthesis, metabolism, and bioactivity. J Clin Pharmacol 28:530–549, 1988.

5. Lewis RA, Austen KF, and Soberman RJ: Leukotrienes and other products of the 5-lipoxygenase pathway: Biochemistry and relation to pathobiology in human diseases. N Engl J Med 323:645–655, 1990.

6. Wilson TW, Kaushal RD, and Dubois M: Prostaglandins, the kidney, and hypertension. West J Med 153:168–172, 1990.

7. Sammuelsson B: An elucidation of the arachadonic acid cascade. Drugs 32(Suppl 1):2–9, 1987.

8. Oates JA, FitzGerald GA, Branch RA, et al: Clinical implications of prostaglandin and thromboxane A$_2$ formation: I. N Engl J Med 319:689–698, 1988.

9. Marcus AJ: Eicosanoids: Transcellular metabolism. *In* Gallin JI, Goldstein IM, and Snyderman R (eds): Inflammation: Basic Principles and Clinical Correlates. New York, Raven Press, 1988, p 131.

10. Delby C: Metabolism of polyunsaturated fatty acids, precursors of eicosanoids. *In* Curtis-Pryor PB (ed): Prostaglandins: Biology and Chemistry of Prostaglandins and Related Eicosanoids. New York, Churchill Livingstone, 1988, p 16.

11. Yamamoto S: Characterization of enzymes in prostanoid synthesis. *In* Curtis-Pryor PB (ed): Prostaglandins: Biology and Chemistry of Prostaglandins and Related Eicosanoids. New York, Churchill Livingstone, 1988, pp 37–45.

12. Goldstein IM: Agents that interfere with arachidonic acid metabolism. *In* Gallin JI, Goldstein IM, and Snyderman R (eds): Inflammation: Basic Principles and Clinical Correlates. New York, Raven Press, 1988, p 935.

13. Vane J: The evolution of non-steroidal anti-inflammatory drugs: Their mechanisms of action. Drugs 33(Suppl 1):18–27, 1988.

14. Oates JA, FitzGerald GA, Branch RA, et al: Clinical implications of prostaglandin and thromboxane A$_2$ formation: II. N Engl J Med 319:716–767, 1988.

15. Zurier RB: Prostaglandins and inflammation. *In* Curtis-Pryor PB (ed): Prostaglandins: Biology and Chemistry of Prostaglandins and Related Eicosanoids. New York, Churchill Livingstone, 1988, p 596.

16. Chignard M and Vargaftig BB: Blood platelet activation. *In* Curtis-Pryor PB (ed): Prostaglandins: Biology and Chemistry of Prostaglandins and Related Eicosanoids. New York, Churchill Livingstone, 1988, pp 205–216.

17. Von Euler US: Biology of prostanoids. *In* Curtis-Pryor PB (ed): Prostaglandins: Biology and Chemistry of Prostaglandins and Related Eicosanoids. New York, Churchill Livingstone, 1988, pp 1–7.

18. Austen KF: The role of arachidonic acid metabolites in local and systemic inflammatory processes. Drugs 33(Suppl 1):10–17, 1987.

19. Lewis RA and Austen KF: Leukotrienes. *In* Curtis-Pryor PB (ed): Prostaglandins: Biology and Chemistry of Prostaglandins and Related Eicosanoids. New York, Churchill Livingstone, 1988, pp 121–128.

20. Weksler BB: Platelets. *In* Curtis-Pryor PB (ed): Prostaglandins: Biology and Chemistry of Prostaglandins and Related Eicosanoids. New York, Churchill Livingstone, 1988, pp 543–557.

21. Rainsford KD: Eicosanoids in arthritis. *In* Curtis-Pryor PB (ed): Prostaglandins: Biology and Chemistry of Prostaglandins and Related Eicosanoids. New York, Churchill Livingstone, 1988, pp 647–653.

22. Higgs GA and Moncada S: Leukotrienes in disease: Implications for drug development. Drugs 30:1–5, 1985.

23. Feldberg W and Kellaway CH: Liberation of histamine and formation of lysolecithin-like substances by cobra venom. J Physiol (London) 94:187–226, 1938.

24. Bigby TD and Nadel JA: Asthma. *In* Gallin JI, Goldstein IM, and Snyderman R (eds): Inflammation: Basic Principles and Clinical Correlates. New York, Raven Press, 1988, pp 685–689.

25. Deby C: Metabolism of polyunsaturated fatty acids: Precursors of eicosanoids. *In* Curtis-Pryor PB (ed): Prostaglandins: Biology and Chemistry of Prostaglandins and Related Eicosanoids. New York, Churchill Livingstone, 1988, p 27.

26. Rainsford KD: Inhibitors of eicosanoid metabolism. *In* Curtis-Pryor PB (ed): Prostaglandins: Biology and Chemistry of Prostaglandins and Related Eicosanoids. New York, Churchill Livingstone, 1988, p 63.

27. Nathan C and Yoshida R: Cytokines: Interferon-gamma. *In* Gallin JI, Goldstein IM, and Snyderman R (eds): Inflammation: Basic Principles and Clinical Correlates. New York, Raven Press, 1988, pp 229–251.

28. Alvaro-Garcia JM, Zvaifler NJ, and Firestein GS: Cytokines in chronic inflammatory arthritis: V. Mutual antagonism between interferon-gamma and tumor necrosis factor-alpha on HLA-DR expression: Proliferation, collagenase production, and granulocyte macrophage colony-stimulating factor production by rheumatoid arthritis synoviocytes. J Clin Invest 86:1790–1798, 1990.

29. Lipsky PE: The control of antibody production by immunomodulatory molecules. Arthritis Rheum 32:1345–1355, 1989.

30. Dinarello CA: Cytokines: Interleukin-1 and tumor necrosis factor (cachectin). *In* Gallin JI, Goldstein IM, and Snyderman R (eds): Inflammation: Basic Principles and Clinical Correlates. New York, Raven Press, 1988, pp 195–208.

31. Dower SK and Urdal DL: The interleukin-1 receptor. Immunol Today 8:46–51, 1987.

32. Moissec P, Dinarello CA, and Ziff M: Interleukin-1: Lymphocyte chemotactic activity in rheumatoid arthritis synovial fluid. Arthritis Rheum 29:461–470, 1986.

33. Korn JH: Cellular and biochemical interactions in the rheumatoid joint. *In* Utsinger PD, Zvaifler NJ, and Ehrlich GE (eds): Rheumatoid Arthritis. Philadelphia, JB Lippincott, 1985, pp 90–105.

34. Arner EC and Pratta MA: Independent effects of interleukin-1 on proteoglycan breakdown, proteoglycan synthesis, and prostaglandin E$_2$ release from cartilage in organ culture. Arthritis Rheum 32:288–297, 1989.

35. McCachren SS, Greer PK, and Niedel JE: Regulation of human synovial fibroblast collagenase messenger RNA by interleukin-1. Arthritis Rheum 32:1539–1545, 1989.

36. Pacifici R, Carano A, Santoro SA, et al: Bone matrix constituents stimulate interleukin-1 release from human blood mononuclear cells. J Clin Invest 87:221–228, 1991.

37. O'Hanley P: Treatment of Septicema. *In* Ground Rounds Lecture Series. San Jose, CA, San Jose Medical Center, April 14, 1991.

38. Dinarello CA: Interleukin-1 and other growth factors. *In* Kelley WN, Harris ED, Ruddy S, et al (eds): Textbook of Rheumatology, Vol. 1, 3rd ed. Philadelphia, WB Saunders, 1989, pp 285–299.

39. Greene WC: Cytokines: Interleukin-2 and its receptor. *In* Gallin JI, Goldstein IM, and Snyderman R (eds): Inflammation: Basic Principles and Clinical Correlates. New York, Raven Press, 1988, pp 209–228.

40. Mills GB, Benedict S, Mellors A, et al: Transmembrane signaling by interleukin 2. *In* Smith, KA (ed): Interleukin 2. San Diego, Academic Press, 1988, pp 113–135.

41. Rubin LA and Nelson DL: The soluble interleukin-2 receptor: Biology, function, and clinical application. Ann Intern Med 113:619–627, 1990.

42. Pauza CD: Interleukin-2 binding induces transcription of a novel set of genes: Implications for T-lymphocyte population dynamics. *In* Smith KA (ed): Interleukin 2. San Diego, Academic Press, 1988, pp 163–177.

43. Tigges MA, Casey LS, and Koshland ME: Mechanism of interleukin-2 signaling: Mediation of different outcomes by a single receptor and transduction pathway. Science 243:781–786, 1989.

44. Golde DW and Gasson JC: Cytokines: Myeloid growth factors. *In* Gallin JI, Goldstein IM, and Snyderman R (eds): Inflammation: Basic Principles and Clinical Correlates. New York, Raven Press, 1988, pp 253–261.

45. Harris ED: Pathogenesis of rheumatoid arthritis. *In* Kelley WN, Harris ED, Ruddy S, et al (eds): Textbook of Rheumatology, Vol 1, 3rd ed. Philadelphia, WB Saunders, 1989, pp 905–942.

46. Meyer FA, Yaron I, and Yaron M: Synergistic, additive, and antagonistic effects of interleukin-1 β, tumor necrosis factor α, and γ-interferon on prostaglandin E, hyaluronic acid, and collagenase production by cultured synovial fibroblasts. Arthritis Rheum 33:1518–1525, 1990.

47. Tracey KJ, Morgello S, Koplin B, et al: Metabolic effects of cachectin/tumor necrosis factor are modified by site of production: Cachectin/tumor necrosis factor–secreting tumor in skeletal muscle induces chronic cachexia, while implantation in brain induces predominantly acute anorexia. J Clin Invest Vol. 86:2014–2024, 1990.

48. Heremans H and Billiau A: The potential role of interferons and interferon antagonists in inflammatory disease. Drugs 38:957–972, 1990.

49. Nathan C and Yoshida R: Cytokines: Interferon-gamma. *In* Gallin JI, Goldstein IM, and Snyderman R (eds): Inflammation: Basic Principles and Clinical Correlates. New York, Raven Press, 1988, pp 229–251.

50. Harris ED: Pathogenesis of rheumatoid arthritis: A disorder associated with dysfunctional immunoregulation. *In* Gallin JI, Goldstein IM, and Snyderman R (eds): Inflammation: Basic Principles and Clinical Correlates. New York, Raven Press, 1988, pp 756–757.

51. Bunning RAD and Russell RGG: The effect of tumor necrosis factor α and γ-interferon on the resorption of human articular cartilage and on the production of prostaglandin E and of caseinase activity by human articular chondrocytes. Arthritis Rheum 32:780–784, 1989.

52. Schumacher HR, Klippel JH, and Robinson DR (eds): Mediators of inflammation. *In* Primer on the Rheumatic Diseases, 9th ed. Atlanta, Arthritis Foundation, 1988, p 29.

53. Pinckard RN, Ludwig JC, and McManus LM: Platelet-activating factors. *In* Gallin JI, Goldstein IM, and Snyderman R (eds): Inflammation: Basic Principles and Clinical Correlates. New York, Raven Press, 1988, pp 139–167.

54. Mayer MM: The complement system. *In* Burnet FM (ed): Immunology: Readings from Scientific American. San Francisco, WH Freeman, 1975.

55. Muller-Eberhard HJ: Complement: Chemistry and pathways. *In* Gallin JI, Goldstein IM, and Snyderman R (eds): Inflammation: Basic Principles and Clinical Correlates. New York, Raven Press, 1988, pp 21–53.

56. Goldstein IM: Complement: Biologically active products. *In* Gallin JI, Goldstein IM, and Snyderman R (eds): Inflammation: Basic Principles and Clinical Correlates. New York, Raven Press, 1988, pp 55–74.

57. Moxley G and Ruddy S: Elevated C3 anaphylatoxin levels in synovial fluids from patients with rheumatoid arthritis. Arthritis Rheum 28:1089–1095, 1985.

58. Wasserman SI: Mediators of inflammation. *In* Stites DP and Terr AI: Basic and Clinical Immunology. San Mateo, CA, Appleton & Lange, 1991, pp 154–155.

59. Robins SL and Cotran RS: Inflammation and repair. *In* Pathologic Basis of Disease. Philadelphia, WB Saunders, 1979, pp 55–106.

60. Schumacher HR, Klippel JH, and Robinson DR (eds): Mediators of inflammation. *In* Primer on the Rheumatic Diseases, 9th ed. Atlanta, Arthritis Foundation, 1988, pp 30–32.

61. White MV and Kaliner MA: Histamine. *In* Gallin JI, Goldstein IM, and Snyderman R (eds): Inflammation: Basic Principles and Clinical Correlates. New York, Raven Press, 1988, pp 169–194.

62. Kozin F and Cochrane CG: The contact activation system of plasma: Biochemistry and pathophysiology. *In* Gallin JI, Goldstein IM, and Snyderman R (eds): Inflammation: Basic Principles and Clinical Correlates. New York, Raven Press, 1988, pp 101–120.

63. Guyton AC: Hemostasis and blood coagulation. *In* Textbook of Medical Physiology, 5th ed. Philadelphia, WB Saunders, 1981, pp 92–102.

64. Klebanoff SJ: Phagocytic cells: Products of oxygen metabolism. *In* Gallin JI, Goldstein IM, and Snyderman R (eds): Inflammation: Basic Principles and Clinical Correlates. New York, Raven Press, 1988, pp 391–444.

65. Bainton DF: Phagocytic cells: Developmental biology of neutrophils and eosinophils. *In* Gallin JI, Goldstein IM, and Snyderman R (eds): Inflammation: Basic Principles and Clinical Correlates. New York, Raven Press, 1988, pp 265–280.

66. Malech HL: Phagocytic cells: Egress from marrow and diapedesis. *In* Gallin JI, Goldstein IM, and Snyderman R (eds): Inflammation: Basic Principles and Clinical Correlates. New York, Raven Press, 1988, pp 297–308.

67. van Furth R: Phagocytic cells: Development and distribution of mononuclear phagocytes in normal steady state and inflammation. *In* Gallin JI, Goldstein IM, and Snyderman R (eds): Inflammation: Basic Principles and Clinical Correlates. New York, Raven Press, 1988, pp 281–295.

68. Schumacher HR, Klippel JH, and Robinson DR (eds): The role of immunologic mechanisms in the pathogenesis of rheumatic disease. *In* Primer on the Rheumatic Diseases, 9th ed. Atlanta, Arthritis Foundation, 1988, pp 36–44.

69. Adams DO and Hamilton TA: Phagocytic cells: Cytotoxic activities of macrophages. *In* Gallin JI, Goldstein IM, and Snyderman R (eds): Inflammation: Basic Principles and Clinical Correlates. New York, Raven Press, 1988, pp 471–492.

70. Welgus HG, Campbell EJ, Curry JD, et al: Neutral metaloproteinases produced by human mononuclear phagocytes. J Clin Invest 86:1496–1502, 1990.

71. Stobe JD: Lymphocytes: Development and function. *In* Gallin JI, Goldstein IM, and Snyderman R (eds): Inflammation: Basic Principles and Clinical Correlates. New York, Raven Press, 1988, pp 599–612.

72. Weiss A: Structure and function of the T-cell receptor. J Clin Invest 86:1015–1022, 1990.

73. Siraganian RP: Mast cells and basophils. *In* Gallin JI, Goldstein IM, and Snyderman R (eds): Inflammation: Basic Principles and Clinical Correlates. New York, Raven Press, 1988, pp 513–542.

74. Weksler BB: Platelets. *In* Curtis-Pryor PB (ed): Prostaglandins: Biology and Chemistry of Prostaglandins and Related Eicosanoids. New York, Churchill Livingstone, 1988, pp 543–557.

75. Junqueira LC, Carneiro J, and Contopoulos AN: Blood cells. *In* Basic Histology, 2nd ed. Los Altos, CA, Lange Medical Publications, 1977, pp 228–243.

76. Schumacher HR, Klippel JH, and Robinson DR (eds): Mediators of inflammation. *In* Primer on the Rheumatic Diseases, 9th ed. Atlanta, Arthritis Foundation, 1988, pp 6–15.

77. Jaffe EA: Endothelial cells. *In* Gallin JI, Goldstein IM, and Snyderman R (eds): Inflammation: Basic Principles and Clinical Correlates. New York, Raven Press, 1988, pp 559–576.

78. Junqueira LC, Carneiro J, and Contopoulos AN: Blood cells. *In* Basic Histology, 2nd ed. Los Altos, CA, Lange Medical Publications, 1977, p 85.

79. Postlethwaite AE and Kang AH: Fibroblasts. *In* Gallin JI, Goldstein IM, and Snyderman R (eds): Inflammation: Basic principles and clinical correlates. New York, Raven Press, 1988, pp 577–597.

80. Herberman RB: Lymphocytes: Cytotoxic activities. *In* Gallin JI, Goldstein IM, and Snyderman R (eds): Inflammation: Basic Principles and Clinical Correlates. New York, Raven Press, 1988, pp 615–617.

81. Robins SL and Cotran RS: Inflammation and repair. *In* Pathologic Basis of Disease. Philadelphia, WB Saunders, 1979, pp 269–270.

82. Harris ED: Pathogenesis of rheumatoid arthritis: A disorder associated with dysfunctional immunoregulation. *In* Gallin JI, Goldstein IM, and Snyderman R (eds): Inflammation: Basic Principles and Clinical Correlates. New York, Raven Press, 1988, p 764.

83. Rugstad HE: The Norway study: Plasma concentrations, efficacy, and adverse events. Am J Med 81(Suppl 5B):11–14, 1986.

84. Abramson SB and Weissmann G: The mechanisms of action of nonsteroidal anti-inflammatory drugs. Arthritis Rheum 32:1–9, 1989.

85. Utsinger PD and Katz WA: Rheumatoid arthritis: Diagnosis. *In* Katz WA (ed): Diagnosis and Management of Rheumatic Diseases, 2nd ed. Philadelphia, JB Lippincott, 1988, pp 345–348.

86. Rothenberg RJ and Sufit RL: Drug-induced peripheral neuropathy in a patient with psoriatic arthritis. Arthritis Rheum 30:221–224, 1987.

87. Brahn E, Helfgott SM, Belli JA, et al: Total lymphoid irradiation therapy in refractory rheumatoid arthritis: Fifteen- to forty-month followup. Arthritis Rheum 27:481–488, 1984.

88. Hanly JG, Hassan J, Moriarty M, et al: Lymphoid irradiation in intractable rheumatoid arthritis. Arthritis Rheum 29:16–25, 1986.

89. Paulus HE, Machleder HI, Levine S, et al: Lymphocyte involvement in rheumatoid arthritis. Arthritis Rheum 20:1249–1262, 1977.

90. Hemler ME, Glass D, Coblyn JS, et al: Very late activation antigens on rheumatoid synovial fluid T lymphocytes. J Clin Invest 78:696–702, 1986.

91. Burkhardt H, Schwingel M, Menninger H, et al: Oxygen radicals as effectors of cartilage destruction. Arthritis Rheum 29:379–386, 1986.

92. Malone DG, Wilder RL, Saavedra-Delgado AM, et al: Mast cell numbers in rheumatoid synovial tissues. Arthritis Rheum 30:130–137, 1987.

93. Wasserman SI: The mast cell and synovial inflammation. Arthritis Rheum 28:841–844, 1984.

94. Carnemolla B, Cutolo M, Castallani P, et al: Characterization of synovial fluid fibronectin from patients with rheumatic inflammatory diseases and healthy subjects. Arthritis Rheum 27:913–921, 1984.

95. Stecher VJ, Kaplan JE, Connolly K, et al: Fibronectin in acute and chronic inflammation. Arthritis Rheum 29:394–399, 1986.

96. Van de Putte LBA, Hegt VN, and Overbeek TE: Activators and inhibitors of fibrinolysis in rheumatoid and nonrheumatoid synovial membranes. Arthritis Rheum 20:671–678, 1977.

CHAPTER 4

Advances in Wound Healing

Michael S. Weingarten, M.D.

The evaluation and treatment of wounds have undergone many changes in the past few years. Wound-healing techniques in the past relied on passive attempts at altering the wound-healing environment. With more recent advances in molecular biology, various stages of wound repair and the factors that promote or interfere with healing have been understood on a molecular level. This knowledge has allowed clinicians to manipulate these factors to actively promote wound repair. This chapter attempts to summarize current understanding of the molecular basis of normal wound healing and how different pathologic conditions interfere with these processes. The chapter concludes with a summary of active and passive approaches to the care of nonhealing wounds.

NORMAL WOUND HEALING

The healing of wounds after injury is a continuous process involving the interaction of multiple cell types and the equilibration of many biochemical processes. To characterize and study wound healing more precisely, the wound-healing process is divided into different phases: substrate, proliferative, and remodeling.[1] These arbitrary divisions of linear events describe different aspects of wound healing.

Substrate Phase

The substrate phase, also referred to as the *inflammatory phase,* predominates during the first 3 or 4 days after wounding. During this phase, cellular and other interactions take place and prepare the wound for subsequent stages.

The initial event in any injury is the damage to blood vessels in the wound. Hemostasis is obtained partly by active vasoconstriction of the smooth muscle cells of the injured vessels. Vasoconstriction initially results from circulating catecholamine and is prolonged by serotonin, released by mast cells and platelets at the site of injury.[2] More important, agents released by platelets produce local vasoconstriction at the site of injury. This release is triggered by platelet adhesion and activation. Platelets adhere to the injured blood vessel walls and are activated. Platelet adhesion depends on the exposure of platelets to collagen types IV and V, found in the subendothelium of the damaged vessels. Specific receptor sites on the platelet membrane, in conjunction with von Willebrand factors, allow the platelet to bind to the

exposed collagen. Adherent platelets release a variety of products from both α granules and dense granules contained within the platelet itself, a process called *degranulation.* These products include adenosine diphosphate (ADP), thromboxane A_2 (TXA$_2$), and platelet-activating factor (PAF); they stimulate further platelet aggregation and activation. Serotonin and calcium are also released during platelet degranulation. Along with TXA$_2$ and ADP, they produce continued vasoconstriction of the injured blood vessels. Additional von Willebrand factor is released and permits continued platelet binding to the injured tissue. Various growth factors, including platelet-derived growth factor (PDGF) and transforming growth factors α and β (TGF-α and TGF-β), are also released from activated platelets in anticipation of new tissue formation.[3]

Activated platelets bind clotting factor V on their surface membrane and then interact with and activate clotting factor X in the blood. Clotting factor XII, Hageman factor, is also activated in areas of tissue injury. Activated factor XII is the first step in the intrinsic clotting system and leads to activation of factor X. Factor X is also activated as the end result of the extrinsic clotting system. This system is stimulated by lipoproteins and calcium released at the site of injury.[4] Activated factor X leads to increasing production of thrombin through activation of prothrombin. Thrombin directly activates more platelets and catalyzes the formation of fibrin monomers from fibrinogen. Fibrin monomers polymerize and form a mesh with the aggregated platelets. Red blood cells are trapped in the mesh, and a stable clot is formed.[5] This entire sequence of events is counterbalanced by mediators produced by or bound to the intact vascular endothelium. Prostacyclin made by endothelial cells inhibits platelet aggregation and causes vasodilatation of the blood vessels. Protein C, bound to the endothelial cell surface, is activated and degrades clotting factors V and VIII. Thrombin is also degraded by surface-bound inactivators.[3]

At the same time hemostasis is being achieved, leukocytes are emigrating into the area of injury. Three types of blood-borne leukocytes are neutrophils, monocytes, and lymphocytes. Blood-borne neutrophils first adhere to the capillary endothelium in the area of the wound. The neutrophils then migrate between the endothelial cells and enter the site of injury, where they are activated. This complex series of events is controlled by various mediators, directly or indirectly produced by platelets, endothelial cells, and the leukocytes themselves.[6] Neutrophil adhesion is stimulated by

PAF, interleukin-1 (IL-1), and tumor necrosis factor (TNF), produced by the endothelial cells. C3a and C5a, proteins produced by activation of the complement cascade at the site of injury, increase neutrophil adherence. Other leukocyte chemoattractants include PDGF and platelet factor IV. Serotonin, histamine, and bradykinin are released from activated platelets. Along with vasoactive agents and enzymes from the neutrophils, they facilitate passage of the neutrophils through the endothelial cells into the wound.

The main function of the neutrophil is to clear the wound of bacteria and foreign debris. Neutrophils accomplish this using both intracellular and extracellular mechanisms. Hydrogen peroxide generated by enzyme systems in the neutrophil cell membrane and the cytoplasm interact with myeloperoxidase and chloride to form hypochlorous acid, a potent bactericidal agent. The hydroxyl radical ($\cdot$OH), also formed as a product of oxygen metabolism in the neutrophil, has bactericidal activity. These oxidants may be released into the extracellular fluid or into the phagosome within the neutrophil.[7]

Neutrophils also produce a variety of antimicrobial proteins that kill bacteria independent of oxygen metabolites. Collagenase and elastase are also released by the neutrophil into the extracellular space during degranulation.[8] Although they effectively clean the wound of bacteria and necrotic tissue, neutrophils contribute little to wound healing. Wounds heal normally in neutropenic animals.[9]

Monocytes are the most important of the leukocytes migrating from the blood into the wound site. Monocytes enter the wound and are transformed into macrophages.[10] Monocytes are attracted to the wound by a number of chemotactic agents present in the wound site at low concentration. One of the most important of these is TGF-β, produced by platelets, neutrophils, other monocytes, and lymphocytes. TGF-β also activates monocytes in higher concentrations.[8] Macrophages continue such work of neutrophils as removal of bacteria and necrotic debris. This continues for weeks after injury, long after the neutrophils have died.[11]

The main function of the macrophage is the release of biologic mediators that regulate the actions of other inflammatory cells and the wound-healing process. These factors are termed *monokines* and include IL-1 tumor necrosis factor–α/cachectin (TNF-α), TGF-α and TGF-β, a PDGF-like substance, and several colony-stimulating factors.[12]

Both TNF and IL-1 have different effects on various cells present in the wound.[12] Both interact with endothelial cells and may be regulators of angiogenesis at the earliest stages of wound healing. IL-1 induces synthesis of a PDGF-like molecule by fibroblasts. This in turn stimulates collagen synthesis. Under different circumstances IL-1, as well as TNF, inhibits collagen synthesis. Other monokines produced by macrophages attract fibroblasts and stimulate their proliferation.[13] Monocyte-macrophages are vital to wound healing. Animals depleted of monocytes do not heal wounds normally.[14]

Only recently has the importance of lymphocytes in wound healing been appreciated. T lymphocytes migrate into the wound at the same time as macrophages.[15] These lymphocytes make a number of secretory products called *lymphokines.* Certain lymphokines regulate fibroblastic migration, proliferation, and collagen synthesis. Other lymphokines affect macrophage as well as endothelial cell activity.

A number of lymphokines have been identified, including interferon-γ TGF-β, fibroblast-activating factor, and IL-2 through IL-8. Two different types of T lymphocytes may be involved at this stage—a T-helper and a T-suppressor population. The regulation of early wound healing may be due to a balance between the effects of these two lymphocyte subgroups and the lymphokines that they produce.[13]

The appearance of fibroblasts in the wound is another important step in the substrate phase. In uninjured tissue, fibroblasts are found in an inactivated state scattered throughout the connective tissue matrix. The sequence of events set off by tissue injury (outlined earlier) results in the appearance of powerful chemotactic agents that attract fibroblasts. PDGF released from the α granules of activated platelets, as well as a PDGF-like substance produced by activated macrophages, induces the migration of fibroblasts into the wound and their subsequent proliferation. Collagen fragments and fibrin-related peptides, products of the inflammatory response, also stimulate fibroblast migration. It has been hypothesized that new fibroblasts may be recruited from smooth muscle cells near the wound.[1]

The stimulation of fibroblast proliferation by PDGF appears to be only an initial step. Progression of deoxyribonucleic acid (DNA) synthesis within the cell, with subsequent cell division, depends on other growth factors in the wound. Epidermal growth factor (EGF) is found in a variety of tissues.[16] Circulating insulin-like growth factor–1 is made primarily by the liver under the regulation of growth hormone.[17] TGF-β, as discussed earlier, is released from the α granules of activated platelets. All three growth factors, in the presence of PDGF, are involved in fibroblast replication.[18] Epithelial cells, also called *keratinocytes,* are found in the epidermal compartment of the wound. Keratinocytes have been found to produce a variety of soluble factors that induce fibroblast activation and proliferation in the dermal compartment.[16]

Other cytokines inhibit fibroblast proliferation and are vital in regulating the wound-healing process. These include TNF-α, produced primarily from macrophages, and interferon-β, produced in part by the fibroblasts themselves. The effect of these cytokines on the fibroblast may change according to the circumstances. TGF, while a growth stimulator of fibroblasts, may also inhibit fibroblastic proliferation under certain conditions.[19]

Proliferative Phase

The proliferative phase begins within 2 days of the initial injury and lasts up to 3 weeks in wounds healing by primary intention. The processes taking place during this stage focus on filling the wound with new tissue.[20] The cells and material necessary to complete the proliferative phase have been assembled at the wound site through a complex series of interactions taking place in the substrate phase, described earlier. The principal activities taking place during the proliferative stage include epidermal regeneration, neoangiogenesis, collagen synthesis, and wound contraction. Key participants in this phase of wound healing include the fibroblasts recruited to the wound, the epithelial cells around the wound, endothelial cells in capillaries at the wound's edge, and the all-important macrophage. Collagen, produced by the fibroblast, is the principal structural protein of the dermal tissue; collagen accounts for approximately 70% of the dry weight of the skin.[21]

Epidermal Regeneration. The epidermal layer covering the mammalian body consists of a multilayered stratified columnar epithelium. This outer layer is vital to the survival of the organism because it provides protection against physical trauma, electromagnetic radiation, fluid loss or gain, and invasion of toxic chemicals or bacteria.[22] Temperature regulation in mammals is based on changes in blood flow to this layer. The basement membrane of the epidermal layer provides structural support and attaches the epidermis to the underlying dermis. The actual attachment of the epidermis to the dermis depends on anchoring fibrils in the basement membrane binding to collagen fibrils in the extracellular matrix of the dermis.[23] The proteins involved in this binding are type IV collagen and laminin.[24]

Injury to the epidermis exposes the underlying dermis to the environment. Fluid loss, heat loss, and bacterial invasion can occur through the wound. The initial stage in the response to injury is clot formation, which provides a temporary protective barrier over the wound. Epidermal cells soon begin to migrate either from the periphery of the wound or from residual epidermal structures in the wound itself.

Early wound coverage is accomplished through migration rather than by replication of the epidermal cells.[25] The initiator of epidermal cell movement is unknown. Epidermal cell migration is supported by a number of substances contained within the wound itself. Two of the most important of these substances are the glycoproteins fibronectin and vitronectin. Fibronectin is made by fibroblasts, macrophages, hepatocytes, and keratinocytes.[26] Control of fibronectin synthesis involves the interaction of these cells with EGF, found in the serum, and TGF-β, released from activated platelets and macrophages. Vitronectin is found in the serum and is present in the ground substance of the wound.[27] In the normal skin, as mentioned earlier, the epidermal attachment to the dermis depends on the adhesive properties of type IV collagen and laminin. In wounds in which the basement membrane is damaged and these proteins are no longer available, a provisional matrix of fibronectin and vitronectin provides adhesion.[28] This adhesive property is dependent on receptors on the cell membranes of the epidermal cells interacting with specific amino acid sequences in the fibronectin-vibronectin molecule.[26] Fibronectin also adheres to fibrin, collagen, and other fibronectin molecules. Cross-linkages between fibronectin molecules further strengthen this matrix.

Keratinocytes in or at the periphery of the wound attach to this extracellular matrix via fibronectin receptors. Once attached, the keratinocytes begin to migrate over the wound and use the initial attachment point for traction. The epithelial cells also migrate along the fibronectin matrix as it covers the de-epithelialized surface. Epithelial cells actually pull themselves along this matrix by using contractile proteins in their cytoplasm (actin filaments). These actin filaments are linked to the fibronectin matrix through the epithelial cell membrane fibronectin receptor.[29]

Migration occurs over viable tissue at an optimal rate of 12 to 21 μm/hr (2 to 3 cell diameters/hr). The rate of migration is directly proportional to the oxygen tension of the tissues and increases under hyperbaric conditions.[30] Epithelial cell migration requires a moist environment and may occur under crusts.[11] Injury may change the normal electrical voltage found across skin. Changing voltage gradients may affect epithelial migration rates.[31] Electric current applied to the skin surrounding superficial wounds in pigs has been shown to increase the rate of epithelialization.[32]

Epithelial cell proliferation begins 1 to 2 days after migration. Epithelial cell division does not begin at the edge of the migrating sheet of epithelial cells.[23] Proliferation begins at the original edge of the wound or within the wound itself in such residual skin appendages as hair follicles. Epithelial cell proliferation is influenced by a number of different substances in the wound, including fibroblastic growth factor (FGF), calcium, EGF, keratinocyte growth factor, PDGF, IL-1, TGF-α, and TGF-β.

Both new and migrating epidermal cells begin to produce fibronectin, laminin, and type IV collagen. The fibronectin facilitates further epidermal cell migration, whereas the laminin and type IV collagen form the new basement membrane. The new basement membrane is formed from the margins of the wound inward. The new epidermis is bound to the dermis, fibrinectin receptors diminish, and the epidermal cells revert back to their normal state.[33]

Neoangiogenesis. If a wound is to heal, blood flow and, therefore, oxygen and nutrient delivery must be restored quickly. The process of neoangiogenesis begins within 24 hours of injury and involves endothelial cell migration and proliferation from blood vessels at the wound's edge.[34] The proliferation and migration of endothelial cells in humans normally occur over decades. Exceptions to this include embryologic development, ovulation, menstruation, inflammation, and wound healing.

Various stimuli are present in injured tissue; they trigger a chain of events leading to new blood vessel formation. Two types of angiogenic factors have been isolated. The direct angiogenic factors stimulate endothelial cell migration and proliferation. Indirect angiogenic factors have no direct effect on the endothelial cell in vitro but seem to affect angiogenesis by regulating other cell types. This process in turn releases direct angiogenic factors.[35]

Angiogenic factors released by macrophages in areas of hypoxia trigger angiogenesis. If the macrophage is made anoxic or if the medium is fully oxygenated, these factors are not produced.[36] Lactic acid may also stimulate angiogenesis factor release.[37] Direct-acting angiogenic factors, produced by macrophages, include TNF-α, FGF, and other partially identified factors that stimulate endothelial cell migration such as angiotropin.[38] PDGF released by platelet α granules stimulates both angiogenesis and growth of vascular smooth muscle cells.[39] Platelets also produce indirect angiogenic factors. Platelet-derived TGF-β attracts monocytes and macrophages to the wound. Other indirect platelet angiogenic factors act on basement membranes to release direct angiogenic factors.[40] Finally, a number of angiogenic factors have been isolated in the extracellular matrix. These are found in deposits bound to the matrix and are released at the time of tissue injury. FGF is bound to heparin molecules in the basement membrane and is released by heparin-degrading enzymes at the time of injury. TGF-α is a potent direct angiogenic factor secreted by tumor cells. This factor may play a role in wound healing as well.[35]

As a result of the stimulation by these angiogenic factors, new capillary formation begins with outgrowths from venules at the wound edge.[35] Endothelial cells in these venules produce enzymes referred to as *metalloproteinases*,[41] which degrade the venule basement membrane on the side of the angiogenic stimulus. Within 24 hours, these endothelial cells migrate out of the venule toward the source of the angiogenic factors. Migration may be facilitated by the fibronectin matrix previously laid down.[26] Other endothelial cells follow and form tubular lumina by subsequent division. These eventually connect with other sprouting lumina to form new capillaries. New basement membranes form, and maturation of the new capillaries takes place.[42] As blood flow is restored to the wound, the hypoxic stimulus to angiogenic factor release decreases. Angiogenesis is also slowed by the release of metalloproteinase inhibitors.[41]

Collagen Synthesis. Collagen is the most common protein found in extracellular tissue and is responsible for maintaining the structure of the organism.[43] On a molecular level, collagen consists of chains of amino acids arranged in a triple helix. The amino acid sequence in the chains is arranged in triplets, with glycine located at the first position of each triplet. The production of collagen begins in the rough endoplasmic reticulum (RER) with the release of procollagen.[44] Modification of the procollagen leads to the formation of the triple helix. The procollagen is then transported to the cell membrane via the Golgi apparatus and released into the extracellular space. Proteolytic enzymes convert the procollagen to collagen monomers. The collagen monomers then self-assemble into collagen. Cross-linkage stabilizes the collagen and gives these fibrils tremendous tensile strength and insolubility.[45] This ability of collagen to self-assemble into extracellular aggregates and to provide supporting structure is one of the distinctive features of collagen.

Thirteen different collagen types, composed of as many as 25 unique polypeptide chains, have been discovered.[43] Research in wound care to date largely has been focused on collagen types I through V.

The regulation of collagen synthesis by the fibroblast occurs at a number of levels. Monokines released by macrophages act on fibroblasts to regulate collagen synthesis at the level of gene expression. TGF-β, insulin-like growth hormone, TNF-α, and IL-1 all act to modulate collagen synthesis.[44] Ascorbic acid stimulates collagen production and is a cofactor for many steps in collagen metabolism.[46]

Collagen synthesis is also dependent on the amount of oxygen in the wound. Oxygen is incorporated directly into the collagen peptide chain during the process of proline hydroxylation. Proline hydroxylation is a critical rate-limiting step in the formation of the collagen molecule and is required if the triple helix is to remain stable. Collagen accumulation increases in wounds as the arterial P_{O_2} rises. Collagen synthesis is impaired in wounds with a mean oxygen tension of less than 20 mm Hg.[47] Clinically, tensile strength of bowel anastomoses in rabbits has been found to correlate with oxygen tension in the perianastomotic tissue.[48]

Lactate levels in wounded tissue also affect collagen synthesis. Lactate levels tend to increase in wounded tissue both as a result of wound hypoxia and as a normal product of wound macrophages.[47] Rising lactate levels result in an increase in collagen synthesis in the early hypoxic stage of wound healing and after oxygen is resupplied.[49]

The continued synthesis of collagen depends on a stable supply of nutrients to the wound. A lack of critical nutrients such as glucose may depress collagen production.[48]

In addition to collagen, fibroblasts produce the "ground substance" of the wound, the proteoglycans.[1] The proteoglycans consist of large polysaccharides made of repeating disaccharide units attached to a protein moiety. Included in the proteoglycans are hyaluronic acid, chondroitin sulfate, heparan sulfate, and keratan sulfate. The proteoglycans are found both intracellularly and extracellularly. They act as adhesive agents, as a transport medium for proteins, and as structural supports. Proteoglycans also bind salt and water and therefore control the microenvironment of the wound.[50] Hyaluronic acid, found in the wound in the first 4 to 5 days after injury, stimulates fibroblast proliferation and migration.[51]

Wound Contraction. Wound contraction begins in the proliferative phase of healing within 7 to 14 days of injury.[11] Wound coverage restores the barrier to infection and fluid and heat loss. The effects of contraction in scar tissue, however, can be extremely deforming and lead to cosmetic and functional problems.[52]

Many theories have been proposed to account for wound contraction.[53–56] One theory proposes that wound contraction occurs as a result of specialized myofibroblasts or fibroblasts interacting with collagen. Myofibroblasts, first found in healing wounds in electron-microscopy studies, share characteristics of both fibroblasts and smooth muscle cells.[53] These cells contain microfilaments similar to the actin and myosin filaments found in smooth muscle. In early stages of wound healing, these filaments lie within the cytoplasm parallel to the long axis of the cell. As contraction proceeds, the bundles increase in size and extend to the cell membrane.[54] Specialized structures in the myofibroblast allow these cells to interconnect with neighboring cells. These connections and the presence of contractile fibers in the cells allow the myofibroblasts to generate isometric contractile forces as a multicellular unit.[55] The observation that contracture may occur in the absence of myofibroblasts has led many to question this theory.[56] Another theory accounts for wound contraction as a result of the movement of individual fibroblasts in the wound matrix, thus producing isotonic tension.

Clinically, wound contraction may actually occur as a result of both individual fibroblast movement and myofibroblast interaction.[56] Isotonic forces may be sufficient to close some wounds. In wounds in which the normal elastic tissue at the wound edge tends to pull the edges apart, isometric forces may be necessary to achieve contracture.

Wound contraction is regulated by both fibronectin and growth factors. Fibronectin, as discussed earlier, is vital as a provisional matrix for fibroblasts. Fibronectin also may serve as the link between the intracellular actin filaments of the myofibroblasts and the extracellular collagen fibrils, creating a contractile unit called a *fibronexus*.[57] Studies have suggested that fibronectin itself may stimulate wound contraction.[56] The effect of two growth factors, TGF-β and PDGF, on myofibroblasts and granulation tissue has been studied in an animal model.[58] Application of these growth factors resulted in more granulation tissue and smaller numbers of myofibroblasts in the treated wounds than in the controls. These two factors act to inhibit fibroblasts directly or through stimulation of granulation tissue. Infection and necrotic tissue impede wound contraction.

Unwanted wound contraction may be completely inhibited by full-thickness skin grafts containing the upper dermis and partially inhibited by split-thickness skin grafts.[59] Active range-of-motion exercises may stretch the contracting wound and result in collagen remodeling. Pressure applied to contracting scar tissue may slow the process, possibly by decreasing scar tissue hypoxia.[60]

Remodeling Phase

The remodeling phase of wound repair begins approximately 3 weeks after injury. The remodeling phase is a dynamic process involving synthesis and cross-linkage of new collagen and breakdown of existing collagen fibrils. The process proceeds rapidly for the first 4 months after injury but continues at a slower rate for as long as 1 or 2 years.[61]

The degradation of older collagen is accomplished by various collagenases produced by fibroblasts and macrophages in the wound.[62] These enzymes are collectively part of the metalloproteases, a family of extracellular enzymes capable of degrading connective tissue.[41] Collagenases require calcium and zinc to function. These enzymes are inhibited by extremely small levels of glucocorticoids, levels well below those known to effect protein synthesis.[63] Growth factors have a number of effects on these enzymes.[64] PDGF stimulates procollagenase synthesis by fibroblasts. TGF-β and EGF inhibit procollagenase synthesis and thereby increase collagen deposition.[62] Collagenase production is also stimulated by IL-1. Finally, the same cells that produce the collagenases, the fibroblasts, also make inhibitors of the collagenases. These are called tissue inhibitors of metalloproteins (TIMPs).[65] At critical concentrations these inhibitors bind to the collagenase molecule and completely block its activity. The result is the regulation of collagen formation and breakdown in specific areas.[62]

As a result of this continued process of collagen synthesis and breakdown, the composition of a healing wound changes over time. Type III collagen appears within 24 to 48 hours after injury in children.[66] Type I collagen is synthesized by more mature fibroblasts and is associated with fiber-rich scar tissue.[67] The appearance of type V collagen seems to parallel the development of capillaries, whereas type IV collagen is associated with the rebuilding of the basement membrane attaching the reformed epidermal layer to the dermis.[43] Also involved in this attachment is type VII collagen containing the anchoring fibrils.

An increase in wound strength is the final result of this remodeling process. Determinants of wound strength include the type and amount of collagen, the degree of cross-linkage of the collagen molecules, and the balance between synthesis and degradation.[34]

Changes in the ground substance—the proteoglycans—also occur in the mature wound and contribute to tensile strength by their intrinsic binding properties, as well as their control of tissue salt and water content.[68] Wound tensile strength continues to increase for years after the injury but never regains the strength of uninjured tissue.[61]

DISEASE STATES PREDISPOSING TO CHRONIC WOUNDS

A number of diseases commonly predispose the patient to the development of chronic wounds. Patients with diseases such as diabetes mellitus, chronic venous disease, connective tissue disorders, and cancer constitute the majority of patients presenting to centers caring for nonhealing wounds.

Diabetes Mellitus

The far-reaching effects of diabetes predispose the patient with diabetes to injury, subsequent infection, and delayed healing. Patients with diabetes develop atherosclerosis at a younger age than do nondiabetic patients.[69] Morphologically, atherosclerosis in the patient with diabetes is the same as in the nondiabetic patient; however, the distribution of the occlusive lesions differs. The infrapopliteal arteries are more often involved in diabetes; total occlusion of two of the three tibial vessels is often seen. Patients with diabetes also develop neuropathy. About 12% of patients with diabetes have clinical neuropathy at the time of the diagnosis of their diabetes. The incidence of neuropathy increases with the duration of the diabetes, with 50% of patients developing neuropathy after 25 years.[70] Diabetic neuropathy affects sensory, motor, and autonomic innervation throughout the body but is most dangerous to the patient when the feet are involved.[71] Abnormalities in the autonomic nervous system of the foot lead to a decrease in perspiration with resultant scaling of the skin. This allows a portal of entry for bacteria. Loss of sympathetic nerve regulation leads to an increase in blood flow in the foot. This has been implicated as a cause of bone absorption in the diabetic foot, leading to Charcot's joint.[72] Motor nerve dysfunction produces changes in gait and, therefore, the development of new pressure points. Sensory nerve loss leaves the diabetic foot insensate. With the loss of sensation as a protective mechanism, even minor mechanical trauma can produce major injuries.[73] Finally, patients with diabetes suffer from multiple disorders in their host-defense mechanisms. Defects in cell-mediated immunity, neutrophil chemotaxis and phagocytosis, serum opsonic activity, as well as lymphocyte function, all have been described.[74]

The combination of ischemia, neuropathy, and an increased vulnerability to bacterial infection leads to the development of chronic, deep ulcers in the diabetic foot. Healing of these wounds is extremely difficult because of the same conditions that predisposed the patient to injury. In addition, many of the processes involved in wound healing are impaired in diabetes.[75] Macrophage function and fibroblast synthesis of collagen seem to be impaired to varying degrees in diabetes. Collagen, exposed to high levels of glucose, may undergo nonenzymatic glycation, leading to abnormal changes in the wound matrix. Limb loss is often the result; an estimated 10,000 lower extremity amputations are performed each year for diabetic gangrene.[69]

Chronic Venous Insufficiency

Chronic ulceration due to venous disease is extremely common in the United States. It is estimated that 27% of the population has venous disease, that 1.5% has or has had ulceration, and that one third of these patients are unable to work because of this problem.[76] The ulcers associated with venous disease are usually found in the gaiter region of the leg, the area extending from the malleoli to the level of the lower edge of the gastrocnemius muscle.[77] Venous ulcers have also been described by both this author and others as occurring on the upper calf and the foot. The skin surrounding a venous ulcer is thickened, fibrotic, and usually stained with hemosiderin. The term *lipodermatosclerosis* has been applied to this tissue.

Venous ulceration appears to result from failure of the calf muscle pump to lower venous pressure in the leg during exercise.[78] At rest, dorsal foot vein pressure is 80 to 100 mm Hg. During exercise in the patient without venous disease,

   57

the pumping action of the calf muscles lowers this pressure to 0 to 20 mm Hg, the normal ambulatory venous pressure (AVP). At the completion of exercise, with the subject standing still, dorsal foot vein pressure returns to the baseline value slowly, usually over 20 seconds or more. In patients with venous insufficiency, there is little change in the ambulatory venous pressure with exercise. The return to baseline of the dorsal foot vein pressure at the end of exercise occurs in less than 20 seconds.[79]

The cause of calf pump failure in most of patients with venous ulcers is usually unknown.[79] Deep venous thrombosis leading to valvular insufficiency, the postphlebitic syndrome, can be documented in only 22% of patients.[76] Venous valvular incompetence, leading to venous reflux, may occur as a result of aging, a genetic defect in the veins, or subclinical episodes of deep venous thrombosis. Chronic venous thrombosis, leading to partial occlusion of the venous outflow tract, has also been postulated. In 403 limbs with venous ulcers or venous insufficiency examined by this author using duplex scanning, only four limbs (3.6%) had evidence of chronic deep venous obstruction.[80] Venous reflux in multiple venous segments in both the superficial and deep systems was associated with venous ulceration in this study. Reflux time in the common femoral vein, as determined by spectral analysis, correlated with the duration of the venous ulcer and the ulcer area. In this study, only 18 limbs with venous ulcers were found to have venous reflux isolated to the superficial system, a finding confirmed by others.[76]

Although there is uniform agreement that chronic venous insufficiency leads to venous ulcers, there is no agreement about the exact mechanism of ulcer formation. Three theories have been postulated. The arteriovenous shunting theory proposes that as a result of elevated venous pressure, arteriovenous fistulae in the dermis open up and divert blood away from the skin.[81] The ''fibrin cuff'' theory was first proposed by Browse in 1982.[82] It has been postulated that the failure of venous pressure to drop with exercise leads to an elevation of capillary pressures in the dermis. This causes an increase in the loss of plasma proteins through the capillary walls. Fibrinogen, the most abundant of these proteins in venous insufficiency, polymerizes around the capillary and forms a fibrin cuff, which interferes with oxygen diffusion to the skin.[83]

The latest theory of venous ulcer formation has been termed the *white blood cell trapping theory*.[84] White blood cells are much larger than red blood cells and on entering a capillary bed take 1000 times longer to deform. In areas of elevated capillary pressures and reduction in flow rates, white blood cells entering the capillary lumen lead to its occlusion. These cells, once in contact with the capillary endothelium, are activated. Activated macrophages and polymorphonuclear leukocytes release proteolytic enzymes, free oxide radicals, and cytokines such as IL-1 and TNF-α. This sets up a low-grade inflammatory response, which leads to the eventual destruction of the tissues around the capillary bed.

Although pure venous disease rarely leads to limb loss, the prevalence of this problem and the cost to the patient and society in lost time and wages have stimulated interest in the cause and treatment of this condition.

Inherited Disorders of Wound Healing

Various genetic disorders lead to an inability of the patient to make normal components necessary for healing.[79] These patients are more vulnerable to injury and may develop chronic ulcers. Patients with Ehlers-Danlos syndrome have very soft, friable skin. The genetic abnormality in these patients is an inability to make normal collagen. In epidermolysis bullosa, there is an inherited failure of the epidermis, the dermis, and the basement membrane to adhere to one another. Skin breakdown is common. Patients with Marfan's syndrome and osteogenesis imperfecta have inherited abnormalities in collagen maturation and cross-linking. Accelerated atherosclerosis with tissue ischemia occurs in homocystinuria, progeria, and Werner's syndrome.

Malignancy

Carcinoma may arise in chronic wounds, even without predisposing factors such as irradiation. Malignant degeneration has been described in burn scars, after frostbite, in areas of chronic osteomyelitis, and in scars occurring after trauma.[86] The clinician must evaluate each patient presenting with a nonhealing wound. A biopsy of the lesion must be done if there is any question as to the cause of the wound. In approximately 550 patients presenting to the Graduate Hospital Wound Care Center (Philadelphia, PA) over a 12-month period, two squamous cell and two basal cell carcinomas were discovered on biopsy of four patients.[87] Three of the carcinomas were in patients treated elsewhere for venous ulcers; the fourth carcinoma was in a patient with osteomyelitis in a bullet tract through the tibia present for 45 years. Over a 3-year period in which 1700 patients were evaluated, a total of 12 carcinomas were found at this facility. Distant malignancy may interfere with wound healing through the tumor's impact on the nutrition of the patient.[88]

Connective Tissue Disorders

This broad category of disease states includes a wide variety of disorders that affect wound healing in several different ways. The disabling effects of osteoarthritis and rheumatoid arthritis also make these patients more susceptible to injury, especially on weightbearing areas. The vasculitides encompass a variety of autoimmune disorders affecting the arterial and, in some patients, the venous circulation.[89] End-organ ischemia can occur; in the extremities this can lead to digital gangrene. (The inherited disorders of connective tissue were discussed earlier.)

Scleroderma, or systemic sclerosis, is a disorder characterized by inflammation, fibrosis, and vascular occlusion.[90] The pathogenesis of scleroderma may involve imbalances of the same mediators and cell types that participate in wound healing.[91] Scleroderma patients may present with nonhealing ulcers of the digits but can also present with wounds unrelated to the scleroderma, such as venous ulceration.

Hematologic Disorders Leading to Chronic Wounds

A number of hematologic disorders are associated with chronic ulcers. The underlying mechanism is related to an increase in blood viscosity, leading to low flow and thrombosis of small vessels.[92] Thrombosis may occur in the digital arteries of the extremities and may lead to digital ischemia and gangrene. Thrombosis of the cutaneous arteries can result in arterial ulcers of the skin. Involvement of the venous system results in chronic deep venous insufficiency and ulceration. These disorders include the hemoglobinopathies, such as sickle cell disease and thalassemia. A number of serum protein abnormalities may lead to hyperviscosity and vascular occlusion. Included are myeloma, cryoglobulinemia, myeloid metaplasia, and macroglobulinemia.

Lymphedema

Lymphedema may be either primary or acquired.[93] Primary lymphedema may present in the infant, the adolescent, or the adult, although symptoms usually begin between the ages of 5 and 20 years. Fifteen per cent of patients with lymphedema have a familial history of this disorder. Acquired lymphedema may occur after lymphatic surgery or infection. The massive swelling and fibrosis of lymphedema may lead to infection and ulceration. Aggressive compression therapy and elevation are the most important factors in the treatment and prevention of ulceration.

Miscellaneous Conditions

Nonhealing ulcers may be manifestations of other diseases. Pyoderma gangrenosum may be found in association with ulcerative colitis. Nonhealing ulcers are rarely associated with hypertension. Ulcerative necrobiosis lipoidica is usually found in patients with diabetes, but it can also be associated with venous insufficiency or arteritis.[94]

TREATMENT OF NONHEALING WOUNDS

Initial Evaluation

The initial evaluation of a nonhealing wound must start with an examination of the patient as a whole. A complete history, including a thorough review of systems, should be done. The initial cause of the wound and its duration are recorded. Current treatments of the wound, as well as past therapies, are noted. Occupation and daily activities, exercise habits, pain tolerance, and smoking history are recorded.

A physical examination, including a complete vascular examination, is performed. This should include the recording of blood pressures in both arms, auscultation for neck bruits, and recording of the pulses in the femoral, popliteal, posterior tibial, and dorsalis pedis vessels. The abdomen must be palpated for the presence of an abdominal aortic aneurysm. In upper extremity wounds, the presence of axillary, brachial, and radial pulses should be recorded. A complete neurologic examination should also be performed, including a thorough sensory examination using Semmes-Weinstein monofilament threads.[95] In wounds of the lower extremities, particularly the feet, the patient's shoes should also be examined.

Nutrition status should be assessed as part of the initial history and physical as well as through appropriate laboratory tests. A complete cardiac evaluation is mandatory in high-risk groups such as patients with diabetes who have peripheral vascular disease.

Wound evaluation must be done quantitatively. A number of wound-grading scales based on location, depth, and degree of infection have been developed.[96, 97] Each wound should be graded at every visit and a photograph taken. Wound size,

including length, width, depth, and degree of undermining, should be recorded. The efficacy of any particular treatment will be determined by the rate of wound healing. The accurate measure of wound area and volume is critical in assessing the results of different therapies. A number of methods for measuring wounds using planimetry, ultrasonography, direct tracing, and stereophotogrammetry have been developed.[98]

The location and type of the wound often determine the need for further studies. Wounds over bony prominences may extend down to and involve the underlying bone. This is particularly important in weightbearing areas of the diabetic foot. Nonweightbearing and weightbearing plain radiographs of the foot should be performed routinely in patients with foot ulcers. Radiographs may reveal the presence of unsuspected fractures as well as Charcot's changes. Osteomyelitis can also be detected on plain radiographs, but when associated with Charcot's changes may not be clear. The use of radionuclide scans has allowed the clinician to strongly suspect osteomyelitis in previously unsuspected cases or in patients with associated Charcot's bone changes.[99]

Cultures of the wound should be taken to determine the presence of a predominating organism. Open wounds soon become colonized with a mixed flora of bacteria but may not be infected. Cultures of the wound surface may show this colonization and may mislead the clinician. Wound cultures of the deep tissues should be taken at the time of débridement or with percutaneous needle aspiration using sterile technique.[100]

Noninvasive vascular testing is useful in determining the cause of wounds. Arterial insufficiency can be quantified using segmental pressure measurements and pulse-volume recordings.[101, 102] In the patient with diabetes who has calcified, noncompressible vessels, or in the patient with an ankle ulcer, preventing the placement of an ankle cuff, these measurements cannot be performed. Using a small cuff and the pencil continuous-wave Doppler device, a toe pressure can be obtained. Usually the digital arteries of the feet are not severely calcified and can be compressed. A toe/brachial index greater than 0.6 to 0.7 is considered normal.[103] Arterial evaluation is supplemented by the determination of the transcutaneous oxygen ($TcPo_2$) levels at the area of the ulcer.[104] The $TcPo_2$ is determined both at the site of the wound and at the chest wall. An absolute $TcPo_2$ value of 30 mm Hg or a Po_2 index of 0.2 or greater is predictive of healing, if infection and repeated trauma are dealt with. Values less than 0.2 suggest that the wound will not heal unless more oxygen is supplied.

The noninvasive evaluation of chronic venous insufficiency has been simplified by the use of color-assisted duplex scanning. Both anatomic and hemodynamic data can be obtained quickly and with reproducible results. Techniques for detecting and quantifying venous reflux using duplex scanning have also been developed and may assist the surgeon in selecting patients for venous surgery.[105] Volume changes of venous blood in the extremity can also be measured directly by using air plethysmography.[106] This technique provides a noninvasive method of measuring ambulatory venous pressure. $TcPo_2$ determinations of the limbs of patients with venous ulcers reveal areas of hypoxia surrounding the ulcer.[107] Unlike in arterial disease, the $TcPo_2$ levels obtained in venous disease have not proved useful either in classifying venous ulcers or in predicting the response to therapy.

Based on the initial assessment, a determination is made as to the most likely etiology of the nonhealing wound, and treatment is directed accordingly (Fig. 4–1).

Specific Therapies

Débridement of Necrotic Tissue. Aggressive débridement of necrotic and infected tissue is the first step in healing the chronic wound. Necrotic tissue with high bacterial levels interferes with the initial steps in wound healing and may itself lead to more tissue damage. Deep tissue cultures should be taken at the time of biopsy. Often, the definitive diagnosis of osteomyelitis is based on direct biopsy and culture. Wound staging may have to be reassessed after débridement. Because chronic wounds may undergo malignant degeneration, all débrided tissue must be sent for pathologic examination. This is especially important in wounds occurring in old burn scars or in areas of previous irradiation.[86] In patients with arterial insufficiency and wounds that are not suppurative, débridement should be delayed until after arterial reconstruction. Sepsis secondary to wound infection, a problem often seen in patients with diabetes, is a true surgical emergency. Necrotic tissue must be completely removed, and all areas of pus must be drained. In the septic diabetic foot, emergency amputation of parts of the foot, or even emergency guillotine amputation of the entire foot at the malleolar level, may be necessary.[108]

Correction of Arterial Insufficiency. In patients with arterial insufficiency as the basis of the nonhealing wound, vascular reconstruction is necessary to promote healing. A complete angiographic study should be performed of the involved area. In the lower extremity, particularly if foot ulcers are present, visualization of the pedal arch must be a routine part of the arteriogram. Aggressive bypass surgery in the lower extremities, with direct grafting into the pedal vessels, has been successful in perfusing a wound long enough for healing to occur.[109] A combination of distal reconstruction and microvascular free tissue transfer may provide both reperfusion and wound coverage and has also been successful in preventing amputation.[110]

Treatment of Venous Ulceration. The treatment of chronic venous ulceration is approached on two fronts. (Treatment of the ulcer itself is discussed later.) Just as important as ulcer care is the treatment of the underlying chronic venous insufficiency. Conservative therapy for chronic venous insufficiency is based on compression therapy. Graded elastic stockings providing 30 to 40 mm Hg pressure at the ankle are recommended.[111] Below-the-knee stockings are preferred, because patient compliance is better, and correction of the calf pump is considered the key to lowering ambulatory venous pressure. Unna's boots have also been used in treating this condition, but the most important effect of the Unna's boot appears to be compression.[112] Sequential pneumatic compression devices have also been used to treat chronic venous insufficiency. Patients are usually asked to use these devices 3 to 4 hr/day at pressures of 30 to 40 mm Hg. Sequential pumping has been shown to be effective in healing of venous ulcers, but the mechanism of action is not clear.[113] Pumping has been shown to decrease edema, but this has not led to an expected increase in oxygen diffusion to the ulcer.[114] Compression pumping has been found to increase fibrinolytic activity in the venous system and may affect the formation of the fibrin cuff found around capillaries in patients with venous ulcers.[115] Patients wear compression stockings when ambulatory. Elevation of the affected limb is also recommended.

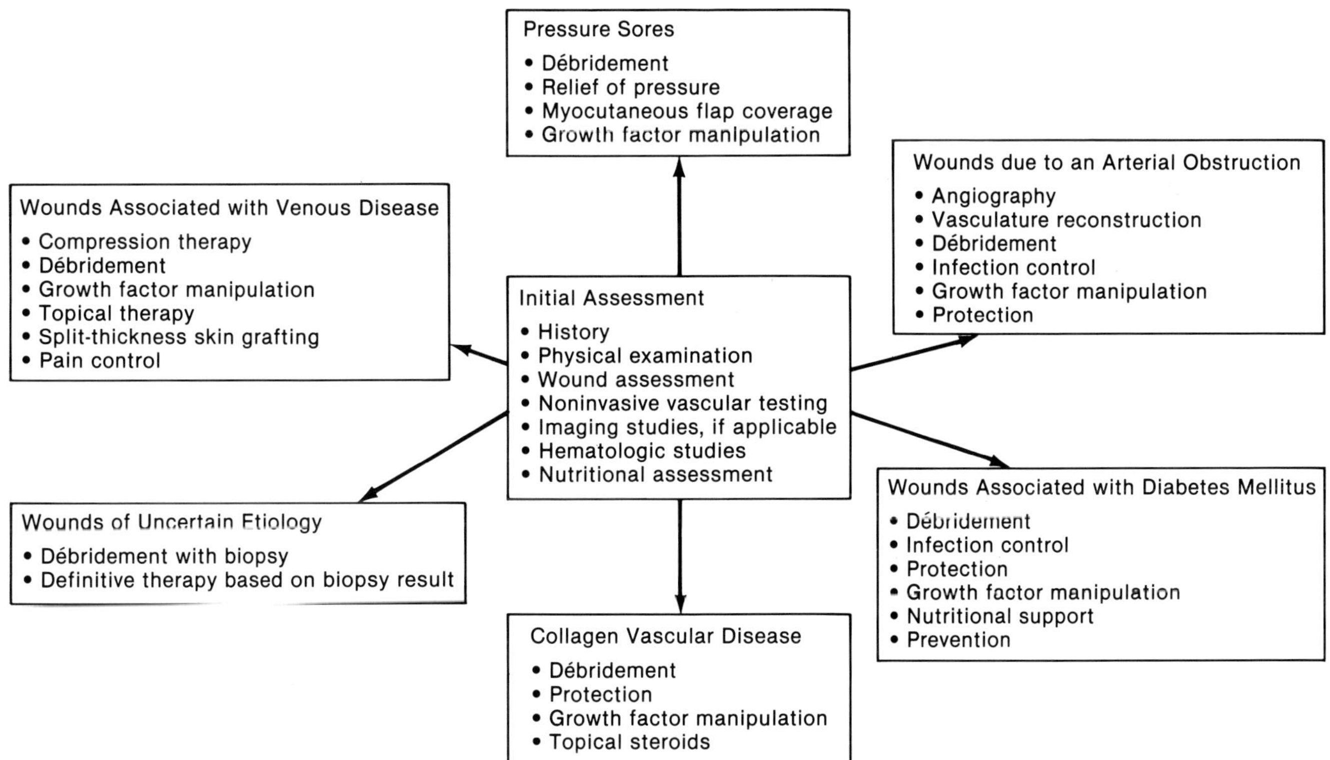

FIGURE 4–1. Algorithm for the evaluation and treatment of chronic wounds.

Pharmacologic treatment of chronic venous ulcers using pentoxifylline (Oxpentifylline) has also been reported with favorable results when compared with placebo.[116] Pentoxifylline has been found to inhibit the effects of TNF-α and IL-1 on neutrophils and therefore to decrease neutrophil adhesion and activation.[117] The drug may be useful in preventing white blood cell trapping in capillaries, with the subsequent release of inflammatory mediators thought to lead to venous ulceration.[78]

Direct Wound Care

The treatment of chronic ulcers can be classified into two broad categories—passive methods and active methods. The passive dressings alter the wound environment through the application of various topical agents such as antiseptics, débriding agents, or moisture. The actual process of wound healing is facilitated but not altered. Active agents are applied to the wound in an attempt to stimulate the wound-healing process directly. These agents may be in the form of cytokines or antibodies to cytokines. The clinical development of these active agents has been possible only with the advances in understanding of the wound-healing process on a cellular level.

Passive Wound-Healing Treatments

Antibacterial and Antiseptic Agents. Bacterial counts in the wound of 100,000/g of tissue or more will delay and possibly prevent wound closure. Wound sepsis usually does not occur until the bacterial count exceeds this level.[118] A number of agents such as silver sulfadiazine, bacitracin zinc, and topical triple antibiotic solution (bacitracin zinc, polymyxin B, and neomycin) have become popular in the care of wounds.[85] Although effective in lowering bacterial counts, these topical antibacterial agents are not a substitute for surgical débridement. Patients placed on these agents should be watched for the development of resistant bacterial strains.

Antiseptic agents such as hydrogen peroxide, povidone-iodine, and chlorhexidine, although toxic to bacteria, also damage leukocytes and interfere with granulation tissue formation.[119] These agents, in addition to Dakin's solution and Hibiclens, also delay epidermal resurfacing.[120] Their main role probably is to physically loosen necrotic tissue, an activity that can be performed just as well with normal saline.

Débriding Agents. Perhaps the most effective débriding agent used in wound care is the wet-to-dry dressing.[85] Saline-moistened gauze applied to a wound will dry, trapping wound exudate in the dressing. On removal of the gauze every 6 to 8 hours, nonviable tissue is removed with the dressing. Topical proteolytic agents have been developed to actively digest necrotic tissue in the ulcer. These topical agents have been found, however, to arrest neutrophil phagocytosis.[121] Long-term use of these agents probably should be avoided.

Wound Dressings. The principal goal of a wound dressing is to provide a moist environment at the surface of the wound with adequate oxygen tension to permit healing.[120] A moist wound environment promotes re-epithelialization. Wounds left open to the air dry out and form a thick eschar. Re-epithelialization is delayed, because the migrating epithelial cells must migrate under the dry crust. In one study, wounds left open to air re-epithelialized in 25 to 30 days, whereas wounds kept in a moist environment took 12 to 15 days to heal.[122] Wounds kept covered in a moist environment are also less painful, perhaps because exposed nerve endings are protected.[118] Autolysis of necrotic tissue is also facilitated by keeping the wound bathed in its own enzyme-containing fluid. Heat loss from a wound is decreased with an occlusive dressing, thereby decreasing the amount of vasoconstriction of the capillary bed supplying the wound. Finally, an occlusive dressing may serve as a barrier to infection, particularly if the wound pH is kept in the 5.8 to 6.6 range.[123] The moist conditions existing under an occlusive dressing may also lead to bacterial growth. Totally occlusive dressings should not be used on infected wounds until proper débridement is performed; they should be used with caution in the patient who is immunocompromised.[118]

Many different types of occlusive dressings are currently available.[124] Hydrocolloids contain hydrophilic colloidal materials such as karaya, gelatin, and pectin. These dressings absorb excess fluid slowly and therefore must be changed frequently in draining wounds. Adhesives incorporated into the dressings allow them to conform to and seal the wound edges. These dressings are useful in areas of constant motion or pressure. Hydrogels are complex lattices of a cross-linked polymer and are composed of 80% to 99% water. A semipermeable membrane over the lattice allows excess moisture to evaporate while preserving wound hydration. These dressings do not adhere to the wound edge and must be held in place by other dressings.

Dressings impregnated with a wide variety of medications thought to promote wound healing are available. The zinc oxide incorporated into the popular Unna's boot dressing is supposed to enhance epithelialization.[118] Dressings are made nonadherent to wound surfaces by impregnating petroleum jelly or paraffin into the gauze, thereby reducing injury to the newly formed epidermal layer.

Absorptive powders, which absorb excess wound drainage, may also be added to dressings. Dextranomer powder (Debrisan) adheres to necrotic tissue and absorbs excess wound fluid.[125] Unfortunately, the beads of dextranomer powder also lead to disruption of the granulating bed if allowed to dry. If left in the wound, these beads tend to form the nidus of granulomas. Thorough removal of the beads after each application is necessary.

Active Wound-Healing Treatments

Oxygen Therapy. As discussed in the review of the stages of wound healing, oxygen plays a vital role in the wound-healing process. A number of approaches have been developed to stimulate wound healing through the use of supplemental oxygen. Topical oxygen has been used to promote epithelialization and suppress superficial infection.[126] Topical oxygen does not penetrate into the wound, however, and should have much the same effect on wound healing as topical antibiotics have on deep infections.[127] Supplemental oxygen given through a nasal cannula to patients with ischemic foot pain or tissue necrosis raises the TcPo$_2$ by 12 mm Hg, suggesting that supplemental inspired oxygen might promote wound healing.[128] The use of hyperbaric oxygen (HBO) in the treatment of certain nonhealing wounds has been the subject of many studies in the last few years. HBO therapy is defined as the treatment of a patient who is entirely enclosed within a pressure vessel and breathing oxygen at a pressure greater than sea level (1 atm absolute).[129] The purpose of HBO as used in wound healing is to deliver blood with a higher oxygen content to tissue beds. This increase in arterial oxygen content is primarily in O_2 dissolved in the plasma. Dissolved oxygen content may reach a high of 6.8 ml/dl of blood with a resultant arterial P_{O_2} of 1900 to 2100 mm Hg at 3 atm of pressure, the highest pressure used clinically in HBO. The oxyhemoglobin dissociation curve is unchanged. Tissue P_{O_2} will generally be less than arterial P_{O_2} owing to increasing arteriolar vasoconstriction, which increases as arterial P_{O_2} rises. Supernormal tissue P_{O_2} levels are reached clinically with HBO.

Higher tissue oxygen pressures may promote wound healing in a number of ways. Oxygen appears to be bactericidal to anaerobic bacteria and bacteriostatic to many aerobes and facultative bacteria. Improvement of tissue oxygen levels in hypoxic wounds may promote phagocytosis of bacteria by white blood cells, which depend on oxygen radicals to kill the bacteria. As reviewed earlier, increasing levels of tissue P_{O_2} stimulate collagen synthesis by fibroblasts. HBO has been shown to induce angiogenesis in previously irradiated tissue.[130]

Based on reports from the Undersea and Hyperbaric Medical Society, the National Blue Cross/Blue Shield Society has approved reimbursement for the use of HBO therapy for only certain conditions.[131] HBO therapy has proved useful in the direct treatment of tissue necrosis in irradiated fields through the stimulation of angiogenesis. Refractory osteomyelitis may respond to HBO. This effect depends on the increase in white blood cell phagocytosis of bacteria as well as the increased activity of osteoclasts, necessary to remove dead bone.[132] HBO may also be helpful as an adjunct to flaps and grafts used to cover an ischemic area such as an irradiated field. HBO may also be used in the treatment of deep wounds of the diabetic foot, but only after proper débridement is performed and arterial inflow problems are corrected.[133]

Electrical Stimulation. The use of electrical stimulation for the healing of bone fractures has been an accepted therapy for many years.[134] It has been suggested that the effect of electrical stimulation on bone is at a cellular level, primarily through alterations in the ionic microenvironment as well as stimulation of DNA synthesis. Nonhealing wounds have also been exposed to a variety of types of electrical stimuli with various results.[135, 136] As in fracture healing, the effect of electrical stimulation on wound healing has been hypothesized to occur at a cellular level.[137] Electrical stimulation of skin tissue has been found to stimulate adenosine triphosphate (ATP) production through its effects on the mitochondrial membrane. Currents applied to tissues may stimulate epidermal, macrophage, and fibroblast migration. These same currents have been found to increase cutaneous circulation, leading to an increase in TcP_{O_2}. Electrical currents have also been reported to be bactericidal.

Ultrasonography and Light. The use of ultrasonography and light in the treatment of nonhealing wounds has been studied. Thermal energy generated by ultrasound beams has been used to treat pain. Ultrasonography in vitro stimulates fibroblastic production of collagen and may have some potential benefits if administered during the proliferative phase of wound healing.[138] Low-energy laser light also affects collagen synthesis by the fibroblast. Anecdotal reports of the acceleration of wound healing with low-intensity laser energy have been published.[139]

Growth Factor Therapy. The use of growth factors to regulate and improve wound healing has been studied intensively in the last few years. TGF-β, PDGF, and PAF have all been found to increase wound-breaking strength in the incisional rat model.[140] EGF has been shown to increase the rate of epithelialization in mice skin defects.[141] In a trial of EGF, applied topically to a variety of types of chronic wounds in nine humans, healing was accomplished in eight.[142] Preparations of growth factors have been extracted from bovine platelets and found to increase the rate of wound healing in humans.[143]

Platelet-derived wound-healing factors (PDWHFs) have been derived from pooled human platelets (homologous PDWHF) as well as from the patient's own platelets (autologous PDWHF).[144] PDWHF has been found to contain at least five active growth factors including PDGF, platelet-derived angiogenesis factor, platelet-derived EGF, TGF-β, and platelet factor-4.[145] A small randomized study involving PDWHF versus placebo applied topically to chronic wounds showed that wound healing was accelerated with PDWHF.[146]

Individual growth factors can now be made using recombinant technology.[147] Recombinant PDGF, used as part of a randomized, placebo-controlled study in humans, was found to increase wound-healing rates significantly.[148] Altering specific stages of the wound-healing cycle has been possible through the control of the levels and activities of individual growth factors. Scar tissue formation in a rat incisional wound model was blocked by injecting neutralizing antibody to TGF-β into the edge of the wound.[149]

Testing Wound Treatments

The complexity of the wound-healing process and the many variables present in any given patient make it difficult to design one wound-healing model to test the effects of these various agents. The efficacy of any one treatment must be demonstrated quantitatively in both in vitro and in vivo models.[150] Research into wound healing in the mammalian fetus provides another model for testing different treatment modalities. In evaluating wound healing clinically in humans, it is imperative that conclusions as to the efficacy of any given treatment be drawn from large randomized prospective trials.[151]

References

1. Hunt TK: Basic principles of wound healing. J Trauma 30(Suppl 12):S122–S128, 1990.
2. Kloth CL and Miller KH: The inflammatory response to wounding. *In* Kloth LC, McCulloch JM, and Feedar JA (eds): Wound Healing: Alternatives in Management. Philadelphia, FA Davis, 1990, pp 3–12.
3. Clark RAF: Cutaneous wound repair: A review with emphasis on integrin receptor expression. *In* Janssen H, Rooman R, and Robertson JIS (eds): Wound Healing. Petersfield, UK, Wrightston Biomedical, 1991, pp 7–17.
4. Bowie EJ and Owen CA: The hemostatic mechanism. *In* Kwaan HC and Bowie EJW (eds): Thrombosis. Philadelphia, WB Saunders, 1982, pp 7–22.
5. Knighton DR, Hunt TK, Thakral KK, et al: Role of platelets and fibrin in the healing sequence. Ann Surg 196:379–388, 1982.
6. Malech HL: Phagocytic cells: Egress from marrow and diapedesis. *In* Gallin JI, Goldstein IM, and Snyderman R (eds): Inflammation: Basic Principles and Clinical Correlates. New York, Raven Press, 1988, pp 297–308.
7. Klebanoff SJ: Phagocytic cells: Products of oxygen metabolism. *In* Gallin JI, Goldstein IM, and Snyderman R (eds): Inflammation: Basic Principles and Clinical Correlates. New York, Raven Press, 1988, pp 391–441.
8. Wahl LM and Wahl SM: Inflammation. *In* Cohen IK, Diegelmann RF, and Lindblad WJ (eds): Wound Healing: Biochemical and Clinical Aspects. Philadelphia, WB Saunders, 1992, pp 40–62.
9. Simpson DM and Ross R: The neutrophilic leukocyte in wound repair: A study with antineutrophilic serum. J Clin Invest 51:2009–2023, 1972.

10. Riches DWH: The multiple roles of macrophages in wound repair. *In* Clark RAF and Henson PM (eds): Molecular and Cellular Biology of Wound Repair. New York, Plenum Press, 1988, pp 213–239.

11. Zitelli J: Wound healing for the clinician. Adv Dermatol 2:243–268, 1987.

12. Rappolee DA, Mark D, Banda MJ, et al: Wound macrophages express TGF and other growth factors in vivo: Analysis of mRNA phenotyping. Science 241:708–711, 1988.

13. Barbul A: Immune aspects of wound repair. Clin Plast Surg 17:433–442, 1990.

14. Leibovich SJ and Ross R: The role of the macrophage in wound repair: A study with hydrocortisone and antimacrophage serum. Am J Pathol 78:71, 1975.

15. Regan MC and Barbul A: Regulation of wound healing by the T cell–dependent immune system. *In* Janssen H, Rooman R, and Robertson JIS (eds): Wound Healing. Petersfield, UK, Wrightson Biomedical, 1991, pp 21–31.

16. Nicolas JF, Gaucherand E, Delaporte E, et al: Wound healing: A result of coordinate keratinocyte-fibroblast interactions. *In* Janssen H, Rooman R, and Robertson JIS (eds): Wound Healing. Petersfield, UK, Wrightson Biomedical, 1991, pp 71–80.

17. Baxter RC: The somatomedins: Insulin-like growth factors. Adv Clin Chem 25:49–115, 1986.

18. Morgan CJ and Pledger J: Fibroblast proliferation. *In* Cohen IK, Diegelmann RF, and Lindblad WJ (eds): Wound Healing: Biochemical and Clinical Aspects. Philadelphia, WB Saunders, 1992, pp 63–76.

19. Gottlieb AB, Khong Chang C, Posnett DN, et al: Detection of transforming growth factor alpha in normal, malignant, and hyperproliferative human keratinocytes. J Exp Med 167:670–675, 1988.

20. Norris S, Provo B, and Stotts NA: Physiology of wound healing and risk factors that impede the healing process. AACN Issues Crit Care Nurs 1:545–552, 1990.

21. Stewart WD, Danto JL, and Maddin S: Dermatology. St. Louis, CV Mosby, 1974.

22. Serafin D: The skin: Functional, metabolic, and surgical considerations. *In* Sabiston DC (ed): Textbook of Surgery. Philadelphia, WB Saunders, 1991, pp 1382–1402.

23. Stenn KS and Malhotra R: Epithelialization. *In* Cohen IK, Diegelmann RF, and Lindblad WJ (eds): Wound Healing: Biochemical and Clinical Aspects. Philadelphia, WB Saunders, 1992, pp 115–127.

24. Woodley DT: Importance of the dermal-epidermal junction and recent advances. Dermatologica 174:1–10, 1987.

25. Marks R and Nishakawa T: Active epidermal movement in human skin in vitro. Br J Dermatol 86:481–490, 1973.

26. Brotchie H and Wakefield D: Fibronectin: Structure, function, and significance in wound healing. Aust J Dermatol 31:47–56, 1990.

27. Suzuki S, Oldberg A, Hayman EV, et al: Complete amino acid sequence of human vitronectin deduced from cDNA: Similarity of cell attachment sites in vitronectin and fibronectin. EMBO J 4:2519–2524, 1984.

28. Grinnell F, Billingham RE, and Burgess L: Distribution of fibronectin during wound healing in vivo. J Invest Dermatol 76:181–189, 1981.

29. Bereiter-Hahn J: Epidermal cell migration and wound repair. *In* Bereiter-Hahn J, Matoltsky AG, and Richards KS (eds): Biology of the Integument. Vol 2: Vertebrates. Berlin, Springer-Verlag, 1986, pp 443–471.

30. Pai MP and Hunt TK: Effect of varying oxygen tension on healing in open wounds. Surg Gynecol Obstet 135:756–757, 1972.

31. Jaffe LF and Vanable JW: Electric fields and wound healing. Clin Dermatol 2:34–44, 1984.

32. Alvarez OM, Mertz PM, Smerbveck RV, et al: The healing of superficial skin wounds is stimulated by external electric current. J Invest Dermatol 81:144–148, 1983.

33. Clark RAF, Lanigan JM, Delle Pelle P, et al: Fibronectin and fibrin provide a provisional matrix for epidermal cell migration during wound epithelialization. J Invest Dermatol 79:264–269, 1982.

34. LaVan FB and Hunt TK: Current concepts in wound healing. Adv Plast Reconstr Surg 7:43–64, 1991.

35. Whalen GF and Zetter BR: Angiogenesis. *In* Cohen IK, Diegelmann RF, and Lindblad WJ (eds): Wound Healing: Biochemical and Clinical Aspects. Philadelphia, WB Saunders, 1992, pp 77–95.

36. Knighton D, Silver IA, and Hunt TK: Regulation of wound healing angiogenesis: Effect of oxygen gradients and inspired oxygen concentration. Surgery 90:262, 1981.

37. Daly TJ: The repair phase of wound healing—re-epithelialization and contraction. *In* Kloth LC, McCulloch JM, and Feedar JA (eds): Wound Healing: Alternatives in Management. Philadelphia, FA Davis, 1990, pp 14–30.

38. Hockel M, Sasse J, and Wissler JH: Purified monocyte-derived angiogenic substance (angiotropin) stimulates migration, phenotypic changes, and tube formation but not proliferation of capillary endothelial cells in vitro. J Cell Physiol 133:1–13, 1987.

39. Ross R, Raines EW, and Bowen-Pope DF: The biology of platelet-derived growth factor. Cell 46:155–169, 1986.

40. Knighton DR, Hunt TK, Thakral KK, et al: Role of platelets and fibrin in the healing sequence: An in vivo study of angiogenesis and collagen synthesis. Ann Surg 196:379–388, 1982.

41. Banda MJ, Howard EW, Herron GS, et al: Regulation of connective tissue turnover by metalloproteinase inhibitors. *In* Janssen H, Rooman R, and Robertson JIS (eds): Wound Healing. Petersfield, UK, Wrightson Biomedical, 1991, pp 61–70.

42. Ausprunk DH and Folkman J: Migration and proliferation of endothelial cells in preformed and newly formed blood vessels during tumor angiogenesis. Microvasc Res 14:53–65, 1977.

43. Miller EJ and Gay S: Collagen structure and function. *In* Cohen IK, Diegelmann RF, and Lindblad WJ (eds): Wound Healing: Biochemical and Clinical Aspects. Philadelphia, WB Saunders, 1992, pp 130–151.

44. Phillips C and Wenstrup RJ: Biosynthetic and genetic disorders of collagen. *In* Cohen IK, Diegelmann RF, and Lindblad WJ (eds): Wound Healing: Biochemical and Clinical Aspects. Philadelphia, WB Saunders, 1992, pp 152–176.

45. Burgeson RE: The collagens of the skin. Curr Prob Dermatol 17:61–75, 1987.

46. Murad S, Grove D, Lindberg KA, et al: Regulation of collagen synthesis by ascorbic acid. Proc Natl Acad Sci USA 78:2879–2882, 1981.

47. Niinikoski J, Gottrup F, and Hunt KA: The role of oxygen in wound repair. *In* Janssen H, Rooman R, and Robertson JIS (eds): Wound Healing. Petersfield, UK, Wrightson Biomedical 1991, 165–174.

48. Shandall A, Lowndes R, and Young HL: Colonic anastomotic healing and oxygen tension. Br J Surg 72:602–609, 1985.

49. Hussain MZ, Ghani QP, and Hunt TK: Inhibition of prolyl hydroxylase by poly (ADP-ribose) and phosphoribosyl-AMP. J Biol Chem 264:7850–7855, 1989.

50. Weitzhandler M and Bernfield MR: Proteoglycan glycoconjugates. *In* Cohen KI, Diegelmann RF, and Lindblad WJ (eds): Wound Healing: Biochemical and Clinical Aspects. Philadelphia, WB Saunders, 1992, pp 195–208.

51. Hopwood JJ and Dorfman A: Glycosaminoglycan synthesis by cultured human skin fibroblasts after transformation with simian virus 40. J Biol Chem 252:4777–4785, 1977.

52. Rudolph R: Contraction and the control of contraction. World J Surg 4:279–287, 1980.

53. Gabbiani G, Hirschel BJ, Ryan GB, et al: Granulation tissue as a contractile organ: A study of structure of function. J Exp Med 135:719–734, 1972.

54. Rudolph R, Guber S, Suzuki M, et al: The life cycle of the fibroblast. Surg Gynecol Obstet 145:389–394, 1977.

55. Majno G, Gabbiani G, Hirschel BJ, et al: Contraction of granulation tissue in vitro: Similarity to smooth muscle. Science 173:548–550, 1971.

56. Rudolph R, Vande Berg J, and Pierce GF: Changing concepts in myofibroblast function and control. *In* Janssen H, Rooman R, and Robertson JIS (eds): Wound Healing. Petersfield, UK, Wrightson Biomedical, 1991, pp 103–115.

57. Singer IL, Kawka DW, Kazazis DM, et al: In vivo co-distribution of fibronectin and actin fibers in granulation tissue: Immunofluorescence and electron microscope studies of the fibronexus at the myofibroblast surface. J Cell Biol 98:2106, 1984.

58. Pierce GF, Mustoe TA, Lingelbach J, et al: PDGF and TGF-beta enhance tissue repair activities by unique mechanisms. J Cell Biol 109:429–440, 1989.

59. Rudolph R: Inhibition of myofibroblasts by skin grafts. Plast Reconstr Surg 63:473–480, 1979.

60. Berry RB, Tan OT, Cooke ED, et al: Transcutaneous oxygen tension as an index of maturity in hypertrophic scars treated by compression. Br J Plast Surg 38:163–173, 1985.

61. Madden JW and Arem AJ: Wound healing: Biological and clinical features. *In* Sabiston DC (ed): Textbook of Surgery, 14th ed. Philadelphia, WB Saunders, 1991, pp 164–177.

62. Jeffrey JJ: Collagen degradation. *In* Cohen KI, Diegelmann RF and Lindblad WJ (eds): Wound Healing: Biochemical and Clinical Aspects. Philadelphia, WB Saunders, 1992, pp 177–194.

63. Bauer EA, Kronberger A, Valle KJ, et al: Glucocorticoid modulation of collagenase expression in human skin fibroblast cultures: Evidence for pre-translational inhibition. Biochem Biophys Acta 825:227–235, 1985.

64. Chua CC, Geiman DE, Keller GH, et al: Induction of collagenase secretion in human fibroblast cultures by growth promoting factors. J Biol Chem 260:5213–5216, 1985.

65. Welgus HG, Jeffery JJ, Roswit WT, et al: Human skin fibroblast collagenase: Interaction with substrate and inhibitor. Collagen Rel Res 5:167–179, 1985.

66. Gay S, Viljanto J, Raekallio J, et al: Collagen types in early phases of wound healing in children. Acta Chir Scand 144:205, 1978.

67. Gay S and Miller EJ: Collagen. *In* The Physiology and Pathology of Connective Tissue. New York, Stuttgart, 1978, p 75.

68. Alexander SA and Donoff RB: The glycosaminoglycans of open wounds. J Surg Res 29:422–429, 1980.

69. Stemmer EA: Influence of diabetes mellitus on the patterns and complications of vascular occlusive disease. *In* Moore W (ed): Vascular Surgery: A Comprehensive Review. New York, Grune & Stratton, 1986, pp 543–558.

70. Pfeifer MA, Schumer M, Jung S, and Pohl SL: Diabetic neuropathy. *In* Bergman M and Sicard GA (eds): Surgical Management of the Diabetic Patient. New York, Raven Press, 1991, pp 119–123.

71. Blair VP, Drury DA, and Levin ME: Diabetic foot care. *In* Bergman M and Sicard GA (eds): Surgical Management of the Diabetic Patient. New York, Raven Press, 1991, pp 195–207.

72. Boulton AJM, Scarpello JHB, and Ward JD: Venous oxygenation in the diabetic neuropathic foot: Evidence of arterial venous shunting. Diabetologia 22:6–8, 1982.

73. Mathews RE: The insensitive foot. *In* Gould JS (ed): The Foot Book. Baltimore, Williams & Wilkins, 1988, pp 280–290.

74. Hewlett D: Syndromes of infections in diabetic patients. *In* Bergman M and Sicard GA (eds): Surgical Management of the Diabetic Patient. New York, Raven Press, 1991, pp 83–95.

75. Goodson WH: Wound healing in diabetics. *In* Bergman M and Sicard GA (eds): Surgical Management of the Diabetic Patient. New York, Raven Press, 1991, pp 39–50.

76. Mayberry JC, Moneta GL, Taylor LM, and Porter JM: Nonoperative treatment of venous stasis ulcer. *In* Bergan JJ and Yao JST (eds): Venous Disorders. Philadelphia, WB Saunders, 1991, pp 381–395.

77. Browse NL, Burnand KG, and Thomas ML: Diseases of the Veins: Pathology, Diagnosis, and Treatment. London, Edward Arnold, 1989, pp 349–441.

78. Coleridge Smith PD, and Scurr JH: Current views on the pathogenesis of venous ulceration. *In* Bergan JJ and Yao JST (eds): Venous Disorders. Philadelphia, WB Saunders, 1991, pp 36–51.

79. Schanzer H and Pierce EC: Pathophysiology evaluation of chronic venous stasis with ambulatory venous pressure studies. Angiology 33:183, 1982.

80. Weingarten MS, Czeredarczuk M, Branas C, et al: Quantification of venous reflux utilizing duplex scanning. J Vasc Surg, in press.

81. Ryan TJ and Copeman PMW: Microvascular patterns and blood stasis in skin disease. Br J Dermatol 8:563, 1970.

82. Browse NL and Burnand KG: The cause of venous ulceration. Lancet 2:243–245, 1982.

83. Partsch H: Investigations on the pathogenesis of venous leg ulcers. Acta Chir Scand 544 [Suppl]:25–29, 1988.

84. Coleridge Smith PD, Thomas P, Scurr JH, and Dormandy JA: Causes of venous ulceration: A new hypothesis. Br Med J 296:1726–1772, 1988.

85. Lawrence WT: Clinical management of non-healing wounds. *In* Cohen IK, Diegelmann RF, and Lindblad WJ (eds): Wound Healing: Biochemical and Clinical Aspects. Philadelphia, WB Saunders, 1992, pp 541–561.

86. Kaplan RP: Cancer complicating chronic ulcerative and scarifying mucocutaneous disorders. Adv Dermatol 2:19–46, 1987.

87. Weingarten MS, Monteiro D, Charland K, and Paz K: Carcinoma arising from chronic wounds: A report of four cases and a review of the literature. J Vasc Surg, in press.

88. Shike M and Brennan MF: Supportive care of the cancer patient. *In* DeVita VT, Hellman S, and Rosenberg SA (eds): Cancer: Principles and Practice of Oncology. Philadelphia, JB Lippincott, 1989, pp 2029–2059.

89. Cupps TR and Fauci AS: The Vasculitides: Major Problems in Internal Medicine, XXI. Philadelphia, WB Saunders, 1981.

90. LeRoy EC: Scleroderma (systemic sclerosis): Comparison with wound healing. *In* Cohen KI, Diegelmann RF, and Lindblad WJ (eds): Wound Healing: Biochemical and Clinical Aspects. Philadelphia, WB Saunders, 1992, pp 510–522.

91. LeRoy EC, Smith EA, Kahaleh MB, et al: A strategy for determining the pathogenesis of systemic sclerosis—is transforming growth factor-beta the answer? Arthritis Rheum 32:817–823, 1989.

92. Taylor LM and Porter JM: Nonatherosclerotic vascular disease. *In* Moore WS (ed): Vascular Surgery: A Comprehensive Review. New York, Grune & Stratton, 1986, pp 117–158.

93. Lynch JB and Franklin JD: Lymphatic disorders of childhood. *In* Dean RH and O'Neill JA (eds): Vascular Disorders of Childhood. Philadelphia, Lea & Febiger, 1983, pp 159–169.

94. Markey AC, Tidman MJ, Rowe PH, et al: Aggressive ulcerative necrobiosis lipoidica associated with venous insufficiency, giant-cell phlebitis, and arteritis. Clin Exp Dermatol 13:183–186, 1988.

95. Gould JS: Ancillary studies: Neurologic. *In* Gould JS (ed): The Foot Book. Baltimore, Williams & Wilkins, 1988, pp 8–14.

96. Knighton DR, Ciresi KF, Fiegel VD, et al: Classification and treatment of non-healing wounds: Successful treatment with autologous platelet derived wound healing factors. Ann Surg 204:322–330, 1986.

97. Pecoraro RE and Reiber GE: Classification of wounds in diabetic amputees. Wounds 2:65–73, 1990.

98. Walsh MS and Goode AW: A scientific approach to wound measurement: The role of stereophotogrammetry. *In* Janssen H, Rooman R, and Robertson JIS (eds): Wound Healing. Petersfield, UK, Wrightson Biomedical, 1991, pp 189–201.

99. Newman LG, Waller J, Palestro C, et al: Unsuspected osteomyelitis in diabetic foot ulcers. JAMA 266:1246–1251, 1991.

100. Blair VP, Drury DA, and Levin ME: Diabetic foot care. *In* Bergman M and Sicard GA (eds): Surgical Management of the Diabetic Patient. New York, Raven Press, 1991, pp 195–207.

101. AbuRahma AF and Diethrich EB: The arterial leg Doppler examination: Segmental limb pressures and analysis of the analog wave tracing. *In* AbuRahma AF and Diethrich EB (eds): Current Noninvasive Vascular Diagnosis. Littleton, MA, PSG Publishing, 1988, pp 199–210.

102. Raines JK and Walburn FJ: The pulse volume recorder in the diagnosis of peripheral arterial disease. *In* AbuRahma AF and Diethrich EB (eds): Current Noninvasive Vascular Diagnosis. Littleton, MA, PSG Publishing, 1988, pp 219–235.

103. Vincent D, Salles-Cunha S, Bernhard V, and Towne J: Noninvasive assessment of toe systolic pressures with special reference to diabetes mellitus. J Cardiovasc Surg 24:22–28, 1983.

104. Alden PB and Sicard GA: Vascular surgery. *In* Bergman M and Sicard GA (eds): Surgical Management of the Diabetic Patient. New York, Raven Press, 1991, pp 215–240.

105. Strandness DE: Duplex Scanning in Vascular Disease. New York, Raven Press, 1990.

106. Nicolaides AN and Christopoulos DC: Methods of quantification of chronic venous insufficiency. *In* Bergan JJ and Yao JST (eds): Venous Disorders. Philadelphia, WB Saunders, 1991, pp 77–90.

107. Nemeth AJ, Eaglstein WH, and Falanga V: Clinical parameters and transcutaneous oxygen measurements for the prognosis of venous ulcers. J Am Acad Dermatol 20:186–190, 1989.

108. McGraw DJ and Allen BT: Lower extremity amputation in the diabetic patient. *In* Bergman M and Sicard GA (eds): Surgical Management of the Diabetic Patient. New York, Raven Press, 1991, pp 263–277.

109. Harrington EB, Harrington ME, Schanzer H, et al: The dorsalis pedis bypass: Moderate success in difficult situations. J Vasc Surg 15:409–416, 1992.

110. Cronenwett JL, McDaniel MD, Zwolak RM, et al: Limb salvage despite extensive tissue loss: Free tissue transfer combined with distal revascularization. Arch Surg 124:609–615, 1989.

111. Eldrup-Jorgensen J: Conservative management of lower extremity chronic venous insufficiency. Semin Vasc Surg 1:86–91, 1988.

112. Kikta MJ, Schuler JJ, Meyer JP, et al: A prospective, randomized trial of Unna's boots versus hydrostatic dressing in the treatment of venous stasis ulcers. J Vasc Surg 7:478–486, 1988.

113. Mulder G, Robison J, and Seeley J: Study of sequential compression therapy in the treatment of non-healing chronic venous ulcers. Wounds 2:111–115, 1990.

114. Nemeth AJ, Falanga V, Alstadt SP, et al: Ulcerated edematous limbs: Effect of edema removal on transcutaneous oxygen measurements. J Am Acad Dermatol 20:191–197, 1989.

115. Allenby F, Boardman L, Pflug JJ, et al: Effects of external pneumatic intermittent compression on fibrinolysis in man. Lancet 2:1412–1414, 1973.

116. Colgan M, Dormandy JA, Jones PW, et al: Oxypentifylline treatment of venous ulcers of the leg. Br Med J 300:972–975, 1990.

117. Sullivan GW, Carper HT, Novick WJ, et al: Inhibition of the inflammatory action of interleukin-1 and tumor necrosis factor (alpha) on neutrophil function by pentoxifylline. Infect Immun 56:1722–1729, 1988.

118. Wiseman DM, Rovee DT, and Alvarez OM: Wound dressings: Design and use. *In* Cohen IK, Diegelmann RF, and Lindblad WJ (eds): Wound Healing: Biochemical and Clinical Aspects. Philadelphia, WB Saunders, 1992, pp 562–579.

119. Pollack AV: The treatment of infected wounds. Acta Chir Scand 156:505–513, 1990.

120. Alvarez O, Rozint J, and Wiseman D: Moist environment for healing: Matching the dressing to the wound. Wounds 1:35–51, 1989.

121. Rodeheaver G, Wheeler CB, Rye DG, et al: Side effects of topical proteolytic enzyme treatment. Surg Gynecol Obstet 148:562–566, 1979.

122. Leipziger LS, Glushko V, DiBernardo B, et al: Dermal wound repair: Role of collagen matrix implants and synthetic polymer dressings. J Am Acad Dermatol 12:409–419, 1985.

123. Hutchinson JJ and Lawrence JC: Wound infection under occlusive dressings. J Hosp Infect 17:83–94, 1991.

124. Krasner D: Wound care products. Ostomy/Wound Manage 33:47–60, 1991.

125. Freeman BG, Cardwell GR, and McGraw JB: The quantitative study of the use of dextranomer in the management of infected wounds. Surg Gynecol Obstet 153:81–86, 1981.

126. Fischer BH: Treatment of ulcers on the legs with hyperbaric oxygen. J Dermatol Surg 1:55–58, 1975.

127. Davis JC: Hyperbaric oxygen therapy. J Intens Care Med 4:55–57, 1989.

128. Johnson WC, Grant HI, Baldwin D, et al: Supplemental oxygen and dependent positioning as adjunctive measures to improve forefoot tissue oxygenation. Arch Surg 123:1227–1230, 1988.

129. Thom SR: Hyperbaric oxygen therapy. J Intens Care Med 4:58–74, 1989.

130. Marx RE: A new concept in the treatment of osteoradionecrosis. J Oral Maxillofac Surg 41:351–357, 1983.

131. Mader JT: Hyperbaric oxygen therapy: A committee report. Bethesda, MD, Undersea and Hyperbaric Medical Society, 1989.

132. Kindwall EP, Gottlieb LJ, and Larson DL: Hyperbaric oxygen therapy in plastic surgery: A review article. Plast Reconstr Surg 88:898–908, 1991.

133. Baroni G, Porro T, Faglia E, et al: Hyperbaric oxygen in diabetic gangrene treatment. Diabetes Care 10:81–86, 1987.

134. Behari J: Electrostimulation and bone fracture healing. Crit Rev Biomed Engineer 18:235–254, 1991.

135. Griffin JW, Tooms RE, Mendius RA, et al: Efficacy of high-voltage pulsed current for healing of pressure ulcers in patients with spinal cord injury. Phys Ther 71:433–441, 1991.

136. Gogia PP, Marquez RR, and Minerbo GM: Effects of high voltage stimulation on wound healing. Ostomy/Wound Manage 38:29–35, 1992.

137. Kloth LC and Feedar JA: Electrical stimulation in tissue repair. *In* Kloth LC, McCulloch JM, and Feedar JA (eds): Wound Healing: Alternatives in Management. Philadelphia, FA Davis, 1990, pp 221–256.

138. Dyson M: Role of ultrasound in wound healing. *In* Kloth LC, McCulloch JM, and Feedar JA (eds): Wound Healing: Alternatives in Management. Philadelphia, FA Davis, 1990, pp 259–283.

139. Cummings J: Role of light in wound healing. *In* Kloth LC, McCulloch JM, and Feedar JA (eds): Wound Healing: Alternatives in Management. Philadelphia, FA Davis, 1990, pp 287–301.

140. Cromack DT, Porras-Reyes B, and Mustoe TA: Current concepts in wound healing: Growth factor and macrophage interaction. J Trauma 30:S129–S133, 1990.

141. Pessa ME, Bland KI, and Copeland EM: Growth factors and determinants of wound repair. J Surg Res 42:207–217, 1987.

142. Brown GL, Curtsinger L, Jurkiewicz MJ, et al: Stimulation of healing of chronic wounds by epidermal growth factor. Plast Reconstr Surg 88:189–194, 1991.

143. Carter DM, Balin AK, Gottlieb AB, et al: Clinical experience with crude preparations of growth factors in healing of chronic wounds in human subjects. *In* Hunt TK, et al (eds): Growth Factors and Other Aspects of Wound Healing: Biological and Clinical Implications. New York, Alan R Liss, 1988, pp 303–317.

144. Knighton DR, Fiegel VD, Austin LL, et al: Classification and treatment of chronic non-healing wounds. Ann Surg 204:322–330, 1986.

145. Knighton DR, Fiegel VD, Doucette MM, et al: The use of topically applied growth factors in chronic nonhealing wounds: A review. Wounds 1:71–77, 1989.

146. Knighton DR, Ciresi K, Fiegel VD, et al: Stimulation of repair in chronic non-healing cutaneous ulcers using platelet derived wound healing formula. Surg Gynecol Obstet 170:56–60, 1990.

147. Pierce GF, Mustoe TA, and Altrock BW: Role of platelet derived growth factor in healing. J Cell Biochem 45:319–326, 1991.
148. Robson MC, Phillips LG, Thomason A, et al: Platelet derived growth factor BB for the treatment of chronic pressure sores. Lancet 339:23–25, 1992.
149. Shah M, Foreman DM, and Ferguson MWJ: Control of scarring in adult wounds by neutralizing antibody to transforming growth factor-beta. Lancet 339:213–214, 1992.
150. Cohen IK and Mast BA: Models of wound healing J Trauma 30:S149–S155, 1990.
151. Steed DL, Moosa HH, and Webster MW: The importance of randomized prospective trials in evaluating therapy for wound healing. Wounds 3:111–115, 1991.

CHAPTER 5

Biomechanics

PART I

Biomechanics of Musculoskeletal Diseases

Jack L. Morris, D.P.M., Richard Berenter, D.P.M.,
and Daniel K. Kosai, D.P.M.

Walking is a repeated performance of a sequence of events in the lower extremities to advance the body forward. Locomotion depends on an interaction of many systems that support, coordinate, and control this forward motion. Normal gait is achieved with relative ease and at a low energy requirement by the physiologic systems of the body. However, in the presence of various disease states, the body makes adjustments that result in an increase in energy expenditure. Consequently, assisted types of support may be necessary during locomotion to reduce fatigue or other symptoms produced as a result of increased energy expenditure. This chapter presents the effects on the lower extremities of various disease states involving the neurologic, muscular, and skeletal systems.

To appreciate the activity of normal gait, the biomechanics of various tissues of the musculoskeletal system are discussed, followed by the definition of normal gait and the effects of various pathologic entities on the normal gait cycle.

BONE

Biomechanics of Bone

The innate anatomic structure of bone, in addition to its inorganic and organic content, imparts the strength and stiffness required for specialized daily activities. These properties of bone, along with muscle attachments and motion about joints, provide the needed mechanical framework for locomotion. Hardness and strength are mechanical properties of bone that make it unique in function. These qualities enable bone to resist external loading forces. The various forces that act on bone include compression, bending, and torsion.

A compression force is a force that is applied from one end of a bone to the other end, parallel to the longitudinal axis. The ability of a bone to resist fracturing in the presence of compression forces is equal to the square of the radius of that bone. The main cause of bone failure is bending forces. The bending force in bone is calculated to the true axis of the bone. The bone's resistance to fracturing in the presence of bending force is equal to the fourth power of the radius of the bone. Torsional forces are twisting forces around a centroid axis. The centroid axis is located in the central part of the bone. For example, fractures of the long bones of the leg tend to occur in the medial cortex, because the longitudinal axis of the bone is located medially. The closer the cortical wall is to the axis, the more prone the cortex is to fracturing.[1]

These forces are all capable of stressing the bone to the point of fracture. When sufficient bending and torsional forces are combined, a fracture occurs in the medial cortex, enters into the centroid axis, then spirals off in either one direction or the other. In addition to specific forces, the absorption of bone during the initial phase of training activities, referred to as *osteoionization,* seems to play a part in the pathogenesis of fractures. Resorption of bone and the period of osteoionization may be compared to the osteopenia seen in the elderly, who may be affected by many diseases. Loss of mineralization and diminished radial width makes bone more vulnerable to fracture by external forces.

CARTILAGE (see Chapter 2)

Biomechanics of the Components of Articular Cartilage

Articular cartilage may be viewed biomechanically as a biphasic material composed of a collagen-proteoglycan solid matrix (25% by weight) surrounded by freely movable interstitial fluid (75% by weight).[2] The compressive modulus of articular cartilage is directly related to the percentage of proteoglycan present (i.e., the stiffer the cartilage, the higher the concentration of glycosaminoglycans). The electrostatic and osmotic properties of proteoglycans also contribute to cartilage elasticity. The negatively charged glycosaminogly-can molecules repel one another as proteoglycan aggregates disperse in an attempt to occupy the largest possible domain. Proteoglycans hold water in the cartilage matrix osmotically and impede the loss of water from loaded cartilage both osmotically and by controlling matrix permeability.

Collagen provides the structural framework for articular cartilage.[3] The tangential orientation of the fibers in the gliding zones allows them to resist shear and surface wear. The more random orientation of deeper fibers permits them to resist compressive loading yet allows for resiliency. The radial orientation of the deepest fibers allows them to resist compressive loading also, and their attachment to the subchondral bone permits them to resist shearing forces between the articular cartilage and underlying subchondral plate. The fiber network also serves to counteract the swelling pressure generated by the proteoglycans, which contributes to the stiffness of the cartilage matrix.

Proteoglycans and collagen each help cartilage to resist the load placed on it. The proteoglycans resist the load by retaining water in the matrix osmotically and by impeding the loss of water from the loaded matrix by reducing its permeability. The collagen resists the load by maintaining the proteoglycans in place. The amount of load that the cartilage is capable of sustaining requires the simultaneous function of both the proteoglycans and the collagen components.

The fluid phase of cartilage is characterized by a high, negatively charged fixed density.[4] The negatively charged proteoglycans lead to a swelling pressure within the cartilage. As a result of the swelling pressure, 65% to 80% of cartilage is relatively noncompressible fluid that absorbs most of the axial load crossing the joint. This contributes to the high initial stiffness of cartilage on impact loading. A prolonged mechanical load causes fluid to flow laterally or be extruded throughout the cartilage matrix. This property of cartilage is partly responsible for its viscoelastic response to compressive loads.

The equilibrium of articular cartilage may be disrupted in two ways.[5] The stress-strain state of articular cartilage may change owing to alterations in the loading conditions of the joint. If the disruption in equilibrium is prolonged, there will be a gradual change in both the structure and the mechanical properties of articular cartilage, as well as changes in the underlying structural components of the system (i.e., the cancellous and compact bones). The second change in structural and mechanical properties of articular cartilage may be caused by alterations in its biochemical composition. When the stress-strain state is altered, pathologic degenerative changes may develop within the cartilage (Fig. 5–1).

SKELETAL MUSCLE

Biomechanics of Skeletal Muscle

Skeletal muscle performs both dynamic and static work to provide locomotion, maintain bony segments in space, and ensure proper posture. What makes muscle unique in its ability to carry out these functions is its properties of excitability and contractility. Skeletal muscle is composed of single cells referred to as *muscle fibers.* Muscle fibers are multinucleated cells between 10 and 100 μm in diameter. These fibers are surrounded by electrically polarized membranes

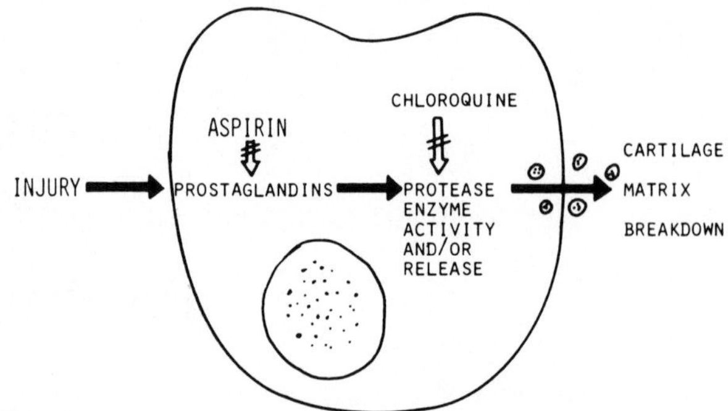

FIGURE 5–1. The vicious cycle of degenerative joint disease. (From Albright J and Brand R: The Scientific Basis of Orthopedics. East Norwalk, CT, Appleton & Lange, 1987, p 366.)

known as *sarcolemma* and are divided into subunits known as myofibrils (Fig. 5–5).[8] Three distinct muscle fiber types have been identified in skeletal muscle: the slow-twitch oxidate or type I, the fast-twitch oxidative glycolytic or type IIA, and the fast-twitch glycolytic or type IIB. The percentage of each of the fiber types varies among different muscles, as well as different people. Individual variations in fiber type proportion may explain why certain athletes are more efficient in a particular type of sport (e.g., speed vs. endurance).[1]

A twitch is the phenomenon whereby a single stimulus of a motor nerve causes a mechanical response of a muscle. When mechanical responses to successive stimuli are added to the initial response, the resultant effect on muscle is called *summation* (Fig. 5–2). Tetany is a sustained contraction of muscle that occurs when maximum tension is maintained as a result of summated action potentials (Fig. 5–3).[1, 8]

Following a stimulus, a latency period of a few milliseconds occurs before tension in the muscle fiber begins to rise. The interval from when tension starts to develop until peak tension is achieved is the contraction time for the muscle. Relaxation time is the time from peak tension until no tension is produced. The refractory or latency period is the time in which a muscle is incapable of any additional response to a second stimuli.[2]

The frequency of stimulation is controlled by individual muscle units. The amount of tension produced by a given muscle is directly proportional to the frequency of stimulation of that muscle. However, there is a limit or maximum frequency. Consequently, no additional tension is produced if a muscle fires at a greater rate than the maximum frequency.[2]

Muscle tension is the amount of force exerted by a contracting muscle onto the lever (i.e., bone) to which that muscle is attached. If the tension produced by a given muscle is greater than the resistance or load of the body segment, then the muscle shortens, producing joint movement. This is known as a *concentric muscle contraction.* However, if the external load outweighs the tension produced by the muscle, then the muscle will progressively lengthen. This type of contraction is known as *eccentric muscle contraction.* Eccentric muscle contractions are useful when the body is attempting to decelerate motion at a given joint. Other types of muscle contractions include isometric, isokinetic, isoinertial, and isotonic. *Isometric contractions* are defined as muscle contractions without motion; therefore, no mechanical work

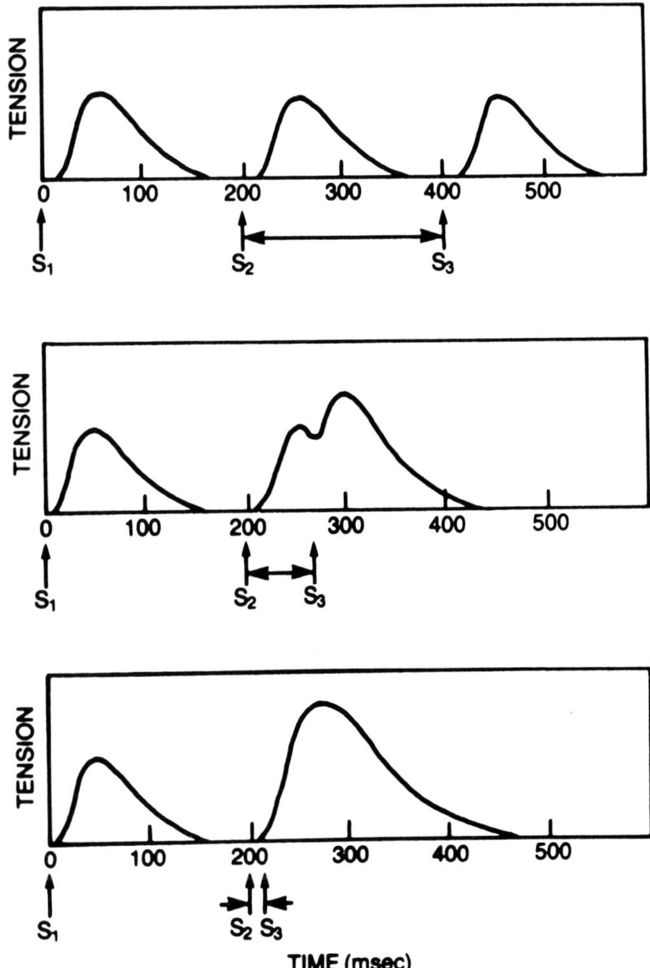

FIGURE 5–2. Summation in muscle at constant length. *Upper,* Three stimuli (S) at 200 msec: no summation. *Middle,* S_2 and S_3 60 msec apart: greater response. Lower, S_2 and S_3 at 20 msec: peak tension is greater than the middle panel. (From Nordin M and Frankel VH: Basic Biomechanics of the Skeletal System. 2nd ed. Philadelphia, Lea & Febiger, 1989, p 97. Reprinted with permission.)

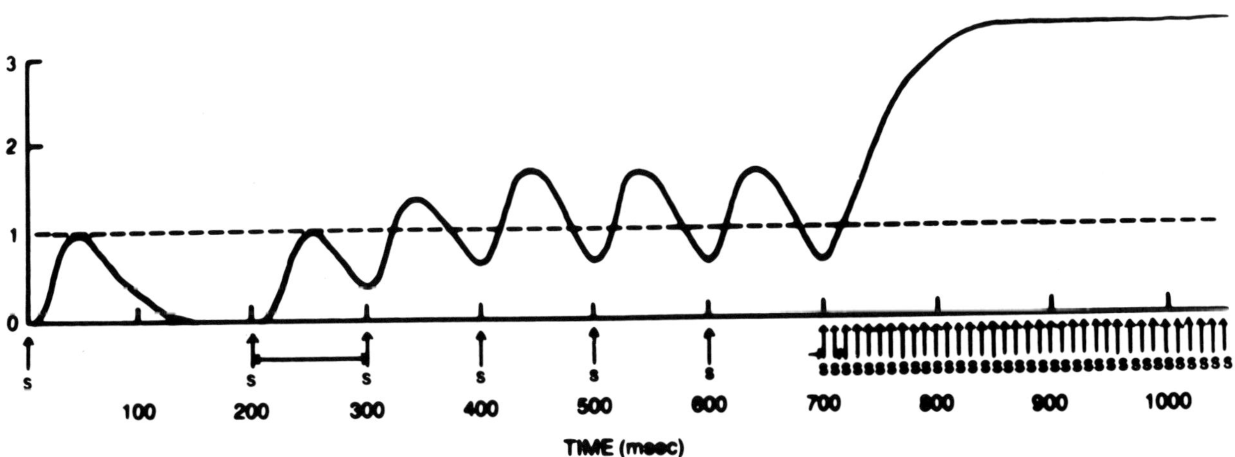

FIGURE 5–3. Tetany—stimuli at 100 msec with sustained peak tension. (From Nordin M and Frankel VH: Basic Biomechanics of the Skeletal System. 2nd ed. Philadelphia, Lea & Febiger, 1989, p 98. Reprinted with permission.)

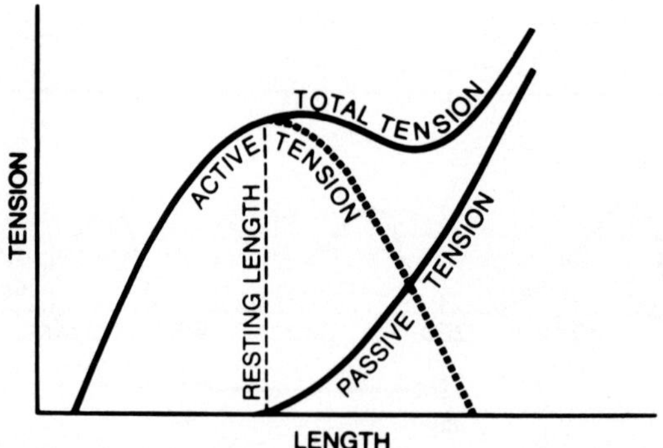

FIGURE 5–4. Active and passive tension of a muscle against its length. (From Nordin M and Frankel VH: Basic Biomechanics of the Skeletal System. 2nd ed. Philadelphia, Lea & Febiger, 1989, p 100. Reprinted with permission.)

is performed. Instead, static work is performed as energy is expended and heat is produced. *Isokinetic contraction* is defined as constant velocity of contraction. Because the velocity remains constant, no acceleration is possible. As a result, all the muscle energy is converted into resisting movement. The amount of force exerted by a muscle during an isokinetic contraction varies according to changes in the length of the lever arm that occur throughout the joint range of motion. An isoinertial contraction occurs when the muscle is working against a constant load or resistance. When joint position is at either extreme, the muscles crossing that joint must overcome the inertia of the load to initiate movement. *Isotonic contraction* is defined as a muscle contraction performed with a constant force or tension.[2, 6, 7]

Alterations in joint position affect the length of the muscle's lever arm and cause changes in the amount of muscle tension produced. The total force produced is a direct result of the muscle's mechanical properties. The principal factors that influence force production include the muscle's temperature and state of fatigue. A muscle that is slack or at its resting length is capable of generating the maximum tension for that muscle because the actin and myosin filaments overlap along their entire length with the greatest possible number of cross bridges. The Blix curve describes the combination of active and passive tension within a muscle. Muscles that cross only one joint usually are not stretched enough for passive tension to develop significantly. However, muscles that span two joints typically function with a significant amount of passive tension (Fig. 5–4).[2]

The relationship between load and velocity is inversely proportional; consequently, the greatest velocity of shortening for a given muscle is when the external load is zero. The force of a given muscle is inversely proportional to the time of contraction for that muscle, so that the longer the contraction time, the greater the force generated, up to a maximal tension. This effect is a result of the contractile elements having time to transmit the tension through the elastic components of the muscle to the tendon. The muscle's ability to perform work is increased when contraction is preceded by warm-up or prestretching. When the temperature of a muscle goes up, the conduction velocity across the sarcolemma increases. This causes the frequency of stimulation to increase and results in a greater force of contraction. Elevation in

temperature also increases the enzymatic activity of a muscle, thus improving the muscle's contraction as well as enhancing the extensibility of the muscle-tendon unit. The temperature may be elevated by increasing the blood flow to the muscle or through the release of heat energy generated by the metabolism of the muscle. Muscles depend on oxygen and adenosine triphosphate (ATP) as energy sources to contract and relax. The body's muscles have three sources of ATP: creatine phosphate, substrate phosphorylation during anaerobic glycolysis, and mitochondrial oxidative phosphorylation. Fatigue affects contractility when the frequency of muscle stimulation increases to a level at which the breakdown rate of ATP is greater than the muscle's capacity to replenish the molecule. The effect of disuse and immobilization is a rapid decrease in the size (i.e., atrophy) and aerobic capacity of the muscle fibers. Type I fibers have been shown to be most affected by the decrease in the cross-sectional diameter of the muscle fiber. Early motion of an injured muscle may prevent this process from occurring. The reason for this may be that there is an increase in afferent impulses from the intrafusal muscle spindle when the muscle is placed under tension, causing an increase in stimulation of type I fibers. However, isometric exercises have not clinically demonstrated an ability to reverse the atrophy that takes place. Physical training or subjecting the muscle to greater than normal use has been shown to increase the cross-sectional diameter of muscle fibers (i.e., hypertrophy), which explains the resultant increase in muscle bulk and strength.[2]

Muscle-stretching programs before an activity are encouraged to prevent injury as well as to improve performance. Stretching exercises increase muscle flexibility, help maintain and augment joint range of motion, and increase the flexibility of the muscle-tendon unit. The control of muscle stretching is a function of the muscle's spindle fibers and Golgi apparatus. The Golgi apparatus responds to increases in muscle tension, and the spindles respond to changes in muscle length. It is theorized that increases in muscle tension prompt the Golgi apparatus to signal the muscle to relax, allowing an increase in length to take place (Fig. 5–5).[2, 6]

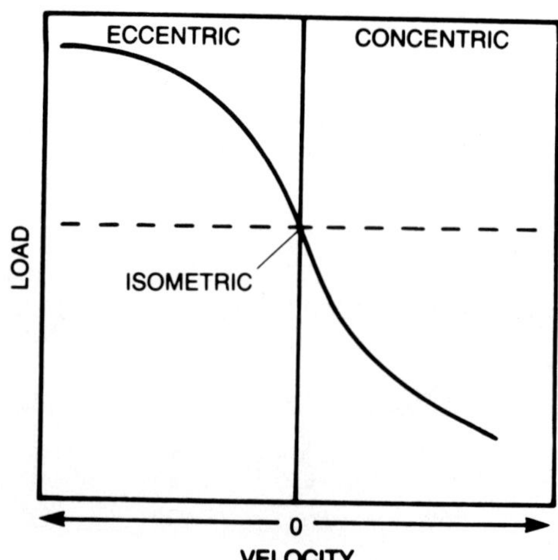

FIGURE 5–5. Concentric and eccentric response in an isometric contraction. (From Nordin M and Frankel VH: Basic Biomechanics of the Skeletal System. 2nd ed. Philadelphia, Lea & Febiger, 1989, p 101. Reprinted with permission.)

BIOMECHANICS OF GAIT

Forces and Lever Arms

The skeleton is the body's framework, to which muscles attach and help bring about movement. This movement occurs in the joints between adjacent bones. The arrangement of how the muscles are attached to the bony segments may be described through engineering principles governed by levers. A lever is a rigid structure rotating about a fixed axis or fulcrum to lift or sustain a weight (i.e., resistance) on one end through the application of force at the other end. The distance between the weight or resistance to the axis and the axis is known as the *resistance arm,* and the distance between the force and the axis is referred to as the *force arm.* The ratio between the force arm and the resistance arm of a lever describes the mechanical advantage of that lever. The functions of levers are to increase either the mechanical advantage to lift a load or the velocity of movement of the load. Lever systems accomplish one of these functions at the expense of the other.[7, 8]

Levers are divided into three different classes depending on the relative positions of the resistance, fulcrum, and applied force (Fig. 5–6). Any of the three lever classes are considered balanced or in equilibrium when the force torque equals the resistance torque. Force torque is equivalent to the product of the force and the length of the force arm; the resistance torque is the product of the resistance and the length of the resistance arm.

The fulcrum of class I levers is located somewhere between the resistance load and the force. As a result of this arrangement, the two arms of the lever move in opposite directions. A class II lever is defined as having placed the resistance between the fulcrum and the force. Class II levers enhance the force at the expense of range of motion. The class III lever has the force situated between the fulcrum and the resistance. Most muscles are of this class. Class III levers allow the muscles that insert close to joints to produce distance and speed of movement with minimal muscle shortening. Another important consideration for the mechanics of muscle contraction is the effect of the angle of pull that the muscle has on the lever arm.[8]

Normal Gait Cycle

Normal gait is a repetitive sequence of events involving the interaction of lower extremity segments to provide the body with locomotion (see Chapter 5, Part II). Each limb goes through two basic phases: swing and stance (Fig. 5–7). The stance phase can be broken down further into the heel-contact, midstance, and propulsive phases.[8] There is also a period during which both feet are on the ground; this is the *double-support phase of stance.* The double-support phase represents approximately 10% of the stance phase for each limb. Locomotion is achieved by the controlled forward falling of the body and the propulsive activity of the stance-phase limb. For normal locomotion to occur, the joints of the lower extremities must be free to move and respond to loading and unloading as changes occur in the positions of the lower limbs in space. Pathologic conditions influence these mechanisms and produce abnormal gait patterns.

Phases of Gait

The swing phase of gait is the period between when the toes leave the ground following propulsion until heel contact of the same limb is made. The stance phase is the period between when the foot strikes the ground at heel contact until toe-off occurs (see Fig. 5–7). The stance phase can be further broken down to the heel-contact, early midstance, late midstance, and propulsive periods. At heel contact the ankle joint is slightly dorsiflexed, the knee is slightly flexed, and the hip is flexed. Following heel strike, the foot plantarflexes toward the floor. When the entire foot contacts the floor, the early midstance period starts, and the foot and leg begin to accept body weight. At this point midstance begins, and the foot must become a stable adaptor so that it can accept the weight of the body being transferred from the opposite limb. The knee and hip are slightly flexed as weight is being carried

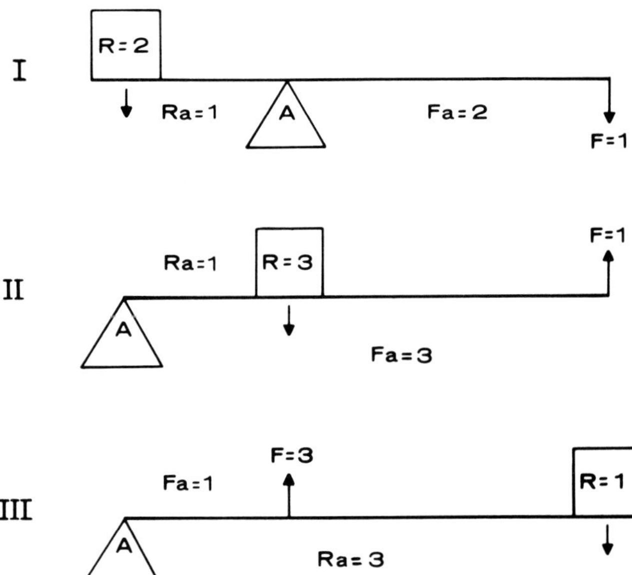

FIGURE 5–6. Lever arms: classes I, II, and III. R, resistance; Ra, resistance arm; F, force; Fa, force arm; A, fulcrum. (From Rasch P: Kinesiology and Applied Anatomy. 7th ed. Philadelphia, Lea & Febiger, 1989, p 91. Reprinted with permission.)

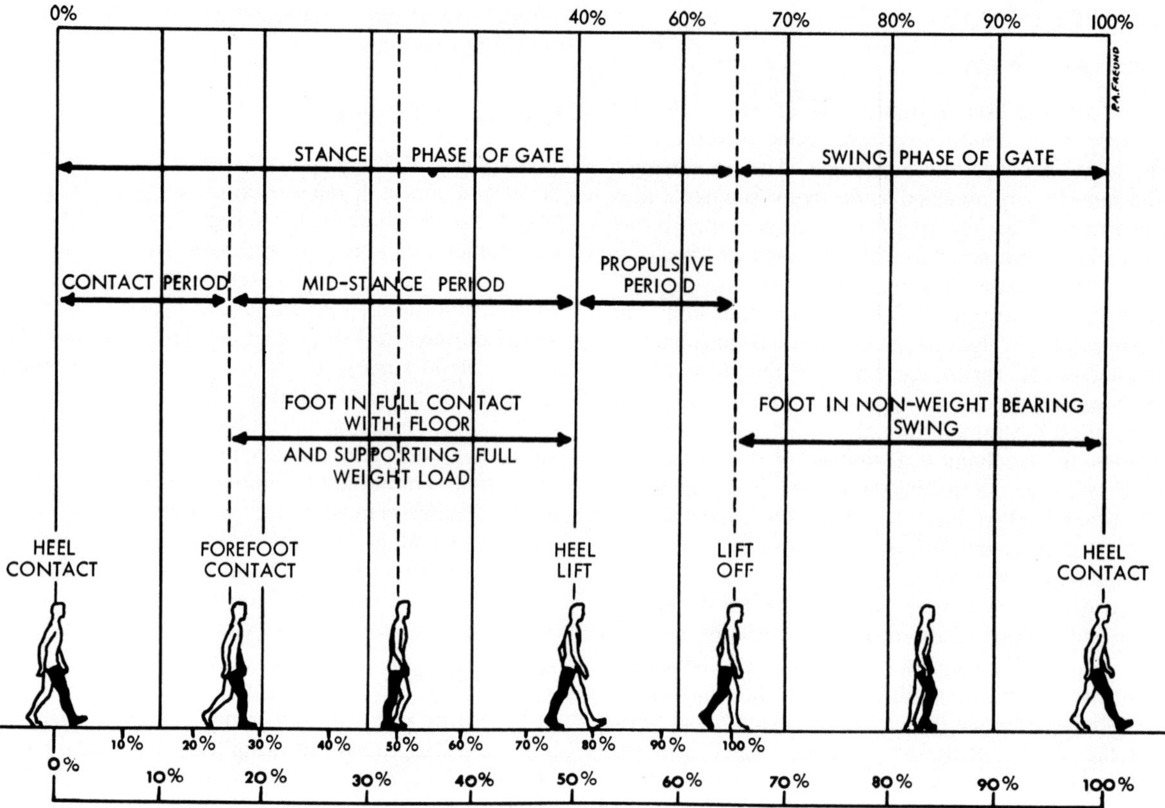

FIGURE 5–7. One complete gait cycle of the right limb. (From Sgarlato T: Compendium of Podiatric Biomechanics. San Francisco, California College of Podiatric Medicine, 1971, p 116.)

over the top of the weightbearing foot. The midstance period is reached when forward progression of the body is over the top of the foot. The body is erect, the ankle joint is at an angle of approximately 90 degrees, the knee is extended and stable, and the hip is in its neutral position. The ankle joint begins to dorsiflex as the body moves forward, thus allowing the tibia to move forward. In addition, quadriceps activity brings the femur forward but at a slower rate than the tibia. The late midstance period begins when the body weight is transferred to the forefoot. The body weight continues to be shifted to the forefoot as the heel rises off the floor, thus beginning the propulsive period of gait. During the propulsive period of stance phase, the swing activity of the contralateral leg and the propulsive activities of the ipsilateral leg propel the body forward (see Fig. 5–7).[9–11]

Hip Joint

The hip joint is a diarthrodial ball-and-socket joint composed of the head of the femur and the acetabulum of the pelvis.[12] The hip possesses three degrees of freedom of motion: flexion and extension in the sagittal plane, abduction and adduction in the frontal plane, and internal and external rotation in the transverse plane.

Motion is greatest in the sagittal plane, where the range of flexion is from 0 to 140 degrees, and extension is from 0 to 15 degrees.[2] The muscles primarily responsible for flexion of the hip joint are the psoas major and the iliacus. Secondary hip flexors include the tensor fasciae latae, rectus femoris, sartorius, and the adductor muscle group. The extensor group

of the hip consists of the gluteus maximus and hamstring muscles. The gluteus maximus is referred to as a one-joint extensor, because the muscle crosses only the hip joint. The hamstring muscles (i.e., semimembranosus, semitendinosus, and biceps femoris) cross both the hip and knee joints and are therefore known as *two-joint extensors* (Fig. 5–8).

The range of abduction is from 0 to 30 degrees, and the range of adduction is from 0 to 25 degrees.[2] Primary hip abductors include the gluteus medius and minimus muscles. The tensor fasciae latae and piriformis muscles function as weak abductors. The adductor muscle group (i.e., adductor longus, adductor brevis, adductor minimus, adductor magnus, gracilis, and pectineus) has little functional significance in the study of normal gait, but it plays a significant role in certain pathologic diseases.

Transverse rotation about the hip joint includes external and internal rotation. External rotation of the hip ranges from 0 to 90 degrees, and internal rotation ranges from 0 to 70 degrees when measured with the hip flexed.[2] The transverse rotation of the hip joint decreases when the hip is extended owing to increased tautness of the muscles and ligaments that surround and support the joint. The rotator musculature of the hip is of minimal importance in normal gait. The anterior fibers of the gluteus minimus and medius appear to be the primary internal rotators, and the obturator externus and quadratus femoris seem to be the primary external rotators (Fig. 5–9).

At heel contact, ground-reactive force is anterior to the hip joint, producing a flexion moment in the sagittal plane. Both the hamstrings and gluteus maximus are active to decelerate

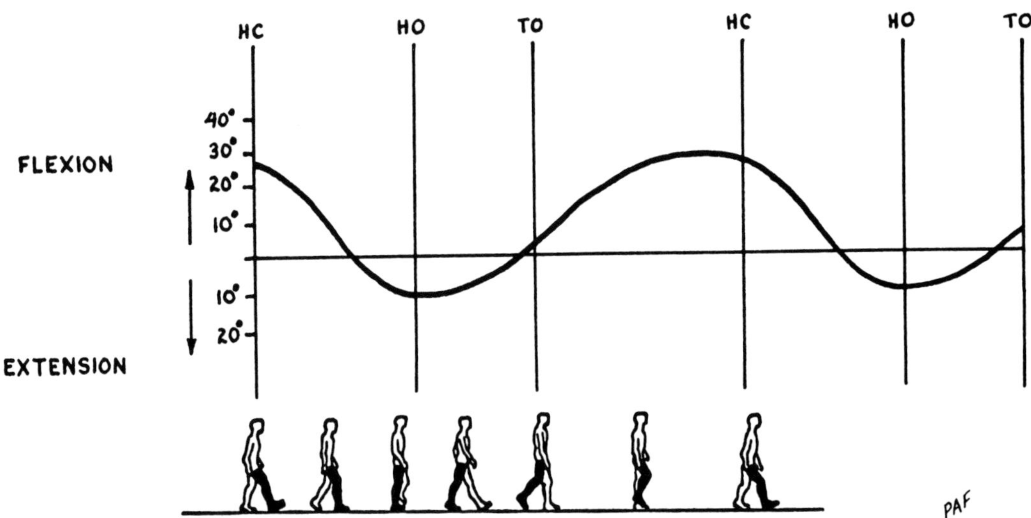

FIGURE 5–8. Hip joint range of motion (sagittal plane motion) during the gait cycle. (From Sgarlato T: Compendium of Podiatric Biomechanics. San Francisco, California College of Podiatric Medicine, 1971, p 81.)

flexion. In the frontal plane, the abductors act eccentrically to resist the adduction moment created by the body's mass across the hip joint. The adductor magnus of the stance limb functions to extend the hip and externally rotate the pelvis on the femur.[13]

During midstance, ground-reactive force passes posterior to the hip, creating an extension moment in the sagittal plane. Hyperextension of the hip is prevented by the iliofemoral ligament, thus obviating the need for muscle action. The

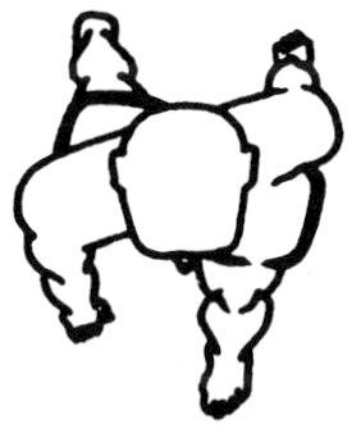

TRANSVERSE PLANE ROTATION OF PELVIS & TRUNK AS PELVIS ROTATES CLOCKWISE, LEFT LEG FORWARD; TRUNK ROTATES COUNTER CLOCKWISE WITH RIGHT ARM SWINGING FORWARD. AS PELVIS ROTATES COUNTER CLOCKWISE, TRUNK ROTATES CLOCKWISE.

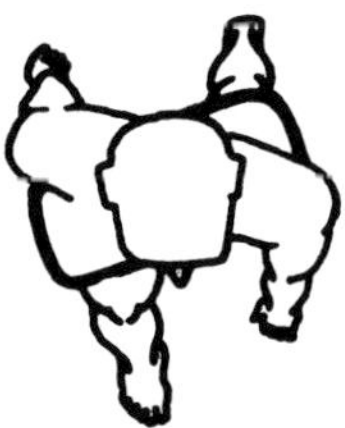

FIGURE 5–9. Transverse plane motion of the pelvis. (From Sgarlato T: Compendium of Podiatric Biomechanics. San Francisco, California College of Podiatric Medicine, 1971, p 120.)

adductor moment created by body weight causes the pelvis on the unsupported limb to fall about 5 degrees in the frontal plane. The abductor group and tensor fasciae latae are active to counteract the adductor moment. Rotation in the transverse plane occurs as a result of inertia; therefore, no muscle action is required.[14]

The hip flexors fire concentrically before toe-off to accelerate the thigh as well as to create a flexion force at the knee. In the frontal plane, the hip abductors become inactive as body weight is transferred rapidly to the opposite limb. In the transverse plane, the pelvis of the trailing limb rotates forward as the contralateral thigh externally rotates.

Knee Joint

The knee joint is composed of the femur, tibia, patella, and related structures, and it is the largest joint in the human body. The knee is considered to be a compound joint. The articular surfaces between the femoral and the tibial condyles are not congruent; however, the presence of cartilaginous menisci assists in adapting the opposing surfaces. The lateral condylar joint surface is almost circular, whereas the medial condylar surface is larger, more oval, elongated anteroposteriorly, and curved. The movements that take place at the knee joint are a result of the unique shape of the articular facets. Close-packing, or maximum congruency of the joint surfaces, is obtained when the knee joint approaches full extension.[15]

Active motion about the knee joint includes flexion, extension, internal rotation, and external rotation. Although flexion and extension are by far the largest ranges of motion, there are two reasons why the knee joint is not a true hinge joint. First, the axis of motion is not fixed. As a result of the spiral configuration of the femoral condyles, the axis shifts in a superior and anterior direction during extension of the leg on the thigh and in an inferior and posterior direction with leg flexion. Second, when the foot is on the ground, the final 30 degrees of knee extension is associated with medial rotation of the femur due to the shape of the joint structures. Therefore, the first 30 degrees of knee flexion exhibit lateral rota-

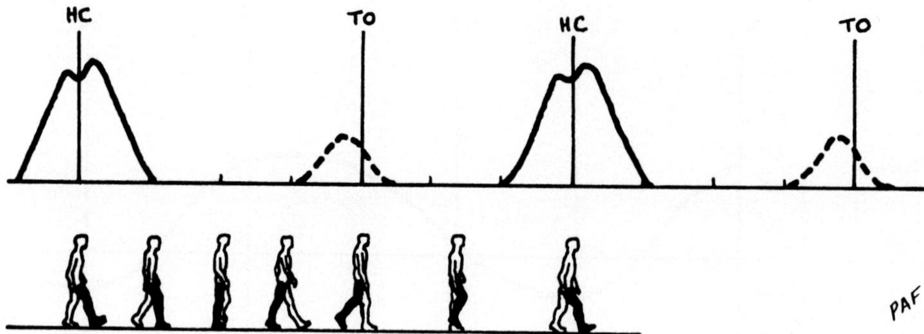

FIGURE 5–10. Phasic activity of the hamstrings. (From Sgarlato T: Compendium of Podiatric Biomechanics. San Francisco, California College of Podiatric Medicine, 1971, p 140.)

tion of the femur when the foot is planted on the ground. In open kinetic chain motion, which occurs when the foot is off the ground, the tibia rotates laterally with the last 30 degrees of knee extension and medially during the first 30 degrees of flexion. The end points of knee joint range of motion for flexion and extension are from approximately 120 to 140 degrees of flexion (maximum flexion depends on hip position) to 5 to 10 degrees of hyperextension. The amount of transverse-plane rotation about the knee joint during gait is approximately 20 degrees. During the later stages of knee extension, the femur rotates medially on the tibia, providing a locking mechanism and increased stability in the joint. Full extension of the knee joint causes maximum compression, surface contact, and congruency between the articular surfaces of the tibia and femur. In addition, maximum tautness and spiralization of the ligaments occur to support the knee joint. Flexion of the knee joint produces a reversal of the events seen in extension. Electromyographic studies have indicated the importance of contraction of the popliteus muscle in bringing about smooth flexion of the joint while avoiding traumatic compression of the menisci.[15]

Muscles that cross the knee joint have a profound effect on joint function during gait. The quadriceps are active only during the early part of the stance phase during walking. The function of this muscle group is to decelerate flexion of the knee joint. When the center of mass passes anterior to the knee joint, the quadriceps muscle activity falls to zero. During running or high-velocity walking, the knee joint extensors may actively contract to initiate knee joint extension after toe-off, as well as to prevent abnormal knee joint flexion. The hamstrings become active at the end of swing phase and decelerate extension at the knee joint. Depending on the speed of walking, the hamstrings may be slightly active during toe-off to assist in knee flexion (Fig. 5–10).[9, 16]

Ankle Joint

The ankle joint is a ginglymus, or hinge-type, joint.[15] The axis of the ankle joint passes through lateral, plantar, posterior to medial, dorsal, and anterior positions. The axis deviates approximately 6 degrees from both the transverse and frontal planes as it passes in an anteromedial direction. The primary motion of the ankle joint is in the sagittal plane and consists of dorsiflexion and plantarflexion. A small amount of supination and pronation is present with ankle motion as a result of the joint's axis angle to the body planes. Consequently, ankle joint supination occurs with plantarflexion of the foot, and ankle joint pronation occurs with dorsiflexion

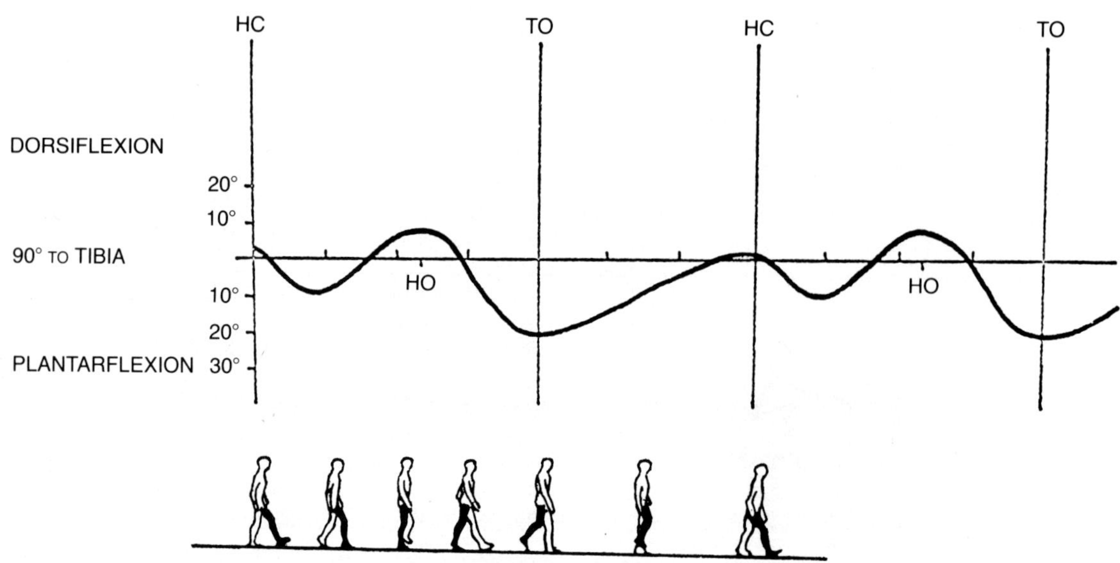

FIGURE 5–11. Ankle joint range of motion (sagittal plane motion) during the gait cycle. (From Sgarlato T: Compendium of Podiatric Biomechanics. San Francisco, California College of Podiatric Medicine, 1971, p 141.)

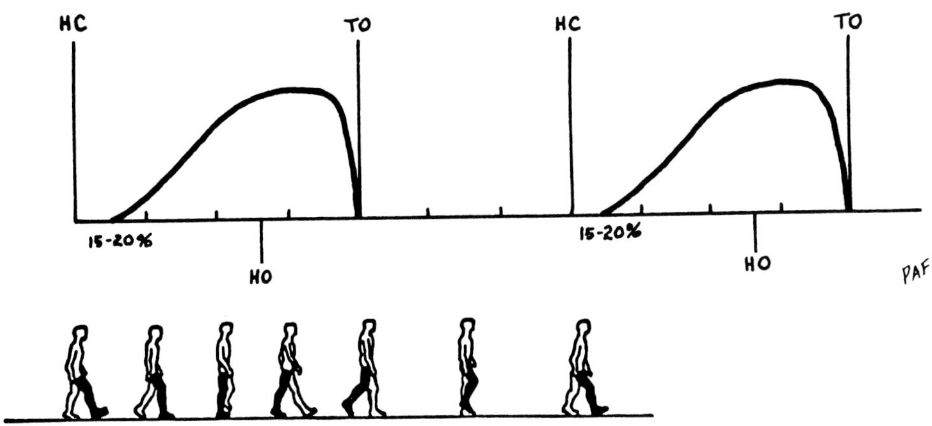

FIGURE 5–12. Triceps surae and posterior muscle group phasic activity. (From Sgarlato T: Compendium of Podiatric Biomechanics. San Francisco, California College of Podiatric Medicine, 1971, p 142.)

of the foot. The range of motion of the ankle joint is approximately 80 degrees. Normal gait requires about 10 degrees of ankle joint dorsiflexion and 20 degrees of plantarflexion (Fig. 5–11).[9, 16, 17]

Muscle Action on the Ankle Joint. The muscles of the lower leg function to stabilize, decelerate, and create propulsion around the ankle joint. The phasic activity of the muscles are coordinated with the joint motion required during gait. The triceps surae (i.e., gastrocnemius and soleus) are active from 20% of stance phase to toe-off (Fig. 5–12). The deep muscles of the leg (i.e., peroneus longus, peroneus brevis, posterior tibialis, flexor digitorum longus, and flexor hallucis longus) have phasic activity similar to the triceps surae.

The anterior muscle group (i.e., anterior tibialis, extensor digitorum longus, extensor hallucis longus, and peroneus tertius) is active at heel contact and during swing (Fig. 5–13).[9, 11] In normal gait, the ankle joint is slightly dorsiflexed at heel contact but immediately plantarflexes as the foot reaches for the floor. The anterior muscle group controls and decelerates the plantarflexion of the foot on the leg. The foot contacts the floor at approximately 15% to 20% of stance. At this point of the gait cycle, the anterior muscle group becomes inactive as the posterior muscle group (i.e., triceps surae and deep posterior group) contracts in an effort to stabilize the ankle and subtalar joints and provide propulsion to the weightbearing limb. The function of the posterior muscle group during stance is crucial in maintaining balance,

because the center of gravity is positioned anterior to the knee and ankle joint axes, thus creating a dorsiflexion moment or force at the ankle joint and an extension moment at the knee. In addition, the ankle is plantarflexed approximately 10 degrees and begins to dorsiflex at 15% to 20% of stance. At heel-off of the contralateral limb at 60% of stance, the ankle is maximally dorsiflexed to 10 degrees, and the leg is swinging forward to bring the body ahead of the weight-bearing foot. Next, the tibia moves forward at the ankle joint. This motion is controlled primarily by the soleus muscle and to a lesser extent by the gastrocnemius. At heel-off, the trunk begins to move forward, resulting in ankle joint plantarflexion. The ankle joint is maximally plantarflexed to 20 degrees when the toes leave the ground. At toe-off, the posterior muscle group becomes inactive, and the anterior leg muscles begin to contract. The anterior muscle group stabilizes the foot to the leg and dorsiflexes the ankle throughout swing from 20 degrees of plantarflexion back to approximately 90 degrees to achieve toe clearance. By the completion of swing phase, the leg and foot are in their proper positions to begin the next heel-contact period.[9–11, 16]

Subtalar Joint

The subtalar joint (i.e., talocalcaneal articulation) is made up of two or three facets and is classified as an arthrodial joint. The position of the subtalar joint axis in space is variable and depends on the relative positions of the bones of the

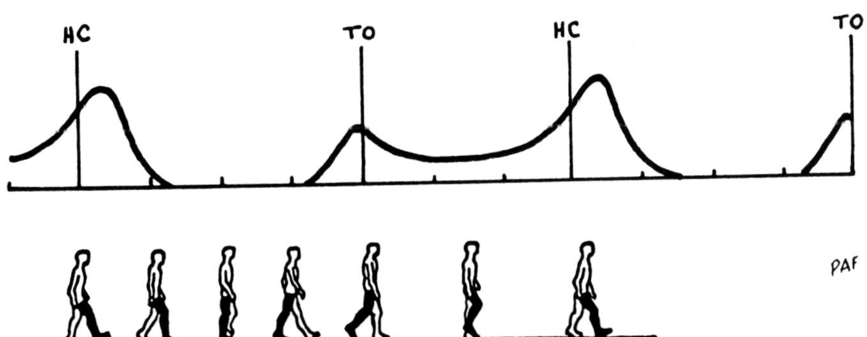

FIGURE 5–13. Phasic activity of the leg's anterior muscle group (anterior tibialis, extensor digitorum longus, extensor hallucis longus, and peroneus tertius). (From Sgarlato T: Compendium of Podiatric Biomechanics. San Francisco, California College of Podiatric Medicine, 1971, p 143.)

rearfoot. An infinite number of axis positions may be averaged to form a helical axis for the subtalar joint. The mean axis for the subtalar joint is deviated 42 degrees from the transverse plane and 16 degrees from the sagittal plane of the foot. The axis begins at the posterolateral-plantar aspect of the calcaneus and exits through the dorsomedial surface of the talar neck in an anteromedial-dorsal direction.[9, 11] Engineering principles state that motion around an axis occurs in one plane, and the subtalar joint is no exception to this rule. However, because the position of the subtalar joint axis is oblique to the three cardinal planes of the body, the bones of the rearfoot will move in an oblique fashion with regard to all three body planes. In other words, movement about the subtalar joint axis translates into motion in all three body planes. The triplanar motions about the subtalar joint axis are referred to as *pronation* and *supination*. In open kinetic motion (non-weightbearing), the calcaneus everts, abducts, and dorsiflexes during pronation and inverts, adducts, and plantarflexes during supination. In closed kinetic chain pronation (i.e., weightbearing), the calcaneus everts, the talus adducts with internal leg rotation, and both tarsal bones plantarflex. The amount of plantarflexion is governed by the stability or laxity present in the midtarsal joint. In closed kinetic chain supination of the subtalar joint the calcaneus inverts, and the talus abducts with external leg rotation. In addition, both the talus and calcaneus dorsiflex during closed kinetic chain supination. The subtalar joint axis, talus, and calcaneus dorsiflex and plantarflex around the ankle joint axis as a single unit. The amount of motion is governed by the mobility or lack of mobility in the midtarsal joint. The motion of the subtalar joint during gait is seen in Figure 5–14. In normal gait, the subtalar joint is supinated at heel contact, and the anterior muscle group provides stability, control, and deceleration to the foot.

After heel strike, ground-reactive forces cause the subtalar joint to pronate and the leg to internally rotate. At this time, the ankle is plantarflexing with supination. Muscle stability provided by the anterior tibialis, extensor digitorum longus, and peroneus tertius is important at this time to prevent excessive subtalar joint pronation. As the foot accepts body weight at 25% of stance phase, ground-reactive forces and muscle activity should be in equilibrium.

At this point in the gait cycle, the contralateral limb starts to toe-off, thus initiating the single-support phase. Consequently, it is important for the stance foot to achieve stability for the body to maintain balance. Inertia created by the swing limb produces a force moment that causes external leg rotation and subtalar joint supination of the stance limb. The subtalar joint supinates until the heel approaches approximately 4 degrees inverted at toe-off. Conversion of stance foot function from a mobile adaptor to a rigid lever is accomplished through supination of the subtalar joint.

As the contralateral foot prepares for heel strike, the tibialis anterior muscle causes the subtalar joint to supinate and be supinated for heel contact. After the contralateral limb strikes the ground, the posterior muscle group of the limb that is toeing-off is no longer active.[9–11, 17]

Midtarsal Joint

The midtarsal joint is formed by the talonavicular and calcaneocuboid joints. The two joints making up the midtar-

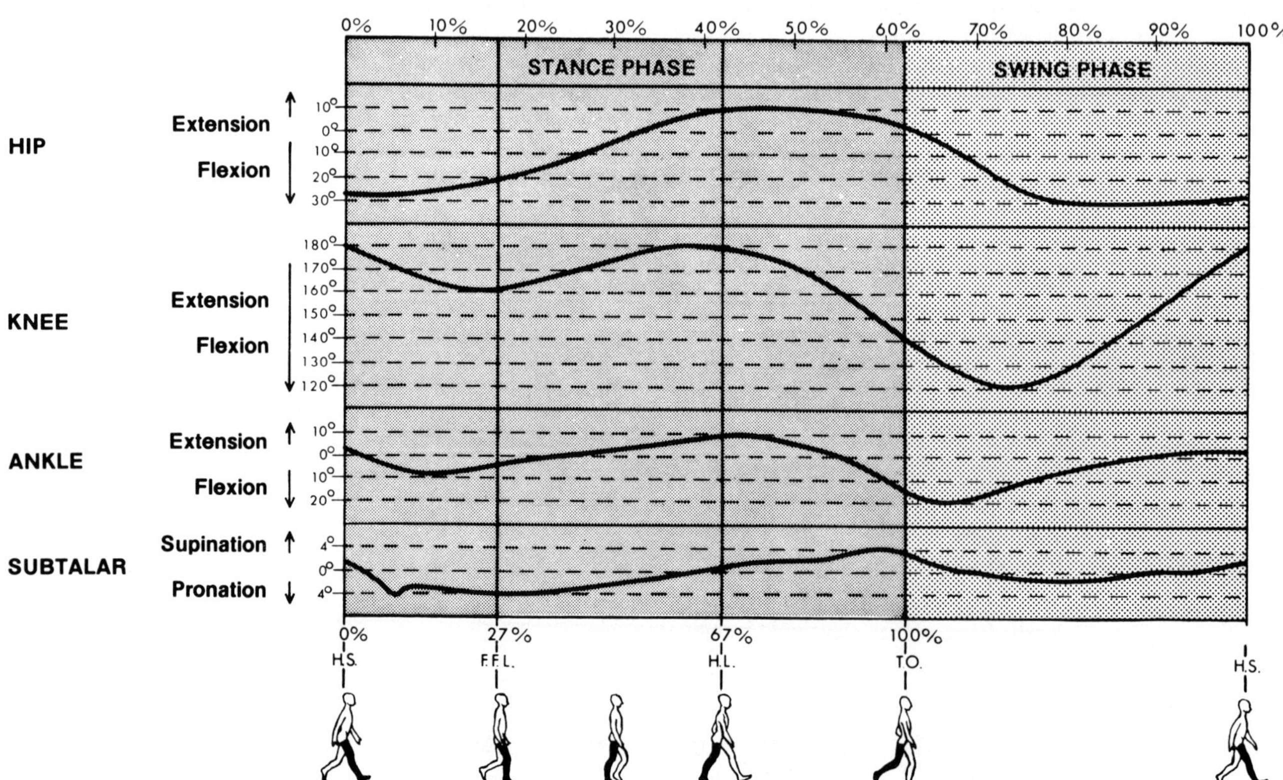

FIGURE 5–14. Subtalar joint and proximal joint range of motion in the sagittal plane during gait. (From Root ML, et al: Normal and Abnormal Function of the Foot. Los Angeles, Clinical Biomechanics Corporation, 1977, p 270.)

sal joint are described as one functional joint with two independent axes of motion. Consequently, one axis may pronate while the other is supinating. The talonavicular joint may be described as a ball-and-socket joint with 3 degrees of freedom, and the calcaneocuboid joint as a saddle-shaped joint with 2 degrees of freedom. The longitudinal axis courses in an anteromedial-distal direction, deviating 15 degrees from the transverse plane and 9 degrees from the sagittal plane. This axis nearly approaches a true anteroposterior direction, creating predominantly inversion-eversion motion. The average oblique axis rises up from the transverse plane anterodorsally about 52 degrees and is directed anteromedially 57 degrees from the sagittal plane.[9] This axis nearly parallels that of the subtalar joint, and the majority of motion is in the sagittal and transverse planes (Fig. 5–15).

The range and direction of motion at the midtarsal joint is dependent on the position of the subtalar joint. The range of motion of the midtarsal joint increases with subtalar joint pronation and decreases with subtalar joint supination. The accepted explanation of this phenomenon is as follows: With pronation of the subtalar joint, the major axis of the talonavicular joint is parallel to the major axis of the calcaneocuboid joint. This allows the forefoot to move freely on the hindfoot without further subtalar joint motion. Conversely, when the subtalar joint is supinated, the two major axes diverge, limiting the motion of the forefoot on the rearfoot (Fig. 5–16).

In open kinetic chain pronation of the midtarsal joint, the navicular and cuboid dorsiflex, abduct, and evert against the rearfoot. Conversely, these two bones plantarflex, adduct, and invert with open kinetic chain midtarsal joint supination.[9]

In closed kinetic chain pronation, the following motions take place at the midtarsal joint: The rearfoot adducts and plantarflexes on the forefoot at the oblique axis. Because the tibia moves with the talus, internal rotation of the leg occurs in conjunction with rearfoot adduction. In addition, the longitudinal axis supinates in response to eversion of the calcaneus, thus allowing the forefoot to remain parallel with the ground.

At heel contact the forefoot is supinated around the longitudinal axis primarily owing to the action of the anterior tibial muscle. The oblique axis is maximally pronated but is in a relatively supinated position owing to the supinated position of the subtalar joint.[18] Once the forefoot contacts the floor, ground reactive force places a strong pronation force against both midtarsal joint axes. However, eccentric contraction of the anterior tibial muscle decelerates the pronation around the longitudinal axis so that the metatarsal heads can contact the ground smoothly from lateral to medial. At the end of contact period the subtalar joint is left approximately 4 degrees pronated, and the oblique axis is maximally pronated. The longitudinal axis is still supinated, permitting the forefoot to remain in full contact with the ground. The posterior tibial muscle is firing eccentrically to pronate the oblique axis and decelerate subtalar joint pronation.[13]

Forward swing of the contralateral leg causes resupination

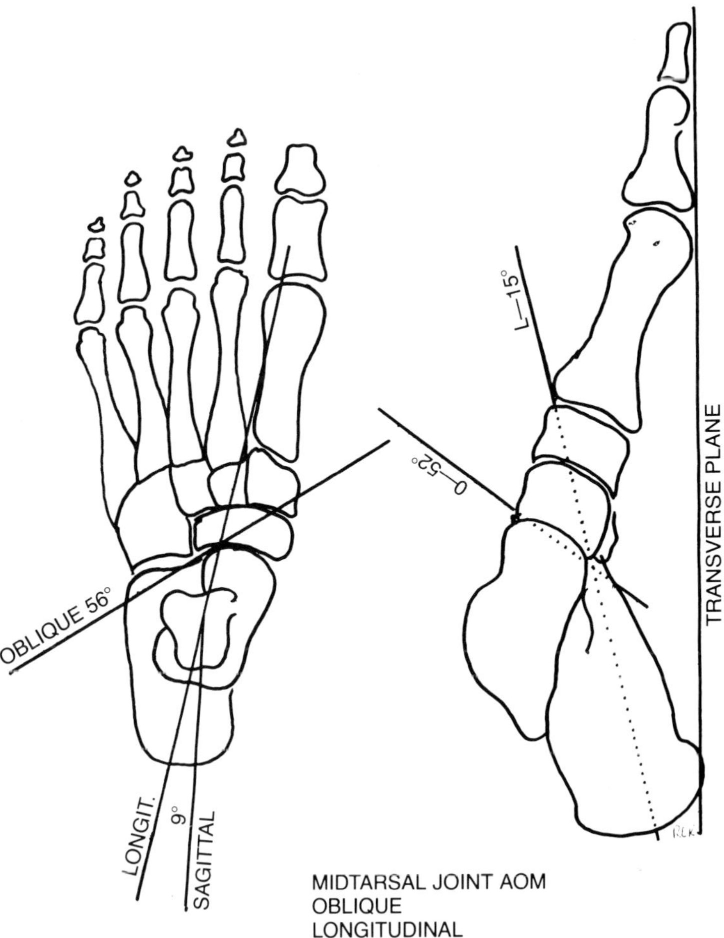

FIGURE 5–15. Diagram of the midtarsal joint axis. (From Sgarlato T: Compendium of Podiatric Biomechanics. San Francisco, California College of Podiatric Medicine, 1971, p 69.)

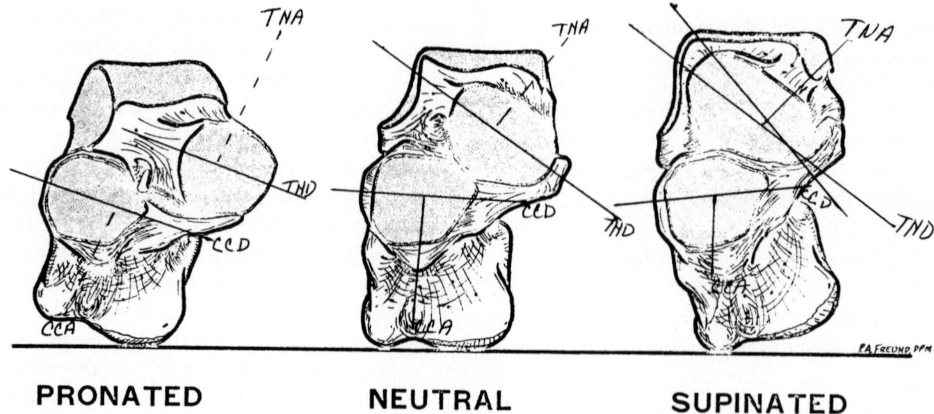

FIGURE 5–16. Frontal plane view of the midtarsal joint and axes. (From Sgarlato T: Compendium of Podiatric Biomechanics. San Francisco, California College of Podiatric Medicine, 1971, p 67.)

of the subtalar joint and marks the beginning of the midstance period.[18] The oblique midtarsal joint remains maximally pronated yet becomes less abducted, everted, and dorsiflexed in response to subtalar joint supination. At this time in the gait cycle, external leg rotation and concentric contraction of the posterior tibial muscle with assistance from the long flexors occur. Subsequently, the longitudinal midtarsal joint pronates to keep the forefoot in contact with the surface, while the oblique midtarsal joint and subtalar joint supinate. The peroneus longus provides the supinatory moment about the subtalar joint, whereas the peroneus brevis counters with a pronatory force to stabilize the longitudinal midtarsal joint during late midstance.

The propulsive phase of gait begins with both midtarsal joint axes in maximally stable positions. The Achilles tendon, which had previously been contracting eccentrically to decelerate the anterior migration of the tibia, now begins firing concentrically. The longitudinal axis stays maximally pronated, but the oblique midtarsal joint may supinate further if the subtalar joint continues to supinate.

PATHOLOGIC GAIT

When types of pathologic gaits are discussed, it is helpful to distinguish between an antalgic versus a short-limb gait pattern. An *antalgic gait* refers to a painful condition that leads to decreased weightbearing on the affected extremity. This requires body weight to remain on the nonpainful limb for a longer period, thus creating unequal timing between the two legs.[19] In addition, the gait is characterized by hip and knee flexion, foot plantarflexion, and excessive lateral displacement of the head and upper trunk toward the painful side (Fig. 5–17). The *short-limb gait* differs from an antalgic gait in that an equal amount of time is spent on both extremities when ambulating.[20] Characteristically, every time weight is borne on the shorter side, the upper body leans toward that side, thus producing a limp without disrupting the timing.

Hip Joint

Alterations in normal hip mechanics may result from muscle imbalance, pain either within the hip joint or elsewhere in the same limb, or other structural abnormality.[10, 21]

At the onset of stance, momentum produces a flexion moment about the hip joint. Under normal circumstances the hip extensors contract eccentrically as a means to decelerate this flexion moment. If the hip extensors are weak, this flexion moment is unimpeded and the trunk falls forward. Compensation for extensor weakness may be achieved by leaning backward, thus increasing the amount of lumbar lordosis and shifting the center of gravity behind the hip joint axis. People incapable of arching their back may require a cane or crutch for support. Weakness of the hip flexors results in a decreased ability to advance the affected limb forward during the swing phase. Compensation for weak hip flexors is achieved by using the abdominal muscles to generate the momentum necessary to flex the swing limb.[10]

A Trendelenburg gait results from weakness in the hip abductors during the midstance period. At the time of single limb support, the abductors of the stance limb actively contract to achieve toe clearance of the non-weightbearing limb through swing. Conditions that bring about weakness or dysfunction to the hip abductors (such as dislocated hip and

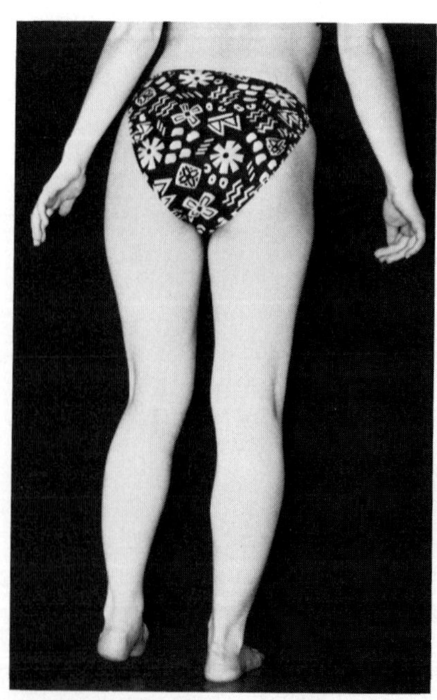

FIGURE 5–17. Gluteus medius limp.

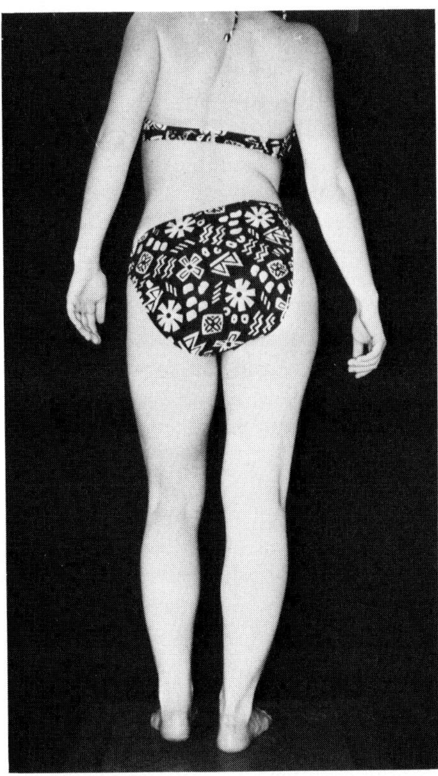

FIGURE 5–18. Trendelenburg gait. Note the drop of the hip on the swing leg due to weak hip abductor function on the stance leg. The trunk leans toward the affected hip to maintain balance.

Common causes of excessive knee flexion as a primary deformity include hamstring spasticity or other soft tissue contractures. Increased knee flexion inhibits normal progression and places excessive demands on the ankle and foot.

Limited flexion may be the result of quadriceps spasticity, voluntary avoidance in the presence of quadriceps weakness, or a fixed ankle equinus. The consequences of limited knee flexion include poor shock absorption and lack of ground clearance. Limited knee extension results from similar mechanisms that cause excessive flexion deformities. One such cause may be related to the soleus muscle. The soleus muscle functions during midstance to decelerate forward progression of the tibia; therefore, weakness of that muscle secondarily causes inadequate knee extension. In midstance, the inability of the support limb to extend the knee places the trunk behind the weightbearing foot, thus requiring compensation in the form of increased dorsiflexion at the ankle or a premature heel-off. In the absence of compensation, forward progression of the limb and body during late stance phase stops. Lack of extension toward the end of swing phase leads to a short stride length and failure to prepare the limb for stance. Knee hyperextension at any moment of the stance phase is pathologic and results from compensation of a deformity at another level. Substitution for quadriceps weakness, quadriceps spasticity, and rigid ankle equinus are the most common causes.

Frontal plane deformities occur during the single support phase when alignment of the body over the knee joint deter-

muscular dystrophies) cause a noticeable downward drop of the contralateral hip. In addition, the trunk will lean toward the weakened stance limb to maintain balance (Fig. 5–18).[22, 23]

When the hip abductors (iliotibial band or gluteus medius muscle) are shortened or contracted, a gait pattern results that avoids any hip drop in the contralateral swing leg. This type of walking style is referred to as a *gluteus medius limp* and differs from a Trendelenberg gait by the rise of the hip on the non-weightbearing limb (see Fig. 5–17).[21]

Knee Joint

Pathologic conditions may affect the knee joint in gait by causing problems related to inadequate extension or flexion, hyperextension or excessive flexion, or a varus or valgus attitude. When investigating knee dysfunction, it is important to differentiate primary disorders from compensatory changes. In addition, certain conditions cause characteristic gait changes at particular times within the gait cycle. The ability of the knee joint to flex and extend with some amount of rotation is essential in keeping with a smooth, coordinated walking style. Knee flexion is required at heel contact for shock absorption and during early swing for toe clearance. Likewise, extension of the knee joint is required during late swing phase to prepare the extremity for contact phase and during midstance to assist in toe clearance of the contralateral limb.

Excessive knee flexion at heel contact is the result of a primary deformity, but when seen during swing is usually a compensatory mechanism (i.e., steppage gait) (Fig. 5–19).

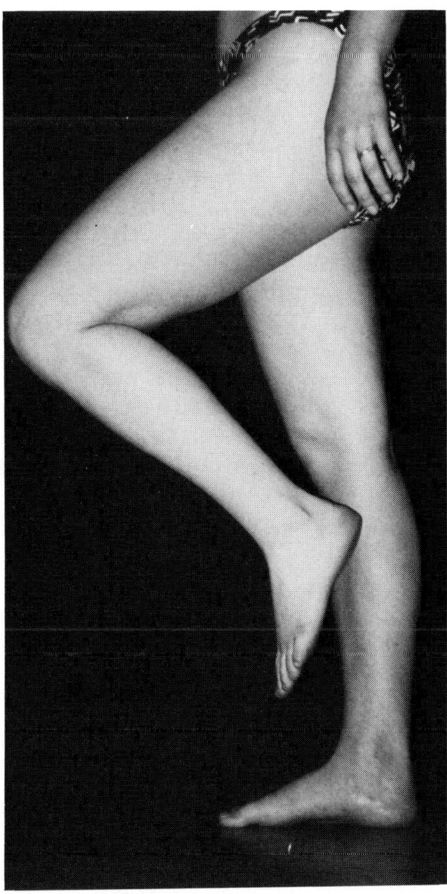

FIGURE 5–19. Steppage gait.

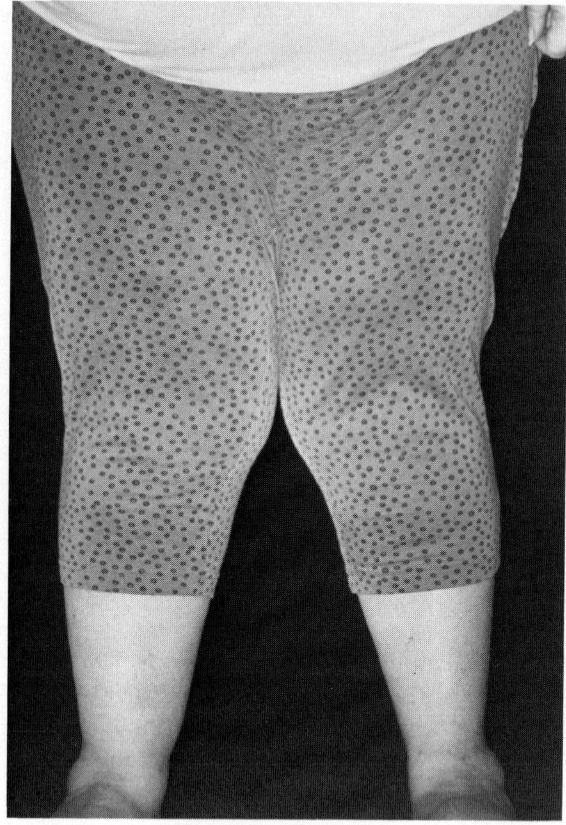

FIGURE 5–20. Genu valgum.

mines which soft tissues are stressed. Unlike sagittal plane knee abnormalities, all frontal plane knee deformities are compensatory in nature. Genu valgum is caused by excessive lateral deviation of the trunk or valgus instability of the foot. These situations are common in patients with hip abductor weakness or rheumatoid arthritis. Varus knee deformity is less common and may be due to a developmental malalignment, osteoarthritis of the knee, or postural compensation for quadriceps weakness (Fig. 5–20).[10, 21]

Ankle Joint

Numerous disease states affect the muscles acting on the ankle joint. These diseases involve the upper motor neurons, lower motor neurons, cerebellum, basal ganglia, spinal cord, nerve root and peripheral nerve, myoneural junction, and primary muscle diseases. Alterations in muscle function cause characteristic changes during gait.

The three groups of leg muscles that may be affected are the (1) posterior group, which is subdivided into the superficial posterior group (i.e., gastrocnemius and soleus) and deep posterior group (i.e., flexor digitorum longus, flexor hallucis longus, and posterior tibialis); (2) anterior group (i.e., extensor digitorum longus, extensor hallucis longus, tibialis anterior, and peroneus tertius); and (3) lateral group (i.e., peroneus longus and peroneus brevis). Phasic activities for these muscle groups were discussed under normal gait.

The superficial posterior group is responsible for approximately 70% of propulsive activity generated by ankle plantarflexion. The gastrocnemius-soleus muscle group also contributes to stability by controlling anterior movement of the tibia. Therefore, muscle diseases that affect the superficial posterior group will result in defects of stability and propulsion. When the superficial group is weak or absent, the activity of propulsion is attempted by the deep flexor group, which normally accounts for 30% of propulsion. Consequently, the deep posterior group exhibits flexor substitution, and depending on the antagonistic activity of the other muscle groups, may develop into a cavus foot. The cavus foot forms as a result of the long flexors (i.e., flexor digitorum longus and flexor hallucis longus) plantarflexing the forefoot on the rearfoot. In the total absence of propulsion, the foot will appear severely abducted with the body weight rolling off the medial forefoot, and the foot will come down flat with the knees flexed. Knee flexion and extension will substitute for the lack of propulsion activity at the ankle joint.[9, 10, 24]

Equinus is a commonly seen foot pathologic condition most often associated with the superficial posterior muscle group (i.e., gastrocnemius and equinus). *Equinus* may be defined as a lack of ankle joint dorsiflexion required for normal walking. This condition may be caused by acquired or congenital tightness of the gastrocnemius, soleus, the gastrocnemius and soleus, osseous ankle joint pathologic condition, a cavus foot (functional equinus), suprapedal compensation (i.e., hamstring or iliopsoas contracture), or hyperreflexia of the plantarflexors. Compensation for an equinus deformity results in either the development of a flatfoot, an early heel-off, or both. The early heel rise associated with an equinus deformity causes the gait pattern to appear bouncy. Heel lift normally occurs just before heel contact of the opposite limb.[9, 11] In equinus, the heel rises off the supporting surface either prior to or when the opposite limb is at midswing. In a severe equinus the heel may remain off the supporting surface throughout the gait cycle. The weight-bearing foot plantarflexes at the ankle joint and lifts the body prematurely, creating a bouncy ''up and down'' gait pattern (Fig. 5–21).

The deep posterior group of leg muscles is composed of the tibialis posterior, the flexor digitorum longus, and the flexor hallucis longus. Weakness or absence of these muscles causes the foot to collapse and diminishes propulsive activity. The medial longitudinal arch of the foot collapses within 6 to 12 weeks when the tibialis posterior muscle is weak or absent.

Loss of propulsion and lack of toe purchase on the ground occur when the flexor digitorum longus or flexor hallucis longus is weak or absent. The ''collapsed'' foot comes off the floor from a pronated position and remains pronated throughout the gait cycle. The gait pattern described is referred to as an *apropulsive gait.*

The classic disease associated with peroneal muscle weakness is called *Charcot-Marie-Tooth* (CMT) *disease* or peroneal muscle atrophy. The gait pattern seen in patients with CMT disease is characterized by a wobbly appearance in the leg and foot. The foot is more supinated than usual at heel strike and pronates as a result of ground reactive force. At forefoot loading the peroneals cannot plantarflex the first ray, and the foot further pronates, then rapidly supinates, causing the lower leg to move in the frontal plane and become unstable. The change in direction of rearfoot motion along with leg position produces the wobbly appearance that is characteristic of peroneal muscle weakness. Weakness of the lateral

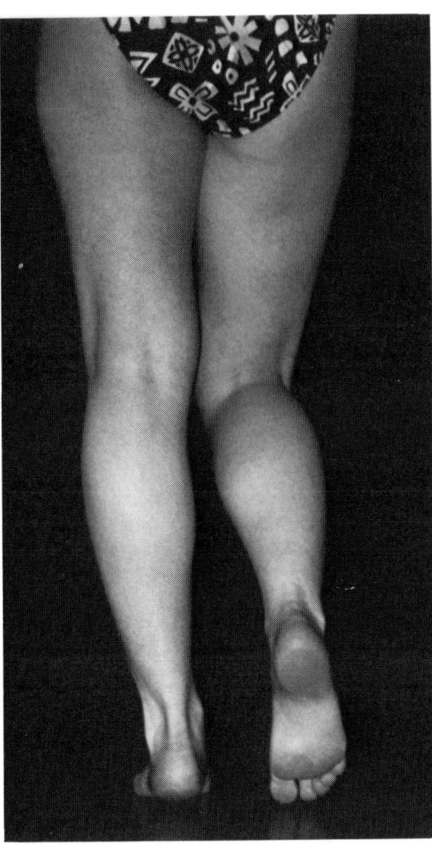

FIGURE 5–21. Gait in equinus deformity. Bouncy, early heel-off indicates that the deformity is uncompensated.

extensor digitorum longus, extensor hallucis longus, and the peroneus tertius. Weakness in the anterior group is seen in many diseases that affect the upper motor neurons (cerebrovascular accident), nerve roots, peripheral nerve units, as well as viral and metabolic diseases of the spinal cord. A drop foot, or equinus deformity, ensues if the posterior leg muscles develop contractures in the presence of a weak or absent anterior muscle group (Fig. 5–22). Compensation for a dysfunctional anterior muscle group produces a characteristic-appearing steppage gait. In a steppage gait excessive hip and knee flexion lift the whole foot off the floor at the end of propulsion. The foot angles down to the floor during swing phase, because the ankle joint stays maximally plantarflexed. The first part of the foot to touch the ground is the toes. This is followed by dorsiflexion of the ankle joint until the rearfoot reaches the floor. The knee extends and the body leans forward causing the center of gravity to move more anterior to both the knee and ankle joint axes. Unopposed contraction of the posterior muscle group leads to the development of an equinus deformity, thus preventing the rearfoot from contacting the floor. Disease entities may affect individual muscles within the anterior leg group in differing patterns. For example, the extensor digitorum longus and extensor hallucis longus are often lost in polio, but the tibialis anterior is spared. The strength of the tibialis anterior muscle along with increased activity in the posterior leg muscles results in an equino-adducto-varus foot similar in shape to a clubfoot.[9, 11] The gait pattern for the equino-adducto-varus

muscle group causes overpowering by the antagonistic deep flexors on the medial side of the foot. The imbalance of muscle function that ensues results in progressive development of a high-arch foot with lateral instability during midstance and frequent episodes of lateral ankle injury.

Hyperactivity of the lateral muscle group may occur in upper motor neuron disease or secondary to pain in the rearfoot. Increased muscle tone of the peroneus longus due to upper motor neuron spasticity causes plantarflexion of the first ray and stabilization of the medial column of the forefoot, thus resulting in a cavus foot deformity. Painful rearfoot conditions such as arthritis and tarsal coalition may result in spasm of the peroneus brevis muscle. The increased tone and overpowering by the peroneus brevis muscle result in abduction of the forefoot with the development of a peroneal spastic flatfoot. The pronatory force imparted by the peroneus brevis causes the foot to remain in a maximally pronated position throughout gait. The foot is lifted straight off the ground rather than rolling off the medial forefoot during propulsion. This apropulsive gait is characterized by contraction of the hip abductors that results in elevation of the opposite extremity. As the opposite limb rises, the corresponding foot is lifted off the ground. At the end of swing phase the limb comes down to the supporting surface, placing the whole foot flat on the ground in a maximally pronated position. At contact period the ankle dorsiflexes and the knee excessively flexes. This results in a waddling or side-to-side pendulum-like gait.[10]

The anterior muscle group consists of the tibialis anterior,

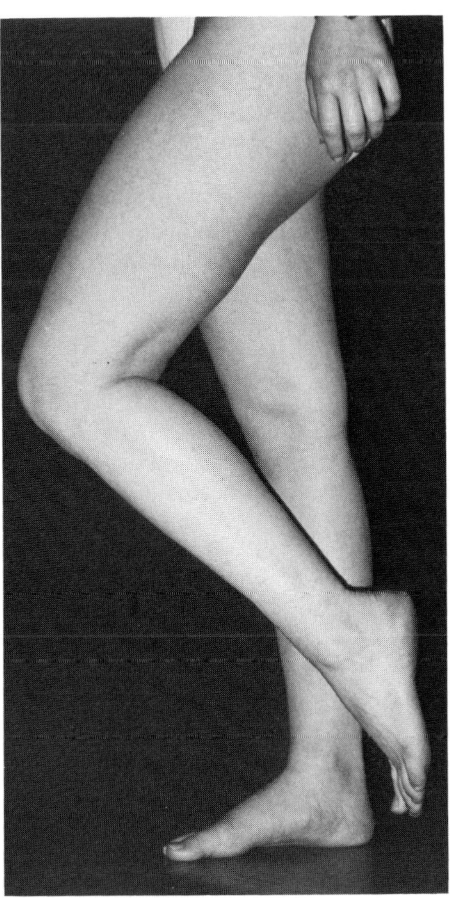

FIGURE 5–22. Drop foot.

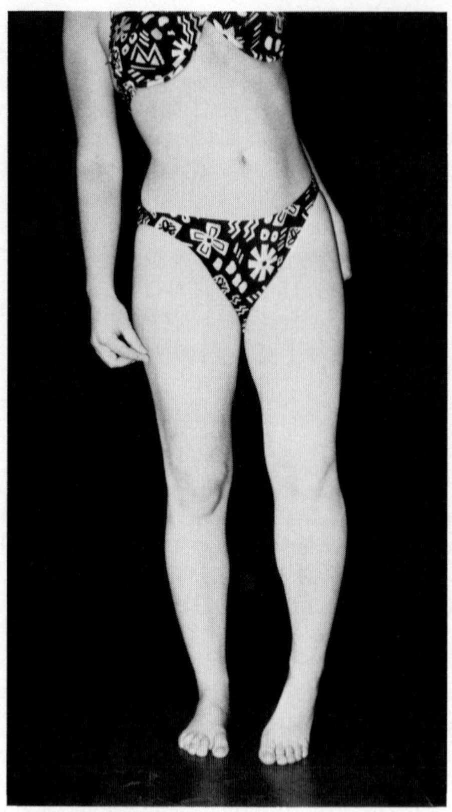

FIGURE 5–23. Toe-to-heel gait.

grees. Motion needed for normal gait is 10 degrees of dorsiflexion and 20 degrees of plantarflexion. The joint range of motion may vary from none to a normal amount. The inability to dorsiflex is discussed under equinus. Intrinsic ankle joint pathology limiting the amount of dorsiflexion available is known as an *osseous equinus.* Loss of ankle joint motion creates a bouncy gait with an early heel-off or collapse of the medial longitudinal arch producing a severe flatfoot. Loss of plantarflexion in the pathologic ankle joint is rare but may be seen in severe trauma or when the ankle has been fused. The gait pattern seen in the absence of ankle joint plantarflexion demonstrates excessive knee flexion along with anterior displacement of the leg.[10, 17] These characteristic events begin after heel contact and continue until midstance in an attempt to lower the heel to the ground. The knee extends and the hip flexes to a neutral position, thus bringing the entire body over the foot. The body weight moves forward, thus resulting in pronation of the subtalar joint and total collapse of the midtarsal joint. The midtarsal joint becomes the primary focus of dorsiflexion within the foot. In severe cases of midtarsal joint subluxation, a rocker bottom flatfoot develops. Providing a rocker bottom shoe prevents excessive knee flexion and provides a fulcrum for the foot at the midtarsal joint. This shoe modification diminishes the force on the midfoot during propulsion, preventing collapse of the arch and secondary degenerative change in the midtarsal joint.

Subtalar Joint

Pathologic conditions of the subtalar joint are due to the same entities as listed for the ankle joint. Joints affected by an inflammatory process tend to be painful, and motion occurring within an inflamed joint aggravates the process. Therefore, motion is limited or restricted by maintaining the joint at the end of its available range of motion through muscle spasm. A painful subtalar joint makes ambulation difficult because ''normal'' walking requires subtalar joint motion, yet any movement by the joint exacerbates the pain. Consequently, a short, shuffling gait develops to reduce motion at the subtalar joint. The entire foot is lifted from the floor, then placed back down following a short swing phase. Limited motion in the subtalar joint most often occurs secondary to arthritis and trauma. Two clinical scenarios may develop when subtalar joint motion is limited. The more common gait pattern results in an increase in angle of gait, decrease in stride length, and an increase in the percentage of stance phase. Body weight moves over the foot in stance, and the person rolls off the inside of the foot rather than propelling off the forefoot. The legs are externally rotated at the hip, and the whole body rocks back and forth in the frontal plane. This gait pattern, previously mentioned, is referred to as a *pendulumlike* or a *waddling gait.*[9, 21] The other gait pattern recognized when subtalar joint motion is limited consists of adduction of the foot to an in-toed position. Forward movement of the torso over the support limb causes the transfer of forces within the foot to the middle phalanges. The force created by gravity acting on body weight travels through the toes from medial to lateral during propulsion. This type of gait pattern is referred to as a *short-lever push-off.* This walking style is also characterized by an exaggerated amount of transverse plane pelvic rotation and forward lean of the body at the waist. The pelvic rotation that occurs

foot is as follows: the lateral forefoot strikes the ground first, followed by dorsiflexion of the ankle joint, eversion of the subtalar joint, and heel contact. The foot maintains a supinated position in stance. The foot comes off the floor as an entire unit at the end of stance phase, thus eliminating propulsion (Fig. 5–23). The extensor digitorum longus and extensor hallucis longus become the prime dorsiflexors when the tibialis anterior is weak or absent. Excessive activity of the extensor digitorum longus and extensor hallucis longus is known as *extensor substitution.*[16] The direction that these muscles cross the subtalar joint axis produces a pronatory force, causing the foot to remain pronated from toe-off to forefoot loading. The position of the foot to the floor is dependent on the subtalar joint range of motion.

Excessive activity in the anterior group is usually seen in spastic conditions such as cerebrovascular accidents and other causes of upper motor neuron disease. Feet with these conditions ultimately develop hammertoe deformities of the digits. A fixed supinated deformity of the medial column of the foot may be seen after a stroke owing to the increased tone of the tibialis anterior muscle. The gait pattern is heel to toe, but the propulsive period is shortened with little or no digital activity.

JOINT DISEASES

Ankle Joint

Different disease entities may cause pathologic conditions of the ankle joint. These include metabolic, congenital, infectious, inflammatory, neoplastic, or mechanical disorders. The normal range of ankle joint motion is approximately 80 de-in a short-lever push-off gait gives the appearance of the whole body moving around the foot (Fig. 5–24).

The muscles acting on the subtalar joint are the same as described for the ankle joint. The subtalar joint axis traverses in an anteromedial-dorsal direction and is angulated approximately 42 degrees from the transverse plane and 16 degrees from the sagittal plane of the foot. The muscles that cross the subtalar axis function as supinators or pronators of the foot owing to the direction of the axis in space. The total range of motion for the subtalar joint averages 25 to 35 degrees. The neutral position of the subtalar joint is located one third the distance from the maximally pronated position, or two thirds the distance from its maximally supinated position. Consequently, there is twice the amount of supination versus pronation available when the subtalar joint is in the neutral position.[9, 11, 15, 16] The supinators include the tibialis anterior and the posterior muscle groups. The anterior muscle group and the peroneus brevis function to pronate the subtalar joint. The peroneus longus functions as a supinator in a closed kinetic chain environment.

Increased activity of the deep leg flexors occurs during the propulsive period as compensation for a nonfunctioning superficial posterior muscle group. Substitution of the superficial posterior muscles by the deep flexor group creates an increased supinatory force on the subtalar joint and, eventually, to the development of a cavus foot deformity. Ultimately, the outcome of foot architecture also depends on function of the other muscle groups as well as the range of motion available in the subtalar joint.

Increased activity of the superficial posterior muscle group produces an equinus deformity. The effect that the equinus has on the subtalar joint is to pronate the joint to the end of its range of motion. The explanation for this is that the foot attempts to compensate for the equinus by dorsiflexing the oblique midtarsal joint, thus allowing the heel to contact the floor. However, midtarsal joint motion is directly related to the position of the subtalar joint.[9] When the subtalar joint pronates, the amount of motion within the midtarsal joint increases, and conversely when the subtalar joint supinates the motion about the midtarsal joint decreases.[9, 18] Subtalar joint pronation shortens the lever arm of the Achilles tendon and increases dorsiflexion of the midtarsal joint. As previously discussed, the gait is bouncy, or the foot collapses into a severe flatfoot.

In the deep posterior muscle group, special attention should be directed to the decreased function of the tibialis posterior. The function of the tibialis posterior is to pronate the longitudinal midtarsal joint, thus stabilizing the medial arch of the foot. Loss of function of the tibialis posterior muscle results in midfoot collapse and pronation of the subtalar joint, possibly causing subluxation of the subtalar joint beyond its normal range of motion. The end result is a severe flatfoot.

Functional loss of the flexor digitorum longus and flexor hallucis longus was discussed under the ankle joint. The resultant changes on the subtalar joint include loss of propulsion, extensor contraction, and hammertoe deformities. Pathologic changes of the flexor digitorum longus also affect the lumbrical muscles, because the flexor digitorum longus is the site of origin for the lumbricales. As a result, the lumbricales lose their ability to plantarflex the proximal phalanges at the metatarsophalangeal joints. The gait changes that result when the deep posterior leg muscles are dysfunctional include lack of propulsion, exaggerated knee flexion, and an increased forward lean of the upper body at the hip to make up for the loss of active propulsion. The subtalar joint is usually maximally pronated throughout gait.

Peroneal loss or weakness has been described under the ankle joint. Reduction of peroneal brevis function results in overpowering by the supinators, causing the subtalar joint to function more inverted at heel contact. The supinated position of the subtalar joint results in lateral instability during gait.

A common clinical entity referred to as *peroneal spastic flatfoot* occurs when a painful rearfoot condition such as tarsal coalition is present. The most common coalitions found in the tarsal region include the facets of the talocalcaneal and calcaneonavicular joints. Other coalitions found in the rearfoot are the talonavicular, calcaneocuboid, and cuboid-cuneiform. Coalitions may be fibrous, cartilaginous, or bony in nature. A *synostosis* refers to a solid osseous fusion between two bones. As a rule, rearfoot coalitions limit the range of motion within the subtalar joint. Limited motion is sometimes accompanied by joint pain that results in spasm of the peroneus brevis. The peroneus brevis attempts to eliminate rearfoot motion that could potentially aggravate the symptoms. The peroneus brevis achieves this function by maintaining the joints of the rearfoot in a maximally pronated position. The foot gradually collapses at the midtarsal joint and fully pronates at the subtalar joint, producing a peroneal spastic flatfoot. The gait pattern is apropulsive with a wide angle and base and short strides, and the foot rolls off the medial border of the forefoot in propulsion.[9, 11]

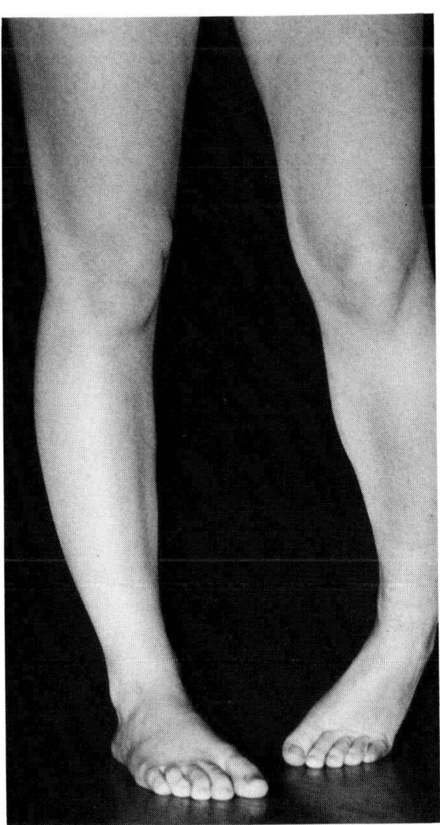

FIGURE 5–24. Short-lever push-off.

When the anterior group is weak or absent, the effect on the subtalar joint is dependent on which muscles in the group are most affected. The extensor hallucis longus, extensor digitorum longus, and peroneus tertius function to pronate the subtalar joint. The extensor hallucis longus exerts the least amount of force about the subtalar joint axis, because the muscle either runs parallel with or just to the side of the axis. The tibialis anterior muscle functions to supinate the subtalar joint. If the tibialis anterior muscle is weak, the other anterior leg muscles will function to pronate the subtalar joint during swing phase. When the tibialis anterior muscle is stronger than the other muscles of the anterior group, the foot becomes supinated.

Loss of the entire anterior muscle compartment results in a drop foot. The gait in drop foot is discussed under the ankle joint and is a toe-heel gait.

Midtarsal Joint

The midtarsal joint serves as a link between the forefoot and the rearfoot; consequently, pathologic conditions associated with the midtarsal joint result in secondary changes involving more proximal joints and vice versa. For instance, equinus at the ankle joint causes the oblique midtarsal joint to dorsiflex in the presence of subtalar joint pronation. Full compensation for an equinus results in midtarsal joint subluxation with a maximally pronated subtalar joint.[25] Instead of being a stable rigid lever, the foot "peels" off the supporting surface during propulsion.

As mentioned previously, posterior tibial dysfunction leads to midfoot collapse. Without posterior tibial function, the foot rapidly supinates around the longitudinal midtarsal joint and pronates around the oblique midtarsal joint until the navicular collapses and hits the supporting surface. The end result is a flat foot that is very inefficient in gait.

Peroneal loss or weakness leads to lateral instability, as mentioned earlier. The peroneal muscles play an important role in lifting the lateral side of the foot off the ground during propulsion. In addition to pronating the oblique midtarsal joint, the peroneus brevis also acts as a brake against the resupinatory force generated by the posterior tibial muscle and the contralateral swing leg. Osseous coalitions involving the midtarsal joint limit the ability of the forefoot to adapt to changes in rearfoot position and vice versa.[26] As a result, compensation takes place at the subtalar joint or other proxi-

mal joints. When pain is present, the rearfoot assumes a valgus position in an effort to reduce the intra-articular pressure in the subtalar joint and reduce symptoms.[27, 28]

References

1. Milgrom C, Giladi M, Stein M, et al: A prospective study of the effect of a shock-absorbing orthotic device on the incidence of stress fractures in military recruits. Foot Ankle 6:101–106, 1985.
2. Nordin M and Frankel VH: Basic Biomechanics of the Skeletal System. Philadelphia, Lea & Febiger, 1989.
3. Soderberg GL: Kinesiology: Application to Pathologic Motion. Baltimore, Williams & Wilkins, 1986.
4. Hall BK: Cartilage. Vol 1: Structure, Function and Biochemistry. San Diego, Academic Press, 1983.
5. Helminon HJ: Joint Loading: Biology and Health of Articular Structure. Bristol, Wright, 1987.
6. Siegel I: Muscle and Its Diseases: An Outline Primer of Basic Science and Clinical Method. Chicago, Year Book Medical Publishers, 1986.
7. Stedman's Medical Dictionary, 22nd ed. Baltimore, Williams & Wilkins, 1972.
8. Rasch P: Kinesiology and Applied Anatomy. Philadelphia, Lea & Febiger, 1989.
9. Root ML, Weed J, and Orien W: Normal and Abnormal Function of the Foot. Los Angeles, Clinical Biomechanics Corporation, 1977.
10. Perry J: Normal and Pathologic Gait: American Academy of Orthopaedic Surgeons Atlas of Orthotics, 2nd ed. St. Louis, CV Mosby, 1985, pp 76–111.
11. Sgarlato T: Compendium of Podiatric Biomechanics. San Francisco, California College of Podiatric Medicine, 1971.
12. Lehmkuhl LD and Smith L: Brunnstrom: Clinical Kinesiology, 4th ed. Philadelphia, FA Davis, 1983.
13. Gage JR: An Overview of Normal Walking. American Academy of Orthopaedic Surgeons Instructional Course Lectures, No. 39, Taunton, MA, Rand McNally, 1990.
14. Perry J: The mechanics of walking. Phys Ther 47:778, 1967.
15. Williams P and Warwick R: Gray's Anatomy, 36th ed. Philadelphia, WB Saunders, 1980.
16. Inman VT: Human Walking. Baltimore, Williams & Wilkins, 1981.
17. Sarrafian SK: Anatomy of the Foot and Ankle. Philadelphia, JB Lippincott, 1983.
18. Phillips R: Biomechanics of the Lower Limb: Principles and Practice of Podiatric Medicine. New York, Churchill Livingstone, 1990.
19. Smidt GJ: Clinics in Physical Therapy: Gait in Rehabilitation. New York, Churchill Livingstone. 1990.
20. Lee DG: Disorders of the Hip. Philadelphia, JB Lippincott, 1983.
21. Perry J: Pathologic Gait. American Academy of Orthopaedic Surgeons Instructional Course Lectures No. 39, Taunton, MA, Rand McNally, 1990.
22. Perry J: Control Dysfunction: I. Pathomechanics. Phys Ther 47:827, 1967.
23. Perry J: Gait Analysis; Normal and Abnormal Function. Thorofare, NJ, Slack, 1992.
24. Sutherland DH: Gait Analysis in Neuromuscular Diseases. American Academy of Orthopaedic Surgeons Instructional Course Lectures No. 39, Taunton, MA, Rand McNally, 1990.
25. Burns MJ: Biomechanics. *In* McGlamary ED (ed): Fundamentals of Foot Surgery. Baltimore, Williams & Wilkins, 1987.
26. Perry J: Structural Insufficiency: I. Pathomechanics. Phys Ther 47:848–852, 1967.
27. Keenan MAE, Peabody TD, Gromley JK, and Perry J: Valgus Deformities of the Feet and Characteristics of Gait in Patients Who Have Rheumatoid Arthritis. J Bone Joint Surg 73A:237, 1991.
28. Locke M, Perry J, Campbell J, and Thomas L: Ankle and subtalar motion during gait in arthritic patients. Phys Ther 64:504, 1984.

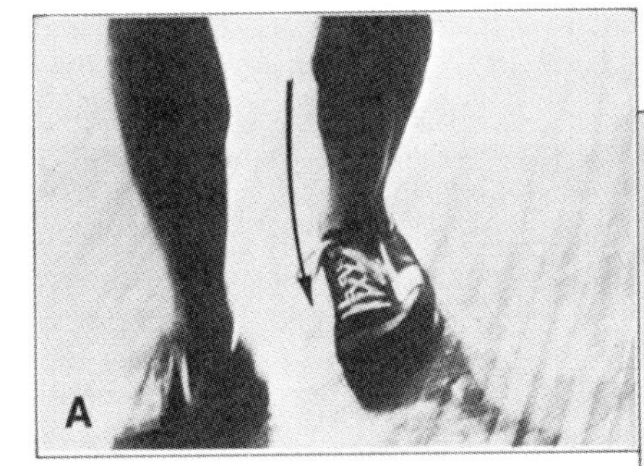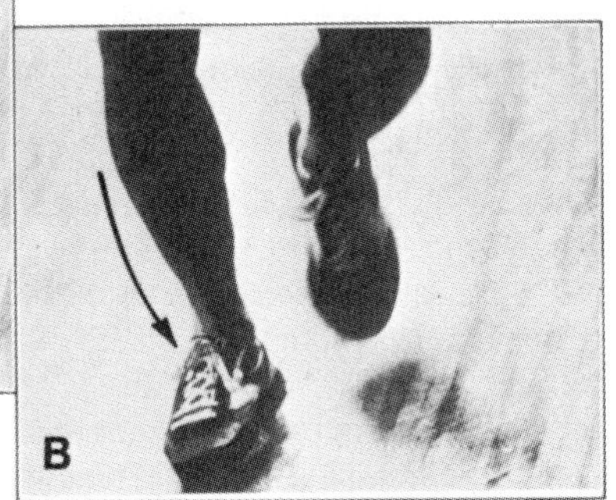

FIGURE 5–27. Schematic diagram of the effect of a banked track on the foot and knee. The downside foot will be supinated, resulting in stress on the lateral aspect of the knee and increased tension across the iliotibial band. (From Kulund DN: The Injured Athlete. Philadelphia, JB Lippincott, 1988, p 444.)

epicondyle. This changing force vector is thought to be responsible for the pivot shift phenomenon that occurs in the anterior cruciate–deficient knee.

The constant motion of the ITB across the lateral femoral epicondyle can lead to irritation and inflammation in this region with repetitive flexion and extension activities (Fig. 5–26). This ITB friction syndrome is seen most commonly in runners and cyclists, although it has been described in skiers, weight lifters, and football players as well.[24, 25]

The etiology of this syndrome is believed to be due to a tight ITB or a prominent lateral femoral epicondyle. However, radiographic evaluation of patients with this syndrome rarely reveals an increased prominence of the epicondyle. Most commonly, a tight ITB can be demonstrated. Factors that tend to increase the tension in the ITB predispose to this syndrome. Thus, any medial displacement of the insertion of the ITB will stretch the band and increase friction across the epicondyle. This can be caused by training errors such as running on a banked track (downslope leg–varus stress),[25] improper bicycle pedal–cleat adjustment (internally rotated),[26] or inadequate stretching of the iliotibial tract prior to running (Fig. 5–27). Anatomic features that can contribute are contractures of the hip abductors, particularly the tensor fasciae latae muscle, genu varus, and excessive internal tibial torsion.

The relationship of foot mechanics to this syndrome is thought by most authors to be related to the effect of foot pronation on internal tibial torsion.[27–30] As mentioned previously, runners with hyperpronation will have an increase in internal tibial torsion during the early ground contact phase of running. This increase in internal tibial torsion will displace Gerdy's tubercle medially and tighten the ITB across the epicondyle. Although this explanation is theoretically sound, it should be kept in mind that no scientific data are available to support this theory or to verify the effectiveness of orthotics in decreasing tension in the ITB or friction across the epicondyle.

Interestingly, Lutter believed that ITB friction syndrome was caused by an abnormal *cavus* foot position.[10] This may be explained by the fact that a cavus foot tends to cause a varus stress at the knee even though internal tibial torsion is reduced. The varus position of the knee stretches the ITB as well and causes increased friction over the epicondyle. It is important to bear this in mind when prescribing orthotics for the patient with ITB friction syndrome, because the reflex prescription of a medially posted orthotic to a patient with a varus knee and cavus foot will obviously make this patient worse.

SHIN SPLINTS AND MEDIAL TIBIAL STRESS SYNDROME

Pain along the posteromedial aspect of the tibia is common in runners. This syndrome has been given many names and probably has multiple causes. Periosteal inflammation at the tibial attachment site of the posterior tibialis[31] or medial soleus muscle[32] is considered by many authors to be the source of this pain. A study by Viitasalo and Kvist demonstrated that runners with hyperpronation may be more predisposed to this syndrome.[33] After evaluating 35 runners with medial tibial stress syndrome and 13 normal runners, they were able to demonstrate a significantly greater Achilles tendon angle at foot strike in the runners with medial tibial stress syndrome, which suggests greater pronation.[33]

STRESS FRACTURES

A stress fracture is another possible cause for posteromedial tibial pain. Stress fractures are caused by excessive cyclic loading of bone either by repetitive concentrated muscular action or by direct axial loading in the presence of muscle fatigue.[34, 35] In each case, repetitive submaximal mechanical insults are thought to result in focal bone resorption, which outstrips lamellar bone formation and results in a cortical defect.

Alterations in the external environment or anatomic abnormalities that increase the loading of the lower extremity predispose to a stress fracture. External factors that have been shown to be important are shoewear, playing surface, and technique.[36] Anatomic factors of significance are foot arch structure[37] and foot alignment[38] as well as body weight and osteoporosis. In normal running, shock dissipation occurs as the foot makes contact with the ground by an unlocking of the midfoot, flattening of the longitudinal arch, and an overall increase in the suppleness and thus elasticity of the foot. In a relative cavus foot, normal pronation cannot occur, which is thought to impair the shock-absorbing capacity of the foot and transmit greater loads to the lower extremity. This may predispose to a stress fracture by the direct loading mechanism.[37, 39]

There appears to be agreement in the literature that a cavus foot is more common in athletes with stress fractures of the femur.[38, 40] However, disagreement exists about the type of foot pattern associated with stress fractures of the tibia. In a retrospective review of athletes with stress fractures, Matheson and associates, using subjective criteria to evaluate foot type, found that pronated feet were more common in athletes with stress fractures of the tibia.[38] The most likely mechanism in this scenario is increased stretch on the posterior tibialis and soleus muscles with resultant secondary overload at the muscle attachment site on the medial tibia. Hyperpronation is also thought to lead to fibula stress fractures.[38, 41] Simkin and associates, on the other hand, in a prospective radiographic study, found that tibial stress fractures were more common in military recruits with radiographically high arches (cavus feet).[37]

Although there is some conflict in the literature, there appears to be agreement that a cavus foot is a predisposition to a femoral stress fracture and that hyperpronation may predispose to fibula stress fractures. Both the cavus and pronated foot have been linked to tibial stress fractures. The lesson is that subtle alterations in mechanical loading can lead to disruption of normal bone remodeling dynamics and result in stress fractures.

CUSHIONING

Just as a rigid cavus foot can lead to increased loading of the lower extremity, improperly cushioned shoewear can result in excessive loads that can lead to stress fractures and knee and hip pain. A study of military recruits demonstrated a lower incidence of femoral stress fractures in those wearing a shock-absorbing orthotic.[42] A later study, however, found that the protective effect of the orthotic was significant only in recruits who had an anatomically high arch and that the incidence of tibial stress fractures was not affected by the use of orthotics.[37] Lutter has recommended the use of a flexible longitudinal orthotic for the cavus foot in runners to improve shock absorption as well.[43] A number of studies have been done using force plates and accelerometer measurements to determine the effect of various shoe conditions.[44, 45] However, forces at the knee can be calculated only roughly, and these methods have not been considered to be accurate.[46]

Although little data are available on the effect of shoe or orthotic cushioning on knee pain, it is a common orthopedic practice to recommend these devices to patients with arthritic knee pain. Shoes with viscoelastic inserts have been reported to reduce the amplitude of tibial deceleration at heel strike.[47] Rooser and associates showed that a 20-mm–thick polyurethane heel significantly lowered the amplitude of tibial impact in patients with rheumatoid arthritis following total knee arthroplasty.[48] In our own practice, we have had only marginal success with this treatment and reserve the use of cushioning devices for patients with mild degenerative changes and no significant limb malalignment. An important factor to keep in mind when prescribing cushioned shoewear or orthotics is the rapid loss of cushioning effect with use. Running shoes, for example, lose as much as 30% of their cushioning capacity after 500 miles of use (Fig. 5–28).[49] Orthotics may decompensate even faster, depending on the material that they are made from.

LEG-LENGTH INEQUALITY

Another area in which a simple shoe modification can prevent or relieve more proximal symptoms in the lower limb and spine is in the patient with a leg-length discrepancy. Minor amounts of leg-length inequality (LLI) are common and can occur in approximately 60% to 95% of people.[50, 51] Although small discrepancies are often unnoticed, the presence of subtle limb asymmetry in situations in which cyclic loading occurs (e.g., in runners) can cause multiple problems.

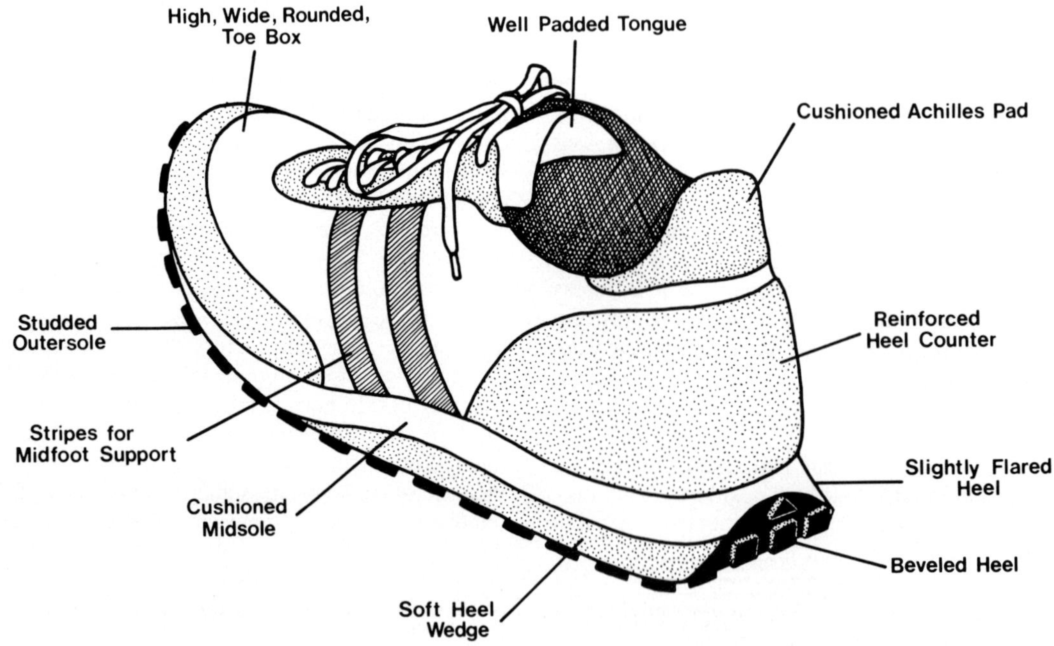

FIGURE 5–28. Running shoes lose as much as 30% of their cushioning capacity after 500 miles of use. (From Shereff MJ: Calzado para el deporte: Modifications y depositerios ortésicos. *In* Viladot R, et al: Ortesis y Prótesis del Aparato Locomotor. 1: Extremidad Inferior. Barcelona, Masson SA, R1991, pp 281–285.)

Typically, the short limb is affected and may experience stress fractures, ITB syndrome, problems related to genu valgum (e.g., lateral knee joint impingement), or medial knee strain. Hyperpronation problems may also occur, such as plantar fasciitis and patellofemoral pain.[39, 41] Other problems that may affect the short limb are trochanteric bursitis, sacroiliac discomfort, Achilles tendinitis, and cuboid syndrome.[50] The longer limb may develop flank pain or degenerative arthritis of the knee or hip. Back pain is also quite common.[50] This constellation of symptoms in runners has been given the name *short leg syndrome.*

True LLI is structural or anatomic shortening of the actual bone length. This can be caused by previous limb trauma affecting epiphyseal growth, fracture malunions, or congenital deformities. Apparent or functional LLI is even more common and may be caused by pelvic obliquity; flexion contractures of the knee or hip; genu varum, valgum, or recurvatum; calcaneovalgus; equinovarus; and rearfoot pronation.[50] A "low talus" appears to be associated with 17% to 50% of patients with LLI.[50, 51]

Identification of functional inequalities is important, because their treatment is different from structural inequalities. For example, a patient with a functional LLI due to hyperpronation should correct the discrepancy and achieve a level pelvis with the talus placed in a neutral position. This patient would benefit more from an orthotic to control pronation than from a simple heel lift. On the other hand, a patient with a congenitally short femur should do well with a simple heel lift, and the patient with genu varum may benefit from a lateral heel wedge. Patients with limb length discrepancies due to flexion contractures of the knee or hip should have those areas directly addressed with stretching exercises or surgical release.

In one of the few scientific studies to address the effect of LLI in runners, Kujala and associates found a significant correlation between LLI and patella displacement, patella alta, and patella symptoms in male runners.[52] The simple addition of a heel lift or buildup of the shoe often relieves knee and back symptoms in runners with short leg syndrome. Gross and associates reported a complete cure or great improvement in 76.7% of runners with LLI with the use of orthotics.[11]

In nonrunners, the significance of a small LLI is less clear. In an evaluation of 247 patients, Soukka and associates found no association between mild LLI (<5 mm) and the presence of low back pain (LBP).[53] Giles and Taylor, on the other hand, found a higher incidence of LLI of 10 mm or greater in patients with LBP (18.3%) than in normal people (8%).[54] In general, most clinical studies using radiologic measurements to verify LLI have found a correlation with LBP, whereas those without radiographic measurement have not.[54–57] Specht and de Boer reported scoliosis or abnormal lordotic curves in patients with greater than 6 mm of LLI.[58] Hoikka found good correlation between pelvic tilt, moderate correlation of sacral tilt, and poor correlation of scoliosis with smaller degrees of LLI.[59] Schuit and associates reported a high incidence of asymptomatic sacroiliac joint malalignment in the presence of LLI.[60]

In one of the more extensive studies, Friberg performed standing radiographic leg-length evaluations on 798 patients with chronic low back or hip symptoms and 359 asymptomatic controls.[55] LLI of 5 to 10 mm was found in 75% of patients with LBP versus 43% of controls. Shoe lift correction resulted in complete relief of symptoms in 75% of patients, alleviation in 15.6%, and no relief in 9.4%. For patients with sciatica, the long leg was most commonly affected (78.5%).

Leg-Length Inequality and Back Pain

The effect of LLI on back pain appears to be related to the creation of pelvic tilt and functional scoliosis, with resultant increased torsional and compressive forces on the spinal motion segments.[55] An LLI results in a compensating functional scoliosis with lumbar convexity toward the short-leg side (Fig. 5–29).[66] This serves to balance the center of gravity. Lateral bending of the spine is often accompanied by axial rotation, causing compressive and torsional forces on the lumbar discs particularly on the concave side of the curve.[55, 62] This explains the increased frequency of sciatica on the long leg side (concave side of the curve). The normal smooth lumbar motion during gait becomes asymmetrical and subjects the lumbosacral spine to repeated bending and torsional forces with ambulation.[63]

Another cause of LBP in LLI may be related to the paraspinous musculature. LLI of 10 mm has been shown by electromyography to lead to a significant asymmetrical increase in muscle activity, which may prevent spinal muscle balance even in a resting position.[64] Similarly, Vink and Huson found that in artificially induced LLI, a shoe elevation

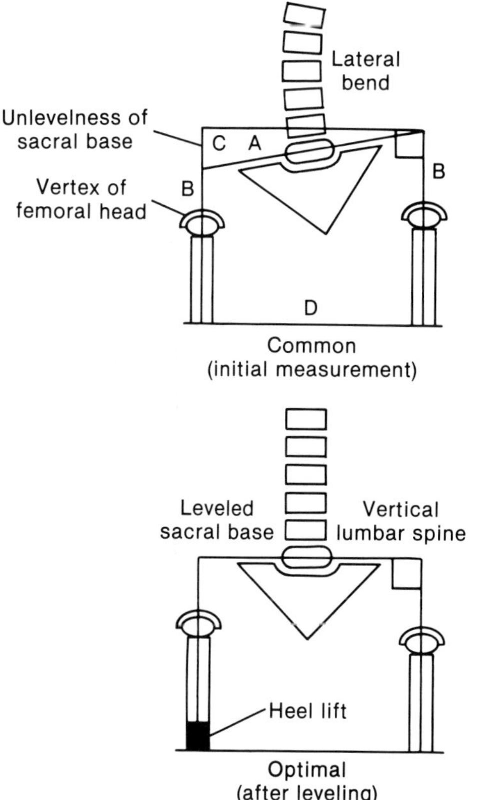

FIGURE 5–29. Leg-length inequality results in compensatory functional scoliosis with lumbar convexity toward the short-leg side that will correct with a heel lift. (From Irvin R: Reduction of lumbar scoliosis by use of a heel lift to level the sacral base. J Am Osteopath Assoc 91:37, 1991.)

of 40 mm increased the activity time of the intrinsic lumbar musculature at heel strike.[65]

Although LLI does appear to play some role in the cause of LB, it is important to emphasize that a small discrepancy of less than 5 mm has not been found by most authors to be significant and that 10 mm may be a more reliable indicator.[54, 55, 65–67] In addition, the accurate measurement of LLI is difficult clinically, and observer error of as much as 10 mm is common.[68–72] Careful radiographic measurement is recommended before prescribing heel lifts for the most accurate and effective treatment.

It is likely that small degrees of LLI (<5 mm) will be asymptomatic in the general population. Runners and other athletes may have a lower threshold for the appearance of symptoms owing to the repetitive loading and may require adjustment of heel height for minor discrepancies.

A number of studies support the benefit of heel lifts in the treatment of patients with LLIs and LBP. Irvin demonstrated that the use of a heel lift can level the sacral base in patients with mild lumbar scoliosis.[61] Interestingly, Schuit and associates reported that although a heel lift levels the pelvis, it also results in increased ground reaction forces that may increase joint stresses in the lower extremity.[60] Most authors recommend correcting only part of the inequality initially to allow the patients to accommodate.[50, 55, 73–75] In our practice, we intentionally undercorrect by 1 cm for large discrepancies and correct half the discrepancy for small length inequalities. Heel lifts greater than 1/4 in. do not fit comfortably into most shoes.[51] Discrepancies greater than this amount should be corrected by additional elevation added to the heel and sole of the shoe to prevent equinous deformity. Surgical procedures to either shorten the long limb or lengthen the short limb are considered only for true structural discrepancies of more than 2.5 cm.

Leg-Length Inequality and Hip Pain

A number of studies suggest an association between unilateral hip pain or coxarthrosis and LLI.[55, 68, 76] Of 254 patients with chronic hip pain, 88.9% had symptoms on the long side. Of 27 patients with arthrosis of the hip, 24 were affected on the longer side as well.[55]

The cause of hip pain and arthrosis from LLI is thought to be related to pelvic tilt. Elevation of the pelvis on the long side causes a varus shift of the pelvis and a relative uncovering of the femoral head in the acetabulum. This leads to a decrease in the articular contact area (Wiberg's angle) of the femur in the acetabulum, increasing the weightbearing load per unit area and resulting in articular degeneration and arthrosis (Fig. 5–30).[68, 70, 77] Of 79 patients with hip symptoms and LLI treated with a shoe lift, 70.8% were reported as symptom free, 15.2% were alleviated, and 13.9% obtained no relief at a mean of 18 months.

OSTEOARTHRITIS OF THE KNEE

Pedal Considerations

Patients with osteoarthritis of the knee typically develop genu varus and, more rarely, genu valgus. With increasing deformity, the weightbearing axis shifts toward the involved compartment of the knee, increasing the load on that com-

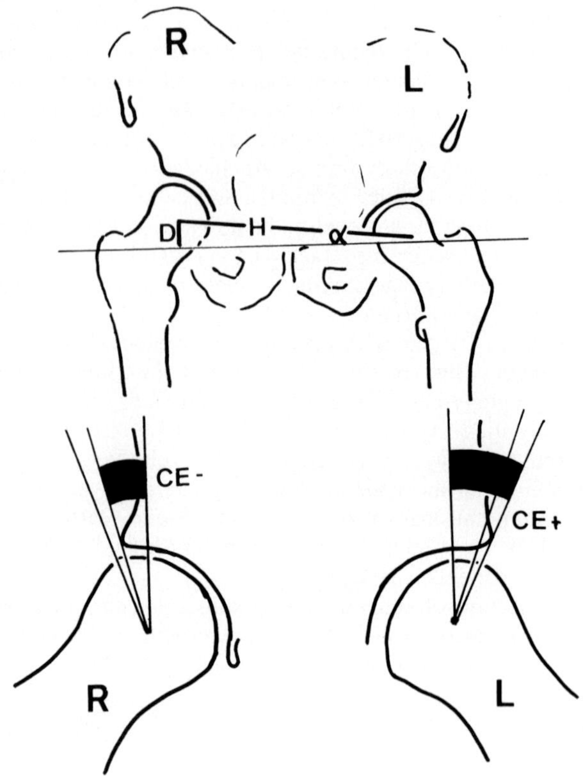

FIGURE 5–30. Leg-length inequality results in adduction (varus) of the longer leg. This decreases articular contact area at the joint, resulting in a greater weightbearing load per unit area and accelerated articular degeneration. (Adapted from Morscher E: Etiology and pathophysiology of leg length discrepancies. Progr Orthop Surg 1:13, 1977.)

partment and causing pain and progression of the disease. Tibial osteotomy and occasionally knee bracing can balance the weightbearing axis to unload the involved compartment and relieve symptoms.[78]

A number of studies have shown that heel wedging can provide similar relief. Tohyama and associates evaluated 62 patients with early medial compartment osteoarthritis of the knee who were treated with lateral heel wedges.[79] At long-term follow-up, patients treated with heel wedges and analgesics showed significantly greater improvement in pain score compared with those treated with analgesics alone, although no effect was demonstrated on the radiographic progression of the disease.[79] Similarly, Wolfe reported good results using a program of heel wedges, nonsteroidal anti-inflammatory drugs, and a simple exercise program.[80] Yasuda and Sasaki found that a wedged insole obtained by prescription was more effective in patients with mild osteoarthritis of the knee than in those with advanced osteoarthritis, with a significant increase in knee score.[81] An earlier biomechanical study by the same authors demonstrated that a 5-degree lateral heel wedge significantly altered the spatial oppositions of the lower limb and changed the calcaneus to a more valgus position, which reduced loading on the medial joint surface according to a two-dimensional analysis (Fig. 5–31).[82]

The use of a well-cushioned heel may also be effective in the alleviation of symptoms in osteoarthritic knees. Normal gait has been shown to generate bone vibration of 25 to 100 cycles/sec at heel strike.[83, 84] Improperly attenuated impact

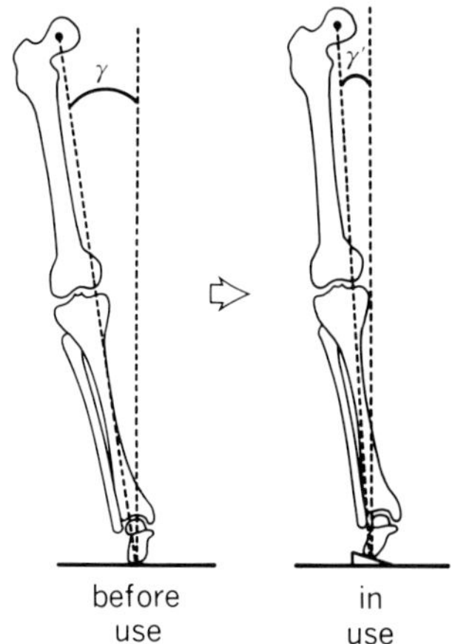

FIGURE 5–31. A schematic diagram of the proven effects of the wedged insole. The wedged insole changes the spatial position of the femur, tibia, and calcaneus. These changes together cause the extended mechanical axis of the lower limb, which connects the center of the femoral head with the calcaneal point of heel strike, to become more upright (decreased angle). Note that no change occurs in the femorotibial angle and that the calcaneus changes to the valgus direction at the subtalar joint. (From Yasuda K and Sazaki T: The mechanics of treatment of the osteoarthritic knee with a wedged insole. Clin Orthop 215:169, 1987.)

loading has been shown to lead to joint overload, microfractures, and degenerative joint disease.[85, 86] Even prolonged walking on concrete floors has been shown to lead to changes in weightbearing articular cartilage and subchondral bone.[87] Rooser and associates demonstrated a decreased tibial deceleration at heel strike in rubber-heeled shoes of 20-mm thickness and recommended cushioning for patients with osteoarthritis or joint implants to decrease joint loads.[48] Using accelerometry, Voloshin and Wosk found a 42% reduction in the amplitude of shock measured at the tibial tubercle with the use of a viscoelastic insert.[88] Clinically, 89% of patients with osteoarthritis of the knee reported good or satisfactory improvement with the use of inserts. In our practice, we often recommend a running shoe with a well-cushioned heel to our patients with mild or moderate osteoarthritis, and we have had some improvement in the milder cases. A soft viscoelastic orthotic would be another option.

BACK PAIN

Orthotics are often prescribed for the treatment of LBP. We have already discussed the effectiveness of heel lifts for LLI-induced back pain (see earlier). The effectiveness of orthotics in the absence of LLI is more controversial.

During normal walking, compressive load measured at the L3–L4 interspace is maximal at toe-off and is related linearly to walking speed and to walking traits.[89] Increasing trunk flexion causes an increase in compressive loading.[89] As mentioned previously, normal gait generates bone vibration of 25 to 100 cycles/sec at heel strike. Running generates force plate values of as much as 275% body weight[39] and generates much greater vibratory stress. Yoganandan and associates were able to demonstrate the presence of microfractures of the vertebral end plates in a cadaver study after submaximal axial loading, suggesting that repetitive loading even below the maximum threshold can be detrimental.[90] Micheli was similarly concerned about the effect of repetitive loading and has cautioned about the effect of dancing on a hard floor surface as a cause of back pain in the dancer.[91]

Recommendations abound for the use of well-cushioned running shoes and a soft track to prevent back injuries from running.[92–94] Basford and Smith studied the effectiveness of viscoelastic insoles in the workplace on 96 women who stand most of the day.[93] The incidence of back pain was significantly reduced ($P = .02$).[93] Tooms and associates reported a similar benefit with the use of viscoelastic shoes in nursing students.[94] In contrast, Garbutt and coworkers showed no correlation between spinal height shrinkage induced by running and complaints of back pain,[95] suggesting that at least in the short term the compressive effects of impact loading on the spine do not appear to be detrimental. We concur with the findings of most authors that repetitive impact loading to the spine can be detrimental, and we strongly advocate the use of well-cushioned running shoes as well as soft running surfaces to our patients.

HIP JOINT

The deleterious effect of LLI on the hip has already been discussed, and the prescription of a heel lift is recommended to avoid or treat hip pain in this situation.

Another area in which modifications at the foot may help prevent hip injury is the use of cushioned inserts for the patient with a rigid cavus foot to prevent stress fractures about the hip. In a review of 320 cases of stress fractures in athletes, Matheson and associates found that a cavus foot was more common in athletes with stress fractures of the femur, although not of the tibia.[38] Runners with snapping hip syndrome may also be benefited by the use of orthotics. Snapping hip is usually due to either the snapping of the abductor tendons over the greater trochanter or, more rarely, snapping of the iliopsoas tendon over the lesser trochanter.[96] Along with a stretching program to increase flexibility, orthotics may be useful to help to control hip rotation and alleviate the snapping.

References

1. Halbrecht JL and Jackson DW: Acute dislocation of the patella. *In* Fox J (ed): The Patellofemoral Joint. New York, McGraw-Hill, 1993.
2. Outerbridge RE and Dunlop J: The problem of chondromalacia patellae. Clin Orthop 110:177–196, 1975.
3. Sims DS and Cavanagh PR: Selected foot mechanics related to the prescription of foot orthoses. *In* Jahss MH: Disorders of the Foot. Philadelphia, WB Saunders, 1991, pp 469–483.
4. Buchbinder MR, Napora NJ, and Biggs EW: The relationship of abnormal pronation to chondromalacia of the patella in distance runners. J Am Podiatr Assoc 69:159, 1979.
5. James SJ: Chondromalacia of the patella in the adolescent. *In* Kennedy JC (ed): The Injured Adolescent Knee. Baltimore, Williams & Wilkins, 1979.
6. Larson RL: Subluxation dislocation of the patella. *In* Kennedy JC (ed): The Injured Adolescent Knee. Baltimore, Williams & Wilkins, 1979, pp 161–195.
7. Paulos L, Rusche K, Johnson C, and Noyes FR: Patella malalignment: A treatment rationale. Phys Ther 60:16–24, 1980.
8. Tiberio D: The effect of excessive subtalar joint pronation on patellofemoral mechanics: A theoretical model. J Orthop Sports Phys Ther 9:160, 1987.
9. Mann RA: Overview of foot and ankle biomechanics. *In* Jahss MH: Disorders of the Foot. Philadelphia, WB Saunders, 1991, pp 385–408.
10. Lutter LD: Foot-related knee problems in the long distance runner. Foot Ankle 1:112–116, 1980.
11. Gross ML, Davlin LB, and Evanski PM: Effectiveness of orthotic shoe inserts in the long distance runner. Am J Sports Med 19:409–412, 1991.
12. D'Ambrosia RD: Orthotic devices in running injuries. Clin Sports Med 4:611–618, 1985.
13. Dugan RC and D'Ambrosia RD: The effects of orthotics in the treatment of selected running injuries. Proceedings of the Sixteenth Annual Meeting of the American Orthopedic Foot and Ankle Society. Foot Ankle 6:313, 1986.
14. Bates BT, Ostering LR, Mason B, et al: Foot orthotic devices to modify selected aspects of lower extremity mechanics. Am J Sports Med 7:338–342, 1979.
15. Scranton PE, Pedegania LR, and Whitesel JP: Alterations in support phase forces using supporting devices. Am J Sports Med 10:6–10, 1982.

16. James SL, Bates BT, and Ostering LR: Injuries to runners. Am J Sports Med 6: 40–50, 1978.
17. Sims DS: The effect of a balanced foot orthosis on muscle function and foot pronation in compensated forefoot varus [Master's Thesis]. Iowa City, University of Iowa, 1983.
18. Rodgers MM and LeVeau BF: Effectiveness of foot orthotic devices used to modify pronation in runners. J Orthop Sports Phys Ther 4:86, 1982.
19. Smith LS, Clarke TE, Hamill CL, and Antropietro F: The effects of soft and semi-rigid orthoses upon rearfoot movement in running. J Am Podiatr Assoc 76: 227, 1986.
20. Taunton JE, Clement DB, Smart GW, et al: A triplanar electrogoniometer investigation of running mechanics in runners with compensatory overpronation. Can J Appl Sports Sci 10:104, 1985.
21. Cavanagh PR, Clarke T, Williams K, and Kalenak A: An evaluation of the effect of orthotics on force distribution and rearfoot movement during running. Presented at the American Orthopedic Society for Sports Medicine Meeting, Lake Placid, NY, 1978.
22. Clarke TE, Frederick EC, and Hlavac HF: Effects of a soft orthotic device on rearfoot movement in running. Podiatr Sports Med 1:20, 1983.
23. Grood ES, Noyes FR, Butler DL, et al: Ligamentous and capsular restraints preventing straight medial and lateral laxity in intact human cadaver knees. J Bone Joint Surg 63A:1257–1269, 1981.
24. Martens M, Librecht P, and Burssens A: Surgical treatment of the iliotibial band friction syndrome. Am J Sports Med 17:651–654, 1989.
25. Orava S: Iliotibial band friction syndrome in athletes. Br J Sports Med 12:69, 1978.
26. Holmes J, Pruitt A, and Whalen N: Iliotibial band syndrome in the cyclist. Orthop Trans J Bone Joint Surg 16:45, 1992.
27. McNicol K, Tauton JE, and Clement DB: Iliotibial band friction syndrome in athletes. Can J Appl Sports Sci 6:76–80, 1981.
28. Sutker AN, Jackson DW, and Pagliano JW: Iliotibial band syndrome in distance runners. Phys Sports Med 9:69–73, 1981.
29. Lindenberg G, Pinshaw R, and Noakes TD: Iliotibial band friction syndrome in runners. Phys Sports Med 12:118–130, 1984.
30. Noble CA: Iliotibial band friction syndrome in runners. Am J Sports Med 8:232–234, 1980.
31. Mubarak SJ, Gould RN, Fon Lee Y, et al: The medial tibial stress syndrome: A cause of shin splints. Am J Sports Med 10:201–205, 1982.
32. Michael RH and Holder LE: The soleus syndrome. Am J Sports Med 13:87–94, 1985.
33. Viitasalo JT and Kvist M: Some biomechanical aspects of the foot and ankle in athletes, with and without shin splints. Am J Sports Med 11:125–130, 1983.
34. Stanitski CL, McMaster JH, and Scranton PE: On the nature of stress fractures. Am J Sports Med 6:391–396, 1978.
35. Clement DB: Tibial stress syndrome. Athletes J Sports Med 2:81–85, 1974.
36. Cook SD, Brinker MR, and Poche M: Running shoes: Their relationship to running injuries. Sports Med 10:1–8, 1990.
37. Simkin A, Leichter I, Giladi M, et al: Combined effect of foot arch structure and an orthotic device on stress fracture. Foot Ankle 10:25–29, 1989.
38. Matheson GO, Clement DB, Mckenzie DC, et al: Stress fractures in athletes: A study of 320 cases. Am J Sports Med 15:46–58, 1987.
39. Mann RA, Baxter DE, and Lutter LD: Running symposium. Foot Ankle 1:190–223, 1981.
40. Cornwell G: Sports medicine and the pes cavus foot. Br Columbia Med J 26:573–574, 1984.
41. Baxter DE: Running injuries. In Jahss MH: Disorders of the Foot. Philadelphia, WB Saunders, 1991, pp 2446–2465.
42. Milgrom C, Giladi M, Kashtan H, et al: A prospective study of the effect of a shock-absorbing orthotic device on the incidence of stress fractures among Israeli infantry recruits. Foot Ankle 6:101–104, 1985.
43. Lutter LD: Cavus foot in runners. Foot Ankle 1:225–228, 1981.
44. Nigg BM: Biomechanical aspects of running. In Nigg BM (ed): Biomechanics of Running Shoes. Champaign, IL, Human Kinetic Publishers, 1986.
45. Clarke TE, Frederick EC, and Cooper LB: Effect of shoe cushioning upon ground reaction forces in running. Int J Sports Med 4:247, 1983.
46. Denoth J: Load on the locomotor system and remodeling. In Nigg BM (ed): Biomechanics of Running Shoes. Champaign, IL, Human Kinetics Publishers, 1986, p 63.
47. Light LH, McLellan G, and Klenerman L: Skeletal transients on heel strike in normal walking with different footwear. J Biomech 13:477–480, 1979.
48. Rooser B, Ekbladh R, and Lidgren L: The shock absorbing effect of soles and insoles. Int Orthop 12:335–338, 1988.
49. McMahon JO: Proper footwear for play and the fitting of painful deformed feet. In Kiene RH and Johnson KA (eds): American Association of Orthopedic Surgeons: Symposium on the Foot and Ankle, No. 50. St Louis, CV Mosby, 1983.
50. Baylis WJ and Rzonca EC: Functional and structural limb length discrepancies: Evaluation and treatment. Clin Podiatr Med Surg 5:509–520, 1988.
51. Beal MC and Grant JH: Standing foot x-rays. J Am Osteopath Assoc 46:306, 1947.
52. Kujala UM, Friberg O, Aalto T, et al: Lower limb asymmetry and patellofemoral incongruence in the etiology of knee exertion injuries in athletes. Int J Sports Med 8:214–220, 1987.
53. Soukka A, Alaranta H, Tallroth K, and Heliovaara M: Leg-length inequality in people of working age: The association between mild inequality and low back pain is questionable. Spine 16:429–431, 1991.
54. Giles LGF and Taylor JR: Low back pain associated with leg-length inequality. Spine 6:5610–5621, 1981.
55. Friberg O: Clinical symptoms and biomechanics of lumbar spine and hip joint in leg-length inequality. Spine 8:643–651, 1983.
56. Grundy PF and Roberts CJ: Does unequal leg length cause back pain? Lancet 2:256–258, 1984.
57. Hult L: The Munkfors investigation. Acta Orthop Scand 16(Suppl):1–76, 1954.
58. Specht DL and De Boer KF: Anatomical leg-length inequality, scoliosis and lordotic curve in unselected clinic patients. J Manipulat Physiol Ther 14:368–375 1991.
59. Hoikka V, Ylikoski M, and Tallroth K: Leg-length inequality has poor correlation with lumbar scoliosis: A radiological study of 100 patients with chronic low back pain. Arch Orthop Trauma Surg 108:173–175, 1989.
60. Schuit D, Adrian M, and Pidcoe P: Effect of heel lifts on ground reaction force patterns in subjects with structural leg-length discrepancies. Phys Ther 69:663–670, 1989.
61. Irvin R: Reduction of lumbar scoliosis by use of a heel lift to level the sacral base. J Am Osteopath Assoc 91:34–44, 1991.
62. White AA and Punjabi MM: Clinical Biomechanics of the Spine. Philadelphia, JB Lippincott, 1978.
63. Edinger A and Biedermann F: Kurzes Bein: Schiefes Becken. Fortschr Geb Rontgenstr Nuklearmed 86:754–762, 1957.
64. Taillard W and Morscher E: Die Beinlangeunterschiede. Basel, S Karger, 1965.
65. Vink P and Huson A: Lumbar back muscle activity during walking with a leg inequality. Acta Morphol Neerl Scand 25:261–271, 1987.
66. D'Aubigne RM and Duboussed J: Surgical correction of large leg-length discrepancies in the lower extremity of children and adults: An analysis of 20 cases. J Bone Joint Surg 53A:61–69, 1968.
67. Gross RH: Leg-length discrepancy: How much is too much? Orthopedics 1:307–310, 1978.
68. Clarke GR: Unequal leg length: An accurate method of detection and some clinical results. Phys Med 11:385–390, 1972.
69. Friberg O: Length asymmetry of lower extremities: An etiologic factor of stress fractures. Ann Milit Fenn 55:149–154, 1980.
70. Morscher E: Etiology and pathogenesis in leg-length discrepancies. Prog Orthop Surg 1:9–19, 1977.
71. Morscher E and Figner G: Measurement of leg length. Prog Orthop Surg 1:21–27, 1977.
72. Nichols PJR: The short leg syndrome. Br Med J 1:1863, 1960.
73. Beal MC: A review of the short leg problem. J Am Osteopath Assoc 50:109–121, 1951.
74. Beal MC: The short leg problem. J Am Osteopath Assoc 76:745–751, 1977.
75. Heilig D: Principles of lift therapy. J Am Osteopath Assoc 77:466–472, 1978.
76. Denslow JS, Chase JA, Gutenshohn OR, and Kumm MG: Methods in taking and interpreting weight-bearing x-ray films. J Am Osteopath Assoc 54:663–670, 1955.
77. Gofton JP: Studies in osteoarthritis of hip and leg-length disparity. Can Med Assoc J 104:791–799, 1971.
78. Horlick S and Loomer R: Valgus knee bracing for medial gonarthrosis. Orthoped Trans J Bone Joint Surg 16:108, 1992.
79. Tohyama H, Yasuda K, and Kaneda K: Treatment of osteoarthritis of the knee with heel wedges. Int Orthop 15:31–33, 1991.
80. Wolfe SA and Brueckmann FR: Conservative treatment of genu valgus and varum with medial/lateral heel wedges. Indiana Med 84:614–615, 1991.
81. Yasuda K and Sasaki T: Clinical evaluation of the treatment in osteoarthritic knees using a newly designed wedged insole. Clin Orthop 221:181–187, 1987.
82. Sasaki T and Yasuda K: The mechanics of treatment of the osteoarthritic knee with a wedged insole. Clin Orthop 215:163–172, 1987.
83. Voloshin A and Wosk J: Shock-absorbing capacity of the human knee (in vivo properties). Proceedings of the Special Conference of the Canadian Society of Biomechanics: Human Locomotion, I. London, Ontario, Canada, October 27 to 29, 1980, p 104.
84. Munro MB, Abernathy PJ, et al: Peak dynamic forces in human gait and its attenuation by the soft tissues. Orthop Res Soc 21:65, 1975.
85. Radin EL, Parker HG, Pugh JW, et al: The response of joints to impact loading: III. Relationship between trabecular microfractures and cartilage degeneration. J Biomech 6:51, 1973.
86. Radin EL, Ehrlich MG, Chernack R, et al: Effect of repetitive impulse loading on the knee joints of rabbits. Clin Orthop 131:288, 1978.
87. Radin EL, Eyre D, et al: Effect of prolonged walking on concrete floors on the joints of sheep. Arthritis Rheum 22:649, 1980.
88. Voloshin A and Wosk J: Influence of artificial shock absorbers on human gait. Clin Orthop 160:52–56, 1981.
89. Capposso A: Compressive loads in the lumbar vertebral column during normal level walking. J Orthop Res 1:292, 1984.
90. Yoganandan N, Maiman DJ, Pintar F, et al: Microtrauma in the lumbar spine: A cause of low back pain. Neurosurgery 23:162–168, 1988.
91. Micheli LJ: Back pain in dancers. Clin Sports Med 2:477, 1983.
92. Liemohn W: Exercise and arthritis: Exercise and the back. Rheum Dis Clin North Am 16:945–970, 1990.
93. Basford JR and Smith MA: Shoe insoles in the workplace. Orthopedics 11:285–288, 1988.
94. Tooms RE, Griffin JW, Green S, and Cagle K: Effect of viscoelastic insoles on pain. Orthopedics 10:1143–1147, 1987.
95. Garbutt G, Boocock MG, Reilly T, and Troup JD: Running speed and spinal shrinkage in runners with and without low back pain. Med Sci Sports Exerc 22:769–772, 1990.
96. Sammarco GJ: The dancer's hip. Clin Sports Med 2:495, 1983.

CHAPTER 6

Biomaterials: Soft Tissue and Bone Reaction to Implants

Vincent J. Hetherington, D.P.M., and Joyce M. Senick, D.P.M.

A biomaterial was best described by the National Institutes of Health Biomaterials Consensus Conference in 1982. The conference defined a biomaterial as ''any substance other than a drug or combination of substances, synthetic or natural in origin, which can be used for any period of time as a whole or as part of a system which treats, augments, or replaces any tissue, organ, or function of the body.''

Biomaterials may be transient or permanent implants or devices.[1] Transient implants include suture materials, synthetic dressings such as polyurethane dressings, temporary fixation devices that may be the traditional metallic devices or the newer absorbable devices. Permanent implants are implants intended for long-term implantation and permanent usage within the body; these include devices such as joint replacements and heart valves.

The success of a biomaterial or an implant is dependent on three factors: (1) properties and biocompatibility of the implant; (2) health of the recipient; and (3) competency of the surgeon who implants and monitors the progress.[1]

Implants have played a prominent role in podiatric surgery. Examples of various types of implants used by podiatrists are presented in Table 6–1. It is readily seen how biomaterials in various forms have been and currently are being used on a regular basis.

BIOCOMPATIBILITY

The biocompatibility of a material is a description of the response of the organism toward the implant. Prior to clinical application, materials are evaluated for their biocompatibility. Biocompatibility must be evaluated mechanically and biologically.

Biologic compatibility is tested by in vitro methods using tissue culture, toxicity testing, and in vivo testing in animal implantation studies.

These methods are described in detail by standards published by the American Society of Testing Materials (Table 6–2).[2]

MECHANICAL COMPARABILITY

Tensile Testing

The most widely used test of mechanical properties of a material is the tensile test. In this form of material testing, a material is stretched at a constant rate, and the force being applied and the elongation of the test specimen are measured. Materials may also be tested in torsion and compression.

Stress is defined as the ratio of force per cross-sectional area. Strain is equal to the change in length less the original length of the test material, divided by the original length. For any material, a stress-strain curve can be constructed that will show the material's change in shape (deformation), or strain, for any applied force, or stress. This stress-strain curve can be divided into an elastic region, a plastic region, yield point (YP), ultimate tensile strength (UTS), and fracture strength (FS) (Fig. 6–1).

The elastic region of the stress-strain curve is the initial straight portion of the curve where deformation of the material occurs; it is elastic in nature so that the material can readily return to its original shape.

The YP is the dividing point between the elastic and plastic portions of the stress-strain curve. This demonstrates the upper limit of elastic behavior beyond which permanent deformation will occur.

The plastic portion of the curve is that area where permanent, or plastic, deformation occurs. Plastic deformation is best described as a change that occurs within a material so that it can no longer return to its original shape. The change in structure occurs on an atomic level, with sliding of the atomic layers over one another and maintenance of the deformed position.

UTS is the point at which the material is able to absorb the highest amount of stress. After this point, with increased load, the material breaks down and proceeds to the point of material fracture or the point measured as fatigue strength.

The slope of the elastic region of the curve is known as the *modulus of elasticity*. Measuring the modulus of elasticity, or stiffness of a material, allows comparison of different materials to one another and estimation of their mechanical interaction. The mechanical properties of certain materials are outlined in Table 6–3.

Materials can be characterized according to their stress-strain curves. Ductile-tough material, which includes metals, can undergo considerable plastic deformation as compared with a hard, brittle material, such as ceramics, that can resist high stresses but does not have the capacity for deformation. Ductile-soft materials, such as plastics, can withstand only low stresses, but they have a high capacity for deformation

TABLE 6–1

DEVICES USED IN PODIATRIC MEDICINE AND SURGERY

Materials	Application and Examples	General Characteristics
Metals		
Stainless steel (SS)	Fixation	High mechanical strength
Cobalt–chromium (CC)	Pins	High modulus of elasticity
Titanium (T)	Staples	High yield point
	Screws	No viscoelasticity
	AO	Subject to corrosion
	Cannulated	Stiff and resilient
	Plates	
	Joint replacement	
	Metatarsal component	
	Richards Manufacturing Co. Inc. total first MPJ replacement (SS)	
	Biomet (Koenig) total toe system first MPJ replacement (T) (also phalangeal tray)	
	Depuy first metatarsophalangeal surface replacement (SS)	
	Dow-Corning-Wright titanium great toe implant, Swanson design	
	Dow Corning Wright titanium toe joint grommets	
Polymers		
Ultra–high molecular weight polyethylene (UHMWPE)	Suture materials	Resilience
Silicone rubber (SIL)	Absorbable	Low mechanical strength
Nylon	Nonabsorbable	Time-dependent degradation
Dacron	Phalangeal components to total first MPJ replacements listed above (Richards, Biomet, Depuy) (UHMWPE)	Bearing material
Polyglycolic acid	Implant arthroplasty	Exhibits viscoelasticity
Polylactic acid	Dow Corning Wright hemi and total double stem hinged Swanson design (SIL)	Susceptible to abrasion
Polydiaxanone (PDS)	Sutter Biomedical hinged great toe MPJ implant (SIL)	Low modulus of elasticity
Polyurethane	Lawrence design	Frictional qualities
Collagen	La Porta design	
Biologic materials (B)	Sutter Biomedical lesser toe metatarsal cap implant Zang design (SIL)	
	Sutter phalangeal cap, Zang design (SIL)	
	Sutter lesser toe proximal interphalangeal implant double stem, Sgarlato design (SIL)	
	Dow Corning Wright hammer toe implant	
	Weil design and Swanson type (SIL)	
	Dow Corning Wright STA–PEG (Smith design)	
	Subtalar arthrosis implant (UHMWPE)	
	Corin Medical, Helal universal joint spacer (silicone-Dacron–reinforced composite)	
	Dressings	
	EPI-Lock polyurethane foam dressing, Calgon Corp.	
	Mitraflex semi-occlusive polyurethane dressing, Polymedica Industries, Inc.	
	Sorbsan topical wound dressing, calcium alginate fibers (B), Dow B. Hickam, Inc.	
	Duoderm hydrocolloid dressing, Squibb	
	Hemopad homostatic agent, bovine collagen, Astra Pharmaceutical Products, Inc.	
	Dow Corning Wright Silastic tissue expander	
	Absorbable fixation	
	Johnson and Johnson Orthosorb absorbable fixation pin (PDS)	
	Acufex, Biofix absorbable fixation pins (self-reinforced polyglycolic acid)	
Ceramics		
Hydroxyapatite	Potential for applications on:	Good biocompatibility
Carbon	Implant fixation and bone substitute and filler	Corrosion resistance
	Joint replacements	High tensile strength
		No viscoelasticity
		Brittle

SS, stainless steel; CC, cobalt chromium; T, titanium; AO, ankle orthosis; MPJ, metatarsophalangeal joint; UHMWPE, ultra–high molecular weight polyethylene; SIL, silicone rubber; PDS, polydiaxanone; B, biologic materials.

TABLE 6–2

ASTM MATRIX OF DEVICE APPLICATIONS AND POTENTIALLY APPLICABLE BIOCOMPATIBILITY TEST PROCEDURES

Classification of Material or Device and Application	Cell culture cytotoxicity (6.2)	Skin irritation (6.3)	Intramuscular implantation (6.4)	Blood compatibility (6.6)	Hemolysis (6.7)	Carcinogenicity (6.8)	Long-term implant (6.9)	Mucous membrane irritation (6.10)	Systemic injection acute toxicity (6.11)	Intracutaneous injection (irritation) (6.12)	Sensitization (6.13)	Mutagenicity (6.14)	Pyrogen Test (6.15)
External devices (5.2)													
Intact surfaces		X									X		
Breached surfaces	X	X							X	X	X		
Externally communicating devices (5.3), with:													
Intact natural channels								X			X		
Body tissues and fluids													
Intraoperative	X							X	X	X			X
Short term	X		X					X	X	X			X
Chronic	X		X					X	X	X	X		X
Blood path, indirect	X		X	X	X				X	X	X		X
Blood path, direct, short-term	X		X	X	X				X	X	X		X
Blood path, direct, long-term	X		X	X	X				X	X	X		X
Implanted devices (5.4) principally contacting:													
Bone	X					X	X		X		X	X	X
Tissue and tissue fluid	X		X			X	X		X	X	X	X	X
Blood	X		X	X	X	X	X		X	X	X	X	X

From 1989 Annual Book of ASTM Standards, Section 13, Medical Devices, p 228. Philadelphia, ASTM, 1989. Copyright ASTM. Reprinted with permission.

(Fig. 6–2). The area under each curve (force × deformation) is the energy a material absorbs prior to failure, or the toughness of the material.

Viscoelasticity describes the viscous and elastic properties typical of polymers and biologic materials. When a load or stress is applied, the initial deformation is the elastic component of viscoelasticity. The ability to fully recover from the applied force is due to this elastic element.

With viscosity there is no elastic return. When the force is removed, the deformation is permanent. With the continued application of a force, the deformation will increase continuously for as long as the force is applied, and thus is time dependent. In addition, the rate of deformation varies directly with the magnitude of the force.

Creep is the slow deformation of a material over time and under constant stress. It is a manifestation of viscoelasticity. Initially, an instantaneous deformation occurs in proportion to the stress; this is referred to as the *elastic element*. Simultaneously, a slow deformation begins; this is known as the *viscous element*. With a sudden removal of the stress, the elastic deformation recovers, but the viscous deformation remains. Creep has no lower threshold and therefore begins with minimal stress or stresses within the elastic portion of the stress-strain curve.

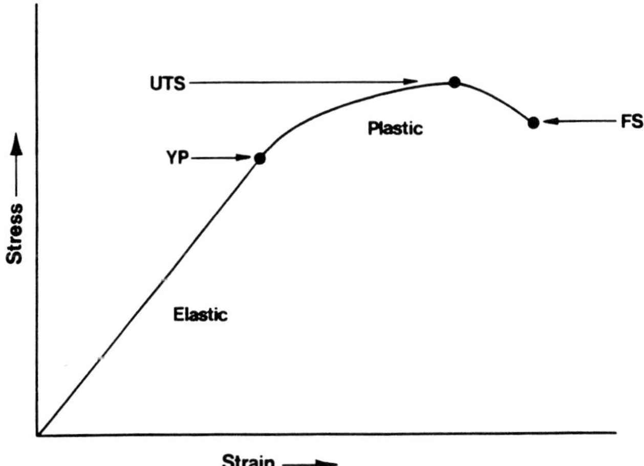

FIGURE 6–1. Stress-strain curve. UTS, ultimate tensile strength; YP, yield point; FS, fracture strength. (From Park JB: Biomaterials: An Introduction. New York, Plenum Press, 1979.)

Fatigue Testing

Another aspect of biomaterial testing is the area of fatigue testing. Certain materials under static load can withstand great stress for prolonged periods. However, submitting the same material to a cyclical load leads to much greater failure, and hence the term *fatigue failure*.

Fatigue failure depends on the combination of the stress

TABLE 6–3

MECHANICAL PROPERTIES OF SELECTED METALS, POLYMERS, AND CERAMICS

Material	Modulus of Elasticity (gPa)	Yield Point (mPa)	Ultimate Tensile Strength (mPa)	Elongation (%)
Titanium alloy 6AL4V	105	970	1000	12
Stainless steel 316 (Aneaded)	200	176	400	45
Stainless steel 316 (cold worked)	200	690	860	12
Cobalt-chromium F-75 (cast)	200	—	450	8
Bone cortical	18–20	—	8–150	1.5
Silicone	0.03		10	800
Hydroxyapatite	114–130		100	0.001
Pyrolytic carbon	17–28		275–550	2
PMMA	2.8		75	3.5
UHMWPE	0.5		30	800
	0.03		10	800

mPa, megapascal (10^6); gPa, gigapascal (10^9); 1 mPa, 145 PSI; PMMA, polymethylmethacrylate; UHMWPE, ultra–high molecular weight polyethylene.

applied and the number of loading cycles. The greater the stress, the lower the number of cycles needed to induce failure. Applied cyclical stresses within the elastic region of the stress-strain curve of a material are less detrimental than those above the YP. Fatigue failure results from the initiation and propagation of cracks. This is especially intensified in the presence of physiologic fluids. Therefore, the testing for fatigue failure in vitro is quite different from in vivo evaluation of strength. Manufacturing of the implant itself or damage occurring in surgical handling can cause imperfections creating focal sites of crack formation and propagation. Consequently, the material may fail even though it is not exposed to its maximal stress. The endurance limit of a material is the stress applied to a cyclically loaded material for 10^6 or 10^7 cycles without breaking (Fig. 6–3).

Hardness Testing

Hardness testing relates directly to the wear of materials. The hardness of a material is determined by measuring the indentation made in a flat surface of material by a known force. The ratio of load to cross-sectional area of the impres-

sion gives an empiric hardness measurement that determines the dimensions of stress. This is especially important in joint replacement devices wherein materials of different hardnesses may be placed against each other. An example is in joint replacement applications in which metal and polyethylene may be used together in a device.

As a result of use, wear occurs on materials. *Wear,* defined as removal of the surface material by mechanical action, can be divided into several forms: Adhesive, abrasive, corrosive, and fatigue wear.

Adhesive wear is dislodging and transfer of a material from the surface against which another material glides (Fig. 6–4). *Abrasive wear* occurs when one material plows through another material more ductile or softer in nature (see Fig. 6–4). *Corrosive wear* occurs at the point of contact between metals wherein an electrochemical effect takes place, leading to wear of the materials. Corrosion may occur in surface imperfections or crevices or may be the result of mechanical damage to the passivation layer, which is known as *fretting corrosion.*

Metals may be protected from corrosion by the process of passivation, which results in a protective adherent oxide coat. This coating reduces chemical reactivity between the metal and its surrounding environment, thus reducing the implant's

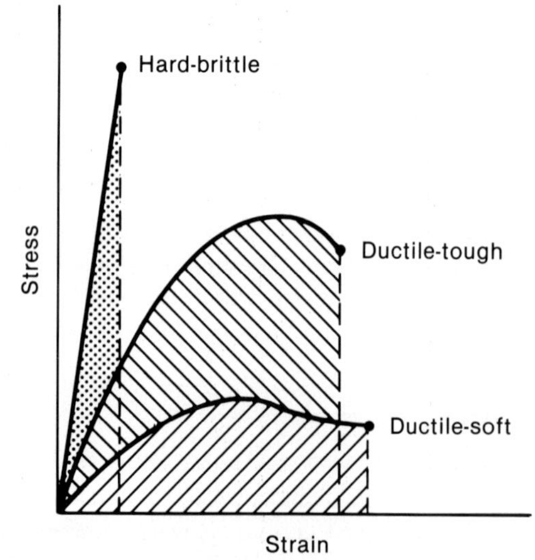

FIGURE 6–2. Stress-strain curves of different types of materials. The area under the curve is the measure of toughness. (From Park JB: Biomaterials: An Introduction. New York, Plenum Press, 1979.)

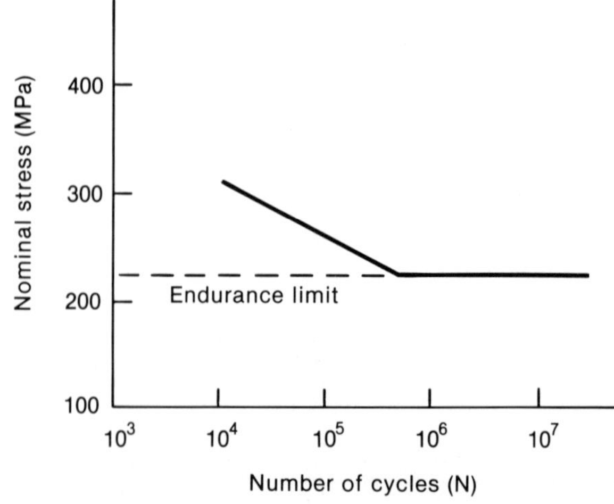

FIGURE 6–3. Typical curve of a fatigue test plotted in stress versus number of cycles. (From Park JB: Biomaterials: An Introduction. New York, Plenum Press, 1979.)

tendency to corrode in static conditions. However, in dynamic conditions motion may disrupt the oxide films, causing fretting corrosion to occur.

For the oxide coat to maintain its ability to function, it must be evenly distributed over the entire implant. Any disruption of the oxide coat, such as the motion of individual components of the implant against each other (e.g., the point of contact between a bone screw and plate) leads to the formation of anodic and cathodic portions of the metal implant. This sets the stage for corrosive activity to begin. The passivation layer can repair itself in body fluids, particularly where there is a high Po_2 level. If the material is unable to restore this passive layer, the metal is then able to corrode, resulting in a self-perpetuating corrosion between the screw and the plate.

Fatigue wear occurs on the surfaces of two materials in articulation with each other under conditions of cyclical loading. This results in surface or subsurface cracks owing to shear forces generated with function, which leads to material loss, fragmentation, and, ultimately, failure.

Summary

The properties of materials are discussed in greater detail in several available texts.[1, 3–6] It is important to realize that no single material is suitable for all applications and that biomaterial requirements will be dictated by the individual functional demands of the tissue the implant is designed to replace.

BIOLOGIC REACTION

A problem arising from the wear of materials is that debris formed can interact with the body locally or systemically. An example is the development of silicone granulomas around particulate material generated from the wear of silicone implants, especially in the hemi type of design (Fig. 6–5).

Metallic implants release corrosion products, some of which are locally bound to tissue, whereas others enter the systemic circulation. Polymeric implants release their components via degradation by hydrolysis or depolymerization, elution, or enzymatic attack. Ceramic implant materials are mainly released by dissolution.

Implanted biomaterials release their degradation products continually and at extremely low rates. Therefore, there is always the possibility of long-term or delayed effects that may be local and systemic in nature and may include carcinogenic, metabolic, immunologic, and bacteriologic disorders.[7]

These products may also enter into metabolic processes of the body. Of the principal metals used in implant alloys, all but titanium and some of the refractory metals are known to have effects on both mammalian and bacterial metabolism.

Wear products may lead to sensitization of a patient to a material.[8, 9] This may be seen clinically as dermatitis or radiographically as an osseous involvement, such as osteolysis, that may be mistaken for osteomyelitis. Allergic dermatitis associated with metal implants is usually attributed to *some* component of the metal, such as chromium or nickel in stainless steel. Nickel allergies have been reported and can be detected clinically by patients who complain of sensitivity to the underside of a stainless steel watch or earring posts.

The method for sensitization appears not to be from metal ions directly but rather from the combination of these ions with a patient's body proteins. During the process of corrosion, metal ions are released into the tissue surrounding the implant. Wear products remain localized in the area or are eliminated in the urine or perspiration. Metal ions behave as haptens and link to proteins, inducing a response shown mainly as type IV delayed-hypersensitivity reaction. Common type IV skin lesions are eczematous dermatitis, bullous dermatitis, and vasculitis.[7–9]

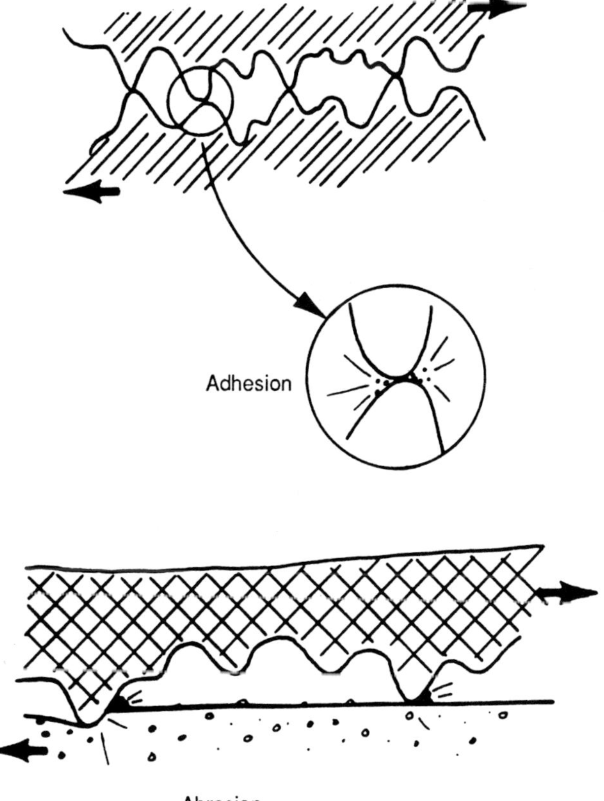

FIGURE 6–4. Comparison of adhesive and abrasive wear. (Adapted from Cochran GVB: A Primer of Orthopaedic Biomechanics. New York, Churchill Livingstone, 1982, p 139. © GVB Cochran.)

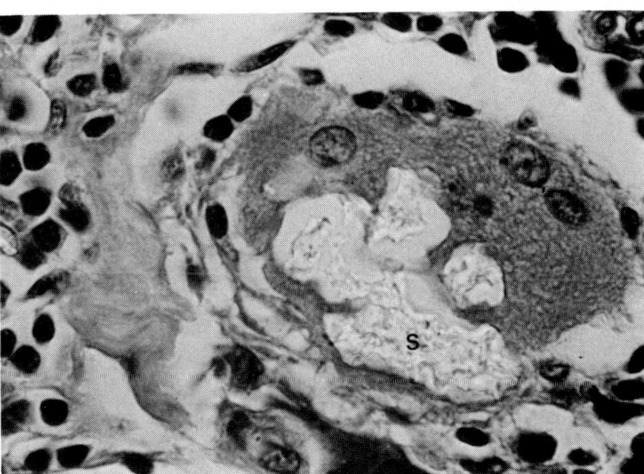

FIGURE 6–5. Histologic section of a lymph node biopsy in a patient 10 years after the insertion of a silicone great toe implant, demonstrating silicone particulate debris (S) contained within a multinucleated giant cell. (Courtesy of David Mazza, M.D., Chula Vista, CA.)

The inflammatory response to implants has been reviewed by Anderson.[10] It consists of acute inflammation, chronic inflammation, and foreign body giant cell interactions. Inflammation occurs as a response to a traumatic or surgical injury inflicted on the body. Clot formation and contraction, which initiate the acute inflammatory phase, are influenced by the intrinsic and extrinsic coagulation systems, the kinin system, the complement system, the fibrinolytic system, and platelets.

Monocytes and lymphocytes are the primary cells of the acute inflammatory phase. Anderson suggested that the accepted idea of acute inflammation followed by chronic inflammation "may be erroneous in regard to biocompatibility studies and the inflammatory response to implants." There is evidence that shows monocytes and macrophages are present at their highest concentrations when polymorphonuclear neutrophils are also present at their highest concentrations, that is, in the acute inflammatory phase.

Chronic inflammation results when macrophages become the predominant cell type. The continuous stimuli from implanted biomaterials and medical devices lead to chronic inflammation. The development of granulation tissue is considered a part of chronic inflammation. Anderson differentiated chronic inflammation from foreign body reaction, which has granulation tissue development, including macrophages, fibroblasts, and capillary formation, in varying amounts depending on the form and topography of the implanted device, the surface properties of the biomaterial, the relationship with the surface area of the biomaterial, and the volume of the implant. Even though a material may be considered biocompatible, the shape or form of the device may alter the tissue reaction and the inflammatory response.

In his evaluation of retrieved human implants, Anderson consistently found the presence of macrophages and foreign body giant cells at or on the surface of the devices. The macrophage, therefore, seems to be the key cell in determining the biocompatibility of an implanted device.

In a review by Pizzoferrato and associates, the following observations are made.[11] Histologic reaction in periprosthetic tissue to polymers and metals involves macrophage and giant cell reactions. Polymer materials such as polyethylene of a particle size of 3 to 5 μm are found in the cytoplasm of macrophages or undergo phagocytosis by multinucleated giant cells (see Fig. 6–5). Large particles are surrounded by fibrous tissue. The intensity of the reaction is dose related. Ceramics develop less of a foreign body reaction than metals and polymers unless they are associated with other debris.

The implant reaction to an articular prosthesis may be differentiated into the following inflammation types histologically based on cellular reactions[11]:

1. Subacute allergic inflammation—eosinophils
2. Subacute infective inflammation—polymorphonuclear neutrophils
3. Chronic infective inflammation—lymphocytes and plasma cells
4. Chronic inflammation from wear debris—histiocytic or giant cell reaction

Their reported frequency, in order of occurrence, is weardebris, infection, and mixed and allergic inflammation. Healing in the presence of debris is characterized by attempts at physiologic healing and disposal of wear particles. As mentioned earlier, wear particles are disposed of by phagocytic cells and, subsequently, reticular cells of the lymph nodes. Particles too large to be eliminated by these processes may remain, delaying tissue healing and propagating reactive tissue. This reactive tissue, including formation of granulation tissue, alters the periprosthetic tissue, leading to osteolysis. The microphage also plays a major role in this process (Fig. 6–6).

MATERIALS

The materials used in podiatric surgery can be metallic alloys, polymers, or ceramics (see Table 6–1).

Metal alloys currently used are stainless steel, titanium, and cobalt chromium alloys (Vitallium). These materials are easily obtained and have an excellent in vivo corrosion resistance. The composition of these metals is outlined in Table 6–4.

Stainless steel consists of approximately 60% iron, 17% to 19% chromium, 12% to 14% nickel, and 3% molybdenum with trace amounts of carbon, manganese, and other elements. There are different types of stainless steel, depending on the proportion of the elements used.

The primary use of stainless steel is in transient or temporary devices. Corrosion-resistant cobalt alloys and titanium are more widely used in joint replacement applications.

Polymers that may be used are ultra–high molecular weight polyethylene, polymethylmethacrylate, and silicone. Silicone rubber is a synthetic polymer (dimethylsiloxane)

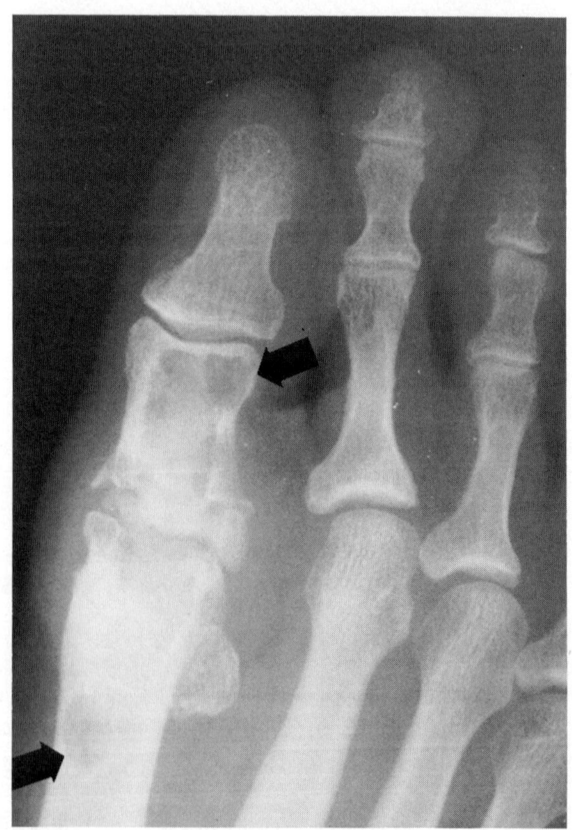

FIGURE 6–6. Osteolysis and cystic bone changes (*arrows*) associated with silicone implant arthroplasty.

TABLE 6–4

CHEMICAL COMPOSITION OF SURGICAL ALLOYS

Stainless Steel F138	Cobalt F75	Cr MP35N	Ti	
			CpTi	*Ti64*
Cr 17–19	27–30	19–21	—	—
Ni 13–15.5	<1	33–37	—	—
Mo 2–3	5–7	9–10.5	—	—
C 08/<0.03	<0.35	<0.025	<0.1	<0.08
N <0.1	—	—	0.03–0.35	<0.05
O —	—	—	0.18–0.40	<0.13
Al —	—	—	—	5.5–6.5
V —	—	—	—	3.5–4.5

F, fluorine; MP, mercaptopurine; CpTi, copper-titanium; Ti, titanium; C, carbon; Cr, chromium; Ni, nickel; Mo, molybdenum; N, nitrogen; O, oxygen; V, vanadium; Al, aluminum.

with a wide range of applications. It is best known in foot surgery for its application in implant arthroplasty.

Ultra–high molecular weight polyethylene is a straight-chained hydrocarbon polymer. It is tough, ductile, resistant to wear, and has low friction and the highest wear resistance of polymers. However, it is also susceptible to abrasion and fatigue cracking, has a low modulus of elasticity, and exhibits viscoelastic behavior and thus undergoes creep.

Polymethylmethacrylate is commonly known as bone cement because it is used to anchor two materials together, usually prostheses into bone. It consists of a powder of methacrylate polymer and a compatible amount of liquid acrylic monomer. The two ingredients are mixed together, and the entire mass polymerizes. An exothermic reaction takes place, and heat is released.

Ceramics include hydroxyapatite, alumina, and carbons.

A composite material is a combination of two or more materials, such that their performance together is significantly enhanced. Examples of composites are matrix material and a fiber material used together. Some examples that best fit this description are resorbable fixation devices of self-reinforced polyglycolic acid, carbon fiber–reinforced plastic for use in bone plates, and Dacron fiber–reinforced silicone.

With regard to biomaterials used in bone and joint replacement, certain priorities need to be addressed. These include the ability to withstand cyclical loading, adaptability to allow rapid fixation of the device, maintenance of a modulus of elasticity similar to bone, and possession of high wear resistance.[12]

IMPLANT FIXATION

Types of implant fixation include cement, direct interference fit, mechanical fasteners, adhesion, and biologic fixation. In recent years, research in implant fixation has intensified with increased interest in biologic fixation.

Biologic Fixation

For biologic fixation to occur, the implant may be porous or nonporous. Biologic fixation occurs by the process of osteoconduction[13] or osseointegration.[14]

Osteoconduction is the process of the ingrowth of vascular tissue and osteoprogenitor cells from a recipient bone bed into a three-dimensional structure of an implant. Biologic

fixation of implants by bone ingrowth has been investigated and applied clinically as an alternative to cement fixation. Porous-coated implants are currently used for hip, knee, and ankle joint replacements. The stages in biologic fixation by bone ingrowth include hematoma formation, cellular infiltration and differentiation, calcification, maturation, and remodeling.[15]

Bone ingrowth for attachment of implantable devices can be accomplished by two mechanisms: (1) macroscopic surface undulations such as grooves, and (2) microscopic interconnecting porosity.

Homsy and associates[16] emphasized that microporosity is an alternative to surface irregularity. The advantages of microporosity are greater surface area for mechanical interdigitation between implant and bone, improved vascularity of the tissues immediately in contact with the implant, and a more rapid fixation.

Homsy and associates also demonstrated that tissue will grow into an open structure with a pore diameter of 20 μm. The depth of ingrowth is enhanced by including pore size of greater than 100 μm (Fig. 6–7A).

Bobyn and associates[17] found that implants with a multiple particle layer configuration developed a greater fixation strength than implants with a single layer. Pore size is important in the fixation of implants by osteoconduction. The researchers also evaluated metallic porous implants of a cobalt alloy in an attempt to determine optimal pore size.[18] Four pore sizes were evaluated: 20 to 50 μm, 50 to 200 μm, 200 to 400 μm, and 400 to 800 μm. Their results by mechanical testing revealed the least fixation to occur with the middle two pore sizes. This range in pore size provided a maximal fixation strength of 17 mPa in the shortest time—8 weeks.

The optimal pore size for ingrowth has been determined to be between 150 and 400 μm. Initial stable fixation of the implant is necessary if ingrowth is to occur. Micromovement at the bone implant interface results in a fibrous tissue fixation similar to nonunion of a fracture.[19] Major factors affecting bone ingrowth include proper design and sizing of an implant, healthy bone, adequate press fit or interference fit of the implant into the bone canal, and the reduction of load bearing in the early postoperative period.[19–22] With a properly designed and implanted porous-coated prosthesis, bone ingrowth occurs in 4 to 6 weeks, followed by a remodeling phase lasting at least 1 year.

Osseointegration is defined as a direct structural connection between ordered living bone and the surface of a load-carrying implant.[23, 24] The clinical aspect refers to lack of clinical mobility, lack of radiolucency around the implants, and a functional connection between living bone and the surface of a load-carrying implant. The histologic aspect refers to a lack of a connective tissue interposition at the implant-bone interface at a light microscopic level (Fig. 6–7B).

Linder and associates[25] studied 25 titanium implants that were inserted into 11 volunteer patients, four with rheumatoid arthritis and seven with osteoarthritis. The implants were removed 5 weeks to 24 months later. The implants were found to be osseointegrated by Branemark's definition. Only one of the 21 implants implanted for longer than 5 months did not show evidence of osseointegration, believed to be the result of inadequate primary contact with bone. They demonstrated that osseointegration can be attained even in porotic bone and in patients with rheumatoid arthritis. They cau-

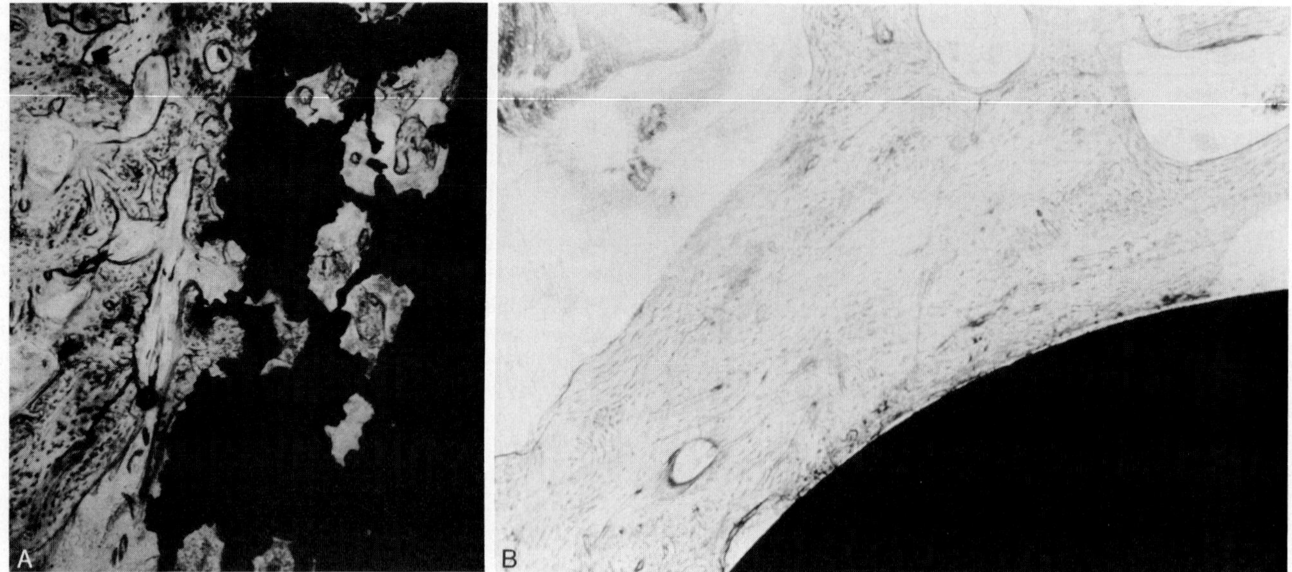

FIGURE 6–7. *A,* Demonstrates fibrous and hard tissue ingrowth in a porous titanium implant. *B,* Demonstrates direct bone apposition to a carbon implant.

tioned, however, that although osseointegrations may occur in patients with either osteoarthritis or rheumatoid arthritis, the bone differs greatly in its ability to carry load, perhaps thereby increasing the risk of failure in rheumatoid arthritis.

The success of implants for biologic fixation are dependent on (1) implant design, (2) anatomic constants, (3) surgical techniques, (4) postoperative management, (5) patient health, and (6) loading conditions.

The last form of biologic fixation can be considered chemical and has been given the term *biointegration.* This is the use of hydroxyapatite coatings of metallic or other materials. Concern has been expressed about the processing and coating of devices with hydroxyapatite in regard to long-term biologic performance, such as its resorption after implantation. Clinical applications of biologic ingrowth include total ankle arthroplasty and first metatarsophalangeal joint arthroplasty.

Flexible or Less Rigid Internal Fixation

A controversy is surfacing about the need for absolutely rigid internal fixation of fractures.[26–29] Several disadvantages of the use of rigid internal fixation have been identified as follows:

1. Elimination of external callus formation
2. Prolonged dependence on a device
3. Slow healing by the process of primary bone union
4. Occurrence of stress-shielding
5. Unreliable radiographic demonstration of healing

Movement, even if it is micromovement, has proved to be of benefit for improving conditions for fracture healing.[30] The use of devices that provide semirigid fixation are under investigation.

Flexible or less rigid fixation is an example of the application of biomaterials for internal fixation. Less rigid internal fixation is based on the principle that rigid internal fixation in the form of plates results in the process of stress-shielding, which may be detrimental to long-term bone healing and remodeling. With increased stiffness of the device, callus formation decreases.

Tayton and associates[26] supported the use of less rigid fixation and stated that "semi-rigid fixation is not only desirable theoretically but also works well in practice." In their study, tibial fractures in sheep using single or double osteotomy to produce an avascular segment of bone between the osteotomy sites were found to heal rapidly with abundant external callus and regain normal strength in 20 and 25 weeks, respectively. They also reported promising results in human clinical trials. The plates used by Tayton and associates were carbon fiber–reinforced plastic (CFRP, epoxy resin), which was described as having the same UTS when compared with osteosynthesis of similar design. However, their fatigue strength was greater and their elasticity, as reflected by Young's modulus, was one third that of steel. Skirving and associates[31] also reported successful results in both animal tests and human clinical trials.

These authors demonstrated that accurate juxtaposition of the fragments is not essential and no radiographic evidence of osteoporosis is present. Unthoff and Finnegan[32] added that less rigid plates permit radiographic assessment of union to allow one to determine the optimal time for removal of the device.

Several areas need to be addressed regarding semirigid fixation with CFRP.[26]

1. What is the appropriate stiffness required of the device for clinical application? Tayton and Bradley[33] reported the occurrence of nonunion with the use of more flexible plates.
2. Stiffness changes in vivo may potentially affect plate performance.
3. Prebending of devices may be a problem.
4. Stiffness of the plates varies, requiring greater standardization in the manufacturing process prior to clinical usage.

The investigation of other materials continues, including metallic plates of less stiffness and other polymers or composites including absorbable materials.

Brown and associates[34] defined flexible fixation as the use of an implant that will maintain fragment apposition and prevent angulation and displacement without shielding the bone from the mechanical stimulus necessary for callus formation. Healing in the flexible environment is by periosteal callus as opposed to primary bone union. With less rigid or flexible fixation, the neutral axis is maintained in a portion of the bone, as opposed to rigid fixation in which the neutral axis is located close to the plate. In the former the bone participates in loading, resulting in periosteal callus formation.

Materials that may be used in the development of less rigid internal fixation include metals and polymers. Metals may be used by controlling the thickness of the plate to allow some degrees of bending, where the stiffness of the device is defined by both geometry and material properties and not just elastic modulus.[35]

With regard to the long-term effects of metal versus plastic, Leo's law is best defined as a bone responding to rigid fixation as "with you there, why should I?"[34] With rigid fixation, there is stress protection and stress transfer. This interferes with the remodeling process of bone governed by Wolff's law, which states the amount of bone is dependent on the need for it. The need for the bone is dependent on the stress applied to the area. The disadvantages of rigid fixation include the elimination of external callus formation, which is a more efficient and stronger method of bone healing, dependence on a device, and the slowness of primary union complicated by stress-shielding, with radiographic evaluation of bone healing being unreliable.

The goal of less rigid internal fixation is to allow the presence of bone callus, which can be detected radiographically, to show evidence of fracture healing. There is no apparent stress-shielding, and fracture union strength is higher than that with rigid internal fixation.

Absorbable Fixation

The last 5 to 10 years have seen enthusiastic research in the development of absorbable devices for orthopedic applications, especially in the area of internal fixation devices. Current research is being aimed at the production of absorbable rods, screws, and plates manufactured from currently marketed absorbable materials. Table 6–1 lists several materials available for this application. Those with current clinical application include polyglycolic acid, polylactic acid, polydioxanone, and copolymers of polyglycolic and polylactic acid.

Parsons[36] described several advantages to the use of absorbable fixation, including (1) the lack of need for secondary intervention to remove implanted devices and (2) a reduction in stress-shielding as the device mechanically degrades. Concerns regarding the rate of degradation and mechanical strength of the device are still being investigated. A recent review of biodegradable polymers and composites described the ideal material to have the initial biocompatibility, strength, stiffness, and ductility of stainless steel with the ability to maintain these properties for several weeks or months, finally undergoing complete and benign biodegradation, absorption, or excretion.[37] No material currently reaches this ideal. They also pointed out that low implant stiffness might be expected to allow too much bone movement to permit fixation; however, unreinforced and reinforced devices (pins) have been used successfully in clinical applications.

Parsons[36] also pointed out that the rate of resorption of polyglycolic acid is generally considered too rapid for use in fracture fixation devices. Poly-L-lactic acid is sufficiently long-lived in vitro, but unfortunately the mechanical strength of the polymer alone may be insufficient for fixating a long bone fracture. Several alternatives to improve the performance of this biodegradable material are being investigated.[38–41] These include the following:

1. Controlling the amount of the racemic form of lactic acid used in the formation of the polymer. Polymers containing 100% L-lactide are extremely resistant to degradation. Inclusions of increasing amounts of D-lactide produce polymers with increasing rates of degradation.
2. Reinforcement of the poly-L-lactic acid polymer with high-strength carbon fibers and absorption of the matrix, leaving the carbon fibers, may present a biocompatibility problem.
3. Alteration of implant geometry.
4. Self-reinforcement of the absorbable materials, which consist of an absorbable polymeric matrix reinforced with fibers of the same material.

Tormala and other investigators[42, 43] have concluded that self-reinforced biodegradable polymers possess sufficient mechanical properties to be applied to the manufacturing of biodegradable fixation devices. This statement has been supported by both experimental and clinical trials. Their primary indications are for the fixation of cancellous bone when external plaster cast fixation is applied for additional support. With regard to cortical bone fixation, further study is indicated. In animal studies, polyglycolic acid proved to be biocompatible and was readily degraded in cancellous bone but to a lesser extent in cortical bone. It degraded over a 12-week period without identified inflammation or foreign body reaction. The biodegradation starts peripherally on absorbable implants and continues with subsequent replacement by the new bone.[44]

Polyglactin 910, a combination of polyglycolic (90%) and polylactic acid (10%), rods were also studied for their effect on epiphyseal plates in the rabbit model.[45] The disappearance of the polyglactin 910 implant and its replacement by a cancellous bone bridge resulted in a growth disturbance similar to that after a drill hole of equal bore of 3.2 mm. This suggested that a biodegradable fixation device may be developed for use in growing bone for the application of epiphysiodesis. In a subsequent study from the same institution, the effect of a polydioxanone implant was investigated for penetration of the growth plate in immature rabbits. Transepiphyseal implants of 2-mm diameter did not result in permanent growth disturbance. An implant of 3.2 mm did result in a growth disturbance similar to a hole made by an equal-sized drill.[46]

Fixation of mandibular fractures in an animal model has also shown promising results with the use of poly-L-lactic acid plates.[47] One study reported that the use of a polydioxanone device also showed satisfactory results in the fixation of osteochondral fragments in the knee of the animal model.[48] All studies appear to show biocompatibility in both soft tissue and bone.

Results of clinical studies on the use of biodegradable fixation for displaced ankle fractures have been reported. Several studies from the Department of Orthopedics and Traumatology, University of Central Hospital, Helsinki, Finland, have demonstrated successful fixation of displaced bimalleolar ankle fractures.[49–52] Hirvensalo[53] also reported promising results in more complex ankle fractures with disruption of the distal tibiofibular syndesmosis and fracture of the posterior tibia requiring reduction and fixation. The rods used in the studies mentioned earlier were of either poly-L-lactic acid, polyglycmolic, polymers alone, or with reinforcement by fibers of the same polymers, self-reinforced polyglycolic acid, or self-reinforced polyglycolic acid with a thin coating of polydioxanone applied to lengthen the hydrolyzation time within bone tissue. All studies reported formation of sterile wound sinuses or accumulation of an inflammatory exudate. However, this did not appear to influence either the radiographic or clinical results. The reaction was described as a nonspecific foreign body response with abundant giant cells.

The foreign body reaction occurred in 41 (7.9%) of 516 patients.[54–55] It was characterized by a fluctuant swelling at the implantation site occurring an average of 12 weeks postoperatively. The sterile exudate contains liquid remnants of the degrading implants. The reaction was believed to be directly related to the local tissue capacity to remove or clear the polymeric debris.

At the same institution, a total of 449 patients has been operated on using biodegradable implants for a variety of traumatic and elective procedures.[56] The postoperative course was uneventful in 408 patients. The complications included failure of fixation in five, clinically insignificant displacement in 13, superficial wound infection in 6, and sterile sinus formation in 17 patients.

In a study on the chevron osteotomy for hallux valgus, 56 osteotomies were performed on 48 patients.[57] Radiologic follow-up was performed at 6 weeks, 6 months, and 1 year postoperatively. The osteotomy was secured in position with a 2-mm $\times$ 25- to 30-mm cylindrical polydioxanone-coated self-reinforced polyglycolic acid rod. Postoperative care also included the use of a medially placed short metallic splint for 2 weeks. Thirty-five of the 56 osteotomies that were followed at 3 months or more showed no failures of the fixation. Bone union proceeded uneventfully in all patients.

Complications included one superficial infection, and in two patients a sinus was formed in the scar without bacterial growth. This occurred in one patient at 4 weeks and the other at 10 weeks after the operation. The sinuses healed within a few weeks without sequelae.

A second report from the same institution further supported the use of absorbable polyglycolic acid rods (Biofix) in this application. The average follow-up time was 14 months; two cases of effusion were reported.[58]

Clinical trials using a bioabsorbable pin of polydioxanone (ORTHOSORB) for the fixation of Austin osteotomies has shown the effectiveness of this form of fixation in this application.[59] No evidence of exudate or foreign body reaction has been described to date. ORTHOSORB pins have also been described as a viable alternative to stainless steel pins for digital arthrodesis.[60]

Research in the area of resorbable internal fixation devices for orthopedic surgery holds great promise. As further study in the biocompatibility and mechanical properties of the devices is done, favorable results and further applications will certainly be developed.

Collagen

Glutaraldehyde cross-linked collagen has been used in the management of painful hyperkeratotic lesions of the toes and plantar aspect of the foot. The collagen is injected subdermally to provide a cushion to relieve pain and reduce the need for palliative care. The subdermal cushion replaced collagen and other structural elements lost as a result of the development of the lesion and resulted in better resolution of local stress forces, temporarily relieving the symptoms associated with the lesion.[61] Local and immune hypersensitivity reactions are of concern with the use of this implant.

Hydroxyapatite

With regard to bone replacement, hydroxyapatite is being investigated as a bone substitute.

In general, the calcium phosphate ceramics include hydroxyapatite and tricalcium phosphate. Hydroxyapatite is available in adequate volume, can easily be contoured, has sufficient mechanical strength for a bone substitute, and allows rapid bone ingrowth. The brittle nature of these ceramics, however, may be a liability.[62]

Whether the implant is resorbed or actually replaced by bone still needs to be clarified. Hydroxyapatite may be used as a filling agent for bony defects. However, some problems associated with nonresorbable bone substitute may include migration, extrusion, and adverse effects on surrounding tissues.

Ceramics for reconstruction of the musculoskeletal system include products based on several materials. The ceramics with the most applications are aluminum oxide, hydroxyapatite, and tricalcium phosphate. Lemons[63] identified the areas of applications of ceramics for bone and joint surgery as (1) bone substitutes and fillers and (2) structural forms and surface coatings.

IMPLANT FAILURE

Implant failure can occur in biologic, mechanical, and structural fashion (Table 6–5).[64]

Early biologic failure may be related directly to infection and soft tissue necrosis associated with the surgical procedure. Later failure, in addition to infection, is the result of the inflammation and sensitivity associated with wear-debris or breakdown of the implanted device and also the subsequent bone involvement in osteolysis and cystic degeneration.

Bacteria resulting in infection may be introduced at the time of implantation or may arise as a result of transient bacteremia. The bacteria have been shown to be encased in a protective biofilm or glycocalyx that was adherent to the biomaterial surface. Because of the adherent nature of the organism, culture and identification may be difficult. The biofilm may also be a resistance mechanism to antibiotic therapy and host-defense reactions. This may explain the chronicity of this type of infection, which ultimately necessitates removal of the biomaterial.[65]

Initial mechanical failures are due to technical problems of

TABLE 6–5

MODES OF FAILURE WITH BIOMATERIAL AND IMPLANT ARTHROPLASTY

Modes of Implant Failure	Early	Late
Biologic	Skin/soft tissue necrosis	Infection
	Infection	Inflammation
		Sensitivity (allergy)
		Osteolysis
		Cystic degeneration
		Ectopic bone formation
		Corrosion
Mechanical	Osteotomy/implant	Dynamic imbalance
	Bed preparation	Wear
	Complications	Loosening
	Malalignment	Migration
	Instability	Sinking
	Dynamic imbalance	
Structural	Bone fracture	Bone fracture
		Implant fracture

Modified from Mollan RAB: Failed joint replacement, diagnosis (i) clinical. Curr Orthop 1(1):7–132, 1986.

insertion of the implant and poor preoperative evaluation. This may lead to early dynamic imbalance that may be present in the perioperative phase.

Late mechanical failures are due to dynamic imbalance of loading around the device, sinking and loosening of the material, and ultimate wear. Wear, although initially a mechanical problem, may lead and contribute to late biologic failure. Structural failure is somewhat mechanically related; it is concerned with failure of the bone or of the component material itself.

More studies need to be done in preimplantation parameters, including research, development, and manufacturing. Peri-implantation (such as surgical technique) and postimplantation parameters also require further evaluation.

Care must be taken in the selection of materials for use in patients. For example, fixation of osteotomies in osteoporotic bone may best be obtained with smooth, nonthreaded Kirschner wires as opposed to screw fixation because of the likelihood of the decreased bone density to interface appropriately with the screw threads to allow compression and maintain alignment. Similarly, resorbable fixation devices that lose their strength in 6 weeks should not be used in situations when prolonged bone healing may be expected or in patients with decreased density of cancellous bone. Implant modifications based on personal preference should be avoided, for example, in the insertion of implants in untested circumstances, the trimming of silicone implants (e.g., removal of a stem in a dual-stemmed hinged device), or use of only one component of a dual-component prosthesis. The choice of the appropriate implant or device should be based on the clinical, patient-appropriate circumstances and not the need to make the procedure more technically challenging.

References

1. Park JB: Biomaterials Science and Engineering. New York, Plenum Press, 1984, pp 1–5.
2. American Society of Testing Materials: 1989 Annual Book of ASTM Standards, Vol 13.01, medical devices, F748–87. Philadelphia, ASTM, 1989.
3. Swanson SAV and Freeman MAR (eds): The Scientific Basis of Joint Replacement. New York, John Wiley & Sons, 1977.
4. Park JB: Biomaterials Science and Engineering. New York, Plenum Press, 1984.
5. Von Recum AF (ed): Handbook of Biomaterials Evaluation: Scientific, Technical and Clinical Testing of Implant Materials. New York, Macmillan, 1986.
6. Cochran GVB: A Primer of Orthopaedic Biomechanics. New York, Churchill Livingstone, 1982.
7. Black J: Systemic effects of biomaterials. Biomaterials 5:11–18, 1984.
8. Massone L, Anonide A, Borghi S, and Isola V: Positive patch test reactions to nickel cobalt and potassium dichromate in a series of 576 patients. Cutis 47(2):119–122, 1991.
9. Rostaker G, Robin J, and Binet O, et al: Dermatitis due to orthopedic implants. J Bone Joint Surg 69A(9):1408–1412, 1987.
10. Anderson J: Inflammatory response to implants. ASAIO, 11(2):101–107, 1988.
11. Pizzoferrato A, Caipetti G, Stea S, and Toni A: Cellular events in the mechanism of prosthesis loosening. Clin Materials 7:51–81, 1991.
12. Jacobs AM and Oloff LM: Podiatric metallurgy and the effects of implanted materials on living tissues. Clin Podiatr 2(1):121–141, 1985.
13. Urist MR: Practical applications of basic research on bone graft physiology. AAOS Instruction Course Lectures 25:1–26, 1976.
14. Albrektsson T, Branemark P, Hansson H, and Lindstrom J: Osseointegrated titanium implants. Acta Orthop Scand 52:155–170, 1981.
15. Habermann ET: Total joint replacement: An overview. Semin Roentgenol 21:7–19, 1986.
16. Homsy CA, Cain TE, Kessler FB, et al: Porous implant systems for prosthesis stabilization. Clin Orthop 89:220–234, 1972.
17. Bobyn JD, Pilliar RM, Cameron HU, et al: The effect of porous surface configuration on the tensile strength of fixation of implants by bone ingrowth. Clin Orthop 149–291, 1980.
18. Bobyn JD, Pilliar RM, Cameron HU, and Weatherly GC: The optimum pore size for the fixation of porous surfaced metal implants by the ingrowth of bone. Clin Orthop 150:263–270, 1980.
19. Collier LP, Major MB, Chae JC, et al: Macroscopic and microscopic evidence of prosthetic fixation with porous coated materials. Clin Orthop 235:173–180, 1988.
20. Spector M: Historical review of porous-coated implants. J Arthroplasty 2:163–177, 1987.
21. Haddad RJ, Cook SD, and Thomas KA: Biological fixation of porous coated implants. J Bone Joint Surg 69A:1459–1466, 1987.
22. Cameron HU, Pilliar RM, and McNab I: The rate of bone ingrowth into porous metal. J Biomed Materials Res 10:295–302, 1976.
23. Albrektsson T and Albrektsson B: Osseointegration of bone implants. Acta Orthop Scand 58:567–577, 1987.
24. Szmulker-Moncler S and Dubruille JN: Is osseointegration a requirement for success in implant dentistry? Clin Materials 5:201–208, 1990.
25. Linder L, Carlsson A, Marsal L, et al: Clinical aspects of osseointegration in joint replacement. J Bone Joint Surg 70B(4):550–555, 1988.
26. Tayton K, Johnson-Nurse C, McKibbin B, et al: The use of semi-rigid carbon-fibre-reinforced plastic plates for fixation of human fractures. J Bone Joint Surg 64B:1, 105–111, 1982.
27. McKibbin B: The biology of fracture healing in long bones. J Bone Joint Surg 60B:2, 150–162, 1978.
28. Sarmiento MA, Latta LL, and Tarr RR: Principles of Fracture Healing: Part II, The effects of function in fracture healing and stability. AAOS Instructional Course Lectures, pp 83–106, 1984.
29. Muller ME, Allgower M, Schneider R, and Willenegter H: Manual of Internal Fixation. Berlin, Springer-Verlag, 1979.
30. Goodship AE and Kenwright J: The influence of induced micromovement upon the healing of experimental tibial fractures. J Bone Joint Surg 67B:4, 650–655, 1985.
31. Skirving AP, Day R, MacDonald W, and McLaren R: Carbon fiber reinforced plastic (CFRP) plates versus stainless steel dynamic compression plates in the treatment of fractures of the tibiae in dogs. Clin Orthop 224:117–124, 1987.
32. Unthoff HK and Finnegan M: The effects of metal plates on post-traumatic remodeling and bone mass. J Bone Joint Surg 65B:1, 66–71, 1983.
33. Tayton K and Bradley J: How stiff should semi-rigid fixation of the human tibia be? J Bone Joint Surg 65B:3, 312–315, 1983.
34. Brown S, Gillett NA, and Broaddus TW: Flexible versus nonflexible fracture fixation. In Lane JM (ed): Fracture Healing. New York, Churchill Livingstone, 1987, pp 191–202.
35. Skinner HB: Isoelasticity and total hip arthroplasty. Orthopedics 14(3):323–328, 1991.
36. Parsons J: Resorbable materials and composites: New concepts in orthopaedic biomaterials. Orthopedics 8:7, 904–915, 1985.
37. Daniels AU, Chang MKO, Andriano KP, and Heller J: Mechanical properties of biodegradable polymers and composites proposed for internal fixation of bone. J Appl Materials 1:57–78, 1990.
38. Christel P, Chabot F, Leray JL, et al: Biodegradable composites for internal fixation. In Winter GD, Gibbons DF, Plenk M (eds): Biomaterials. London, John Wiley & Sons, 1980, pp 271–280.
39. Vainionpaa S, Majola A, Mero M, et al: Biodegradation and biocompatibility of the polylactic acid in bone tissue and mechanical properties in vitro (abstract). Transactions of the Third World Biomaterials Congress, Kyoto, Japan, April 21–25, 1988, p 500.
40. Pellinen M, Ponjonen T, Tamminmaki M, et al: The in vitro degradation of biodegradable self-reinforced (SR) polyglycolide rods (abstract). Transactions of the Third World Biomaterials Congress, Kyoto, Japan, April 21–25, 1988, p 562.

41. Laiho J, Mikkonen T, and Tormala P: A comparison of in vitro degradation of biodegradable polyglycolide (PGA) sutures and rods (abstract). Transactions of The Third World Biomaterials Congress, Kyoto, Japan, April 21–25, 1988, p 564.

42. Tormala P, Vainionpaa S, Pellinen M, et al: Totally biodegradable polymeric self-reinforced (SR) rods and screws for fixation of bone fractures (abstract). Transactions of The Third World Biomaterials Congress, Kyoto, Japan, April 21–25, 1988, p 501.

43. Tormala P, Vasenius J, Vainionpaa S, et al: Ultra-high-strength self-reinforced polyglycolide (SP-PGA) composite rods for internal fixation of bone fractures: In vitro and in vivo study. J Biomed Materials Res 25:1–22, 1991.

44. Vainionpaa S: Biodegradation of polyglycolic acid in bone tissue: An experimental study on rabbits. Arch Orthop Trauma Surg 104:333–338, 1986.

45. Maketa E, Vainionpaa S, Vihtomen K, et al: The effects of penetrating biodegradable implant on the epiphyseal plate: An experimental study on the growing rabbits with special regard to polyglactin 910. J Pediatr Orthop 7(4):415–420, 1987.

46. Makela EA, Vainionpaa S, Vihtonen K, et al: The effect of a penetrating biodegradable implant on the growth plate. Clin Orthop 241:300–308, 1989.

47. Rozema FDR, Bos RRM, Boering G, et al: Resorbable plates and screws of poly (L-Lactide) fixation of bone fractures: An animal study (abstract). Transactions of The Third World Biomaterials Congress, Kyoto, Japan, April 21–25, 1988, p 191.

48. Greve H and Holste J: Refixation of osteochondral fragments via absorbable plastic rods. Acta Traumatol 15:145–149, 1985.

49. Rokkanen P, Bostman O, Vainionpaa S, et al: Biodegradable internal fixation in displaced ankle fractures (abstract). Transactions of The Third World Biomaterials Congress, Kyoto, Japan, April 21–25, 1988, p 192.

50. Bostman O, Vainionpaa S, Hirvensalo E, et al: Biodegradable internal fixation for malleolar fractures. J Bone Joint Surg 69B(4):615–619, 1987.

51. Bostman O, Hirvensalo E, Vainionpaa S, et al: Ankle fractures treated using biodegradable internal fixation. Clin Orthop Rel Res 238:195–203, 1989.

52. Bostman O, Hirvensalo E, Vainionpaa S, et al: Degradable polyglycolide rods for the internal fixation of displaced bimalleolar fractures. Int Orthop 14:1–8, 1990.

53. Hirvensalo E: Fracture fixation with biodegradable rods. Acta Orthop Scand 60:601–606, 1989.

54. Bostman O, Hirvensalo E, Makinen J, and Rokkanen P: Foreign-body reactions to fracture fixation implants of biodegradable synthetic polymers. J Bone Joint Surg 72B(4):592–596, 1990.

55. Santavirta S, Kodttinen YT, Tomoyuki S, et al: Immune response to polyglycolic acid implants. J Bone Joint Surg 72B(4):597–600, 1990.

56. Rokkanen P, Bostman O, Hirvensalo E, et al: Biodegradable osteofixation in orthopaedic surgery (abstract). Transactions of The Third World Biomaterials Congress, Kyoto, Japan, April 21–25, 1988, p 502.

57. Rokkanen P, Hirvensalo E, Bostman O, et al: Biodegradable fixation in metatarsal osteotomy for hallus valgus (abstract). Transactions of The Third World Biomaterials Congress, Kyoto, Japan, April 21–25, 1988, p 194.

58. Hirvensalo E, Bostman O, Tormala P, et al: Chevron osteotomy fixated with absorbable polyglycolide pins. Foot Ankle 11(4):212–218, 1991.

59. Brunetti V, Trepal MJ, and Jules KT: Fixation of the Austin osteotomy with bioresorbable pins. J Foot Surg 30(1):56–65, 1991.

60. Patton GW, Shaffer MW, and Kostakos DP: Absorbable pin: A new method of fixation for digital arthrodesis. J Foot Surg 29(2):122–127, 1990.

61. Collagen Podiatric Investigation Group: Report on the clinical evaluation of glutaraldehyde cross-linked collagen (Keragen) implant treatment of heloma durum and heloma molle. J Am Podiatr Med Assoc 25(6):427–435, 1986.

62. Jarcho M: Calcium phosphate ceramics as hard tissue replacements. Clin Orthop 157:259–276, 1981.

63. Lemons JE: Bioceramics. Clin Orthop 261:153–158, 1990.

64. Mollan RAB: Failed joint replacement, diagnosis (i) clinical. Curr Orthop 1(1):7–132, 1986.

65. Gristina AG and Costerton JW: Bacterial adherence to biomaterials and tissue. J Bone Joint Surg 67A(2):264–273, 1987.

Clinical Features of Articular Disease

CHAPTER 7

Rheumatoid Arthritis

Richard D. Roth, D.P.M.

In 1800, Landre-Beauvais provided the first clear description of a symmetrical, inflammatory, chronic, and deforming arthritic disorder consistent with rheumatoid arthritis.[1] In 1876, Sir Alfred Garrod was the first to use the term *rheumatoid arthritis* (RA) in an attempt to differentiate gouty rheumatism from nongouty rheumatism.[2] RA was not accepted as a valid diagnostic entity until 1922 in Europe and 1941 in the United States.[3] From the time that Garrod first used the term until its acceptance, a wide variety of distinct arthritic disorders formerly included under the umbrella of RA had been differentiated and appropriately given distinct names.

Many different disorders present with similar or identical clinical and histopathologic findings in joints. Until diagnostic advances allow for their differentiation, they will be considered the same disorder. There are few places in the history of medicine where this is more true than with RA. In the past 125 years, more than 50 distinct disorders that were formerly diagnosed as RA have been identified. Recognition of these entities has often been complicated by unknown causes and overlap of symptoms and clinical findings. The situation is further complicated by variable disease presentations, courses, and responses to identical treatments in similar patients with identical diagnoses.[4] There is little doubt that many of these factors in RA will prove to be due to the presence of different and distinct disorders that are as yet labeled RA.

RA usually presents with symmetrical, inflammatory, chronic, and destructive joint findings, but it is also associated with systemic findings that can affect any body tissue or organ system. Its diagnosis, although based on clinical and laboratory findings, is established only after exclusion of other known causes of synovitis and related findings. Most patients with RA present with insidious onset, chronic course

of disease, fluctuating disease activity, spontaneous partial or complete remissions, progressive joint destruction, deformity, and disability. Although it has long been known that RA is associated with a general increase in morbidity in other areas (e.g., increased incidence and severity of unrelated infections), the belief that RA did not affect life expectancy was long held. Recent research has confirmed both increased morbidity and mortality in RA.[5]

ETIOLOGY AND INCIDENCE

The etiology of RA has eluded extensive research and remains unknown. Research has, however, uncovered substantial relevant information. A genetic predisposition appears to be related to the histocompatibility genetic marker HLA-DR4, especially in those patients who maintain high titers of immunoglobulin M (IgM) rheumatoid factor.[6] The lack of 100% concordance in monozygotic twins confirms that the cause is not strictly related to or governed by genetic factors.[7]

As the autoimmune nature of RA has been established, it is possible to observe that RA results from a continuing antigenic challenge by an infectious or noxious agent, a portion of such an agent remaining in articular tissues after the initial agent has been cleared, or tissue that has been altered by a formerly present agent that acts as a persistent antigen. Many findings in RA are similar to those in other forms of arthritis with known infectious causes, but exhaustive research has failed to identify and confirm any specific noxious, bacterial, mycoplasmal, spirochetal, fungal, yeast, or viral-inciting agent.

The spread of syphilis from the Americas to Europe provides a classic example of the potential spread of an infectious disease. This may also be true for RA. Skeletal remains dated earlier than 1500 A.D. in Europe have shown findings consistent with osteoarthrosis, tuberculous and septic arthritis, and spondyloarthropathies, but have failed to exhibit any findings consistent with RA. Recent findings (as yet to be confirmed) show rheumatoid arthritic destructive changes in the skeletal remains of pre-Columbian Indians from North America and what is now Mexico.[3] The incidence of RA in the United States is between 0.3 and 1.5%.[8] An incidence of 3.4% in a Yakima Indian population of women between the ages of 18 and 79 years has been shown in one study.[9] A second study has documented an incidence of 5.3% in a Chippewa Indian population.[10] The Chippewa population also had an HLA-DR4 prevalence of 68%, which is considerably higher than that found in the general European or American populations. All Chippewa Indians found to have RA maintained HLA-DR4 histocompatibility antigen. These Indian tribes would be expected to have closer genetic ties to the pre-Columbian Indian population than would be expected in the European or American populations. These findings tend to support a potential infectious cause and genetic predisposition in RA.

RA may also represent an aberration in joints' normal cyclical pattern of injury, inflammation, and repair. The initial inflammation noted in joints affected by RA closely resembles that noted following trauma. It is also possible that tissues found within joints with potential for immunoglobulin production become altered so as to continually produce an antigen that causes RA. Elucidation of the etiology of RA will have to await further advances in diagnostic capabilities. In all probability, this etiology will be multifactorial.

RA affects people from all geographic areas, racial origins, and ethnic groups; however, it is rare in blacks. Onset has been noted in young children and after the seventh decade, but it is most commonly noted in the fourth and fifth decades.[11] Females are affected two to three times more than males, but this difference is minimized when only those with IgM rheumatoid factor are considered.[12] Onset is more common in winter months, with twice as many experiencing onset between October and March than in the other 6 months of the year in North America.[13] Onset also commonly follows other situations that can substantially increase emotional or physical stress.[14]

PATHOGENESIS

The changes noted in joints afflicted with RA have two stages. An acute, exudative, inflammatory stage is noted initially with an influx of plasma proteins and cellular elements into articular tissues and joint fluid. The chronic inflammatory stage is associated with an influx of monocellular infiltrate into subsynovial tissues, local antibody production and distribution throughout local tissues and joint fluid, immune complex reactions, and progressive formation of destructive, inflammatory granulation tissue (pannus). Both of these stages are simultaneously found in joints and related tissues once the disease is established.[15]

The earliest findings involve the small blood vessels in the joint capsule and synovial tissues. Initially, these vessels become obliterated by thrombi and accumulations of inflammatory cells. Endothelial injury occurs, and exudation of plasma proteins and white blood cells into adjacent tissue and synovial fluid progresses. With perpetuation of the primary inflammation, synovial tissues proliferate and form villous projections that extend into the joint cavity. Synovial lining that is normally 1 to 3 cells thick further thickens and becomes 6 to 10 cells thick. Segmental inflammatory changes are noted in the local blood vessels with thrombosis, venous distention, capillary blockage, local hemorrhage, and mononuclear cell infiltration throughout local tissues. These monocytes and dendritic synovial cells produce substantial amounts of IgG that acts against other IgG found in synovial tissue, cartilage, and joint fluid.[16]

Immune complex and inflammatory activity attract phagocytic cells into the area. These cells ingest immune complexes and subsequently release lysosomal enzymes and proteases that attack cartilage and elastic fibers. Oxygen free radicals released in the inflammatory process initiate the arachidonic acid pathway by activation of the cyclooxygenase and lipoxygenase pathways, resulting in the production of products inducing further inflammation. The inflammatory activity thus becomes self-perpetuating.[17]

Chronic inflammation in a joint promotes proliferation of synovial tissues resulting in the formation of continually expanding, inflammatory granulation tissue (pannus). Inflammatory processes continue to occur within, and be propagated by, this pannus. The physical advancement of pannus over cartilage cuts off synovial fluid nutrition from this avascular tissue. The physical pressure from the advancing pannus, action of destructive enzymes within it, and similar action from identical enzymes in the joint fluid lead to the further destruction of articular cartilage, ligaments, tendons, and bone that is seen in RA.[18]

Cartilage consists of a network of collagen fibers filled with proteoglycans (disaccharide molecules linked to a protein core) that retain large quantities of water. In the early stages of inflammation, proteases initially cause loss of proteoglycans and their water shells from the cartilage matrix. The triple-helical configuration of collagen protects it from damage by these proteases. Although this loss of proteoglycans is reversible, it decreases the ability of cartilage to withstand deformation from mechanical stresses. At this stage of the inflammatory process, mechanical stresses can cause permanent damage to cartilage.

Among the released lysosomal enzymes are collagenases that are capable of destroying the collagen matrix of cartilage. These enzymes in synovial fluid and advancing pannus produce irreversible cartilage destruction. As the exudative phase progresses to the inflammatory granulation tissue phase, ingress of blood vessels, fibroblasts, and inflammatory cells further propagates pannus formation and advancement. Within the advancing granulation tissue, synovial cells continually secrete proteases, collagenases, and a factor known as catabolin. Chondrocytes exposed to catabolin secrete an enzyme that directly degrades cartilage.[19] These destructive processes along with the exudative and granulomatous phases can be seen in any synovial joint that is receiving sustained trauma or microtrauma. Perpetuation of the trauma is associated with the release of antibodies and soluble substances by macrophages and lymphocytes in synovial tissues and synovial fluid; they induce dendritic synovial cells to produce more proteases, collagenases, and antibodies.

Discontinuation of the traumatic stimulus is associated with the cessation of the exudative phase and regression of the inflammatory granulation tissue.[20] Suppressor cells and other factors have been identified in synovial tissues. They are at least partially responsible for the cessation of traumatically induced synovitis on removal of the traumatic stimulus. Related substances have been shown to stabilize cellular membranes, inhibit protease and collagenase release, and directly inhibit activity of these enzymes.[21, 22] Early histologic findings in RA are identical to those noted earlier. Known facts about the patterns of onset and disease activity associated with RA indicate that the same mechanisms are at least in part responsible for the disease activity noted in this disorder. When a joint has been paralyzed prior to the onset of RA, that joint is completely spared from disease activity.[23] Joints that become paralyzed after onset of RA show reduced levels of inflammatory synovitis and reduced degrees of joint destruction.[24] Explanted inflamed synovial tissue from joints affected by RA demonstrate protease, collagenase, and antibody release from dendritic cells that is stimulated by exposure to aggregates of fragmented immunoglobulins, collagen, and even plant lectins.[25, 26] It is possible that a genetically based or induced defect in normal suppressor mechanisms is responsible for the persistent production by synovial tissues of the antigen(s) that perpetuate the inflammatory rheumatoid synovitis.

PATHOLOGY

The granulomatous, inflammatory, invasive synovitis of RA is responsible for the destructive findings that are predominantly noted in diarthrodial (synovial) joints and less often in related tendons, tendon sheaths, ligaments, bursae, bone, and subcutaneous tissues. Extensive cartilage destruction is an early finding in joints affected by RA. Bony destruction begins in periarticular bone through direct contact with advancing, destructive, inflammatory granulation tissue and by advancement of this tissue through vascular foramina into epiphyseal bone.

As osteolytic destruction occurs around joints, new bone formation and remodeling occur under the influence of mechanical forces acting on those joints. These new bone formations are usually less prominent than similar findings associated with other forms of arthropathy. An osteoclast-stimulating substance secreted by rheumatoid arthritic synovium is most likely responsible for this finding. The decrease in bone mass frequently seen in RA is primarily due to disuse atrophy. With advancement of the disease, dense fibrous connective tissue replaces cartilage and periarticular tissues. This connective tissue has the potential to mature and differentiate into hyaline or fibrous cartilage, synovial tissue, fibrous scar tissue, or bone. Limitation of functional joint capacities, restriction of joint motion, or bony ankylosis can ultimately result in any joint.

Extra-articular damage and destruction of tissues are usually less frequent and less severe than are the articular findings in RA. Tendons, tendon sheaths, and bursae can be damaged by contact with advancing pannus from afflicted joints or from inflammatory activity within their own synovial tissues. Periostitis may be noted along the shafts of long bones, especially along phalanges and metatarsals, owing to proximity to reflections of involved joint capsules.

Spinal Involvement

Vertebral involvement in RA can occur at spinal disci, apophyseal joints, and their supporting structures. It occurs in 30% to 40% of those diagnosed with RA and can occasionally be seen in the absence of peripheral joint findings.[27] Disease activity in these areas is usually less frequently noted and is less severe in intensity than that noted in peripheral joints. Rheumatoid damage to cervical spinal joints and their supporting structures can produce substantial disability and even death. The five types of cervical involvement that can be noted either individually or in combination in RA are shown in Table 7–1. Destruction by inflammatory granulation tissue can involve joints, bony structures, and supporting tissues in the cervical spine.

In the first type of cervical involvement, disease activity in the synovial joints between the atlas and skull and between the atlas and axis causes erosion, thinning, or total destruction of the atlas. Unless the dens has been simultaneously destroyed, it is pressed upward into the foramen magnum. Resultant damage to the spinal cord or even to the brain stem can be associated with nerve damage, paralysis, and even sudden death. Disease activity in the joint surrounding the dens can lead to destruction of the transverse ligament of the atlas. Unless the dens is simultaneously destroyed, the second type of rheumatoid cervical involvement may result, in which forward flexion of the head on the neck results in the dens being driven backward into the spinal cord causing injury, potential paralysis, and possible death. Lateral radiographs of the head flexed on the neck show a space no larger than 3 to 4 mm (averaging 2.5 mm in females and 3 mm in males) between the dens and the anterior atlas if the ligament is intact.[28] Periorbital radiographs can be used to evaluate the degree of destruction in the dens when the ligament has been stretched or destroyed.

A third type of cervical involvement in RA is noted when disease activity involves the apophyseal joints between the vertebral arches. Posterior cervical pain and muscle splinting may be noted on neck flexion, extension, rotation, and lateral bending with disease activity in these joints.

The fourth type of cervical involvement is noted with advanced degrees of destruction involving these apophyseal joints. Advanced destruction of these joints and their supporting structures can result in forward displacement of one

TABLE 7–1

TYPES OF CERVICAL SPINAL INVOLVEMENT SEEN IN RHEUMATOID ARTHRITIS

Description of Involvement	Results
Collapse of the atlas, with potential impingement of the dens on the spinal cord or brain stem through the foramen magnum	Nerve damage, paralysis, sudden death
Destruction of the transverse axial ligament, with impingement of the dens on the spinal cord with flexion of the head and atlantoaxial subluxation	Nerve damage, paralysis, possible death
Primary disease activity in the vertebral apophyseal joints, without subluxations	Stiffness, pain, and limitation of neck motion
Vertebral apophyseal joint destruction with subluxation(s)	Sensory, motor, or sensorimotor neuropathy (primarily in upper extremities)
Thinning or destruction of spinal disci and space-occupying lesions (synovitis, rheumatoid nodules)	Sensory, motor, or sensorimotor neuropathy (primarily in upper extremities)

or more of the upper vertebrae on lower vertebrae with subsequent pinching of the spinal cord and accompanying neurologic symptoms and deficits in the upper extremities. The most common site of such subluxations is between C3 and C4.

A fifth type of cervical involvement is seen with compression of nerve roots that arise within and exit through these vertebrae. Disease activity in the spinal disci can lead to their thinning. Thinning of the disci, apophyseal synovitis, and rare nodule formations in proximity to nerve roots can result in compression of those roots with accompanying neurologic symptoms and signs.[27]

Cervical spinal involvement in RA is often present in the absence of significant signs and symptoms and may be easily overlooked. It should be evaluated before the initiation of physical therapy programs that might involve the head and neck, before surgical procedures requiring intubation, and even before advising use of extra pillows in the presence of congestive heart failure or peripheral vascular disease.[29]

Rheumatoid Nodules

Rheumatoid nodules are subcutaneous lesions that are noted in 20% to 35% of patients with RA.[30] They are noted primarily at periarticular locations subject to excessive external pressure, often occurring on the weightbearing surfaces of the forefoot, elbow, posterior heels, toes, fingers, ankles, and occipital areas. These nodules are nonencapsulated, frequently lobulated structures measuring up to several centimeters in diameter. An outer envelope of granulation tissue surrounds an inner, radially arranged area of connective tissue with a central core of necrosis high in lipid content. The nodules may occur before, during, or even in the complete absence of articular disease. The presence of nodules in areas of increased pressure on the skin, often from underlying bony prominences, is often associated with symptoms of pain on application of pressure. Continued application of excessive pressure on these areas can result in subcutaneous hemorrhage and skin ulceration. The lack of encapsulation makes dissection from adjacent and even incorporated periosteum, bursae, tendons, skin, and other soft tissues quite difficult. Recurrence is common after excision, especially when excessive pressure on the involved area is not alleviated and bony underlying prominences are insufficiently excised.

Inflammation and Vasculitis

Tendons and ligaments are often affected by RA owing to their proximity to inflamed synovial tissues of joints. They can also be primarily involved in the inflammatory processes of RA. Necrosis, nodule formation, formation of adhesions, partial loss of integrity, and even complete rupture can be noted. Tenosynovitis, tendon entrapment, and even tendon ruptures can be associated with rheumatoid synovitis in tendon sheaths. Diffuse atrophy of striated muscle is noted in RA to a much greater extent than would be anticipated due solely to disuse atrophy. Immunoglobulins have been identified in RA within the walls of blood vessels supplying muscle tissue and those within muscle tissue. Histologic studies have confirmed vasculitis in the blood vessels supplying striated muscles in 10% of an unselected sample of patients

with RA.[31] Nodules can also occasionally be found in muscle tissue in RA.

Clinical presentation of vasculitis is usually noted only in patients with high IgM rheumatoid titers, severe and chronic disease, and subcutaneous nodules. Although there has been widespread belief that vasculitis is caused by steroid therapy, many patients with RA who have never received steroid therapy develop vasculitis.[31] No studies have documented any definite causal relationship between steroid use and vasculitis.[31] Lesions are noted primarily in limited, noncontiguous segments of small and terminal arteries. Histologic examination confirms signs of acute and chronic inflammation, and immunofluorescent staining techniques confirm the presence of immune complex depositions in the intima and tissues of involved vessel walls.[32] Lesions are predominantly noted in vessels supplying and within skin, muscle, and nerve tissue, but they may be noted in vessels supplying or within any tissue. Involvement can range from mild segmental arteritis without necrosis to fulminant necrosis and destruction of the entire length of a vessel, as seen in periarteritis nodosa.[33]

Clinical presentation of vasculitis in RA can be noted in one or a combination of patterns, as shown in Table 7–2. These include superficial dermal vasculitis, digital arteritis, peripheral neuropathy, myositis, visceral arteritis, pericarditis, pleuritis, and acro-osteolysis. Early, dermal, vasculitic lesions usually appear as erythematous, sharply defined, macular lesions that often show central clearing (target lesions). Sharply defined, erythematous to purpuric, fine blood vessels often border or are found within these lesions. The lesions are usually asymptomatic, but they can present with considerable pruritus. Their appearance is often fleeting and recurrent, but individual lesions can remain for days to weeks. Similar lesions can be seen in disorders as diverse as infectious mononucleosis and other infections and allergic reactions.[34] Their presence in RA tends to correlate with extensive and severe flares in disease activity.

Small hemorrhagic areas only a few millimeters in diameter, as seen in Figure 7–1, may appear on the nail fold, the nail bed, the skin adjacent to the free margin of nails, or any other digital site in digital arteritis. They represent thrombosis of small blood vessels associated with immune complex

TABLE 7–2

VASCULITIS AND ITS MANIFESTATIONS IN RHEUMATOID ARTHRITIS

Type of Arteritis	Manifestation
Subcutaneous vasculitis	Palmar erythema
	Erythema marginatum
Digital arteritis	Subcutaneous hemorrhage
	Ulceration
	Gangrene
	Acro-osteolysis
Vasa nervorum vasculitis	Sensory neuropathy
	Sensorimotor neuropathy
Vasa musculi vasculitis	Myositis
	Muscle atrophy
Vasa visceri vasculitis	Visceral infarction
	Visceral ulceration
	Visceral gangrene
Pericardial vasculitis	Pericarditis
Pulmonary vasculitis	Pleuritis

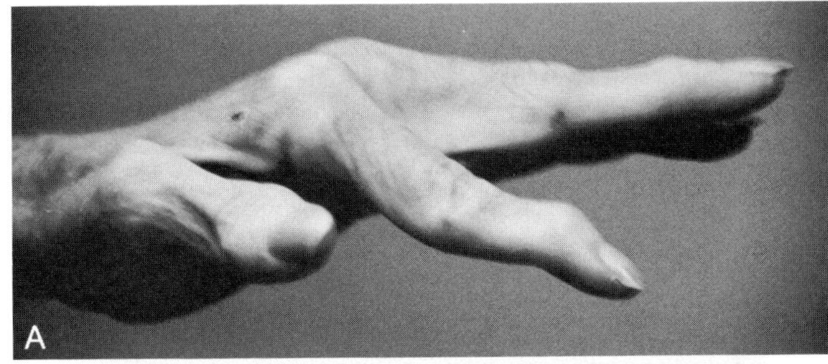

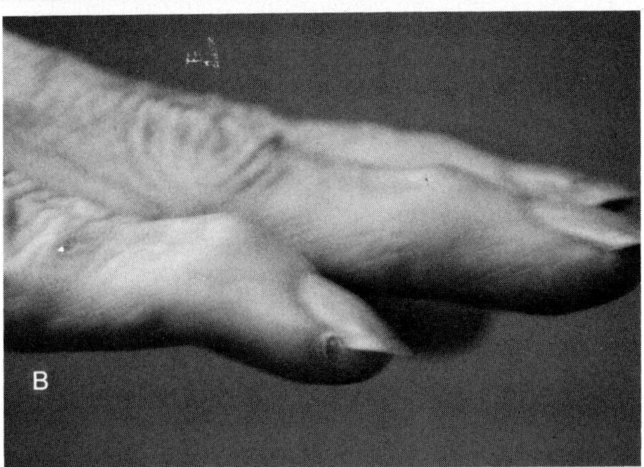

FIGURE 7–1. *A,* Spontaneous subcutaneous hemorrhage medial to the second and third metacarpophalangeal joints and ulcerations medial to the second metacarpophalangeal joint and at the second finger, medial nail fold secondary to rheumatoid digital vasculitis. *B,* Close-up view of ulceration at the second finger, medial nail fold.

deposition and subsequent inflammatory reaction. Thin, transverse, erythematous to purpuric lines across the most distal portion of the nail bed can be a related finding. These lesions are often brought on or exacerbated by physical or thermal trauma, but lesions also are seen in the absence of trauma. Lesions frequently undergo spontaneous ulceration and may be associated with gangrene. Breaks in skin integrity in the presence of digital arteritis significantly increase the risk of infection, delayed healing, failure to heal, and gangrene.

Peripheral (usually mild), distal, sensory neuropathy or more profound sensorimotor neuropathy may be the only presenting sign or symptom of vasculitis in RA. Rheumatoid sensory neuropathies usually begin distally in the toes and progress proximally to involve the forefoot and sole, the rearfoot, the ankle, and the lower leg. Involvement of the fingers and hands is less commonly noted and tends to occur only after onset in the feet. Sensory neuropathy involving loss of dull, sharp, vibratory, and joint position sensations is the most common type of neuropathy presenting in association with RA.[35] Often sensory neuropathy causes a subjective sensation of burning in the soles, worse on weightbearing, and most severe at circumscribed areas of intensified, excessive pressure. Sensorimotor neuropathy can result in weakness, footdrop, and paralysis either unilaterally or bilaterally. Drug-induced neuropathies can also be seen in RA in association with remissive, cytotoxic, and other drugs frequently used in the treatment of this disease.

Other types of neuropathy can be seen in RA in addition to those associated with vasculitis. These neuropathies are secondary to mechanical irritation that may be caused by impingement on and traction over nonyielding deformed surfaces. Entrapment neuropathies can be associated with synovitis, inflammation of local tissues, and progressive advance of inflammatory granulation tissue.

Mechanically induced neuropathy in some instances can be seen with severe pes planus acquired as a result of RA, wherein the medial and lateral plantar nerves are stretched over and pressed against the medial wall of the tarsal tunnel. Under these circumstances, tarsal tunnel syndrome can be noted in the absence of space-occupying lesions within the tunnel. Carpal and tarsal tunnel syndromes can also be seen in instances when reactive joint, tendon sheath, or bursal synovitis and subsequent pannus formation cause space-occupying lesions within these spaces. Additional symptoms of these and other neuropathies can be associated with direct pressure due to rheumatoid nodules or other inflamed tissues impinging on nerves traversing over or through them. Rarely, neuropathy can be associated with nodule formation within a nerve sheath.

Claudicatory and other muscle pains in RA can be associated with vasculitis affecting small vessels that supply muscle tissue. This vasculitis is frequently associated with myalgias that are present during rest, exacerbated by initial activity, and somewhat relieved with continued activity. Sudden onset of persistent, severe, boring abdominal pain in RA may be associated with visceral infarction. This type of pain heralds the onset of surgical emergency. Gangrene rapidly develops in the involved organ if the infarction is not quickly treated.[36]

Pericarditis is noted at autopsy in as many as 50% of those with RA.[37] It may be the only clinical symptom associated with vasculitis in a patient with RA. Pleuritis is similarly common in RA with vasculitis. Both of these conditions are frequently present in patients in whom other significant signs and symptoms of rheumatic vasculitis fail to develop.[37] In more severe forms of vasculitis, especially digital vasculitis, resorption of the ungual tufts of the distal phalanges may be noted.[38]

Several other forms of cardiac involvement in RA may be seen in addition to pericarditis. Rheumatic heart disease is noted in 6% to 10% of patients with RA.[39] Interstitial myocarditis, coronary arteritis, and calcareous aortic stenosis are noted with greater frequency in RA than in the general population. Rheumatoid granuloma-like formations in the heart are rare but can occur in any cardiac tissue. Aortic and mitral valve insufficiency can be associated with rheumatoid vasculitis or nodule formation. Vasculitis at the base of the aorta in RA can lead to occlusion of the coronary arteries at their source. Other related cardiac disorders noted in RA may include myocarditis, mitral valve and aortic valve incompetence, conduction defects, and coronary arteritis with and without myocardial infarction.[40]

Pulmonary interstitial fibrosis presenting with a diffuse reticular pattern on chest radiographs is frequently noted in RA. Pleuritis, diffuse rales throughout the lung fields, and impairment of alveolar gas exchange are often present. Pulmonary granulomatous nodules, occasionally noted on chest radiographs of patients with RA, rarely cause symptoms or clinical problems, but occasionally they need to be differentiated from those noted in sarcoidosis, tuberculosis, and cancer. Diffuse interstitial pneumonia presents in 2% of patients with RA.[41] In rare instances, a rapidly progressive and often fatal pneumonitis is noted in patients with RA. Unusually large silicotic nodules (Caplan's syndrome) are occasionally noted in the lungs of anthracite coal miners with RA.[42] Pulmonary hypertension can be noted in some patients with RA who have vasculitis affecting the pulmonary vessels.

Most patients with RA of significant duration have a normocytic, hypochromic anemia of chronic disease resulting from impaired red blood cell production; the anemia is unresponsive to iron supplementation. The severity of anemia usually parallels disease activity in RA. Hemoglobin values are usually higher than 10 gm/100 ml unless other causes of bleeding or anemia are present. Ulcerogenic medications (i.e., steroids) used in the treatment of RA are often responsible for dramatically lowering hemoglobin values. Eosinophilia and thrombocytosis are also commonly noted in RA.[43, 44] Eosinophilia greater than 5% is associated with more severe disease.[43] Prominent thrombocytosis tends to be associated with more severe disease activity and a greater degree of extra-articular involvement.[44] Enlargement of lymph nodes draining areas of chronic, active disease is also commonly noted.

A relatively small percentage of those afflicted with RA present with Felty's syndrome. Some authorities consider this a distinct disease entity, but others consider it a manifestation of RA. The syndrome consists of enlargement of the spleen and neutropenia in the presence of rheumatoid arthritic joint disease. Rheumatoid arthritis is usually associated with mild leukocytosis. Patients with Felty's syndrome often have white blood cell counts of less than 3000/mm³. These patients also may present with cutaneous hyperpigmentation, leg ulcerations, lymphadenopathy, significant recent weight loss, and substantially increased risk of infection.[45]

Sjögren's syndrome may represent a distinct entity or a variant of RA. It involves autoimmune destruction of lacrimal and salivary gland tissues in the presence of inflammatory, destructive arthritis. Almost all patients with this syndrome maintain IgM rheumatoid factor, and one third present with classic findings of RA.[46] Other significant gastrointestinal tract involvement in RA can include decreased esophageal motility, gastric ulceration secondary to related medications, and visceral infarctions.

Ocular manifestations are often noted in RA. Immune complex infiltration followed by chronic inflammation can cause chronic episcleritis and scleritis.[47] Subsequent keratitis and dramatic thinning of the sclerae may be noted. Occasionally, the sclerae are reduced to paperlike thinness and take on a bluish coloration similar to that noted in osteogenesis imperfecta. Subsequent scleral ulceration and perforation can result in blindness. Rheumatoid nodules can form in the sclerae and adjacent tissues. Steroids are often used to control severe, acute, or persistent rheumatoid synovitis and vasculitis. Long-term administration of steroids is associated with development of posterior subcapsular cataracts in 42% of patients with RA receiving them.[48]

Renal lesions are rarely a direct result of rheumatoid disease. Medications used to treat RA, however, can cause both significant and substantial renal damage. Remissive therapy with gold salts can be associated with membranous glomerulonephritis. Substantial intake of aspirin and phenacetin can be associated with renal papillary necrosis.[49]

PATTERNS OF ONSET AND DISEASE COURSE

Insidious, acute, and intermittent patterns of onset are seen in RA. Insidious onset is most frequently noted, with 55% to 70% experiencing prolonged periods of generalized or protean symptoms of fatigue, malaise, and diffuse musculoskeletal pain followed by joint pain and inflammatory arthritis.[50] Symmetrical initial involvement of joints is most commonly seen. Asymmetrical initial joint involvement is also common, with increased symmetry noted with time. Morning stiffness often precedes joint pain. Symptoms present in one set of joints rarely regress or remit as additional joints become involved. Periarticular muscle atrophy and weakness are usually far more prominent than would be anticipated with reported pain levels.

Acute onset is least commonly seen, with 8% to 15% of involved patients being able to pinpoint the exact moment of onset.[51] Asymmetrical involvement of single joints is common with this type of onset. Misdiagnoses are frequently made when initial involvement is limited to a single joint, bursa, or tendon sheath. Progression of disease activity with increased symmetry of joint involvement and increased numbers of sites involved aids in establishing a correct diagnosis.

An intermittent form of onset occurs in 15% to 20% of patients with RA.[52] These patients usually experience onset of symptoms over a period of several days to weeks. Patients with intermittent onset of RA usually demonstrate more widespread and severe systemic involvement.

Initial onset and ultimate joint involvement are most commonly seen in the metacarpophalangeal, wrist, and proximal interphalangeal joints of the hand. The next most frequently involved sites are the metatarsophalangeal (MTP) joints and the ankle. With the exception of the shoulder, joints on the right side of the body tend to be more frequently involved than those on the left.[51, 52] More than 75% have bilateral joint involvement. Large joints tend to become involved before small joints. Joints with the highest ratio of synovial membrane area to cartilage surface area tend to be most frequently involved in RA.[53]

Onset is most frequently noted in the fourth and fifth decades and is more common in women (2:1 to 3:1). Onset after the fifth decade, and without nodule formation, tends to result in milder disease. Insidious onset and sustained slow progression of disease activity are associated with the worst prognosis. More severe and rapidly destructive disease is associated with onset involving the first, second, and third MTP joints.[50]

Onset and exacerbation of symptoms have historically been associated with increases in humidity, temperature, and vapor pressure and decreases in barometric pressure. Repeated studies have failed to confirm any such relationship, although onset during winter months is far more frequently noted (2:1 to 3:1) than in the months of April through September.[54] Other significant increases in physical stress (accidental or surgical trauma, vaccinations, and infections) and emotional trauma (such as divorce, death of a close relative or spouse, and loss of job) have been noted frequently to precede the onset of RA.

Complete remissions are experienced by 10% to 20% of patients after fairly brief episodes of disease activity in multiple joints.[52] In many of these patients, the original diagnosis of RA may have been made in error. Most of the remainder of those diagnosed with RA have disease activity characterized by intermittent involvement of relatively few joints, generally milder and more fluctuating disease, and periods of clinical remission. Of those who experience partial or complete remissions, 50% have remissions of 1 year or longer. In one study, a group of patients with RA experienced remissions for as long as 31 years (mean 12 years).[55] Erythrocyte sedimentation rates often remain elevated during periods of clinical remission, indicating ongoing subclinical inflammatory activity.

Slowly or rapidly progressive, persistent disease activity in RA is associated with significantly greater and more rapid joint destruction and associated disabilities. In one study of 75 patients at 9-year intervals, almost all had increased degrees of joint destruction, decreased functional capacities, and increased rates of mortality.[56] No recent studies show that early diagnosis and initiation of treatment result in any reduction in morbidity or mortality in those with 2 years or more of sustained disease activity.[3]

Most patients with RA have episodic exacerbations and partial remissions of disease activity with gradual progression of deformity and disability. After 10 to 15 years of disease activity, 50% remain employed and only 10% are incapacitated.[57] The factors associated with the poorest prognoses include symmetrical polyarthritis with nodule formations and high IgM rheumatoid factor titers, more than 1 year of sustained disease activity, onset under age 30 years, and extra-articular disease. These factors and female gender are related to substantially increased morbidity and mortality. Increased morbidity and mortality in RA has also been associated with less than 5 years of formal education and lower income.[58]

RADIOGRAPHIC FINDINGS

A thorough review of radiographic findings in RA is beyond the scope of this chapter. Excellent reviews of early, intermediate, and late radiograph, computed axial tomography, and magnetic resonance imaging findings in RA are presented in Chapters 19, 22, and 23. Several specific points, however, do warrant review. Early findings are usually limited to signs of joint effusion and periarticular swelling. Pathognomonic erosions in all four quadrants of the fourth and fifth metatarsophalangeal joints involving both feet may often be noted early in the course of the disease. Frequently, this diagnostic finding can be seen before significant symptoms are encountered. Juxta-articular osteoporosis in affected joints and even in some unaffected joints may be apparent only weeks after onset of clinical signs and symptoms of RA.

Other changes involving erosive destruction of periarticular bone are usually noted only after several months of sustained disease activity. The erosive involvement in all four quadrants of the fourth and fifth MTP joints discussed earlier tends to occur early in RA. In the hand, similar findings are noted in the second and third metacarpophalangeal (MCP) joints. Advanced joint destruction, deformity, subluxations, dislocations, and ankyloses are late findings.

IMMUNOGLOBULINS AND RHEUMATOID FACTOR

Immunoglobulins are proteins produced by the immune system that are responsible for the recognition, destruction, and elimination of foreign substances. Although five classes of different immunoglobulins are recognized, the basic structural configuration of all immunoglobulins is similar (Figure 7–2A). Each immunoglobulin consists of a two-pair of polypeptide chains. The smaller ''light chain'' is linked at its carboxyl terminal end through disulfide bonds to the central region of the larger ''heavy chain.'' Two usually identical pairs of these light and heavy chains are linked through disulfide bonds at the central, hinge, or variable segment of each of the heavy chains to form an immunoglobulin.

The enzyme pepsin divides an immunoglobulin at the hinge section into Fab and Fc fragments. The four amino terminal ends of the Fab fragment form the site of antibody interaction with a foreign substance or antigen. The carboxyl terminal ends of the Fc fragment can act as an antigen in the stimulation of antibody production by tissues in the immune system.

Five classes of immunoglobulins have been identified based on genetically induced structural changes in the heavy chains: IgG, IgA, IgM, IgD, and IgE. IgG represents the major immunoglobulin class. It accounts for most of the antibody response to, and activity against, substances recognized as foreign. IgA represents the second most common form of immunoglobulin. It is primarily present in the secretions of the gastrointestinal, pulmonary, salivary, lacrimal, and genitourinary systems. It can be found as single units or in the form of more than one unit linked together. It is responsible for the normal immune competence maintained in the presence of high bacterial levels usually present in secretory tissues; it maintains the immune competence against frequent antigenic challenges posed to secretory tissue by external agents.

IgM represents the next most common immunoglobulin. It is present in serum and tissues as single units and as pentameric units in which five individual IgM units are linked

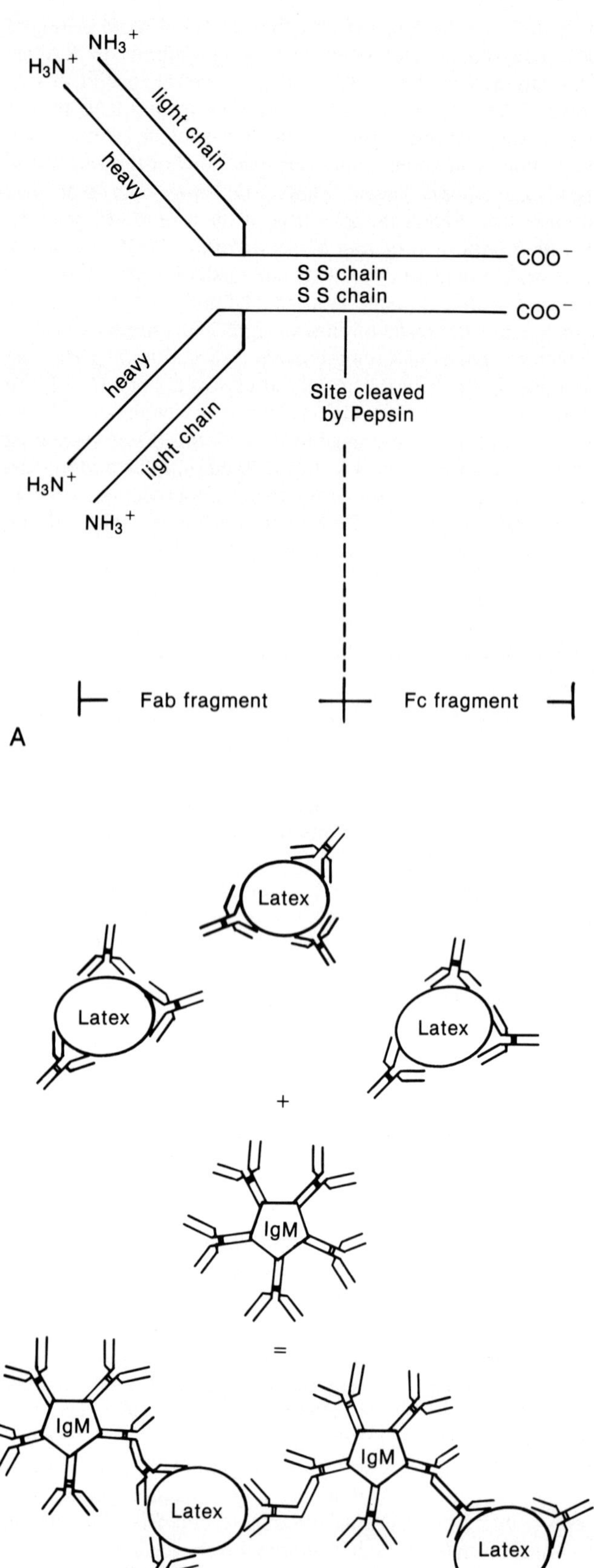

FIGURE 7–2. *A,* Structural configuration of an immunoglobulin. *B,* Relationship of latex particles covered with immunoglobulin G (IgG) and IgM rheumatoid factor in the agglutination test.

together into a single mass. IgM can represent the primary immunoglobulin in many immune responses and can be the sole antibody in long-term reactions, as seen with cold agglutinins. The test for rheumatoid factor identifies the presence of pentameric IgM reacting against IgG (see Fig. 7–2*B*).

In the test for rheumatoid factor, latex particles coated with IgG are mixed with serum. If the pentameric form of IgM capable of reacting against IgG is present, it will bind with that IgG, forming a sediment of interlocked pentameric and latex particles.

IgD represents an immunoglobulin that is found primarily on the surface of lymphocytes and is absent in the serum of primates. Its presence, along with IgM, on the surface of lymphoid tissue is believed to be associated with antigen-antibody reactions at these sites triggering or suppressing antibody production. IgE is found primarily at extravascular sites. It is associated with allergic reactions, wherein its interactions with antigens are related to release of vasoactive amines responsible for clinical manifestations of allergic reactions.

LABORATORY FINDINGS

Anemia and other hematologic findings associated with RA and Felty's syndrome have been described earlier in regard to pathologic changes noted in RA. Initial anemia tends to be normochromic and normocytic, but with prolonged disease activity anemia tends to become hypochromic and microcytic. Erythrocyte sedimentation rate (ESR) is elevated in virtually all patients with RA. The degree of elevation is related to both the extent and severity of active inflammation at any moment in the course of the disease. Sudden dramatic increases in the ESR may herald the onset of marked exacerbation of disease activity. Sudden substantial decreases in ESR may precede periods of spontaneous or therapeutically induced remissions.

Immunoglobulins of the IgG, IgM, and IgA classes reactive against fragmented, complete, or aggregated immunoglobulin IgG have been identified in RA. As reviewed earlier, rheumatoid factor specifically refers to a pentameric form of IgM reactive against IgG. There is no specific test for RA. A positive result on a test for rheumatoid factor only confirms the presence of this form of IgM antibody.

Rheumatoid factor is present in about 5% of the general population.[59] It is present at dilutions of 1:80 or greater in 70% of patients with RA.[60] Those testing positive for rheumatoid factor are considered seropositive, whereas others with RA are considered seronegative. Most seronegative patients with RA maintain immunoglobulins of the IgG class that are reactive against other IgG immunoglobulins in the body. Rheumatoid factor is also associated with connective tissue, hepatic, and infectious disease. Its presence may be noted after multiple inoculations. The frequency of positive results on tests for rheumatoid factor increases with age in the general population.

Eosinophilia and thrombocytosis also can be noted secondary to RA. Occasionally, leukocytosis also can be related to the presence of RA. Elevation in the ESR, the degree of anemia, leukocytosis, eosinophilia, and thrombocytosis, and the dilution at which the rheumatoid factor is positive vary in the same patient during the course of RA. Generally, fluctuations in these values tend to parallel the severity and extent of articular and extra-articular disease. Occasionally, their fluctuations herald a marked change in disease activity.

DIAGNOSIS

Few situations in the practice of modern medicine require more thorough application of clinical expertise than in establishing a diagnosis of RA. An accurate, early diagnosis of this disorder is often quite difficult and occasionally impossible. Overlap of clinical signs and symptoms with similar disorders is commonly noted. Concurrent presence with diseases and disorders that can modify clinical presentation is frequently seen. Individual variations within any patient population are generally the rule rather than the exception. In addition, RA as currently defined certainly includes a number of diverse and distinct arthropathies that as yet cannot be diagnostically differentiated. Often, only a presumptive diagnosis of RA can be established. Patients meeting the criteria for a diagnosis of definite and even classic RA at a given time may quite often prove later to have a different disorder.

Most patients with RA present with a history of insidious onset of generalized weakness, fatigue, loss of appetite, and prolonged stiffness in involved joints. This stiffness usually persists for several hours, improving with continued use of the affected joints. Occasionally, patients present with a history of either a chronic, unabated or intermittent, low-grade fever (38°C). Often symptoms are related to antecedent viral or other debilitating infection or a period of excessive psychological stress or depression.

If weightbearing joints are involved early in the course of RA, conspicuous atrophy of the quadriceps and calf muscles and an apropulsive, fully pronated gait are often seen. Excessive pronation during weightbearing frequently causes irritation from shoes around the tuberosity of the navicular bone and the posterolateral calcaneus. It is associated with "unlocking" of the tarsal joints, resultant splaying of the forefoot, and notation of previously comfortable shoes becoming too snug. Patients may report that their shoes have recently become too snug in the morning but seem to fit better during the afternoon and evening.

The combination of continued, excessive weightbearing pronation and inadequate room within shoes can result in acute onset of hammertoe, hallux valgus, bunion, and tailor's bunion deformities, and accompanying signs and symptoms of local irritation. Generalized weakness, atrophy of intrinsic and extrinsic muscles of the feet, and excessive weightbearing pronation result in inadequate support and "unlocking" of the tarsal joints, resulting in substantial depression of arch structure. This depression of the arch structure causes elongation of the feet. The resultant increase in overall length of the feet may have necessitated the patient's purchasing larger sized shoes in the weeks or months preceding clinical presentation. When it is present and longer shoes have not been purchased, ingrowth of the medial borders of the great toenails may be seen. Tenderness and pain in the area of the distal medial great toe may also be reported. Under these circumstances, excessive tightness of shoes can result in deformities, as described earlier.

Hands and wrists that are normally exposed are easily observed and examined. Palmar erythema and symmetrical involvement of the second and third MCP, wrist, and proximal interphalangeal (PIP) joints of the hands frequently are early clinical findings. Muscle wasting out of proportion to the intensity and duration of reported symptoms is usually seen around involved joints. Marked venous prominence over the dorsum of the hand is a related finding. Involved joints usually show fusiform swelling, local increase in dermal temperature without notable local erythema, and limited active and passive ranges of motion with soft end points. Occasionally, small, poorly differentiated, soft nodules can be noted on the surfaces of the forearm, elbow, posterior heel, medial arch, or metatarsal pad. Occasionally, erythema multiforme (target lesions) are reported or seen on the skin of the palms or other areas. Involvement of the distal interphalangeal joints of the hand is rare in RA. Pre-existent post-traumatic degenerative joint disease is often present at these sites, especially with onset of RA later in life.

There has been a continuing effort in rheumatology to formulate a satisfactory set of criteria for establishing a diagnosis of RA. In 1958, the American Rheumatism Association (ARA) revised a set of criteria presented the previous year that served as a foundation for most clinical diagnoses and related research for the next 30 years.[61,62] The 1958 ARA classification shown in Table 7–3 relied on 11 signs, symptoms, and laboratory features with specific exclusions. Classifications of classic RA, definite RA, and probable RA were established based on an individual patient meeting seven, five, or three criteria, respectively.

The authors of this classification recognized the limitations

---

TABLE 7–3

1958 CRITERIA FOR DIAGNOSTIC CLASSIFICATION OF RHEUMATOID ARTHRITIS

Diagnostic Classification	Criteria Met
Classic RA	7
Definite RA	5
Probable RA	3

Criteria

1. Morning stiffness*
2. Pain on motion or tenderness in at least one joint*†
3. Swelling of one joint representing soft tissue or fluid*†
4. Swelling of at least one other joint (soft tissue or fluid) with an interval free of symptoms of no more than 3 months*†
5. Symmetric joint swelling (bilateral symmetry)*†
6. Subcutaneous nodules over bony prominences, extensor surfaces, or near joints†
7. Typical x-ray changes that must include demineralization of periarticular bone as an index of inflammation
8. Positive test for rheumatoid factor in serum
9. Poor mucin clot formation on adding synovial fluid to dilute acetic acid (indicative of intra-synovial inflammation)
10. Synovial tissue histologic examination consistent with rheumatoid arthritis; marked villous hypertrophy, synovial cell proliferation, subsynovial lymphocyte/plasma cell infiltrate, and fibrin deposition on or around microvilli
11. Rheumatoid nodules biopsied from any site having characteristic histologic findings

---

*Must be present for a minimum of 5 weeks (criteria 1–5).
†Must be observed by a physician (criteria 2–6).
Diagnosis of possible RA requires that for at least 3 weeks, three of the following factors be present—criteria 1, 2, 3, 6, an elevated sedimentation rate, or an elevated C-reactive protein level.
If a given patient meets the criteria for diagnosis of an arthropathy that might mimic RA, the diagnosis of classic RA is excluded.
RA, rheumatoid arthritis.
Adapted from Ropes MW, Bennet GA, and Cobb S: Revision of diagnostic criteria for rheumatoid arthritis. Arthritis Rheum 2:16, 1959.

TABLE 7–4

1987 REVISED ARA CRITERIA FOR CLASSIFICATION OF RHEUMATOID ARTHRITIS

1. Morning stiffness lasting at least 1 hour around joints*
2. At least three or more areas have simultaneous soft tissue swelling or joint effusion observed by a physician. The seven possible areas include bilateral PIP (hand), MCP, wrist, elbow, MTP, ankle, and knee joints*
3. Joint swelling involving at least one joint in a wrist, MCP or PIP (hand) joint*
4. Bilateral involvement symmetrically when wrist, elbow, knee and ankle joints are involved. With bilateral involvement of the PIP (hand), MCP, and MTP joints, absolute bilateral symmetry is not required*
5. Rheumatoid nodules observed by a physician over bony prominences, extensor surfaces, or in periarticular areas
6. Demonstration of positive amounts of rheumatoid factor in serum at levels that are not present in at least 5% of the general population (titer 1:80 or greater)
7. Radiographic changes on AP hand and wrist views that must include juxta-articular osteoporosis and/or erosions consistent with those seen in RA

*Criteria 1–4 must be present for at least 6 weeks to be valid.

For classification purposes, a patient is said to have RA if at least four of the seven criteria have been met.

PIP, proximal interphalangeal; MCP, metacarpophalangeal; MTP, metatarsophalangeal; AP, anteroposterior; RA, rheumatoid arthritis.

From Arnett FC, Edworthy SM, Bloch DA, et al: The American Rheumatism Association 1987 revised criteria for the classification of rheumatoid arthritis. Arthritis Rheum 31:315, 1988.

inherent in it. They advised using the categories of "probable" and "definite" RA for research and reporting and the category of classic RA only for establishing individual patient diagnosis.[62] A duration of unabated symptoms of at least 6 weeks was required to help eliminate erroneous inclusion of infectious, traumatic, or other acute arthropathies. Even with this sophisticated form of classification, a significant number of patients with probable and even definite RA were shown in time to have other rheumatic disorders and not RA.

The cumbersome nature and limitations of the 1958 criteria led to a proposal of a new set of criteria in 1987, which was again refined in 1988.[63] In the 1988 revised ARA criteria, seven criteria were established with no exclusions (Table 7–4). As long as criteria one to four are satisfied by unabated symptoms of at least 6 weeks' duration, any patient who satisfies four of the seven criteria is said to have RA. Distinc-

tions of classic, definite, and probable types have been discontinued.

In the 1988 criteria, the first criterion is morning stiffness in and around affected joints lasting a minimum of 1 hour. The second criterion involves arthritis with soft tissue swelling or joint effusion present in a minimum of three joints. These joints must be either individual PIP or MCP joints, wrist, elbow, knee, ankle, or MTP joints. To meet the third criterion, at least one joint in a hand or wrist must be affected. The fourth criterion requires that synovitis be present symmetrically on both sides of the body, although absolute bilateral symmetry in involvement of the PIP, MCP, and MTP joints is not required. The fifth criterion requires that a physician observe rheumatoid nodules over the extensor surfaces, juxta-articular areas, or bony prominences. The sixth criterion requires that serum rheumatoid factor be present in quantities not found in 5% of normal control subjects. Although IgM rheumatoid factor is present in about 5% of the general population and an even greater percentage of the elderly, it is usually not present in these groups in titers greater than 1:80 dilutions. The seventh and final criterion requires that radiographic findings in the hand and wrist demonstrate erosive changes or pronounced juxta-articular osteoporosis. These criteria will identify appropriately 91% to 94% of the population with RA.[63] When four of the seven criteria are met, there is an 89% chance that the person actually has RA.[63]

DIFFERENTIAL DIAGNOSIS

The similarity in presenting symptoms in a variety of rheumatic disorders requires that even though the criteria in Table 7–4 are met, exclusion of other arthropathies must be ensured whenever possible. Table 7–5 shows a number of arthritic disorders that may be commonly, uncommonly, and rarely seen, but when noted can frequently be confused with RA. The most common confusion is encountered with degenerative or traumatic arthritis, arthritis related to infection, gout, calcium pyrophosphate dihydrate deposition disease, seronegative spondyloarthropathies and enteric disease, Behçet's disease, diffuse connective tissue diseases, polymyalgia rheumatica, giant cell arteritis, and Parkinson's disease. Less

TABLE 7–5

DISORDERS AND THEIR RELATIVE FREQUENCY OF CONFUSION WITH RHEUMATOID ARTHRITIS

Common	Uncommon	Rare
Traumatically induced arthritis	Thyroid disease	Malignancy
Degenerative joint disease	Complications with use of oral contraceptives	Lyme disease
Infectious arthritis		Multicentric
Gout	Hemoglobinopathies	reticulohistiocytosis
Calcium pyrophosphate deposition disease (pseudogout)	Hemochromatosis	Angioblastic lymphadenopathy
Seronegative spondyloarthropathies	Hemophilia	
Ankylosing spondylitis	Hyperlipoproteinemia	
Reiter's syndrome	Polychondritis	
Psoriatic arthritis	Sarcoidosis	
Enteric disease–related arthritis		
Diffuse connective tissue disease		
Polymyalgia rheumatica		
Giant cell arteritis		
Parkinson's disease		
Behçet's syndrome		

common errors in diagnosis are seen with arthritis associated with thyroid disease, use of oral contraceptives, hemoglobinopathies, hemochromatosis, hemophilia, hyperlipoproteinemia, polychondritis, and sarcoidosis.

Degenerative or Traumatic Arthritis

Structural or functional anatomic abnormalities and malalignments can produce chronic, excessive, biomechanical stress and strain, especially in weightbearing joints. Repetitive obvious or occult trauma to joints can have similar results. These findings are often concurrently noted with RA. They can intensify the clinical signs, symptoms, and severity of disease in already involved joints. They can also occasionally produce disease involvement in joints that would probably otherwise be spared.

In the absence of RA, the presence of continuing destructive forces on joints that already have significant degenerative changes can often result in inflammatory arthritis within those joints. When this type of inflammatory arthritis presents in sustained, bilateral symmetry, it can be confused with RA.

In the absence of systemic arthropathy (e.g., RA), identification and appropriate control of aberrant, repetitive, biomechanical, and traumatic forces on arthritic joints usually reduce and occasionally eliminate the arthritis present. Radiographic studies of such joints usually show findings consistent with osteoarthrosis or traumatic arthritis. Findings include subchondral sclerosis, uneven loss of joint space, and osteophyte formation; erosions tend to be limited in extent with corticated borders.

In the absence of systemic arthropathy, stiffness on use of rested joints is of shorter duration (usually less than 1 hour). Pain tends to increase with continued use. Bouchard's nodes (symmetrical PIP joint enlargements) in osteoarthrosis can be confused with the symmetrical arthritis of these joints seen in RA.

Arthritis Related to Infections

Synovitis of proximal and peripheral joints following bacterial and viral infections can mimic early RA. Postinfectious synovitis has been reported[64, 65] following infections with *Salmonella, Shigella, Brucella, Neisseria,* and *Yersinia.* Arthritis similar to that seen in RA has been reported after intestinal infection with *Yersinia.*[64] In Europe, Reiter's syndrome has frequently occurred after severe intestinal infections with *Salmonella* and *Shigella,* whereas in the United States it seems to be spread by venereal contact.[65] Peripheral arthritis in Reiter's syndrome can mimic that of RA (see earlier).

Arthritis associated with gonorrhea can occasionally mimic that of RA, but it tends to be seen with asymmetrical, migratory patterns not common in RA. In 30% of patients with subacute bacterial endocarditis, myalgias, arthralgias, and arthritis are noted.[66] This form of arthritis usually involves one or more proximal joints, presents with concurrent high fever and heart murmur, and may be due to circulating immune complexes.

In rheumatic fever, a symmetrical, additive polyarthritis affecting mainly large joints in the lower extremities may be seen in adults. Chronic inflammation in the wrists and hands associated with rheumatic fever can result in ulnar deviation at the MCP joints and PIP joint involvement (Jaccoud's arthritis) that can be quite similar to hand deformities in RA. The erythema marginatum, chorea, and subcutaneous nodules seen in the pediatric form of this disorder are rare in the adult form. Antecedent streptococcal infection (high antistreptolysin-O titers), severe tenosynovitis, and dramatic response to salicylates help differentiate this form of arthritis from RA. Also, the tendency for fevers to remit or be quotidian in juvenile RA is not noted in rheumatic fever, wherein fevers tend to remain both high and constant.

In familial Mediterranean fever, monoarticular or oligoarticular pain and inflammation are commonly noted in proximal and large joints. Symptoms are acute, usually accompanied by fever and abdominal pain. Juxta-articular osteopenia without joint erosions can be seen, especially when the arthritis that usually lasts only for days to weeks continues for months.[67]

Gout and CPPD

An explosive pattern of onset, severe intensity of reported pain, dramatic erythema and swelling, characteristic radiographic findings, serum uric acid determination, and synovial fluid analysis usually allow for rapid differentiation of acute episodes of gout and calcium pyrophosphate dihydrate deposition disease (CPPD). Confirmed dietary and ethanol excesses and use of thiazide diuretics or low-dose salicylates can also aid in the differentiation of a gouty attack.

Chronic tophaceous gout can at times be quite difficult to differentiate from RA. Recurrent subacute attacks can present with subcutaneous nodules, symmetrical polyarthritis, fusiform swelling, and bony erosions quite similar to those seen in RA.[68] Rheumatoid factor is found in 30% of those with chronic tophaceous gout in the absence of any clinical or radiographic signs of RA.[69] Coexistence of gout and RA appears to be extremely rare. A review of medical literature from 1881 through 1978 revealed that only 10 cases of concurrent gout and RA had been reported.[70] Patients with concurrent RA and hyperuricemia have been noted to have substantial reductions in serum uric acid with the onset of flares in RA disease activity.[71]

CPPD is seen in approximately 1 in 1000 people, being about one half as common as gout in the general population.[72] Other studies have shown prevalence as high as 15% between the ages of 65 and 74 years, increasing to 44% in those older than 84 years of age.[73] CPPD is characterized by calcification of joint and periarticular structures and release of calcium pyrophosphate dihydrate crystals into these joints.

Attacks frequently mimic those of acute or chronic gout and can be confused with RA.[74] For this reason, CPPD is commonly referred to as "pseudogout." The knee is the most commonly affected joint, whereas the joints of the great toe are rarely involved. Ankle involvement is also commonly seen. Approximately 5% of patients with CPPD have a chronic, symmetrical, erosive polyarthritis that can be quite difficult to differentiate from RA.[75] The small joints of the hands and feet are infrequently involved in this form of CPPD. Radiographs of the wrists and knees may reveal calcification of cartilages. Synovial fluid analysis may demonstrate dull-ended, rhomboid-shaped, positively birefringent (under compensated polarized light), calcium pyrophosphate dihydrate crystals. Their presence is diagnostic for this disorder.

Spondyloarthropathies and Enteric Disease–Related Arthritis

Peripheral arthritis mimicking rheumatoid arthritis is frequently seen in the seronegative spondyloarthropathies, including ankylosing spondylitis, Reiter's syndrome, psoriatic arthritis, and inflammatory bowel disease–related arthritis.[3] Peripheral arthritis is occasionally seen in each of these disorders prior to onset of spinal, skin, or enteric signs and symptoms. Unlike the symmetrical patterns of RA, such peripheral involvement often begins and remains in asymmetrical patterns. Inflammatory involvement of the insertion areas of ligaments and tendons (enthesopathies) are much more common in these disorders than in RA. Any of these disorders can present concurrently with RA.

Presence of the histocompatibility antigen HLA-B27, although not pathognomonic for any of these disorders, can assist in their differentiation from RA. Familial history of ankylosing spondylitis may be of assistance in differentiating it from RA. History of recent travel to Europe with severe intestinal infection or of conjunctivitis, urethritis, or a genital ulcerative lesion can be of assistance in differentiating Reiter's syndrome. Previous history and the presence of extensive digital swelling in a sausage shape, insertional tendinitis or plantar fasciitis, periostitis, peri-insertional osteoporosis and juxta-articular erosions can assist in differentiating Reiter's syndrome and psoriatic arthritis from RA. The presence of psoriatic skin lesions can be helpful in differentiating psoriatic arthritis from RA.

Intestinal pain, cramping, malabsorption, and hemorrhage associated with ulcerative colitis or regional enteritis (Crohn's disease) can precede, accompany, or follow the onset of an associated peripheral arthritis that may be confused with RA. Peripheral arthritis mimicking and occasionally confused with that of RA can be seen in Behçet's disease.[76] This disorder is associated with oral and genital ulcerations and central nervous system involvement that are rarely noted in RA. Spondyloarthropathy similar to that described earlier can also be seen in this disorder in association with HLA-B27.

Peripheral arthritis mimicking that of RA can also be noted several weeks after gastrointestinal infections, especially after that with *Yersinia enterocolitica*.[64] Intestinal lipodystrophy (Whipple's disease) can also be associated with peripheral arthritis that can occasionally be confused with RA.[4] Peripheral arthritis associated with these intestinal disorders usually tends to be oligoarticular or polyarticular, migratory, of limited duration, and nondestructive.

Diffuse Connective Tissue Disease

Systemic lupus erythematosus, polymyositis, dermatomyositis, mixed connective tissue disease, scleroderma (progressive systemic sclerosis), and forms of vasculitis often present initial peripheral, inflammatory arthritis that can be difficult to distinguish clinically from that of RA.[77] Although chronic, progressive joint deformity is seldom seen in these disorders, it is occasionally noted in the latter course of systemic lupus erythematosus, progressive systemic sclerosis, and mixed connective tissue disease. Systemic lupus erythematosus can present deformities in the hands identical to those seen in RA. Erosive joint destruction is also rare in all of these disorders, with the exception of mixed connective tissue disease. A number of patients initially diagnosed with RA go on to develop mixed connective tissue disease. Any of these disorders can present concurrently with RA.

Soft tissue and muscle inflammation occasionally lead to dislocation of specific tendons and associated deformities in systemic lupus erythematosus and polymyositis. Soft tissue contractures in progressive systemic sclerosis, polymyositis, and dermatomyositis can also cause deformities. In most of these disorders, characteristic involvement of multiple organ systems is noted with disease progression, aiding in differentiation from RA. Tissue biopsies from involved areas can often be valuable early in the course of these disorders before clinical involvement has become apparent.

Polymyalgia Rheumatica and Giant Cell Arteritis

Polymyalgia rheumatica is a syndrome consisting of pain and weakness primarily in the shoulder and pelvic regions, marked elevations in the ESR of 100 mm/hr (Westergren method), and dramatic, prompt response to corticosteroids. It occurs more commonly in women, is rare in non-whites and has an onset usually after age 60 years and rarely before age 50 years. Onset of severe pain and profound weakness can occur literally overnight.[78]

Affected patients may suddenly be unable to arise without assistance. They may experience severe pain in the hips, shoulders, upper arms, and neck with attempted use of joints in these areas. Pain and stiffness are worse after periods of rest, as seen with inflammatory articular disorders, and occasionally patients report "hurting all over." Examination in the presence of these symptoms is remarkably normal, with no significant synovitis or swelling around affected joints. Electromyographic studies, serum muscle enzyme levels, and biopsies of muscle tissue are normal as compared with abnormal findings in polymyositis.[78] In an older adult, acute onset of severe, symmetrical joint and periarticular pain of polymyalgia rheumatica can mimic the onset of RA. Absence of rheumatoid factor, peripheral arthritis, and notable synovitis helps differentiate these disorders, as does a rapid and dramatic response to low-dose corticosteroids.

Diagnostic differentiation of RA from polymyalgia rheumatica is important, because the latter is usually a manifestation of giant cell arteritis (cranial arteritis and temporal arteritis). Giant cell arteritis involves immune complex deposition with subsequent inflammation, exudation, and potential thrombosis in larger arteries. Local manifestations are limited to the tissues supplied by an involved artery. Jaw claudication resulting from facial artery involvement is pathognomonic for giant cell arteritis. Systemic manifestations include polymyalgia rheumatica, fever, anemia, weight loss, and general malaise. As with polymyalgia rheumatica the ESR shows substantial elevation. Alkaline phosphatase levels may be elevated, but liver biopsies are normal.[78] The diagnosis is established through histologic examination of a section of an involved artery. The temporal artery is usually selected for this biopsy.

Parkinson's Disease

People with Parkinson's disease have a predilection for development of swan-neck deformities in the hands.[4] These include flexion contractures of the MCP and distal interphalangeal (DIP) joints and extension deformity of the PIP joint of the same finger. Bilaterally symmetrical swan-neck deformities of the fingers are usually seen in RA and less frequently in spondyloarthropathies.

Although the rigidity and tremors of Parkinson's disease can be obvious, they are often absent in patients receiving medication to control this disease. When symptoms are few or absent, notation of bilaterally symmetrical swan-neck deformities in the hands of patients with symmetrical arthritis in joints of the lower extremities can lead to a misdiagnosis of RA. The concurrent presence of Parkinson's disease and RA is possible.

CLINICAL FINDINGS

Upper Extremities

Hand. The frequent tendency to disregard symptoms in the lower extremities, which are usually covered by clothing, makes presentation of clinical features in RA more obvious in the upper extremities. Even in the clothed patient, the findings in the hand are readily visible. Minimal functional deficits are readily noted in the hands because of their primary use in almost all daily living, occupational, and avocational activities.

Although DIP joint involvement is rarely a prominent clinical finding early in the course of RA, ultimate involvement of these joints has been confirmed in most patients with RA. Multiple DIP joints had tenderness in 80% of a sample of RA patients in one extensive study.[79] Bulging of the long extensor tendon insertion and associated area of the dorsal joint capsule can be noted, with occasional rupture of the insertion and subsequent flexion deformity of the joint. Fusiform swelling in these areas is almost never seen. Two systematic studies have documented DIP joint erosions in the fingers of 16% to 37% of involved patients.[80, 81]

Symmetrical, fusiform swelling of the PIP joints in the fingers is frequently a prominent presenting sign of RA. The joints demonstrate anticipated inflammatory signs, including prolonged stiffness after rest, tenderness to light palpation, pain on movement, and increased overlying dermal temperature. Flexion deformities can result from either tenosynovitis of the long flexor tendon and subsequent tendon contracture or rupture of the central slip of the extensor tendon. The latter can occur abruptly, resulting in a marked, fixed flexion contracture of the PIP joint with dislocation of the proximal phalangeal head. The head passes upward between the two lateral bands of the long extensor tendon, much like a button through a buttonhole, to show prominently under the dorsal skin. In recognition of the mechanism of this deformity, it has been termed a *boutonnière (buttonhole) deformity* (Fig. 7–3).

Flexor tenosynovitis is often overlooked in the examination of the hand in RA because of more dramatic dorsal, digital, and wrist findings. However, it is common in RA, being noted in 55% of patients in one meticulous study.[81] In this study an average of approximately 3 flexor tendons per patient were involved with significant disease activity. The flexor to the third finger was most commonly involved, followed by the second, fourth, fifth, and first flexor tendons, in order of frequency.

Contracture of the extensor tendons or of the intrinsic muscles (interossei and lumbricales) can lead to flexible or fixed extension deformities of the PIP joint. If the DIP joint has a simultaneous flexion deformity, the overall deformity is sometimes referred to as a "grasshopper" deformity. DIP and MCP joint flexion contractures in the presence of a PIP joint extension contracture are referred to as "swan-neck"

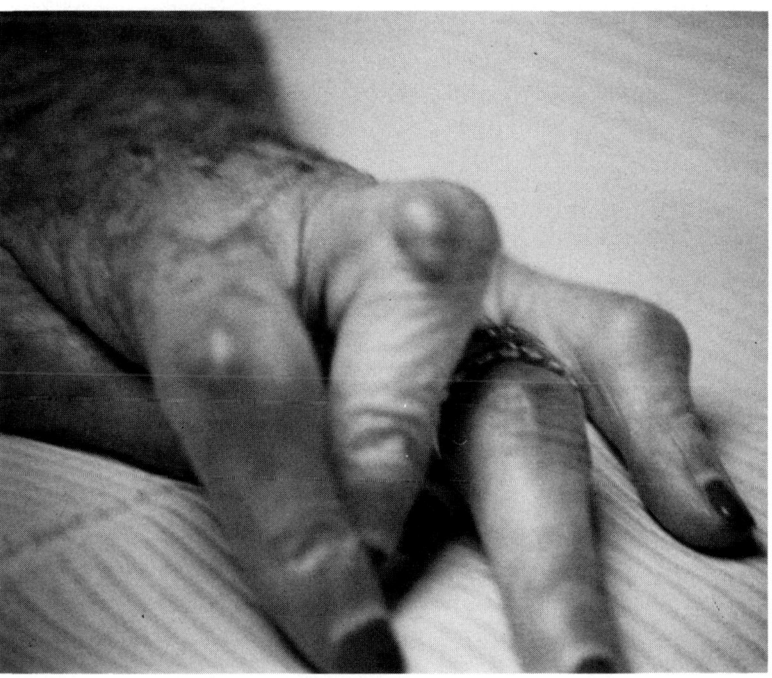

FIGURE 7–3. Boutonnière deformity of the proximal interphalangeal joint in rheumatoid arthritis.

deformity. Each of these deformities can be disabling. Stenosing tenosynovitis of the thumb (de Quervain's tenosynovitis) is also occasionally noted.

Inflammatory, destructive synovitis in the MCP joints is an early finding in most patients with RA. One of the earliest signs of RA may be a decrease in, or total loss of, the dells between the second, third, and fourth MCP joints that are normally visualized when a fist is made. This finding is demonstrated in Figure 7–4. It is noted because most MCP swelling tends to appear dorsally owing to the presence of the flexor plate on the volar aspects of these joints. Doughy synovitis tends to be somewhat less prominent early in the disease. It usually begins at the second and third MCP joints and progresses laterally across the MCP joints.

Progressively erosive synovitis resulting in loss of ligamentous integrity at the MCP joints allows the volar fibrocartilaginous plate (similar to that along the plantar surfaces of the MTP joints) to drift. The proximal phalangeal base resting on this plate subsequently becomes subluxed and even dislocated volarly. Prolonged synovitis also commonly results in rupture of the first dorsal interosseus muscle, causing a notable dell on the dorsal surface between the thumb and second finger. Similar loss of other interossei and lumbricales results in the marked depressions in the dorsal skin overlying areas between the metacarpals seen in Figure 7–5A. In combination with dermal atrophy from accompanying vasculitis and increased blood flow to the inflamed synovial tissues, marked venous prominence becomes apparent over the dorsa of the hands.

The extensor tendons become stretched with progressive MCP volar subluxation.[82] Disease at the wrist can alter the alignment of these tendons, leading to classically noted ulnar deviation of the fingers and subcutaneous prominence of the metacarpal heads seen in Figure 7–5B. Grip strength is reduced dramatically in patients with RA secondary to both guarding from pain and extensive muscle atrophy. Subluxation of the thumb can occur early in the course of RA. Rupture of the first MCP joint medial collateral ligament leads to volar subluxation of the thumb, referred to as "game-

keeper's thumb." This subluxation is occasionally the first clinical sign of RA.

Wrist. The ulnar bursa lies within the distal recess of the ulna. It communicates with the distal radioulnar synovial cavity. Erosive synovitis in this bursa is frequently responsible for destruction of the ligament holding the radius and ulna together. Destruction of this ligament results in dorsal migration of the ulna so that it comes to ride over the radius. This marked dorsal prominence of the ulna, termed *caput ulnae syndrome,* is shown in Figure 7–6. Its presence is responsible for the ulnar deviation of the carpus at the wrist.[83] After the ulna dislocates, light manual pressure over it is capable of reducing the deformity. This is known as the "piano key" sign. Late dislocations are rarely reducible in this manner.

If tenosynovitis is present in the extensor tendons of the hand, it becomes aggravated by dislocation of the ulnar head. Resnick[84] has demonstrated that the ulnar styloid becomes eroded from synovitis in structures at its end, inferior to it, and dorsolateral to it. Erosive synovitis in the radiocarpal joint is also frequently noted. Although rupture of the flexor tendons is most common at the MCP joint level, rupture of the extensors of the hand is most common at the wrist where the most extensive synovitis is present dorsally. Ability to fully extend the wrist is lost early in RA with synovitis in this area. The degree of loss is proportional to the severity and extent of local disease activity. Rheumatoid nodules are often seen on the dorsa of the fingers and wrist and posterior to the elbow. They tend to accompany more severe disease but are occasionally noted in its absence.

Elbow and Shoulder. Erosive synovitis of RA frequently affects both the ulnohumeral and radiohumeral joints and can occasionally be seen involving the olecranon bursa. Flexion contractures are seen early in the course of elbow involvement. Progression of disease activity in this area is associated with progressively greater flexion deformity. Swelling from synovitis tends to displace the fat pads anterior and posterior to the humerus. This, combined with occasional olecranon bursitis and use of the proximal ulna to push off in arising from seated positions, tends to produce signs of skin irritation and tenderness over the proximal ulna. Rheumatoid nodules are also commonly seen in this area.

Shoulder involvement is less commonly noted. When seen, it usually does not present with extensive, erosive destruction. Patients often report pain in the acromioclavicular joint when they lie in bed on the arm of that side. Synovitis is occasionally seen in the tendon sheath of the biceps and is most frequently noted near the muscle insertion. Patients with severe or advanced disease may be unable to raise their forearms up and over their heads. This is usually because of generalized muscle weakness and guarding from the pain of myositis, not from primary disease involvement of the shoulder.

Cervical Spine

The five types of cervical involvement seen in RA have been reviewed in the section on pathology. The clinical findings in relation to disease activity in this area can include tenderness, pain, joint laxity, and neurologic disturbances. The ultimate neurologic disturbance that may be noted with cervical disease in RA is death. The severity of cervical

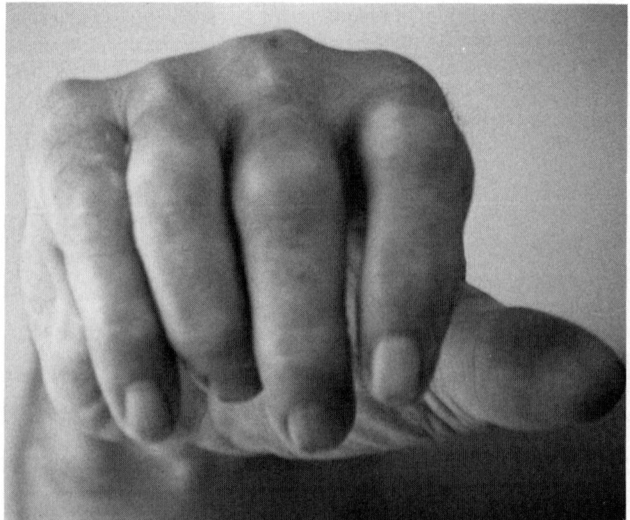

FIGURE 7–4. Synovitis of the second and third metacarpophalangeal joints in rheumatoid arthritis resulting in loss of the dells usually noted between the second, third, and fourth metacarpal heads on the dorsum of the hand.

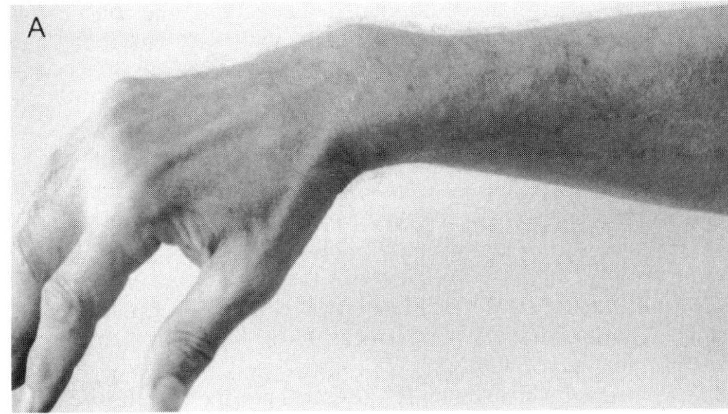

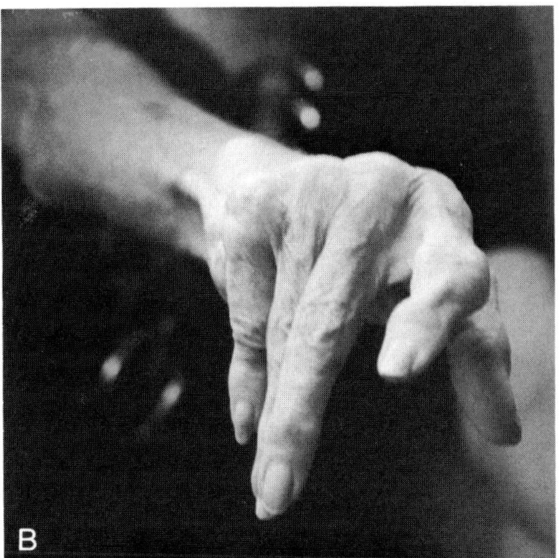

FIGURE 7–5. *A,* Wasting of the interossei and lumbricale muscles results in dells between the metacarpal bones on the dorsa of the hand of this patient with long-term rheumatoid disease. *B,* Advanced rheumatoid disease in the metacarpophalangeal joints and wrist resulting in ulnar deviation of the second through fourth fingers.

erosions strongly correlates with the severity of peripheral erosive disease.[85] Several post mortem studies of rheumatoid arthritis found atlantoaxial subluxation in 11% to 46% of patients with RA.[86] Its presence tends to correlate with seropositivity, subcutaneous rheumatoid nodules, history of glucocorticoid therapy, and the presence of severe, mutilating disease.[87] It is more commonly noted in males.

Stiffness, pain, and crepitus are typically noted in the occipital and cervical areas. Pain is reproduced in this area by placing anterior pressure against C2 with the head flexed and simultaneously extending the head (Sharp-Purser test). An occipital headache may be noted. Pyramidal tract involvement can result in pathologic reflexes. When the basilar artery is occluded, symptoms including double vision and other visual disturbances, tinnitus, and vertigo may be seen. Early signs of potentially fatal bulbar involvement may include changes in the voice and difficulty in swallowing. Occasionally, urinary retention followed by urinary incontinence is noted.

Lower subluxations in the cervical area are more commonly associated with sensorimotor disturbances, usually limited to the arms, shoulders, and neck. Partial or complete numbness, paresthesias, or alteration in perception of hot and cold can be seen. Occasionally, these findings are noted within dermatomal patterns. Motor symptoms of weakness are difficult to differentiate from weakness associated with muscle atrophy, active myositis, and intentional guarding of painful joints and periarticular structures. Once present, these neurologic symptoms tend to advance with significant progression of peripheral articular disease.

Lower Extremity

Foot. Comprehensive studies of the degree of pedal involvement in RA have yet to be reported. Few of the studies currently available differentiate between pedal involvement directly attributable to invasive, proliferative synovitis of RA

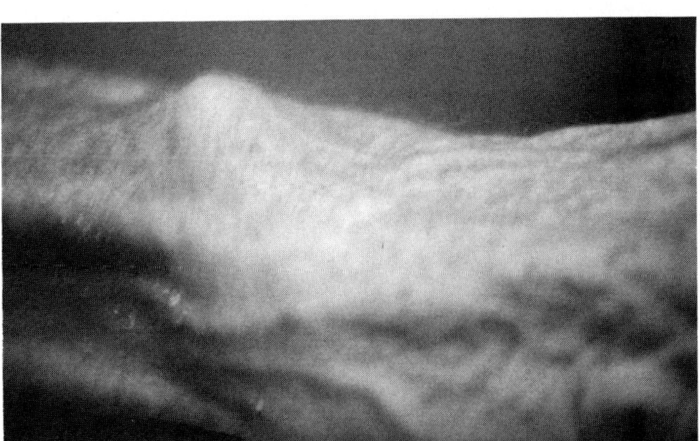

FIGURE 7–6. Marked subcutaneous prominence of the ulnar styloid following its dislocation caused by erosive rheumatoid synovitis.

and symptoms attributable to unrelated structural, and functional aberrations in the feet of patients with RA. The foot has been reported to be the site of initial symptoms in 17% to 20% and is ultimately involved in 90% of all patients with RA.[88] The foot has been described as second only to the knee, and more frequently than the hand, as a site of initial, symptomatic joint disease in RA.[89] In another series, initial involvement was seen in the right MTP joints (48%), the left MTP joints (47%), and bilateral MTP joints (43%).[50] In the same report, initial involvement was seen in the right ankle (25%), left ankle (23%), and bilateral ankles (18%). Another study reported ultimate involvement in the MTP joints and ankle at the rate of 48% and 53%, respectively.[51] A study of 50 hospitalized patients with RA revealed erosive findings in the forefoot in 84%, in tarsal areas in 68%, and in ankles in 16%, with 92% having foot involvement.[90]

Structural and functional aberrations within the foot are among the most commonly noted causes of pain and disability in RA. Anatomic and biomechanical abnormalities present before disease onset can be aggravated by disease activity. They can also exacerbate extant disease activity in any joint. Proliferative synovitis can cause extensive deformity, destruction, and disability within the foot and related structures. This can result in anatomic and biomechanical aberrations that create abnormal stress on involved joints. Rheumatoid disease activity beyond the foot can have significant influence on pedal structural and functional integrity. Unrelated diseases with manifestations both within and beyond the feet can further influence the presentation and course of findings in the feet of patients with RA. Obesity and patterns of use can place additional abnormal stresses on the joints of the feet.

Signs and Symptoms. Signs and symptoms of rheumatoid arthritic involvement in patients' feet are primarily dependent on a number of variables. Disease activity in specific areas and joints is generally more apparent and severe at sites of intensified pressure, stress, and strain. Comprehension and evaluation of findings and their progression in the foot affected by RA require familiarity with the biomechanical implications of normal and abnormal alignments in the foot. An almost endless number of variations is possible.

Some general findings in the feet are frequently seen early in RA. The most common early findings include unaccustomed fatigue in muscles of the legs; generalized soreness in the feet, ankles, and legs; metatarsalgia, aching in the arches, and shoes that have recently become excessively snug. Occasionally, persistent aching and soreness in the fifth, and less commonly fourth, MTP joints are noted early in RA. Symptoms directly attributable to proliferative, erosive synovitis in other pedal joints are rarely noted early in the disease course. Any synovial structure has the potential to present with disease activity, including joints, tendon sheaths, and bursae. Rheumatoid nodules can present in any subcutaneous site, including tendons.

Progressive deformities in the feet are seen with prolonged disease. Although many potential mechanisms for these deformities have been presented, most lack a fundamental understanding of biomechanical considerations in the feet. Deformities in the rheumatoid foot usually follow loss of the integrity of the talonavicular (TN) joint.

Talonavicular Joint Involvement. The structural integrity of the TN joint serves as a key to maintenance of the medial longitudinal arch of the foot. Loss of this integrity leads to collapse of the arch structure. This often occurs early in the course of RA and without notable, symptomatic erosive disease in any pedal joints. The only muscle capable of assisting in the maintenance of normal alignment of the TN joint is the tibialis posterior. Significant, prolonged weakness of this muscle predisposes to collapse of the joint. Loss of TN joint integrity is often seen before significant synovitis in the foot is noted. Subclinical involvement, however, may be present. Tenosynovitis involving the tibialis posterior can further weaken its ability to assist in supporting the TN joint. Chronic or repetitive inflammation may ultimately lead to tendon rupture. Sudden reduction of inflammation within the TN joint, as seen with use of anti-inflammatory medication and in periods of disease remission, can result in significant instability of the joint.

Synovial joints have internal mechanisms that pump excessive internal fluids out of them during their use. This is seen with a stiff elbow that is "freed up" through brief repetitive motion. In this manner, fluid within a joint is expressed without stretched, supportive, soft tissue structures having sufficient time to contract and provide appropriate support. This mechanism probably plays a significant role in the loss of integrity of the TN joint commonly seen early in the course of RA. In addition, synovitis in local bursae and in the middle and anterior compartments of the subtalar joint can weaken the spring ligament. Support by this ligament is essential for maintenance of normal TN joint alignment.

Any loss of normal structural alignment and integrity of the TN joint causes the talus to migrate downward. The structure of the subtalar joint dictates that this movement be accompanied by medial displacement of the talus and concurrent valgus rotation of the calcaneus. The tarsal joints of a normal, skeletal foot structure bound together by normal ligaments have an inherent locking mechanism that maintains a medial longitudinal arch. This locking mechanism allows maintenance of normal arch structure with application of weight to the talar dome only so long as the calcaneus functions in a direction either vertical or inverted to the ground surface (Harford GE: Personal communication, 1977).

Loss of TN joint integrity and secondary eversion of the calcaneus with rearfoot pronation unlock the tarsal joints. This leads to further collapse of the TN joint, medial migration of the talus, and collapse of the medial arch. With pronation of the rearfoot, motion around the oblique axis of the midtarsal joint leads to abduction of the forefoot on the rearfoot. In the presence of rearfoot pronation, intensified pressure is produced under the medial forefoot as it is driven downward against the ground surface. With progressive pronation, inability of the medial forefoot to push downward through the ground surface results in relative supination of the foot distal to the midtarsal joint in relation to the calcaneal and talar positions shown in Figure 7–7.

The base of the second metatarsal is locked into the tarsal bones along three sides of its base. This makes the second metatarsal resistant to dorsiflexion at its tarsometatarsal articulation. The first metatarsal is significantly more mobile. Prolonged, excessive weightbearing pressures under the medial forefoot force this bone upward at the first metatarsocuneiform joint. Motion at this joint is limited to combined dorsiflexion and medial angulation. Progressive rearfoot pronation, therefore, is usually accompanied by adduction and elevation of the first metatarsal. Simultaneous unlocking of the navicular and medial cuneiform articulation tends to aug-

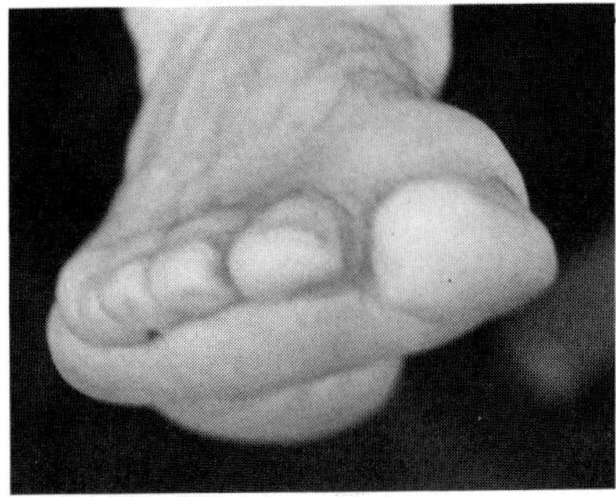

FIGURE 7–7. Relative supination of the forefoot in rheumatoid arthritis secondary to excessive subtalar joint pronation during weightbearing.

ment this deformity. In RA, it can be further augmented by primary weakness in the peroneus longus muscle and by related tenosynovitis. This widening of the forefoot in RA is shown in Figure 7–8.

Hallux Valgus and Bunion Formation. Etiology of concomitant hallux valgus has been attributed to erosive synovitis affecting the abductor hallucis muscle in RA.[91] It is also frequently attributed to the use of shoes with excessively narrow toe box areas. In fact, excessive pronation solely due to anatomic abnormalities and in the absence of synovitis or use of shoes has been shown to result in severe hallux valgus and bunion deformities. The medial and dorsal angulation of the first metatarsal combined with valgus drift of the calcaneus causes the short flexor and short extensor of the great toe to pull it into an abducted and everted (valgus) position. The transverse and oblique portions of the adductor hallucis muscle produce similar deforming forces on the great toe. With abduction of the great toe, its flexor and extensor tendons come to lie lateral to the center of the first MTP joint. Subsequent function of these muscles tends to pull the great toe into further abduction. The great toe often proceeds to move to a position under the second, third, and even the fourth toe.

Irritation of soft tissues between the bunion area and the inside of shoes results in local erythema, tenderness, and swelling and occasional bursitis. With prolonged irritation, reactive periostitis at the dorsomedial first metatarsal head can cause deposition of additional bone. This can substantially increase the size of the bunion deformity. Continued

excessive pressure on the soft tissue structures between the bunion and the inside of shoes can result in marked tenderness, prominent bursitis, rheumatoid nodule formation, subcutaneous hemorrhage, ulceration, and sinus tract formation, as seen in Figure 7–9.

The lateral drift of the great toe pushes the lesser toes into an abducted position with regard to their respective metatarsals. Simultaneously, the collapse of the medial longitudinal arch elongates the foot. This tends to compress the toes against the ends of shoes, causing extension deformity at the MTP joints and flexion deformities at the PIP joints. Additional related flexion deformity at the DIP joints can be seen in many instances.

Digital Deformities. The fifth toe usually comes to underlay the fourth toe. Friction and pressure between crowded and overlapping toes result in interdigital areas of skin irritation. This irritation is most intense between the normally flared heads and bases of the phalanges. Persistent irritation in these areas is accompanied by hypertrophy and exostosis formation, which further intensify tissue irritation. Excessively tapered and snug toe box areas in stylish shoes (high heels) further aggravate this situation. Persistent irritation often produces painful interdigital corns, subcutaneous hemorrhage, ulceration, and sinus tract formation.

In instances in which patients have had all toes amputated and have maintained propulsive gait patterns, recurrent ulcerations under multiple metatarsal heads are common. The intrinsic and extrinsic flexors of the toes function to help relieve weightbearing pressure under the metatarsal heads during propulsion. Initially in RA, metatarsalgia is seen because weakness in these muscles diminishes their functional capacity. Extension deformities of the MTP joints further weaken the functional capacity of these muscles, inducing more severe metatarsalgia.[92]

Extension of each toe at the MTP joint also depresses its respective metatarsal head and tends to pull the fat pad plantar to the metatarsal head forward. Even in the absence of notable synovitis, progressive deformity of the toes frequently results in their complete dorsal dislocation at the MTP joints with proximal migration of the proximal phalan-

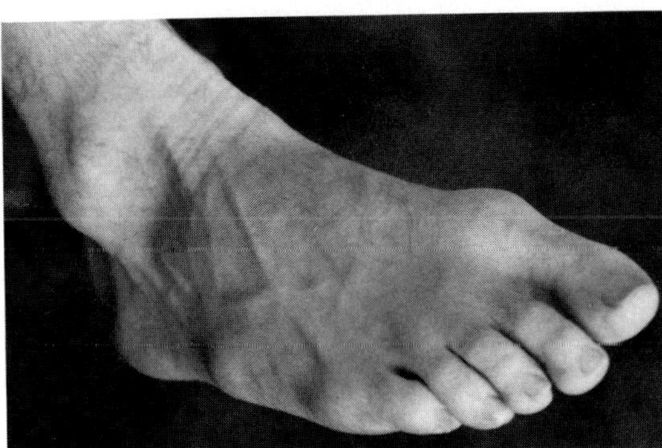

FIGURE 7–8. Widening of the forefoot seen early in the course of rheumatoid arthritis secondary to dorsiflexion and adduction of the first metatarsal and dorsiflexion and abduction of the fifth metatarsal associated with loss of functional integrity of the talonavicular joint and secondary excessive subtalar joint pronation during weightbearing.

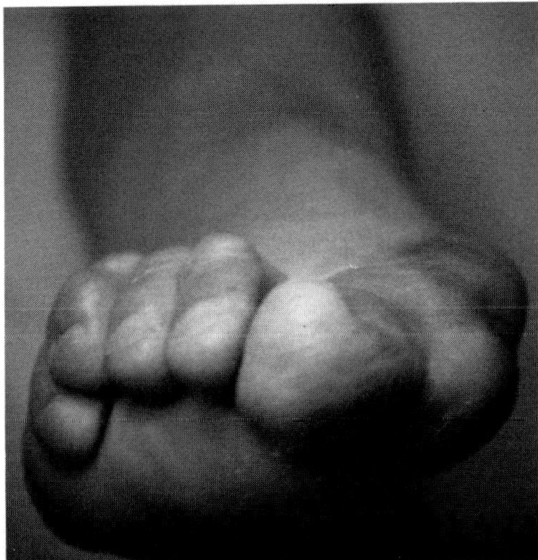

FIGURE 7–9. Rheumatoid nodule formation at the plantar medial base of the great toe. Associated hallux abductovalgus, bunion, and first metatarsal angulation deformities are also noted.

geal base. This serves to further depress involved metatarsal heads. Marked plantar prominence of the metatarsal heads is frequently noted. These findings are demonstrated in Figure 7–10. Irritation in these areas can be associated with rheumatoid nodule formations, erythema, marked tenderness, subcutaneous hemorrhage, and ulceration.

Arch Collapse and Plantar Fasciitis. Early collapse of the TN joint often leads to medial prominence of the tuberosity of the navicular bone. Skin caught between it and the inside of shoes often shows erythema and tenderness secondary to irritation. Occasionally, rheumatoid nodules are noted in this area. Prolonged progression of this deformity can be associated with ulceration of overlying skin. Similar findings can be seen over the posterior, dorsolateral calcaneus with excessive pronation in shoes during the gait cycle and with pre-existent Haglund's deformity.

Progressive collapse of the joints in the medial longitudinal arch causes stretching of the plantar fascia. Increasing valgus deviation of the calcaneus places additional pull on the plantar fascia, as does dorsal subluxation of the toes at the MTP joints. The plantar fascia is firmly and extensively anchored anteriorly and has a limited area of attachment posteriorly at the anterior margin of the inferior calcaneal tuberosities. Plantar fasciitis, with pain reported centered at the posterior insertion of the plantar fascia, is seen much less frequently than would be anticipated throughout the course of RA. It does occasionally present in association with a fairly rapid collapse of arch structure early in the course of RA. It is occasionally the first presenting symptom of this disease.

Although insertional tenderness is noted in many patients with advanced, erosive joint disease, symptoms related to active synovitis and even to secondary osteoarthrosis usually overshadow those of plantar fasciitis. Reproduction of pain is established on direct palpation of the insertional area. This maneuver usually elicits greater pain medially than laterally. Passive, simultaneous, full dorsiflexion of the toes and foot with simultaneous palpation of the insertional area usually elicits intensified discomfort.

Pre-existent pathomechanical problems can predispose to, induce, or exacerbate pedal symptoms noted in RA.[92] Proper evaluation of any RA patient's foot requires that the pre-existent status of that foot be thoroughly delineated and understood.[93] In rearfoot varus and compensated forefoot val-

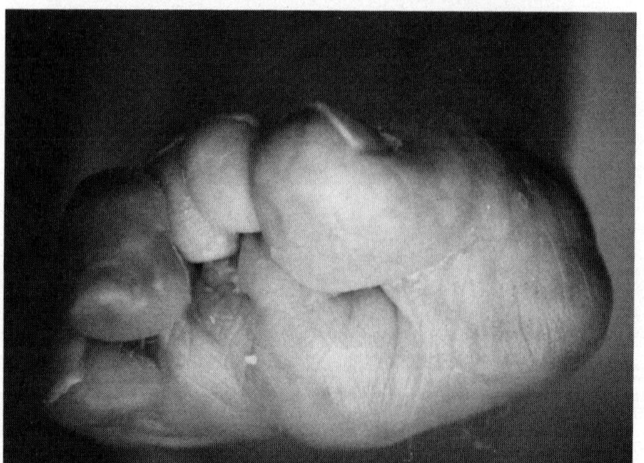

FIGURE 7–10. Spontaneous dorsal dislocation of the second, third, and fourth metatarsophalangeal joints in rheumatoid arthritis.

gus deformities, the subtalar joint functions in a supinated position, preventing medial displacement of the center of gravity in the foot and consequent unlocking of the tarsal joints. Similarly, these factors are prevented in feet that have functional or structural rigidity of the subtalar joint that holds the heel either in varus or perpendicular to the ground surface. In such feet, the aforementioned deformities tend to present less frequently and with less severity.

Forefoot Splaying. "Splaying of the forefoot" is one of the most commonly cited findings in the foot affected by RA. Many authors have attributed it to erosive destruction of intermetatarsal ligaments and to MTP joint synovitis. In fact, clinical and radiographic examinations confirm that splaying of the central three metatarsals and toes is extremely rare in RA. Prior to notation of significant first and fifth metatarsal deformity, intermetatarsal bursitis and MTP joint synovitis can be responsible for mild to moderate widening of the forefoot. Adduction of the first metatarsal and abduction of the fifth metatarsal account for the moderate to severe splaying or overall widening of the forefoot that is usually seen in advanced cases of RA. This splaying has sequelae, an example of which is seen with the fifth metatarsal. Initially, irritation of skin between the prominent dorsolateral fifth metatarsal head and the shoes causes erythema and tenderness, callus formation, and swelling. Prolonged friction in this area between the skin and bone causes reactive periostitis, bony hypertrophy, and exostosis formation in this area. Their presence intensifies irritation and can cause severe local pain, bursitis, rheumatoid nodule formation, subcutaneous hemorrhage, and ulceration, as seen with medial bunion deformities.

Loss of Transverse Arch. Another related misconception that is widely held in medical and orthopedic literature is that RA is associated with collapse of the "transverse metatarsal arch" in the region of the metatarsal heads. This has been widely reported to result in plantar depression of the central three metatarsal heads with resulting excessive, concentrated weightbearing under them. In fact, the normal foot has no transverse arch in the frontal or coronal plane at the metatarsal head area. Simple examination of shoe insoles reveals that all metatarsal heads are weightbearing in a normal foot. Normally, the first metatarsal bears approximately one half the pressure in the ball of the foot, with the remainder equally divided among the lesser metatarsals. In actuality, instability and dorsiflexed positioning of the first and fifth metatarsals commonly seen in RA cause intensified weightbearing under the central three metatarsals. Functional incapacity and dorsal subluxation and dislocation of the three central toes exacerbate excessive weightbearing pressures in these areas.

Progressive Joint Deformity. Synovitis in the first MTP joint can be noted early in the course of a rare form of RA. It is most commonly seen in seropositive males with accompanying rheumatoid nodules and severe, aggressive, rapidly progressive, and destructive erosive joint disease.[52] Proliferative, inflammatory, erosive synovitis involving the tarsometatarsal and intertarsal joints is rarely seen in early RA. Later in the course of RA, rearfoot involvement can equal or surpass that seen in the forefoot. One study in Europe that relied primarily on radiographic evaluations and that failed to differentiate between osteoarthrosis and true rheumatoid joint disease indicated that the TN joint was the most common site of pedal involvement in the rheumatoid foot.[94] Extensive clinical experience and observation have subsequently confirmed that this joint is much less frequently a site of erosive rheumatoid involvement when compared with the lateral MTP joints.

Symptoms of strain in the TN joint associated with collapse of the medial longitudinal arch, with occasional concurrent plantar fasciitis, are common in both early and late RA. Frequently, patients report that this pain emanates from the medial ankle area. Palpation directly over the TN joint with simultaneous inversion and eversion of the midtarsal joint confirms that symptoms are arising from the TN joint. Although 42% of one series of patients reported some rearfoot symptoms, only 16% reported that rearfoot involvement significantly interfered with their walking.[95]

Progressive collapse of the rearfoot structure and its valgus angulation produces frequent pain in the subtalar joint. Involvement in this area is associated with significant pain reported on attempts to walk on any uneven terrain. This pain is often referred to the lateral heel area, or more specifically to the lateral, plantar weightbearing margin of the heel. With subtalar joint involvement, palpation over the sinus tarsi usually elicits soreness. Similar reproduction of symptoms is achieved with forced pronation of the calcaneus combined with palpation over this area or over the anterior and posterior margins of the lateral malleolus. Occasionally, erosive disease is seen in the posterior, middle, or anterior facets of the subtalar joint. Erosive involvement of the subtalar joint in RA is usually severely painful and disabling.

Erosive disease in the subtalar, TN, calcaneocuboid, or ankle joints is rarely noted in RA in the absence of significant collapse of the arch structure or valgus deformity of the rearfoot. Marked valgus deformity of the rearfoot can be associated with traumatic synovitis associated with pinching of the lateral subtalar and calcaneocuboid joint capsules, peroneal tendons, and dorsal TN joint capsule. Symptoms are perceived in the anterolateral ankle area. They can be associated with compressive irritation and even damage to these structures and subsequent post-traumatic synovitis. Because post-traumatic synovitis is caused by excessive stress in an area that simultaneously is predisposed to inflammatory synovitis in active RA, it is often impossible to determine the extent to which each is present or responsible for presenting symptoms in a patient.

Tenosynovitis. Tenosynovitis of the long flexors and extensors of the toes is occasionally a presenting complaint or is noted on initial examination in RA. It can be confirmed through notation of tenderness on palpation, active motion, and especially resisted active motion of the toes. Occasionally, grating can be noted on palpation where the extensors pass under the cruciate ligaments or in the region of the tarsal tunnel. Tenderness at insertional areas also may be noted.

Tenosynovitis involving the tibialis posterior, peroneus longus, and Achilles tendons can be seen early in the disease course. It is less commonly seen involving the tibialis anterior tendon. Involvement is occasionally seen early in the disease course but is more commonly noted with progression of the disease and deformity of the foot. Pain in the TN joint caused by inflammatory synovitis or strain associated with collapse of the joint can cause spasm of the peroneus brevis.[96] This spasm can induce or aggravate valgus deformity of the rearfoot and collapse of the arch structure. To test for it, adductory pressure is rapidly applied a few times to the lateral fifth metatarsal head and released. If peroneal spasm is present, sudden abduction of the forefoot will be immediately noted on ceasing repetitive pressure application.

Tenosynovitis of the tibialis posterior is most frequently noted as the tendon courses through its sheath behind and beneath the medial (tibial) malleolus. It also can be seen when severe valgus deformity causes irritation of the tendon between the head of the talus and inside of shoes. Occasionally, strain placed on this tendon accompanying rapid early collapse of the medial arch is associated with tenosynovitis as a presenting symptom of RA. Although the tibialis anterior is normally a swing-phase muscle, tenosynovitis involving it can occasionally be seen under the same circumstances. More frequently, it is noted in association with contracture deformity or profound weakness of the gastrocnemius-soleus complex.

Tenosynovitis of the peroneal tendons occasionally is seen because of impingement of these tendons along the lateral calcaneus. A marked valgus deformity of the heel can cause these tendons to be caught between the lateral side of the calcaneus and the inside of the shoe. More frequently, tenosynovitis of the peroneus longus is seen where it courses in its tendon sheath behind and under the lateral (fibular) malleolus. Rarely, collapse of the lateral longitudinal arch, combined with an inverted weightbearing position of the foot, can be associated with tenosynovitis of this tendon as it passes under the cuboid. Occasionally, rapid progression of dorsiflexion deformity of the first metatarsal can be associated with tenosynovitis in either of these areas.

Tenosynovitis of the Achilles tendon in RA is most commonly associated with strain placed on the gastrocnemius-soleus complex secondary to unlocking of the tarsal joints. One of the primary functions of the foot is to act as a rigid lever during propulsion. The muscle complex is responsible for acting on this rigid lever in a manner so as to elevate total body weight and propel it forward with each stride.

Unlocking of the tarsal joints results in structural incompetence of the normal rigid lever formed by the tarsus and metatarsus. Significantly greater effort, therefore, is required to achieve reasonably normal patterns of ambulation. This strain can be associated with tendinitis at the insertional area and within the substance of the Achilles tendon. Inflammatory erosive bursitis in the retrocalcaneal and retro-Achilles bursae can also cause both forms of tendinitis.

Abnormal pronation of the calcaneus in shoes can cause irritation of the Achilles tendon between it and the internal counter of shoes. This irritation, pre-existent hypertrophy of the posterosuperior calcaneus (Haglund's deformity), and pressure from enlarged retrocalcaneal or retro-Achilles bursae, can also predispose to Achilles tendinitis. Granulomatous, inflammatory synovitis or rheumatoid nodules can also occur within the substance of the tendon and induce similar tendinitis.[97]

Tarsal tunnel syndrome is seen with far greater frequency in patients with RA than in the general population. In one series of 30 patients with confirmed, erosive rheumatoid disease, 4 (13%) had electrodiagnostically confirmed tarsal tunnel syndrome.[98] Because these tests were not performed with the involved feet weightbearing and fully pronated, the actual number involved may have been substantially higher.

Extra-Articular Involvement. Extra-articular findings in RA are frequently noted in the feet. Rheumatoid nodules can potentially be noted in any subcutaneous or other soft tissue location. They are most commonly seen under the central three metatarsals, medial to the navicular bone or medial cuneiform, and over the posterior heel area. Their presence usually correlates with structural or functional deformities that induce excessive pressures at these sites.

A rare, but often misdiagnosed, finding in RA involves fistula formations through the skin into bursae, periarticular soft tissue, bone cysts, or joints. They are primarily noted in seropositive patients with long-standing disease. Although the fistulas are occasionally septic in origin, quite often they are sterile.[99] Cultures of these areas frequently yield only normal skin flora. These fistulas tend to be nontender and usually form at sites of intensified, abnormal pressure.

Skin and joint infections are present with increased frequency and intensity in the feet of those with RA compared with the general population. Recent research has confirmed that there is no increased incidence of bronchopulmonary or genitourinary infections either before or after onset in RA patients when compared with those with osteoarthrosis. This is true only in uncomplicated and untreated disease. Treatment with glucocorticoids and immunosuppressive drugs in RA is associated with substantially increased incidence, severity, and resistance to treatment of infections.[100]

Although the initial and probably primary lesions in RA involve vasculitis in the synovium, vasculitis affecting skin, muscle, and nerve vasculature often presents distinct additional signs of this disease in the feet. These extra-articular forms of vasculitis are more commonly seen in men with high titers of rheumatoid factor and severe, extensive, rapidly destructive arthropathy. Signs and symptoms of cutaneous vasculitis presenting in the feet include splinter hemorrhages, cutaneous ulcerations, and gangrene. They are most common on the distal toes and at sites of intense pressure on skin. Rarely, erythematous, frequently pruritic, sharply marginated, macular or slightly raised lesions (erythema marginatum, target lesions) are seen on the soles and palms. Related palpable purpura has been reported.[101] Skin lesions in the presence of vasculitis show delayed healing and often complete failure to heal.

Neurovascular manifestations are commonly the only vasculitic findings in RA. The two most commonly seen patterns are a slowly progressive, distal, sensory neuropathy and a more seriously debilitating mononeuritis multiplex (sensorimotor neuropathy).[102] In distal sensory neuropathy, decreased soft and sharp touch are noted; temperature, vibratory, and joint position sensation normally remain intact. Those patients with sensorimotor neuropathy usually present with similar, although more profound, sensory neuropathy accompanied by substantial loss of muscle strength. Occasionally, involvement of anterior leg compartment muscles in this latter form of neuropathy results in footdrop.

A wide variety of diseases and disorders can present concurrently with RA in any given patient. Signs and symptoms of associated diseases can be similar and may be confused with those of RA. Peripheral vascular disease and neuropathies associated with diabetes and other causes are typical examples. Whenever possible, diagnostic distinction between the symptoms of each disorder should be attempted. Too often, such distinctions prove impossible.

Ankle. Although granulomatous, erosive, inflammatory synovitis rarely presents in the ankle early in the course of RA, ankle symptoms early in the disease are common. Most patients with TN joint involvement perceive and report associated pain emanating from the ankle joint. With severe valgus positioning of the calcaneus, imposition of body weight on the rearfoot causes valgus torque at the ankle. The three-sided mortise of an intact ankle joint does not allow this torque to be accommodated by motion within the ankle joint. The extent of misconceptions throughout the medical literature warrants stressing that the eversion and pronation of the foot in RA almost always precedes disease involvement in the ankle joint.

Throughout medical (especially rheumatologic and orthopedic) literature, ankle pain noted in RA has been related to "pronounced affectation of the fibular part of the talocrural joint" or loss of the integrity of the inferior tibiofibular ligaments and syndesmosis.[103, 104] In fact, it is the integrity of the distal tibiofibular ligaments and syndesmosis that prevents lateral migration of the fibula from mitigating the excessive pressure produced in the lateral portion of the joint in association with weightbearing on a rearfoot deformed into a valgus position. Continued, intense, localized pressure at this site can ultimately result in stress fractures of the distal tibia or fibula.[104]

Erosive ankle joint synovitis is noted ultimately in approximately 10% to 16% of those with a prolonged course of RA.[51, 52] It should be differentiated from tenosynovitis involving muscles passing behind and under the malleoli, as described earlier. Clinical differentiation between ankle joint enlargement due to synovitis and that due to joint effusion is possible with palpation around the joint. With true ankle joint effusions, pressing into a swollen area adjacent to one malleolus with simultaneous palpation of the joint capsule adjacent to the other malleolus or anteriorly allows for notation of a fluid wave across the joint. Palpation in the presence of significant synovitis reveals a doughy, firm but fluctuant consistency in the joint capsule. Traumatic effusions and synovitis are common in the absence of significant inflammatory, erosive rheumatoid synovitis in the ankle. Both types of synovitis can be concurrently or sequentially present in the ankle of any patient with RA. Occasionally, tenosynovitis involving the peroneal tendons causes ankle joint effusion owing to communication of the tendon sheaths with the joint interior. This communication is normally present in less than 20% of all people.

Knee and Hip. The medial and lateral femorotibial, patellofemoral, and proximal tibiofibular joints are frequently involved in RA. Dramatic weakness of the quadriceps is often seen early in the course of the disease and may be a presenting complaint. Erosive synovitis also often occurs in the knees early in the course of the disease. Joint effusions are frequently visualized superior, inferior, medial, and lateral to the patella. Mild downward pressure exerted over the patella with the knee relaxed, supported, and fully extended reveals that the patella is floating on a bed of fluid with significant effusion in the joint. With significant inflammatory rheumatoid synovitis in the knee joint, boggy synovial consistency usually can be palpated along the borders of the patella. It can occasionally be palpated at the proximal tibiofibular joint when active disease is present at this site.

With progression of the disease, mild to moderate flexion contractures of the knee develop. Although full extension of the knee is normal in gait, it is associated with the tautest position of the joint. Ligamentous structures within the knee are in their loosest possible position with 20 degrees of flexion. Although it requires substantially more effort from already weakened muscles, patients with RA involvement of the knee often ambulate with the joint intentionally flexed to this degree to lessen pressures of internal effusions, tension on internal ligaments, and pressures between articular surfaces. Knees with active synovitis are also more comfortable when rested in a position of about 20 degrees of flexion. In time, the flexion deformity of the knee can become fixed.

The excessive pronation of the rearfoot seen in RA produces both abnormal internal rotation of the limb and a valgus torque at the ankle joint. This internal rotation tends to malalign the patella. This causes excessive compression between it and its corresponding, lateral, articular surface on the distal femur. These abnormal forces are often sufficient to produce a complaint of significantly increased pain along the lateral border of the patella and in the lateral compartment of the knee. Often, treatment that effectively decreases the valgus deformity of the rearfoot is accompanied by substantial improvement of such knee pain.

As discussed earlier, the ankle mortise usually remains intact in RA. The ankle, therefore, is unable to compensate for the valgus torque placed on it during weightbearing. This torque acts proximally on the knee to induce and exacerbate its own valgus deformity. Prolonged and advanced disease tends to be associated with increasingly greater degrees of valgus deformity of the knee joint. Many patients who have undergone surgical replacement of knee joints ultimately may have less than anticipated and desired results from surgery if the rotary and valgus components of foot deformity are not concurrently and appropriately addressed.

Increased pressure within the knee can result in posterior synovial cyst (Baker's cyst) or ganglion formation. These cysts may present with tenderness and swelling behind the knee. Rarely, they dissect through tissues distally, progressing down the back of the leg. Occasionally, such growths can be confused with phlebitis in the calf or even with ankle involvement in RA when they reach that area. If a patient is receiving glucocorticoid therapy, prominent enlargement of the fat pad inferior to the patella may be noted. This may occur because this is one of the areas involved in redistribution of body fat that often accompanies glucocorticoid therapy.

Occasionally, proliferative synovitis at the proximal tibiofibular joint causes entrapment of the superficial peroneal nerve as it courses around this area. Sensory deficits in the lateral leg and over the dorsum of the foot and partial or complete paralysis of the peroneal muscles may be noted. Formation of rheumatoid nodules in this area, or stress fracture of the proximal fibula, can be associated with similar findings. Rarely, Baker's cysts or rheumatoid nodules can cause additional compression neuropathies that may involve the posterior tibial, deep peroneal, or superficial peroneal nerves.

Significant clinical involvement of the hip joint in RA is far less commonly noted than involvement of the foot, knee, and ankle. Proliferative, granulomatous synovitis in the hip joint can slowly erode the adjacent cartilaginous surfaces, leading to loss of joint space. Even with almost complete loss of joint space, some patients with RA continue to function with few symptoms referable to the hip joint. Supratrochanteric bursitis is much more commonly the cause of symptoms in the hip area, especially early in the disease course. Occasionally, advanced destruction of the hip joint in combination with significant osteoporosis causes protrusion of the acetabular cup into the pelvis and profound disability with or without pelvic fracture.

An interesting clinical finding frequently seen in the presence of significant limb-length discrepancy is greater symptomatic involvement of the knee on the short side and the hip on the long side. Considering that the knee of the short leg would have a greater tendency to be fully extended, this finding would be anticipated. On the long side, body weight has to be lifted higher as it passes forward during weightbearing on that side, if a contralateral drop of the pelvis is to be avoided. Because the center of body weight is four times the distance medial to the center of the hip than the insertion of the hip abductors are lateral to it, the force necessary to maintain proper alignment of the pelvis by these muscles is magnified considerably. As the contralateral leg passes through swing phase, the compressive force on the dorsum of the hip joint is equal to five times body weight (actual body weight plus the abductors producing a compressive force four times its value). This force results in substantially increased compressive forces across the dorsal hip joint during unilateral stance on the long lower extremity.

MANAGEMENT

General Considerations

Optimally efficacious treatment of any disease or disorder must be directed at management of presenting signs and symptoms. These are unusually variable in RA, and they can be determined and modified by many factors. They include, but are not limited to, the patient's genetic inheritance, age, sex, body build, health status, mental status, pre-existing illness, and congenital or acquired structural and functional abnormalities. This disease is characterized by chronic, intermittent, and progressive destruction of body tissues. Signs and symptoms tend to be continually evolving. All these variables mandate that treatment regimens be tailored individually for each patient.

Disease activity in RA can affect every body system and every facet of the patients' lives. The enormity of the fund of currently available, relevant information in different medical specialties makes it impossible for any single physician to render complete and appropriate care. Comprehensive evaluation of signs, symptoms, and functional incapacities is required to establish appropriate treatment regimens. During and after such evaluation a health care team approach offers the only hope of establishing and implementing an optimal, individualized treatment plan.[105] Appropriate team management usually requires inclusion of a family practitioner or internist, rheumatologist, psychiatrist or psychologist, social worker, physical therapist, occupational therapist, and orthopedist. RA involving the lower extremities should mandate inclusion of a skilled and knowledgeable podiatric physician and surgeon.[105]

Once a tentative diagnosis of RA is confirmed and a patient has been thoroughly evaluated, individualized and realistic therapeutic goals can be established. These goals must take into account the previous course, current severity, and extent of joint and systemic disease. Demands of desired and realistic lifestyle and vocational and avocational activities have to be considered. Functional incapacities have to be recognized. They should be reduced and, wherever possible, eliminated. Permanent incapacities need to be accepted and dealt with realistically. After all preliminary data are accumulated and assessed, the anticipated disease course should be considered in establishing individual treatment goals.

Patients' mental attitudes, personal desires, and individual needs should be elicited and given appropriate consideration. Recognition of their disease as one of unknown cause, with chronic, progressive destruction and disability and without a known cure, often is accompanied by depression, frustration, loss of motivation, feelings of helplessness, and despair. Patients who maintain positive attitudes and high levels of motivation appear to have substantially higher overall quality of life. Interaction with physicians and extensive patient education play a key role in sustaining these positive attitudes. They can be rapidly destroyed by failure to set appropriate, realistic, and attainable therapeutic goals or by inadequate patient education.

The goals of any treatment plan in RA should include four objectives (Table 7–6). Signs and symptoms of disease activity should be managed to reduce their effects. Efforts should be made to stem the course of, and if possible eradicate, underlying disease processes. Existing structural and functional integrity needs to be preserved and protected. Structural and functional capacities that have become diminished or lost need to be optimally rehabilitated. These goals are usually best achieved through a combination of pharmacologic, conservative, and surgical therapeutic regimens.

Pharmacologic Management

Oral Medications. Overall pharmacologic management of RA is usually beyond the scope of expertise of those physicians concentrating their skills on management of lower extremity disorders. They should, however, have familiarity with medications that are specifically directed at management of signs and symptoms of disease throughout the body, including the lower extremities. They should also be aware of these agents' potential side effects and their implications.

Salicylates. The first line of therapeutic agents used in RA is usually the salicylate drugs. Recent availability of ibuprofen without prescription has led to its frequent use as a first-line medication. Patients have usually begun intake of salicylates or ibuprofen prior to their initial presentation. Both agents are associated with potential gastritis, gastrointestinal ulceration, hemorrhage, and increased coagulation times.

A wide variety of salicylate preparations is available. Many patients can take inexpensive acetylated salicylates without significant gastrointestinal problems. Buffered preparations and enteric-coated preparations tend to be better tolerated by many patients with ''sensitive'' stomachs. Overall absorption of enteric-coated preparations is equal to that of uncoated forms of salicylates.[106] Time-release preparations tend to have increased efficacy with regard to morning stiff-

ness. A minimum of 3.6 grains of salicylates daily, and often as much as 4.2 grains, taken in divided doses, is necessary to achieve anti-inflammatory efficacy.

Onset of RA primarily after the fourth decade, combined with the chronicity of the disease, results in a large proportion of patients being elderly. Elderly patients may have significant intolerance of salicylates.[107] They tend to experience tinnitus as a sign of overdose at lower levels of intake. This tinnitus is rapidly reversible by lowering dosages. Occult gastrointestinal hemorrhage can be related to salicylate intake. Patients on long-term therapy with these agents should be advised to monitor the color of their stools. Black and tarry stools may be the only accompanying sign of gastrointestinal hemorrhage. Substantial, and occasionally sudden, fluctuations in plasma levels of salicylates may be seen. Renal excretion fluctuates in dehydrated states, with use of concurrent medication (glucocorticoids, probenecid), and in the presence of diseases affecting the kidneys. Renal effects are significant but are neither chronic nor cumulative.

Many patients who have intolerance of salicylates can take a number of nonacetylated forms of salicylate currently available. These preparations are considerably more expensive than most forms of acetylated salicylates, but they do offer more convenient dosing schedules. Nonacetylated forms of salicylates do not acetylate plasma proteins. This makes their concurrent use with a wide variety of protein-bound medications considerably safer than is seen with the use of acetylated salicylates. It also provides for less effect on coagulation mechanisms.

Avoidance of excessive bleeding tendencies can be achieved with discontinuation of nonacetylated salicylates 1 or 2 days before elective surgical procedures. Discontinuation of acetylated salicylates is advisable 2 weeks or more before such surgery. Low-level intake of salicylates is associated with renal retention of urate; it can aggravate existent hyperuricemia. At higher plasma levels, salicylates are uricosuric, tending to reduce serum uric acid concentration.

The antiinflammatory activity of salicylates is insufficient to significantly mask signs of infection.[108] Sodium salicylate is equally efficacious in reducing inflammation when compared with acetylated salicylates. Sodium salicylate does not block the cyclooxygenase pathway.[109] Although it is believed that salicylate's antiinflammatory efficacy is primarily related to this area of arachidonic acid metabolism, this finding further indicates that the basis of this efficacy may still be unknown.

Nonsteroidal Antiinflammatory Drugs. Nonsteroidal antiinflammatory drugs (NSAIDs) are widely used in the treatment of the inflammation and accompanying pain and disability seen in RA. They are currently frequently used as first-line agents in the control of inflammatory symptoms. Currently available agents are discussed thoroughly in Chapter 24. Response of patients with RA to specific agents tends to be highly individualized. Often one patient recurrently experiences dramatic relief with one agent, whereas another patient presenting with clinically similar disease experiences no effect. When a specific agent fails to provide satisfactory relief, trial of an agent from another class should be attempted.

Potential side effects of any specific NSAID should be considered before it is prescribed. All agents in this class have potential gastrointestinal side effects similar to those seen with acetylated salicylates. The incidence of these side

TABLE 7–6

TREATMENT GOALS IN RHEUMATOID ARTHRITIS

1. Manage and control signs and symptoms of disease activity
2. Control, minimize, and, if possible, eliminate underlying disease activity
3. Protect and conserve existing structural and functional integrity
4. Optimally rehabilitate diminished or lost structural and functional capacities

effects appears to be less than that seen with acetylated salicylates, but it is probably greater than that seen with nonacetylated salicylates.

Prescription of NSAIDs in any patient with a history of frequent gastritis, abdominal pain, or gastrointestinal ulceration and hemorrhage should be made with caution. Even with such a past history, these agents can often be safely prescribed for extended periods with concurrent use of medication that blocks gastric acid production. Similar safety can be attained with newer (although quite expensive) agents that fortify the normal protective barrier in the gastric mucosa. Prescription of indomethacin should be avoided in elderly patients with histories of chronic headaches or mental confusion. Similarly, meclofenamate should be avoided in patients with histories of frequent bouts of diarrhea.

Glucocorticoids. Glucocorticoid therapy is commonly used to help control the inflammation in RA. Prednisone in doses of 10 mg/day and higher is associated with significant suppression of the pituitary-adrenal-hypophyseal axis and associated side effects. Capillary fragility, increased incidence of infection, delayed healing, and redistribution of the fat pads in the body are also seen with similar doses. Chronic suppression of the adrenal glands with such intake can result in severe disease exacerbation whenever dramatic increases in physical or psychic stress are unaccompanied by substantial increases in oral glucocorticoid intake.[110] Signs of adrenocortical insufficiency can be seen following elective surgery in patients taking oral glucocorticoids who have not had their daily doses substantially increased during the postoperative period.

Research indicates that most of these side effects can be avoided with use of a single, daily, low dose (7.5 mg or less) of prednisone.[110] Although such doses have limited obvious anti-inflammatory efficacy, significant symptomatic improvement can occasionally be seen at this dose level. Sudden withdrawal of even low-dose prednisone therapy is often associated with dramatic flares in disease activity that can last 1 or 2 months or longer. Even at these low daily doses, supplemental glucocorticoids may be required during any time of substantially increased stress.

Combined Therapeutic Agents. A decade ago, it was considered generally unwise to prescribe combinations of acetylated salicylates, nonacetylated salicylates, NSAIDs, and glucocorticoids. Significant additive benefits were generally found to be insufficient to outweigh the additive side effects seen, especially those in the gastrointestinal tract. With the advent of use of medication to concurrently protect from gastrointestinal irritation and injury, the use of combinations of therapeutic agents is becoming more common. With the widespread individual variability in disease presentation and response to individual therapeutic agents seen in RA, these combinations allow for an almost infinite variety of individualized therapy.

Disease-Modifying Agents and Remissive Drugs. The third class of therapeutic agents used in the treatment of RA are the disease-modifying agents and remissive drugs (DMARDs). These medications tend to have the greatest toxicities but also may offer the most substantial long-term benefit. All of these agents can have side effects including dermatitis and significant gastrointestinal complications. A significant lag time usually exists between the initiation of treatment and initial signs of effectiveness.

Sulfasalazine and hydroxychloroquine are agents that tend to decrease the intensity of inflammatory synovitis and possibly erosive disease. Their potential side effects can include gastrointestinal ulceration, dermatitis, and potential permanent blindness (hydroxychloroquine).[111] Chloroquine was once somewhat popular for such use, but permanent blindness was far too frequently a side effect of its use.

Orally administered and injectable gold salts are more expensive, have more serious potential side effects, and may induce periods of reduction in disease severity and potential remission. Side effects can include severe renal damage and hematologic disorders. Similar benefits may result from treatment with penicillamine. This agent is the most toxic of the DMARDs. Its use can result in myasthenia, myositis, dermatitis, and renal damage. Methotrexate is another drug that may reduce disease severity or achieve remission of disease activity. Currently, its use is becoming fairly widespread in the presence of chronic disease. Potential side effects can include occlusive bronchiolitis, pulmonary fibrosis, and hepatitis.

The DMARDs continue to be used because there is no better treatment available. Extensive studies of control populations of patients with erosive RA and populations treated with individual DMARDs have failed to document any definitive benefit over limited but fairly long terms. In fact, placebo controls and untreated patients often show approximately the same degree of disease progression or remission as is noted in the treated populations. No studies published as of this date clearly demonstrate that the overall destructive and disabling course of RA can be significantly modified by use of any currently available oral or parenteral agent.

Injection Therapy. Local erosive, inflammatory, symptomatic disease often responds well to injections of glucocorticoids. Before using these agents, one must understand their mechanisms of action and therapeutic limitations if significant short- and long-term harm are to be avoided.

Glucocorticoids are the most potent antiinflammatory, therapeutic agents currently available. Use of injectable glucocorticoids often provides dramatic, almost immediate, and sustained relief of inflammatory pain. Their continuing presence in involved structures also simultaneously blocks the normal defensive mechanism that inflammation can serve. Prior to injection of glucocorticoids, patients should be advised of the potent antiinflammatory activity the drugs provide, giving both simultaneous relief and the risk, with overuse, of damage to involved structures without inflammatory warning signs. One needs to be cognizant of the fact that painful inflammation noted on use of a structure may be the only way the body has of warning an individual to cease further use before potentially extensive, irreversible damage occurs. Injected joints should be splinted and supported to provide protection from ''silent'' damage after instillation of glucocorticoids. Injected tendons should be given similar protection. Patients should be advised as a general rule to do no more than 75% to 80% of what would have been reasonably comfortable use of involved structures prior to these injections. The duration of this restriction will depend on the half-life of the specific agent injected. Use of elastic braces and adhesive strappings can be beneficial in providing support and protection to areas that have been injected with glucocorticoids.

Conservative Management

General Considerations. Conservative management of manifestations of RA in the lower extremities can provide substantial therapeutic relief of symptoms and associated disability. Maintenance of functional capacity is a primary goal of all treatment in RA. Symptomatic disease in the lower extremities can be associated with substantial functional impairment. Appropriate care of symptoms and deformities in the lower extremities can substantially increase ambulatory comfort and abilities. It can also dramatically increase, prolong, and even restore functional independence.

Insoles, Orthotics, and Shoe Therapy. Early in the course of RA, many symptoms in the feet, ankles, and knees often result from stresses and strains produced by abnormal structural or functional alignments in the foot. Trial strappings and paddings on the feet and temporary modifications of shoes can mimic support and realignment that can be offered by insoles, permanent shoe modifications, and orthotics. These measures often provide substantial and almost immediate relief. When this is noted, prefabricated insoles, permanent shoe modifications, or orthotics can be prescribed. Usually, orthotics composed of rigid materials are far less well tolerated initially and in the long term in RA than less rigid bracing and support devices. Flexible orthotics offer an advantage of replacing some of the shock absorption provided by the supinatory-pronatory motion seen in the normal rearfoot. The normal foot also undergoes a graded depression of the arch on loading that offers additional shock absorption during gait. Both of these intrinsic mechanisms of shock absorption are substantially diminished or absent in the presence of many structural and functional deformities seen in rheumatoid feet. Loss of such shock absorption produces constant microtrauma in all lower extremity joints that can be affected by RA.

Graded depression of the medial longitudinal arch of orthotics due to their inherent flexibility affords additional shock absorption during the gait cycle. Even more shock absorption can be achieved by lining heel areas or entire orthotics with shock-absorptive covers, use of shock-absorptive insoles, and recommendation of shoes with greater than average shock-absorbing capacities. Examples would include sneakers, jogging-style shoes, and shoes with crepe or rubber soles. Some care must be taken in prescribing shoes with rubber or crepe soles to elderly patients owing to the tendency for these soles to ''catch'' on carpeted surfaces. People who work prolonged hours on hard concrete or similar surfaces often complain about foot fatigue, even with relatively normal feet and in the absence of rheumatic disease. These complaints are more common in patients with rheumatoid disease and are compounded by structural and functional pedal deformities like those shown in Figure 7–11. When the dictates of style, fashion, or occupational factors allow for the use of jogging-style shoes, they should be advised. Considering the goals of protection and conservation of remaining structural and functional integrity in the patient with RA, use of these shoes whenever possible is wise, even in the absence of specific symptoms.

Supportive insoles or orthotics are also indicated for delaying or preventing progressive collapse of the arch structure usually seen in RA. Accommodative supportive insoles should also be used to alleviate, and where possible eliminate, excessive pressures noted at plantar locations. Accommodative modifications of, or additions to, orthotics can similarly be prescribed. Medial and lateral flanges can be added to insoles and orthotics to alleviate excessive pressure at bunion, tailor's bunion, navicular tuberosity, and other prom-

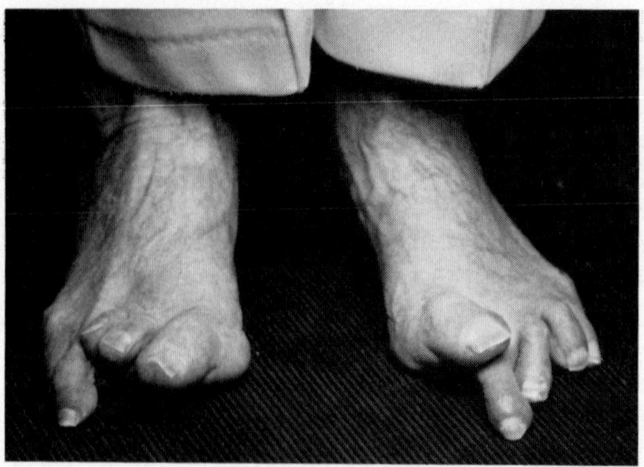

FIGURE 7–11. Extensive foot deformities in rheumatoid arthritis, including collapse of the medial longitudinal arch, hallux valgus, dislocation of lesser toes, and bunion and tailor's bunion deformities. These deformities, weakness, and destruction of joint and periarticular tissues cause substantial pain and disability during weightbearing attempts.

inent, irritated, and symptomatic areas. Similarly, posterior flanges can be added and pocketed out to protect prominences (Haglund's deformity) in the heel area.

Clinical observations have shown that five types of feet are seen in RA. These include relatively normal feet, stiff feet, hyperflexible feet, normal feet with rheumatoid disease, and previously abnormal feet with superimposed rheumatoid disease. The normal foot in RA tends to show signs of excessive fatigue and generalized soreness after prolonged ambulation. These are most likely the result of generalized muscle fatigue and weakness seen with the disease. Prescription of supportive and shock-absorptive shoes and insoles often provides substantial relief. These symptoms tend to be seen in the other four foot types but are often overshadowed by other far more conspicuous symptoms. Occasionally, they may represent presenting symptoms in the foot of a patient with RA.

In relatively stiff feet, the use of regular shoes and shoes with increased flexibility is accompanied by substantial discomfort that is noted primarily during the propulsive phase of gait. These foot types are also quite intolerant of even minimal functional or structural depressions of the arch structure. Increase in the rigidity of the soles of shoes and use of supportive insoles usually result in significantly increased comfort during ambulation.

Use of stiffer-soled shoes increases the lever arm of the foot during the propulsive phase of ambulation. Sole stiffness tends not to be a problem in patients with apropulsive gaits. In those with propulsive gait patterns, it causes increased demand on the gastrocnemius-soleus complex and Achilles tendon and may be associated with symptoms in these areas. These are usually alleviated with use of a rocker-bottom forefoot sole that allows for propulsive function without as great a lengthening of the lever arm. Relatively stiff soles with rocker-bottom additions also negate the need for extension of the MTP joints during propulsion. When these joints present with disease activity, this type of sole usually offers dramatic relief of associated symptoms during gait. With stiffness and soreness in the ankle and subtalar joint, a high-topped boot often provides substantial relief.

Flexible foot types tend to present with greater discomfort on prolonged standing. Supportive and shock-absorptive insoles usually provide relief. Occasionally, flexible orthotics are necessary to alleviate symptoms. These feet tend to be more symptomatic in stiff-soled shoes, and they feel better with shoes that have flexibility in their anterior portion. Patients with excessive flexibility or disease activity at the naviculocuneiform articulations tend to have increased discomfort with use of rigid-soled shoes and orthotics, especially when symptoms in these areas are secondary to excessively taut Achilles tendons. In such feet, relative collapse of the involved joint occurs as a result of dorsiflexion of the foot to the rear of the joint induced by the Achilles tendon. This "buckling" increases as the foot goes into propulsion and is actually rising off any orthotic present. Usually, a shock-absorptive heel lift alone, or incorporated into supportive devices, provides substantial relief.

Feet with pre-existing deformities and biomechanical aberrations tend to present the greatest degree of symptoms in RA. The ability to delineate, quantitate, and understand deformities is essential if significant symptomatic relief and minimization of progressive deformities is to be achieved. To achieve optimal relief in these feet, orthotic control; alterations in shoe styles; modification of shoes; use of shields, strappings, elastic bracing; and occasional use of more supportive braces may be necessary.

In some instances, active rheumatoid disease is seen superimposed on existing biomechanical problems. The combination of these findings usually is associated with the most severe symptoms and disability noted in the feet of patients with RA. These concurrent findings are also most commonly associated with symptoms that either partially or completely fail to respond to extensive conservative therapeutic measures. Oral medications; judicious use of injectable glucocorticoids; use of physical therapy modalities; elastic bracing, strapping, and padding; use of orthotics; bracing; and prescription of special and specially modified shoes are often indicated in the ongoing treatment of these feet. Special shoes with removable insoles (inlay depth), high toe boxes, and soft upper materials can be prescribed when indicated. Velcro shoe closures or elastic shoe laces are often of considerable benefit with disabling upper extremity disease (Fig. 7–12). Occasionally, assistive devices, including canes, crutches, forearm crutches, walkers, and even wheelchairs, are required in the treatment of these patients.

When structural or functional aberrations are present in the feet of patients with rheumatoid disease, it is essential to recognize the effect that they have on more proximal structures. Feet functioning in severe valgus can cause significant irritation and damage to ankle, knee, and hip joints. Appropriate management of these disorders can substantially improve, and occasionally eliminate, more proximal symptoms and disabilities.

Muscle Testing, Evaluation, and Treatment. Manual muscle testing of the intrinsic and extrinsic muscles of the feet usually reveals weakness in multiple muscles in the presence of RA. More complete Cybex or similar evaluations of all lower extremity muscle groups are often warranted and beneficial in assessing functional capacities in the lower extremities. These tests often reveal weakness in specific muscles that may not be appreciated on physical examination, and they can be crucial in determining areas that require protection owing to lack of support or altered muscle balance. They are often valuable in formulating optimal treatment regimens.

Extrinsic flexors and extensors of the feet and toes can be

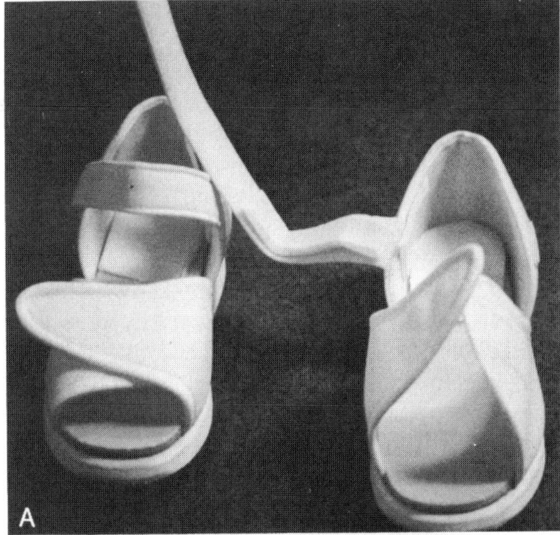

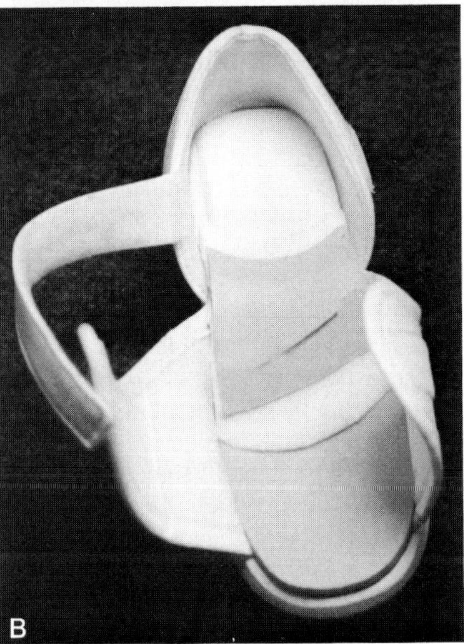

FIGURE 7–12. *A,* Sandals specifically designed for patients with advanced arthritic deformities of the feet. They feature soft upper materials, open toe box areas, cushioned insoles, shock-absorptive soles, and adjustable straps with Velcro closures. *B,* Additional accommodative and supportive modifications to insoles can achieve substantial increases in comfort and functional abilities.

strengthened with active resisted exercises and exercises with attachable weights moved against gravity. Intrinsic flexors of the foot can be exercised with gripping against a giving material (rolled towel, shoebox three-fourths filled with sand), repetitive picking up and squeezing of objects (marbles), or walking on surfaces that allow plantar flexion of the toes on propulsion (soft sand on beaches). Patients should be cautioned to avoid overexertion and exhaustion both in their daily lives and in their exercise programs. When possible, exercise regimens for maintenance of or increasing muscle strength and tone should be designed so as to avoid excessive and unnecessary stress to weightbearing joints. Swimming, use of bicycles, and sitting or reclining positions can help achieve this goal.

Bracing. When deformities and disease activity resulting in significant pain and disability persistently progress or fail to adequately respond to treatment, temporary or permanent bracing can be used. When possible, braces should limit the function of involved joints and tendons while allowing the greatest possible degree of function in the remaining structures. Flexible, molded ankle-foot orthoses fit these criteria. By allowing continued function of those structures in the forefoot, midfoot, and ankle, disuse atrophy in these areas can be minimized. Simultaneously, these braces can be used to limit subtalar joint motion and instability.

When restrictive bracing is used, it should be removed regularly to allow for range-of-motion exercises that encourage desired mobility in specific joints. Any braces that are prescribed should be as cosmetically acceptable as possible. Molded ankle-foot orthoses can be worn under socks and slacks and are often unnoticed. Rarely, bracing with outer irons attached to shoes may be indicated. For those patients who require only temporary bracing or who are unable to afford expensive prescription braces, a number of commercially available products may suffice.

Hygiene and Skin Care. Painful hyperkeratotic lesions overlying areas of excessive pressures should be débrided regularly. Often patients can keep them under control for extended periods with the use of pumice stones, emery boards, or sandpaper. Deformities of the toes and other areas of the feet frequently cause these painful hyperkeratoses by rubbing the skin against areas in shoes. When this is noted, it is often possible to stretch or spot-stretch the shoes.

Removable shields can be used to further decrease or eliminate localized excessive pressures. Shields can occasionally be designed to help straighten flexible digital deformities associated with these types of lesions or ones that cause problems with shoe fitting. When digital deformities present difficulty with fitting shoes, shoes specifically designed with wider toe boxes and greater toe box height can be prescribed. Shoes with removable, thicker than average insoles (inlay depth) can be of considerable assistance in allowing for the use of shock-absorptive and prescription insoles and orthotics. They often give satisfactory internal room for extensive digital deformities. Occasionally, these deformities require use of open-toed sandal styles.

Patients should be made aware of appropriate hygienic care of the feet. The patient's functional incapacities of the upper extremities may limit the ability to care for the feet. Assistive devices (such as long-handled bath brushes) can aid in maintaining functional independence. Occasionally, it is necessary to assign hygienic supervision and care of a patient's feet to a spouse, relative, or other caregiver.

Wounds in the lower extremities of patients with RA should be recognized early and treated aggressively to promote rapid resolution and prevent infection. Patients should be advised to keep involved areas free of all bath or shower water to prevent potential contamination with fecal or other bacteria. Topical antiseptics and antibiotics should be appropriately prescribed. Excessive weightbearing and other compressive forces should be alleviated and, where possible, eliminated. When ulceration occurs secondary to such excessive pressures, as in Figure 7–13, permanent relief of pressure from involved areas is essential if rapid resolution is to be achieved and repetitive problems are to be avoided.

Similarly, patients with neuropathy should be advised to have all surfaces of their feet checked daily. This includes all interdigital areas. Any problem areas noted should be reported immediately to a physician. In the presence of neuropathy, patients must be made to understand that pain can no

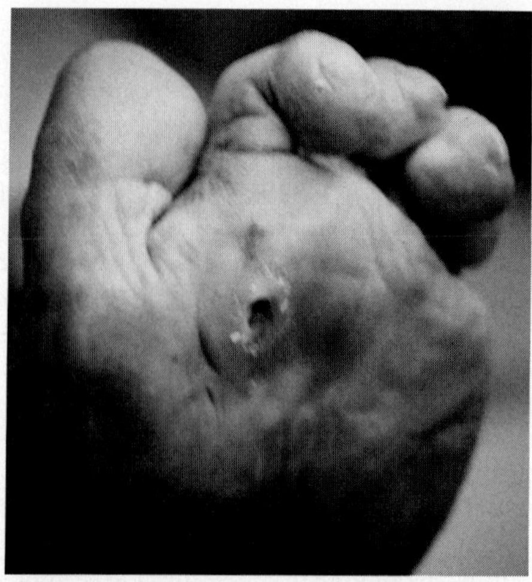

FIGURE 7–13. Ulceration under the second metatarsal head in a patient with rheumatoid arthritis of 12 years' duration. Associated hallux abducto-valgus, dorsal dislocation and hammertoe deformities involving the lesser toes, and dorsiflexion of the first metatarsal are contributory factors.

longer be used as an accurate barometer of the severity of, or danger posed by, injuries or infections.

When indicated, instruction in appropriate basic pedal hygiene should be given. Patients with active vasculitis, significant neuropathy, bleeding diatheses, substantially decreased immunity, peripheral vascular disease, significant loss of visual acuity, substantial mental deficits, and marked limitations in manual strength and dexterity should not attempt to cut their own toenails. All patients with RA should be discouraged from using sharp instruments on or around their feet in attempts to trim hyperkeratotic lesions. In the presence of significantly impaired immunity, vascular supply, and neurologic status, all surfaces of the feet must always be observed daily and in good lighting. Appropriate antisepsis and protection of injured areas should be maintained at all times. Skin infections, such as tinea pedis, should be attended to immediately. Any bacterial or resistant fungal infections should be presented to a physician at the earliest opportunity.

Surgical Management

Before any pedal surgery in the rheumatoid foot is planned, it is incumbent on the surgeon to thoroughly evaluate the anticipated benefits, attendant risks, and ramifications of both the surgery and anticipated aftercare. Any such surgery should be planned and coordinated within an overall framework of realistic treatment goals. Anticipated benefits are directly governed by the therapeutic goals established for any surgery. The anticipated benefits should far outweigh attendant risks before any elective surgery is undertaken. When possible and appropriate, the goals of surgical procedures should include return of both structural and functional capacities. Usually, surgery alone cannot provide these benefits. Postoperative regimens should be designed to enhance overall benefits. Surgical procedures and postoperative regimens should be carefully designed within the framework of each individual patient's active and anticipated disease and current and anticipated incapacities. Supplemental measures can include prescription of temporary home assistance, physical therapy, shoe inserts, orthotics, shoes, shoe modifications, and assistive devices (such as canes, crutches, forearm crutches, wheelchairs, and braces). Substantial relief of disabling pain is often an accompanying goal of surgery; in advanced disease, it is usually the primary or even the sole goal of such surgery.

The anticipated functional status of the foot after surgery must be carefully considered. Patients with advanced, chronic, and severe forefoot deformities rarely have propulsive gaits. They often have a minimally functional foot, extensive forefoot deformity, and associated disabling pain. Surgical procedures involving numerous joint resections and replacement with implants to re-establish a functional forefoot in patients who will never have propulsive gaits is usually ill-conceived. What is commonly referred to as "forefoot reconstruction" in RA is in fact a partial forefoot internal ablation designed solely to alleviate pain and deformity. This procedure is seldom designed to produce a functional forefoot, nor can it be expected to. Careful consideration should be made before placing single or multiple implants into the feet of patients with decreased overall immunity, limited functional prognoses, potential vascular compromise, and possible delayed healing.

Significant structural and functional deficits remaining after surgical procedures can often be improved with changes in shoe styles, shoe modifications, orthoses, removable shields, shoe fillers, elastic support, bracing, and prostheses. Substantial increase in functional capacity through shoe modification after a forefoot reconstruction is seen with the prescription of a rocker-bottom forefoot sole and balanced heel. The closer that foot-shoe unit functions approximate normal, the less abnormal stresses and strains are placed on extrapedal structures. Use of this forefoot sole allows the shoe to maintain an inflexible sole that splints the afunctional MTP area while it provides a potentially more normal heel-to-toe gait pattern.

Some patients with RA maintain a significant functional neuromuscular status in the foot and good bone stock but may require multiple MTP joint arthroplasties. In these patients, first MTP joint fusions or implant arthroplasties can be considered. These procedures yield better structural and functional integrity of the foot when compared with excisional arthroplasties. Concomitant fusion of related interphalangeal joints almost always has to be performed simultaneously, because advanced atrophy of intrinsic muscles to toes usually has essentially eliminated any hope of their postoperative normal functional capacity. A shoe with a rigid, rocker-bottom sole also can be of substantial benefit to patients in whom fusions of the MTP and interphalangeal joints have been performed during and after healing of the surgery.

Patients with RA who are receiving glucocorticoid medication orally, or who have received significant amounts within the previous 6 months, should have increased steroid coverage considered perioperatively. No consensus exists on any formula or dosage that should be given in all instances. The overall stress that any specific surgery is anticipated to create should be the main factor in determining any one patient's specific perioperative coverage. It is usually best to consult the patient's internist or rheumatologist to determine exactly what supplemental regimen should be followed.

Many patients with advanced deformity and disability associated with RA require extensive reconstructive surgery. Any combination of hand, wrist, elbow, cervical spine, hip, knee, ankle, foot, or soft tissue repair or reconstruction may be indicated in any specific patient. Usually, bilateral procedures are required. Coordinating and staging surgical intervention are usually in the best interest of these patients.

In staging multiple surgical procedures in a patient with RA, forefoot "rehabilitative" surgery often should be performed initially. The minimal disability and pain associated with these procedures, rapid return to ambulatory status, relief of pain, and substantial increases in ambulatory ability all help motivate patients to pursue other needed surgery.

It is usually essential to consider the interrelationship of multiple joint disease in patients with RA when planning any surgery. Extensive forefoot surgery in any patient with RA is indicated only when more proximal joints can be expected to allow sufficient short- and long-term functional capacity to afford substantial overall benefit postoperatively. It is rarely, if ever, indicated in those patients whose more proximal joint disease precludes any significant ambulation or when such ambulation would endanger the overall remaining viability of those joints. It is also important to ensure preoperatively that the patient will be capable of using assistive devices that may be needed postoperatively. Patients with advanced elbow, wrist, and hand deformity and active disease at these sites are often unable to effectively use walkers, crutches, forearm crutches, or even canes.

Any surgery in a patient with RA should be designed so as to minimize periods of bed rest and inactivity. When prolonged bed rest is required, physical therapy should be ordered at the bedside. Patients should be ambulated at the earliest reasonable opportunity. Even relatively brief periods of inactivity and bed rest can be accompanied by profound weakness, muscle atrophy, and disuse atrophy of bone.

To save patients considerable time, expense, and multiple periods of postoperative disability when possible, several surgical procedures on different sites can be performed at one time. Often, simultaneous surgery can be performed in the upper and lower extremities. Occasionally, multiple surgical procedures can be performed at one time in the same extremity. This also limits risks associated with multiple exposures to anesthetic agents.

Reconstructive surgery of joints, repair of tendons and joint capsules, and excision of functionless, painful deformities can provide dramatic improvement in the functional capacities and overall quality of life for many patients with RA. Current restrictions imposed by governmental, insurance, and peer review organizations are beginning to limit the availability of the highest quality care to these patients. Expenses involved in providing optimal care are approaching prohibitive levels. In rendering surgical, pharmacologic, and conservative care, the goal of providing the best possible service and care at the most reasonable cost needs to be strictly adhered to.

References

1. Parish LC: An historical approach to the nomenclature of rheumatoid arthritis. Arthritis Rheum 6:158, 1963
2. Garrod AB: A Treatise on Gout and Rheumatic Gout (Rheumatoid Arthritis). London, Longman Greene, 1876.
3. McCarty DJ: Clinical picture of rheumatoid arthritis. *In* McCarty, DJ (ed): Arthritis and Allied Conditions, 11th ed. Philadelphia, Lea & Febiger, 1989, p 175.
4. Harris ED: Rheumatoid arthritis: The clinical features of rheumatoid arthritis. *In* Kelley WN, Harris ED, Ruddy S, and Sledge CB (eds): Textbook of Rheumatology, 3rd ed. Philadelphia, WB Saunders, 1989, p 946.
5. Mitchell DM, Spitz PW, Young DY, et al: Survival, prognosis, and causes of death in rheumatoid arthritis. Arthritis Rheum 29:706, 1986.

6. McMicheal AJ, Sasazuki T, McDevitt HO, and Payne RO: Increased frequency of HLA-Cw3 and HLA-Dw4 in rheumatoid arthritis. Arthritis Rheum 20:1037, 1977.

7. Aho KM, Koskenvuo M, Touminen J, and Kaprio J: Occurrence of rheumatoid arthritis in a nationwide series of twins. J Rheumatol 13:899, 1986.

8. Wolfe AM: The epidemiology of rheumatoid arthritis: A review. Bull Rheum Dis 19:518, 1968.

9. Beasley RP, Willkens RF, and Bennett PH: High prevalence of rheumatoid arthritis in Yakima Indians. Arthritis Rheum 16:743, 1973.

10. Harvey J, Lotze M, Arnett FC, et al: Rheumatoid arthritis in a Chippewa band: II. Field study with clinical, serologic, and HLA-D-correlation. J Rheumatol 10:28, 1983.

11. Lawrence JS: Prevalence of rheumatoid arthritis. Ann Rheum Dis 20:11, 1961.

12. Plotz CM and Singer JM: The latex fixation test: II. Results in rheumatoid arthritis. Am J Med 21:893, 1956.

13. Sibley JT: Weather and arthritis symptoms. J Rheumatol 12:707, 1985.

14. Lawrence JS: Rheumatoid arthritis—nature or nurture. Ann Rheum Dis 29:357, 1970.

15. Zvaifler NJ: The immunopathology of joint inflammation in rheumatoid arthritis. Adv Immunol 16:265, 1973.

16. Winchester RJ: Characterization of IgG complexes in patients with rheumatoid arthritis. Ann NY Acad Sci 256:73, 1975.

17. Cecere F, Lessard J, McDuffy S, and Pope RM: Evidence for the local production and utilization of immunoreactants in rheumatoid arthritis. Arthritis Rheum 25:1307, 1982.

18. Ridge SC, Oronski AL, and Kerwar SS: Induction of the synthesis of latent collagenase and latent neutral protease in chondrocytes by a factor synthesized by activated macrophages. Arthritis Rheum 23:448, 1980.

19. Dingle JT, Skatvala J, and Hembry R: A cartilage catabolic factor from synovium. Biochem J 184:177, 1986.

20. Yoghami I, Rookoamini SM, and Faunce HF: Unilateral rheumatoid arthritis: Protective effects of neurologic deficits. Am J Roentgenol 128:299, 1977.

21. Ohlsson K and Laurell CB: The disappearance of enzyme inhibitors in human plasma. Surgery 83:323, 1978.

22. Reynolds JJ, Murphy G, Sellers A, and Cartwright E: A new factor that may control collagen resorption. Lancet 2:333, 1977.

23. Glick EN: Asymmetrical rheumatoid arthritis after poliomyelitis. Br Med J 3:26, 1967.

24. Thompson M and Bywaters EGL: Unilateral rheumatoid arthritis following hemiplegia. Ann Rheum Dis 21:370, 1961.

25. Dayer JM, Krane SM, Russell RGG, and Robinson DR: Production of collagenase and prostaglandins by isolated adherent rheumatoid synovial cells. Proc Natl Acad Sci USA 73:945–949, 1971.

26. Dayer JM, Robinson DR, and Krane SM: Prostaglandin production by rheumatoid synovial cells: Stimulation by a factor from human mononuclear cells. J Exp Med 145:1399–1404, 1977.

27. Nakano KK: Neurologic complications in rheumatoid arthritis. Orthop Clin North Am 6:861, 1975.

28. Decker JL and Plotz PH: Extra-articular rheumatoid disease. In McCarty, DJ (ed): Arthritis and Allied Conditions, 9th ed. Philadelphia, Lea & Febiger, 1979, p 479.

29. Roth RD: The rheumatic patient—special considerations in foot surgery. In McGlamry ED (ed). Fundamentals of Foot Surgery. Baltimore, Williams & Wilkins, 1987, p 393.

30. Hurd ER: Extra-articular manifestations of rheumatoid arthritis. Semin Rheum Dis 8:151, 1979.

31. Hough AJ Jr and Sokoloff L: Pathology of rheumatoid arthritis and allied disorders. In McCarty, DJ (ed): Arthritis and Allied Conditions, 11th ed. Philadelphia, Lea & Febiger, 1989, pp 674–697.

32. Prillamin WW: Intestinal complications in rheumatoid arthritis and their relationship to corticosteroid therapy. J Chronic Dis 27:475–481, 1974.

33. Fernandez-Diez J: General pathology of necrotizing vasculitis. Clin Rheum Dis 6:279–295, 1980.

34. Soter NA: The skin and rheumatic disease. In Kelley WN, Harris ED, Ruddy S, and Sledge CB (eds): Textbook of Rheumatology, 3rd ed. Philadelphia, WB Saunders, 1989, pp 597–607.

35. Martel W, Hayes JT, and Duff IF: The pattern of bone erosion in the hand and wrist in rheumatoid arthritis. Radiology 84:204, 1965.

36. Schmid FR, Cooper NS, Ziff M, and McEwen C: Arteritis in rheumatoid arthritis. Am J Med 30:56, 1961.

37. Geirsson AJ, Sturfelt G, and Truedsson L: Clinical and serologic features of severe vasculitis in rheumatoid arthritis: Prognostic implications. Ann Rheum Dis 46:727, 1987.

38. Bonfiglio T and Atwater E: Heart disease in patients with seropositive rheumatoid arthritis: A controlled autopsy study and review. Arch Intern Med 127:714, 1969.

39. Turner R, Collins R, and Vomeir AM: Extra-articular manifestations of rheumatoid arthritis. Bull Rheum Dis 29:986–990, 1979.

40. Lebowitz WB: The heart in rheumatoid arthritis: A clinical and pathological study of 62 cases. Ann Intern Med 58:102, 1963.

41. Cerrantes-Perez P, Toro-Perez AH, and Rodriquez-Jurado P: Pulmonary involvement in rheumatoid arthritis. JAMA 243:1715–1719, 1980.

42. Benedek G: Rheumatoid pneumoconiosis: Documentation of onset and pathogenic considerations. Am J Med 55:515–524, 1973.

43. Winchester RJ, Litwin SD, Koffler D, and Kunkel HG: Observations on the eosinophilia of certain patients with rheumatoid arthritis. Arthritis Rheum 14:650, 1971.

44. Hutchinson RM, Davis P, and Jayson MIV: Thrombocytosis in rheumatoid arthritis. Ann Rheum Dis 35:138, 1976.

45. Goldberg J and Pinals RS: Felty's syndrome. Semin Arthritis Rheum 10:52, 1980.

46. Fox RI, Robinson CA, Curd JG, et al: Sjögren's syndrome: Criteria for classification. Arthritis Rheum 29:577, 1986.

47. Watson PG and Hayreh SS: Scleritis and episcleritis. J Ophthalmol 60:163–191, 1976.

48. Kenkind P and Gold DH: Ocular manifestations of rheumatic disorders. Rheumatology 4:13–59, 1973.

49. Hardon LD, Sellars L, Morley AR, et al: Hematuria in rheumatoid arthritis: An association with mesangial glomerulonephritis; a role for immune complex dissociative techniques. J Rheumatol 11:342, 1984.

50. Fleming A, Crown JM, and Corbett M: Early rheumatoid disease. I: Onset. Ann Rheum Dis 35:357, 1976.

51. Jacoby RK, Jayson MIV, and Cosh JA: Onset, early stages, and prognosis of rheumatoid arthritis: A clinical study of 100 patients with 11-year follow-up. Br Med J 2:96, 1973.

52. Fleming A, Bean RT, Corbett M, and Wood HN: Early rheumatoid disease: II. Patterns of joint involvement. Ann Rheum Dis 35:357, 1976.

53. Mens JMA: Correlation of joint involvement in rheumatoid arthritis and in ankylosing spondylitis with the synovial:cartilaginous ratio in various joints. Arthritis Rheum 30:359, 1987.

54. Short CL: Rheumatoid arthritis: Types of course and prognosis. Med Clin North Am 52:549, 1968.

55. Short CL and Bauer W: The course of rheumatoid arthritis in patients receiving simple medication and orthopedic measures. N Engl J Med 238:142, 1948.

56. Pincus T, Callahan LF, Sale WG, et al: Severe functional declines, work disability, and increased mortality in 75 RA patients studied over 9 years. Arthritis Rheum 27:864, 1984.

57. Yelin E, Henke C, and Epstein W: The work dynamics of the person with rheumatoid arthritis. Arthritis Rheum 30:507, 1987.

58. Pincus T and Callahan LF: Taking mortality in RA seriously—predictive markers, socioeconomic status, and comorbidity. J Rheumatol 13:841, 1986.

59. Dresner E and Trombly P: The latex fixation reaction in nonrheumatic diseases. N Engl J Med 26:891, 1959.

60. Carson DA: Rheumatoid factor. In Kelley WN, Harris ED, Ruddy S, and Sledge CB (eds): Textbook of Rheumatology, 3rd ed. Philadelphia, WB Saunders, 1989, p 198.

61. Ropes MW, Bennet GA, and Cobb S: Proposed diagnostic criteria for rheumatoid arthritis. Ann Rheum Dis 16:118, 1957.

62. Ropes MW, Bennet GA, and Cobb S: Revision of diagnostic criteria for rheumatoid arthritis. Arthritis Rheum 2:16, 1959.

63. Arnett FC, Edworthy SM, Bloch DA, et al: The American Rheumatism Association 1987 revised criteria for the classification of rheumatoid arthritis. Arthritis Rheum 31:315, 1988.

64. Ahvonen P, Sievers K, and Ano K: Arthritis associated with *Yersinia enterocolitica* infection. Acta Rheumatol Scand 15:232, 1969.

65. Ford DK: The etiology of non-gonococcal urethritis and Reiter's syndrome. Excerpta Medica Int Congress Series 165:227, 1969.

66. Churchill MA, Geraci JE, and Hunter GG: Musculoskeletal manifestations of bacterial endocarditis. Ann Intern Med 87:754, 1977.

67. Heller JT, Ganfi J, and Michaeli JG: Arthritis of familial Mediterranean fever (FMF). Arthritis Rheum 9:1, 1966.

68. Rappoport AS, Susman JL, and Weissman BN: Lesions resembling gout in patients with rheumatoid arthritis. Am J Roentgenol 126:41, 1976.

69. Kozin F and McCarty DJ: Rheumatoid factor in the serum of gouty patients. Arthritis Rheum 20:1559, 1977.

70. Wallace DJ, Klinenberg JR, Morbain D, et al: Co-existent gout and rheumatoid arthritis: Case report and literature review. Arthritis Rheum 22:81, 1979.

71. Agudelo CA, Turner RA, Panwetti M, and Pisko E: Does hyperuricemia protect from rheumatoid inflammation? A clinical study. Arthritis Rheum 27:443, 1984.

72. O'Duffy JD: Clinical studies of acute pseudogout attacks: Comments on prevalence, predisposition, and treatment. Arthritis Rheum 19(Suppl):394, 1976.

73. Wilkens E, Dieppe P, Maddison P, and Evison G: Osteoarthritis and articular chondrocalcinosis in the elderly. Ann Rheum Dis 42:280, 1983.

74. Moskowitz RW and Katz D: Chondrocalcinosis and chondrocalsynovitis (pseudogout syndrome)—analysis of 24 cases. Am J Med 43:322, 1967.

75. McCarty DJ: Diagnostic mimicry in arthritis—patterns of joint involvement associated with calcium pyrophosphate crystal deposits. Bull Rheum Dis 25:804, 1967.

76. O'Duffy JD: Behçet's disease. In Kelley WN, Harris ED, Ruddy S, and Sledge CB (eds): Textbook of Rheumatology, 3rd ed. Philadelphia, WB Saunders, 1989, p 1209.

77. Bennett M: Mixed connective tissue disease and other overlap syndromes. In Kelley WN, Harris ED, Ruddy S, and Sledge CB (eds): Textbook of Rheumatology, 3rd ed. Philadelphia, WB Saunders, 1989, p 1147.

78. Harley LA: Polymyalgia rheumatica and giant cell arteritis. In Wyngaarden JB and Smith LH (eds): Cecil's Textbook of Medicine, Vol 2, 16th ed. Philadelphia, WB Saunders, 1982, p 1981.

79. McCarty DJ and Gatter RA: A study of distal interphalangeal joint tenderness in rheumatoid arthritis. Arthritis Rheum 9:325, 1966.

80. Halla JT, Fallahi S, and Hardin JG: Small joint involvement: A systematic radiographic study in rheumatoid arthritis. Ann Rheum Dis 45:327, 1986.

81. Jacob J: Distal interphalangeal joint involvement in rheumatoid arthritis. Arthritis Rheum 29:10, 1986.

82. Kellgren JH and Ball J: Tendon lesions in rheumatoid arthritis. Ann Rheum Dis 9:48, 1950.

83. Ranawat CS and Straub LR: Volar tenosynovitis of the wrist in rheumatoid arthritis. Arthritis Rheum 13:112, 1970.

84. Resnick D: Rheumatoid arthritis of the wrist: Why the ulnar styloid? Radiology 112:29, 1974.
85. Winfield J, Cooke D, Brook AS, and Corbett M: Prospective study of radiologic changes in hands, feet, and cervical spine in adult rheumatoid arthritis. Ann Rheum Dis 42:613, 1983.
86. Lipson SJ: The cervical spine. *In* Kelley, WN, Harris ED, Ruddy S, and Sledge CB (eds): Textbook of Rheumatology, 3rd ed. Philadelphia, WB Saunders, 1989, p 2004.
87. Weissman BN, Aliabadi P, Weinfield MS, et al: Prognostic features of atlantoaxial subluxation in rheumatoid arthritis. Radiology 144:745, 1982.
88. Black JR, Cahalin C, and Germaine BF: Pedal morbidity in rheumatic disease. J Am Podiatr Assoc 72:360, 1982.
89. Calabro JJ: A critical evaluation of the diagnostic features of the feet in rheumatoid arthritis. Arthritis Rheum 5:19, 1962.
90. Minaker K and Little H: Painful feet in rheumatoid arthritis. Can Med Assoc J 109:724, 1973.
91. Tillman K: Mutual interplay between forefoot and hindfoot affections and deformities in rheumatoid arthritis. *In* Hagena FW (ed): Rheumatoid Arthritis Surgery of the Complex Hand and Foot. Basil, Karger, 1987, p 98.
92. D'Amico JC: The pathomechanics of adult rheumatoid arthritis affecting the foot. J Am Podiatr Assoc 66:227, 1976.
93. Taylor PM: A review in changes in the hand and feet in rheumatoid arthritis. J Am Podiatr Assoc 68:817, 1978.
94. Vaino K: The rheumatoid foot: A clinical study with pathological and roentgenological comments. Ann Chir Gynaecol 1(Suppl): 45, 1978.
95. King J, Burke D, Freeman MAR: The incidence of pain in the rheumatoid hindfoot and the significance of calcaneo-fibular impingement. Int Orthop 2:255, 1978.
96. Harris RI, Beath T: Etiology of peroneal flatfoot. J Bone Joint Surg 30B:50, 1948.
97. Rask MR: Achilles tendon rupture owing to rheumatoid disease. JAMA 239:435, 1978.
98. McGuigan L, Burke D, and Fleming A: Tarsal tunnel syndrome and peripheral neuropathy in rheumatoid arthritis. Ann Rheum Dis 42:128, 1983.
99. Bassett LW, Gad RH, and Mirra JM: Rheumatoid arthritis extending into the clavicle and to the skin surface. Ann Rheum Dis 44:336, 1985.
100. Baum J: Infection in rheumatoid arthritis. Arthritis Rheum 14:135, 1971.
101. Fischer M, Miekle H, Glaefke S, and Deicher H: Generalized vasculopathy in finger blood flow abnormalities in rheumatoid arthritis. J Rheumatol 11:33, 1984.
102. Schmid FR, Cooper NS, Ziff M, and McEwen G: Arteritis in rheumatoid arthritis. J Clin Invest 56:725, 1975.
103. Vahvanen V: Arthrodesis of the talocalcaneal joint or pantalar joints in rheumatoid arthritis. Acta Orthop Scand 40:642, 1969.
104. Kirkup JR: Ankle and tarsal joints in rheumatoid arthritis. Scand J Rheumatol 3:50, 1974.
105. Roth RD: The role of the podiatrist in the rheumatology team approach. *In* Ehrlich GE (ed): Rehabilitation Management of Rheumatic Conditions, 2nd ed. Baltimore, Williams & Wilkins, 1986, p 285.
106. Orozco-Alcala JJ and Baum J: Regular and enteric-coated aspirin: A re-evaluation. Arthritis Rheum 22:1034, 1979.
107. Grigor RR, Spitz DW, and Furst DE: Salicylate toxicity in elderly patients with rheumatoid arthritis. J Rheumatol 14:60, 1987.
108. Robinson HJ, Phares HF, and Gaessle OE: Prostaglandin synthetase inhibitors and infection. *In* Robinson HJ and Vane JR (eds): Prostaglandin Synthetase Inhibitors. New York, Raven, 1974.
109. Abramson S, Korchak H, Ludewig R, et al: Modes of action of aspirin-like drugs. Proc Natl Acad Sci USA 82:7227, 1985.
110. Myles AB, Schiller CFB, Glass D, and Daly JR: Single-dose corticosteroid treatment. Ann Rheum Dis 35:73, 1976.
111. Pullar T, Hunter JA, and Capell HA: Effect of sulphasalazine on the radiologic progression of rheumatoid arthritis. Ann Rheum Dis 46:398, 1987.

CHAPTER 8

Seronegative Spondyloarthropathies

James L. McGuire, M.D., and Wilfred Laine, D.P.M.

The seronegative spondyloarthropathies are a group of disorders that share a number of factors in common, namely (1) an increased frequency of the gene human leukocyte antigen (HLA)-B27, (2) arthritic involvement of the sacroiliac joint, (3) variable arthritic involvement of the joints of the lower extremity and spine, (4) negative blood test for rheumatoid factor (RF), and (5) maximal expression and severity in males.[1] In general, four distinct clinical entities exist:

1. Ankylosing spondylitis (AS) predominantly involves the spine with minimal peripheral joint or extra-articular involvement, such as skin and mucous membranes.
2. Reiter's syndrome (RS) consists of a classic triad of conjunctivitis, nongonococcal urethritis, and arthritis, which involves both the spine and peripheral joints of lower extremities.
3. Psoriatic arthritis (PA) has multiple presentations including a rheumatoid-like pattern in a patient with psoriasis. Another variant is a spondyloarthropathy, which is similar to RS.
4. Inflammatory bowel disease (IBD), especially in males with HLA-B27, may be associated with spondylitis that resembles AS. Undifferentiated spondyloarthropathy may have overlapping clinical features. For instance, the presentation of spondylitis may precede the onset of either psoriasis or IBD. There may be other patients who have a course that always remains unclassified.[2] HLA-B27 is found in as many as 90 per cent of males with AS; lesser frequencies are observed in PA, RS, and IBD.[3, 4]

CLINICAL FEATURES

Ankylosing Spondylitis

AS characteristically begins in males in their late teens and usually presents as an insidious low backache associated with morning stiffness. The symptoms improve during the remainder of the day and after exercise. Over time, the disease tends to progress at variable rates to involve the entire spine, which results in progressive limitation of motion as a result of ligamentous calcification and spinal joint involvement. In some young men, the disease remains localized to the low back. Peripheral joint involvement, especially in the hips, may lead to flexion deformities and further aggravates the posture. Inflammation of attachments of ligaments and the

tendons, also known collectively as the *entheses*, accounts for symptoms of pain and tenderness without dramatic swelling. This enthesopathy often affects the knees, ankles, and heels. This classic pattern of AS is characteristic in males with HLA-B27. However, females with AS usually have milder back symptoms.[5] Moreover, prominent lower extremity complaints may delay the diagnosis and can be confused with rheumatoid arthritis (RA).

Extra-articular manifestations are relatively uncommon in AS but may be potentially serious. First, all patients with HLA-B27 are susceptible, albeit in an unpredictable manner, to acute uveitis. This painful red eye is obvious to the patient. Second, inflammatory involvement of the aortic arch extending to the aortic valves can result in aneurysms and valvular insufficiency. Auscultation for the diastolic murmur of aortic insufficiency should be done at 6-month intervals. Third, an interstitial fibrosis of the upper lobes of the lung has been described. Although usually found on routine chest radiograph, it can be confused with prior infection with tuberculosis, which also has an apical pattern.

Reiter's Syndrome

RS usually presents in young men with arthritis of the lower extremities and low back in the setting of nongonococcal urethritis. The urethritis may be mild, and the culture for gonococcus is negative. However, infection with *Chlamydia* is common. The conjunctivitis is usually transient and may be remembered only after close historical scrutiny. RS is considered a reactive arthritis. This implies that an infection that occurs in a genetically susceptible host (i.e., HLA-B27 positive) can initiate the inflammatory process. Moreover, this inflammation of the joints and entheses persists after the original infection is eliminated. It is now clear that pathogens that cause both urethritis and dysentery can initiate RS. These include *Chlamydia, Salmonella, Shigella, Yersinia,* and *Campylobacter.*[6] Although certain HLA-B27–positive patients with acquired immunodeficiency syndrome have an RS-like disease, it is not clear that human immunodeficiency virus initiates the inflammatory cycle.[7, 8]

RS has been expanded from the original triad. Three additional mucocutaneous lesions should be included. First, a psoriasiform rash on the soles of the feet is called *keratoderma blennorrhagicum* (KB). KB may start with small clusters of papules, which coalesce into the scaly lesion that is typical of the later phase of this rash. Second, a circular rash of the penis, usually just below the corona, is called *circinate balanitis.* Third, oral lesions, which are usually painless, can occur on the buccal mucosa and tongue. Involvement of the latter can produce the ''geographic tongue'' appearance.

The peripheral arthritis of RS is both acute and chronic. The acute syndrome is usually dramatic and presents with involvement of the low back and lower extremity. Large knee effusions, often asymmetrical, are characteristic. In the feet, the dramatic swelling and tenderness of the Achilles tendons and plantar fascia in these young men resulted in the description of the term *lover's heels* in early clinical descriptions of RS (Fig. 8–1). Additionally, a ''sausage toe'' phenomenon can appear rapidly with or without metatarsophalangeal (MTP) involvement[3] (Fig. 8–2). The ankles and hips may be affected by either true joint effusions or an enthesopathy.

The spinal involvement in RS is less predictable than in AS. Inflammation of the sacroiliac joints may be asymmetrical. The disease may skip the thoracic spine and affect the cervical spine, even in the acute phases.[9] This is contrasted with the relatively orderly progression of AS, which proceeds with caudal-rostral involvement over years.

The acute arthritis characteristically continues after the initial precipitating infection has been eliminated. In some patients, the entire arthritis totally resolves over several weeks. In others, probably the majority of patients, the peripheral synovitis becomes chronic and occasionally progressive. Some degree of chronicity involving the spine is the general rule in HLA-B27–positive patients. Finally, appropriate treatment of the initiating infection with antibiotics neither stops the acute phase nor prevents the chronic sequelae.

Psoriatic Arthritis

PA is actually a group of syndromes that occur in patients with psoriasis.[10] Although overlap of the arthritis symptoms may be present, several relatively distinct subsets exist: (1) a symmetrical arthritis similar to RA involving large and small joints; (2) a distal arthritis of the distal interphalangeal (DIP)

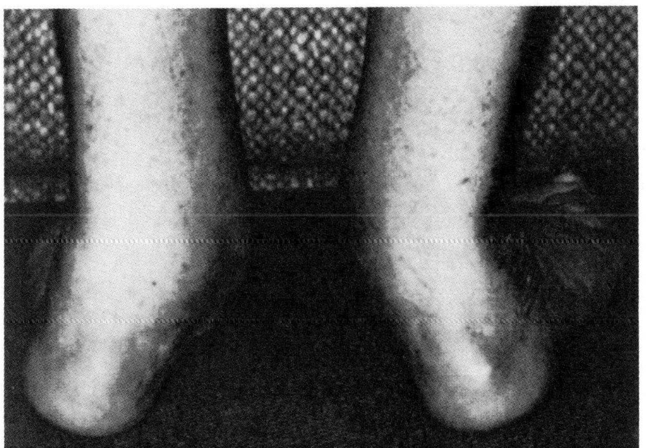

FIGURE 8–1. ''Lover's heels.'' Dramatic swelling and tenderness of the Achilles tendons and plantar fascia. (From Saltzman CL and Johnson KA: The ankle and foot. *In* Kelley WN, Harris ED Jr, Ruddy S, and Sledge CB [eds]: Textbook of Rheumatology, Vol 2, 4th ed. Philadelphia, WB Saunders, 1992, p 1857.)

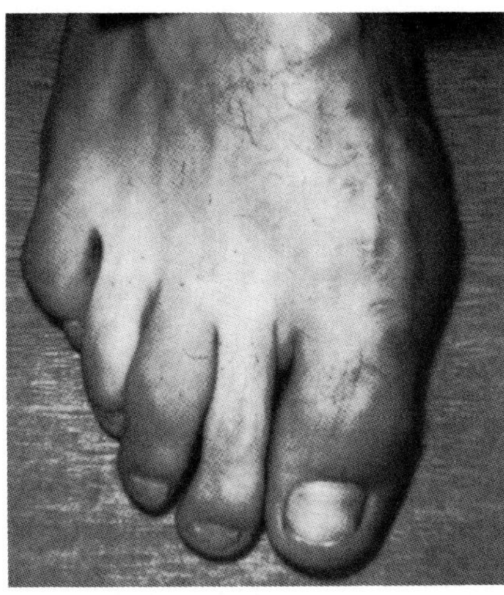

FIGURE 8–2. Sausage toe phenomenon. (From Saltzman CL and Johnson KA: The ankle and foot. *In* Kelley WN, Harris ED Jr, Ruddy S, and Sledge CB [eds]: Textbook of Rheumatology, Vol 2, 4th ed. Philadelphia, WB Saunders, 1992, p 1858.)

joints of hands and, to a lesser extent, the feet; (3) an RS-like arthropathy with sausage toes, plantar fasciitis, and Achilles tendinitis; (4) a spondyloarthropathy, especially in males with HLA-B27; and (5) a rapidly destructive arthropathy, which is fortunately rare, called *arthritis mutilans.* Abnormalities of the nails, including pitting and oncholysis, are observed in all groups. Although all these subsets are usually easily identified, the psoriasis itself may not be found without a careful search. In general, the extent of the psoriasis does not correlate with the pattern or severity of the arthritis. Furthermore, improvement of the skin disease does not result in similar remissions of the arthropathy.[11] Additionally, the arthritis may even precede the onset of psoriasis.[12] These patients are initially classified as a nonspecific seronegative polyarthritis or seronegative RA in those with a symmetrical arthritis.

Psoriasis is a common skin problem. Some sources estimate that 2 per cent of the population may have this condition.[9] However, PA is relatively rare, even within this potentially large reservoir of patients.[13] Moreover, diagnostic confusion may occur in patients who have psoriasis and who acquire one of the more common arthropathies such as inflammatory osteoarthritis with Heberden's nodes (DIP joints of hands) and seropositive RA.

The spondyloarthropathy of PA is also similar to RS. Asymmetry of sacroiliitis, early involvement of the cervical spine, and nonmarginal syndesmophytes are shared features of PA and RS. On the other hand, circinate balanitis, KB, oral lesions, urethritis, and conjunctivitis are not characteristically seen in patients with PA. The prevalence of HLA-B27 in RS approaches 80%, whereas in PA with spondylitis it is variably estimated between 40% and 60%.[14]

In addition to the skin, extra-articular manifestations of PA are rare. The patient with PA who is HLA-B27 positive has a higher risk for the development of acute uveitis than does the general population.

Inflammatory Bowel Disease

The spondyloarthropathy associated with an IBD is similar to AS. Although both ulcerative colitis and Crohn's disease are IBDs with different intestinal and extraintestinal manifestations, the arthropathies are almost identical. In general, the IBD-associated spondylitis also affects males who are usually HLA-B27 positive. There are two types of peripheral arthritis. First, a nonerosive arthritis occurs in the lower extremities and characteristically parallels the intestinal activity of the respective IBD. Additionally, the appearance of joint symptoms may even herald an exacerbation of the colitis. This arthritis is usually well controlled with nonsteroidal antiinflammatory drugs (NSAIDs). Second, patients with spondylitis also have a lower extremity arthritis that is similar to other HLA-B27–associated arthropathies. Heel and Achilles tendon involvement is common, whereas sausage toes are unusual. Although one form of peripheral arthritis parallels disease activity in the intestine, the spondyloarthropathy, once initiated, often proceeds in the caudal-rostral manner characteristic of AS. Moreover, a colectomy, which cures the bowel disease in ulcerative colitis, does little to alter the course of the spondylitis.

Extra-articular manifestations of an IBD include a variety of mucocutaneous problems. Erythema nodosum and pyoderma gangrenosum characteristically involve the lower legs. Several types of oral lesions are also observed. In a manner similar to other HLA-B27 spondyloarthropathies, acute uveitis can occur.

The first presentation of IBD may be arthritis. Patients presenting with a seronegative arthritis of the lower extremity or unexplained inflammatory enthesopathy of the heel and Achilles tendon should be questioned for any change in bowel habits. If any suggestive symptoms are uncovered, a barium enema that includes the right colon and the terminal ileum, should be performed. Flexible sigmoidoscopy, usually in association with colonoscopy, may confirm a diagnosis of IBD in those patients who are minimally symptomatic.

PHYSICAL FINDINGS

The articular manifestations of the seronegative spondyloarthropathies are characteristically similar in all four types. Lumbar rigidity and sacroiliac pain, especially on palpation, are observed in active disease. The restriction of lumbar motion is tested by the Schober test.[15] Most clinicians place two midline points (separated by 10 cm) on the skin of the low back when the patient is standing upright. The first mark is at the level of the ''dimples'' caused by the posterior iliac spines. The second mark is 10 cm above. The patient is then asked to bend forward, keeping the knees as extended as possible, in an attempt to touch the fingers to the toes. This movement reverses the usual lumbar lordosis. As the skin over the now kyphotic lumbar spine stretches, the distance between the marks increases. Normally, this difference should be at least 5 cm, having a total expansion between 16 and 22 cm. Methods to elicit sacroiliac tenderness include direct palpation, iliac wing compression, and several pelvic-tilt/straight-leg maneuvers. The sensitivity is excellent, but the specificity for the sacroiliac joint is low because other abnormalities of the lumbar spine, hips, and deep pelvis may also result in pain with these maneuvers.

Inflammation of the peripheral joints in the spondyloarthropathies can present with either dramatic effusions of the joints and digits or tenderness at tendon and ligament insertions with minimal objective signs of swelling. True arthritis, especially of the knee, is often asymmetrical. Involvement of the heel and ankle is usually the result of Achilles tendinitis or plantar fasciitis. The Achilles tendon is often swollen and tender at the insertion on the calcaneus. To detect plantar fasciitis, deep pressure must be applied to the heel pad to elicit pain. Although a sausage digit is observed more commonly in RS and PA, this finding can occur in any of the spondyloarthropathies. The entire digit, usually a toe, is involved, and the companion toes on either side may be totally normal. This phenomenon is usually the result of a true arthritis involving the MTP and proximal interphalangeal joints in addition to a tenosynovitis.

Inflammation of the hips and shoulders is another manifestation of axial disease. The hips must be carefully examined for flexion deformities. Involvement of these joints will result in more forward flexion of the spine.

The joints of the upper extremity may be involved later in the disease, usually after the lower extremity has been prominently affected. The exception is certain forms of PA that can have either an RA-like pattern or well-localized swelling of the DIP joints of the fingers in association with nail pitting and onycholysis. Similar nail abnormalities may be noted on the toes.

Some patients with seronegative spondyloarthropathy complain of sciatica. Characteristically, both the neurologic examination and imaging studies for lumbar disc herniation are negative. Nevertheless, these symptoms should be investigated carefully because a cauda equina syndrome may be found.[16]

The extra-articular manifestations often involve the skin, including the oral mucosa, and the eyes.[3–5] The skin is a major component of PA and RS, a variable component of IBD, and an almost nonexistent feature of AS. The most common mucocutaneous signs were discussed under Clinical Features. It is important to realize that the skin lesions may precede or follow the arthritis.[10–13]

The inflammation of the eyes is usually acute and symptomatic. This is especially characteristic of an anterior uveitis, which presents with a painful red eye and visual changes.[17] On the other hand, the conjunctivitis may be transient and characteristically does not affect vision. Most patients do, however, recall the episode of conjunctivitis.

LABORATORY TESTS

The laboratory tests assist in the confirmation of the diagnosis and the monitoring of the disease activity. The erythrocyte sedimentation rate (ESR) is an acute-phase reactant and may reflect the degrees of systemic inflammation. Practically, an elevated ESR is consistent with the diagnosis of a seronegative spondyloarthropathy, but a normal ESR neither rules out this diagnosis nor implies a mechanical alteration as the only cause for the back pain. An elevated ESR during disease activity may normalize when clinical quiescence occurs. In these patients demonstrating this pattern, this test may be helpful to monitor disease activity during future exacerbations.

A positive result for HLA-B27 can be difficult to interpret. The frequency of the gene in the white population in the United States is estimated to be between 5% and 10% of the population.[4, 5] Moreover, low back pain, both acute and chronic, is very common in young males. Therefore, the risk of a false-positive test result could be expected to occur relatively frequently if used for all forms of back pain.[4] This may result not only in misdiagnosis but in a less favorable insurability status for some young males. In summary, the test is often ordered when a positive result can serve to unify a set of early, or atypical, symptoms within the group of seronegative spondyloarthropathies. It is probably prudent not to order this test in cases of acute back pain and in patients who do not relate a pattern of morning stiffness. Additionally, HLA-B27 testing can be ordered in certain undiagnosed cases of peripheral arthritis of the lower extremity that have features of sausage toe, plantar fasciitis, or inflammatory Achilles tendinitis.[4] A positive test result may help to strenghten the clinician's resolve to try an alternative or more aggressive therapeutic approach, even if the final diagnosis (AS, PA, IBD, or RS) has not been established.

Obviously, an RF is characteristically negative in this group of disorders. Low titers of RF may be seen in a small percentage of the population. Occasionally, this will confuse the certainty of the diagnosis of spondyloarthropathy. In a similar manner, antinuclear antibody positivity is not expected to be found at a higher frequency than in the general healthy population. This test, unlike the RF, does not have to be routinely ordered in young males with low back pain and peripheral arthritis.

White blood cell counts in the inflammatory range are found in synovial fluid taken from involved peripheral joints. White blood cell counts can range from a few thousand to as high as 75,000/mm.[3] Neutrophils often account for up to 90% of the white blood cell differential. Glucose levels are normal, and crystals are not found. Culture of the synovial fluid is always negative, especially in the reactive arthritis group (RS). Currently, the mucin clot test is not used as an indicator of inflammatory joint fluid, but, historically, the fluid would be expected to show a fair to poor clot. A Wright's stain on the fluid reflects the preponderance of neutrophils, although some patients with RS have monocytes that have ingested other monocytes called *Reiter's cells*. These cells are not specific for RS and can be seen in other inflammatory joint diseases.

IMAGING

The most important image is the plain radiograph of the pelvis with or without sacroiliac views (see Chapter 19 for further information about imaging). The changes of sclerosis, pseudowidening, and obliteration of the sacroiliac joint can be seen in both men and women at various stages of sacroiliitis.[18] In AS and IBD, the sacroiliac involvement is usually bilateral, whereas in PA and RS asymmetry is common. Radiographs of the lumbar spine may be normal during early disease. Squaring of the vertebral body may occur in some patients before obvious ligamentous calcification. These calcifications are called *syndesmophytes* and are classified as marginal or nonmarginal, depending on the origins and insertions. In general, IBD and AS have marginal syndesmophytes, whereas PA and RS have nonmarginal syndesmophytes.[9] In later disease, the entire spine may become encased in ligamentous calcification and give the appearance of a ''bamboo'' spine. Despite the excess calcium in the ligaments around the vertebrae, the bone density within the vertebral body may be low.

The peripheral joints may have radiographs that suggest both articular and entheses involvement. Bony erosions and periarticular demineralization is not as common as in RA. However, erosions do occur in long-standing cases. Calcific periostitis can be seen in the small bones of the feet and hands. The prominent calcaneal spurs along the Achilles tendon insertion and the plantar fascia occur in chronic cases. These spurs may first appear months to years after the onset of symptomatic heel pain.

Imaging of the soft tissues has advanced rapidly in this disease, especially with respect to the inflammation of the entheses, which can rarely be detected by plain radiographs. Occasionally, swelling of the entire digit in a sausage toe or an enlarged Achilles tendon could be detected. In the 1970s, bone scans using technetium 99 helped to detect localized increases of blood flow, reflective of inflammation, in symptomatic joints with negative radiographs. Bone scans were proposed to help differentiate mechanical versus inflammatory joint disease. Unfortunately, the false-positive and false-negative rates were numerous. Attempts at transferring mammographic techniques (xeroradiography) to the soft tissue of the feet, especially the Achilles tendon, provided better structural definition. The anatomic limits of the tendon could now be visualized. In the 1980s, computer tomography followed by magnetic resonance imaging (MRI) helped define both structure and function. With MRI, inflammation and fluid in joints, tendon sheaths, and deep bursae of the feet could now be visualized. MRI cannot always answer the mechanical versus inflammatory questions, but it provides a pattern that may suggest one instead of another. This is especially helpful in differentiating early seronegative disease involving the feet in which the plain radiographs are normal.

DIFFERENTIAL DIAGNOSIS

The process of establishing the diagnosis of seronegative spondyloarthropathy and then determining which one is present is relatively straightforward when the classic signs and symptoms are present. Low back pain in an inflammatory pattern (morning stiffness), abnormal sacroiliac joint radiographs, sausage toes, acute uveitis, chronic heel pain, and HLA-B27 positivity help establish the general category. The extra-articular signs of psoriasis, KB, circinate balanitis, colitis, oral mucosal lesions, and conjunctivitis suggest a specific type (PA, AS, IBD, or RS). Diagnostic problems occur when the inflammation is confined to the entheses without obvious swelling. Similarly, the extra-articular features can occur after or out of sequence with the joint disease, which adds to the diagnostic dilemma. In general, disease confined to the back and maybe the heel, without obvious synovitis of the knees, is called *AS*. When peripheral joints of the lower extremities are more prominently affected, a search for PA, RS, and IBD is often undertaken. However, a positive HLA-B27 and a negative RF does not distinguish the type of seronegative spondyloarthropathy.

The diagnosis of AS involving the spine alone is usually obvious during the physical examination and confirmed by the radiographs demonstrating syndesmophytes. In the spine, a condition called *diffuse idiopathic skeletal hyperostosis* (DISH) can produce thick syndesmophyte-like bridges. Patients with DISH are usually older and HLA-B27 negative.[19] Moreover, the physical examination of the back is less restricted, and pelvic radiographs demonstrate normal sacroiliac joints. Interestingly, tendinous and ligamentous calcification can occur in DISH, especially in the patella and calcaneus, which may add to the diagnostic difficulty.

PA and RS pose a most difficult diagnostic problem. They are commonly confused with each other. First, RS has a specific skin lesion, KB, that has close similarities to psoriasis. Second, both conditions commonly have sausage toes. Third, RS may be incomplete. The arthritis can occur without a history of conjunctivitis or urethritis. Finally, the arthritis of PA may precede the skin disease. In other patients, the psoriasis is so limited that it goes undetected. In a similar manner, both PA and RS can be confused with early RA, especially in seronegative cases. This diagnostic dilemma is made more difficult if the arthritis of PA and RS is symmetrical and low back involvement is not prominent.

AS, presenting in the teenage years, is usually classified as a form of juvenile polyarthritis and is also referred to as a type of *juvenile RA* (JRA) by some investigators. When patients are in their 20s, most of the cases with pure AS emerge, and the spinal restriction may progress. Furthermore, some cases of JRA, unlike adult RA, may involve the cervical spine and have radiographic features similar to AS. However, involvement of the lumbar spine, sacroiliac joint, and heel is not typical of JRA.

IBD may be clinically silent. Some patients do not present with bloody diarrhea or abdominal pain. Any bowel abnormality in patients with articular signs or symptoms suggestive of spondyloarthropathy should be pursued diagnostically. Both IBD and sarcoidosis can present with the skin lesion erythema nodosum involving the lower legs. Inflammation of the ankle and Achilles tendon may also be seen in both disorders. However, the bowel symptoms usually distinguish the two.

THERAPY

In most patients, the back and peripheral joint symptoms respond to NSAIDs. Usually, potent NSAIDs such as indomethacin and tolmetin, in maximal doses, are required. Historically, salicylates have not been effective in the spondyloarthropathies. On rare occasions, phenylbutazone has been used for patients with persistent synovitis. This is one of the very few indications for this medication because of the rare but unpredictable association with aplastic anemia. In general, the potent NSAIDs, used to control seronegative spondyloarthropathy, can result in gastric mucosal ulceration. These NSAIDs should be given with food. Other patients may require additional gastric cytoprotection with prostaglandins, such as misoprostol, to prevent ulceration. Misoprostol should be avoided in women of childbearing age and in patients with IBD.

The concept disease-modifying antirheumatic drugs in these diseases is less clear than for RA. Sulfasalazine has been effective in some patients with AS and PA.[20, 21] Methotrexate (MTX) is the drug of choice for patients with PA and peripheral joint involvement. MTX may be less effective for the spondylitis of PA. Injectable gold has been shown to help the peripheral joint involvement in PA.[22] MTX is effective in some patients with RS and should be tried in patients not responding to NSAIDs alone.

Local glucocorticoid injections can be extremely effective in controlling the active arthritis and enthesopathy, especially when one or two sites persist after systemic therapy has been initiated. As with any steroid injection of tendon sheaths and ligamentous insertions, the smallest effective dose with a short-acting preparation should be used. The clinician must carefully avoid injecting the ligament and tendon itself.

Historically, irradiation was used to treat the spine affected with inflammatory arthritis. Although temporary relief was afforded, it usually did not stop the disease, and an excess mortality rate was observed over time.[23] Nevertheless, low-dose irradiation to the heel has been done in certain patients with intractable inflammation of the Achilles tendon and plantar fascia.

FOOT SURGERY IN THE SERONEGATIVE SPONDYLOARTHROPATHIES

A patient with an established diagnosis of seronegative spondyloarthropathy with peripheral arthritis and enthesopathy of the feet (i.e., plantar fasciitis, synovitis of the MTP joints, Achilles tendinitis, and synovitis of the subtalar joint) who is unresponsive to conservative measures may be a candidate for a variety of surgical procedures. As with other inflammatory arthritides, medical and local conservative measures (such as NSAIDs, corticosteroid injections, heel lifts, and the wearing of quality athletic shoes and well-fabricated orthoses) are tried before undertaking surgical alternatives. In our experience, the use of shoes, padding, and orthoses have had limited value except in milder pathological cases (e.g., the use of heel lifts to reduce the pull on the Achilles tendon in tendinitis and soft metatarsal pads incorporated onto an orthotic for MTP joint synovitis). The symptomatology of the variants of seronegative spondyloarthropathies are quite similar, and, once recalcitrance has been established, we would consider some potentially helpful surgical procedures.

Before surgical procedures can be considered in the seronegative arthropathies, some preoperative considerations must be reviewed.[24, 25] Seronegative spondyloarthropathy patients are predisposed to additional surgical risks as a consequence of the characteristics of their disease process. General factors to be considered are as follows: obesity, which should be energetically treated to reduce stress on weightbearing joints; anemia of chronic disease; low serum albumin levels; impaired vascularity; osteoporosis; cardiac involvement in AS and RD; and increased risk of infection in IBD from a focus of bowel infection or bacterial spread from a colostomy. The administration of anesthesia is often complicated by a rigid spine. Intubation in patients with fixed flexion deformities of the cervical spine is challenging even to the most experienced anesthesiologist. Furthermore, spinal anesthesia may be extremely difficult by the conventional midline approach through the calcified ligaments of the posterior lumbar spine. A lateral approach is usually successful in avoiding these ligamentous calcifications. It is probably prudent to obtain new radiographs of the cervical and lumbar spine before administering anesthesia, even if the previous radiographs are only several years old.

Wound healing is of importance in this group of patients because of the use of immunosuppressive drugs and the potential for hematoma formation secondary to NSAIDs. Careful dissection and hemostasis are important to lessen the incidence of postoperative complications in this patient population. Preoperative prophylactic antibiotics administered intravenously 15 to 30 minutes before the procedure are advised because this patient population constitutes a higher risk group. In the psoriatic patient, Koebnerization (i.e., an isomorphic effect whereby there is a phenomenon of induction by physical trauma or by other noxious influence of lesions of the very same form that is characteristic of the disease) of the surgical site may be a possibility. The presence of psoriatic outbreaks along the incision increases the risk of infection and dehiscence. In our experience, and fortunately so, Koebnerization is not commmon.

The following procedures have been deemed valuable or potentially valuable for the indicated foot pathologic conditions.

Valuable Procedures

1. Sectioning of the plantar fascia for plantar calcaneal enthesopathy.
2. Panmetatarsal head resection and fusion of the toes for synovitis of the MTP joints.
3. Modified Keller procedure for joint disease of the first MTP joint.

Potentially Valuable Procedures

1. Tendo-Achilles lengthening or gastrocnemius recession for Achilles tendinitis.
2. Fusion of the interphalangeal joints and tenotomy for sausage digit.
3. Fusion of the subtalar joint for subtalar synovitis.

In the potentially valuable group, insufficient procedures have been performed or inadequate follow-up has occurred to determine long term benefits; however, the results to date have been promising and warrant further investigation.

Valuable Procedures

Plantar Fascial Sectioning. Release of the plantar fascia has been advocated in recalcitrant cases of heel pain. This same approach has been successfully applied to selective patients with seronegative spondyloarthropathy. We have applied this approach to those patients in whom pharmacologic and local measures have been unsuccessful and the patients have been left significantly dysfunctional as a result. Until further information is available, this approach should not be universally applied. The surgical approach differs somewhat in seronegative patients in comparison to the nonarthritis population. In seronegative patients, sectioning of the fascia versus release is advised to lessen the chance for recurrence.

The technique we have used with these patients is as follows. A lateral preoperative non-weightbearing radiograph of the foot is obtained, and the distance from the plantar skin surface to the plantar calcaneal spur is measured. These measurements are translated on the operating table to the medial surface of the heel, with the two intersecting lines marking the approximate site of the plantar fascial insertion into the calcaneus (Fig. 8–3). A 3-cm skin incision is made horizontal to the floor on the medial side of the heel directly over the intersecting lines. Using blunt dissection, a channel is created both dorsal and plantar to the plantar fascia at its calcaneal insertion. A straight Kelly clamp is used to grasp the plantar fascia immediately distal to its insertion, and a meniscotome is directed medial to lateral, proximal, and dis-

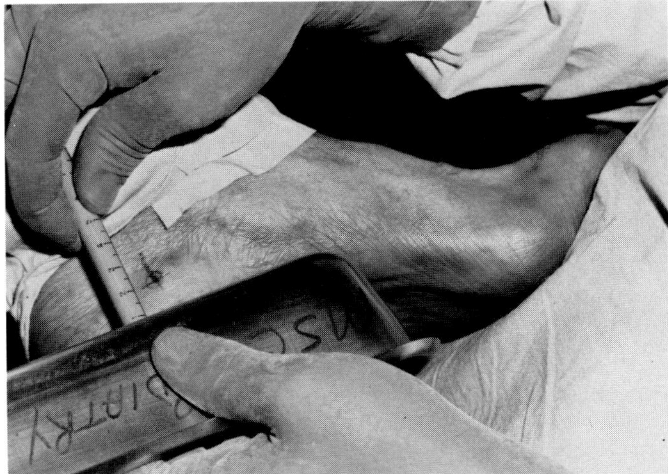

FIGURE 8–3. Intersecting lines for plantar fascial resection.

tal to the Kelly clamp, thereby removing a section of the plantar fascia and reducing the possibility of reapposition. Weightbearing is allowed the following day to tolerance.

Panmetatarsal Head Resection. Panmetatarsal head resection has a time-honored respect in the management of the arthritic forefoot. Initial and ongoing emphasis has been applied primarily to the rheumatoid forefoot, but occasional application exists in the seronegative spondyloarthropathy patient. This procedure is used in the seronegative patient basically because of the disease patterns. For example, cases of RS may be remitting, cautioning against extensive surgical approaches. There are instances when disease is more extensive, is unremitting, and is unresponsive to conservative measures. Hoffman[26] first described the excision of the metatarsal heads through a transverse plantar incision: "The single plantar incision is preferable to any dorsal incision because the heads which are pushed into the sole by the dorsally displaced phalanges are superficial and very accessible there" (p. 1911). Clayton[27] approached the heads through a transverse dorsal incision, resecting the bases of the proximal phalanges as well as the metatarsal heads. The excision of the phalangeal bases was necessary because they obscured the metatarsal heads for resection. Lipscomb and colleagues[28] used a dorsal approach through three longitudinal incisions to resect the phalangeal bases and metatarsal condyles. Dwyer[29] proposed many modifications to impart stability to the foot. He fused the first MTP joint and interposed the long extensor tendon of each of the lesser digits in the space created by the resection of the metatarsal heads. He also fused all the lesser digits. Hodor and Dobbs[30] used the five-dorsal-incisions approach for better exposure and decreased trauma from excessive retraction. Refer to Chapter 30 for more detailed information on this procedure.

The question as to whether this procedure is appropriate depends in part on the experiences of the individual surgeon. Diffuse and extensive MTP joint destruction and pain suggest this approach. As previously mentioned, seronegative spondyloarthropathies often involve only a few joints. Even in these instances, one might want to consider panmetatarsal resection because of the transfer problems brought about by disturbance of the metatarsal parabola when two or more metatarsal heads are resected. We have used a panmetatarsal

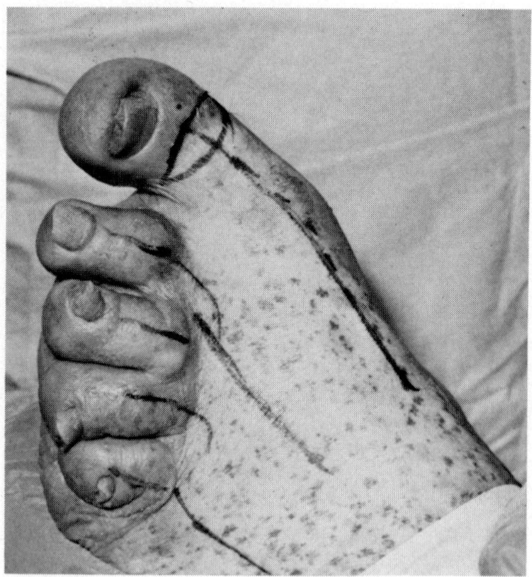

FIGURE 8–4. Proposed skin incisions for panmetatarsal head resections and fusion of the toes.

head procedure that has evolved from the work of many previous authors, as well as our own, over more than 15 years with numerous modifications. We believe this facilitates the surgery and provides a surprisingly functional foot for the long term. The patient with seronegative spondyloarthropathy can be successfully treated with this procedure.

Procedure Considerations. A cutaneous longitudinal incision is directed over the first MTP joint and extended distally to the hallux interphalangeal joint (Fig. 8–4). If the hallux

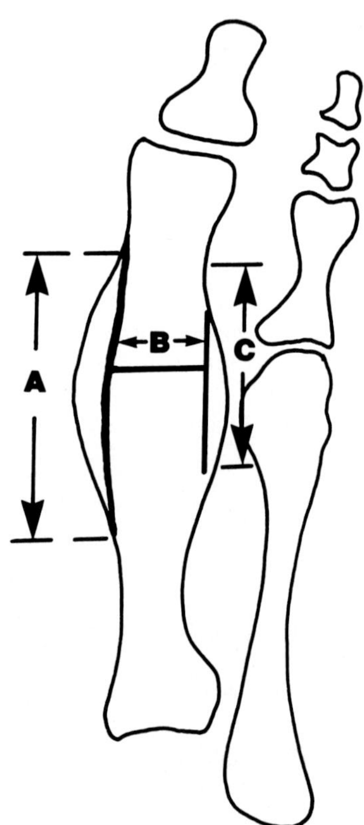

FIGURE 8–5. Dorsal H-shaped capsulotomy.

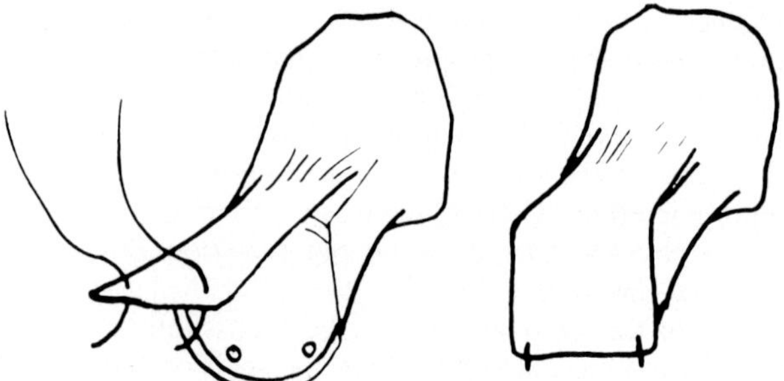

FIGURE 8–6. Capsular interposition of first metatarsal.

interphalangeal joint is to be fused, two transverse elliptical incisions are made over the joint and, after excision of the appropriate bones, fusion is performed with either a 4.0 cancellous screw or a 0.062-in. Kirschner wire. A dorsal medial capsular incision is made (Fig. 8–5, line A). A transverse dorsal capsular incision, line B, is made from line A to the proposed line C through the MTP joint, and a final capsular incision is made on a dorsal lateral side of the first MTP joint (line C). This creates an H-shaped dorsal flap for the covering of the raw bone surface of the first metatarsal after resection of the head (see Fig. 8–5). A medial capsular flap is fashioned to prevent transverse plane drift of the hallux.

The head of the first metatarsal and the sesamoids are excised, and the first metatarsal is cut in a beveled manner so as to avoid irritation on the plantar surface. The dorsal flap is interposed into the joint space and sutured at the distal plantar corners of the remaining metatarsal shaft (Fig. 8–6). A 0.062-in. Kirschner wire is used to stabilize the hallux and metatarsal. The medial capsular flap is sutured into a drill hole in the first metatarsal shaft (Fig. 8–7).

The second metatarsal head is approached before closure of the first incision, which allows the surgeon to calculate the level of resection of the second metatarsal head without the need for visualizing all the metatarsal heads on subsequent dissection. This provides for a smooth 2–1–3, 4,5 parabolic configuration.

Each lesser metatarsal head is excised in a step-by-step manner from step 2 through step 5, and the extensor digitorum longus tendon (Fig. 8–8) is cut as far proximal as possible and interposed into the MTP joint space.

The PIP joints of toes 2, 3, 4, and 5 are excised and fixated end to end with 0.045-in. Kirschner wires, which are directed into the metatarsals. A TLS drain is inserted medially or laterally to prevent postoperative hematoma formation.

Modified Keller Procedure. The Keller bunionectomy has been a standard procedure for the treatment of hallux limitus and hallux abductovalgus with or without associated

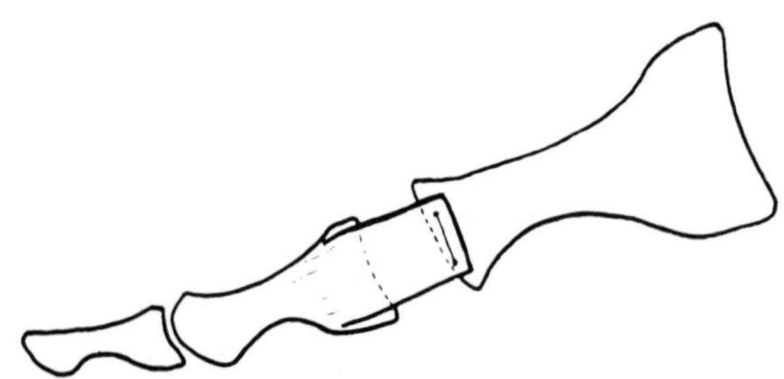

FIGURE 8–7. Medial capsular flap.

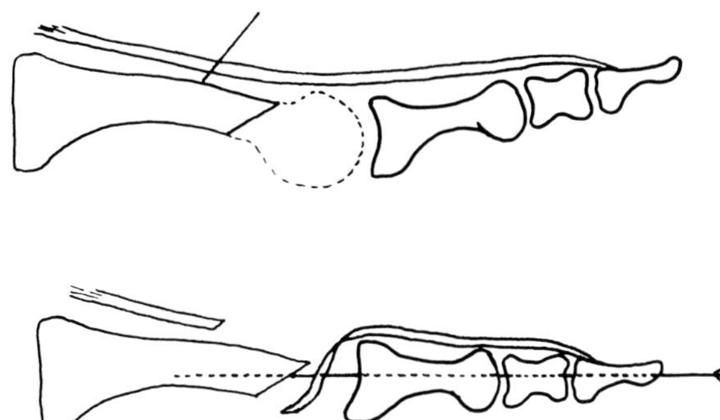

FIGURE 8–8. Interposition of extensor digitorum longus in the metatarso-phalangeal joint.

arthritis. Although this procedure has been accepted as a joint-destructive intervention, it is not without complications. Complications and sequelae include flail toe, excessive shortening, recurrence of hallux abductovalgus and hallux limitus, hyperextension of the hallux, and lack of toe purchase, resulting in excessive biomechanical trauma to the second metatarsal head. Because of these sequelae, the Keller procedure prompted review, and alternate procedures were sought. The use of interpositional implants was favored for years in the arthritic population. More recently, concerns about implant-mediated risks and complications have prompted review of these procedures. Arthrodesis remains a viable alternative, especially in the younger patient whose gait is more propulsive. As an alternative, Keller bunionectomy may be considered if appropriate modifications are undertaken to balance and reestablish supporting soft tissue structures of the first MTP joint. The reattachment of the flexor hallucis brevis was advocated by McGlamry and co-workers, as was the medial capsular flap.[31] The author (WL) used an interpositional capsular flap since the late 1960s in response to failed Stone bunionectomies in an attempt to gain range of motion in the stiff first MTP joint. Many modifications of capsular flaps were used until finally a dorsal-to-plantar flap on the proximal phalanx was standardized. The following modifications, used by the author (WL) the last 25 years, address the same concerns.

Procedure. The longitudinal skin incision is made medial to the extensor hallucis longus tendon, extending from the hallux interphalangeal joint to the neck of the first metatarsal. An H-shaped capsulotomy (see Fig. 8–5) is performed similar to the panmetatarsal head resection capsulotomy on the

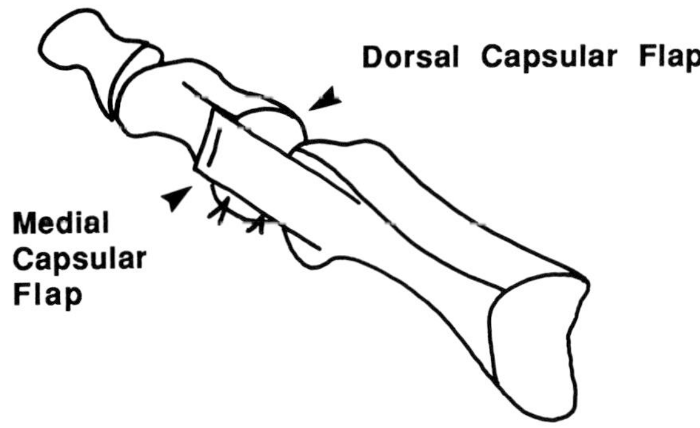

FIGURE 8–9. Medial capsular flap for Keller procedure.

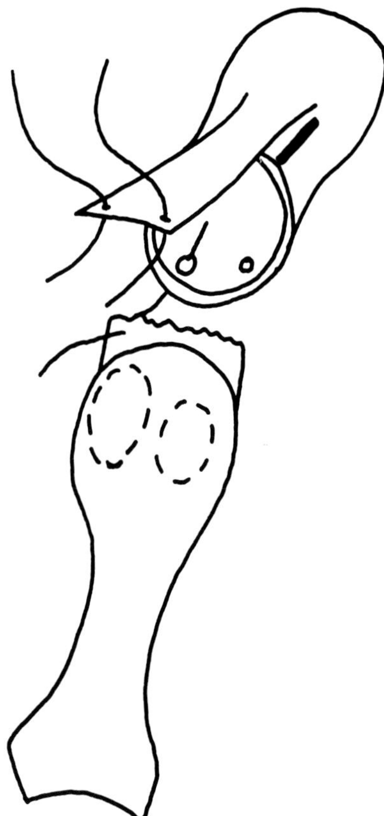

FIGURE 8–10. Suturing of the flexor hallucis brevis tendon and the capsular flap.

dorsal surface of the first MTP joint. A medial capsular flap (see Fig. 8–7) is fashioned with the base of the flap at the neck of the first metatarsal and attached ultimately to the amputated stump of the base of the proximal phalanx (Fig. 8–9). The capsular flaps are retracted, and the proximal one third of the proximal phalanx and the medial eminence of the first metatarsal head are resected. The sesamoidal apparatus is inspected for adherence to the metatarsal head and is freed, if necessary. Three drill holes are created in the stump of the proximal phalanx. One is plantar lateral, the second is plantar medial, and the third is a dorsal plantar hole in the medial cortex of the base of the proximal phalanx. The proximal articular set angle is evaluated, and, if beyond normal limits, a Reverdin-Green osteotomy may be performed at the metatarsal head for correction. The intermetatarsal angle can be substantially reduced by the elimination of the retrograde force of the hallux, and it need not be addressed. The flexor hallucis brevis tendon, which was detached during the excision of the base of the proximal phalanx, is now reattached to the plantar medial hole using O–O Ethibond or comparable suture (Fig. 8–10). This allows function of the flexor hallucis brevis and prevents lack of hallux purchase, which is a common problem with the Keller procedure. On occasion, the long flexor tendon can be used in a similar manner if the flexor hallucis brevis is not viable. The dorsal capsular flap, which is attached to the proximal phalanx distally, is now used to cover the raw bone surface of the base of the proximal phalanx. This capsular flap prevents bone-to-bone contact and becomes integrated into a fibrocartilaginous articular surface at the base of the proximal phalanx. The medial capsular flap is attached with tension through the previously drilled holes in the cortex of the base of the proximal phalanx using a nonabsorbable suture such as O–O Ethibond. This controls the transverse plane drift of the hallux. The proximal portion of the H-shaped capsular flap is sutured to the dorsal surface of the capsule of the proximal phalanx. The extensor hallucis longus tendon is usually lengthened to weaken it slightly and to prevent overpowering of the flexor apparatus but is repaired under physiologic tension.

In the first week postoperatively, aggressive range of motion is initiated using a continuous passive motion device, or, if not available, passive range of motion by the patient, walking on tiptoe and squatting with heels raised.

Potentially Valuable Procedures

In the potentially valuable series of surgeries for foot problems such as Achilles tendinitis, sausage digit, and subtalar synovitis, sufficient data have not been gathered to come to a firm conclusion; however, encouraging results have been forthcoming from the few procedures that have been done. In Achilles tendinitis of Reiter's disease, a tendo-Achillis lengthening has been performed, and, after 1 year, the results are still satisfactory, with total patient relief. The sausage digit that is absolutely intractable to conservative measures has been fused at the interphalangeal joints with satisfactory results. For recalcitrant subtalar synovitis, fusion of the subtalar joint seems to be a satisfactory answer coupled with synovectomy of the sinus tarsi.

References

1. Masi AT: Do sex hormones play a role in ankylosing spondylitis? Rheum Dis Clin N Amer 18:153–196, 1992.
2. Zeidler H, Mau W, and Khan MA: Undifferentiated spondyloarthropathies. Rheum Dis Clin North Am 18:187–202, 1992.
3. Calin A: Reiter's syndrome. *In* Kelley WN, Harris ED, Ruddy S, and Sledge CB (eds): Textbook of Rheumatology, 3rd ed. Philadelphia, WB Saunders, 1989, pp 1038–1052.
4. Arnett FC: Seronegative spondylarthropathies. Bull Rheum Dis 37:1–12, 1987.
5. Calin A: Ankylosing spondylitis. *In* Kelley WN, Harris ED, Ruddy S, and Sledge CB (eds): Textbook of Rheumatology, 3rd ed. Philadelphia, WB Saunders, 1989, pp 1021–1052.
6. Keat A: Reiter's syndrome and reactive arthritis in perspective. N Engl J Med 309:1606–1615, 1983.
7. Espinoza LR, Java LJ, Espinoza CG, et al: There is an association between human immunodeficiency virus and spondyloarthropathies. Rheum Dis Clin North Am, 18:257–267, 1992.
8. Clark MR, Solinger AM, and Hochberg MC: Human immunodeficiency virus infection is not associated with Reiter's syndrome. Rheum Dis Clin North Am, 18:267–276, 1992.
9. McEwen C, Tata D, Lingg C, et al: Ankylosing spondylitis and spondylitis accompanying ulcerative colitis, regional enteritis, psoriasis and Reiter's disease. Arthritis Rheum 14:291–302, 1971.
10. Gladman DD: Psoriatic arthritis: Recent advances in pathogenesis and treatment. Rheum Dis Clin North Am 18:247–256, 1992.
11. Wright V: Psoriatic arthritis. Arch Dermatol 80:27, 1959.
12. Wright V, Roberts MC, and Hill AGS: Dermatological manifestations in psoriatic arthritis: A follow up study. Acta Dermatol 59:235, 1979.
13. Stern RS: The epidemiology of joint complaints in patients with psoriasis. J Rheumatol 12:315, 1985.
14. Kingsley G, and Panayi G: Antigenic responses in reactive arthritis. Rheum Dis Clin North Am 18:49–66, 1992.
15. Moll JMH, and Wright V: Normal range of spinal mobility: An objective clinical study. Ann Rheum Dis 30:281, 1971.
16. Russell ML, Gordon DA, and Ogryzlo MA: The cauda equina syndrome in ankylosing spondylitis. Ann Intern Med 78:551, 1973.
17. Rosenbaum JT: Acute anterior uveitis and spondyloarthropathies. Rheum Dis Clin North Am 18:143–151, 1992.
18. Gran JT, Husby G, and Hardvik M: Radiological changes in men and women with ankylosing spondylitis. Ann Rheum Dis 43:570–575, 1984.
19. Resnick D, and Niwayama G: Radiographic and pathological spinal involvement in diffuse idiopathy skeletal hyperostosis (DISH). Radiology 119:559, 1976.
20. Dougados M, Boumier P, and Amor B: Sulfasalazine in ankylosing spondylitis. Br Med J 293:911, 1986.
21. Farr M, Kitas GD, Waterhouse L, et al: Sulphasalazine in psoriatic arthritis. Br J Rheumatol 29:46–49, 1990.
22. Dorwart BB, Gall EP, and Schumacher HR: Chrysotherapy in psoriatic arthritis. Arthritis Rheum 21:513, 1978.
23. Radford EP, Doll R, and Smith PG: Mortality among patients with ankylosing spondylitis not given x-ray therapy. N Engl J Med 297(11):572–576, 1977.
24. Beddow F: The Surgical Management of Rheumatoid Arthritis. London, Butterworth Co., 1988, pp 43–44.
25. Moll JMH: Management of Rheumatic Disorders. New York, Raven Press, 1983, pp 252–255.
26. Hoffman P: An operation for severe grades of contracted or clawed toes. Am J Orthop Surg 9:441–449, 1911–1912.
27. Clayton ML: Surgery of the lower extremity in rheumatoid arthritis. J Bone Joint Surg. 45A:1517, 1963.
28. Lipscomb PR, Benson GM, and Sones DA: Resection of proximal phalanges and metatarsal condyles for deformities of the forefoot due to rheumatoid arthritis. Clin Orthop 82:24, 1972.
29. Dwyer AE: The correction of severe toe deformities. J West Orthop Assoc 7:19, 1970.
30. Hodor L and Dobbs BM: Panmetatarsal head resection. J Am Podiatr Assoc 73:287, 1983.
31. McGlamry ED, Kitting RW, Butlin WE: Keller bunionectomy and hallux valgus correction: Appraisal and current modifications sixty-six years later. J Am Podiatr Assoc 70:161–167, 1970.

CHAPTER 9

Crystalline Deposition Disease

Divyang Patel, D.P.M., and James Stavosky, D.P.M.

CRYSTAL-INDUCED ARTHROPATHIES

An acute attack of gout of the first metatarsophalangeal (MTP) joint is such a striking event that it was the main form of arthritis recognized by the ancient Greeks. The disease was originally called *podagra*, a Greek definition from *pous* (foot) and *agra* (attack). Hippocrates, Seneca, Galen, Sydenham, and other masters of ancient medicine wrote a number of aphorisms about gout. The current term is adapted from the Latin word *gutta* (drop), referring to the early belief that the disease was a result of ''malevolent humor'' dropping on the joint.[1] The classic description of the disorder was set forth by Thomas Sydenham in the seventeenth century, and his description has never been surpassed:

> The victim goes to bed and sleeps in good health. About two o'clock in the morning he is awakened by a severe pain in the great toe; more rarely in the heel, ankle, or instep. This pain is like that of a dislocation . . . then follow chills and a little fever. The pain . . . becomes more intense. . . . Now it is a violent stretching and tearing of ligaments—now it is a gnawing pain and now a pressure and tightening. So exquisite and lively meanwhile is the feeling of the part affected, that it cannot bear the weight of the bed-clothes nor the jar of a person walking in the room. The night is passed in torture.[2]

In 1859, Garrod suggested that crystals were the cause of the inflammation, and in 1901 Freudweiler supported this hypothesis by demonstrating the phlogistic potential of urate crystals in vivo.[1] However, it was not until the early 1960s that the relationship between acute gout and crystal deposition became established.[3] It was then revealed that monosodium urate crystals were always present in the synovium of joints during acute attacks of gout. Later, it was shown that injection of these crystals into normal joints caused acute inflammation.[4]

Today, gout is probably the best understood rheumatic disorder. It is defined as a heterogeneous group of genetic and acquired diseases that are manifest in different ways. It is generally regarded as hyperuricemia and is displayed as a characteristic acute inflammatory arthritis induced by monosodium urate crystals. Some patients develop aggregated deposits of these crystals(tophi) in and around joints of extremities that can be severely disabling and deforming. Other patients develop uric acid nephrolithiasis, which is common in gout; rarely, some develop chronic interstitial nephropathy.

These manifestations of gout can occur in different combinations, but the term *gout* should be reserved only for inflammatory arthritis or tophaceous disease and not essential hyperuricemia. Elevated levels of serum uric acid are seen in more than 90% of gout patients, and hyperuricemia is considered the precursor of gout. However, most persons with elevated serum or uric acid levels do not have gout, and most never experience an episode of gout.[5, 6]

Prevalence and Incidence

Gout is the most common form of inflammatory joint disease in men older than 40 years of age, and it accounts for 5% of all arthritis patients. Its prevalence, which is increasing, varies from about 0.13% to 0.37% in Europe and the United States. An unusually high prevalence of the disease is found among certain racial groups, including the Maori of New Zealand, the inhabitants of the Mariana Islands, and Filipinos in the United States.

It is not surprising that gout primarily affects men in the fifth decade of life. Only about 5% of cases are found in women, largely in the postmenopausal group. Onset before the age of 30 years in a male and in any premenopausal female is associated with either an enzyme defect leading to marked uric acid overproduction or renal disease. A family history of gout is obtained in 6% to 18% of patients.[7]

Pathophysiology and Classification

Classification. Traditionally, gout has been classified as primary or secondary. Primary gout is the result of an inborn error of metabolism or idiopathic gout, when the basic metabolic defect is unknown. About 90% of cases fall into this category of primary gout. *Secondary gout* refers to those cases in which the hyperuricemia is a consequence of other acquired or genetic disorders. In these patients, gout is not the main clinical disorder (Table 9–1).

Pathophysiology. In normal subjects, two thirds of the uric acid, which is an end product of purine metabolism, is excreted unchanged by the kidneys, whereas one third is excreted by bacteria in the gut. In the event of overproduction, enteric uricolysis is enhanced and renal excretion is increased. However, in most patients with idiopathic gout, renal excretion continues at normal levels in spite of overproduction of uric acid. In some patients, renal clearance of uric acid is inefficient in spite of normal production. This lack of efficiency of the kidneys in idiopathic gout may possibly be due to (1) an increased reabsorption of urate crystals, (2)

TABLE 9–1

CLASSIFICATION OF GOUT AND HYPERURICEMIA

Clinical Category	Metabolic Defect
Primary Gout (90% of cases)	

Idiopathic (>94% of primary gout)	Overproduction of uric acid
	   Normal excretion (majority)
	   Increased excretion (minority)
	Underexcretion of uric acid with normal production

Known metabolic or enzyme defects (<1% of primary gout)	
Increased activity of pyrophosphate ribose-P-synthetase	Overproduction of uric acid
''Partial'' HGPRT deficiency	Overproduction of uric acid
Secondary Gout (10% of cases)	
Associated with increased nucleic acid turnover such as in hemolysis, polycythemia vera and myeloid metaplasia	Overproduction of uric acid
Associated with increased purine synthesis	
''Complete'' HGPRT deficiency	Overproduction of uric acid
Glucose-6-phosphatase deficiency (glycogen storage disease, type 1; Lesch-Nyhan syndrome)	Overproduction of uric acid Underproduction of uric acid
Associated with decreased renal clearance (such as that caused by drugs, toxins, endogenous metabolic end products, and diabetes)	Reduced excretion of uric acid with normal production

HGPRT, hypoxanthine guanine phosphoribosyl transferase.

reduced secretion of urate per nephron, or (3) an inhibitory effect of some metabolic products produced elsewhere. No matter what the mechanism proposed, uric acid begins to accumulate and becomes deposited as sodium urate in tissues (Table 9–2).

The depositions of sodium urate are dependent on the solubility of urate in plasma and body fluids; the solubility is dependent on the pH and temperature. In the physiologic state, i.e., at pH 7.4 and 37°C, the solubility of urate is 6.4 to 6.8 mg/dl in plasma. About 0.4 mg/dl is bound to protein α_1- and α_2-globulin. Therefore, under physiologic conditions (with normal body temperature and normal pH), the solubility limit of urate in plasma is 7 mg/dl. However, solubility is considerably less in the foot and ankle region, where temperatures may be about 29°C.[8] As a result, in hyperuricemic conditions, there is a tendency for urate to crystallize in peripheral joints. The reason why crystals precipitate in some patients and not in others is unknown.

The complexity of the pathogenesis of urate crystallization is illustrated by two observations. First, most people with hyperuricemia do not have gout. Second, some patients with normouricemia also may have gout. Therefore, aside from the generalized metabolic predisposition, local factors in addition to pH and temperature may play a more important role in pathologic crystal formation. Some evidence shows that local changes in tissue biochemistry are important in crystal deposition.[9] It has been suggested that pathologic crystal deposition may occur owing to a loss of inhibitors of crystallization, the presence of nucleation and growth promoters on the cartilage matrix, or excess concentrations of ions.[10] Crystals may form in cartilage and tendons without causing symptoms, and direct trauma (either frank trauma or microtrauma) may displace these crystals into the synovial fluid. Changes in the local metabolic environment, as may occur with resorption of the synovium at night, may either displace these crystals or increase their concentration. Thus, local tissue factors may be as important, if not more so, than a generalized metabolic predisposition.

In regard to metabolic predisposition, genetic factors appear to play some role (fewer than 15% of the patients with overproduction of uric acid) in the predisposition of gout and

hyperuricemia. Lesch-Nyhan syndrome is an example of an inherited case of ''overproduction gout.'' This rare syndrome is characterized by hyperuricemia, mental retardation, self-mutilation, choriathetosis, and uric acid nephrolithiasis. It is the result of a total deficiency of the enzyme hypoxanthine guanine phosphoribosyl transferase (HGPRT) and is transmitted by a recessive gene on the X chromosome; hence, it occurs in male children. Down's syndrome is also associated with hyperuricemia.[11] Lesch-Nyhan and Down's syndromes are examples of secondary gout. In both syndromes, gouty arthritis is neither common nor a prominent clinical feature. On the other hand, partial HGPRT deficiency may present clinically with severe gout beginning in adolescence and thus is classified as primary gout.

Environmental factors such as high-protein diets contribute to the development of gout. During World Wars I and II

TABLE 9–2

CAUSES OF HYPERURICEMIA AND GOUT

Overproduction (10–15%)	
Genetic	HGPRT deficiency
	Pyrophosphate ribose-P-synthetase overactive
	Glucose-6-phosphatase deficiency
Acquired	
Increased cell turnover	Malignant disease
	Lymphoproliferative disorders
	Nonmalignant disease (such as hemolytic anemias and psoriasis)
Increased purine catabolism	Alcohol induced
Increased purine intake	
Decreased Efficiency of Excretion (85–90%)	
Genetic	Possible intrinsic renal tubular defect
	Possible effect of some metabolic end products
	Down's syndrome
Acquired	Drug induced (diuretics; low-dose salicylates; alcohol, laxative abuse)
	Abnormal metabolic states (starvation, dehydration)
Mixed	Alcohol

HGPRT, hypoxanthine guanine phosphoribosyl transferase.

acute gouty arthritis was uncommon in Europe, but when dietary protein became ample again, the frequency of gout increased to prewar levels. Starvation and obesity can also be risk factors for hyperuricemia and gout. Occupational and environmental lead exposure may increase the risk of gout by causing renal insufficiency and decreased solubility of synovial fluid uric acid.

The association of alcohol and gout has long been documented. It is said that ''in youth wine goes to the head; in old age it goes to the feet.'' It is suggested that alcohol ingestion increases uric acid levels by inhibiting the clearance of uric acid via lactate, one of the end products of alcohol metabolism. It has also been suspected that an increased catabolism of purine nucleotides occurs with alcohol ingestion.[8] Tainted alcohol, consisting of high levels of lead (saturnine gout), is another mechanism that causes gout and hyperuricemia.

Medications also induce gout. Potential problems include low-dose aspirin intake, certain diuretic agents, and pyrazinamide. Low-dose aspirin, thiazides, ethacrynic acid, acetazolamide, and furosemide inhibit the clearance of uric acid in susceptible persons whereas pyrazinamide, used for treating tuberculosis, causes an increased production of uric acid.

Secondary gout can also result from other conditions. Secondary gout associated with excessive production of uric acid results from conditions in which there is an increased breakdown of cells and increased nucleic acid turnover. These include polycythemia vera, myeloid metaplasia, psoriasis, chronic myeloid leukemia, acute myelogenous and lymphocytic leukemia, sarcoidosis, starvation, myocardial infarction, and Gaucher's disease.[12]

More local factors also may precipitate gout. Local trauma to the joint, such as from overuse and occult or obvious trauma, or surgery, such as bunionectomies, may cause gouty attacks.

Pathogenesis of Gouty Attacks. Acute gouty arthritis takes the form of acute inflammatory synovitis that is always accompanied by the deposition of monosodium urate crystals in the joint effusion. In order of frequency, the joints most commonly involved in the body include the first MTP joint (90% of patients), the talonavicular joint, the subtalar joint, the ankle joint, the knee joint, and the wrist.

The inflammatory response in the joints is initiated by the monosodium urate crystals in the synovium. The crystals directly or indirectly activate a number of humoral and cellular inflammatory responses.[13] The humoral mediators in gout include factors in the complement and coagulation systems; in the latter system, these include activation of the Hageman factor. A multitude of cellularly derived mediators are involved in gout, but neutrophils play a central role in acute gouty inflammation.

Monosodium urate crystals are chemotactic, thereby triggering a neutrophilic response.[13] Phagocytosis of the monosodium urate crystals, which is dependent on microtubular function, leads to rapid destruction of the phagolysosome membrane. This results in the release of hydrolytic enzymes into the cell, which eventually destroys the leukocyte, thus pouring the lysosomal and cytoplasmic contents into the joint fluid. The lysosomal contents stimulate a potent inflammatory response that is capable of destroying the collagen and elastin of the joint. Urate crystals also activate Hageman factor and the contact system of coagulation, leading to the generation of kallikrein, bradykinin, plasmin, and other inflammatory mediators.[13, 14] As a result of the inflammatory process, the synovial membranes are congested, swollen, and heavily infiltrated with neutrophils, platelets, mast cells, macrophages, and lymphocytes. When the formed crystals are resolubilized, the acute attack remits.

Crystal cell interactions may be augmented and modulated by glycoproteins adherent to the crystals. Crystals in gout patients are coated with immunoglobulin G (IgG), and studies have shown that IgG coating enhances neutrophil accumulation and phagocytosis of urate crystals.

Three theories have been advanced to explain the events leading to an acute attack of gout. The first theory postulates the shedding of crystals from pre-existing cartilaginous tophi into the synovial fluid, such as may occur with trauma (frank, chronic, or surgical). The second theory suggests that an additional release of urate into the synovial fluid, resulting in crystallization, occurs when disruption or increased turnover of the cartilage proteoglycans occurs. It is believed that the proteoglycans of cartilage absorb urate crystals. The third theory postulates that the effusion of a traumatized joint at some point undergoes a rapid rate of reabsorption of water and then solute, resulting in the supersaturation of synovial fluid with urate and the precipitation of crystals.[2]

These theories may all have some merit and may explain why the first MTP joint is the joint most prone to gout. This joint is exposed to the greatest amount of pressure per unit area of any joint in the body during gait and therefore is susceptible to trauma. Any limitation of motion of the first MTP joint predisposes the joint to undue stress and increases the chance and recurrence of gouty attacks in susceptible patients.

Disease Association with Gout

Gout has important associations with other diseases. In studies of patients with gout, the prevalence of hypertension, coronary artery atherosclerosis, hyperlipidemia, alcohol abuse, obesity, and calcium urolithiasis is impressive.[15, 16] With the exception of calcium urolithiasis, there is no evidence that abnormal uric acid metabolism is a causative factor in these disorders or that correction of the hyperuricemia affects the course of these diseases.

Treatment of associated disorders may significantly affect uric acid metabolism, causing hyperuricemia and occasionally inciting gouty attacks. The use of diuretics in the treatment of hypertension is a prime example.[17] This is not to say that concerns with hyperuricemia or gout should deter appropriate treatment of potentially more serious metabolic diseases.

Gout also has important associations with other rheumatic diseases—some positive and some negative. The association of gout and calcium pyrophosphate deposition disease has been known for years. Apatite deposition also sometimes occurs in patients with gout. Unlike the positive association with other rheumatic disorders, gout appears to have a negative association with rheumatoid arthritis, explained by genetic, immunologic, and biochemical factors.[18]

Clinical Manifestations

Clinically, gout has four typical stages: (1) asymptomatic hyperuricemia gout; (2) acute gouty arthritis; (3) the intercritical gout; and (4) chronic tophaceous gout.

Stage 1: Asymptomatic Hyperuricemia Gout. In this

stage there is an absence of clinical manifestations, although the serum uric acid level is elevated. Asymptomatic hyperuricemia begins at puberty in males but is delayed in females until after menopause, probably owing to the uricosuric effect of estrogen.[8] Twenty percent of these persons develop acute gouty arthritis or renal calculi. The onset of either or both of these complications marks the end of this phase of the disease.

Stage 2: Acute Gouty Arthritis. Acute gouty arthritis usually is the first manifestation of gout. Early in the course of gouty arthritis, the disorder is asymmetrical and monoarticular (75% to 90%) or oligoarticular. However, polyarticular acute gout is increasingly seen in hypertensive patients with alcohol abuse and in postmenopausal women.[19, 20] Acute gout is predominantly a disease of the lower extremity. At least 50% of the first attacks involve the first MTP joint, and 90% of patients have involvement of the first MTP joint at some time. Next in order of frequency as sites of initial involvement are the talonavicular joint, the ankle joint, the heel, the knee, the wrist, the interphalangeal joints of the feet and hands, and the elbow.[8, 12, 21]

The first episode of acute gouty arthritis frequently begins at night or early morning with excruciating, incapacitating pain and swelling. Several factors may have precipitated the acute gouty arthritis, including local trauma, high purine diet or alcohol intake, surgery (usually third to fifth day postoperative), uricosuric agents, acute medical illness (e.g. myocardial infarction, infection, and stroke), emotional stress, or corticosteroid withdrawal. Attacks may follow a long walk or run, a round of golf, or a hunting trip (e.g., ''pheasant hunter's toe''). Gout flares postoperatively are thought to be a result of mild dehydration, emotional stress, lactic acidosis, and discontinuation of uric acid–lowering medications.[22] These situations cause an increase in serum uric acid levels.

Patients report a variety of symptoms and signs, including debilitating pain, swelling, erythema, locally increased temperature, and, occasionally, malaise, fever, and chills. Light pressure or weightbearing is intolerable. Rarely, patients report low-grade, chronic symptoms of insidious onset. More often, the first attack occurs with dramatic onset. Within minutes to hours of onset, the first MTP joint becomes hot, erythematous, and exquisitely tender. The systemic signs of inflammation include fever, tachycardia, leukocytosis, and elevated erythrocyte sedimentation rate. Lymphangitis may be present. Thus, the inflammatory reaction suggests cellulitis or septic arthritis.

The course of untreated gouty attack is variable, with initial attacks subsiding spontaneously over days to weeks. Mild attacks subside rapidly within hours to a few days, whereas severe attacks may last many days to several weeks. Once the gouty attack episode has subsided, the patient enters an asymptomatic phase called the *intercritical stage*.

Stage 3: Intercritical Gout. This stage refers to the intervals between attacks. Uric acid crystals can be aspirated from previously involved joints, but no symptoms are reported. Some patients may never have a second attack of gout, whereas others never fully recover from the first stage and experience exacerbations leading to chronic tophaceous gout. More often, however, a pattern of recurrences develops. In the first year 62% of the patients report a recurrence.[12] An asymptomatic period may last from months to years partly depending on the adequacy of treatment. Without prophylaxis several attacks may occur each year. With time, recurring attacks occur more frequently, become polyarticular in distribution, and last longer. Eventually, the recovery period between acute attacks becomes incomplete.

Stage 4: Chronic Tophaceous Gout. The incidence of tophaceous gout ranges from 5% to 25% of patients with gout. Before the advent of effective hyperuricemia therapy, however, more than half of the gouty patients developed visible tophi. The more frequent and more severe the gout, the higher the degree of renal involvement, and the greater the duration of gout, the higher the likelihood for tophaceous deposits to occur. The average duration from the initial attack to the development of visible tophaceous gout is approximately 12 years.[8]

Tophaceous deposits most commonly occur in the articular cartilages and erode the cartilage and underlying bone. Initially, the deposits are superficial, probably originating from the adjacent synovial fluid.[23] Following nonspecific cartilage degenerative changes, such as fibrillation, fragmentation, and erosion, the urate deposits penetrate deeper into the cartilage and subchondral bone. These deposits cause destruction of the subchondral bone and proliferation of marginal bone; sometimes, fibrous and bony ankylosis develops. Pannus formation can also occur as a result of deposition of crystals on synovial membrane. The punched-out lesions, which are apparent on radiographs in patients with chronic gout, represent marrow tophaceous deposits that communicate with the urate deposits in the defective articular cartilage.[12]

The extra-articular subcutaneous manifestations of gout resemble rheumatoid nodules and, indeed, the location of both lesions is the same. The subcutaneous deposits in gout, however, may be visible as chalky, yellowish-white infiltrates that are irregular and hard and occasionally ulcerate the overlying skin. Rarely, they present as draining sinuses (of urate crystals) resembling pus, but culture results are negative. More often, the drainage is dry and chalklike. These ulcerations may become secondarily infected, however, and can lead to osteomyelitis.

Gouty tophi in the foot and ankle often present a physical problem for the patient. There may be complete joint destruction, deformity, and disability. The deposits in the feet particularly involve the first MTP joint, and the patient may present with a bunion deformity or hallux limitus. Smaller joints of the feet are also affected,[24] although fusiform or nodular enlargements of the Achilles tendons are more common. Tophaceous deposits in the foot are particularly seen periarticularly, in bursae, in tendon sheaths, or at areas of chronic excessive dermal pressure. As the tophi become larger, they may cause underlying osseous erosion, become ossified or calcified, and cause entrapment neuropathies or tendon ruptures. Hence, these deposits can cause marked disability. They can mechanically interfere with weightbearing surfaces of the foot and cause pain when shoes are worn.[25] The patient may present to the podiatrist with a classic ''gout shoe''—a window cut out in the shoe to accommodate the tender, swollen joint (often around the first MTP joint).

Gouty tophi may also involve a variety of other tissues, including the heart valves, cardiac conducting system, vocal cords, epiglottis, eyelids, cornea of the eye, and nasal cartilage. However, they do not affect the liver, spleen, central nervous system, and lungs. In rare circumstances, tophaceous deposits occur in the feet in the absence of previous articular involvement.[26] When this occurs, they are difficult to differentiate from benign and malignant neoplasms.[26]

Tendon ruptures, such as those of the Achilles and quadriceps, have been reported in patients with chronic gout and can be extremely debilitating. As with rheumatoid arthritis, synovial popliteal cysts may also develop and can mimic deep venous thrombosis. A clinical syndrome of gout has been described in elderly women, unlike the classic form that affects middle-aged men. Most of these women have renal impairment and receive diuretics. These women have developed tophaceous deposits most commonly around osteoarthritic interphalangeal joints in the upper extremities. The tophi in this group of patients, unlike those in the typical patient with chronic gout, develop rapidly and precede typical gouty arthritis.[27]

CLINICAL EVALUATION

The podiatrist's role in the clinical evaluation of patients suspected of having gout in the foot should be based on ruling out septic arthritis and determining the possible cause of gout. It may seem trivial to investigate whether patients overproduce or underexcrete uric acid, but this information may be important for long-term therapy.

With this caveat in mind, the podiatric medical practitioner should obtain a history with emphasis on the following: age of onset, duration and time of onset, prior personal history of other possible manifestations of gout (renal calculi, hematuria, and soft tissue masses), previous attacks of arthritis, locations of previous joint involvement, trauma, surgery, recent symptoms of possible underlying disease, and especially alcohol intake.

If gout is suspected in a preadolescent male, in a male younger than 25 years of age, or in a premenopausal female, special attention to family history should be given. The family history should have an emphasis on gout and neurologic associations (enzyme defects) and renal status.

On physical examination, the first presentation of a gouty joint typically shows signs of acute infection with marked periarticular swelling, warmth, redness, and exquisite tenderness. The overlying skin often appears shiny, tense, and erythematous. These findings most commonly occur over the first MTP joint, and occasionally findings vary depending on the time of presentation, the nature of the attack, and the site affected. With involvement of gout in the foot, the patient is noted to have an antalgic gait, and any passive or active motion of the involved joint is limited, severely painful, and guarded. Even light touch elicits severe pain.

Presentation of gout is typically asymmetric and monoarticular. Examination for the presence of soft tissue masses must be performed, particularly around subcutaneous and periarticular structures such as the joint capsule, tendons, ligaments, and bursae; the soles, Achilles, prepatellar, olecranon regions, ears, palms, and fingertips. Lesser toes should also be evaluated for deposits on flexor or extensor tendons and deformity of interphalangeal joints. Gout rarely exhibits in the shoulder, sacroiliac, sternoclavicular joints, or cervical spine.

Tophaceous deposits may be the initial presentation in chronic, untreated gout. These may appear to ulcerate or may have already ulcerated and can cause secondary infection. The physical examination also reveals marked deformities in the feet in patients with chronic gout. These include digital contractures, pes planus, and bunion deformities.

Finally, the physical examination should also emphasize the signs of possible underlying disease (e.g., myeloproliferative or lymphoproliferative disorder) or signs of neurologic abnormalities and of associated cardiovascular or metabolic disorders (e.g., hypertension). It is not uncommon for gout patients to have a mildly elevated oral temperature, lymphangitis, and tachycardia. These findings make it difficult to completely rule out a septic joint. Hence, further diagnostic studies are needed.

Radiographic Findings. The radiographic findings of gouty arthritis vary with the clinical stage of gout. In the early stages of gout, radiographs are helpful in ruling out destructive changes associated with septic arthritis, chondrocalcinosis, and calcific periarthritis and in assessing the presence of bony tophi. During the initial or early attacks, no abnormalities of articular structures are evident. An increase in the mass and density of the soft tissue and effusion of the joint may be the only findings. These findings coincide with the presence of synovitis, distention of the joint, and inflammation. The soft tissue or periarticular swelling of acute gout is eccentric, not fusiform as seen in rheumatoid arthritis. Osteopenia is *not* a feature of gout. Osseous changes occur with subsequent and frequent attacks of gout; however, rarely, initial attacks may present with erosive changes. Generally, however, as the initial acute attack subsides, the soft tissue or periarticular radiographic changes disappear.

Following years of recurrent attacks, the first erosive changes are seen, namely at the dorsal and medial aspects of the first metatarsal head and at the base of the first proximal phalanx. These are sites of capsular attachments. Eventually, these punched-out areas become larger; their internal borders become sclerotic with time.[12] Erosions are often evident without joint destruction. Remarkably, the joint space is often well preserved until late in the course of the disease.

Erosions are also seen in rheumatoid arthritis, but in gout the "rat bite" erosions are eccentric, frequently with sclerotic margins, with some overhanging bone (Martel's sign)[28] near the erosions (which is a sign of a secondary repair process). In rheumatoid arthritis, the erosions tend to be marginal at the attachment of synovium to the subchondral bone (i.e., in the "gutter" area). In gout the erosions are remote from the articular surface, which is a key distinguishing feature. The gouty erosions vary in size and shape, progressively increasing with uncontrolled disease and additional attacks. Rarely, erosions of the sesamoids are seen with advanced gout; the erosive changes may be so extensive as to produce a mutilating arthritis seen in rheumatoid and psoriatic patients.[29]

The lesser MTP joints, interphalangeal joints of the hallux, and lesser toes all may reveal abnormalities similar to those seen at the first MTP joint. The erosive destructive changes may also be evident in the talonavicular joint, the ankle joint, the intertarsal joints, the tarsometatarsal joints, and the talocalcaneal joints.[30] Involvement of these joints, except for the ankle, is unusual in rheumatoid arthritis. Other areas of involvement in the foot include the posterosuperior aspect of the calcaneus at the insertion of the Achilles tendon and the plantar inferior aspect of the calcaneus at the insertion of the plantar fascia. With multiple or prolonged subclinical attacks in these structures as well as bursae in the feet, hyperemic resorption of the underlying bone may be evident. Proliferative changes have also been observed in areas of the plantar fascia and tendinous insertions and appear as irregular bony spicules.

"Mushrooming" of the ends and shaft of the metatarsal and phalangeal heads can also occur. Secondary osteoarthritic changes then become common in gouty joints with subchondral sclerosis and osteophytosis becoming apparent. This is a common finding in the first MTP joint, the talonavicular joint, and the interphalangeal joint of the hallux. Joint malalignment and subluxation then become manifest as hammertoe, hallux abductovalgus, and pes planus deformity.

In time, multiple joint involvement occurs, and at this stage gout can be confused with rheumatoid arthritis because of the large amount of destruction. However, polyarticular gout has normal joint spaces with typical punched-out lesions at the ends of small bones. Moreover, the polyarticular disease remains asymmetric, unlike rheumatoid arthritis.

Rarely, distal phalangeal resorption can occur. In rare instances, growth disruption can occur with juvenile gout owing to physeal injury. Intraosseous calcific deposits have been reported in 6% of patients with chronic gout, and radiographic findings resemble enchondromas or bone infarctions.[12]

In summary, chronic gout can have a spectrum of radiographic presentations that can mimic other diseases. In general, it is characterized by marked deformities that are evident on radiographs but rarely manifest as bony ankylosis of the joint.

Laboratory Analysis. The definitive diagnosis of gout depends on identifying uric acid crystals in joint aspirate. Even if the clinical appearance strongly suggests gout, the diagnosis should be confirmed by needle aspiration of joints or of tophaceous deposits. Examination of the aspirate under polarized light reveals typical negatively birefringent needle-shaped monosodium urate crystals in the leukocytes. A monosodium urate crystal appears blue when its long axis is perpendicular to the axis of the lens and yellow when its long axis is parallel to the axis.

The technique for evaluation of joint aspirate is most applicable for the first MTP joint. It is less useful when the interphalangeal or tarsal joints are involved or when the foot and ankle are diffusely swollen. In such situations, an attempt may be made at aspiration, but finding the exact location of the urate crystals may be difficult because it is obscured.

When the first MTP joint is aspirated, an 18- or 20-gauge needle is inserted in the inflamed area and the plunger withdrawn. This is performed through either a dorsomedial or dorsolateral approach. Distraction of the hallux eases entry into the joint. Before the first MTP joint is aspirated, the site of the arthrocentesis should be anesthetized by performing a field block. The arthrocentesis should then be performed using sterile technique.

Aspiration of the joint may not reveal gross fluid; extremely small amounts of fluid are sufficient for analysis. The fluid can be expressed onto a slide, and the wet specimen may be analyzed. The glass slide and coverslip should be clean and free of scratches because dust particles are positively birefringent. Tophi can also be examined microscopically after needle aspiration. Synovial fluid cell counts are elevated from 2000 to 60,000/mm³.[31] Effusions appear cloudy owing to leukocytes and crystals and occasionally produce a chalky or pasty joint fluid. Joint fluid must be cultured if there is any question. A Gram's stain should always be obtained to evaluate for infection, which may

coexist. The synovial fluid yields a friable, poor mucin clot when added to dilute acetic acid.

Crystal examination does have pitfalls. The failure to visualize crystals does not mean the patient has no gout but only that crystals were not seen. However, absence of crystals in an inflamed joint aspirate makes the diagnosis of gout highly unlikely. Technique of aspiration and preparation of the wet field may affect the results.

Occasionally, crystals may be obtained from a quiescent, asymptomatic MTP joint and can aid in the diagnosis after an episode of gout has subsided.

Polarized light microscopy may not be practical for many reasons, including lack of equipment and unfamiliarity with the procedure. Most diagnoses may be established clinically on the basis of the typical picture of an acute attack coupled with hyperuricemia. However, as many as one third of the patients may have uric acid levels in the normal range. The key to diagnosis, therefore, depends on the strict adherence of the clinical picture of gout.[32] Serum uric acid levels may not be elevated during acute gouty attack; hence, repeat serum uric acid measurements may be useful for diagnostic accuracy. If crystalline examination is difficult to achieve, clinical diagnosis can also be inferred if appropriate criteria have been met (Table 9–3). Some physicians believe that a rapid resolution of a red, hot, swollen joint also is pathognomonic for gouty arthritis.

Once gout is suspected, a serum uric acid level should be obtained. Probably the most common mistake leading to misdiagnosis is equating an elevated serum uric acid level and joint pain with gout, particularly when noncharacteristic joints such as those in the axial skeleton, upper extremities, and knee are involved. Additionally, during an acute attack, the serum uric acid levels can be low, because sudden lowering of uric acid with hypouricemic therapy or with the cessation of alcohol intake commonly precipitates an acute gouty attack.[33] Warfarin, high doses of aspirin, phenylbutazone, and radiographic contrast dyes may also lower uric acid levels.[8] In spite of the limitations of uric acid levels in the diagnosis of gout, serum uric acid always is elevated at some time in the course of the disease, and a repeat measurement may be used for diagnostic accuracy.

TABLE 9–3

CRITERIA FOR THE DIAGNOSIS OF GOUT

I. Presence of characteristic urate crystals in the joint fluid
   and/or
II. Tophus proved to contain urate crystals
   and/or
III. Six of 12 clinical, laboratory, or radiographic features
   1. More than one attack of acute arthritis
   2. Maximum inflammation developed within 1 day
   3. Monoarthritis attack
   4. Redness observed over joints
   5. First metatarsophalangeal joint painful or swollen
   6. Unilateral first metatarsophalangeal joint attack
   7. Unilateral tarsal joint attack
   8. Tophus (proven or suspected)
   9. Hyperuricemia
   10. Asymmetric swelling within a joint on x-ray
   11. Subcortical cysts without erosion on x-ray
   12. Joint fluid culture negative for organisms during attack

Adapted from Wallace SL, Robin H, Masi AT, et al: Preliminary criteria for the classification of acute arthritis in primary gout. Arthritis Rheum 20:895–900, 1977.

The normal values for uric acid vary by the technique used. The normal value using the calorimetric technique is under 6 mg/dl. Using the enzymatic (uricase) method, this normal value may be below 7 mg/dl, whereas with the automated technique the value is below 8 mg/dl. Premenopausal women tend to have lower amounts of urate, although this increases to values found in males after women become menopausal.

A complete blood cell count is useful in all patients with acute gout to evaluate total leukocyte, differential count, hemoglobin, and hematocrit levels. The erythrocyte sedimentation rate is elevated. An electrolyte panel should also be obtained to show the patient's renal function status. A urinalysis may reveal uric acid crystals and signs of renal disease.

In the past, considerable emphasis was placed on a 24-hour urinary uric acid measurement to determine if the patient was overproducing or underproducing uric acid. In our opinion, this is helpful in new cases of gout. However, those patients already diagnosed with gout and receiving allopurinol prophylaxis are overexcreting uric acid. The samples ideally should be collected after 3 days of moderate purine restriction during an interventional stage. Values greater than 600 mg/1.72 m^2/day indicate overproduction, whereas values greater than 750 mg/day necessitate ruling out enzymatic deficiency or a myeloproliferative disorder. Additionally, higher levels of uric acid signify that the patient may be at risk for renal stones. Finally, patients on uricosuric agents have lower levels of uric acid in the urine.

If a 24-hour uric acid sample cannot be obtained, a uric acid:creatinine ratio greater than 75% obtained from a single specimen can help suggest overproduction.

Differential Diagnosis

Acute gout must be differentiated from a variety of arthritic conditions.[12] Septic arthritis may be confused with an acute gout attack, but culture of the synovial fluid demonstrates bacteria. Pseudogout may also mimic gout, although it demonstrates positively birefringent crystals and a milder clinical course. Gout and pseudogout, however, may coexist. In young persons, acute rheumatic fever with joint involvement and juvenile rheumatoid arthritis may simulate gout. Palindromic rheumatism may also mimic acute gout in middle-aged or elderly men. Acute gout must also be differentiated from traumatic arthritis, osteoarthritis, sarcoidosis, psoriatic arthritis, Reiter's syndrome, cellulitis, and acute bursitis.

Treatment

The goals in treating gout are (1) termination of the acute gouty attack as soon as possible; (2) prevention of recurrent attacks; (3) prevention and reversal of complications resulting from deposits of sodium urate, such as in joints, kidneys, or other sites; and (4) prevention or reversal of associated features, such as hypertriglyceridemia, obesity, and hypertension.[8, 34–37] The podiatrist should be part of a multidisciplinary approach in treating the patient with the main goals of stopping the acute attack quickly and preventing recurrent attacks. After the diagnosis has been properly made and the acute attack treated, the podiatrist should then refer the patient to a family practitioner or rheumatologist.

The treatment of gouty arthritis depends on the stage and severity of the disease.

Acute Gouty Arthritis. The mainstay of treatment during an acute gout attack is the administration of nonsteroidal anti-inflammatory drugs (NSAIDs). NSAIDs have largely replaced colchicine in the management of acute gout. Unlike colchicine, they can be taken by mouth without significant diarrhea. However, both colchicine and NSAIDs may be particularly toxic in the presence of renal disease and during diuretic administration. In elderly patients, intra-articular steroid injections and cool compresses may be more beneficial.

Indomethacin is the NSAID most commonly used in the treatment of acute gout. Dosages of 50 mg orally three or four times daily should be given until there is significant improvement, usually in about 2 days. When pain is relieved, the dosage is tapered to 25 mg orally three or four times daily until there is total resolution of the acute arthritis. The side effects of indomethacin include dizziness, headache, hyperkalemia, azotemia, fluid retention, confusion, and gastrointestinal disturbances.[34] Other NSAIDs may not have as many neurologic side effects and may be equally efficacious. These agents include naproxen, ibuprofen, sulindac, fenoprofen calcium, and piroxicam. With all NSAIDs, renal function should be monitored, because these agents may cause life-threatening hyperkalemia in patients whose renal blood flow is prostaglandin dependent.

Phenylbutazone was the first NSAID used for the treatment of gout; its efficacy is comparable to that of indomethacin. However, phenylbutazone has severe and significant hematologic side effects, including agranulocytosis and aplastic anemia. Therefore, it is no longer recommended for gout owing to the severity of these potential side effects.

There are many other NSAIDs with proven efficacy in the treatment of gout; dosages of NSAIDs commonly used are listed in Table 9–4. These regimens are not fixed, and treatment with NSAIDs typically lasts about 1 week. However, the key to effective treatment is to begin with maximum dosages initially and then to reduce the dosage as the gouty attack subsides. The reason to choose one NSAID instead of another is the differences in toxicity. For example, indomethacin should be avoided in the elderly owing to a higher incidence of central nervous system side effects. Sulindac can be used in patients with moderately compromised renal function, hypertension, or fluid retention states. Agents with prolonged half-life and onset should be avoided. Additionally, care must be taken in dealing with patients on warfarin when contemplating the use of NSAIDs.

Colchicine has a success rate of 75% to 95% when treatment is started within 12 hours of a gouty attack.[36] It is traditionally given orally, and the response of gouty attack is so dramatic that the colchicine response also may be of diagnostic value. The initial dose of colchicine is 0.6 mg orally every hour for 8 hours, then every 2 hours until a response is obtained or until abdominal cramps, diarrhea, or vomiting appear. In severe cases, as much as 4 to 8 mg may be needed. No more than 8 mg should be taken in 48 hours.[8, 34–37] In most patients, dramatic relief of pain and the onset of gastrointestinal side effects occur simultaneously, and the diarrhea may be treated with paregoric.

Colchicine may also be given intravenously. This may be considered if the gastrointestinal tract is intolerant of oral medications. This route is also useful for treatment or prophylaxis perioperatively when patients cannot take medica-

TABLE 9–4

TREATMENT OF ACUTE GOUT WITH NSAIDS

Drug	Dosage (mg)
Indomethacin (Indocin)	Initially 50 po TID or QID, then 25 po TID or QID as maintenance dose
Phenylbutazone	Initially 100 po QID, then 100–200 po QD for maintenance
Naproxen (Anaprox, Naprosyn)	Initially 500 po, then 250 po TID
Ibuprofen (Motrin and others)	800 po TID
Sulindac (Clinoril)	200 po BID
Fenoprofen calcium (Nalfon Pulvules)	800 po TID or QID
Piroxicam (Feldene)	20 po QID
Tolmetin	400 po TID or QID
Ketoprofen	50 po QID
Meclofenamate	100 po TID

tions orally. When given parenterally, the usual initial dose is 1 to 2 mg in 20 ml of saline solution given slowly over 10 minutes. Doses may be repeated at 6-hour intervals, but not more than 4 mg should be given in a 24-hour period.[34, 38] The most frequent toxic manifestation of intravenous colchicine is local chemical thrombophlebitis. Subcutaneous infiltration can cause tissue necrosis and slough. The parenteral use of colchicine reduces the risk of gastrointestinal side effects but does not eliminate it. Life-threatening intravenous colchicine toxicity and sudden death have been described when the drug has been inappropriately administered, particularly when dosages have been too large, in elderly patients, or in the presence of renal, liver, or heart disease.[35] The patient who is given full doses of colchicine orally or intravenously must have normal renal and hepatic function. Dose-related toxic effects include alopecia (reversible), bone marrow suppression, and hepatocellular damage. It is because of these concerns that colchicine is now rarely used to treat acute gout.

Antihyperuricemic therapy should not be initiated during acute attacks of gout. When initiated, therapy should begin with low dosages to avoid sudden excretion of urate (especially with uricosuric agents) and should be gradually increased weekly to maintenance levels. High fluid intake should be recommended. Colchicine prophylaxis may be used when hypouricemic therapy is initiated. As long as 3 months of colchicine prophylaxis without gouty attacks may be necessary, or colchicine may have to be used as long as tophi are present.

Arthrocentesis followed by injection of corticosteroid in or around the joint is beneficial, especially after the diagnosis of gout is certain. This should be considered in patients with low tolerance for NSAIDs and colchicine. The injection of corticosteroid is contraindicated in the presence of actual or potential sepsis. The podiatrist should consider this approach to managing gout because it has the potential for definitive diagnosis and the ability to provide dramatic and immediate relief. A mixture of a short- and long-acting corticosteroid is preferred. The short-acting corticosteroid relieves synovitis rapidly, whereas the longer-lasting agent delays future crystalline-induced synovitis. Injections of corticosteroid can be performed intra-articularly or periarticularly. The latter technique may be considered if the gout is limited to a bursa or if entry into the first MTP joint is difficult as a consequence of degenerative changes.

In joints not amenable to intra-articular corticosteroid injections or in patients in whom colchicine or NSAIDs are contraindicated, or in patients with severe polyarticular gout, adrenocorticotropic hormone (ACTH) and systemic corticosteroids have been employed.[36] Unfortunately, although both agents can be effective, rebound attacks are frequent, which necessitates the use of low-dose colchicine or nonsteroidal agents.[39]

General measures such as elevation, application of ice, and rest can also be used in this stage of gout. Postoperative or wooden shoes may also provide symptomatic relief.

Intercritical Phase. During this phase patients should be advised to lose weight if they are obese, to avoid high-purine foods (i.e., sweetbreads, fish, liver, kidney, roe, and tinned fish), refrain from alcohol consumption, and control hypertension and hypertriglyceridemia. Gradual weight reduction is recommended because sudden weight reduction may precipitate gout attacks. Diets should consist of low fat and moderate protein content. Hypertension should be managed by the patient's primary physician and should be treated vigorously even if antihypertensive agents worsen the hyperuricemia. The hyperuricemia can be managed with antihyperuricemic agents.

Colchicine or NSAIDs can be used as prophylaxis against recurrent attacks of gouty arthritis. NSAIDs should be prescribed at lower doses than those used for acute attacks, whereas colchicine may be given in a dose of 0.5 to 2 mg/day. The use of colchicine as prophylaxis against recurrent attacks might be particularly beneficial in the first months or year after institution of allopurinol or uricosuric agents. Indomethacin is not recommended as a prophylactic agent for chronic gout because of other side effects previously discussed.

Although useful in preventing recurrent attacks of gout, colchicine does not retard joint damage produced by tophi. However, damage to the joints can be prevented by resolution of the tophaceous deposits and maintenance of a low serum uric acid level.

Chronic Gouty Arthritis. Many physicians believe that the first attack of gout should require treatment with an antihyperuricemic agent. Seventy-eight percent of patients will have a second attack of gout within 2 years.[40] The biochemical abnormality in gout is hyperuricemia. Reduction of the serum uric acid level has the benefit of reducing risks of nephrolithiasis, development of tophi, and further gouty attacks. Antihyperuricemic therapy may be accomplished either by using a uricosuric agent such as probenecid and sulfinpyrazone or by blocking uric acid production (i.e., with a xanthine oxidase inhibitor such as allopurinol). The antihyperuricemic therapy of gout should be managed by the patient's primary physician or rheumatologist.

Before the patient's hyperuricemia is treated, the cause of the attack should be determined. This can be done using methods previously described—namely, by collecting a 24-hour urine sample for uric acid analysis. Hyperuricemia is most commonly due to a primary renal mechanism abnormality in which there is an underexcretion of uric acid. This is most often caused by diuretics but can also be caused by low-dose aspirin, hypertension, decreased renal function, lactic acidosis, and lead intoxication as noted previously.

If the cause of hyperuricemia is an underexcretion of uric acid, uricosuric agents should be used. These agents interfere with tubular reabsorption of filtered urate. Probenecid is the drug of choice in this category. It should be used in patients with adequate renal function but who underexcrete urate. It is started at a dose of 250 mg orally twice daily, then slowly increased up to 2 g daily to maintain a serum uric acid level of less than 6.4 mg/dl.[34, 39] Sulfinpyrazone is another potent uricosuric agent and is similarly used. The former drug may produce gastrointestinal upsets, headaches, or skin rash; sulfinpyrazone may cause untoward reactions similar to its related phenylbutazone. Sulfinpyrazone, however, seems to be generally better tolerated than probenecid.[34] Salicylates in high doses (more than 3 g) can be uricosuric, but few patients can tolerate these doses, whereas low doses may interfere with the uricosuric action of probenecid and sulfinpyrazone.

Allopurinol is the drug of choice in the treatment of chronic gout in terms of convenience. Moreover, it is the best drug to lower serum urate levels in patients with uric acid overproduction, stone formation tendencies, advanced renal disease, and tophaceous deposits elsewhere. A single morning dose is adequate for treatment in most instances. It can be started at 300 mg and then increased to 800 mg if needed. In advanced renal failure, 100 mg doses may be used. Toxicity of allopurinol can occur if the dosage is not adjusted. Hence, some physicians favor using uricosuric agents in underexcretors to avoid allopurinol toxicity. The most common side effects include skin rash, followed by gastrointestinal intolerance, headache, and diarrhea. The most serious side effects of allopurinol include life-threatening toxic epidermal necrolysis, systemic vasculitis, bone marrow suppression, granulomatous hepatitis, and renal failure.[41, 42] Allopurinol has been particularly useful in metabolic gout (i.e., that caused by enzyme deficiencies or cancer chemotherapy or allergic reaction to probenecid and sulfinpyrazone).

Surgical intervention may also be necessary in patients with chronic gout. Several authors have reported on the benefits of surgery in this stage.[43–46] Surgery is indicated when (1) tophi interfere with weightbearing and shoe gear; (2) tophi are painful because of their location; (3) draining sinus tracts associated with tophi or infection are present; (4) tophi interfere with the movement of joints or tendons; (5) further destruction of bone, joints, and soft tissue is to be prevented; (6) tophi cause deformities such as prominent bunions, pes planus, digital deformities, and arthritic changes that interfere with normal gait; and (7) nerves have become impinged by tophi.

Prophylaxis should be initiated about 2 to 3 days before surgery is performed on patients predisposed to gouty attacks. Postoperatively, an acute attack of gouty arthritis can be further prevented if prophylaxis is continued for several days.

Procedures described for management of tophaceous gout have ranged from amputation of digits to partial excision of tophi. Amputations are rarely indicated,[46] and when performed, patients have extensively damaged osseous structures. Most often, amputation of an involved lesser toe results in little functional loss. Partial or total excision of tophi has also been performed; the removal hastens the mechanical and functional rehabilitation of the involved joint or tendon. Total excision is not always indicated because a tophus may be the only supporting framework of the joint or bone and total excision might destroy function; additionally, the tophi may encircle vital structures that need to be preserved. Therefore, in such instances, excision and curettage can be carried out only to a limited degree.

Excision of entire cartilaginous and osseous structures can be performed if function of the foot is not compromised. Procedures for the first MTP joint that can be used include the Keller procedure, arthroplasty with total artificial joint replacement, and arthrodesis. Synovectomy may be adjunctive to these procedures.[47, 48] Partial excision of osseous and cartilaginous structures can also be performed in milder cases of chronic gout, particularly if the tophus is localized eccentrically as it is when it mimics a bunion deformity. In such situations, resection of the involved medial eminence with synovectomy or resection of pannus tissue offers great relief. Occasionally, tophi can be found incidentally during bunionectomy, especially in elderly patients.

Asymptomatic Hyperuricemia. Treatment of nongouty asymptomatic hyperuricemia is controversial. Most physicians do not treat asymptomatic hyperuricemia in otherwise healthy people. However, some clinicians have suggested treating patients younger than 40 years of age with uricosuric agents if they have persistent hyperuricemia of 9 mg/dl or higher with normal 24-hour urinary urate excretion.

CALCIUM PYROPHOSPHATE DIHYDRATE DEPOSITION DISEASE

Calcium pyrophosphate crystal is the most common form of calcium crystal–producing articular disease.[50] The crystal may be deposited in articular cartilage, menisci, synovia, and closely associated tendinous and articular structures. Calcium pyrophosphate dihydrate (CPPD) crystal deposition disease encompasses an array of disorders including pseudogout and chronic arthropathy. The spectrum of CPPD disease has been clinically subdivided into (1) pseudogout, (2) pseudorheumatoid arthritis, (3) pseudo-osteoarthritis, (4) asymptomatic joint disease, and (5) pseudoneuropathic arthritis.[49] The disease has been further classified as sporadic, familial, and secondary. Sporadic cases make up most of the cases, whereas familial cases present in young persons. In the elderly, the disease has been associated with various metabolic conditions, most commonly hyperparathyroidism, gout, hemochromatosis, amyloidosis, and myxedema. The cause of CPPD disease remains unknown.

CPPD deposition disease was initially described as *chondrocalcinosis articularis* based on the characteristic radiographic appearance of intra-articular calcium deposits. In 1962[50] the condition was termed *pseudogout* when acute inflammatory goutlike attacks were noted in elderly patients who had CPPD crystals rather than expected urate crystals in the synovial fluid and articular cartilage. Three presentations of CPPD deposition disease are now commonly recognized: asymptomatic chondrocalcinosis, acute pseudogout, and chronic pyrophosphate arthropathy.

Asymptomatic Chondrocalcinosis

Most patients with chondrocalcinosis remain asymptomatic. Sixty percent of people older than 80 years of age may have this disease.[49, 50] Chondrocalcinosis is the radiographic description of calcification in the cartilage. The most common site of involvement is the knee, followed by the wrist and symphysis pubis, but any joint may be involved. Involvement of joints in the foot is rare. Chondrocalcinosis usually is the result of CPPD deposition but may also be produced by other crystalline deposition, such as calcium hydroxyapatite, calcium oxalate, and dicalcium phosphate dihydrate. The findings of chondrocalcinosis are usually coincidental, and if joints are asymptomatic, no specific therapy is required. However, any associated metabolic condition should be treated.

Acute Pseudogout

Acute pseudogout is the most dramatic clinical manifestation of CPPD deposition disease and is the major cause of acute monoarticular or oligoarticular arthritis in the elderly. Males and females are affected with equal frequency, unlike gout. The attack most commonly occurs in the knee (58%), followed by the wrist (33%) and then the ankle joint. When it involves the foot (5% of cases), it mainly involves the talonavicular joint. It presents like gout with a sudden onset of severe pain, swelling, redness, and localized heat of the affected joint. It may also mimic acute septic arthritis in its presentation. Diagnosis is based on demonstration of weakly birefringent rhomboid-shaped crystals in the the synovial fluid. The synovial fluid reveals an inflammatory reaction with white blood cell counts ranging from 2000 to 80,000/mm^3 and neutrophils predominating.[52] Identification of CPPD crystals does not exclude other causes of joint inflammation such as gout, rheumatoid arthritis, and infection because these diseases can coexist with pseudogout.

There are clues that help differentiate gout from pseudogout. Differentiation can sometimes be difficult because pseudogout may be present in joints that are commonly involved in gout. Pseudogout does not respond as dramatically as gout to colchicine. Additionally, pseudogout patients tend to be older and do not usually have as excruciating pain. However, as in gout, pseudogout can be precipitated by trauma, surgery, or acute medical illnesses such as stroke and myocardial infarction. Patients may similarly present with fevers, chills, leukocytosis, and elevated erythrocyte sedimentation rate.

Laboratory evaluation should be the same as for gout patients and should also include evaluation of thyroxine, calcium, phosphorus, magnesium, and uric acid levels. Acute pseudogout attacks are self-limiting, but attacks can be rapidly controlled with NSAIDs. Indomethacin is the drug of choice, but other NSAIDs can also be effective. Oral colchicine has not been as dramatically effective as in gout, although intravenous colchicine has been quite effective. It is usually effective in a dose of 1 to 4 mg. Long-term, low-dose colchicine helps decrease the number of recurrent attacks of pseudogout. The intra-articular administration of corticosteroid, along with aspiration of synovial fluid, can also be effective.

Chronic Arthropathy

About 50% of patients with CPPD deposition disease present with clinical and radiographic features identical to those of osteoarthritis, but the joints involved are different from those involved in osteoarthritis. The joints include the knees, wrists, MTP joints, shoulders, elbows, and hips. Any joint may be involved, although chronic arthropathy of the foot is rare. The patient is typically elderly and has complaints of stiffness and limited motion in the involved joint. Examina-

tion reveals synovitis with limited motion, crepitus, and mild pain. The disease may overlap with osteoarthritis. Chronic pyrophosphate arthropathy can be distinguished from osteoarthritis by having more severe destruction of the joints and adjacent bone. The talonavicular joint is the most commonly involved joint of the foot with chondrocalcinosis, and calcification of nearby capsules, tendons, and ligaments is not uncommon.

Occasionally, chondrocalcinosis may cause a pseudorheumatoid-type disorder, with subacute joint inflammation lasting several months. Radiographs reveal erosive changes, and demonstration of rhomboid, positively birefringent crystals helps differentiate CPPD deposition disease from rheumatoid arthritis. Some of these patients with chondrocalcinosis have a positive rheumatoid factor, however.

Rarely, pseudotophaceous or bursal para-articular deposition of CPPD crystals can be the only manifestation of the disease. Achilles tendinitis and retrocalcaneal bursitis have been reported.[51, 52] Diffuse calcification of retrocalcaneal bursa is seen. The deposition of CPPD crystals along the Achilles tendon is characteristically linear and extensive. This can be distinguished from the more nummular calcification of apatite crystals.[12]

CPPD deposition disease can also mimic ankylosing spondylitis.[53] Occasionally, the disease can be associated with marked joint destruction with fragmentation and instability similar to a Charcot's joint. However, the patient has no neurologic deficit. Instances have also been described in which the disease has mimicked rheumatic fever, traumatic arthritis, polymyalgia rheumatica, and fibrositis.[49, 50, 54] The radiographic manifestations may vary, and findings can mimic other rheumatic diseases.

Treatment of chronic pyrophosphate arthropathy is similar to that of the disease that it mimics. Analgesics, NSAIDs, physical therapy, intra-articular corticosteroid injections, ankle foot orthoses, and surgical replacement of destroyed joints all may be used to alleviate the patient's pain.

CALCIUM HYDROXYAPATITE CRYSTAL DEPOSITION DISEASE

Calcium hydroxyapatite crystal deposition disease is a rare disorder that mainly affects periarticular soft tissues but can also affect joints. It is caused by the deposition of hydroxyapatite crystals. Hydroxyapatite crystals are frequently detected in osteoarthritic joints and are now recognized as possibly contributing to advanced osteoarthritis. They are also believed to be responsible for calcinosis associated with chronic renal failure, hypercalcemia, myositis ossificans, polymyositis, hyperphosphatemia, and scleroderma.

Hydroxyapatite deposition disease may mimic gouty arthritis, traumatic arthritis, and septic arthritis. Radiographic fluffy calcification is seen at the joint versus the linear pattern present in CPPD deposition disease. The disease has been associated with a rapidly destructive form of shoulder arthritis most commonly found in elderly women. Its occurrence in the foot is extremely rare, but when it occurs, it involves the first MTP joint, the ankle joint, and the insertion of the Achilles tendon.[55, 56]

References

1. Rodnan GP: Early theories concerning etiology and pathogenesis of the gout. Arthritis Rheum 8:599–610, 1965.

2. Kelley WN and Fox IH: Gout and related disorders of purine metabolism. *In* Kelley WN, Harris ED, Ruddy S, and Sledge CB (eds): Textbook of Rheumatology, 2nd ed. Philadelphia, WB Saunders, 1985, pp 1359–1398.

3. McCarty DJ and Hollander JL: Identification of urate crystals in gouty synovial fluid. Ann Intern Med 54:452–460, 1961.

4. Nakagawa Y, Abram V, Kezdy FJ, et al: Purification and characterisation of the principal inhibitor of calcium oxalate monohydrate crystal growth in human urine. J Biol Chem 258:12594–12600, 1983.

5. Levinson DJ: Clinical growth and pathogenesis of hyperuricemia. *In* McCarty DJ (ed): Arthritis and Allied Conditions: A Textbook of Rheumatology, 11th ed. Philadelphia, Lea & Febiger, 1989, pp 1645–1676.

6. Lawrence RC, Hochberg MC, Kelsey JL, et al: Estimates of the prevalence of selected arthritic and musculoskeletal diseases in the United States. J Rheumatol 16:427–441, 1989.

7. Masi AT and Medsger TA: Epidemiology of the rheumatic diseases. *In* McCarty DJ (ed): Arthritis and Allied Conditions: A Textbook of Rheumatology, 11th ed. Philadelphia, Lea & Febiger, 1989, pp 16–54.

8. Wyngaarden JB: Gout. *In* Wyngaarden JB, Smith LH, and Bennett JC (eds): Cecil Textbook of Medicine, 19th ed. Philadelphia, WB Saunders, 1992, pp 1107–1115.

9. Fiddis RW, Vlachos N, and Calvert PD: Studies of urate crystallization in relation to gout. Ann Rheum Dis 42(Suppl): 12–15, 1983.

10. Dieppe P and Calvert P: Crystals and Joint Disease. London, Chapman and Hall, 1983.

11. Pallela TD and Fox IH: Hyperuricemia and gout: *In* Scriver CR, et al (eds): The Metabolic Basis of Inherited Disease, 6th ed. New York, McGraw Hill, 1989, p 965.

12. Resnick D and Niwayama CT: Gouty arthritis: *In* Resnick D and Niwayama CT (eds): Diagnosis of Bone and Joint Disorders. Philadelphia, WB Saunders, 1981, p 1465.

13. Terkeltaub RA and Ginsberg MH: The inflammatory reaction to crystals. Rheum Dis Clin North Am 14(2): 353–364, 1988.

14. Ginsberg MH, Jaques B, Cochrane CG, et al: Urate crystal-dependent cleavage of Hageman factor in human plasma and synovial fluid. J Lab Clin Med 95:497–506, 1980.

15. Klein R, Klein BE, Coroni JC, et al: Serum uric acid—its relationships to coronary heart disease risk factors and cardiovascular disease: Evans County, Georgia. Arch Intern Med 132: 401–410, 1973.

16. Berger L and Yu T-F: Renal function in gout: An analysis of 524 gouty subjects, including long-term follow-up studies. Am J Med 59:605, 1975.

17. Horwitz L, Liebman J, and Carolo D: Thiazide-induced hyperuricemia and gout. J Am Podiatr Med Assoc 72:511–516, 1982.

18. Spector A and Christman R: Coexistent gout and rheumatoid arthritis. J Am Podiatr Med Assoc 79:522 558, 1989

19. Doherty M and Dieppe P: Crystal deposition in the elderly. Clin Rheum Dis 12:97–114, 1985.

20. Yu T-F: Some unusual features of gout in females. Semin Arthritis Rheum 6:247–255, 1977.

21. Marcinko D (ed): Rheumatology and associated connective tissue disorders. *In* Medical and Surgical Therapeutics of the Foot and Ankle. Baltimore, Williams & Wilkins, 1991, pp 716–720.

22. Zier BG: Essentials of Internal Medicine in Clinical Podiatry. Philadelphia, WB Saunders, 1990.

23. Jaffe HL: Metabolic, Degenerative, and Inflammatory Diseases of Bones and Joints. Philadelphia, Lea & Febiger 1972, p 479.

24. Addante A and Paicos P: Tophaceous gout involving the fourth toes bilaterally. J Am Podiatr Med Assoc 78:599–603, 1988.

25. Smith L, Adelman H, and Black J: Gouty arthritis: A case study. J Am Podiatr Med Assoc 78:642–644, 1988.

26. Lerman R, Danna A, and Boykoff T: Tophaceous deposition in the absence of known antecedent gout. J Am Podiatr Med Assoc 81:273–275, 1991.

27. McFarlane D and Dieppe P: Diuretic-induced gout in elderly women. Br J Rheumatol 24:155–159, 1985.

28. Martel W: Overhanging margin of bone: A roentgenographic manifestation of gout. Radiology 95:775, 1986.

29. Martel W: Radiology of the rheumatic diseases. *In* Hollander JL and McCarty DJ Jr (eds): Arthritis and Allied Conditions: A Textbook of Rheumatology, 8th ed. Philadelphia, Lea & Febiger, 1972, p 115.

30. Lacey PG and Harrison RB: Case report 178. Skeletal Radiol 7:225, 1981.

31. McCarty DJ: Arthritis and Allied Conditions: A Textbook of Rheumatology, 9th ed. Philadelphia, Lea & Febiger, 1979, p 1221.

32. Wallace SL, Robin H, Masi AT, et al: Preliminary criteria for the classification of acute arthritis in primary gout. Arthritis Rheum 20:895–900, 1977.

33. Steele TH and Oppenheimer S: Factors affecting urate excretion following diuretic administration in man. Am J Med 47:564, 1969.

34. Emmerson BT: Therapeutics of hyperuricemia. Med J Aust 141:31–36, 1984.

35. Wallace SL and Singer JZ: Therapy in gout. Rheum Dis Clin North Am 14: 441–457, 1988.

36. Gutman AB: Medical management of gout. Postgrad Med 51:61–66, 1972.

37. Thompson CP, Duff IF, and Robinson WD: Long-term uricosuric therapy in gout. Arthritis Rheum 5:384–396, 1962.

38. Neal RW, Liang HM, and Stern SH: Colchicine in acute gout: Reassessment of risk and benefits. JAMA 257:1920–1922, 1987.

39. Reginato AS, Paul H, and Schumacher HR: Crystal-induced arthritis. Arch Phys Med Rehabil 63:401–408, 1982.

40. Gutman AB: The past four decades of progress in the knowledge of gout, with an assessment of the present status. Arthritis Rheum 16:431–445, 1973.

41. McInnes GT, Lawson DH, and Jick H: Acute adverse reactions attributed to allopurinol in hospitalized patients. Ann Rheum Dis 40:245–249, 1981.

42. Singer JZ and Wallace SL: Allopurinol hypersensitivity syndrome: Unnecessary morbidity and mortality. Arthritis Rheum 29:82–87, 1986.

43. Woughton HW: Surgery of tophaceous gout. J Bone Joint Surg 41A:116, 1959.

44. Larmon WA, and Kurtz JF: The surgical management of chronic tophaceous gout. J Bone Joint Surg 40A:743, 1958.

45. Levy LA: Arthritis. *In* Levy LA and Hetherington, VJ: Principles and Practice of Podiatric Medicine. New York, Churchill Livingstone, 1990, p 374.

46. Rana NA: Gout. *In* Jahss MH: Disorders of the Foot and Ankle, 2nd ed. Philadelphia, WB Saunders, 1991, pp 1716–1717.

47. Landry JR and Schilero J: The medical/surgical management of gout. J Foot Surg 25:160–175, 1986.

48. Caputi RA: Synovectomy. Clin Podiatr Med Surg 5:249–257, 1988.

49. McCarty DJ: Calcium pyrophosphate dihydrate crystal deposition disease—1975. Arthritis Rheum 19 (Suppl):275, 1976.

50. McCarty DJ Jr, Kohn NN, and Faires JP: The significance of calcium phosphate crystals in the synovial fluid of arthritis patients: The ''pseudogout'' syndrome. Ann Intern Med 56:711–737, 1962.

51. Gerster JC, Baud CA, Lagier R, et al: Tendon calcification in chondrocalcinosis: A clinical, radiologic, histologic, and crystallographic study. Arthritis Rheum 20:717, 1977.

52. Gerster JC, Lagier R, and Boivin G: Achilles tendinitis associated with chondrocalcinosis. J Rheumatol 7:82–88, 1980.

53. Reginato AJ, Schiapachasse V, Zmijewski CM, et al: HLA antigens in chondrocalcinosis and ankylosing chondrocalcinosis. Arthritis Rheum 22:928, 1979.

54. Moskowitz RW, and Katz D: Chondrocalcinosis coincidental to other rheumatic diseases. Arch Intern Med 115:680, 1965.

55. Gruneberg R: Calcifying tendinitis in the forefoot. Br J Radiol 36:378, 1963.

56. Kernohan J, Dakin PK, and Helal B: Dolorous calcification of the lateral sesamoid bursa of the great toe. Foot Ankle 5:545, 1984.

CHAPTER 10

Connective Tissue Diseases

Charles A. Eiser, D.P.M., and Marley M. Taylor, D.P.M.

The generally accepted constituents of the connective tissue diseases (CTDs) are rheumatoid arthritis (RA), systemic lupus erythematosus (SLE), scleroderma, polymyositis, dermatomyositis, Sjögren's syndrome, the various vasculitic diseases, and mixed CTD. Although a common etiologic agent is highly suspected, a proven etiologic agent is lacking. Despite sharing many of the clinical findings that these diseases manifest, rheumatic fever is excluded on the basis of its known streptococcal pathogenicity. The genetically acquired or so-called heritable connective tissue disorders, such as Ehlers-Danlos syndrome, are similarly excluded from this classification.

What remains are a group of rheumatic diseases with no proven cause and no cure and whose immunologic pathophysiology is ethereal at best. Clinical features are frequently subacute, maturing and undergoing metamorphosis seemingly so as to defy diagnosis. The nature of these CTDs is so protean that proper description and classification are often based on conjecture.

SYSTEMIC LUPUS ERYTHEMATOSUS

SLE is gaining increasing recognition as being an archetypical autoimmune disease. Numerous independent researchers are developing the likely suspicion that unlocking the cause and pathogenicity of this disorder will produce a quantum advance in the understanding of not only the other connective tissue disorders but perhaps the larger family of rheumatic diseases as well.

SLE is a chronic inflammatory syndrome of unknown cause that may be acute and fulminating (a rarity now) or slowly progressive, with typical remissions and exacerbations. Pathologic changes are manifest in many organs and organ systems, most likely owing to vascular effects on the viscera. More particularly, SLE is characterized by the widespread production of autoantibodies to deoxyribonucleic acid (DNA), ribonucleic acid, and a plethora of other cell nuclear components functioning as antigens. Although the effects of disease on the cardiopulmonary system, renal system, and central nervous system (CNS) are most significant to the morbidity and mortality profile, the most frequent manifestations of SLE are those producing skin and joint disease. Historically, the term *lupus* (from the Latin for "wolf") has been associated since the Middle Ages with the characteristic ulcerative facial erosions. Since 1982, a revision of the 1971

criteria for the classification of SLE has been in existence (Table 10–1). To be considered as having SLE, a patient must exhibit 4 or more of these 11 criteria at one time or another.[1]

SLE is a disease once thought to be quite rare. Historical demographic studies are revealing an increasing prevalence in the general population, with some reports as high as 1 case in 8000.[2] This increasing incidence over the years the disease has been studied may be real and linked to an unknown environmental agent or perhaps is a reflection of the increased interest in this fascinating and malicious syndrome. There is also the undeniable effect of our increasing and widespread use of highly sensitive diagnostic testing, such as antinuclear antibody (ANA) testing. There is a substantial preponderance of female patients, roughly 10:1, with an incidence of 1 female for every 1000 persons. Some authors recently described a higher incidence in women of African-American descent.[3] Diagnosis is most often made between the ages of 15 and 35 years; however, onset has been reported in both elderly and adolescent populations (Fig. 10–1).

Hughes[4] reviewed a number of previous studies and reported substantiating the prevalence for this syndrome to affect the female and African-descendant patient, particularly in the United States and West Indies. He documented that the prevalence of SLE on the island of Jamaica may approach 1 in 250 women.[4] Siegel and Lee[2] performed extensive epidemiologic research and likewise documented an incidence of 80.9 per 100,000 persons or just under 1 in 1000 females. Fessel[5] reported an extensive review of cases in San Francisco and found a rate of nearly 1 in every 2000 females. When race was factored in, incidence in African-American females decreased to 1 in 245.[5]

Pathology

Circulating complexes of ANAs and their antigens, notably anti-DNA bound to DNA, are believed to be responsible for the major pathologic abnormalities seen on the cellular level.[6] Such antibodies and cellular nuclear antigens are observed in glomerular capillary basement membranes and at the skin's dermal-epidermal junction. Atkins and colleagues, in 1972, described the presence of gamma globulin deposition in the brain's choroid plexus of patients who died of CNS lupus.[7] Antigen-antibody complexes deposit, followed

TABLE 10–1

REQUIRED CRITERIA FOR DIAGNOSIS OF SYSTEMIC LUPUS ERYTHEMATOSIS

Criterion	Definition
1. Malar rash	Fixed erythema, flat or raised, over the malar eminences, tending to spare the nasolabial folds
2. Discoid rash	Erythematous raised patches with adherent keratotic scaling and follicular plugging; atrophic scarring possible in older lesions
3. Photosensitivity	Skin rash as a result of unusual reactions to sunlight, found by patient history or physician observation
4. Oral ulcers	Oral or nasopharyngeal ulceration, usually painless, found by physician observation
5. Arthritis	Nonerosive arthritis involving two or more peripheral joints, characterized by tenderness, swelling, or joint effusion
6. Serositis	Pleuritis: convincing history of pleuritic pain or rub heard by physician or evidence of pleural effusion or pericarditis documented by electrocardiogram, rub, or evidence of pericardial effusion
7. Renal disorder	Persistent proteinuria >0.5 g per day or >3+ if quantitation not performed or cellular casts (may be red cell, hemoglobin, granular, tubular, or mixed)
8. Neurologic disorder	Seizures or psychosis in the absence of offending drugs or known metabolic derangements (uremia, ketoacidosis, electrolyte imbalance, and so on)
9. Hematologic disorder	Hemolytic anemia with reticulocytosis, leukopenia, lymphopenia, or thrombocytopenia in the absence of offending drugs
10. Immunologic disorder	Positive lupus erythematosus cell preparation or anti-deoxyribonucleic acid or anti-SM or false-positive serologic test for syphilis known to be positive for at least 6 months and confirmed by *Treponema pallidum* immobilization or fluorescent antibody absorption test
11. Antinuclear antibody	An abnormal titer of antinuclear antibody by immunofluorescence or an equivalent assay at any point in time and in the absence of drugs known to be associated with ''drug-induced lupus'' syndrome

Adapted from Tan EM, Cohen AS, Fries JF, et al: The 1982 revised criteria for the classification of systemic lupus erythematosus. Arthritis Rheum 25(11):1271–1282, © Williams & Wilkins, 1982.

by fixation of complement and thus the activation of the complement system and its cascade of inflammatory events, leading to chemotaxis, increased vascular permeability, and enhanced phagocytosis. As the process progresses, histologic changes can begin to be appreciated, most notably the presence of fibrinoid necrosis in the walls of capillaries, arterioles, and small arteries.[8] Presumably, this necrotizing vasculitis represents the localized effect of the antigen-antibody complement system deposition. With time, the vessels show fibrous thickening and a narrowed lumen. Similarly, the deposition of fibrinoid affects the interstitial collagen and membranes such as those found in the visceral pleura and, of particular interest for this occasion, joints and joint capsules of the musculoskeletal system.

Clinical Features

Unfortunately for diagnostic purposes, there is no characteristic pattern to the clinical features at the onset of SLE, and the course of the disease rarely shows any consistent patterns emerging. The clinical spectrum displayed can be very broad and complicated, with one or perhaps many organs involved. The first signs of illness are often insidious and constitutional: weakness and general malaise, weight loss, fever, and depression. A great advance in diagnosis is the recognition of milder subclinical forms of SLE. As with many other rheumatologic disorders, the astute, alert, and suspicious clinician can document such ''nonspecific'' complaints many years in advance of more recognizable and classic disease features. In many instances, it may require the cumulative gathering of laboratory and multidisciplinary clinical findings to appreciate the underlying picture of the emerging disease. In a young female patient with a classic butterfly facial rash (Fig. 10–2), fever, pain, joint pain but no deformity, photosensitivity, and pleuritic chest pains, the diagnosis may be obvious. Table 10–2 contains the principle clinical features associated with SLE. The most common diagnosis for patients who ultimately are correctly diagnosed as having SLE are RA and nonspecific arthritis.[6] One study revealed that as many as 25% of SLE patients were incor-

rectly diagnosed as having RA or nonspecific arthritis for a full year before positive disease identification.[9] Other differential diagnoses include rheumatic fever, Sjögren's syndrome, chronic discoid lupus erythematosus, idiopathic thrombocytopenic purpura, Raynaud's phenomenon, seizure disorder, anemia, and other CTDs.[10] As with any presentation of articular inflammation, infections and neoplasm must be entertained as a possibility and appropriately addressed.

The presentation of SLE in the lower extremity typically involves those features associated with the musculoskeletal or dermatologic systems (see Table 10–2), although a neurovascular component may be present. Peripheral neuropathies in SLE, although not frequent, have in fact been described and may be an early clinical feature.[4] Such neuropathies are usually sensory but can be sensorimotor as well. One study reported an incidence of 14% of lupus pa-

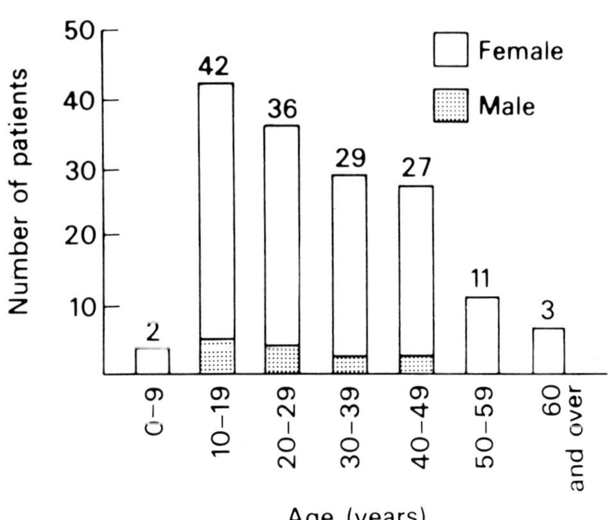

FIGURE 10–1. Age distribution at the onset of disease in systemic lupus erythematosus. (From Estes D and Christian CL: The natural history of systemic lupus erythematosus by prospective analysis. Medicine 50[Mar]:85–96. © Williams & Wilkins, 1971.)

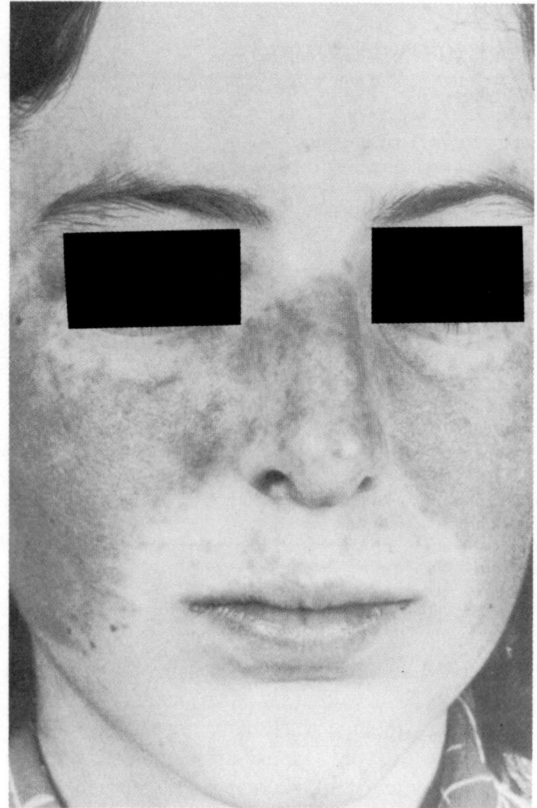

FIGURE 10–2. Characteristic butterfly rash of systemic lupus erythematosus. (From Currey HLF [ed]: Mason and Currey's Clinical Rheumatology, 4th ed. Edinburgh, Churchill Livingstone, 1986, p 179.)

tients with peripheral neuropathy.[3] Frequently, the underlying hallmark of this syndrome, namely vasculitis, exacts a toll on the peripheral vasculature and is noted as Raynaud's phenomenon. The most frequent cutaneous features of SLE consist of an erythematous rash, often symmetrical and evident on the face, neck, or extremities, especially the dorsal and distal aspects of the fingers, elbows, and palms. The classic characteristic butterfly rash (see Fig. 10–2) is not universally present: Many studies reported it in the minority of cases. Even fewer patients manifest the characteristic periungual erythema. The skin lesions of subacute cutaneous lupus erythematosus are more widespread but less persistent and erosive than those of chronic discoid lupus erythematosus.[9] The later lesions are more common in patients with SLE and may occur at any point in the course of the disease. Pruritic papules appear in isolation or clusters and progress to coalesce and form bright erythematous plaques with edema and central induration. Hyperkeratosis and follicular plugging may be noted, as well as histologic findings of perivascular infiltrate with lymphocytes, plasma cells, and fibrinoid necrosis in the dermis.[8] A typical central depression and atrophy will be noted to the lesion. As the plaque enlarges, the margins remain edematous and erythematous while central clearing takes place, hence the discoid appearance. The lesion therefore progresses through three distinct chronologic states: erythema, hyperkeratosis, and atrophy, with the resultant "burned out" lesion usually hypopigmented.

Vasculitic skin lesions are usually found at the distal digits (upper and lower extremeties) on the extensor surface of the forearms or about the malleoli. The lower extremity lesions frequently ulcerate, are usually painful, and are quite slow to heal.[11] Splinter hemorrhages may be seen around the nails as may periungual erythema (Fig. 10–3A–D). A mild form of vasculitis referred to as livedo reticularis is a quite common dermal finding on the lower extremities of patients with SLE. Alopecia is common as well.

By far, the most frequent complaints and clinical findings in SLE are peripheral arthritis and arthralgia. Most studies have reported an incidence of 90% or greater. Characteristic of joint pain in this disorder is a symmetrical, polyarticular, episodic presentation, with symptoms waxing and waning even without therapeutic intervention. Specialists in this field frequently report finding their SLE patients' symptoms out of proportion to the degree of synovitis and other objective findings, albeit less so than with reflex sympathetic dystrophy and without the vasomotor pathology associated with the latter. Synovial effusions and hypertrophy are rare and the joint deformities that do exist usually reveal an absence of osseous erosions.[12] When joint effusions do occur, a class I (noninflammatory) fluid is usually produced. The joint fluid from these patients usually reveals a low level of complement, as does joint fluid analysis on patients with RA. In SLE, however, this reflects a systemic reduction in circulating serum complement levels, whereas in RA the lessening of complement in the synovial fluid is due to local depletion.[9] Histologically, the synovium of lupus reveals little cellular inflammation, occasional hematoxylin bodies, and nonspecific vasculitis and perivasculitis.[13]

The joint deformations associated with SLE occur as a result of muscle-tendon imbalances directly related to the more prominent tenosynovitis. This deforming but nonerosive arthritis—so-called Jaccoud's arthritis—may be clinically reminiscent of RA. A patient may present with symmetric ulnar-fibular deviation and joint subluxations; however, radiographic examination would reveal the absence of juxta-articular erosions resulting from the more aggressive permeative effects of rheumatic pannus. The tendon contractures of SLE alone are responsible for the hyperextension deformities at the proximal-interphalangeal joints that produce the almost pathognomonic "Z thumb", "hitchhiking thumb," and swan-neck deformities. These contractures and deviation deformities occur more frequently in the hands than in the lower extremities. The lupus foot, however, shows a predilection for splayfoot deformities, with mild to moderate hallux abductovalgus and flexion digital contracture deformities.[14, 15]

The effects on the musculature in SLE are less well understood. Morning stiffness may be reported but is unusual. Although 30% to 50% of lupus patients exhibit myalgia, muscle weakness, or tenderness, most do not feature a concomitant myositis. The clinical picture is often further clouded by the possibility of myopathy associated with the therapeutic use of oral corticosteroid preparations.[16]

Treatment

As with all CTDs, the absence of an identifiable etiologic agent leaves treatment protocols targeted to the symptomatic relief of affected organ systems. Given this managed approach, the type and intensity of treatment are based on the severity of the patient's illness. It should be noted again that

TABLE 10–2

CLINICAL FEATURES OF SYSTEMIC LUPUS ERYTHEMATOSUS

System	Approx. Cum. (%)	System	Approx. Cum. (%)
Musculoskeletal		***Renal***	
Arthralgia/arthritis	90	Hematuria	10
Tenosynovitis	20	Proteinuria	60
Myalgia	50	Casts	30
Myositis	5	Serum albumin <35 g/L	30
		Serum creatinine >125	30
Cardiopulmonary		24-hr creatinine clearance >0.1 g	35
Shortness of breath	40		
Pleurisy	35	***Cerebral***	
Pleural effusions	25	Depression	15
Lupus pneumonitis	5	Psychosis	12
Interstitial fibrosis	5	Seizures	20
Pulmonary function abnormalities	85	Hemiplegia	10
Cardiomegaly	20	Cranial nerve lesions	10
Pericarditis	15	Cerebellar signs	5
Cardiomyopathy	10	Meningitis	1
Myocardial infarction	5	Migraine	40
Gastrointestinal		***Hematologic***	
Anorexia	40	Anemia (iron deficiency)	30
Nausea	15	Anemia (chronic disease)	75
Vomiting	<10	Autoimmune hemolytic anemia	15
Diarrhea	<10	Leukopenia	60
Abdominal pain	30	Lymphopenia	60
Ascites	<10	Thrombocytopenia	25
Hepatomegaly	25	Circulating anticoagulants	15
Splenomegaly	10		
Dermatologic			
Butterfly rash	40		
Erythematous maculopapular eruption	35		
Discoid lupus	20		
Relapsing nodular nonsuppurative panniculitis	<5		
Vasculitic skin lesion	25		
Livedo reticularis	20		
Purpuric lesions	40		
Alopecia	70		

Adapted from Morrow J and Isenberg D: Autoimmune Rheumatic Disease. Oxford, England, Blackwell Scientific, 1987.

there is a high rate of spontaneous remission in SLE, and such patients with mild signs and symptoms may require little or no treatment. Although not all patients with SLE display photosensitivity, the use of sunscreens on exposed extremities to block ultraviolet light is recommended. A number of environmental sensitizing agents (e.g., hair color, insecticide sprays, immunizations) have been recognized, and patients are advised to avoid or minimize their exposure. Penicillins and sulfonamides have also been cited by many as being well-known potentiating factors for patients with SLE.

Depending on the severity and involvement of more active cases of SLE, there are four groups of pharmacologic agents that are used: nonsteroidal antiinflammatory drugs (NSAIDs), antimalarials, corticosteroids, and cytotoxic drugs. Of these, NSAIDs and pulsed or tapered systemic corticosteroids (prednisone) have been the mainstay of treatment. The antimalarials, such as hydroxychloroquine (Plaquenil), are usually reserved for those patients with greater dermal involvement. More fulminant disease with renal and CNS involvement has required the use, either alone or in combination, of pulsed methylprednisolone or immunosuppressants (such as cyclophosphamide or azathioprine).

Surgical management of the SLE patient is indicated when musculoskeletal deformities have not responded to noninvasive management techniques. Pedal digital contractures, although less frequent than upper extremity digital deformities, have nevertheless benefited from appropriate and timely intervention. As with RA, the deforming forces governing the progressive joint contractures and deviations are frequently poorly controlled. Proximal interphalangeal joint arthrodesis rather than arthroplasty is therefore often indicated. As with RA, when deformity is substantial and plantar adipose tissue is atrophied, panmetatarsal head resection with digital arthrodesis can result in substantial relief of symptoms and provide for necessary forefoot stabilization. The presence of systemic corticosteroids or immunosuppressive agents requires that the surgeon be diligent in regard to the increased risk of infection in these patients.[17] Similarly, long-term use of corticosteroids has also been implicated in an increased incidence of avascular necrosis, atherosclerosis, hypertension, psychosis, diabetes mellitus, and myopathy. Lower extremity myopathy can be particularly disabling, and, in this regard, quadriceps strengthening and other forms of physical therapy have proved very beneficial.

SCLERODERMA (SYSTEMIC SCLEROSIS)

Scleroderma (systemic sclerosis) is a connective tissue disorder of unknown cause characterized by widespread and

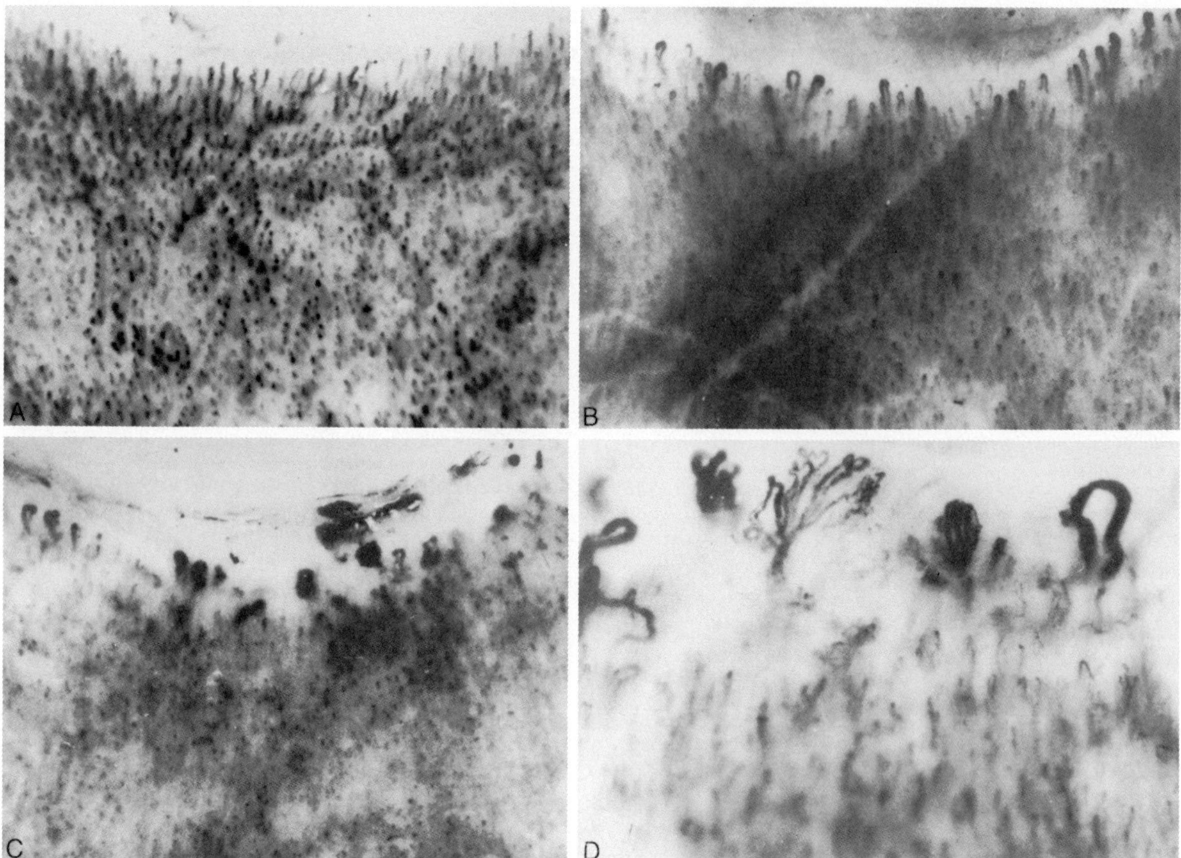

FIGURE 10–3. Appearance of the nail fold capillary bed viewed with emulsion oil and an ophthalmoscope. *A,* Normal; *B,* Enlarged capillary loops and zones of avascularity in Raynaud's disease; *C,* Enlarged capillary loops and wider zones of avascularity in systemic sclerosis; and *D,* Extremely large capillary loops with budding and branching in dermatomyositis. (*A* through *D* from Maricq HR and Maize JC: Nailfold capillary abnormalities. Clin Rheum Dis 8:455–478, 1982.

excessive fibrosis affecting the gastrointestinal system, heart, smooth and striated muscles, and especially the skin. Although the liver is frequently spared, pulmonary and renal involvement is not uncommon. Some authors used the term *progressive systemic sclerosis* for this disorder; however, many cases show either a plateau effect or a remission of symptoms. Hence, this terminology is falling out of favor. Although skin involvement is the usual presenting symptom, the overwhelming morbidity and mortality result from visceral pathology.

The pathophysiology of scleroderma is not completely understood and is cause for some debate as to the classification and subgrouping of this disease or, as some argue, set of diseases. Whether vascular changes precede or result from excessive collagen deposition is unknown. Others propose that neither is the primary event, but rather the disease is a reflection of an underlying immunologic disorder.[18] The observation that scleroderma is frequently complicated by Sjögren's syndrome reinforces a commonality to autoimmune dysfunction.[19] The subgrouping of scleroderma based on the extent of dermal pathology has been proposed.[20] Alper and Leroy (1988)[21] differentiated between diffuse cutaneous and limited cutaneous forms of generalized systemic sclerosis. The diffuse variety displays greater truncal skin involvement, widespread visceral disease, rapid progression, and a poorer prognosis. Limited cutaneous systemic sclerosis includes the CREST syndrome: *c*alcinosis (usually subcutaneous and often in the fingers), *R*aynaud's phenomenon, *e*sophageal hypermobility, *s*clerodactyly, and *t*elangiectasias. It had been believed that these CREST patients presented less visceral disease involvement and therefore a more protracted, indolent cause of illness.[20] Although this may be a legitimate generalization, these patients are not exempt entirely from visceral complications such as pulmonary fibrosis and hypertension later in the course of disease. Of great significance, Furst and colleagues reported on a carefully controlled comparison of 17 well-matched patients with the CREST syndrome and systemic sclerosis. Their study found no significant differences between these groups in regard to gastrointestinal, cardiovascular, or renal involvement.[22] The patients with systemic sclerosis were, in fact, distinguished by the presence of antiribonucleoprotein antibodies and more frequent and extensive involvement of muscle and skin pathology. More recent studies bear out the notion that the CREST variant is less benign than was previously believed. A more significant distinction must be made between the systemic generalized entities of systemic sclerosis and CREST syndrome and the more limited and less destructive variant of scleroderma: morphea and linear scleroderma. Scleroderma-associated syndromes and scleroderma-like illness induced by drugs, environmental agents, and activity round out this rather ill-defined classification system (Table 10–3).

Scleroderma has a predilection for women, who are in-

TABLE 10–3

CLASSIFICATION OF SCLERODERMA

Generalized Scleroderma (Systemic Sclerosis)

Diffuse scleroderma: acute and chronic; bilateral, symmetrical, "classic" involvement of skin (face, extremities, trunk) and early visceral pathology

Limited scleroderma: CREST syndrome (*c*alcinosis, *R*aynaud's phenomenon, *e*sophageal hypomotility, *s*clerodactyly, *t*elangiectasia)

Localized Scleroderma

Morphea: plaque-like, guttate, or generalized; subcutaneous morphea or keloid morphea

Linear scleroderma: with or without melorheostosis

Scleroderma en coup de sabre: linear scleroderma seen in children, involving frontoparietal area of forehead and scalp

Scleroderma-Associated or -Like Syndrome

Undifferentiated overlap or mixed connective tissue syndrome: sclerolupus, sclerodermatomyositis, scleromyxedema, primary biliary cirrhosis, Sjögren's syndrome

Indurated/atrophic: porphyria cutanea tarda, acromegaly, Werner's syndrome, lichen sclerosis, amyloid, carcinoid syndrome, phenylketonuria, progeria

Eosinophilic fasciitis

Graft-versus-host reaction

Scleroderma of Buschka: often postinfectious

Environmental/drug induced: vinyl chloride disease, pentazocine, bleomycin, tryptophan, toxic oil, silicosis, vibration induced ("jackhammer disease")

volved three to five times more frequently. The disease shows a peak onset between the ages of 30 and 50 years. It is a relatively uncommon illness; retrospective studies demonstrate an incidence of 2.7 to 12 cases per 1 million persons per year.[23] It is seen in all geographic areas, shows no predilection for any racial or ethnic group, and can develop at any age, although adolescent cases are quite rare. The female to male ratio is even higher in this premenopausal age group, which, some believe, may point to a possible hormonal element in the disease's pathogenicity. Although there have been a few rare reports of familial clustering of scleroderma, no conclusive evidence exists for specific human leukocyte antigen (HLA) haplotyping.

Pathology

The variety of features manifest in scleroderma typically shows vascular disease as an underlying agent. Such findings as Raynaud's phenomenon, digital pitting, ulceration, and gangrene are reflective of morbidity associated with the small arteries and arterioles.[24] These vessels display thickening of the intima and adventitial fibrosis without disruption of the internal lumina. This adventitial fibrosis develops as a cuff of collagen without fibroblastic proliferation. It is hypothesized by numerous authors that, as the vessels narrow and occlude with fibrosis, those smaller vessels and capillaries involved in providing collateralization dilate and become readily visible on the skin as telangiectasias; periungual erythema, subungual splinter hemorrhages (Fig. 10–3C); and edema. As the arterioles further narrow and occlude, the edema resolves but the localized tissue ischemia results in atrophy and further tissue fibrosis. Similar vascular and microvascular changes to the viscera, notably the renal, hepatic, and gastrointestinal vascular beds, reflect the substantial morbidity associated with this disease. Cell-mediated immunity, humoral immunity, and defects in the collagen-collagenase

balance itself are also proposed in explaining the pathologic changes seen in all affected organ systems. Histologic examination of the skin shows a dramatic increase in dermal type I and type III collagen notably associated with the hyalinization and occlusion of small blood vessels. There is a noted atrophy of the epidermis with loss of normal dermal appendages. A diffuse mononuclear cell infiltrate is found in about 50% of untreated cases. Roumm and associates found this to be mostly consisting of activated thrombocytes with an increased ration of T helper to T suppressor cells.[25]

The histologic effects on the internal organs are overtly similar to those findings in the skin, with commonality of pathogenicity likely. The kidneys typically show glomerular involvement with focal areas of endothelial cell proliferation and thickening of the basement membrane. Renal arterioles and microvessels narrow, serum proteins clog channels, and heavy deposits of immunoglobulin, especially IgM, with or without complement are seen on microscopic examination. Although fewer than half of all patients display clinical features of kidney disease, histopathologic renal changes are found in roughly 90% of these patients. In the lungs, interstitial fibrosis is the most common finding of systemic sclerosis. Increased collagen deposition and arteriolar thickening often lead to pulmonary hypertension. Focal fibrosis of the myocardium is seen in approximately 50% of patients; however, the seemingly universal vascular changes noted in scleroderma spare the coronary vessels. The gastrointestinal tract shows atrophy of the smooth muscle layer with replacement by fibrosis.

Clinical Features

Scleroderma's pseudonym, systemic sclerosis, hints at the widespread, system-wide manifestation of clinical pathology (see Table 10–4). For the purposes of addressing lower extremity concerns, our focus is on the skin and musculoskeletal organ systems.

Raynaud's Phenomenon. More than 90% of all patients with scleroderma display Raynaud's phenomenon as a prominent feature.[21] The presence of Raynaud's phenomenon is usually unequivocal and helps clinicians differentiate scleroderma from other CTDs in which Raynaud's phenomenon is quite unusual. A clinical aphorism frequently cited is that the sudden appearance of Raynaud's phenomenon in a patient older than 40 years is due to scleroderma unless and until proved otherwise. LeRoy stated,

> A high proportion of patients with Raynaud's phenomenon, when followed carefully for several years, eventually develop scleroderma or an overlapping variant of scleroderma. Because Raynaud's syndrome may precede scleroderma by months or years, we consider patients with Raynaud's syndrome as the nearest thing to an identifiable population with a high incidence of scleroderma in whom observations can be made and therapies considered before the appearance of fibrosis.[26]

Skin. Late cutaneous pathologic changes in scleroderma are usually easily recognizable as thickened, tight, shining hidebound skin. However, most patients' disease progresses through three cutaneous stages: edematous, fibrotic, and atrophic. During the early inflammatory, edematous state, the involved skin displays nonpitting edema. The patient may complain of swollen fingers and, less frequently, toes, as well as morning stiffness. Involvement of truncal skin is a later

TABLE 10–4

MAJOR CLINICAL FEATURES SEEN IN SCLERODERMA

System	Features
Lungs	Pulmonary hypertension
	Pleurisy
	Pleural effusion
	Diffuse interstitial fibrosis
	Bronchitis
Heart	Pericarditis
	Dysrhythmias
	Secondary effects from pulmonary disease
Liver	Portal hypertension leading to biliary cirrhosis
Gastrointestinal	Esophagus: hypomobility plus incompetence of lower esophageal sphincter, resulting in dysphagia, hiatal hernia, esophageal stricture
	Duodenum: hypomobility leading to malabsorption
	Colon: hypomobility, dilatation, constipation, and fecal impaction
Muscle	Simple myopathy, inflammatory myositis
Joints	Symmetrical, nonerosive, seronegative polyarthropathy
Neurologic	Trigeminal neuralgia
	Peripheral neuropathy
Skin	Edema (early)
	Raynaud's phenomenon
	Telangiectasias
	Ulcerations
	Alopecia
	Dermal calcification with thickening, tightening, atrophy
	Hyperpigmentation
	Regions of vitiligo

feature. With time, the skin gradually becomes fibrotic, resulting in a tight, hidebound appearance. Sclerodactyly (tight skin distal to the proximal interphalangeal joints) may be the full extent of skin pathologic changes with limited disease. Otherwise, those patients with diffuse scleroderma experience widespread cutaneous changes that have come to be widely recognized as characteristic of the disease. The forehead is usually smooth, free of wrinkles, and immobile. Tautness of the skin around the nose suggests a birdlike appearance. The skin around the mouth becomes drawn, wrinkled, and pinched, giving a mouselike appearance to the face (Fig. 10–4). Alopecia can occur with widespread generalized scleroderma, although not as frequently as is seen with SLE. Pigmentary changes are frequently noted in this stage.

The tightly bound skin is usually responsible for the flexion contractures seen in the fingers and toes. The fingertips, distal pulp of toes, and extensor surfaces such as contracted proximal interphalangeal joints in the toes are subject to subcutaneous calcification. Combined with the increased friction, shearing, and pressures assumed by these areas, the skin is likely to break down. Radiographs at this stage would indeed show evidence of this abnormal calcification and in some instances, distal phalangeal erosions (Fig. 10–5). Patients with limited cutaneous systemic sclerosis are more apt to experience severe calcinosis. This variant is associated with greater local anatomic morbidity with a cycle of contracted skin over proliferating calcifications, leading to ulceration, secondary infection, and distal phalangeal resorption. Telangiectasias are often observed on the hands, face, and less frequently the malleoli of those patients with limited disease. During the later course and stages of scleroderma, the skin may assume a thinned-out or atrophic appearance, with some softening but not resolution of the more pathologic changes. Despite the widespread dermatopathologic and vascular insults, surgical incisions in sclerodermic skin typically heal remarkably well with few complications.

Musculoskeletal System. More than 90% of patients with scleroderma report musculoskeletal complaints during the course of their disease.[27] Relapsing, intermittent arthralgias in the extremities are frequently reported early in the onset of disease. Active, progressive arthritis with joint erosions is typical of RA but highly unusual in scleroderma. The synovium and synovial fluid of scleroderma are typically noninflammatory. Fibrosis of joints and tendon sheaths, with dermal thickening and rigidity, is mainly responsible for the loss of joint range of motion. Crepitus from this periarticular fibrosis is often found in the patella, wrists, and hindfoot. On close physical examination, most patients will exhibit some degree of proximal muscle weakness. In combination with the fibrotic changes in joints and tendons, this leads to disuse atrophy associated with scleroderma, which is indolent and rarely progresses to severe weakness. This variety shows no abnormalities on electromyography (EMG) and only mild elevations of serum muscle enzymes and generally requires no specific therapy. In contrast, a smaller percentage of patients experience a more aggressive myopathy with histologic and clinical findings similar to those of primary inflammatory

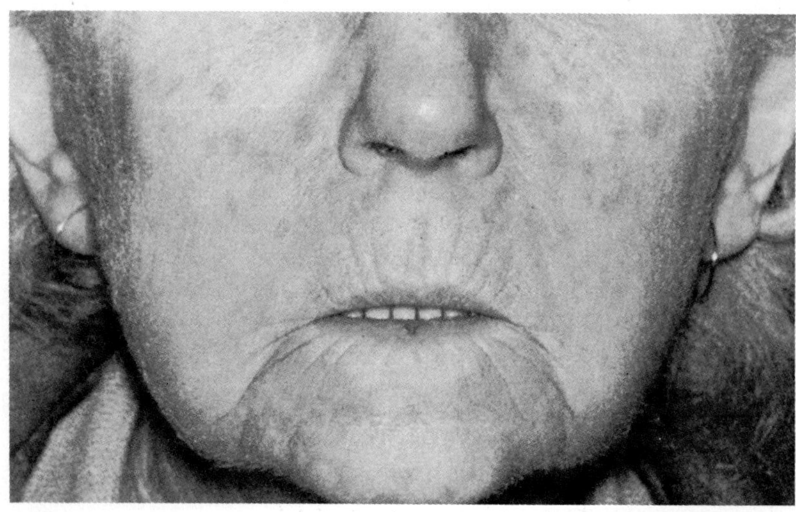

FIGURE 10–4. Periorbital skin puckering and tight nasal skin in scleroderma. (From Wright V and Harvey A: Diagnostic Picture Tests in Rheumatology. London, Wolfe Medical, 1987, p 17.)

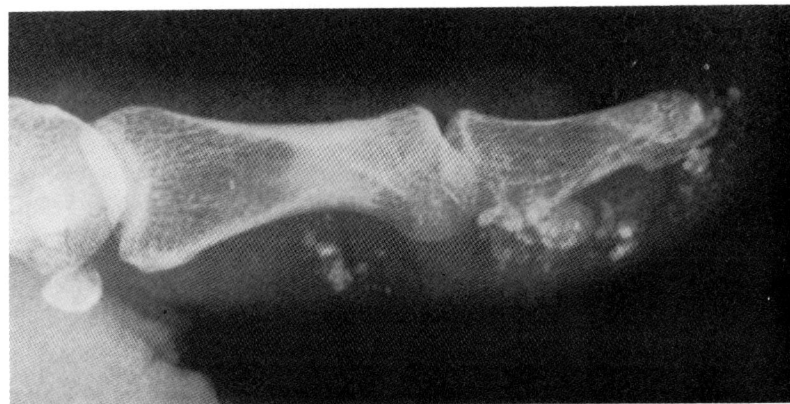

FIGURE 10–5. Subcutaneous calcinosis of the thumb in a patient with scleroderma. (From Currey HLF [ed.]: Mason and Currey's Clinical Rheumatology, 4th ed. Edinburgh, Churchill Livingstone, 1986, p 196.)

myositis, such as in polymyositis. EMG studies and muscle biopsies of this variant show pathologic changes consistent with inflammatory myositis. Treatment with corticosteroids is indicated and generally is successful in retarding progressive muscle weakness.

The presence of trigeminal neuralgia, carpal tunnel syndrome, tarsal tunnel syndrome, and peripheral neuropathies has been reported in patients with scleroderma, but these disorders are far less frequent.[28] Autonomic dysfunction has been reported as a feature of systemic sclerosis.[29] With parasympathetic impairment and marked sympathetic overactivity being so common, especially early in the disease course, the role of autonomic dysfunction in the pathogenicity of Raynaud's phenomenon and systemic sclerosis is of great interest.[30]

Treatment

An old aphorism is that "no drug has been proved totally useless until it has been tried in treating scleroderma." There is universal frustration among physicians and patients alike regarding the helplessness in attempting to treat this disease. Pharmacologic intervention is mostly aimed at reducing cutaneous fibrosis, diminishing any inflammatory component, and improving the quality of life. In recent years, some limited success has been reported using antimalarials and immunosuppressive agents. Some early reports of relief with colchicine have not stood up to later investigations. In 1992, Alain Rook and associates from the Department of Dermatology at the University of Pennsylvania reported on the results of a promising clinical trial.[30a] The group reported retardation and possible reversal of cutaneous sclerosis using extracorporeal photochemotherapy (or photophoresis) as compared with D-penicillamine alone. The deleterious effects of Raynaud's phenomenon can be diminished with the avoidance of cold exposure and the use of warm gloves and socks and less successfully via surgical sympathectomy and vasoactive drugs. Certainly, the NSAIDs have a prominent role in avoiding inflammation and providing analgesia if there are no contraindications from the visceral effects of the disease. Short, tapered courses of oral corticosteroid therapy may be required during episodes of myositis when more aggressive treatment is necessary. Local musculoskeletal pathologic changes need to be carefully evaluated and treated. Physical therapy, especially the application of moist heat, has proved beneficial. Tenosynovitis not responding to oral medication

may sometimes be quickly and comfortably managed with judicious local injection of corticosteroids. Surgical management in the lower extremities is primarily aimed at symptom relief and preservation of function if possible. Arthroplasty and, quite frequently, arthrodesis prove most rewarding, especially if the patient has experienced prolonged arthralgia unrelieved by more conservative initial management.

POLYMYOSITIS AND DERMATOMYOSITIS

Polymyositis and dermatomyositis are acquired, chronic, inflammatory muscle diseases of unknown cause. Dermatomyositis is distinguished from polymyositis by the presence of a characteristic skin rash. Although there appears to be a bimodal peak age of onset of between 5 and 15 years and 50 and 60 years, either disease can be diagnosed at any age. Females are affected two to three times more often than males, except when in the presence of an accompanying neoplasm, in which case the incidence favors males 2:1. Polymyositis and dermatomyositis occur less frequently than most other acquired CTDs, with an incidence of approximately 1 in 200,000. Because there is a four times greater incidence among black females, ethnic and racial cofactors may be involved.[31–33]

Several theories have been offered as to the pathogenesis of this disease. Areas of investigation currently focus on the role of cell-mediated immune response, the role of infectious agents, and the association of polymyositis with malignant disease. The reported incidence of malignancy varies between 9% and 15%; the most frequently reported tumors are carcinoma of the breast and lung.[34, 35] Patients with dermatomyositis are at greater risk for the development of carcinoma than are those with polymyositis.[36]

Various schemes have been suggested for the classification of patients with myositis, none of which has been uniformly adopted. Given the uncertainty of cause, any grouping would aptly subtype patients by clinical presentation with specific regard to age of onset, presence of skin rash, presence of neoplasms, and ancillary features associated with other CTDs or overlap syndromes (Table 10–5).

Pathology

Histologic examination of skeletal muscle reveals widespread, diffuse degeneration of myofibers, with necrotic muscle fibers being actively phagocytized. There may be chronic

TABLE 10–5

CLASSIFICATION OF MYOSITIS

Idiopathic polymyositis
Idiopathic dermatomyositis
Adolescent myositis
Myositis with neoplasm
Myositis with associated connective tissue disorders (e.g., systemic lupus
  erythematosus, scleroderma, rheumatoid arthritis, Sjögren's syndrome,
  overlap syndromes)

inflammatory cell infiltration between muscle fibers, with some in reparative stages. The hallmark of disease is the perivascular infiltrate often associated with an increase in collagen fibers and connective tissue, particularly in patients with chronic disease. In later stages of myositis, the inflammatory component may lessen, with a predomination of muscle fiber atrophy, fibrosis, and deposition of lipid.[37] Table 10–6 summarizes the frequency of muscle biopsy findings. The demonstration of inflammatory myopathy by histologic examination of muscle biopsy is diagnostic of polymyositis and dermatomyositis. However, it should be stressed that false-positive results may occur from biopsies obtained from sites of previous muscle trauma such as contusions, EMG needles, injections, or surgery. Rates of false-negative results as high as 17% have been reported.[31]

Clinical Features

Although acute presentations are possible, most patients with polymyositis or dermatomyositis present with an insidious onset of muscle weakness and wasting developing over months or years. This loss of muscle strength is the usual major finding at first presentation, and, although all skeletal muscle groups may be so affected, symmetrical weakness of the proximal lower extremity and then the upper extremity is most frequent.[39] Patients often present with initial complaints of vague soreness, fatigue, or weakness, with reports of reduced tolerance for ambulation and difficulty climbing stairs and rising from a seated position. With progression of the disease, there is further difficulty in walking, and noticeable alterations in the patient's gait may begin (e.g., a widening of the base and angle of gait with increasing apropulsion). Standing, balancing, and toe walking are frequently helpful in discerning subtle changes and progression of disease in the lower extremities. Tendon reflexes are usually intact and well preserved until late in the course of disease. This be-

TABLE 10–6

FREQUENCY OF BIOPSY FINDINGS IN POLYMYOSITIS AND DERMATOMYOSITIS

Findings	Percentage
Interstitial and perivascular inflammation with myofiber atrophy	46
Interstitial and perivascular inflammation with minor myofiber atrophy	19
Myofiber atrophy without inflammation	8
Myofiber atrophy with other nonspecific findings	11
Normal	17

Adapted from DeVere R and Bradley WG: Polymyositis: Its presentation, morbidity, and mortality. Brain 98:637, 1975; by permission of Oxford University Press.

comes quite significant as one attempts to distinguish polymyositis or dermatomyositis from muscular dystrophies.

With involvement of anterior cervical and trunk muscles, lifting the head from the pillow and rising from a supine position become increasingly difficult. As intercostal muscles and the diaphragm become involved, respiration may become labored; therefore, pulmonary function requires close serial monitoring. In more widespread disease, pharyngeal musculature is affected, resulting in a nasal voice tone. On rare occasions, an individual localized muscle may be solely affected, presenting a substantial challenge to even the most astute diagnostician. Focal myositis of the gastrocnemius may, in fact, easily simulate thrombophlebitis.[38, 39]

The characteristic, virtually pathognomonic rash of dermatomyositis is seen as a dusky lilac discoloration of the upper eyelids, sometimes accompanied by periorbital edema (heliotrope rash). Patchy involvement of the scalp, neck, chest, and extensor surfaces of the upper extremity and, rarely, the lower extremity can also be seen. The violaceous erythematous rash over the joints is known as Gottren's papules. With time and advancement of disease, these cutaneous lesions scale, fibrose, and atrophy, producing an almost scleroderma-like appearance to the skin. These lesions may ulcerate and become quite problematic. Subungual splinter hemorrhages are sometimes seen in the hands and feet, more noteworthy in the child than in the adult (see Fig. 10–3D). More common in the adolescent variant is calcinosis of subcutaneous tissue and connective tissues of muscles (Fig. 10–6). This latter calcification of muscular fascia can severely

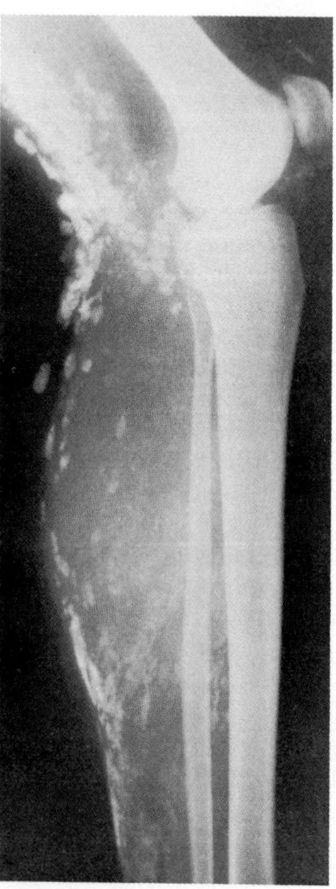

FIGURE 10–6. Lower extremity calcifications in polymyositis. (From Hughes GRV: Connective Tissue Diseases, 3rd ed. Oxford, Blackwell Scientific, 1987, p 177.)

limit motion and may also lead to superficial extrusions, erosions, and draining ulcerations.

Treatment

Rehabilitation in the form of occupational and physical therapy can be of enormous benefit to those with polymyositis and dermatomyositis. Passive range of motion and stretching exercises are quite useful in the prevention of contracture deformities, especially if begun early in the course of the disease. Because polymyositis and dermatomyositis are characterized by periods of remission and exacerbation, the course of disease in each patient must be carefully followed. The status of disease is measured by correlating clinical findings (rash, arthralgia, myalgia, and telangiectasias) with laboratory findings (serum glutamic oxaloacetic transaminase, serum glutamic pyruvic transaminase, and creatine phosphokinase, enzyme levels, serum myoglobin, and erythrocyte sedimentation rate). During periods of active inflammation, rest is advised. Combination functional and accommodative orthoses can be of benefit in managing gait anomalies and reducing stress in the lower extremities.

Pharmacologically, corticosteroids remain the mainstay of treatment. Tapered courses of prednisone, initially in the range of 40 to 80 mg per day, are the usual practice; some patients require low-dosage maintenance when recalcitrant symptoms persist. Management is further complicated by the long-term side effects of steroid use.

Life-threatening or unresponsive disease may also require the addition of immunosuppressive or cytotoxic agents such as azathioprine, methotrexate, cyclophosphamide, and cyclosporinc. Plasmaphcrcsis has also bccn tricd with mixcd and uncertain results.[40]

Given the reported frequency of malignancy in adult myositis (especially dermatomyositis in the fifth and sixth decades of life), a search for concurrent neoplasms is often undertaken in these susceptible patients. If such a tumor is found and removed, complete remission of the disease may follow.

SJÖGREN'S SYNDROME

Sjögren's syndrome is a chronic inflammatory disorder characterized by the triad of (1) keratoconjunctivitis sicca (dry eyes); (2) xerostomia (dry mouth); and (3) an associated CTD. By far, RA is the most frequently associated CTD; however, occasionally, SLE, polymyositis, or scleroderma may accompany the syndrome.

Mikulicz first described a case history of massive enlargement of both lacrimal and salivary glands with associated histologic changes more than 100 years ago, but it was Sjögren in 1931 who detailed the syndrome's presentation.[41] When only the ocular or oral disease is observed (although a rarity), the term *primary Sjögren's sicca complex* or *sicca syndrome* has been used. In the more common presentation, an underlying CTD exists, and secondary Sjögren's syndrome is described. In recent years, a desire to move away from eponyms such as Sjögren's syndrome has led some authors to use the more descriptive term *autoimmune exocrinopathy*. The syndrome is far from rare, occurring more often than SLE but less frequently than RA. The disease shows no racial predilections, is more common in females than males, and is diagnosed at the mean age of 50 years.[42]

Pathology

Keratoconjunctivitis and xerostomia are a direct result of an intense infiltration of lymphocytes and macrophages into the lacrimal and salivary glands. No etiologic agent has yet been found to trigger this destructive, cell-mediated, autoimmune reaction. In fact, Sjögren's syndrome is second only to SLE in its multiplicity of serum autoantibodies. The most common autoantibody isolated is rheumatoid factor. This is present in patients with Sjögren's syndrome whether or not RA is pre-existing. As expected, there is an elevation in serum immunoglobulin levels. This is primarily noted in the IgG component line; however, to a lesser degree, IgA and IgM fractions show an elevation as well.[43] Approximately 70% of patients demonstrate ANAs,[44] and 60% to 80% show circulating immune complexes.[45, 46] Many other autoantibodies have also been identified, such as those to gastric parietal cells, thyroglobulin, thyroid microsomes, salivary duct cells, lacrimal duct cells, pancreatic duct cells, vaginal mucosal cells, mitochondria, and other autologous antigens.

Genetic factors may also play an important role in the pathogenicity of Sjögren's syndrome because it represents one of several autoimmune diseases associated with histocompatibility antigens. An association with HLA-DR3 has been found and is currently the focus of much research.[47]

Clinical Features

Ocular symptoms occur when secretory epithelium of the lacrimal gland atrophies, resulting in drying (loss of tears), inflammation, erosion, and, if not treated, ulceration of the cornea and conjunctiva. Initially, the most frequent complaint is that of a foreign body sensation; the eye is described by patients as feeling ''gritty'' or ''sandy.'' Later symptoms may include burning, decreased tearing, fatigue, redness, photosensitivity, and itching. A characteristic symptom is the presence, especially on awakening, of a ropy strand of material at the inner canthus of the eye (Fig. 10–7). Occasional blurring or a filmy sensation may interfere with vision. Secondary bacterial infection is common.

Parotid gland enlargement occurs in approximately one third of patients, and submaxillary gland enlargement is less common still. When glandular enlargement occurs, it is usually unilateral and is firm, smooth, slightly tender, and episodic in nature. It may also be accompanied by erythema and fever. Luminal narrowing in the parotid duct may eventually lead to the formation of compact cellular conglomerates called *epimyothelial islands*. As salivary glands atrophy, production of saliva decreases and the resultant xerostomia (dryness of the mouth) can be quite troublesome. Chewing and swallowing become difficult. Speech may be affected because of the extreme dryness of the tongue, buccal membranes, and lips. Fissures of these areas may develop and lead to ulcerations. The loss of saliva often leads to rampant dental caries and tooth/gingival decay.[48] Dryness may also affect the membranes in the nose, pharynx, larynx, and tracheobronchial passages. This may lead to respective bouts of epistaxis, laryngitis, otitis media, bronchitis, and pneumonia.[44, 49]

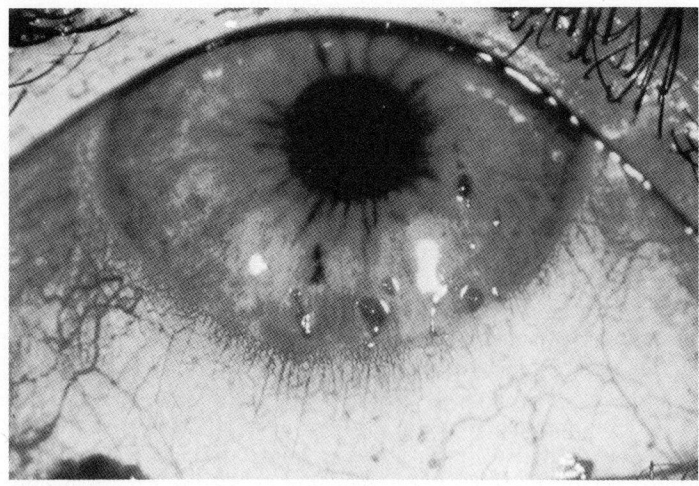

FIGURE 10–7. Corneal vascularization and keratitis filamentosa in Sjögren's syndrome. (From Hughes GRV: Connective Tissue Diseases, 3rd ed. Oxford, Blackwell Scientific, 1987, p 85.)

Gastrointestinal effects, including chronic atrophic gastritis, are the direct result of mucosal and submucosal atrophy from cellular infiltration.[50] Hepatobiliary disease has been associated with Sjögren's syndrome, as has pancreatitis. Investigators, however, have been unable to demonstrate that diabetes mellitus is any more likely in Sjögren's syndrome than in the general population.[43] Approximately 20% of patients experience renal tubular acidosis. Secondary amyloidosis and nephropathy may also develop, and interstitial nephritis is a frequent finding.[51] There is a greatly increased risk of lymphoma in patients with parotid enlargement, splenomegaly, and lymphadenopathy.

Peripheral neuropathy especially has been associated with the concomitant presence of polyarteritis nodosa.[52] No reports of specific lower extremity peripheral neuropathy are found in the literature.

Treatment

Treatment of Sjögren's syndrome is largely symptomatic and supportive in nature. The deleterious effects of the sicca components can best be combated with frequent use of artificial tear and artificial saliva solutions. Such methylcellulose agents are usually helpful in the management of dry eyes and mouth. Patients must be alert to using only sugar-free gums or lozenges and are best kept under close dental supervision. Normal saline drops for nasal passages and lubricants such as K-Y jelly for the vagina are effective.

Connective tissue involvement of the musculoskeletal system is usually mild, and therefore corticosteroids and immunosuppressants are rarely required. An increased incidence of toxic reactions to injectable gold salts and other drug allergies has been reported in patients with Sjögren's syndrome.[44, 47] Therefore, care must be taken, especially when treating an underlying CTD such as RA.

VASCULITIS

Vasculitis includes a broad spectrum of disorders that are not easily classified but are characterized by inflammation and necrosis of blood vessels. The terms *vasculitis* and *angiitis* are used interchangeably to imply inflammation of veins, arteries, or capillaries. *Arteritis* implies specific inflammation of arteries and arterioles. The clinical effects depend on the specific vessels involved, and the disease manifest is an anatomic reflection of the specific vascular obstruction. Prognosis is quite variable, from the relatively benign dermal effects of hypersensitivity vasculitis to the morbidity and sometimes rapid mortality associated with polyarteritis nodosa. Vasculitis may present as a primary disorder, or it may be secondary to other CTDs such as SLE, RA, and scleroderma (Fig. 10–8). Several attempts at classification on the basis of histopathology, size of vessels involved, or clinical presentation have been offered but with no universal agreement.[53–55]

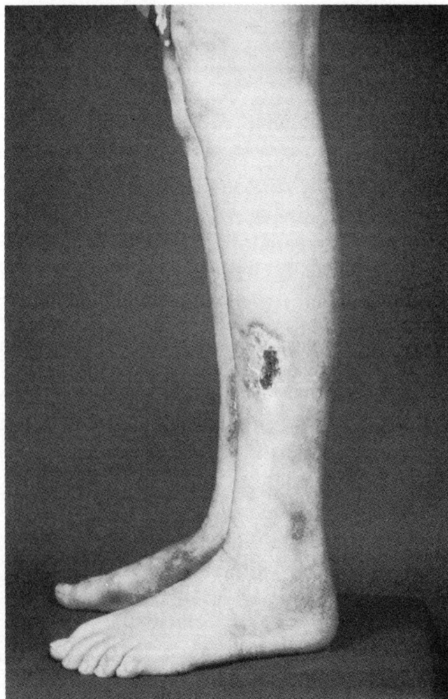

FIGURE 10–8. Lower extremity ulceration in a patient with cutaneous vasculitis. (From Hughes GRV: Connective Tissue Diseases, 3rd ed. Oxford, Blackwell Scientific, 1987, p 236.)

Pathology

The vascular damage associated with vasculitis may follow a number of pathogenic mechanisms. It has been associated with a history of infectious disease such as hepatitis B or bacterial endocarditis and high-dose antibiotic therapy. It is theorized that high levels of circulating antigens initiate the formation of antigen-antibody complexes.[53] A type III hypersensitivity reaction ensues because these complexes, unable to be cleared by the reticuloendothelial system, are deposited in blood vessel walls. The complement cascade system is activated by these deposited complexes, which results in the chemotaxis of neutrophils. Neutrophils release lysosomal enzymes, which damage vessels, leading to thrombosis, embolization, occlusion, necrosis, hemorrhage, and ischemia.[56] Cell-mediated (T cell) immune response also explains vascular damage via the antigenic attraction of lymphocytes and macrophages. As inflammation becomes more chronic, granulation tissue may form, and the giant cells and patchy areas of fibrinoid necrosis may be seen, which are associated with granulomatous vasculitides.

Clinical Features

Within the context and scope of this book, what is presented here is intended as an overview of the pathophysiology and presentation of several of the recognized vasculitis syndromes.

Polyarteritis (Nodosa). This is a multisystem disease and is the prototype of necrotizing vasculitis. The disease is characterized by acute inflammation and fibrinoid necrosis of small and medium-sized arteries. Lesions tend to be segmental, occur at the branchings and bifurcations of arteries, and spread distally to arterioles. Especially severe lesions may involve adjacent veins. *Periarteritis nodosa* is the older term that stems from the occasional subcutaneous visceral nodules seen along the outer walls of arteries. Involvement of the arteries or the intestinal tract, heart, kidney, and brain poses an emergency, life-threatening situation. Renal involvement in polyarteritis accounts for the highest mortality rate.[54] General signs and symptoms at onset include fever, malaise, weakness, abdominal pain, hypertension, chest pain, headache, myalgia, and arthralgia. Diagnosis is made on the basis of symptoms history, elevated sedimentation rate, leukocytosis, anemia, thrombocytosis, decreased C3 complement, rheumatoid factor greater than 1:60, circulating immune complexes, and a tissue biopsy positive for necrotizing vasculitis.

The myalgias and arthralgias seen in polyarteritis are evident in more than 50% of patients. These are typically the earliest complaints, often preceding other more visceral complaints by months. Arthritis may be monoarticular and migratory, resembling gout, or it may present in a polyarticular symmetrical pattern easily confused with RA. There is a strong predilection of severe myalgia for the gastrocsoleus complex muscles, with the tissue biopsy revealing typical polyarthritis histology.[57]

Involvement of the peripheral nerves occurs in most patients and is also usually evident early in the course of the disease. Lesions and occlusion of the small arteries supplying peripheral nerves (vasa nervorum) produce an acute onset of simultaneous peripheral mixed nerve disease. Symptoms and findings of this so-called mononeuritis multiplex include paresthesias, hyperesthesia, and muscle weakness supplied by a peripheral nerve and must be distinguished from nerve root distribution. With time, this progresses to muscle atrophy and associated functional disability. In the lower extremity, typical involvement is peroneal nerve atrophy with the development of footdrop. Stocking and glove–type peripheral neuropathy is a less frequent (12%) finding.[58]

Dermatologic findings are also of great interest in the lower extremities, evident in at least 25% of cases. Tender, movable, firm, subcutaneous nodules are evident in 15% of patients, most often in the legs. There is usually overlying erythema, and at times a slight increase in local skin temperature may be present. Other cutaneous findings include bullae, vesicles, purpura, livedo reticularis, splinter hemorrhages, superficial ulcerations, and gangrene (Fig. 10–9).[57]

Wegener's Granulomatosis. The vessels most frequently affected by Wegener's granulomatosis are those of the respiratory tract and kidney. Clinical pathologic changes are therefore most manifest in the nasopharyngeal mucosa, paranasal sinuses, respiratory tract, pulmonary parenchyma, and kidneys.[53] Signs and symptoms include pulmonary congestion or cough, fever, malaise, weight loss, polyarthralgia, and mild to moderate hematuria. The classic presentation is that of purulent sinusitis, with malodorous discharge, persistent pneumonia, and kidney failure. Erosion of the nasal septum by granulomatous necrosis eventually may lead to the development of a secondary saddle-nose deformity. Joint pathology has been reported in two thirds of patients with Wegener's granulomatosis. Overall, symmetrical polyarthritis is slightly less frequent than polyarthralgia, with synovitis, fibrinoid necrosis, and granuloma formation reported on histologic examination.[59] There is evidence to support an association of Wegener's granulomatosis with HLA antigens.[60]

Temporal Arteritis. The synonyms cranial arteritis and giant cell arteritis also describe this form of vasculitis with a predilection for medium- to large-sized arteries, most commonly seen in branches of the carotid artery.[61] Histologic examination reveals disruption of the internal elastic lumina, infiltration of the arterial wall by lymphocytes (mainly T helper cells), and granulomatous formation with multinucleated giant cells.[62] Constitutional symptoms include fever, malaise, myalgia, and weight loss. Clinical findings directly

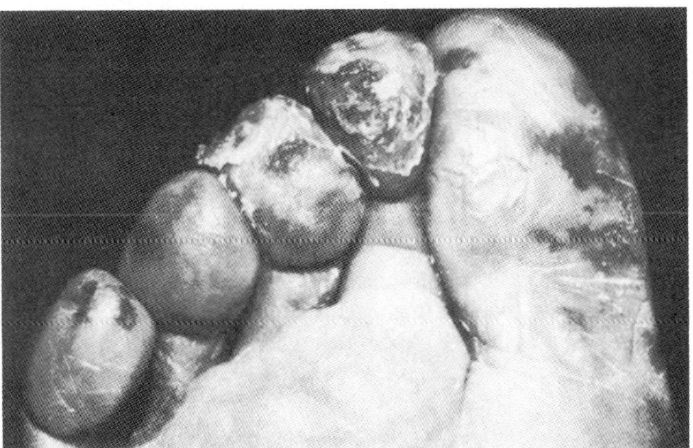

FIGURE 10–9. Distal digital infarction seen in polyarteritis. (From Hickling P and Golding JR: An Outline of Rheumatology. Oxford, Butterworth-Heinemann, 1984, p 97.)

related to the involved arteries include headache, tenderness, visual enlargement of the artery, visual changes or loss of vision, and pain in the muscles of mastication during chewing. Temporal artery biopsy confirms the diagnosis. There is a strong association between temporal arteritis and polymyalgia rheumatica, a relatively more common syndrome characterized by severe aching of the neck, shoulder, and pelvic girdle.

Takayasu's Arteritis. Other than the eponym Takayasu's arteritis, this disease is also known as *pulseless disease, aortic arch arteritis, aortic arch syndrome, brachial arteritis,* and *reverse coarctation,* among others. It affects medium- to large-sized arteries, particularly the aortic arch and its branches. Symptoms are typically insidious and include general complaints of headache, dizziness, fatigue, fever, nausea, tinnitus, night sweats, paresthesias of the extremities, arthralgia, and arthritis. Transient ischemia may lead to local claudication, blurred vision, dyspnea, syncope, paresthesias, and angina. An important physical finding is the absence or diminution of peripheral pulses, mostly in the upper extremity but possibly with associated bruits in the narrowed femoral, popliteal, and tibial arteries. It is almost pathognomonic to find absent blood pressures in the arms, with elevated pressures in the lower extremities. Raynaud's phenomenon is a frequent secondary finding, with cool distal extremities likely. Arteriography will demonstrate smooth narrowing, occlusion, poststenotic dilatation, and extensive collateralization. Laboratory findings include the presence of leukocytosis, decreased hemoglobin levels, and an elevated erythrocyte sedimentation rate. Tissue biopsy shows inflammation of adventitia and intima of vessels and thickening of vessel walls. HLA antigenic association has been found,[63] as has a strong incidence in Asians, with a 90% prevalence for females.[64]

Hypersensitivity Vasculitis. These most common forms of vasculitis are distinguished from polyarteritis primarily by their unique histopathology. Unlike the vascular lesions of polyarteritis, which are found in all stages of evolution and progression, the lesions of hypersensitivity vasculitis appear in the same stage of development. The inference is made that hypersensitivity vasculitis represents an immune-mediated response to an antigen at a specific time exposure, whereas the immune reaction of polyarteritis is in response to a more continuous exposure to some antigenic agent. Histologic examination demonstrates a pathologic picture known as *leukocytoclastic angiitis.* This is manifest as polymorphonuclear cell infiltration of vessel walls with leukocytosis (nuclear debris), extravasation of erythrocytes, endothelial swelling, fibrinoid necrosis, and occasionally complement and immunoglobulin deposits.[53] Because small arterioles, vessels, and capillaries are the targeted vessels, most disease is confined to the skin. Patients may demonstrate palpable purpura or hemorrhagic infarcts with localized superficial necrosis, especially in the lower legs. Other presentations include urticaria, vesicles, bullae, nodules, or superficial ulcerations. Occasionally, the patient may complain of arthralgias, and, less frequently, renal and gastrointestinal complications of vasculitis are present.

There are several distinct clinical syndromes characterized by this picture of leukocytoclastic angiitis. These subvarieties of hypersensitivity vasculitis, originally described as hypersensitivity reaction caused by drugs or serum sickness, include Schönlein-Henoch purpura (also known as anaphy-

lactoid or allergic purpura), mixed cryoglobulinemia, hypocomplementemic vasculitis, and the vasculitis associated with RA, SLE, and Sjögren's syndrome. These last entities have been previously described.

Mucocutaneous Lymph Node Syndrome. Also known as Kawasaki disease, this entity was first described in 1967.[65] However, it is likely that many cases of infantile polyarteritis have been confused with it, given the many similarities. Presumably of infectious origin, its incidence has been increasing worldwide and is in epidemic proportions in Japan.[66, 67] Mostly striking children younger than 5 years, Kawasaki disease is characterized by fever unresponsive to antibiotics, cervical lymphadenitis, edema of the hands and feet, conjunctival infection, and skin and mucous membrane disease. Kawasaki disease seems to progress in three phases. The first, an acute febrile phase, lasts approximately 2 weeks and is characterized by a spiking fever, conjunctival injection, and frequently an erythematous, desquamating perianal eruption.[67] This is followed by oropharyngeal manifestations including a diffuse red throat, erythema, dryness and fissuring of the lips, and the characteristic enlarged erythematous papillae known as "strawberry tongue." By the beginning of the second, or subacute, phase, there is evidence of cervical lymphadenopathy, indurative edema of the hands and feet, and an intensely erythematous rash on the extremities. With progression through the subacute phase and into the convalescent phase, the rash may spread onto the trunk, and, as the edema subsides, there is resolution of the palmar and plantar erythema, with residual desquamation, especially at the distal fingers and toes. The arthralgias and arthritis found in as many as half of the patients in the subacute phase are mostly gone in the convalescent phase. A late finding may be the presence of transverse grooves in the finger- and toenails. Generally self-limiting and responsive to high-dose gamma globulin and aspirin, Kawasaki disease does claim a 1% to 2% mortality rate as a result of myocardial infarction in the apparent recovery phase of the illness.[68, 69]

Behçet's Syndrome. The prominent vasculitic features of Behçet's syndrome allow for its inclusion in this vascular group of CTDs; however, this is a multisystem disorder frequently classified separately by many authors. Its cause is unknown; however, the histopathologic vascular changes common to all affected organs suggest a common autoimmune response to a viral or environmental agent. The probability of genetic mediation is strong, given the demographic profile. Although uncommon in the West, an incidence of 1 in 10,000 has been found in Japan, with not quite so high a prevalence also seen in other parts of Asia and the eastern Mediterranean area.[70] Usually first diagnosed in the third decade of life, the disease affects predominantly men, with ratios of between 2:1 and 5:1.[71] Behçet's syndrome is typically characterized clinically by the triad of oral and genital ulcerations and ocular inflammation (Fig. 10–10). The syndrome is chronic, with frequent episodic flares and remissions. Although it is by and large benign, occasional blindness, paralysis, or embolic events may complicate the course of disease.[72] Fatalities, when they occur, are usually related to late episodes of neurologic (CNS), vascular, or gastrointestinal involvement. Arthralgias are present in approximately 50% of cases, are usually associated with a mild synovitis, and are most often seen in the hands, knees, and ankles. Degenerative erosive joint changes are not typical.

Thrombophlebitis occurs in approximately 25% of pa-

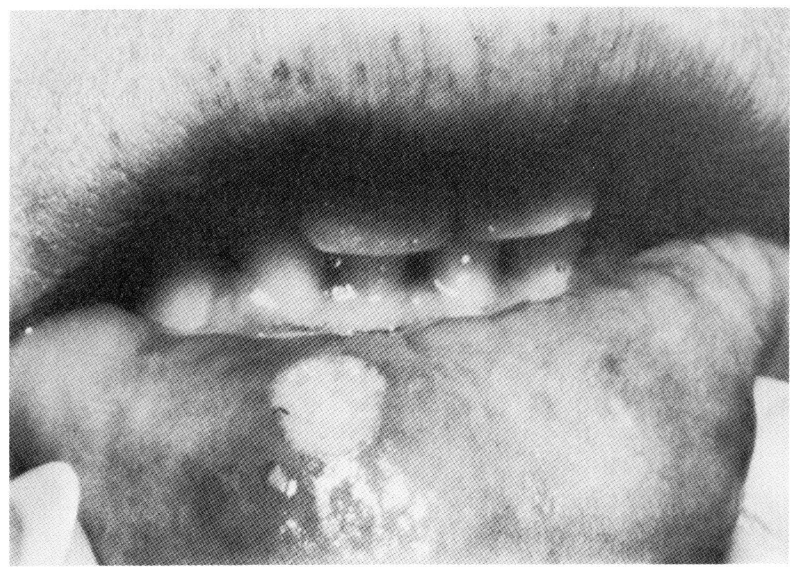

FIGURE 10–10. Buccal ulceration in Behçet's syndrome. (From Currey HLF [ed]: Mason and Currey's Clinical Rheumatology, 4th ed. Edinburgh, Churchill Livingstone, 1986, p 320.)

tients. There is evidence to support decreased fibrinolytic activity, decreased levels of prostaglandin I, and increased platelet aggregation as possible mechanisms in thrombus formation. More recently, there is great interest in the possibility that, like SLE or Sjögren's syndrome, there may be an elevation of anticardiolipin antibody levels in Behçet's syndrome.[73, 74] The use of corticosteroids has been the mainstay of treatment.

MIXED CONNECTIVE TISSUE DISEASE/ OVERLAP SYNDROMES

As we acquire knowledge, things do not become more comprehensive, but more mysterious.

ALBERT SCHWEITZER

Many patients with various rheumatic disorders do not fit neatly into a prescribed classification system. If the clinical and laboratory features of the previously detailed CTDs were not already sufficiently protean in nature, these mixed or overlap syndromes present a veritable conundrum for the diagnostician. One entity, mixed CTD, seems to offer a unique distinct presentation and can therefore be considered separately. The remainder of the so-called overlap syndromes, although amorphous in character, nevertheless lend

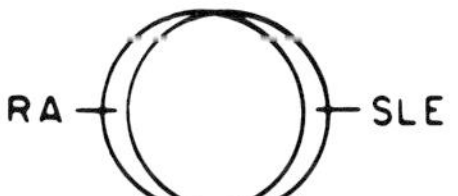
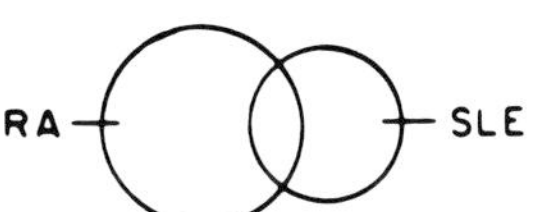
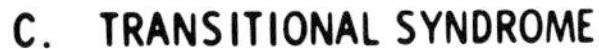
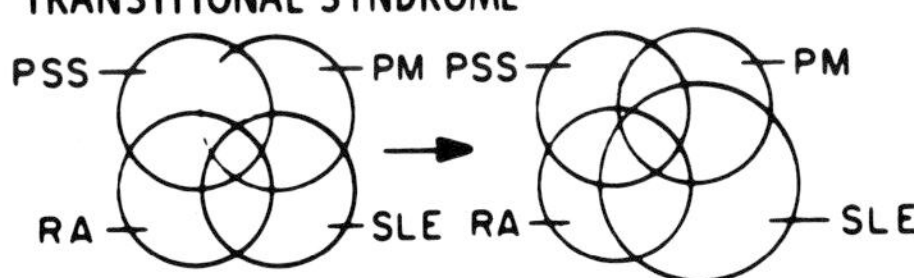
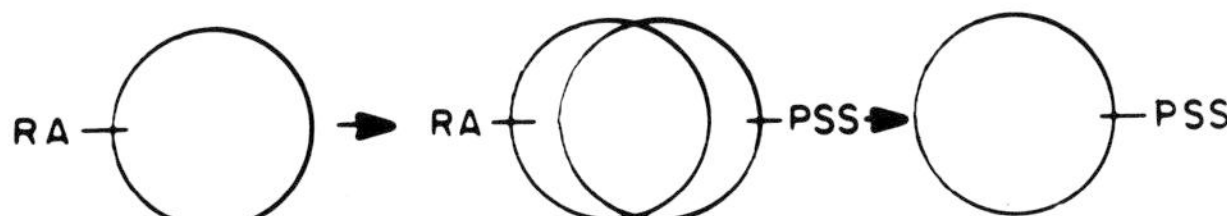
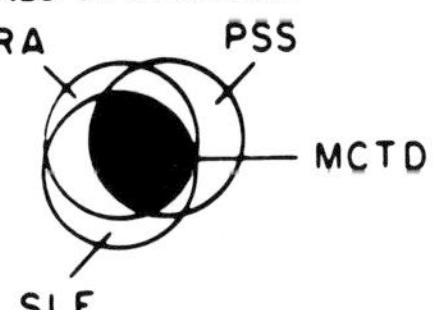

FIGURE 10–11. Overlapping connective tissue diseases—some possible syndromes. RA, rheumatoid arthritis; SLE, systemic lupus erythematosus; PSS, progressive systemic sclerosis; PM, polymyositis; MCTD, mixed connective tissue disease. (From Katz WA [ed]: Diagnosis and Management of Rheumatic Diseases, 3rd ed. Philadelphia, JB Lippincott, 1988, p 531.

TABLE 10–7

CLINICAL MANIFESTATIONS OF MIXED CONNECTIVE TISSUE DISEASE

Clinical Manifestation	Percentage
Arthritis/arthralgia	85–100
Raynaud's phenomenon	75–91
Cutaneous eruptions	35–40
Sclerodactyly	85–90
Other skin features	5–30
Myopathy	35–80
Pulmonary involvement (pleurisy, interstitial fibrosis, pulmonary hypertension)	68–85
Cardiac	25–35
Mitral valve prolapse	25
Renal	28
Neurologic	10–50
Hematologic	30–35
Gastrointestinal	80–85
Esophageal hypomotility	80

From Katz WA (ed): Diagnosis and Management of Rheumatic Diseases, 3rd ed. Philadelphia, JB Lippincott, 1988, p 531.

TABLE 10–8

OVERLAPPING PATHOLOGIC MANIFESTATIONS OF DISEASES AND THEIR IMMUNOLOGIC FEATURES*

Disease	Myositis	Glomerulo-nephritis	Lymphocytic Infiltration of Solid Organs	Lymphoid Hyperplasia	Perivascular Inflammation	Vasculitis	Necrotizing Arteritis
Systemic lupus erythematosus	+	+ +	+	+ +	+	+	±
Discoid lupus erythematosus	—	—	—	±	+	—	—
Rheumatoid arthritis	+	—	±	+	+	+	±
Sjögren's syndrome	±	—	+ +	+	+	+	±
Systemic sclerosis	+	±	—	±	+	+	—
Polymyositis	+ +	—	±	—	+	+	±
Polyarteritis	+	+	—	±	+ +	+ +	+ +

*Estimations of approximate frequency are as follows: + +, >50%; +, >10%; ±, <10%; and —, not present.

Adapted from Townes AS and Stevens MB: Multisystem disease as a problem in differential diagnosis. *In* Harvey AM, Johns RJ, et al: The Principles and Practice of Medicine, 18th ed. New York, Appleton-Century-Crofts, 1972, p 1271.

themselves to a spectral pattern in regards to their temporal and natural history (Fig. 10–11).

Mixed Connective Tissue Disease

This diagnosis features the presence of two or more coexisting CTDs such as RA, SLE, scleroderma, and polymyositis. Initial diagnosis of only one CTD is usually made first; however, with time, additional clinical and laboratory findings demonstrate the emergence of the distinct pattern of mixed CTD. Although the prevalence is unknown, mixed CTD occurs less frequently than SLE but more often than polymyositis/dermatomyositis. Approximately 80% of patients are female.

Pathology. The primary distinguishing serologic characteristic of this disease is the presence of very high titers (greater than 1:100,000) of circulating ANAs to an extractable nuclear antigen, specifically ribonucleoprotein antigen.[75] This finding is quite uncommon in SLE and more rare in the other CTDs and therefore is of great diagnostic significance in early undifferentiated presentations. Histopathology is primarily a picture of an obstructive vasculopathy with internal proliferation of the dermal and pulmonary vascular beds rather than an inflammatory necrotizing vasculitis. However, EMGs show typical inflammatory myopathy, with biopsies revealing muscle fiber degeneration. Interstitial and perivascular infiltration of lymphocytes, immune complexes, and other plasma cells is common. A mild to moderate normochromic, normocytic anemia and leukopenia appear in approximately one third of patients. Elevation of the erythrocyte sedimentation rate is a more frequent finding, as is diffuse hyperglobulinemia and a positive rheumatoid factor.[76]

Clinical Features. The clinical features most often seen in mixed CTD are summarized in Table 10–7. As can be seen, and of great importance to the examiner of the lower extremities, Raynaud's phenomenon, arthritis, and arthralgias are frequent manifestations. Raynaud's phenomenon is a particularly early finding, often preceding other findings by months or years.[77] More than two thirds of patients experience edema of the hands, with sausage-like swelling of the fingers and a mild sclerodactyly.

Diffuse sclerodermatous pathology is less frequently observed and, as with scleroderma, is more commonly seen in the upper, not lower, extremities.[78] Other cutaneous findings include those common to SLE: malar rash, diffuse erythematous lesions, and discoid eruptions. Additional cutaneous presentations include alterations in pigmentation, erythema nodosum, alopecia, and periungual telangiectasia.[76]

Almost all patients with mixed CTD have polyarthralgia and 75% have frank arthritis. Early arthritic changes are

TABLE 10–9

SOME OF THE OVERLAPPING CLINICAL MANIFESTATIONS OF DISEASES THAT HAVE IMMUNOLOGIC FEATURES*

Disease	Fever	Erythematous Skin Eruption	Muscle Weakness	Rheumatoid-Like Arthritis	Sicca Syndrome	Pleurisy or Pericarditis	Pulmonary Fibrosis	Myocardial Disease	Hypertension	Raynaud's Phenomenon	Altered Esophageal or Intestinal Motility	Nephritis	Focal Brain Involvement	Leukopenia	Hemolytic Anemia
Systemic lupus erythematosus	+ +	+ +	+	+	±	+ +	—	+	+	+	±	+ +	+	+ +	+
Discoid lupus erythematosus	—	+ +	—	±	—	—	—	—	—	±	—	—	—	±	—
Rheumatoid arthritis	±	—	+	+ +	+	+	±	±	—	+	±	—	—	±	—
Sjögren's syndrome	—	—	±	+ +	+ +	±	±	—	—	+	±	—	—	±	±
Systemic sclerosis	—	—	+	+	±	+	+	+	+	+ +	+ +	+	—	—	±
Polymyositis	+	+ +	+ +	+	±	—	±	—	—	±	+	—	—	—	—
Polyarteritis	+ +	±	+	+	±	±	±	+	+	±	±	+ +	+	—	—

*Estimations of approximate frequency are as follows: + +, >50%; +, >10%; ±, <10%; and —, not present.

Adapted from Townes AS and Stevens MB: Multisystem disease as a problem in differential diagnosis. *In* Harvey AM, Johns RJ, et al: The Principles and Practice of Medicine, 18th ed. New York, Appleton-Century-Crofts, 1972, p 1271.

TABLE 10–10

OVERLAPPING SEROLOGIC MANIFESTATIONS OF DISEASES THAT HAVE IMMUNOLOGIC FEATURES*

Disease	Hyper-gamma-globulinemia	Antinuclear Antibodies	Rheumatoid Factor	Positive Coombs' Test	Biological False-Positive Reaction	Thyroid Antibodies	Reduced Serum Complement
Systemic lupus erythematosus	+ +	+ +	+	+	+	+	+ +
Discoid lupus erythematosus	±	+	±	—	±	±	—
Rheumatoid arthritis	+	+	+ +	—	±	±	—
Sjögren's syndrome	+ +	+	+ +	±	±	+	±
Systemic sclerosis	±	+	+	—	±	±	—
Polymyositis	+	±	±	—	—	—	—
Polyarteritis	±	—	+	—	—	—	—

*Estimations of approximate frequency are as follows: + +, >50%; +, >10%; ±, <10%; and —, not present.

Adapted from Townes AS and Stevens MB: Multisystem disease as a problem in differential diagnosis. *In* Harvey AM, Johns RJ, et al: The Principles and Practice of Medicine, 18th ed. New York, Appleton-Century-Crofts, 1972, p 1271.

indistinguishable from those of RA. However, the joint erosions, pannus invasion, articular deformation, deviation, and subcutaneous nodules so evident with advanced RA are only occasionally seen in mixed CTD. Myopathy of the upper and lower extremities is frequently found and commonly restricted to proximal muscle groups. Myalgia and loss of muscle strength may or may not be present.

Other organ disease and related clinical features of mixed CTD reflects the relative recruitment of underlying syndromes. Pulmonary, renal, cardiac, gastrointestinal, and hematologic disorders may all be manifest, depending on whether SLE, scleroderma, polymyositis, dermatomyositis, or RA is active. Other findings may include features common to Sjögren's syndrome, Hashimoto's thyroiditis, fever, splenomegaly, hepatomegaly, and lymphadenopathy. Neurologic findings are infrequent, but reports of peripheral neuropathy have been made.[79]

Treatment and Prognosis. General medical management and pharmacologic therapy are similar in nature to those used in the treatment of SLE. The usual precautions regarding exposure to cold are given to those patients suffering the effects of Raynaud's phenomenon. Otherwise, appropriate treatment is usually targeted to those organ systems most extensively involved, whether related to SLE or the other frequently present CTDs. Most patients respond well to corticosteroids, especially if given early in the course of disease activity. There is also a role for NSAIDs, although renal disease may limit their use. Severe major organ disease may require larger doses of corticosteroids or the use of cytotoxic or antimalarial agents. It is interesting to note that those patients with clinical features most expressive of scleroderma respond least well to steroids and have the poorest prognoses.[78] If there is renal, hepatic, pulmonary, or diffuse vascular disease, mortality rates climb as high as 15%. This is roughly the equivalent of SLE.

Overlap Syndromes. A variety of patients have CTD but no readily available pattern of symptoms that permits a confident diagnosis. These patients may manifest features of multiple CTDs at a given time or may reveal clear evidence of one CTD that changes to another with the passage of time (see Fig. 10–3). Tables 10–8 to 10–10 summarize the overlapping pathologic, clinical, and serologic manifestations that make identifying the components of overlapping CTDs so difficult. Disorders intermingle, and occasionally a predominance of one disorder over another is displayed. Transitional syndromes may emerge, or conversion disorders may be expressed as one CTD literally metamorphoses into another. The future discovery of the antigens responsible for so many of the CTDs as well as an increased understanding of immunology and the advancement of HLA genetic mapping will undoubtedly clear up the present mystery of these overlap syndromes.

References

1. Tan EM, Cohen AS, Fries JF, et al: The 1982 revised criteria for the classification of systemic lupus erythematosus. Arthritis Rheum 25:1271–1277, 1982.
2. Siegel M and Lee SL: The epidemiology of systemic lupus erythematosus. Semin Arthritis Rheum 17:1, 1988.
3. Rothfield NF: Clinical features of systemic lupus erythematosus. *In* Kelley WN, Morris ED Jr, Roddy S, and Sledge CB (eds): Textbook of Rheumatology, Vol 2. Philadelphia, WB Saunders, 1981, pp 1106–1132.
4. Hughes GR: Connective Tissue Diseases, 3rd ed. Oxford, England, Blackwell Scientific Publications, 1987.
5. Fessel WJ: Systemic lupus erythematosus in the community. Arch Intern Med 134:1027, 1974.
6. Vitto J and Perejda AJ: Connective Tissue Disease—Molecular Pathology of the Extracellular Matrix. New York, Marcel Dekker, 1987.
7. Atkins CJ, Kondon JJ, Quismorio FP, and Friou CJ: The choroid plexus in systemic lupus erythematosus. Ann Intern Med 76:65, 1972.
8. Robbins S, Angell M, and Kumar V: Basic Pathology. Philadelphia, WB Saunders, 1981, p 199.
9. Parke A and Rothfield NF: Systemic lupus erythematosus. *In* Katz WA (ed): Diagnosis and Management of Rheumatic Diseases, 2nd ed. Philadelphia, JB Lippincott, 1988.
10. Morrow J and Isenberg D: Autoimmune Rheumatic Disease. Oxford, England, Blackwell Scientific Publications, 1987.
11. Martel W: Acute and chronic arthritis of the foot. Semin Roentgenol 5:391, 1970.
12. Russell AS, Percy JS, Rigal WM, and Wilson GL: Deforming arthropathy in systemic lupus erythematosus. Ann Rheum Dis 33:204–209, 1974.
13. Labowitz R and Schumaker MR: Articular manifestations of systemic lupus erythematosus. Ann Intern Med 74:911–921, 1971.
14. Mizutani W and Quismorio FP: Lupus foot: Deforming arthropathy of the feet in systemic lupus erythematosus. J Rheumatol 11:80, 1984.
15. Morley KD, Leung A, and Rynes RI: Lupus foot. Br Med J 284:557, 1982.
16. Askari A, Vignos PJ, and Moshowitz RW: Steroid myopathy in connective tissue disease. Am J Med 61:485–492, 1977.
17. Cogen J, Pinching AJ, Rees AJ, and Peters DK: Infection and immunosuppression (a study of the infective complications of 75 patients with immunologically-mediated disease). Q J Med 201:1, 1982.
18. Fleischmajer R: The pathophysiology of scleroderma. Int J Dermatol 1666:310–318, 1977.
19. Alarcon-Segovia D and de Lasep GI: Features of Sjögren's syndrome and scleroderma. *In* Black LM, Myers AR (eds): Current Topics in Rheumatology, Systemic Sclerosis. London, Gower Medical Publishing, 1985, pp 42–46.
20. Rodnan GP, Jablonska S, and Medsger TA Jr: Classification and nomenclature of progressive systemic sclerosis (scleroderma). Clin Rheum Dis 5:5, 1979.
21. Alper J and Leroy EL: Scleroderma (systemic sclerosis). *In* Katz WA (ed): Diagnosis and Management of Rheumatic Diseases. Philadelphia, JB Lippincott, 1988, pp 467–480.
22. Furst DE, Clements PJ, Saab M, et al: Clinical and serological comparison of 17 chronic progressive systemic sclerosis (PSS) and 17 CREST syndrome patients matched for sex, age, and disease duration. Ann Rheum Dis 43:794–801, 1984.
23. Medsger TA Jr and Masi AT: Epidemiology of progressive systemic sclerosis. Clin Rheum Dis 5:15, 1979.

24. Campbell PM and LeRoy EL: Pathogenesis of systemic sclerosis: A vascular hypothesis. Semin Arthritis Rheum 4:351, 1975.

25. Roumm AD, Whiteside TL, Medsger TA Jr, and Rodnan GP: Lymphocytes in the skin of patients with progressive systemic sclerosis. Quantification, subtyping, and clinical correlations. Arthritis Rheum 27:645–653, 1984.

26. LeRoy EC: Scleroderma. *In* Hughes GRV (ed): Topics in Rheumatology. London, Heinemann, 1976.

27. Blocka KLN, Bassett LW, Furst DE, et al: The arthropathy of advanced progressive systemic sclerosis: A radiographic survey. Arthritis Rheum 24:874, 1981.

28. Lee P, Bruni J, and Sukenik S: Neurological manifestations in systemic sclerosis (scleroderma). J Rheumatol 11:480, 1984.

29. Klimiuk PS, Taylor L, Baker RD, and Jayson MIV: Autonomic neuropathy in systemic sclerosis. Ann Rheum Dis 47:542–545, 1988.

30. Dessein PH, Joffe BI, Metz RM, et al: Autonomic dysfunction in systemic sclerosis: Sympathetic overactivity and instability. Am J Med 93:143–150, 1992.

30a. Rook AH, Freundlich B, Jegasothy BV, et al: Treatment of systemic sclerosis with extracorporeal photochemotherapy: Results of a multicenter trial. Arch Dermatol 128:337–346, 1992.

31. DeVere R and Bradley G: Polymyositis: Its presentation, morbidity and mortality. Brain 98:637, 1975.

32. Medsger TA, Dawson WN, and Masi AT: The epidemiology of polymyositis. Am J Med 48:7815, 1970.

33. Pearson CM: Polymyositis. Annu Rev Med 17:63, 1966.

34. Bohan A, Peter JB, Bowman RL, et al: A computer assisted analysis of 153 patients with polymyositis and dermatomyositis. Medicine 56:255, 1977.

35. Callen JP: Dermatomyositis. Int J Dermatol 18:423, 1979.

36. Callen JP: Myositis and malignancy. Clin Rheum Dis 10:117–130, 1984.

37. Schwarz HA, Slavin G, Ward P, et al: Muscle biopsy in polymyositis and dermatomyositis—A clinicopathological study. Ann Rheum Dis 39:500, 1980.

38. Heffer RR and Barron SA: Polymyositis beginning as a focal process. Arch Neurol 38:439, 1981.

39. Kalyanaraman K and Kalyanaraman UP: Localized myositis presenting as pseudothrombophlebitis. Arthritis Rheum 25:1374, 1982.

40. Bennington JA and Dau PC: Patients with polymyositis and dermatomyositis who undergo plasmaphoresis therapy: Pathologic findings. Arch Neurol 38:535, 1981.

41. Morgan WS and Castleman B: A clinicopathologic study of ''Mikulicz's disease.'' Am J Pathol 29:471, 1953.

42. Shearn MA: Sjögren's syndrome. *In* Smith LH (ed): Major Problems in Internal Medicine, Vol II. Philadelphia, WB Saunders, 1971.

43. Whaley K, Webb J, McAvoy BA, et al: Sjögren's syndrome: Clinical association and immunological phenomena. Q J Med 42:513, 1973.

44. Bloch KJ, Buchanan WW, Wohl MJ, and Bunim JJ: Sjögren's syndrome: A clinical, pathological and serological study of 62 cases. Medicine 44:187, 1965.

45. Lawley T, Moutsopolos HM, Katz SE, et al: Demonstration of circulating immune complexes in Sjögren's syndrome. J Immunol 123:1382, 1979.

46. Moutsopolos HM, Chused TM, Mann DL, et al: Sjögren's syndrome (sicca syndrome): Current issues. Ann Intern Med 92 (Part 1): 212, 1980.

47. Panay GS, Wooley P, and Batchela JR: Genetic basis of rheumatoid disease: HLA antigens, disease manifestation and toxic reactions to drugs. Br Med J 2:1326, 1978.

48. Henkin RI, Talal N, Larson AL, and Mattern CFT: Abnormalities of taste and smell in Sjögren's syndrome. Ann Intern Med 76:375, 1972.

49. Strimlan CV, Rosenow EC, Divertie MB, and Harrison EG: Pulmonary manifestations of Sjögren's syndrome. Chest 70:354, 1976.

50. Adams JF, Glen AI, Kennedy EH, et al: The histological and secretory changes in the stomach in patients with autoimmunity to gastric parietal cells. Lancet 1:401–403, 1964.

51. Tu WH, Shearn MA, Lee JC, and Hopper J: Interstitial nephritis in Sjögren's syndrome. Ann Intern Med 69:1163, 1968.

52. Atwood W and Poser CM: Neurologic complication of Sjögren's syndrome. Neurology 11:1034–1041, 1961.

53. Fauci AS, Haynes BF, and Katz P: The spectrum of vasculitis: Clinical, pathologic, immunologic, and theraputic considerations. Ann Intern Med 89:660, 1978.

54. Alarcon-Segovia D and Brown AL: Classification and etiologic aspects of necrotizing angiitides: An analytical approach to a confused subject with a critical review of evidence for hypersensitivity in polyarteritis nodosa. Mayo Clin Proc 39:205, 1964.

55. Zeek PM: Periarteritis nodosa and other forms of necrotizing angiitis. N Engl J Med 248:764, 1953.

56. Savage COS, Winearls CG, Jones S, et al: Prospective study of radioimmunoassay for antibodies against neutrophil cytoplasm in diagnosis of systemic vasculitis. Lancet 1:1037, 1987.

57. Borrie P: Cutaneous polyarteritis nodosa. Br J Dermatol 87:87, 1972.

58. Sigal LH: The neurologic presentation of vasculitic and rheumatologic syndromes. Medicine 66:157, 1987.

59. Fauci AS, Haynes BF, Katz P, and Wolff SM: Wegener's granulomatosis: Prospective clinical and theraputic experience with 85 patients for 21 years. Ann Intern Med 98:76, 1983.

60. Papiha SS, Murty GE, Ad'Hia A, et al: Association of Wegener's granulomatosis with HLA antigens and other genetic markers. Ann Rheum Dis 51:246–249, 1992.

61. Wilkinson IM and Russell RW: Arteries of the head and neck in giant cell arteritis: A pathologic study to show the pattern of arterial involvement. Arch Neurol 27:378–391, 1972.

62. Fauchald P, Rygvold B, and Oystease B: Temporal arteritis and polymyalgia rheumatica: Clinical and biopsy findings. Ann Intern Med 77:845–852, 1972.

63. Isohisa I, Numano F, Maczawa H, and Sasazuki T: HLA-Bw52 in Takayasu's disease. Tissue Antigens 12:246, 1978.

64. Ishikawa K: Natural history and classification of occlusive thromboaortopathy (Takayasu's disease). Circulation 57:27, 1978.

65. Kawasaki T, Kosaki F, Osawaz S, et al: A new infantile acute febrile mucocutaneous lymph node syndrome (MLNS) prevailing in Japan. Pediatrics 54:271–276, 1974.

66. Shiokawa Y: Vascular Lesions of Collagen Diseases and Related Conditions. Baltimore, University Park Press, 1977.

67. Fritter BS, et al: The perianal eruption of Kawasaki syndrome disease. Arch Dermatol 124:1805, 1988.

68. Newburger JW, Takahashi M, Burns JC, et al: The treatment of Kawasaki syndrome with intravenous gamma globulin. N Engl J Med 315:341, 1986.

69. Rowley AH, et al: Prevention of giant coronary artery aneurysms in Kawasaki disease by intravenous gamma globulin therapy. J Pediatr 113:290, 1988.

70. Shimizu T, Ehrlich GE, Inaba G, et al: Behçet disease (Behçet syndrome). Semin Arthritis Rheum 8:223–260, 1979.

71. Lehner T and Barnes CG: Criteria for diagnosis and classification of Behçet's syndrome. *In* Lehner T, Barnes CG (eds): Behçet's Syndrome: Clinical and Immunological Features. London, Academic Press, 1979.

72. Cakir N, Yazici H, Chamberlain MA, et al: Response to intradermal injection of monosodium urate crystals in Behçet's syndrome. Ann Rheum Dis 50:634–637, 1991.

73. Efthimio J, Cambridge G, et al: Anticardiolipin antibodies and vascular complications. *In* Lehner T, Barnes CG (eds): Behçet's Syndrome: Clinical and Immunological Features. London, Academic Press, 1986.

74. Asherson RA, Fei HM, Staub HL, et al: Antiphospholipid antibodies and HLA associations in primary Sjögren's syndrome. Ann Rheum Dis 51:495–499, 1992.

75. Sharp GC, Irvin WS, Tan EM, et al: Mixed connective tissue disease—An apparently distinct rheumatic disease syndrome associated with a distinct antibody to an extractable nuclear antigen (ENA). Am J Med 52:148, 1972.

76. Bernhard GC: Mixed connective tissue disease and other overlap syndromes. *In* Katz WA (ed): Diagnosis and Management of Rheumatic Diseases, 2nd ed. Philadelphia, JB Lippincott, 1987, p 530.

77. Sharp GC: Mixed connective tissue disease. Bull Rheum Dis 25:828, 1975.

78. Wolfe JF, Kingsland L, Lindberg D, and Sharp GC: Disease pattern in patients with antibodies only to nuclear ribonucleoprotein [Abstract]. Clin Res 25:488A, 1977.

79. Bennett RM and O'Connell DJ: Mixed connective tissue diseases. A clinicopathologic study of 20 cases. Semin Arthritis Rheum 10:25–51, 1980.

CHAPTER 11

Cutaneous Signs of Systemic Disease

Todd S. Anhalt, M.D.

Most clinicians see skin disease every day. The diagnosis and treatment of dermatologic disorders of the lower extremity are an important part of the practice of podiatry. There are a number of dermatologic diseases that are, in fact, manifestations of underlying internal or systemic disorders. When the signs or symptoms occur on the lower extremity, the podiatrist may well be the first physician to see them. An understanding of the spectrum of skin lesions encountered during the evaluation of such a patient may lead to the early diagnosis of an underlying illness. This is virtually always to the advantage of the patient and may occasionally be lifesaving. This chapter is an overview of a number of skin diseases that reflect underlying disease and that may be seen during a podiatric examination. The major dermatologic manifestations of these diseases may or may not be limited to the skin of the lower extremity. Recognition of the clues should lead the physician to elicit further history from the patient and to foster examination of the skin elsewhere on the body. Appropriate laboratory tests may be ordered by the podiatrist, and patients should be referred to the internist or other specialist if necessary.

The rather heterogeneous group of diseases covered in this chapter is divided into a number of categories, including connective tissue/autoimmune diseases, endocrine and metabolic disorders, infectious diseases, keratodermas, miscellaneous skin disorders associated with systemic disease, and nail changes in systemic disease. Some of these groups overlap, and the aforementioned categorization is used merely to facilitate the understanding of these diseases.

The purpose of this chapter is to describe the lesions of the skin that may appear on the lower extremity and that may be associated with underlying systemic disease. Many, but not all, of these diseases have rheumatologic manifestations. Systematic and complete descriptions of these diseases are not the goal of this chapter. Rather, the detailed description of skin manifestations is given, and the systemic illnesses associated with them are enumerated and described briefly. A more detailed and explicit description of these individual diseases can be found elsewhere in this book or in any major dermatology textbook.

EXAMINATION OF THE SKIN OF THE LOWER EXTREMITY

The examination of the integument of the lower extremity should be guided by the type, degree, and distribution of the skin lesions. Of course, all aspects of the foot should always be examined, including all toenails. If lesions arise on the foot and extend up the leg, the entire lower extremity up to and including the inguinal area needs to be evaluated. For example, the presence of inguinal lymphadenopathy may be an important clue betraying an underlying inflammatory, infectious, or neoplastic process. Many diseases affecting the skin of the feet also affect the hands. Examination of the hands and fingernails can therefore add valuable diagnostic information.

CONNECTIVE TISSUE/AUTOIMMUNE DISEASE

Raynaud's Syndrome

Raynaud's syndrome is characterized by episodic attacks of digital ischemia associated with vasospasm of the peripheral blood vessels on exposure to cold and sometimes to emotional stress. Typically, the patient gives a history of changes in color, temperature, and sensation involving acral areas, most often the fingers and toes. It may affect one, all, or any combination of the digits. The affected digits often, but not always, show a characteristic pattern of progression and regression through the phases of pallor, cyanosis, and erythema (Fig. 11–1). There is well-demarcated blanching or cyanosis extending proximally from the tip of the digit. Distal to the line of ischemia, the skin is white or blue and cold. The fingers or toes may be completely or partially affected. The proximal skin is pink and warmer. Patients often describe numbness of the affected digits during this phase of decreased blood flow. On rewarming, the digits may remain or become cyanotic owing to sluggish blood flow. After the attack, the digits either return to normal color or become hyperemic and bright red. This phase may be associated with pain or discomfort in the affected digits.

When no associated internal disease can be found, the disease is considered to be idiopathic and is called *Raynaud's disease*. When the episodes are secondary to or associated with another underlying illness it is called *Raynaud's phenomenon*. In Raynaud's phenomenon, patients may experience persistent vasospasm that is more often associated with a painful recovery phase. The idiopathic variety is more common and affects women approximately five times more frequently than it affects men. Connective tissue disease is the most common cause of secondary Raynaud's phenomenon (Table 11–1). Most of these diseases are discussed in

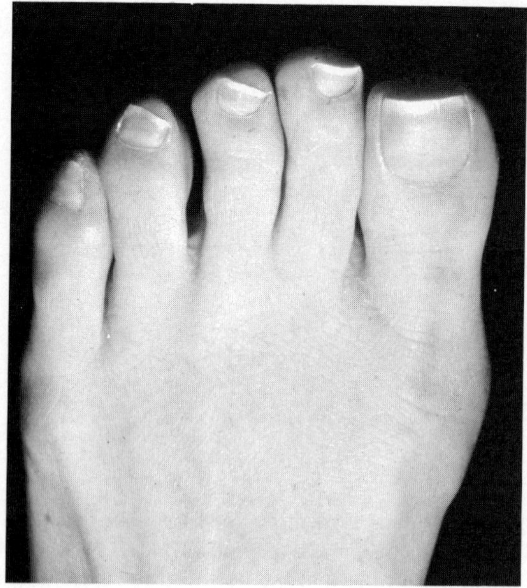

FIGURE 11–1. Raynaud's disease. There is well-demarcated proximal blanching and distal cyanosis of the digits.

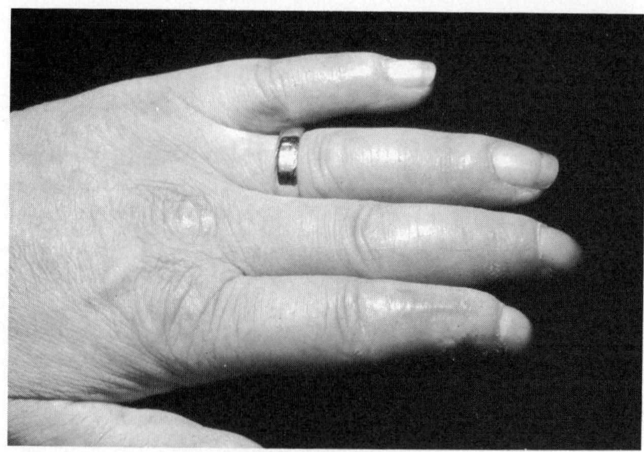

FIGURE 11–2. CREST syndrome. Sclerodactyly is present as well as calcinosis cutis of the distal index finger.

more detail in this chapter. Raynaud's phenomenon may also be seen in hematologic disorders including malignancies (e.g., lymphomas) or associated with cryoglobulinemias. Hypothyroidism, obstructive arterial disease, and multiple sclerosis have also been associated with Raynaud's phenomenon. Certain drugs and medications may trigger or exacerbate Raynaud's phenomenon in patients. In particular, patients must be persuaded to stop cigarette smoking.

Scleroderma and Variants

Scleroderma, or *progressive systemic sclerosis,* is a chronic multisystem disease leading to sclerosis and dysfunction of the affected tissues. It may occur as a disease localized only to skin and is then called *morphea.* Common sites of more generalized or systemic involvement are the skin, esophagus, kidneys, and vascular system. Approximately 80% to 90% of patients with scleroderma may be affected with Raynaud's phenomenon. It may be the presenting symptom in one third of patients and may precede other manifestations of scleroderma by years. The skin of the toes and fingers in scleroderma appears smooth, bound down, and occasionally swollen (Fig. 11–2). The digits take on a "sausage shape," especially the fingers. If the disease is aggressive, there may be loss of the distal digits. Patients with scleroderma may also present with chronic and recalcitrant ulcers of the foot and ankle. Scleroderma may also be associated with the *c*alcinosis cutis (Fig. 11–3), *R*aynaud's, *e*sophageal dysmotility, *s*clerodactyly, *t*elangiectasia (CREST) syndrome. Morphea is usually not associated with the CREST syndrome. Both localized and systemic forms appear to be more common in women. A full physical examination and appropriate laboratory studies, including blood counts, renal function tests, serologic studies, and chemistry screenings, are essential. A skin biopsy may also help in making a diagnosis.

Systemic Lupus Erythematosus

Lupus erythematosus (LE) is a chronic inflammatory autoimmune disease of unknown etiology. It is characterized

TABLE 11–1

CONDITIONS ASSOCIATED WITH RAYNAUD'S PHENOMENON

Connective Tissue Diseases	**Drugs**
Progressive systemic sclerosis	Tobacco
CREST syndrome	β-adrenergic blockers
Rheumatoid arthritis	Ergot alkaloids
Systemic lupus erythematosus	Methysergide
Dermatomyositis	Bleomycin
Polyarteritis nodosa	Clonidine
Sjögren's syndrome	
Leukocytoclastic vasculitis	**Neurologic Disorders**
	Carpal tunnel syndrome
Hematologic Disorders	Multiple sclerosis
Cryoglobulinemia	Thoracic outlet syndrome
Polycythemia	
Macroglobulinemia	**Endocrine Disorders**
	Hypothyroidism
Obstructive Arterial Disease	
Arterial emboli	**Trauma**
Arteriosclerosis obliterans	Vibratory tools
Thromboangiitis obliterans	Pianists and typists

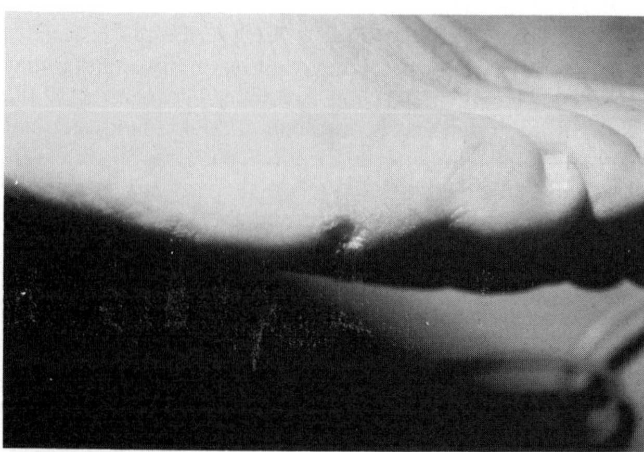

FIGURE 11–3. Calcinosis cutis. Extrusion of calcific material is seen from the skin of the lateral proximal fifth digit.

by the abnormal production of immunoglobulins that may bind to various tissues and lead to their destruction via poorly understood mechanisms. Cutaneous disease may occur with or without systemic disease or vice versa. Skin is involved in the different forms of LE in about 70% to 85% of patients, ranks only second to joint symptoms as an initial presenting symptom, and is commonly a major feature of the disease. Lupus may present as a purely cutaneous disease. Discoid LE is commonly seen in a photodistribution and is not usually seen on the foot, although the sun-exposed areas of the lower leg in some patients may be involved. Lesions of discoid LE are typically annular and show cutaneous atrophy, follicular plugging (except palms and soles), and scarring (Fig. 11–4). Subacute cutaneous LE is only occasionally associated with systemic disease. It usually presents as a papulosquamous eruption often in a photodistribution.

Systemic LE (SLE) is a multisystem disease that can affect virtually every organ in the body. It is usually associated with various serologic abnormalities. Most commonly it affects skin, joints, kidneys, lungs, and the central nervous system (CNS). Vasculitis is a common denominator in many of these manifestations (see Fig. 11–15). Approximately 10% to 35% of patients with SLE also have Raynaud's phenomenon. Cutaneous manifestations of SLE include the classical facial "butterfly" rash on the cheeks (Fig. 11–5) and diffuse maculopapular, bullous, erythema multiforme–like, and toxic epidermal necrolytic types. The eruption of acute SLE on the dorsum of the fingers tends to be localized over the interarticular skin as opposed to over the articulations as seen with Gottron's papules of dermatomyositis (Fig. 11–6). Diffuse or localized cutaneous vasculitis is also fairly common. A patient with palpable purpura (leukocytoclastic vasculitis until proved otherwise) or hemorrhagic bullous lesions on the lower extremity should be investigated for abnormal serologic studies, and SLE should be included in the differential diagnosis. Biopsies of lesions suspected of being caused by SLE and other connective tissue diseases should be sent for both standard hematoxylin-eosin stains and for evaluation by direct immunofluorescence techniques (Fig. 11–7).

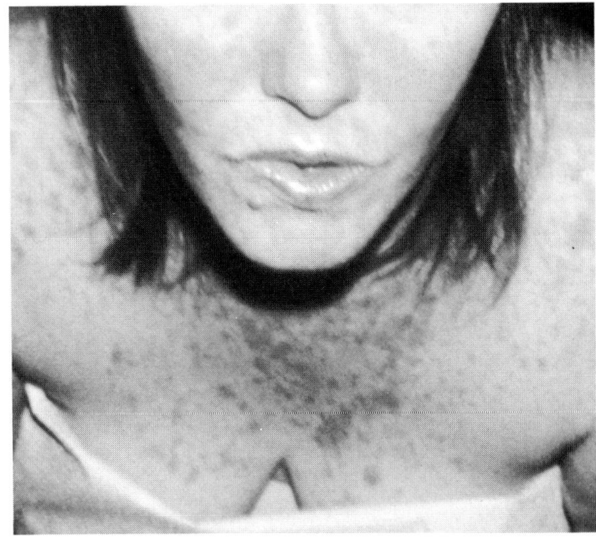

FIGURE 11–5. Acute systemic lupus erythematosus. The typical "butterfly rash" is present as well as a macular erythematous eruption. Note the photodistribution.

Dermatomyositis/Polymyositis

Dermatomyositis/polymyositis (DM/PM) is a disease complex that combines an inflammatory myopathy with characteristic skin lesions. Dermatomyositis is closely related to polymyositis in which an identical myopathy is present, but without typical skin disease. The specific cause is unknown, but myositis is thought to be immunologically mediated. Both DM and PM may be associated with other connective tissue diseases in overlap syndromes. DM/PM have been reported with SLE, Sjögren's syndrome, scleroderma spectrum disease, rheumatoid arthritis (RA), and other vasculitides. For years, DM was thought to be associated with a higher risk of internal malignancy. Although this assumption has not been supported or refuted, more recent studies seem to indicate an increased association of DM with internal malignancy, and enough data exist to suggest the usefulness of a general history and complete physical examination in these patients. The disease affects women twice as often as men, with a peak incidence in the fifth and sixth decades.

Clinical cutaneous manifestations include the classical *heliotrope rash* and *Gottron's papules* (Figs. 11–8 and 11–9).

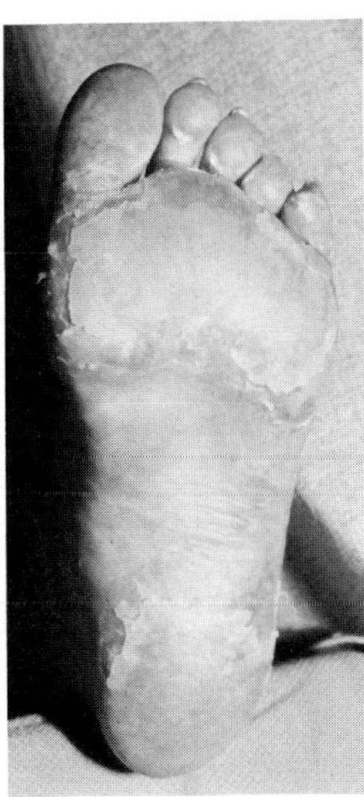

FIGURE 11–4. Discoid lupus erythematosus. The plantar surface shows cutaneous atrophy and scarring.

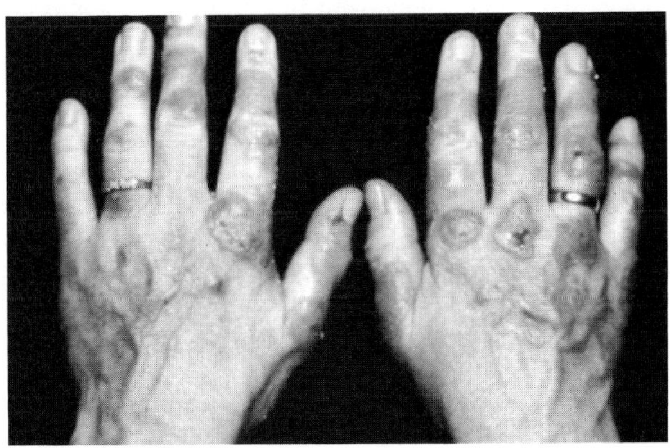

FIGURE 11–6. Systemic lupus erythematosus. Erythematous scaly plaques appear over the dorsal fingers and hands.

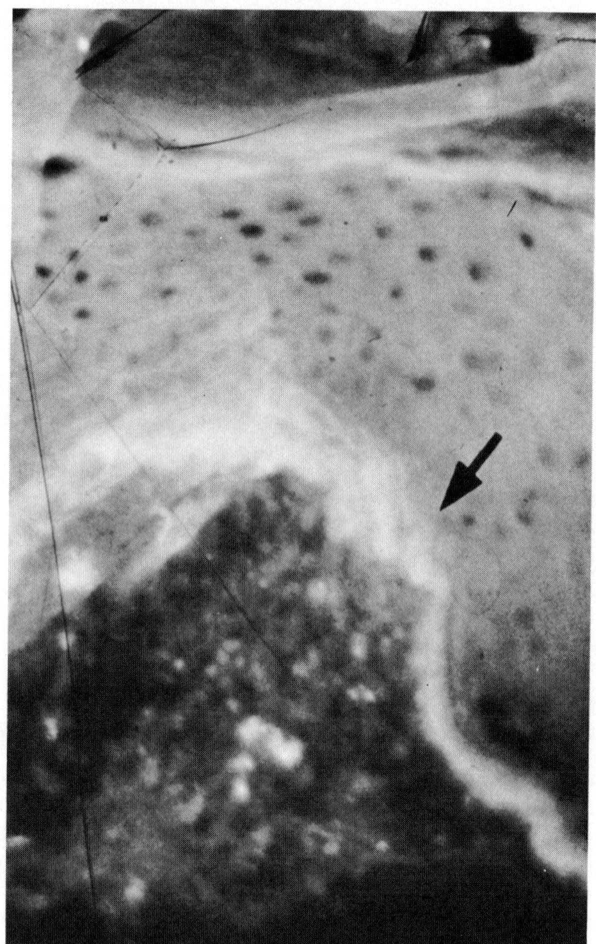

FIGURE 11–7. Lupus erythematosus—direct immunofluorescence micrograph. The deposition of immunoreactants (e.g., IgG and IgM) and complement at the basement membrane zone (*arrow*) between the dermis and epidermis is demonstrated.

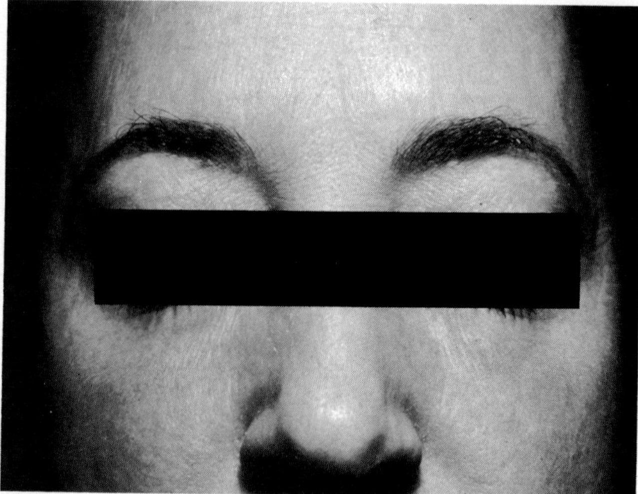

FIGURE 11–8. Dermatomyositis-heliotrope rash. Erythematous to lilac-colored patches involve the upper eyelids.

The heliotrope rash is named after the flower that has a characteristic violet to lilac hue and follows the sun during the course of the day. The lesions are lilac, violaceous to dusky erythematous patches, with or without edema in a symmetrical periorbital distribution on the face. In patients with more subtle forms of the disorder, the rash affects only the eyelid margins. Podiatrists are more likely to recognize Gottron's papules, which are violaceous to dusky erythematous slightly raised lesions with superimposed telangiectatic blood vessels found over the bony prominences of the extremities. Most commonly, they can be seen on the skin directly overlying the metacarpophalangeal and proximal interphalangeal joints. They may be found on the elbows, knees, and toes. The lesions may also be hypopigmented or hyperpigmented and some cutaneous atrophy may be present (Fig. 11–10). Nail fold changes, although not specific to DM, are present as periungual telangiectasias, hypertrophy of the cuticle, and small hemorrhagic infarcts (Fig. 11–11). These changes may also be seen in LE, vasculitides, and the scleroderma spectrum of diseases. Biopsies of the various skin lesions are not specific for DM but are occasionally helpful. Myositis associated with DM/PM is predominantly a proximal limb girdle weakness, but all muscle groups may be affected in severe cases. The muscles are generally weak but

are not tender or painful. The symptoms progress over weeks or months. Patients who have difficulty with swallowing (dysphagia) may have a poorer prognosis.

DM/PM may also be associated with arthralgias, usually as morning stiffness of the small joints. Arthritis, when present, is usually symmetrical and noninflammatory. Lung and esophageal disease, myocarditis, and pericarditis have been reported. In younger patients, calcinosis cutis is common.

A laboratory evaluation must include serum muscle enzymes such as creatine kinase, lactate dehydrogenase, serum glutamic-oxaloacetic transaminase, and serum and urinary aldolase.

Rheumatoid Arthritis

The pathophysiology and clinical description of RA are covered in great detail elsewhere in this book. Except for skin ulcerations, the skin manifestations of RA are seen only

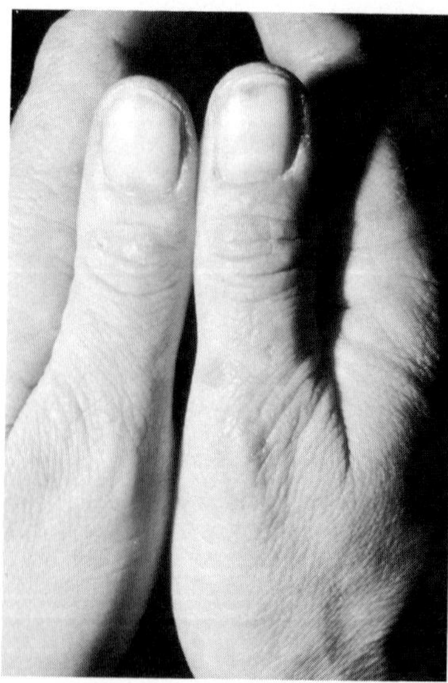

FIGURE 11–9. Dermatomyositis—Gottron's papules. Erythematous scaly plaques are seen over the joints of the dorsal thumbs.

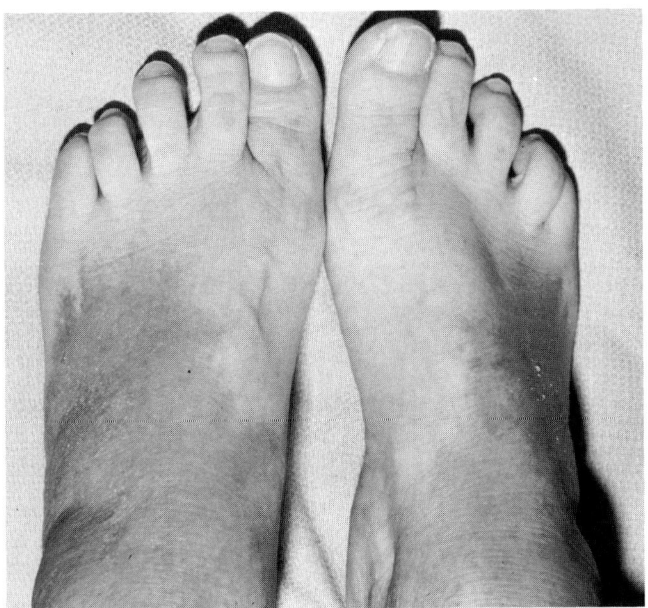

FIGURE 11–10. Dermatomyositis. Symmetrical erythematous patches are seen over the lower legs and dorsal feet.

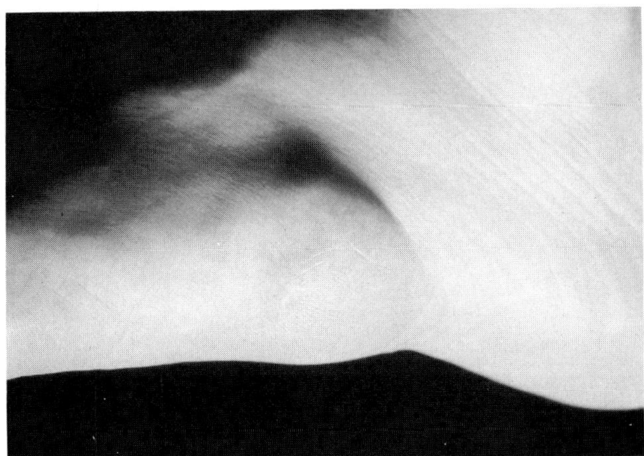

FIGURE 11–12. Rheumatoid nodule. A nontender periarticular subcutaneous nodule has developed on the lateral foot in this patient with rheumatoid arthritis.

in patients with detectable levels of the immunoglobulins known as *rheumatoid factor*. These include vasculitis, periarticular subcutaneous nodules (Fig. 11–12), ulcerations, and even pulp atrophy and gangrene. In mild cases, nail ridging caused by vascular lesions limited to the nail beds may be the only apparent cutaneous sign. Vasculitis, which may be seen in RA, is probably secondary to the deposition of immunoglobulin in the vessel walls and the subsequent activation of complement. The sine qua non of cutaneous vasculitis is palpable purpura (see leukocytoclastic vasculitis). Vasculitis may also present as necrotic ulcers (Fig. 11–13), digital infarcts, bullae, nonpalpable purpura, livedo reticularis, and less specific cutaneous lesions. Periarticular subcutaneous nodules of RA are generally firm, fairly mobile, usually nontender masses adjacent to or overlying articulations. The nodules are not particularly red or inflamed. Aspiration of these nonfluctuant nodules reveals no fluid or chalky (tophaceous)

material and is not helpful in making a diagnosis. A biopsy of these nodules may be useful when making a diagnosis. Severely affected patients may have actual gangrene, with loss of digits or acral extremities.

Livedo Reticularis

This is reddish-blue mottling of the skin in a fish net (reticular) pattern (Fig. 11–14). The skin within the lines of the net appears normal or pale in color. As a normal reaction to cold, this is called *cutis marmorata*. If the pattern persists despite rewarming, or is present with no history of cold exposure, it is called *livedo reticularis*. The pattern is most commonly seen on the lower extremity. In more diffuse cases, it affects the trunk as well as the upper and lower extremities. The association of livedo reticularis with systemic disease is seen in a number of diseases. Vasospastic conditions such as Raynaud's phenomenon may be present in patients with livedo reticularis. The spectrum of systemic diseases associated with Raynaud's phenomenon is discussed earlier. Vasculitis may appear in a livedo pattern, so-called *livedo vasculitis*. This particular pattern may be associated with the *anticardiolipin syndrome* in which patients produce

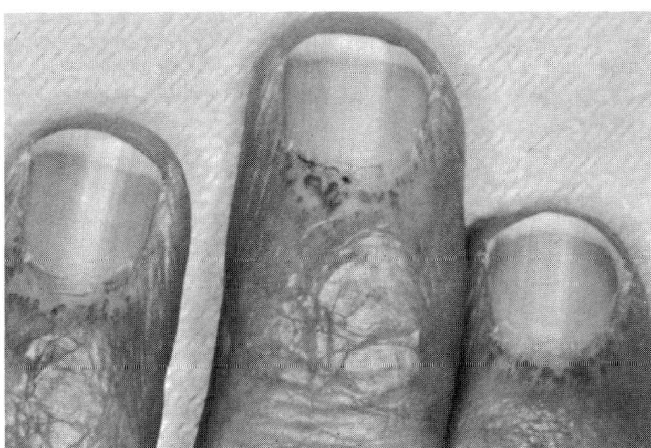

FIGURE 11–11. Dermatomyositis—nail fold changes. Cutaneous atrophy and prominent capillary loops alternating with areas of sclerosis at the proximal nail fold are typical of dermatomyositis and other connective tissue diseases.

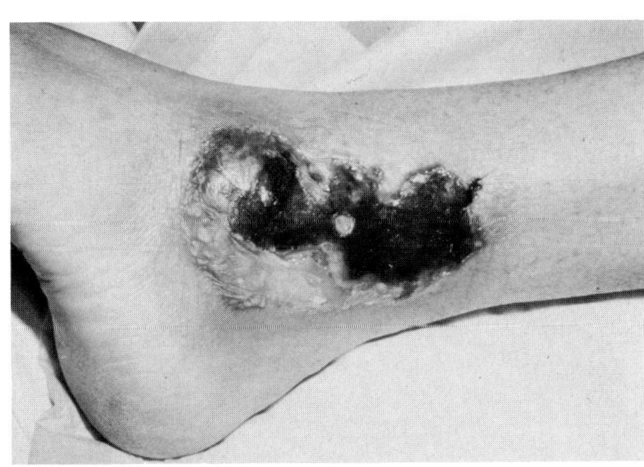

FIGURE 11–13. Rheumatoid arthritis—leg ulcer. This chronic cutaneous ulcer developed rapidly in this patient with rheumatoid vasculitis.

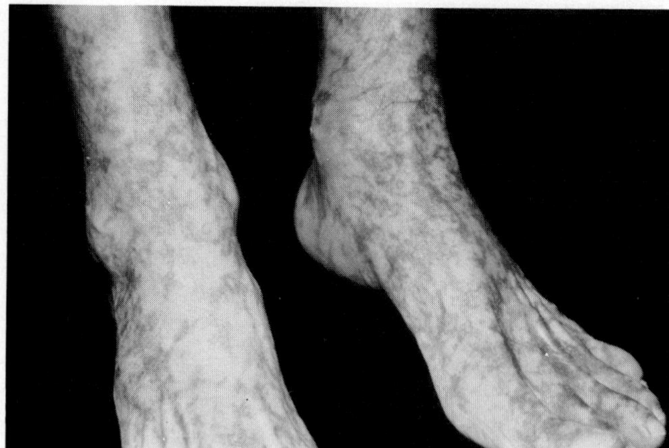

FIGURE 11–14. Livedo reticularis. Reddish-blue and hyperpigmented net-like mottling of the skin of the lower extremity may be associated with vasospastic or vasculitic conditions.

an abnormal immunoglobulin that appears to be involved in thrombotic disease affecting skin, coronary arteries, and the CNS. Livedo reticularis is also occasionally seen in the context of obstructive arterial disease, such as atheromatous microembolization; hematologic disorders including hyperviscosity syndromes; drug eruptions due to amantadine; and various other connective tissue diseases.

Leukocytoclastic Vasculitis

The term *leukocytoclastic vasculitis* is actually a histopathologic term that describes the association of an acute neutrophilic infiltrate involving the vessel wall of postcapillary venules, fibrin clots in the vascular lumina, and the presence of ''nuclear dust'' around and in the affected vessels. Extravasated red blood cells are often seen as well. The term *rheumatic vasculitis* is used by some authors when referring to vasculitis in a patient with any one of the connective tissue disorders, such as RA, Sjögren's syndrome, LE, dermatomyositis, or progressive systemic sclerosis. The clinical sine qua non of cutaneous vasculitis is palpable purpura (Fig. 11–15). These are nonblanching, usually 3- to 8-mm discrete or confluent bright red papules (raised above the surface of the surrounding skin). The nonblanching character of the lesions is caused by the extravasation of red blood cells through the vessel wall into the surrounding dermis. Occasionally, lesions are seen that are nodular, bullous, pustular, ulcerated, necrotic, in a livedo pattern, or any combination thereof (Figs. 11–16 to 11–18). An unusual variant is *urticarial vasculitis* seen in infections such as hepatitis B. These are similar to typical hives, but individual lesions persist for more than 48 hours on the skin. Patients with such an eruption should always be evaluated for hepatitis B, including serologic studies, liver function tests, and physical examination. *Henoch-Schönlein purpura* is a syndrome associated with a variant of leukocytoclastic vasculitis, which is usually seen in young men (Fig. 11–19). These patients present with vasculitis, most often presenting as palpable purpura of the lower legs, arthralgias, abdominal pain and diarrhea, and evidence of renal dysfunction. This condition generally is glomerulonephritis; thus, patients have hematuria and proteinuria. The renal involvement may occasionally be

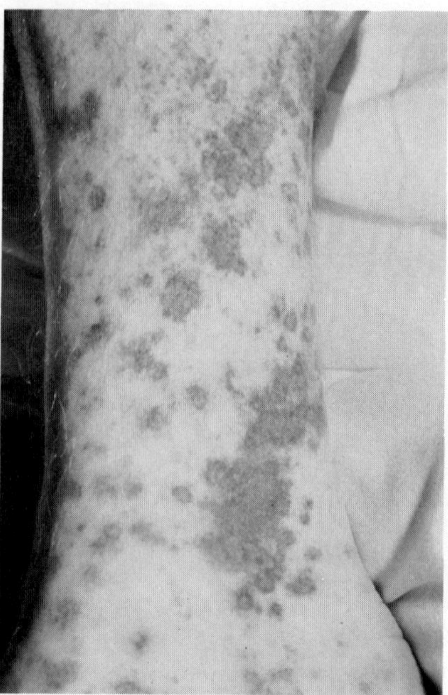

FIGURE 11–15. Leukocytoclastic vasculitis—palpable purpura. Nonblanching discrete and coalescent papules are the sine qua non of leukocytoclastic vasculitis.

severe. The diagnosis of Henoch-Schönlein purpura is usually clinical and is confirmed on skin or renal biopsy if necessary. The differential diagnosis includes other types of cutaneous and systemic vasculitis, such as those mentioned elsewhere in this chapter. Cutaneous vasculitis may also be associated with drug reactions, chronic bacterial infections, or as sequela to β-streptococcal infections. Infrequently, cutaneous vasculitis may be seen in the context of carcinoma or hematologic malignancies such as lymphoma and leukemia. Approximately 50% of cases are idiopathic and are not associated with any other discernible disease.

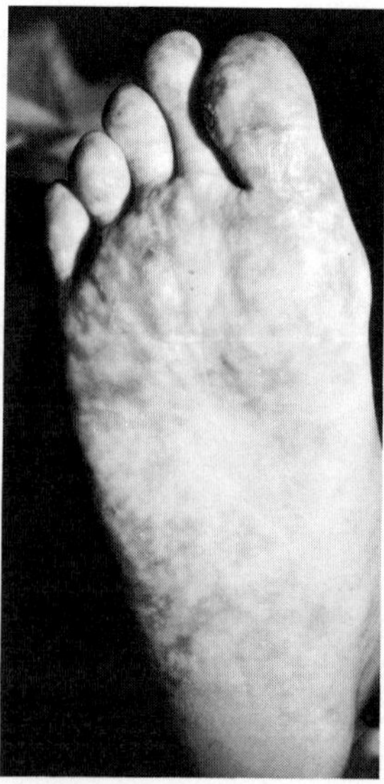

FIGURE 11–16. Leukocytoclastic vasculitis. Palpable purpura and ecchymotic plaques on the plantar surface may be exquisitely tender in some patients.

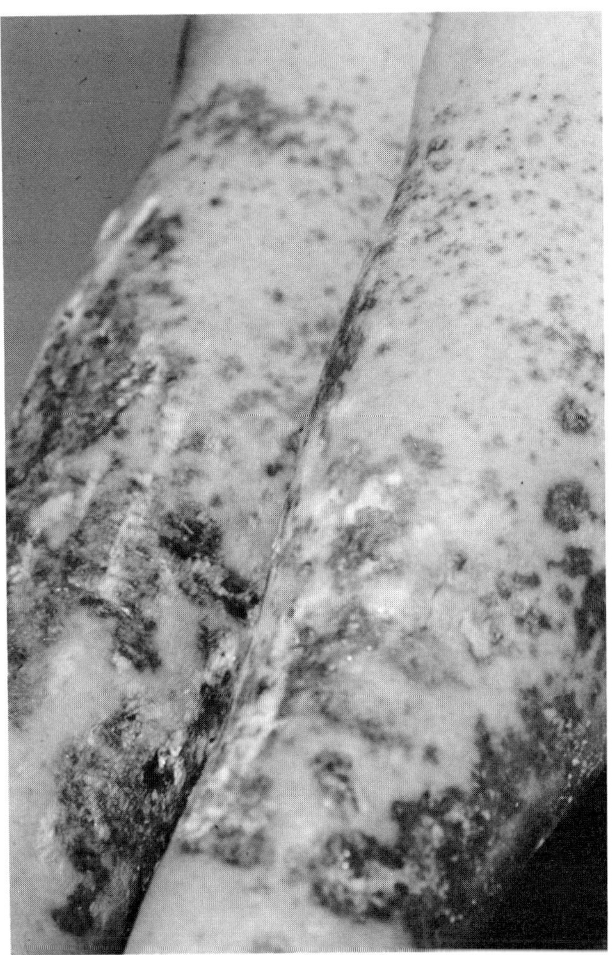

FIGURE 11–17. Leukocytoclastic vasculitis. Patients may present with or evolve toward hemorrhagic or necrotic plaques or bullae. Note the palpable purpura at the upper part of the photograph.

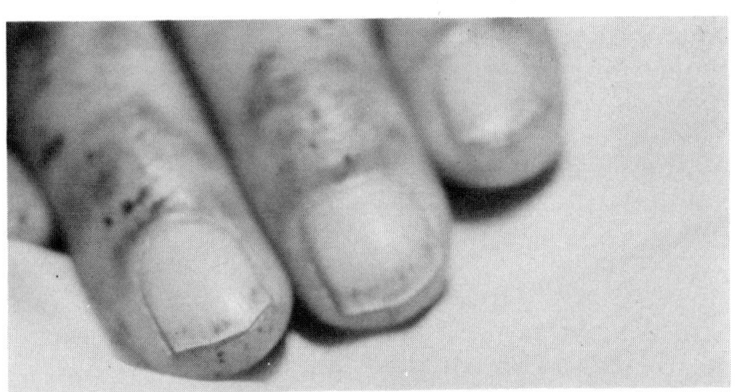

FIGURE 11–18. Leukocytoclastic vasculitis. Palpable purpura associated with cutaneous infarctions and subungual splinter hemorrhages are present in this patient with infective endocarditis.

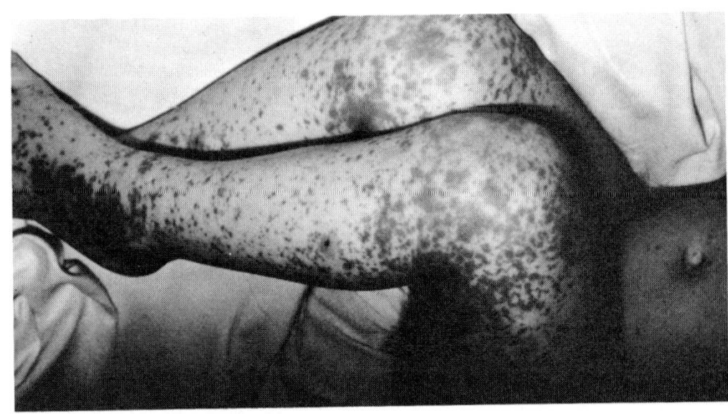

FIGURE 11–19. Henoch-Schönlein purpura. Palpable purpura is often restricted to the lower extremities and inferior trunk. Biopsy shows leukocytoclastic vasculitis.

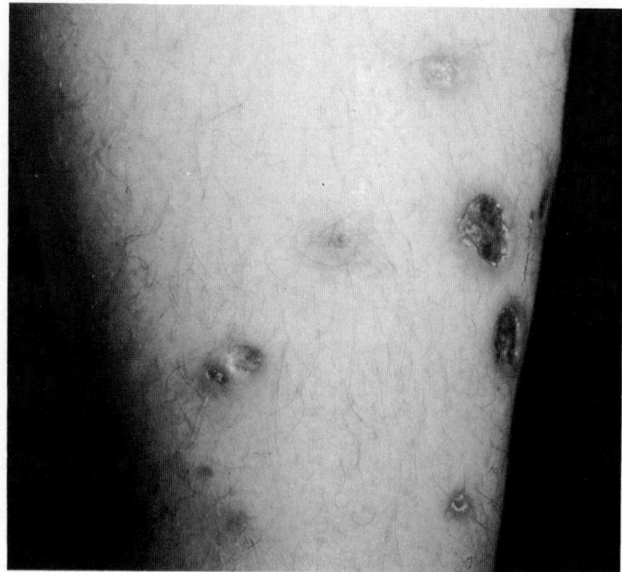

FIGURE 11–20. Cutaneous polyarteritis nodosa. Typical lesions include tender erythematous nodules and ulcerations.

Polyarteritis Nodosa

Cutaneous polyarteritis nodosa (PAN) is seen as tender or painful erythematous to skin-colored 2- to 20-mm deep subcutaneous nodules. These are most often found on the lower extremity, usually below the knee. Flares are often associated with myalgias, arthralgias, and occasionally fever, but nodules may occur anywhere on the trunk or extremities. Lesions may become ulcerated, hemorrhagic, or necrotic resulting from vasculitis-induced ischemia of the skin (Figs. 11–20 and 11–21). Biopsies of the lesions should be done by inci-

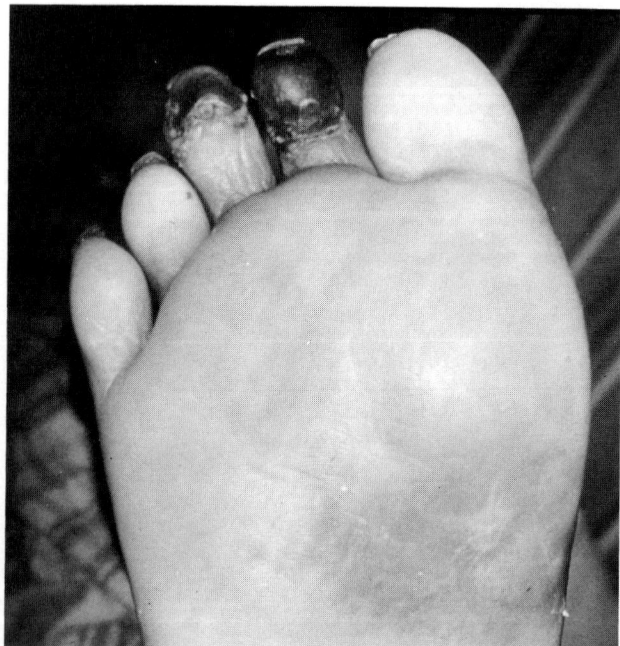

FIGURE 11–21. Cutaneous polyarteritis nodosa. Tender, painful nodules may appear on the plantar surface. Note the infarcted digits caused by vascular occlusion.

sional technique and not by punch technique, because the histologic changes occur in the medium- and small-sized arteries at the dermosubcutaneous junction. Punch biopsies often do not contain enough subcutaneous tissue to make a diagnosis. Biopsy is needed to differentiate PAN from other panniculitides such as erythema nodosum.

Cutaneous PAN is generally considered to be a benign variant of systemic PAN. In the systemic form, necrotizing inflammation involves the noncapillary blood vessels in single or multiple organs leading to vascular occlusion or aneurysm formation. Lesions may be seen in any organ except the lung and are not generally associated with cutaneous disease.

Cryoglobulinemia

Cryoglobulins are abnormal, circulating immunoglobulins. Detectable plasma titers may be seen in autoimmune diseases and in malignancies such as multiple myeloma. These proteins are soluble at body temperature and tend to precipitate as the local temperature is lowered. Precipitation occurs usually in acral and thus cooler structures such as fingers, toes, nose, and earlobes (Fig. 11–22). The presence of these precipitated immunoglobulins causes an increase in the viscosity of the blood leading to "protein plugs" in the small vessels. This causes ischemia, secondary hemorrhage, and eventually necrosis. Gangrene and loss of digits may occur. Skin ulcers on the lower leg are also occasionally seen. A search for underlying neoplasms and autoimmune disorders such as SLE is warranted if cryoglobulins are detected in the patient's blood. Occasionally, cryoglobulinemia may be idiopathic.

Reiter's Syndrome

Reiter's syndrome or *Reiter's disease* is classically defined as the triad of nongonococcal urethritis, conjunctivitis, and arthritis. Mucocutaneous lesions are seen commonly enough to support the notion of a clinical "tetrad." The American Rheumatologic Association, however, has adopted the definition of Reiter's syndrome as "an episode of peripheral arthritis greater than one month's duration occurring in association with urethritis and/or cervicitis." It is currently

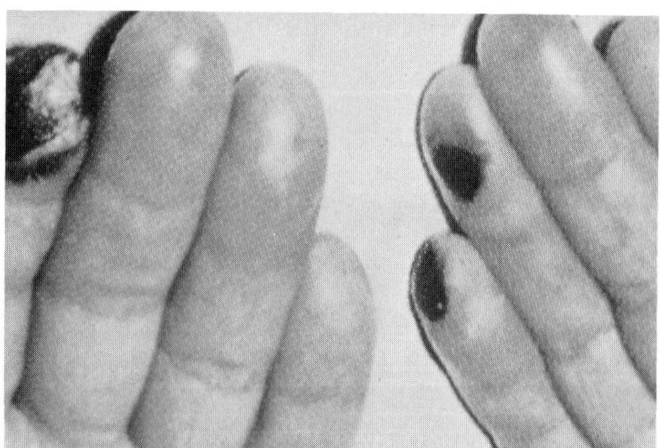

FIGURE 11–22. Cryoglobulinemia. Precipitation of abnormal immunoglobulins in small acral vessels leads to infarction and gangrene.

believed that the arthritis is of a reactive nature, possibly in response to sexually transmitted diseases such as chlamydia in a genetically predisposed population. There is a higher frequency of the presence of the HLA-B27 histocompatibility antigen in patients with Reiter's syndrome. It affects men more frequently than women. These men are usually from 15 to 35 years of age.

In addition to the mucocutaneous lesions seen in conjunctivitis and urethritis, the cutaneous manifestations of Reiter's include *keratoderma blennorrhagicum* (Fig. 11–23). This disorder is usually thick, scaling, often erythematous plaques distributed over a portion of most of the plantar surfaces, palmar surfaces, and occasionally over the ankles. The lesions may closely resemble those of palmoplantar pustular psoriasis and may be severe or debilitating. More extensive lesions are sometimes found in a psoriasiform distribution: elbows, knees, groin, scalp, or penis *(circinate balanitis)*. Pathologically, these lesions may be indistinguishable from psoriasis.

Sjögren's Syndrome

Since being described by Sjögren in 1933, the triad of *keratoconjunctivitis sicca, xerostoma,* and *RA* has been termed *Sjögren's syndrome.* The sicca complex (xerostoma and keratoconjunctivitis) can be seen in many of the autoimmune diseases. The syndrome is most common in middle-aged women. Clinical manifestations of Sjögren's syndrome appear to be the result of abnormally decreased function of the body's exocrine glands. The glands of the oral and ocular mucosa are the most commonly and severely affected, but almost any mucosal or mucocutaneous surface can be involved as may the exocrine pancreas. Cutaneous manifestations also include itchy, dry skin and decreased sweating; itchy, dry "gritty" eyes; and light sensitivity. Patients may present with the sicca complex and Raynaud's syndrome (see Fig. 11–1) or cutaneous vasculitis that is often evident on podiatric examination. Vasculitis of the foot or lower leg may first come to the podiatrist's attention as an ulcer that will not heal. Cryoglobulinemia (see Fig. 11–22) has also been reported with Sjögren's syndrome. A full history and physical examination should be performed as well as laboratory evaluation of serologic studies, chemistries, and complete blood count. Thus, a patient who presents with lower leg ulcers, a history of arthritis, and, on further questioning, dry eyes and dry mouth should be suspected of having either isolated Sjögren's syndrome or some overlap syndrome involving other connective tissue diseases.

METABOLIC AND ENDOCRINE DISORDERS

Metabolic diseases are those in which specific metabolic abnormalities of cells, tissues, organs, or organ systems have been identified or suspected. Endocrine disorders are those that are primarily caused by defects in endocrine glandular tissue and hormone transport or activity. Endocrine and metabolic diseases may also overlap, because endocrine function is intimately involved in metabolic processes in almost all organ systems. A number of metabolic and endocrine diseases have cutaneous manifestations. The skin of the lower extremity, and the foot in particular, is frequently affected. Certain endocrinopathies such as diabetes mellitus may first present to the podiatrist as a neuropathic foot even before the patient has been identified as diabetic. Myxedema affecting the lower leg might be recognized by the podiatrist in a patient with undiagnosed thyroid disease. Gout is frequently seen in general practice. The podiatrist must work closely with other specialists to offer patients the best and broadest therapeutic approaches to these sometimes devastating diseases. Hyperlipidemia syndromes can be identified clinically in patients with xanthomas, leading to potentially lifesaving intervention.

Diabetes Mellitus

Diabetes is the most common serious endocrine-metabolic disorder. Long-term complications of diabetes may affect virtually every organ system. The skin is commonly affected in patients with diabetes. The pathogenesis of some of the cutaneous diseases associated with diabetes is poorly understood and is still considered idiopathic. Other disorders of the skin in diabetic patients are directly attributable to specific pathologic processes such as neuropathy, microangiopathy, vascular insufficiency, increased susceptibility to certain infections, and abnormal processes such as lipid transport and metabolism.

The basic description of the pathophysiology, chemistry, and metabolic and mechanical abnormalities seen in diabetic foot disease is beyond the scope of this chapter. It is aptly presented in other sections of this book. This chapter deals only with the clinical cutaneous lesions associated with diabetes mellitus. These include diabetic ulcers of the foot, necrobiosis lipoidica diabeticorum, bullous diabeticorum, angiopathy leading to skin disease, and infections of the diabetic foot. More purely metabolic disorders such as xanthomas in the hyperlipidemic diabetic patient are described elsewhere in this chapter.

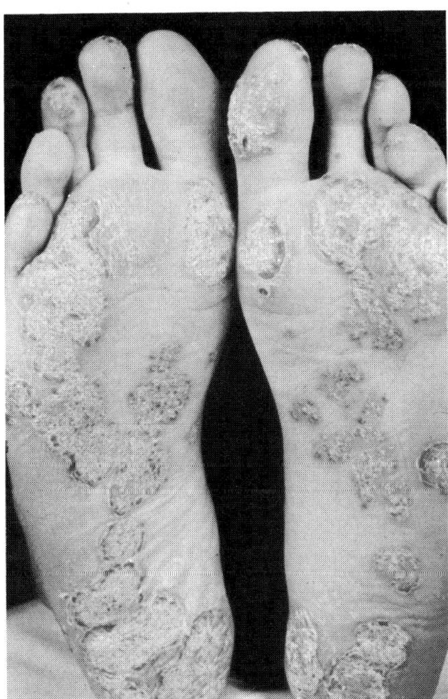

FIGURE 11–23. Reiter's syndrome—keratoderma blennorrhagicum. Typical symmetrical, thick, scaling, discrete, and coalescent psoriasiform plaques are present on the plantar surfaces.

The neuropathy of the diabetic foot is the cause of extensive disability in affected patients. It may be motor, sensory, or both in origin; it predisposes to trauma and ulceration of the foot. These ulcerations are often chronic, deep lesions of the skin that are commonly refractory to most therapies currently available. Lesions may appear anywhere on the foot but commonly occur in areas predisposed to local trauma such as the heel, plantar metatarsal areas, and toes. Custom-made footwear is essential in these patients to reduce mechanical trauma and to redistribute weight in the foot. Ulcers are of varying size but may eventually involve large areas of the foot. They are generally nontender due to the underlying sensory neuropathy that contributes to the chronicity of the lesions. The depth of the ulcers ranges from superficial dermal ulceration in earlier or uncomplicated cases to the all too common deep ulcerations extending to fascia, muscle, or even bone. Aggressive attempts to heal these lesions with sophisticated biologically active dressings may result in complete resolution of the ulcer. Often, however, the healing does not progress beyond the stage of granulation tissue. Ulcers are commonly secondarily infected with bacterial pathogens. These typically include organisms such as *Staphylococcus aureus*, coliforms, and *Pseudomonas*. More unusual organisms are found in some patients either as the dominant infecting bacteria or as part of mixed flora in the wound. Diabetic patients also have an abnormally high incidence of fungal infections compared with the nondiabetic population. *Candida*, which can be isolated from the ulcers, may identify the patient as diabetic even before the demonstration of hyperglycemia.

Necrobiosis lipoidica diabeticorum (NLD) is an eruption that may be seen in diabetics. Of the well-defined cutaneous disorders associated with diabetes, NLD is perhaps the best documented. It occurs in women three times more commonly than in men. About one third of patients have clinically obvious diabetes mellitus; one third have only abnormal glucose tolerance but normal fasting glucose; and about one third of patients have no clinical or laboratory evidence of diabetes, although some of these patients later develop diabetes. All patients with NLD should be evaluated for the presence of diabetes. The characteristic distribution is on the pretibial surfaces of either one or both lower legs (Fig. 11–24). Lesions may be single or multiple and discrete or confluent. Lesions on the trunk and upper extremities can also occur but are distinctly less common. Early lesions usually appear as well-defined dusky erythematous papules or nodules. The lesions enlarge slowly, and the borders become more irregular. As the lesions develop, they become well-circumscribed yellow to brown patches that show pronounced atrophy and depression of the skin. The peripheral borders are often erythematous and sometimes raised. The lesions tend to become more brownish yellow as they mature. The characteristic yellow hue and red border remain to some extent and are useful diagnostic signs for NLD. Over time, the patches of NLD may ulcerate and become tender and painful. The ulcers are usually shallow and generally progress slowly. In more severely affected patients, the spectrum of lesions may spread to involve most of the anterior lower leg. Histologically, the lesions of NLD show sclerosis of the dermal collagen surrounded by inflammatory infiltrate. The dermal collagen appears as characteristically acellular, eosinophilic areas called *necrobiosis*. The fully formed le-

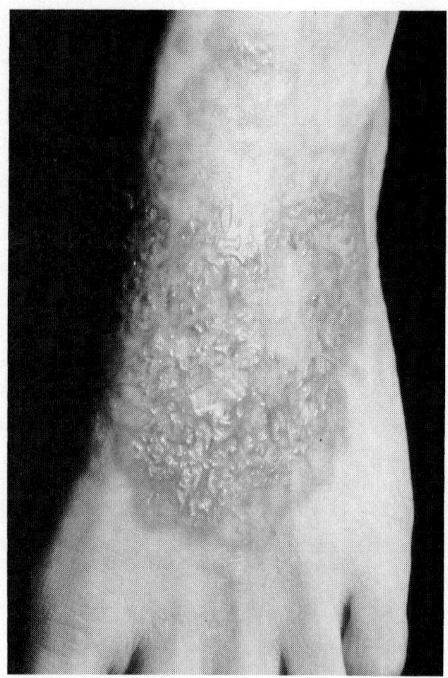

FIGURE 11–24. Necrobiosis lipoidica diabeticorum. Lesions are typically on the pretibial area but may extend onto the dorsal feet. Note the yellowish, atrophic, depressed central region and erythematous, irregular, advancing inferior border.

sions show pallisading granulomas, dermal sclerosis, and destruction of adnexal structures such as hair follicles and sweat glands.

Lesions of NLD do not seem to improve significantly with better control of blood glucose levels in diabetic patients. There are currently no well-studied effective therapies for NLD. Intralesional or ultrapotent topical corticosteroid seems to have some benefit in preventing the progression of the lesions. There is anecdotal evidence of the effectiveness of aspirin and dipyridamole or pentoxifylline (Trental) in these patients. Semipermeable and bio-occlusive dressings such as DuoDerm, Restore, Op-Site, Vigilon, and others have been used with some success in treating the ulcerated lesions of NLD. Surgical excision of the lesions is not advisable and is often followed by a recurrence.

Bullosis diabeticorum, or diabetic bullae, is seen primarily on the lower extremities, especially the feet. They appear spontaneously as tense bullae. The underlying cause of this uncommon condition is not currently well understood, although abnormalities of the basement membrane zone have been suggested. Neither immunologic mechanisms nor trauma have been demonstrated in the pathogenesis of these lesions. Most patients with diabetic bullae also have retinopathy. Therapy should be conservative and directed toward facilitating re-epithelialization of existing lesions as well as good control of hyperglycemia.

Diabetic dermopathy, although not specific for diabetes, occurs in elderly diabetic patients. Men are affected about twice as often as women. It is characterized by the presence of generally asymptomatic, hyperpigmented, atrophic patches predominantly on the anterior lower legs (Fig. 11–25). These may start as grouped erythematous, occasionally scaly papules that slowly coalesce. Individual lesions tend to appear in crops and resolve in 1 to 3 years. The fairly constant

FIGURE 11–25. Diabetic dermopathy. Lesions may be hyperpigmented and atrophic, as seen on the lateral foot of this patient with insulin-dependent diabetes.

appearance of new lesions gives the impression of relatively static disease. Diabetic dermopathy can look like post-traumatic scarring, but patients fail to give a history of actual trauma to the area. Histologically, these lesions show thickening of the vessel walls associated with a lymphocytic infiltrate. They are distinguishable from lesions of NLD, which they may resemble clinically, by the absence of distinctive changes in dermal collagen. About half of patients with diabetic dermopathy also have evidence of microangiopathy elsewhere, such as retinopathy, nephropathy, and neuropathy.

Vascular changes in diabetics may take the form of microangiopathy or large vessel disease. Changes due to small vessel disease are described earlier (e.g., diabetic dermopathy and NLD). Large vessel disease and microangiopathy associated with atherosclerosis may lead to dry gangrene (Fig. 11–26). Peripheral vascular pathology also leads to leg and foot ulcers. Even minor local infection with *Tinea* or *Candida* in macerated toe web spaces may initiate an inexorable progression toward cutaneous bacterial infection, osteomyelitis, and eventually amputation of the affected foot or even the leg. Patients with intermittent claudication or foot pain at rest are at high risk for this kind of scenario and need to be evaluated carefully. Consultation with a vascular surgeon may be necessary.

Skin infections in the diabetic foot are all too common. Poorly controlled or undiagnosed diabetics appear to have a significantly increased risk of certain bacterial and fungal infections. The well-controlled diabetic may be at somewhat greater risk for these infections, but conclusive studies have not been done. Acute mucocutaneous candidal infections are difficult to control and recur in these patients. *Candidal paronychia* is seen more frequently in poorly controlled diabetics (Fig. 11–27). It presents as chronic nail matrix dystrophy leading to nail ridging and loss of the cuticle. More acute candidal paronychias tend to be proximal in location as opposed to dermatophyte and bacterial paronychias that are more lateral or distal. In addition to scrupulous and aggressive local care, treatment often requires systemic antifungal therapy with imidazole antifungals (e.g., ketoconazole or fluconazole) and is greatly enhanced by control of the hyperglycemia. Secondary infection with gram-positive or gram-negative organisms may occur. Dermatophyte infection in the diabetic foot may be devastating by facilitating the entry of more dangerous organisms into the skin. Primary *pyodermas* due to *Staphylococcus aureus* and β-hemolytic *Streptococcus* may progress rapidly and be difficult to control owing to local inhibition of neutrophil function. *Impetigo, erysipelas, cellulitis, folliculitis, and furunculosis* are common. Antistaphylococcal antibiotics such as erythromycin, certain cephalosporins, and the newer quinolones are usually the drugs of choice. Intravenous antibiotic therapy may be necessary. Patients may be chronic carriers of *Staphylococcus aureus* in the nasopharynx. *Erythrasma* is a superficial infection of the skin caused by the gram-negative bacteria *Corynebacterium minutissimum* (Fig. 11–28). It typically occurs in the web spaces of obese diabetic patients. Wood's lamp examination shows a highly characteristic coral-pink fluores-

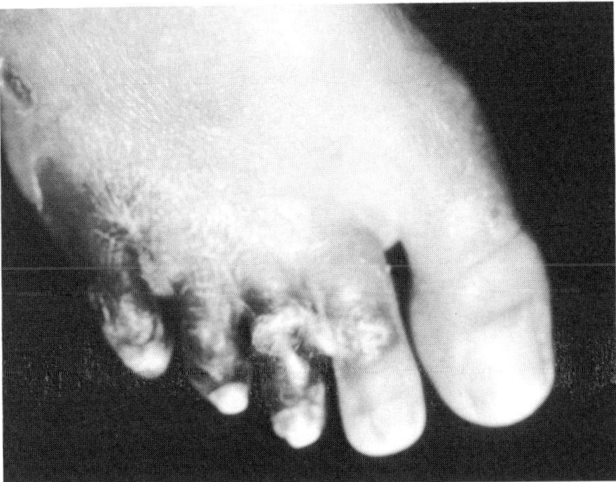

FIGURE 11–26. Diabetic dermopathy. Notice the peripheral erythema and scaling associated with the more distal inflammation, infarction, and gangrene.

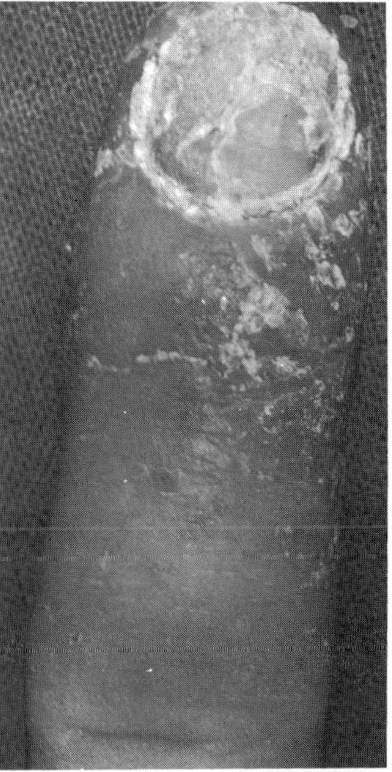

FIGURE 11–27. Candidal paronychia. The distal digit, proximal nail fold, and the entire nail plate are infected by *Candida albicans* in this patient with diabetes. Similar changes may be seen on the toes.

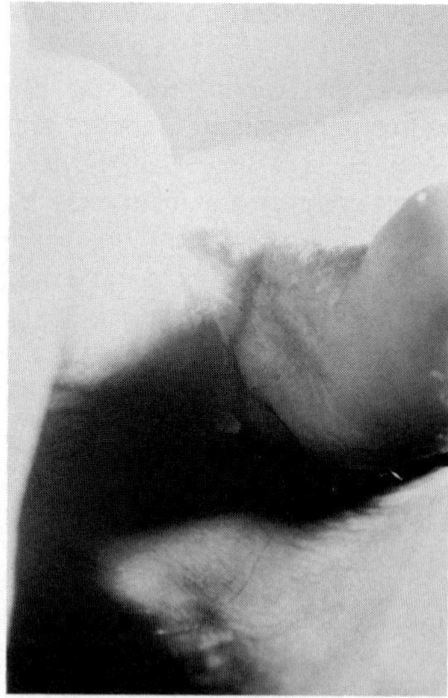

FIGURE 11–28. Interdigital erythrasma. Although clinically similar to or associated with interdigital tinea pedis, lesions tend to be more macerated and odoriferous than tinea alone.

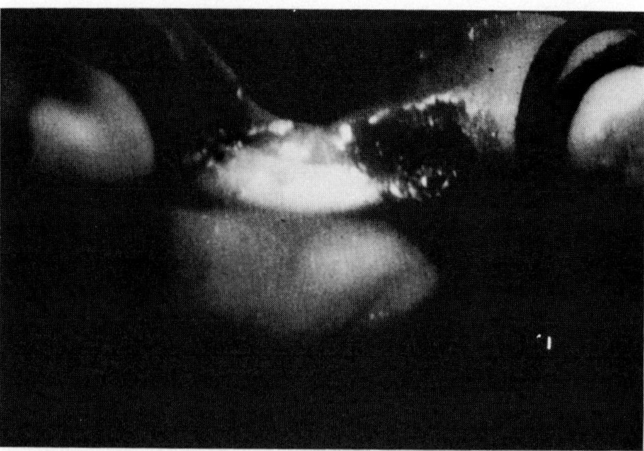

FIGURE 11–29. Interdigital erythrasma—Wood's lamp examination. Shining a Wood's lamp on the infected area reveals the typical coral red-orange fluorescence of *Corynebacterium minutissimum.*

cence owing to a porphyrin produced by the bacteria (Fig. 11–29). Treatment with topical or oral erythromycin or topical clindamycin is usually effective. In general, the concept of tight control of hyperglycemia, newer antibiotics, and better understanding of foot care and prevention of infection have significantly decreased morbidity and mortality in these patients.

Thyroid Disease

Abnormalities in the functioning of the thyroid gland or any part of the hypothalamic-pituitary-thyroid axis may lead to cutaneous manifestations of thyroid disease. Various abnormalities of skin, hair, and nails may be seen in both hypothyroidism and hyperthyroidism.

Hypothyroidism is caused by decreased availability of thyroid hormone. Like hyperthyroidism, it is more common in women, generally in their fifth to seventh decades. Systemic symptoms include weakness, fatigue, lethargy, weight gain, cold intolerance, and constipation. The skin is generally cold, dry, rough, coarse, and pale. Bogginess and edema are also seen. Primary deposition of acid mucopolysaccharides such as hyaluronic acid in the dermis leads to nonpitting edema called *myxedema* (Fig. 11–30). This accumulation is most obvious in the skin but also occurs in internal organs. The typical distribution of myxedema is in the pretibial area, tongue, lips, around the eyes, and acral regions. Pretibial myxedema may be easier to feel than to see. Enlarged follicular openings impart a "pig skin" appearance to the skin-colored plaques (Fig. 11–31). These lesions are most often initially asymptomatic but may become pruritic as they enlarge. The entire lower leg may be involved followed by verrucous hyperplasia at the dependent limits of the plaques. Patients may present with papules, nodules, or plaques limited to the feet or legs. Pretibial myxedema is also seen in patients with a history of Graves' disease, with or without

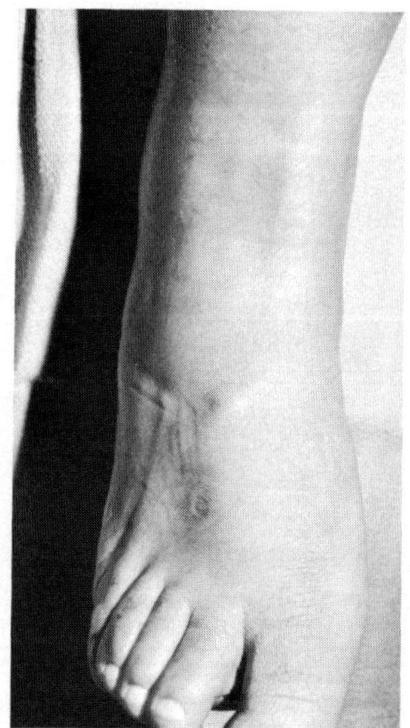

FIGURE 11–30. Pretibial myxedema. Boggy nonpitting edema is apparent over the pretibial area and extends onto the dorsal foot in this hypothyroid patient.

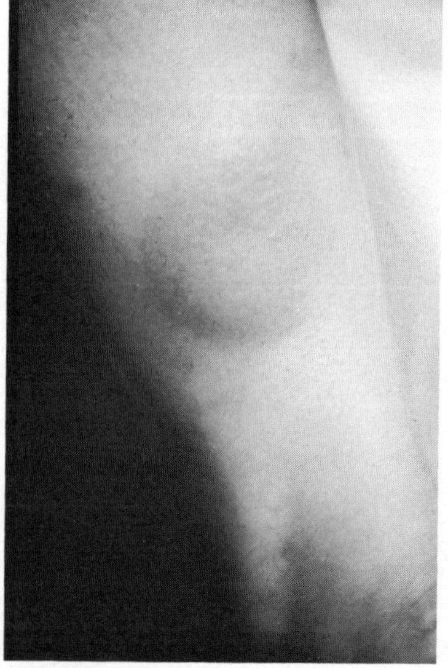

FIGURE 11–31. Pretibial myxedema. Patulous follicular openings in infiltrated areas of skin lead to a "pig skin" appearance in this patient with hypothyroidism.

concurrent hyperthyroidism. Ichthyosis and palmoplantar hyperkeratosis may be severe in addition to generally dry skin. Ichthyosis of the skin of the lower extremity is commonly found in patients with severe hypothyroidism. Patients may also present with easy bruisability due to capillary fragility. Infrequently, eruptive xanthomas may occur in hypothyroid patients with hyperlipidemia. The hair in hypothyroidism tends to be dull, coarse, brittle, and dry. Hair grows slowly and may be lost in certain areas such as the lateral third of the eyebrows. Nails in these patients are thin, dry, brittle, striated, and slow growing.

Patients with *hyperthyroidism* may also have abnormalities of the skin, hair, and nails. *Graves' disease* accounts for more than 85% of hyperthyroid disease. Other causes include toxic multinodular goiter, subacute thyroiditis, autoimmune thyroiditis, and ectopic production of thyroid hormone by nonthyroid tumors. General systemic effects of hyperthyroidism include nervousness, tremor, weight loss, heat intolerance, hyperhidrosis, emotional lability, muscle weakness, and palpitations. Graves' disease is quite common and may affect as much as 2% of the general female population. It consists of diffuse enlargement of the thyroid gland associated with elevated levels of thyroid hormone and, occasionally, pretibial myxedema. Pretibial myxedema is uncommon in Graves' disease, occurring in only 1% to 3% of cases. It may be seen in patients weeks to years after surgical or radioactive iodine therapy for the hyperthyroidism. Patients may be euthyroid at the time of onset of pretibial myxedema. The skin of patients with hyperthyroidism tends to be fine, velvety or smooth, and warm and moist. Localized hyperpigmentation, vitiligo, pruritus, urticaria and dermatographism, palmar erythema, and facial flushing may also be seen. Hyperhidrosis of the palms and soles occurs despite generally dry skin. The hair in hyperthyroid patients is thin, fine, and straight. Alopecia areata and mild diffuse hair loss have been described in these patients. Nail abnormalities include onycholysis, koilonychia, and clubbing.

Gout

Gout is a systemic metabolic disorder due to abnormal metabolism and excretion of purines and their metabolites. This results in elevated serum uric acid levels and, eventu-

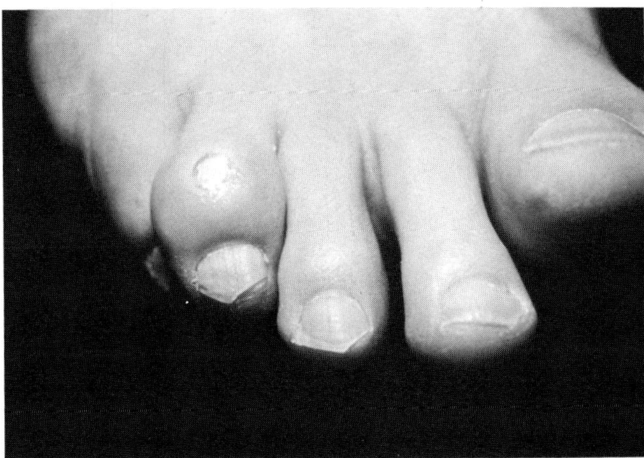

FIGURE 11–33. Gout—tophus on the toe. This typical tophus has begun to break down and extrude chalky material containing crystals of monosodium urate.

ally, the deposition of monosodium urate crystals in various tissues, particularly joints, periarticular tissues, skin, kidneys, and bones (Fig. 11–32). Hyperuricemia may result from increased production or decreased excretion of uric acid. The major clinical consequences of monosodium urate crystal deposition occur as a result of inflammation and eventual destruction of the affected tissues. This leads to episodes of acute arthritis and to the production of tophi and end-organ disease such as nephropathy.

An acute attack of gout is typically seen in men 30 to 40 years of age who give a history of the sudden onset of several hours of acute severe articular pain, usually involving a peripheral joint. In classic *podagra,* the arthritis appears in the first metatarsophalangeal joint. The area is erythematous, swollen, and exquisitely tender. Aspiration of joint fluid reveals the presence of uric acid crystals showing the typical negative birefringence pattern under the polarizing microscope. Local inflammation may resemble cellulitis, although no infection is present. If left untreated, the symptoms disappear spontaneously over several weeks, leaving no apparent sequelae. It remains in remission from months to years. If the patient's hyperuricemia is not treated, the symptoms will return. The natural history of gout is one of recurrent attacks in different joints more and more frequently. The overlying skin may become violaceous, hyperpigmented and scaly. Eventually, the interval between episodes becomes shorter and shorter until the patient has *chronic tophaceous gout* with no intercritical periods. By this stage, the inflammation has begun to erode bone and cartilage and cause renal disease, which further reduces excretion of already chronically elevated serum uric acid.

The primary cutaneous lesions seen in gout are nontender, intradermal, or subcutaneous nodules called *tophi* (Fig. 11–33). The tophaceous deposit often shows a salmon-pink coloration of the overlying skin. On palpation they may appear somewhat fluctuant or firm. These commonly appear in tissue over the helix of the ear, olecranon surface of the elbow, and prepatellar bursae. Tophi may also occur in acral sites over tendons of the hands or feet (Fig. 11–34). When these lesions are large, they may have a white chalky discharge that consists of monosodium urate crystals with the typical anisotropic birefringence under polarization microscopy. Speci-

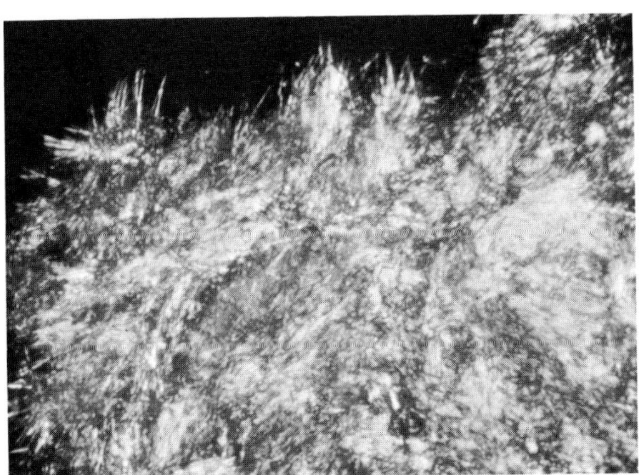

FIGURE 11–32. Gout—polarized microscopy of monosodium urate crystals. The typical negative birefringence of the crystals taken from a tophaceous lesion is evident.

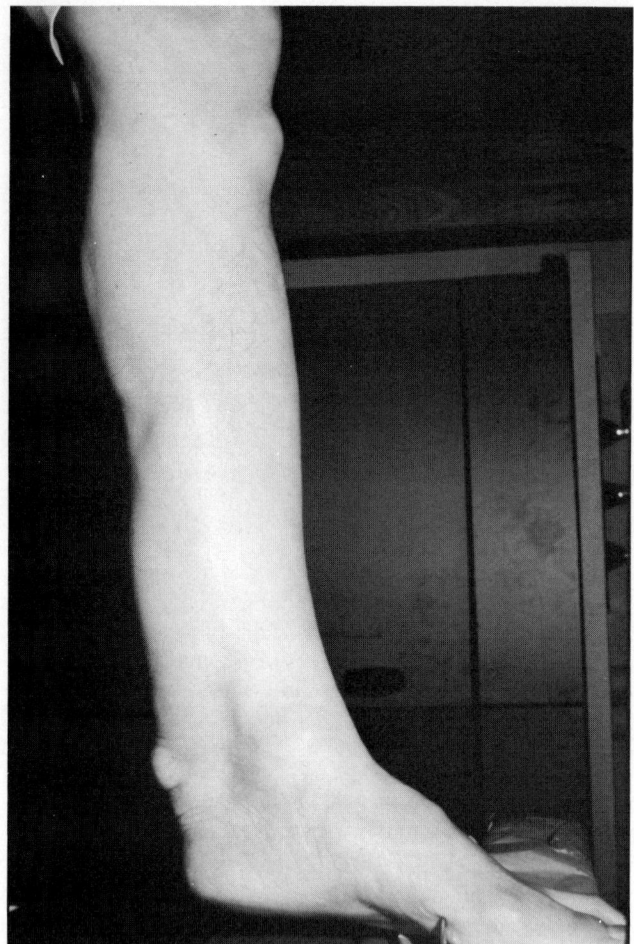

FIGURE 11–34. Gout. Tophi may appear on the lower extremities, usually in a periarticular location, and occasionally over tendons. These must be differentiated from the lesions of tuberous xanthomas or rheumatoid nodules.

mens must be fixed in alcohol and not formalin to preserve the crystals. Tophi must be differentiated from other periarticular subcutaneous nodules, including rheumatoid nodules and xanthomas.

Patients may also present with fever, malaise, leukocytosis, proteinuria, and elevated sedimentation rate. Elevated serum uric acid is a constant. Abnormal renal function (gouty nephropathy) may be seen in long-standing chronic gout.

Therapy in gout is directed toward terminating the acute attack, preventing recurrences, and avoiding complications of chronic tophaceous gout. Colchicine is the most frequently used medication in acute gouty arthritis. Agents such as indomethacin and other nonsteroidal anti-inflammatory drugs are also useful. Occasionally, oral or intra-articular corticosteroids may be indicated. Neither allopurinol nor uricosuric drugs are useful in the treatment of acute gouty arthritis. Prophylaxis of attacks of acute gouty arthritis may be achieved with colchicine, although this does not reduce serum uric acid and thus does not prevent the manifestations of chronic tophaceous gout and associated organ system disease. Antihyperuricemic drugs are used to lower serum uric acid levels. These include probenecid, sulfinpyrizone, and allopurinol. Hydration and alkalinization of the urine are also helpful in patients with gouty nephropathy.

Xanthomas

Xanthomas are a manifestation of abnormal lipid metabolism and transport. They are localized accumulations of "foamy" histiocytes containing abnormal lipids (Fig. 11–35). The underlying metabolic diseases that are associated with most xanthomas are called *dyslipoproteinemias*. A frequent clinical expression of dyslipoproteinemia is deposits of lipoprotein components in the skin, subcutaneous tissues, and tendons. These are termed *xanthomas*. A detailed description of the specific hereditary syndromes of dyslipoproteinemias, dyslipidemias, and xanthomatoses is beyond the scope of this chapter.

Xanthomas associated with the dyslipoproteinemias are generally classified into tendinous, tuberous, eruptive, and palmoplantar or planar types. The major lipid, cholesterol ester, is stored intracellularly except in tendinous xanthomas, which frequently contain extracellular cholesterol crystals. Specific syndromes are classified according to the particular type of lipid-lipoprotein abnormality, the associated type of xanthoma, and the associated risk of early cardiovascular or pancreatic disease. Table 11–2 lists the major syndromes associated with xanthomas.

The presence of any xanthomatous lesions should alert the clinician to search for underlying abnormalities in plasma lipids or lipoproteins as well as evidence of cardiovascular disease. Patients may occasionally have normal total cholesterol and fasting triglyceride levels but will have abnormal cholesterol subtype distribution on serum electrophoresis, which the clinician should always order when evaluating these patients.

Tendinous xanthomas are caused by the infiltration of lipid in tendons, ligaments, and fascia (Fig. 11–36). Most often they affect the extensor tendons of the hands, elbows, knees, and Achilles tendons. The lesions tend to be nontender, smooth, firm, subcutaneous nodules. The overlying skin is normal and is not fixed to the underlying xanthoma. Elevated cholesterol is the major lipid abnormality in tendinous xanthomas, which may be associated with other xanthomatous lesions of the skin such as xanthalasma and tuberous xanthomas. *Cerebrotendinous xanthomatosis* is a rare disease in which tendinous xanthomas are associated with an accumulation of lipids in the brain and tissues other than the skin.

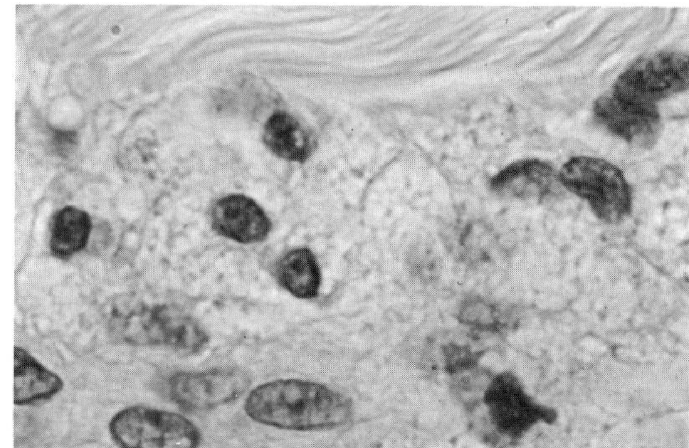

FIGURE 11–35. Xanthoma—histopathology. Numerous "foamy histiocytes" are seen in this xanthomatous lesion. The "foam" consists of microglobules of lipid within the cells.

TABLE 11–2

MAJOR SYNDROMES ASSOCIATED WITH VARIOUS XANTHOMAS

Syndrome	Associated Xanthoma	Predominant Lipoprotein	Incidence	Clinical Features
Homozygous atherosclerotic familial hypercholesterolemia	Xanthelasma Tendinous Tuberous	LDL	1/1,000,000	Onset in first or second decade
Familial dys-β-lipoproteinemia type III	Palmar Tuberoeruptive Tuberous Xanthelasma	Chylomicron VLDL	1/10,000	Premature atherosclerosis Peripheral vascular disease
Heterozygous familial hypercholesterolemia	Tendinous Tuberous Xanthelasma	LDL	1/500	Premature atherosclerosis
Familial hyperlipoproteinemia type V	Eruptive	VLDL Chylomicron	1/7500	Pancreatitis Diabetes mellitus Hypertension Hyperuricemia Polyneuropathy Premature atherosclerosis?
Lipoprotein lipase deficiency	Eruptive	Chylomicron	Rare	Lipemia retinalis Hepatosplenomegaly Pancreatitis

LDL, low-density lipoprotein; VLDL, very low-density lipoprotein.

Adapted from Cruz PD Jr, East C, and Bergstresser PR: Dermal, subcutaneous and tendon xanthomas: Diagnostic markers for specific lipoprotein disorders. J Am Acad Dermatol 19(1):95–111, 1988.

Patients exhibit progressive cerebellar ataxia, dementia, subnormal intelligence, and cataracts.

Tuberous xanthomas appear most often on the extensor surfaces of the body (Fig. 11–37). Elbows, knees, and buttocks are common sites. Lesions initially appear as small (1 to 3 mm), nontender, soft, skin-colored to red-yellow papules. The lesions may eventually coalesce into large globular masses, especially over bony prominences. Lipid abnormalities include elevated plasma cholesterol and may involve elevated levels of triglycerides as well. Tuberous xanthomas may be seen in patients with poorly controlled diabetes mellitus associated with hypertriglyceridemia. This particular syndrome is found in patients who have a highly significant risk of premature and severe atherosclerotic cardiovascular disease.

Eruptive xanthomas usually appear suddenly as crops of small (1 to 4 mm), soft, yellow papules surrounded by an erythematous halo around their base (Fig. 11–38). Most commonly they are found over the extensor surfaces of the arms, legs, and buttocks. Occasionally they may be more diffusely distributed over the mucous membranes and truncal skin. The predominant abnormal lipid found in these lesions is triglyceride.

Palmoplantar or *planar xanthomas* are the most common type of xanthomas. They may be seen as *xanthelasmas* (Fig. 11–39), *xanthoma striatum palmare* (Fig. 11–40), and *diffuse plane xanthomas*. In general, they are smooth, soft, yellowish, flat to slightly palpable lesions. Xanthelasmas occur on or around the eyelids. Approximately half of patients with

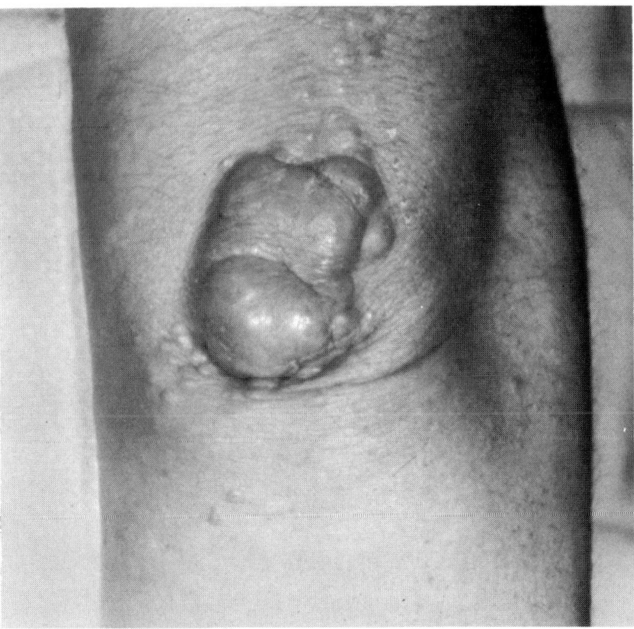

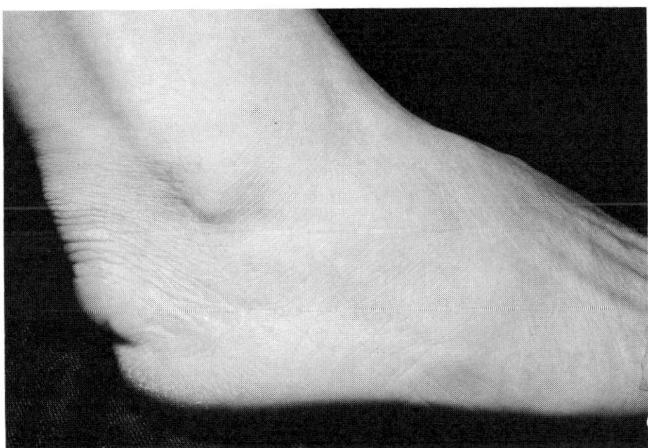

FIGURE 11–36. Tendinous xanthoma. These lesions are commonly found over the Achilles tendons.

FIGURE 11–37. Tuberous xanthomas. These lesions are usually seen over the extensor surfaces of the elbows and knees. Note the smaller satellite lesions.

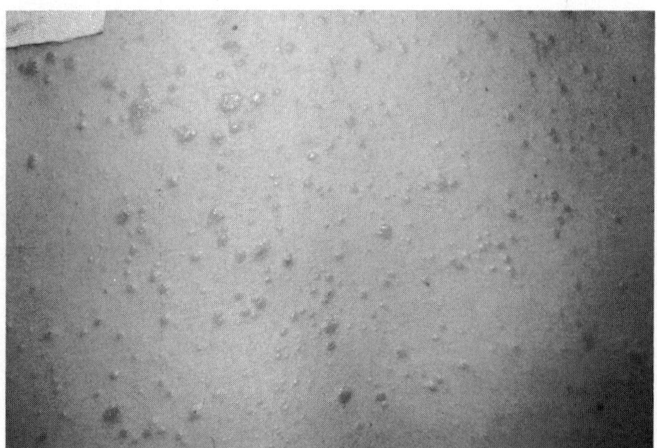

FIGURE 11–38. Eruptive xanthomas. Multiple 1- to 4-mm soft yellow papules appear as crops of lesions on the trunk and extremities.

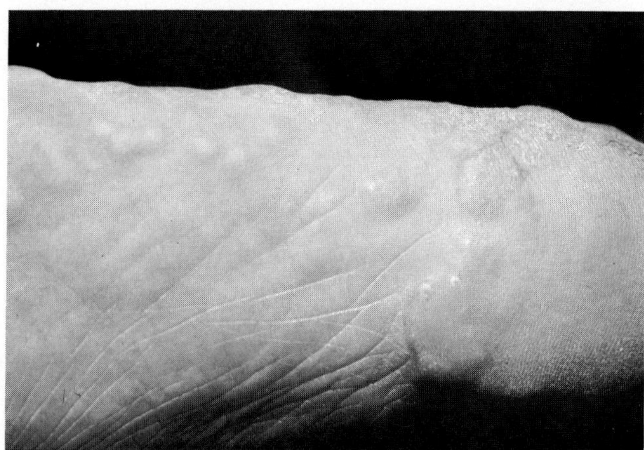

FIGURE 11–40. Plantar xanthomas. Flat-topped yellowish papules and plaques appear over the lateral foot and plantar surface.

xanthelasmas have normal total cholesterol levels. Fractionation of the cholesterol reveals distribution abnormalities in some of these patients. When the lipid profile is abnormal, cholesterol is generally elevated. Only patients with lipid abnormalities have xanthomas in the palmar or plantar creases. Termed *xanthoma striatum palmare,* these are usually flat, yellow-orange lesions associated with both elevated triglycerides and cholesterol. Patients with *diffuse plane xanthomas* have similar lesions on the face, neck, arms, and upper trunk. Not all of these patients have abnormal lipid profiles. However, this syndrome has been reported to be associated with various types of underlying hematolymphoid malignancies, such as multiple myeloma and leukemia.

Therapy for these syndromes is directed toward lowering plasma lipids either through dietary manipulation or medications that decrease abnormal lipid levels. Because these are probably genetically inherited diseases, family members of affected patients should be examined and their lipid profiles should be evaluated.

Blue Toe Syndrome

Blue toe syndrome occurs when a cholesterol or atheromatous microembolus usually arising from the iliac or femoral vessels breaks free and lodges in a small artery, arteri-

oles, or capillaries of a toe, most often the hallux, and leads to acute digital ischemia (Fig. 11–41). The toe appears blue to violaceous and cool. More than one toe may be affected. The foot appears otherwise well perfused. An arteriogram typically reveals atherosclerotic peripheral vascular disease. Patients may eventually require arterial bypass surgery or other intervention to prevent further embolization. Prompt evaluation to find the source of the embolus and its eradication is necessary to restore the vascularization of the toe. Blue toe syndrome is an indication for "limb salvage" surgery. These patients may also be at increased risk for severe atherosclerotic cardiovascular disease.

INFECTIOUS DISEASES

Many systemic infectious diseases may present with cutaneous manifestations. Patients with some of these diseases have cutaneous signs and symptoms involving the foot or lower extremity. In certain cases the findings may be specifically localized or limited to the foot. Examples to be discussed include hand-foot-and-mouth disease, Rocky Mountain spotted fever, syphilis, gonorrhea, filarial disease, and human immunodeficiency virus (HIV)-associated disease. Early detection and diagnosis of these infections may be made by the podiatrist.

Hand-foot-and-mouth disease is a distinctive clinical syndrome caused by an enterovirus called Coxsackie virus, usually type A16, occasionally A5, A9, and others. The virus is

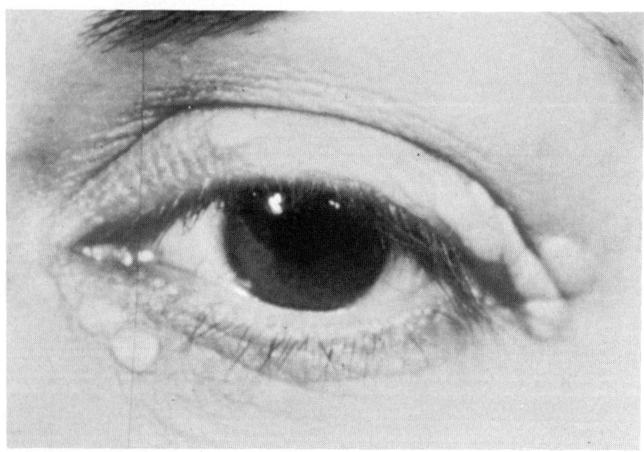

FIGURE 11–39. Xanthelasma. These lesions appear as yellowish discrete or confluent papules around the eyes or on the lids.

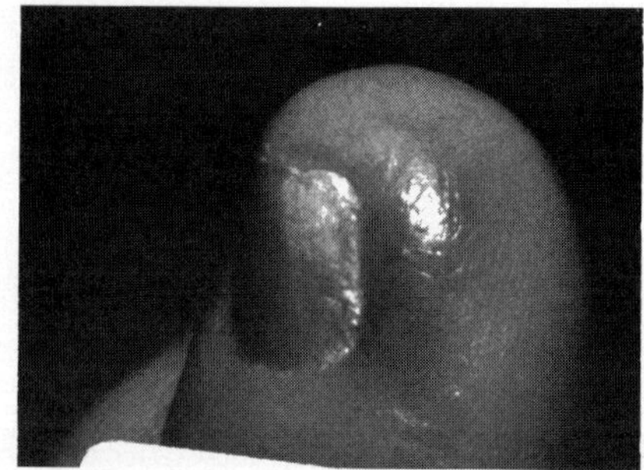

FIGURE 11–41. Blue toe syndrome. Vascular occlusion by an upstream atheromatous or cholesterol embolus leads to cyanosis or even ulceration or gangrene of the ischemic digit.

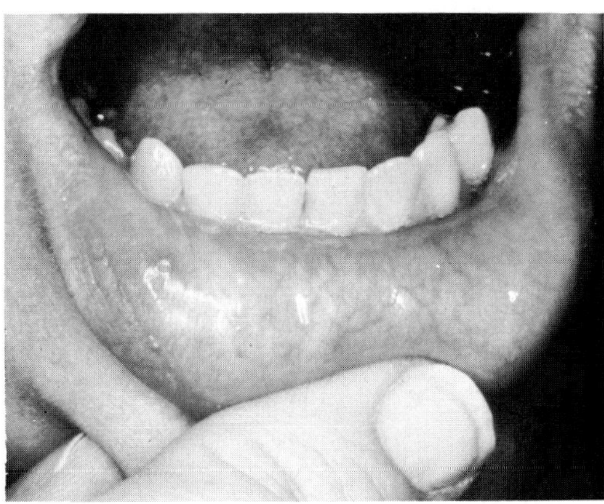

FIGURE 11–42. Hand-foot-and-mouth disease. Infection by the Coxsackie virus leads to vesicles or eroded, shallow ulcers of the buccal, gingival, and lingual mucosa. Oral lesions are present in 95% of patients with hand-foot-and-mouth disease.

transmitted by orofecal contamination. The incubation period is from 3 to 6 days. Patients, most often children and young adults, may present with a mild viral syndrome consisting of low-grade fever, malaise, and abdominal pain. Lesions then appear as tender oral vesicles or eroded gray shallow ulcers on the tongue, lips, palate, and buccal or gingival mucosa (Fig. 11–42). Simultaneously or shortly thereafter, lesions appear on the dorsal and lateral surfaces of the fingers, hands, toes, and feet (Fig. 11–43). These start as erythematous papules and progress to vesicles with an erythematous flare around the base. They may be asymptomatic or somewhat tender. All lesions eventually crust over and resolve over a 7- to 10-day period, usually without scarring. Rare sequelae include myocarditis, meningoencephalitis, aseptic meningitis, and paralytic disease. Hand-foot-and-mouth disease may be easily differentiated from herpetic disease using a Tzanck smear, viral culture, or direct immunofluorescence. The disease is quite contagious but is self-limited and requires no therapy other than symptomatic relief of fever and malaise.

Rocky Mountain spotted fever is caused by the intracellular parasite *Rickettsia rickettsii*, is transmitted by the bite of certain ticks, and is the most serious and potentially fatal of the rickettsial diseases. The syndrome may range from an

essentially asymptomatic form to a fulminant, often fatal illness if not treated promptly. The vector for the microorganism is the *Dermacentor,* or brown wood tick. Despite the name, ticks are found more commonly in the eastern United States than in the Rocky Mountains. The history of a tick bite in a patient having been in an endemic region is helpful but is not a constant finding. The incubation period is from 3 to 12 days, and the onset of symptoms is usually abrupt with fever, chills, headache, myalgias, and arthralgias. The disease goes through a well-described, regular, and unique progression. Pink macules appear first on the volar wrist, forearms, and ankles. After 6 to 18 hours the rash appears on the palms and soles of the feet and then extends centrally (Fig. 11–44). Systemic signs and symptoms may be severe. Delirium, renal failure, and irreversible shock may occur. After 3 to 4 days, papules appear along with the macules and the color of the lesions becomes a deeper red. Petechiae may arise in these lesions. A diagnosis is made on clinical and serologic grounds using complement fixation techniques. Therapy consists of antibiotic therapy with chloramphenicol or tetracycline and supportive care.

Syphilis is a multisystem infection caused by the spirochete *Treponema pallidum*. The disease is almost always transmitted sexually. Recent statistics show that syphilis is increasing in frequency in the United States. Like most spirochetal diseases, syphilis has several successive stages. These stages may be separated by symptom-free intervals, or the stages may clinically overlap. Primary syphilis is characterized by the syphilitic chancre. This appears at the site of inoculation, most often, but not always, the genitalia. The chancre is a shallow, often firm ulcer that is classically described as painless and indurated. However, lesions are not infrequently tender or painful, perhaps owing to the presence

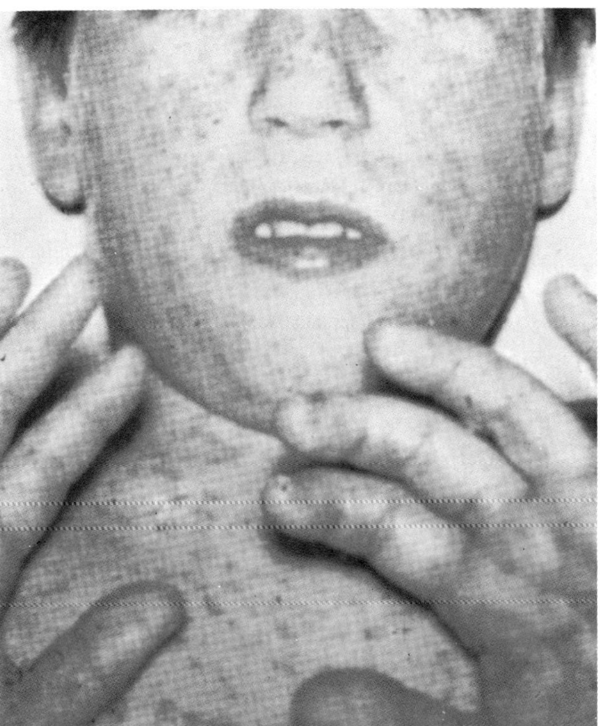

FIGURE 11–44. Rocky Mountain spotted fever. Pink to erythematous macules first appear on the volar wrists, forearms, and ankles. Lesions rapidly spread to affect the palms, soles, and face and then spread more centrally.

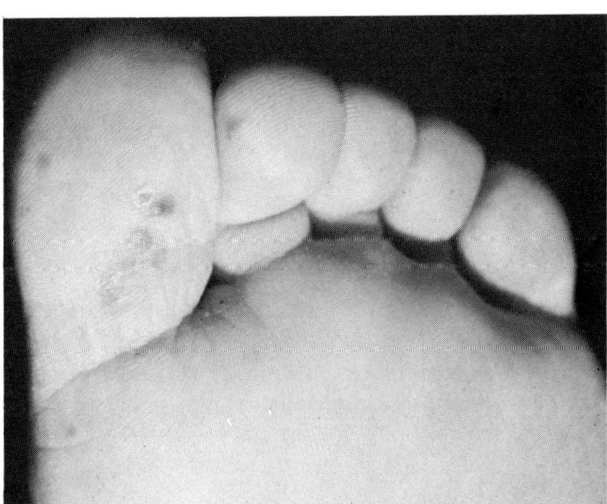

FIGURE 11–43. Hand-foot-and-mouth disease. Erythematous papules progress to papulovesicles on the palmar surface.

of secondary bacterial infection. This primary lesion appears from 6 days to 6 weeks after inoculation and may be single or multiple. After 1 or 2 weeks, the chancres resolve spontaneously, usually without scarring. Primary syphilitic chancres are unnoticed in approximately 30% of patients. The lesions of secondary syphilis, a generalized cutaneous eruption, usually appear 6 to 8 weeks after the primary lesion is visible. Occasionally, the rash of secondary syphilis appears while the chancre is still active or may not appear until 6 months after the chancre disappears. The secondary stage recedes without scarring over the course of 4 to 12 weeks. As many as three discrete relapse episodes may occur during the first year after the disease is contracted in as many as 25% of patients. Generalized symptoms of fever and malaise and generalized lymphadenopathy may occur. The disease may affect any organ system in addition to the skin. Almost any morphologic type of skin lesion may be seen in secondary syphilis. For this reason syphilis has been called ''the great imitator.'' Macular, papular, papulosquamous, follicular, pustular, or nodular variants or any combination of these morphologic forms may appear successively or simultaneously in secondary syphilis. Most often, however, secondary syphilis presents as brawny to copper colored, scaly, round, or oval patches on the trunk and extremities. Lesions commonly occur on the palmar and plantar surfaces and may bring the patient to the podiatrist (Figs. 11–45 and 11–46). Although the lesions do occasionally itch, they are generally nonpruritic, oval, erythematous, scaly macules or papules. Primary and secondary lesions may contain large numbers of spirochetes that can be seen on dark-field examination. Tertiary syphilis is quite uncommon in the United States today. When the disease affects the posterior columns of the spinal tract, *tabes dorsalis* occurs if the disease is not treated in a timely manner. Patients lose spinal proprioceptor and sensory tracts, which leads to the development of unnoticed repeated mechanical trauma to the lower extremity. Neurotrophic ulcers and Charcot's joints result from sustained and repeated trauma in these patients with spinal neuropathy. Syphilis can be cured in the primary and secondary phases of the disease. Once tertiary syphilis has evolved the progression may be halted but not reversed. A diagnosis of syphilis should be suspected in sexually active (past and present) patients with suspicious clinical lesions. Laboratory evaluation of these

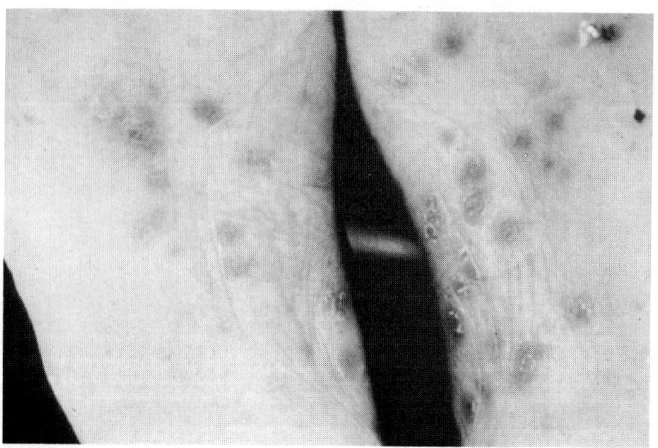

FIGURE 11–45. Secondary syphilis. Erythematous to brawny scaling macules are commonly seen on the trunk and are typically seen on the palms and soles.

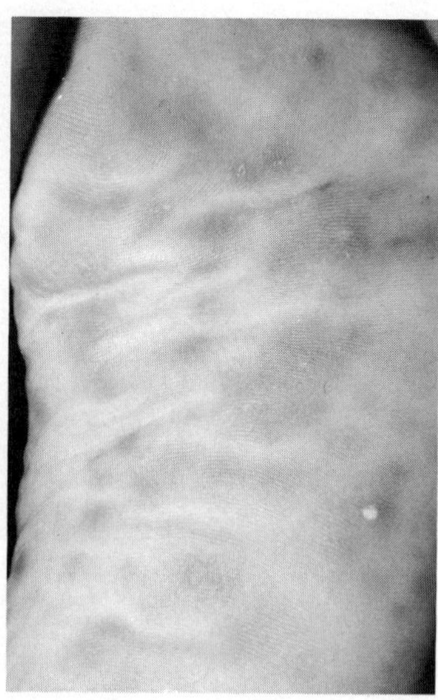

FIGURE 11–46. Secondary syphilis. Plantar lesions may appear as salmon-colored to erythematous, discrete, and confluent papules and plaques. Focal scaling may be present as well.

patients with serologic tests specific for syphilis are both sensitive and specific. These include Venereal Disease Research Laboratory (VDRL) titers, rapid plasma reagin test, and fluorescent treponemal antibody test. Proper interpretation of these tests is extremely important in determining whether the results indicate current versus previous disease activity. Syphilis can be cured, but infection does not confer immunity against subsequent reinfection. Acute and convalescent titers are essential in following the effects of therapy on the disease. Lumbar puncture for cerebrospinal fluid sampling and evaluation is necessary if neurosyphilis is suspected. In immunocompromised patients, such as those infected with HIV, lumbar puncture is often recommended even in apparently early and uncomplicated cases. A biologically false-positive result on a serum VDRL test may be seen in normal persons and in certain conditions such as the anticardiolipin syndrome. Therapy for syphilis is generally administration of intramuscular penicillin. Oral erythromycin or tetracyclines may be used in penicillin-allergic patients who are not immunocompromised. The specific type and regimen of antibiotic therapy depend on the stage at which syphilis is being treated.

Gonorrhea is a sexually transmitted disease caused by the gram-negative diplococcus *Neisseria gonorrhoeae*. In men, gonorrhea is usually limited to urethritis (''the clap''), although other presentations may occur. In both men and women, pharyngeal and rectal gonorrhea are becoming more and more common. In women, the infection is often asymptomatic. Dysuria, vaginal discharge, dyspareunia, and infection of the vaginal Bartholin's glands are the most common clinically symptomatic presentations. In women with long-standing undiagnosed gonorrhea, the infection progresses to pelvic inflammatory disease. If the infection is not treated, chronic inflammation of the pelvic organs leads to salpingitis (infection of the fallopian tubes) and eventually to sterility.

Gonococcal arthritis-dermatitis syndrome is probably the most common cause of acute septic arthritis in sexually active young adults. Its relevance in podiatric medicine arises from the acute septic arthritis that develops when untreated

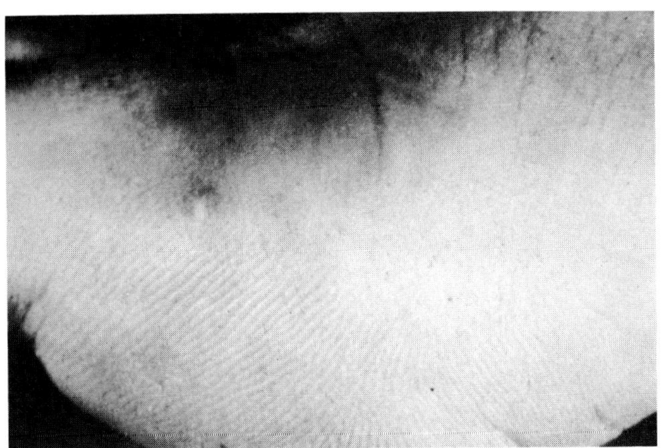

FIGURE 11–47. Gonococcal dermatitis-arthritis syndrome. Acute infectious arthritis of the first metatarsophalangeal joint is associated with overlying papulopustules containing *Neisseria gonorrhoeae* bacteria.

patients become bacteremic and seed peripheral joints with the gonorrheal pathogen. Two thirds of these cases are in women. The arthritis is usually monoarticular or pauci-articular and has all the hallmarks of acute septic arthritis. Patients present with purulent arthritis affecting one or two joints. Fever and polyarthralgias are usually described. Skin lesions may be the most prominent symptom in addition to the arthritic joint. Pustular, papular, petechial, or necrotic lesions may be seen (Fig. 11–47). These are often periarticular in location and may be limited to one or a few lesions. Wrists, fingers, knees, and ankles are the most frequently affected joints. Occasionally, no symptoms other than arthritis are present. If the diagnosis is not made and treatment is delayed, purulent material accumulates and progressively destroys the joint. Diagnosis of acute septic arthritis is made by Gram's stain and by culturing the joint aspirate. Acute gonococcal arthritis should also be suspected in patients known to have disseminated gonococcal disease. Cultures must be planted on Thayer-Martin agar for optimal growth of the organism. If gram-negative diplococci are seen on Gram's stain, treatment for gonorrheal infection must be started immediately to avoid irreversible sequelae.

Female and male patients must be evaluated for the primary and other secondary sites of infection. The particular sites involved may determine the specific therapy indicated. Hospitalization and intravenous antibiotic therapy are generally indicated in patients with disseminated disease, septic arthritis, and bacteremia. Remember also that patients with one sexually transmitted disease often have other sexually transmitted diseases and should be screened for both syphilis, gonorrhea, and possibly chlamydia. Until recently, the drug of choice for all foci of gonorrheal infection had been oral penicillin or ampicillin with probenecid. Penicillinase-producing *Neisseria gonorrhoeae* is now occasionally encountered and requires other antibiotic regimens. Cefotaxime, ceftriaxone, ceftazidime, cefuroxime, and the newer quinolone antibiotics are used in penicillin-allergic patients and other patients with complicated gonorrheal disease, especially if a penicillinase-producing strain of *N. gonorrhoeae* has been identified. Occasionally, patients fail to experience defervescence, and arthritis persists despite apparently appropriate antibiotic therapy. These patients may require repeated closed joint irrigations with saline before resolution of the infection occurs.

Elephantiasis caused by chronic lymphedema is a common final pathway for diseases producing long-standing stasis of local or regional lymphatic systems. Chronic infection and inflammation, which occur in the inguinal, femoral, and iliac lymph nodes, may be caused by bacteria such as in granuloma inguinale, but is more frequently caused by parasitic diseases such as filariasis, deep fungal infections such as chromoblastosis, or surgical lymphostasis. Long-standing stasis dermatitis of the lower extremity may also lead to elephantiasis. Patients living in or having visited endemic areas of filariasis who develop severe lymphostasis and elephantiasis should be evaluated for infection by such parasites as *Wuchereria bancrofti*, *Brugia malayi*, or *Loa loa*. Patients give a history of the short self-limited episodes of fever, chills, sweats, headache, photophobia, and muscle pain. The involved lymphatic vessels are often palpable, tender, and painful. The overlying skin is erythematous and swollen. These acute symptoms subside after a few days only to recur at regular intervals of weeks or months. Chronic lymphedema occurs as the lymphatic tracts become scarred and obstructed (Fig. 11–48). Diagnosis of these diseases is made in patients with a history of exposure who have laboratory evidence of eosinophilia. An examination of blood smears by a qualified parasitologist or pathologist confirms the diagnosis of filariasis. Because different filaria appear in the

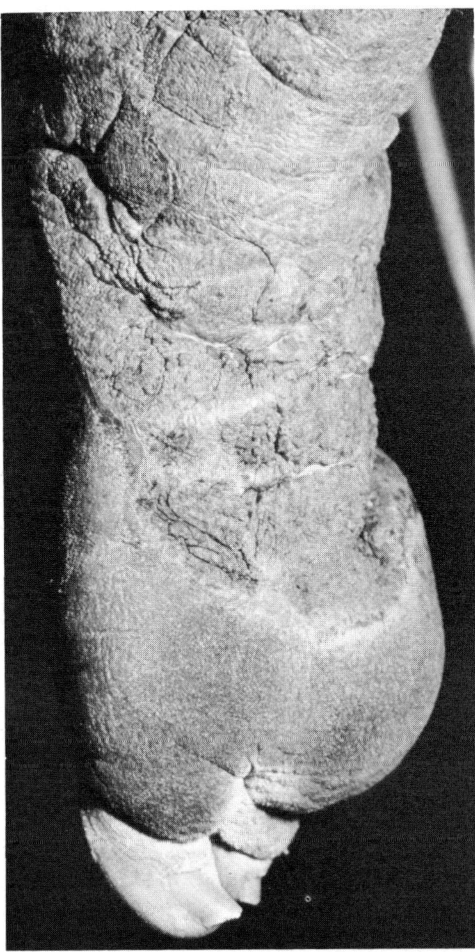

FIGURE 11–48. Elephantiasis—chronic lymphedema. As chronic lymphatic obstruction progresses, the skin of the affected limb becomes thickened and indurated, and develops thick verrucous hyperplasia and hyperpigmentation.

peripheral blood at specific and different times of the day or night, it is imperative to obtain blood samples in patients with suspected filariasis at the appropriate time, depending on which organism is to be isolated and identified. Therapy is directed at eliminating the organism with antiparasitic agents such as diethylcarbamazine for 3 to 4 weeks. The chronic lymphedema and elephantiasis is usually irreversible due to scarring. The skin of the lower extremity needs to be kept clean and should be regularly cleansed with antibacterial soaps. Bacterial and fungal superinfection should be treated aggressively with topical and systemic medications. In some patients the application of ultrapotent topical corticosteroids may help to reduce the extent of thickening of the skin in elephantiasis but is generally only mildly effective. Compression stockings and elevation of the affected extremity should be encouraged. Reinfection may occur if the patient is reinoculated with the organisms.

Patients with *HIV infection* may present with infectious, neoplastic, or inflammatory lesions of the lower extremity. Skin lesions may be the first evidence of HIV infection. Fungal infections, particularly *Candida* or unusually severe and recalcitrant dermatophyte infection may signal the onset of profound immunologic suppression. This may present as paronychia or even as interdigital candidal infection. The severe moccasin distribution of tinea pedis has also been described. Bacterial superinfection with *Pseudomonas*, coliform, or other gram-negative bacteria may complicate simple tinea infection. Usually nonpathogenic organisms such as *Staphylococcus epidermidis* may cause severe local or even systemic disease. These bacterial and fungal infections often do not respond to standard treatments. Patients with HIV infection often have a psoriasiform dermatitis characterized by erythematous scaly plaques that may be generalized or localized to the lower extremities. Plantar hyperkeratosis may be part of this syndrome. Patients with HIV also have a higher than normal incidence of certain neoplasms. In addition to lymphomas, patients have an increased frequency of basal cell carcinoma. These often occur in non–sun-exposed areas and may include the lower extremity or plantar surface, which is an extremely unusual site for this tumor in otherwise healthy persons. Kaposi's sarcoma that is associated with HIV infection differs from classic Kaposi's sarcoma by virtue of its multicentric distribution, rapid progression, and systemic lesions that are not limited to the skin. Patients describe tender violaceous nodules on the plantar surface as well as on other sites (Fig. 11–49). Any patient suspected of having Kaposi's sarcoma must be evaluated for the presence of HIV infection. If lesions on the foot or elsewhere are symptomatic, Kaposi's sarcoma may require systemic chemotherapy or local injection with chemotherapeutic agents. Cryotherapy with liquid nitrogen may offer these patients temporary symptomatic relief and cosmetic improvement of individually treated lesions.

KERATODERMAS

Diffuse or localized thickening of the stratum corneum, primarily of the palms or soles, is termed *keratoderma*. The condition may be limited to the hands or feet or may be part of a more generalized phenomenon. Keratodermas may be part of the expression of hereditary or acquired disorders. The term *tylosis* is sometimes used as a synonym for kerato-

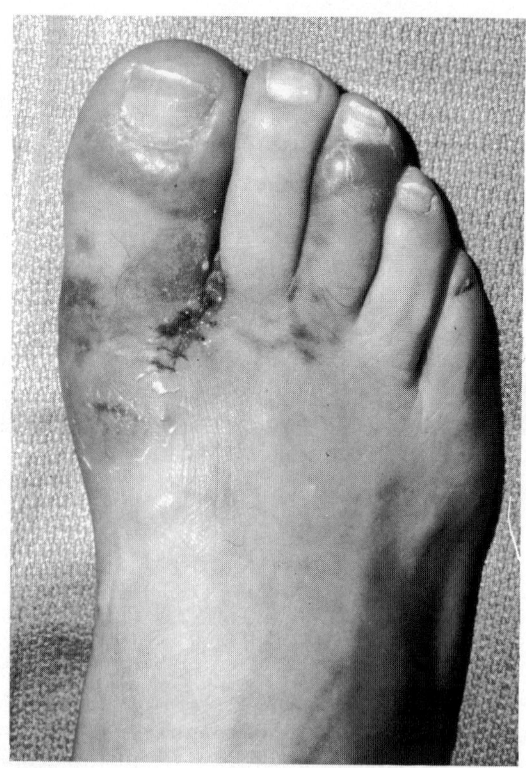

FIGURE 11–49. Kaposi's sarcoma—human immunodeficiency virus associated. Partially blanchable purplish plaques and nodules are commonly seen on the skin, including the lower extremities. The lesions may be tender and eventually ulcerate if not treated.

derma. Numerous syndromes may include keratoderma within their clinical spectrum (Table 11–3). A brief description of the more important of these disorders that may be associated with systemic disease follows.

Howel-Evans syndrome is a diffuse keratoderma of the palms and soles associated with carcinoma of the esophagus in most, but not all, affected people. The syndrome was described in two possibly related English families and was believed to be dominantly inherited. The hyperkeratosis appeared in patients between the ages of 5 and 15 years. Patients with this syndrome report symptoms of dysphagia (difficulty with swallowing) and may have signs of tarry or occult blood in the stool. Patients presenting with keratoderma and with a history of dysphagia or changes in the stool suggestive of an upper gastrointestinal hemorrhage should be referred for an evaluation of the upper gastrointestinal tract.

Papillon-Lefèvre syndrome is an autosomal recessive disorder characterized by the onset of palmoplantar hyperkera-

---

TABLE 11–3

SYSTEMIC DISEASES ASSOCIATED WITH KERATODERMAS

Arsenical toxicity
Bazex's syndrome
Keratoderma climactericum (?)
Howel-Evans syndrome
Papillon-Lefèvre syndrome
Reiter's syndrome
Richner-Hannert syndrome
Syphilis
Yaws

tosis during the first 6 months of life. The affected areas appear erythematous and puffy. Gingivitis and changes in periosteal alveolar bone occur. Calcification of the falx cerebri and tentorium in the brain are seen on radiograph. Permanent and deciduous teeth are lost. A psoriasiform dermatitis is occasionally seen on the dorsa of the hands, feet, elbows, and knees.

Richner-Hannert syndrome is an autosomal recessive disorder associated with tyrosinemia. The clinical manifestations include prepatellar and palmoplantar keratodermas, corneal dystrophy, oligophrenia, and brachyphalangia. If levels of tyrosine ingested are restricted in the diet, the ocular and cutaneous lesions resolve.

Keratoderma climactericum has been described as an acquired keratoderma that can occur in women during menopause. Patients are often obese. Lesions tend to occur in areas of trauma, and painful fissures may be troublesome. The extent of lesions may vary from discrete hyperkeratotic areas that may become confluent. The term *keratoderma climactericum* may be a misnomer, because similar lesions are seen in male patients in the same age range and therefore may not be a distinct pathologic entity. Therapy is directed toward keeping the skin soft and pliable with emollients. Topical corticosteroids may be of some benefit.

Bazex's syndrome (acrokeratosis paraneoplastica) is a paraneoplastic disease that by definition is associated with an underlying malignancy. The syndrome progresses through three identifiable phases. Initially, acral areas begin to develop erythematous to violaceous poorly marginated psoriasiform scaly macules and patches. Typically, the fingers, toes, ears, and nose are affected. As the disease progresses to the second phase, keratoderma appears and the initial lesions become more generalized. The third phase is essentially the persistence of the keratoderma and the generalized violaceous acral lesions. Plantar surfaces may be involved in as many as 50% of cases of Bazex's syndrome. The underlying malignancies are most often squamous cell carcinomas of the upper airways and gastrointestinal tract. The progression of the cutaneous lesions may parallel the development of the underlying malignancy, and lesions may regress if the tumor is treated successfully. Bazex's syndrome is considered to be a true cutaneous sign of internal malignancy.

Reiter's syndrome is another disorder that is associated with keratoderma. As described elsewhere in this chapter, keratoderma blennorrhagicum is a well-circumscribed hyperkeratosis of the palms and soles of patients with Reiter's syndrome.

Spirochetal diseases such as syphilis and yaws may be associated with keratoderma.

In the past, punctate keratoses of the palms and soles were thought to be associated with an increased risk of internal malignancy, although evidence is scant. These are discrete skin-colored hyperkeratotic papules. The papules may have a depressed center or a central hyperkeratotic plug. Lesions remain discrete and do not coalesce. Similar lesions may be seen in Howel-Evans syndrome as described earlier. Otherwise, punctate keratoses of the palms and soles are probably not indicators of internal malignancy. Although not identical histopathologically, arsenical keratoses are clinically indistinguishable from punctate keratoses. The arsenical keratoses are found in patients with a history of excessive arsenic ingestion, and these keratoses are usually caused by well water. Patients living near industrial sites, such as smelting plants where arsenic is a byproduct of the smelting process, may develop these palmoplantar hyperkeratoses or pits after years of exposure. Chronic exposure to arsenic can also cause Mees' lines (see the section on nail changes in systemic disease). Evaluation of the patient's hair or nails is valuable in determining the level of heavy metal exposure. Chronic arsenic exposure has been implicated in the pathogenesis of cutaneous and internal squamous cell malignancies.

MISCELLANEOUS SKIN DISORDERS ASSOCIATED WITH SYSTEMIC DISEASE

Erythema Multiforme

Erythema multiforme (EM) is an acute, usually self-limited eruption of the skin and mucous membranes characterized by the distinctive target or iris lesion (Fig. 11–50). When present, the mucocutaneous lesions are often accompanied by a systemic serum sickness–like syndrome. The term *erythema multiforme* refers to the cutaneous lesions. However, the disease can either be limited to or affect primarily the mucosal and mucocutaneous surfaces. It may also rarely affect internal organ systems. This is termed *erythema multiforme major* or *Stevens-Johnson syndrome* and may be a severe and sometimes fatal disease with mortality approaching 15% to 30% when the process progresses to toxic epidermal necrolysis (TEN). The precise limits of what clinically constitutes EM is poorly defined. EM minor in of itself is not a cause of significant morbidity. Infection and medications are the most common underlying causes of EM, implicating hypersensitivity as a major mechanism involved in the pathogenesis of this eruption. Common causes for the minor form of EM include drug reactions, herpes simplex infections, mycoplasmal pneumonia, infections by various other viruses such as adenoviral infection, infectious mononucleosis, and Coxsackie B5 infection. Deep fungal infections and leukemia have also been described in association with EM. Elimination of the infection or withdrawal of the offending medication leads to the disappearance of the eruption. Neoplasia, radiation therapy, and connective tissue disease may also be associated with EM. No cause is found in approximately 50%

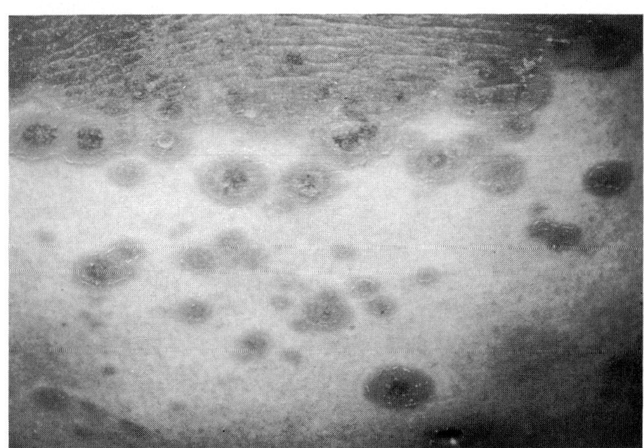

FIGURE 11–50. Erythema multiforme. Typical iris, or target, lesions may coalesce to form larger plaques. The central gray areas of the target correspond to keratinocyte necrosis in the epidermis. These are surrounded by the erythema of more peripheral inflammatory infiltrate.

of cases. The name *multiforme* indicates the diversity of the clinical lesions seen in this disease. The classic cutaneous lesion seen in EM is the target, or iris, lesion. These lesions are usually bilaterally symmetrical and acral and often occur on the palmar and plantar surfaces. The lesions are a dull-red macule or patch that expands to approximately 2 cm in diameter. The periphery of the lesion stays erythematous, while the center of the lesion becomes dusky gray, cyanotic, or purpuric. There may be a small rim of pink skin around the center of the lesion, giving it a "targetoid" appearance. The center of the lesion corresponds to necrosis of the epidermal cells, whereas the more erythematous areas are associated with a less locally advanced or aggressive inflammatory response. Lesions may be polycyclic or arcuate in shape in some patients. The cutaneous eruptions of EM minor tend to persist for 1 or 2 weeks and fade, leaving some degree of postinflammatory hyperpigmentation. In some patients, lesions may persist for as long as 4 weeks. A small number of mucosal or mucocutaneous lesions may be seen in EM minor. The early lesions of EM may be primarily urticarial plaques. This urticarial stage of EM tends to differ from typical urticaria or hives by the persistence of any individual urticarial lesion longer than 24 to 48 hours. Vesicles and bullae are rarely seen but may occur within already existing target or urticarial lesions (Fig. 11–51). This occasionally portends the transition to the major form of EM, or Stevens-Johnson syndrome. Patients may have fever, arthralgias, and myalgias. This end of the clinical spectrum is characterized by more generalized diffuse lesions, especially on the trunk. These lesions tend to be less targetoid and more confluent. Vesiculobullous lesions may be large, flaccid, and fragile giving the appearance of TEN. If these areas become confluent, distinguishing between EM major and TEN becomes difficult (Fig. 11–52). Patients with severe systemic disease as part of Stevens-Johnson syndrome may have hepatitis, bronchopulmonary disease, or renal failure, which in unusu-

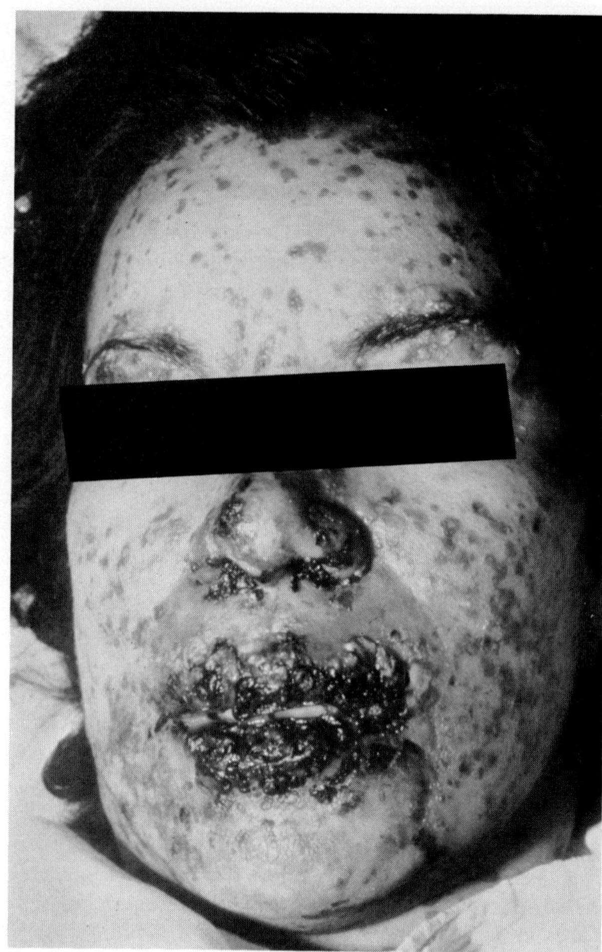

FIGURE 11–52. Stevens-Johnson syndrome (erythema multiforme major). Patients with this form of erythema multiforme may develop extensive mucocutaneous lesions as well as lesions of internal organs such as the lung and gastrointestinal tract. The periorificial hemorrhagic crusting is typical.

ally severe cases may result in death. Patients with severe TEN require treatment at specialized burn centers because the large areas of denuded skin have the same infectious and metabolic problems as those with severe burns (Fig. 11–53). The most common cause of TEN is a drug reaction.

Erythema Nodosum

Erythema nodosum is characterized by distinctive painful subcutaneous nodules, which are usually located on the pretibial areas (Fig. 11–54). Erythema nodosum may be associated with infectious and inflammatory causes, including mycobacterial and other granulomatous processes. Drug reactions may also be implicated. In the common form of erythema nodosum, oval subcutaneous nodules develop on the pretibial areas of one or both lower extremities. These nodules are exquisitely tender, uniform 1 to 5 cm in size, and range from several to a dozen lesions. Initially, they appear as bright red, hot, and raised. Over the course of several days the nodules may flatten and become a more dusky brown to purple. These are sometimes mistaken for ecchymoses. The most common causes of erythema nodosum are streptococcal infections; pregnancy; oral contraceptives; drug reactions; and deep bacterial, fungal, and parasitic infec-

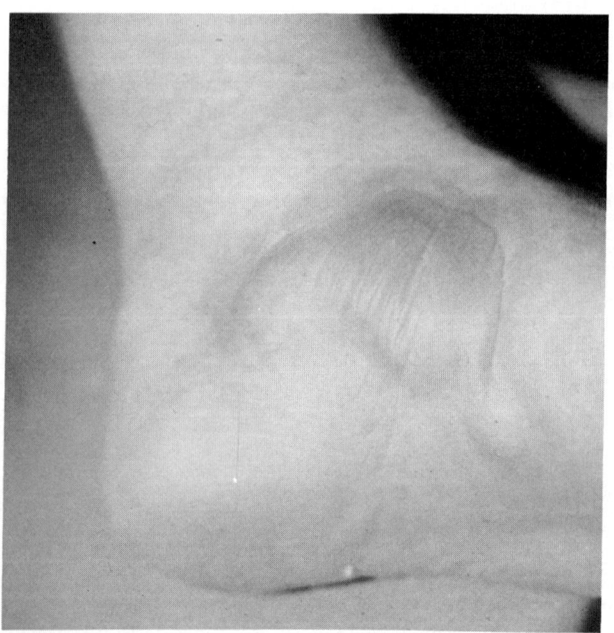

FIGURE 11–51. Bullous erythema multiforme. An unusual variant of erythema multiforme, bullous lesions may develop alone or in association with the more typical target lesions.

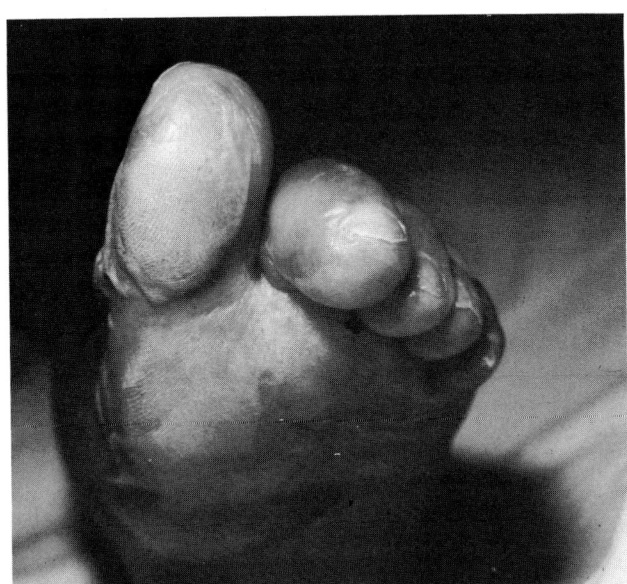

FIGURE 11–53. Toxic epidermal necrolysis. Partial- to full-thickness necrosis of the epidermis leads to sloughing of the skin similar to that seen in large-area second-degree burns.

tions. Other systemic causes of erythema nodosum include sarcoidosis, inflammatory bowel disease, rheumatic fever, tuberculosis, and Behçet's syndrome. Histopathologically, erythema nodosum is a septal panniculitis, that is, inflammation of the fibrous septae and its blood vessels within the subcutaneous fat lobules. Lesions usually resolve spontaneously over 3 to 6 weeks but may persist for months. Because erythema nodosum is associated with multiple underlying conditions, it is thought that these processes are responsible for circulating immune complexes that are deposited in the septal blood vessels in the fibrous septae of the subcutaneous fat lobules. Patients may present with a serum sickness–like illness with fever, arthralgias, and myalgias. Recurrent episodes are not uncommon and appear in as many as one third of patients, especially if they are rechallenged with the offending antigen. *Erythema nodosum leprosum* is considered to be a reactional type of erythema nodosum that occurs in patients with Hansen's disease (leprosy). Patients with erythema nodosum leprosum tend to be at the lepromatous pole of the leprosy spectrum. Lesions may be in atypical locations and have unusual clinical morphology.

Treatment of erythema nodosum is directed toward the underlying condition if one can be identified. Most patients are uncomfortable enough to require therapy. Nonsteroidal anti-inflammatory drugs are useful. Oral potassium iodide may be helpful in more resistant cases. Rarely systemic corticosteroids may be used. It is necessary to identify and adequately treat any underlying infections in these patients, especially if systemic corticosteroids are being considered. In general, patients need to be evaluated carefully for any of the possible underlying diseases that may be associated with erythema nodosum. The work-up should be directed by the history and physical examination.

Sarcoidosis

Sarcoidosis is an idiopathic noninfectious multisystem disorder characterized histologically by the presence of epithe-

lioid granulomas in affected tissues. Sarcoidosis is usually seen in young adults, in women more frequently than men and in blacks more than whites. Patients present most commonly with skin or eye lesions, diffuse or localized lymphadenopathy, and bilateral pulmonary hilar adenopathy on a chest radiograph. Actual pulmonary parenchymal infiltrates usually indicate more serious disease. In order of decreasing frequency, sarcoidosis affects intrathoracic tissues; eye, skin, liver, heart, and musculoskeletal tissues; neural tissues; and endocrine organs. A diagnosis is most definite when there are clinicoradiologic findings supported by histopathologic confirmation of epithelioid granulomas in more than one organ. A positive result on a Kveim-Siltzbach skin test is also helpful if the antigens are available to identify the presence of a delayed hypersensitivity reaction. Immune system abnormalities have been implicated in the pathogenesis of this disease. These include depression of cell-mediated immunity and increased or abnormal immunoglobulin levels. It is not clear whether these are important in the actual cause of the disease or are just an epiphenomenon. Most studies indicate that approximately 30% of patients with sarcoidosis have cutaneous involvement. Sarcoid may be limited to the skin, without involvement of any other organ systems. Skin lesions of sarcoid may be specific or nonspecific. Specific lesions are histologically noncaseating epithelioid granulomas and are similar to granulomas in other affected organs. These occur in about 25% to 30% of patients with systemic sarcoidosis and are commonly associated with chronic disease. The variable morphology of the skin lesions may have some significance in determining the course of the disease. Erythematous to violaceous papules are frequently found around the eyelids, nose, mouth, and occipital region of the head and neck. A more diffuse papular form may herald the onset of the disease. The nodular or plaque form of cutaneous sarcoidosis is deeper, more chronic, and more widely distributed (Fig. 11–55). *Lupus pernio* is a form of plaque type sarcoidosis that tends to be insidious and chronic and resolves with fibrosis and scarring. The nonspecific lesions of

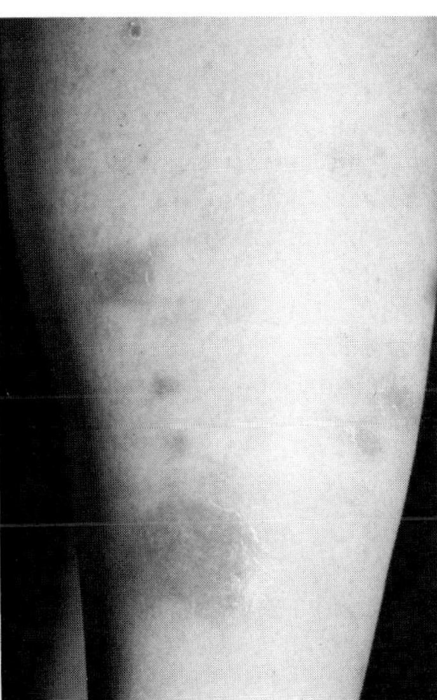

FIGURE 11–54. Erythema nodosum. Tender, painful erythematous subcutaneous nodules are classically found on the pretibial area but may appear elsewhere on the skin. Lesions are usually but not always multiple.

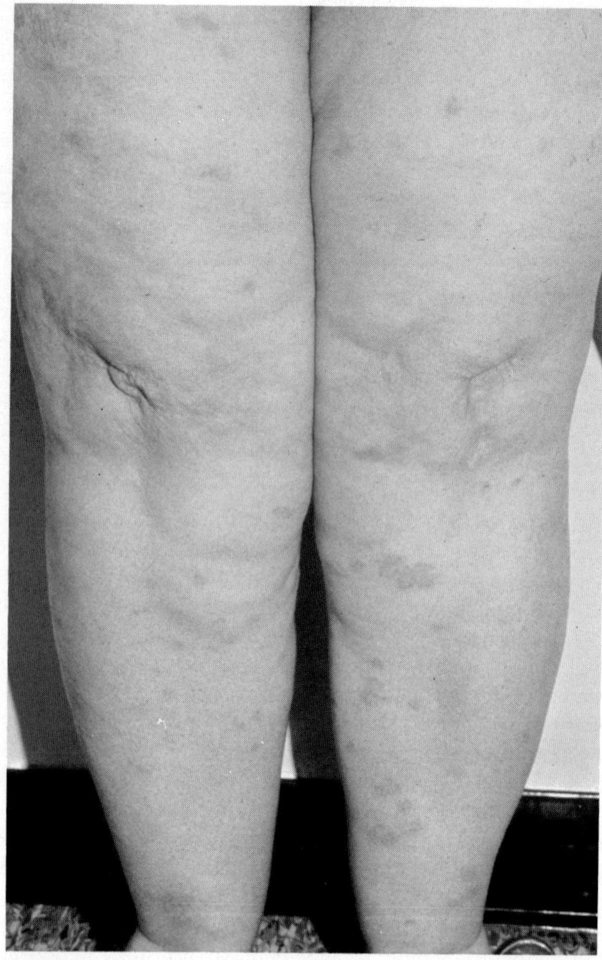

FIGURE 11–55. Sarcoidosis. Erythematous, somewhat indurated nodules and plaques may be chronic and result in scarring of the affected skin.

sarcoidosis are not granulomas and are associated with the disease elsewhere in the skin. The most common of these is erythema nodosum (see Fig. 11–54). It appears in approximately 20% of patients and may be the first clinical symptom of the disease. Conversely, approximately 20% of patients with erythema nodosum have sarcoidosis. Other nonspecific lesions are quite rare. When sarcoidosis presents within the constellation of fever, uveitis (inflammation of the uveal tract of the eye), erythema nodosum, and peripheral and bilateral pulmonary hilar lymphadenopathy, it is termed *Löfgren's syndrome*. It resolves spontaneously in more than 90% of affected patients. An unusual manifestation of sarcoidosis is lesions arising in tattoos or pre-existing scars. Previously normal scars that become livid and inflamed may reveal noncaseating epithelioid granulomas. Although granulomas can commonly be found in skeletal muscle, this is not a common cause of morbidity. Bone cysts are seen in approximately 10% of patients and are also usually asymptomatic. Podiatrists may see a typical syndrome of heel pain in patients with systemic sarcoidosis. Hypercalciuria with or without hypercalcemia secondary to renal involvement may be present. Serum angiotensin-converting enzyme (ACE) may be elevated in some patients with systemic sarcoidosis. ACE levels do not correlate well with cutaneous disease.

Once a diagnosis of sarcoidosis is made by biopsies of affected tissue and radiologic confirmation is made, the pa-

tient should have a complete physical examination, ophthalmologic evaluation, and appropriate laboratory tests to evaluate serum calcium and ACE levels. The result of the electrocardiogram may be abnormal in patients with cardiac involvement. Pulmonary function testing may be one of the earliest detectors of sarcoidal pulmonary disease. Acute sarcoidosis with limited disease is often self-limited. Many specialists do not believe that this form of the disease needs to be treated aggressively. Nonsteroidal anti-inflammatory agents and ophthalmic corticosteroids may be indicated. Chronic sarcoid may require systemic corticosteroids, antimalarials, allopurinol, methotrexate, and other chemotherapeutic agents that have been tried with variable success. Absolute indications for aggressive therapy include hypercalcemia or CNS or cardiac sarcoidosis. Mortality is estimated at 3% to 6% and is usually associated with CNS or cardiac disease.

Pyoderma Gangrenosum

Pyoderma gangrenosum (PG) is an uncommon destructive inflammatory skin disease in which painful nodules or pustules break down to form a rapidly enlarging ulcer with characteristically raised, tender, violaceous undermined borders (Fig. 11–56). The lesions may be solitary or multiple and discrete or coalescent. Lesions are commonly found on the upper and lower extremities. PG may be limited to the skin or may be associated with a number of underlying systemic diseases. Most authors consider PG to be a manifestation of disordered immunity but the precise cause is still unknown. The phenomenon of ''pathergy,'' trivial trauma evoking new lesions or aggravating existing ones, is seen in association with PG in approximately 20% of patients. PG is not primarily infectious. Lesions may become secondarily infected with bacteria, but early lesions are virtually always sterile. Biopsy examination of the lesions may be detrimental because it may induce progression or enlargement of the lesion being evaluated. This suggests an altered, exaggerated, and uncontrolled inflammatory response to nonspecific stimuli. No specific and constant pattern of abnormal immune response has been identified to date. Laboratory abnormalities are nonspecific. Elevated erythrocyte sedimentation rate and leukocytosis are usually present. Histopathologic find-

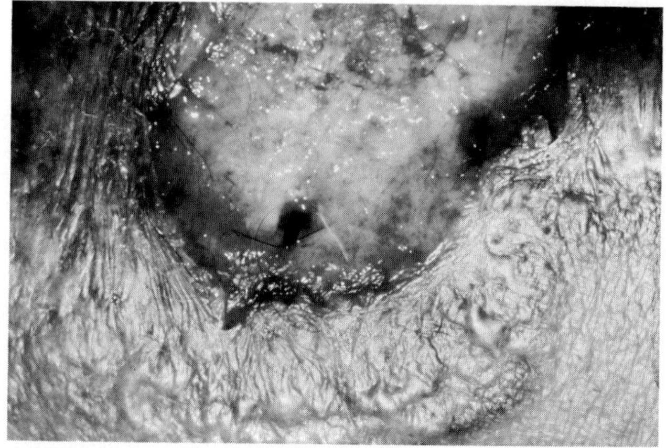

FIGURE 11–56. Pyoderma gangrenosum. Ulcers with ragged undermined violaceous borders develop and progress rapidly. Trauma to the ulcer (e.g., a biopsy) may accelerate the progression.

ings are not diagnostic. Therefore, the diagnosis of PG is generally made on clinical grounds: a rapidly enlarging ulcer with the typical violaceous undermined borders.

PG is idiopathic in about half of cases. Patients with associated systemic disease most often have one of the following conditions: RA or polyarthritis, inflammatory bowel disease (Crohn's disease, ulcerative colitis), chronic active hepatitis, hematolymphoid disorders and malignancies (granulocytic leukemias, polycythemia vera, myeloid metaplasia, multiple myeloma), and rarely, Behçet's syndrome. In most of these diseases, the appearance of PG follows the onset of the primary systemic disease in question. PG occasionally precedes the clinical symptoms of inflammatory bowel disease or leukemia. In general, the underlying condition determines the final prognosis. In the idiopathic form the prognosis for complete recovery is good. Scarring is a common sequela.

Because there are no specific laboratory or histologic findings, clinical impression is the basis on which PG is generally diagnosed. The differential diagnosis includes cutaneous gangrene, ecthyma gangrenosum, atypical mycobacterial infections, deep mycoses, amebiasis, and noninfectious tropical ulcers. Demonstration of a known associated underlying disease should be a strong consideration in making the diagnosis of PG.

Therapy is directed both toward the underlying disease, if present, and the ulcers themselves. Topical therapy alone is usually insufficient. Control of secondary infection and general wound care is essential. Surgical débridement of the ulcers is not advised as it may worsen the lesion. High-dose systemic corticosteroids, dapsone, sulfapyridine, and sulfasalazine (Azulfidine) may be beneficial. These may also be helpful in treating the underlying disease in patients with inflammatory bowel disease. Because the natural history of PG is one of spontaneous regression, the efficacy of sulfa drugs has not been conclusively established. Clofazimine and immunosuppressants such as azathioprine, cyclophosphamide, and more recently, cyclosporine have been used with some success.

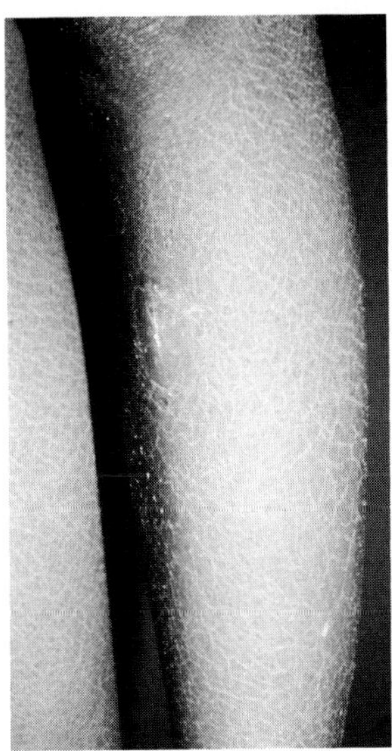

FIGURE 11–57. Acquired ichthyosis. Onset of extremely dry skin with typical rhomboidal ''fish scales'' may be seen in patients with underlying illnesses such as lymphoreticular malignancies.

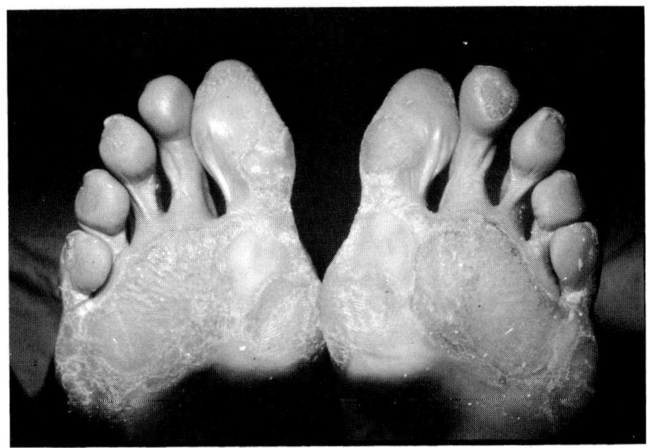

FIGURE 11–58. Acquired ichthyosis. Patients with more widespread ichthyosis may also have a scaly palmoplantar keratoderma.

Ichthyosis

Ichthyosis may be inherited or acquired. Acquired ichthyosis is clinically similar to the genetically transmitted ichthyosis vulgaris. Patients present with thick rhomboidal scales with free edges that may be lifted off the skin (Fig. 11–57). The entire body may be affected, but most commonly the extremities and trunk are involved (Fig. 11–58). Patients may have a long history of dry skin but then develop the characteristic scales. Acquired ichthyosis is occasionally associated with an underlying malignancy. Most of these tumors are lymphoreticular malignancies, such as Hodgkin's disease and lymphocytic lymphomas. Other diseases have also been associated with acquired ichthyosis including thyroid disease and sarcoidosis. In general, the diagnosis of the underlying malignancy is made before the appearance of the typical ichthyotic skin changes. Treatment of ichthyosis should be directed toward the resolution of the underlying disease if possible and the use of emollients such as urea-containing lotions or α-hydroxy acid lotions.

Psoriasis and Psoriatic Arthritis

Psoriasis is a chronic and relapsing skin disease with variable expression of clinical lesions. The disease is classified as papulosquamous or erythrosquamous. Lesions are classically raised red papules and plaques with a typical silvery white scale. These arise in a typical bilaterally symmetrical distribution on the body. The morphology and distribution of the lesions may be highly variable and different types of psoriasis may be found even in the same patient. A detailed description of psoriasis is beyond the scope of this chapter and can be found in any textbook on general dermatology. Psoriasis may be associated with a seronegative arthritis that ranges from mild arthritis of the digits to arthritis mutilans with severe disability. This section deals with the clinical lesions of psoriasis that may be seen by the podiatrist or other specialist of the foot and lower extremity.

Psoriasis affects approximately 1% to 2% of the U.S. population and may begin any time from infancy to old age. Most patients first show clinical signs in the third decade. Approximately 30% of psoriatic patients have relatives who

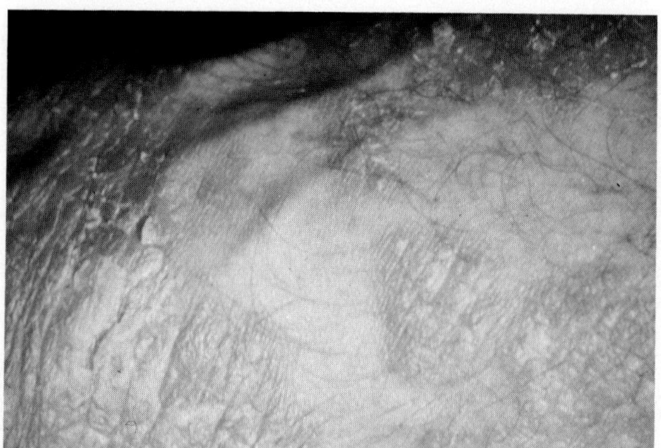

FIGURE 11–59. Psoriasis vulgaris. Typical psoriatic plaques may vary in thickness and usually have an overlying white to silvery scale.

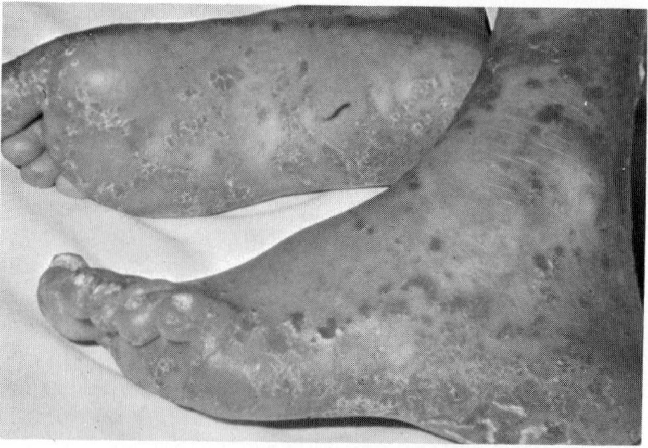

FIGURE 11–61. Pustular psoriasis. Patients may present with an acute febrile systemic illness. Multiple pustules superimposed on highly inflammatory psoriatic patches or plaques on the feet are associated with psoriatic arthritis in this patient.

have psoriasis. The specific mode of inheritance of psoriasis is poorly understood at this time.

The most common clinical pattern of psoriasis is *psoriasis vulgaris.* Lesions are typically red and scaly as described earlier and remain stationary over the course of years if they are not treated. The distribution of psoriasis vulgaris usually includes the elbows, knees, scalp, and nails. The scale may be thin or thick. Truncal lesions are also seen frequently and may coalesce to affect large areas called *geographic plaques.* Lesions of the palms and soles are common (Fig. 11–59).

Inverse psoriasis affects the flexural folds such as antecubital, popliteal, and inguinal areas. Scaling is often absent in these lesions. Patients may have lesions on both extensor and flexural surfaces concomitantly or sequentially.

Palmoplantar psoriasis should be included in the differential diagnosis of keratodermas. Psoriasis is limited to the palms and soles of certain patients. Both palmar or both plantar surfaces are generally affected. The bilateral symmetry is highly characteristic of essentially all psoriatic disease (Fig. 11–60). The differential diagnosis should include contact dermatitis, dyshidrosiform eczema, pityriasis rubra pilaris, and other conditions associated with keratodermas.

Generalized pustular psoriasis (von Zumbusch's psoriasis) is an acute, sometimes severe, and occasionally fatal variant

of psoriasis. It is characterized by fever and by the eruption of 2- to 4-mm sterile pustules over a variable amount of skin surface. The lesions may affect the trunk, palm, soles, and nail beds. The skin on which the pustules arise is bright red. Affected areas may coalesce to form large confluent areas of pustular psoriasis (Fig. 11–61). Patients may be acutely ill with malaise and prostration.

Guttate psoriasis is seen as small 0.5- to 3-mm erythematous scaly macules or thin plaques that usually begin on the trunk or lower extremity. This form of psoriasis is most common in young adults. Streptococcal infection or even chronic asymptomatic carriage of streptococcal bacteria may induce episodes of guttate psoriasis, and patients must be questioned for a history of recent sore throat or other localized infection. A throat culture is a cost-effective test to rule out pharyngeal streptococcal infection or colonization. Treatment of an underlying infection may lead to resolution of the guttate psoriasis, but these patients seem predisposed to further episodes of guttate psoriasis or progression to psoriasis vulgaris or other variants.

Localized pustular psoriasis may present as palmoplantar pustular psoriasis in which lesions are confined to the palms and soles. These lesions are chronic and recurrent, and remissions last from weeks to months.

Acrodermatitis continua of Hallapeau is a rare variant of pustular psoriasis that starts on the fingers or toes and extends slowly proximally. Destruction of the nail unit and atrophy of the distal digit may be seen. As in other types of pustular psoriasis, lesions may occur elsewhere on the body.

Nail changes are quite common in patients with psoriasis. Fingernails appear to be affected in 50% of patients and toenails in about 35%. Lesions range from isolated nail plate pits to complete destruction of the nail unit (Fig. 11–62). The degree and type of changes depends on the particular size and location of the psoriatic lesion within the nail unit. Specific changes include pits, ''oil spots,'' onychodystrophy, and subungual pustules. Patients with psoriatic nail changes may have a higher incidence of psoriatic arthritis than do those without nail disease.

Nail pits are the most common morphologic pattern seen in nail psoriasis and consist of 0.2- to 0.5-mm discrete or confluent pits on the superficial nail plate. Pits may be the

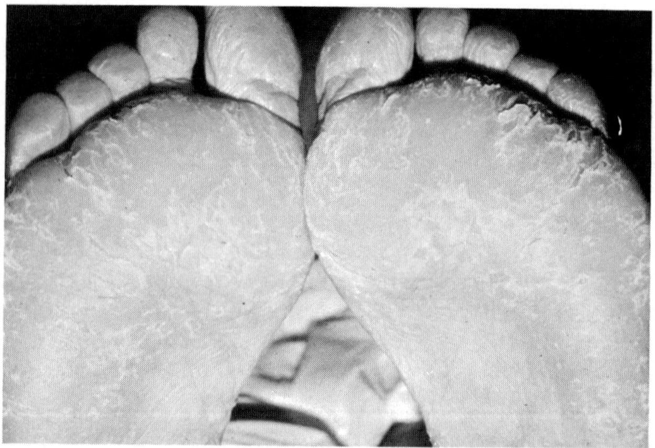

FIGURE 11–60. Psoriasis. Psoriatic plantar keratoderma may be associated with more widespread psoriasis vulgaris or with palmar keratoderma. Note the typical bilateral symmetry of the lesions.

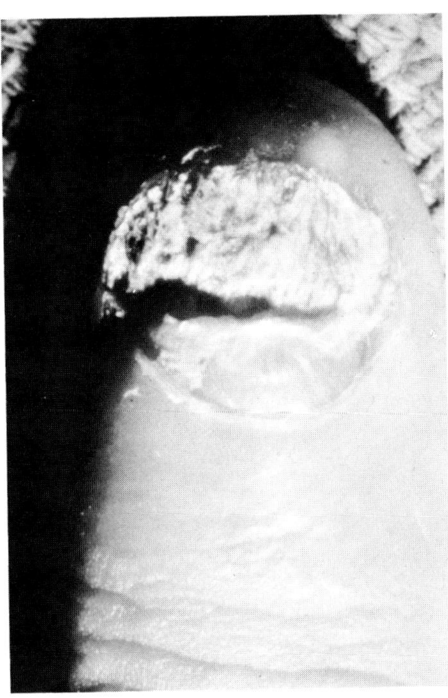

FIGURE 11–62. Psoriatic nail changes. Onycholysis and nail plate dystrophy may affect single, multiple, or all nails of the fingers and toes.

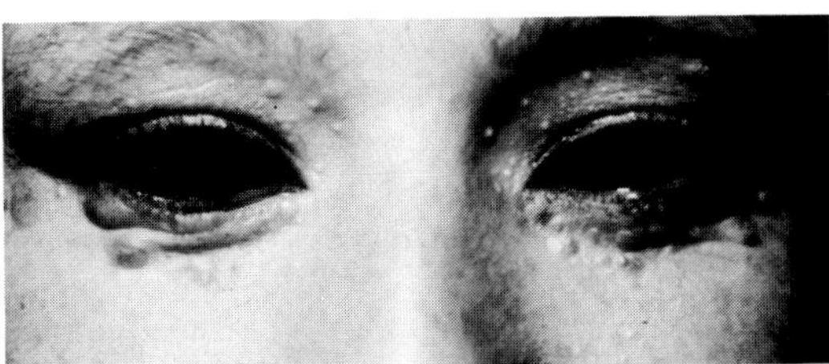

FIGURE 11–63. Basal cell nevus syndrome. This young patient has multiple basal cell carcinomas on the face. Lesions are typical of most basal cell carcinomas and are usually pearly, violaceous papules or nodules with superimposed telangiectasias.

only evidence of psoriasis in some patients. The presence of pits should lead the clinician to ask about a family history of psoriasis.

Oil spots are a brownish discoloration of the nail bed beneath the nail plate. These spots usually appear close to the distal nail fold.

Onychodystrophy in the psoriatic patient can range from mild distal onycholysis to complete destruction of the nail plate. Nails are often thickened, yellow, and crumbly with variable amounts of subungual debris.

The association of psoriasis with identifiable underlying systemic disease is essentially limited to psoriatic arthritis and pustular psoriasis.

The treatment of psoriasis depends on many factors. The type and distribution of the lesions, severity, thickness of the plaques, presence or absence of pustules, and response to previous therapy all are important. Topical therapies include topical corticosteroids, emollients, keratolytics, anthralin, phototherapy (ultraviolet B and ultraviolet A plus psoralen [PUVA]), and topical vitamin D. Systemic therapy is indicated in patients who do not respond to topical regimens or phototherapy. Methotrexate is an extremely effective and relatively safe therapy in psoriatic patients with severe or recalcitrant disease and patients with severe psoriatic arthritis. Cyclosporine is currently being used with success but requires considerable expertise in managing these patients. Some patients with severe arthritis have also been treated with other potent immunosuppressants such as cyclophosphamide and azathioprine. Only clinicians with significant experience with these systemic medications should attempt to use them.

Basal Cell Nevus Syndrome

The basal cell nevus syndrome is an inherited multisystemic, progressively degenerative disease characterized by the early onset of multiple basal cell carcinomas, facial bone deformities such as frontal bossing, and mandibular cysts. The term *nevus* in this designation does not refer to melanocytic or any other type of true nevus but derives from antiquated medical terminology meaning any well-defined lesion arising from genetic influences.

Diagnosis of the syndrome may be suspected at an early age, long before the appearance of any skin manifestations. An examination of the palms or soles reveals the presence of minute pitting of the epidermis. Congenital blindness or hydrocephalus may be noted at birth or during early infancy. Patients usually have characteristic facies including frontal bossing (prominence of the frontal bone of the skull) and prominent supraorbital ridges and lower jaw, a broad nasal root, and widely set eyes. Patients develop multiple basal cell carcinomas, usually as young adults (Fig. 11–63). Besides the early age of onset, the basal cell carcinomas in this syndrome are somewhat unusual in their distribution because they appear in sun-protected areas. Multiple cutaneous basal cell carcinomas have been noted in regions of previous exposure to x-ray or other radiation therapy. In addition, affected patients have a significantly higher than normal incidence of internal neoplasms, such as tumors of the head and neck, brain, and genitalia. Multiple jaw cysts are present in most patients. The palmoplantar pits that are so characteristic of this syndrome occur in approximately 50% of patients but are not pathognomonic for basal cell nevus syndrome (Fig. 11–64); they are due to a defect in the production of keratin in the epidermis of the palms and soles. Pits are also found on the lateral surfaces of the fingers and toes. Other cuta-

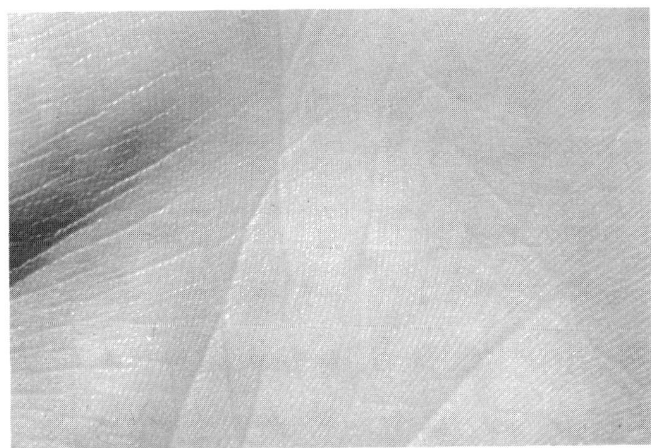

FIGURE 11–64. Palmar pits—basal cell nevus syndrome. Multiple small palmar and plantar pits may be seen in association with multiple cutaneous basal cell carcinomas, bone cysts of the facial structures, and intracranial calcifications.

neous signs of the syndrome include multiple cutaneous cysts, lipomas, and fibromas. Teeth may be abnormal. Occasionally, mental retardation is associated with this syndrome. An interesting clinical and radiologic abnormality found in basal cell nevus syndrome is called *Albright's sign,* which is an abnormally short fourth metacarpal bone.

The finding of palmoplantar pits in the general population is most often not an indication of this disease. Pits may be found in conditions such as arsenical keratoses due to chronic arsenic ingestion or pitting keratolysis (a corynebacterial infection of the epidermis). Pits may be idiopathic.

Acrolentiginous and Subungual Melanomas

Melanoma is the most dangerous of all cutaneous malignancies. The incidence of melanoma has risen alarmingly during the past several decades. Melanoma may appear in four distinct forms: *nodular, superficial spreading, lentigo maligna, and acrolentiginous melanoma.* The vertical tumor thickness (Breslow thickness) and whether the tumor extends into the epidermis, dermis, or subcutaneous tissue (Clark level), along with where on the body the melanoma is found are important prognostic factors in the short-term and long-term survival of patients with melanoma. In general, melanomas arising on the scalp, trunk, hands, and feet appear to have a worse prognosis than elsewhere on the body.

The superficial spreading and nodular melanomas are the most common types and may arise anywhere on the body (Fig. 11–65). The most common sites appear to be the upper back in men and the lower legs in women. Lentigo maligna (Hutchinson's freckle) usually arises on sun-exposed areas of the head and neck. It tends to be a more indolent and slowly progressive tumor, taking as long as 30 years or more to become metastatic. Acrolentiginous melanoma is found on the palms, soles, or digits and accounts for approximately 14% of melanomas. They may be mistaken initially for benign, longitudinal, pigmented nail bands. The specific histology of acral and subungual melanomas may vary, but they are all potentially lethal tumors. The biologic behavior of acrolentiginous melanomas is thought to be similar to that of superficial spreading melanoma with a high potential for widespread metastasis. When broken down into demographic

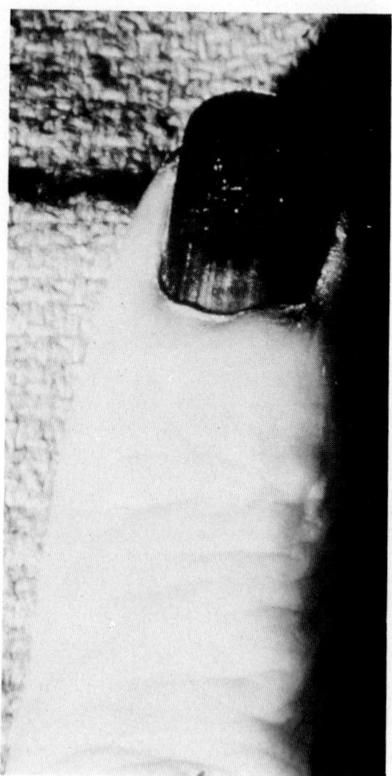

FIGURE 11–66. Subungual acrolentiginous malignant melanoma. Dark, irregular pigmentation completely obliterates the nail bed and extends onto the lateral nail folds (Hutchinson's sign). This lesion first appeared as an irregular longitudinal pigmented nail band.

subsets, subungual melanoma accounts for 2% to 3% of melanomas in whites but as many as 20% in blacks and 30% in Japanese and southwestern Indians. These statistics must be viewed somewhat critically because many melanomas are not reported and are therefore not used in these statistical analyses. Tumors under the nails of the hallux and thumb account for most subungual melanomas. These patients are generally slightly older than are patients with other cutaneous malignant melanomas.

Subungual melanomas may present as longitudinal pigmented nail bands or as a dark tan, brown, black, or red discoloration under the nail plate or at a nail fold (Fig. 11–66). Twenty-five percent of subungual melanomas are amelanotic, that is, with little or no visible pigment in the tumor (Fig. 11–67). This may delay the diagnosis and have catastrophic consequences. Therefore melanoma—both pigmented and amelanotic—must be considered in the differential diagnosis of all subungual tumors or discolorations. Hutchinson's sign, the presence of pigmentation at the proximal nail fold involving both subungual and periungual tissue, is helpful when present and is highly suggestive of subungual melanoma.

The clinical staging of subungual melanoma is divided into stages I, II, and III. Stage I signifies local disease only; stage II indicates the presence of regional metastases; and stage III is used for patients with distant metastases. Nodal involvement may skip the epitrochlear or popliteal lymph node groups while affecting the axillary or inguinal nodes first. An examination of the inguinal region is therefore extremely important when these patients are evaluated.

The 5-year survival rate for patients with subungual melanoma is from 21% to 48%. Primary sites on the feet may be associated with a poorer prognosis, perhaps because of delay

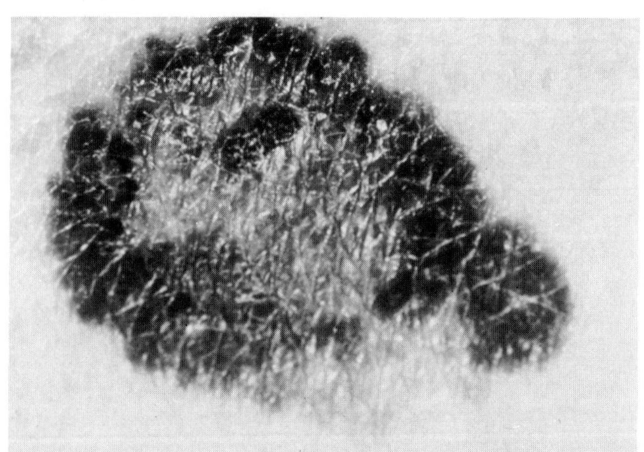

FIGURE 11–65. Superficial spreading malignant melanoma. Irregularly pigmented lesions with irregular borders and focal regression of the tumor (lower border in this photograph) characterize melanoma.

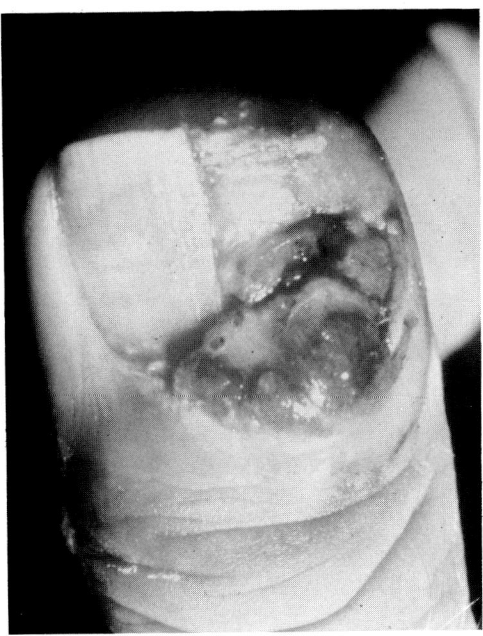

FIGURE 11–67. Amelanotic subungual malignant melanoma. This mostly nonpigmented tumor has destroyed the proximal nail fold and nail bed.

in diagnosis and a slightly older population of affected patients.

A biopsy of any suspicious subungual or cutaneous lesion is mandatory. If the nail plate needs to be avulsed prior to biopsy, this should not delay the evaluation. Care must be taken when a biopsy of the proximal nail fold region is performed so as to minimize destruction of the nail matrix, although this should not be a factor in determining whether or not to perform a biopsy. Therapy is initially surgical with the extent of the excision dependent on the histology and stage of the disease. Amputation of a digit or even a portion of the extremity may be necessary. The presence of regional nodal involvement may require wide excision of the affected lymph node groups, although this is still somewhat controversial. Chemotherapy and immunotherapy are currently being used with some success in patients with metastatic disease. Selective limb perfusion and intralymphatic injection protocols are also being investigated.

Malignant tumors of the nail unit other than melanoma may present as longitudinal pigmented bands and subungual masses. These include pigmented basal cell carcinoma and squamous cell carcinoma in situ.

NAIL CHANGES IN SYSTEMIC DISEASE

Changes in toenails and fingernails are seen in many different primary dermatologic diseases. Abnormal nails are also sometimes evidence of underlying systemic disease, with or without associated skin lesions. Most of these nail conditions are more striking in or limited to the fingernails. A small number of diseases, however, may present with changes in the toenail plate or unit. These are usually, but not always, associated with similar abnormalities in the fingernails. This section is limited to changes seen in the toenails of patients with associated underlying disease. It is always prudent to examine the fingernails when toenail abnormalities are observed. In certain patients, such as those

with 20-nail syndrome, the diagnosis cannot be made without a careful evaluation of all 20 digits. Most of the well-described nail changes are not specific for one particular disease. However, a few are specific and may be extremely helpful in making a correct diagnosis. In general, a search for underlying systemic disease is warranted in only a few of these patients, and these are cases in which the nail changes are fairly specific.

Transverse White Bands

Transverse white bands of the nail plates are quite common. Most result from local trauma to the nail matrix. There are a few points that may help differentiate trauma-induced transverse white bands from white bands associated with underlying disease. In the latter group the changes tend to occur in multiple nails and on both fingernails and toenails when the toenails are involved. The bands usually spread across the entire breadth of the nail bed or plate and tend to be more homogeneous and have smoother borders than trauma-induced lesions. The absence of a history of trauma is helpful, and a history of systemic insult may be elicited.

Another common cause of smaller or incomplete transverse white bands is mild to moderate zinc deficiency. Oral zinc supplements eliminate further appearance of these lines. These may be clinically indistinguishable from trauma-induced lines. Both types of lesions grow out with the nail plate.

Mees' lines may be single or multiple transverse white lines that occur in the nail plate and also move distally as the nail grows (Fig. 11–68). The lines do not disappear when the distal digit is squeezed. Mees' lines are not specific for any one disease and may be associated with a number of conditions (Table 11–4). Mees' lines are no longer produced when the underlying condition is resolved.

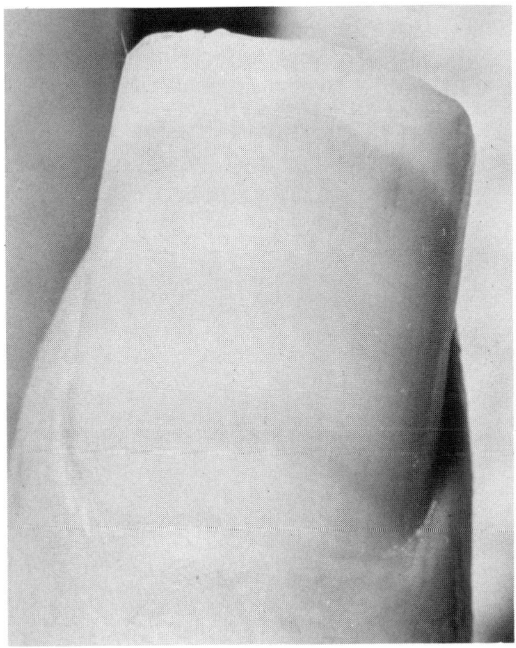

FIGURE 11–68. Mees' lines. The nail plate shows multiple transverse white lines or bands that do not disappear when the nail and distal digit are squeezed.

TABLE 11–4

CONDITIONS ASSOCIATED WITH MEES' LINES

Arsenic toxicity
Chemotherapeutic agents
Hansen's disease
Hodgkin's disease
Hemoglobinopathies
Labor and delivery
Malaria
Myocardial infarction and heart failure
Pellagra
Pulmonary disease
Renal failure

Adapted from Scher RK and Daniel CR: Nails: Therapy, Surgery, Diagnosis. Philadelphia, WB Saunders, 1990.

Beau's Lines

Beau's lines are one of the most common and least specific nail changes associated with systemic disease. Temporary cessation of nail plate growth or decreased deposition of the nail plate results in a transverse groove or depression that extends from one lateral nail fold to the other (Fig. 11–69). Multiple nails are usually affected. An estimation of the time of systemic trauma can be made by approximating the fraction of nail length intervening between the proximal nail fold and Beau's line. For example, given that it takes about 1 year for a toenail to grow from the proximal to distal nail groove, Beau's line at the midnail would reflect a systemic insult approximately 6 months earlier. Beau's lines may be seen in patients who have experienced conditions such as febrile illnesses, major surgery, and organ system failure such as myocardial infarction. Beau's lines have been seen in patients who have acute hypocalcemia resulting from parathyroidectomy. It is not clear whether the surgical procedure itself was contributory in the production of the lesions, but when calcium metabolism was normalized the changes resolved. In fact, any significant insult can lead to Beau's lines. Occasionally, patients may present with Beau's lines that result from emotional trauma. In some patients, no clear history of physical or emotional trauma can be elicited.

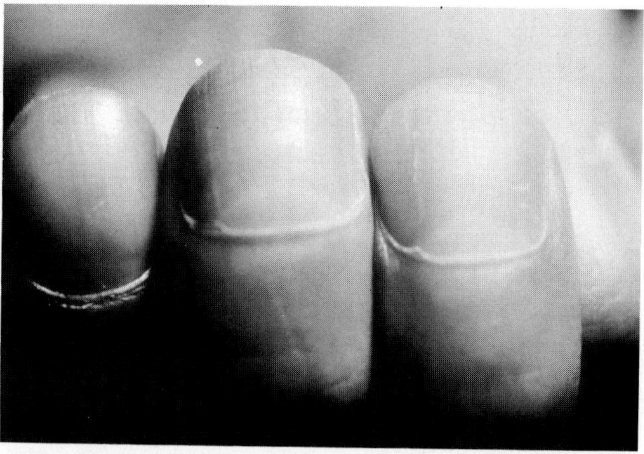

FIGURE 11–70. Clubbing—pulmonary osteoarthropathy. Increased longitudinal curvature of the nail plate, opening of the angle formed by the proximal nail fold area and the nail plate, and increased sponginess of the distal dorsal digit near the nail fold constitute simple clubbing.

Clubbing is most often idiopathic but may be associated with congenital, systemic, or local disease. Clubbing may be divided into three morphologic types. The *Hippocratic finger* has increased bilateral curvature of the nail plate and enlargement of the soft connective tissue limited to the distal phalanges. It is uncommon and may be associated with local or systemic suppurative and cyanotic disease. A second type of clubbing is called *hypertrophic osteoarthropathy* (Fig. 11–70). This usually appears on the toes as simple clubbing. The longitudinal curvature of the nail plate is increased, and the nail may curve over the distal tip of the finger or toe. The obtuse angle formed by the junction of the proximal nail fold and the nail plate is opened and becomes a flat line or greater than 180 degrees. The dorsal distal digit just proximal to the nail fold is spongy and occasionally enlarged. About 80% of simple clubbing is associated with respiratory ailments. Hypertrophic osteoarthropathy may also present with considerable distal digital hypertrophy, extensive periosteal thickening, articular pain, and gynecomastia. The third type of clubbing, *pachydermoperiostosis,* is rare and most often id-

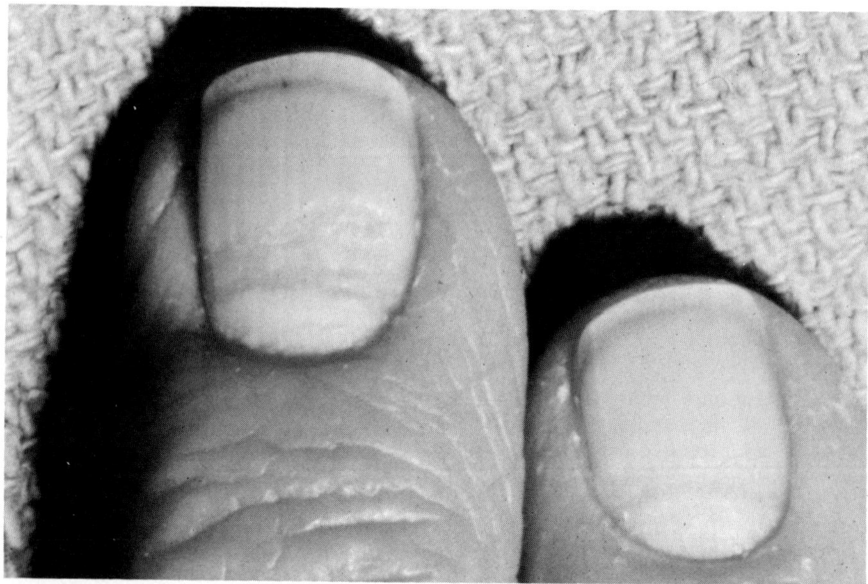

FIGURE 11–69. Beau's lines. Transverse grooves or indentations across the nail plate represent periods of slowed nail matrix activity that correspond to periods of systemic illness or emotional stress.

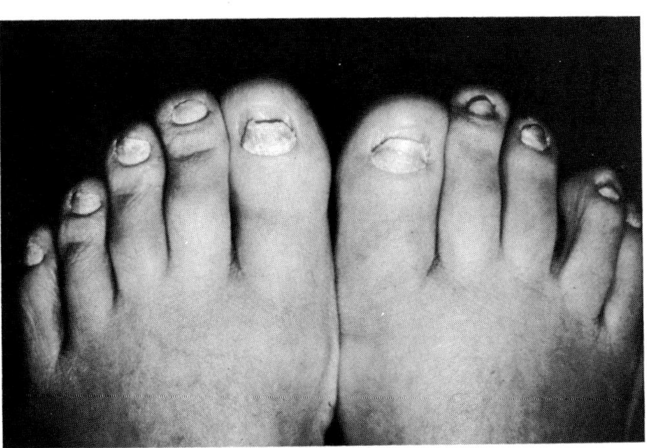

FIGURE 11–71. Yellow nail syndrome. All 20 nails show significantly slowed growth, yellowish discoloration of the plates that are thickened and excessively curved transversally, absent lunulae, variable onycholysis, and swelling of the periungual tissues. Yellow nail syndrome may be associated with pleural effusions and lung disease, including malignancy.

iopathic. In this disorder, there is clubbing of the terminal phalanges and pawlike or spadelike enlargement of the hands, thickening of the legs and forearms involving both bone and soft tissue. Symmetrical periosteal bone ossification may also be seen and may clinically resemble acromegaly.

Probably the most specific and potentially significant nail changes associated with underlying systemic disease is the *yellow nail syndrome*. All 20 nails are usually affected. The

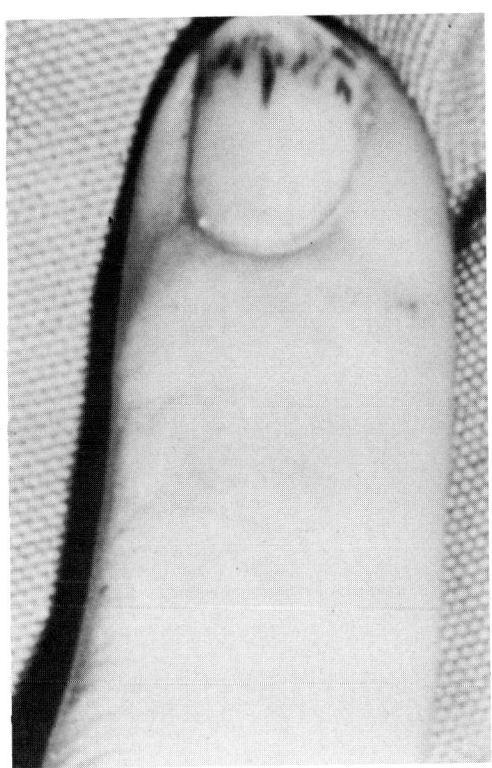

FIGURE 11–72. Subungual splinter hemorrhages. Small longitudinal red, brown, or black focal hemorrhages under the nail plate are usually caused by trauma but may represent hemorrhage due to microemboli lodged in the capillaries of the nail bed.

TABLE 11–5

CAUSES OF SUBUNGUAL SPLINTER HEMORRHAGES

Trauma	Peptic ulcer disease
Infectious endocarditis	Psoriasis
Cirrhosis	Radiodermatitis
Dialysis	Rheumatoid arthritis
Drug reactions	Scurvy
Fungal infection	Tetracycline
Systemic illness	Thyrotoxicosis
Mitral stenosis	Trichinosis
Mycosis fungoides	Vasculitis

Adapted from Scher RK and Daniel CR: Nails: Therapy, Surgery, Diagnosis. Philadelphia, WB Saunders, 1990.

nail plates show a significantly slowed rate of growth. There is yellowish discoloration of the plate that is thickened and excessively curved from one side to another. The lunulae are absent, as are the cuticles. There is swelling of the periungual tissue and a variable degree of onycholysis (Fig. 11–71). The yellow nail syndrome has been described in patients with a number of pulmonary diseases, including malignancies. Pleural effusions (the collection of fluid in the pleural cavity between the chest wall and the lung) may be seen. A search for systemic and particularly pleuropulmonary disease is mandatory because a large percentage of patients will have underlying pathologic changes. A chest radiograph will reveal many of these conditions. Less common associations include thyroid disease, tuberculosis, and congenital lymphedema.

Splinter hemorrhages are extremely common in both fingernails and toenails. By far, the most common cause of splinter hemorrhages is local trauma to the distal digit and nail bed. The hemorrhages appear as thin linear black, brown, or dark red lines parallel with the long axis of the digit (Fig. 11–72). They may appear at any area of the nail bed and are caused by the extravasation of blood into the parenchyma of the nail bed. They are linear because they correspond to the distribution of the small blood vessels in the dermal papillae of the skin of the nail bed. In trauma-induced splinter hemorrhages, usually one or only a few nails are affected. The location of the lesions may be proximal or distal. Patients often do not recall the inciting trauma. If the splinter hemorrhages are present on multiple nails, nails of more than one extremity, and both fingernails and toenails, infective endocarditis (an infection of the heart valves) may be the cause. Small emboli break off from the infected heart valve and become lodged in the capillaries of the distal nail bed. This leads to infarction of the vessels and extravasation of the blood into the nail bed tissue leading to splinter hemorrhages. Other causes and diseases associated with splinter hemorrhages are shown in Table 11–5.

For a discussion of psoriatic nail changes, see the section on psoriasis. For a discussion of subungual malignant melanoma, see the section on melanoma.

The author thanks the Department of Dermatology, Stanford University Medical Center, Stanford, California, for the kind use of their photographic library.

Bibliography

Baran R and Dawber R (eds): Diseases of the Nails and Their Management. Oxford, Blackwell Scientific, 1984.

Bernstein JE, Medenica M, Soltani K, and Griem SF: Bullous eruption of diabetes mellitus. Arch Dermatol 115:324–325, 1979.

Braunwald E, et al (eds): Harrison's Principles of Internal Medicine, 11th ed. New York, McGraw-Hill, 1987.

Braverman I: Skin Signs of Systemic Disease, 2nd ed. Philadelphia, WB Saunders, 1981.

Callen P and Jorizzo J: Dermatologic Signs of Internal Disease. Philadelphia, WB Saunders, 1988.

Cruz PD Jr, East C, and Bergstresser PR: Dermal, subcutaneous, and tendon xanthomas: Diagnostic markers for specific lipoprotein disorders. J Am Acad Dermatol 19(1):95–111, 1988.

Fitzpatrick T, et al: Dermatology in General Medicine, 3rd ed. New York, McGraw-Hill, 1987.

Howel-Evans W, McConnell RB, Clarke CA, and Sheppard PM: Carcinoma of the oesophagus with keratosis palmaris et plantaris (tylosis): A study of two families. Q J Med 27:413–429, 1958.

Jacobs PH and Anhalt TS: Handbook of Skin Clues of Systemic Diseases, 2nd ed. Philadelphia, Lea & Febiger, 1992.

Mindel A, Tovey SJ, Timmins DJ, and Williams P: Primary and secondary syphilis, 20 years experience: Clinical features. Genitourin Med 65:1–3, 1989.

Mitchell DM and Fries JF: An analysis of the American Rheumatism Association criteria for rheumatoid arthritis. Arthritis Rheum 25:481, 1982.

Rigel D (ed): Melanoma/skin cancer update 1991. Dermatol Clin 9:4, 1991.

Scher RK and Daniel CR: Nails: Therapy, Surgery, Diagnosis. Philadelphia, WB Saunders, 1990.

Sigurgeirsson B, Lindelöf B, Edhag O, and Allander E: Risk of cancer in patients with dermatomyositis or polymyositis: A population-based study. N Engl J Med 326(6):363–367, 1992.

Sjögren H: Zur Kenntnis der Keratoconjunctivitis sicca (Keratitis filiformis bei Hypofunktion der Trandendrusen). Acta Ophthalmol 11 (Suppl 2) 1933.

Tomecki KJ (ed): Systemic Mycoses and Parasitic Diseases. Dermatol Clin 7(2):192–402, 1989.

Vascular Manifestations of Articular Disease

David Mullens, D.P.M.

Arthritis is often envisioned solely as a joint-based disease. In fact, the extra-articular manifestations of arthritis carry greater risks for the patient. The vascular manifestations of arthritis are one such example.

The three separate vascular problems associated with arthritis that are discussed in this chapter include (1) vasculitis associated with connective tissue disease; (2) Raynaud's phenomenon associated with connective tissue disease; and (3) neurologically mediated vasodilatation associated with (diabetic) Charcot's arthropathy. Each of these problems has a separate etiology, and it is the mechanism of disease to which we pay particular attention. An understanding of the pathophysiology of each disease process allows us to make better decisions when treating patients with that disease process. In addition, as we examine each of these three disease processes, we will try to answer the threshold question: Does the arthritis precede or cause the vascular problem, or does the vascular problem precede or cause the arthritis?

VASCULITIS

Rheumatoid arthritis is used as the example of a connective tissue disease associated with vasculitis. But before we discuss rheumatoid vasculitis, we shall discuss the basic disease mechanism responsible for rheumatoid arthritis. An understanding of the immunologic aspects of rheumatoid arthritis is fundamental to an understanding of the pathophysiology of vasculitis. The immunologic considerations of this disorder are summarized as follows:

1. Blood contains three separate groups of proteins: albumins, globulins, and fibrinogen.
2. All of the antibodies are globulins. These antibodies can be divided into the following types: immunoglobulin G (IgG), IgA, IgM, IgD, and IgE.
3. In rheumatoid arthritis, something happens to the IgG. For whatever reason(s), the patient begins to manufacture structurally altered IgG.[1, 2]
4. The altered IgG is recognized by the patient's body as antigen.
5. Anti-IgG antibodies are formed against altered IgG.
6. Anti-IgG antibodies are called *rheumatoid factors.*

7. Altered IgG combines with rheumatoid factor to become a soluble immune complex.
8. Intra-articular soluble immune complex attracts polymorphonuclear neutrophils (PMNs) and activates the complement system.
9. Activated complement dilates local blood vessels and draws more inflammatory cells into the joint.
10. The inflammatory cells (PMNs) engulf the immune complexes.
11. The PMNs, after engulfing the immune complex, release lysosomal enzymes into the joint.
12. The lysosomal enzymes
    a. Destroy cartilage.
    b. Activate complement (causing a repeat of step 9).
    c. Stimulate synovial cell hypertrophy and hyperplasia, which results in pannus formation.
    d. Attack the phospholipid portion of the PMN cell membrane to release prostaglandins, which stimulate more inflammation.

Although this sequence of events translates into joint inflammation, it may likewise mediate vascular disease. In rheumatoid vasculitis, the soluble immune complex (mentioned earlier in step 7) is trapped in the small vessel walls. (The term *small vessels* refers to the small arteries, arterioles, venules, and small veins). This trapped soluble immune complex "fixes" complement that is floating by in the blood stream. Graphically stated, the soluble immune complex has an almost magnetic attraction for complement, and the reaction between the two sets off a chain reaction of inflammatory events.

The area of complement fixation within the blood vessel wall becomes the target for a massive inflammatory attack. As a result, the blood vessel wall and all of the surrounding soft tissue, including the adjacent skin, may be destroyed in the process.

Usually, the vasculitis associated with rheumatoid arthritis is relatively mild, and the patient develops little more than refractory ulcers of the legs and feet. Although the morbidity associated with rheumatoid vasculitis should not be minimized, the point remains that rheumatoid vasculitis is not typically associated with the extensive and even life-threat-

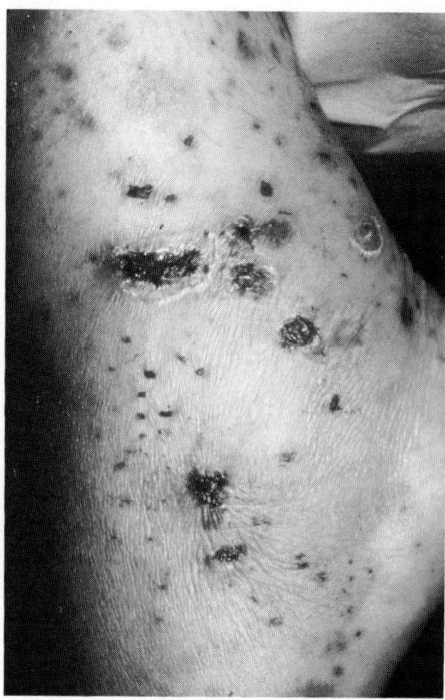

FIGURE 12–1. Palpable purpura, the cutaneous hallmark of vasculitis.

plement takes place in the vessels of the superficial dermis. At first the lesion is small, maculopapular, and erythematous. This is what you would expect from a small nidus of inflammation within the wall of a cutaneous blood vessel. With continued inflammatory destruction of the blood vessel wall, the patient bleeds into this piece of skin and the maculopapular spot of erythema now becomes petechial. In other words, there has been an actual bleed into the skin. This petechial lesion may grow larger if the underlying inflammation continues. If there are other similarly expanding petechial lesions in the same area of skin, these lesions may coalesce to become purpuric.

The cutaneous hallmark of vasculitis is palpable purpura (Fig. 12–1). These lesions are actually raised above the skin surface, and you can tell this by simply running your finger over the lesions and feeling the elevation of the lesion. Discoloration due to intracutaneous hemorrhage does not disappear when a glass slide is pressed against the skin. (On the other hand, if the discoloration is due to erythema or cyanosis, the discoloration temporarily disappears with the pressure of the glass slide. Why? Because the glass slide temporarily squeezes the blood out of the skin venules and into the veins. Release of the glass slide pressure allows the blood to flow back into the venules.)

If the purpuric lesions continue to enlarge, they may coalesce to become *hemorrhagic bullae* (Fig. 12–2). If the blood supply to the soft tissue under a hemorrhagic bulla remains intact, the bulla will crust and then heal over. If the blood supply to the soft tissue under a hemorrhagic bulla is lost owing to continued inflammation, the bulla may become gangrenous. This is the explanation for the progression from an erythematous macule/papule to a petechia to purpura to hemorrhagic/gangrenous bullae.

Livedo Reticularis. Another skin lesion associated with arthritis vasculitis is livedo reticularis (Fig. 12–3). The physiologic variant of livedo reticularis occurs in young women who have fair skin and who develop a blotchy or fishnet-like pattern of skin discoloration in response to cold exposure.

Livedo reticularis can be described in the following way.

ening vasculitis seen with other diseases that have a vasculitic component.

Skin Lesions Associated with Vasculitis

A discussion of the pathophysiology of the basic skin lesions associated with vasculitis of any type is appropriate.[3] These basic skin lesions consist of hemorrhagic papules, livedo reticularis, infarcts, and nodules.[4] The topic of vasculitis and vasculitic lesions can be confusing, and the following discussion should help clarify these issues.

Hemorrhagic Papules. Hemorrhagic papules occur when the interaction between soluble immune complex and com-

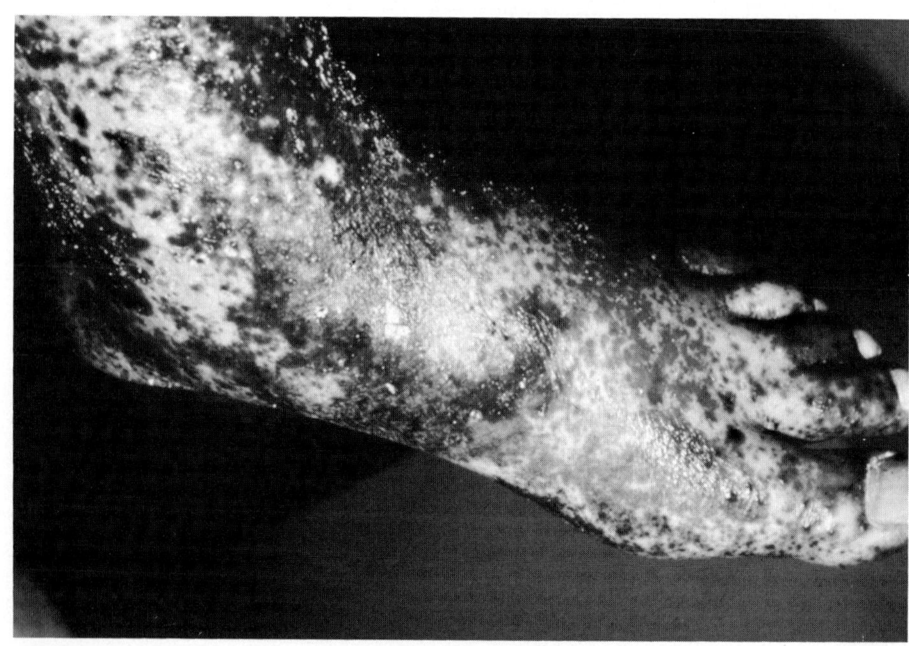

FIGURE 12–2. As purpuric lesions enlarge, they may coalesce to form hemorrhagic bullae, as illustrated.

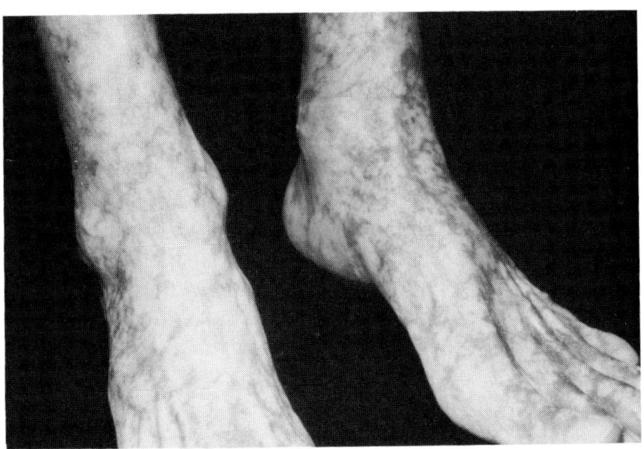

FIGURE 12–3. One form of arthritic vasculitis is livedo reticularis. Note the fishnet-like pattern.

Anatomically and physiologically, the skin venous network may be thought of as a wheel with a central hub and a peripheral tire with connecting spokes. The central hub represents the central collecting vein, the spokes represent the connecting veins, and the tire represents the peripheral venules that feed into the central vein through the connecting veins. Livedo reticularis associated with connective tissue disease is due to sympathetically mediated constriction of the central vein and the connecting veins while the peripheral venules are dilated. The peripheral venules are dilated because the venules are responsive to the locally accumulating metabolic waste products from the adjacent tissue cells. As these waste products accumulate, they will directly cause the smooth muscles in the walls of the venules to relax. The central and connecting veins, however, are under the "complete" control of the sympathetic nervous system and continue to constrict as long as the sympathetic nerves innervating their walls continue to fire.

As the patient is exposed to a warmer environment, the rate of sympathetic impulses tapers off, and the skin blood vessels under sympathetic control are allowed to dilate. As a result of the reduced sympathetic tone, the peripheral venular blood flows through the connecting and central veins into the proximal veins. As a result of this venous dilation, the fishnet-like pattern of the cutaneous veins disappears.

Although livedo reticularis is most commonly discussed as an arterial disorder, this presentation simply "fits" better and is easier to use.

Infarcts. Infarcts associated with cutaneous vasculitis occur when the inflammatory reaction destroys a small artery supplying a piece of the skin. There is tremendous overlap of arterial supply to any piece of skin, but for the purpose of explanation, we are going to assume that each piece of skin has a single small artery responsible for bringing the nutrient arterial inflow to that piece of skin. If that single small artery is lost due to the inflammation associated with vasculitis, the overlying piece of skin fed by that artery will die. This is the reason and explanation for cutaneous infarct association with vasculitis.

Nodules. Nodules associated with vasculitis are clinically dramatic and academically straightforward. Each nodule represents a nidus of vasculitis within a muscle belly. Because the nodules occur in the deeper tissues, there is no overlying skin loss. However, the patient, as expected, has significant pain at the side of each nodule as long as the vasculitis process is active in the area of the nodule.

RAYNAUD'S PHENOMENON

"Raynaud's phenomenon may be defined as an episode of constriction of the small arteries and arterioles which results in intermittent changes in skin color."[5] The color changes, in order, consist of pallor, cyanosis, and erythema (Fig. 12–4). So the obvious questions are: how and why do Raynaud's phenomena occur?

Other than stating that people who exhibit Raynaud's phenomenon are "more sensitive to cold," we really do not have an adequate answer as to why. As to how Raynaud's phenomenon occurs, we can at least give a compelling explanation regarding the physiologic steps that accompany the color changes.

Cutaneous Arteriospasm

Before discussing the step-by-step events in a typical attack of Raynaud's phenomenon, the broader topic of cutaneous arteriospasm should be reviewed. The term *cutaneous arteriospasm* is commonly used to describe the clinical finding of cold feet, despite the presence of palpable pulses. And if we are fairly certain the patient has no significant upstream arterial obstruction, we assume the cutaneous arteriospasm represents a profound state of constriction of the skin blood vessels. Finally, we assume this vasoconstriction is due to increased sympathetic tone in response to a heightened sensitivity to cold.

Additionally, cutaneous arteriospasm means that blood flow through the small arteries and arterioles supplying a piece of skin temporarily comes to a halt. Cutaneous arteriospasm is a functional change and is analogous to turning off a faucet; cutaneous arteriospasm is due to increased resistance to blood flow through the small arteries and arterioles that supply the skin of the foot.

The two primary determinants of resistance to flow through the small arteries and arterioles supplying the skin of the foot are the viscosity of the blood and the radii of the blood vessels. The viscosity of blood is determined by the

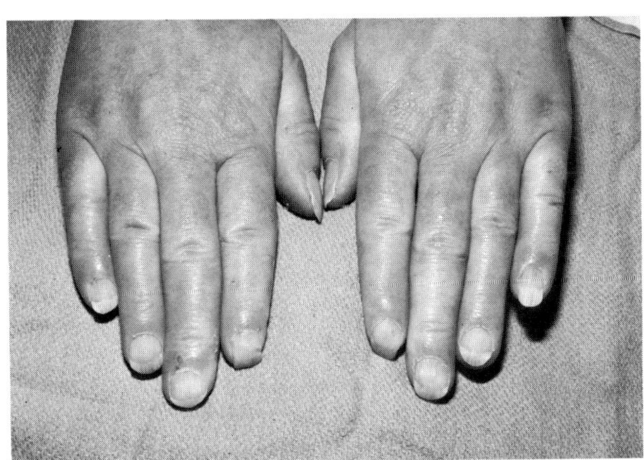

FIGURE 12–4. Note the varying stages of pallor and rubor in this patient with Raynaud's phenomenon.

protein concentration of the blood, by the hematocrit level, and by the extent of capillary filtration. The radii of these blood vessels supplying the skin of the foot are determined by the presence or absence of organic arterial occlusive disease, by the withdrawal of sympathetic tone, and by the amount of sympathetic constriction.

Which of these determinants is important when cutaneous arteriospasm is discussed? Clinically, the only important determinant of blood viscosity is the protein concentration of the blood. Practically, this means that the patient with a connective tissue disorder must produce cryoglobulins (which are macroglobulins) or cold agglutinins to precipitate an attack of Raynaud's phenomenon on the basis of increased blood viscosity, and Raynaud's phenomenon on the basis of increased blood viscosity is clinically uncommon.

Control of vessel radius is the most important determinant of the resistance of blood flow through the small arteries and arterioles, and the amount of sympathetic constriction is the most important determinant of vessel radius. In summary, cutaneous arteriospasm is most commonly caused by sympathetic vasoconstriction. This understanding will lend itself to an academic model explaining Raynaud's phenomenon.

Sympathetic Versus Local Control

The term *sympathetic control* is used to signify which of the small blood vessels is innervated by sympathetic nerve fibers. The term *local control* signifies which of the small blood vessels is responsive to the accumulation of metabolic waste products. In other words, local control means that as the local tissue cells become anoxic secondary to local vasoconstriction, the anoxic cells begin to release chemicals into the surrounding extracellular fluid. These chemicals have a direct dilating effect on the small arterioles, precapillary sphincters, and venules in the immediate area.

We can list the small blood vessels and whether they are under sympathetic control or local control, as follows:

A. Small arteries and large arterioles: sympathetic control (only)
B. Small arterioles: sympathetic control and local control
C. Precapillary sphincters: local control (only)
D. Venules: sympathetic and local control
E. Veins: sympathetic control (only)

Using this list, Raynaud's phenomenon can be broken down into the following order of events:

Pallor
1. Sympathetic firing produces constriction of vessels A, B, D, and E.
2. Metabolic waste products accumulate around vessels A, B, C, D, and E.
3. The precapillary sphincters, which are devoid of sympathetic nerve fibers, dilate owing to the accumulation of metabolic waste products. However, this is to no avail, because the small arteries and arterioles are still constricted.

Cyanosis
4. The small arterioles dilate, allowing a small amount of blood into the precapillary sphincters and capillaries. Because the precapillary sphincters are massively dilated, the flow of blood is very slow. In addition, be-

cause the oxygen gradient is very large, the hemoglobin level in the red blood cells is rapidly reduced. This change in the oxygenation of hemoglobin produces frank cyanosis of the tissues.

Erythema
5. The sympathetic tone of the small arteries and arterioles diminishes while the metabolic waste products are increasing. As a result, these vessels dilate, which produces a reactive hyperemia, lasting until the normal tissue values for oxygen and cellular metabolites have been re-established.

CHARCOT'S ARTHROPATHY

Before we can discuss the underlying disease process in Charcot's arthropathy, we need to review some basic information regarding the autonomic nervous system control of blood flow through peripheral (extremity) blood vessels. First, there are no parasympathetic nerve fibers running from the central nervous system to the peripheral blood vessels. Thus, stimulation of the parasympathetic nerve fibers in the central nervous system does not produce peripheral dilatation. We are therefore left with the inescapable conclusion that all the autonomic nerve fibers to the blood vessels of the lower extremity are sympathetic nerve fibers.

These sympathetic (postganglionic, adrenergic) nerve fibers normally innervate the smooth muscles in the walls of the blood vessels and the sweat glands in the skin. The smooth muscles in the walls of the blood vessels are oriented in a circular fashion around the lumen of the vessel. Stimulation of the sympathetic nerve fibers causes the smooth muscles to contract, and this results in profound constriction of the blood vessels (and loss of lumen size). Stimulation of the sympathetic nerve fibers to the sweat glands of the skin induces contraction of the smooth muscles surrounding the glands. This squeezing of the sweat gland pushes the sweat gland contents through the sweat gland ducts to the surface of the skin.

In Charcot's arthropathy, the sympathetic nerve fibers cease to work, and the foot becomes massively vasodilated and dry to the touch. There is abundant evidence to support the statement that blood flow to the foot with Charcot's arthropathy is at least normal, if not greater than normal, including observations by constant-wave Doppler technique,[6, 7] venous occlusion plethysmography,[8–10] skin temperature studies,[10, 11] bone scan,[12] and arteriography.[13]

The patient with Charcot's arthropathy is typically diabetic and has a mixed sensory and motor distal polyneuropathy. This neuropathy wipes out the sensory and sympathetic nerves to the foot. As a result, the bones of the foot become soft and fracture (Fig. 12–5A and *B*). The ensuing repair process is exuberant but ineffectual, because the abnormally increased arterial inflow allows for significant collagen scaffolding without adequate mineralization. Thus, the patient forms a lot of new soft bone at the fracture site, and this new bone is also vulnerable to fracture as the patient bears weight.

In addition, the normal sensory feedback information that allows bone remodeling to occur along lines of stress is absent, resulting in a piece of bone that becomes very soft and that fractures under the pressure of weightbearing. The patient forms an excessive amount of new bone at the frac-

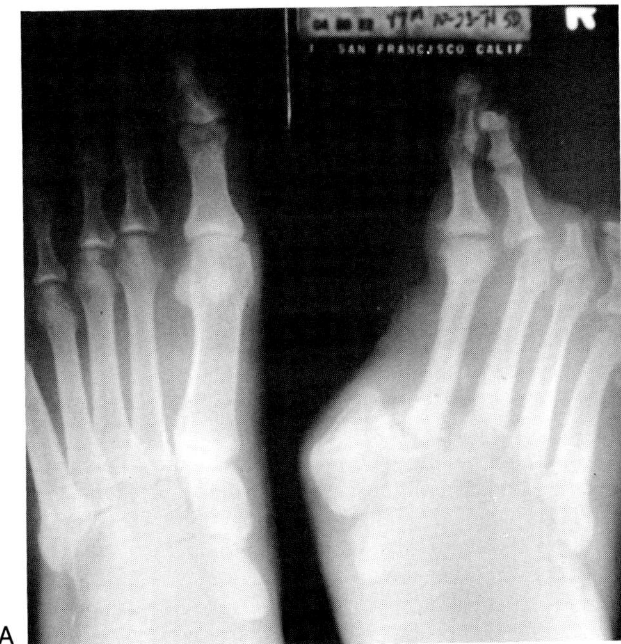

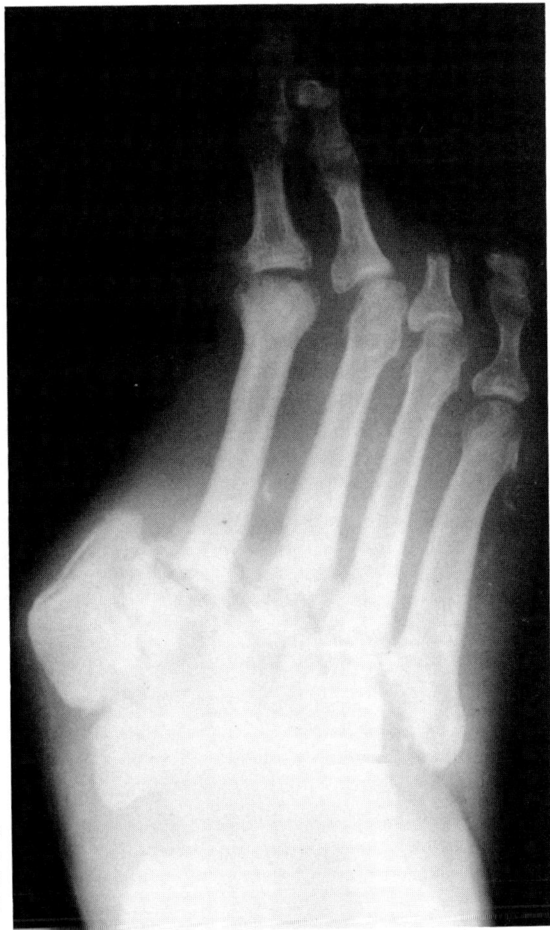

FIGURE 12–5. *A,* This diabetic patient underwent amputation of the first ray owing to osteomyelitis that developed from an ulceration. Malposition of the first ray was the cause, which developed from Charcot's arthroplasty. *B,* Close-up view of the same patient displays widespread osseous disruption of Lisfranc's joint.

ture site. This new bone may also fracture, owing to inadequate mineralization. However, the new bone formed at the fracture site or sites fails to be remodeled, so that the initial site of injury remains massively deformed.

This process of Charcot's arthropathy stops if the local blood flow is reduced. In fact, a published case history documents a diabetic patient who developed Charcot's arthropathy that stopped with the onset of significant arteriosclerosis obliterans and started again after the ischemic limb was revascularized.[14]

The natural history of Charcot's arthropathy is as follows:

1. The foot becomes numb.
2. The bones become soft.
3. The patient walks on the numb foot with soft bones.
4. The soft bones fracture.
5. The fractures heal with malposition of the fragments and deposition of bone fragments in the adjacent joint capsule.
6. This process repeats.
7. The foot becomes shorter and wider and develops angular bony prominences.
8. The foot becomes ulcerated and infected as the patient walks on the angular prominences.

The pathophysiology of Charcot's arthropathy requires two basic clinical events. First, the patient must have well-developed diabetic neuropathy. Second, the patient must have at least normal arterial inflow to the already neuropathic foot so that the loss of sympathetic control will allow for a massive increase in blood flow through the bones of the foot. This increase in blood flow allows for a "washing-out" and softening of the bones, and it is this increase in blood flow that allows for a massive attempt at repair after each of the fractures.

TREATMENT

Vasculitis

The treatment of vasculitis is simple and straightforward. When the underlying "inflammation" associated with the connective tissue disease process is successfully controlled or suppressed, the vasculitis ulcers will heal. Until the inflammation is reduced, the ulcers will continue to expand, despite the use of antibiotics and diligent wound care.

The most commonly prescribed drug for suppressing the inflammation associated with vasculitis is prednisone. It makes no difference what the cause of the vasculitis is. Once the patient has vasculitis ulcers, the common pathway of inflammation must be suppressed before the ulcers will heal.

Raynaud's Phenomenon

The treatment of Raynaud's phenomenon is interesting in that the emphasis has been on changing the response of the patient's blood vessels to cold rather than on preventing the exposure of the blood vessels. Simply stated, the best way to treat Raynaud's phenomenon is to prevent the precipitating event, cold exposure, from occurring.

Raynaud's phenomenon affects women far more frequently than men. By employing common-sense measures such as wearing pants instead of dresses, socks instead of stockings, high-collared sweaters instead of open-neck blouses, long-sleeved tops instead of short sleeves, and gloves when going out into cold weather, women with this disease may avoid repeated episodes of cutaneous arteriospasm. This is important, because with each episode of severe constriction, the skin vessels are more and more likely to undergo permanent damage from scarring and fibrosis of the blood vessel walls. This will eventually lead to a fixed reduction in lumen size and a loss of the ability of the vessel to dilate. Over time, the functional response of arteriospasm changes to permanent narrowing or closure of the small arteries and arterioles.

When the patient is doing the best he or she can to avoid cold exposure and still is experiencing symptomatic Raynaud's phenomenon, we can use an oral vasodilating agent. The only oral vasodilating agent commonly used at this time is nifedipine (Procardia),[15] which blocks the movement of calcium ions (Ca^{2+}) across the cell membrane of vascular smooth muscle cells. Specifically, nifedipine blocks the transport of Ca^{2+} through the L channels, which are present in the cell membrane of smooth muscle cells. By preventing the movement of Ca^{2+} from the extracellular compartment into the intracellular smooth muscle compartment, contraction of the smooth muscle is inhibited. Nifedipine selectively dilates the arterioles without affecting the venules or veins. As a result, it can be used to stop peripheral arteriospasm before it starts.

Nifedipine should be given at the lowest dose that will achieve the goal of peripheral dilatation. Because the dose of nifedipine varies from 10 to 20 mg given once, twice, or three times a day, this drug should be administered and monitored by the patient's family physician. This recommendation has to do with the fact that surgical subspecialties just do not do an adequate job of monitoring long-term medications.

For the patient who fails to respond to the common-sense measures and the use of an oral-vasodilating agent (or agents), lumbar sympathectomy can be considered. Although cervical sympathectomy has been an abysmal failure when used for arteriospasm of the upper extremity, lumbar sympathectomy has been successful in the relief of arteriospasm of both the upper and the lower extremities.

Charcot's Arthropathy

The treatment of Charcot's arthropathy is not yet well defined. Treatment had been limited to orthotic/molded-shoe support, cast immobilization with varying periods of non-weightbearing, and surgical débridement. Recently, however, more emphasis has been given to fusion stabilization of the involved Charcot's joints with concomitant tendon lengthening when the patient has a significant equinus along with a midfoot Charcot's arthropathy.

The following clinical question must be addressed: If the Charcot's arthropathy is due to sympathetic denervation, which results in a localized hyperemia of bone, and if the hyperemia produces a localized demineralization of bone, which results in fracture fragmentation of the bone with weightbearing, then why would the Charcot's arthropathy stop after fusion (with or without tendon lengthening)? After all, the underlying disease process consists of denervation of the sympathetic and sensory nerve fibers to a given area of a foot. If this disease process is still present after the fusion procedure, one should anticipate a recurrence of the arthropathy after surgery. Ultimately, long-term studies are necessary to demonstrate which, if any, patients with Charcot's arthropathy will do well with fusion procedures.

References

1. Brower AC and Allman RM: Pathogenesis of the neurotrophic joint: Neurotraumatic vs. neurovascular. Radiology 139(2):349–354, 1981.
2. Edmonds J and Hughes G: Lecture Notes on Rheumatology. Oxford, Blackwell Scientific, 1985, p 33.
3. Roenigk H and Young J: Leg Ulcers. New York, Harper & Row, 1975, p 116.
4. Fitzpatrick TB, et al: Dermatology in General Medicine. New York, McGraw-Hill, 1971, pp 1485–1486.
5. Allen EV, Barker NW, and Hines EA Jr: Peripheral Vascular Diseases, 3rd ed. Philadelphia, WB Saunders, 1962, pp 125–162.
6. Scarpello JH, Martin TR, and Ward JD: Ultrasound measurements of pulse-wave velocity in the peripheral arteries of diabetic subjects. Clin Sci Mol Med 58(1):53–57, 1980.
7. Edmonds ME, Roberts VC, and Watkins PJ: Blood flow in the diabetic neuropathic foot. Diabetologia 22(1):9–15, 1982.
8. Sknitizsky R: Spontaneous rhythm of peripheral blood supply. Z Gesamte Inn Med 32:310–313, 1977.
9. Partsch H: Neuropathies of the ulceromutilating types: Clinical aspects, classification, circulation measurements. Vasa 6(Suppl):1–48, 1977.
10. Archer AG, Roberts VC, and Watkins PJ: Blood flow patterns in diabetic neuropathy. Diabetologia 27:563–567, 1984.
11. Ward JD: The diabetic leg. Diabetologia 22:141–147, 1982.
12. Edmonds ME, Clarke MB, Newton S, et al: Increased uptake of bone radiopharmaceutical in diabetic neuropathy. Q J Med 57(224):843–855, 1985.
13. Seignon B, Menanteau B, Hibon J, et al: Ulcero-mutilating acropathy and the arthropathy of diabetes mellitus: II. Arteriographic study. Rev Rhum Mal Osteoart 41:341–347, 1974.
14. Edelman SV, Kosofsky EM, Paul RA, and Kozak GP: Neuro-osteoarthropathy (Charcot's joint) on diabetes mellitus following revascularization surgery: Three case reports and a review of the literature. Arch Intern Med 147(8):1504–1508, 1987.
15. Gilman A, Rall T, Nies A, and Taylor P: Goodman & Gilman's The Pharmacological Basis of Therapeutics. New York, Pergamon Press, 1990, pp 774–780.

CHAPTER 13

Septic Arthritis

John J. Stienstra, D.P.M., Christopher J. Lamy, D.P.M.,
and Warren S. Joseph, D.P.M.

Septic arthritis is an infrequent, albeit important disease due to its morbidity and mortality. When treatment is delayed, the prognosis is generally poor. A surprising number of infections result in death. Since the advent of antibiotics, the morbidity and mortality have decreased.[1] The prevalence and clinical characteristics, however, have changed little over the last 10 to 20 years.[2] The diminished capacity for repair in the diarthrodial joint increases the morbidity of the destructive changes associated with joint sepsis. Destructive changes occur within hours of the onset of septic arthritis.[3] Preservation of normal anatomic structure by prompt interruption of the infectious process and the degenerative cascade that follows is the appropriate role of the physician. If appropriate therapy is rendered within a few days of onset, a full recovery can be anticipated in most patients.[4] Prompt diagnosis and treatment are crucial to improving the likelihood of a favorable outcome. For these reasons, septic arthritis is considered a medical emergency. Other consequences include chronic degenerative arthritis and osteomyelitis.

CLINICAL PRESENTATION

Septic arthritis usually presents as a monoarticular arthritis in one of the large joints of the lower extremity. Ninety percent of cases are monoarticular.[14] When polyarticular arthritis occurs, it most often is in elderly patients with a history of rheumatoid arthritis or who are receiving systemic corticosteroids. Any diarthrodial joint may be involved; however, the joints of the lower extremity are the most commonly involved. The knee joint has the highest incidence, occurring in 40% to 50% of cases.[14] The hip and ankle are involved in 20% to 25% and 10% to 15% of cases, respectively.[14] The symptoms and signs of this disease are nonspecific. Recognizing the possibility of this disease as part of the differentials for a painful joint is important. Critical early clinical suspicion, with eventual diagnosis and treatment of septic arthritis, gives the patient the best chance for a favorable result.

The classic presentation of bacterial septic arthritis is a patient complaining of a painful, swollen joint. On physical examination, the involved joint is usually tensely edematous, erythematous, and hot with restricted painful range of motion. Eighty percent of patients have fever, usually low-grade.[5] Rigors are present in fewer than 25% of patients and correlate often with positive blood cultures.[7] Patients with prosthetic septic joints present with pain and fever.

PREDISPOSING FACTORS

Most patients with septic arthritis have some type of identifiable predisposing factor.[2] In general, these predisposing factors are alterations that inhibit the immune system either systemically or locally. Diseases and treatments producing immune compromise, such as intravenous drug abuse, connective tissue disease, malnutrition, and chronic disease states are examples of commonly associated conditions. The ability to extend life has increased the numbers of patients with joint sepsis.

Conditions that affect the immune system and that have been associated with joint sepsis constitute a variety of disorders. Rare, inherited immune system diseases, such as complement deficiencies, are associated with joint sepsis. More common than the diseases that directly affect immunocompetence are systemic diseases that interfere with or indirectly affect the immune system. The interference can be from either the disease itself or the treatment of a disease. Some of the diseases reported in the literature include sickle cell anemia, diabetes mellitus, cancer, liver disease, and chronic renal disease. Cancer patients undergoing immunosuppressive therapy are particularly prone to septic arthritis involving gram-negative bacilli, atypical *Mycobacterium*, or fungi.[2] It would be logical that patients with renal transplants would have a higher incidence of septic arthritis; however, in reality this has been reported infrequently.[6] Human immunodeficiency virus (HIV) disease is associated with an increased incidence of opportunistic infections not otherwise seen in the unaffected population. Fungal infection and mycobacterial infection are more frequent in patients with HIV disease.[91] Diagnosis of fungal or mycobacterial bone or joint infection should cause the clinician to consider concomitant HIV infection.

Septic arthritis is most common in infants and in the elderly. These two age groups are prone to septic arthritis for the same reason—both often have defects in their immune system.[2] Infants have immature immune systems. Between the ages of 1 to 24 months, there is a period of time in which the maternal antibodies have been lost and the infant has not acquired natural antibodies. In the elderly, most patients who acquire septic arthritis have serious underlying chronic diseases.[7] The immune system is weakened by these illnesses, making it less effective in protecting the host. The elderly are not only predisposed to septic arthritis but also have a greater chance of having an unfavorable outcome.[2]

Joint diseases can also predispose a joint to septic arthritis. Both systemic and local joint diseases are associated with an increased incidence of joint infection. Rheumatoid arthritis and the related connective tissue diseases are examples of systemic diseases predisposing a patient to septic arthritis. The predominant local disease predisposing a joint to septic arthritis is osteoarthritis. Osteoarthritis can result from previous trauma or from a number of other disease processes. A history of pre-existing arthritis or trauma can be found in approximately 30% of patients with septic arthritis.[14] Multiple animal studies have shown that arthritic and traumatized joints are more likely to develop septic arthritis.[8]

There are several proposed reasons cited for the incidence of septic arthritis in patients with rheumatoid arthritis. Local factors in rheumatoid arthritis produce defects in phagocytic function and antibacterial activity. Mahowald and associates[9] proposed that chronic arthritis produces neovascularization that may become obstructed with bacteria. They believe this would lead to subchondral osteonecrosis in patients with rheumatoid arthritis. Treatment of rheumatoid arthritis using systemic or intra-articular steroids is an additional factor predisposing the joints to septic arthritis. The weakening of the immune system, increasing the susceptibility to infection in general with this disease, is well known.

Most of the patients with rheumatoid arthritis who develop septic arthritis have had seropositive erosive disease for many years' duration.[2] A significant number of these patients tend to have multiple affected joints. Approximately 75% of the infections in this group are due to *Staphylococcus aureus*.[7] Rheumatoid arthritis is important as a predisposing factor because patients with both rheumatoid arthritis and septic arthritis concurrently have a poor prognosis. This may be the result of delayed diagnosis and initiation of therapy due to the similarity of symptoms between rheumatoid arthritis and septic arthritis. Complete recovery with therapy is reported in only one third of patients. More important is that 15% to 20% of these patient die of sepsis.[7]

Arthritides other than rheumatoid arthritis and osteoarthritis have been associated with septic arthritis. These diseases include the crystal-induced arthritides, sickle cell arthropathy, hemarthrosis, and Charcot's arthropathy. Many types of bacteria are recovered from septic joints in patients with gout and pseudogout.[2] The knee is the most common joint affected in these crystal-induced arthritides. Septic arthritis may increase the likelihood of urate crystals precipitating within the joint. The bacterial infection increases the lactic acid. The bacterial infection lowers the pH, which then decreases the solubility of urate. Patients with gout who contract septic arthritis usually have a prior history of gouty arthritis. Alternatively, patients with pseudogout usually are not similarly affected.

The incidence of septic arthritis in intravenous (IV) drug abusers has been increasing. This predisposing factor is of particular importance in urban centers, where most patients with septic arthritis present as IV drug abusers. Between 1973 and 1982, 10% of patients with septic arthritis were IV drug abusers. Recent reports have stated that this incidence is closer to 50%.[2] These patients are, at least in part, suscep-

tible to developing sepsis from the recurrent and multiple self-inflicted injections with contaminated needles. Sepsis predisposes these individuals to developing infectious arthritis. Septic arthritis in these patients often involves unique joints and organisms. The sternoclavicular and sacroiliac joints are not typically involved in septic arthritis. However, in IV drug abusers, these joints are infected frequently.[14] It is also interesting to note that IV drug abusers are prone to developing osteomyelitis of the vertebrae and pubic symphysis, which are usually sites for this disease.[2] Septic arthritis in IV drug abusers is often caused by gram-negative organisms and methicillin-resistant *Staphylococcus aureus* (MRSA).[10] Geographic differences make gram-negative arthritis or MRSA more common. The reason for this is unknown. *Pseudomonas* and *Serratia* organisms are also particularly common gram-negative organisms infecting these patients.[2] IV drug abusers tend to fully recover from their gram-negative septic arthritis, whereas other patients with the same disease remain symptomatic.

Invasive procedures increase the potential for joint sepsis. Injection of the joint for diagnostic or therapeutic purposes is associated with an increased yet small risk. It is estimated that the occurrence of septic arthritis following intra-articular injections is between 1:500 and 1:5000 cases.[7] Patients with central venous lines are predisposed to septic arthritis, most likely due to bacteremia.[2] Infections tend to occur near access points. For example, the sternoclavicular joint is prone to septic arthritis in patients with subclavian catheters. Patients undergoing hemodialysis have a high incidence of sternoclavicular, acromioclavicular, and sacroiliac joint involvement.

The source of bacteria can also be considered another type of predisposing factor. This may be identifiable by history, such as a history of an intra-articular injection or surgery. Alternatively, the source may be identified by physical examination, such as a patient with an abscess or pharyngitis. There is an identifiable extra-articular site of infection in as many as 50% of adults with septic arthritis.[14] Although bacteremia is a common event preceding septic arthritis, it is important to note that bacteremia is much more common than septic arthritis. This illustrates the point that bacteremia alone is not enough to produce septic arthritis.

CAUSATIVE AGENTS

Virtually any agent capable of causing an infection can produce septic arthritis. Bacteria, viruses, and fungi have all been implicated. Bacterial septic arthritis is the most common type, chiefly nongonococcal septic arthritis and gonococcal septic arthritis.

Gonococcal Arthritis

Because of the frequency of occurrence and the unique treatment considerations, gonococcal (GC) joint sepsis is usually considered as a separate entity. GC joint sepsis is the most frequent type of joint sepsis seen today.[11] GC joint sepsis should be considered in any sexually active person with an acute monoarticular or oligoarticular joint effusion. GC joint sepsis is usually considered as part of a complex associated with disseminated gonococcal infection (DGI). Hematogenous spread of *Neisseria gonorrhoeae* with resultant dermatitis, tenosynovitis, and arthritis occurs at a rate of

2.8 per 100,00 population.[12] Patients of either low socioeconomic status or with a larger number of sexual partners are at greatest risk.

The last sexual contact may vary from 2 days to 2 months prior to the onset of symptoms. Both men and women are at risk, although there are conflicting opinions as to the frequency in these groups. The knee and ankle joints are frequently involved in this disease. Patients usually present with polyarthralgia or monoarthralgia lasting 2 to 3 days prior to presentation. Genitourinary symptoms are frequently absent. Fever and chills, mild leukocytosis, elevations of the erythrocyte sedimentation rate, with associated tenosynovitis or dermatitis, are frequent findings. Joint aspiration reveals a purulent synovial fluid with frequent intracellular gram-negative diplococci.

Differential diagnoses include nongonococcal arthritis, hepatitis, rheumatic disorders, and acute rheumatic fever. Patients with suspected GC arthrosepsis or DGI should have urethral cultures performed because they are more productive than peripheral sites, including the joint fluid. Pharyngeal, rectal, or cervical cultures should also be taken when indicated by history. Synovial fluid cultures are positive in about 25% to 30% of patients with DGI.[13] Synovial fluid should be plated on warm chocolate agar medium and placed in carbon dioxide (CO_2) for incubation. Aseptic arthritic processes related to cell wall–induced inflammation or circulating immune complexes may account for the difficulties in culturing synovial fluid.

Nongonococcal Arthritis

Gram-positive organisms are the most common bacteria causing nongonococcal septic arthritis. Of these infections, *Staphylococcus* is responsible for 40% to 70% of the cases of purulent arthritis.[14] *Staphylococcus aureus* represents approximately 80% of the infections in patients with rheumatoid arthritis.[15] *S. aureus*, as well as *S. epidermidis*, are the most common organisms involved in prosthetic joint infection.[7] *Streptococcus* is also a common etiology of septic arthritis. It accounts for approximately 25% of the cases of nongonococcal septic arthritis.[14] Thus, almost all cases of gram-positive septic arthritis are due to either staphylococcal or streptococcal organisms. *Pneumococcus*, although once an organism frequently involved in septic arthritis, has become relatively rare during the last 25 years.[7]

Approximately 5% to 7% of nongonococcal infections of joints were due to gram-negative bacteria in the 1940s and 1950s.[7] Recently, up to one third of joint infections have been due to gram-negative bacilli.[7] The predisposing factors for this type of bacterial arthritis are similar to those for gram-negative bacteremia. Most of the patients with this disease are either seriously ill, elderly, or are IV drug abusers. In the elderly patients, *Escherichia coli* urosepsis is a common source of these infections.[14] IV drug abusers frequently have pseudomonal septic arthritis.[16] Another important group predisposed to gram-negative joint infections is patients with sickle cell disease or other hemoglobinopathies. These patients are particularly susceptible to *Salmonella* infections. *Haemophilus influenzae* joint infections are common in children. The frequency of *H. influenzae* joint infections in adults is increasing.[14]

Recently, polymicrobial septic arthritis has been frequently reported in the literature.[17] Some studies have reported a frequency as high as 10%.[18] Many of these cases have mixed infections consisting of both anaerobic and aerobic organisms. Underlying host immune defects are common, and the sources are often from intra-abdominal and intrapelvic infections.[7]

Anaerobic infections have also been reported with an increasing frequency. It is thought that the increase is due to improved culturing techniques rather than a true increase in the frequency of the disease itself.[7] *Fusobacterium necrophorum*, *Peptococcus anaerobius*, and *Bacteroides fragilis* have been the most common bacteria isolated. Most anaerobic infections have been in patients after total joint replacement, with postoperative sepsis in the presence of an extremity wound or injury, or in patients with chronic debilitating illnesses.[7]

Tuberculous Arthritis

Tuberculous arthritis and mycotic infections of joints are rare causes of arthritis but are of importance due to the increasing incidence of tuberculosis (TB) in the immunosuppressed and acquired immunodeficiency syndrome (AIDS) populations. The continuing influx of immigrants from third-world countries with endemic disease increases the incidence of TB in the United States.[19]

Joint sepsis with *Mycobacterium tuberculosis* is the most common form of granulomatous arthritis.[20] As with other septic arthritis, the route of infection is direct, hematogenous, or lymphatic seeding. The most common form of tubercular arthritis is Pott's disease or spinal tuberculosis. Peripheral joint involvement is rare, but it should be considered when monoarticular arthritis appears in a patient with a history of pulmonary tuberculosis, other tubercular infection, or positive purified protein derivative (PPD) test. Diagnosis is made by recovery of caseous or granulomatous material from the joint at arthrotomy or aspiration. Acid-fast stains and cultures should be routinely performed on suspicious joints and on patients with a known history of immune compromise. The clinical picture is of monoarthritis of long duration, loss of range of motion, effusion, and in the later stages overt joint collapse. Radiographs may demonstrate joint space narrowing and osteopenia. PPD is usually positive, and chest radiograph may be consistent with TB pneumonia, but not necessarily.

Rare non-tubercular strains of *Mycobacterium* are becoming more common with the increasing population of immunocompromised patients. *Mycobacterium avium-intracellulare*, *kansasii*, and *marianum* have been reported most frequently. *Mycobacterium leprae* is known to affect the joint but its frequency appears rare.[21] A negative acid-fast stain of joint fluid does not rule out active *Mycobacterium* infection. Clinically, all *Mycobacterium* strains are frequently indistinguishable until speciated at culture.[22] Diagnosis of any tubercular infection should cause the clinician to consider concomitant HIV infection.

Treatment is joint decompression and antitubercular agents. The treatment regime is similar to that of active pulmonary infection. Usually a combination therapy of two drugs, isonicotine hydrazine (INH) and rifampin, is recommended.[20]

Arthritis Due to Spirochetal, Mycobacterial, Fungal, Viral, and Parasitic Infections

Although arthritis is sometimes reported with active syphilis, actual *Treponema pallidum* infection of joints is rare but has been reported.[23] This spirochete can be found in nearly every tissue in secondary syphilis. The ankle and the knee are the most frequently involved joints.[24] The patient's history and the local incidence of syphilis should be taken into consideration because this is part of the differential diagnosis.

One spirochetal infection gaining recent prominence is Lyme disease. Lyme disease is noted in geographic areas of the world where the *Ixodes dammini*, *I. ricinus*, and *I. pacificus* ticks are vectors for the spirochete *Borrelia burgdorferi*. These ticks are endemic parasites of deer, birds, and small mammals in three areas of the United States: The northeast (New Jersey, New York, Connecticut, Rhode Island, and Massachusetts), the midwest (Minnesota and Wisconsin), and the southwest (California, southern Oregon, and western Nevada).

Clinically, Lyme disease is divided into three stages. The first stage is characterized by flu symptoms and a typical rash at the bite site known as erythema chronicum migrans. This stage may last several days to several weeks. The second stage of Lyme disease is characterized by cardiac and neurologic symptoms expressing themselves in the third through twelfth weeks. Although quite variable, atrioventricular block and headache are the most common symptoms in the second stage. Mental status changes, Bell's palsy, and meningitis-like symptoms may also be noted. The third stage is an arthritis that may present as early as 1 week following the first stage but is usually seen 3 to 4 weeks after the onset of Lyme disease. The infectious organism, *B. burgdorferi* has been demonstrated in the joint fluid of a knee.[25] Whether this is the proximate cause of the arthritis or perhaps a related arthritic antigen-antibody reaction is the subject of some debate. Lyme arthritis is generally a recurrent asymmetrical migratory oligoarthropathy of short duration (1 to 12 weeks). The joints affected include the knee, shoulder, elbow, temporomandibular joint, and small joints of the fingers and toes. Episodic involvement of these joints is known to occur for years.

The diagnosis of spirochetal infection is made by serologic identification of the organism from the tissue. In the late stages of Lyme disease, Lyme serology testing is very sensitive, with good specificity. In the early stages, serology is sensitive but not specific because there is some overlap with other treponemal diseases including syphilis, yaws, and pinta, which may need to be ruled out by further serology testing or by history.[2, 26]

Fungal infections of joints are infrequent except in areas endemically predisposed. Coccidioidomycosis in the southwest and histoplasmosis in the midwest and south are usually acquired from pulmonary infection. Blastomycosis is found in the north and south central United States and may be acquired from either direct infection from soil or pulmonary extension. *Blastomyces dermatitidis* in the yeast form has been recognized in synovial fluid.[27] Although there is increasing reporting of other fungal joint infections including *Candida*, *Sporothrix*, and *Cryptococcus* species, active infection is very rare in the peripheral joints. As with tubercular infection, consideration of concomitant HIV infection or other immunocompromising disorder should be explored when fungal joint infection is discovered.

Viral infections of joints are recognized causes of acute and chronic arthritis in humans. Hepatitis B, rubella, and mumps, among others, are commonly associated with both acute and prolonged joint inflammation.

Parasitic infection has been recognized as a cause of seronegative arthritis. Among others, nematodes, flatworms, and protozoa may be associated with arthritis. Clinical and immunologic response to antihelmintics has been reported.[28]

CLASSIFICATION BY SOURCE

The etiology of septic joint infections can also be classified by the source of the infection. Generally, the sources are classified as hematogenous, direct, and contiguous. These categories are not rigid and overlap may occur between them.

Hematogenous inoculation of bacteria into the joint is the most common event leading to septic arthritis.[14] These infections are initiated by a distant infection that produces bacteremia and eventually seeds the synovium. Hematogenous infections are most common in young and old individuals. In part, the distribution is due to the immune-system and disease-related factors mentioned earlier.

Surgically induced septic arthritis can occur from any surgery in which the joint is opened or penetrated with surgical instrumentation. Infections following arthroscopy also are included in this category. Surgically induced septic arthritis can occur indirectly. The joint can be seeded with bacteria from an adjacent soft tissue or bone infection.

Direct inoculation of bacteria into the joint can be from intra-articular injections, traumatically induced wounds, or surgery. Infections can result from intra-articular injections, with or without use of steroid medications. Puncture wounds are infrequent yet regular causes of joint sepsis. A traumatic wound can be a simple puncture wound or severe soft tissue injury with the joint exposed.

Prosthetic joint infections are a unique type of infection and should be considered separate from other surgically induced joint infections. The natural history and treatment consideration of this disease can be different from other types of septic arthritis. These infections are also usually more insidious and difficult to diagnose.[7] Prosthetic joint infections have been classified by their time of onset, starting with the time of surgical implantation of the artificial joint.[7] Infections that occur within 3 months of the time of surgery are termed ''acute.'' In acute infections *S. epidermidis*, *S. aureus*, and anaerobes are most often recovered. ''Chronic'' infections are those that occur more than 1 year after surgery. *S. aureus* has been recovered from these chronic infections. Infections occurring between the time period of 3 months to 1 year are referred to as ''subacute.''

The source of bacteria in a joint infection may come from either infected bone or soft tissue adjacent to the joint. This is considered to be a contiguous source of infection. An example of this type would be an infected diabetic foot ulcer near a joint, which consequently infects the joint.

In contiguous infection, there are important anatomic considerations in infants and children regarding the relationship between septic arthritis and osteomyelitis. The incidence of septic arthritis in infants is approximately twice as high as osteomyelitis. In adolescents and adults the incidence of these two diseases is approximately equal. Septic arthritis can result from osteomyelitis in infants, less often in the adult.[2] However, children are protected by the epiphyseal plate from this source of bacteria. During the first year of life the metaphyseal blood supply penetrates the epiphyseal plate.[29] This allows the bacteria to enter the joint, thus promoting septic arthritis. Before the end of the first year of life, the avascular epiphyseal plate forms an impenetrable barrier separating the metaphyseal blood supply from the epiphyseal blood supply.[30] This prevents bacteria from crossing from the metaphysis into the joint, thus resisting the development of septic arthritis. The hip and shoulder joints are exceptions because the metaphysis is intracapsular.[30] In the adult, the circulation between the metaphysis and epiphysis is restored. This again will allow seeding of the joint via the metaphyseal blood supply. Septic arthritis and osteomyelitis are closely related in several ways, other than both being infections of the musculoskeletal system. They usually occur as individual and separate processes. However, they can be present at the same time, in which one may precede and be the cause of the other.

PATHOPHYSIOLOGY

In 1924, Phemister demonstrated that enzymes from polymorphonuclear neutrophils (PMNs) were capable of cartilage destruction.[31] Later, Curtiss and Klein were able to show in an in vitro study that proteolytic enzymes diminished the proteoglycan content of articular cartilage.[32, 33] They stated that loss of collagen is necessary for gross cartilage destruction.

Animal studies have provided most of the pathophysiologic knowledge regarding nongonococcal bacterial arthritis.[2] The bacteria may arrive at the joint by the hematogenous route, by direct inoculation, or from a contiguous source, as previously mentioned. The synovial membrane has no basement membrane and, thus, substances including bacteria can easily enter the joint space. Although the modes by which the bacteria may arrive at the joint are different, the pathophysiology resulting in articular cartilage destruction remains essentially the same. The time sequence is somewhat variable. The infection may destroy the synovium, which is replaced by granulation tissue, and then cartilage and bone destruction follow. Alternatively, the infection may originate from the bone, as in osteomyelitis. The bone and cartilage destruction may occur with late seeding of the joint. The end result of the pathologic process is determined by the inflammation-induced damage.

Important differences in the characteristics of bacterial joint infections do occur from individual to individual. These differences are based on the same variables that occur in other infections. The number of bacteria injected or implanted and the virulence of the specific bacteria will have effects on how an infection will manifest itself.[2] The host response or lack of response will also be important in the development of infections. These factors will not only determine the characteristics of the infection of the joint but will also determine whether a clinical infection occurs at all.

Septic arthritis originating from a hematogenous source in animals begins with the introduction of virulent bacteria into the blood. The bacteria are found, within 1 to 2 hours, scattered throughout the outermost layer of the synovium.[2] The infiltration of PMNs occurs and synovial lining cells phagocytize bacteria. Approximately 90% of the bacteria are engulfed by the synovial lining cells.[34] At this stage, if the host resolves the initial assault by the bacteria, infection will not occur. Alternatively, if the host fails to rid the joint of bacteria, a joint infection will result.

Articular cartilage destruction begins with the breakdown of glycosaminoglycans. Collagen depletion follows and begins within 8 hours. The prognosis resulting from the septic process is intimately dependent on the extent of collagen loss.[2, 32, 33] In nongonococcal bacterial arthritis, collagen loss cannot be prevented by antibiotic treatment alone. Studies in rabbits have demonstrated that the only way to effectively prevent collagen loss with antibiotics alone is to pretreat the host before bacteria are introduced into the joint.[35] Collagen loss may be reduced or prevented by lavage of the joint.[36] The morbidity of joint infection is due in large degree to the destructive nature of the bacterial enzymes and the inflammatory response of the body to the joint sepsis. Destructive proteolytic enzymes are liberated from both the infecting agent and the host.[27, 28]

Of considerable interest is the hormone catabolin. Catabolin induces chondrocyte-mediated proteoglycan degradation. This substance, normally involved with homeostatic controls, is liberated in large quantities from synovium in response to inflammation.[37, 38] This enzyme is most likely a common mediator of articular cartilage degeneration in all forms of joint inflammation. Degradation of articular cartilage is also noted with exposure of the joint to lymphokines, interleukin-1, and lymphocytic protease. In addition, lipopolysaccharides of gram-negative cell walls are known to directly cause cartilage breakdown.[39]

During the period between 24 to 48 hours following introduction of bacteria to the joint, synovial hypertrophy and the accumulation of large amounts of inflammatory cells occur.[2] Both acute and chronic inflammatory cells are present within the joint and the synovium. These cells within the joint produce a purulent effusion that becomes evident within this period. Cells within the synovium may coalesce to form synovial abscesses. Viable bacteria are generally present within the joint for at least 48 hours. At the conclusion of the 48-hour period, the glycosaminoglycan (GAG) content of the cartilage is reduced by 20% to 40%.[40]

After 7 days, chronic synovitis progresses and pannus invades the cartilage.[2] Pannus is a thin layer of very well vascularized granulation tissue that overlies the articular cartilage. Some of the synovial changes that occur are irreversible.[14] If necrosis occurs as a result of direct pressure from the arthritic process, it will contribute to the damage of local tissues. Bacteria can be identified by electron microscopy at 7 to 10 days, although viable bacteria are usually not recoverable from the joint.[41, 42] Viable bacteria are not necessary for the destruction to continue. Cartilage and bone destruction will progress long after the joint fluid becomes sterile. Pannus and exudate may be present as well as erosions of the articular cartilage.

By the third week, the GAG content of the cartilage is depleted by 60% to 70% and cartilage destruction begins.[3] Gross cartilage destruction is dependent on the degradation of collagen. The persistence of the inflammatory process is primarily responsible for the damage to cartilage, which occurs as a result of a joint infection. However, the exact enzymatic pathway leading to the cartilage destruction remains unknown. Various studies have demonstrated that enzymes from PMNs[27, 28] synovial lining cells,[32] chondrocytes,[43, 44] and sometimes bacteria[45] themselves contribute significantly to the degradation of cartilage. Specifically, neutral and acid proteases, as well as collagenase, have been investigated.

The immune system plays a role in the development of inflammatory arthritis. This is of particular interest when considering the persistence of synovial inflammation following antibiotic treatment and sterilization of the joint fluid or reactive arthritis. It has been postulated that this inflammation may be the result of cartilage antibodies.[46] This could also be explained by systemic bacterial antigens.

DIAGNOSIS

Aspiration

Early joint aspiration, also called arthrocentesis, is important for both diagnostic and treatment purposes in all clinically suspect joints. The approach that most easily allows entry into the joint is best advised (Table 13–1). Fluoroscopy should be available to guide access to difficult or small joints. When it is necessary to verify that the tip of the needle is in the joint, arthrography may be helpful. Aspiration should be performed with sterile technique in order to minimize chances for contamination of the joint or the sample for culture.

Gram's stain, crystal analysis, white blood cell count with percentage of polymorphonuclear cells, and a synovial fluid analysis can be performed within hours of patient presentation. The synovial fluid should be cultured for both aerobic and anaerobic bacteria. Mycobacterial and fungal cultures should be made when there is suspicion of exposure or when the presentation is that of a low-grade illness or "cold" process. Although confirmative growth occurs less than 50% of the time, a smear should be made on chocolate agar whenever *N. gonorrhoeae* is suspected. Presumptive diagnosis of bacterial arthritis leads to initiating and selecting appropriate antibiotic therapy and consideration for repeated aspiration or surgical drainage of the joint.

In cases in which there is no preliminary evidence of bacterial infection, the joint should be observed while considering other causes of joint symptoms. Other considerations include crystalline synovitis (gout and pseudogout), acute degenerative joint disease, rheumatoid arthritis, and reactive arthritis (seronegative spondyloarthropathies and immune-related diseases). Less frequent diagnoses to consider are par-

asitic diseases; viral arthritis (especially hepatitis B); mycobacterial, fungal, Lyme, and other spirochetal arthritides. Acute rheumatic fever and other diseases causing arthralgia also should be considered.

Laboratory Studies

Several laboratory studies are useful in the diagnosis of septic arthritis. Most of these tests involve the examination of the synovial fluid. The synovial fluid examination provides the most important diagnostic laboratory data. Synovial fluid tests can be divided into microbiologic, hematologic, and chemical tests. Other tests provide nonspecific information and may reflect disease processes elsewhere in the body. Also, certain blood tests are useful. A white blood cell count, blood cultures, and erythrocyte sedimentation rate are often used.

The microbiologic tests performed on the synovial fluid are a Gram's stain and cultures. It is important that the first specimen be acquired before antibiotics are started. Also, it has been recommended that Gram's stain be performed either on purulent fluid or from a centrifuged pellet of synovial fluid.[47] This enhances organism identification. The Gram's stain results confirm the diagnosis and are positive in 65% of cases of septic arthritis.[48] The positive Gram's stain yield depends on which organism is responsible for the infection. For example, in staphylococcal infections, recovery of the etiologic organism occurs in 75% of cases,[49] whereas in gram-negative bacilli infections recovery occurs only in 50% of cases.[49] Thus, Gram's stain helps determine the probable bacteriologic source and guide initial antibiotic therapy. Anaerobic and aerobic cultures should always be obtained in cases when septic arthritis is suspected. In general, all specimens should be plated on blood agar. A chocolate agar plate should be incubated in 5% to 10% CO_2 when the infection is suspected as due to *N. gonorrhoeae* or *H. influenzae*.[7] The cultures are particularly important when Gram's stain is negative for organisms. In bacterial nongonococcal septic arthritis, the majority of cultures are positive.[14] Culture results and sensitivities identify the etiologic organism and further specify antibiotic treatment.

A synovial fluid white blood cell count with differential contributes nonspecific data. This test helps differentiate inflammatory from noninflammatory arthritides. Of the potential inflammatory arthritides, septic arthritis typically produces very large values. The synovial leukocyte count in 70% of patients will be greater than 50,000 cell/mm[3].[49] The leukocyte count usually approaches 100,000 cell/mm[3] with polymorphonuclear cells comprising greater than 85%.[50, 51]

Examination for crystals is very important because septic arthritis and an acute gout attack have very similar clinical presentations. It is important to realize that the presence of crystals, whether of urate or calcium pyrophosphate, does not rule out septic arthritis within a given joint. The coexistence of these two diseases is not unusual. The association between these two diseases was discussed earlier in this chapter.

Laboratory examination of the synovial fluid serves two purposes. The Gram's stain and culture are done to confirm a diagnosis of septic arthritis and determine the etiologic organism. The hematologic examination is utilized to determine whether the process occurring in the joint is inflammatory or noninflammatory.

TABLE 13–1

ASPIRATION OF THE JOINTS OF THE FOOT

Joint	Recommended Approach for Aspiration
Ankle	Anterior/medial
Subtalar joint	
(Posterior facet)	Sinus tarsi or posterior
(Anterior facet)	Sinus tarsi or medial
Talonavicular	Dorsomedial
Calcaneocuboid	Lateral
Intertarsal	Dorsal
Metatarsophalangeal and digital	Dorsal

The utility of synovial fluid glucose and protein levels is controversial. It has been suggested that these tests are irrelevant when trying to determine the nature of the joint disease—inflammatory or noninflammatory—due to a lack of consistency and reliability.[52] Some recommend ordering a glucose level in the presence of septic arthritis and using the result to monitor the disease process. Others believe that a glucose level may be useful in the diagnosis of septic arthritis.[52]

Other attempts have been made to correlate chemical changes in the joint fluid with septic arthritis. These changes include elevation of lactate dehydrogenase, elevation of bacterial fatty acids using liquid chromatography, and detection of bacterial cell wall antigens in synovial fluid using counterimmunoelectrophoresis.[7, 52] Tests for lactate dehydrogenase and bacterial fatty acids lack both specificity and sensitivity. They can, however, be useful in evaluating patients who have previously received antibiotics. Detection of cell wall antigens can be helpful in the diagnosis of septic arthritis due to *N. meningitidis*, *H. influenzae*, and *Streptococcus pneumoniae*. In general, the above tests are nonspecific and serve no purpose in the evaluation of patients with septic arthritis due to gram-positive cocci or *N. gonorrhoeae*.

In the small joints of the foot it is frequently difficult to gather enough aspirate to run a complete synovial fluid examination. Priority should be given to culture, Gram's stain, and crystal examination. If sufficient synovial fluid is available, glucose levels and cell counts should be obtained.

Although examination of the joint fluid is important, other tests can contribute pertinent data. These tests include a peripheral white blood cell count, blood cultures, erythrocyte sedimentation rate, serum glucose level, and cultures of possible primary infection sources. The white blood cell count is elevated in approximately one half of the patients presenting with septic arthritis.[48] Elevation of the erythrocyte sedimentation rate also frequently occurs. The serum glucose level is used for comparison to the joint fluid glucose level, when one is performed. The specimens should be obtained at the same time, if the comparison is to be accurate. Blood cultures should be drawn in all patients with suspected septic arthritis. These cultures are positive in 50% of patients with nongonococcal septic arthritis.[48] If other infections are present, which may be the source of the bacteria, these sources should likewise be cultured. Possible sources include skin, urine, throat, and sputum. These cultures are especially useful in determining antibiotic treatment, when joint fluid cultures are negative.

Radiographic Studies

Plain films, bone scans, and computed tomography all have useful purposes in the diagnosis of septic arthritis. Plain films and bone scans are used to rule out osteomyelitis.[1, 7] Plain films are also used to follow the destructive changes that result from the disease. Computed tomography and bone scans may be useful in examining joints, such as the hip and axial joints, in which diagnosis may be difficult. It is important to realize that arthrocentesis does not necessarily interfere with bone scan interpretation.[1]

When septic arthritis is suspected, baseline plain radiographs should always be taken to rule out osteomyelitis. Plain-film radiographic signs are initially vague. There may be joint effusion and a slight amount of juxta-articular osteoporosis present. It takes 10 to 20 days for radiographic changes to take place. Resnick and Niwayama[53] described the radiographic abnormalities that occur with septic arthritis and the pathologic changes that correlate with these abnormalities. Initial joint effusion and soft tissue swelling are associated with increased synovial fluid production and soft tissue edema and hypertrophy. Osteoporosis appears as the hyperemic processes resulting from inflammation occur. Loss of joint space and osseous erosions correspond to continued destruction due to the inflammatory pannus. Bony ankylosis correlates radiographically to the same process occurring pathologically.

TREATMENT

The basic treatment protocol of arthrosepsis includes appropriate antibiotics and adequate drainage and débridement of pus and the reactive byproducts of the defensive response to the infective process (Table 13–2). Following adequate initial care, the joint should be monitored carefully for response to therapy by repeated examination, serial synovial fluid analysis, and regular hematologic and chemical profiles. Supportive care including protective mobilization, rehabilitation, and gradual return to function are dictated by the individual circumstance. Patients with poor outcome face the same alternatives as the patient with arthritis—medical and surgical management of the condition, lifestyle changes, and orthotic bracing. Chronic or acute osteomyelitis may result from joint sepsis and is treated according to principles of managing infective osteitis.

TABLE 13–2

INITIAL DIAGNOSTIC AND TREATMENT GUIDELINES IN BACTERIAL ARTHRITIS

Step 1.	Immediate aspiration of suspicious joint. If unable to obtain fluid, consider aspiration with fluoroscopic guidance or proceed with further assessment (radiography, joint scintigraphy, computed tomography, magnetic resonance imaging)
Step 2.	Send synovial fluid for routine culture (and anaerobic, gonococcal, mycobacterial, and fungal cultures when indicated). Perform a complete synovial fluid analysis (white blood cells, % polymorphonuclear cells, glucose with simultaneous blood glucose, Gram's stain and crystal analysis)
Step 3.	A. If the synovial fluid is suggestive of sepsis ("pus," very high white blood cell level, low glucose), start antibiotics based on likelihood of the specific infection
	B. If the result of a synovial fluid Gram's stain is positive, start appropriate antibiotics
	C. If the synovial fluid is not suggestive of bacterial arthritis, observe while awaiting results of the culture
Step 4	A. If culture is positive, readjust antibiotics on basis of sensitivities, if necessary
	B. Drain the joint as dry as possible
	C. Each time the joint is drained obtain a small aliquot for culture and analysis
Step 5.	If the joint is not adequately responding, consider:
	A. Inadequate antibiotic activity: obtain bacteriocidal levels on serum and synovial fluid
	B. Inadequate drainage: consider arthroscopy or surgical drainage

Adapted from Goldenberg DL: Nonsurgical treatment of bacterial arthritis. *In* Espinoza L, Goldenberg DL, Arnett FC, and Alarcon GS (eds): Infections in the Rheumatic Diseases: A Comprehensive Review of Microbial Relations to Rheumatic Disorders. Orlando, FL, Grune & Stratton, 1988, p 58.

Antibiotics

Antibiotic selection should be made once the diagnosis is made or strongly suspected. Antibiotic selection should be based on the history and the clinical presentation in light of the objective laboratory evidence that can be gathered. Due to many factors, antibiotic selection is often made on empiric evidence instead of the patient presentation and the likelihood of certain bacteria in the population associated with the socioeconomic status of the patient (Table 13–3).

Antibiotic selection should be carefully adjusted to the cultured bacterial sensitivities (Table 13–4). Synovial fluid concentrations of antibiotics are uniformly adequate if sufficient serum levels are obtained. IV antibiotics are favored for septic arthritis, because appropriate bacteriocidal concentrations are reliably achieved and monitored. There is no place in treatment for irrigating the joint with antibiotics. Addition of antibiotics to joint irrigants provokes a chemical synovitis with associated inflammatory response. This will only serve to exacerbate the inflammation of the joint, accelerating the deterioration of the joint. Hospitalization for administration and monitoring of the response is recommended in most cases of suspected suppurative arthritis. Oral antibiotic therapy is considered acceptable only for follow-up therapy. Antibiotic administration alone is not sufficient therapy for septic arthritis.[54] Concurrent decompression of the joint by aspiration or surgical intervention is required in all types of joint sepsis.

TABLE 13–3

EMPIRIC ANTIBIOTIC SELECTION BASED ON PATIENT PRESENTATION

Patient Presentation	Probable Organism	Antibiotic Selection
IV drug user	Methicillin-resistant *Staphylococcus* *Pseudomonas aeruginosa*	Vancomycin + quinolone
IV drug user "Greasing" (licking) needle	Above organisms *plus* anaerobes	Vancomycin + imipenem Vancomycin + ticarcillin/clavulanic acid
Sexually active young adult	Gonococcus	Ceftriaxone or other third-generation cephalosporin
Rheumatoid arthritis	*Staphylococcus aureus*	See *Staphylococcus* guidelines
Sickle cell (hemoglobinopathy)	*Salmonella* + other gram-negatives	Third-generation cephalosporin or quinolone
Diabetes	*Staphylococcus, Streptococcus,* anaerobes	Ticarcillin/clavulanic acid Ampicillin/sulbactam Imipenem Clindamycin/quinolone
Prosthetic joint implant	Coagulase-negative *Staphylococcus*	Vancomycin
Lyme disease	*B. burgdorferi*	Ceftriaxone or third-generation cephalosporin (14 days) Parenteral penicillin (14 days) Oral doxycycline (30 days) Oral amoxicillin (30 days)

IV = intravenous.

Variables Affecting Treatment

Many variables affect morbidity, treatment selection, and the prognosis in septic arthritis. The nature of the infecting organism with respect to its virulence and its capacity to injure the joint, factored with the host's ability to mount a defensive and reparative response, all affect the prognosis of this disorder.

Staphylococcal sepsis is notably destructive in all tissues, including articular cartilage and the supporting structures of the joint. Staphylococcal species liberate 25 to 30 extracellular toxins that are known to be proteolytic. In addition, staphylococcal species also liberate a proteoglycan-liberating factor that may cause loss of as much as 85% of cartilage proteoglycan content.[55] In contrast, GC joint sepsis is rarely associated with joint destruction and usually responds rapidly to aspiration and appropriate antibiotics. Surgical débridement is rarely necessary in GC joint sepsis.[56] Because of these factors, most of these patients have an excellent recovery. Other gram-negative infections are associated with greater degrees of joint destruction. Joint infections caused by viruses, fungi, and spirochetes are less destructive than bacterial infections if caught in the early stages. *Brucella* and *Mycobacterium* joint infections are also less destructive than other bacterial infections.[57, 58]

The duration of the infection affects the outcome of the infection more than any other variable in most cases of joint sepsis.[59] Nongonococcal bacterial joint sepsis is associated with poor results if left untreated for longer than 5 to 7 days.[60–63] Animal studies seem to indicate that even a delay of 24 hours is important.[64] Early initiation of treatment is the most important significant variable associated with a favorable prognosis (Table 13–5).

Once the diagnosis of joint sepsis has been positively established, a definitive treatment plan must be initiated rapidly. A hospital admission is indicated to appropriately decompress the joint, to administer IV antibiotics and to monitor and adjust the therapeutic response. In many acute cases, in the large joints of the foot, ankle, knee, or hip, declaring an operative emergency is completely appropriate.

Drainage

The goal of débridement of the septic joint is removal of organisms, necrotic material, and other byproducts of infectious inflammation. The degree of invasion and surgical exposure must be balanced by the need to preserve normal anatomy and to maximize functional recovery of the part. Drainage can be accomplished by needle aspiration, arthroscopy, or by open arthrotomy. The procedure chosen involves the clinical setting, the joint involved, and the surgical abilities of the physician. A great deal of controversy regards the optimal means of drainage. Because of the large number of variables presenting in this clinical situation, it is difficult to unequivocally recommend a particular approach. No large controlled study has been reported to date. A composite view of the current literature seems to indicate that repeated aspiration of infected superficial joints is adequate (Table 13–6).[65, 66] In these series the ankle joint and the knee joint were included as superficial joints.

Needle Aspiration. Needle aspiration should be performed daily or more frequently if the effusion is recurring.

TABLE 13–4

ANTIBIOTIC SELECTION IN SEPTIC ARTHRITIS

Organism	Parenteral Agent	Dosage (Adult)	Oral Agent	Dosage
Staphylococcus aureus				
Penicillinase-positive	Nafcillin	1–2 g q 6 hr	Dicloxacillin	500 mg qid
Methicillin-sensitive	Cefazolin	1–2 g q 8 hr	Cephalexin	500 mg qid
	Cefuroxime	1.5 g q 12 hr	Cefuroxime axetil	500 mg bid
	Vancomycin[1]	1 g q 12 hr	Clindamycin	300 mg bid
	Clindamycin[1]	600–900 mg q 8 hr		
S. aureus				
Methicillin-resistant	Vancomycin	1 g q 12 hr	TMP/SMX	1 DS[2] bid
	TMP/SMX[2]	160 mg q 8–12 hr	Minocycline	100 mg bid
			Quinolone[3] + rifampin	300 mg bid
Staphylococcus coagulase-negative (CNS)	Same guidelines as with *S. aureus.* CNS may have high incidence of methicillin resistance			
Streptococcus groups A and B	Penicillin	1–4 million U q 4 hr	Penicillin V	500 mg qid
	Cefazolin	1 g q 8 hr	Cephalexin	500 mg qid
	Vancomycin	1 g q 12 hr	Cefuroxime axetil	500 mg bid
	Clindamycin	600–900 mg q 8 hr	Clindamycin	300 mg bid
Enterococcus	Ampicillin	2 g q 6 hr	Amoxicillin	500 mg tid
	Vancomycin[4]	1 g q 12 hr		
N. gonorrhoeae (gonococcus)	Ceftriazone[5]	1 g q 12 hr	Quinolones	
	Ciprofloxacin	400 mg q 12 hr	Cefuroxime axetil	
			Cefixime	400 mg every day
Group 1 Gram-negative rods				
Proteus mirabilis	Cefazolin	1 g q 8 hr	Cephalexin	500 mg qid
Escherichia coli	Cefuroxime	1.5 g q 12 h	Cefuroxime axetil	
Salmonella	TMP/SMX	160 mg 1 8–12 hr	Quinolone	
			TMP/SMX	1 DS bid
Group 2 Gram-negative rods				
Enterobacter	Ciprofloxacin	400 mg q 12 hr	Quinolones	
	Third-generation cephalosporins[5]		TMP/SMX	1 DS bid
Citrobacter				
Serratia	Aztreonam	1 g q 8 hr		
Morganella	Imipenem	500 mg q 8 hr		
Proteus vulgaris	Aminoglycoside + ESP[6]			
Pseudomonas aeruginosa	Ceftazidime	2 g q 12 hr	Quinolones	
	Ciprofloxacin	400 mg q 12 hr		
	Aminoglycoside + ESP[6]			
Xanthomonas maltophila	TMP/SMX	160 mg q 8–12 hr	TMP/SMX	1 DS bid
Pseudomonas cepacia	Ceftazidime	2 g q 12 hr		
Bacteroides fragilis	T/C[7]	3.1 g q 6–8 hr	A/C[8]	500 mg tid
	A/S[9]	3.0 g q 6 hr	Clindamycin	300 mg bid
	Imipenem	500 mg q 8 hr	Metronidazole	500 mg tid
	Clindamycin	600–900 mg q 8 hr		
	Cefoxitin	2 g q 6 hr		

Agent	Dosage (Adult) Oral Agent
Mycobacterium tuberculosis	Isoniazid (INH) + rifampin × 9 months or longer. Add ethambutol or streptomycin if strain is INH-resistant
Nontubercular *Mycobacterium*	Rifampin + ethambutol × 3 months ± ciprofloxacin or as per sensitivity testing results
Fungal infection	Amphotericin B[10], oral ketoconazole, fluconazole There are little to no data regarding treatment of fungal joint sepsis

1. Use should be reserved for patients with documented allergy to penicillins and cephalosporins.
2. Trimethoprim/sulfamethoxazole. Dosing is given by the amount of trimethoprim. 1 DS = Double Strength = 160 mg trimethoprim/800 mg sulfamethoxazole.
3. Quinolones can be either Ciprofloxacin 750 mg bid *or* Ofloxacin 400 mg bid.
4. Aminoglycosides can be added to vancomycin or ampicillin for synergy against *Enterococcus.* The necessity for this in septic arthritis has not been clearly shown.
5. Or other third-generation cephalosporins. Cefotaxime 1–2 g q 8 hr, ceftizoxime 1–2 g q 8 hr, ceftazidime 2 g q 12 hr.
6. Extended-spectrum penicillins. Ticarcillin, mezlocillin, piperacillin. Because of aminoglycoside toxicities, these agents should be reserved for the most refractory cases.
7. Ticarcillin/clavulanic acid.
8. Amoxicillin/clavulanic acid.
9. Ampicillin/sulbactam.
10. Infectious disease consultation is a must due to multiple drug toxicity and dosing difficulties.
11. Not all antibiotics have "official" Food and Drug Administration (FDA) approval for use in septic arthritis. This indication usually falls under the vague classification of "bone and joint infections." The selections in this chart are based on in vitro activity and indicate at least a theoretical efficacy. Accepted clinical data are not available for all antibiotics.
12. Oral forms are given for the purpose of "follow-up" therapy following a course of parenteral treatment. They are not meant to be used as initial, sole therapy. Only the quinolones may be efficacious for this purpose.

TABLE 13–5

OUTCOME OF TREATMENT BY DURATION OF SYMPTOMS

Clinical Status	Complete Recovery	Poor Results
Patients with symptoms <7 days	46	26
Patients with symptoms >6 days	6	22

Data from Goldenberg DL and Reed JI: Bacterial arthritis. N Engl J Med 312:764–771, 1985; Goldenberg DL, Brandt KD, Cohen AS, et al: Treatment of septic arthritis. Arthritis Rheum 18:83–90, 1975; and Goldenberg DL and Cohen AS: Acute infectious arthritis: A review of patients with nongonococcal joint infections. Am J Med 60:369–377, 1976.

Needle aspiration should be performed until the joint is free from effusion. The joint should be aspirated with a large-bore (18-gauge) needle in all but the smallest joints of the foot. Anesthesia is optional. A rapid puncture of an effused joint is frequently better tolerated than trying to establish a field block in an infected area. Aspiration should be performed with sterile technique to avoid contamination of the joint or the aspirate with new bacteria. Joints that are difficult to drain due to viscous pus can be cautiously injected with sterile irrigant in order to dilute the exudate. Irrigating with sterile Ringer's solution or saline must be balanced against the risks of mechanical injury or of spreading the infection to the supporting structures of the joint. An egress portal is helpful in diminishing this risk. Encountering loculations, as evidenced by feeling the needle encounter fibrous tissues or by noting a sudden increase in pus production while aspirating multiple areas of the joint, is an indication that aspiration alone may be inadequate. Arthroscopy or arthrotomy of the joint should be considered in these cases.

When volume is appropriate, the serial aspirates should be examined for response to therapy. The joint should be sterile in 2 to 4 days with substantial improvement in synovial fluid leukocytosis in 5 to 7 days.[4] Achieving a sterile aspirate rapidly is a key parameter of successful therapy.[67] Persistence of joint sepsis in the face of appropriate antibiotic therapy and regular aspiration of the joint is an indication for open arthrotomy or arthroscopic débridement. Poor results can be expected if bacteria continue to be recovered after 6 days of appropriate therapy. Objective improvement usually correlates well with clinical signs.

Arthrotomy. Open surgical débridement is indicated in septic arthritis that is unresponsive to antibiotic therapy and aspiration, when sepsis is prolonged, and when extensive loculation or secondary abscess formation are suspected. In addition, deep and complex joints may need arthrotomy when arthroscopic techniques fail or are inadequate. Recovery of certain types of resistant strains of bacteria, including MRSA, may indicate a need for surgical débridement as initial therapy to control the infective process.[68] Open surgical drainage is necessary in most postoperative infections and in all cases of implant or retained foreign body. Access of pus to the extracapsular tissue planes requires open débridement of these ''noncontained'' areas of the extremity.

Surgical débridement of the septic joint allows for direct visual inspection of the joint cavity and the supporting structures of the joint. Care should be taken to limit the degree of dissection and exposure to that which is needed to perform the task. Arthrotomy allows for removal of all infectious material including the organism and the necrotic and devitalized tissues, as well as reactive and suppurative proteolytic enzymes and hormones. Arthrotomy also facilitates débridement of loculations and occult abscesses. The joint is irrigated with copious amounts of nontoxic fluid; drains are easily placed. The biologic price to be paid is the addition of tissue injury from the surgical dissection of already injured tissue. The poor outcome of surgical therapy compared to aspiration therapy may well be due to the difference in tissue injury and repair.

The surgical approach to the joint should be performed in such a fashion as to minimize damage to the supporting structures of the joint while entering the most advantageous portions of the joint for surgical manipulation. The ideal approach allows for inspection and débridement of all structures, capsular pouches, and reflections. The articular surface must be protected against mechanical or surgical injury. Most articular surface injury is permanent. Avoidance of injury to the supporting structures of the joint including ligaments, capsule, and normal synovial folds improves the prospect for functional recovery of the joint. In some cases many small incisions are preferred to a single long one.

Routine aerobic and anaerobic cultures and Gram's stain should be obtained in all cases. Acid-fast stains, fungal culture, fungal stains, and mycobacterial culture are obtained when the clinical picture is not consistent with bacterial infection or crystalline arthropathy. Fungi and *Mycobacterium* are difficult to culture from synovial fluid. Synovial biopsy and culture is frequently necessary to confirm or diagnose disease when fungal or mycobacterial infection is present.

Synovium frequently harbors bacteria in its villous structures. In well vascularized synovium, immune processes and antibiotics are generally able to overwhelm bacteria. In cases when the infection is established or chronic, significant débridement of the synovium is necessary to resolve the infec-

TABLE 13–6

ANALYSIS OF OUTCOME IN SPECIFIC JOINTS ACCORDING TO TYPE OF TREATMENT (NUMBER OF JOINTS)

Joint	Good	Fair	Failed	Died	Total
Medical Therapy (Aspiration/Antibiotics)					
Knee	45	10	2	3	60
Hip	2	—	3	—	5
Shoulder	13	3	1	—	17
Wrist	16	1	1	1	19
Elbow	5	—	—	3	8
Ankle	9	—	—	1	10
Total	91	14	7	8	120
Percent (%)	75	12	6	7	100
Surgical Therapy (Arthroscopy or Arthrotomy/Antibiotics)					
Knee	35	13	5	1	54
Hip	2	—	5	—	7
Shoulder	2	2	—	—	4
Wrist	11	8	4	1	24
Elbow	—	—	—	—	—
Ankle	1	—	—	1	2
Total	51	23	15	3	91
Percent (%)	56	25	15	3	100

Adapted from Broy SG and Schmid FR: A comparison of medical drainage (needle aspiration) and standard surgical drainage (arthrotomy and arthroscopy) in the initial treatment of infected joints. Clin Rheum Dis 12:501–522, 1986.

tion. In chronic synovitis when fibrous proliferation and scarring limit the exposure of the bacteria to humoral influences, débridement of the synovium is frequently necessary to eliminate the occult reservoir of the infecting agent. Débridement of the synovium should be performed cautiously to minimize scarring and interference with the blood supply of adjacent bone. Bleeding is generally significant and frequently requires drains to prevent hematoma.

The use of ingress/egress drainage systems for septic arthritis is controversial, at best. Proponents argue that continuous irrigation allows for continuing removal of the destructive byproducts in the joint that may be responsible for articular cartilage destruction.[69, 70] In addition, proponents argue that the intense boggy hypertrophic synovitis and hyperemic nature of the synovium during joint sepsis preclude adequate drainage by aspiration. No long-term studies exist documenting any clear advantage to this or other approaches. Opponents of irrigation systems argue that bacteriocidal concentrations of antibiotic in the synovium and synovial fluid are more than adequate and that egress drains alone are frequently a satisfactory approach.[63] Drains themselves may allow access of bacteria to the joint interior and must be handled with sterile precautions. Drains should be removed as soon as the course allows to avoid nosocomial contamination and infection.

Arthroscopy. Arthroscopy was initially developed in the 1920s as a method of treating tuberculous arthritis of the knee by Takaji.[71] Since the late 1970s, arthroscopic examination and débridement of the septic joint have gained significant popularity because they combine the advantages of traditional arthrotomy and aspiration.[72–75]

Arthroscopy of the septic knee is frequently reported.[76, 77] There is as of this date no published report on the specific aspects of ankle arthroscopy for septic arthritis. Most of the joints of the ankle and foot are amenable to arthroscopy (Fig. 13–1). I (J.J.S.) have had successful experience with arthroscopic intervention in septic arthritis of the great toe and the ankle joints.

Arthroscopy allows for direct visual inspection of the joint

in a wet environment under magnification. The synovium in joint sepsis has a characteristic appearance that can be distinguished from other conditions, including rheumatoid arthritis, crystal synovitis, and pigmented villonodular synovitis. These conditions can be confused with a septic joint in the clinical setting. Septic synovium appears inflamed and friable with degenerating villi and occasional masses of necrotic synovium floating in the synovial fluid. A gray fibrous exudate is frequently noted forming strands in areas of focal involvement. Loculations and abscess pockets may be sequestered by organizations of these fibrous strands. The cartilaginous surface may appear normal if examined early in the disease. As the course of the disease progresses, a characteristic loss of color and surface texture occurs as the cartilage degenerates.

Arthroscopy is especially helpful in diagnosing cases of granulomatous or fungal arthritis. These usually present as monoarticular arthritis with less intense inflammatory symptoms than bacterial or crystalline arthritis; the appearance in blastomycosis is the exception. In many cases infection is not initially suspected until arthroscopy is performed. The diagnosis is made by appearance, synovial fluid culture, and by synovial biopsy and culture of the specimen. Synovial biopsy and culture of infected tissue is significantly more sensitive than culture of synovial fluid alone.[78, 79] Arthroscopy is regarded as the diagnostic method of choice for obtaining synovial tissue for confirming fungal infection.[80] Arthroscopy allows surgical débridement of the infected synovium, excision of necrotic and nonviable debris, removal of pus, and mechanical lysis of adhesions and loculation. The same principles and goals of open débridement guide the arthroscopic surgeon. Depending on the joint affected and skill of the surgeon, arthroscopic débridement can approach the magnitude of a traditional arthrotomy. Drains can be placed under arthroscopic guidance without difficulty.

The great advantage of arthroscopy is the limitation of injury to the surrounding structures of the joint. This limitation diminishes morbidity to the joint and allows early return of motion and function. The limitations of arthroscopy are due to the limitations of the surgeon and the anatomic constraints of individual joints that place physical limitations on where the instrument and the surgical instrumentation can reach. Failures are also known to occur when sepsis is both intra-articular and extra-articular.[81] Lastly, arthroscopy is not without complication, nor has its efficacy in the treatment of septic arthritis been proven in large studies. Judgment in case selection and technique is recommended.

Aftercare

Whether to immobilize or mobilize the infected joint has been the matter of much controversy through the ages.[82, 83] Immobilization of the joint is known to cause deleterious effects in the homeostasis and repair of hyaline articular cartilage in joints.[84–86] Periods of immobilization following aspiration or surgery were once thought necessary to protect the joint tissues from noxious stimuli and to allow healing of the joint and supporting structures. Once the infection was resolved, cautious active and passive motion exercises were instituted to help restore functional movement and strength of the part. The need to immobilize infected and injured joints has been based on empiric dogma of British orthopedic

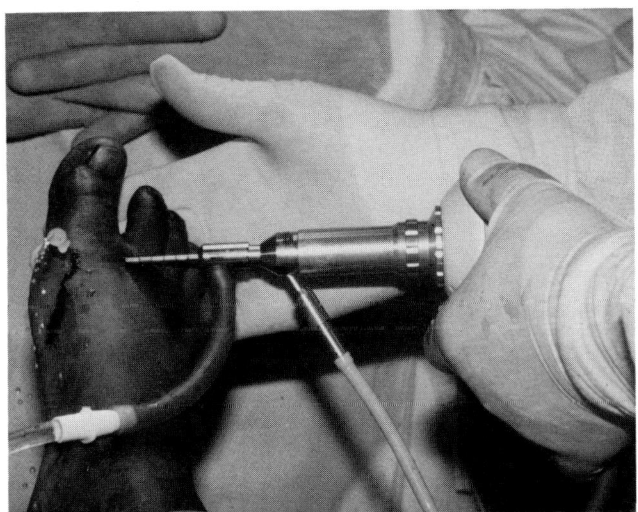

FIGURE 13–1. Arthroscopy of the great toe joint for joint sepsis. The toe joint of a 14-year-old boy who stepped on a nail and developed joint sepsis from a contiguous site.

surgeons of the 1900s. There is no evidence that immobilization is necessary or beneficial once treatment has been initiated. Motion in a joint with a significant effusion may mechanically increase the intra-articular pressure and cause pain and spasm and risk rupture of the infected joint fluid from the constraints of the joint capsule. Once the joint is decompressed, there is no longer a need to restrain motion.

There is growing evidence that mobilization is helpful in treating joint sepsis. Continuous passive motion (CPM) has been shown to have a protective effect on rabbit knee joints with septic arthritis.[87] Early clinical reports on CPM in joint sepsis including three cases of ankle joint sepsis seem to confirm the rabbit studies.[88] CPM can also be applied to the small joints of the foot.[89] The efficacy of CPM when applied to septic arthritis in the lower extremity is yet to be determined in a large prospective study. Although there is evidence to suggest that CPM should be applied for no less than 8 hr/day, no other optimal parameters of therapeutic application of CPM are known.

Following the resolution of the infective process, the joint should be managed with regular motion, guarded loading, and strengthening of the supporting musculature and soft tissue structures. Local edema and joint symptoms may persist depending on the nature of the infection, the duration of the infection, and the destruction associated with the process.

Patients with histories of prolonged or destructive infections should expect continued degenerative changes over time. In addition to the degenerative changes due directly to the infection and mechanical deterioration of the joint, sterile postinfectious arthritis is a frequent finding.[90] The proximate cause of the postinfectious "reactive" arthritis is likely to be mediated by circulating immune complex. The antigen may be the cell wall, infective toxin, or any component of the infecting agent. Similar arthritic symptoms and causation are also associated with other nonarticular infections including other bacteria (*Brucella*, *Salmonella*, *Streptococcus*, *N. gonorrhoeae*), spirochetes (Lyme, syphilis), and viruses (hepatitis B, rubella, mumps, and varicella-zoster).[4]

Septic Arthritis and Osteomyelitis. Infection of adjacent bone tissue is a rare complication of joint sepsis if treated promptly. Several anatomic barriers impair rapid spread of joint sepsis to surrounding tissues. The dense fibrous capsule generally contains the infection to the joint space. The articular cartilage and underlying bone plate are a significant barrier to bacterial spread to bone. Chronicity of joint sepsis, especially in the face of appropriate treatment, should lead the clinician to consider the diagnosis of osteomyelitis. Osteomyelitis due to the spread of joint infection can occur with all bacteria, fungi, mycoplasma, and spirochetes discussed in this chapter. Once bone infection is established, appropriate measures for the treatment of osteomyelitis should be undertaken. Bone infection and its treatment are beyond the scope of this chapter.

Joint Sepsis Following Arthroplasty. Infection following any invasive procedure on a joint is a likely disaster. Not only does it put the joint at risk from early and late destructive change, but the patient is also exposed to all the problems associated with joint infection, including life-threatening sepsis and endocarditis. Adjacent reconstructive bone procedures are at risk of being disturbed in the treatment of the infected joint. Exposure of reconstructive osteotomy to bacteria makes osteomyelitis a serious concern. Implants and other retained foreign material associated with joint surgery

further complicate the diagnosis and treatment of iatrogenic joint sepsis.

The goals and principles of treatment for postoperative joint sepsis are similar to those of a virgin pyarthrosis—rapid sterilization of the joint with removal of destructive byproducts of the inflammatory process, decompression, débridement, and antibiotic therapy. The bacteria that are likely to be encountered are *Staphylococcus* and *Streptococcus* species. The infection may be intra-articular, extra-articular, or both. For this reason simple aspiration or arthroscopic drainage is not recommended. Timely open surgical drainage, débridement, irrigation, bacterial identification, and appropriate IV antibiotic therapy are recommended to diminish the morbidity of this disorder. A complete discussion of postoperative wound sepsis is beyond the scope of this chapter. The reader is recommended elsewhere.

References

1. Shaw BA and Kasser JR: Acute septic arthritis in infancy and childhood. Clin Orthop Rel Res 257:212, 1990.
2. Goldenberg DL: Pathophysiology—nongonococcal bacterial arthritis. *In* Espinoza L, Goldenberg DL, Arnett FC, and Alarcon GS (eds): Infections in the Rheumatic Diseases: A Comprehensive Review of Microbial Relations to Rheumatic Disorders. Orlando, FL, Grune & Stratton, 1988, p 3.
3. Smith RL and Schurman PJ: Comparison of cartilage destruction between infectious and adjuvant arthritis. J Orthop Res 1:136–143, 1983.
4. Swartz MN and O'Hanley P: Current update, infectious arthritis. *In* Rubenstein E and Federman DD (eds): Scientific American Medicine, Section 7. New York, Scientific American, 1987, pp 1–7.
5. Sharp JT, Lidsky MD, Duffy J, and Duncan MW: Infectious arthritis. Arch Intern Med 139:1125, 1979.
6. Bomalaski JS, Williamson PK, and Goldstein CS: Infectious arthritis in renal transplant patients. Arthritis Rheum 29:227–232, 1986.
7. Goldenberg DL: Infectious arthritis: Bacterial. *In* Schumacher, HR (ed): Primer on the Rheumatic Diseases, 9th ed. Atlanta, Arthritis Foundation, 1988, pp 181–185.
8. Lewis GW and Cluff LE: Synovitis in rabbits during bacteremia and vaccination. Bull Johns Hopkins Hosp 116:175–190, 1965.
9. Mahowald ML, Gerding D, Majeski P, and Peterson L: Microvascular changes in arthritic joints infected with *S. aureus* (abstract). Arthritis Rheum 29:S80, 1986.
10. Ang-Fonte GZ, Rozboril MB, and Thompsen GR: Changes in non gonococcal septic arthritis: Drug abuse and methicillin resistant *Staphylococcus aureus*. Arthritis Rheum 28:210–213, 1985.
11. O'Brien JP, Goldenberg DL, and Rice PA: Disseminated gonococcal infection: A prospective analysis of 49 patients and a review of the pathophysiology and immune mechanisms. Medicine 62:395–406, 1983.
12. Koss PG: Disseminated gonococcal infection. Cleve Clin Q 52:161–173, 1985.
13. Goldenberg DL: Gonococcal arthritis. *In* Espinoza L, Goldenberg DL, Arnett FC, and Alarcon GS (eds): Infections in the Rheumatic Diseases: A Comprehensive Review of Microbial Relations to Rheumatic Disorders. Orlando, FL, Grune & Stratton, 1988, pp 43–52.
14. Simpson ML: Septic arthritis in adults. *In* Gustilo RB, Gruninger RP, and Tsukayama DT (eds): Orthopedic Infection: Diagnosis and Treatment. Philadelphia, WB Saunders, 1989, p. 284.
15. Mitchell WS, Brooks PM, Stevenson RD, and Buchman WW: Septic arthritis in patients with rheumatoid disease: A still underdiagnosed complication. J Rheumatol 3:124, 1976.
16. Gifford DB, Patzakis M, Ivler D, et al: Septic arthritis due to *Pseudomonas* in heroin addicts. J Bone Joint Surg 57A:361, 1975.
17. Hall BB, Rosenblatt JE, and Fitzgerald RH Jr: Anaerobic septic arthritis and osteomyelitis. Orthop Clin North Am 15:505, 1984.
18. Petty BG, Sowa DT, and Charache P: Polymicrobial polyarticular septic arthritis. JAMA 249:2069, 1983.
19. Kutzbach AG: Tuberculous arthritis. *In* Espinoza L, Goldenberg DL, Arnett FC, and Alarcon GS (eds): Infections in the Rheumatic Diseases: A Comprehensive Review of Microbial Relations to Rheumatic Disorders. Orlando, FL, Grune & Stratton, 1988, pp 138–139.
20. Evanchick CC, Davis DE, and Harrington TM: Tuberculous arthritis: An often-missed diagnosis. J Rheumatol 13:187–189, 1986.
21. Guedes Barbosa LS and Scheinberg MA: Articular manifestations of leprosy. *In* Espinoza L, Goldenberg DL, Arnett FC, and Alarcon GS (eds): Infections in the Rheumatic Diseases: A Comprehensive Review of Microbial Relations to Rheumatic Disorders. Orlando, FL, Grune & Stratton, 1988, pp 159–163.
22. Yangco BG, Espinoza CG, and Germain BF: Nontuberculous myobacterial joint infections. *In* Espinoza L, Goldenberg DL, Arnett FC, and Alarcon GS (eds): Infections in the Rheumatic Diseases: A Comprehensive Review of Microbial Relations to Rheumatic Disorders. Orlando, FL, Grune & Stratton, 1988, pp 139–155.

23. Reginato AJ, Schumacher HR, and Jimenez S: Synovitis in secondary syphilis: Clinical, light, and electron microscopic findings. Arthritis Rheum 22:170–176, 1979.
24. Reginato AJ and Falasca G: Immunologic and musculoskeletal manifestations of syphilis. *In* Espinoza L, Goldenberg DL, Arnett FC, and Alarcon GS (eds): Infections in the Rheumatic Diseases: A Comprehensive Review of Microbial Relations to Rheumatic Disorders. Orlando, FL, Grune & Stratton, 1988, pp 215–228.
25. Snydman DR, Schenkein DP, and Berardi VP: *Borrelia burgdorferi* in joint fluid in chronic Lyme arthritis. Ann Intern Med 104:798–800, 1986.
26. Bartlett JC: Lyme arthritis. *In* Espinoza L, Goldenberg DL, Arnett FC, and Alarcon GS (eds): Infections in the Rheumatic Diseases: A Comprehensive Review of Microbial Relations to Rheumatic Disorders. Orlando, FL, Grune & Stratton, 1988, pp 229–233.
27. Espinoza LR and Bergen-Losee LL: Arthritis due to mycobacteria, fungi, spirochetes and miscellaneous arthritides: Basic pathogenetic considerations. *In* Espinoza L, Goldenberg DL, Arnett FC, and Alarcon GS (eds): Infections in the Rheumatic Diseases: A Comprehensive Review of Microbial Relations to Rheumatic Disorders. Orlando, FL, Grune & Stratton, 1988, pp 125–129.
28. Bocanegra T, Espinoza LR, and Bridgeford P: Reactive arthritis induced by parasitic infestation. Ann Intern Med 94:206–209, 1981.
29. Trueta J: The three types of acute hematogenous osteomyelitis. J Bone Joint Surg 41B:671, 1959.
30. Nade S: Acute septic arthritis in infancy and childhood. J Bone Joint Surg 65B:234, 1983.
31. Phemister DB: The effects of pressure on the articular surfaces in pyogenic and tuberculous arthritides and its bearing on treatment. Ann Surg 80:481–500, 1924.
32. Curtiss PH and Klein L: Destruction of articular cartilage in septic arthritis. I: In vitro studies. J Bone Joint Surg 45A(4):797–806, 1963.
33. Curtiss PH and Klein L: Destruction of articular cartilage in septic arthritis: II. In vivo studies. J Bone Joint Surg 47A(8):1595–1603, 1965.
34. Johnson AH, Campbell WG, and Callahan BC: Infection of rabbit knee joints after intraarticular injection of *Staph. aureus.* Am J Pathol 60:165, 1970.
35. Smith RL, Schurman DJ, Kajiyama GMM, and Gilkerson E: The effects of antibiotics on the destruction of cartilage in experimental infectious arthritis. J Bone Joint Surg 69A:1063, 1987.
36. Dale D, Akeson W, Amiel D, et al: Lavage of septic joints in rabbits: Effect of chondrolysis. J Bone Joint Surg 58A:393, 1976.
37. Dingle JT, Saklatvala J, Hembry R, et al: A cartilage catabolic factor from synovium. Biochem J 184:177–180, 1979.
38. Fell HB and Jubb RW: The effect of synovial tissue on the breakdown of articular cartilage in organ culture. Arthritis Rheum 20:1359–1371, 1977.
39. Jasin HE: Bacterial lipopolysaccharides induce in vitro degradation of cartilage matrix through chondrocyte activation. J Clin Invest 72:2014–2019, 1983.
40. Smith RL and Schurman DJ: Comparison of cartilage destruction between infectious and adjuvant arthritis. J Orthop Res 1:136, 1983.
41. Bhawan J, Tardon HD, and Roy S: Ultrastructure of synovial membrane in pyogenic arthritis. Arch Pathol 96:155, 1973.
42. Goldenberg DL, Chisholm PL, and Rice PA: Experimental models of bacterial arthritis: A microbiologic and histopathologic characterization of the arthritis after the intraarticular injections of *Neisseria gonorrhoeae, Staphylococcus aureus*, group A streptococci, and *Escherichia coli.* J Rheumatol 10:5, 1983.
43. Steinberg J, Sledge CB, Nobel J, and Sirrat CR: A tissue culture model of cartilage breakdown in rheumatoid arthritis. Biochem J 180:403–412, 1979.
44. Sapolsky AI, Altman RD, Woessner JF, and Howell DJ: The action of cathepsin D in human articular cartilage on proteoglycans. J Clin Invest 52:624–632, 1973.
45. Smith RL, Merchant TC, and Shurman DJ: In vitro cartilage degradation by *Escherichia coli* and *Staphylococcus aureus.* Arthritis Rheum 25:441, 1982.
46. Bobechko WP and Mandell L: Immunology of cartilage in septic arthritis. Clin Orthop 108:84–89, 1975.
47. Goldenberg DL: Nonsurgical treatment of bacterial arthritis. *In* Espinoza L, Goldenberg DL, Arnett FC, and Alarcon GS (eds): Infections in the Rheumatic Diseases: A Comprehensive Review of Microbial Relations to Rheumatic Disorders. Orlando, FL, Grune & Stratton, 1988, pp 57–63.
48. Goldenberg DL and Cohen AS: Acute infectious arthritis: A review of patients with nongonococcal joint infections (with emphasis on therapy and prognosis). Am J Med 60:369–377, 1976.
49. Goldenberg DL and Reed JI: Bacterial arthritis. N Engl J Med 312:764–771, 1985.
50. Fries JF and Mitchell DM: Joint pain or arthritis. JAMA 235:199–204, 1976.
51. Cohen AS: Synovial fluid. *In* Cohen AS (ed): Laboatory Diagnostic Procedures in the Rheumatic Diseases, 3rd ed. New York, Grune & Stratton, 1985, pp 5–53.
52. Shmerling RH, Delbanco TL, Tosteson ANA, and Trentham DE: Synovial fluid tests: What should be ordered? JAMA 264:1009–1014, 1990.
53. Resnick D and Niwayama G: Osteomyelitis, septic arthritis and soft tissue infection: The mechanisms and situations. *In* Resnick D and Niyawama G (eds): Diagnosis of Bone and Joint Disorders, 2nd ed. Philadelphia, WB Saunders, 1988, pp 2524–2618.
54. Riegels-Nelson P, Frimodt-Mueller N, Sorenson M, and Jenson JS: Antibiotic treatment insufficient for septic arthritis. Acta Orthop Scand 60(1):113–115, 1989.
55. Smith RL and Schurman DJ: Bacterial arthritis: A staphylococcal proteoglycan releasing factor. Arthritis Rheum 29:1378–1386, 1986.
56. Goldenberg DL: Gonococcal arthritis. *In* Espinoza L, Goldenberg DL, Arnett FC, and Alarcon GS (eds): Infections in the Rheumatic Diseases: A Comprehensive Review of Microbial Relations to Rheumatic Disorders. Orlando, FL, Grune & Stratton, 1988, pp 43–52.
57. Gotuzzo E and Carril C: Brucella arthritis. *In* Espinoza L, Goldenberg DL, Arnett FC, and Alarcon GS (eds): Infections in the Rheumatic Diseases: A Comprehensive Review of Microbial Relations to Rheumatic Disorders. Orlando, FL, Grune & Stratton, 1988, pp 31–41.
58. Yangco BG, Espinoza CG, and Germain BF: Nontuberculous mycobacterial joint infections. In Espinoza L, Goldenberg DL, Arnett FC, and Alarcon GS (eds): Infections in the Rheumatic Diseases: A Comprehensive Review of Microbial Relations to Rheumatic Disorders. Orlando, FL, Grune & Stratton, 1988, pp 139–155.
59. Goldenberg DL and Reed JT: Bacterial arthritis. N Engl J Med 312:764–771, 1985.
60. Nade S: Acute septic arthritis in infancy and childhood. J Bone Joint Surg 65B:234–241, 1983.
61. Paterson DC: Acute suppurative arthritis in infancy and children. J Bone Joint Surg 52B: 474–482, 1970.
62. Kelly PJ: Bacterial arthritis in the adult. Orthop Clin North Am 6:973–981, 1975.
63. McGuire NM and Kauffman CA: Septic arthritis in the elderly. J Am Geriatr Soc 33:170–174, 1985.
64. Orchard RA and Stump WG: Early treatment of induced suppurative arthritis in rabbit knee joints. Clin Orthop 59:280–293, 1968.
65. Goldenberg DL, Brandt KD, Cohen AS, et al: Treatment of septic arthritis. Arthritis Rheum 18:83–90, 1975.
66. Broy SB and Schmidt FR: A comparison of medical drainage (needle aspiration) and standard surgical drainage (arthrotomy or arthroscopy) in the initial treatment of infected joints. Clin Rheum Dis 12:501–522, 1986.
67. Ho G and Su EV: Therapy for septic arthritis. JAMA 247:797–800, 1982.
68. Harris JM: Orthopedic aspect of septic arthritis. *In* Espinoza L, Goldenberg DL, Arnett FC, and Alarcon GS (eds): Infections in the Rheumatic Diseases: A Comprehensive Review of Microbial Relations to Rheumatic Disorders. Orlando, FL, Grune & Stratton, 1988, pp 65–75.
69. Daniel D, Akeson W, Amiel D, et al: Lavage of septic joints in rabbits: Effects of chondrolysis. J Bone Joint Surg 58A:393–395, 1976.
70. Goldstein WM, Gleson TF, and Barmada R: A comparison between arthrotomy and irrigation and multiple aspirations in the treatment of pyogenic arthritis. Orthopedics 6(10):1309–1314, 1983.
71. Takaji K: The classic arthroscopy. Clin Orthop 167:6–8, 1982.
72. Broy SB, Stulberg SD, and Schmid FR: The role of arthroscopy in the diagnosis and management of the septic joint. Clin Rheum Dis 12:489–500, 1986.
73. Jarrett MP, Grossman L, Sadler AH, et al: The role of arthroscopy in septic arthritis. Arthritis Rheum 24:737, 1981.
74. Gainor BJ: Installation of continuous tube irrigation in the septic knee at arthroscopy: A technique. Clin Orthop 183:96–98, 1984.
75. McGinty JB: Editorial. J Bone Joint Surg 65A: 287, 1983.
76. Jackson RW: The septic knee: Arthroscopic treatment. Arthroscopy 1(3): 194–197, 1985.
77. Smith MJ: Arthroscopic treatment of the septic knee. Arthroscopy 2(1):30–34, 1986.
78. Wallace R and Cohen AS: Tuberculous arthritis: A report of two cases with a review of biopsy and synovial fluid findings. Am J Med 61:277–282, 1976.
79. Hoffman GS: Mycobacterial and fungal infections in bones and joints. *In* Kelly WN, Harris ED Jr, Ruddy S, and Sledge CB (eds): Textbook of Rheumatology. Philadelphia, WB Saunders, 1985, pp 1527–1540.
80. Koster FT and Galgiani JN: Coccidioidal arthritis. *In* Espinoza L, Goldenberg DL, Arnett FC, and Alarcon GS (eds): Infections in the Rheumatic Diseases: A Comprehensive Review of Microbial Relations to Rheumatic Disorders. Orlando, FL, Grune & Stratton, 1988, pp 165–171.
81. Kohn D: Unsuccessful arthroscopic treatment of pyarthrosis following anterior cruciate ligament reconstruction. Arthroscopy 4(4):287–289, 1988.
82. Willems C: The treatment of purulent arthritis by wide arthrotomy followed by immediate active immobilization. J Surg Gynecol Obstet 20:546, 1919.
83. Salter RB: Motion vs. rest: Why immobilize joints? Presidential address to Canadian Orthopedic Association. J Bone Joint Surg 64B:251–254, 1982.
84. Ekholm R: Articular cartilage nutrition: How gold reaches the cartilage in rabbit knee joints. Acta Anat (Suppl 11):1–69, 1951.
85. Troyer H: The effect of short-term immobilization on the rabbit knee joint cartilage: A histochemical study. Clin Orthop 107:249, 1975.
86. Hall MC: Cartilage changes after experimental immobilization of the knee joint in the young rat. J Bone Joint Surg 45A:36, 1963.
87. Salter RB, Bell RS, and Keeley F: The protective effect of continuous passive motion on living articular cartilage in acute septic arthritis. Clin Orthop 159:223, 1981.
88. Mooney V and Stills M: Continuous passive motion with joint fractures and infections. Orthop Clin North Am 18(1):1–9, 1987.
89. Stienstra JJ: Continuous passive motion: A podiatric overview. J Foot Surg 26(1):41–45, 1987.
90. Goldenberg DL: "Postinfectious" arthritis: New look at an old concept with particular attention to disseminated gonococcal infection. Am J Med 74(6):925, 1983.
91. Kaye BR: Rheumatologic manifestations of infection with human immunodeficiency virus (HIV). Ann Intern Med 111:158–167, 1989.

CHAPTER 14

Laboratory Testing in Arthritic Disease

Thomas J. Kaschak, D.P.M.

The diagnostic laboratory plays an important role in the management of inflammatory joint diseases. Its role, however, is limited by the lack of specificity that characterizes many diagnostic tests. In general, the information gained through testing the arthritides chronicles the effects of the inflammatory processes rather than specifics of the disease itself. Facts gathered through patient history and clinical examination may prove more important to the diagnosis and management of arthritis. The laboratory then becomes a useful tool for obtaining supplemental information important to establishing the course of care.

The numerous tests available to the diagnostician are best taken in the aggregate to lend support to disease identification and to follow its management. The laboratory is also widely used to monitor those physiologic systems that may be adversely affected by the many toxic agents used to treat arthritis. In this latter role, laboratory testing enjoys a greater specificity because disorders of each organ system known to be affected by these therapeutics produce measurable characteristic changes in the organ's function.

Multiple tissue sources may be sampled in the course of arthritis care. These sources include blood, joint fluids, soft tissue, and bone. Each tissue sample may hold clues essential to the elucidation of the disease, and they may provide witness to the progression or control of the disease process.

HEMATOLOGIC STUDIES

Blood is the most easily accessible and most commonly analyzed of all tissues. Just about any disease state will alter the normal chemistry and physical composition of the tissue. These alterations can be readily evaluated by most diagnostic laboratories.

Erythrocyte Sedimentation Rate

The erythrocyte sedimentation rate (ESR) is one of the most common laboratory tests used to determine inflammatory activity. The test is an indirect measurement of the acute-phase response.[1] Its clinical usefulness is quite varied and broad, reflective of the nonspecificity of this test.

The increased rate of red blood cell settling in certain disease states has been recognized for years.[2] A complex chain of events involving the reaction of blood proteins to the inflammatory process may partly explain the sedimentation phenomenon.[3] The settling is probably related to cell adherence and rouleaux formation, causing the aggregation of the red blood cells. The greater and faster the aggregate formation, the higher the ESR. Factors that govern cell settling include cell-surface free energy, cellular electrical charge, and the dielectric constant.[1, 4] Changes in the rate of settling may be caused by alteration of plasma proteins, especially fibrinogen, and, to a lesser extent, α_2-globulins.[5]

The two methods of ESR measurement are the Westergren and the Wintrobe methods. The Westergren method appears to be the more dependable of the two.[2] Sodium citrate or ethylenediaminetetraacetic acid (EDTA) with a saline diluent is used as an anticoagulant for collected venous blood. The specimen is agitated and placed in a commercially available Westergren tube filled to the 200-mm mark. In 1 hour, the difference in millimeters between the top of the plasma and the top of the erythrocyte column is measured.[3]

Possibly less sensitive, the Wintrobe method may fail to reflect accurately the presence of active disease in situations that would have been revealed by the Westergren method.[4] Most types of anemias falsely increase the ESR as measured by this method.[5] The technique of measurement and the equipment needs are also less favorable to the Wintrobe ESR.[3]

The Wintrobe method uses less than 1 ml of blood for measurement. This simple procedure, which is used mostly in small laboratories and physician offices, requires no diluent. Anticoagulated blood is simply placed in a graduated tube, and the results are read directly in 1 hour. The tube is half the length of that used in the Westergren method, making values greater than 60 mm/hr difficult to measure.[4]

There are three major limitations to the clinical usefulness of the ESR. First, the test is nonspecific. Second, the ESR is sometimes measured as normal in disease states in which elevation should be expected. Last, technical factors can greatly influence the results of this test.[5] These technical factors include use of an excessive amount or inadequate amounts of anticoagulant; failure to agitate the specimen adequately; and tilting of the sedimentation tube away from vertical. In addition, the test should be performed within 2 hours if sodium citrate is used as the anticoagulant (within 12 hours for EDTA); it should be performed at precisely 20°C; and the number, size, and shape of the red blood cells should be recorded.[3] Any of these latter details may influence the accuracy of the results.

There are many conditions in addition to rheumatic disease that influence the ESR. The test can be elevated in pregnancy, in certain lymphoproliferative disorders, and with chronic renal failure. Acute and chronic infection raises ESR values, and its return to normal reflects successful resolution. Tissue necrosis, infarction, well-established malignancy, abnormal serum proteins, and certain physiologically stressful conditions such as obesity also elevate the ESR. Conversely, the ESR may be reduced in congestive heart failure, probably because of decreased fibrinogen synthesis by the passively congested liver, and in rheumatic carditis. The ESR may be low or normal during viral infection.[3, 5]

In rheumatoid arthritis (RA), the ESR may achieve values exceeding 80 mm/hr. Such high levels may also occur with systemic lupus erythematosus (SLE), renal disease associated with azotemia, malignant lymphoma, multiple myeloma, and polymyalgia rheumatica.[3] The inflammation of gout and septic arthritis elevate the ESR, but noninflammatory musculoskeletal disorders and osteoarthritis generally do not cause the ESR to rise.[2, 3]

There is a general correlation between activity of RA and ESR levels. As the affected joints begin to show inflammatory activity, the ESR begins to increase. When the disease becomes quiescent or when therapeutic suppression of inflammation is successful, the ESR will gradually return to normal. At times, however, levels remain elevated despite subsiding inflammation, presumably because of continued elevation of serum proteins.[3, 4]

The test may be predictive of the course of RA. When the disease onset is acute and accompanied by a high ESR, the course is generally mild. Conversely, high ESR levels without acutely active disease portend a more severe course with poor functional results.[3]

The normal values for ESRs may vary considerably from one laboratory to another. It is important to check the normal ranges from the testing laboratory before making decisions on the basis of reported results. Normal results also vary with age. In general, the accepted Westergren values for adults younger than 60 years are 0 to 15 mm/hour for males and 0 to 20 mm/hour for females[6], but values of 0 to 30 mm/hour for either sex have also been reported as normal.[7] It has been suggested that 10 mm/hour be added to normal values for young adults and for patients older than 60 years. A formula based on the Westergren method is also available that accounts for all age variations[3]:

$$\text{ESR for men} = \frac{\text{age in years}}{2}$$

$$\text{ESR for women} = \frac{\text{age in years} + 10}{2}$$

As mentioned earlier, the presence of anemia, common in patients with RA, falsely elevate the ESR. It is important for the treating physician to determine the status of anemia before relying on the ESR to guide therapy. A formula has been developed for the Westergren method that accounts for the presence of anemia and provides reasonable correction[3]:

$$\text{Corrected ESR} = \text{ESR} - [(\text{standard hematocrit} - \text{actual hematocrit}) \times 1.75]$$

where standard hematocrit is 45 ml/dl for males and 42 ml/dl for females.

C-Reactive Protein

C-reactive protein (CRP) is a normal constituent of human plasma.[8] The protein is quite ancient in its derivation, having been conserved through hundreds of millions of years of evolution. A similar protein is present in the horseshoe crab, an arthropod that has remained structurally unchanged for more than 500 million years.[9] The protein was named for its ability to precipitate *Pneumococcus* somatic C-polysaccharide.[5, 9]

Although the exact function of this protein is unknown, CRP is suspected to play an important role in the inflammatory process. Levels of CRP increase more than 1000-fold after severe inflammatory stimulation.[1, 9] The protein has the propensity to bind to a constituent of the cell walls of bacteria and cell membranes of damaged eukaryotic cells, perhaps targeting these cells for clearance by inflammatory processes. Other qualities attributed to CRP include its ability to activate complement and to inhibit superoxide production by neutrophils. CRP may also have direct antitoxant activity.[9, 10]

CRP imposes several effects on cells and cell constituents. The protein inhibits platelet aggregation and can modulate the activities of phagocytic cells. It has been observed to bind to nuclear chromatin and small ribonucleoproteins, suggesting a pathophysiologic role.[9] Although synovium does not synthesize CRP, it has been identified bound to certain synovial nuclei in patients with RA.[10]

The indications for testing CRP are essentially the same as those for ESR. The advantage of CRP over the latter is its lack of interference by an anemic state or by serum protein changes. In addition, fewer technical problems plague the test as compared with the ESR. The CRP demonstrates a greater sensitivity to the inflammatory state as well. The test is performed by incubating CRP antiserum with the patient's serum inside a capillary tube. The column of precipitate measured in millimeters is the reported value. Normal levels range from 0 to 6 mm.[3, 5] Newer, more sophisticated testing procedures have been developed that can provide true quantitative CRP measurement (reported in milligrams per deciliter).[5, 9] By these methods, the protein is measured in blood at low levels (580 ng/ml for adults) in the normal state.[8]

CRP is almost always elevated during the early stages of rheumatic fever[3], and levels subside with clinical improvement. Substantial elevations occur in patients with SLE, and it rises significantly during bacterial infections. CRP levels are high during active RA but decrease as inflammation is brought under control. There is no evidence, however, that normalizing either the ESR or the CRP in arthritis protects the joint from destruction.[9, 10]

Although CRP measurement is a more sensitive indicator of inflammation, its use is usually withheld in favor of the ESR because of the familiarity of the latter, technical simplicity, and lower cost.[11]

Rheumatoid Factors

Rheumatoid factors (RFs) make up a heterogeneous group of antiglobulin antibodies found primarily in patients with RA. These antibodies react to specific antigenic determinants on the crystallizable fragment of human immunoglobulin G (IgG). RF has been found in all classes of immunoglobulins,

TABLE 14–1

METHODS FOR DETECTION OF RHEUMATOID FACTORS

Method	Particulate Carrier	Coating	Specificity for Rheumatoid Arthritis	Sensitivity
Latex fixation	Latex particles	Human IgG	75	75
Bentonite flocculation	Bentonite particles	Human IgG	75	75
Sensitized human D cell agglutination	Human Rh positive erythrocytes	Human IgG	75	75
Sensitized sheep cell agglutination	Sheep erythrocytes	Rabbit IgG	90	50
Sensitized human O cell agglutination	Human group O erythrocytes	Rabbit IgG	90	50

but those of class IgG and class IgM appear to hold the most clinical significance.[11, 12] The IgM-RF is the principal antibody measured in clinical practice.[3]

RF is produced mainly by lymphocytes of the synovial membrane. Bone marrow, lymph nodes, subcutaneous nodules, the spleen, and synovial fluid lymphocytes are also important sites for the production of RF in RA patients. Circulating lymphocytes probably do not represent a significant source of RF.[13] The stimulatory events that provoke the production of RF have not been clearly defined, but several mechanisms have been postulated.

IgG is produced by the synovium of RA patients, directed against as yet unknown antigens. The immunoglobulins produced by the synovial tissues appear to differ both qualitatively and quantitatively from IgG produced in the serum. RF from the synovial fluid reacts against the altered synovial IgG, which serves as the antigenic stimulus. The reaction between these molecules forms immune complexes that activate complement and initiate the inflammatory response. Alone, free circulating IgM-RF causes no observable harm.[12]

A variety of laboratory techniques have been devised to identify the presence of RF. The Norwegian pathologist Erik Waaler first characterized RF in 1937. While working on a diagnostic test for syphilis, Waaler discovered that sheep red blood cells sensitized with rabbit IgG antibodies would agglutinate when mixed with serum from a patient with RA. The clinical usefulness of the test was identified a decade later by H. M. Rose.[12, 14] Thus, the Rose-Waaler test was conceived and continues to enjoy clinical application.

From the Rose-Waaler, or sheep cell agglutination test, other agglutination tests were derived. The sensitized human O cell agglutination test replaces human group O erythrocytes for sheep red blood cells. The latex fixation test (LFT) and the bentonite flocculation test use latex particles and bentonite respectively coated with human and rabbit immunoglobulin to identify the presence of RF. Of these, the sheep cell agglutination test has been identified as the most specific but least sensitive test for the diagnosis for RA, whereas the LFT is considered the most sensitive but least specific.[14] Table 14–1 compares these methods for detecting RF.

Other more sophisticated tests for RF have been developed. The rheumatoid rosette assay is seldom used because of a high frequency of false-positive reactions. Immunofluorescent and immunoabsorbent techniques have likewise fallen from favor because of the difficulty associated with their use. Radioimmunoassay (RIA) can accurately identify RF activity but has the disadvantage of requiring radioactive reagents for testing. Enzyme-linked immunosorbent assay (ELISA) shows more promise than RIA for routine quantitation of RF because the test is not associated with radioactivity and is less expensive.[12] Figure 14–1 compares RIA and ELISA techniques.

A variation on ELISA was studied that measured serum RFs that simultaneously bind and cross-link human and sheep IgG.[15] The sensitivity and specificity results were compared with those of LFT, a test that continues to enjoy clinical favor. The ELISA double-binding test was about as sensitive to the presence of RF (36% for ELISA versus 38% for

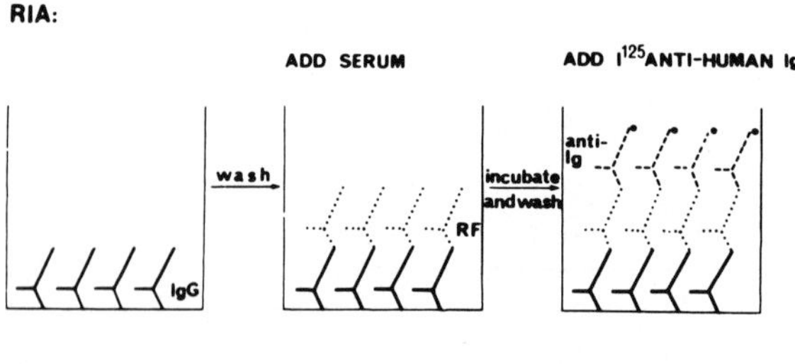

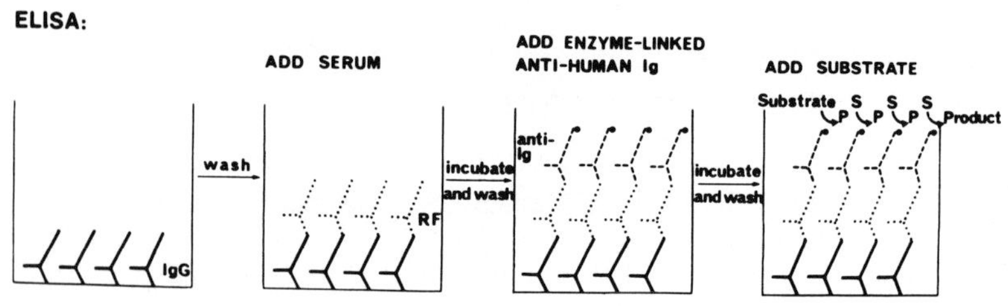

FIGURE 14–1. Principles of radioimmunoassay (RIA) and enzyme-linked immunosorbent assay (ELISA) for detecting human rheumatoid factor (RF). (From Egeland T and Munthe E: Rheumatoid factors. Clin Rheum Dis 9:148, 1983.)

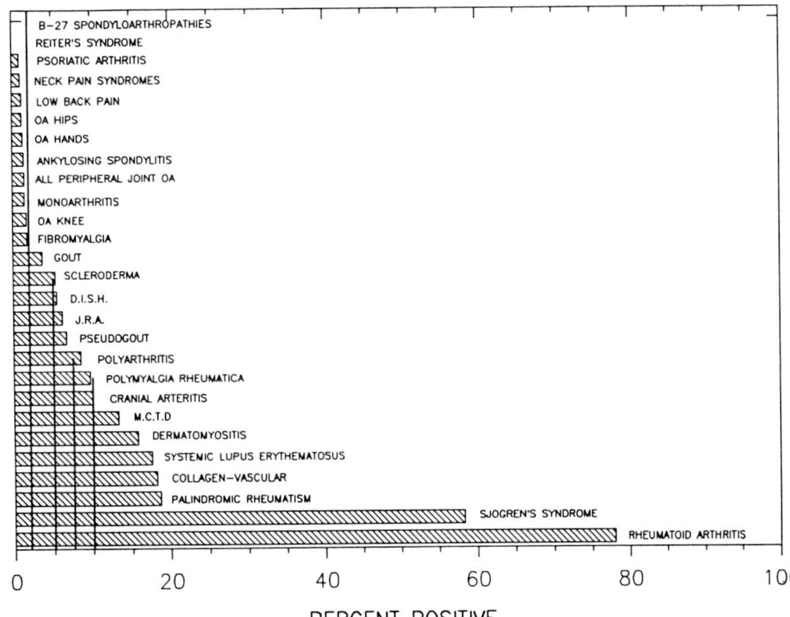

FIGURE 14–2. Diseases and conditions with rheumatoid factor positivity. OA, osteoarthritis; DISH, diffuse idiopathic skeletal hyperostosis; JRA, juvenile rheumatoid arthritis; MCTD, mixed connective tissue disease. (From Wolfe F, Cathey MA, and Roberts K: The latex test revisited. Arthritis Rheum 34:954, 1991.)

LFT) but was significantly more specific (99.2% versus 94%).

RF occurs in a number of rheumatic disorders, including Sjögren's syndrome, palindromic rheumatism, SLE, dermatomyositis, in a variety of other arthritic and nonarthritic conditions, and in situations such as advanced age and pregnancy (Fig. 14–2).[3, 14, 15] Its appearance in the serum of RA patients can precede clinical symptoms by years.[16] The occurrence of RF before clinical disease happens more often in men than in women.

The RF tests cannot and should not be used to diagnose RA; rather, these tests should be used to support clinical impressions. Often, patients with musculoskeletal disorders other than RA who test positive for RF are labeled with a diagnosis of RA and are therapeutically treated as such. If RF tests are used as a screening tool in general practice in which the prevalence of RA is quite low, most patients with a positive RF will probably not have the disease. When used more properly in instances in which the physician's suspicion for disease is at least 10%, a positive RF test indeed correlates with disease more than 70% of the time, whereas a patient with a negative test result will contract the disease less than 3% of the time.[14]

ciation of Clq with the disease state suggests a role for this protein in the pathogenesis of RA, and the appearance of this easily measurable marker in the serum may be a useful prognostic indicator of the future course of the disease.[19]

Many of the complement proteins can be measured directly through immunochemical and immunodiffusion techniques.[3] Normal serum levels of individual complement proteins are listed in Table 14–3.

Complement activity can be measured by assaying the system's biologic function of cell lysis.[20] The activity tests use sheep erythrocytes sensitized by rabbit antisheep erythrocyte antibody. The degree of cell lysis is proportional to the overall function of the complement system or of an individual complement protein if all other components are added under controlled conditions. The end point of the test is reached when 50% of a predetermined amount of sensitized sheep cells are lysed (a total of about 1×10^8 cells). This represents one unit of activity and is reported as 50% hemolytic units per milliliter of fluid tested (CH_{50} U/ml). Components of the complement system are quite labile, so specimens should be tested within 2 hours of collection, or the specimen should be frozen at 20°C until testing can be performed.[3, 20]

Complement

Immune complexes formed by the interaction of RF with altered synovial IgG are important activators of the complement cascade. Many of the products of this cascade are chemotactic for immune cells and potent mediators of inflammation in other ways (see Chapter 3). Biologic activities of some of the complement proteins are listed in Table 14–2.

Serum levels of complement protein Clq have been shown to correlate well with the erosive joint changes characteristic of RA.[17] Likewise, a strong correlation has been made between absolute levels of Clq within the first 5 years of the disease and the development of joint destruction.[18] The asso-

TABLE 14–2

BIOLOGICAL ACTIVITIES OF COMPLEMENT

Biological Function	Components Involved
Phagocytosis	C3b
Anaphylatoxic activity	C3a, C5a
Chemotaxis	C3bBb, C5a
Inhibition of macrophage migration	Bb
Clearance of immune complexes	C4b, C3b
Lysis of immune complexes	C4-binding activity
Membrane damage and cell lysis	C5b-9
Viral neutralization	C1, C3, C4

From George D and Glass D: Quantitation of complement proteins. Clin Rheum Dis 9(1):180, 1983.

TABLE 14–3

SERUM LEVELS OF COMPLEMENT COMPONENTS

Protein	Range or Mean Serum Concentration
C1q	35–56 mg/dl
C1r	3.4 mg/dl
C1s	3.1 mg/dl
C4	26–83 mg/dl
C2	1.58–3.02 mg/dl
C3	91–198 mg/dl
P	2.5 mg/dl
D	0.2 mg/dl
B	24.0 mg/dl
C5	11–23 mg/dl
C6	6.0 mg/dl
C7	5.5 mg/dl
C8	8.0 mg/dl
C9	16.0 mg/dl
C1 INH	16–34 mg/dl
C4-BP	—
I	35 mg/dl
H	36 mg/dl

George D and Glass D: Quantitation of complement proteins. Clin Rheum Dis 9(1):182, 1983.

Antinuclear Antibodies

The antinuclear antibodies (ANAs) are a heterogeneous group of antibodies specific for many nuclear constituents including deoxyribonucleic acid (DNA), deoxynucleoprotein (DNP), histone, ribonucleic acid (RNA), and for antigen in the soluble nuclear extract of the cell known as *extractable nuclear antigen*.[21] Other groups of ANA have been identified for antibodies to nonhistone proteins (NHP) and to complexes of NHP bound to RNAs (NHP-RNA), and antibodies to nucleolar antigens.[22]

It is uncertain whether DNA–anti-DNA complexes cause disease and promote associated tissue damage or whether these complexes arise secondarily as part of the immune reaction.[23] They were first discovered in the mid-1960s in the sera of patients with SLE. They now serve as useful diagnostic markers for SLE and other autoimmune disorders and are of prognostic significance, especially for SLE in which a strong correlation exists between the presence of ANA and tissue destruction.[23]

SLE can be considered the prototypical autoimmune disorder. The disease seems to result from disturbances in immune regulation leading to, or resulting from, a polyclonal activation of B cells. The activated B cells exaggerate production of autoantibodies which causes the disease. It is theorized that genetic, environmental, and hormonal factors may be responsible for this immunoregulatory abnormality.[24]

Several antibodies in addition to those native to DNA may occur in SLE. These include antiperinuclear factor, antibodies to histones, and antibodies to Sm and nuclear ribonucleoprotein. The usual SLE patient displays an average of three circulating antibodies simultaneously.[25] The immune deposits that characterize the disease may arise through one of three proposed mechanisms: (1) Circulating DNA–anti-DNA immune complexes deposit in the target tissues, (2) anti-DNA antibody binds directly to tissue DNA in situ, or (3) anti-DNA antibody binds directly to target tissue components. Most research has focused on the first proposed mechanism;

however, circulating anti-DNA antibodies have proved difficult to demonstrate.[23]

In a similar manner, ANA to various cellular structures has been suspected to cause a variety of disorders including RA. Studies using monoclonal anti-DNA have shown that antibodies to DNA circulate freely in both normal and autoimmune persons.[23] What triggers the pathologic reaction to develop between anti-DNA antibodies and their tissue targets has yet to be elucidated. ANA specificities and their disease associations are listed in Table 14–4.

RA has been associated with the presence of several ANA types. Antiperinuclear factor was thought to be a useful diagnostic tool for RA, occurring in 59% of patients with seropositive RA and in 36% of those with seronegative RA. Subsequently, this factor was discovered in SLE, Sjögren's syndrome, and systemic sclerosis and thus was shown to lack the specificity to establish a diagnosis of RA.[26] Antibodies to laminae, the major components of nuclear envelopes, have been discovered in patients with RA.[27] These also lack specificity because they have been observed in patients with a variety of other autoimmune disorders as well. A new ANA has been discovered, however, that may indeed be highly specific for RA.[28] This antibody, currently designated *anti-RA33* by virtue of its association with RA and its molecular weight of 33,000, has been found to occur in 36% of RA patients studied and in only 1 of 170 control patients.

TABLE 14–4

ANTIGENIC SPECIFICITIES OF ANTINUCLEAR ANTIBODIES AND CONDITIONS IN WHICH THEY ARE FOUND

Antigenic Specificity (Synonyms)	Conditions
Nucleoprotein	SLE, RA, CAH, isoniazid ingestion
dsDNA	SLE, MCTD, MG
ssDNA	SLE, discoid LE, RA, juvenile RA, anticonvulsant treatment, CAH
Histones	SLE, RA?, procainamide or hydralazine treatment and drug-related SLE
dsRNA	SLE
ssRNA (uracil-specific)	Diffuse scleroderma
Centromere	CREST syndrome
Nuclear matrix	SLE, RA
nRNP (Mo)	MCTD, SLE
rRNP (TM, MU)	SLE, SS, MCTD
Sm	SLE, CAH, RA
Ro (SS-A)	SLE, RA, SS
LA (SS-B, Ha)	SLE, RA, SS
RANA (SS-C)	RA, Normal subjects
PM-1	DM/PM
Mi	DM/PM
Jo (1)	DM/PM
Scl-70 (Scl-1, & Og)	Scleroderma
MA	SLE
Proliferating cell nuclear antigen (Ne)	SLE
Ki	SLE
Ku	Scleroderma/PM overlap
Nucleosomal protein HMG-17	SLE-MCTD

CAH, chronic active hepatitis; MG, myasthenia gravis; SS, Sjögren's syndrome; SLE, systemic lupus erythematosus; RA, rheumatoid arthritis; MCTD, mixed connective tissue disease; LE, lupus erythematosus; CREST, *c*alcification, *R*aynaud's phenomenon, *e*sophageal dysfunction, *s*cleroderma, and *t*elangiectasia; DM/PM, dermatomyositis/polymyositis; DNA, deoxyribonucleic acid; RNA, ribonucleic acid; RNP, ribonucleoprotein.

Adapted from Alarcon-Segovia D: Antibodies to nuclear and other intracellular antigens in the connective tissue diseases. Clin Rheum Dis 9(1):163, 1983.

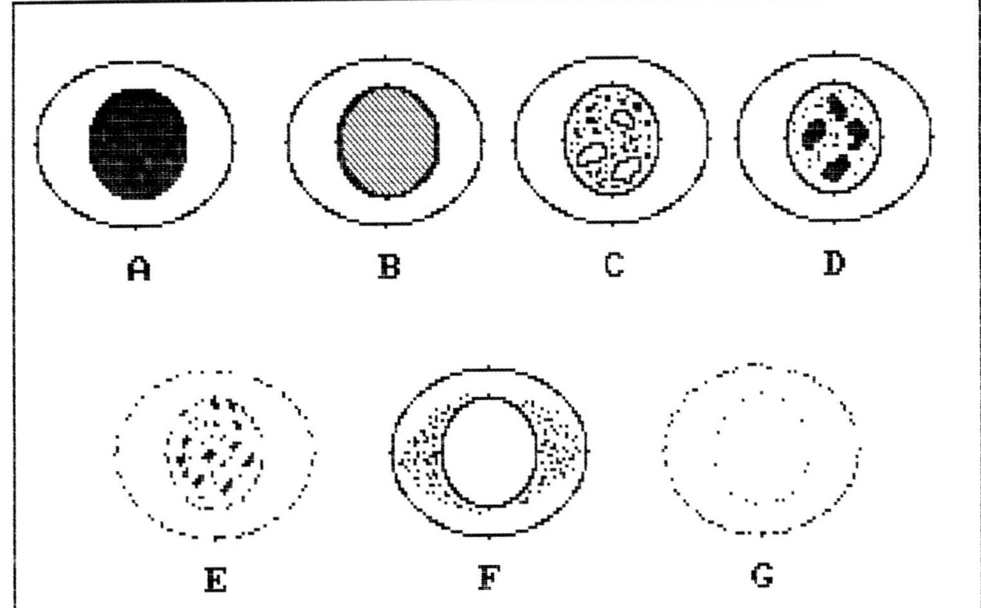

FIGURE 14–3. Patterns of antinuclear antibody fluorescence. A, solid (homogeneous); B, peripheral (rim); C, speckled; D, nucleolar; E, anticentromere; F, antimitochondrial; G, normal (nonreactive). (Adapted from Ravel R: Clinical Laboratory Medicine, 5th ed. Chicago, Year Book Medical Publishers, 1989, p 376.)

Assay techniques have been developed to detect specific autoantibodies. The oldest is the Farr method, an RIA technique that uses radioactive tritium (^{3}H) or carbon 14 as the radioisotope. Variations of this technique use the more traditional radioactive iodine isotope. Another method has been developed that uses the protozoan *Crithidia luciliae*. Patient serum is added to prepared slides of the dead organism, and any anti-DNA antibodies attach to the kinetoplast of the organism. A fluorescent antihuman globulin antibody is added that causes the kinetoplast to fluoresce if antibody has attached.[5]

The ANA test is similar to the *C. luciliae* test just described. Patient serum is incubated with a sample of nucleated cells and is later tagged with antigamma globulin antibody to detect patient ANA coating the sample cell nuclei. The antibody tag may be fluorescent (FANA test) or may be an enzyme (EANA test).[5]

Results of the ANA test report both antibody titer and pattern of antibody distribution. Several patterns of distribution, which are thought to be associated with certain of the autoimmune disorders, can occur (Fig. 14–3). These patterns include (1) the rim (peripheral) pattern, (2) the solid (homogeneous) pattern, (3) the speckled pattern, (4) the nucleolar pattern, and (5) the centromere pattern. Table 14–5 reviews the association between patterns and disease.[5]

Lupus Erythematosus Cell Test

The lupus erythematosus (LE) cell test (or LE prep) is the most widely used diagnostic test for SLE. The test is a visualization of the LE phenomenon caused by the reaction between autoantibody and DNP.[3]

A source of nuclei from laboratory-damaged tissue or white blood cells is incubated with patient serum. ANA against DNP, designated *LE factor*, complexes with nuclear antigens in disrupted cells, producing a homogeneous, amorphous mass that stains basophilic with Wright's stain. The mass is then phagocytized by undamaged polymorphonuclear

TABLE 14–5

ANTINUCLEAR ANTIBODY TEST PATTERNS

Pattern	Description	Specificity	Disease Associations
Rim	Fluorescence around nuclear border	dsDNA, ssDNA, sNP, histones	SLE
Solid	Fluorescence uniform throughout nucleus	dsDNA, ssDNA, sNP, histones	SLE, rheumatoid-collagen diseases, drug-induced ANA
Speckled	Small, fluorescent dots throughout nucleus, sparing nucleolus	Sm, RNP, SS-A [Ro], SS-B, Scl-70, advanced age	MCTD, SLE, RA, drug-induced ANA, SS, PSS, scleroderma
Nucleolar	Fluorescence in nucleoli	n-RNA	PSS
Centromere	Fluorescent speckles smaller and fewer than speckled pattern	Centromere antigen	CREST syndrome
Mitochondrial	Fluorescence in cytoplasm along poles of nucleus	Antimitochondrial	CAH, primary biliary cirrhosis, cryptogenic cirrhosis

DNA, deoxyribonucleic acid; PSS, progressive systemic sclerosis; RNP, ribonucleoprotein; SLE, systemic lupus erythematosus; RA, rheumatoid arthritis; ANA, antinuclear antibody; SS, Sjögren's syndrome; CREST, *c*alcification, *R*aynaud's phenomenon, *e*sophageal dysfunction, *s*cleroderma, and *t*elangiectasia; CAH, chronic active hepatitis; MCTD, mixed connective tissue disease.

Adapted from Ravel R: Clinical Laboratory Medicine, 5th ed. Chicago, Year Book Medical Publishers, 1989, pp 375–377 and Betts Carpenter A and Rabin BS: Autoimmunity and immunopathy. Clin Lab Med 3(4):745–762, 1983.

neutrophils, producing the characteristic LE cell (Fig. 14–4). The presence of the cell indicates a positive test result and is strongly suggestive of SLE. The test can be positive as well for drug-induced SLE-like syndrome, RA, some forms of hepatitis and cirrhosis, and other collagen-vascular diseases.[3, 5]

Histocompatibility Antigens

The human major histocompatibility complex consists of a series of genes located at position 21 on chromosome 6. These genes encode two sets of glycoproteins that have come to be known as the *human leukocyte antigen* (HLA) molecules. Two classes of cell-surface antigens have been identified and are found to occur on human white blood cells and other nucleated tissue cells. Class I genes encode the HLA-A, B, and C antigens and have wide tissue distribution. Class II genes (sometimes designated as *class Ia*) encode for the HLA-D region, which includes the five family members HLA-DR, DQ, DO, DN, and DP antigens. The class II antigens have a more restricted tissue distribution.[29–31]

The occurrence of surface antigens on lymphocytes and other tissue cells is determined by testing the cells against a variety of antisera of known HLA specificity. More recently, DNA typing using sequencing techniques or restriction fragment length polymorphism and protein typing using monoclonal antibodies have been used to identify the antigen.[32, 33]

The presence of certain HLAs has been associated with the development of disease or with an individual's response to a disease process (Tables 14–6 and 14–7).[29] The most

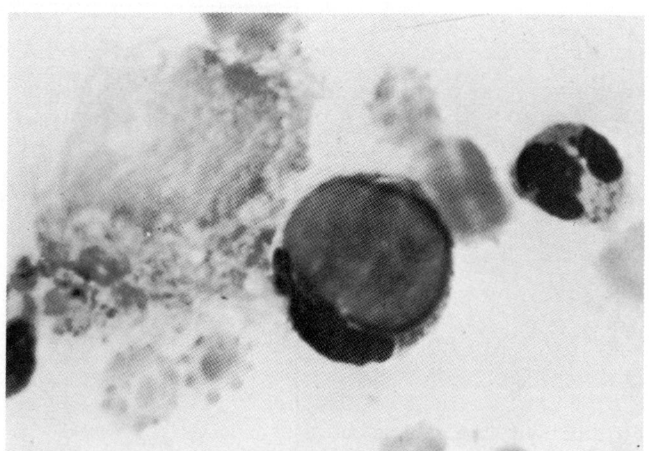

FIGURE 14–4. The lupus erythematosus cell. (From D'Angelo WA: Diagnostic procedures and tests. *In* Halsted JA: The Laboratory in Clinical Medicine: Interpretation and Application, 1st ed. Philadelphia, WB Saunders, 1976, p 525.)

widely known of these associations occurs between HLA-B27 and ankylosing spondylitis. Just how the presence of surface antigen confers disease susceptibility is not yet fully understood. However, investigations have shown that the association is not strict (i.e., a considerable number of patients who are not positive for HLA-B27 can still contract the disease, whereas others who are positive can remain disease free). The antigens, then, may not be directly related to the

TABLE 14–6

SUMMARY OF COMMON ASSOCIATIONS OF MAJOR HISTOCOMPATIBILITY COMPLEX CLASS I ALLELES WITH RHEUMATIC DISEASES

Disease	HLA allele	Relative risk	Patients (% positive)	Controls (% positive)
Seronegative				
Spondylarthropathy				
Ankylosing spondylitis	B27	69.1	89	9
Pauciarticular peripheral arthritis	B27	15.6	69	9
Isolated sacroiliitis	B27	20.4	62	9
Reiter's syndrome	B27	37.1	80	9
Reactive arthritis				
Salmonella species	B27	35.5	85	10
Shigella flexneri	B27	28.7	85	14
Campylobacter jejuni	B27	13.8	71	14
Yersinia species	B27	21.4	77	11
Inflammatory bowel disease	B27	10.2	52	10
Psoriatic arthritis				
Axial arthropathy	B13	3.9	16	5
Axial arthropathy	Bw16	7.8	26	5
Axial arthropathy	B17	2.2	13	7
Axial arthropathy	B27	10.8	47	8
Axial arthropathy	B38	10.3	23	3
Peripheral arthropathy	B13	2.4	12	7
Peripheral arthropathy	Bw16	2.1	10	7
Peripheral arthropathy	B17	5.1	25	7
Peripheral arthropathy	B27	2.0	14	10
Peripheral arthropathy	B38	5.5	15	3
Behçet's syndrome				
"East"	B5(W51)	7.2	69	23
"West"	B5(W51)	3.8	31	12
Whipple's disease	B27	4.6	30	8

HLA, human leukocyte antigen.

From Schumacher HR, Klippel JH, and Robinson DR: Immunogenetics. *In* Primer on the Rheumatic Diseases, 9th ed. Atlanta, Arthritis Foundation, 1988, p 47. Used by permission of the Arthritis Foundation.

TABLE 14–7

SUMMARY OF COMMON ASSOCIATION OF MAJOR HISTOCOMPATIBILITY COMPLEX CLASS II ALLELES WITH RHEUMATIC DISEASES

Disease	HLA allele (haplotype)	Relative risk	Patients (% positive)	Controls (% positive)
Rheumatoid arthritis	DR1	1.4	20	17
	DR2	−2.2	13	25
	DR3	−1.4	16	21
	DR4	2.7	47	25
	DR5	−3.1	7	19
	DRw6	−3.1	2	6
	DR7	−1.7	14	22
After recalculation for DR4 increase	DR1	1.7	20	13
Systemic lupus erythematosus	DR2	2.3	44	25
	DR3	2.5	40	21
Sjögren's syndrome	DR2	5.2	73	33
	DR3	3.6	56	26
Takayasu's arteritis	B5	3.3	63	36
	DRw52	5.0	45	14
	DR2	2.4	60	36

HLA, human leukocyte antigen.

From Schumacher HR, Klippel JH, and Robinson DR: Immunogenetics. *In* Primer on the Rheumatic Diseases, 9th ed. Atlanta, Arthritis Foundation, 1988, p 47. Used by permission of the Arthritis Foundation.

disease but may instead be markers for another gene that does indeed determine susceptibility to disease.[34] Alternative explanations are reviewed in Chapter 3.

Another antigen-disease association has been recognized between certain HLA-D and HLA-C antigens and RA. HLA-DR4 has been associated with a risk for the development of RA.[35] There is also an increased frequency of HLA-Dw4 (36%) and HLA-Cw3 antigens in patients with RA, but the latter antigen-disease association appears to be less significant.[33, 36] Only a small percentage of patients carrying these genetic markers for RA actually contract disease, suggesting that the disease is probably multifactorial and susceptibility is polygenic.[33]

The value of HLA typing for establishing a diagnosis is limited and costly. Physicians must carefully consider the test's cost versus benefit profile before relying on this or any other test for diagnosis, particularly when the test offers only vague diagnostic information. HLA typing may prove most useful when used as an aid in controlled clinical trials of new treatment regimens in diseases with known HLA associations to ensure appropriate test and control group distributions. Also, typing may be useful in helping predict the effect or response to treatment of patients in an HLA-related disease group.[30] For example, a mild association occurs with the presence of HLA-DR3 antigen and the development of toxic reactions to gold therapy (21.1%), whereas decreased toxicity may be observed in patients carrying the DR2 gene.[37]

Serum Uric Acid

Measurement of serum uric acid is helpful in establishing the diagnosis of hyperuricemia but not gout. Uric acid is synthesized by the body de novo and also originates from the metabolic breakdown of purine nucleoproteins. Total daily uric acid production is in the range of 600 to 700 mg, and dietary protein adds another 600 mg. Serum levels reflect an equilibrium between the rate of uric acid produced and the rate excreted.[3]

Retained uric acid produces the condition of hyperurice-

mia, which may lead to gout. The hyperuricemia may be of three forms, any one of which elevates uric acid levels through either increased production or decreased excretion of the metabolite. Primary hyperuricemia reflects an inborn error of metabolism that directly alters uric acid metabolism, whereas secondary hyperuricemia refers to a genetic or acquired condition that indirectly increases uric acid levels. Any disease characterized by high cell turnover, such as myeloproliferative disorders, is a typical cause of secondarily elevated uric acid. Idiopathic hyperuricemia cannot be directly attributed to any systemic cause. Gout and hyperuricemia are discussed further in Chapter 9.

OTHER HEMATOLOGIC STUDIES

The presence of various other substances in blood or synovial fluids has been related to arthritic diseases, but these again are more reflective of the inflammatory process rather than specific for the diseases themselves. For instance, blood and synovial fluid concentrations of the neuropeptide substance P become elevated in different forms of arthritis and in post-traumatic states. This suggests that specifically the unmyelinated articular neurons may play a role in mediating or modulating intra-articular inflammation.[38] Serum hyaluronate levels also increase in early RA and may be reflective of ongoing joint destruction or predictive of subsequent joint damage.[39–41] Although these tests are of significant academic interest, their diagnostic usefulness is not of great value.

Other more established blood tests continue to hold great value in the course of patient care. Complete blood counts, cell morphology tests, liver and kidney function tests, and others are essential for monitoring organ function while the patient with arthritis undergoes drug therapy. Although not diagnostic of the primary disease, they may be prognostic for complications that may arise from the disease or from treatment. In addition, monitoring indicators of inflammation may be helpful in determining the effectiveness of drug therapy.[42] Likewise, monitoring serum levels of some therapeutic agents may be helpful in achieving proper dosage, as with salicylates. Other agents, however, do not show any useful correlation between serum drug levels and efficacy or toxicity.[43]

Some of the common laboratory findings for RA are listed in Table 14–8.

Synovial Fluid Studies

The evaluation of synovial fluid (SF) can be of great value in monitoring the course of inflammatory joint diseases. It is useful diagnostically in conditions such as gout and septic arthritis. Some common synovial fluid parameters in health and disease are listed in Table 14–9.

Joint aspiration is not always an innocuous procedure. The possibility of joint contamination (i.e., introducing pathogens into a sterile joint) requires a preaspiration sterile preparation of the area surrounding the joint and use of sterile technique for the procedure. For patient comfort, the area proximal to the aspiration site should first be anesthetized with a local anesthetic of the physician's choice, taking care not to introduce the anesthesia into the joint. The anesthetic should be injected deep because superficial deposit does not adequately anesthetize the joint capsule and results in a painful aspiration. Besides patient consideration, it is important to have the patient as comfortable as possible during the procedure to avoid joint contamination, inadequate sampling volume, or iatrogenic hemarthrosis and blood in the sample. A 19- or 20-gauge needle should be used for the aspiration to ensure ease and completeness of sampling.

The most commonly aspirated joints of the foot are the ankle and first metatarsophalangeal (MTP) joints. Besides the lesser MTP joints, most other joints of the foot are so tightly fit even in the inflamed state that sampling is difficult and prone to poor sample collection.

The best approach to the ankle joint is through the anterolateral aspect of the ankle. The needle should be directed posteromedially and in a slightly cephalic direction. The skin should be pierced between the lateral aspect of the extensor digitorum brevis tendons and just medial and anterior to the lateral malleolus. Care must be taken to avoid the intermediate dorsocutaneous nerve, which courses just medial to the point of puncture. The joint can be accessed medially as well, puncturing the skin between the anterior tibial and extensor hallux brevis tendons. The needle should be aimed posterolaterally and slightly cephalic. The saphenous nerve and veins course through this area and must be avoided.

The MTP joints may present a challenge to aspiration, especially the lesser joints. For accessing the first MTP joint, the joint should be distracted by pulling the hallux distally. This will cause a transverse dimple to form at the level of the joint. The needle should be held at approximately a 45-degree angle to the skin and should penetrate the skin medial or lateral to the extensor tendons and just at the proximal point of the dimple. A similar technique can be used to gain access to the lesser MTP joints.

When the joint capsule is punctured, an attempt should be made to extract all fluid present in the joint. This may be easy in larger joints and in those extended by inflammatory

TABLE 14–8

LABORATORY FINDINGS IN RHEUMATOID ARTHRITIS

Test	Characteristic Results
Blood Elements	
Erythrocytes	Moderate normochromic or hypochromic, normocytic anemia; low plasma iron; moderately decreased bone marrow iron stores; normal use of plasma iron; slightly decreased survival time; inadequate release of iron from tissue stores; normal transferrin levels; decreased total iron binding capacity; increased plasma volume
Leukocytes	Normal or slightly elevated polymorphonuclear leukocytes; leukocytosis possible in severe disease; leukopenia rare (Felty's syndrome); eosinophilia with severe disease and systemic complications; thrombocytosis during active disease; normal nitroblue tetrazolium test results; reduced chemotaxis; lymphocytes—normal B, T, and null cell distribution; decreased blastogenic transformation
Acute-Phase Reactants and Immunoglobulins	
Erythrocyte sedimentation rate	Increased
C-reactive protein	Usually positive
Serum amyloid protein	Slightly elevated
Serum proteins	Alpha-2, fibrinogen, and gamma globulins increased; albumin decreased
Immunoglobulins	IgG increased (seropositive patients mostly); IgA and IgM increased; IgD normal or low
Cryoglobulins	Rare
Urinary gamma globulin	Increased IgG, IgA, and free light chains
Ceruloplasmin	Elevated
Fibronectin	Normal serum levels
Immune Factors	
Lupus erythematosus factor	Present in 10% of patients
Antinuclear antibody	Present in 15%; associated with more severe disease and rheumatoid factor positivity
Rheumatoid factor	Usually present in adults
Biological false-positive serologic test for syphilis	Present in 5 to 10% of patients
Complement	Normal or slightly elevated levels; hypocomplementemia rare and associated with vasculitis and severe disease

Adapted from Baum J and Ziff M: Laboratory findings in rheumatoid arthritis. *In* McCarty DJ: Arthritis and Allied Conditions, 11th ed. Philadelphia, Lea & Febiger, 1989, p 745.

TABLE 14-9

SYNOVIAL ANALYSIS IN THE ARTHRITIDES*

Condition	Viscosity	Cell Count (per cu mm)	% PMN	Glucose Level	Mucin Clot	Other Tests or Findings
Normal	Normal (high)	0–200 (0–600)	0–25	Normal	Good	—
Trauma with hemorrhage/coagulation abnormalities	Normal	>5,000	50 (25–50)	Normal	Good	Many RBCs
Osteoarthritis/osteochondritis dissecans/trauma without hemorrhage	Normal	500 (200–2,000)	25	Normal	Good	Cartilage fragments
Acute rheumatic fever	Low	2,000–15,000 (0–60,000)	50 (50–60)	Occasional small decrease	Good to poor	—
SLE	Normal or low	2,000–5,000 (0–10,000)	25 (10–30)	Normal to 20 mg below blood glucose level	Good to fair	LE prep
RA RA variants	Low	2,000–50,000† (200–100,000)	70–85 (25–85)	Normal to 30 mg below blood glucose level	Fair, 50% Poor, 45%	RA latex test
Gout (acute attack)	Low	2,000–50,000‡ (100–100,000)	75 (40–90)	Normal to 30 mg below blood glucose level	Fair, 50% Poor, 40%	Urate crystals
Pseudogout	Low	2,000–50,000‡ (100–100,000)	75 (35–85)	Normal	Fair, 40% Poor, 35%	Calcium pyrophosphate crystals
Acute bacterial arthritis	Low	>50,000§ (2,500–300,000)	90 (75–95)	More than 40 mg below blood glucose level‖	Poor (85% of cases)	Culture Gram's stain**

*Parentheses indicate ranges from the literature.
†More than 50,000/mm^3 in 4% of cases; 2500 in 6% of cases.
‡More than 50,000/mm^3 in 12% of cases; 1000 in 15% of cases.
§Less than 50,000/mm^3 in 30% of cases; 20,000 in 11% of cases.
‖More than 40 mg/100 ml below blood glucose level in 40 to 50% of cases.
**Gram's stain reported positive in 55 to 95% of gram-positive and 30 to 55% of gram-negative infections.
SLE, systemic lupus erythematosus; RA, rheumatoid arthritis; RBCs, red blood cells; LE, lupus erythematosus; PMN, polymorphonuclear leukocytes.
Adapted from D'Angelo WA; Diagnostic procedures and tests. *In* Halsted JA: The Laboratory in Clinical Medicine, Interpretation and Application, 2nd ed. Philadelphia, WB Saunders, 1981, pp 514–515 and Ravel R: Clinical Laboratory Medicine, 5th ed. Chicago, Year Book Medical Publishers, 1989, p 388.

fluids, but the procedure is difficult in small or mildly swollen joints. The joint fluid should be examined promptly after arthrocentesis.[44]

Traditionally, the appearance of joint fluid has been classified into three or more groups: normal, noninflammatory, inflammatory, septic, and hemorrhagic.[45] These classifications are not universally followed but may still be useful (Tables 14–10 and 14–11). Identifying the SF as either inflammatory or noninflammatory and determining the cause of inflammation are the more important messages from laboratory evaluation.

Normal joint fluid is transparent, almost colorless, and present in small quantities in normal diarthrodial joints. Larger volumes may be indicative of inflammation but not

TABLE 14-10

JOINT FLUID CHARACTERISTICS

	Normal	Group I (Noninflammatory)	Group II (Inflammatory)	Group III (Septic)
Volume (knee, in ml)	<3.5	>3.5	>3.5	>3.5
Viscosity	Very high	High*	Low	Variable
Color	Clear	Xanthochromic	Xanthochromic to opalescent	Variable with organisms
Clarity	Transparent	Transparent	Translucent, opaque at times	Opaque
Mucin clot	Firm	Firm	Friable	Friable
WBC/mm^3	200	200–2000	2000 100,000	>50,000† usually >100,000
PMN (%)	<25	<25	>50	>75†
Culture	Negative	Negative	Negative	Usually positive

*Rapid accumulation of fluid will lower viscosity.
†May be lower with partially treated or low-virulence organism.
WBC, white blood cell; PMN, polymorphonuclear neutrophils.
From Gatter RA and Schumacher HR: Practical Handbook of Joint Fluid Analysis. Philadelphia, Lea & Febiger, 1991.

TABLE 14–11

DIFFERENTIAL DIAGNOSES BY JOINT FLUID GROUPS*

Group I (Noninflammatory)	Group II (Inflammatory)	Group III (Septic)	Group IV (Hemorrhagic)
Osteoarthritis	Rheumatoid disease	Bacterial infections	Trauma with or without fracture
Traumatic arthritis	Crystal-induced synovitis		Charcot's arthropathy
Avascular necrosis	Gout		Hemorrhagic diathesis
Internal derangement	Pseudogout		Anticoagulant therapy
Osteochondritis dissecans	Hydroxyapatite		Von Willebrand
Osteochondromatosis	Corticosteroid injection		Hemophilia
Charcot's arthropathy	Psoriatic arthritis		Scurvy
Subsiding inflammation	Reactive arthritis		Thrombocytopenia
Villonodular synovitis	Reiter's syndrome		Hemangioma
Hypertrophic pulmonary osteoarthropathy	Regional enteritis		Tumor
Systemic lupus erythematosus†	Ulcerative colitis		Pigmented villonodular synovitis
Rheumatic fever†	Postileal bypass		Synovioma
Scleroderma†	*Yersinia*		
Amyloidosis†	*Campylobacter*		
Myxedema	Whipple's disease		
Acromegaly	Connective tissue disease		
Hemochromatosis	Systemic lupus		
Gaucher's disease	Polyarteritis		
Ochronosis	Scleroderma		
Paget's disease of bone	Polymyositis		
Sickle cell disease	Vasculitis (nonspecific)		
	Polymyalgia rheumatica		
	Polychondritis		
	Sarcoidosis		
	Behçet's syndrome		
	Ankylosing spondylitis		
	Juvenile rheumatoid arthritis		
	Rheumatic fever		
	Agammaglobulinemia		
	Infectious arthritis (low-virulence)		
	Viral		
	Fungal		
	Bacterial		
	Mycobacterial		
	Mycoplasmal		
	Hypersensitivity		
	Serum sickness		
	Erythema multiforme		

*Partial listing.
†May be Group I or II.
From Gatter RA and Schumacher HR: Practical Handbook of Joint Fluid Analysis. Philadelphia, Lea & Febiger, 1991.

necessarily. Clarity is lost with inflammation, and the fluid may become yellow to yellow-green depending on the protein content and other cellular debris. The more inflamed the joint becomes, the more opaque and purulent it will appear. The cloudiness is not always due to pus but can be caused by crystals or other debris. Rice bodies (named for their resemblance to polished rice), consisting primarily of fibrin, fibronectin, and collagen, are sometimes seen in inflammatory fluids, particularly in patients with RA.[45, 46]

Normal joint fluid is highly viscous owing to its hyaluronic acid content. A drop of SF delivered from the tip of the aspiration needle produces a long, intact string often several inches long. This viscosity is lost in inflammation; the sample becomes more like water.

Normal SF does not clot owing to the absence of fibrinogen and other clotting factors.[46] Inflamed SF forms a firm clot (mucin clot test) when added to 5% acetic acid. The clot resists fragmentation on agitation, and the size of the clot is roughly proportional to the degree of inflammation. Small clots may occupy about 25% of the volume and may take several hours to form, whereas large clots, occupying more than 50% of the sample volume, develop almost instantly.[46]

All SF samples should be sent to the laboratory for white blood cell count and differential. Normal joint fluid contains fewer than 300 white blood cells/mm^3, with up to 2000/mm^3 present in normal joints or in joints with noninflammatory diseases. The presence of more than 50,000/mm^3 is characteristic of a septic joint. Levels ranging from 5000 to 75,000/mm^3 may be observed in RA, ankylosing spondylitis, connective tissue diseases, and other seronegative spondyloarthropathies.[47] In general, the white blood cell count elevates as does the degree of inflammation.

The differential may add more clues to the diagnosis of joint disease. Noninflamed SF has neutrophil counts less than 50%, whereas inflamed joints have neutrophil counts greater than 50%. Septic joints have neutrophil counts greater than 95% total; RA has neutrophil counts less than 90%. Crystal-induced effusions will have neutrophil percentages in the higher range.[45] Whenever infection is suspected, Gram's stain should be performed immediately and the fluid sampled for culture and sensitivity.

Normal joint fluid contains no crystals. When crystals are suspected, the fluid should be collected in tubes containing EDTA or heparin (avoid crystalline anticoagulants so as not to confuse examination) and submitted for crystal examination under a polarizing microscope.

Gout is diagnosed when monosodium urate crystals are present in joint fluid. These are needle-shaped crystals that display negative birefringence when observed under a polarizing microscope (Figs. 14–5A and B). Weakly positive birefringent crystals of calcium pyrophosphate are found with pseudogout or chondrocalcinosis.[48] Basic calcium phosphate crystals, formerly known as hydroxyapatite, are associated with periarticular diseases such as periarthritis and tendinitis. Individual basic calcium phosphate crystals are needle or plate shaped and are too small to be resolved by the light microscope. Aggregates may be visible as shiny, laminated "coins."

The glucose content of SF may be of limited value for making a diagnosis. Generally, glucose content is about 80% of plasma concentrations. Lower levels in the face of an elevated white blood cell count may indicate an infective process because these cells and bacterial organisms use joint glucose as a source of energy. SF lactic acid levels are usually elevated under these same conditions.[11, 45]

No convincing evidence supports examining SF for protein or immune complexes other than for academic or research interests. Noninflamed joints usually contain less than 3.5 g/dl protein, whereas inflamed joint fluid may show concentrations of up to 6 to 8 g/dl.[3, 5] Immune complexes can activate complement within the rheumatoid joint. Normally, complement concentration in SF is 10% of serum complement, but with inflammation this level is decreased.[45]

Synovial Tissue Examination

A biopsy of synovial tissue may at times provide definitive diagnostic information, but again many times histologic examination shows only the effects of a generalized state of inflammation. Still, useful information can be gained for many joint disorders that cannot otherwise be obtained. If joint structure biopsy is performed, the expected diagnostic benefit should be worth the risk of the procedure.

Joint structure biopsy is most useful to diagnose conditions with distinctive findings such as granulomatous infections; sarcoidosis; bacterial or fungal infections; pigmented villonodular synovitis; synovial, cartilaginous, or bone neoplasms; crystal deposition diseases; and others.[48] Depending on the technique, bone, cartilage, and synovial membrane can all be accessed percutaneously. Common synovial tissue biopsy findings are listed in Table 14–12.

The tissue retrieved should be immediately preserved to prevent desiccation or other changes that would make examination difficult. A good general-purpose preservative is formaldehyde. For crystal analysis, the tissue, or a portion, should be preserved in absolute alcohol to prevent crystal

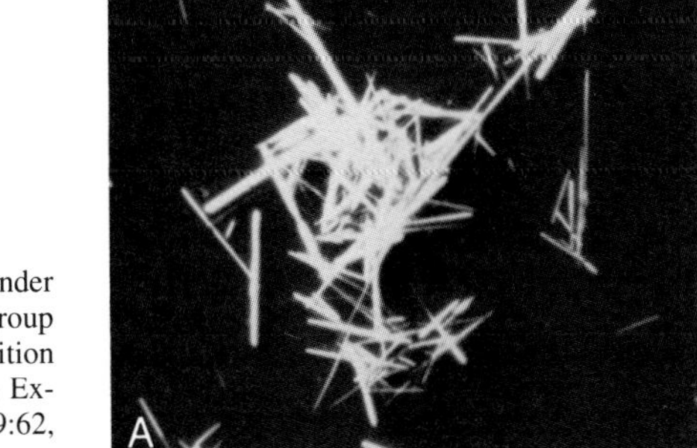
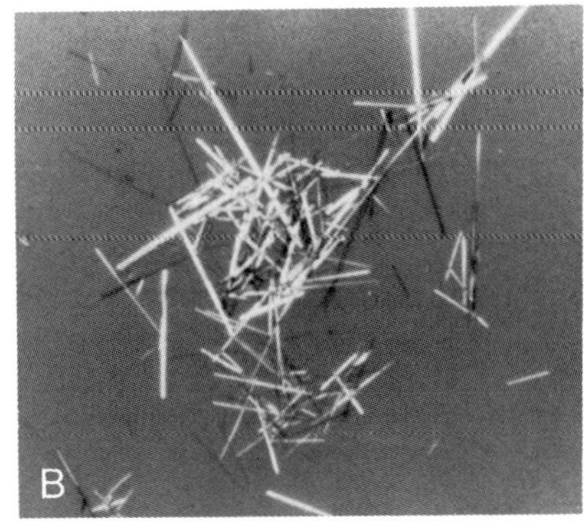

FIGURE 14–5. Uric acid crystals. *A,* Seen under crossed polarized light (× 400). *B,* Same group shown using a first-order red compensator in addition to the crossed polarized lenses. (From Platt PN: Examination of synovial fluid. Clin Rheum Dis 9:62, 1983.)

TABLE 14–12

SPECIFIC HISTOPATHOLOGIC CHARACTERISTICS DEMONSTRATED IN CERTAIN RHEUMATIC DISEASES

Rheumatic Disease	Characteristic
Bacterial and fungal arthritis	Demonstrate organism in sections or with culture
Tuberculosis	Demonstrate organisms in section or culture; caseating granuloma with giant cells
Hemochromatosis	Iron in synovial lining cell
Ochronosis	Fragments of pigmented cartilage
Pigmented villonodular synovitis	Villous hypertrophy, hemosiderin deposits with numerous giant cells
Primary and metastatic cancer	Malignant cells in the synovium
Gout	Monosodium urate crystals
Pseudogout	Calcium pyrophosphate dihydrate crystals

From Goldenberg DL: Synovial membrane biopsy. *In* Cohen AS (ed): Rheumatology and Immunology. New York, Grune & Stratton, 1979, p 90.

dissolution. If sepsis is suspected, or if immunofluorescence procedures are to be ordered, the specimen should be transported immediately in saline solution without a bacteriostat. The laboratory should be advised of the suspected diagnosis before the tissue is submitted and the tests requested before the tissue is processed. This allows the laboratory to plan proper tissue-handling techniques.

Larger joints, such as the knee and ankle, may be entered and tissue sampled via an arthroscope. This allows the surgeon to visualize sample sites directly for retrieval of tissue most representative of the disease process. The disadvantage is that small joints cannot be accessed in this manner, and the procedure must be performed with the use of special facilities and equipment. Anesthesia services are also required.

Many pedal joints can undergo biopsy in an office setting. The biopsy should be treated as a surgical procedure and proper precautions observed. As for arthrocentesis, the area proximal to the biopsy site must be anesthetized, taking care to inject deep enough to numb the joint structures. Again, anesthesia should not be introduced into the area undergoing biopsy.

Percutaneous needle biopsy can be achieved through the use of a Parker-Pearson biopsy needle (Fig. 14–6). The skin is first prepared and draped in the usual manner for surgical procedure. Under sterile technique, the joint is entered as described for arthrocentesis with the outer needle and trocar. The trocar is removed and the joint aspirated. The fluid should be sent to the laboratory for analysis. The joint can then be injected with several milliliters of 1% or 2% lidocaine. The biopsy needle is then inserted with the hooked edge against the synovium. A large sterile Luer-Lok syringe is attached and suction applied. Six to eight samples are collected from different areas of the joint.[48] On completion of the procedure, anesthesia with epinephrine can be instilled to control hemarthrosis formation if no contraindications to the vasoconstrictor are present. Bone and cartilage can undergo similar biopsy using a small-bore trephine through a stab incision.

The surgeon should be prepared to submit the patient for open biopsy should percutaneous technique fail to produce representative specimens. If problems occur during percuta-

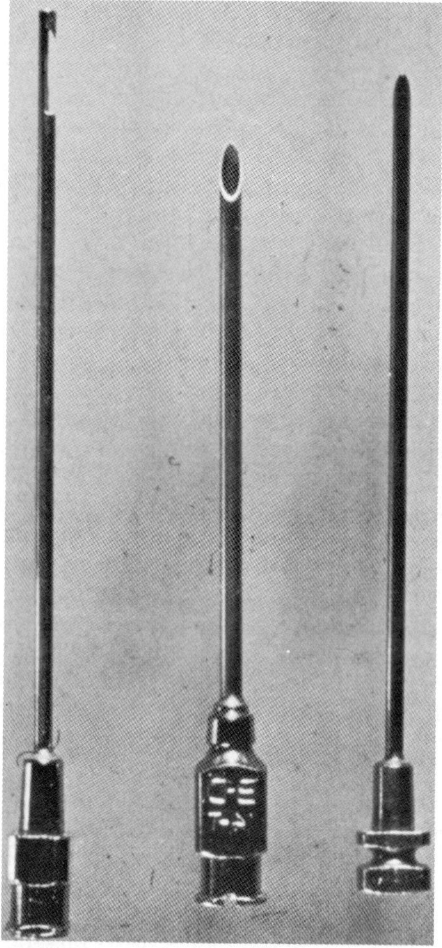

FIGURE 14–6. Parker-Pearson biopsy needle. (From Schumacher RH Jr: Synovial fluid analysis and synovial biopsy. In Kelley WN, Harris ED, Ruddy S, et al [eds]: Textbook of Rheumatology, 3rd ed. Philadelphia, WB Saunder, 1989, p 644.)

neous attempts, the procedure should be stopped immediately. If facilities permit, open biopsy should then proceed; otherwise, the procedure should be rescheduled. After the biopsy procedure, patient care should be the same as for any other similarly invasive procedure.

References

1. Carr WP: Acute-phase proteins. Clin Rheum Dis 9:227–239, 1983.
2. Baum J and Ziff M: Laboratory findings in rheumatoid arthritis. *In* McCarty DJ (eds): Arthritis and Allied Conditions, 10th ed. Philadelphia, Lea & Febiger, 1985, pp 643–659.
3. D'Angelo WA: Diagnostic procedures and tests. *In* Halsted JA (ed): The Laboratory in Clinical Medicine: Interpretation and Application, 2nd ed. Philadelphia, WB Saunders, 1981, pp 510–512.
4. Kelley WN, Harris ED, Ruddy S, et al: Textbook of Rheumatology, Vol 1, 2nd ed. Philadelphia, WB Saunders, 1985.
5. Ravel R: Cardiac, pulmonary, and miscellaneous diagnostic procedures. *In* Clinical Laboratory Medicine, 5th ed. Chicago, Year Book Medical Publishers, 1989, pp 330–331.
6. Ravel R: Appendix: A compendium of useful data and information. *In* Clinical Laboratory Medicine, 5th ed. Chicago, Year Book Medical Publishers, 1989, p 706.
7. Hockett RD and Green ED: Barnes Hospital Laboratory Reference Values. *In* Woodley M and Whelan A (eds): The Washington Manual: Manual of Medical Therapeutics, 27th ed. Boston, Little, Brown, pp 517–523.
8. Claus DR, Osmand AP, and Gewurz H: Radioimmunoassay of human C-reactive protein and levels in normal sera. J Lab Clin Med 87:120–128, 1976.
9. Kushner I: C-reactive protein in rheumatology. Arthritis Rheum 34(8): 1065–1068, 1991.

10. Gitlin JD, Gitlin JI, and Gitlin D: Localization of C-reactive protein in synovium of patients with rheumatoid arthritis. Arthritis Rheum 20 (8): 1491–1499, 1977.
11. Kaschak J and Edworthy S: Laboratory testing in arthritic disease. Clin Podiatr Med Surg 5(1):17–23, 1988.
12. Egeland T and Munthe E: Rheumatoid factors. Clin Rheum Dis. 9(1): 135–160, 1983.
13. Hoffman WL, Jump AA, and Smiley JD: Synthesis of specific IgG idiotypes by rheumatoid synovium. Arthritis Rheum 33(8): 1196–1204, 1990.
14. Wolfe F, Cathey MA, and Roberts FK: The latex test revisited. Arthritis Rheum 34(8): 951–960, 1991.
15. Noritake DT, Colburn KK, Chan G, et al: Rheumatoid factors specific for active arthritis. Ann Rheum Dis 49:910–915, 1990.
16. Aho K, Palosuo T, Raunio V, et al: When does rheumatoid disease start? Arthritis Rheum 28(5):485–489, 1985.
17. Ochi T, Yonemasu K, Iwase R, et al: Serum Clq levels as a prognostic guide to articular erosions in patients with rheumatoid arthritis. Arthritis Rheum 27:883–887, 1984.
18. Ochi T, Iwase R, Yonemasu K, et al: Natural course of joint destruction and fluctuation of serum Clq levels in patients with rheumatoid arthritis. Arthritis Rheum 31:37–43, 1988.
19. Olsen NJ, Ho E, and Barats L: Clinical correlations with serum Clq levels in patients with rheumatoid arthritis. Arthritis Rheum 34(2): 187–191, 1991.
20. George D and Glass D: Quantitation of complement proteins in rheumatic disease. Clin Rheum Dis 9(1):177–198, 1983.
21. Akizuki M, Schacter BZ, Hochberg MG, et al: Comparative study of immunologic methods for demonstration of antibodies to soluble nuclear antigens. Arthritis Rheum 20:693–701, 1977.
22. Nakamura RM and Tan EM: Recent advances in laboratory tests and the significance of autoantibodies to nuclear antigens in systemic rheumatic diseases. Clin Lab Med 6(1):41–53, 1986.
23. Emlen W, Pisetsky DS, and Taylor RP: Antibodies to DNA, a perspective. Arthritis Rheum 29(12):1417–1426, 1986.
24. Schumacher HR, Klippel JH, and Robinson DR (eds): Systemic lupus erythematosus. *In* Primer on the Rheumatic Diseases, 9th ed. Atlanta, Arthritis Foundation, 1988, pp 96–100.
25. Nakamura RM and Tan EM: Update of autoantibodies to intracellular antigens in systemic rheumatic diseases. Clin Lab Med 12(1): 1–23, 1992.
26. Vivino FB and Maul GG: Histologic and electron microscopic characterization of the antiperinuclear factor antigen. Arthritis Rheum 33(7):960–969, 1990.
27. Lassoued S, Oksman F, Fournie B, et al: Antibodies to lamins in rheumatoid arthritis. Arthritis Rheum 33(6): 877–879, 1990.
28. Hassfeld W, Steiner G, Hartmuth K, et al: Demonstration of a new antinuclear antibody (anti-RA33) that is highly specific for rheumatoid arthritis. Arthritis Rheum 32(12): 1515–1520, 1989.
29. Petersdorf EW and Deeg HJ: Diagnostic use of molecular probes before and after marrow transplantation. Clin Lab Med 12(1): 113–128, 1992.
30. Dewar PJ: HLA antigens. Clin Rheum Dis 9(1): 93–116, 1983.
31. Ravel R: Immunohematology: Antibody detection, blood group antigens, and pretransfusion tests. *In* Clinical Laboratory Medicine, 5th ed. Chicago, Year Book Medical Publishers, 1989, pp 126–128.
32. Schumacher HR, Klippel JH, and Robinson DR (eds): mmunogenetics. *In* Primer on the Rheumatic Diseases, 9th ed. Atlanta, Arthritis Foundation, 1988, pp 44–48.
33. McMichael AJ, Sasazuki T, McDivitt HO, et al: Increased frequency of HLA-Cw3 and HLA-Dw4 in rheumatoid arthritis. Arthritis Rheum 20(5): 1037–1042, 1977.
34. Khan A, Kushner I, and Braun WE: Comparison of clinical features in HLA-B27 positive and negative patients with ankylosing spondylitis. Arthritis Rheum 20(4): 909–912, 1977.
35. Stastny P: Association of the B-cell alloantigen DRw4 with rheumatoid arthritis. N Engl J Med 298:869–871, 1978.
36. Gao X, Olsen NJ, Pincus T, et al: HLA-DR alleles with naturally occurring amino acid substitutions and risk for development of rheumatoid arthritis. Arthritis Rheum 33(7): 939–946, 1990.
37. Barger BO, Acton RT, Koopman WJ, et al: DR antigens and gold toxicity in white rheumatoid arthritis patients. Arthritis Rheum 27(6): 601–605, 1984.
38. Marshall K, Chiu B, and Inman RD: Substance P and arthritis: Analysis of plasma synovial fluid levels. Arthritis Rheum 33(1): 87–90, 1990.
39. Goldberg RL, Huff JP, Lenz ME, et al: Elevated plasma levels of hyaluronate in patients with osteoarthritis and rheumatoid arthritis. Arthritis Rheum 34(7):799–807, 1991.
40. Paimela L, Heiskanen A, Kurki P, et al: Serum hyaluronate level as a predictor of radiologic progression in early rheumatoid arthritis. Arthritis Rheum 34(7): 815–821, 1991.
41. Woessner JF Jr: Serum hyaluronan: A status report from the joint [Editorial]. Arthritis Rheum 34(7): 927–930, 1991.
42. Cush JJ, Jasin HE, Johnson R, et al: Relationship between clinical efficacy and laboratory correlates of inflammatory and immunogenic activity in rheumatoid arthritis patients treated with nonsteroidal antiinflammatory drugs. Arthritis Rheum 33(5): 623–633, 1990.
43. Dahl SL, Coleman ML, Williams HJ, et al: Lack of correlation between blood gold concentrations and clinical response in patients with definite or classic rheumatoid arthritis receiving auranofin or gold sodium thiomalate. Arthritis Rheum 28(11):1211–1218, 1985.
44. Kerolus G, Clayburne G, and Schumacher HR Jr: Is it mandatory to examine synovial fluids promptly after arthrocentesis? Arthritis Rheum 32(3):271–278.
45. Schumacher HR, Klippel JH, and Robinson DR: Arthrocentesis and synovial fluid analysis. *In* Primer on the Rheumatic Diseases, 9th ed. Atlanta, Arthritis Foundation, 1988, pp 55–60.
46. Platt PN: Examination of synovial fluid. Clin Rheum Dis 9(1): 51–67, 1983.
47. Calin A: Diagnosis and Management of Rheumatoid Arthritis. Menlo Park, CA, Addison-Wesley, 1983, p 124.
48. Schumacher HR. Biopsy. *In* Kelley WN, Harris ED, Ruddy S, et al (eds): Textbook of Rheumatology, Vol. 1, 2nd ed. Philadelphia, WB Saunders, 1985, pp 256–269.

CHAPTER 15

Athletic Injuries

Richard T. Bouché, D.P.M.,
Katrina Sullivan, D.P.M., and Douglas J. Ichikawa, D.P.M.

The role of the sports podiatrist is to provide comprehensive care for foot, ankle, and foot-related suprastructural problems of the lower extremity. Comprehensive care includes evaluation, diagnosis, education, treatment, rehabilitation, and prevention of lower extremity disease. In addition, the podiatrist serves as a resource person on general issues related to sports medicine. Background knowledge in the following areas is recommended: first aid, emergency care, general conditioning, exercise physiology, taping, rehabilitation principles, physical therapy modalities, nutrition, sports psychology, footwear evaluation/modification, orthotics and bracing, videotape/motion analysis, and foot and ankle surgery. Knowledge of sports is helpful, especially those that have a high incidence of lower extremity injury. Appreciation for sports is best accomplished by becoming an active participant.

The purpose of this chapter is to acquaint the reader with common and interesting sports medicine problems that would likely be encountered in a general podiatric medical practice.

FRICTION BLISTER

Anyone who has provided medical care at a marathon or road race can attest to the fact that the friction blister is the most common running malady. This relatively minor injury warrants appropriate care to avoid potential complications that could adversely affect athletic performance.

A blister is a circumscribed elevation of skin containing clear or bloody fluid between the layers of epidermis. The elevated portion of skin comprises the roof, and the remaining skin layers comprise the base. Although any area of the foot can be involved, the most prevalent areas are the posterior heel, plantar forefoot, and digits.

Blisters incurred by athletes are mechanically induced. Three factors are involved in their formation: friction, moisture, and heat. Friction is common at the shoe-foot interface because the superficial skin of the foot is relatively thicker and susceptible to rapidly applied shearing forces.[1] Extremes of dryness and wetness decrease friction, whereas intermediate degrees of moisture (e.g., in an athletic shoe) tend to increase friction.[2] Skin that is hot will form blisters more quickly than skin that is cold.[3] Predisposing factors for blister formation may include poor-fitting shoes, hyperhidrosis, structural deformities (bunions, hammertoes, posterior heel

prominence, and so on), and functional disorders (such as hyperpronators and muscle imbalances).

Treatment of blisters depends on the extent of involvement and whether the blister is painful. If a blister is asymptomatic, treatment is not indicated. Blisters larger than 1 in. in diameter may warrant treatment to avoid potential infection. "Hot spots" require application of a protective barrier (i.e., moleskin, mole foam, adhesive tape, Spenco second skin [Spenco Medical Corporation, Waco, TX]) to prevent blister formation. Second skin is an inert, transparent gel sheeting consisting of 96% water and 4% polyethylene oxide. Benzoin tincture compound spray or solution is a good skin preparation and provides a sticky surface on which a protective barrier can be applied. Second skin must be secured in place with adhesive tape, paper tape, or Spenco adhesive knit. Once a painful blister has formed and the roof is intact, the treatment of choice is to drain fluid and apply a sterile protective dressing. The area is cleansed with an antimicrobial skin cleanser (povidone-iodine solution or Hibiclens). Skin refrigerant sprays can be used for topical anesthesia. The blister is punctured at multiple sites around its border with a sterile needle or surgical blade, thus allowing adequate drainage. The blister roof is left intact, acting as a protective covering over the exposed base.[3] Antibiotic cream or povidone-iodine solution can then be applied to the blister. After preparing the surrounding skin with benzoin tincture compound, protective dressings or an accommodative moleskin patch can be applied. The area is then covered with tape or adhesive knit, both of which work well on the digits. It is important not to apply tape or moleskin directly to the blister roof to avoid deroofing.

Blister prevention includes the following points: (1) ensure that the athletic shoe fits appropriately (it should match the patient's sport and biomechanical needs), (2) allow an adequate break-in period for new shoes and be aware of hot spot formation, (3) socks can be helpful in preventing blister formation, especially those constructed with acrylic fibers,[4] (tube socks should be avoided because of increased potential for blister formation, especially in the digital area), (4) Spenco and PPT (Langer Biomechanics Group, Inc., Deer Park, NY) insoles are excellent for preventing plantar blister formation; (5) hyperhidrosis is addressed with astringent foot soaks (Domeboro solution, Epsom salts, tea, and so on), absorbent powders, drying agents (antiperspirant sprays,

Drysol), and alternating shoes, (6) structural and biomechanical abnormalities should be recognized and treated, and (7) recurrent blister formation should be suspect for a mechanobullous disease (e.g., epidermolysis bullosa simplex).[5]

NEUROMA

Several nerve-related injuries of the lower extremity are seen in athletic individuals. The most common is interdigital nerve entrapment syndrome known as Morton's neuroma. This is an inflammatory condition of the plantar intermetatarsal nerve, resulting in perineural fibrosis. The third interspace is most commonly affected, followed by a combination of the second and third interspaces and rarely an isolated second interspace.

The medial and lateral plantar nerves send off common plantar digital nerves, which course distally, plantar to the deep intermetatarsal ligament, and divide at the web space to form the proper digital nerves[6, 7] (Fig. 15–1). It is the communication branches that typically make the third interspace unique and contribute to the prevalence of this site.

Interdigital nerve entrapment is probably due to repetitive microtrauma of the common digital nerve. Abnormal pronation and a hypermobile first ray are seen as contributing factors in the development of this condition. Pathologic findings include perineural fibrosis and fibrinoid degeneration, which are consistent with compressive neuropathy. Athletes with this condition complain of cramping, burning, tingling, and sharp pain radiating into the involved digits. Pain is exacerbated by weightbearing or with the use of constricting shoe gear, (e.g., cycling cleats or alpine ski boots). Physical findings include interspace pain on palpation (with or without distal paresthesia), positive Mulder's click sign of involved interspace (with reproduction of symptoms), and Sullivan's sign (splaying of involved toes). Swelling is not apparent.

Differential diagnosis of interdigital nerve entrapment includes capsulitis, bursitis, flexor or extensor tendinitis, plantar plate injury, plantar forefoot neuritis, osteochondral lesion, stress fracture, lateral plantar nerve entrapment, tarsal tunnel syndrome, and growth plate injury in adolescents.

Radiographic examination of the patient with Morton's neuroma is unremarkable. Diagnostic ultrasonography and magnetic resonance imaging (MRI) have been used but are nonspecific. To confirm Morton's neuroma, a diagnostic injection of 2 ml of 1% lidocaine into the interspace will temporarily relieve pain. Although this may not necessarily be diagnostic, it does serve to separate articular from extra-articular diseases.

Treatment addresses contributing causes and symptoms, including change in shoe gear (i.e., lower heel height and additional forefoot width) and shoe modifications (i.e., change padding in ski boots or removal of a soccer cleat). Abnormal pronation and hypermobility of the first ray need to be addressed biomechanically. The use of metatarsal pads proximal to the level of the metatarsal heads will relieve the pressure at the involved interspace. A series of two to four local anesthetic/steroid injections can be effective in alleviating symptoms. Excellent results have been achieved with a combination of 1 ml of betamethasone phosphate-acetate mixture (6 mg/ml) and 1 to 2 ml of 1% lidocaine infiltrated into the interspace given at 4-week intervals.[8] Additional treatments can include sclerosing injections.[7] If these conservative measures fail, the athlete can choose to live with the condition or have the neuroma excised. Excision is usually performed through a dorsal approach. We recommend keeping the patient non-weightbearing for 2 weeks postoperatively to prevent excessive scar formation and the subjective feeling of a lump.

PLANTAR FOREFOOT NEURITIS

Forefoot neuritis has been seen with increasing frequency in two groups of active people: long-distance cyclists and stair climbers. These athletes present with pain or numbness of the plantar forefoot.

Medial and lateral plantar nerves send off common plantar digital nerves, which course distally and plantar to the deep intermetatarsal ligament and, at that level, are vulnerable to abnormal pressure.

Cause is related to mechanical shear and compressive forces on the forefoot, but it is unclear as to which one plays a larger role. Faulty biomechanics coupled with activities that concentrate pressure on the forefoot play a role in this symptom complex.

Patients complain of burning pain and may experience numbness of the entire plantar forefoot. This is at times difficult to distinguish from tarsal tunnel syndrome. Symptoms worsen as activity is continued. Physical examination reveals no neurologic deficits and often an inability to reproduce the symptoms.

This is a diagnosis of exclusion after all other causes of forefoot pain have been considered. Differential diagnosis should include interdigital nerve entrapment, flexor tendinitis, capsulitis, bursitis, metatarsal stress fracture, distal plantar fasciitis, tarsal tunnel syndrome, chronic compartment syndrome of the leg (deep posterior), radiculopathy, and peripheral neuropathy of systemic cause.

Treatment consists of providing support for biomechanical imbalances of the foot and padding to reduce compressive and shear forces. Treatment for plantar forefoot neuritis

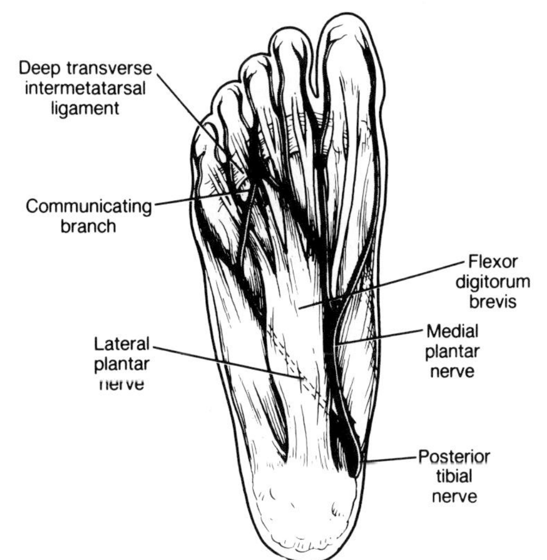

FIGURE 15–1. Anatomy of the plantar aspect of foot showing the classic location of Morton's neuroma. (From Miller SJ: Morton's neuroma: A syndrome. *In* McGlamry ED [ed]: Comprehensive Textbook of Foot Surgery. Baltimore, Williams & Wilkins, 1987, p 45. © 1987, the Williams & Wilkins Co., Baltimore.)

should also include activity modification. Spenco insoles are excellent and can be used alone or can be incorporated into an orthotic. Correct shoe gear for the intended sport is another important consideration. Several running, cross-training, and aerobic shoes are available that offer superior forefoot cushioning, which is helpful for stair climbers. Women with wide feet may need to switch to a men's model for proper fit. Cyclists' shoes and shoe-pedal interface require evaluation. Repositioning the foot forward on the pedal will usually relieve symptoms. Riding style and previous injuries are considered before changing shoe position. A change in shoe style that allows more room in the forefoot or the addition of forefoot padding may also help.

METATARSALGIA

Metatarsalgia is a general term referring to pain localized to the lesser metatarsophalangeal (MTP) joints and represents inflammation of the joint structures (i.e., synovitis, capsulitis, or periarticular structures).

The cause of metatarsal pain is complex. A simplified approach consists of two categories: primary and secondary metatarsalgia. Primary metatarsalgia includes structural, functional, traumatic, and iatrogenic causes of pain.[9, 10] Structural causes are foot imbalances (such as discrepancy in metatarsal length/declination and fat pad atrophy). Functional causes are due to muscle imbalance, leading to conditions such as claw and hammertoe formation and equinus deformity. Acute trauma can cause direct damage to the capsular structures, leading to pain and disability. Overuse injury to the lesser MTP joints may be independent of structural or functional problems and may be due to excessive use, poor equipment, or improper surfaces. There are numerous examples of iatrogenic causes of pain at the MTP joint level (e.g., second MTP joint transfer pain after Keller bunionectomy).

Secondary metatarsalgia refers to pain at the MTP joint level secondary to a systemic disturbance. This includes rheumatoid arthritis, gout, seronegative arthritis, and neuromuscular disorders.[9]

The history typically reveals pain of insidious onset with gradual progression, exacerbated by weightbearing activity and relieved by rest. Shoes and soft surfaces are better than bare feet. Physical examination of the forefoot includes determination of vascular and neurologic status. Musculoskeletal examination includes joint compression and distraction, passive and active joint range of motion (ROM), active resistance to flexors and extensors, and palpation of surrounding soft tissue structures. There is pain and swelling of the capsular structures. Clinical classification is based on physical findings and activity limitations. Grade I has mild pain without effusion and no limitation of activity. Grade II has moderate pain, minimal effusion, and some limitation of activity. Grade III has moderate to severe pain, joint effusion, and restriction of weightbearing. Grade IV is subluxation and dislocation of the MTP joint.

Differential diagnosis includes avascular necrosis of a metatarsal head (Freiberg's disease), subluxation and dislocation MTP joint, metatarsal stress fracture, interdigital nerve entrapment (Morton's neuroma), plantar forefoot neuritis, plantar bursitis, distal plantar fasciitis, growth plate injury in children, tarsal tunnel syndrome, vascular abnormalities, inflammatory joint disease, peripheral neuropathy, and osteoarthritis.

Diagnostic tests include radiographs to rule out bone disease followed by bone scans in equivocal cases when clinically indicated. Diagnostic injections of 1% lidocaine may be of value in differentiating confusing presentations. MRI and computed tomography (CT) are used in patients whose cases defy definitive diagnosis.

Treatment of metatarsalgia is based on severity of symptoms. Grade I responds well to accommodative orthotics, shoe gear changes, nonsteroidal anti-inflammatory drugs (NSAIDs), application of ice with activity, ROM exercises, and curtailment of offending activities.[11] Grade II metatarsalgia requires specific relief padding with the use of walking cast or brace or postoperative shoe, NSAIDs, ice, and cessation of painful activity for the acute phase. Two to three intra-articular steroid injections (i.e., ½ ml dexamethasone phosphate) may be given at 4-week intervals. Repeated injections should be avoided. Joint mobilization and strengthening are begun after the acute pain and inflammation are controlled. Return to full activity is permitted only when the patient is pain free and may require shoe gear accommodations. Grade III metatarsalgia may require several weeks of non-weightbearing for initial control of symptoms. The remainder of the treatment course follows that for grade II. Grade IV, symptomatic subluxation and dislocation, requires open anatomic reduction. Steroid injections are not recommended because of compromised joint capsule. The immobilization and progressive therapy are similar to that for grade III injury.

Preventive measures include the use of appropriate shoes for activity, padded or accommodative insoles and orthotics, and appropriate surfaces for activity (i.e., suspended wood floor versus concrete for aerobic dance). An external rocker-bottom sole applied to existing shoe gear has proved helpful for some athletes.

SESAMOIDITIS

Sesamoiditis is an inflammatory condition involving the hallucal sesamoid bones, resulting in pain and disability. The tibial sesamoid bone is involved more often than the fibular bone; however, in rare instances, both can be symptomatic. The condition can be acute or chronic.

The sesamoid bones of the first MTP joint are located within the flexor hallucis brevis tendon just proximal to the joint level and articulate with the metatarsal head, separated by a crista on the plantar aspect of the metatarsal. The tibial sesamoid receives attachments from the medial head of the flexor brevis and abductor hallucis as well as the medial joint capsule. The fibular sesamoid receives attachments from the lateral head of the flexor brevis and the oblique and transverse heads of the adductor hallucis under the intermetatarsal ligament. An intersesamoid ligament connects the two bones. There is a constant bursa on the plantar aspect of the sesamoid on the tibial side. An interphalangeal sesamoid is present in approximately 13% of the population. Sesamoids ossify from multiple ossification centers, which may or may not coalesce, giving rise to bipartite or multipartite sesamoids. The reported incidence of bipartite sesamoids varies from 10% to 33% of the population; the tibial side is affected more frequently.[12, 13]

Sesamoiditis is due to repetitive microtrauma to the first ray. It presents as acute at 2 weeks of symptom duration, as subacute 2 to 6 weeks of symptom duration, and as chronic after 6 weeks of symptom duration. Rigid plantarflexed first ray and pes cavus feet are cited as contributing factors to the development of sesamoiditis; the theory is that plantarflexion and eversion of the first metatarsal head place the tibial sesamoid in a more vulnerable position. This may account for the increased incidence of tibial sesamoid injuries compared with the fibular side.[14] The theoretical role of the sesamoids is to (1) protect the interposed flexor hallucis longus tendon, (2) act as a fulcrum for the flexor hallucis brevis tendon to increase its mechanical advantage, and (3) protect the first metatarsal head from trauma. Activities that place weight on the forefoot (e.g., ballet, aerobic dance, running, and stair climbing) are often aggravating factors.

History reveals gradual, insidious onset of pain localized to the sesamoid apparatus aggravated by forefoot activity and relieved with cushioning and shoes. Physical examination reveals guarded ROM with no pain on joint compression and distraction. Pain is present with passive dorsiflexion, especially at end range, with resistance to active contraction of flexor hallucis brevis, palpation of sesamoid and flexor hallucis brevis tendon, and tiptoe position. Gait is apropulsive and antalgic, with the first ray held in an inverted position to compensate for the painful area.

Differential diagnosis of sesamoiditis includes avascular necrosis, osteoarthritis, stress fracture, fracture, osteomyelitis, gouty arthritis, traumatic neuritis of the medial plantar digital nerve, flexor longus or brevis tendinitis, bursitis, and osteochondral lesion.[15]

Diagnostic tests include radiographs to rule out other bone and joint disease. Bone scans are usually negative. Diagnostic injections are useful to localize the problem.

Classification of sesamoid pain and disability aids the practitioner in developing a rational treatment plan. Grade I sesamoiditis has minimal pain to palpation, with activity, or swelling. Pain is easily relieved by a change in shoe gear or accommodative padding. NSAIDs and ice after activity are used, and few restrictions of activity are needed. Grade II sesamoiditis has moderate pain to palpation and passive ROM, weightbearing, and mild to moderate swelling of the MTP joint. Pain is relieved by restricting weightbearing activities and using an orthotic with accommodation. NSAIDs, physical therapy, and activity modification are needed to relieve symptoms. Time loss from activity ranges from 2 to 6 weeks. Grade III sesamoiditis has exquisite tenderness to palpation and guarded first MTP joint ROM, preventing weightbearing. There is moderate to severe swelling. Pain is relieved by non-weightbearing immobilization, intra-articular steroid injection, and NSAIDs. Patients progress to weightbearing in a walking brace with accommodation and physical therapy to accommodated orthotics. Time loss from activity often exceeds 6 weeks. Return to activity is permitted when all symptoms have subsided and injured structures are adequately protected. Failure to achieve symptom-free activity or the presence of sesamoid degenerative changes may necessitate surgical intervention.[16]

Prevention involves the use of properly fitted shoes and adequate insole padding for the intended activity. Surface selection and activity modification can also prevent recurrence of this condition.

FIRST METATARSOPHALANGEAL JOINT SPRAIN

First MTP joint injuries have become a common problem since the advent of artificial playing surfaces requiring flexible shoe gear. Most of these cases are hyperextension injuries, known as *turf toe*; however, there are also hyperflexion, abduction, and adduction injuries.[17]

The most common mechanism of injury is hyperextension of the MTP joint with the toes fixed on the playing surface and the heel raised. The leg is forced forward, causing hyperextension of the joint (Fig. 15–2). Injuries range from capsular tears, volar plate disruption, and sesamoid fracture to dislocation with the metatarsal head button-holing through the plantar joint capsule. Dorsal impingement or avulsion fracture may also occur. Hyperflexion and adduction injuries are more common in martial arts, whereas abduction injuries are commonly seen in soccer. Long-term sequelae of turf toe include calcification of the ligaments, metatarsalgia, bunion formation, and hallux limitus.

Patient history reveals an acute traumatic event. It is important to obtain information regarding mechanism of injury, presence of an audible pop or snap, type of shoe gear, playing surface at time of injury, and ability to continue participation. Physical examination reveals presence of hyperemia, effusion, exquisite tenderness to palpation of the first MTP joint, significant guarding to passive ROM, especially end-range dorsiflexion, and resistance to active ROM. Gait is antalgic and apropulsive.

We use a classification previously described for turf toe based on the extent of injury.[18] Grade I is a mild sprain of

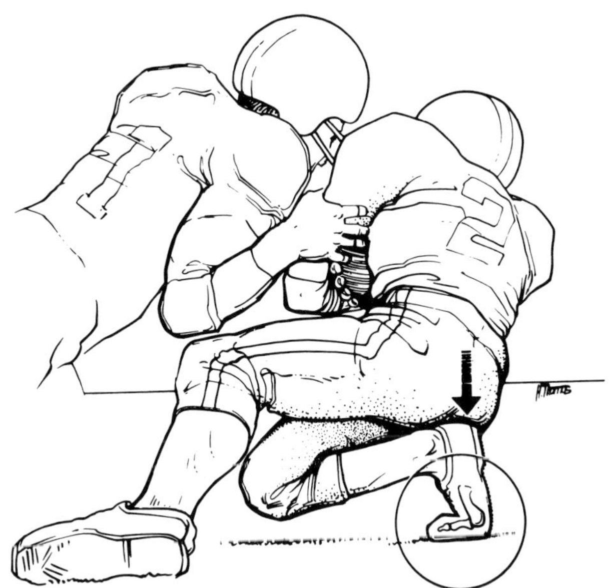

FIGURE 15–2. The most common mechanism of injury of first metatarsophalangeal joint sprain is hyperextension of the joint. (From Rodeo SA, O'Brien S, Warren RA, et al: Turf-toe: An analysis of metatarsophalangeal joint sprains in professional football players. Am J Sports Med 18:284, 1990.)

the joint capsule caused by stretching of the capsuloligamentous complex with localized tenderness, minimal swelling, and no ecchymosis. Grade II involves partial rupture of capsuloligamentous structures with diffuse tenderness, mild to moderate swelling and ecchymosis, and pain restricting motion. There is no articular injury. Time loss from activity ranges from 2 to 6 weeks. Grade III injury involves partial rupture of the capsule and ligaments with articular injury (i.e., avulsion fracture or cystic changes in subchondral bone). Severe tenderness is demonstrated, along with considerable swelling, ecchymosis, and marked restriction of joint motion. Time loss from activity ranges from 6 to 12 weeks. Grade IV is subluxation or dislocation with the metatarsal head button-holing through the plantar capsule. There is possible interposition of the plantar plate into the joint and a high likelihood of articular injury. Time loss from activity often is in excess of 12 weeks.

Differential diagnosis includes collateral ligament sprain, dorsal joint compression with chondral lesion, plantar plate avulsion, sesamoid fracture, avulsion fracture of the proximal phalanx base, metatarsal fracture, and dislocation of MTP joint.

Diagnostic testing involves radiographs to rule out bone and joint changes and possibly an arthrogram to assess joint capsule integrity.

Treatment can be broken down into three main components: (1) acute phase to control inflammation, (2) rehabilitation phase to restore ROM and increase strength, and (3) return to function, which includes appropriate shoe gear modifications and protection. The inflammatory phase is controlled with rest, ice compression, elevation, and administration of NSAIDs. A walking brace or non-weightbearing in a posterior splint with a toe extension is used, depending on the severity of the injury. Although the joint is still protected from unwanted motion, physical therapy gradually introduces ROM and progresses to strengthening exercises as tolerated.

Grades II to IV injuries may require 6 or more weeks of immobilization. Gradual return to activity can be facilitated by turf toe strappings and shoe gear modifications (i.e., stiff material placed in the forefoot to restrict motion at the MTP joint level).[18] Return to full activity is permitted when the athlete is pain free.

JONES FRACTURE

Jones fracture is a proximal diaphyseal fracture of the fifth metatarsal. It deserves special attention because of its high incidence of painful delayed union and nonunion. It should be distinguished from styloid avulsion fractures of the fifth metatarsal base (Fig. 15–3). The Jones fracture is proximal in the metatarsal diaphysis approximately 2 cm from the tuberosity. The mechanism of injury is either overuse or indirect trauma. The fracture results from a combination of ground-reactive forces (axial loading of the forefoot and overload of the fifth ray)[19] and tension force from the pull of the short peroneal muscle.

Jones fractures are classified as stress fracture, acute fracture, subacute fracture, delayed union, and nonunion.[20, 21] A high index of suspicion is needed for stress fractures, which may not be evident on plain film. A bone scan will elucidate the diagnosis. Acute fractures present radiographically as an obvious fracture line extending from the plantar cortex. Subacute fractures present with a 1- to 2-week prodrome of discomfort in this region. Periosteal reaction and a widened lucent fracture line are seen on radiograph.

Presenting symptoms include pain, swelling, and difficulty running. There is a variable amount of edema and tenderness on palpation of the proximal fifth metatarsal and pain with resisted plantarflexion-eversion of the foot. Symptoms are reproduced with repeated forefoot loading.

Treatment of this fracture should be aggressive from the onset to avoid complication. Non-weightbearing, below-knee

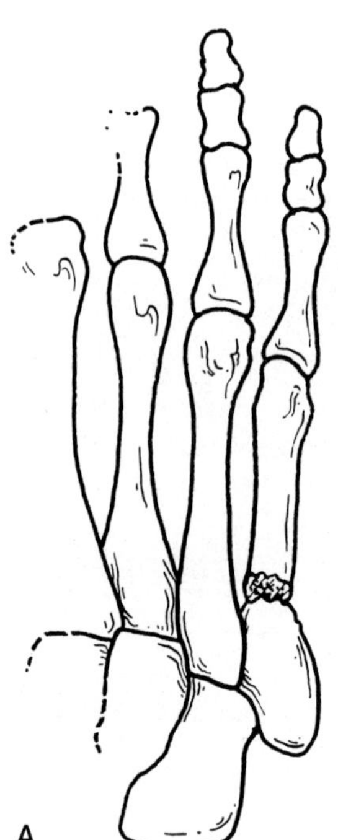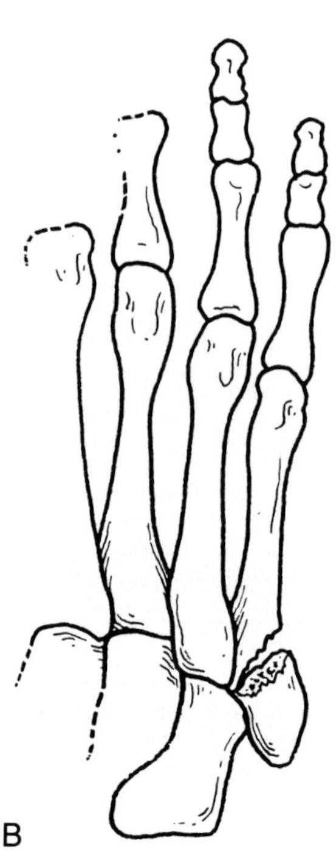

A   B

FIGURE 15–3. Jones fracture (*A*) compared with an oblique fracture of the styloid process (*B*). (Adapted from McGlamry ED [ed]: Comprehensive Textbook of Foot Surgery, Vol 2. Baltimore, Williams & Wilkins, 1987. © 1987, the Williams & Wilkins Co., Baltimore.)

cast immobilization is used in all cases except nonunions.[21] Delayed unions and nonunions may require electrical bone stimulation.[22] The average time to heal is 8 weeks but may extend much longer. After clinical tenderness has subsided, and there is evidence of bony union, casting may be discontinued. At this time, custom-molded orthoses and supportive footwear are recommended.[23] Return to full activities should be reserved until radiographic union is evident. Nonunions, some delayed unions, and displaced acute fractures may require surgery. This involves an axially placed screw or pin guided distally through the styloid process.[24] Visualization is best aided by the use of the newer generation minifluoroscopy units. The fracture site should first be drilled and curetted through all sclerotic bone. Acute displaced fractures are treated with fixation alone. Delayed unions may need a small amount of cancellous bone grafting. For nonunions, an onlay corticocancellous graft is placed in a trough created across the fracture site.[21] Non-weightbearing casting postoperatively for 2 to 3 months is generally required.

The Jones fracture is a serious injury to the competitive and casual athlete alike. Prompt recognition and aggressive non-weightbearing casting are necessary to prevent complications.

OS NAVICULARIS SYNDROME

Os navicularis syndrome is a symptom complex involving the accessory navicular (or prominent ''cornuated'' navicular). Synonyms for this accessory bone are the os tibiale externum or prehallux. The os naviculare arises as a secondary center of ossification posterior and medial to the body of the navicular in 14% of the population, and it becomes radiographically apparent by age 9 to 11 years.[25]

Symptoms arise for two reasons: (1) The medial aspect of the navicular will be prominent and susceptible to shoe irritation (especially in the flexible flatfoot) and (2) application of a tension force may disrupt the attachment of the os naviculare to the navicular body. Secondary soft tissue inflammation (e.g., posterior tibial tendinitis) is also commonly encountered.

There are three types of accessory navicular.[26] Type I is an ossicle enveloped in the substance of the posterior tibial tendon, type II is a synchondrosis of the accessory bone, and type III is a cornuated or prominent navicular tuberosity.

The patient presents with complaints of activity-induced pain and swelling around the navicular, both in and out of shoes. This syndrome is often seen after an inversion ankle sprain. Palpation in this area is painful, as is resistance to active plantarflexion and inversion of the foot.

Differential diagnosis includes tarsal coalition, plantar fasciitis, stress fracture of the navicular, posterior tibial tendinitis, osseous tumor, osteochondritis of the lesser tarsus, talonavicular joint arthritis, and sprains of the midfoot.

Anteroposterior and lateral oblique radiographs are usually sufficient to identify the accessory bone. Triphasic bone scan may be helpful. For better elucidation of the attachment site, CT and MRI may be used (Fig. 15–4).

Conservative treatment should include NSAIDs, strapping, orthotics, and shoe gear modification to prevent irritation in this area. Cast immobilization may be needed.

Surgical treatment involves excision of the accessory ossicle through a medial incision. It is not necessary to reroute the PT tendon plantarly as described by Kidner.[27–29] The athletic individual may be adequately served by removing the enlarged navicular or accessory ossicle that is making the athletic shoe gear uncomfortable. Occasionally, removal of a large ossicle or disruption of the tendon during excision will require advancement. Postoperatively, the patient is placed in a short-leg non-weightbearing cast for 1 to 2 weeks. Additional immobilization up to 1 to 6 weeks may be required, depending on the amount of tendon disruption.

MIDFOOT SPRAIN

Midfoot sprains are defined as injuries to ligamentous and capsular structures of the midfoot joints including midtarsal (Chopart's), intertarsal, and tarsometatarsal (Lisfranc's) joints. These injuries are not uncommon but are often neglected, being considered a minor injury not requiring specific treatment. Our experience with this injury suggests that care be taken in evaluation and treatment to avoid morbidity (joint instability, degenerative arthritis, and so on), which can affect athletic performance. A review of the literature reveals a paucity of articles concerning midfoot sprains.[30–32] Most articles pertain to overt trauma involving fractures and dislocations of midtarsal and tarsometatarsal joints.

Midfoot sprains are usually caused by indirect trauma; many mechanisms of injury are possible. The most common mechanism involves axial loading of the forefoot with midfoot hyperplantarflexion (demi-pointe position). Sudden medial and lateral loading of the forefoot in this position may also cause injury. Additional mechanisms of injury involve hyperplantarflexion of the entire foot in a loaded (pointe position in ballet) and unloaded (kicking a soccer ball with the dorsum of the foot) situation. A hyperplantarflexion injury may also occur when the forefoot is fixed (foot straps on a windsurfer or toe clips on a cyclist) and the leg is forced backward. Inversion and eversion ankle sprains are also described by patients with midfoot injury.

As with other sprains of the body, midfoot sprains can be classified into three grades depending on severity. Grade 1 involves a stretching injury with few ligamentous fibers disrupted. Grade 2 indicates partial disruption. Grade 3 denotes

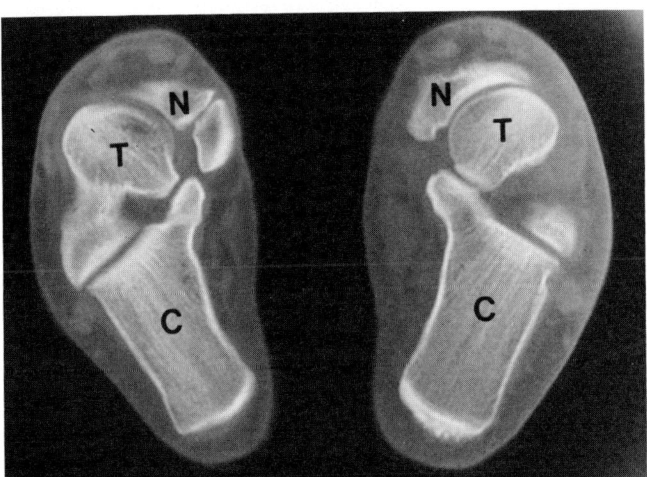

FIGURE 15–4. Bilateral computed tomography scan views in the long axial (transverse) plane. Right foot exhibits os navicularis in relation to navicular (N), talus (T), and calcaneus (C).

complete ligamentous rupture. Associated injuries (e.g., joint subluxation or avulsion fracture) are denoted with an asterisk after the injury grade.

Clinically, patients with midfoot sprains present with localized pain, erythema, and swelling. Ecchymosis is evident usually in grade 2 or grade 3 sprains. Manual forefoot loading with or without frontal plane stress is painful, and patients will usually exhibit an antalgic, apropulsive gait. Joint instability (e.g., first-ray hypermobility) may be present and should be evaluated in comparison to the contralateral side. A change in the shape of the foot (increased flattening or abduction of the forefoot) may also occur, depending on the nature of the injury.

Differential diagnosis should include overt fracture/dislocation, avulsion fracture, stress fracture, chondral/osteochondral fracture, joint subluxation, first- or second-ray diastasis, tendon attenuation/rupture, and so on.

Diagnostic testing includes weightbearing radiographs and stress views of the midfoot (adduction, abduction, and plantarflexion) to assess joint stability (Fig. 15–5). To assess occult subluxations and fractures, CT scans can be helpful.[33] In chronic midfoot injuries, a collimated bone scan may be helpful as a screening tool in elucidating bone and joint involvement.

Accurate diagnosis is critical in dealing with midfoot sprains, because grade of injury will dictate specific treatment. All grades of midfoot sprain need to be treated aggressively. Acutely, all sprains are treated with ice, compression, elevation, and NSAIDs (if indicated). Grade 1 injuries usually require up to 1 week of protected weightbearing in a functional walking brace. Additional protection (i.e., taping) may be necessary for a period after the use of the walking brace. Grade 2 injuries are treated with 2 weeks of nonweightbearing followed by 1 to 2 weeks of protected weightbearing (functional walking brace or walking cast). The treatment of grade 3 injuries is controversial, and they can be treated conservatively or surgically, depending on the clinical situation. Conservative treatment consists of 3 weeks of nonweightbearing followed by 3 weeks of protected weightbearing (walking cast). Surgical treatment involves open stabilization of the involved joint with the use of wires or screws followed by 3 weeks of non-weightbearing and 3 weeks in a walking cast. After the immobilization period is complete, physical therapy can be initiated, with gradual progression to

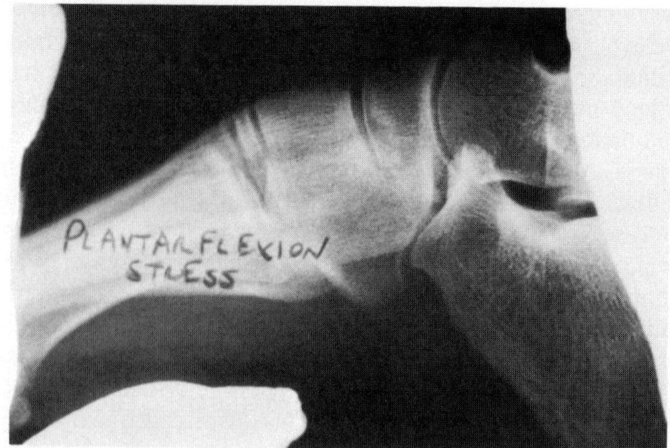

FIGURE 15–5. Plantarflexion stress view of the forefoot revealing instability of the first metatarsal-cuneiform joint, with dorsal gapping evident.

functional activity. Orthotics may be helpful for protection and prevention of further injury. In our experience with these injuries, early mobilization and premature weightbearing can inhibit healing, resulting in prolonged return to athletic activity.

The sequelae from unrecognized midfoot sprains can be devastating to the athlete, significantly affecting performance. These sequelae include prolonged pain, first- and second-ray diastasis, occult fracture/subluxation joint instability, degenerative arthritis, and progressive flatfoot deformity.

PLANTAR FASCIITIS

Plantar fasciitis, the most common cause of foot pain in the athlete, is an inflammatory process involving the plantar fascia. The symptoms vary from mild to severe and are found in a wide range of age groups.

The plantar fascia is a tough, fibrous band superficial to the muscle layers of the foot extending from the medial and lateral tubercle of the calcaneus distal to the level of the MTP joints (Fig. 15–6). A plantar calcaneal spur, when found, is deep to the fascia associated with the first muscle layer.

Plantar fasciitis is due to overuse involving a repetitive tension force applied to the fascia to the point of fatigue.

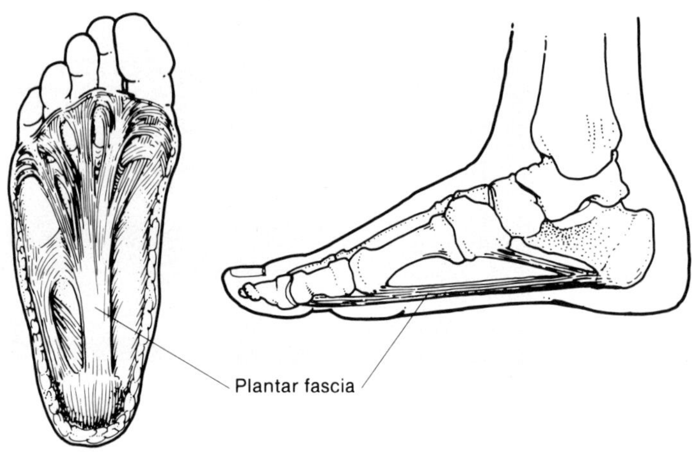

FIGURE 15–6. Anatomy of the plantar fascia.

Training errors, inappropriate shoes, change in training surface, biomechanical imbalances, and faulty technique are all factors associated with the development of plantar fasciitis. Excessive pronation, causing a functional tension on the fascia, and rigid pes cavus, with a tight fascia, are contributing factors.[34] Excessive pronation allows elongation of the foot during midstance, creating a functional tension force on the fascia, and is helped by orthotics. With pes cavus, the disease is found at propulsion when hallux dorsiflexion increases the tension on an already tight fascia and is more difficult to control with orthotics.

Evaluation of the athlete with plantar fasciitis reveals a classic history of heel pain (i.e., ''stone bruise'') in the morning on arising and after a period of rest. Symptoms lessen after walking for a short period of time and return again depending on activity level. Onset is insidious, with no history of injury or trauma. Swelling is rarely present. Physical examination reveals pain with palpation of the medial or central bands of the fascia (extending to the calcaneal tubercle), exacerbated by toe extension and ankle dorsiflexion. Patients may also experience pain with repeated loading (jumping) on the forefoot. Paresthesias may be elicited on palpation of the plantar medial arch as well as tenderness of the abductor muscle belly. Concurrent Achilles tendinitis is common. Classification is based on duration of symptoms, acute case symptoms last fewer than 2 weeks, subacute case symptoms last between 2 and 6 weeks, and chronic case symptoms last longer than 6 weeks.

Differential diagnosis includes fascial strain or rupture, stress fracture, subcalcaneal bursitis, tarsal tunnel syndrome, nerve entrapment, fat pad atrophy, systemic arthritis, calcaneal apophysitis, and posterior heel pathology.

Diagnostic methods include radiographs to rule out bony disease. The radiographic presence of a plantar calcaneal exostosis has not been proven to correlate with the severity of symptoms or resistance to treatment.[35] Appropriate laboratory studies are indicated in athletes with a history suggestive of a nonmechanical cause of pain or in those whose cases fail conservative treatment. Triphasic bone scan can be confusing, and we have encountered three patterns consistent with planter fasciitis. Delayed phase findings are (1) normal scan without increase in uptake, (2) localized uptake at fascial insertion to calcaneal tubercle, and (3) diffuse uptake of the heel, not just at insertion of fascia. These findings should not be confused with calcaneal stress fracture. Diagnostic injections of 1% lidocaine are used to determine the role of surrounding nerves in heel pain.

Treatment includes restricting activity, controlling inflammation, and addressing biomechanical imbalances. Athletic participation is restricted initially to non-weightbearing activity (swimming, bicycling), progressing to select weightbearing activity as tolerated. Severe cases may initially require immobilization and physical therapy modalities to control inflammation. NSAIDs, moist heat, and stretching before activity and icing after activity are helpful. Static stretching of the Achilles tendon and plantar fascia is emphasized. Low dye strapping of the foot, temporary orthotics, or custom orthotics are used to neutralize the tension forces.[36–38] Pes cavus foot type with plantar fasciitis has a better response to orthotic control when a fascial groove is incorporated into the device and cushioned top covers are used. Transverse friction massage and strengthening exercises of the plantar

fascia are helpful once acute symptoms subside. A series of two to four steroid/local anesthetic injections given at 4-week intervals, with 1 ml of betamethasone phosphate and acetate mixed with 2 ml of 1% lidocaine injected via a plantar approach at the point of maximum tenderness, is effective. Oral steroids, immobilization, and the use of a night splint have helped in resistant cases. A night splint is fabricated from thermoplastic material to hold the foot and ankle at a 90-degree angle while the patient sleeps. After conservative measures have been exhausted and a systemic cause has been eliminated, a fascial release with or without spur excision is considered.

CALCANEAL APOPHYSITIS

Calcaneal apophysitis, or Sever's disease, is inflammation of the open apophysis of the os calcis and is a self-limiting condition seen in active children. Age at presentation is between 8 and 15 years, with a median age of 10 to 11 years. Boys are more commonly affected than girls.[39] Calcaneal apophysitis is the most common sports injury in children we encounter.

The calcaneus is the first of the tarsal bones to begin ossification, with the primary center appearing during the fifth and sixth fetal month.[40] The apophysis of the os calcis begins to ossify at 4 to 6 years of age in girls and at 5 to 9 years of age in boys. The apophysis fuses with the main body of the calcaneus around 16 years in females and 20 years in males.[40] The Achilles tendon insertion extends from the middle third of the posterior calcaneus plantarly to encompass the apophysis.

The apophysis is most susceptible to injury during rapid growth phases, when it is subject to traction from the Achilles tendon and plantar fascia.[41] Symptoms are activity induced; however, faulty biomechanics (i.e., excessive pronation and gastrocsoleus equinus) are contributing factors.

History reveals posterior and plantar heel pain associated with activity. Patients will complain of pain during and after activity, which subsides with activity restriction. Palpable pain is present at the Achilles tendon insertion in the posterior calcaneus and extends plantarly. Some children will walk on their tiptoes to prevent the painful heels from contacting the ground. Severe cases may present with mild hyperemia and edema, which must be differentiated from a more severe condition.

Differential diagnosis includes hematogenous osteomyelitis, osteomyelitis from local extension, bone tumor, rheumatic fever, juvenile rheumatoid arthritis, fracture of the apophysis, and heel contusion.

Diagnostic tests include radiographic examination to rule out bony disease. Normal apophysis may appear sclerotic and fragmented; thus, radiographic changes are not diagnostic of apophysitis.[42] Laboratory tests are used to rule out systemic causes of pain.

Treatment involves limiting activity until symptoms subside. Use of heel lifts and orthotics to reduce traction at the apophysis may hasten healing. Achilles tendon/plantar fascia stretches with moist heat application before activity and ice after activity are helpful. NSAIDs are used to control severe pain but do not take the place of activity restriction in young athletes. Severe cases may require immobilization until ambulation without pain is possible.

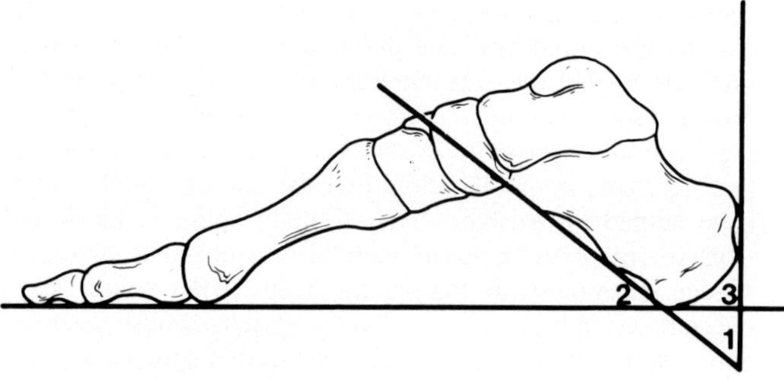

FIGURE 15–7. Relationship among (1) the Fowler and Philip angle, (2) the calcaneal inclination angle, and (3) the combined angle. The combined angle represents the additive effect of the posterosuperior aspect of the calcaneus and the calcaneal inclination angle. (From Malay DS and Duggar GE: Heel surgery. *In* McGlamry ED [ed]: Comprehensive Textbook of Foot Surgery. Baltimore, Williams & Wilkins, 1987, p 272. © 1987, the Williams & Wilkins Co., Baltimore.)

Prevention includes an examination of shoes for problems such as abnormal wear pattern, spike placement, and heel rigidity.

POSTERIOR HEEL DISORDERS

Haglund's deformity (enlargement of the posterosuperior calcaneal process) and enlargement of the posterolateral calcaneus are the two most common causes of posterior heel pain. Haglund's deformity is associated with development of retrocalcaneal bursitis, whereas adventitious bursitis is encountered with posterior lateral enlargement. Athletes with these conditions experience pain secondary to shoe gear irritation.

The Achilles tendon inserts into the middle one third of the posterior calcaneus (posterior tuberosity), whereas the superior posterior border (bursal projection) is free of soft tissue attachments. A retrocalcaneal bursa separates the Achilles tendon from the bursal projection, and an adventitious bursa is located between the tendon and overlying skin.[43]

Posterior heel pain results from inflammation of the posterior heel structures. This may be due to enlargement of the posterosuperior or posterolateral calcaneus or may be secondary to compensated abnormal subtalar joint motion (rigid forefoot valgus, hindfoot varus), or a combination of both,

producing excessive shear forces.[44, 45] Both causes result in chronic irritation from heel counters of shoes.

Athletes complain of pain associated with shoe gear, especially rigid heel counters. Bare feet and open-heel footwear (i.e., sandals and clogs) are rarely associated with discomfort. Pain is insidious in onset and gradually worsens to the point of activity limitation. Physical examination reveals an enlargement at either the posterosuperior or posterolateral aspect of the calcaneus, often accompanied by skin changes (i.e., callus, blister, erythema, and so on). Palpable pain and bursal enlargement are evident in more severe cases.

Differential diagnosis includes insertional Achilles tendinitis, insertional spurring, retrocalcaneal bursitis, adventitious bursitis, enthesitis caused by systemic disease and osteomyelitis.

Diagnostic tests include radiographs to rule out bony disease. Calcaneal inclination angle is determined from lateral weightbearing radiographs and used in combination with the Fowler-Philip angle to assess the extent of the bursal projection.[43, 44] The criterion of a Fowler-Philip angle greater than 75 degrees is rarely met by symptomatic athletes; thus, a combined angle (Fowler-Philip plus calcaneal inclination) greater than 90 degrees or a positive parallel pitch line may provide better diagnostic criteria when evaluating this condition[43–45] (Figs. 15–7 and 15–8). Posterolateral prominence of the calcaneus is difficult to demonstrate by radiograph be-

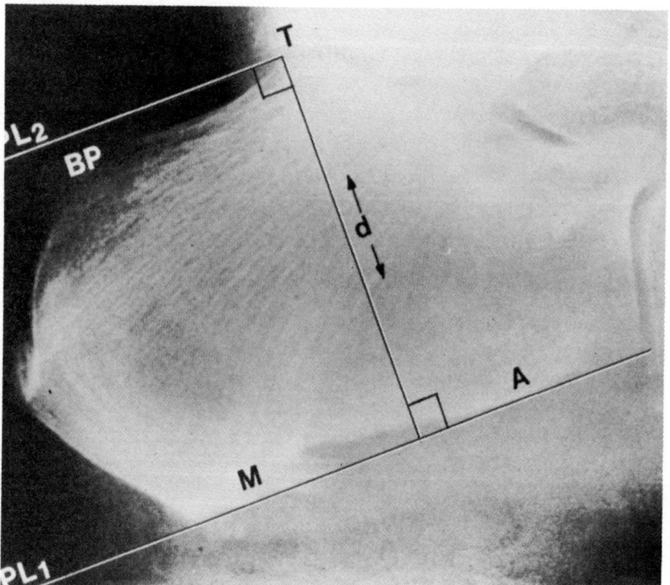

FIGURE 15–8. Use of parallel pitch lines (PL) to determine the prominence of the bursal projection (BP). Lower PL (PL₁) is the baseline, the line tangent to the anterior tubercle (A) and the medial tubercle (M) of the posterior tuberosity. A perpendicular line (d) is drawn between the posterior lip of the talar articular facet (T) and PL₁. Upper PL (PL₂) is drawn parallel to PL₁ at distance (d). (From Malay DS and Duggar GE: Heel surgery. *In* McGlamry ED [ed]: Comprehensive Textbook of Foot Surgery. Baltimore, Williams & Wilkins, 1987, p 273. © 1987, the Williams & Wilkins Co., Baltimore.)

cause it is superimposed over the posterior aspect of the calcaneus on normal views but on occasion is visible on a rotated calcaneal axial image.[46]

Conservative treatment of posterior heel pain involves padding to reduce pressure from the heel counter of shoes or change to open-heel shoes, heel cups, or heel lifts. Modifications of shoes to relieve pressure can also be implemented. Orthotic control of abnormal subtalar joint motion will reduce shear forces generated by compensation for rigid forefoot valgus and hindfoot varus. Icing after activity, physical therapy modalities, and NSAIDs are helpful in controlling the inflammatory response. Steroid injection is not indicated because of the close proximity of the Achilles tendon insertion. Surgical management of posterior heel pain is indicated when conservative measures fail. A demonstrable posterolateral prominence is amenable to remodeling of the involved area by a posterolateral approach. A Fowler-Philip angle greater than 75 degrees, large combined angle, long calcaneus, and positive parallel pitch line are diagnostic criteria used when determining the indication for a Keck and Kelly osteotomy.

POSTERIOR ANKLE IMPINGEMENT

Posterior impingement of the ankle may arise from two sources: soft tissue or bone. Pain is present with plantarflexion of the ankle, most often associated with athletic activity.

Soft tissue impingement may be due to synovitis, adhesions secondary to previous injury, hypertrophied transverse tibiofibular ligament, or meniscal lesions (marsupial meniscus).[47] Anatomically, the transverse tibiofibular ligament runs obliquely from its distal fibular origin to the posterior tibia at the junction of the medial malleolus and may be a separate slip from the posterior inferior tibiofibular ligament.[47] Bony impingement is due to an enlarged tubercle or presence of a separate ossicle (os trigonum). The lateral tubercle arises from a separate ossification center at approximately 8 to 11 years and fuses to the main bone approximately 12 months later. Incidence of unfused ossicle ranges from 3 to 11% and is bilateral 50% of the time.[48, 49]

The pathomechanics of bony posterior impingement involves compression of the posterior tubercle, or os trigonum, between the calcaneus and the tibia during full plantarflexion. There is not a good correlation between the size of the tubercle (os trigonum) and degree of symptoms. Small os trigonums can produce activity-limiting pain, whereas impressively large ossicles may limit motion but remain asymptomatic. The ossicle may be subject to contusion (cystic bone changes), extrusion, compression fracture, or fracture of the lateral tubercle of the posterior process from the body of the talus. Posterior ankle pain in the absence of bony disease may be due to soft tissue impingement. Synovitis, adhesions, and hypertrophied transverse tibiofibular ligament can be caught between the posterior tibia and calcaneus during full plantarflexion. A marsupial meniscus, when present in the posterior ankle, is subject to trauma and tears, which can render it symptomatic.

Evaluation reveals a history of pain at the posterior ankle, particularly with full plantarflexion. Athletes report an inability to extend the foot completely compared with the uninvolved side. The pain may have an insidious onset or may follow trauma. Pain is reproducible on examination with end-range plantarflexion of the foot or by having the athlete assume the pointe or demi-pointe position. Pain associated with os trigonum is usually located posterolateral and is present with deep palpation of the interval between the Achilles and peroneal tendons.

Differential diagnosis includes os trigonum fracture, fracture of the lateral tubercle, hypertrophied lateral talar tubercle, flexor hallucis stenosing tenosynovitis, peroneal tendinitis, posterior tibial tendinitis, Achilles tendinitis, marsupial meniscus syndrome, ankle joint instability after trauma, chondral/osteochondral lesion of the ankle subtalar joint, and subtalar joint arthritis.

Diagnostic tests include radiographs to rule out bony disease. Lateral weightbearing radiographs will give the best views of a hypertrophied tubercle or os trigonum. On occasion, a weightbearing plantarflexion (demi-pointe position) radiograph is indicated to demonstrate bony impingement. Triphasic bone scan will be positive when bone disease is present. Diagnostic injections with 1% lidocaine from a lateral approach will relieve the pain of an os trigonum. Absence of radiographic and bone scan findings in the presence of continued posterior ankle joint pain may indicate soft tissue impingement. Arthrograms and diagnostic ankle arthroscopy are useful in determining soft tissue disease.[47]

Treatment involves control of inflammation by restricting offending activities, administering NSAIDs, implementing physical therapy modalities, and using orthotic devices. Dancers, in particular, need to understand that they must discontinue the aggravating activities until symptoms subside. Recalcitrant cases may require injection with corticosteroids. Soft tissue impingement is amenable to ankle arthroscopy. Bony impingement that fails to respond to conservative treatment may warrant surgical excision, which is best accomplished via a lateral approach.

ANKLE SPRAINS

The ankle sprain is the most common traumatic injury seen in sports medicine, and it deserves a thorough discussion of diagnosis and treatment philosophies. The lateral collateral ankle ligaments are the most frequently injured structures in the body. Ankle sprain alone accounts for 10% to 20% of time loss injury in the adolescent and professional athlete.[50] It is undertreated by many physicians who may be unaware of the potential for long-term sequelae of the unstable ankle.[51] Inversion ankle sprain involves injury primarily to the lateral collateral ligaments: the anterior talofibular ligament (ATFL), calcaneofibular ligament (CFL), and posterior talofibular ligament. Of primary importance is the CFL, which is the only extracapsular ligament and does not uniformly respond as well to simple immobilization if ruptured or attenuated.

Inversion ankle sprain most commonly occurs when the foot is in a plantarflexed position. Ground-reactive forces cause inversion of the ankle/subtalar complex until the end ROM of these joints is realized. Ligaments and lateral soft tissue structures then attempt to absorb these forces. The ATF ligament is oriented most in line with the inversion forces when the foot is plantarflexed. It is also the weakest of the three ligaments, and a midbody rupture of this ligament is usually the first injury to occur. The CFL is oriented more oblique to the inversion forces of the plantarflexed foot and is often the next ligament to be injured. Attenuation of this ligament will often occur as opposed to frank rupture.

History should include mechanism of injury, area of discomfort, associated injury, previous ankle injury, and treatment rendered. Physical examination focuses on extent of injury to lateral soft tissue structures by palpation and passive motion. Specific areas of tenderness and edema should be noted. Palpation should be performed over the entire fibula, malleoli, anterior inferior tibiofibular ligament, posterior talar process, anterior calcaneus, styloid process, and so on. Edema, ecchymosis, and erythema are useful in judging severity of injury, but they must be evaluated in conjunction with the time of injury and previous treatment.

Three radiographic views of the ankle and a medial oblique view radiograph of the foot are taken to rule out fracture. Radiographs of the proximal fibula should be taken if clinical signs are suggestive of injury. Screening for talar dome lesions should be made at this time. Fracture of the fifth metatarsal styloid process, anterior superior process of the calcaneus, and posterior process of the talus are specific areas in which fracture must be ruled out. If no fracture exists, a systematic approach should be taken for further work-up, taking into account the severity of injury and the patient's future functional needs (Fig. 15–9).

Traditionally, ligament sprains have been graded as I, II, and III for intact ligament, partial rupture, and total rupture, respectively.[52] Diagnosis is based on the level of pain, edema, and ecchymosis. Treatment plans have been established relative to this grading system. Unfortunately, this grading system cannot determine the integrity of the ligament, and the physical findings will vary greatly depending on previous treatment.

Stress testing is a more objective method of classifying ligament injury. Quantitative and objective data can be ob-

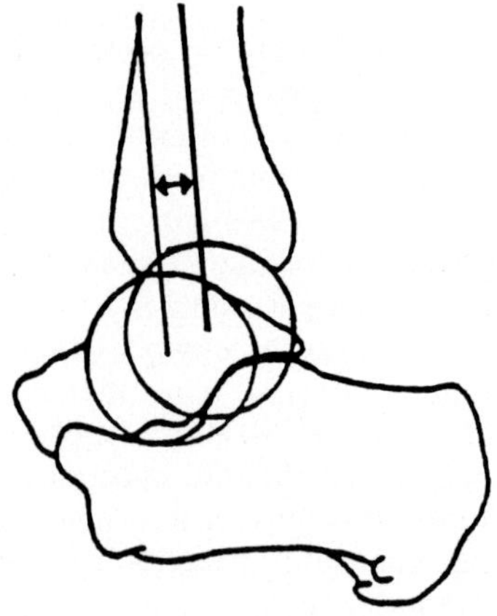

FIGURE 15–10. The method of Lindstrand and Mortensson to measure anterior displacement of the talus in an anterior drawer test. The displacement of centers is taken as a percentage of the overall tibia plafond length. (Adapted from Lindstrand A and Mortensson W: Anterior instability in the ankle joint following acute lateral sprain. Acta Radiol Diagn 18:529–539, 1977.)

tained to differentiate between functional and nonfunctional injury of the ligaments. A higher degree of accuracy is obtained by use of a Telos apparatus (Telos Corporation, Grieshein, Germany).[53] This instrument is designed to apply a reproducible force and position while stress views are being taken. This is combined with common peroneal and infiltrative blocks to aid in patient comfort and muscle relaxation. Inversion (talar tilt) tests the CFL and values are considered positive when they are greater than 5 degrees compared with the contralateral side.[53] Anterior drawer tests the ATFL and is positive when greater than 10 mm[53] compared with the contralateral side. The method of Lindstrand and Mortensson[54] is used to measure this value, taken as a percentage of the overall length of the tibial plafond (Fig. 15–10). Positive stress testing means that structural damage to the ligaments has occurred and is nonspecific for rupture or attenuation of the ligaments.

If the Telos test result is negative, then symptomatic treatment will suffice. This includes rest, ice, compression, and elevation (RICE) therapy, with gradual return to activity as tolerated. If the test result is positive, more aggressive treatment is indicated. This includes a regimen of immobilization or primary surgical repair of the ligaments. Surgical repair is warranted only in the young athlete with at least a two-ligament injury.[55, 56] A tenogram or arthrogram is used to differentiate one-ligament versus two-ligament injury and is indicated only if surgery is contemplated. Communication between the peroneal tendons and the ankle joint indicates a rent in the tendon sheath, joint capsule, and CFL. This communication is regarded as abnormal and is strongly suggestive of a CFL tear. These tests are also useful in identifying talar dome lesions, diastasis injury, and ATFL injury.[57]

Recommended casting protocol involves non-weightbearing in a compression cast until acute symptoms subside (about 1 week). This is followed by an additional 2 to 5 weeks of weightbearing immobilization and physical therapy.

Surgical repair is performed through an anterolateral curvilinear incision within the skin lines. An arthrotomy is performed to evaluate the articular surfaces of the ankle. A high

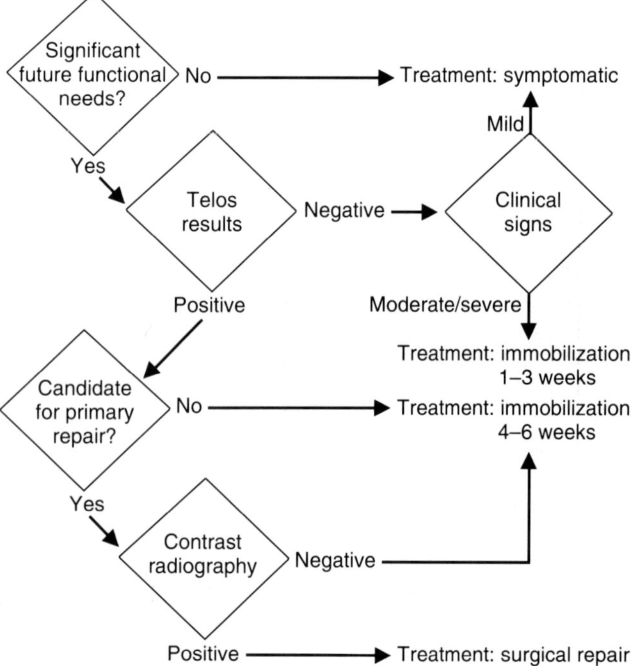

FIGURE 15–9. Treatment algorithm for ankle sprain with no osseous pathologic changes.

incidence of anterolateral dome lesion has been associated with inversion values greater than 18 degrees.[58] Ligaments are repaired with a combination of absorbable and nonabsorbable suture. If the CFL is attenuated, a portion is resected at midbody and the ligament is shortened. Postoperatively, the ankle is casted for 4 to 6 weeks.

Graduated physical therapy is initiated in the casted and surgically repaired ankle. Week 1 focuses on electrical stimulation, massage, cryotherapy, and gentle ankle ROM exercises. Week 2 includes weightbearing exercises and workouts on the exercycle, and tiltboard. The third and fourth weeks focus on strengthening through isokinetic exercise and continued use of the cycle and tiltboard. A rehabilitation program will ensure full ROM, strength, and proprioceptive function, thus helping to prevent future ankle injury.

ANKLE SPRAIN SEQUELAE

Regardless of treatment, several sequelae may occur after an ankle sprain (Table 15–1). Most sequelae can be prevented through careful diagnosis of the original injury. Acute sprains will present with diffuse pain and edema, making localization of tenderness impractical. A follow-up examination is necessary after a week of immobilization and nonweightbearing. The sequelae consist of chronic instability of the ankle/subtalar joints and a variety of lesions involving soft tissue and osseous structures of the ankle.

Recurring ankle sprains are due to structural, functional,[59] and mechanical causes. Structural causes include a rigid plantarflexed first metatarsal or rigid forefoot valgus. Functional cause refers to a lack of proper proprioceptive capacity of the lateral soft tissue supporting structures. Mechanical cause suggests laxity of the ligaments, which may arise from either congenital hypermobility syndromes or previous injury. Improper treatment of ankle ligament injury may result in the healing of these structures in an attenuated and dysfunctional state, predisposing the ankle to frequent sprains. Chronic spraining can lead to synovitis, fibrosis, and eventual arthrosis of the ankle.[60]

Prevention of chronic sprains must be tailored to the cause of the instability. If a forefoot valgus or plantarflexed first ray is causing compensatory hindfoot inversion during midstance, then orthotics with forefoot posting should be implemented. If proprioception is deficient, then a rehabilitation program with emphasis on the tiltboard is indicated. If ligamentous laxity is present, conservative bracing and taping should be tried. Lace-up and Velcro braces have been found

to be most effective for prevention of sprains during athletic activity because they can be retightened throughout the activity.[61, 62] Peroneal strengthening and proprioceptive exercises are adjunctive methods of prevention. Stretching of tight heel cords may help because the Achilles tendon is a closed-chain supinator of the subtalar joint.

The goal of surgical treatment of the chronic unstable ankle is best decided by addressing the particular cause. If the cause is structural, existing deformities are addressed. For example, heel position is evaluated preoperatively and an uncompensated heel varus is corrected through calcaneal osteotomy.

Surgical treatment of the chronic, unstable ankle resulting from mechanical causes reinforces the injured ankle ligaments anatomically. Our preferred method of stabilization is the split peroneus brevis free graft. This procedure uses a transverse drill hole through the fibula at the level of the ankle joint. The graft is threaded through the hole and undergoes tenodesis to the point of original insertion of the CFL and ATFL (lateral calcaneus and anterolateral talar body).

The awareness of subtalar joint instability is becoming increasingly apparent in recent literature. Subtalar joint instability is manifested by chronic pain and dysfunction of the talocalcaneal and calcaneofibular ligaments. Evaluation parameters of stress radiographs are being developed. Conservative and surgical treatment parallels that of ankle instability, with subtalar instability responding well to orthotic treatment.

Chronic synovitis of the ankle may occur as a result of frequent sprains or impingement.[60] Anterior impingement of the ankle may be due to bony or soft tissue impingement. Bony impingement is easily ruled out by a lateral radiograph. Soft tissue impingement will be painful when the patient assumes the skier's position (in which the heels are on the ground and the knees are flexed forward as far as possible). Pain may also be elicited with passive ankle dorsiflexion with the knee flexed. Bone scan and radiographs will usually be negative in soft tissue impingement. Anterior impingement is successfully treated by heel lifts, cortisone injection, or arthroscopic débridement. Sources of impingement include accessory bands of the anterior inferior tibular/fibular ligament, nonspecific synovitis, fibrous bands, synovial lesions, and meniscal lesions. Posterior impingement, especially from the os trigonum, may also occur after ankle sprain (see Posterior Ankle Impingement).

Sinus tarsi syndrome may develop after ankle sprain.[63] The sinus tarsi will be painful during activity, with the patient relating a feeling of instability. The sinus tarsi will be tender on palpation, and pain may be elicited with passive inversion of the subtalar joint. This is probably due to chronic synovitis and talocalcaneal ligament injury. Interestingly, the syndrome is also seen in the excessively pronated foot. Resolution is seen with cortisone injections and, if necessary, sinus tarsi synovectomy.

Subluxing peroneals may occur after ankle sprain.[63] Diagnosis is made clinically with resisted eversion of the foot while the ankle is put through a full ROM. Ankle x-ray films may show an avulsion fragment. This injury occurs as the result of tear of the peroneal retinaculum, which is often overlooked with the acute injury. An ankle brace may prove helpful. If not, surgical considerations include groove reconstruction or tenodesis.

TABLE 15–1

POTENTIAL SEQUELAE FROM ANKLE SPRAIN

Soft Tissue	Osseous
Synovitis	Avulsion fifth metatarsal styloid
Anterior impingement	Avulsion of extensor digitorum brevis
Posterior impingement	Anterior calcaneal process fracture
Sinus tarsi syndrome	Osteochondral lesion
Ligamentous insufficiency	Posterior talar process fracture
Neuropraxia of common and	Avulsion fragments of malleoli
superficial peroneal nerves	Os navicularis syndrome
Subluxing peroneal tendons	
Anterior inferior tibiofibular	
ligament sprain	

Chronic pain may also be due to occult osseous trauma. This includes talar dome lesion, small avulsion fragments from the extensor digitorum brevis or off the malleoli, and posterior process fracture of the talus. Diagnostic injections, triphasic bone scan, and CT are helpful in diagnosing these lesions.

Talar dome lesions are classically caused by inversion mechanisms and are inherent sequelae to the "simple" ankle sprain. They are most commonly found on the anterolateral and posteromedial quadrants of the dome, depending on the sagittal plane attitude of the foot during injury. Staging of talar dome lesions by Berndt and Harty[63a] is based on morphology of the fracture: Stage I is a compression of cartilage and subchondral bone, stage II is a partial fracture, stage III is a complete fracture through subchondral bone, and stage IV is a displaced fragment. Diagnosis is made from plain radiographs, bone scan, and CT. Double contrast (with air and diluted dye) may be beneficial in identifying smaller lesions. Treatment is immobilization, open reduction and internal fixation, or surgical curettage of the lesion. Arthroscopy or open arthrotomy is used to visualize the lesion. With use of the newer, smaller arthroscopes and ankle distraction units, access to the posterior ankle has greatly increased. Larger fragments are fixed with pins, nails, or screws. Most chronic lesions will be too small for fixation and are excised with drilling or curettage of the subchondral bone to promote fibrocartilage replacement. Continuous passive motion, a device that facilitates gentle constant passive ROM, may be used postoperatively.

Styloid avulsion fracture of the fifth metarsal may occur from an inversion injury and is easily seen on plain x-ray films of the foot.[63] If displaced, and with involvement of the fifth metatarsal cuboid joint, open reduction and internal fixation is indicated. Otherwise, a short period of weightbearing immobilization (2 to 4 weeks) is recommended.

Extensor digitorum brevis avulsion fracture and calcaneal anterior process are seen after ankle sprain. The appropriate x-ray views will help with diagnosis: For extensor digitorum brevis avulsions, anteroposterior foot and anteroposterior ankle films are used; for anterior process fractures, a lateral projection with the central ray coming from slightly anterior and inferior is helpful.

ACHILLES RUPTURE

Rupture of the Achilles tendon is a commonly encountered traumatic sports injury, accounting for one fifth of all tendon ruptures and being the third most commonly ruptured tendon behind rotator cuffs and quadriceps tendons.[64] The classic presentation of Achilles tendon rupture is in a 30- to 50-year-old male recreational athlete involved in ballistic sports activities (e.g., baseball, basketball, racquet sports). The mechanism is usually a quick plantarflexion push-off maneuver.[65] Pain in the area of injury is surprisingly variable.[65]

Rupture of this tendon has been associated with previous steroid injection, oral corticosteroid use,[65] equinus deformity, rheumatoid arthritis, tuberculosis, syphilis, and gout.[66] A prodrome of Achilles tendinitis has been documented as early as 3 months before acute rupture.[66] Histopathologic examination has shown chronic degenerative and inflammatory changes to the tendon substance indicating that even an acute injury may stem from chronic disease. Ruptures consistently occur 2 to 6 cm proximal to the calcaneal insertion because of the decreased vascularity in this area, as demonstrated by Lagergren and Lindholm.[67]

Patients commonly present believing they have incurred only an ankle sprain. Ecchymosis and edema may surround the Achilles tendon. Obvious weakness will be present with plantarflexion, and a palpable defect in the tendon substance will often be found. The Thompson/Doherty test result will be positive in complete ruptures of the tendon. This test involves squeezing the calves of the patient in the prone position. A positive test result will reveal little or no plantarflexion of the involved foot relative to the uninjured side. Most authors believe that this is adequate for diagnosis, with an accuracy of 95%.[68]

Additional diagnostic tests include lateral plain radiographs of the distal leg and ankle, looking for irregularities in Kayger's triangle, or an increase in Toygar's angle less than 150 degrees. Kayger's triangle is composed of the posterior cortex of the tibia, the superior aspect of the calcaneus, and the anterior aspect of the Achilles. Any change in the homogeneity of this triangle could indicate ruptured fibers of the Achilles tendon. Toygar's angle is the representation of the posterior contour of the distal leg overlying the Achilles tendon. Any depression in this area is diagnostic of a rupture of the tendon. MRI and ultrasonography have been found to be good adjunctive measures in diagnosis. A high clinical suspicion, good history, and thorough physical examination account for the majority of the diagnoses of a ruptured Achilles tendon.[69] Authors report as much as a 25% rate of missed diagnoses.[70]

Few classification schemes have been proposed in this injury. Puddu, in 1976, classified Achilles tendon disease into three stages: stage I, tenosynovitis; stage II, frank tendinitis; stage III, an actual rupture. Other forms of classification have simply distinguished between partial and total rupture and acute and chronic rupture.

As with primary repair of ankle ligaments, there is a great debate in the literature as to the most beneficial way to treat a ruptured Achilles tendon. The casting regimen involves a gravity equinus (above knee or below knee) cast applied for 4 weeks' duration. Ultrasonography can be used to determine optimum plantarflexion of the ankle joint.[72] The imaging is used to allow for proper coaptation of the ruptured tendon ends by varying ankle position before initial casting. This is followed with additional casting of 4 weeks in a less plantarflexed cast. A 2- to 3-cm heel lift is then dispensed for an additional 4 weeks. Total non-weightbearing time is usually 4 to 8 weeks.[72]

If the patient is a suitable candidate, surgical repair is recommended because of the much lower rerupture rate[73] and the more predictable outcome. Our preferred method of surgical treatment is end-to-end repair after debriding the "mop ends" at the rupture site. This is done with the appropriate lengthening procedure (e.g., a proximal tongue and groove, to obtain additional tendon length if necessary.) The plantaris is used to augment the repair either as a cord-like structure or fanned out as a sheath-like structure. Stay sutures are used, coursing from the proximal tendon to the plantar heel area to relieve tension on the repair site and to keep tension on the muscle.[71] Our postoperative course is aggressive, using a gravity equinus cast for 1 week followed by a non-weight-bearing neutral below-knee cast for 1 to 2 weeks, then progressing to a walking brace for 3 to 4 additional weeks. Aggressive physical therapy should begin 1 to 2 weeks postoperatively and consist of passive ROM progressing to isokinetic and proprioceptive training. This last point is often neglected and can make the difference in the overall outcome.

SUPERFICIAL PERONEAL NERVE NEUROPRAXIA

Neuropraxia of the superficial peroneal nerve (SPN) is an uncommon cause of leg and foot pain in the athlete. Injury can occur at any place along the course of the nerve; however, it is more common for the distal sensory nerve to be involved. Stretch injuries of the SPN have been reported as sequelae to ankle sprains, and compression injuries are seen at the deep fascial exit and on the dorsum of the foot.[74]

The common peroneal nerve divides near the proximal fibular neck into the superficial and deep peroneal nerves. Classically described, SPN descends within the lateral compartment in contact with the proximal fibula, piercing the origin of the peroneus longus muscle to lay superficial to the peroneus brevis muscle in relation to the middle portion of the fibula.[75] SPN supplies motor branches to the peroneus longus and brevis muscles and then exits the deep fascia of the lateral compartment approximately 8 to 10 cm proximal to the anterior ankle joint. From this point on, it is a sensory nerve supplying the distal leg, dorsum of the foot, and dorsal aspect of the first four toes, with the exception of the first web space. SPN usually divides into its terminal branches— medial-dorsal cutaneous nerve and intermediate dorsal cutaneous nerve—before exiting the deep fascia. These two nerves are superficial for the remainder of their course. Variations of the SPN are common, with the nerve contained in the anterior compartment, both compartments, and so on[76] (Fig. 15–11).

SPN is subject to several types of trauma resulting in pathologic changes and symptoms. Ankle sprains involving plantarflexion and inversion may cause a stretch injury to the nerve, which is tethered proximally at the fibular neck and distally at its fascial exit.[74] The nerve is also subject to compression at the fascial exit, especially in the presence of a taut fascial band, muscle hernia, or space-occupying lesion. Chronic compartment syndrome of the leg can also affect the SPN at its fascial exit.[76] Distal nerve branches can become irritated secondary to shoe pressure. Ski boots and toe clips for cycling are notorious for causing neuropraxia of the inter-

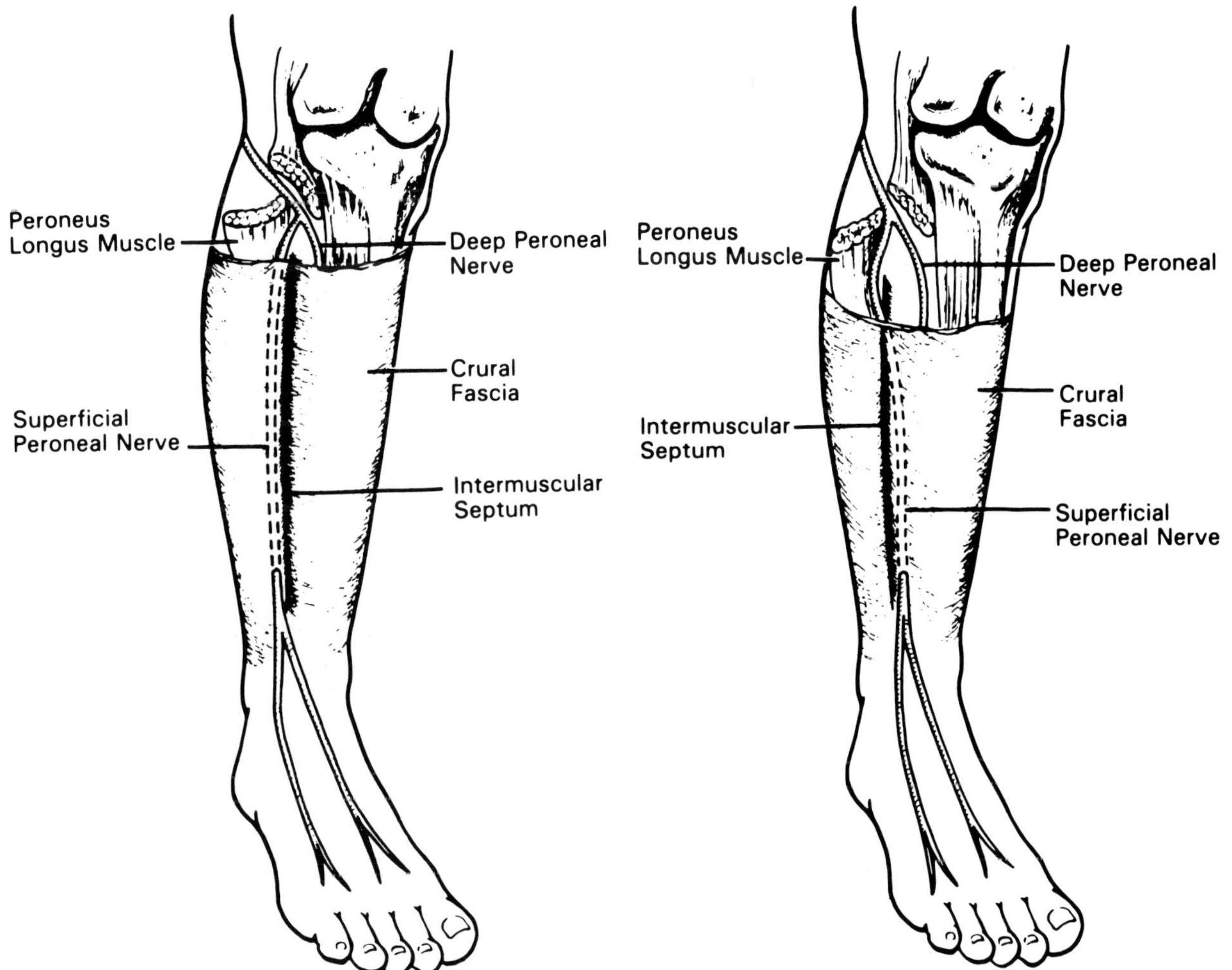

FIGURE 15–11. The left diagram is the most common course of the superficial peroneal nerve (SPN). It travels inferiorly in the lateral muscle compartment until it pierces the crural fascia 3 to 18 cm proximal to the lateral malleolus. On the right, the SPN courses inferiorly within the anterior muscle compartment until it passes through the crural fascia. (From Adkison DP, Bosse MJ, Gaccione DR, and Gabriel KR: Anatomic variations in the course of the superficial peroneal nerve. J Bone Joint Surg 73A:113, 1991.)

mediate or medial-dorsal cutaneous nerves on the dorsum of the foot, especially in patients who lack subcutaneous fat.

Evaluation of SPN injury requires a complete history to determine onset, duration, location, and nature of symptoms. Inciting events such as ankle sprains, start of hiking or ski season, change in shoe gear, or appearance of a lump on the anterolateral leg deserve attention. Physical findings include change in sensation (hyperesthesia, hypoesthesia, and anesthesia) in an anatomic distribution along the course of the nerve. This will differ from an L4 to L5 or S1 nerve root distribution of sensory changes. The entire course of the nerve is palpated: the proximal fibular neck, the exit point from the deep fascia (approximately 8 to 10 cm proximal to the lateral malleolus), and the two terminal branches on the dorsum of the foot. Fusiform enlargement of the nerve or a positive Tinel's sign may be present. The anterolateral leg is examined for anatomic defects (i.e., fascial herniation, space-occupying lesion, and so on). Isolated weakness of the peroneal muscles with sensory changes to the dorsum of the foot indicate proximal SPN disease, whereas sensory changes alone indicate disease from the fascial exit or a point more distal. Provocative maneuvers may include plantarflexion and inversion of the ankle, percussion of the nerve at its fascial exit, exercise, or application of the offending shoe gear. Diagnostic blocks with 1% lidocaine will eliminate pain and can be used to localize the damaged portion of the nerve.

Differential diagnosis of SPN neuropraxia includes L4 to L5 or S1 nerve root injury, chronic compartment syndrome, bony entrapment from trauma, peripheral neuropathy of systemic cause, peroneal tendinitis, and fibular stress fracture.

Diagnostic tools for the evaluation of SPN neuropraxia include selective local anesthetic blocks, radiographs to rule out underlying bony disease, nerve conduction, and electromyographic studies.

Treatment of SPN neuropraxia is dependent on the cause and location of the nerve injury. Neuropraxia resulting from ankle sprains requires protection from further stretch and adequate time for recovery of nerve function. Entrapment neuropraxia at the exit from the deep fascia occasionally responds to conservative measures (i.e., a series of steroid injections); however, limited release of the fascia is curative when performed early. Chronic compartment syndromes require appropriate fasciotomy. Localized pressure from ski boots is treated with boot modification to relieve pressure points or boot change from a front-entry to a rear-entry boot. Toe clip pressure is treated with either a change in the clip and strap position or a switch to a "step in" pedal-binding system.

Prevention involves use of appropriate shoe gear that is well fitted. Symptoms need to be addressed early to prevent further damage that may prove to be irreparable.

TIBIAL STRESS SYNDROME (SHIN SPLINTS)

Tibial stress syndrome (TSS) is an inflammatory condition characterized by exercise-induced pain localized to the posteromedial or anterior crest of the tibia, or both (Fig. 15–12). Clement coined the term TSS[77] but other names have been used including medial tibial syndrome,[78] and medial tibial stress syndrome.[79] This condition is the most common cause of leg pain in the athlete and is prevalent in running sports, especially at the beginning of the season. Although often

considered a minor problem that one can "run through," this condition can become serious, resulting in significant disability.

This condition is caused by unaccustomed and excessive exertional exercise (overuse) typically associated with running sports, resulting in fatigue failure at deep fascial attachment sites of the tibia anteriorly and more commonly posteromedially. Fatigue failure commences as a fasciitis, progressing to periostitis, and eventually developing endosteal activity if the leg continues to be stressed. This inflammatory response is due to tension force applied to the fascia by eccentrically contracting muscle-tendon units of the involved compartment. Pressure exerted by tendons on the fascia is directed to the fascial-periosteal attachment site on the tibial crest, where stress reaction can occur.[80] Pronatory foot disorders and exercising on hard surfaces will also accentuate eccentric contractions of leg muscles and must be considered when discussing pathomechanics of this condition.[81] Foot pronation can also cause a direct tension force on the deep fascia via the "soleus bridge" (soleus muscle and fascia).[82]

TSS is classified by duration, location, and severity of symptoms. Duration of symptoms is arbitrarily broken down into acute (less than 2 weeks), subacute (2 to 6 weeks), and chronic (more than 6 weeks). Location of symptoms will be posteromedial, anterior, or combined. Symptoms are classified as grades 1 through 4 in severity. Grade 1 is characterized by pain to palpation of involved tibial crest, with no symptoms during daily activity or running. Grade 2 indicates

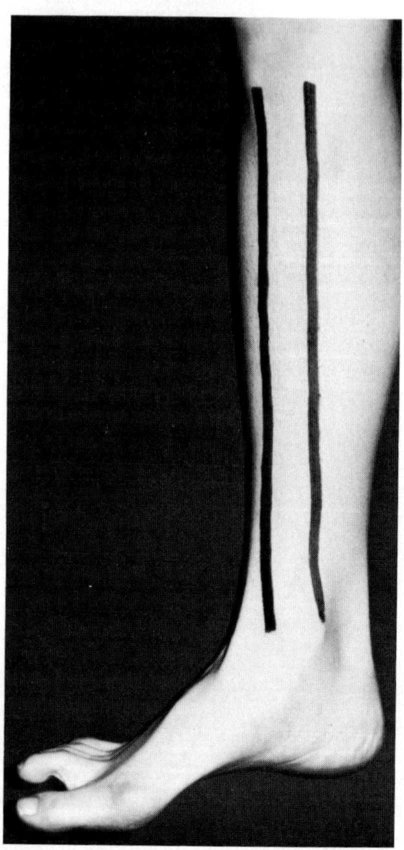

FIGURE 15–12. Lines indicating location of the anterior and posteromedial crests of the tibia.

discomfort mainly after running but not during running. Some mild discomfort may be present initially but subsides with continued exercise. Grade 3 patients have pain during running and residual discomfort after running. Grade 4 patients are symptomatic with walking and are unable to run comfortably.

Clinically, patients will present with exercise-induced symptoms of a gradual, insidious onset that improve with rest. Pain is the chief complaint and may vary from dull to intense. Tightness and cramping may also be related, especially if patients attempt to ''run through'' their discomfort. Training programs should be scrutinized for training errors because a sudden increase in existing activity and participation in a new activity are extremely common inciting factors. Examination reveals tenderness to palpation and induration of the anterior or, more commonly, the posteromedial tibia. No symptoms can be elicited on specific muscle testing, and neurovascular status is normal. Loading the involved extremity with a one-legged hop test can usually be performed without problems in grades 1 through 3. Grade 4 patients can perform the test, but symptoms become apparent with increased repetitions.

Radiographs are usually negative for overt bony changes, but localized cortical hypertrophy may be seen. Triphasic bone scanning has been helpful in differentiating TSS from stress reaction and stress fracture. A specific scintigraphic pattern has previously been reported for TSS.[83] Radionuclide angiograms and blood-pool images are normal, with delayed images revealing longitudinal uptake, with variable tracer uptake along the involved tibial crest (Fig. 15–13). This bone scan finding indicates localized periostitis. Two other scintigraphic findings have been apparent in our patients presenting with TSS. Normal findings on bone scan indicate fasciitis without bone involvement, and diffuse tracer uptake not localized just to the tibial crests indicates diffuse periostitis. Endosteal activity can be documented with use of single-photon emission computed tomographic imaging, which essentially has bone scan and CT scan capabilities.

Differential diagnosis includes stress reaction, stress fracture, tendinitis, muscle strain, chronic compartment syndrome, and claudication syndromes.

Treatment programs should be individualized to meet the needs and expectations of each athlete, and a 4-phase program is recommended. At what phase the athlete will enter the program depends primarily on accurate injury classification and the findings of diagnostic testing. The aim of phase 1 is to decrease acute pain and inflammation. This is accomplished with the use of relative rest (avoiding offending activity for a period of time), absolute rest (crutches in severe cases), cryotherapy, anti-inflammatory medication, and immobilization in the form of removable walking braces and casting. Phase 1 can last a few days to weeks and is critical in the treatment of this injury. Phase 2 focuses on decreasing and preventing scar tissue and decreasing tension forces acting on the bone with the purpose of further decreasing pain. Scar tissue can be treated with the use of moist heat followed by deep transverse friction massage, local anesthetic/steroid injections, and phonophoresis. Tension forces can be decreased with use of taping, orthotics, stretching exercises, and neoprene sleeves. The objective of phase 3 is to strengthen the fascial-bone interface. This is accomplished by exercising deep compartment muscles, which direct a

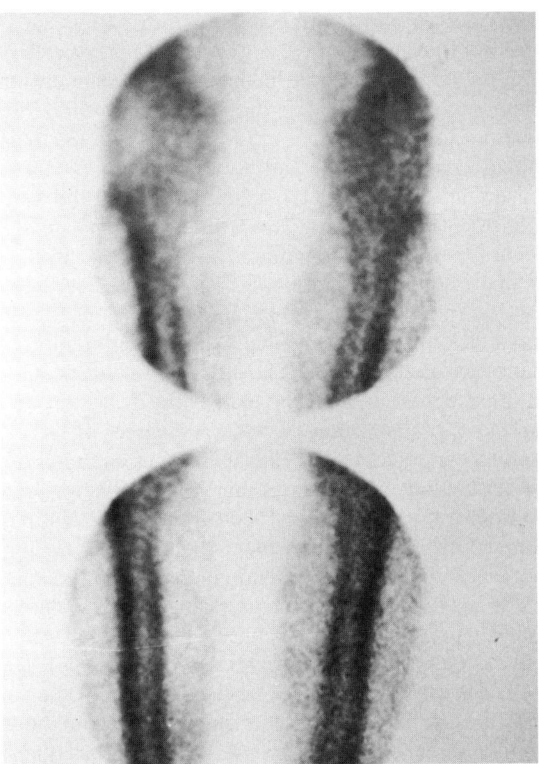

FIGURE 15–13. Delayed-phase bone scan of a patient with bilateral combined anterior and medial tibial stress syndrome.

tension force to the deep fascial insertion. Strengthening should be performed only after pain is adequately controlled. A graduated strengthening program is initiated with isometric exercises followed by isotonic and variable resistance exercises and progressing to isokinetic exercises. Controlled functional exercises should be performed when symptoms are not present. Phase 4 is designed to return the athlete to the desired activity. This phase is based on many factors including level of fitness, previous training program, and personal injury pattern. This phase should be gradual, systematic, and to tolerance. If pain is experienced and sustained, this phase of treatment should be discontinued and the patient re-evaluated. Conservative treatment is successful, but some cases become resistant to all conservative measures. In these situations, surgical release of the deep fascia should be considered. Our results in a limited series of patients have been excellent, although surgery is not a panacea.

TSS can be prevented by (1) determining proper shoes for the biomechanical demands of each patient, (2) maintaining flexibility and ROM through specific stretching exercises, (3) strengthening deficient muscle groups, (4) temporary and permanent orthotic therapy when indicated, and (5) a proper training program consistent with the abilities and goals of the athlete. The last factor is the most important prevention measure.

PATELLOFEMORAL PAIN SYNDROME

Disorders of the patellofemoral joint represent one of the most common and controversial athletic injuries. The term *patellofemoral pain syndrome* (PPS) is used generically to describe this group of conditions localized to the patellofemoral articulation and contiguous structures. PPS can be divided into four categories[84, 85] (Table 15–2). In the past, patellofemoral pain was attributed to either chondromalacia patella or patellar dislocation, but, with the advent of arthroscopy, it became evident that most patients with the diagnosis of chondromalacia patella had no articular injury.[86] This led to the emphasis on patellar malalignment as the cause of discomfort in many of the PPS conditions. This review focuses on the role of malalignment as it relates to PPS.

An understanding of normal function of the patellofemoral joint is essential to any evaluation involving patellofemoral dysfunction.[87, 88] Biomechanically, the patellofemoral joint contains two complex mechanisms for ameliorating forces transmitted across it, namely increasing the extensor lever arm in the important range of 30 to 70 degrees of flexion and increasing the contact area with increasing amounts of flexion. With the knee in full extension, the patella lies proximal to the trochlea, resting against the supratrochlear fat pad. As flexion begins, the patella enters the trochlea at approximately 20 degrees of flexion and centralizes in the sulcus at approximately 30 to 45 degrees. Until it is well seated, patellar stability depends solely on muscle tension. Because of the quadriceps or Q angle (the angle between the line of application of the quadriceps force and the direction of the patellar tendon), the patella always enters the trochlea from the lateral side. Once patellar-trochlear contact is made, resultant flexion compresses the patella against the femur. The congruence of the patellofemoral joint and this compression force provide considerable stability irrespective of restraining ligaments. Up to 80 degrees of flexion, only the articular surface of the patella makes contract with the trochlea. After 90 degrees, however, the broad tendinous band of the quadriceps begins to share in load transmission from the extensor mechanism. After 90 degrees, the patella is beginning to contact the condylar facets of the femur. From 20 to 90 degrees, the entire articular surface of the patella with the exception of the ''odd'' facet has come in contact with the trochlea. After 135 degrees of flexion, the ''odd'' facet of the patella contacts the medial femoral condyle. The increased area available for loadbearing with increasing flexion is an important factor in offsetting the increasing load to be borne with increasing flexion. This is not sufficient, however, to completely offset the increase; therefore, the load per unit area increases. With extension against resistance, the area for weightbearing actually decreases, even though force significantly increases. This information is important when designing a rehabilitation program. If keeping patellofemoral compression forces to a minimum is desired, straight leg raising with weights is recommended because this exercise maximally stresses the quadriceps muscle with minimal patellofemoral compression force exerted because the patella is out of contact, proximal to the trochlea.

The cause of PPS appears to be multifactorial and can be secondary to acute trauma, overuse injury, muscle weakness, muscle inflexibility, or a result of patellar malalignment (static or dynamic). Of particular interest to podiatrists is lower extremity malalignment and its effect on patellofemoral function. James and associates described the ''miserable malalignment syndrome'' to include internal hip position (femoral anteversion), squinting patellas, external tibial torsion, tibia varum, and excessive foot pronation.[89] It has been suggested that athletes with this particular alignment may be prone to PPS and, empirically, foot orthoses have been used successfully in reducing the symptoms of malalignment-related PPS conditions.[90, 91] In reviewing the literature, it becomes evident that PPS and biomechanical abnormalities have been documented only in patients who are symptomatic. The role of foot pronation and its effects on patellofemoral function has not been established as a marker for PPS in a prospective manner. Despite this fact, foot orthoses have become an integral part of the conservative approach to certain PPS conditions. Why, then, are orthotics effective? Although many theoretical models have been proposed to account for foot pronation–induced PPS, no theory has been biomechanically proven.[92–94] The functional knee valgus theory is proposed and is explained as follows: Prolonged subtalar joint pronation (extending into midstance and propulsion) is accompanied by prolonged internal leg rotation, proximal leg adduction, and knee flexion, also causing excessive internal femoral rotation and adduction. This results in a dynamic valgus positioning of the knee, which we believe is responsible for functional malalignment and the pathologic force (Fig. 15–14). Previous theories have stressed the importance of the quadriceps angle, which is measured by two lines transecting the middle of the patella, one from the anterior superior iliac spine and the other from the tibial tubercle. This angle is measured statically and in our experience correlates poorly with a functional situation. In addition, internal leg rotation, which accompanies subtalar joint pronation, decreases the quadriceps angle on a theoretical basis. In comparing walking and running, there is a significant increase in the amount of knee flexion required with running, resulting in increased patellofemoral compression forces and quadriceps tension forces (eccentric contraction). This fact alone can account for PPS related to overuse. Add to this scenario excessive subtalar joint pronation (which results in even more knee flexion, leg-femur internal rotation and, most important, knee adduction) and a significant valgus force is produced, resulting in abnormal quadriceps tension force on the patella with increase in lateral patellar compression. Orthotics limit excessive subtalar joint pronation and appear to limit this functional valgus positioning during gait. This can be appreciated on slow-motion videotape analysis. In our experience, no change can be appreciated in the amount of internal leg rotation and knee flexion occurring in these pa-

TABLE 15–2

CATEGORIES OF PATELLOFEMORAL PAIN SYNDROME

Articular Cartilage Injury
Chondromalacia (patellofemoral arthralgia)
Osteoarthritis
Patellar subluxation/dislocation
Osteochondral fracture

Soft Tissue Injury
Patellar tendinitis (jumper's knee)
Fat pad irritation
Patellar bursitis
Media/lateral retinaculitis
Peripatellar synovitis
Plica syndrome

Lower Extremity Malalignment
Patellar compression syndrome

Miscellaneous Conditions
Reflex sympathetic dystrophy
Pain dysfunction syndrome

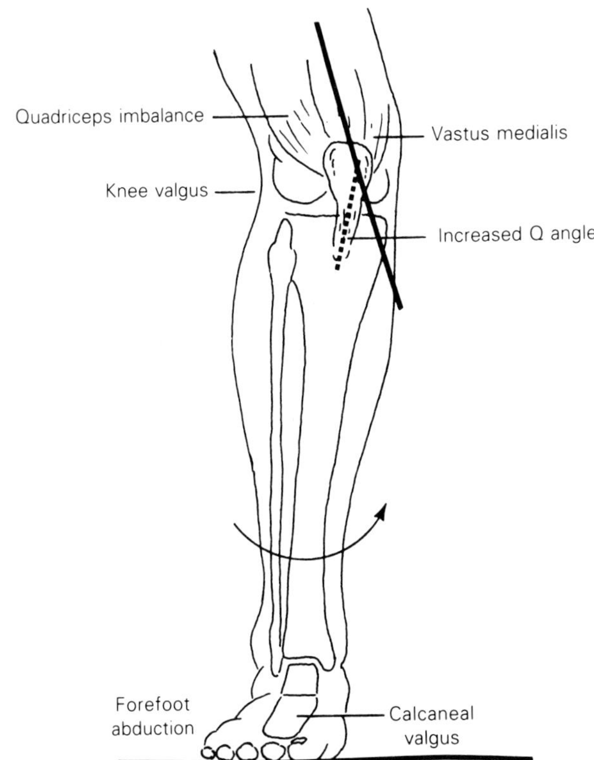

FIGURE 15–14. Excessive valgus position of the knee during midstance in a patient with a hyperpronated foot type and an increased "VQ" angle. (From Subotnick SI: Normal biomechanics. *In* Subotnick SI (ed): Sports Medicine of the Lower Extremity. Churchill Livingstone, New York, 1989, p 152.)

tients with or without orthotics. Further biomechanical studies are needed to determine the role of foot pronation and orthotics in PPS. Patellar malalignment may be caused by abnormalities of the patellofemoral joint itself or by abnormalities of supporting soft tissue structures. In these situations, excessive foot pronation may have nothing to do with the disease involved. Thus, the challenges for the podiatrist are as follows: Is the PPS caused by malalignment? Is the malalignment caused or aggravated by excessive foot pronation?

Evaluation of PPS involves a thorough history and complete lower extremity examination. Diagnosis should be firmly established because treatment protocols for different types of PPS can vary. It can be difficult to differentiate the types of PPS because their clinical presentation can be quite similar. PPS is exacerbated by activity, especially those requiring increased knee flexion (e.g., running, biking, skiing), and is improved with rest. Symptoms include pain of variable description usually behind or around the patella that is aggravated by stair climbing, cycling, and prolonged sitting with the knee in a flexed position (movie sign).

Asymptomatic crepitation (described as crackling or grating) with active knee motion is also described. Stiffness and tightness are related early in the activity and diminish with continued use. Locking or catching occurs when the patient attempts knee extension and must be differentiated from true locking as found in meniscal lesions. The symptoms of buckling or giving way are usually associated with walking or running stairs or down an incline. Localized swelling should

be differentiated from an effusion. Physical examination includes static and dynamic evaluation specifically evaluating ROM (hip, knee, and ankle), lower extremity alignment (such as "miserable malalignment," patella alta, genu valgum, and genu recurvatum), muscle flexibility (quadriceps and hamstrings), muscle atrophy, (especially of vastus medialis obliquus by resisting knee extension at 45 degrees of flexion), patellar mobility (testing for soft tissue tightness), and areas of discomfort determined by palpation. Provocative testing is performed and includes repeated deep knee bends or squats from a standing position, patellar compression test (compressing the patella against the femoral condyles at 30, 60, and 90 degrees of flexion), patellar grinding or Clark's test (pushing the patella distally into the trochlea and resisting quadriceps contraction at 20 degrees of flexion), and patellar apprehension test (test for lateral instability of the patella by attempting to sublux the patella mediolaterally). Diagnostic testing (radiographs, CT scans, arthroscopy, and so on) is often required for elucidation of the problem. Radiographs, in addition to being a good screening tool, can provide documentation for patella alta, patellar instability, and patellar compression syndrome (Fig. 15–15). CT scanning is being used to study the dynamics of the patellofemoral joint, and different patterns of malalignment have been determined.[95, 96] Arthroscopy provides direct visualization of the joint and can be diagnostic for chondromalacia, osteochondral lesions, and plica syndromes.

Differential diagnosis should include meniscal and articular injuries, ligamentous disorders, and common overuse injuries affecting the medial, lateral, and posterior aspects of the knee. In differentiating PPS, four categories should be considered (as mentioned at the beginning of this chapter):

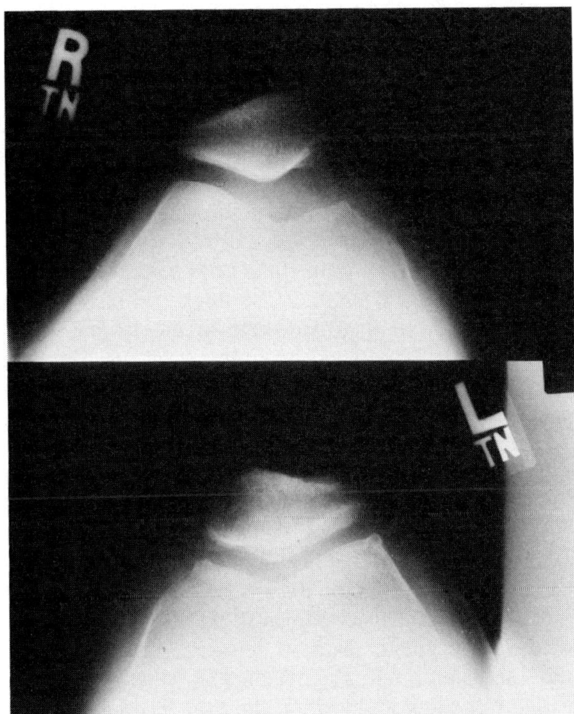

FIGURE 15–15. Bilateral sunrise views of patellofemoral articulation in a patient with lateral patellar compression syndrome involving the right knee. Note the opening of the medial joint space.

patellofemoral joint disorders, soft tissue abnormalities, malalignment, and miscellaneous conditions. A systematic evaluation should differentiate these disorders and establish a specific diagnosis.

Once a diagnosis has been established, an individualized treatment plan is determined. This is one disorder that warrants a multidisciplinary diagnostic and treatment approach. Empiric treatments, such as orthotics for generalized knee pain, should be avoided. Primary treatment is conservative, with all etiologic factors taken into consideration. The patient is progressed from the acute phase to the functional phase in an efficient manner. The mainstay of the rehabilitation program is isometric and short-arc quadriceps-strengthening exercises supplemented by a comprehensive lower extremity stretching program, temperance of aggravating activity, cryotherapy, NSAIDs, patellar mobilization techniques, and so on. Patellar malalignment can be addressed therapeutically and diagnostically with taping and patellar bracing. Foot orthotics are considered early in the treatment program when indicated. Appropriate footwear and temporary supports are initially prescribed followed by custom orthotics pending therapeutic response. In our experience, patients with foot pronation–related PPS respond best to a combined rehabilitation-orthotic therapy treatment program. Orthotic therapy alone is not a panacea for this disorder. Surgery can be considered on exhaustion of conservative measures, and appropriate referral is suggested with continued symptoms. Three procedures are considered: lateral release, arthroscopic shaving, and open patellar realignment.

Prevention is an extension of the rehabilitation program addressing etiologic factors as necessary. Emphasis is placed on maintaining strength and flexibility of involved muscle groups, using good judgment when designing training programs, and wearing shoes (and orthotics) that are appropriate for biomechanical needs.

ILIOTIBIAL BAND SYNDROME

Iliotibial band (ITB) syndrome is an inflammatory condition secondary to overuse involving the lateral aspect of the knee. This injury is second only to PPS as the most common knee problem we encounter and is prevalent in runners and cyclists.

The anatomy of the iliotibial tract has been well described by Kaplan.[97] The ITB or tract is a thickened strip of fascia lata extending from the iliac crest to the lateral tibial or Gerdy's tubercle. This band receives partial insertions from the tensor fascia lata and the gluteus maximus muscles, and, as it courses distally along the lateral aspect of the thigh, fibers extend to the lateral intermuscular septum and lateral patella (Fig. 15–16). Over the lateral femoral epicondyle, the ITB is free to glide anteriorly and posteriorly. The band acts as a stabilizing ligament of the knee between the lateral femoral condyle and the tibia. When the hip is flexed, the tensor fascia lata pulls the ITB anteriorly, and when the hip is extended, the gluteus maximus shifts the band posteriorly. In knee flexion greater than 30 degrees, the ITB lies on or behind the lateral femoral epicondyle, whereas when the knee is in an extended position the ITB lies anterior to the lateral femoral epicondyle. Repeated flexion and extension movements of the knee under stress can produce an inflammatory reaction at the level of the lateral femoral epicondyle

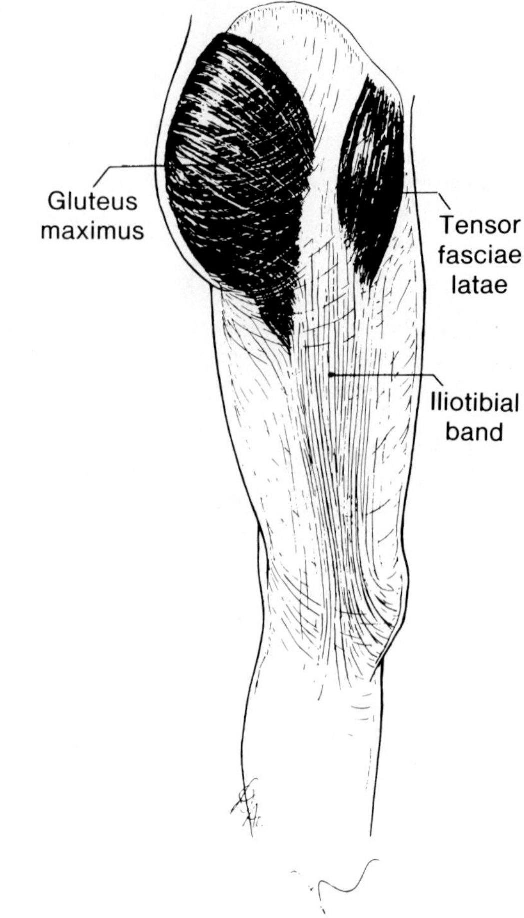

FIGURE 15–16. Diagram depicting the location of the iliotibial band with proximal contributions from the gluteus maximus and tensor fascia lata muscles. (From Kendall FP and McCreary EK: Muscle Testing and Function, 3rd ed. Baltimore, Williams & Wilkins, 1983, p 175. © 1983, the Williams & Wilkins Co., Baltimore.)

from friction, resulting in ITB irritation, bursitis, or periostitis of the femoral epicondyle.[98] An enthesitis can also occur at Gerdy's tubercle as a result of tension forces applied to this area.

The cause of ITB syndrome is multifactorial.[99–102] Training errors (high mileage and intense workouts) and inappropriate bicycle fit (seat too high) can precipitate symptoms. In runners, many factors have to be considered including shoes (excessively worn), surfaces (canted road, banked track), training routines (hills, intervals, increased mileage), excessive foot pronation, and anatomic factors that include prominent lateral femoral epicondyle, contracture of the hip abductors, genu varum, internal tibial torsion, and limb length discrepancy. The role of excessive foot pronation in ITB syndrome can be theorized as follows. Subtalar joint pronation results in obligatory internal tibial rotation. Prolonged or excessive subtalar joint pronation results in prolonged or excessive internal tibial rotation (more transverse plane rotation), thus drawing the ITB anteromedially and increasing the distance between Gerdy's tubercle and the lateral femoral epicondyle. This movement tightens the ITB, producing excessive friction across the femoral epicondyle and resulting in a localized inflammatory reaction.[99]

Clinically, patients present with localized lateral knee pain, although commonly proximal symptoms are related involving the greater trochanter and iliac crest. Pain is exacerbated by knee flexion activity (especially downhill running and cycling) and relieved with rest. Walking is usually without pain, especially with the knee extended. A complete lower extremity physical examination should be performed including biomechanical assessment, motion analysis, and footwear evaluation. Alignment abnormalities and inflexible muscle groups should be identified. Regional examination reveals tenderness to palpation localized either to the lateral femoral epicondyle approximately 2 cm proximal to the lateral joint line or more commonly at Gerdy's tubercle. Inflammatory signs are usually minimal. Two provocative tests are performed after the athlete exercises. The one-legged hop test requires the patient to repeatedly load the affected extremity with the knee maintained in a 30- to 40-degree flexed position. Pain will be reproduced in the lateral knee. The ITB compression test is performed with the patient in a supine position and the knee flexed to 90 degrees. The knee is slowly extended, and, as the knee approaches 30 degrees of flexion, pressure is applied to the ITB at the level of the femoral epicondyle. Pain and occasional snapping can be elicited. Ober's test is helpful for evaluating ITB tightness. The patient is placed in a lateral decubitus position with the affected leg raised. The contralateral hip is flexed to stabilize the pelvis. The affected knee is flexed to 90 degrees, and the hip is extended and adducted. Inability to adduct the limb to the level of the table is considered a positive test result. Hamstring and quadriceps tightness should also be evaluated.

Occasionally, diagnostic testing may be indicated. Tests include screening x-rays (for bone disease), ultrasonography, and MRI (for soft tissue disease).

Differential diagnosis for ITB syndrome includes degenerative joint disease, torn/cystic lateral meniscus, lateral collateral ligament sprain/avulsion, PPS, and popliteal and biceps femoris tendinitis.

Conservative treatment is effective and individualized for each athlete on the basis of assessment of involved etiological factors. Generally, a period of relative rest is indicated, consisting of a decrease in participation of the offending activity or substitution with other aerobic activities. Good activities to substitute for running and cycling are using the Stairmaster and swimming. Icing, compression (neoprene compression sleeves with patellar accommodation), NSAIDs, and physical therapy modalities are helpful. A balanced stretching/strengthening program for quadriceps, hamstrings, and hip abductors is paramount. Resistant cases may require prolonged rest from offending activity, local steroid injections, functional foot orthotics, and surgical intervention involving a partial resection of the ITB over the lateral femoral epicondyle.[103] In our experience, orthotics have generally been helpful in the treatment of this condition. Care must be taken when prescribing orthotics for patients with significant genu varum deformity because symptoms can be exacerbated with orthotic therapy as a result of overcorrection.

Prevention of ITB syndrome includes wearing appropriate footwear for biomechanical needs, participating in sensible training programs, and performing stretching exercises for tight muscle groups. Cyclists are encouraged to have their bicycle professionally fitted (i.e., Fit-Kit [New England Cycling Academy, Lebanon, NH]), if riding comfort or recurrent injuries are a problem.

MUSCLE STRAIN

Muscle strains are among the most common and often disabling injuries incurred by athletes. When excessive tensile force is applied to muscle, the muscle becomes overstretched (causing muscle fiber disruption), thus resulting in a strain.[104] Although this discussion emphasizes injury to muscle, the entire muscle-tendon unit is susceptible to injury. The musculotendinous junction appears to be the most vulnerable site of injury, but strain can also occur at the muscle origin, within the muscle substance, or at the tendon-bone junction.[105] Strain injuries are most common in sports requiring rapid accelerations and sudden bursts of speed (i.e., court sports, sprinting, and so on). Muscles at risk for strain injury are those that have a high percentage of type II or fast-twitch muscle fibers and cross two or more joints.[105] Two-joint muscles are susceptible to stretch at more than one joint and cannot allow full ROM at all joints simultaneously.

Muscle strain occurs in response to stretching a muscle forcibly either passively or more commonly when the muscle is activated during an eccentric contraction (e.g., by a sudden uncoordinated movement when the muscle is maximally contracted).[106] Injury can result from a single tensile force that exceeds the critical limit of the muscle or from repetitive submaximal force, producing a cumulative fatigue failure of the muscle.[107] When muscle contracts eccentrically, it lengthens while producing force as opposed to a concentric contraction in which muscle shortens while producing tension. There is greater force production during an eccentric contraction; therefore, greater stress is exerted on the muscle-tendon unit with greater potential for injury.[108] Factors that predispose a muscle-tendon unit to injury include lack of or insufficient warm-up,[109] muscle fatigue,[106] muscle weakness,[110] muscle tightness,[111] and previous injury (with scar formation).[112]

Our classification of muscle strain is a modified version of previously published classification schemes.[104, 113] A mild or type I strain is a stretch injury with few muscle fibers being disrupted (less than 5%). A type I strain is considered a muscle pull in which the limits of the muscle have not been exceeded. A moderate or type II strain is a partial muscle tear. If the perimysium and fascia remain intact a local hematoma will form (type IIA). If the perimysium and fascia are disrupted, a diffuse ecchymosis will be evident (type IIB). A severe or type III strain is a complete disruption of the muscle and fascia.

An athlete with a muscle strain presents with localized pain (especially in type I, more diffuse in type II and III) and swelling (minimal in type I, significant in types II and III) of an acute onset with an inability to use the involved muscle. A causal event is related, usually involving eccentric contraction activity. Depending on the type of injury, localized hematoma formation or diffuse ecchymosis can develop and is usually evident a day or more after the initial event. A muscle tear can be present even without obvious bleeding.[114]

Physical examination reveals localized pain on palpation and swelling (minimal or absent in type I). The involved muscle will be maintained in a position of least tension, and the athlete will exhibit significant muscle guarding and splinting on attempted joint ROM. Pain is elicited on passive stretch and resistance to active contraction of the involved muscle. A palpable defect may be evident in a type II or type III strain. Depending on the length of time since the injury, bleeding may be evident.

Diagnosis can usually be established clinically with a thorough history and physical examination. Radiographs are obtained for suspected bony disease. Ultrasonography,[115] soft tissue CT scanning,[116] or MRI[117, 118] can be obtained when the diagnosis is in doubt or when additional information is desired. In differentiating type I from type II strains, muscle enzyme levels can be obtained. There is no elevation observed with a muscle pull but there is an elevation in proportion to the extent of injury witnessed with a muscle tear. Maximal enzyme levels are realized 2 to 3 days after the injury.[114]

The regeneration potential of injured muscle fibers is limited; disrupted fibers are being replaced by inelastic scar tissue.[104] The goal of treatment is a small, painless, supple scar not limiting muscle elasticity. Most of the muscle strains we encounter are type I, less commonly type II, and rarely type III. Type III injuries generally require open surgical repair to avoid a painful, extensive, nonfunctional scar. Type I and type II injuries are treated similarly with a systematic progression from the acute phase to the rehabilitation phase and then to the functional phase. Once the patient has returned to activity, a preventive phase is entered, thus completing formal treatment. Phase duration varies depending on the type of injury, with treatment programs being individualized to accommodate the needs of each patient. Acute-phase treatment consists of relative rest, protection of the involved muscle, application of ice, compression, elevation, and the use of NSAIDs. Interferential electrical stimulation can be used if swelling is present. Gentle muscle contraction to tolerance can also be started at this time. During the acute phase, massage is contraindicated to avoid further muscle injury. Patients with type I strains can usually walk with protection (i.e., taping, neoprene compression sleeve, and so on). Type II injuries require non-weightbearing with crutch ambulation for a period of time. During the rehabilitation phase, the degree of pain is used to determine efficacy and rate of progression of treatment. All treatment should be performed within limits of pain, and if pain is present, treatment should be discontinued and the patient re-evaluated. Initially, passive ROM exercises are performed followed by active ROM exercises. When ROM is pain free, gentle, passive stretching exercises are initiated. A strengthening program is then started, progressing from isometric to isotonic (first concentric and then eccentric exercises) to isokinetic exercises. Physical therapy modalities and massage are also used during this phase. The functional phase consists of a variety of supervised therapeutic exercises stressing sport-specific activities and preparing the patient for return to activity. A final assessment of the patient is performed with consideration of strength, flexibility, general conditioning, biomechanics, and ability to perform sport-specific activities. In the prevention phase, the athlete is counseled on the beneficial effects of warm-up,[109, 110] proper stretching,[119] and strengthening exercises.[110]

Strains we commonly encounter involve the gastrocne-

mius, tibialis anterior, and abductor hallucis muscles and the plantar fascia.

The most common strain we have seen involves a type I injury to the gastrocnemius muscle at the musculotendinous junction. Activities involving repetitive eccentric loading are usually responsible. These injuries respond well to conservative treatment. Type II and type III injuries of the gastrocnemius muscle at the musculotendinous junction are known as "tennis leg".[120–123] Previously, this injury was thought to represent a rupture of the plantaris muscle, but there is no evidence that a plantaris rupture has ever occurred and its existence is in doubt.[124] The onset of tennis leg is sudden, with sharp pain localized to the calf. Patients describe a sensation of being struck on the back of the leg and sometimes relate an audible snap. Patients are unable to support themselves while standing on their toes. The mechanism usually involves knee extension with foot dorsiflexion associated with a stretching or lunging maneuver. This injury must be differentiated from deep vein thrombophlebitis and infection. Type III strains of the gastrocnemius muscle usually involve the medial head and may require surgery for optimal strength and minimal scar formation. Further study is needed in this area.

Injuries to the anterior tibial muscle are commonly seen in cyclists (using toe clips), swimmers (training with fins), runners (excessive downhill running), and cross-country skiers (using the skating technique). All of these activities can load the anterior tibial tendon excessively, resulting in muscle strain. Type I injuries predominate, and this injury must be differentiated from other exercise-induced conditions of the leg including TSS (anterior), tibial stress fracture, and chronic anterior compartment syndrome.

We have only encountered type I abductor hallucis muscle injuries, and in our small series of patients with this injury no correlation could be made with a specific activity or foot type. There is a paucity of information in the literature on this entity, and further study and research are needed. This injury must be differentiated from plantar fasciitis, plantar fascial strain, tarsal tunnel syndrome, deep flexor tendinitis, calcaneal stress fracture, and chronic compartment syndrome of the foot.

Although neither a muscle nor a tendon, the plantar fascia is a structure constantly exposed to tensile forces, and the principles that apply to muscle strains also apply to the plantar fascia. Type II and type III injuries have been reported.[125, 126] We have mainly encountered type I strains, but a few type II injuries have also been seen. Patients present with severe plantar heel pain and significant swelling usually at the insertion of the medial and central fascial bands into the medial calcaneal tubercle, sometimes extending into the medial longitudinal arch. A causal event is usually identified. Passive stretch of the fascia with ankle joint dorsiflexion and toe extension reproduces the pain. A palpable defect may be appreciated in type II injuries. Gait is antalgic and apropulsive. Differential diagnosis includes calcaneal stress or overt fracture, fractured heel spur, periostitis secondary to bone contusion, systemic arthritis, and so on. Treatment for type I sprains involves an initial 1- to 2-week period of immobilization in a functional walking brace combined with a physical therapy program. Type II strains require a period of non-weightbearing immobilization for 2 to 4 weeks followed by the use of a functional brace for an additional 2 to 4 weeks. A progressive physical therapy program is also followed until full function is attained. We have found the initial period of immobilization to be critical in the treatment of fascial strains.

STRESS FRACTURE

Stress fractures of the lower extremity are common and potentially serious overuse injuries prevalent in athletes and military personnel who participate in strenuous activity (especially running) (Fig. 15–17). Stress fracture must be differentiated from insufficiency and pathologic fracture.[127] Stress or fatigue fracture implies a disruption in the continuity of normal bone in response to repeated subthreshold forces. Insufficiency fracture occurs when normal stress is applied to abnormal bone (i.e., rheumatoid arthritis and osteoporosis). Pathologic fracture refers to any bone weakened by pre-existing neoplasm.

Two theories have been set forth to explain the cause of stress fracture.[128, 129] The first theory hypothesizes that muscular fatigue secondary to stress overload causes a loss of shock absorption function, which allows excessive forces to be transmitted to the underlying bone. The second theory contends that repeated muscular forces acting on a bone can produce a stress fracture. The second theory is supported by the fact that stress fractures can occur in non-weightbearing bones (i.e., humerus).[13] It is likely that both mechanisms play a role, but the relative contribution of each is unknown.

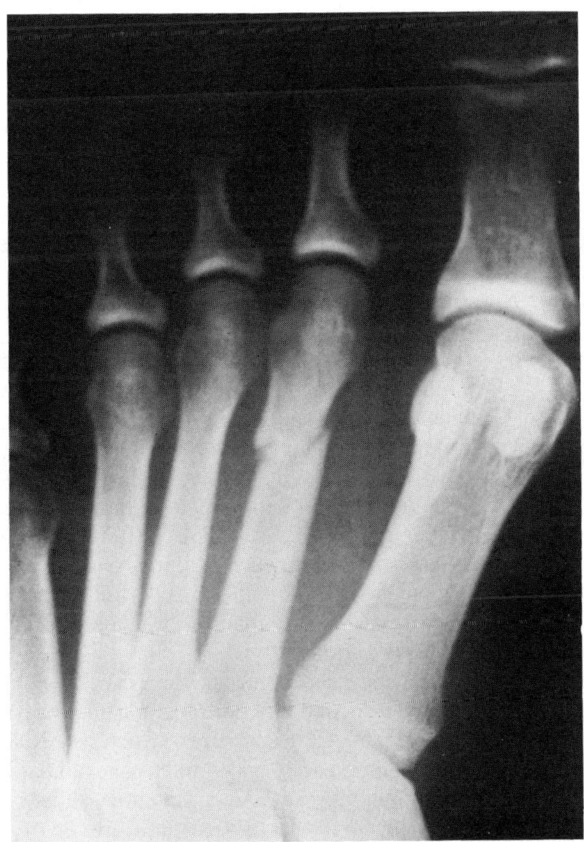

FIGURE 15–17. Overt fracture secondary to previous misdiagnosed stress fracture of the second metatarsal.

Clinical evaluation of stress fracture includes history, physical examination, and diagnostic testing. Typically, an athlete will present with localized pain and swelling exacerbated with weightbearing and improved with rest. Onset is gradual and insidious, with no history of overt trauma. Historically, the athlete relates participating repeatedly in a strenuous activity that is either new or different. Recurrent stress fractures may indicate osteoporosis, and an in-depth history should be performed. Physical examination reveals a discrete area of pain on palpation, percussion pain, localized swelling and erythema, and an inability to perform the one-legged hop test because of pain. Significant muscle splinting and guarding may also be evident. Initial screening x-rays should be obtained, although they are frequently negative. We have found radiographs to be insensitive early and late in the course of stress-fracture healing. When positive, radiographs are specific for stress fracture and exhibit characteristic findings including periosteal new-bone formation, intracortical lucency, and endosteal new-bone formation, although these findings may take weeks to months to be evident. The bone scan provides the most useful information. Technetium bone scan is highly sensitive but not specific for stress fracture because other disease processes can cause similar bone scan findings. Bone scan findings for stress fracture reveal a sharply marginated dense fusiform uptake correlated to the area of involvement (Fig. 15–18). The bone scan becomes positive within days of the stress fracture and can stay positive for more than 1 year despite clinical healing. Asymptomatic areas of uptake may be found on bone scan, indicating subclinical sites of bone remodeling.[132] False-negative findings have also been reported.[133] Triphasic or triple-phase bone scans consist of angiographic, blood-pool, and delayed phases and can provide additional information (acute versus chronic, soft tissue versus bone involvement, stress fracture versus stress reaction).[134] In cases in which bone scan is positive and radiographs are negative, tomography and CT scanning may be helpful to elucidate the disease involved. Patients suspected of being osteoporotic with a history of recurrent stress fractures are candidates for bone mineral content studies. A relatively new technique called single- and dual-photon absorptiometry is available for measuring cortical and cancellous bone, respectively.[135]

The classification we use takes into consideration clinical symptoms, radiograph, and bone scan findings and is based on the concept of bone stress being part of a continuum that can vary from accelerated bone remodeling (stress reaction) to bone fatigue and exhaustion (stress fracture).[136] Grade 0 indicates normal bone remodeling with no symptoms, negative radiographs, and negative bone scan findings. Grade I represents an asymptomatic stress reaction, with negative x-ray and positive bone scan. Grade II represents a stress reaction, with pain present, negative x-rays, and positive bone scans. Grade III is characterized by marked pain, positive x-rays, and positive bone scan findings indicating stress fracture. Most of the injuries we see are actually symptomatic stress reactions (grade II) but may represent occult stress fractures that are not evident on x-ray. Tomography or CT scanning[137] may better elucidate grade II injury.

Differential diagnosis for stress fracture should include stress reaction, tendinitis, soft tissue or bone infection, and neoplasm (i.e., osteogenic sarcoma, osteoid osteoma, and so on).

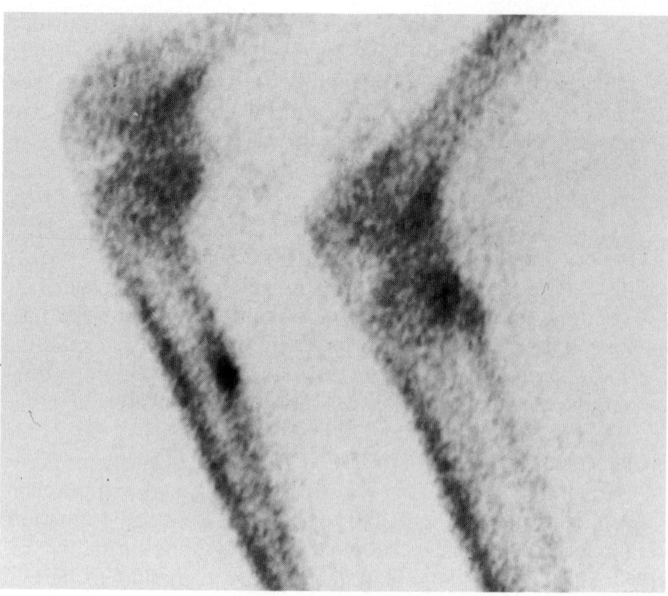

FIGURE 15–18. Delayed-phase bone scan (oblique view) depicting a stress fracture involving the proximal metaphysis of the posteromedial cortex of the right tibia.

Treatment of stress fractures consists of relative or absolute rest depending on the clinical situation. The offending activity must be avoided for a period of time to prevent further injury. Cross-training emphasizing non-weightbearing activity (i.e., swimming, bicycling, and water running with a wet vest) is recommended. If walking is painful, immobilization with a cast or functional leg brace may be indicated for a period of time. Certain at-risk fractures may require a period of non-weightbearing with use of crutches. Acute phase treatment (ice, compression, elevation) and use of NSAIDs may be helpful. Specific time frames concerning fracture healing should be specifically and thoroughly discussed with the patient. The patient's short- and long-term goals should be realized. When the "rest period" of the treatment program has been completed and the patient has been pain free for a 2-week period, being able to load the involved extremity without pain, a supervised rehabilitation program is initiated. The most common problem we encounter in patients with recurrent pain secondary to stress fracture involves an inadequate period of rest with a premature return to weightbearing activity. A gradual, progressive return to full activity is recommended, allowing adequate rest periods between workouts. Care should be taken, especially in the first 4 weeks after the reintroduction of activity, because bone is most vulnerable to reinjury during this period. During this time, bone resorption is greater than bone replacement.[130] Prevention involves identifying etiological factors that may potentiate injury (e.g., inappropriate footwear, muscle imbalances, and structural abnormalities). Training programs should be thoroughly reviewed and altered as necessary, being consistent with the athlete's goals. Pronated feet and pes cavus feet have been associated with stress fractures of specific bones,[128, 138] but the role of orthotics has not been elucidated.[139–141] Further research is needed in this area.

Stress fractures of the lower extremity we most commonly encounter involve the tibia, fibula, metatarsals (internal), and the hallucal sesamoids. One report listed tarsal navicular stress fractures as the second most commonly involved bone in a large series of athletes.[138]

Stress fractures of the tibia are the most common, usually involving the posteromedial crest at the junction of the middle and distal thirds of the leg. Healing time can take up to 12 weeks with this injury, but usually 8 to 10 weeks is adequate. Differential diagnosis should include periostitis secondary to contusion, TSS, deep flexor tendinitis, muscle strain, chronic compartment syndrome, claudication syndromes, and thrombophlebitis (superficial and deep). Radiographs for this injury should include the standard anteroposterior and lateral as well as oblique views. When obtaining a bone scan, it is also important to order oblique views to avoid a false-negative finding, which we have seen numerous times. Tibial stress fractures occur less commonly at the proximal third (posteromedial crest) and medial tibial plateau. Anterior midshaft tibial stress fractures have been associated with delayed union, nonunion, and complete fracture.[142, 143] These injuries should be treated aggressively with a prolonged period of rest and electrical bone stimulation for a minimum of 3 to 6 months before considering surgical intervention (fracture excision with bone grafting).[144] Medial malleolar stress fractures have previously been reported.[145] We have also encountered this fracture in four patients. All patients in our series responded well to a 3- to 6-week period in a functional leg brace.

Fibular stress fractures usually involve the distal third of the fibula. These injuries respond well to a period of rest, taking 6 to 8 weeks for complete healing. Differential diagnosis includes periostitis, peroneal tendinitis, chronic compartment syndrome, and disorders of the superficial peroneal nerve. Stress fracture of the proximal third of the fibula can also occur but is less common.

Stress fractures of the internal metatarsals (two, three, and four) are common; the second and third metatarsals are most often involved. Distal metaphyseal stress fractures usually heal without a problem in 6 weeks with relative rest. Diaphyseal and proximal metaphyseal stress fractures should be treated cautiously, especially if two cortices are involved. These should initially be treated non-weightbearing to prevent overt fracture and potential displacement. These injuries must be differentiated from periostitis secondary to contusion, extensor tendinitis, metatarsalgia, and growth plate injuries in the adolescent.

Stress fractures of the hallucal sesamoids require early recognition and proper treatment to avoid chronic disability. In addition to the standard anteroposterior and lateral x-ray views, oblique and axial sesamoid views may be helpful. Bone scans should include a plantar view of the forefoot and a collimated view of the first MTP joint. Differential diagnosis should include bipartite or multipartite sesamoid, avascular necrosis, chondral/osteochondral lesion of the first metatarsal head, long- or short-flexor tendinitis, traumatic arthritis, and sesamoiditis. In differentiating bipartite sesamoid from a fractured sesamoid, a dorsiflexion stress view of the first MTP joint may be helpful. Acute stress fractures with an obvious fracture line are treated non-weightbearing with the hallux in an equinus position for 3 to 4 weeks followed by a weightbearing functional leg brace with sesamoid accommodation for an additional 3 to 4 weeks. Acute stress reactions and stress fractures without an obvious fracture line are treated in a weightbearing functional leg brace with sesamoid accommodation for 4 to 6 weeks. Chronic sesamoid stress fractures are treated with an intra-articular local anesthetic/steroid injection and a weightbearing cast or functional leg brace for 6 weeks. After the initial period of immobilization, an accommodative orthotic is fabricated and appropriate footwear is recommended. A formal rehabilitation program is initiated, and a gradual return to full activity is advised. If the injury is unresponsive to conservative treatment, surgical excision may be indicated.

Tarsal navicular stress fractures can be difficult to diagnose, and a high index of clinical and radiographic suspicion is required because the fracture is rarely evident on radiograph or standard tomograms. If initial screening radiographs are negative, a bone scan is obtained, including plantar and collimated views of the midfoot. A positive bone scan should be followed by an anatomic anteroposterior tomogram or CT scan to elucidate the disease involved. Anatomic positioning of the foot allows the central beam to be tangential to the talonavicular joint (by supinating and elevating the forefoot), thus allowing better resolution of the central third of the navicular, which is the site of fracture.[146] Stress fractures and nondisplaced fractures are treated with non-weightbearing cast immobilization for 8 weeks. Displaced fractures and stress fracture nonunions are treated by open reduction and internal fixation, possibly requiring a bone graft.

References

1. Spence WR and Shields MN: Prevention of blisters, callosities and ulcers by absorption of shearing forces. J Am Podiatr Med Assoc 58:428–434, 1968.
2. Sulzberger MB, Cortese TA, Fishman L, et al: Studies of blisters produced by friction: I. Results of linear rubbing and twisting technics. J Invest Dermatol 47:456–465, 1966.
3. Cortese TA, Fukuyama K, Epstein W, et al: Treatment of friction blisters. An experimental study. Arch Dermatol 97:717–721, 1968.
4. Herring KM and Richie DH: Friction blisters and sock fiber composition: A double-blind study. J Am Podiatr Med Assoc 80:63–71, 1990.
5. DeLauro T: Pedal vesiculobullous diseases. In McCarthy DJ (ed): Podiatric Dermatology. Baltimore, Williams & Wilkins, 1986, pp 192–193.
6. Miller SJ: Surgical technique for resection of Morton's neuroma. J Am Podiatr Assoc 71:181–188, 1981.
7. Miller SJ: Morton's neuroma: A syndrome. In McGlamry ED (ed): Comprehensive Textbook of Foot Surgery, Vol 1. Baltimore, Williams & Wilkins, 1987, pp 38–57.
8. Greenfield J, Rea J, and Ilfeld FW: Morton's interdigital neuroma: Indications for treatment by local injections versus surgery. Clin Orthop 185:142–144, 1984.
9. Scranton PE: Metatarsalgia: Diagnosis and treatment. J Bone Joint Surg 62A:723–732, 1980.
10. Scranton PE: Metatarsalgia: A clinical review of diagnosis and management. Foot Ankle 1:229–234, 1981.
11. Doxey GE: Management of metatarsalgia with foot orthotics. J Orthop Sports Phys Ther 6:324–333, 1985.
12. Helal B: The great toe sesamoid bones: The lus or lost souls of Ushaia. Clin Orthop 157:82–87, 1981.
13. Jahss MH: The sesamoids of the hallux. Clin Orthop 157:88–97, 1981.
14. Van Hal ME, Keene JS, Lange TA, et al: Stress fractures of the great toe sesamoids. Am J Sports Med 10:122–128, 1982.
15. Resnick D, Niwayama G, and Feingold ML: The sesamoid bones of the hands and feet: Participators in arthritis. Diagn Radiol 123:57–62, 1977.
16. Scranton PE and Ruikowski R: Anatomic variations in the first ray: II. Disorders of the sesamoids. Clin Orthop 151:256–264, 1980.
17. Rodeo SA, O'Brien S, Warren RA, et al: Turf-toe: An analysis of metatarsophalangeal joint sprains in professional football players. Am J Sports Med 18:280–285, 1990.
18. Clanton TO, Butler JE, and Eggert A: Injuries to the metatarsophalangeal joints in athletes. Foot Ankle 7:162–176, 1986.
19. Kavanaugh J, Brower T, and Mann R: The Jones fracture revisited. J Bone Joint Surg 60A: 776–782, 1978.
20. Torg J: Fractures of the base of the fifth metatarsal distal to the tuberosity. Orthopedics 13:731–737, 1990.
21. Torg J, Balduini F, Zelko R, et al: Fractures of the base of the fifth metatarsal distal to the tuberosity. J Bone Joint Surg 66A:209–214, 1984.
22. Hulkko A, Orava S, and Nikula P: Stress fracture of the fifth metatarsal in athletes. Ann Chir Gynaecol 74:233–238, 1985.
23. Zogby R and Baker B: A review of nonoperative treatment of Jones fracture. Am J Sports Med 15:304–307, 1987.
24. Delee J, Evans P, and Julian J: Stress fracture of the fifth metatarsal. Am J Sports Med 11:349–353, 1983.
25. Bennett G, Weiner D, and Leighley B: Surgical treatment of symptomatic tarsal navicular. J Pediatr Orthop 10:445–449, 1990.
26. Sella E, Lawson J, and Ogden J: The accessory navicular synchondrosis. Clin Orthop 209:280–285, 1985.
27. Kidner FC: The prehallux (accessory scaphoid) in its relation to flatfoot. J Bone Joint Surg 11:831, 1929.
28. Grogan D, Gasser S, and Ogden J: The painful navicular: A clinical and histopathological study. Foot Ankle 10:164–169, 1989.
29. MacNicol MF and Voutsinas S: Surgical treatment of the symptomatic accessory navicular, J Bone Joint Surg 66B:218–226, 1984.
30. Norfray JF, Geline RA, Steinberg RI, et al: Subtleties of Lisfranc fracture—dislocations. Am J Roentgenol 137:1151–1156, 1981.
31. Faciszewski T, Burks RT, and Manaster BJ: Subtle injuries of the Lisfranc joint. J Bone Joint Surg 72A:1519–1522, 1990.
32. Turco VJ and Spinella AJ: Occult trauma and unusual injuries in the foot and ankle. In Nicholas JA and Hershman EB (eds): The Lower Extremity and Spine in Sports Medicine. St. Louis, CV Mosby, 1986, pp 547–551.
33. Goiney RC, Connell DG, and Nichols DM: CT evaluation of tarsometatarsal fracture-dislocation injuries. Am J Roentgenol 144:985–990, 1985.
34. Kwong PK, Kay D, Voner RT, et al: Plantar fasciitis: Mechanics and pathomechanics of treatment. Clin Sports Med 7:119–126, 1988.
35. McBryde AM: Plantar fasciitis. In AAOS Instructional Course Lectures: Running Injuries. pp 278–282, 1984.
36. D'Ambrosia RD: Conservative management of metatarsal and heel pain in the adult foot. Orthopedics 10:137–142, 1987.
37. Hlavac HF: Wraps, straps and pads. In Hlavac HF (ed): The Foot Book: Advice for Athletes. Mountain View, CA, World Publishers, 1977, pp 298–304.
38. Newell SG and Miller SJ: Conservative treatment of plantar fascial strain. Physician Sports Med 5:68–73, 1977.
39. McCrea JD: Osteochondroses of the foot. In McCrea JD (ed): Pediatric orthopedics of the lower extremity. Mount Kisco, NY, Futura, 1985, pp 249–251.
40. Tachdjian MO: The Child's Foot. Philadelphia, WB Saunders, 1985, pp 40–44.
41. Jahss MH: Disorders of the Foot, Vol 1. Philadelphia, WB Saunders, 1982, pp 203–204.
42. Tax HR: Orthopedic problems. In Tax HR (ed): Podopediatrics. Baltimore, Williams & Wilkins, 1980, pp 129–130.
43. Pavlov H, Heneghan MA, Hersh A, et al: The Haglund syndrome: Initial and differential diagnosis. Radiology 144:83–88, 1982.
44. Miller AE and Vogel TA: Haglund's deformity and the Keck and Kelly osteotomy: A retrospective analysis. J Foot Surg 28:23–29, 1989.
45. Malay DS and Duggar GE: Heel surgery. In McGlamry ED (ed): Comprehensive Textbook of Foot Surgery, Vol 1. Baltimore, Williams & Wilkins, 1987, pp 264–287.
46. Mann RA: Miscellaneous afflictions of the foot. In Mann RA (ed): Surgery of the Foot. Princeton, NJ, CV Mosby, 1986, pp 247–253.
47. Guhl JF: Soft Tissue (synovial) pathology. In Guhl JF (ed): Ankle Arthroscopy, Pathology, and Surgical Techniques. Thorofare, NJ, Slack, 1988, pp 87–94.
48. Hamilton WG: Stenosing tenosynovitis of the flexor hallucis longus tendon and posterior impingement upon the os trigonum in ballet dancers. Foot Ankle 3:74–80, 1982.
49. Quirk R: Talar compression syndrome in dancers. Foot Ankle 3:65–68, 1982.
50. Garrick J: The frequency of injury, mechanism of injury, and epidemiology of ankle sprains. Am J Sports Med 5:241–242, 1977.

51. Brand R, Black H, and Cox J: The natural history of inadequately treated ankle sprain. Am J Sports Med 5:248–249, 1977.

52. Lassiter T, Malone T, and Garrett W: Injury to the lateral ligaments of the ankle. Orthop Clin North Am 20:629–640, 1989.

53. Scheuba G: Telos Stress Device User's Manual. Grieshein, Germany, Telos Corporation, 1989.

54. Lindstrand A, and Mortensson W: Anterior instability in the ankle joint following acute lateral sprain. Acta Radiol Diagn 18:529–539, 1977.

55. Brostrom L: Sprained ankles: V. Treatment and prognosis in recent ligament ruptures. Acta Chir Scand 132:537–550, 1966.

56. Rijke A, Barrington J, and Vierhout P: Injury to the lateral ankle ligaments of athletes: A posttraumatic follow-up. Am J Sports Med 16:256–259, 1988.

57. Downing J, Oloff L, and Jacobs A: Radiologic diagnosis and assessment of lateral ankle ligamentous injuries. J Foot Surg 18:135–146, 1979.

58. Hutchinson B, and Wardle D: Diagnosis and treatment of talar tilt and its relationship to the occurrence of transchondral fractures: A retrospective study. J Foot Surg 30:151–155, 1991.

59. Freeman M, Dean M, and Hanham W: The etiology and prevention of functional instability of the foot. J Bone Joint Surg 47B:678–685, 1965.

60. Larsen E and Aru A: Synovitis in chronically unstable ankles. Acta Orthop Scand 60:340–344, 1989.

61. Bunch R, Bednarski K, and Holland D: Ankle joints support: A comparison of reusable lace-on braces with taping and wrapping. Physician Sports Med 13:59–62, 1985.

62. Rovere G, Clarke T, and Yates C: Retrospective comparison of taping and ankle stabilizers in the prevention of ankle injuries. Am J Sports Med 16:228–233, 1988.

63. Perlman M, Leveille D, DeLeonibus J, et al: Inversion lateral ankle trauma: Differential diagnosis, review of literature, and prospective study. J Foot Surg 26:95–135, 1987.

63a. Berndt AL and Harty M: Transchondral Fractures (osteochondritis dissecans) of the talus. J Bone Joint Surg 41A:996, 1959.

64. Goldman J, Linschdid RL, and Bickel WA: Disruption of tendo Achillis: Analysis of 53 cases. Mayo Clin Proc 44:28, 1969.

65. Kellam J, Hunter G, and McElwain M: Review of the operative treatment of Achilles tendon rupture. Clin Orthop 201:80–83, 1985.

66. Beskin J, Sanders R, Hunter S, et al: Surgical repair of Achilles tendon ruptures. Am J Sports Med 15:1–8, 1987.

67. Lagergren C and Lindholm A: Vascular distribution in the Achilles tendon. Acta Chir Scand 116:491–495, 1959.

68. Thompson TC and Doherty JH: Spontaneous rupture of tendon of Achilles: A new clinical diagnostic test. J Trauma 2:126–129, 1962.

69. Hattrup S and Johnson K: A review of ruptures of the Achilles tendon. Foot Ankle 6:34–38, 1985.

70. Wills C, Washburn S, Caiozzo V, et al: Achilles tendon rupture: A review of the literature comparing surgical vs. nonsurgical treatment. Clin Orthop 207:156–163, 1986.

71. Haggmark T, Leidberg H, Eriksson E, et al: Calf muscle atrophy and muscle function after non-operative vs operative treatment of Achilles tendon ruptures. Orthopedics 9:160–164, 1986.

72. Lea R and Smith L: Non-surgical treatment of tendo Achillis rupture. J Bone Joint Surg 54A:1398, 1972.

73. Andersen E and Hvass I: Suture of Achilles tendon rupture under local anesthesia. Acta Orthop Scand 57:235–236, 1986.

74. Schon LC and Baxter DE: Neuropathies of the foot and ankle in athletes. Clin Sports Med 9:489–509, 1990.

75. Sarrafian SK: Anatomy of the foot and ankle: Descriptive, topographic, functional. Philadelphia, JB Lippincott, 1983, pp 317.

76. Adkison DP, Bosse MJ, Gaccione DR, et al: Anatomical variations in the course of the superficial peroneal nerve. J Bone Joint Surg 73A:112–114, 1991.

77. Clement DB: Tibial stress syndrome in athletes. J Sports Med 2:81–85, 1974.

78. Puranen J: The medial tibial syndrome. Exercise ischemia in the medial fascial compartment of the leg. J Bone Joint Surg 56B:712–715, 1974.

79. Mubarak SJ, Gould RN, Lee YF, et al: The medial tibial stress syndrome: A cause of shin-splints. Am J Sports Med 10:201–205, 1982.

80. Johnell O, Rausing A, Wendeberg B, et al: Morphological bone changes in shin splints. Clin Orthop 167:180–184, 1982.

81. Richie DH, DeVries HV, and Endo CK: Shin muscle activity and floor surfaces in dance exercise: An electromyographic study. Paper presented at the annual meeting of the American Academy of Podiatric Sports Medicine, Phoenix, AZ, 1989.

82. Michael RH and Holder LE: The soleus syndrome: A cause of medial tibial stress (shin-splints). Am J Sports Med 13:87–94, 1985.

83. Holder LE and Michael RH: The specific scintigraphic pattern of "shin-splints in the lower leg": Concise communication. J Nucl Med 25:865–869, 1984.

84. Insall J: Current concepts review: Patellar pain. J Bone J Surg 64A:147–152, 1982.

85. Kettelkamp DB: Current concepts review: Management of patellar malalignment. J Bone J Surg 63A:1344–1348, 1981.

86. Griffiths I and Pinder I: Chondromalacia patella: A clinical and arthroscopic study. Ann Rheum Dis 40:617, 1981.

87. Hungerford DS and Barry M: Biomechanics of the patellofemoral joint. Clin Orthop 144:9–15, 1979.

88. Woodall W and Welsh J: A biomechanical basis for rehabilitation programs involving the patellofemoral joint. J Orthop Sports Phys Ther 11:535–542, 1990.

89. James SL, Bates BT, and Osternig LR: Injuries to runners. Am J Sports Med 6:40–50, 1978.

90. Rubin BD and Collins HR: Runner's knee. Physician Sports Med 8:49–58, 1980.

91. Newell SG and Bramwell ST: Overuse injuries to the knee in runners. Physician Sports Med 12:81–92, 1984.

92. Bogdan RJ, Jenkins D, and Hyland T: The runner's knee syndrome. In Rinaldi RR and Sabia ML (ed): Sports Medicine '78. Mount Kisco, NY, Futura, 1978, pp 159–177.

93. Buchbinder MR, Napora NJ and Biggs EW: The relationship of abnormal pronation to chondromalacia of the patella in distance runners. J Am Podiatr Assoc 69:159–161, 1979.

94. Tiberio D: The effect of excessive subtalar joint pronation on patellofemoral mechanics: A theoretical model. J Orthop Sports Phys Ther 9:160–165, 1987.

95. Schutzer S, Ramsby G, and Fulkerson J: Computed tomographic classification of patellofemoral pain. Orthop Clin North Am 17:235–248, 1986.

96. Schutzer S, Ramsby G, and Fulkerson J: The evaluation of patellofemoral pain using computerized tomography. Clin Orthop 204:286–293, 1986.

97. Kaplan EB: The iliotibial tract. Clinical and morphological significance. J Bone J Surg 40A:817–832, 1958.

98. Renne JW: The iliotibial band friction syndrome. J Bone J Surg 57A:1110–1111, 1975.

99. McNicol K, Taunton JE, and Clement DB: Iliotibial tract friction syndrome in athletes. Can J Appl Sports Sci 6:76–80, 1981.

100. Sutker AN, Jackson DW, and Pagliano JW: Iliotibial band syndrome in distance runners. Phys Sports Med 9(10):69–73, 1981.

101. Lindenberg G, Pinshaw R, and Noakes TD: Iliotibial band friction syndrome in runners. Phys Sports Med 12(8):118–130, 1984.

102. Noble CA: Iliotibial band friction syndrome in runners. Am J Sports Med 8:232–234, 1980.

103. Martens M, Libbrecht P, and Burssens A: Surgical treatment of the iliotibial band friction syndrome. Am J Sports Med 17:651–654, 1989.

104. Zarins B and Ciullo JV: Acute muscle and tendon injuries in athletes. Clin Sports Med 2:167–182, 1983.

105. Garrett WE: Muscle strain injuries: Clinical and basic aspects. Med Sci Sports Exerc 22:436–443, 1990.

106. Garrett WE, Safran MR, Seaber AV, et al: Biomechanical comparison of stimulated and nonstimulated skeletal muscle pulled to failure. Am J Sports Med 15:448–454, 1987.

107. Solomonow M and D'Ambrosia R: Biomechanics of muscle overuse injuries: A theoretical approach. Clin Sports Med 6:241–257, 1987.

108. Stauber WT: Eccentric action of muscles: Physiology, injury, and adaptation. Exerc Sport Sci 17:157–185, 1989.

109. Safran MR, Garrett WE, Seaber AV, et al: The role of warm-up in muscular injury prevention. Am J Sports Med 16:123–129, 1988.

110. Stone MH: Muscle conditioning and muscle injuries. Med Sci Sports Exerc 22:457–462, 1990.

111. Wiktorsson-Moller M, Oberg B, Ekstrand J, et al: Effects of warming up, massage, and stretching on range of motion and muscle strength in the lower extremity. Am J Sports Med 11:249–252, 1983.

112. Nikolaou PK, Macdonald BL, Glisson RR, et al: Biomechanical and histological evaluation of muscle after controlled strain injury. Am J Sports Med 15:9–14, 1987.

113. Ryan AJ: Quadriceps strain: Rupture and charley horse. Med Sci Sports 1:106–111, 1969.

114. Krejci V and Koch P: Muscle and Tendon Injuries in Athletes. Chicago, Year Book Medical, 1979, p 5.

115. Fornage BD, Touche DH, and Segal P: Ultrasonography in the evaluation of muscular trauma. J Ultrasound Med 2:549–554, 1983.

116. Garrett WE, Rich FR, Nikolaou PK, et al: Computed tomography of hamstring muscle strains. Med Sci Sports Exerc 21:506–514, 1989.

117. Sartoris DJ, Brozinsky S, and Resnick D: MRI's role in assessing musculoskeletal disorders. J Musculoskel Med 4:12–26, 1987.

118. Solomon MA and Oloff-Solomon J: Magnetic resonance imaging in the foot and ankle. Clin Podiatr Med Surg 5:945–965, 1988.

119. Taylor DC, Dalton JD, Seaber AV, et al: Viscoelastic properties of muscle-tendon units: The biomechanical effects of stretching. Am J Sports Med 18:300–309, 1990.

120. Millar AP: Strains of the posterior calf musculature ("tennis leg"). Am J Sports Med 7:172–174, 1979.

121. Miller WA: Rupture of the musculotendinous juncture of the medial head of the gastrocnemius muscle. Am J Sports Med 5:191–193, 1977.

122. Arner O and Lindholm A: What is tennis leg? Acta Chir Scand 116:73–75, 1958.

123. Froimson AI: Tennis leg. JAMA 209:415–416, 1969.

124. Severance HW and Bassett FH: Rupture of the plantaris—Does it exist? J Bone J Surg 64A:1387–1388, 1982.

125. Leach R, Jones R, and Silva T: Rupture of the plantar fascia in athletes. J Bone J Surg 60A:537–539, 1978.

126. Ahstrom JP: Spontaneous rupture of the plantar fascia. Am J Sports Med 16:306–307, 1988.

127. Daffner RH: Stress fracture: Current concepts. Skeletal Radiol 2:221–229, 1978.

128. Taunton JE, Clement DB, and Webber D: Lower extremity stress fractures in athletes. Phys Sports Med 9(1):77–86, 1981.

129. Stanitski CL, Mcmaster JH, and Scranton PE: On the nature of stress fractures. Am J Sports Med 6:391–395, 1978.

130. Sweet DE and Auman RM: RPC of the month from AFIP. Radiology 99:687–693, 1971.
131. Allen ME: Stress fracture of the humerus: A case study. Am J Sports Med 12:244–245, 1974.
132. Matheson GO, Clement DB, McKenzie DC, et al: Scintigraphic uptake of 99m Tc at non-painful sites in athletes with stress fractures: The concept of bone strain. Sports Med 4:65–75, 1987.
133. Milgrom C, Chisin R, Giladi M, et al: Negative bone scans in impending tibial stress fractures. Am J Sports Med 12:488–491, 1984.
134. Rupani HD, Holder LE, Espinola DA, et al: Three-phase radionuclide bone imaging in sports medicine. Radiology 156:187–196, 1985.
135. Benson JW and Hanelin LG: Place of bone density measurement in the management of osteoporosis. Bull Mason Clin 39:61–69, 1985.
136. Roub LW, Gumerman LW, Henley EN, et al: Bone stress: A radionuclide imaging perspective. Radiology 132:431–438, 1979.
137. Yousem D, Magid D, Fishman EK, et al: Computed tomography of stress fracture. J Comput Assist Tomogr 10:92–95, 1986.
138. Matheson GO, Clement DB, Mckenzie DC, et al: Stress fractures in athletes: A study of 320 cases. Am J Sports Med 15:46–58, 1987.
139. Milgrom C, Giladi M, Kashtan H, et al: A prospective study of the effect of a shock-absorbing orthotic device on the incidence of stress fractures in military recruits. Foot Ankle 6:101–104, 1985.
140. Simkin A, Leichter I, Giladi M, et al: Combined effect of foot arch structure and an orthotic device on stress fractures. Foot Ankle 10:25–29, 1989.
141. Milgrom C, Burr DB, Boyd RD, et al: The effect of a viscoelastic orthotic on the incidence of tibial stress fractures in an animal model. Foot Ankle 10:276–279, 1990.
142. Orava S and Hulkko A: Stress fracture of the mid-tibial shaft. Acta Orthop Scand 55:35–37, 1984.
143. Green NE, Rogers RA, and Lipscomb AB: Nonunions of stress fractures of the tibia. Am J Sports Med 13:171–176, 1985.
144. Rettig AC, Shelbourne KD, McCarroll JR, et al: The natural history and treatment of delayed union stress fractures of the anterior cortex of the tibia. Am J Sports Med 16:250–255, 1988.
145. Shelbourne KD, Fisher DA, Rettig AC, et al: Stress fractures of the medial malleolus. Am J Sports Med 16:60–63, 1988.
146. Pavlov H, Torg JS, and Freiberger RH: Tarsal navicular stress fractures: Radiographic evaluation. Radiology 148:641–645, 1983.

Musculoskeletal Manifestations of Specific Systemic Diseases

CHAPTER 16

The Diabetic Foot

Steven J. Palladino, D.P.M.

The diabetic foot has been the topic of a multitude of scientific articles, reflecting its importance in the scheme of diabetic complications. In fact, entire textbooks have been devoted to the subject.[1–8] The emphasis of discussion regarding the diabetic foot has been placed on the major complication of amputation and its antecedents. Therefore, topics such as neuropathy, ulceration, infection, and dysvascularity generally have received detailed attention.

In contrast, the topic of musculoskeletal disorders of the diabetic foot has received only isolated attention. Usually, pedal musculoskeletal deformities are discussed in the context of their relationship to neuropathic ulceration.[9–21] The exception to this generalization is neuropathic arthropathy (Charcot's joint) of the diabetic foot.[22–28]

Despite the relative lack of singular attention in the literature, the topic of musculoskeletal disorders of the diabetic foot remains a critical one to the comprehensive management of the patient with diabetes. It is true that the presence of pedal deformities tends to focus peak environmental stresses and increase the risk of ulceration and amputation.[17, 29, 30] Clearly, this important relationship has implications in the management of the diabetic patient.[11, 12, 15–17, 19, 31–38] Moreover, musculoskeletal disorders affect the diabetic foot in ways other than ulcerogenesis. Patients with diabetes may manifest certain musculoskeletal disorders with increased frequency compared with similar nondiabetic populations.[39–48] Despite the lack of bearing that some of these disorders have on ulcerogenesis, they nevertheless are relevant to comprehensive foot care provided to diabetic patients. Thus, management of these problems as they appear in the feet of patients requires an increased awareness of their existence and of the potentially unique aspects of management of these disorders in diabetes.

Previous reports have addressed musculoskeletal disorders associated with diabetes mellitus[39–48] but only in a general way. The intention in this chapter is to focus specifically on noninfectious musculoskeletal disorders of the diabetic foot. Conditions that may be found in the diabetic foot are described. When applicable, pathogenesis is discussed. The incidence of the disorder and its relationship to diabetes mellitus are explored. Most important, signs, symptoms, and management of selected disorders are addressed. In summary, the aim of this chapter is to increase awareness and recognition of musculoskeletal disorders of the diabetic foot so that comprehensive management of the diabetic foot is facilitated.

NEUROARTHROPATHY

Numerous detailed reviews of neuroarthropathy in diabetes have been published, using varying terminology (such as *Charcot's joint, osteoarthropathy, neuropathic osteoarthropathy,* and *neuropathic joint*) for the disorder.[22–28, 39, 45, 49–60] It is not the goal of this chapter to reproduce these discussions of neuroarthropathy but to review the pertinent aspects of the disorder and place it within the context of musculoskeletal disorders that can affect the diabetic foot.

Neuroarthropathy commonly manifests as periarticular fracture or joint dislocation of one or more of the joints of the foot and ankle. The prevalence of neuroarthropathy among all patients with diabetes is probably 1% or less.[27, 28, 30, 39] However, among those with neuropathic diabetes the prevalence may be as high as 29%.[52] There is no apparent sex predisposition.[27, 39] The condition most frequently has its onset in patients in their fifth through seventh decades of life.[39, 45] Neuroarthropathy generally occurs in patients who have had diabetes for 10 years or more.[28, 39] The tarsometatarsal articulations (Lisfranc's joint) are the most commonly affected (31%), followed closely by the metatarsophalangeal (MTP) joints (29%) (Figs. 16–1 and 16–2).[39] The tarsal articulations are the next most commonly affected (24%), with talonavicular and calcaneocuboid (Chopart's joint) predominating over subtalar sites (Fig. 16–3).[39] The ankle joint (11%) and interphalangeal joints (5%) are relatively less frequently involved (Fig. 16–4).[39]

Pathogenesis

The pathogenesis of these potentially disastrous fracture-dislocations has been a source of debate over the years. However, there is now perhaps a greater degree of agreement over the pathogenesis and contributory risk factors than ever before. The most detailed accounts of risk factors and pathogenesis recently have been by Banks and McGlamry[22] and Sanders and Frykberg.[27] The three most important risk factors are autonomic vasomotor neuropathy, disruptive mechanical forces, and sensory neuropathy.

Autonomic vasomotor neuropathy results in peripheral vasodilatation, bounding pulses, thermal inversion (foot warmer than the leg), increased blood flow to bone, open arteriovenous shunts, and distended pedal veins. The increased blood flow to the bone is generally thought to produce localized osteopenia and increased susceptibility to fracture-dislocation on exposure to deleterious forces. Although patients with diabetes have been shown to be slightly osteopenic,[39] this has not translated to an increase in the risk of fracture.[61] An alternate explanation for the pathogenic role of vasomotor neuropathy may be that the increased blood flow to the bone increases the periarticular intramedullary osseous pressure, potentially creating focal areas of osteonecrosis.[62]

At this point, both exogenous and endogenous mechanical forces may be able to disrupt the periarticular integrity more readily. The magnitude of the forces, therefore, does not necessarily have to be extreme, as is the case for most traumatic fracture-dislocations in normal persons. Exogenous forces such as a minor ''sprain,'' a trivial stubbing injury, and even an excessive period of normal walking activity may be enough to initiate the process. One must not belittle the role that endogenous forces play in pathogenesis. Gastrosoleal equinus, which is often found in patients with diabetic neuroarthropathy, may generate key forces across the joints most frequently involved with neuroarthropathy (Fig. 16–5). Furthermore, sensorimotor neuropathy may create a degree of ataxia, which additionally provides deleterious forces for the articular structures to contend with.

The forces may not produce instantaneous fracture-dislocation but instead may create periarticular inflammation or joint effusion, which further contributes to osteonecrosis by additionally increasing intramedullary osseous pressure. Alternatively, the forces may create only a stress injury to the periarticular bone. Regardless, sensory neuropathy completes

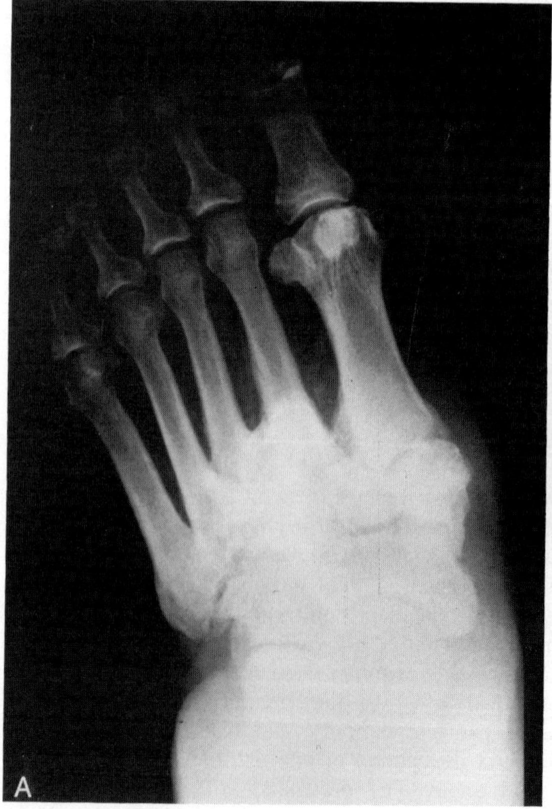

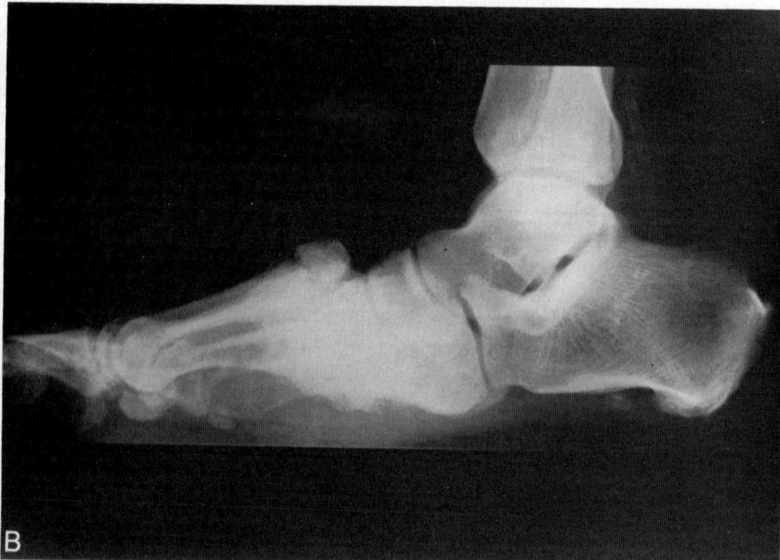

FIGURE 16–1. Anteroposterior *(A)* and lateral *(B)* radiographs of neuroarthropathy affecting the tarsometatarsal (Lisfranc's) joints, which are the most common pedal sites encountered.

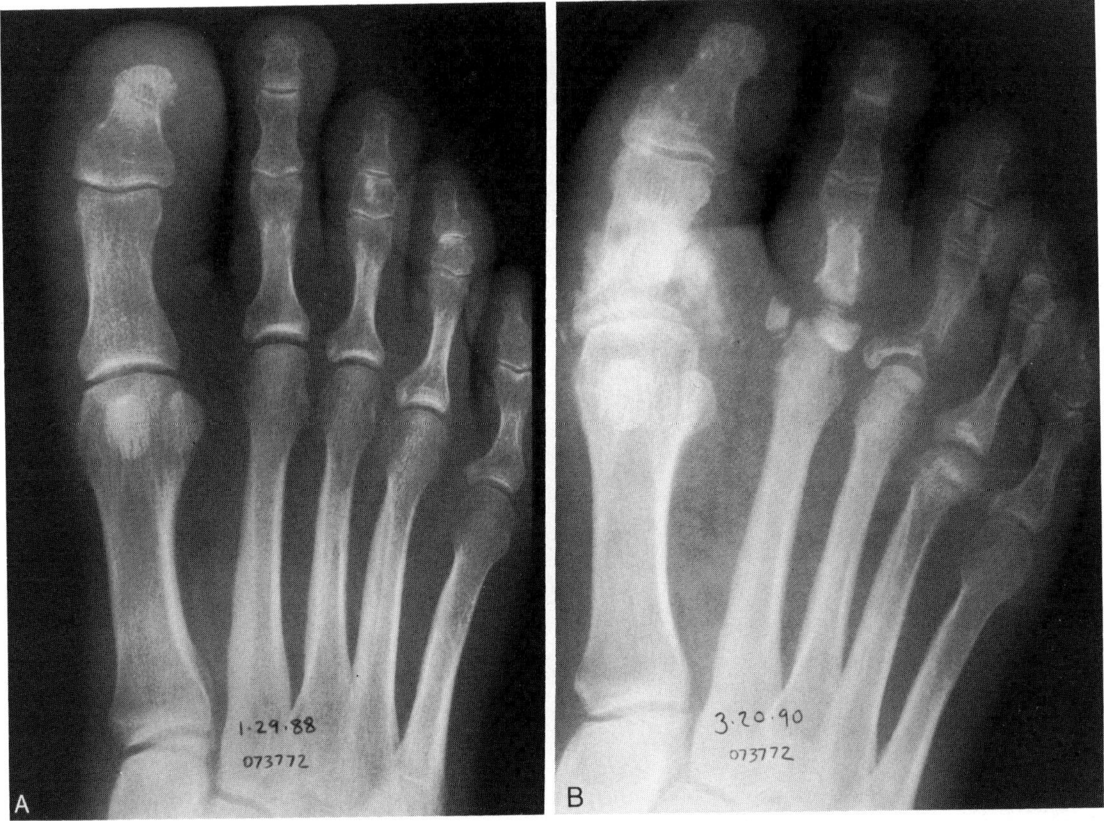

FIGURE 16–2. Before *(A)* and after *(B)* anteroposterior radiographs of neuroarthropathy affecting the first through fourth metatarsophalangeal joints.

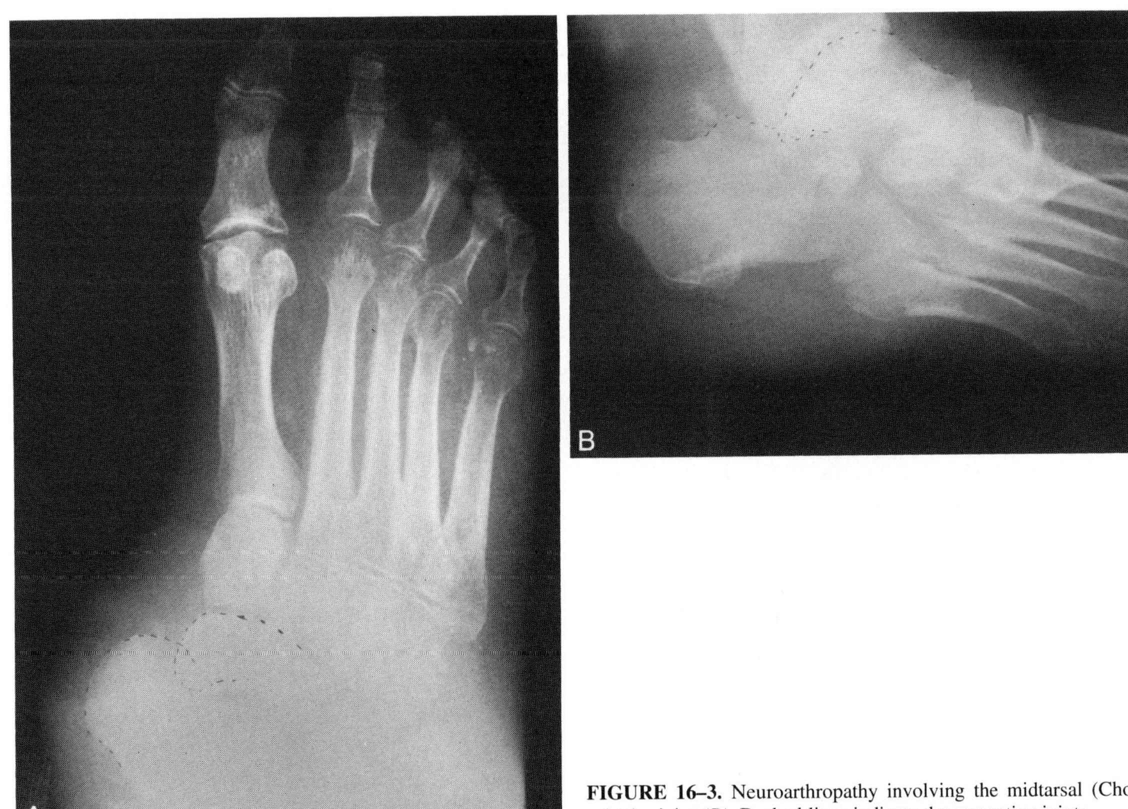

FIGURE 16–3. Neuroarthropathy involving the midtarsal (Chopart's) joint *(A)* and the subtalar joint *(B)*. Dashed lines indicate the respective joints.

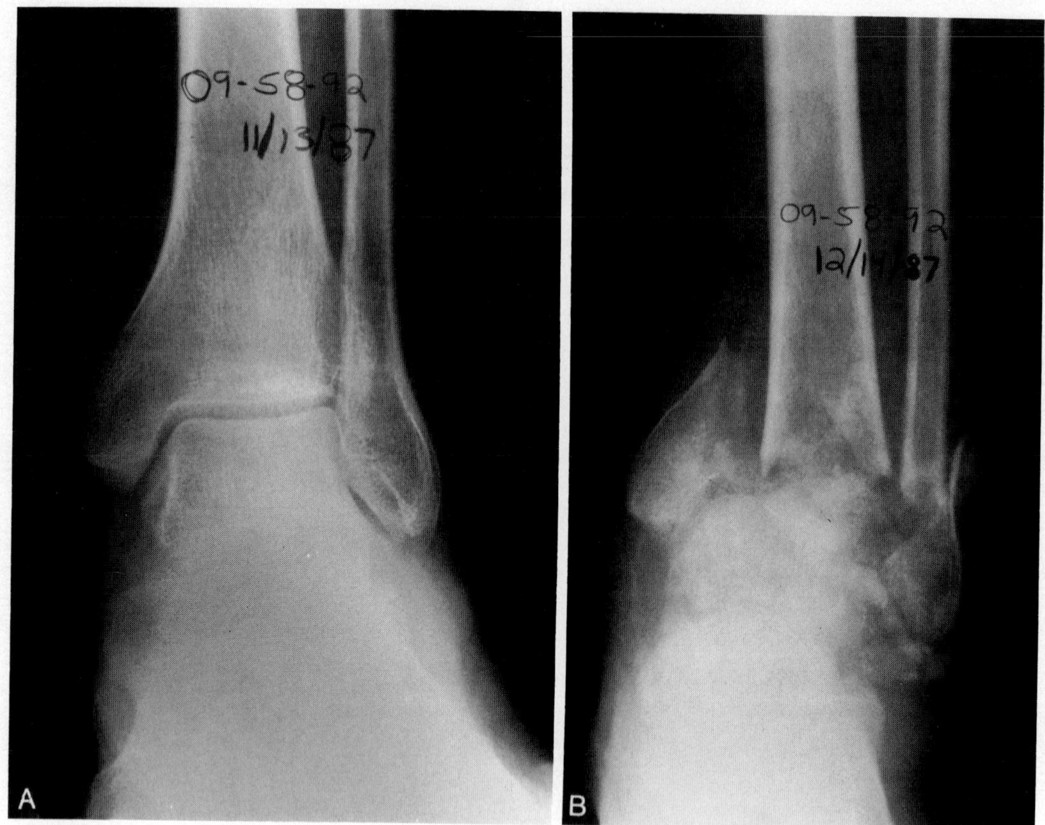

FIGURE 16–4. Before *(A)* and after *(B)* anteroposterior radiographs of neuroarthropathy affecting the ankle joint.

the pathologic scenario by depriving the patient of a protective withdrawal behavior. Without a pain response to the initial periarticular changes, the patient continues with unrestricted activities until overt disruption of the periarticular structures is complete. Chronologically, the pathogenesis may take days to weeks. But, in the absence of rest or even protective limping reflexes, periarticular disruption continues until the displacement of the fracture fragments and joints is striking.

Once periarticular collapse and dislocation have occurred, the ultimate disposition of the joint is dependent on a number of intervening factors. On the one hand, if the foot is either not treated or treated inappropriately, the joint is likely to proceed through a cycle of injury, followed by an incomplete healing attempt, followed by reinjury. During this cycle, the displacement of the osseous structures is likely to progress, resulting in a severely distorted and chronically warm, swollen foot. The foot becomes increasingly difficult to shod.

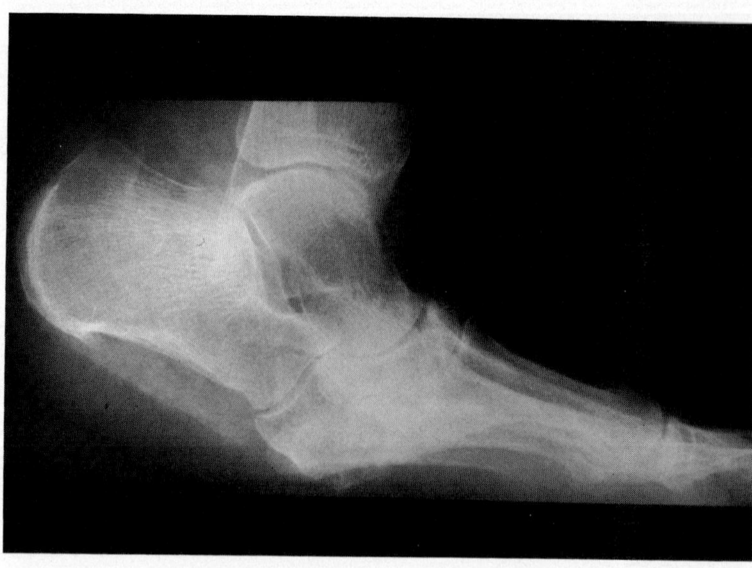

FIGURE 16–5. Neuroarthropathy of the tarsometatarsal and lesser tarsal joints associated with significant gastrosoleal equinus, resulting in an equinus position of the hindfoot and rocker-bottom deformity.

Normal gait is sacrificed as the foot continues to destabilize. Furthermore, bony prominences may develop owing to the subluxation, which in turn are associated with extremely high weightbearing pressures.[63] The extreme focal stresses in the presence of an insensate foot set the scenario for neuropathic ulceration.[17] The untreated or inappropriately treated ulcer may become deeper and infected, eventually resulting in osteomyelitis at the site of the bony prominence. In the end, it is possible that amputation may be required for the neglected foot with neuroarthropathy owing to either diffuse osteomyelitis or intractable shoeing difficulties.

On the other hand, the process may be arrested with appropriate treatment. If the process is arrested in the precollapse phase of development, the foot architecture may be preserved and ultimately maintained with appropriate shoeing, patient education, and activity modification. If the process is arrested after collapse has ensued, osseous healing is still possible. Unfortunately, areas of bony prominence are predisposed to ulceration, but appropriate preventive efforts may be employed. In either instance, the best sign that the process has been successfully arrested is that the temperature of the foot returns to baseline (or symmetrical with the contralateral foot) and swelling resolves. Basing a definition of arrest on radiographic findings may be unreliable. Bone scans remain hot well after arrest has been achieved. Furthermore, it is a misconception that the end result of arrested neuroarthropathy is autofusion of the involved joint. Although autofusion occurs frequently in neuroarthropathy of the spine, it is uncommon in the foot.[39, 45]

Although appropriate treatment and aftercare may guarantee a lasting arrest of the process, as long as the risk factors remain present there is a chance of reactivation. It is impossible to restore a patient's sensory status to an acceptable threshold level at this point. However, proper education may help compensate for the persisting neuropathy. Although vasomotor neuropathy also is unlikely to undergo spontaneous regression, it is possible to observe a reduction in the hypervascular state associated with neuroarthropathy. In instances when atherosclerotic disease progresses, diminishing available blood flow to the foot, it is possible that a lasting arrest may ensue. Ephedrine can effectively reverse the effects of vasomotor neuropathy, although this drug has not been used in the management of neuroarthropathy.[64] Finally, a lasting arrest is often based on a resolution of disruptive mechanical forces. The forces may inherently resolve with collapse of the foot. However, direct intervention, in the form of shoeing and activity modification, is most frequently employed to ensure that disruptive forces are resolved.

Classification

Although pathologically correct classification systems for neuroarthropathy have been presented in other sources, they are generally not management oriented. Therefore, rather than discuss the earlier systems, it may be more useful to present an adapted classification (based on the temporal evolution of neuroarthropathy just discussed) that can also be used to guide management (Table 16–1). The system defines four stages of neuroarthropathy, with an additional designation used in instances when either a preceding or concurrent ulcer is located in the area of the neuroarthropathy. Stage progression often proceeds from I to IV, with patients generally seeking care while in stage II or III. If no treatment is sought or inappropriate therapy is provided, patients may continue the cycle through stages II and III. In instances in which a high index of suspicion is employed, an early diagnosis in stage I may lead to an arrest (stage IV) without progression through stages II and III. Although it is the goal of management to keep the condition arrested in stage IV, it is possible for pathologic changes to be reactivated and return to stage I or II again.

Evaluation

Two keys to effective management of neuroarthropathy are a high index of suspicion and an early diagnosis. The ideal situation would be to identify a process in stage I or early stage II and arrest the process with little or no distortion of the foot architecture (and therefore function). A knowledgeable diagnostic effort is essential.

A history of a recent onset of periarticular swelling should be interpreted as highly suspicious. The patient may complain of a vague ache or there may be no pain at all. The patient may or may not have noticed changes in pedal alignment. Close attention should be given to recent trauma, even trivial episodes. Similarly, any recent changes in activity level or work duties should be explored. The history should also be devoted to investigating other potential causes of swelling, including infection, venous insufficiency, thrombophlebitis, congestive heart failure, renal failure, reflex sympathetic dystrophy, and other arthritic diatheses, such as gout.

Physical Examination. On physical examination, it is important first to verify that intrinsic risk factors for neuroarthropathy are present. Sensory neuropathy should be present. Patients at risk generally fail to recognize the Semmes-Weinstein 5.07 monofilament. Autonomic vasomotor neuropathy should also be present. The examiner should be able to ascertain this by recognizing the aforementioned pedal signs of vasomotor neuropathy, including bounding pulses, thermal inversion, and distended pedal veins. Furthermore, distended veins generally fail to collapse on raising of the foot just above the level of the heart.[66] The clinical manifestations of neuroarthropathy should also be investigated but will vary, depending on the stage in which the patient presents (see Table 16–1). If an associated ulcer is present, it should be fully evaluated, with particular attention to tracking and clinical signs of infection. Finally, the clinical examination should continue with the investigation of potential mimickers, which was started with the history.

Radiographic Examination. Bilateral standard radiographs should be obtained. The contralateral foot serves as a comparison against which subtle changes may be detected. Furthermore, the contralateral radiographs serve as a baseline for that side. It is not uncommon for an unprotected contralateral foot to succumb to neuroarthropathy during the some times long period of enforced non-weightbearing on the originally affected foot.[67] The radiographic findings may be subtle or overt, depending on the stage of disease at which the patient presents (see Table 16–1). In patients with no radiographic evidence of injury or history of neuroarthropathy, a three-phase technetium bone scan may aid in the diagnosis of stage I neuroarthropathy. In patients with a prior history of neuroarthropathy that has arrested and now is suspected of reactivating, the bone scan is of no benefit

TABLE 16–1

CLASSIFICATION, FINDINGS, AND MANAGEMENT ALTERNATIVES FOR THE DIABETIC NEUROARTHROPATHY

Stage*	Findings	Management Alternatives†
I. Precollapse	Bounding pulses Periarticular swelling Thermal inversion Joint effusion Normal clinical alignment Normal radiographic findings, except increased soft tissue density, volume	Below-knee, non-weightbearing cast Alternative immobilization techniques Alternative methods of non-weightbearing Ephedrine? Activity/work restriction Protection of contralateral foot
II. Collapse	Bounding pulses Increased swelling and local temperature Hypermobility Clinical malalignment Fractures, fragmentation, and/or dislocation on radiograph	Below-knee, non-weightbearing cast Electrical bone stimulation? Ephedrine? Activity/work restriction Protection of contralateral foot
III. Healing	Bounding pulses Decreased, but persistent swelling and local hyperthermia Reduction of hypermobility Unchanging clinical alignment Periosteal new bone Hypertrophic bone formation Resorption of finer debris	Below-knee, non-weightbearing cast Walking cast Patellar bearing brace Electrical bone stimulation? Ephedrine? Activity/work restriction Protection of contralateral foot
IV. Arrest	Bounding, normal or decreased pulses Resolved swelling and local hyperthermia Reduced joint motion Unchanging clinical alignment Consolidation of fractures/fragments	Custom-molded or extra-depth shoe Custom-molded insoles Rigid rocker soles Activity/work modification Patient education/inspection Follow-up every 1–2 months Achilles lengthening Partial ostectomy Reconstruction/stabilization

*If an ulcer was associated with the affected joint area prior to the current stage or is present concurrently with the stage, then the stage should have the additional designation of ''u'' (i.e., Iu, IIu, IIIu, IVu). Management may then require a work-up to rule out osteomyelitis, if clinical findings are suggestive.

†Secondary measures are indented.

Adapted from Eichenholtz SN: Charcot Joints, 1966. Courtesy of Charles C Thomas, Publisher, Springfield, Illinois.

diagnostically. Furthermore, confirmation of reactivation of a previously collapsed joint on plain radiographs may be extremely difficult. The examiner may have to rely solely on clinical evidence to make that judgment. An additional imaging dilemma presents itself when the examiner must rule out osteomyelitis in the presence of neuroarthropathy. This dilemma can arise particularly in stage IIu or IIIu. Use of magnetic resonance imaging (MRI) is becoming increasingly important in this scenario.[68] Other options include combinations of a three-phase technetium scan with either a gallium scan or an indium-labeled white blood cell scan.[60, 68] However, the most accurate method of diagnosis is obtaining a bone specimen for culture and microscopic diagnosis. Finally, the examiner should interpret radiographs with the awareness that there may be some pathologic mimicry posed by disorders other than osteomyelitis and septic arthritis, such as diabetic osteopathy and osteolysis, gout, osteoarthritis, diffuse idiopathic skeletal hyperostosis (DISH), and pathologic fractures.

Treatment

If two keys to management of neuroarthropathy are a high index of suspicion and an early diagnosis, then a final key to management is that regardless of stage, some type of attenuation of deleterious forces must be employed. In stages I through III, the ideal method of accomplishing this goal is to employ a non-weightbearing below-knee cast and to severely restrict activities, including work. This therapy should be continued until the condition is clearly in stage IV (signified clinically by the lack of swelling and the return to a baseline, nonelevated local skin temperature), which may take from 6 weeks to 6 months. In stage IV, the goal can be accomplished with the use of extra-depth or custom-molded shoes with custom-molded insoles and a rigid rocker sole. In addition, the patient should be allowed to return only to activities and work that have been modified to significantly reduce the potential for reactivation.

Other universal interventions, regardless of stage, include control of blood glucose levels and protection of the contralateral foot. It is clear that grossly elevated blood glucose levels contribute to delayed healing. Therefore, blood glucose levels should be closely managed to ensure an optimal rate of healing. Protection of the opposite foot is important owing to its inherent predisposition toward neuroarthropathy, given the symmetrical nature of diabetic sensory and autonomic neuropathy and the increased load that the contralateral foot must bear during the off-loading of the originally affected foot. Thus, a supportive shoe with a custom-molded insole should be employed for the contralateral foot from the onset of treatment. Activity and work restriction are important in the protection of the contralateral foot as well.

Although the aforementioned interventions are ideal guidelines, not every patient is always managed in the manner described. Depending on the stage, additional or alternative interventions may be employed. In stage I, the practitioner may use alternative forms of immobilization, such as an Unna's boot, a posterior splint, or a Jones dressing. The demand for absolute immobilization may not be as great in stage I. Alternate methods of off-loading may be employed, such as various commercially available half-shoe designs that off-load the MTP area. Finally, the use of ephedrine may hold promise in the correction of the abnormal blood flow in neuroarthropathy, although the effectiveness of its use in neuroarthropathy has not been established.[64]

In stage II, the practitioner is afforded less latitude in methods of immobilization and off-loading, regardless of site of involvement. Although not tested under the confines of a controlled, double-blind study, adjuncts such as electrical bone stimulation[69] and ephedrine[64] are interesting for their potential use in this stage.

Stage III should be managed essentially in the same manner as stage II. However, based on the clinical judgment of the practitioner, the patient may be converted to protected weightbearing in late stage III. Examples of potentially suitable alternatives to the non-weightbearing below-knee cast (ideal) in late stage III are the walking cast and the patellar-bearing brace.

In addition to the previously described methods of management for stage IV, at least two other aspects of management should be uniformly applied. First, the patient should receive general education for care of the neuropathic foot. Patients should be taught that they are at risk for both reactivation of neuroarthropathy and neuropathic ulceration. Patients should be taught to inspect the skin for signs of breakdown. Most important, patients should be taught to inspect their feet for areas of increased swelling and increased local temperature, because these signs may indicate the beginnings of an ulcer or reactivation of neuroarthropathy. If the signs are observed on inspection, patients must understand that it is imperative that they see the practitioner as soon as possible, so that early preventive care may be provided. Second, it is important to establish regular follow-up visits at 1- to 2-month intervals to ensure that the foot is ulcer free and the condition is remaining in a state of stage IV arrest. This schedule ensures that sequelae are addressed early. In addition, shoes and insoles should be inspected and palliative care provided.

Despite the appropriate management already described, some patients continue to experience sequelae. Examples include (1) recurrent episodes of reactivation and mutilating subluxation; (2) recurrent ulcerations; (3) recalcitrant shoeing problems; and (4) osteomyelitis. Although management of osteomyelitis is beyond the scope of this chapter, the management of the other noninfected, recalcitrant sequelae (1 to 3 above) deserves some discussion. In patients with noninfected sequelae that are recalcitrant to the appropriate-stage management protocols, surgery may be an option that can be evaluated. However, regardless of the type of surgery to be performed, the patient's diabetes should meet at least the following minimum general criteria: Medical and endocrinologic stability, adequate peripheral vascular status, and neuroarthropathy arrested in stage IV.[38]

Surgical Management. For recurrent episodes of reactivation and mutilating subluxation, as well as for recalcitrant shoeing problems, reconstruction and stabilization through arthrodesing procedures may be the only alternatives other than amputation for tarsometatarsal, tarsal, and ankle sites.[22, 58] For MTP sites, local resection arthroplasty or panmetatarsal head resection may be suitable alternatives to transmetatarsal amputation.[22, 58] It is critical to evaluate the patient for gastrosoleal equinus, and if found, to include an Achilles tendon lengthening in the surgical treatment plan.[22] It is important to focus the evaluation on dorsiflexion of the hindfoot, because a rocker-bottom deformity may give the false impression that there is adequate dorsiflexion of the foot to the leg. Failure to correct a significant equinus may directly lead to the failure of the aforementioned reconstructive procedures.

The same reconstructive efforts just described also may be employed for recurrent ulcerations associated with bony prominences. However, in many patients, simple resection of the prominent portion of bone may be ameliorative and thus the preferred mode of treatment.[27] Once again, strong consideration should be given to lengthening the Achilles tendon if gastrosoleal equinus is present.[38]

Regardless of which of the aforementioned surgical procedures are to be employed, it is advisable to incorporate some period of non-weightbearing cast immobilization into the postoperative management. The rationale is threefold. First, the period in the non-weightbearing cast promotes healing in the lesser procedures and is required for healing in the arthrodesis and tendon procedures. Second, surgery may activate the neuroarthropathy process again. The period in a non-weightbearing cast prevents stage advancement and facilitates arrest. Finally, because the patient is neuropathic, there is no painful stimulus to deter full weightbearing as there would be in normal postoperative patients. Without enforcing a non-weightbearing period in a cast, the patient is likely to ambulate excessively on the operated foot, producing a severe deleterious effect on healing. The period that a non-weightbearing cast must be employed varies. For resection procedures, 3 to 6 weeks may be sufficient. When an Achilles tendon lengthening is also performed, the period may increase to 6 to 8 weeks. For reconstructive arthrodesis procedures, the period may last as long as 6 months. Gradual reintroduction of weightbearing forces is advised. Moreover, the patient must be refitted with an appropriate shoe and custom-molded insole. No surgical procedure is intended to supplant appropriate shoeing and insoles.

Although surgical management of recalcitrant cases can be successful, both the surgeon and the patient should be aware of the potential complications. Examples include infection; delayed wound healing; delayed union or nonunion; reactivation of neuroarthropathy; transfer ulcers; transfer neuroarthropathy; and loss of digits, limb, or life. In analyzing the potential risks, the advantage of salvage must be weighed against the alternative of electing amputation. Comparative studies of salvage versus amputation of the foot with recalcitrant sequelae of neuroarthropathy are not available.

In summary, neuroarthropathy is a potentially disastrous manifestation that can occur in the patient with diabetes with sensory and autonomic vasomotor neuropathy. Keys to management include a high index of suspicion, early diagnosis, and attenuation of deleterious forces acting on the foot. Most patients are successfully managed conservatively, using the stage protocols presented here. However, some patients have conditions that are recalcitrant, and surgical intervention may be required.

DIABETIC OSTEOLYSIS

Relatively less is known about diabetic osteolysis, otherwise called *diabetic osteopathy,* than neuroarthropathy. Nevertheless, the condition receives a fair amount of attention in the literature.[23–25, 27, 41, 44, 45, 55, 57, 68, 70–77] The condition presents with sometimes striking resorption of bone from the periarticular regions of the MTP joints, interphalangeal joints, or distal phalangeal tufts, with an almost equally striking capacity in some instances to completely reconstitute the involved bony structure (Fig. 16–6). Although the disorder is undoubtedly associated with the diabetic state, its prevalence has not been clearly established, perhaps because of asymptomatic cases that are not diagnosed or confusion in terminology and a tendency to include diabetic osteopathy-osteolysis with neuroarthropathy as a single entity.[23–25, 27] Nevertheless, true osteolysis is probably less prevalent among patients with diabetes than is neuroarthropathy. In a study of 67 patients with diabetic neuropathy plus bone and joint disorders, true osteolysis was demonstrated in 12 (18%), whereas neuroarthropathy was observed in 54 (81%).[57]

Pathogenesis

The pathogenesis of diabetic osteolysis is not well understood. Most authors believe that the process is caused by

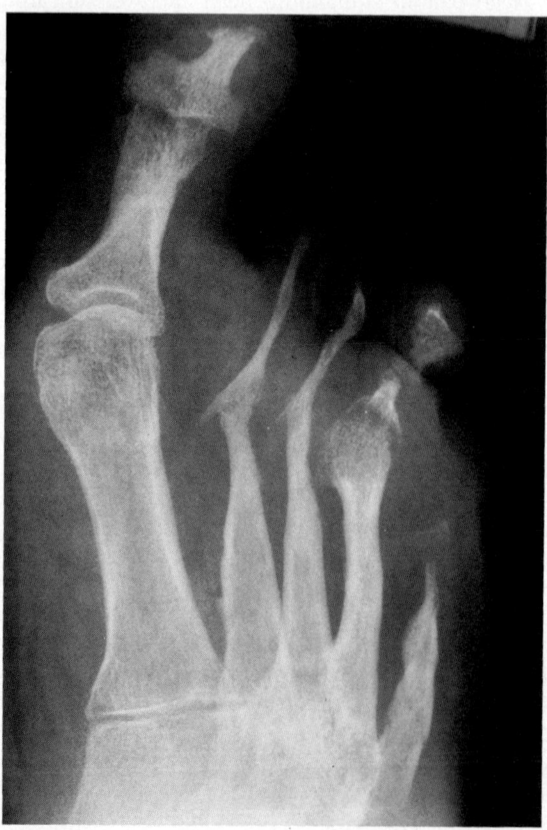

FIGURE 16–6. Anteroposterior radiograph of a foot with marked permanent diabetic osteolysis.

osteoclasis and bone resorption induced by the hypervascular status of bone that arises with autonomic vasomotor neuropathy.[24, 25, 27, 39, 41, 45, 68, 71, 74, 76] Diminished sensitivity to pain has also been cited as a factor.[41, 45, 55, 76] However, the condition can be observed in the absence of sensory neuropathy, which differentiates it from neuroarthropathy.[41, 44, 68, 75] Some authors believe that the changes are secondary to an infectious process.[77] Although the condition can be seen concurrently with an ulcer,[74, 77] osseous changes can be seen in sites where no portal has been known to exist[27] and no prior infection has been noted.[55, 68, 70] Furthermore, bone affected by osteolysis can revert to a normal state spontaneously, without evidence of sequestrum or involucrum, unlike osteomyelitis.[41, 44] Some authors believe that ischemia or microvascular disease may play a role.[45, 55, 73] However, avascular bone remains sclerotic, whereas osteopenia requires adequate vascularity.[55] In addition, osteolysis is generally found in a foot that is not ischemic.[44, 68, 74] Finally, some authors believe that trauma may be a factor.[41, 76]

On further analysis, it may be possible that at least one other process may be involved—a derangement of local prostaglandin metabolism. Prostaglandins, particularly those of the prostaglandin E (PGE) class, are noted to induce significant bone resorption, both in vitro and in vivo.[78] In diabetes, increased synthesis of PGE has been noted in cell systems such as platelets.[79] Increased synthesis can be triggered by a number of inciting factors and perhaps reversed by improved metabolic control.[79]

It is conceivable that the pathogenesis of diabetic osteolysis may be initiated by local inflammation caused by trauma, increased weightbearing forces, ulceration, or even local soft tissue infection. The inflammation, in turn, may trigger an exaggerated synthesis of PGE, which, potentiated by a hypervascular state resulting from vasomotor neuropathy, may produce the characteristic changes seen in diabetic osteolysis. Continued weightbearing on the osteopenic bone may initiate structural damage. In the absence of sensory neuropathy, a painful stimulus may lead to a self-imposed period of rest, which may allow local inflammation to subside and the bone to revert to normal. In the presence of sensory neuropathy, continued exposure to deleterious forces is ensured, allowing more serious and potentially irreversible structural damage to the affected bone.

Evaluation

Evaluation of the patient primarily should be directed at ruling out an infectious process. When giving the history, the patient may or may not report pain.[75] The patient generally does not report findings of swelling or change in foot architecture, as may be the case with neuroarthropathy. A history of trauma or increased weightbearing activities or work should be investigated. The history should also be used to rule out other mimickers of the bone changes besides osteomyelitis, such as Hansen's disease, psoriatic arthritis, and systemic sclerosis.

Physical Examination. On physical examination, sensory neuropathy may or may not be detected.[41, 44, 68, 75] Signs of autonomic vasomotor neuropathy may predominate over those of sensory neuropathy. Pulses are generally present, and signs of ischemia are generally absent.[44, 68, 74] Mild swelling and increased local temperature may be present, but not to the degree seen in neuroarthropathy. Alignment is generally not disturbed in the early stage, but foreshortening of the affected toe may be seen in severe cases.[27, 55] A pre-existing hammertoe may be present. Hyperkeratoses (corns and calluses) may be seen on the distal aspect of the toe, on the dorsal aspect of an interphalangeal joint, or under the metatarsal head, signifying increased mechanical forces acting on the site. Ulcers may be seen adjacent to the involved site.[74, 77] If infection is present, osteomyelitis should be ruled out.

Radiographic Examination. Bilateral standard radiographs of the feet are advisable. Radiographic findings can be classified as physiologic and pathologic. Early findings are physiologic changes in the bone associated with the pathogenic process previously described. Initially, a subtle thinning of the metaphyseal cortices of a phalanx or distal metatarsal may be missed.[44, 55, 74] The osteopenia then extends throughout the metaphyseal region.[44, 45, 55] Early metaphyseal osteopenia may give the appearance of a juxta-articular cortical defect or erosion.[27, 55, 57, 70, 74] Progression of the osteopenia may eventually give the appearance that the entire metaphyseal segment has been washed away.[44, 45, 55] The subchondral bone and diaphysis are relatively spared.[41, 44, 55, 68, 74]

At a critical level of osteopenia, the bone is predisposed to pathologic structural damage. Progression to pathologic radiographic findings may depend on factors such as continued exposure to deleterious forces and timing of initiation of treatment. If structural damage is minimal or absent and the process can be arrested, the bone may reconstitute to normal levels of mineralization and structure.[27, 45, 68, 70, 73, 75] Otherwise, pathologic changes will ensue.

The distal metatarsal bone with mild to moderate damage may partially reconstitute to the appearance of a Freiberg's infraction.[44, 45, 73] With more advanced damage, the end of the metatarsal looks gnawed off,[55] eventually reconstituting to an appearance described as ''sucked candy'' or ''pencil point.''[24, 25, 27, 55, 70, 73, 76] The base of the proximal phalanx may collapse, with the diaphysis telescoping proximally, eventually reconstituting to an expanded cup shape.[27, 70, 74] If the process involves both ends of the phalanx, the final appearance will resemble an hourglass, with the diaphysis appearing narrowed.[24, 25, 27, 74]

In the physiologic stage, joints are preserved.[41, 45] Only in severe cases of destruction will subluxation of the MTP joint be observed.[27, 74] However, ankylosis is generally not observed, even in cases of relative reconstitution.[41, 44]

More than one ray concurrently may be involved.[74] Rarely, if ever, is hypertrophic bone formation seen throughout the process,[39, 41] which additionally distinguishes osteolysis from neuroarthropathy. Nevertheless, the changes of osteolysis may also be seen concurrent with proximal neuroarthropathy.[24, 25] If osteomyelitis cannot be ruled out on a clinical basis, the combination of a three-phase technetium scan with either a gallium scan or an indium-labeled white blood cell scan may be of some diagnostic benefit.[74]

Treatment

The treatment of diabetic osteolysis is especially ill-defined in the literature. Although most authors fail even to comment on therapy, some say that no specific treatment is required.[57, 74] Others simply state that the condition is self-limiting with conservative care.[55] One author lists rest, proper diet, and metabolic control as therapies, however.[73] Improved metabolic control seems prudent, given the potentially beneficial effect this may have on healing in general and on prostaglandin synthesis more specifically.[79] Furthermore, if prostaglandins are, in part, mediating the osteolysis, consideration might be given to the use of inhibitors of arachidonic acid metabolism, such as aspirin and nonsteroidal anti-inflammatory drugs. Specific management of diabetic osteolysis involving the MTP joints is best accomplished by following the primary management guidelines already presented for neuroarthropathy. This form of management improves the potential for anatomic reconstitution and decreases the chances of transfer weightbearing and its sequelae to an adjacent metatarsal. Management of distal osteolysis not involving the MTP joint can be accomplished by placing the patient in a protective healing sandal or postoperative shoe until arrest is achieved. Thereafter, the patient should be placed in appropriately fitting shoes and followed for recurrences.

GENERALIZED OSTEOPENIA

Numerous reports on generalized osteopenia associated with diabetes mellitus have appeared in the literature.[39, 44–46, 55, 57, 61, 73, 74, 80–104] Among these, there is conclusive evidence that a loss of bone mineral content (BMC) is associated with type I diabetes mellitus.[85–97, 99–101, 103] The BMC of type I diabetes typically is approximately an average of 10% lower than that in age- and sex-matched control groups as measured by photon absorption technique.[87, 91–97, 99, 103] The deficit of BMC seen in type I diabetes is usually accounted for within the first few years of onset.[88, 90–93, 96, 99, 103] The rate and severity of BMC loss during this initial period apparently parallel the loss of β cell function in these patients.[93, 94, 96, 97] Although there can be milder expressions of BMC loss during this period, the deficit can be as much as 20%.[94, 97] After approximately 5 years, there is usually no advancement of the BMC deficit, unless the patient demonstrates microangiopathic complications.[91]

In type II diabetes, BMC may be lower than,[81, 89, 92, 98, 102] equal to,[39, 104] or higher than[81] the BMC of age- and sex-matched control groups. The BMC findings of various studies of type II diabetes are more difficult to assess owing to the potential heterogeneity of this population of patients (e.g., body weight, therapy, and β cell function) and the different methodologies employed by the various researchers.[86]

The mechanism for the early loss in BMC is not fully understood, but a multifactorial process involving metabolic and hormonal effects is postulated.[80, 85–87, 93–95, 97, 98, 100, 103] Later mineral loss may be related to the effects of microvascular disease.[91]

Generalized osteopenia of the foot (not associated with disuse) has been described in diabetes.[55, 57, 84] Geoffroy and associates[84] demonstrated generalized osteoporosis on the pedal radiographs of 12.2% of 1501 patients with diabetes. Newman[57] demonstrated similar pedal changes on radiographs in 7 of 67 (10.4%) patients with diabetes.

Whether the magnitude of osteopenia in diabetes is associated with an increased risk of fracture is controversial.[45] Some authors imply that there may be an increased risk,[73, 86] whereas others state that there is not.[44, 61] Authors that present evidence in support of an increased fracture risk generally cite studies in which the percentage of patients with diabetes among patients with femoral neck fracture (10% to 30%) is higher than the percentage of diabetes in the general population (6%).[39, 73] Conversely, the study by Heath and associates[61] serves as the foundation for authors who argue that there is no increased fracture risk.[39, 44] At first glance, the study appears well performed and convincing in its argument against an increased fracture risk in diabetics.[61] However, the patients were not classified according to their diabetes type (type I or II) or by the presence of microvascular complications, which may have influenced the results.

The aforementioned deficiencies notwithstanding, Heath and associates[61] did record a significantly higher rate of ankle fractures among patients with diabetes, in contrast with the general population. In addition, Newman reported two cases of ''spontaneous'' phalangeal fracture among seven patients with generalized osteopenia of the feet (28.6%).[57] Despite the possibility that there may be clinical significance attached to the loss of BMC in patients with diabetes, no specific treatment has been identified.

DIFFUSE IDIOPATHIC SKELETAL HYPEROSTOSIS

DISH is a disorder that encompasses ankylosing hyperostosis of the spine (Forestier's disease), as well as extraspinal ossification of ligamentous and tendinous structures with potential for periosteal new bone formation.[39, 47, 105, 106] DISH appears to occur more frequently in patients with diabetes than in nondiabetics.[39, 43–45, 47, 48, 55, 107] Varying reports have placed the incidence of DISH in diabetic patients between 13% and 49%.[39] In comparison, DISH has been variously found to occur in 1.6% to 13% of nondiabetics.[39] Forgacs[39] reported the prevalence of DISH in 500 patients with diabetes older than 40 years of age to be 23.6%, whereas in 500 age-matched nondiabetic controls, the prevalence was 3.1%. When patients with DISH are examined for the presence of diabetes, between 12% and 32% will be found to have the condition.[39] If both diabetes and abnormal glucose tolerance are evaluated, studies have reported as many as 79% of the patients with DISH have an abnormality of glucose homeostasis.[39]

Pathogenesis

The pathogenesis of DISH in the diabetic patient is not fully understood. However, the condition is not related to the severity or duration of diabetes.[39, 43–45, 107] In contrast, obesity does apparently correlate with DISH.[39, 43–45, 55, 105] In patients both with and without diabetes, the incidence of DISH increases in each decade after 40 years of age; it is relatively unusual before the age of 40 years.[39] However, DISH may appear earlier in patients with diabetes than in nondiabetic patients.[39, 107] Generally, DISH occurs more frequently in males than in females.[44, 47] However, in diabetes, male predominance for the condition is reduced, and studies have failed to show a significant difference in incidence based on gender.[39, 107] DISH appears to occur more frequently in type II diabetes than in type I diabetes.[39, 48] Forgacs[39] found the incidence of DISH in type II diabetes to be 29.3% versus 10.6% in type I diabetes ($P <.001$). In type II diabetes, it is not unusual for DISH to occur just before or after the diagnosis of diabetes.[39] In contrast, the onset of DISH usually occurs years after the diagnosis of diabetes in patients with type I disease.[39] In addition, Forgacs frequently found macroangiopathy in diabetic patients with DISH.[39]

A role in pathogenesis of DISH in patients with diabetes has been postulated for growth hormone and related mediators.[39, 44, 107] It has been established that circulating levels of growth hormone are increased in types I and II diabetes.[108–110] Abnormal levels of growth hormone and its related local mediators have been either demonstrated or postulated to be associated with the pathogenesis of a number of complications of diabetes, including derangement of glucose homeostasis, microvascular disease, and macrovascular disease.[108–110] The incidence of DISH has also been demonstrated to be increased in patients with acromegaly.[107] Furthermore, growth hormone levels have been noted to be significantly higher in patients with DISH than in those without DISH.[39]

It is not unreasonable, therefore, to postulate a permissive role by growth hormone or related local mediators in the pathogenesis of DISH in diabetes. In this scenario, the process may be started by initiating factors at the local level, which may include local trauma or recurrent microtrauma.[39] Growth hormone and related local mediators then may play a role as potentiators.

Evaluation

When evaluating the patient with diabetes, one must remember that DISH is frequently symptomatically silent.[39, 43, 44, 47] However, patients may occasionally complain of stiffness or pain.[39, 43, 44, 47] Among extraspinal sites, the foot and heel may be more frequently associated with symptoms.

Radiographically, DISH can be characterized by ankylosing hyperostosis of the spine, as well as extraspinal involvement.[39, 47] Spinal involvement is confirmed on a lateral radiograph of the spine.[39, 47] Ossification of the anterior longitudinal ligament results in the appearance of flowing ossification along the anterolateral aspect of the vertebral bodies.[39, 47] The diagnosis in the spine is confirmed when at least four contiguous vertebral bodies are involved, whereas the disc spaces are preserved and there is no ankylosis of the sacroiliac or apophyseal joints.[47] The middle and lower thoracic vertebrae are most frequently involved.[47] Thoracic vertebrae are involved more frequently than cervical vertebrae, which in turn are involved more frequently than lumbar vertebrae.[39]

Extraspinal involvement may occur at numerous sites, but the lower extremities predominate.[39, 47, 106] The feet appear to be particularly common extraspinal sites (Fig. 16–7). Radiographic characteristics of DISH in the feet include ossification of the insertions of numerous tendons and ligaments (Achilles tendon, peroneus brevis tendon, plantar fascia, long plantar ligament, unguicular ligaments) and periosteal new bone formation in the metatarsal and phalangeal bones.[39] These findings are often seen in the feet of patients with diabetes.[39, 55, 57, 73, 84, 111]

Treatment

No specific treatment for DISH has been advocated. Pedal symptoms associated with spur formation may be addressed with conservative measures, including padding, shoe modifi-

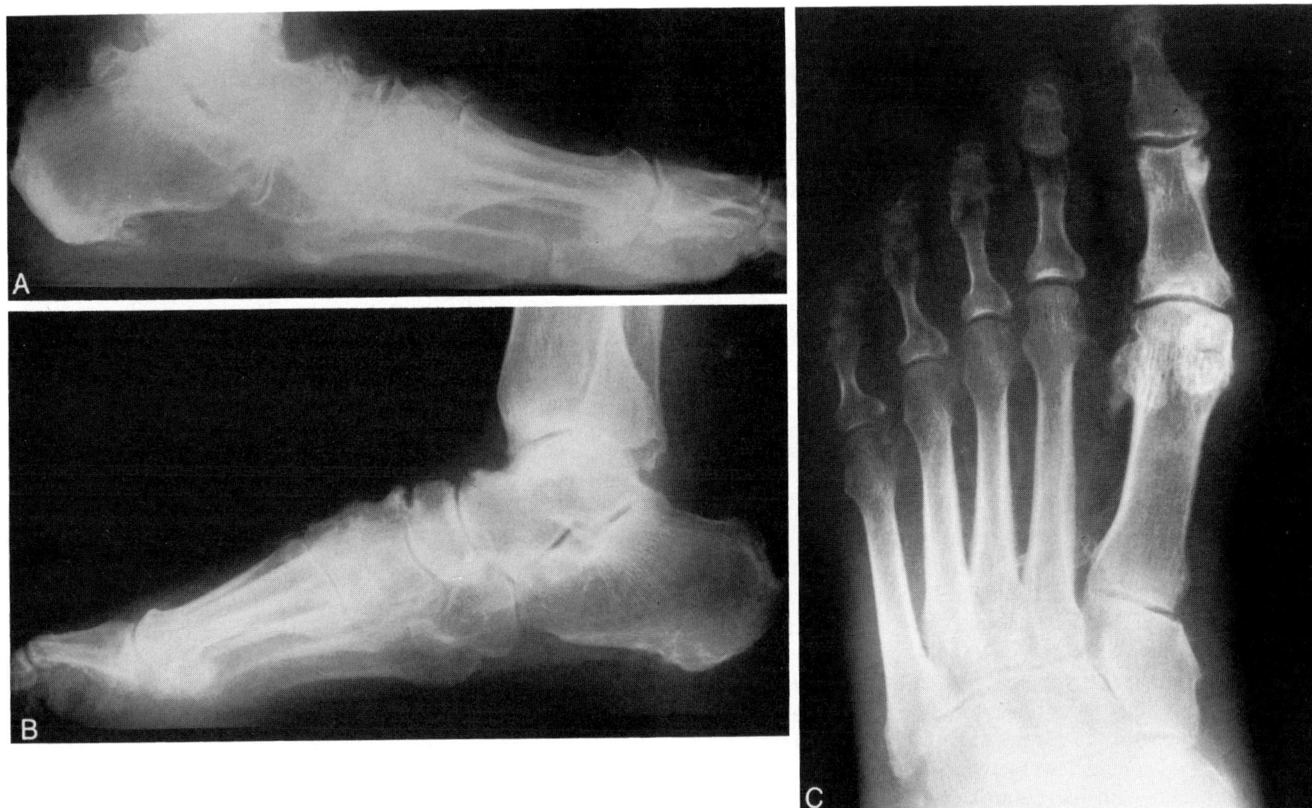

FIGURE 16–7. Examples of pedal manifestations of diffuse idiopathic skeletal hyperostosis in diabetic patients. *A,* Hyperostosis of the plantar fascia insertion and multiple periarticular sites. *B,* Hyperostosis of the plantar fascia insertion, long plantar ligament insertion, Achilles tendon insertion, peroneus brevis insertion, and periarticular sites in the lesser tarsus. *C,* Hyperostosis of peroneus brevis insertion, intrinsic muscle insertion into the fibular sesamoid, first metatarsophalangeal joint collateral ligaments, and unguicular ligaments.

cations, orthoses, injections, and physical therapy. If these measures fail and surgery is contemplated, one must be aware that osseous proliferation can readily recur after removal of the osseous projections in patients with DISH.[47, 112]

LIMITED JOINT MOBILITY

Limited joint mobility (LJM) is a specific condition of progressive reduction of joint mobility in patients with diabetes, which ultimately may be associated with the development of fixed contractures.[42–48, 113–134] Although most references focus on the manifestations of this process in the hands,[42–48, 113–134] LJM also can manifest in the feet,[3, 17, 22, 27, 30, 135–139] as well as other locations.[44, 45, 48, 115, 116, 119, 128, 132]

The prevalence of LJM in diabetes has been reported to be 40% by several secondary sources.[42, 45, 48] However, various studies have demonstrated prevalences for LJM in patients with diabetes ranging from 18% to 55% in type I diabetes[113, 115, 116, 118, 122, 128, 130, 131, 133, 134] and 45% to 76% in type II diabetes.[120, 134] In comparison, the prevalence of LJM in nondiabetic control subjects has been shown to range from 1% to 15%, depending mostly on age.[120, 122, 134] The prevalence of LJM increases with age in patients both with and without diabetes.[123] Thus, in a nondiabetic control group age matched to a young population of patients with diabetes, the prevalence of LJM was 1%,[122] whereas in controls matched to a mixed-age population, the prevalence was 4%,[134] and in control subjects matched to an older population, the prevalence

was 15%.[120] The prevalence of LJM also appears to increase with the duration of diabetes.[113, 118, 128, 130, 131, 133, 134] Costello and associates[118] found that for patients with a type I diabetes duration of 0 to 3 years, the prevalence of LJM was 28%, which increased to 41% in the 4- to 8-year duration group, which in turn increased to 67% in the longer than 8-year duration group. Similarly, Rosenbloom and associates[131] found the prevalence of LJM in patients with type I diabetes for more than 4.5 years to be 49%, compared with a 30% prevalence of LJM in their total test population of patients with type I diabetes. There is no apparent predisposition for LJM, based on the sex[130, 133] or race[130] of the patient.

Pathogenesis

Although the pathogenesis of LJM in diabetes is not fully understood, an important role may be played by nonenzymatic glycosylation of collagen and other proteins in the periarticular region.[17, 22, 27, 42, 44, 45, 116, 139–141] Nonenzymatic glycosylation of a variety of proteins, including collagen, is known to occur in diabetes.[142, 143] This linkage of a sugar to a protein can occur spontaneously, but oxidative stresses also may contribute to the formation of protein glycosylation.[143–145] Proteins, once glycosylated, can undergo further rearrangements, resulting in clinically significant, structurally changed hybrids referred to as *advanced glycosylation end products* (AGEs). In tissues composed of long-lived proteins such as collagen, AGEs tend to accumulate with time (i.e., increasing age and duration of diabetes).[142] Additional factors with potentially direct relationships to AGEs accumulation may include the mean blood glucose levels[142] and oxidative stresses.[143] The structural changes in collagen induced with AGEs formation result in increased cross-linking of collagen, increased stiffness of collagen, AGEs-related fluorescence, entrapment of other soluble proteins, resistance to proteolytic degradation, and potentially increased autoimmunogenicity.[142, 143] Clinically, these changes can lead to increased thickness and stiffness of the periarticular tissues.

A variety of findings associated with LJM suggest that this mechanism, at least in part, plays a pathogenic role. Tight, stiff, thickened, waxlike skin is often associated with LJM.[3, 17, 27, 42, 44–48, 115, 116, 118, 120, 128, 138] As many as 51% of patients with type I diabetes have this finding in conjunction with LJM.[115] Histopathologic studies have revealed that the skin in patients with LJM has alterations of collagen, including increased accumulation in the lower dermis, increased resistance to extraction, and increased cross-linking.[116, 140, 146] Furthermore, nonenzymatic glycosylation of collagen and AGEs formation has been documented in the skin of patients with diabetes and LJM.[116, 140, 141] Monnier and associates[141] measured collagen-linked fluorescence in 41 patients with type I diabetes and 25 control subjects. The amount of fluorescence correlated with both patient age and duration of diabetes, but it was stronger with the former than the latter. Fluorescence levels, adjusted for age, were twice as high in the diabetic group compared with the control group. Finally, increasing fluorescence was found to correlate with LJM.[141]

Nonenzymatic glycosylation of periarticular proteins is consistent with the generalized pathologic process suggested by the diverse sites of involvement associated with LJM, such as multiple upper and lower extremity joints, the skin, and the lungs.[44, 45, 48, 115, 116, 118, 119, 128, 132, 135] Microvascular disease has also been considered by some authors for a potential role in the pathogenesis of LJM.[113, 147] Numerous authors have demonstrated an association between LJM and microvascular disease manifestations, most notably retinopathy.[113, 118–120, 127, 128, 131, 134] However, LJM is often found in the absence of microvascular disease or preceding microvascular changes for years.[44, 118, 119, 123, 131] Specific attempts to demonstrate a microvascular cause for LJM have failed.[147] Therefore, it is unlikely that microvascular disease has a direct pathogenic relationship with LJM. However, the correlation between the two disorders may suggest an independent pathogenic process that is, in part, shared.

Another pathogenic factor in the development of LJM may involve the polyol metabolic pathway.[42, 148] Activation of the polyol pathway can occur in tissues that do not require insulin for glucose transport as a mechanism for diverting excess glucose.[149] Because this is an insulin-independent pathway of glucose metabolism, the process is similar to nonenzymatic glycosylation of proteins.[149] The net accumulation of sugar alcohols, such as sorbitol, produced through the pathway leads to an increased osmotic gradient, among other derangements.[149] Some authors believe that the accumulated sugar alcohols lead to an increase in connective tissue swelling, and thus altered function of the periarticular tissues.[42, 148] In the presence of AGEs collagen, this added insult may produce even more impressive findings.[42] Support for this hypothesis is primarily offered by Eaton and associates,[148] who demonstrated improvement in joint mobility, grip strength, and functional capacity in three patients with severe LJM of the hands after 4 weeks of therapy with an inhibitor of the polyol pathway (aldose reductase inhibitor). Although it is unlikely that this mechanism is the sole pathogenic force in LJM, it is possible that it may contribute to the severity of findings.

Eadington and associates[150] suggested that smoking may be an additional factor that promotes LJM. Cigarette smoking was positively associated with LJM in both type II diabetics and age- and sex-matched control groups. Cigarette smoking may be an oxidative stress that directly contributes by the formation of nonenzymatic glycosylation of tissue proteins or indirectly contributes by the depletion of antioxidants.

Evaluation

Evaluation of the patient with diabetes should be performed with the awareness that LJM may be completely asymptomatic but, despite this, may have considerable podiatric implications. Although generally asymptomatic in the early stages of development, the process can be progressive, eventually leading to symptoms.[42, 48, 128] Symptoms directly related to the LJM may include aching and stiffness.[42, 48] In the hands, LJM can become disabling, with severe immobility, weakness, and in some patients, pain.[42, 48, 148] Hand symptoms may grossly impair activities of daily living, including self-administration of insulin.[148] The feet are generally less symptomatic, more commonly ignored, and may be masked by sensory neuropathy. Nevertheless, LJM in the foot and ankle may play a pathogenic role in foot ulceration as well as neuroarthropathy.[3, 17, 22, 27, 30, 136, 137]

As mentioned earlier, LJM is often associated with overlying skin that is stiff, tight, waxlike, and thickened (Fig. 16–8).[3, 17, 27, 42, 44–48, 115, 116, 118, 120, 128, 138] LJM may also be associated with retinopathy, neuropathy, and perhaps nephropathy.[42, 44–48, 113, 118–120, 127, 128, 131, 134] Carpal tunnel syndrome is more common in patients with diabetes and LJM than in patients with diabetes without LJM.[151] Therefore, it is not unreasonable that this may also be the case for tarsal tunnel syndrome. In LJM, the joints affected may be palpably thickened and display a reduced range of motion.[42, 128] In the hands, patients may not be able to flatten the palmar surfaces together (positive prayer sign), indicating the presence of contractures.[42, 44, 48, 128, 131] As the condition progresses, contractures may first become clinically apparent and then increasingly fixed.[42, 48, 128]

In the feet, joints become increasingly stiff, and as contractures develop, they become increasingly fixed (see Fig. 16–8).[3, 17, 22, 27, 30, 135–139] Joint stiffness may alter gait and loading dynamics, which may contribute to the pathogenesis of ulceration and neuroarthropathy.[3, 17, 22, 27, 30, 136, 137] Sanders and associates[27] have recorded limited subtalar mobility in neuropathic diabetics versus age-matched nondiabetic control subjects. Holewski and associates[30] found that patients with diabetes with a history of ulcer or amputation had a significantly higher prevalence of limited ankle joint dorsiflexion, compared with diabetic patients without a history of those complications. Delbridge and associates[136] demonstrated that in patients with neuropathic disease, those with LJM of the subtalar joint were at greater risk for neuropathic ulceration. Fernando and associates[137] evaluated five groups: patients with diabetes with LJM plus neuropathy (DM + LJM + N), diabetes with LJM alone (DM + LJM), diabetes with

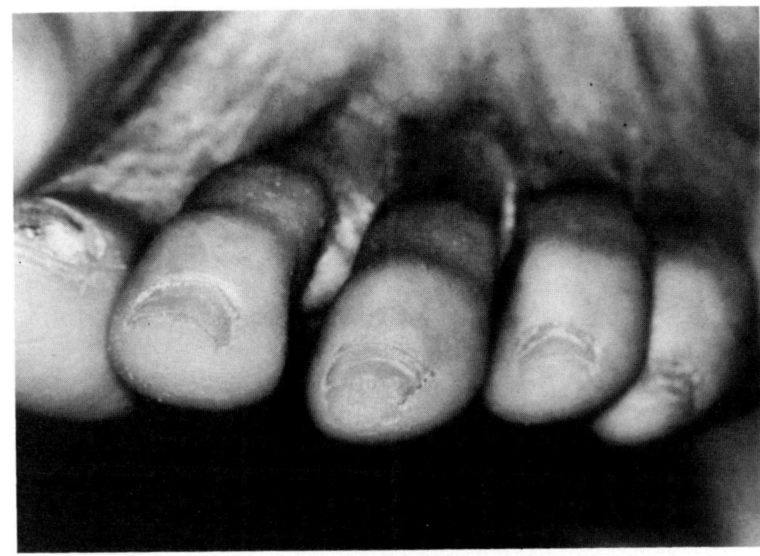

FIGURE 16–8. A foot displaying thickened, bound-down, waxlike skin, stiff joints, and digital contractures, suggestive of the syndrome of limited joint mobility associated with diabetes mellitus.

neuropathy alone (DM + N), diabetes without the two complications (DM-control), and nondiabetics without the two complications (NDM-control). The subtalar (STJ), first MTP, and metacarpophalangeal (MCP) joints were evaluated for range of motion (ROM). Although no difference in joint mobility was detected between the DM + LJM and DM + LJM + N groups, these groups were significantly more restricted than the controls. The STJ ROM correlated well with both MTP and MCP joint ROM, as well as with peak plantar pressures. Peak plantar pressures were found to be significantly higher in patients with restricted motion (DM + LJM and DM + LJM + N) than in those in the DM + N group, which in turn, were significantly higher than in those in the control groups (DM-control and NDM-control). There was no difference in peak plantar pressures between the DM + LJM group and the DM + LJM + N group. The prevalence of plantar foot ulceration was 65% in the DM + LJM + N group, whereas it was only 5% in the DM + N group. It is apparent that not only can LJM manifest in the foot, but it can also contribute to the development of other serious pedal complications.

Radiographs do not typically assist in the diagnosis.[48] However, increased thickness of the periarticular soft tissues may be appreciated on radiograph in some patients.[128] Laboratory test results are generally normal (including antinuclear antibodies and rheumatoid factor), except for serum glucose levels.[42, 48]

Treatment

Once LJM is present, reversal may be difficult.[42] Strict diabetes control (insulin pump therapy) may be of some benefit, as is physical therapy.[42, 48] The use of an aldose reductase inhibitor has produced some reversal of findings, but this therapy warrants further investigation.[42, 48, 148]

Patients with LJM of the feet and neuropathy should be considered to be at higher risk for ulceration[17, 30, 136, 137] and, perhaps, for neuroarthropathy.[22, 27] Therefore, these patients should be placed in a foot complication prevention program consisting of patient education, frequent follow-up, home mobility exercises, appropriate shoeing (extra-depth shoes and custom-molded insoles, or suitable alternative), and perhaps other preventive measures. Preventing advancement of LJM may be possible, but it also deserves further research. Possible avenues for preventing LJM advancement include strict diabetes control, physical therapy, antioxidant therapy (vitamins E and C prevent nonenzymatic glycosylation), and aminoguanidine therapy (prevents AGEs formation).[42, 48, 144, 145, 152]

FASCIAL DISORDERS

Dupuytren's disease of the palmar fascia (DDPF) has long been noted for its association with diabetes mellitus.[40, 42–45, 48, 153–173] Of patients with DDPF, between 10% and 47% have been found to have diabetes.[155, 156, 164, 165] The cumulative prevalence of diabetes in 513 DDPF patients from four studies is approximately 25%.[155, 156, 164, 165] Furthermore, if overt diabetes mellitus and abnormal glucose tolerance are considered together, the prevalence of abnormal glucose homeostasis in patients with DDPF is between 64% and 97%.[164, 165]

Between 3% and 42% of patients with diabetes have DDPF.[156, 158, 160–162, 164, 166, 168–170, 172] The cumulative prevalence of DDPF in 7287 patients with diabetes from 13 studies is approximately 19%.[156, 158, 160–162, 164, 166, 168–170, 172] In comparison, the cumulative prevalence of DDPF in 4735 nondiabetic control subjects from six studies is approximately 4%.[156, 158, 162, 164, 166, 169] In studies that have employed nondiabetic control groups, the prevalence of DDPF has routinely been higher among patients with diabetes than among control subjects: 3% versus 1%,[156] 37% versus 14%,[158] 25% versus 8%,[162] 18% versus 1%,[164] 10% versus 4%,[166] and 21% versus 5%.[169]

Although a larger proportion of studies has been devoted to the study of DDPF, some authors also have noted an association between its related counterpart, plantar fibromatosis, and diabetes mellitus (Fig. 16–9).[22, 174, 175] The relative lack of study of plantar fibromatosis in diabetes patients may be due to the relative lack of symptoms and disfigurement produced by the pedal counterpart.[176, 177] In addition, the presence of neuropathy and failure to examine the feet may

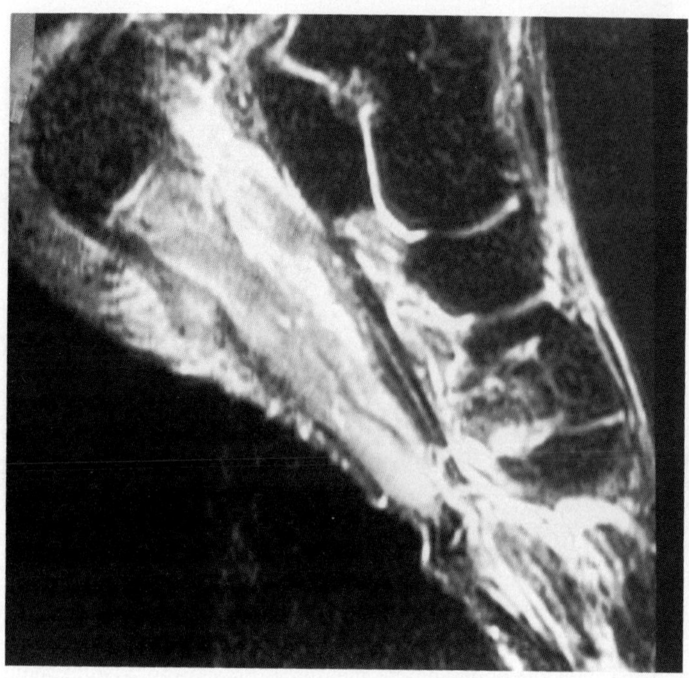

FIGURE 16–9. This STIR magnetic resonance image of a diabetic patient's foot demonstrates a plantar fibroma within the plantar fascia just distal to its calcaneal origin with intramass as well as perimass inflammation or bound water.

contribute to a relative underreporting of plantar fibromatosis in diabetic patients.

Nevertheless, evidence suggests that plantar fibromatosis, like DDPF, may occur more frequently among patients with diabetes than among control groups. This contention has been made by several authors.[22, 174, 175] The pathologic findings are indistinguishable between the palmar fascia and the plantar fascia affected by these disorders, suggesting a similar pathologic process.[175, 179] If the permissive pathogenic effect of diabetes on DDPF is a system-wide derangement, it is likely that plantar fibromatosis may also be manifested either alone or in conjunction with DDPF. In 211 accumulated patients with plantar fibromatosis, DDPF has been found (before, concurrently, or after) in 53%, further suggesting a shared pathologic process.[177, 179, 180] To illustrate these relationships, in a report of three cases of concurrent plantar fibromatosis and DDPF, one patient had diabetes mellitus.[181]

Pathogenesis

It is likely that diabetes plays a permissive role in the pathogenesis of these fascial disorders, resulting in an accelerated appearance of pathologic changes. Like LJM, the occurrence of DDPF increases with age and with duration of diabetes.[48, 159, 161, 164, 169, 170] When compared with patients with diabetes without DDPF, those with DDPF are an average of 10 years older and have had diabetes 5 years longer.[161] Apparently there is no relationship with the type of diabetes that the patient has or the method of metabolic control.[48, 161, 163, 170] There does appear to be an association with retinopathy[153, 158, 159, 163] and possibly neuropathy.[153, 169, 171]

The presence of diabetes probably does not change the predilection of these fascial disorders for whites. The disorders are rare in blacks.[40, 42, 161, 175] DDPF and plantar fibromatosis may occur more frequently in males than in females in the general population,[45, 154, 175, 176, 182] but there may be no sex

predilection in patients with diabetes.[163, 165] This may be consistent with the relative loss of protection against other pathologic changes seen in females with diabetes. In the general population, DDPF tends to occur in males more frequently than in females in younger age groups, whereas in the elderly, the prevalence equalizes between males and females.[42] Perhaps the lack of sex predilection in patients with diabetes points to an acceleration of the aging process.

Genetic factors and environmental factors probably are important pathogenic factors in patients with and without diabetes,[45, 48, 175] but the metabolic derangements associated with diabetes no doubt provide an added pathogenic stress.[48, 158] A number of authors believe that these fascial disorders share with LJM some of the same pathogenic processes, such as AGEs collagen formation.[153, 158, 163] In fact, a clinical association between the two conditions has been demonstrated.[153, 163] Collagen at sites where the fascial disorder is present binds water more avidly, which contributes to connective tissue swelling; this can be demonstrated on MRI.[42]

Evaluation

Plantar fibromatosis presents as single or multiple firm thickenings or nodules either unilaterally or bilaterally along the medial and occasionally central band of the plantar fascia. Symptoms are generally absent in most patients with the disorder.[174, 176–178, 180, 182] The coexistence of neuropathy may contribute to the relative frequency of asymptomatic plantar fibromatosis in diabetes.[153, 169, 171] If symptomatic, patients with plantar fibromatosis generally complain of a localized ache at the site of a nodule, which is exacerbated with weightbearing. Occasionally, neuritic radiations to the medial toes may present when larger masses are impinging on the adjacent medial plantar nerve.

Masses are firm, nonpulsatile, subcutaneous, and rarely adherent to the overlying skin. The mass does not move with motion of adjacent tendons. Tenderness on palpation of nodules may be observed in some patients. In contrast with DDPF, plantar fibromatosis is rarely associated with digital contractures.[175–177] Masses have been reported with their largest dimension measuring 0.5 to 5 cm, but it is uncommon to encounter nodules larger than 2 to 3 cm. The nodule can develop slowly or rapidly but often spontaneously ceases progression over time and may even regress somewhat.[178] Dupuytren's-like fibromatous lesions may be found elsewhere on examination.[175, 177–180] In patients with plantar fibromatosis, the diagnosis of DDPF may occur before, concurrently with, or after the initial pedal diagnosis has been made.[178]

Radiographs occasionally demonstrate a noncalcified soft tissue mass. Because of the occasional misidentification of plantar fibromatosis for fibrosarcoma on percutaneous biopsy,[177–179] MRI is probably a more useful and reliable method of confirming diagnosis in clinically atypical presentations (see Fig. 16–9).

Treatment

Asymptomatic lesions require no treatment other than reassurance for the patient. Conservative therapy, consisting of accommodative insoles with padding, physical therapy, rest, and corticosteroid injection (after MRI verification of diagnosis), should be exhausted before considering surgery for symptomatic plantar fibromatosis in diabetes.[40, 42, 48, 182] Surgical excision of the fibromas is associated with a high complication rate, with recurrence of the mass being the most common complication.[42, 178, 179]

TENDON XANTHOMAS

Tendon xanthomas are masses of lipid-containing histiocytic foam cells surrounded by dense fibrous connective tissue that infiltrate tendons in patients with hyperlipoproteinemia.[183–185] Tendon xanthomas are classically associated with type II familial hyperlipoproteinemia (hypercholesterolemia).[183, 185, 186] However, secondary hyperlipoproteinemia is associated with 20% to 70% of the patients with diabetes mellitus.[110, 185] Therefore, xanthomatous manifestations are also directly associated with the secondary hyperlipoproteinemia found with the diabetic state.[184–186]

Although the most common form of secondary hyperlipoproteinemia in diabetes is type IV (most frequently associated with eruptive xanthomas), type II patterns also can exist.[110, 185] Therefore, tendon xanthomas are among the various xanthomatous manifestations in diabetes mellitus.[184, 185]

The Achilles tendon is one of the most common sites to be affected.[183, 186] The masses are often slow growing and may persist for years.[186, 187] Generally, the masses diffusely infiltrate the Achilles tendon and may escape the confines of the tendon to involve the subcutaneous tissues and skin.[183] Clinically, a deep, firm, smooth, fusiform mass involving the Achilles tendon can be palpated, with freely movable overlying skin.[185, 187] The mass can range from 1 to 3 cm or larger in size.[187] Pain is not frequently associated with the lesion.[183, 187] Achilles tendon xanthomas are often discovered incidentally, but patients may present with complaints of disfigurement or pain related to shoe irritation.[183, 187] As many

as 90% of patients display bilateral involvement of the Achilles tendon.[183]

As many as 80% of patients with Achilles tendon xanthomas may display other manifestations of hyperlipoproteinemia.[183] Most frequently, other tendons may be involved, including the extensor tendons of the hands or feet, patellar tendon, and triceps brachii tendon.[183] In addition, tendon xanthomas may arise from tissues other than tendon, such as ligament and fascia.[183, 185] Thus, the plantar fascia is another site of involvement that can be seen in patients with Achilles tendon xanthomas.[183] Furthermore, patients with Achilles tendon xanthomas may also have other nontendon xanthomatous manifestations, such as tuberous xanthomas, or xanthelasma.[183, 185] Finally, coronary heart disease may be found in as many as 30% of the patients with Achilles tendon xanthomas.[183]

Radiographic evaluation is generally negative except for findings consistent with a soft tissue mass. However, calcifications occasionally may be seen in the mass.[187] MRI may be useful in narrowing the diagnosis.

Patients with suspected xanthoma of the Achilles tendon should be evaluated for serum triglyceride, serum cholesterol, and serum lipoprotein levels. Further evaluation and medical management should be coordinated by the patient's primary care physician or endocrinologist. Medical management should be directed at dietary modification and perhaps pharmacologic intervention to reduce hyperlipidemia. Additional efforts to reduce cardiovascular risk also should be instituted.[110, 185]

Some xanthomatous manifestations, such as eruptive xanthomas, tend to resolve with improved control of serum glucose levels, but this may not be the case for tendon xanthomas. In addition, tendon xanthomas also tend to be resistant to therapy (dietary and pharmacologic) that reduces hyperlipidemia. Nevertheless, improved glycemic and lipidemic control should be a goal in management.[183, 185]

In resistant symptomatic or disfiguring cases, surgical excision of the mass is another treatment alternative.[183, 187] Although excised xanthomas do recur frequently, they do not tend to be symptomatic or disfiguring.[183]

INTRINSIC MINUS FOOT

As diabetic sensorimotor neuropathy progresses to create paresis of the intrinsic musculature of the foot, a condition is in turn created that is often referred to as the *intrinsic minus foot*.[3, 9–22, 29, 63, 139, 188] The stabilizing function of the intrinsic muscles on the MTP joints is progressively lost. As these joints become increasingly destabilized, functional overpowering of the long digital flexors over the digital extensors in the stance phase of gait leads to the development of digital contractures, such as claw toes. Unlike non neuromuscular causes of digital contractures, this process also affects the hallux, resulting in hallux malleus (or hallux hammertoe). The advanced intrinsic minus foot demonstrates intrinsic muscle atrophy and clawing of all the toes (Fig. 16–10).

As the toes become progressively deformed, their function is impaired, resulting in a decreased ability to accept weight-bearing forces in the propulsive period of gait. Dynamic digital ground purchase decreases.[189–192] Forces that cannot be transferred to the toes accumulate under the metatarsal heads in the propulsive period of gait. Furthermore, the de-

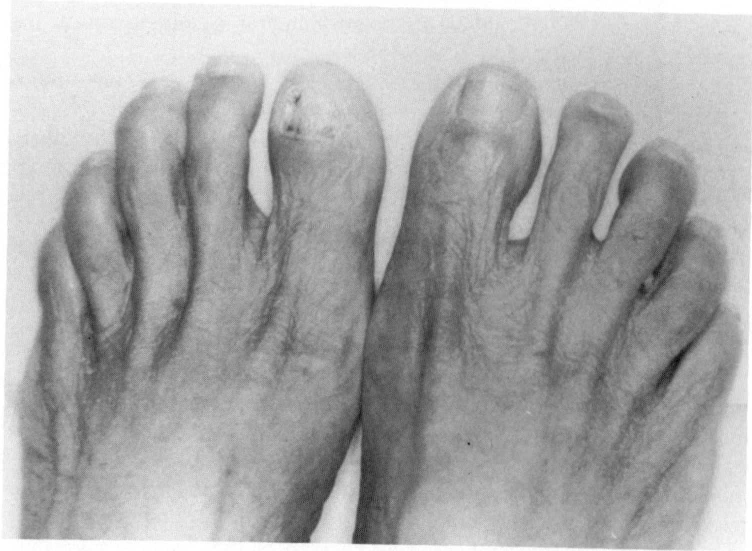

FIGURE 16–10. The feet of this diabetic patient display the manifestations of the intrinsic minus foot, with intrinsic muscle wasting, and clawing of the toes.

formed toe, which has buckled up over the MTP joint, exerts a retrograde force down on the metatarsal head. The net result is increased dynamic weightbearing forces under the metatarsal heads.[189-192]

In neuropathy with loss of sensation beyond a protective threshold, the intrinsic minus foot tends to focus potentially deleterious forces to specific areas of the foot, which results in those areas being placed at higher risk for ulceration.[17] Areas at risk for ulceration in the foot with concurrent loss of sensory protective threshold primarily include the submetatarsal head region, but they also may include the dorsal aspect of the proximal interphalangeal joints and distal aspect of the toes (particularly the hallux). Holewski and associates[30] found that in patients with diabetes and a history of ulceration or amputation, the prevalence of hammertoes (85% versus 23%) was significantly increased compared with patients without a history of ulceration or amputation.

The prevalence of intrinsic minus foot is not well established, but no doubt it increases directly with the severity of sensorimotor neuropathy. The prevalence of hammertoe deformity in diabetes has been variously established at 15%,[193] 31%,[194] and 48%.[195] In a study of 96% of all patients with diabetes age 15 to 50 years from one county, the prevalence of hammertoes in type I (46%) and type II (58%) diabetes was significantly increased, compared with healthy age-matched controls (25%).[195] The prevalence of hammertoes in type I diabetic patients appeared to increase with age and duration of diabetes.[195] However, in a study of veterans age 70 to 90 years, there was no significant difference in the prevalence of hammertoes between patients with and without diabetes.[193]

The severity of the hammertoes in patients with diabetes is increased compared with age-matched healthy control subjects.[195] Compounding the severity of the deformity that develops in the intrinsic minus foot are the potential effects of advanced glycosylation of collagen in the periarticular structures of the MTP and interphalangeal joints. The effect of AGEs collagen formation is progressive stiffness and fixed deformities. Further complicating the intrinsic minus foot is subluxation of the plantar metatarsal head fat pad. The dorsal migration of the toes draws the fat pad distally, rendering it

incapable of providing the viscoelastic buffer that it normally provides between the metatarsal heads and the ground.

Management of the intrinsic minus foot should be initiated with an extra-depth shoe with a custom-molded insole. In many patients, this is effective. However, in patients with preulcerative areas or recurrent ulcers under the metatarsal heads, a rocker sole may be added to the shoe to additionally unweight the forefoot. Shoes may be spot-stretched in areas where dorsal toe lesions continue to be a problem. However, in patients recalcitrant to conservative care, corrective surgery may be required.[38]

Digital arthroplasty may be elected, but consideration should also be given to (1) an effective surgical reduction of the MTP contracture, and (2) transfer of the long flexor tendon to the proximal phalanx. Hallux malleus is best addressed with an interphalangeal joint fusion. In some patients, particularly those with previous obliteration of weight-bearing of one or more metatarsal heads, a panmetatarsal head resection might be considered.[38]

DROP FOOT

Another lower extremity musculoskeletal manifestation of diabetic peripheral neuropathy is drop foot.[3, 10, 13, 17, 20, 139, 196] Paresis and, in severe cases, paralysis of the dorsiflexors of the foot and ankle can occur through two neuropathic mechanisms. Distal symmetrical sensorimotor polyneuropathy may progress proximally in severe cases to involve the motor nerves to the anterior leg muscles. Alternatively, a mononeuropathy may affect peroneal nerve function.

In mild or early cases, anterior leg group weakness may result in accelerated forefoot loading and foot slap. In an effort to decelerate forefoot loading, the long digital extensors increasingly may be recruited. Thus, early in the course of development, extensor substitution may contribute to the formation of digital contractures. Furthermore, because the gastrosoleal group remains relatively strong, the early muscle imbalance between the anterior and posterior muscle groups leads to the development of a contracture that limits ankle joint dorsiflexion.

Later, gait changes are apparent. Progressive weakness of

the anterior leg group interferes with their ability to clear the foot relative to the ground in the swing phase of gait. At first, the drop foot may be subclinical, with the only clue to dysfunction being patient complaints of tripping or ''ankle sprains.'' Finally, the drop foot becomes fully developed clinically with steppage gait. The motor imbalance created early in the course of development may continue to facilitate a more severe equinus contracture.

Although the prevalence of drop foot in the diabetic population has not been clearly established, it is probably true that its prevalence increases with increased duration of diabetes and severity of neuropathy. Drop foot that is attributable to progressive sensorimotor polyneuropathy is probably also accompanied by a relatively insensate dorsal and plantar foot and an increased risk for plantar metatarsal head ulcerations. In contrast, drop foot attributable to mononeuropathy of the peroneal nerve may have intact sensation plantarly, and thus, less risk for plantar metatarsal head ulceration.

Treatment for drop foot in diabetes rarely calls for tendon transfer procedures. In contrast, most cases are amenable to drop foot bracing, either with an ankle-foot orthosis or one of a variety of braces that can be affixed to the shoe.[196] In addition, consideration should be given to prescribing a rocker sole if ankle joint dorsiflexion is restricted. Also, a custom-molded insole should be incorporated in the shoeing of patients with advanced sensorimotor polyneuropathy.

Daily ROM exercises for maintenance of ankle joint dorsiflexion may be helpful to prevent the sequelae of equinus. If the secondary equinus is severe, surgical lengthening of the tendo-Achilles or gastrosoleal complex may be indicated, which is discussed later.

GAIT DISTURBANCES

Although their prevalence has not been established, alterations in smooth, coordinated gait are probably not rare findings in patients with diabetes. Gait changes can arise from sensory or motor neuropathic disturbances, among other mechanisms.[3, 10, 13, 17, 18, 20, 139, 197] Clearly, motor neuropathy can create weakness and gait alterations, such as described with drop foot. Further, sensory deprivation may also alter fine tactile feedback to the control of gait. Particularly when there is a dominant large-fiber component of the peripheral neuropathy, with diminution of proprioceptive function, sensory ataxia may be recognized. In advanced sensory ataxia, a positive Romberg test may be demonstrated.[197] Ambulation in the dark or without visual feedback may be significantly impaired. The patient may sway when standing still.

Still other changes in patients with diabetes may adversely affect their gait. Severe loss of visual acuity or blindness due to retinopathy may cause patients to alter their gait. So, too, do the effects of some strokes.

Regardless of mechanism, gait changes may impart additional ulcer risk in selected patients. Owing to altered loading, and perhaps a more shuffling type of gait, deleterious changes in both vertical and shear forces acting on the foot may be expected. In a patient with existing loss of protective sensory threshold, these additional deleterious forces can become an added risk factor in ulcerogenesis.[17]

Furthermore, loss of sensory protective threshold deprives the patient of natural or inherent protective gait alterations, such as limping, altering the foot loading, or simply resting

in an attempt to avoid further injury to damaged tissues. Thus, the ulcerogenic process is allowed to propagate.

Management of gait changes in diabetes is probably best accomplished by recognizing (1) the presence of the gait alteration; and (2) the risk for it to potentiate ulcerogenesis. Thus, patient education in foot care and inspection, accompanied by frequent professional care and proper shoeing, is essential for patients with diabetes demonstrating gait alterations.

EQUINUS

Equinus, or limited ankle joint dorsiflexion, is another important musculoskeletal abnormality in diabetes that appears to play a pathogenic role in the development of plantar ulceration[12, 17, 20, 30, 139, 198] and neuroarthropathy.[22, 38] Holewski and associates[30] found limited ankle joint dorsiflexion in 57% of the patients with diabetes whom they examined and who did not have a history of foot ulcer. In contrast, among patients with a history of diabetes and foot ulceration, a significantly higher proportion (92%) was noted to have limited ankle joint dorsiflexion.

The etiology of limited ankle joint dorsiflexion in diabetes probably is multifactorial. First, patients probably are not spared from the common causes of equinus in the nondiabetic population, such as congenital or acquired shortness of either the gastrocnemius alone or the entire gastrosoleal complex. Compounding these processes are additional factors seen specifically in diabetes. As subacute paresis of the anterior leg muscle group develops due to motor neuropathy, the posterior muscle group gains a mechanical advantage. The muscle imbalance that develops in these patients can also lead to limited ankle joint dorsiflexion and equinus.[20, 22] The effect of the generalized LJM associated with diabetes mellitus on ankle motion must also be considered to be an important etiologic factor.[12, 22] The common causes of osseous block of ankle joint dorsiflexion found in some nondiabetics may also be present. However, patients with diabetes also may have an osseous block anteriorly at the ankle owing to osseous proliferation associated with neuroarthropathy.[22]

Regardless of cause, it is apparent that limited ankle joint dorsiflexion may in turn play a contributory role in the pathogenesis of plantar forefoot ulceration and neuroarthropathy. In both of these resultant pathologic conditions, however, the patient must have a prerequisite severity of sensory and autonomic neuropathy.[17] The presence of equinus merely increases the deleterious forces acting across the joints in question (particularly the midfoot) and the weightbearing surface under the metatarsal heads, increasing the risk for neuroarthropathy and plantar forefoot ulceration.[12, 17, 22, 139]

For all patients with diabetes, except those with active neuroarthropathy or foot ulceration, it is probably prudent to employ a regular program of preventive gastrosoleal and Achilles tendon stretching exercises. For those patients with insensate feet and equinus, extra-depth shoes with custom-molded insoles should be used. In addition, a rocker-bottom sole may be added to the shoes of those patients with equinus and a history of neuroarthropathy or recurrent plantar forefoot ulcers.

Finally, when surgical procedures to address neuroarthropathy or recurrent ulcerations are contemplated, ankle joint dorsiflexion should be evaluated. If equinus is found, one should then determine if it is either (1) a significant patho-genic contributor to the neuroarthropathy or recurrent ulcers, or (2) a potentially damaging force on the outcome of the primary procedure if left uncorrected. If the equinus is significant in this manner, one must seriously consider the benefits of additionally performing an Achilles tendon lengthening (or suitable alternative) versus its relative risks.[22, 38]

HALLUX VALGUS AND BUNIONS

Hallux valgus, tailor's bunions, and splay foot are all conditions associated with a bunion on the medial or lateral marginal aspect of the forefoot. It is unlikely that these conditions occur any more frequently in patients with diabetes than in age-matched non-diabetic populations.[193] The prevalence of bunions in diabetes has been reported to be 8%,[30] 12%,[193] and 25%[194] by various researchers.

However, bunion deformities, whether medial or lateral, deserve discussion here on the basis of their clinical importance as a potential factor in ulcerogenesis.[3, 12, 17] Insensate feet with a bunion deformity are at risk for ulceration over the bunion when shoe pressure is extreme or is allowed to act on the site for an excessive period (Fig. 16–11).

Therefore, insensate feet with bunions should be restricted to wider shoes with soft, moldable uppers. In selected patients the uppers may be stretched at the bunion site, or protective padding may be used to accommodate larger bunions. When new shoes are purchased, a 2- to 4-week period of gradual break-in should be advised, with no period of use lasting longer than 2 hours initially.

In cases when the bunions are associated with preulcerative lesions that are recalcitrant to conservative therapy, or are associated with recurrent ulcers, surgical correction should be considered.[11, 16, 34, 36–38]

HALLUX LIMITUS

Hallux limitus is often defined as a limitation of dorsiflexion of the proximal phalanx relative to the first metatarsal long axis to less than 65 degrees. However, the function of the first MTP joint in gait must also be considered. Any

functional limitation of first MTP joint dorsiflexion in the propulsive period of gait may produce the same symptoms and associated findings as a structural limitation of dorsiflexion.[199]

Limited dorsiflexion of the first MTP joint, or hallux limitus, is often associated with dorsal jamming and degenerative symptoms of the joint in sensate patients. However, in insensate diabetic patients, these symptoms are usually absent. In addition, owing to the lack of free dorsiflexion of the first MTP joint, loading is increased under the hallux interphalangeal joint during the propulsive period of gait. Consequently, the increased forces transmitted to the plantar aspect of the hallux interphalangeal joint in turn increase the risk for ulceration at this site in the insensate patient (Fig. 16–12).[12, 17, 200–202]

Despite the importance of the association of hallux limitus with selected hallux ulcers in insensate diabetic patients, the prevalence of the condition has not been established in patients with diabetes. There is no doubt that these patients may develop hallux limitus from the same causes as nondiabetic patients, such as dorsiflexed first metatarsal, long first metatarsal, hypermobile first ray associated with abnormal pronation, trauma, or arthridity.[199] However, patients with diabetes also may have additional contributing factors. Most notably, the effects of generalized LJM may contribute to the reduction of first MTP joint dorsiflexion.[10, 12, 136, 137] Dysfunction of the peroneus longus secondary to motor neuropathy also may contribute to the development of hallux limitus in some patients with diabetes.[20] Finally, hallux limitus may develop as a sequela of neuroarthropathy of the first MTP joint (see Fig. 16–12). Therefore, it is not unreasonable to expect hallux limitus to occur more frequently in patients with diabetes than in age-matched nondiabetic patients.

Diabetic patients who are insensate and have hallux limitus ideally should be managed with extra-depth shoes and custom-molded insoles. Strong consideration should be given to the use of rocker-bottom soles, as well. Regular follow-up inspection, palliative care, and preventive education are also practical in the prevention of ulcer sequelae in insensate diabetics with hallux limitus. For recalcitrant cases, surgical correction of the hallux limitus may be quite successful in

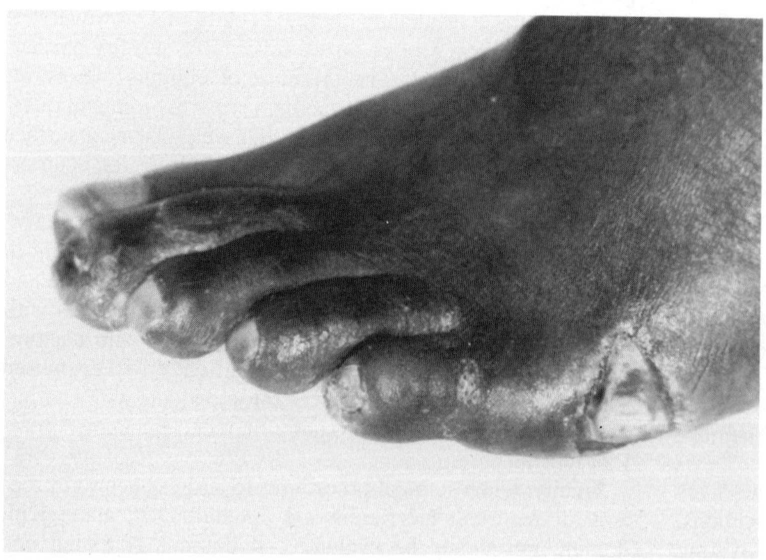

FIGURE 16–11. An ulceration developed over a tailor's bunion in an at-risk diabetic patient. The bony prominence associated with a bunion on either the medial or lateral aspect of the foot may predispose these sites to ulceration in the insensate diabetic patient.

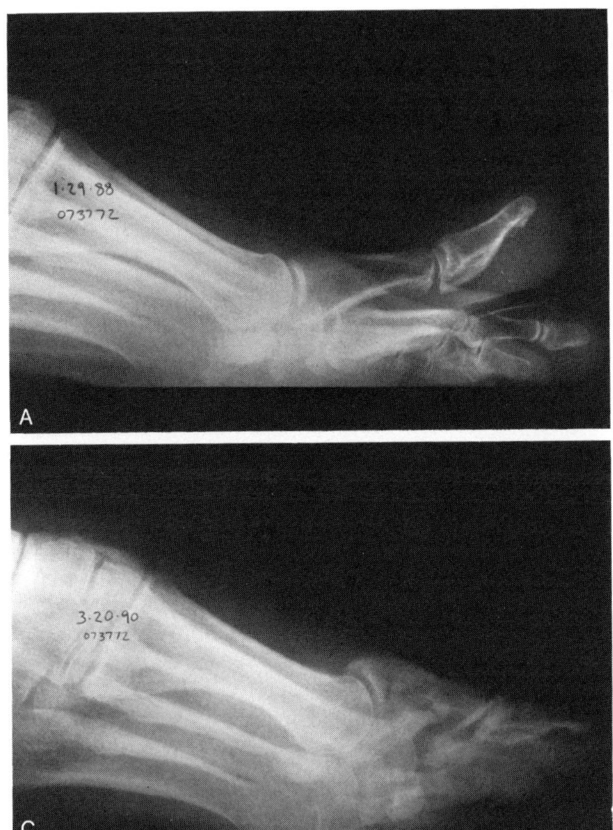

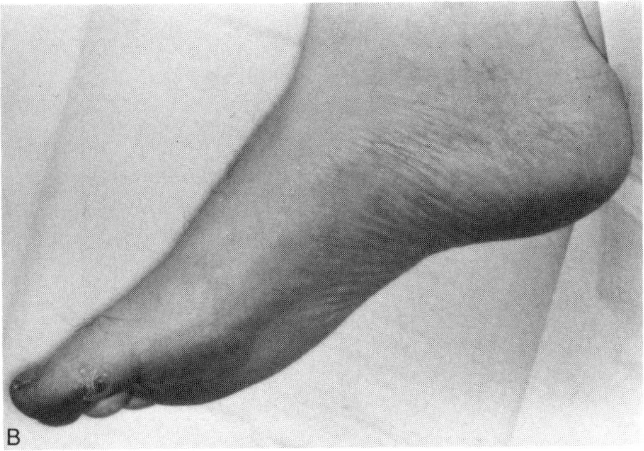

FIGURE 16–12. *A,* This insensate diabetic patient (see also Fig. 16–2) had hallux limitus in 1988. *B,* The limited dorsiflexion of the first metatarsophalangeal joint was the prime cause of an ulcer under the hallux interphalangeal joint, shown here nearly healed. *C,* The later development of metatarsophalangeal joint neuroarthropathy further reduced joint mobility, compounding the hallux limitus.

preventing recurrent ulcers under the hallux interphalangeal joint.[34, 38, 202, 203] Contrary to surgical management of hallux limitus in sensate, nondiabetic patients, the use of a joint replacement implant or arthrodesis of the joint is contraindicated in insensate diabetics.[38] Keller's joint resection arthroplasty may be the best alternative in many patients.[34, 38]

OSTEOARTHRITIS

A number of authors have suggested a possible relationship between diabetes mellitus and osteoarthritis.[40, 42–45, 48, 154, 204–207] In one study comparing 30 patients with diabetes to 30 age- and sex-matched nondiabetic control subjects, osteoarthritis had a higher incidence, earlier onset, and more severe manifestations in diabetics.[207] Furthermore, a study of 200 sternoclavicular joints at autopsy demonstrated a positive correlation between degenerative changes and diabetes.[206] However, a more recent study failed to show a statistically significant relationship. This study found that the prevalence of diabetes in patients with osteoarthritis was 6%, whereas in age- and sex-matched control subjects the prevalence of diabetes was 4%.[41]

It is beyond the scope of this chapter to detail the pathogenesis of osteoarthritis, but the additional possible predisposing factors of diabetes should be mentioned. It is possible that osteoarthritis in diabetes may be related to the additional stresses on the joints that are accompanied by obesity.[45, 48] However, this does not fully explain findings in the sternoclavicular joint.[206] Pathogenic roles may also be played by disturbances in growth hormone and somatomedin and their effect on articular cartilage,[27] decreased formation of glycosaminoglycans from impaired glucose utilization,[43, 44] and the effects of accumulated articular cartilage collagen advanced glycosylation end products.

GOUT

Diabetes and gout often share similar features and risk factors, such as obesity, hyperlipidemia, hypertension, and vascular disease. The shared features suggest that a possible relationship may exist between the two metabolic diseases, but no such association has been clearly established.[39, 40, 42–45, 48, 154, 208] At the root of the problem lies a multitude of studies with differing definitions of gouty arthritis and diabetes mellitus, as well as the lack of suitable control groups.

The prevalence of gout in diabetic patients apparently is low. Furthermore, there apparently is no increase in prevalence of gout in diabetics versus well-matched control groups. In contradistinction, among patients with gout, there appears to be a high incidence of glucose intolerance.

Nevertheless, there may be some links between carbohydrate and urate metabolism. Hyperglycemia apparently has a uricosuric effect. Urate, it seems, has an alloxan type of effect, producing hyperglycemia.

In addition, there are clinical situations when secondary hyperuricemia and gout may be definitely associated with diabetes mellitus, such as in renal failure, ketoacidosis, and concurrent use of thiazide diuretics (which is decreasing). Therefore, the practitioner must remain vigilant to the possibility of acute gout attacks in patients with diabetes, potentially mimicking neuroarthropathy, septic arthritis, pseudogout, reflex sympathetic dystrophy, or neuropathic edema, among other causes of pedal edema (Fig. 16–13).

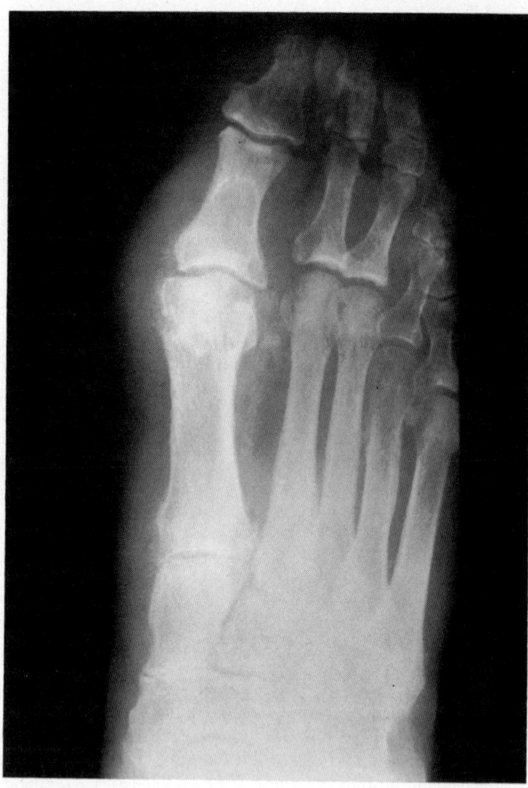

FIGURE 16–13. The presence of gout in this diabetic patient underscores the radiographic mimicry that may be shared among neuroarthropathy, septic arthritis/osteomyelitis, gout, and others.

CHONDROCALCINOSIS AND PSEUDOGOUT

Calcium pyrophosphate dihydrate (CPPD) crystal deposition may occur in various periarticular and articular structures. CPPD crystal deposition in articular cartilage is often referred to as *chondrocalcinosis,* and it is usually asymptomatic. Symptomatic joint inflammation associated with CPPD crystal deposition is also called *pseudogout.* CPPD crystal deposition has been clearly demonstrated to be associated with advanced age.[42, 47]

Among patients with CPPD crystal deposition, the prevalence of diabetes mellitus and glucose intolerance has been reported to be quite high, more than 40% in some studies.[39, 40, 43, 45] However, uncontrolled studies may reflect nothing more than age-related impaired glucose tolerance and diabetes. In fact, when age-matched controls are used, no statistically significant difference is seen in the prevalence of abnormal glucose metabolism in patients with pseudogout (55%) compared with control subjects (45%).[209] Until larger, better controlled studies of the relationship between diabetes and CPPD crystal deposition are available, caution should be used in suggesting an association between the two entities.[39, 40, 42–45, 48, 154]

Nevertheless, the practitioner should be aware that chondrocalcinosis and pseudogout are possible entities in elderly patients with diabetes. It even has been suggested that patients with diabetes and CPPD crystal deposition are more susceptible to pseudogout attacks than are nondiabetics with CPPD crystal deposition.[40, 154] Unfortunately, improved control of blood glucose levels does not usually alter the frequency or severity of pseudogout attacks.[40, 154]

AUTOIMMUNE-RELATED DISORDERS

Associations between diabetes mellitus and a number of autoimmune-related disorders have been suggested, including rheumatoid arthritis, juvenile rheumatoid arthritis, adult-onset Still's disease, systemic lupus erythematosis, and Sjögren's syndrome.[39, 42, 48, 210–218] When found concurrently with diabetes, these various autoimmune disorders are generally associated with insulin-dependent, or type I, diabetes mellitus, which also may demonstrate an autoimmune-related origin.[219, 220]

Type I diabetes mellitus is strongly associated with HLA-DR3 and HLA-DR4 antigens, as well as the HLA-B8 antigen.[219, 220] Similarly, rheumatoid arthritis (HLA-DR4), juvenile rheumatoid arthritis (HLA-DR4), adult-onset Still's disease (HLA-DR4 and HLA-B8), systemic lupus erythematosis (HLA-DR3), and Sjögren's syndrome (HLA-DR3, HLA-B8, and HLA-DR4) are strongly associated with one or more of the same HLA antigens.[47] Thus, linkage between type I diabetes and any of these autoimmune-related disorders may reflect a shared genetic susceptibility. However, this type of linkage remains to be definitively proved.[221]

Another possible linkage between the diseases could be the generation of insulin receptor antibodies by the autoimmune disorder, resulting in insulin-resistant diabetes mellitus.[42, 48, 216–218] Certainly, in patients with insulin resistance, thought should be given to the possibility that one of the various aforementioned autoimmune disorders could be the underlying problem.[42, 48]

References

1. Brenner MA (ed): Management of the Diabetic Foot. Baltimore, Williams & Wilkins, 1987.
2. Connor H, Boulton AJM, and Ward JD (eds): The Foot in Diabetes. New York, John Wiley & Sons, 1987.
3. Faris I: The Management of the Diabetic Foot, 2nd ed. New York, Churchill Livingstone, 1991.
4. Frykberg RG (ed): The High-Risk Foot in Diabetes Mellitus. New York, Churchill Livingstone, 1991.
5. Kozak GP, Hoar CS, Rowbotham JL, et al (eds): Management of Diabetic Foot Problems. Philadelphia, WB Saunders, 1984.
6. Levin ME and O'Neal LW (eds): The Diabetic Foot, 4th ed. St. Louis, CV Mosby, 1988.
7. Rakow R: Podiatric Management of the Diabetic Foot. Mt Kisco, New York, Futura Publishing, 1979.
8. Sammarco GJ (ed): The Foot in Diabetes. Philadelphia, Lea & Febiger, 1991.
9. Boulton AJM: The importance of abnormal foot pressures and gait in the causation of foot ulcers. In Connor H, Boulton AJM, and Ward JD (eds): The Foot in Diabetes. New York, John Wiley & Sons, 1987, pp 11–21.
10. Cavanagh PR and Ulbrecht JS: Biomechanics of the diabetic foot: A quantitative approach to the assessment of neuropathy, deformity, and plantar pressure. In Jahss MH (ed): Disorders of the Foot and Ankle: Medical and Surgical Management, 2nd ed. Philadelphia, WB Saunders, 1991, pp 1864–1907.
11. Frykberg RG: Podiatric problems in diabetes. In Kozak GP, Hoar CS, Rowbotham JL, et al (eds): Management of Diabetic Foot Problems. Philadelphia, WB Saunders, 1984, pp 45–67.
12. Frykberg RG: Diabetic foot ulcerations. In Frykberg RG (ed): The High-Risk Foot in Diabetes Mellitus. New York, Churchill Livingstone, 1991, pp 151–195.
13. Habershaw G and Donovan JC: Biomechanical considerations of the diabetic foot. In Kozak GP, Hoar CS, and Rowbotham JL, et al (eds): Management of Diabetic Foot Problems. Philadelphia, WB Saunders, 1984, pp 32–44.
14. Harkless LB and Dennis KJ: You see what you look for and recognize what you know. Clin Podiatr Med Surg 4:331, 1987.
15. Harkless LB and Dennis KJ: The role of the podiatrist. In Levin ME and O'Neal LW (eds): The Diabetic Foot, 4th ed. St. Louis, CV Mosby, 1988, pp 249–272.
16. Jacobs RL: The diabetic foot; Diabetic neuropathy. In Jahss MH (ed): Disorders of the Foot and Ankle: Medical and Surgical Management, 2nd ed. Philadelphia, WB Saunders, 1991, pp 1908–1925.
17. Jenkin WM and Palladino SJ: Environmental stress and tissue breakdown. In Frykberg RG (ed): The High-Risk Foot in Diabetes Mellitus. New York, Churchill Livingstone, 1991, pp 103–123.
18. Levin ME: The diabetic foot: Pathophysiology, evaluation, and treatment. In

Levin ME and O'Neal LW (eds): The Diabetic Foot, 4th ed. St. Louis, CV Mosby, 1988, pp 1–50.

19. Meggitt BF: Diabetes. *In* Helal B and Wilson D (eds): The Foot. New York, Churchill Livingstone, 1988, pp 710–738.

20. Schoenhaus HD, Wernick E, and Cohen RS: Biomechanics of the diabetic foot. *In* Frykberg RG (ed): The High-Risk Foot in Diabetes Mellitus. New York, Churchill Livingstone, 1991, pp 125–137.

21. Stess RM and Hetherington VJ: The diabetic and insensitive foot. *In* Levy LA and Hetherington VJ (eds): Principles and Practice of Podiatric Medicine. New York, Churchill Livingstone, 1990, pp 523–548.

22. Banks AS and McGlamry ED: Charcot foot. J Am Podiatr Med Assoc 79:213, 1989.

23. Frykberg RG and Kozak GP: The diabetic Charcot foot. *In* Kozak GP, Hoar CS, Rowbotham JL, et al (eds): Management of Diabetic Foot Problems. Philadelphia, WB Saunders, 1984, pp 103–112.

24. Frykberg RG: Osteoarthropathy. Clin Podiatr Med Surg 4:351, 1987.

25. Frykberg RG: Diabetic osteoarthropathy. *In* Brenner MA (ed): Management of the Diabetic Foot. Baltimore, Williams & Wilkins, 1987, pp 75–86.

26. Reiner M, Scurran BL, Karlin JM, and Silvani SH: The neuropathic joint in diabetes mellitus. Clin Podiatr Med Surg 5:421, 1988.

27. Sanders LJ and Frykberg RG: Diabetic neuropathic osteoarthropathy: The Charcot foot. *In* Frykberg RG (ed): The High-Risk Foot in Diabetes Mellitus. New York, Churchill Livingstone, 1991, pp 297–338.

28. Sinha S, Munichoodappa CS, and Kozak GP: Neuroarthropathy (Charcot joints) in diabetes mellitus: Clinical study of 101 cases. Medicine 51:191, 1972.

29. Boulton AJM: The diabetic foot. Med Clin North Am 72:1513, 1988.

30. Holewski JJ, Moss KM, Stess RM, et al: Prevalence of foot pathology and lower extremity complications in a diabetic outpatient clinic. J Rehabil Res Dev 26:35, 1989.

31. Coleman WC: Shoe gear for the insensitive foot. Clin Podiatr Med Surg 4:459, 1987.

32. Coleman WC: Footwear in a management program of injury prevention. *In* Levin ME and O'Neal LW (eds): The Diabetic Foot, 4th ed. St. Louis, CV Mosby, 1988, pp 293–309.

33. Coleman WC: Footwear considerations. *In* Frykberg RG (ed): The High-Risk Foot in Diabetes Mellitus. New York, Churchill Livingstone, 1991, pp 487–496.

34. Gudas CJ: Prophylactic surgery in the diabetic foot. Clin Podiatr Med Surg 4:445, 1987.

35. Miller J: Custom-made shoe therapy for the diabetic foot. *In* Brenner MA (ed): Management of the Diabetic Foot. Baltimore, Williams & Wilkins, 1987, pp 167–173.

36. Nicklas BJ: Prophylactic surgery in the diabetic foot. *In* Frykberg RG (ed): The High-Risk Foot in Diabetes Mellitus. New York, Churchill Livingstone, 1991, pp 513–541.

37. O'Neal LW: Surgical pathology of the foot and clinicopathologic correlations. *In* Levin ME and O'Neal LW (eds): The Diabetic Foot, 4th ed. St. Louis, CV Mosby, 1988, pp 203–236.

38. Palladino SJ and Jenkin WM: Surgery upon the diabetic foot. *In* Complications in Foot Surgery, 3rd ed. Baltimore, Williams & Wilkins, 1992, pp 235–274.

39. Forgacs S: Bones and Joints in Diabetes Mellitus. Boston, Martinus Nijhoff, 1982, pp 13–179.

40. Gray RB and Gottlieb NL: Rheumatic disorders associated with diabetes mellitus: Literature review. Semin Arthritis Rheum 6:19, 1976.

41. Magaro M, Altomonte L, Zoli A, et al: Prevalence of diabetes mellitus in common rheumatic diseases. Panminerva Med 31:11, 1989.

42. McCarty DJ (ed): Arthritis and Allied Conditions: A Textbook of Rheumatology, 11th ed. Philadelphia, Lea & Febiger, 1989, pp 1477–1481, 1588, 1724, 1851–1853.

43. Pastan RS and Cohen AS: The rheumatologic manifestations of diabetes mellitus. Med Clin North Am 62:829, 1978.

44. Podolsky S and Marble A: Diverse abnormalities associated with diabetes. *In* Marble A, Krall LP, Bradley RF, et al (eds): Joslin's Diabetes Mellitus, 12th ed. Philadelphia, Lea & Febiger, 1985, pp 843–866.

45. Resnick D and Niwayama G (eds): Diagnosis of Bone and Joint Disorders, 2nd ed. Philadelphia, WB Saunders, 1988, pp 2292–2299, 3154–3185.

46. Rosenbloom AL: Skeletal and joint manifestations of childhood diabetes. Pediatr Clin North Am 31:569, 1984.

47. Schumacher HR (ed): Primer on the Rheumatic Diseases, 9th ed. Atlanta, GA, Arthritis Foundation, 1988, pp 47–50, 137, 170, 200, 211, 218, 252.

48. Sibbitt WL: Musculoskeletal complications of diabetes mellitus. Mediguide Inflammat Dis 7:1, 1988.

49. Brooks AP: The neuropathic foot in diabetes: II. Charcot's arthropathy. Diabetic Med 3:116, 1986.

50. Brower AC and Allman RM: Pathogenesis of the neuropathic joint: Neurotraumatic vs. neurovascular. Radiology 139:349, 1981.

51. Clouse ME, Gramm HF, Legg M, and Flood T: Diabetic osteoarthropathy: Clinical and roentgenographic observations in 90 cases. Am J Roentgenol 121:22, 1974.

52. Cofield RH, Morrison MJ, and Beabout JW: Diabetic neuroarthropathy in the foot: Patient characteristics and patterns of radiographic change. Foot Ankle 4:15, 1983.

53. Forgacs S: Clinical picture of diabetic osteoarthropathy. Acta Diabetol Lat 13:111, 1976.

54. Goldman F: Identification, treatment, and prognosis of Charcot joint in diabetes mellitus. J Am Podiatr Assoc 72:485, 1982.

55. Hardy DC, Staple TW, Picus D, and Gilula LA: Imaging of the diabetic foot. *In* Levin ME and O'Neal LW (eds): The Diabetic Foot, 4th ed. St. Louis, CV Mosby, 1988, pp 131–150.

56. Harris JR and Brand PW: Patterns of disintegration of the tarsus in the anesthetic foot. J Bone Joint Surg 48B:4, 1966.

57. Newman JH: Non-infective disease of the diabetic foot. J Bone Joint Surg 63B:593, 1981.

58. Sammarco GJ: Diabetic arthropathy. *In* Sammarco GJ (ed): The Foot in Diabetes. Philadelphia, Lea & Febiger, 1991, pp 153–172.

59. Santori FS, Ghera S, Sadeh H, et al: Diabetic neuroarthropathy of the foot. Ital J Orthop Traumatol 10:411, 1984.

60. Zlatkin MB, Pathria M, Sartoris DJ, and Resnick D: The diabetic foot. Radiol Clin North Am 25:1095, 1987.

61. Heath H, Melton LJ, and Chu C-P: Diabetes and risk of skeletal fracture. N Engl J Med 303:567, 1980.

62. Hungerford P (ed): Ischemia and Necrosis of Bone. Baltimore, Williams & Wilkins, 1980.

63. Cavanagh PR and Ulbrecht JS: Plantar pressure in the diabetic foot. *In* Sammarco GJ (ed): The Foot in Diabetes. Philadelphia, Lea & Febiger, 1991, pp 54–70.

64. Edmonds ME, Archer AG, and Watkins PJ: Ephedrine: A new treatment for diabetic neuropathic oedema. Lancet 1:548, 1983.

65. Eichenholtz SN: Charcot Joints. Springfield, IL, Charles C Thomas, 1966.

66. Ward JD, Boulton AJM, Simms JM, et al: Venous distintion in the diabetic neuropathic foot. J R Soc Med 76:1011, 1983.

67. Clohisy DR and Thompson RC: Fractures associated with neuropathic arthropathy in adults who have juvenile-onset diabetes. J Bone Joint Surg 70A:1192, 1988.

68. Kerr R, Sartoris DJ, Fix CF, and Resnick D: Imaging of the diabetic foot. *In* Frykberg RG (ed): The High-Risk Foot in Diabetes Mellitus. New York, Churchill Livingstone, 1991, pp 79–102.

69. Bier RR and Estersohn HS: A new treatment for Charcot joint in the diabetic foot. J Am Podiatr Med Assoc 77:63, 1987.

70. Dean MRE: The role of the radiologist in the diagnosis and treatment of the diabetic foot. *In* Connor H, Boulton AJM, and Ward JD (eds): The Foot in Diabetes. New York, John Wiley & Sons, 1987, pp 33–58.

71. Friedman SA and Rakow RB: Osseous lesions of the foot in diabetic neuropathy. Diabetes 20:302, 1971.

72. Gondos B: Roentgen observations in diabetic osteopathy. Radiology 91:6, 1968.

73. Griffiths HJ: Diabetic osteopathy. Orthopedics 8:401, 1985.

74. Gventer M: Radiological evaluation of the diabetic foot. *In* Brenner MA (ed): Management of the Diabetic Foot. Baltimore, Williams & Wilkins, 1987, pp 48–74.

75. Pogonowska MJ, Collins LC, and Dobson HL: Diabetic osteopathy. Radiology 89:265, 1967.

76. Schwartz GS, Berenyi MR, and Siegel MW: Atrophic arthropathy and diabetic neuritis. Am J Roentgenol 124:17, 1975.

77. Whitehouse FW and Weckstein M: On diabetic osteopathy: A radiographic study of 21 patients. Diabetes Care 1:303, 1978.

78. Dietrich JW and Raisz LG: Prostaglandin in calcium and bone metabolism. Clin Orthop 11:228, 1975.

79. Halushka PV and Colwell JA: Prostaglandins and diabetes mellitus. *In* Ellenberg M and Rifkin H (eds): Diabetes Mellitus: Theory and Practice, 3rd ed. New York, Medical Examination Publishing, 1983, pp 295–308.

80. Auwerx J, Dequeker J, Bouillon R, et al: Mineral metabolism and bone mass at peripheral and axial skeleton in diabetes mellitus. Diabetes 37:8, 1988.

81. DeLeeuw I and Abs R: Bone mass and bone density in maturity-type diabetics measured by the ^{125}I photon-absorption technique. Diabetes 26:1130, 1977.

82. Forgacs S, Halmos T, and Salamon F: Bone changes in diabetes mellitus. Isr J Med Sci 8:782, 1972.

83. Forgacs S, Rosinger A, and Vertes L: Diabetes mellitus and osteoporosis. Endokrinologie 67:343, 1976.

84. Geoffroy J, Hoeffel JC, Pointel JP, et al: The feet in diabetes: Roentgenologic observation in 1501 cases. Diagn Imaging 48:286, 1979.

85. Giacca A Fassina A, Caviezel F, et al: Bone mineral density in diabetes mellitus. Bone 9:29, 1988.

86. Hough FS: Alterations of bone and mineral metabolism in diabetes mellitus: I. An overview. S Afr Med J 72:116, 1987.

87. Hough FS: Alterations of bone and mineral metabolism in diabetes mellitus: II. Clinical studies in 206 patients with type I diabetes mellitus. S Afr Med J 72:120, 1987.

88. Hui SL, Epstein S, and Johnston CC: A prospective study of bone mass in patients with type I diabetes. J Clin Endocrinol Metab 60:74, 1985.

89. Levin ME, Boisseau VC, and Avioli LV: Effects of diabetes mellitus on bone mass in juvenile and adult-onset diabetes. N Engl J Med 294:241, 1976.

90. Mathiassen B, Nielsen S, Ditzel J, and Rodbro P: Does insulin-dependent diabetes itself lead to loss of bone. J Intern Med 227:325, 1990.

91. Mathiassen B, Nielsen S, Johansen JS, et al: Long-term bone loss in insulin-dependent diabetic patients with microvascular complications. J Diabetic Complications 4:145, 1990.

92. McNair P, Madsbad S, Christiansen C, et al: Osteopenia in insulin-treated diabetes mellitus: Its relation to age at onset, sex, and duration of disease. Diabetologia 15:87, 1978.

93. McNair P, Madsbad S, Christiansen MS, et al: Bone mineral loss in insulin-treated diabetes mellitus: Studies on pathogenesis. Acta Endocrinol 90:463, 1979.

94. McNair P, Madsbad S, Christiansen C, et al: Bone loss in diabetes: Effects of metabolic state. Diabetologia 17:283, 1979.

95. McNair P, Christensen MS, Madsbad S, et al: Hypoparathyroidism in diabetes mellitus. Acta Endocrinologica 96:81, 1981.

96. McNair P, Christiansen C, Christensen MS, et al: Development of bone mineral loss in insulin-treated diabetes: A 1 1/2 year follow-up study in sixty patients. Eur J Clin Invest 11:55, 1981.

97. McNair P: Bone mineral metabolism in human type I (insulin dependent) diabetes. Dan Med Bull 35:109, 1988.

98. Pietschman P, Schernthaner G, and Woloszczuk W: Serum osteocalcin levels in diabetes mellitus: Analysis of the type of diabetes and microvascular complications. Diabetologia 31:892, 1988.

99. Rosenbloom AL, Lezotte DC, Weber FT, et al: Diminution of bone mass in childhood diabetes. Diabetes 26:1052, 1977.

100. Saggese G, Bertelloni S, Baroncelli GI, et al: Bone demineralization and impaired mineral metabolism in insulin-dependent diabetes mellitus: A possible role of magnesium deficiency. Helv Paediatr Acta 43:405, 1989.

101. Santiago JV, McAlister WH, Ratzan SK, et al: Decreased cortical thickness and osteopenia in children with diabetes mellitus. J Clin Endocrinol Metabol 45:845, 1977.

102. Seino Y, Ishida H, Imura H, et al: Diabetic osteopenia in central Japan. Diabete Metab 11:216, 1985.

103. Shore RM, Chesney RW, Mazess RB, et al: Osteopenia in juvenile diabetes. Calcif Tissue Int 33:455, 1981.

104. Weinstock RS, Goland RS, Shane E, et al: Bone mineral density in women with type II diabetes mellitus. J Bone Miner Res 4:97, 1989.

105. Forestier J and Rotes-Querol J: Senile ankylosing hyperostosis of the spine. Ann Rheum Dis 9:321, 1950.

106. Resnick D, Shaul S, and Robins J: Diffuse idiopathic skeletal hyperostosis (DISH): Forestier's disease with extraspinal manifestations. Radiology 115:513, 1975.

107. Julkunen H, Karava R, and Viljanen V: Hyperostosis of the spine in diabetes mellitus and acromegaly. Diabetologia 2:123, 1966.

108. Flyvbjerg A: Growth factors and diabetic complications. Diabetic Med 7:387, 1990.

109. Ganda OP: Hormones affecting the secretion and actions of insulin. In Marble A, Krall LP, Bradley RF, et al (eds): Joslin's Diabetes Mellitus, 12th ed. Philadelphia, Lea & Febiger, 1985, pp 158–184.

110. Ganda OP: Pathogenesis of macrovascular disease including the influence of lipids. In Marble A, Krall LP, Bradley RF, et al (eds): Joslin's Diabetes Mellitus, 12th ed. Philadelphia, Lea & Febiger, 1985, pp 217–250.

111. Williams CE, Carey BM, Birtwell AJ, et al: Metatarsal periosteal reactions: A common non-specific finding in radiographs of the diabetic foot. Br Med J 297:1243, 1988.

112. Resnick D, Linovitz RF, and Feingold ML: Postoperative heterotopic ossification as a manifestation of ankylosing hyperostosis of the spine (Forestier's disease). J Rheumatol 3:313, 1976.

113. Beacom R, Gillespie EL, Middleton D, et al: Limited joint mobility in insulin-dependent diabetes: Relationship to retinopathy, peripheral nerve function, and HLA status. Q J Med 56:337, 1985.

114. Benedetti A and Noacco C: Juvenile diabetic cheiroarthropathy. Acta Diabetol Lat 13:54, 1976.

115. Buckingham B, Perejda AJ, Sandborg C, et al: Skin, joint, and pulmonary changes in type I diabetes mellitus. Am J Dis Child 140:420, 1986.

116. Buckingham BA, Uitto J, Sandborg C, et al: Scleroderma-like changes in insulin-dependent diabetes mellitus: Clinical and biochemical studies. Diabetes Care 7:163, 1984.

117. Burton JL: Thick skin and stiff joints in insulin-dependent diabetes mellitus. Br J Dermatol 106:369, 1982.

118. Costello PB, Tambar PK, and Green FA: The prevalence and possible prognostic importance of arthropathy in childhood diabetes. J Rheumatol 11:62, 1984.

119. Fisher I., Kurtz A, and Shipley M: Association between cheiroarthropathy and frozen shoulder in patients with insulin-dependent diabetes mellitus. Br J Rheumatol 25:141, 1986.

120. Fitzcharles MA, Duby S, Waddell RW, et al: Limitation of joint mobility (cheiroarthropathy) in adult noninsulin-dependent diabetic patients. Ann Rheum Dis 43:251, 1984.

121. Garza-Elizondo MA, Diaz-Jouanen E, Franco-Casique JJ, and Alarcon-Segovia D: Joint contractures and scleroderma-like skin changes in the hands of insulin-dependent juvenile diabetics. J Rheumatol 10:797, 1983.

122. Grgic A, Rosenbloom AL, Weber FT, et al: Joint contracture in childhood diabetes. N Engl J Med 292:372, 1975.

123. Haitas B, Jones DB, Ting A, et al: Diabetic retinopathy and its association with limited joint mobility. Horm Metab Res 18:765, 1986.

124. Jennings AM, Milner PC, and Ward JD: Hand abnormalities are associated with the complications of diabetes in type 2 diabetes. Diabetic Med 6:43, 1989.

125. Jung Y, Hohmann TC, Gerneth JA, et al: Diabetic hand syndrome. Metabolism 20:1008, 1971.

126. Rosenbloom AL: Joint contractures preceding insulin-dependent diabetes mellitus. Arthritis Rheum 26:931, 1983.

127. Rosenbloom AL: Limitation of finger joint mobility in diabetes mellitus. J Diabetic Complications 3:77, 1989.

128. Rosenbloom AL: Limited joint mobility in insulin-dependent childhood diabetes. Eur J Pediatr 149:380, 1990.

129. Rosenbloom AL and Frias JL: Diabetes mellitus, short stature and joint stiffness—a new syndrome. Clin Res 22:92A, 1974.

130. Rosenbloom AL, Silverstein JM, Lezotte DC, et al: Limited joint mobility in diabetes mellitus of childhood: Natural history and relationship to growth impairment. J Pediatr 101:874, 1982.

131. Rosenbloom AL, Silverstein JM, Lezotte DC, et al: Limited joint mobility in childhood diabetes indicates increased risk for microvascular disease. N Engl J Med 305:191, 1981.

132. Shinabarger NI: Limited joint mobility in adults with diabetes mellitus. Phys Ther 67:215, 1987.

133. Starkman H and Brink S: Limited joint mobility of the hand in type I diabetes mellitus. Diabetes Care 5:534, 1982.

134. Starkman HS, Gleason RE, Rand LI, et al: Limited joint mobility (LJM) of the hand in patient with diabetes mellitus: Relation to chronic complications. Ann Rheum Dis 45:130, 1986.

135. Campbell RR, Hawkins SJ, Maddison PJ, and Reckless JPD: Limited joint mobility in diabetes mellitus. Ann Rheum Dis 44:93, 1985.

136. Delbridge L, Perry P, Marr S, et al: Limited joint mobility in the diabetic foot: Relationship to neuropathic ulceration. Diabetic Med 5:333, 1988.

137. Fernando DJS, Masson EA, Veves A, and Boulton AJM: Relationship of limited joint mobility to abnormal foot pressures and diabetic foot ulceration. Diabetes Care 14:8, 1991.

138. Huntley AC: Cutaneous manifestations of diabetes mellitus. In Sammarco GJ (ed): The Foot in Diabetes. Philadelphia, Lea & Febiger, 1991, pp 124–144.

139. Sammarco GJ and Stephens MM: Diabetic foot function. In Sammarco GJ (ed): The Foot in Diabetes. Philadelphia, Lea & Febiger, 1991, pp 36–53.

140. Brink SJ: Limited joint mobility as a risk factor for diabetic complications. N Engl J Med 318:1315, 1988.

141. Monnier VM, Vishwanath V, Frank KE, et al: Relation between complications of type I diabetes mellitus and collagen-linked fluorescence. N Engl J Med 314:403, 1986.

142. Brownlee M, Vlassara H, and Cerami A: Nonenzymatic glycosylation and the pathogenesis of diabetic complications. Ann Intern Med 101:527, 1984.

143. Dominiczak MH: The significance of the products of the Maillard (browning) reaction in diabetes. Diabetic Med 8:505, 1991.

144. Ceriello A, Giugliano D, Quatraro A, et al: Vitamin E reduction of protein glycosylation in diabetes: New prospect for prevention of diabetic complications? Diabetes Care 14:68, 1991.

145. Davie SJ, Gould BJ, and Yudkin JS: Effect of vitamin C on glycosylation of proteins. Diabetes 41:167, 1992.

146. Vera M, Shumkov G, and Guell R: Histological and histochemical skin changes in insulin-dependent diabetic patients with and without limited joint mobility. Acta Diabetol Lat 24:101, 1987.

147. Larkin JG, Belch JJ, Flanigan P, et al: Microvascular disease and limited joint mobility in diabetes: A comparison of fibrinolysis and prostacyclin in diabetes and systemic sclerosis. Diabetic Med 5:53, 1988.

148. Eaton RP, Sibbitt WL, and Harsh A: The effect of an aldose reductase inhibiting agent on limited joint mobility in diabetic patients. JAMA 253:1437, 1985.

149. Cohen MP: The Polyol Paradigm and Complications of Diabetes. New York, Springer-Verlag, 1987, pp 1–4.

150. Eadington DW, Patrick AW, and Frier BM: Association between connective tissue changes and smoking habit in type 2 diabetes and in non-diabetic humans. Diab Res Clin Pract 11:121, 1991.

151. Chaudhuri KR, Davidson AR, and Morris IM: Limited joint mobility and carpal tunnel syndrome in insulin-dependent diabetes. Br J Rheumatol 28:191, 1989.

152. Brownlee M, Vlassara H, Loozy A, et al: Aminoguanidine prevents diabetes-induced arterial wall protein cross-linking. Science 232:1629, 1986.

153. Bergaoui N, Dibej K, and el May M: Association of cheiroarthropathy and Dupuytren's disease in diabetes mellitus. Rev Rhum Mal Osteoartic 58:179, 1991.

154. Bland JH, Frymoyer JW, Newberg AH, et al: Rheumatic syndromes in endocrine disease. Semin Arthritis Rheum 9:23, 1979.

155. Borsotti C, Dacatra U, and Giancola R: Dupuytren's disease and diabetes mellitus. Chir Ital 37:559, 1985.

156. Davis JS and Finesilver EM: Dupuytren's contracture with a note on the incidence of the contracture in diabetes. Arch Surg 24:933, 1932.

157. Gunther O and Miosga R: Dupuytren's contracture as a late complication of diabetes. Z Gesamte Inn Med 27:777, 1972.

158. Larkin JG and Frier BM: Limited joint mobility and Dupuytren's contracture in diabetic, hypertensive, and normal populations. Br Med J 292:1494, 1986.

159. Lawson PM, Maneschi F, and Kohner EM: The relationship of hand abnormalities to diabetes and diabetic retinopathy. Diabetes Care 6:140, 1983.

160. Montenero P, Colletti A, and Fabbri G: Dupuytren's disease and diabetes. J Ann Diabet Hotel-Dieu 6:75, 1965.

161. Noble J, Heathcoate JG, and Cohen H: Diabetes in the aetiology of Dupuytren's disease. J Bone Joint Surg 66B:322, 1984.

162. Paeslack V: Dupuytrensche kontraktur und diabetes mellitus. Schweiz Med Wchnschr 92:349, 1962.

163. Pal B, Griffiths ID, Anderson J, and Dick WC: Association of limited joint mobility with Dupuytren's contracture in diabetes mellitus. J Rheumatol 14:582, 1987.

164. Ravid M, Dinai Y, and Sohar E: Dupuytren's disease in diabetes mellitus. Acta Diabetol Lat 14:170, 1977.

165. Revach M and Cabilli C: Dupuytren's contracture and diabetes mellitus. Isr J Med Sci 8:774, 1972.

166. Ricci N and Tovanella B: Malattia di Dupuytren e diabete mellito. Minerva Med 54:3272, 1963.

167. Ruffino C, Berton A, Bonanni F, et al: An elevated incidence in the association of diabetes mellitus and Dupuytren's disease. Minerva Med 80:371, 1989.

168. Schneider T: Dupuytren's contracture in diabetes mellitus [Abstract]. Excerpta Med Int Cong Series 74:75, 1964.

169. Spring M, Fleck H, and Cohen BD: Dupuytren's contracture: Warning of diabetes? NY S J Med 70:1037, 1970.

170. Stradner F, Ulreich A, and Pfeiffer KP: Dupuytren's contracture as a concomitant disease in diabetes mellitus. Wien Med Wchnschr 137:89, 1987.

171. Sturfelt G, Leden E, and Nived O: Hand symptoms associated with diabetes mellitus: An investigation of 765 patients based on a questionnaire. Acta Med Scand 210:35, 1981.

172. Teshemacher V: Ueber das vorkommen der Dupuytrenschen fingerkontractur bei diabetes mellitus. Deutsche Med Wchnschr 30:501, 1904.

173. Wegmann T, Gurtner B, and Munz W: Dupuytren's contracture, diabetes mellitus and chronic alcoholism. Schweiz Med Wchnschr 96:852, 1966.

174. Kashuk KB and Pasternack WA: Aggressive infiltrating plantar fibromatosis. J Am Podiatr Assoc 71:491, 1980.

175. Skoog R: Dupuytren's contracture with special reference to aetiology and improved surgical treatment. Acta Chir Scand 139 [Suppl]:1, 1948.

176. Cavolo DJ and Sherwood GF: Dupuytren's disease of the plantar fascia. J Foot Surg 21:12, 1982.

177. Pickren JW, Smith AG, Stevenson TW, and Stout AP: Fibromatosis of the plantar fascia. Cancer 4:846, 1951.

178. Allen PW: The fibromatoses: A clinicopathologic classification based on 140 cases. Am J Surg Pathol 1:255, 1977.

179. Allen RA, Woolner LB, and Ghormley RK: Soft-tissue tumors of the sole. J Bone Joint Surg 37A:14, 1955.

180. Aviles E, Arlen M, and Miller T: Plantar fibromatosis. Surgery 69:117, 1971.

181. Synder M: Dupuytren's contracture and plantar fibromatosis. J Am Podiatr Assoc 70:410, 1980.

182. Pentland AP and Anderson TF: Plantar fibromatosis responds to intralesional steroids. J Am Acad Dermatol 12:212, 1985.

183. Fahey JJ, Stark HH, Donovan WF, and Drennan DB: Xanthoma of the Achilles tendon. J Bone Joint Surg 55A:1197, 1973.

184. Kozak GP and Krall LP: Disorders of the skin in diabetes. In Marble A, Krall LP, Bradley RF, et al (eds): Joslin's Diabetes Mellitus, 12th ed. Philadelphia, Lea & Febiger, 1985, pp 769–783.

185. Parker F: Xanthomas and hyperlipidemias. J Am Acad Dermatol 13:1, 1985.

186. Samitz MH: Cutaneous Disorders of the Lower Extremities. Philadelphia, JB Lippincott, 1981, pp 106–107, 112–113.

187. Marcinko DE, Miller II, and Read JM: Achilles tendon hypercholesteremic xanthoma. J Foot Surg 23:398, 1984.

188. Lippmann HI, Perotto A, and Farrar R: The neuropathic foot of the diabetic. Bull NY Acad Med 52:1159, 1976.

189. Boulton AJM, Hardisty CA, Betts RP, et al: Dynamic foot pressure and other studies as diagnostic and management aids in diabetic neuropathy. Diabetes Care 6:26, 1983.

190. Boulton AJM, Betts RP, Franks CI, et al: Abnormalities of foot pressure in early diabetic neuropathy. Diabetic Med 4:225, 1987.

191. Ctercteko GC, Dhanendran MK, Hutton WC, et al: Vertical forces acting on the feet of diabetic patients with neuropathic ulceration. Br J Surg 68:608, 1981.

192. Stokes IAF, Faris IB, and Hutton WC: The neuropathic ulcer and loads on the foot in diabetic patients. Acta Orthop Scand 46:839, 1975.

193. Evans SL, Nixon BP, Lee I, et al: The prevalence and nature of podiatric problems in elderly diabetic patients. J Am Geriatr Soc 39:241, 1991.

194. Spencer F, Sage R, and Graner J: The incidence of foot pathology in a diabetic population. J Am Podiatr Med Assoc 75:590, 1985.

195. Borssen B, Bergenheim T, and Lithner F: The epidemiology of foot lesions in diabetic patients aged 15–50 years. Diabetic Med 7:438, 1990.

196. Rubin G, Cohen E, and Rzonca EC: Prostheses and orthoses for the foot and ankle. In Frykberg RG (ed): The High-Risk Foot in Diabetes Mellitus. New York, Churchill Livingstone, 1991, pp 463–486.

197. Thomas PK and Brown MJ: Diabetic polyneuropathy. In Dyck PJ, Thomas PK, Asbury AK, et al (eds): Diabetic Neuropathy. Philadelphia, WB Saunders, 1987, pp 56–65.

198. Mueller MJ, Diamond J, DeLitto A, and Sinacore DR: Insensitivity, limited joint mobility, and plantar ulcers in patients with diabetes. Phys Ther 69:453, 1989.

199. Root ML, Orien WP, and Weed JH: Normal and Abnormal Function of the Foot: Clinical Biomechanics, Vol II. Los Angeles, Clinical Biomechanics, 1977, pp 349–376.

200. Barrett JP and Mooney V: Neuropathic and diabetic pressure lesions. Orthop Clin North Am 4:43, 1973.

201. Birke JA, Cornwall MA, and Jackson M: Relationship between hallux limitus and ulceration of the great toe. J Orthop Sports Phys Ther 10:172, 1988.

202. Dannels E: Neuropathic foot ulcer prevention in diabetic American Indians with hallux limitus. J Am Podiatr Med Assoc 79:447, 1989.

203. Downs DM and Jacobs RL: Treatment of resistant ulcers on the plantar surface of the great toe in diabetes. J Bone Joint Surg 64A:930, 1982.

204. Bianchi V and Ricci G: The role of various factors in the etiology of osteoarthritis: Observations on 500 subjects. Rheumatismo (Milano) 19:146, 1967.

205. Ghanem MH and Said M: Diabetes mellitus and osteoarthritis. Egypt Rheum 4:1, 1967.

206. Siberberg M, Frank EL, Jarrett BS, et al: Aging and osteoarthritis of the human sternoclavicular joint. Am J Pathol 35:851, 1959.

207. Waine H, Nevinny D, Rosenthal J, and Jaffe JB: Association of osteoarthritis and diabetes mellitus. Tufts Folia Med 7:13, 1961.

208. Buchanan KD: Diabetes mellitus and gout. Semin Arthritis Rheum 2:157, 1972.

209. McCarty DJ, Silcox DC, Coe F, et al: Diseases associated with calcium pyrophosphate dihydrate crystal deposition. Am J Med 56:704, 1974.

210. Binder A, Maddison PJ, Skinner P, et al: Sjögren's syndrome: Association with type-1 diabetes mellitus. Br J Rheumatol 28:518, 1989.

211. Fruman LS: Diabetes mellitus, islet-cell antibodies, and HLA-B8 in a patient with systemic lupus erythematosis. Am J Dis Child 131:1252, 1977.

212. Jenkins EA, Hull RG, Gray RE, and Ansell BM: Diabetes mellitus and myasthenia gravis in a patient with systemic onset juvenile chronic arthritis. J R Soc Med 82:368, 1989.

213. Rudolf MC, Genel M, Tamorlane WV, and Dwyer JM: Juvenile rheumatoid arthritis in children with diabetes mellitus. J Pediatr 99:519, 1981.

214. Sattar MA, Al-Sughyer AA, and Siboo R: Coexistence of rheumatoid arthritis, ankylosing spondylitis, and dermatomyositis in a patient with diabetes mellitus and the associated linked HLA antigens. Br J Rheumatol 27:146, 1988.

215. Sibley JT: Concurrent onset of adult onset Still's disease and insulin-dependent diabetes mellitus. Ann Rheum Dis 49:547, 1990.

216. Tsokos GC: Lupus nephritis and other autoimmune features in patients with diabetes due to autoantibody to insulin receptors. Ann Intern Med 102:176, 1985.

217. Tyring SK, Downing P, and Poffenbarger PL: Insulin-insensitive variety of combined types A and B diabetes mellitus progressing to systemic lupus erythematosis. South Med J 80:641, 1987.

218. Weinstein PS: Insulin resistance due to receptor antibodies: A complication of progressive systemic sclerosis. Arthritis Rheum 23:101, 1980.

219. Kaldany A, Busick EJ, and Eisenbarth GS: Diabetes and the immune system. In Marble A, Krall LP, Bradley RF, et al (eds): Joslin's Diabetes Mellitus, 12th ed. Philadelphia, Lea & Febiger, 1985, pp 51–64.

220. Krolewski AS and Warram JH: Epidemiology of diabetes mellitus. In Marble A, Krall LP, Bradley RF, et al (eds): Joslin's Diabetes Mellitus, 12th ed. Philadelphia, Lea & Febiger, 1985, p. 12–42.

221. Hakala M, Ilonen J, Reijonen H, et al: No association between rheumatoid arthritis and insulin dependent diabetes mellitus: An epidemiologic and immunogenetic study. J Rheumatol 19:856, 1992.

CHAPTER 17

Afflictions of Nerves and Muscles

Craig Wargon, D.P.M., Jon R. Risser, D.P.M., and Flair David Goldman, D.P.M.

When neuromuscular diseases that affect the foot and leg are reviewed, it is noted that a variety of conditions confront the podiatric practitioner. We have chosen to look at the two most common neuromuscular diseases we see in our practice: cerebral palsy and poliomyelitis. These diseases are useful models because there are abundant clinical and follow-up experiences with them. Poliomyelitis represents a classic model of paralytic disease; spastic cerebral palsy is a classic model of spastic disease. Just as each patient is an individual, and no one procedure can be used exclusively to treat all patients, so each neuromuscular disease is individual with its own unique characteristics. However, the basic principles discussed in this chapter have broad application for the podiatric surgeon.

POLIOMYELITIS

Prior to the introduction of prophylactic vaccinations for poliomyelitis in the mid-1950s, this acute viral infection was prevalent and endemic in all countries. The western world implemented extensive immunization campaigns, which dramatically decreased the incidence of poliomyelitis. This disease is now limited to underdeveloped third-world countries and isolated cases in highly developed countries.

Prior to widespread immunization, much energy was placed in the training programs on surgical and nonsurgical management of this paralytic disease. Consequently, the eradication of poliomyelitis in developed countries has resulted in the demise of this training. Musculoskeletal management of the rare new cases of polio now is highly dependent on the well-documented principles of the experienced surgeons and physicians who managed poliomyelitis prior to immunization. The principles learned can be appropriately utilized only with an understanding of the anatomy, biomechanics, and normal strength and action of muscles acting on the lower extremity.

Most patients treated for the effects of poliomyelitis today have long-standing deformities that are the residual effects of prior treatment that has resulted in undercorrection or overcorrection. Also included are those patients who have recurrences, progressive secondary deformities, and degenerative arthritis. Many of these deformities affect multiple joints and often require osseous realignment and stabilization in the form of arthrodesis. If surgical treatment is not feasible, some type of external bracing often is required.

Another more recently observed late complication associated with poliomyelitis patients is postpoliomyelitis muscular atrophy. This syndrome is presenting with increased incidence more than 30 years after the initial contraction of the virus. Patients are presenting with increased pain and weakness in both the previously affected and nonaffected muscles, resulting in increased disability. The exact cause is unknown, but its increased incidence is presenting new challenges.[1]

The application of the principles of surgical and nonsurgical management of poliomyelitis is of great value in any paralytic disorder affecting the foot and lower extremity, whether of traumatic, genetic, infectious, or metabolic origin.

Etiology

The target cells of the poliomyelitis virus are the anterior horn cells of the spinal cord and the nuclei of various brain stem motor cells. Necrosis of these cells results in the denervation of the motor units they supply with subsequent partial or complete paralysis of the muscles involved. The muscles affected as they act on the foot and ankle result in an unequal balance of strength in relation to the nonaffected muscles, which causes specific and sometimes predictable deformities of the foot and ankle.

General Principles

Preventing and correcting foot deformities require rebalancing of muscle power around the foot and ankle to compensate for power deficits, to stabilize flail joints, and to correct and stabilize structural deformities. The ultimate decision for a treatment plan should be based on each patient's physical, emotional, occupational, and social potential to give the best possible functional result within the patient's capacity. When treating the foot deformities in poliomyelitis, deformities in the rest of the lower extremity must be considered. Examples include genu recurvatum, genu valgum, leg-length discrepancy, quadriceps and hamstring paralysis, and others. All these factors play an important role in the decision-making process if surgical treatment of the foot and ankle is to be successful.

Restoration of Muscle Balance. Surgical restoration of muscle balance around the foot can be accomplished by (1) reinforcing weak antagonist muscles, (2) transferring a deforming muscle, and (3) lengthening or releasing a deforming muscle. The whole system of foot balance must be well understood and considered. Accurate muscle testing is essential (Table 17–1). Tendon transfers should never be expected to correct existing structural deformities; likewise, stabilization procedures in the presence of significant muscle imbalance may result in recurrent deformities because the deforming forces still act on joints proximal and distal to the joints stabilized.[2, 3] In children affected by poliomyelitis, conservative means to attempt to prevent deformities should be used until skeletal maturity is achieved or until splints, braces, and casts are unsuccessful in preventing deformity.[2–4] In patients in whom deformity has already occurred and conservative attempts at correcting or preventing the deformity have failed, surgical intervention may be necessary. Dynamic deformities that are reducible are appropriate for muscle-rebalancing procedures. Tendon transfers in children can be performed before skeletal maturity is reached, but with caution. Tendon transfers generally should be deferred until children are 5 years of age.[4] The child should be old enough to participate with the physician in eliciting an accurate clinical muscle strength rating examination and in postoperative muscle re-education programs. The deformity must be dynamic and flexible in nature, and it must be determined that the affected muscles have reached their full recuperation after the convalescent phase of the disease has terminated and no further recovery of muscle strength is likely.[3, 4] Muscle-rebalancing procedures are especially important in the growing child because proper rebalancing can affect growth in a positive way. However, skeletal growth after a tendon transfer brings unpredictability because effects of the transfer may change owing to skeletal growth. Lengthening of a contracted Achilles tendon should be performed early to alleviate its severe deforming effects on the foot and ankle.[5]

Fixed Deformities. Fixed foot deformities in poliomyelitis require stabilization procedures to re-establish foot alignment, to produce stability, to prevent progressive or recurrent deformity, and to improve function. Stabilization procedures include either arthrodesis or bone-blocking procedures. Arthrodesis procedures limit the number of joints that the affected muscles must control. Classically, it has been taught that arthrodesis procedures should be performed in children after skeletal maturity owing to (1) the negative effects on growth; (2) the higher incidence of nonunion and pseudoarthrosis; (3) the recurrence in deformities; and (4) the need to resect greater articular surfaces because of the depth of cartilage. In children with rapidly progressive deformities that are resistant to bracing, stabilization of the hindfoot via an extra-articular subtalar joint arthrodesis, as described by Grice, is the procedure of choice because of its minimal effects on growth.[6, 7]

Some studies have challenged these classic teachings. Hill and associates[8] performed a total of 43 triple arthrodeses on children between the ages of 5 and 8 years with a 9.5 year follow-up. Galindo and associates[9] performed 19 triple arthrodeses in children all younger than 10 years of age (average age 8.4 years) and an average follow-up of 4 years. Both studies concluded that the potential complications of increased nonunion, or pseudoarthrosis, severe compromise of foot length, and increased incidence of recurrent deformities were not observed. Once a child reaches skeletal maturity, deformities should be corrected to prevent secondary adaptive changes that are irreversible. If static deformities with adaptive bony changes exist, they should be corrected, or stabilized prior to tendon transfer. This allows for accurate positioning of the tendons and allows them to function on a more anatomic, stable foot.

The most common foot stabilization procedure in paralytic disorders such as poliomyelitis is the triple arthrodesis (talocalcaneal calcaneocuboid, and talonavicular joints). Medial and lateral deformity and instability of the hindfoot are common problems that this hindfoot arthrodesis successfully controls. Triple arthrodesis, when properly planned, can correct most hindfoot and midfoot deformities. Severe deformities require more precision and accuracy of bone resected, which translates into more shortening of the foot. Proper wedge resection of bone can correct hindfoot varus, valgus, equinus, planus, cavus, and calcaneus deformities. The precision required can be more predictably achieved by the use of preoperative templates. The radiographs act as excellent templates for paper cut-outs to assess accurately the amount of bone to be resected. Radiographs of the ankle and leg also should be considered, because deformities above the foot often contribute to what may be perceived purely as a foot deformity. The foot should be considered in three parts: (1) talotibial, (2) calcaneal, and (3) navicular and cuboid, with the remaining midfoot and forefoot. The important goals that should be achieved when correcting a deformity and stabilizing the foot with the triple arthrodesis include the following: (1) bring the hindfoot into neutral position or slight valgus; no varus should be present; (2) the forefoot should be perpendicular to the ground so that weightbearing is evenly distributed over the plantar surface of the foot; (3) any cavus, planus, adductus, or abductus deformities should be corrected at the midtarsal joint. The long axis of the foot should be as close to perpendicular to the ankle joint axis as possible. Triple arthrodesis increases the inversion, eversion, and rotary forces across the ankle joint. Also, compression forces across the ankle joint are increased, because the shock absorption properties that normally occur with pronation at the subtalar joint are lost and are transferred to the midfoot, ankle joint, and more proximal joints in the lower extremity. Degenerative changes present at the ankle joint are likely accelerated and may lead to pantalar fusion. Instability or deformity at the ankle joint is magnified after triple arthrodesis. Pantalar arthrodesis would be a consideration in such cases.

Leg-Length Discrepancies. Leg-length discrepancy is common with poliomyelitis. In children with established leg-length discrepancies, timing and planning of procedures to reduce the inequality must be based on careful radiographic

TABLE 17–1

RATING SYSTEM FOR CLINICAL MUSCLE TESTING[2, 3]

Score	Criteria
0	Absent—no observable contractility
1	Trace—some observable contractility without motion at the joint
2	Poor—full range of motion at the joint involved without gravity
3	Fair—full range of motion at the joints involved against gravity only with no resistance
4	Good—full range of motion at the joint involved with gravity and mild resistance
5	Normal—full range of motion at the joint involved against full resistance

interpretation of skeletal maturity and growth potential. Adults with inadequately treated long-standing leg-length discrepancy have structurally compensated for this inequality.

In some instances, the short leg has developed an equinus attitude at the ankle joint and foot to compensate for length discrepancy. Custom-molded equinus position shoes to re-establish weightbearing force across the whole plantar surface of the foot are an effective, conservative means of reducing the forefoot problems associated with walking in severe equinus.

Untreated leg-length discrepancy, in which the ankle joint and foot of the short leg have not compensated in equinus for the inequality, usually displays structural compensatory changes in the more proximal lower extremity and the spine. These long-standing rigid structural adaptations may preclude the use of shoe lifts to re-establish leg-length equality.

SPECIFIC DEFORMITIES

Equinus Deformity

The most common cause of equinus deformity in poliomyelitis is secondary to a paralytic footdrop from lack of dorsiflexion power. Paralysis of the anterior tibialis muscle, which is the strongest dorsiflexor of the foot, contributes most significantly to drop foot deformities. Transfer of muscle power to regain dorsiflexion can be achieved by transferring synergistic muscles (extensor hallucis longis and extensor digitorum longus) more proximally on the foot,[34, 40] increasing their mechanical advantage for dorsiflexion at the ankle and decreasing the retrograde plantarflexor effects on the forefoot at the metatarsophalangeal (MTP) joints. When synergistic muscles are not available, antagonist muscles can be used to transfer anteriorly. Transfer of the posterior tibial tendon anteriorly through the interosseous membrane to achieve dorsiflexion can be useful but may result in medial instability and a valgus deformity in the presence of strong peroneal muscles.[10–15]

When contracture of the Achilles tendon occurs in children, the tendon should be stretched or surgically lengthened, along with posterior ankle joint capsular and ligamentous release, if needed, to bring the foot into a more neutral position.[16] When the equinus is long-standing, the degree of secondary osseous changes contributing to the deformity should be radiographically determined. If possible, the osseous component should be surgically treated with the soft tissue procedure to achieve adequate correction. Osteophyte proliferation can be surgically excised to increase ankle joint dorsiflexion. In cases when the talus and ankle joint mortise are incongruous, surgical correction is much more difficult. In these cases, ankle joint arthrodesis, triple arthrodesis as described by Lanbrinudi,[17] or in severe cases, talectomy is required to correct the equinus.

Equinus deformity may be secondary to genu recurvatum from lack of muscle power controlling the knee. The knee deformity must be recognized and addressed in such cases if successful treatment of the equinus is to be achieved.

Equinus deformity is usually accompanied by inversion or eversion instability or deformity (Fig. 17–1A to C). In an equinus deformity secondary to dorsiflexor weakness or drop foot the invertor or evertor muscles, when strong, can be used to transfer anteriorly on the foot to achieve dorsiflexion power at the ankle joint. When the invertor or evertor muscles are transferred to become dorsiflexors at the ankle, a loss of lateral stability occurs. Stabilizing the hindfoot may be necessary to prevent varus or valgus instability or deformity (Fig. 17–1D). By stabilizing the hindfoot, the anteriorly transferred muscles can exert their power to achieve dorsiflexion more effectively at the ankle.

Tendon Transfer for Varus Deformities

When the varus deformity is dynamic in nature without structural or osseous changes, transfer of the anterior tibial tendon to a more lateral position on the dorsum of the foot is usually adequate to achieve functional balance of the foot and reduce the varus instability. Lateral transfer of the anterior tibial tendon for varus deformity is one of the most effective transfers in the foot.[2–4] When the peroneus longus and peroneus brevis are the only muscles paralyzed, the anterior tibial tendon should be transferred to the third metatarsal base or adjacent cuneiform. If transferred too far laterally, a valgus deformity may result. If the varus instability is mild owing to only partial weakness of the peroneals, a split anterior tibial tendon transfer may be more appropriate, with the lateral half of the anterior tibial tendon transferred to the fourth metatarsal base or the cuboid.[18–20]

If the anterior tibial tendon and peroneals are weak or paralyzed, dorsiflexion and eversion power of the foot and ankle are compromised. The triceps surae and posterior medial muscle groups become the deforming forces resulting in an equinovarus deformity. Transfer of the posterior tibial tendon through the interosseous membrane to the dorsum of the foot removes a strong deforming force and functions as a tenodesis anteriorly with contractile properties, in some cases.[21, 22] The flexor hallucis longus and flexor digitorum longus can be transferred with the posterior tibialis to increase the strength of the transfer.[23] Because dorsiflexion power is usually low after this transfer, an ankle-foot orthosis or dorsiflexion assist brace may be needed to prevent recurrent deformity.

When subtalar joint varus or calcaneal varus is not accompanied by advanced subtalar joint arthritis, a calcaneal osteotomy to realign the hindfoot should be performed prior to or in concert with the previously discussed tendon transfers (Figs. 17–2A to D).[24–26]

Subtalar joint or triple arthrodesis is usually required in varus instability when (1) the varus instability is too severe to be corrected adequately by a calcaneal osteotomy; (2) advanced secondary degenerative changes have occurred at the subtalar joint; or (3) muscle power around the foot and ankle is inadequate to maintain inversion or eversion stability.

Tendon Transfers for Valgus Deformities

Tendon transfers for valgus deformities are less reliable than those for varus deformities. Often valgus cannot be corrected with tendon transfers alone.[4]

In flexible deformities secondary to an isolated anterior tibial paralysis when there is no significant structural adaptive change, transfer of the peroneus longus to the dorsum of the foot (usually the base of the second or third metatarsal or

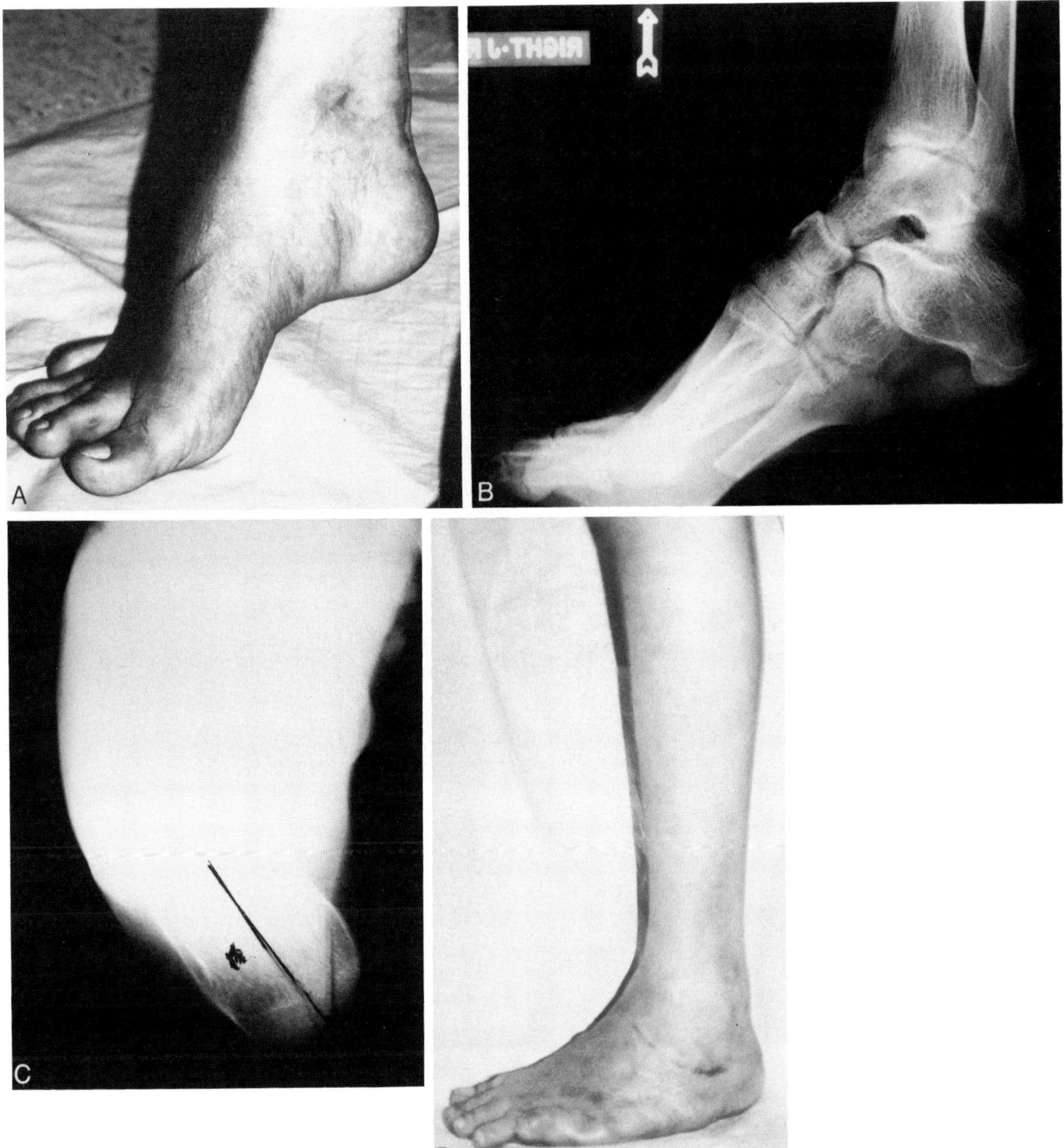

FIGURE 17–1. *A*, Equinovarus deformity secondary to poliomyelitis. *B* and *C*, Weightbearing radiograph after tendo-Achillis lengthening and fifth metatarsal head resection with persistent equinus *B*, and hindfoot varus *C*. *D*, Plantigrade foot after triple arthrodesis.

cuneiforms) can suffice.[2] When the extensor hallucis longus is strong and a hallux hammertoe is present, a Jones tenosuspension wherein the extensor hallucis longus is transferred to the head of the first metatarsal, is used in conjunction with fusion of the hallux interphalangeal joint.[27]

Tendon transfers for isolated paralytic posterior tibial muscle can be achieved by transferring the flexor digitorum longus, flexor hallucis longus, and extensor hallucis longus to the navicular or medial cuneiform.[28] The peroneus brevis can be transferred to the dorsum of the foot further medially to reduce its eversion deforming influences.

Pes planoequinovalgus deformity secondary to paralysis of both the anterior tibial and posterior tibial muscles cannot be adequately controlled with tendon transfers and usually requires some type of osseous stabilization.

For valgus deformities secondary to either an anterior tibial or a posterior tibial paralysis, tendon transfers alone may not be adequate to support the medial column, and a medial column fusion may be required to maintain the support of the arch. We prefer a talonavicular joint arthrodesis through a medial incision.[16] In a combined anterior tibial and posterior tibial paralysis, the tendon transfers and talonavicular fusion may suffice, but the combined paralysis is more likely to result in a recurrent deformity, necessitating a triple arthrodesis at a later date.

Calcaneal Deformities

Calcaneal deformities are associated with partial or complete paralysis of the triceps surae. This is the most difficult

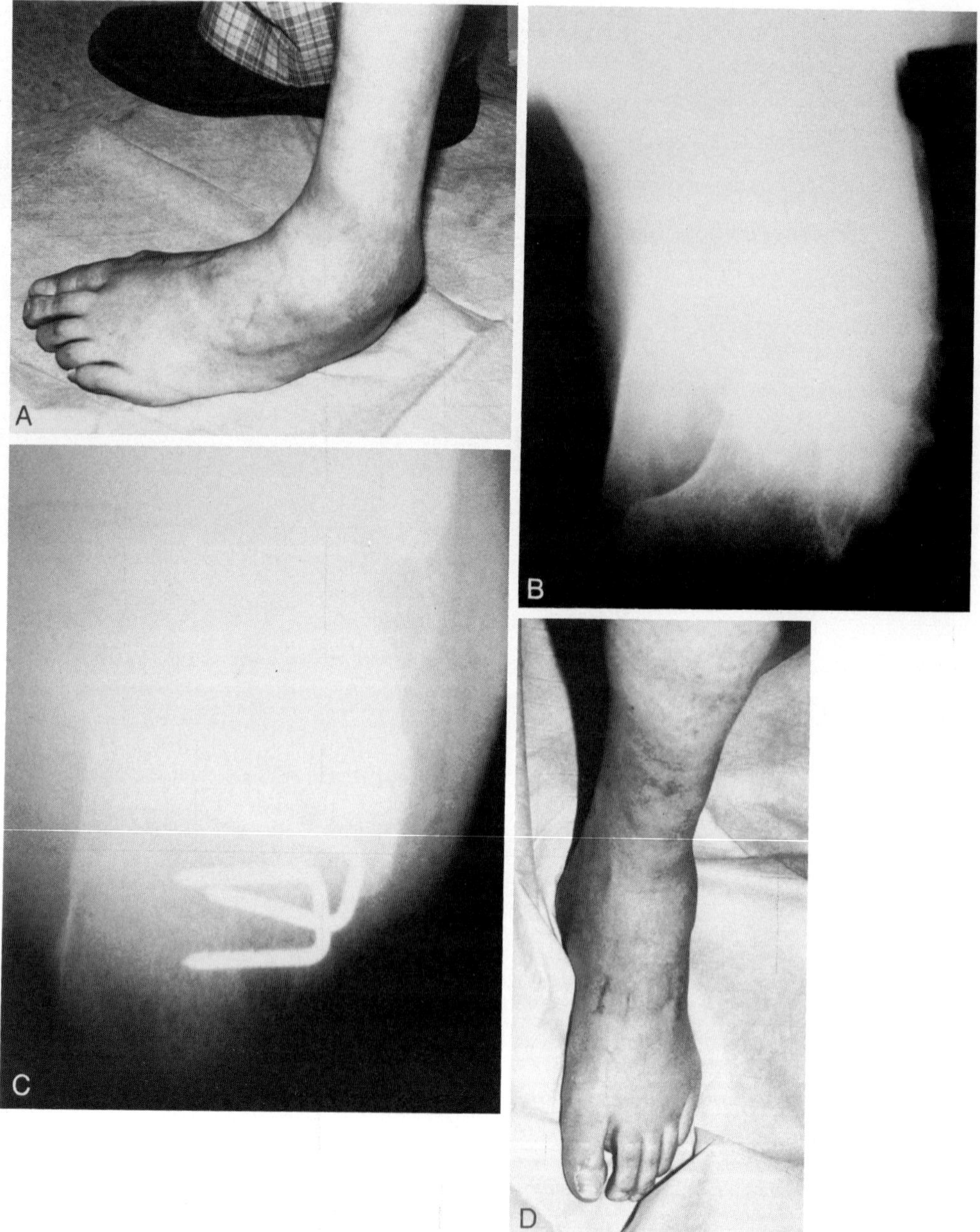

FIGURE 17–2. *A,* Rigid varus deformity secondary to long-standing peroneal muscle paralysis in poliomyelitis. *B,* Weightbearing calcaneal axial radiograph demonstrating calcaneal and subtalar varus. *C,* Weightbearing calcaneal axial radiograph demonstrating improved heel position after a Dwyer osteotomy. Note the slight undercorrection. *D,* Plantigrade foot after a Dwyer osteotomy and lateral transfer of the anterior tibial tendon.

paralytic foot deformity to treat.[4, 5] Calcaneal deformities result in classic, disabling gait. The heel remains on the ground, and the foot maintains a dorsiflexed postion at the ankle joint throughout the full-stance phase of gait. The posterior tibialis, flexor hallucis longus, flexor digitorum longus, and the peroneus longus, when strong, become the compensatory plantarflexors of the foot. The posterior tibialis and peroneus longus plantarflex the forefoot as a result of their more distal insertion, contributing to the anterior cavus component of the deformity. The compensatory action of the flexor hallucis longus and flexor digitorum longus muscles results in the buckling of the toes with retrograde plantarflexory force on the metatarsal heads, also contributing to the anterior cavus (Fig. 17–3*A* and *B*). The progression of the

calcaneus foot is virtually impossible to prevent with bracing. Progression is rapid in children. Early tendon transfer should be considered.[4, 23]

Tendon Transfer for Calcaneal Deformity. When the triceps surae muscle is weak or paralyzed, transfer of more than one muscle to the posterior calcaneus is usually required to regain adequate plantarflexory strength. With complete paralysis of the triceps surae, the posterior tibialis, flexor hallucis longus, and both peroneals can be transferred to the calcaneus. Transfer of the anterior tibialis to the second metatarsal base to prevent a secondary metatarsus primus elevatus should be performed in conjunction with, or within 1 year of, the posterior transfer when the peroneus longus is transferred.[5]

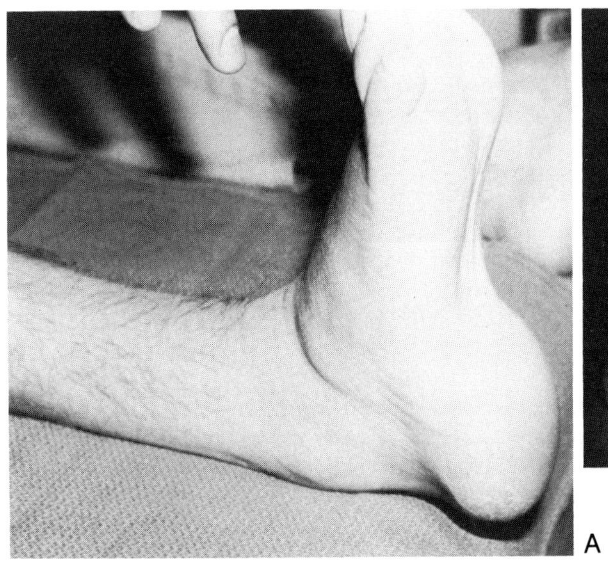

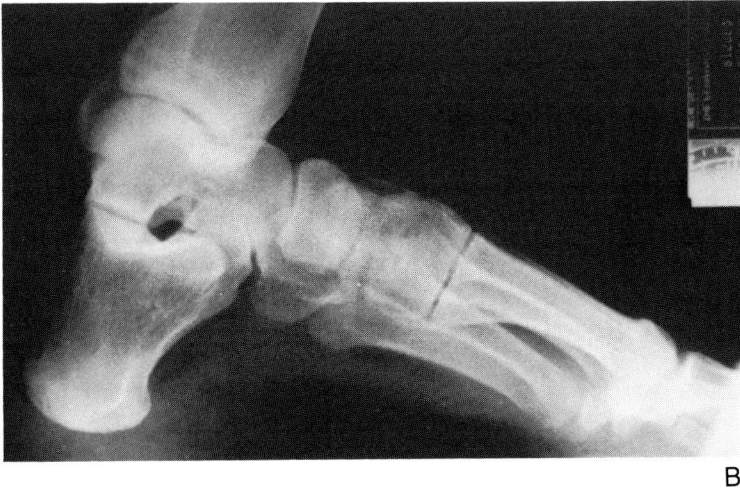

FIGURE 17–3. *A*, Calcaneus foot. *B*, Weightbearing radiograph of a calcaneus foot demonstrating severe posterior cavus component of this deformity.

When the triceps surae is only partially paralyzed (muscle rating of 2 or 3), a transfer of the posterior tibialis and peroneus longus to the calcaneus is preferable.[2, 30] If the peroneal muscles and posterior tibialis muscle are also involved and are too weak to transfer posteriorly, posterior transfer of the anterior tibialis muscle through the interosseous membrane to the calcaneus reduces the strong dorsiflexory deforming force and produces some plantarflexory strength. It is important to remember that tendon transfers for complete paralysis of the gastrosoleus complex may need to be performed in children before they reach 5 years of age if prevention or correction of deformity with growth is to be expected.[4]

Osteotomies for Calcaneal Deformity. Osseous procedures in conjunction with tendon transfers are usually necessary at an earlier age to achieve correction in calcaneal deformities. Osteotomies to reduce the calcaneal component of the deformity include crescentic, slide, and wedge osteotomies at the posterior body of the calcaneus to reduce the posterior cavus. Correction with osteotomies may be highly dependent on the surgical release of the contracted plantar fascia and intrinsics. In some cases when anterior cavus is well advanced, tarsal osteotomies also may be necessary (Fig. 17–4).[31, 32] Osteotomies in the skeletally immature foot should be performed in a way to minimize interference with growth.

Arthrodesis Procedures for Calcaneal Deformity. Severe calcaneal deformities in the skeletally mature foot usually require triple arthrodesis to correct the deformity and stabilize the foot. Posterior tendon transfers also can be used in conjunction with triple arthrodesis to achieve some functional plantarflexory strength at the ankle joint.

Stabilizing the hindfoot greatly enhances the mechanical advantage of posterior muscle transfer on the ankle joint by alleviating the subtalar and midtarsal joint influences. Posterior displacement of the calcaneus during triple arthrodesis also enhances the plantarflexory mechanical properties by increasing the lever arm posteriorly.[5, 33]

Bone-Blocking Procedures. In severe paralytic involvement, calcaneal and equinal deformities cannot be prevented owing to a lack of adequate musculature to transfer anteriorly or posteriorly to achieve dorsiflexory or plantarflexory power. Bone-blocking procedures can prevent progression of deformity by limiting ankle joint motion selectively in either plantarflexion or dorsiflexion. The anterior bone block limits dorsiflexion at the ankle joint, which can prevent progression of a calcaneal deformity. The posterior bone block limits plantarflexion and can prevent progression of an equinal de-

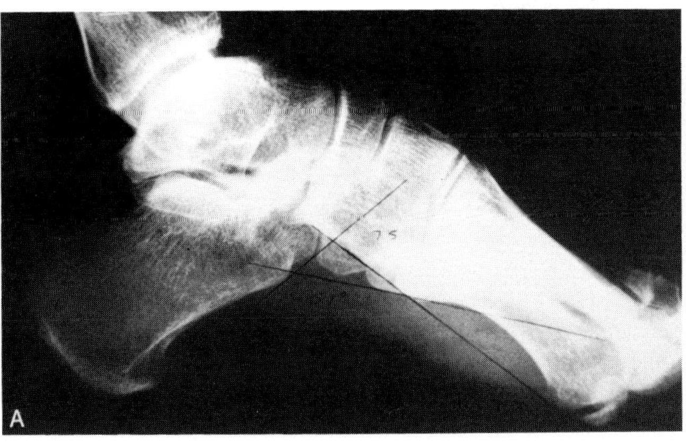

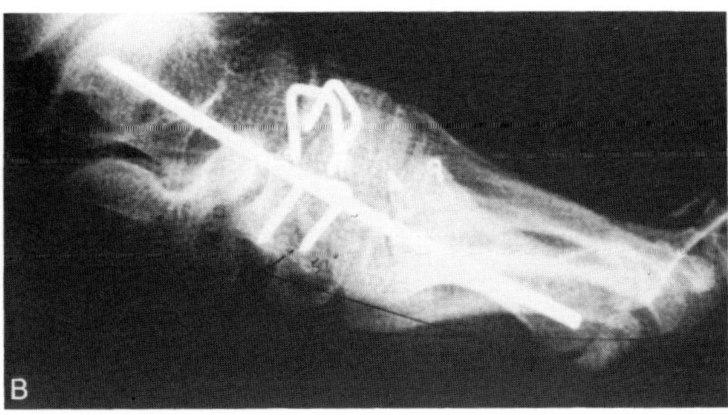

FIGURE 17–4. *A*, Cavus foot. *B*, After a Cole tarsal osteotomy.

formity. Long-term follow-up studies of these bone-blocking procedures have been less than satisfactory owing to a high incidence of recurrent deformities, painful fibrous ankylosis, painful degenerative joint disease of the ankle, and flattening of the talus. These complications often result in ankle joint or pantalar fusions (Fig. 17–5).[34–36]

Metatarsus Primus Elevatus, or Dorsal Bunion

Metatarsus primus elevatus, or dorsal bunion, in paralytic disorders is most commonly secondary to imbalances between the anterior tibialis and the peroneus longus muscles. In this deformity the first metatarsal is dorsiflexed and the hallux is plantarly contracted at the metatarsophalangeal joint (Fig. 17–6A and B). The plantarflexion of the hallux is a compensatory result of the flexor hallucis longus contracting and plantarflexing the hallux at the metatarsophalangeal joint to produce a rigid lever at toe-off. The increased ground-reactive force against the plantarflexed hallux causes dorsiflexion at the hallux interphalangeal joint. The balance of the first ray should always be considered when plans are made to transfer the anterior tibial or the peroneus longus tendons.

A less common cause of metatarsus primus elevatus is paralysis or transfer of the posterior tibial muscle. In this abnormality, pronatory forces result in collapse of the arch and a relative dorsiflexed position of the metatarsal to the midfoot and hindfoot. The flexor hallucis longus also has a strong plantarflexory influence on the hallux in its attempt to compensate for the weak or absent posterior tibial muscle. Usually adductovarus hammertoes occur at the second to fifth digits and accompany the hallux hammertoe owing to an overactive flexor digitorum longus muscle. When transferring the posterior tibial muscle for varus instability, this compensatory effect of the flexor hallucis longus should be considered.

Treatment. Metatarsus primus elevatus secondary to a weak peroneus longus muscle usually requires either a plantarflexory closing or an opening base wedge osteotomy of the first ray or a first metatarsal cuneiform joint arthrodesis where a plantarflexory-based wedge resection is made to correct the deformity (Fig. 17–3C). For more severe defor-

mities, a more proximal medial column fusion may be necessary at either the talonavicular or navicular cuneiform joints. Rebalancing can be achieved with a more proximal transfer of the anterior tibial tendon to the plantar-medial navicular and a transfer of the flexor hallucis longus to the head of the first metatarsal (Fig. 17–5D).[5, 23, 29] When an absent posterior tibial muscle is the cause of the metatarsus primus elevatus, a more proximal medial column fusion (i.e., talonavicular fusion or triple arthrodesis) is likely to be required for stability.

CEREBRAL PALSY

This section presents cerebral palsy (CP) as it relates to the deformities of the developing foot and ankle. CP is defined as a nonprogressive abnormality or lesion in the brain that alters motor control, leading to disorders of movement and posture. The severity and extent of involvement varies widely; it may involve one or all extremities. The deformities associated with CP can become more severe as the patient becomes older as a result of long-standing spasticity, soft tissue adaptation, and diminished elasticity of the tissues, although the cerebral disorder is nonprogressive.[37–42]

A thorough discussion of etiologic factors is beyond the scope of this chapter. The lesion responsible for CP may develop in prenatal, natal, or postnatal periods. Although traditionally most lesions leading to CP were believed to occur in the perinatal period, there is increasing evidence to suggest that prenatal causes occur more often than has been suspected.[43, 44]

Clinical Types

Classification of CP is difficult, as reflected by the numerous classification systems that have been employed over the years. There is no general agreement in this area. Various authors have looked at the state of muscle tone, the presence or absence of involuntary movement, the type of movement, the topographic involvement, the severity, and the etiology.[39, 42–45] The neurologist or pediatrician may use one of numerous classifications; therefore, it is necessary for the

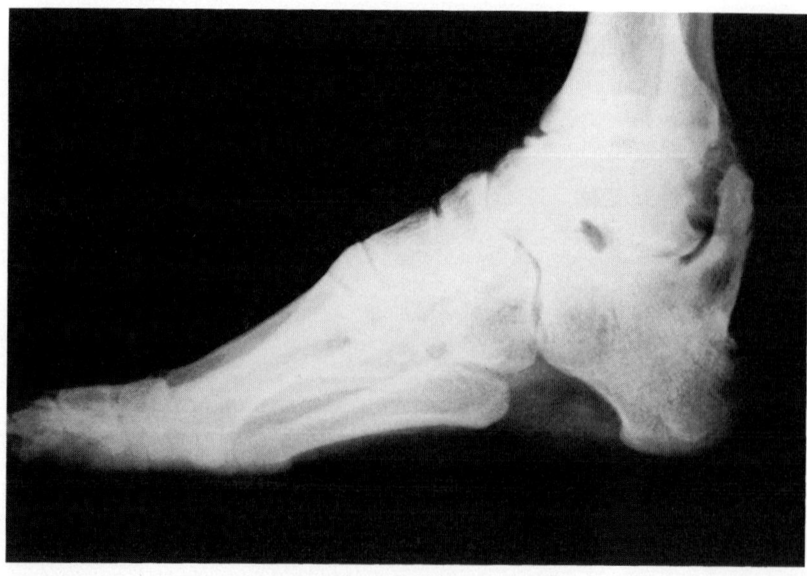

FIGURE 17–5. Posterior bone block for drop foot deformity.

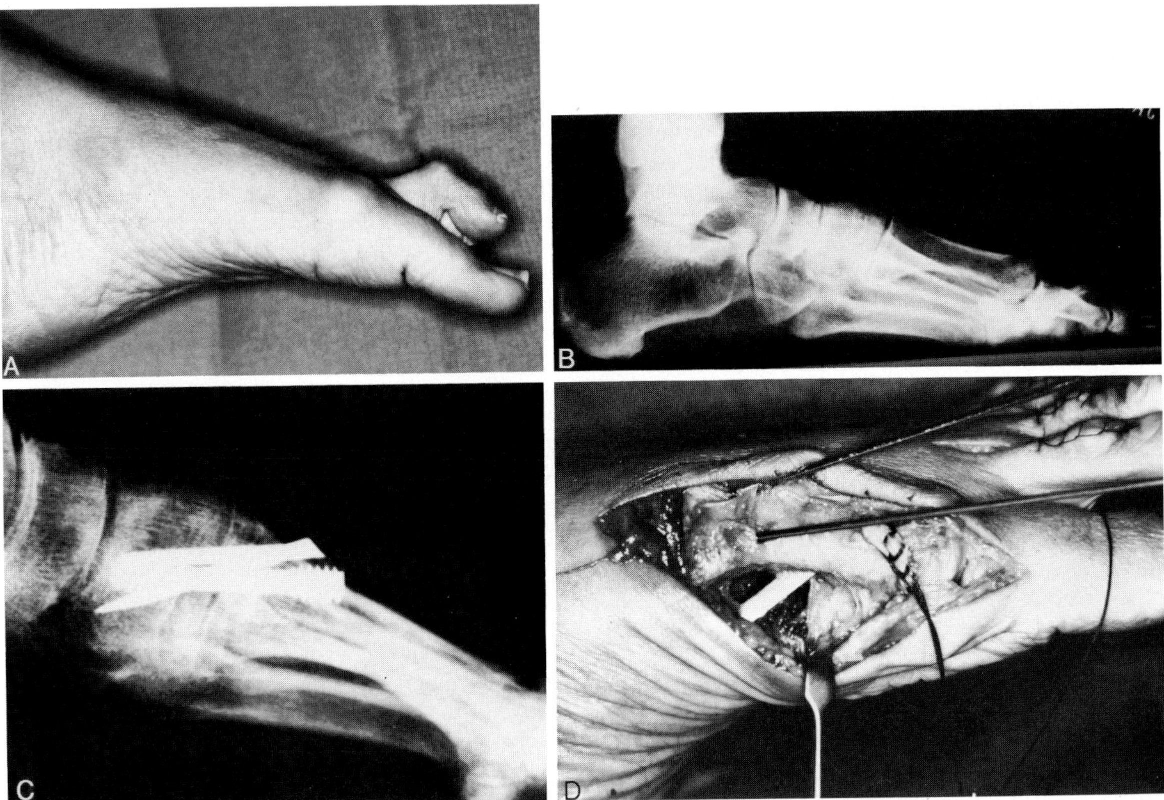

FIGURE 17–6. *A*, Dorsal bunion. *B*, Lateral weightbearing radiograph demonstrating metatarsus primus elevatus and hallux flexus. *C*, First metatarsal-cuneiform arthrodesis with plantarflexor-based wedge resection to correct the metatarsus primus elevatus. *D*, Intraoperative view of the first metatarsal-cuneiform arthrodesis combined with a flexor hallucis longus transfer through the head of the first metatarsal.

practitioner treating the foot and lower extremity to be familiar with the terminology. In this section, clinical presentation by muscle tone and character of involuntary movement are considered separately from the distribution of the disease.

Classification by Clinical Presentation. CP as classified by clinical assessment is characterized into four types: spastic, dyskinetic, ataxic, and mixed. Furthermore, patients with dyskinetic CP are subdivided according to the types of posture or movement: athetosis, tremor, dystonia, choreiform, and rigidity.

Spastic CP occurs in more than one half of the cases. Dyskinetic CP is the next largest group and ataxic CP is the rarest form, claiming fewer than 3% of the cases. As analysis of abnormal movement becomes more sophisticated, more cases than expected fit into the mixed category.[42, 43, 46]

Spasticity. Spasticity is caused by an exaggeration of the muscle stretch reflex, which leads to a state of increased tension of a muscle when it is passively lengthened. Clonus also is often present. Defects in the motor cortex may be the primary cause of spasticity.[41] Resistance is felt to a sudden, fast movement of the muscle, followed by some degree of relaxation. This is often referred to as *cogwheel resistance.* Passive movement performed more slowly does not elicit this type of increase in tension. This is distinguished from rigidity in that rigidity is not velocity dependent. With rigidity, resistance to passive movement is not intermittent. With spasticity, deep tendon reflexes are exaggerated and generally pathologic reflexes, such as Babinski's and Hoffman's signs, are present.

Dyskinesia. Dyskinesia is a disorder characterized by irregular tone and uncontrollable motion of the skeletal mus-

cles. These may be defined as involuntary contractions that are often exacerbated by the patient's attempts at voluntary control. The lesions that account for this type of CP usually lie at the base of the brain; therefore, total body involvement usually results. It is this type of involvement that results in characteristic facial grimacing, drooling, and difficulty with speech. It should be emphasized that these children are not necessarily mentally retarded, although their ability to communicate may be greatly compromised. Chorea, athetosis, and dystonia are similar in nature and are distinguished by a particular tension, rhythm, and speed of abnormal muscle activity. Coordination is often poor, and primitive reflexes are retained. With athetosis voluntary actions to control involuntary movement may lead to increased muscle tension. This may falsely lead the examiner to suspect spasticity. By rapid, repeated passive extension and flexion of the involved joints, the examiner can cause this state of tension to be released when athetosis is the disorder; not so with spasticity.[42, 44–47]

Dystonia. Dystonia is characterized more by increased tension than by abnormal movement; therefore, postural abnormalities are common. The motion is faster in chorea, and there is generally less tension present in the muscles.

Rigidity. Rigidity is characterized by generalized stiffness due to increased muscle tension in both agonist and antagonist muscle groups. Rigid paralysis is generally believed to be caused by a diffuse lesion of the brain. When the resistance is continuous, it is often referred to as a ''lead pipe'' resistance. This is in contradistinction to waxing and waning resistance referred to as cogwheel resistance.

Tremor. A tremor is a small involuntary repetitive movement with a certain amplitude and rhythmicity that often follows encephalitis.

Ataxia. Lesions in the cerebellum produce an inability to coordinate incoming proprioceptive stimuli that leads to a loss of kinesthetic sense. These patients have poor balance and a wide-base staggering gait. Often the muscles are hypotonic, the reflexes diminished, and the joints hypermobile. It is not uncommon for ataxia to improve with time, as the patient learns to apply voluntary control.

Classification by Pattern or Distribution. In assessing patients with CP, it is helpful for the practitioner to be familiar with the nomenclature for the different patterns of paresis (Table 17–2).

Treatment

CP is a condition that results in deformity, static or dynamic muscle power imbalances, and unstable joints. The goal of the podiatric surgeon, therefore, is to establish a stable plantigrade, painless foot that is compatible with ambulation. Correction of dynamic deformities generally involves lengthening of musculotendinous units or weakening of such units by tenotomy and capsulotomy.

Tendon transfers to balance muscle power are difficult in CP. The muscles involved are usually spastic and difficult for the patient to control. This is especially true when the position has been changed or reversed by surgery. Furthermore, spastic muscles retain their spasticity once transferred. For these reasons there is a significant degree of unpredictability when tendons are transferred in this patient population. A more important role for tendon transfers in CP is to remove a dynamic deforming force.[42, 48, 49]

Standard procedures to fuse and stabilize joints continue to be the mainstay of treatment for many children with CP, especially when valgus deformities exist.[50–52]

Equinus Deformity. Equinus is the most common foot deformity encountered when treating spastic CP. This may be present in isolation or in combination with valgus and, less commonly, with varus deformities of the foot.[53] The anterior tibial muscles and other dorsiflexors often appear weak or nonfunctional owing in large part to the overwhelming spasticity of the gastrosoleus muscle complex. The usual

rationale of attempting conservative treatment before surgical alternatives are considered applies when treating these deformities. Many authors have pointed out that even minimal deformities without treatment may become quite marked as the child grows and matures.[42, 46, 51, 52, 54, 55]

Nonoperative Treatment. Conservative measures consist of passive stretching of the gastrosoleus complex, active strengthening of the anterior tibial muscle, and bracing. The patient and parents should be properly taught how to stretch (generally with the knee straight) three times per day. A bivalve, removable above-the-knee fiberglass cast is an excellent means of night splinting. Many authors have recommended continued night splinting until skeletal maturity has been achieved.[42, 46] Serial casting and wedging are often not tolerated by the child with spastic CP. Therefore, a cast to hold correction should be applied comfortably snug, although not with the foot maximally dorsiflexed. The ankle should be held in 0 to 10 degrees of dorsiflexion and the knee in 0 to 15 degrees of flexion. As the equinus deformity lessens, the cast can be made with the ankle held in progressively more dorsiflexion.

Surgical Correction. Surgery may be indicated when conservative therapy does not adequately correct the equinus or the deformity is so severe that conservative therapy is unreasonable. It is important to evaluate the child stationary in stance and dynamically in gait. In stance, if the heel is in marked valgus position with severe pronation with midtarsal joint breakdown, heel cord lengthening should be considered to prevent a rocker-bottom deformity of the foot.[54, 55] In gait, if spasticity exists dynamically with a persistent toe-toe or toe-heel gait, surgery may be indicated, even if the foot can reach neutral position in a static examination. Surgical candidates should be old enough to cooperate with the physician, usually at least 4 to 5 years of age, and they must be able to understand simple commands. A potential for standing or independent walking is a prerequisite to equinus surgery unless gross deformity gives rise to ulcers and infections in the nonambulatory patient. Lengthening of the Achilles tendon continues to be the mainstay of equinus surgery in CP.[42, 46, 54, 56, 57] Other operations include lengthening of the gastrocnemius alone (gastrocnemius recession), advancing of the insertion of the Achilles tendon, releasing the heads of origin of the gastrocnemius, and partial tibial nerve neurectomy, sometimes in combination with gastrocnemius head recession; the latter are additional but less widely used approaches.

In approaches to Achilles tendon lengthening, the currently preferred procedure to correct equinus in CP is the slide lengthening of the heel cord, also known as the *White procedure.*[46, 51, 58] The procedure is predicated on the natural rotation of the fibers of the Achilles tendon. The proximal medial fibers of the Achilles tendon twist laterally as they approach the calcaneus (Fig. 17–7*A* to *D*) so they now lie posterior and lateral to the fibers to which they originally were medial. The tendon is then incised at two levels, noting the rotation of these fibers. The proximal incision is made transversely in the posteromedial two thirds of the tendon, 6 to 9 cm proximal to the calcaneal insertion. The distal incision is made in the anteromedial two thirds of the Achilles tendon. With the knee in extension, the foot is dorsiflexed to the neutral position; as this is done, the fibers slide, and the tendon lengthens. It may be necessary to make a third incision more lateral and central in the tendon if correction was

TABLE 17–2

**GEOGRAPHIC CLASSIFICATION
OF CEREBRAL PALSY**

Geographic Classification	Extremities Involved	Comment
Monoplegia	One extremity (upper or lower)	Rare
Hemiplegia	Two extremities same side	Usually spastic
Paraplegia	Both lower extremities	Usually spastic associated with prematurity
Triplegia	Three of four extremities	Rare
Quadriplegia	All four extremities involved	Spasticity dyskinesia or mixed
Diplegia	Upper extremity less affected than lower	
Double hemiplegia	Lower extremity less affected than upper	Uncommon, usually spastic
Tetraplegia	All four extremities equally involved	Spastic

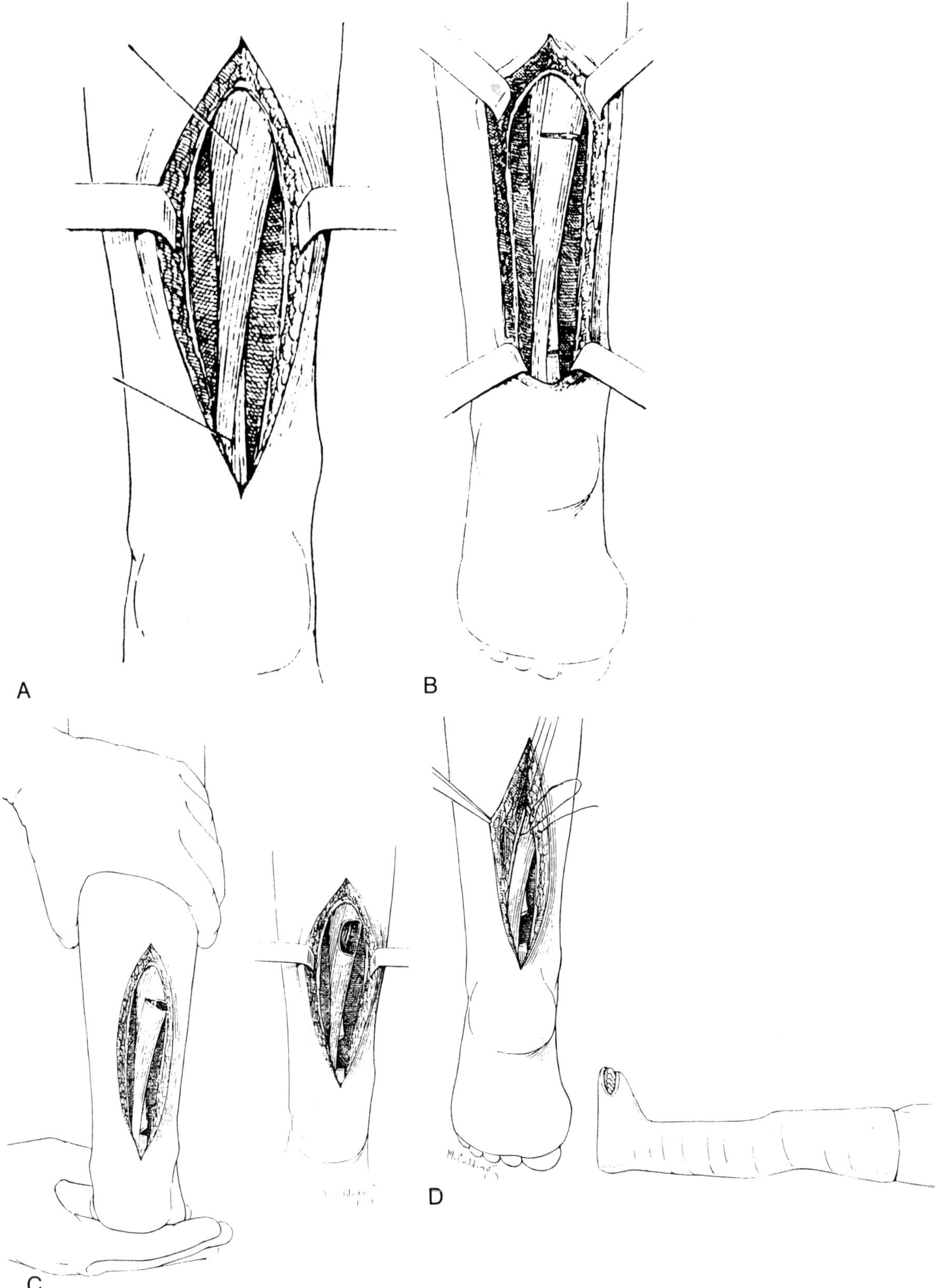

FIGURE 17–7. *A,* The rotation of the fibers is carefully identified so that one half can be divided above and one half below. *B,* The tendon is then incised at two levels, observing the rotation of the fibers. A third incision midway between the others is occasionally indicated. *C,* Passive dorsiflexion of the ankle to 90 degrees results in slight lengthening of the Achilles tendon to the appropriate length and tension. *D,* The sheath must be closed over the lengthened tendon. The limb is immobilized with a toe-to-groin cast with the knee in extension and the foot in neutral dorsiflexion. (*A* to *D* from Banks HH and Green WT: The correction of equinus deformity in cerebral palsy. J Bone Joint Surg 40A:1359, 1958.)

inadequate.[46, 54, 55, 59] The disadvantage of this procedure is the amount of lengthening that can be achieved. When significant length is needed, Z-plasty lengthening under direct visualization is preferred.

Postoperative Care. The limb is immobilized in an above-the-knee cast with the knee fully extended; the ankle joint should rest in neutral position. Care is taken not to dorsiflex the ankle, because this can lead to overcorrection. A long-leg cast with the knee straight is left in place for 3 weeks, and the patient is allowed to bear weight. After this, a short-leg weightbearing cast is applied for another 3 weeks. At 6 weeks, the cast is removed, and the child is fitted with an ankle-foot orthosis with the ankle at 90 degrees. The AFO is worn primarily at night and usually until skeletal maturity has been achieved. If the triceps surae remains spastic with inadequate dorsiflexor strength to overcome the strong pull of the posterior muscles, a daytime AFO may be indicated.[60]

Other Procedures. Posterior capsulotomy of the ankle joint or subtalar joint is rarely needed to address equinal deformities in CP. An exception may be in the equinus of long duration that occurs when the deformity is allowed to persist into adulthood. In such instances, a posterior capsulotomy of the tibiotalar joint may be necessary to allow adequate dorsiflexion.

Advancement of the Insertion of the Achilles Tendon. In the presence of a dynamic equinal deformity, advancement of the Achilles tendon has been shown to be an effective means of treating a child with little or no fixed equinus. Pierrot and Murphy introduced anterior advancement of the Achilles tendon insertion, which effectively decreased the leverage of the triceps surae.[61] This procedure has the advantage of not changing the length, depending on the length of the triceps surae, to effect the correction. Thus, the correction should not be affected by growth. In the resting position with the foot flat, the fulcrum of the triceps surae is functionally at the center of the ankle. In this position, anterior transfer of the Achilles tendon substantially decreases the lever arm, thus decreasing the effective power of the triceps surae, theoretically by 48% (Fig. 17–8, *upper*). During propulsion, the fulcrum is transferred anteriorly, and push-off power is decreased by as little as 15% (Fig. 17–8, *lower*). Thus, this procedure corrects equinus but has less of a weakening action on the posterior muscle group than Achilles tendon lengthening.

With this procedure, the Achilles tendon is detached from the tuberosity of the calcaneus distally, and the tendon is routed anterior to the flexor hallucis longus, passed through a drill hole in the calcaneus, and tied over a button on the plantar surface of the foot with the foot held in slight plantarflexion (Fig. 17–9A to D). The tendon is transferred anterior to the flexor hallucis longus in an effort to prevent it from reattaching to the original insertion site.

The foot is held in a long-leg cast with the foot in slight dorsiflexion for approximately 6 weeks. At this time, the cast and pull-out sutures are removed and therapy is begun to restore ankle joint motion.

Varus Deformity. Varus deformity is a common disorder seen in CP; it is often accompanied by equinus and thus is termed equinovarus. The deformity is most often the result of muscle spasticity. In the young child, the deformity is dynamic and reducible; if left untreated in the growing child, it will become fixed and nonreducible with resultant bone and joint deformities. In a study by Bennett and associates of

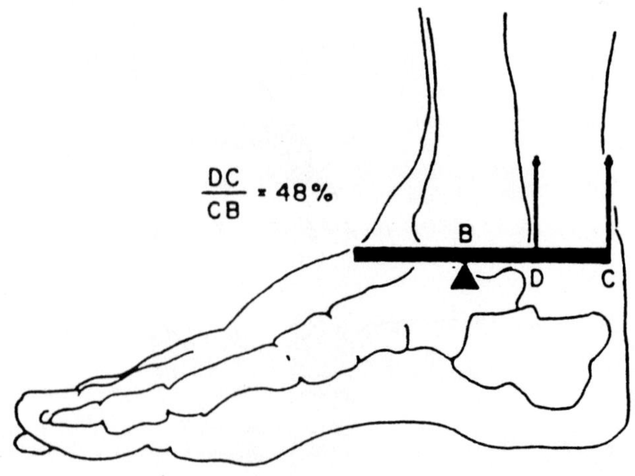

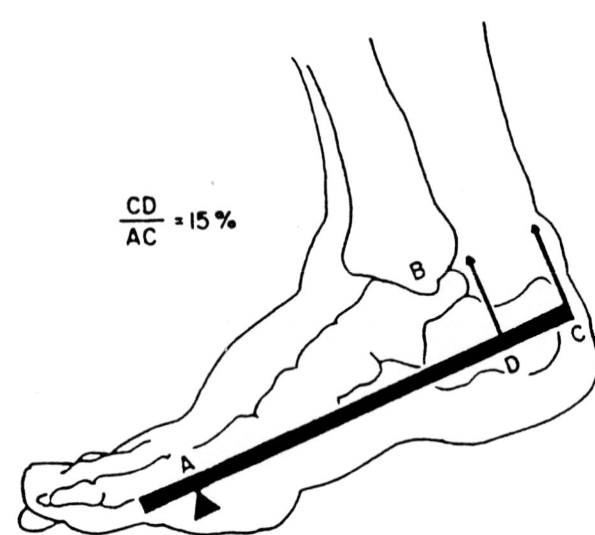

FIGURE 17–8. *Upper,* The power of the gastrosoleus complex is reduced by 48% when the Achilles tendon is transferred from C to D. *Lower,* During propulsion, the power of the Achilles tendon is reduced by only 15% when transferred from C to D. (From Crawford AH, Kucharzyk D, Roy DR, and Bilbo J: Subtalar stabilization at the planovalgus foot by staple arthroereisis in young children who have neuromuscular problems. J Bone Joint Surg 72A:842, 1990.)

230 children, hemiplegia was accompanied by equinus or equinovarus 98% of the time, whereas in diplegia or quadriplegia, varus was present in only 36% of the children; the remainder demonstrated valgus deformities.[56]

Varus deformity is less well tolerated and more disabling than valgus deformities but is considerably easier to treat surgically. Consequently, surgery is done more often and more successfully for varus deformities than for valgus deformities. Many reports have indicated that the posterior tibial muscle tendon unit is the primary deforming force in varus and equinovarus deformities of the foot.[46, 60, 62, 64] Normally, this muscle has no swing phase activity. Dynamic gait studies in children with spastic equinovarus deformities have shown this muscle to be active continuously or, rarely, to demonstrate a complete phase reversal. Other authors believe that the anterior tibial muscle plays a more dominant role in

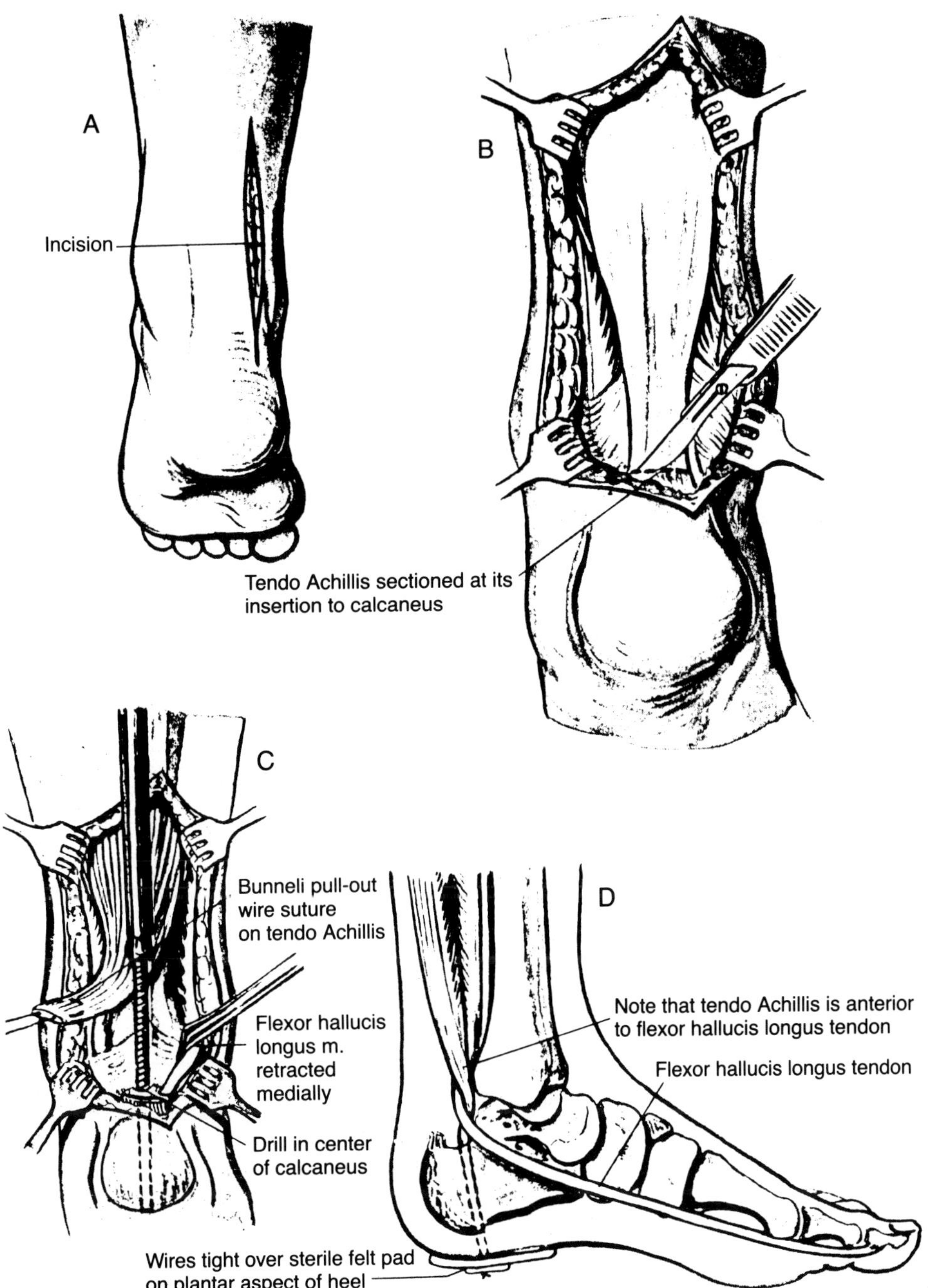

FIGURE 17–9. *A*, The incision is made medial to the Achilles tendon. *B*, The Achilles tendon is detached as far distally as possible to preserve length. *C* and *D*, The Achilles tendon is passed through a drill hole as shown anterior to the flexor hallucis longus tendon. (*A* to *D* from Crawford AH, Kucharzyk D, Roy DR, and Bilbo J: Subtalar stabilization at the planovalgus foot by staple arthroereisis in young children who have neuromuscular problems. J Bone Joint Surg 72A:842, 1990.)

dynamic varus deformities.[65, 66] No one argues that triceps surae spasticity and contracture add considerably to the varus component when the pull is medial to the longitudinal axis of the os calcis (Fig. 17–10).

Initially, mild deformities may be corrected by orthoses or braces. Frequently, the deformity progresses owing to growth and contracture, and orthotics become cumbersome or poorly tolerated. Surgical procedures then may be necessary to correct or improve the deformity. Soft tissue procedures to address the overactive invertor muscles have included posterior tibial tendon lengthening, anterior transfer of the posterior tibial tendon through the interosseous membrane, split posterior transfer of the posterior tibial tendon to the peroneal brevis insertion, anterior tibial tendon transfer, and rerouting of the posterior tibial tendon anterior to the medial malleolus.

As stated previously, transferring spastic muscles can give highly unpredictable results, and the possibility of producing a reverse deformity or an undercorrection always exists. It can be helpful to obtain dynamic electromyography test results before selecting the muscle-tendon unit to be transferred or lengthened, although this is not always practical and often serves to confirm what is observed clinically.[63, 65, 67, 68] When

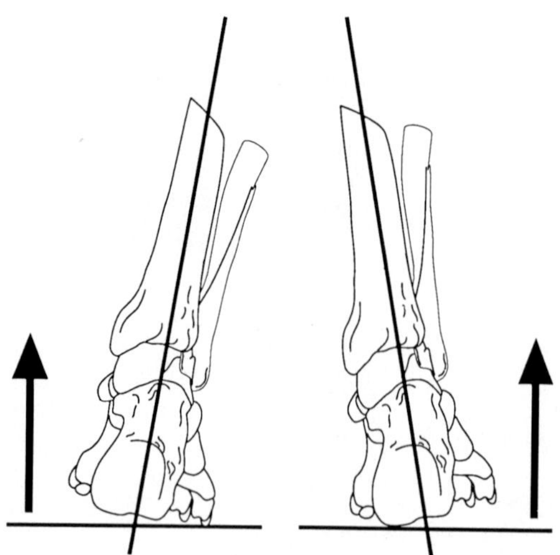

FIGURE 17–10. Spasticity of the triceps surae contributes to varus deformity when the pull is medial to the longitudinal axis of the os calcis.

discussing surgery with the patient and family, we usually present a concept of staged surgery, as indicated earlier. This makes all people involved aware of the unpredictable nature of this type of surgery and the possibility of additional surgery that could include lengthening, transfers, or fusions.

Split Anterior Tibial Tendon Transfer. This procedure has been used widely with a large degree of acceptance.[42, 46, 56, 66, 67] The anterior tibial tendon is split, and the lateral portion is transferred and reattached to the cuboid. Split anterior tibial tendon transfer may be indicated when there is a *dynamic* hindfoot varus and continuous anterior tibial muscle activity. Clinically, the practitioner sees a varus in the swing phase of gait and a clinically apparent functioning anterior tibial muscle-tendon unit.

Hoffer and associates studied dynamic electromyograms in patients with spastic equinovarus deformities and found abnormal hyperactivity of the tibialis anterior tendon in some.[66, 67] In the majority of these feet, there were fixed equinus deformities requiring lengthening of the tendocalcaneus, lengthening of the tibialis posterior tendon, and in a number of cases with fixed varus the medial hindfoot was released. In feet where the deformity was totally dynamic and flexible, the split tibialis anterior transfer was performed in isolation. In only one instance was the procedure unsuccessful. Electromyograms done after the surgery showed sometimes slightly modified results, but not dramatically so. Hoffer and associates recommended that when the gait electromyogram preoperatively shows the tibialis anterior tendon to be neither overactive or nonphasic, and there is a concomitant phase reversal in the tibialis posterior muscle, then and only then should a transfer of the tibialis posterior be considered.[66, 67]

Split anterior tibial tendon transfer is not the procedure of choice when trying to address a drop foot or a steppage gait. Overcorrections are less commonly reported with this procedure; however, undercorrections remain a distinct possibility.[66]

Anterior Transfer of the Tibialis Posterior Tendon Through the Interosseous Membrane. Transfer of the tibialis posterior tibial tendon through the interosseous membrane to the dorsum of the foot has the effect of removing a dynamic deforming force, which can assist in dorsiflexion and eversion of the foot. This procedure commonly has been done in conjunction with heel cord lengthening.

Rerouting a spastic muscle to alter its function can give highly unpredictable results. Once a muscle is transferred, it still retains spasticity. Therefore, once the tibialis posterior muscle is rerouted anteriorly through the interosseous membrane to the dorsum of the foot, it is changed from a spastic invertor and plantarflexor to a spastic dorsiflexor and possibly evertor. Therefore, there is a significant risk of overcorrection. This is supported by review of the literature. Turner and Cooper[69, 70] found only 21% of their results were excellent or good, whereas others (Bisla,[64] Williams,[71] Schneider and Balon[72]) have reported 80% or more excellent or good results from this procedure. In another report, Miller and associates recommended electromyogram gait study because it helps in the proper selection of CP patients with spastic CP for transfer procedures. They advise that patients with posterior tibial activity in swing phase alone are the best candidates for transfer.[63] Other authors have pointed out that failures may be due to (1) overzealous Achilles tendon lengthening, leading to calcaneal deformity; (2) transplantation of the tendon too far laterally, which may lead to excessive valgus; and (3) technical failures leading to an overly taut or perhaps overly loose insertion into the bone, leading to an undercorrection or overcorrection.[72, 73] Many authors now prefer one of the tendon-splitting transfer procedures to correct dynamic varus of the hindfoot and midfoot due to the reports of unpredictability of rerouting of the tibialis posterior tibial tendon.[39, 42, 44]

Split Tibialis Posterior Tendon Transfer. Kling and associates in 1985[73a] described a split tibialis posterior tendon transfer using a four-incision technique wherein half of the tibialis posterior tendon is transferred posterior to the tibia laterally through the sheath of the peroneal brevis and sutured to the base of the fifth metatarsal. This procedure commonly has been done in conjunction with heel cord lengthening. The procedure has similar indications as anterior transfer of the posterior tibial tendon through the interosseous membrane but has fewer reported complications. The authors[73a] reported that the postural deformity was corrected using this procedure in 29 of 30 feet. In no instance did a calcaneal deformity result. A number of other authors have reported excellent or good results with this procedure.[42, 74, 75] It is possible that few calcaneal deformities result because the plantarflexion strength of the tibialis posterior muscle is maintained with the split tibialis posterior tendon transfer (and not so when this muscle is transferred anteriorly through the interosseous membrane) even when heel cord lengthening is carried out at the same time. Furthermore, valgus overcorrection is a rare complication of this procedure. One factor in preventing valgus deformity is preservation of the original insertion of the posterior tibial muscle, which therefore continues to stabilize the medial column and thus the hind part of the foot.

Lengthening of the Tibialis Posterior Tendon. The tibialis posterior tendon may be lengthened by a Z-plasty technique or a slide lengthening of the musculocutaneous junction. The disadvantage of lengthening the tendon by step-cut or Z-plasty procedure is that it may bind down behind the medial malleolus in its tendon sheath and thus may lead to stenosing tenosynovitis. Also, if a deformity recurs, a previously lengthened tendon is less suitable for transfer because it is scarred and may be attenuated. A slide lengthening at the musculotendinous junction, described by Majestro and associates[76] may be a more desirable procedure because there is less possibility of scarring and less trauma done to the tendon sheath.[76, 77] This procedure has been combined with tendocalcaneal lengthening through the same incision.

Valgus Deformity. Pes valgus is generally more common in CP than are varus deformities, particularly in spastic diplegia.[23] Although valgus is less deforming and better tolerated than varus deformities, it is more difficult to correct.

In CP, the primary deforming force leading to valgus deformity most often is contracture of the triceps surae. Obviously, this restricts normal dorsiflexion at the ankle joint. The necessary dorsiflexion during the stance phase of gait is therefore achieved at the midtarsal joint. Retrograde forces push the calcaneus into eversion, thus removing the sustentaculum tali from its supporting position under the head of the talus. The talus adducts and plantarflexes while the forefoot abducts. Valgus deformity may also be a result of a dynamic muscle imbalance between the evertors and invertors of the foot. The peroneal muscles may be spastic and strong while the anterior tibial and posterior tibial muscles are weak.

Treatment. Treatment of the valgus foot initially is conservative with a foot orthosis or a University of California Biomechanics Lab (UCBL) orthosis. Several reports have recommended taking standing anteroposterior and lateral radiographs while the child is wearing the orthosis to determine whether plantarflexion of the talus and sagging of the talonavicular and navicular cuneiform joints have been corrected while wearing the orthotic device.[62, 78] Often the Achilles tendon is so tight that control is not possible with any orthosis, and the foot continues to break at the midtarsal joint; then the first step is to lengthen the Achilles tendon, as described earlier.

Surgery to correct valgus deformity includes Achilles tendon lengthening, lengthening of the peroneal tendons at the musculocutaneous junction, transfer of the peroneal tendons, medial column stabilization, extra-articular subtalar joint arthrodesis, and, in the more mature patient, triple arthrodesis.

Little has been written about peroneal muscle tendon transfers, and thus these procedures have not gained much popularity. Peroneal brevis lengthening at the musculocutaneous junction has some degree of support in mild to moderate cases as an adjunctive procedure to heel cord lengthening and extra-articular subtalar arthrodesis.

If the peroneal tendons are lengthened, there is always a possibility of producing an opposite varus deformity.

If symptomatic pes valgus deformity persists in a child up to 5 to 10 years old, with the child demonstrating poor balance and locomotion, the Grice subtalar arthrodesis has been the mainstay of operative treatment for stabilizing the planovalgus foot.[79] It should be preceded or accompanied by operations to correct soft tissue deformities and to attempt to balance muscle power. The Grice procedure, when done properly, can correct the hindfoot valgus and restore the height of the longitudinal arch; it interferes only slightly with growth of the foot. It does not correct an unstable medial column or fixed deformities of the forefoot.

The equinus deformity should be addressed prior to subtalar joint fusion. We believe that this operation should be staged, the heel cord lengthening taking place first. This allows the calcaneus to be restored underneath the talus—the

position in which it should be fused. Most authors prefer autogenous bone graft to homogeneous bone bank graft.[50, 79–82] The bone graft should be placed in the sinus tarsi so that the longitudinal axis of the cortical strut lies parallel to the long axis of the leg (Fig. 17–11). Furthermore, additional stability is achieved by placement of a cancellous screw dorsally through the subtalar joint. Extremities should be immobilized until the fusion is solid; usually this requires 8 weeks of above-the-knee non-weightbearing cast and 4 weeks in a below-the-knee weightbearing cast. Extreme care should be taken not to fuse the subtalar joint in varus alignment. This is poorly tolerated, and even slight varus seems to increase with age.

The collective results of extra-articular subtalar arthrodesis for the operative treatment of paralytic and spastic planoval-

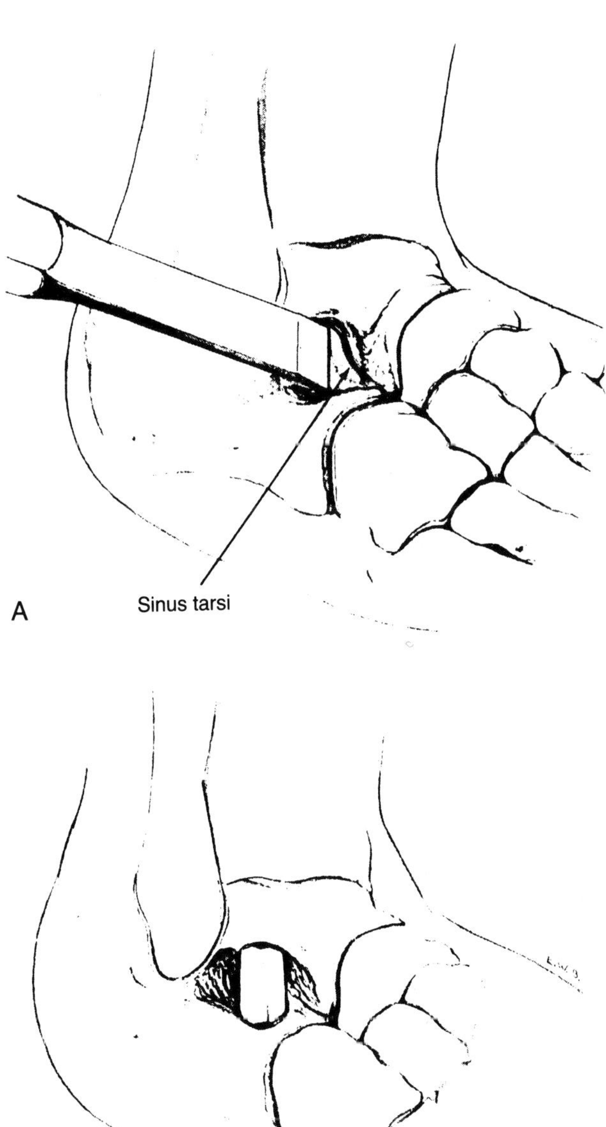

FIGURE 17–11. *A,* The osteotome is shown measuring the length of bone graft to be used. *B,* The longitudinal axis of the cortical bone graft is placed parallel to the shaft of the tibia.

TABLE 17–3

SUMMARY OF VARIOUS AUTHORS' RESULTS WITH GRICE SUBTALAR ARTHRODESIS

Number of feet (procedures)	1188
Age (years)	2–38 (average, 6–8)
Duration of follow-up (years)	1–16 (average, 2–4)
Results (number)	
Good	842 (70.87%)
Bad	346 (29.12%)
Complications (number)	
Valgus position	110 (10.6%)
Varus position	131 (12.6%)
Pseudarthrosis	58 (5.6%)
Infection	5
Tibial fracture	4
Graft slippage	7

From Crawford AH, Kucharzyk D, Roy DR, and Bilbo J: Subtalar stabilization at the planovalgus foot by staple arthroereisis in young children who have neuromuscular problems. J Bone Joint Surg 72A:844, 1990.)

gus feet in growing children have enjoyed a wide degree of acceptance. Table 17–3 gives a summary of various authors' results, looking at 1188 feet, indicating a good outcome in 70.87% of the cases, and also shows cumulative data on the common complications associated with this procedure.

An interesting new approach for the treatment of planovalgus deformities in children younger than 6 years of age with spastic CP involving subtalar joint arthrodesis has been reported by Crawford and associates.[83] This procedure consists of subtalar joint stabilization using a Vitallium staple to limit subtalar joint motion and maintain correction. The authors report an 85% good or excellent outcome with an average follow-up of 4.1 years.

References

1. Perry J and Fleming C: Polio: Long-term problems. Orthopedics 8(7):877, 1985.
2. Reidy J, Broderick TF, and Barr J: Tendon transplantation in the lower extremity: A review of end results in poliomyelitis. J Bone Joint Surg 34A(4):900, 1952.
3. Kuhlmann RF and Bell JF: Clinical evaluation of tendon transplantation for poliomyelitis affecting the lower extremity. J Bone Joint Surg 34A(4):915, 1952.
4. Mortens J and Pilcher MF: Tendon transplantation in prevention of foot deformities after poliomyelitis in children. J Bone Joint Surg 38B(3):633, 1956.
5. Crenshaw AH (ed): Campbell's Operative Orthopedics, Vol 4, 7th ed. St Louis, CV Mosby, 1987, p 2927.
6. Grice S: Extra-articular arthrodesis of the subtalar joint for correction of paralytic flat feet in children. J Bone Joint Surg 34A(4):927, 1952.
7. Dennyson WG and Fulford GE: Subtalar arthrodesis by cancellous grafts and metallic internal fixation. J Bone Joint Surg 58B(4):507, 1976.
8. Hill NA, Hudson WJ, Franslisio C, and Sweterlifsch PR: Triple arthrodesis in the young child. Clin Orthop 70:187, 1970.
9. Galindo MJ Jr, Siff S, Butler J, and Cain T: Triple arthrodesis in young children: A salvage procedure after failed releases in severely affected feet. Foot Ankle 7(6):319, 1987.
10. Hsu JD and Hoffer MM: Posterior tibial tendon transfer anteriorly through the interosseous membrane: A modification of the technique: Clin Orthop 131:202, 1978.
11. Miller GM, Hsu JD, Hoffer MM, and Rentfro R: Posterior tibial tendon transfer for persistent palsy of the common peroneal nerve. J Pediatr Orthop 2:363, 1982.
12. Warren AG: The correction of foot drop in leprosy. J Bone Joint Surg 50B:629, 1968.
13. Watkins MB, Jones JB, Ryder CT, and Brown TM: Transplantation of the posterior tibial tendon. J Bone Joint Surg 36A:1181, 1954.
14. William PF: Restoration of muscle balance of the foot by transfer of the tibialis posterior. J Bone Joint Surg 58B:217, 1976.
15. Tuell JI: Anterior transposition of the posterior tibial tendon muscle in equinovarus. Clin Orthop 23:227, 1962.
16. Jahss MH: Disorders of the foot and ankle. Medical and Surgical Management, Vol 3, 2nd ed. Philadelphia, WB Saunders, 1991, p 2047.
17. Lambrinudi C: New operation on drop foot. Br J Surg 15:193, 1927.
18. Hoffer MH, Reiswig JA, Garrett AM, and Perry J: The split anterior tibial tendon transfer in the treatment of spastic varus hindfoot of children. Orthop Clin North Am 5:31, 1974.
19. McGlamry ED, Ruch JA, and Green DR: Simplified technique for split tibialis anterior tendon transposition (STATT procedure). J Am Podiatr Assoc 65:927, 1975.
20. Fenton CF, Gilman RD, Jassen M, et al: Criteria for selected major tendon transfers in podiatric surgery. J Am Podiatr Assoc 73:561, 1983.
21. Gunn DR and Molesworth DD: The use of the tibialis posterior as dorsiflexor. J Bone Joint Surg 39B:674, 1957.
22. Watkins MB, Jones JB, Ryder CT, et al: Transplantation of the posterior tibial tendon. J Bone Joint Surg 36A:1181, 1954.
23. Tachdjian MO: The Child's Foot. Philadelphia, WB Saunders, 1985, p 465.
24. Dwyer FD: Osteotomy of the calcaneus for pes cavus. J Bone Joint Surg 41B:80, 1959.
25. Silver CM, Simon SD, and Litchman HM: Calcaneal osteotomy for valgus and varus deformity of the foot. Int Surg 58(124):24–30, 1973.
26. Wesley MS and Borenfeld PA: Mechanism of the Dwyer calcaneal osteotomy. Clin Orthop 70:137, 1970.
27. Daniels C and Worthingham C: Muscle Testing, 3rd ed. Philadelphia, WB Saunders, 1972.
28. Fried A and Moyseyev S: Paralytic valgus deformity of the foot: Treatment by replacement of paralyzed tibialis posterior muscle: A long term follow-up study. J Bone Joint Surg 52A:1674, 1970.
29. Lapidus PW: Dorsal bunion: Its mechanics and operative correction. J Bone Joint Surg 22:627, 1940.
30. Makin M and Yassipovitch A: Transposition of the peroneus longus in the treatment of paralytic pes calcaneus: A follow up study of thirty three cases. J Bone Joint Surg 48A:1541, 1966.
31. Cole WH: The treatment of claw foot. J Bone Joint Surg 22:895, 1940.
32. Jappas LM: Surgical treatment of pes cavus by tarsal Y-osteotomy. J Bone Joint Surg 50A:927, 1968.
33. Siffert RS, Forster RI, and Nachamie B: "Beau" triple arthrodesis for correction of severe cavus deformity. Clin Orthop 45:101, 1966.
34. Ingram AJ and Hundley JM: Posterior bone block of the ankle for paralytic equinus: An end result study. J Bone Joint Surg 33A:679, 1951.
35. Gill AB: An operation to make a posterior bone block at the ankle to limit foot drop. J Bone Joint Surg 15:166, 1933.
36. Inclan A: End results in physiological bone blocking of flail joints. J Bone Joint Surg 31A:748, 1949.
37. Ingram TTS: Pediatric Aspects of Cerebral Palsy. Baltimore, Williams & Wilkins, 1964.
38. Balf CL and Ingram TTS: Problems in the classification of cerebral palsy. Br Med J 2:163, 1955.
39. Goldner JL: Cerebral palsy: I. General principles. In American Academy of Orthopaedic Surgeons: Instructional Course Lectures, Vol. 20. St Louis, CV Mosby, 1971.
40. Holm VA: The causes of cerebral palsy: A contemporary perspective. JAMA 247:1473, 1982.
41. O'Reilly DE and Walentynowicz JE: Etiological factors in cerebral palsy: An historical review. Dev Med Child Neurol 23:633, 1981.
42. Sage SP: Cerebral palsy. In Crenshaw AH (ed): Campbell's Operative Orthopaedics, 7th ed. St Louis, CV Mosby, 1987, pp 2855–2875.
43. Dale A and Stanley FJ: An epidemiological study of cerebral palsy in Western Australia, 1956–1975: II. Spastic cerebral palsy and perinatal factors. Dev Med Child Neurol 22:13, 1980.
44. Bax MCO: Terminology and classification of cerebral palsy. Dev Med Child Neurol 6:295, 1964.
45. Hoffer MM, Reiswig JA, Garrett MM, and Perry J: The split anterior tibial tendon transfer in the treatment of spastic varus hindfoot in childhood. Orthop Clin North Am 5:31, 1974.
46. Tachdjian MO: Neuromuscular disease. In Tachdjian MO: The Child's Foot. Philadelphia, WB Saunders, 1972, pp 1601–1626.
47. Capute A and Palmer F: A pediatric overview of the spectrum of developmental disabilities. J Dev Behav Pediatr 1:66, 1980.
48. Samilson RL and Hoffer MM: Problems and complications in orthopaedic management of cerebral palsy. In Samilson RL (ed): Orthopedic Aspects of Cerebral Palsy. Philadelphia, JB Lippincott, 1975, p 258.
49. Root L: Tendon surgery on the feet of children with cerebral palsy. Dev Med Child Neurol 18:671, 1976.
50. Engstrom A, Erikson U, and Hjelmstedt A: The results of extra-articular subtalar arthrodesis according to the Green-Grice method in cerebral palsy. Acta Orthop Scand 45:945, 1974.
51. Baker LD: A rational approach to the surgical needs of the cerebral palsy patient. J Bone Joint Surg 38A:313, 1956.
52. Bleck FE: Orthopaedic Management of Cerebral Palsy. Philadelphia, WB Saunders, 1979.
53. Bennett FC, Chandler LS, Robinson NM, and Sells CJ: Spastic diplegia in premature infants: etiological and diagnostic considerations. Am J Dis Child 135:732, 1981.
54. Banks HH: Equinus and cerebral palsy: Its management. Foot Ankle 4:149, 1983.
55. Banks HH and Grun WT: The correction of equinus deformity in cerebral palsy J Bone Joint Surg 40A:1359, 1958.
56. Bennett GC, Rang M, and Jones D: Varus and valgus deformities of the foot in cerebral palsy. Dev Med Child Neurol 24:499, 1982.
57. Sharrard WJW and Smith TWD: Tenodesis of flexor hallucis longus for paralytic clawing of the hallux in childhood. J Bone Joint Surg 58B:224, 1976.
58. White JW: Torsion of the Achilles tendon: Its surgical significance. Arch Surg 46:784, 1943.

59. Gaines RW and Ford TD: A systematic approach to the amount of Achilles tendon lengthening in cerebral palsy. J Pediatr Orthop 4:448, 1984.

60. Gritzka TL, Staheli LT, and Duncan WR: Posterior tibial tendon transfer through the interosseous membrane to correct equinovarus deformity in cerebral palsy: An initial experience. Clin Orthop 89:201, 1972.

61. Pierrott AH and Murphy OB: Heel cord advancement: A new approach to the spastic equinus deformity. Orthop Clin North Am 5:117, 1974.

62. Root L: Varus and valgus foot in cerebral palsy and its management. Foot Ankle 4:174, 1984.

63. Miller GM, Hsu JD, Hoffer MM, and Rentfro R: Posterior tibial tendon transfer: A review of the literature and analysis of 74 procedures. J Pediatr Orthop 2:363, 1982.

64. Bisla RS, Louis HJ, and Albano P: Transfer of tibialis posterior tendon in cerebral palsy. J Bone Joint Surg 58A:497, 1976.

65. Perry J, Hoffer MM, Giovani P, et al: Gait analysis of the triceps surae in cerebral palsy: A preoperative and postoperative clinical and electromyographic study. J Bone Joint Surg 56A:511, 1974.

66. Hoffer MM and Perry J: Pathodynamics of gait alterations in cerebral palsy and the significance of kinetic electromyography in evaluating foot and ankle problems. Foot Ankle 4:128, 1983.

67. Hoffer MM, Reiswig JA, Garrett AM, and Perry J: The split anterior tibial tendon transfer in the treatment of spastic varus hindfoot of childhood. Orthop Clin North Am 5:31, 1974.

68. Hoffer MM, Barakat G, and Koffman M: 10-year follow-up at split anterior tibial tendon transfer in cerebral palsy patients with spastic equinovarus deformity. J Pediatr Orthop 5:432, 1985.

69. Turner JW and Cooper RR: Anterior transfer of the tibialis posterior through the interosseous membrane. Clin Orthop 83:241, 1972.

70. Turner JW and Cooper RR: Posterior transposition of tibialis anterior through the interosseous membrane. Clin Orthop 79:71, 1971.

71. Williams PF: Restoration of muscle balance of the foot by transfer of the tibialis posterior. J Bone Joint Surg 58B:217, 1976.

72. Schneider M and Balon K: Deformity of the foot following anterior transfer of the posterior tibial tendon and lengthening of the Achilles tendon for spastic equinovarus. Clin Orthop 125:113, 1977.

73. Root L, Miller SR, and Kirz P: Posterior tibial-tendon transfer in patients with cerebral palsy. J Bone Joint Surg 69A:1133, 1987.

73a. Kling TF, Kaufer H, and Hensinger RN: Split posterior tibial-tendon transfers in children with cerebral spastic paralysis and equinovarus deformity. J Bone Joint Surg 67A:186, 1985.

74. Green NE, Griffin PP, and Shiavi R: Split posterior tibial-tendon transfer in cerebral palsy. J Bone Joint Surg 65A:748, 1983.

75. Kling TF Jr and Hensinger RN: The results of split posterior tibial tendon transfer in children with cerebral palsy [Abstract]. Orthop Trans 8:102, 1984.

76. Majestro TC, Ruda R, and Frost HM: Intramuscular lengthening of the posterior tibialis muscle. Clin Orthop 79:59, 1971.

77. Ruda R and Frost HM: Cerebral palsy: Spastic varus and forefoot adductus, treated by intramuscular posterior tibial tendon lengthening. Clin Orthop 79:61, 1971.

78. Baker LD and Hill LM: Foot alignment in the cerebral palsy patient. J Bone Joint Surg 46A:1, 1964.

79. Grice DS: Further experience with extra-articular arthrodesis of the subtalar joint. J Bone Joint Surg 36A:246, 1955.

80. Grice DS: The role of subtalar fusion in the treatment of valgus deformities of the feet. *In* American Academy of Orthopaedic Surgeons: Instructional Course Lectures, Vol 16. St Louis, CV Mosby, 1959.

81. Guttman G: Modification of the Grice-Green subtalar arthrodesis in children. J Pediatr Orthop 1:219, 1981.

82. Williams PF and Menelaus MB: Triple arthrodesis by inlay grafting: A method suitable for the underformed or valgus foot. J Bone Joint Surg 59B:333, 1977.

83. Crawford AH, Kucharzyk D, Ray DR, and Bilbo J: Subtalar stabilization at the planovalgus foot by staple arthroereisis in young children who have neuromuscular problems. J Bone Joint Surg 72A:840, 1990.

CHAPTER 18

HIV Infection and AIDS

Carolyn K. Harvey, D.P.M.

The first cases of acquired immunodeficiency syndrome (AIDS) in the United States were noted by the Centers for Disease Control and Prevention (CDC) in 1981 when a number of young homosexual men in New York City and San Francisco mysteriously presented with the heretofore unusual skin lesions of Kaposi's sarcoma or the opportunistic infection of *Pneumocystis carinii* pneumonia. One hundred twenty-four people are known to have died from AIDS in 1981, with 306 diagnosed with the disease during that year. From this limited beginning, AIDS has become a tremendous health problem in this country—its etiologic agent is estimated to affect 1 to 1.5 million Americans and the number of people infected is growing exponentially. As of November 1993, deaths from AIDS nationally reached 204,390. AIDS was first thought to be limited to homosexual men, intravenous drug users, Haitian refugees, and hemophiliacs. However, it is now understood that the virus that causes AIDS, designated *human immunodeficiency virus* (HIV), is present in body fluids of an infected person and can be passed to any other person through these fluids. Semen and blood have high viral loads, putting at high risk any person having contact with these infected fluids and in whom the skin or mucosal barrier has been interrupted. It is also known that the higher the volume of inoculum, the more likely is the passing of the infection from one person to another. These factors place homosexual males or heterosexual females at particularly high risk. Risk is increased if condoms are not used, if anal intercourse is practiced, if there are ulcerations (e.g., other sexually transmitted disease), and if the HIV-infected partner is late in the course of the disease. Because vaginal fluids contain small numbers of the virus and the inoculum from an infected woman is much less than would be received from an infected male, there is a much higher transmission rate from male to female as compared with female to male. The population experiencing the fastest rate of increase in HIV infection consists of women, and it is predicted that by 2000 as many women as men in the United States will be infected. The fetus of an infected female is at risk both in utero and when passing through the birth canal. Before blood bank screening for HIV was initiated, those receiving transfusions were at grave risk of infection. Needle stick with contaminated blood is also an avenue for infection, and one is at greatest risk if there is repeated exposure, as in intravenous drug users who share needles or if a large inoculum is deposited. Universal precautions are necessary to protect medical practitioners from this lethal disease. As of Septem-

ber 1993, there have been 39 documented cases of occupational transmission of the virus in this country, with 2 cases of *possible* occupational transmission to surgeons.

PATHOGENESIS

HIV has been identified as a lentivirus, which is a retrovirus with a long incubation period and a propensity to affect hematopoietic and nervous system tissues and to depress cell-mediated immunity with an increased, although abnormal, humoral immune response. Two forms of HIV have been identified: HIV-1 (found primarily in the United States, Europe, and central Africa) and HIV-2 (found in western Africa). Although the sequences of nucleotides in HIV-1 and HIV-2 differ by more than 50%, the basic structures of the viruses are similar in that they consist of a core containing the viral genome surrounded by a lipoprotein envelope. Glycoproteins gp 120 and gp 41 protrude from this coat (Fig. 18–1). Gp 120 fits into a CD4 receptor molecule on a target host cell via a key-in-lock mechanism, and gp 41 is thought to facilitate fusion of the virus to the target cell in a similar manner (Fig. 18–2), allowing injection of the contents of the viral envelope into the cell. Host cells most susceptible to infection are those that express the CD4 receptor site. T helper cells (T4 cells) have large numbers of CD4 receptors. Other cells with these receptors are monocytes and macro-

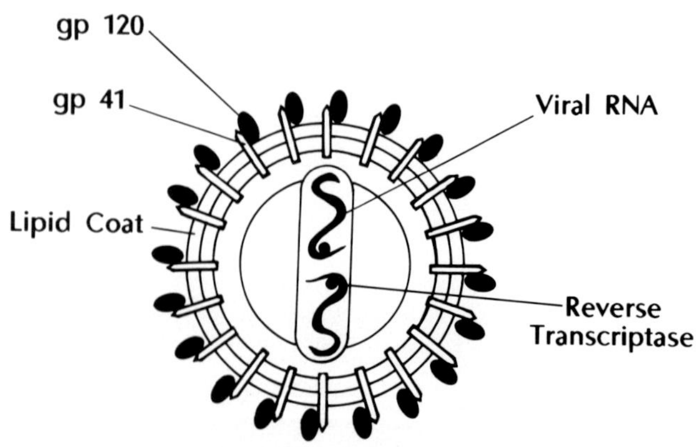

FIGURE 18–1. Diagrammatic representation of the human immunodeficiency virus. RNA, ribonucleic acid. (Reprinted with permission. Levy JA: The pathogenesis of HIV infection. HOSPITAL PRACTICE 25(11):42, 43, 1990. Illustration by Alan D. Iselin.)

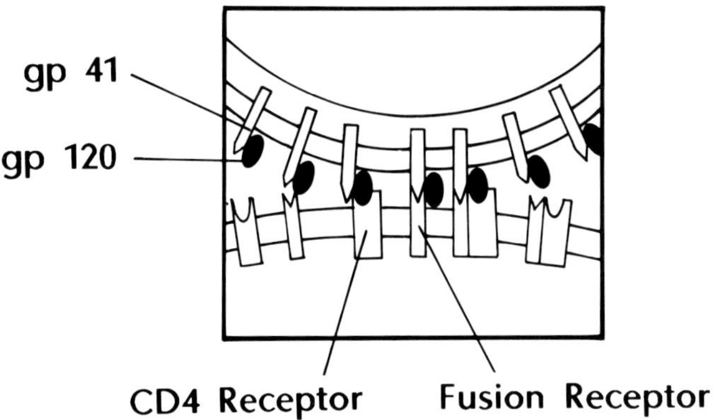

FIGURE 18–2. Diagrammatic representation of key-in-lock mechanism of viral attachment and fusion to a CD4 cell. (Reprinted with permission. Levy JA: The pathogenesis of HIV infection. HOSPITAL PRACTICE 25(11):42, 43, 1990. Illustration by Alan D. Iselin.)

phages. There are, however, other mechanisms of infection, because cells that do not express CD4 receptors, such as astrocytes, skin fibroblasts and bowel epithelial cells, become infected with HIV, albeit less readily than T4 cells. Once the HIV has entered the host cell, the viral ribonucleic acid (RNA) is transformed into deoxyribonucleic acid (DNA) with the aid of the enzyme reverse transcriptase. The double-stranded viral DNA is then incorporated into the host cell DNA and is replicated with any host cell division. The HIV infection may continue in a latent period inside the host cell, or progeny may be produced in the cytoplasm of the host cell and subsequently be extruded through the cell membrane (Fig. 18 3). T4 cells tend to be prolific in their production of viral progeny and often die as these progeny break through the cell, whereas macrophages and monocytes tend to be less prolific and, although injured, survive the HIV infection, subsequently serving as a reservoir of infection.

Destruction of the T4 cells takes place in different ways. Not only can they be lysed, as progeny bud from their surfaces, but also noninfected T cells may form a nonfunctional syncytium, which is a group of 50 to 500 T cells that may be uninfected by the virus but may fuse to gp 120 of the virus envelope that remains expressed on the surface of a single infected T cell. Additionally, infected cells may shed virus gp 120, which can attach to other CD4 receptors. Although these cells do not become infected with the virus, they are now targets for destruction by the immune system, resulting in further depletion of T4 cells via an autoimmune mechanism that may be accelerated, especially early in the disease, by enhancement of humoral immunity secondary to the HIV infection.

There are hundreds of strains of HIV-1 and HIV-2, which may account for differences in the clinical expression of AIDS. For example, some patients with neurologic disease demonstrate normal T4 cell counts that may be attributable to a particular strain of virus that has a propensity to infect macrophages as opposed to T helper cells. Additionally, some strains cause disease rapidly, whereas others may have a latent, asymptomatic period of 10 to 15 years. Strains of HIV in asymptomatic patients have been found to be relatively nonpathogenic, whereas those isolated in patients with advanced disease are virulent. This finding raises the possibility that more pathogenic strains may develop in an HIV-infected patient as the disease progresses.

TESTING

Screening for HIV can be accomplished by enzyme-linked immunosorbent assay (ELISA). This is a sensitive test for anti-HIV antibodies that is capable of identifying approximately 95% of people infected with the virus. The ELISA may show false-negative results, especially early in the infection, and there also is a fairly high false-positive result necessitating that the ELISA be repeated. If the ELISA result is again positive, it is most often confirmed by Western blot assay. This latter test can detect antibodies to specific viral proteins and glycoproteins. If the ELISA result is positive and the Western blot result is negative, some authors suggest the use of a polymerase chain reaction (PCR) test, which confirms the presence of the HIV by detecting and copying a fragment of the genetic code of the virus, thus amplifying it and allowing its identification. The advantage of PCR is that it can aid in the diagnosis of HIV infection prior to the onset of symptoms, signs, or presence of antibodies and may also be applicable in cases of needle stick injury or in newborns of infected mothers who will always show the presence of antibodies whether or not they are actually infected with the virus.

STAGING

The CDC revised its definition of HIV infection in December 1992 to more accurately reflect the severity of immunosuppression in a patient, as well as to serve as a better guideline for treatment. The current classification system uses both laboratory findings (CD4 cell count) and clinical disease in the presence of documented HIV infection. Categories of CD4 cell counts are (1) 500 or more, (2) 200 to 499, and (3) less than 200 or less than 14% of total lymphocytes. Categories of clinical findings are (A) asymptomatic with possible lymphadenopathy or history, or both, of HIV acute flulike illness, (B) symptomatic HIV infection (such as peripheral neuropathy, oral hairy leukoplakia, and pelvic inflammatory disease), and (C) clinical conditions that in previous classification systems resulted in an AIDS diagnosis (Table 18–1). Persons with AIDS are defined as those who

Target Cell

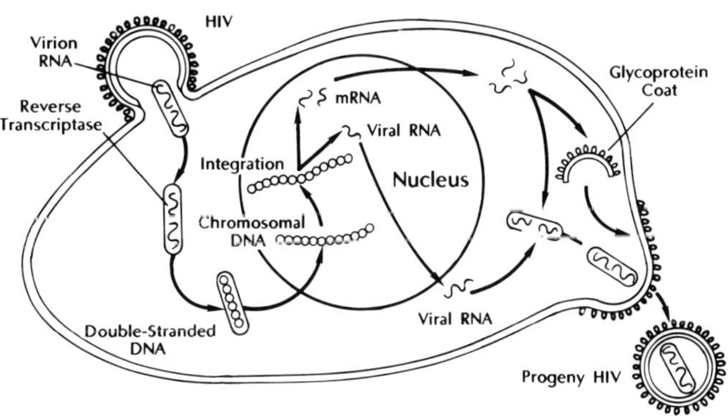

FIGURE 18–3. Diagrammatic representation of human immunodeficiency virus (HIV) infection showing multiplication and extrusion from a host target cell. RNA, ribonucleic acid; DNA, deoxyribonucleic acid. (Reprinted with permission. Levy JA: The pathogenesis of HIV infection. HOSPITAL PRACTICE 25(11):42, 43, 1990. Illustration by Alan D. Iselin.)

TABLE 18–1

AIDS-DEFINING DISEASES AS DESIGNATED BY THE CENTERS FOR DISEASE CONTROL AND PREVENTION

Candidiasis of bronchi, trachea, or lungs
Candidiasis of the esophagus
Cervical cancer, invasive
Coccidioidomycosis, disseminated or extrapulmonary
Cryptococcosis, extrapulmonary
Cryptosporidiosis, chronic intestinal (>1 month's duration)
Cytomegalovirus disease other than liver, spleen, or nodes
Cytomegalovirus retinitis with loss of vision
Encephalopathy, HIV related
Herpes simplex with chronic ulcer(s) (>1 month's duration); or bronchitis, pneumonitis, or esophagitis
Histoplasmosis, disseminated or extrapulmonary
Isosporiasis, chronic intestinal (>1 month's duration)
Kaposi's sarcoma
Lymphoma
   Burkitt's
   Immunoblastic
   Primary, of brain
Mycobacterium avium complex of *Mycobacterium kansasii,* disseminated or extrapulmonary
Mycobacterium tuberculosis, extrapulmonary
Mycobacterium tuberculosis, pulmonary
Mycobacterium, other species or unidentified species, disseminated or extrapulmonary
Pneumocystis carinii pneumonia
Pneumonia, recurrent
Progressive multifocal leukoencephalopathy
Salmonella septicemia, recurrent
Toxoplasmosis of brain
Wasting syndrome due to human immunodeficiency virus

have a CD4 cell count less than 200 regardless of clinical findings or those who have an AIDS-defining illness regardless of CD4 cell count, that is, persons falling into categories 1C, 2C, 3C, 3A, 3B, or 3C.

TREATMENT

Treatment of HIV infection is directed either to the opportunistic infections and malignant lesions that occur with the disease or to the virus. Drugs directed to the virus are designed to interfere with a stage in the life cycle of the virus. Zidovudine (AZT), didanosine (ddI), and dideoxycytidine (ddC) are nucleoside analogues that bind with reverse transcriptase, inhibiting the transcription of viral RNA to DNA, thus reducing the spread of the virus to host cells. The production of progeny in a chronically infected cell is not affected by these drugs.

AZT is considered as the first line of defense against progression of HIV infection to clinical AIDS. It has been associated with weight gain and increased CD4 cell count and improves cognition and neurologic function in patients with AIDS dementia complex. AZT has been shown to reduce the incidence and severity of opportunistic infections in patients receiving it in late-stage disease and in patients who are asymptomatic but who have laboratory evidence of immune dysfunction (a CD4 count <500.) Unfortunately, patients receiving the drug early do not necessarily have a prolonged survival rate, but they may be free of the complications of the disease approximately twice as long as those who do not take the drug.

It can be uncomfortable for a patient to take AZT because of the relatively common and early side effects of headache, nausea, fatigue, and myalgias. Myopathy is not an infrequent side effect of longer-term use of the drug. For those patients who are able to tolerate the drug, a resistance develops so that it is unable to sustain its antiviral activity, resulting in the eventual death of the patient.

ddI is indicated in patients who cannot tolerate AZT or who have developed advanced clinical disease or have demonstrated rapidly decreasing CD4 cell counts while receiving AZT. ddI may be used in conjunction with AZT or alone. ddC is used in the event of a deteriorating clinical scenario or immune function, as in CD4 cell counts lower than 300, and is recommended to be used in conjunction with another nucleoside analogue. Severe sensory peripheral neuropathy is a common toxic effect of these medications that necessitates their discontinuation. Uncommonly, blue-black discoloration of the nails may result from ddI or ddC use.

Other medications (unapproved by the Food and Drug Administration) have promise, such as soluble CD4, which binds to viral gp 120, inhibiting viral attachment to T4 cells; reverse transcriptase inhibitors that are not nucleoside analogues; glycoside inhibitors, which impair the formation of gp 120 on the virus, altering its ability to bind to the CD4 cell; and, finally, inhibitors of proteases, which are necessary to break viral proteins down into smaller functional units essential for viral infectivity.

CLINICAL PRESENTATION

The first indication of possible HIV infection is a flulike illness. This may be followed by years of apparent good health with asymptomatic lymphadenopathy in some patients. Progression to clinical disease correlates somewhat with the duration of infection but even more with the CD4 cell count (Fig. 18–4). Rapid progression of the disease is associated with weight loss (>10% of baseline), unrelenting diarrhea, elevated temperature (>101.5°F) for more than 2 weeks), fatigue, pseudomembranous candidiasis (white, curdlike lesions that can be scraped off an erythematous base and are often symptomatic), oral hairy leukoplakia (white, velvety asymptomatic lesions that cannot be scraped off), multiple dermatomal herpes zoster, and involution of previously enlarged lymph nodes. A CD4 cell count less than 50 is an ominous sign associated with a substantially increased risk of death. HIV infection in women has not been studied as extensively as infection in men, but associated diagnoses include esophageal candidiasis (which may present initially as heartburn), vulvovaginal candidiasis, cervical dysplasia, meningitis, pneumonia, sepsis, tuberculosis, and bacterial endocarditis as well as possibly pelvic inflammatory disease. Generally, HIV infection may be manifest in virtually every organ system (Table 18–2).

Lower extremity manifestations of HIV infection include those due to the direct action of the virus on tissues, including those of the immune system, skin, nerves, and joints; an autoimmune phenomenon; the effects of opportunistic infections; and the side effects of antiviral medications. Because there are innumerable podiatric manifestations, the focus of the following discussion is on those clinical entities that the podiatrist is most likely to be called on to evaluate or those

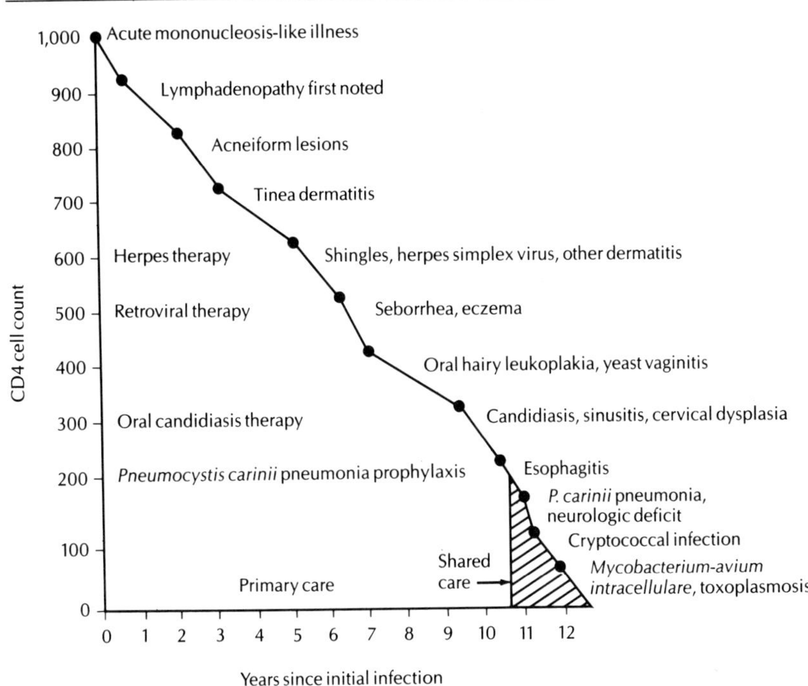

FIGURE 18–4. Typical (not absolute) times for certain human immunodeficiency virus (HIV)-related diseases to occur and their relationship to CD4 cell count. Also shown are typical times for HIV therapies to be initiated. (From Montauk SL and Mandell K: Update on drug therapy for HIV and related infections in adults. Am Fam Physician 46(6):1773, 1992. Reprinted with permission of the publisher, The American Academy of Family Physicians.)

that may present to the podiatric physician in a previously undiagnosed HIV positive patient.

Neurologic Manifestations

Neurologic complications of HIV infection are common, ranging from AIDS dementia complex, cerebral vascular accidents, and ischemic neurologic defects to spinal cord problems and peripheral neuropathy. Spastic paraparesis may occur in vacuolar myelopathy in which spinal cord degeneration results in lower extremity weakness. Examination reveals hyperactive reflexes and may include an abnormal extensor plantar response (Babinski's sign.) This entity is not treatable. On the other hand, cytomegalovirus (CMV) polyradiculopathy is treatable, presenting as a flaccid paraparesis with weakness and hypoactive lower extremity reflexes. This

radiculopathy usually develops late in the disease process in patients with CD4 cell counts less than 100 and is more common now as patients survive longer. Demyelinating polyneuropathy with a Guillain-Barré–type syndrome, such as acute progressive motor neuropathy, can be confused with CMV polyradiculopathy, except that the former occurs early in the disease process in patients with a preserved CD4 cell count. In fact, this demyelinating polyneuropathy may be the first indication of disease in a patient presenting to a podiatrist for evaluation. Symptoms include pain, paresthesias, progressive weakness with hypoactive reflexes, and tenderness on examination. As in Guillain-Barré syndrome, recovery usually occurs in this neuropathy.

Three types of predominantly sensory neuropathy are associated with HIV infection. The first type is a distal symmetrical polyneuropathy common in late-stage disease with

TABLE 18–2

AIDS: CLINICAL MANIFESTATIONS BY ORGAN SYSTEMS

Skin	Respiratory System	Gastrointestinal Tract	Central Nervous System	Hematologic System
Abscesses	Atypical tuberculosis	Chronic diarrhea with wasting	Brain abscesses	Allergic reactions
Erythroderma	CMV	Disease of the appendix	Leukoencephalitis	Anemia
Folliculitis	*Cryptococcus*	Gallbladder disease	Meningitis	Bleeding
Kaposi's sarcoma	Lymphoid interstitial	Necrotizing gingivitis	Myelopathy	Bruising
Molluscum contagiosum	pneumonitis	Oral candidiasis	Peripheral neuropathies	Leukopenia
Seborrheic dermatitis	Other fungal infections	Oral hairy leukoplakia	Primary CNS lymphoma	Lymphadenopathy
Tinea	*Pneumocystis carinii*	Oral Kaposi's sarcoma	Profound dementia	Lymphopenia
Varicella zoster	Pulmonary Kaposi's	Other malignancies and ulcers	Subacute encephalitis	Non-Hodgkin's lymphoma
(shingles)	sarcoma	Periodontitis	Toxoplasmosis of brain	Spontaneous petechiae
		Recurrent *Salmonella* bacterium		Thrombophlebitis

AIDS, acquired immune deficiency syndrome; CMV, cytomegalovirus; CNS, central nervous system.
From Zier BG: Essentials of Internal Medicine in Clinical Podiatry. Philadelphia, WB Saunders, 1990.

paresthesias and pain as well as depressed reflexes and frequently impaired sharp and vibratory sensation in a stocking-glove distribution. The second type is a patchy, asymmetric neuropathy involving nerve trunks that is presumed to have an ischemic cause and resembles mononeuritis multiplex seen in diabetes mellitus. This mononeuritis multiplex of HIV infection is seen early in the disease and is thought to be part of the autoimmune phenomenon that occurs with the increased, although aberrant, humoral immunity of HIV infection.

Finally, painful distal sensory peripheral neuropathy may result, usually within the first 24 weeks of therapy, from the use of ddI or ddC, or both, and is apparently related to the cumulative dose that is administered. In that ddI and ddC are usually given in late-stage disease, it is difficult to distinguish between neuropathy secondary to these medications and to the sensory neuropathy that results from the HIV infection itself. However, patients on ddI and ddC should be monitored closely for the onset of peripheral neuropathy and the drug(s) should be discontinued if signs or symptoms develop. Alternating therapies with AZT and ddI/ddC may minimize this toxic side effect.

Musculoskeletal Manifestations

Rheumatologic manifestations may herald the onset of HIV infection because polymyositis occurs in the flulike syndrome of initial viral exposure or later in the course of the disease. HIV polymyositis appears clinically identical to idiopathic polymyositis unrelated to HIV infection with muscle aches, weakness, and fatigue. Muscle biopsy findings may also be identical. On the other hand, there is a second pattern of pathologic changes in HIV infection in which the biopsy specimen may lack inflammatory changes and nemaline rods may be present. In fact, polymyositis with this biopsy finding should prompt the physician to consider HIV infection in an otherwise healthy person. If the patient is receiving AZT, it may also be the source of the problem, because a myositis-like syndrome has been well documented with long-term use of this drug. Signs and symptoms resolve quickly once AZT is discontinued.

Arthralgias occur in approximately 35% to 40% of patients infected with HIV. Seronegative spondyloarthropathies occur, including Reiter's syndrome and psoriatic arthritis as well as undifferentiated spondyloarthropathies. Additionally, heretofore undiagnosed arthritis confined to the lower extremities, without associated lesions or HLA B27 alleles, has been documented. HIV-infected patients with Reiter's syndrome often do not present with the classic triad of arthritis, conjunctivitis, and urethritis; rather, the more common presentation is oligoarthritis, that is, an asymmetrical arthritis usually involving large joints of the lower extremities (ankles, knees). Enthesopathy at the Achilles tendon insertion, tenosynovitis of the posterior tibial tendon, plantar fasciitis, and dactylitis (sausage digits) may be part of the presentation. Additionally, extra-articular signs, such as keratoderma blennorrhagica, stomatitis, uveitis, and circinate balanitis, may occur. Although Reiter's syndrome often presents late in the course of HIV disease, a significant number of cases have a simultaneous onset with clinical symptoms of AIDS or may precede the onset of these symptoms by as long as 2 years and thus may be the initial complaint of a previously

undiagnosed HIV-infected person. HLA B27 is positive in approximately two thirds of tested patients. Although no specific organism has been linked to Reiter's syndrome in the HIV-positive patient, as in Reiter's syndrome in the general population, it is thought to be a reactive arthritis with possible triggering organisms that include intestinal pathogens such as *Shigella, Yersinia,* and *Campylobacter,* as well as sexually transmitted organisms such as *Chlamydia.* The course of Reiter's syndrome in these patients is variable, ranging from mild, transient symptoms to the more usual scenario of recurring symptoms that is recalcitrant to conventional antiinflammatory therapy. Treatment with systemic steroids may be temporarily effective, although there may be rebound with termination of the drug. There have been reports of patients treated with methotrexate who have subsequently developed full-blown AIDS. Although it is impossible to determine if this would have been the natural course of the disease in these patients, cytotoxic therapy is now avoided in the treatment of seronegative arthritides in HIV-positive patients.

Psoriatic arthritis is associated with HIV infection. There is a less marked association between psoriatic arthritis and positive HLA B27 compared with HIV-infected patients with Reiter's syndrome. Joint pain and inflammation may occur prior to, concomitant with, or after the clinical onset of AIDS. Joint involvement is typically polyarticular and asymmetrical but may be oligoarticular, and there may be distal interphalangeal joint involvement. Enthesopathy and dactylitis occur frequently. The course of psoriatic arthritis in HIV infection is often severe and unremitting. Radiologic changes and deformities may occur relatively quickly. Optimal treatment of psoriatic arthritis has not yet been determined in the HIV-positive patient, although steroid injection therapy has been tried with good response in several patients. Again, use of systemic steroids or cytotoxic drugs is generally to be avoided because of its known adverse effect on the immune system and the possibility that it may exacerbate the underlying viral infection.

Enthesopathy, dactylitis, and oligoarthritis may occur in HIV-positive patients as undifferentiated spondyloarthropathy; that is, there are no associated nail or skin changes consistent with psoriatic arthritis or history and findings consistent with Reiter's syndrome.

There are AIDS-related arthropathies that do not fit into any known classification of arthritis. For the most part, these are severely painful arthralgias often involving the lower extremities, with no extra-articular manifestations or a correlation with HLA B27 allele, and they may or may not demonstrate synovial inflammation. The duration of these arthralgias, which frequently require hospitalization secondary to pain and disability, ranges from 2 hours to several months, with most having an eventual self-limiting 4- to 6-week course. Treatment has consisted of nonsteroidal antiinflammatory drugs and, in unresponsive patients, intra-articular steroids with good, although not necessarily lasting, effect.

Finally, septic joint should be considered, especially if the presentation is a monoarticular inflammatory process. Predisposing factors for a septic joint are intravenous drug use and hemophilia.

Dermatologic Manifestations

There is a myriad of dermatologic manifestations of HIV disease. Kaposi's sarcoma was noted in approximately one third of the first 1000 cases of AIDS reported to the CDC in 1981. Although this percentage has decreased over time, it is still the most common skin problem predictive of HIV infection. This nonmetastasizing tumor of the reticuloendothelium presents in several different forms, including macules, papules, plaques, and nodules. The lesions are generally painless and purple, reddish, or brown. There may be single or few lesions, or they may be widespread and aggressive, involving bone and internal organs in addition to the readily apparent skin lesions. In the lower extremity, they may be associated with edema, especially if there is lymph node involvement, and these hyperpigmented areas may ulcerate, mimicking venous stasis ulcerations. Diagnosis is made by biopsy, although a clinical diagnosis is often made in the known HIV-positive patient. Excisional biopsy may be indicated to eliminate bulky or uncomfortable nodular lesions on the foot. For palliative purposes or cosmesis, radiation therapy or intralesional chemotherapy, such as with vinblastine, may be used for single or localized lesions. For patients with widespread symptomatic lesions or rapidly advancing disease, systemic therapy may be used, including vincristine, bleomycin, and interferon.

Dermatophytosis of skin and nails is an almost universal finding in patients with AIDS and, there may be severe hyperkeratotic palmar and plantar scaling resembling keratoderma blennorrhagicum of Reiter's syndrome. The most commonly isolated organism is *Trichophyton rubrum,* but other dermatophytes or saprophytes may be found, as well as *Candida albicans.* Nail involvement is often of a type unique to HIV-infected patients termed *proximal white onychomycosis.* As its name suggests, it begins at the proximal nail plate and gradually affects the distal aspect of the nail. Dermatophytosis of the foot is often recalcitrant to topical therapy, dictating the use of systemic therapy for eradication. If the patient is receiving ddI, it is important for the podiatrist to be aware of the buffering effect of this drug and the resultant increase in absorption of ketoconazole necessitating that it be given at least 2 hours prior to ddI administration. Recurrence of fungal infection is common once oral medication is withdrawn. Appropriate diagnosis of tinea pedis should be made by culture or potassium hydroxide (KOH) microscopy, or both, in that there are other diseases that mimic dermatophytosis of skin, including eczema (which has an increased incidence in these patients). Systemic fungal infections may manifest in the lower extremities. For example, cryptococcosis has been found in lower extremity ulcerations, and histoplasmosis can cause a maculopapular rash on the palms and soles similar in appearance to molluscum contagiosum (see later).

Viral infections of skin are common in HIV-positive patients. Single or multiple verrucae secondary to the human papilloma virus may occur and seem to be more recalcitrant to therapy than those found in the non–HIV-infected population. These lesions are found not only on the foot but also in areas not normally associated with verrucae, such as the nostrils and palate. Molluscum contagiosum secondary to the virus of the same name may also be found on the feet, although the groin, axillae, and eyelids are the more common sites. This lesion presents as single or multiple pearly white papules that have an indented center and from which keratin can be expressed. The lesions can be totally asymptomatic or may be pruritic. The herpes simplex virus is common in HIV-infected patients and becomes clinically evident as the

immune system becomes compromised. The lesions appear as groups of painful vesicles that are tender and have associated erythema. An entire digit is sometimes involved and when it occurs is termed *herpetic whitlow.* The lesions also commonly involve the anal and genital areas as well as the face. Diagnosis can be made by Tzanck smear, viral culture, or viral antibody testing. Treatment consists of acyclovir, 200 mg five times a day for 10 days (until lesions crust) in mild cases and parenteral acyclovir for more severe cases. Recurrent herpes zoster (shingles) or herpes zoster involving more than one dermatome is also associated with HIV infection. Treatment consists of intravenous or oral acyclovir. The dosage of the latter is 800 mg five times per day for 7 to 10 days.

Severe psoriatic flares or new-onset psoriatic lesions are not uncommon in HIV-positive patients and should prompt a physician to consider the possibility of HIV infection in the otherwise healthy patient. Skin lesions in HIV infection are identical to other psoriatic lesions with, however, a predilection for the groin and axilla. Nail changes, including pitting and lysis, are common. Differential diagnosis may include onychomycosis or paronychia necessitating KOH microscopy or cultures to aid in diagnosis.

Bacterial infections in the HIV-positive patient may include pneumonia and urinary tract infections presenting with spiking fevers with a secondary necrotic pustular rash of the plantar surface of the feet. Syphilis may be reactivated in the HIV-positive patient, resulting in recalcitrant skin lesions, neurosyphilis, or polyarthralgias. Bacillary angiomatosis is a potentially fatal but treatable infection caused by an unknown gram-negative organism in HIV-infected patients. These lesions are often mistaken for pyogenic granulomas or Kaposi's sarcoma. They can appear as dark-red pedunculated lesions, subcutaneous nodules, or, especially in blacks, hyperpigmented plaques. Recommended treatment is erythromycin 250 to 500 mg four times a day for several weeks, with excellent results. Folliculitis, impetigo, furuncles, cellulitis, and paronychia are other bacterial infections that can occur on the lower extremities. When using antibiosis in the treatment of infections in persons who are taking ddI, the physician must be cognizant of the fact that ddI serves as a buffer, resulting in greater absorption of quinolones and tetracycline-related antibiotics, and these should be administered 2 hours prior to ddI.

Vascular Manifestations

Vascular lesions are also more common in the HIV-infected patient. These include telangiectasias (whether associated with the viral infection or topical medications used), lower extremity edema, vasculitis, and idiopathic thrombocytopenia purpura (which may occur along with hemorrhagic herpes zoster). There are several case reports of deep venous thrombosis in HIV positive patients who were active with no known risk factors for venous thromboembolism. Delay in diagnosis was significant in many of these patients, dictating a higher index of suspicion to avoid fatal outcomes. Additionally, there have been reported cases of pseudothrombophlebitis with signs of inflammation along with tender, palpable cords but an intact deep venous system.

SUMMARY

Because the incidence of HIV infection is increasing exponentially, it is imperative that the podiatric physician play a role in its prevention, diagnosis, and treatment. Universal precautions must be adhered to strictly in both office and hospital settings. Education of patients, staff, and communities about the pathogenesis, epidemiology, and prevention of this entity is best accomplished as the physician becomes better informed. Optimal treatment by podiatrists depends on their knowledge of this disease, its diagnosis, staging, and general medical treatment as well as its presentation in the lower extremity.

Bibliography

AIDS and the internist: I. Audio Dig Intern Med 39(17): 1992.

AIDS and the internist: II. Audio Dig Intern Med 39(18): 1992.

Becker M, Saunders TJ, Wispelwey B, and Schain DC: Case report: Venous thromboembolism in AIDS. Am J Med Sci 303:395–397, 1992.

Becker SL: Epidemiology and pathogenesis of HIV infection. J Am Podiatr Med Assoc 80(1):3–8, 1990.

Buehler JW, Hanson DC, and Chu SY: The reporting of HIV/AIDS deaths in women. Am J Public Health 82(11):1500–1504, 1992.

Burns S: Podiatric manifestations of AIDS. J Am Podiatr Med Assoc 80(1):15–20, 1990.

Calabrese LH: The rheumatic manifestations of infection with the human immunodeficiency virus. Semin Arthritis Rheum 18(4):225–239, 1989.

CDC Morbidity and Mortality Weekly Report, U.S. Department of Health and Human Services, CDC, 41(RR-17), December 18, 1992.

Cohen JR, Lackner R, Wenig P, and Pillari G: Deep venous thrombosis in patients with AIDS. NY State J Med 90(3):159–161, 1990.

Corey L and Fleming TR: Treatment of HIV infection: Progress in perspective (Letter). N Engl J Med 326(7):484–485, 1992.

Espinoza LR, Jara LJ, Espinoza CG, et al: There is an association between human immunodeficiency virus infection and spondyloarthropathies. Rheum Dis Clin North Am 18(1):257, 1992.

Golbus J: Rheumatic disease and AIDS: An interesting but mysterious relationship. Postgrad Med 92(4):99–110, 1992.

Goldschmidt R and Dong BJ: Update on drug therapy for HIV and related infections in adults (Letter). Am Fam Physician 48(1):39–40, 1993.

Gordon S: Seroconversion: staging and survival. J Am Podiatr Med Assoc 80(1):9–14, 1990.

Guadara J and Prignano J: Laboratory testing for human immunodeficiency virus. Clin Podiatr Med Surg 9(4):895–899, 1992.

HIV/AIDS: Surveillance Report. US Department of Health and Human Services, CDC, 5(3), October, 1993.

Hoth DF and Myers MW: Current status of HIV therapy: I. Antiretroviral agents. Hosp Pract 26:94–117, 1991.

Keat A and Rowe I: Reiter's syndrome and associated arthritides. Rheum Dis Clin North Am 17(1):25–42, 1991.

Lee RG (ed): Wintrobe's Clinical Hematology. Philadelphia, Lea & Febiger, 1993.

Levy JA: The pathogenesis of HIV infection. Hosp Pract 25:31–38, 1990.

Montauk SL and Mandell K: Update on drug therapy for HIV and related infections in adults. Am Fam Physician 46(6):1772–1781, 1992.

Newlin B: HIV infection control for podiatric practitioners. J Am Podiatr Med Assoc 80(1):21–25, 1990.

Rakel RE: Conn's Current Therapy 1993. Philadelphia, WB Saunders, 1993.

Richman DD: Antiviral therapy of HIV infection. Annu Rev Med 42:69–90, 1991.

Spinosa FA (ed): Clinics in Podiatric Medicine and Surgery. Philadelphia, WB Saunders, 1992.

Webster GF, Cockerell CJ, and Friedman-Kien AE: The clinical spectrum of bacillary angiomatosis. Br J Dermatol 126:535–541, 1992.

Radiologic Evaluation

CHAPTER 19

Radiologic Manifestations of Arthritides Involving the Foot

Richard G. Stiles, M.D., Walter A. Carpenter, Ph.D., M.D., and Donald Resnick, M.D.

Articular disorders commonly involve the foot, and radiologic examination is important in their evaluation. Radiographs are useful in confirming, if not establishing, the appropriate diagnosis; staging the disease process; and following the progression or regression of the disease.[1–5] Furthermore, in this era of surgical intervention for articular disorders, radiographs are important for the evaluation of results and complications in the postoperative foot.

However, one must be aware of the limitations of radiography for evaluating arthritis. The American Rheumatism Association's 1987 revised criteria list radiographic findings as only one of many factors that should be considered in a diagnosis of arthritis.[6] In a recent review article, Dr. Jeremy Kaye has discussed the various roles of radiography in the evaluation of arthritis.[1] These roles are listed in Table 19–1. Although it is beyond the scope of this chapter to discuss these roles and their limitations in detail, one should keep in mind that normal radiographs do not exclude the presence of arthritis. Also, subtle changes in radiographic manifestations of arthritis are difficult to detect visually. Therefore, radiographs are limited in their ability to allow assessment of change with time or therapy.[1, 7, 8] Many staging systems have been developed for evaluation of arthritis, particularly in the hand.[1, 7, 8] However, the systems that are easy to use have generally not had good correlation with clinical status of disease; and the detailed systems, although they have relatively good correlation with the status of a patient's disease, are too tedious for practical clinical use.[1, 7, 8]

This discussion was included at this point to emphasize that standard radiography and all other imaging modalities have limitations in the evaluation of arthritis, particularly in the assessment of progression or regression of disease during therapy. The remainder of this chapter emphasizes the radiologic manifestations of different arthritides.

GENERAL PRINCIPLES

Three basic areas of knowledge are required for accurate interpretation of radiographs in patients with articular disease: (1) an organized understanding of the diseases in question, according to their underlying pathophysiology (Table 19–2); (2) an awareness of the cardinal radiographic signs of each specific articular disease (Table 19–3); and (3) the application of the "target" area approach to analysis of articular disease (Fig. 19–1).[3]

Table 19–2 offers an abbreviated but practical classification of articular disease for the clinician. It should be noted that the classification utilized by the American Rheumatism Association is much more extensive and occupies two full

---

TABLE 19–1

ROLES OF RADIOGRAPHY IN EVALUATION OF ARTHRITIS

Determine if arthritis is present
Establish specific diagnosis
Determine extent of disease
Assess activity of disease
Detect complications
Evaluate progression of disease
Evaluate response to drug therapy
Evaluate for surgical treatment
Aid in surgical procedure choice
Aid in size, design, and fabrication of prostheses
Identify surgical complications

Adapted from Kaye JJ: Arthritis: Roles of radiography and other imaging techniques in evaluation. Radiology 177:601–608, 1990.

TABLE 19–2

CLASSIFICATION OF COMMON ARTICULAR DISEASE BASED ON THE UNDERLYING PATHOPHYSIOLOGY

Synovial inflammatory diseases
  Rheumatoid arthritis
  Seronegative spondyloarthropathies
    Ankylosing spondylitis
    Psoriatic arthritis
    Reiter's syndrome
Degenerative arthritis (osteoarthritis)
Crystal deposition diseases
  Gout
  Calcium pyrophosphate dihydrate
  Crystal deposition disease
  Calcium hydroxyapatite deposition disease
Connective tissue diseases
  Systemic lupus erythematosus
  Scleroderma
  Dermatomyositis
  Mixed connective tissue disease
Infection, septic arthritis
Neuropathic disease

From Stiles RG, Resnick D, and Sartoris DJ: Radiologic manifestations of arthritides involving the foot. Clin Podiatr Med Surg 5:1–16, 1988.

pages in textbooks.[3] Although such a detailed classification is useful, the abbreviated, more practical classification listed in Table 19–2 is adequate for most clinicians and includes the most common arthritic disorders for which standard radiography is helpful.

The cardinal roentgen signs of the arthritides are shown in Table 19–3. Some general principles should be discussed further regarding these radiographic signs. Generally, osteoporosis associated with arthritis of any form is due to hyperemia. Of course, this would be a more prevalent finding in synovial inflammatory diseases than in degenerative diseases. However, one must keep in mind that disuse can be a prominent factor in the development of osteoporosis and may be demonstrated radiographically.

Radiographic joint space narrowing is the classic and most helpful hallmark radiographic finding of arthritis. However, the "joint space" is not really a space at all. This radiolucent area represents the cartilaginous portion of the joints. Usually, if joint space narrowing is not present, one cannot make a radiographic diagnosis of arthritis.

A basic principle of differentiating inflammatory from degenerative arthritis is the identification of bony erosions in inflammatory disease and osteophytosis in degenerative disease. Conversely, the absence of osteophytosis in inflammatory disease and of bony erosions in degenerative disease is helpful in making this differentiation as well. However, one must remember that inflammatory disease, such as rheumatoid arthritis, may show superimposed degenerative changes if the inflammatory component decreases, as might be seen in patients who respond well to treatment. These radiographs usually do not present diagnostic difficulty because the patients are known to have the inflammatory form of arthritis. However, without appropriate history, the radiographs can sometimes be confusing, although usually one can discern that both inflammatory and degenerative radiographic changes are present.

The target area approach makes use of the fact that specific articular disorders predominantly affect certain articulations in patterns that are often sufficiently characteristic to allow for specific diagnoses.[3] These patterns will be discussed with each arthropathy classification specified later. Figure 19–1 is a diagrammatic representation of the application of the target area approach to rheumatoid arthritis, psoriatic arthritis, and Reiter's syndrome adapted from Resnick and Niwayama.[3]

Use of these basic areas of knowledge is of great assistance in accurately appraising the frequently complicated radiologic manifestations of articular disease. If this knowledge is applied to radiographs of the foot, one will generally be able to confirm or establish the diagnosis and have an idea of the extent and activity of disease.

SYNOVIAL INFLAMMATORY DISEASES

As the name implies, the underlying pathophysiology of synovial inflammatory diseases is synovial inflammation. The synovitis produces pathologic changes that are depicted

TABLE 19–3

RADIOGRAPHIC SIGNS IN ARTHRITIS OF THE FOOT

Type	Osteo-porosis	Joint Space Narrowing	Soft-Tissue Swelling	Bony Erosions	Osteophytosis or Proliferation	Bony Sclerosis	Subchondral Cysts	Bony Frag-mentation	Intra-articular Bony Ankylosis	Subluxations and Deformities
Rheumatoid arthritis	+	Early, diffuse	Fusiform	Marginal	−	−	+	−	Carpus, tarsus	+
Reiter's syndrome	In acute phase	Early, diffuse	Fusiform and "sausage digit"	Marginal	Ill-defined proliferation	−	+	−	+	±
Psoriatic arthritis	In acute phase	Early, diffuse	Fusiform and "sausage digit"	Marginal	Ill-defined proliferation	−	+	−	+	±
Osteoarthritis	−	Diffuse	−	−	+	+	+	−	−	−
Inflammatory osteoarthritis	−	Diffuse	+	Central	+	+	−	−	+	−
Gout	−	Late	Lobulated	Eccentric	Overhanging edge	+	±	−	−	−
Infection	+	+	+	+	−	+	+	+	±	−
Neuroar-thropathy	−	±	+	−	−	Extreme	+	+	−	+
Connective tissue disease	±	−	−	−	−	−	−	−	−	+

From Stiles RG, Resnick D, and Sartoris DJ: Radiologic manifestations of arthritides involving the foot. Clin Podiatr Med Surg 5:1–16, 1988.

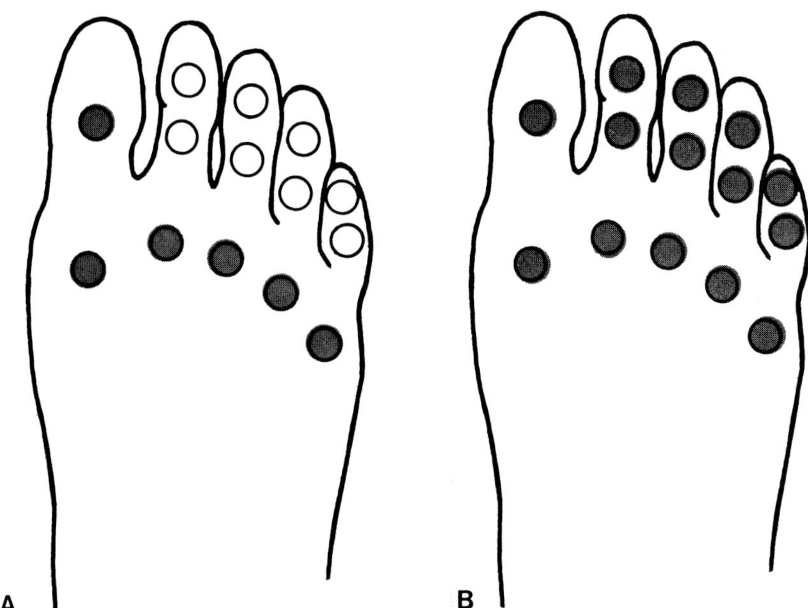

FIGURE 19–1. Target area approach to an evaluation of arthritis. *A,* Distribution of rheumatoid arthritis in the forefoot with predominant involvement of the interphalangeal joint of the great toe and of the metacarpophalangeal joints. *B,* Distribution of psoriatic arthritis and Reiter's syndrome in the forefoot with predominant involvement of the interphalangeal joints. The metacarpophalangeal joint involvement tends to appear later in the course of these diseases. (Adapted from Resnick D and Niwayama G [eds]: Diagnosis of Bone and Joint Disorders, 2nd ed. Philadelphia, WB Saunders, 1988, pp 1921–1922.)

in the radiographs. The classic radiographic signs of a synovial inflammatory disease are typified by those in rheumatoid arthritis (RA), which produces an intense synovitis. These signs include periarticular soft tissue swelling, osteoporosis (secondary to hyperemia), marginal erosions with progression to central erosions, joint space narrowing, deformities, subluxations, and fibrous ankylosis.[3] Bony ankylosis is unusual in RA except in the carpus and the tarsus.[3]

Psoriatic arthritis, ankylosing spondylitis, and Reiter's syndrome are also synovial inflammatory diseases. They are termed *seronegative* because of the characteristic absence of rheumatoid factor in serologic studies. The classic radiographic changes reflecting synovial inflammation are also present in the seronegative diseases, but the morphology in seronegative disorders generally indicates a less intense or less persistent synovitis. Thus, in seronegative diseases, osteoporosis is variable. Synovial proliferation or whiskering occurs adjacent to marginal erosions (related to enthesopathy), and intra-articular osseous ankylosis may develop. These radiographic changes, in conjunction with the differences of disease distribution (target area approach), are usually sufficiently distinctive to allow radiographic differentiation between RA and the seronegative diseases. One should note that the seronegative diseases are also known as *rheumatoid variants* reflecting their similarity to rheumatoid disease. Also, the term *entheseal arthropathies* is sometimes used for the seronegative diseases to emphasize the inflammation of entheses characteristic of these disorders. Entheses are the anatomic sites of tendinous and ligamentous attachments to bone. It is at these entheses that the whiskering and "mouse ear"[9] effect occurs.

Rheumatoid Arthritis

The forefoot is commonly involved in RA. Indeed, clinical and radiographic abnormalities of the forefoot may be the

initial manifestations of RA in 10% to 20% of the patients.[3] The earliest changes are seen at the metatarsophalangeal articulations. Erosions predominate on the medial aspect of the metatarsal heads, except for the fifth head, where the lateral aspect of the bone may be an early and characteristic site of involvement (Figs. 19 2 and 19–3). The interphalangeal joints of the foot are generally spared, with the exception of that in the great toe, which is commonly involved (see Fig. 19–2).

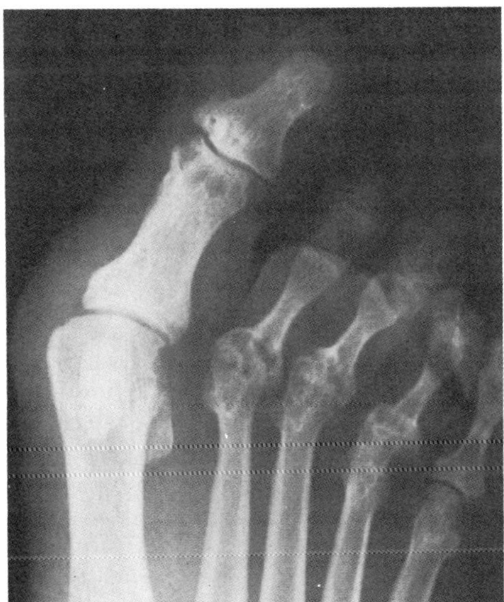

FIGURE 19–2. Classic rheumatoid arthritis with a characteristic distribution in the metatarsophalangeal joints and in the interphalangeal joint of the great toe. Note also the soft tissue swelling at the first metatarsophalangeal joint and mild fibular deviation of the first four digits. (From Stiles RG, Resnick D, and Sartoris DJ: Radiologic manifestations of arthritides involving the foot. Clin Podiatr Med Surg 5:1–16, 1988.)

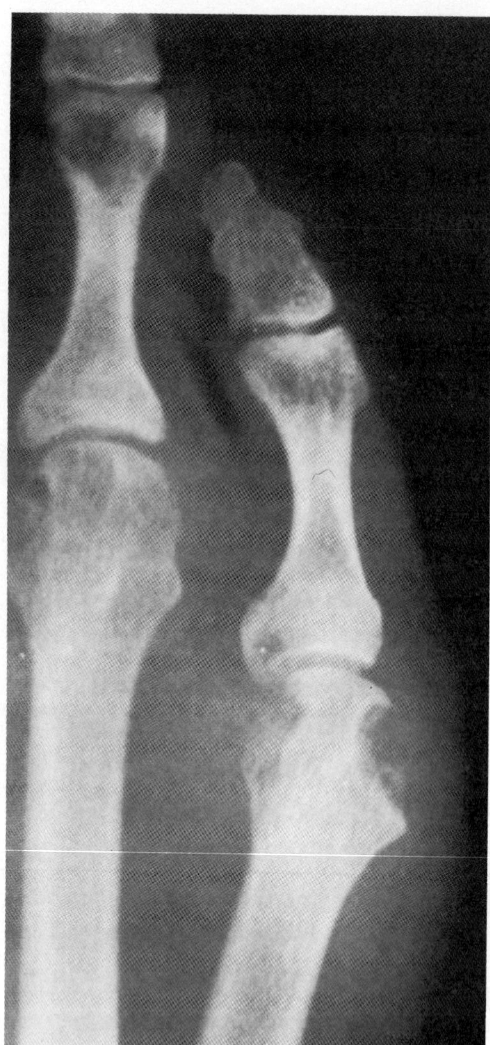

FIGURE 19–3. Demonstration of a characteristic erosion in the lateral aspect of the fifth metatarsal head. (From Stiles RG, Resnick D, and Sartoris DJ: Radiologic manifestations of arthritides involving the foot. Clin Podiatr Med Surg 5:1–16, 1988.)

Generally, the changes of RA in the forefoot are bilaterally symmetrical. This rule, however, does not uniformly apply, especially in early RA. A study by Halla and colleagues[28] indicates that mild asymmetry and even unilateral disease should not discourage the diagnosis of RA if the other findings are indicative of the disease. Our own clinical experience supports this concept.

Abnormalities of the midfoot and hindfoot in RA are not as characteristic as those of the forefoot; however, they can commonly cause clinical problems. The more common radiographic manifestations[10] include talocalcaneal joint sclerosis; articular space loss in any of the intertarsal articulations, particularly the talonavicular joint (Fig. 19–4); osteophytosis (an unusual and late occurrence), pes planovalgus deformity; midfoot collapse[11] (Fig. 19–5); bony ankylosis (Fig. 19–6); and retrocalcaneal bursitis (Fig. 19–7). Also, subtalar dislocation recently has been reported in three patients with longstanding RA.[12]

The pes planus deformity of RA has been reported in as many as 46% of patients.[13] The etiology of this flatfoot deformity is usually attributed to muscle weakness and stretched inflamed ligaments.[3, 11, 14] However, Downy and associates[14] have shown that tibialis posterior tendon rupture may be a more specific cause of rheumatoid flatfoot, analogous to extensor tendon ruptures in the rheumatoid hand. These tendon ruptures may be demonstrable on magnetic resonance examinations.[14]

Calcaneal abnormalities are much more common and more characteristic in seronegative diseases than in RA,[15] although considerable overlap exists in abnormalities among rheumatoid and related disorders. Figure 19–7 demonstrates calcaneal abnormalities in both RA and Reiter's syndrome. The calcaneal abnormalities can be quite similar. However, the morphology generally is somewhat different and allows differentiation between seronegative diseases and RA. Important target areas in the calcaneus include the posterior superior surface adjacent to the retrocalcaneal bursa, the posterior surface above and at the attachment of the Achilles tendon, the plantar surface at the insertion of the plantar aponeurosis, and the plantar surface at the insertion of the long plantar ligament. These areas may exhibit erosions and well-defined spurs (enthesophytes) in RA.

An important association exists between the severity of the RA in the peripheral small joints and that in the cervical spine.[5] Awareness of this association is important whenever operative intervention is contemplated. If changes in the appendicular disease are severe enough to warrant surgery, prominent cervical spine involvement is also likely, including atlantoaxial instability. Therefore, before proceeding with general anesthesia requiring endotracheal intubation, the cervical spine should be evaluated for stability with flexion and extension views of the cervical spine in lateral projection (Fig. 19–8).

Seronegative Spondyloarthropathies

Seronegative spondyloarthropathies include ankylosing spondylitis, psoriatic arthritis, and Reiter's syndrome. Ankylosing spondylitis is not discussed here because it rarely produces foot disease. In contrast, psoriatic arthritis and Reiter's syndrome frequently involve the foot, with Reiter's syndrome demonstrating a predilection for the lower extremity with relative sparing of the upper extremity. This pattern is one of the few radiographic features that may allow practitioners to distinguish Reiter's syndrome from psoriatic arthritis, as the articular manifestations of these diseases are otherwise quite similar.[2]

As suggested earlier, the distribution and morphology of radiographic abnormalities in seronegative diseases are usually distinctive, allowing their differentiation from RA. The most important differentiating feature is the occurrence of bone proliferation or "whiskering" adjacent to the marginal erosions (Fig. 19–9). The whiskering may produce characteristic "mouse ear" deformities.[9] Periostitis also occurs in seronegative diseases and is not usually present in RA. The osseous response in seronegative diseases produces poorly defined, or "fuzzy" marginal erosions, a morphologic feature that is unusual in RA. Other less reliable differentiating features of the seronegative spondyloarthropathies include diffuse soft tissue swelling producing a sausage digit (as opposed to the more focal periarticular swelling in RA), relative absence of osteoporosis reflecting less intense or less persistent synovitis, asymmetrical (as opposed to symmetri-

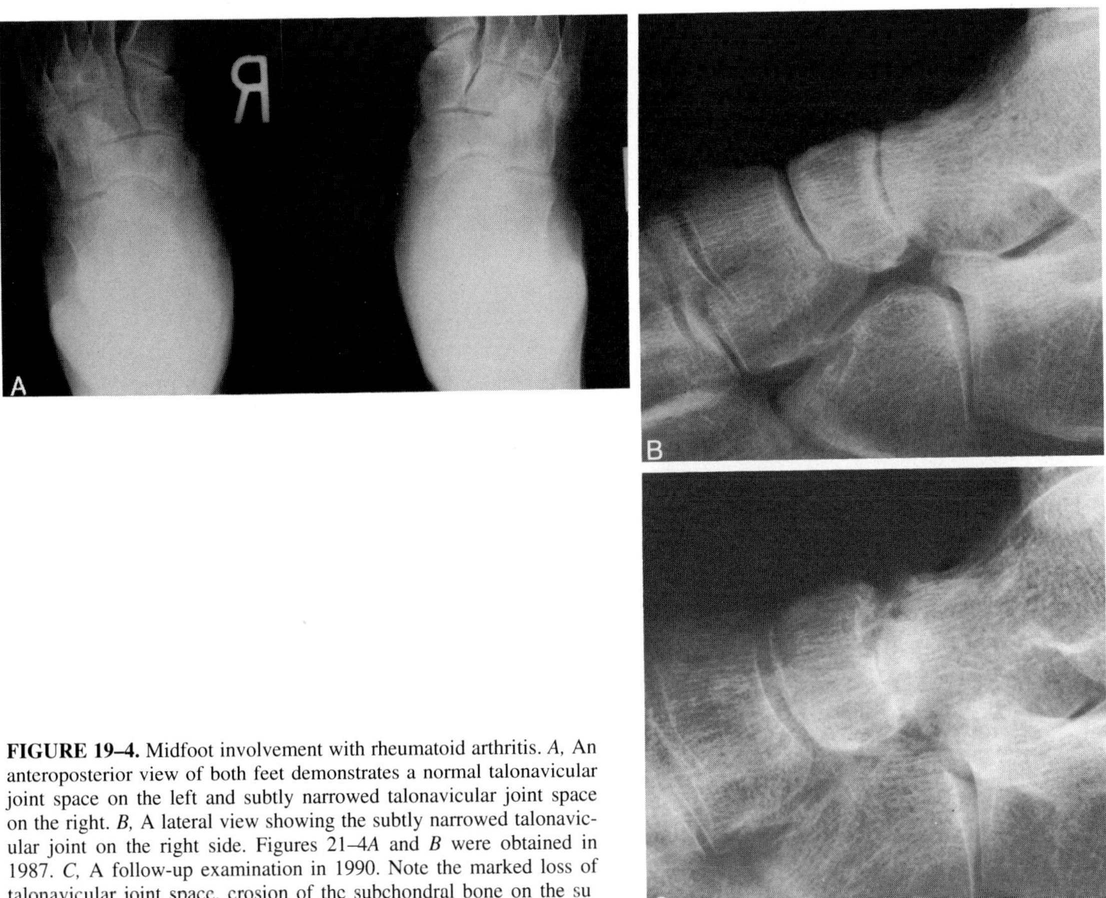

FIGURE 19–4. Midfoot involvement with rheumatoid arthritis. *A,* An anteroposterior view of both feet demonstrates a normal talonavicular joint space on the left and subtly narrowed talonavicular joint space on the right. *B,* A lateral view showing the subtly narrowed talonavicular joint on the right side. Figures 21–4*A* and *B* were obtained in 1987. *C,* A follow-up examination in 1990. Note the marked loss of talonavicular joint space, erosion of the subchondral bone on the su perior aspect of the joint, and diffuse osteopenia.

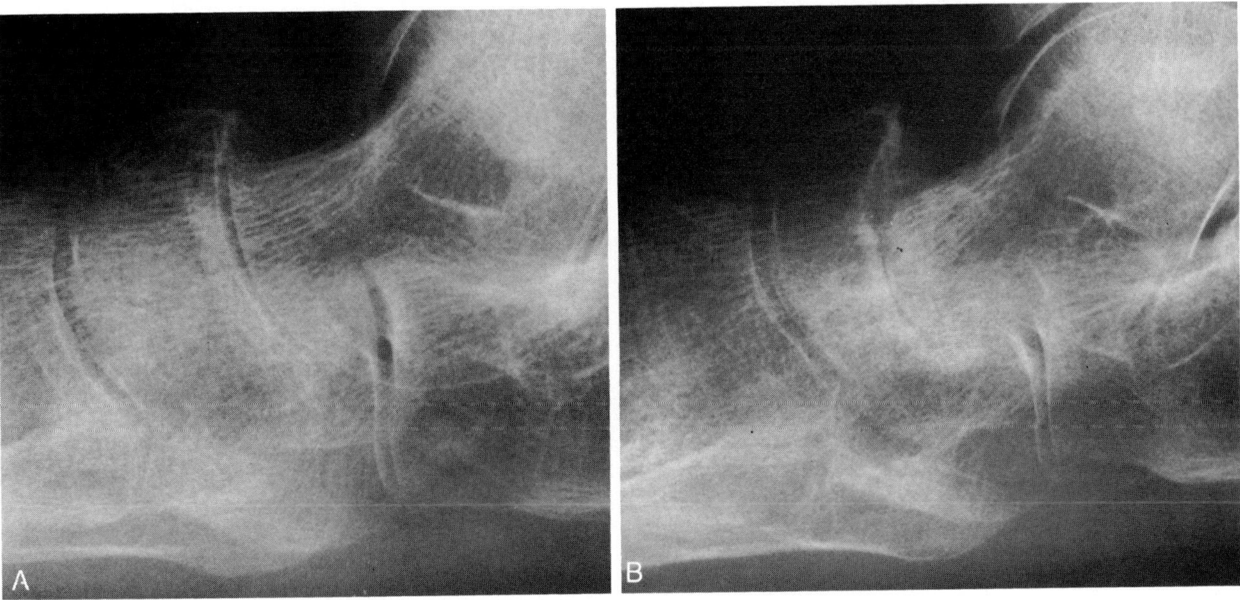

FIGURE 19–5. Midfoot collapse, secondary to talonavicular involvement with rheumatoid arthritis. *A,* On the left side, there is mild joint space narrowing and marked subluxation of the talus relative to the navicular, producing a more vertical orientation of the talus. *B,* The right side shows more severe joint space narrowing and erosive changes in the talonavicular joint, with similar subluxation and midfoot collapse.

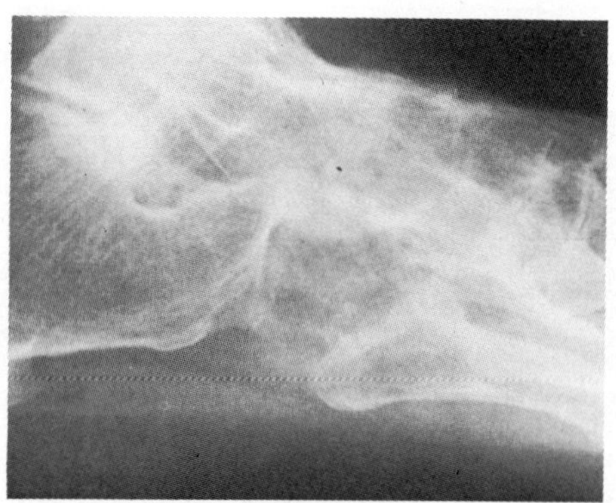

FIGURE 19–6. Lateral view of the foot demonstrating osseous fusion of the tarsus in rheumatoid arthritis (RA). Osseous fusion is unusual in RA except for the tarsus and carpus. (From Stiles RG, Resnick D, and Sartoris DJ: Radiologic manifestations of arthritides involving the foot. Clin Podiatr Med Surg 5:1–16, 1988.)

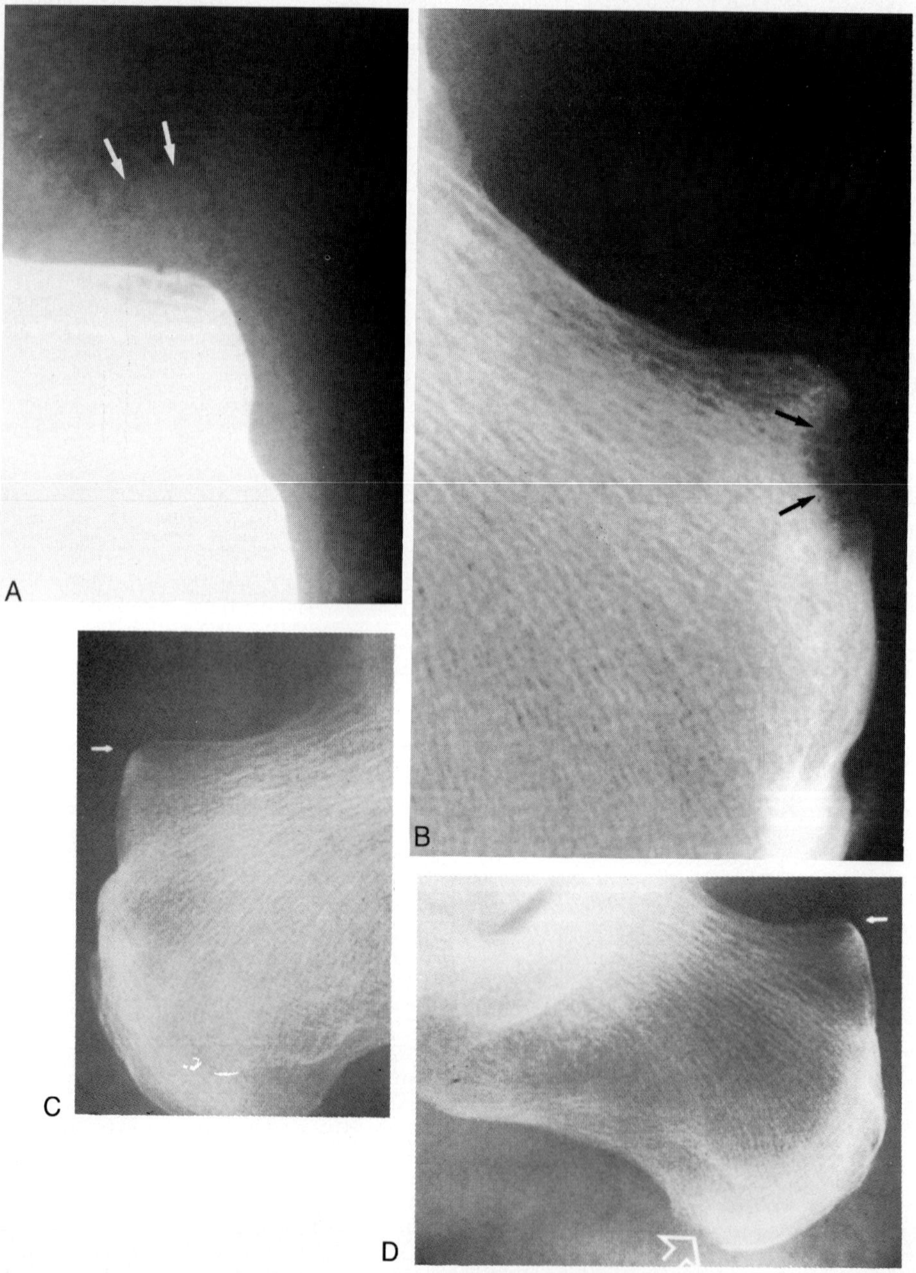

FIGURE 19–7. Calcaneal erosions in the inflammatory arthritides. *A,* Lateral view of the posterosuperior aspect of the calcaneus imaged for soft tissue detail demonstrating rounded soft tissue density occupying the region of the retrocalcaneal bursa, obliterating the normal posteroinferior aspect of the retrocalcaneal fat pad *(arrows). B,* Erosion of the posterosuperior surface of the calcaneus adjacent to the retrocalcaneal bursa with associated soft tissue density obliterating the pre-Achilles fat pad *(arrows). These* findings are consistent with long-standing retrocalcaneal bursitis. The abnormalities are nonspecific and can be seen in other inflammatory diseases. The cause in this case is rheumatoid arthritis. *C* and *D,* Reiter's syndrome involving the calcaneus demonstrating obliteration of the pre-Achilles fat pad *(closed arrow)* and an erosion along the plantar surface of the calcaneus at the insertion of the plantar aponeurosis *(open arrow).* Note that this erosion has relatively indistinct margins compared with the rheumatoid arthritis erosions seen in *B.* (*B* and *C* from Stiles RG, Resnick D, and Sartoris DJ: Radiologic manifestations of arthritides involving the foot. Clin Podiatr Med Surg 5:1–16, 1988.)

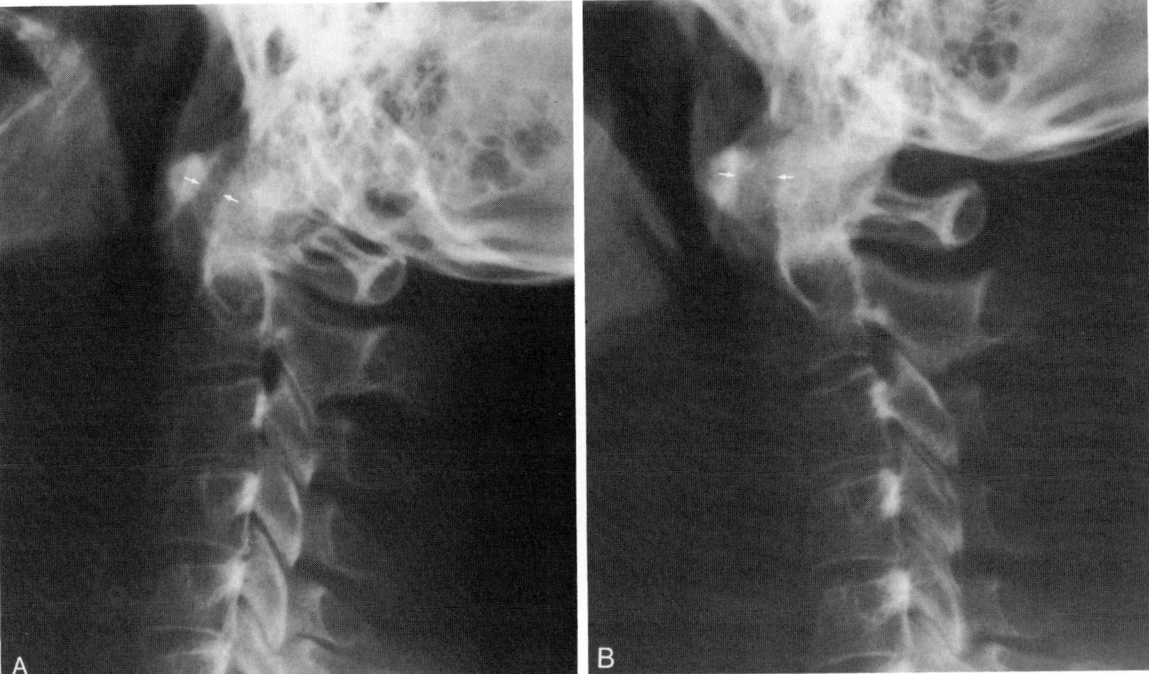

FIGURE 19–8. Atlantoaxial instability in a patient with rheumatoid arthritis. *A,* Extension radiograph of the cervical spine in lateral projection shows increased predental space (space between the *arrows*). Normal space in adults is less than 3 mm. *B,* Flexion radiograph of the cervical spine in lateral projection shows worsening of the atlantoaxial subluxation with further widening of the predental space (space between the *arrows*).

cal) disease, and occurrence of intra-articular bony anky-losis.[11] Distribution of disease in the joints of a single ray and terminal tuftal erosions are especially characteristic of psoriatic arthritis.

The forefoot and calcaneus are the major target sites for seronegative diseases in the foot. Both psoriatic arthritis and Reiter's syndrome can involve any of the interphalangeal or metatarsophalangeal joints.[3, 16] Extensive destruction of the interphalangeal joint of the great toe, however, is more characteristic of psoriatic arthritis than any other disease,[2, 17, 18] although it also may occur in Reiter's syndrome. Alterations of the calcaneus are characteristic of Reiter's syndrome and are frequently present in psoriatic arthritis.[3, 16, 17] Changes occur along both the posterior and plantar aspects of the bone

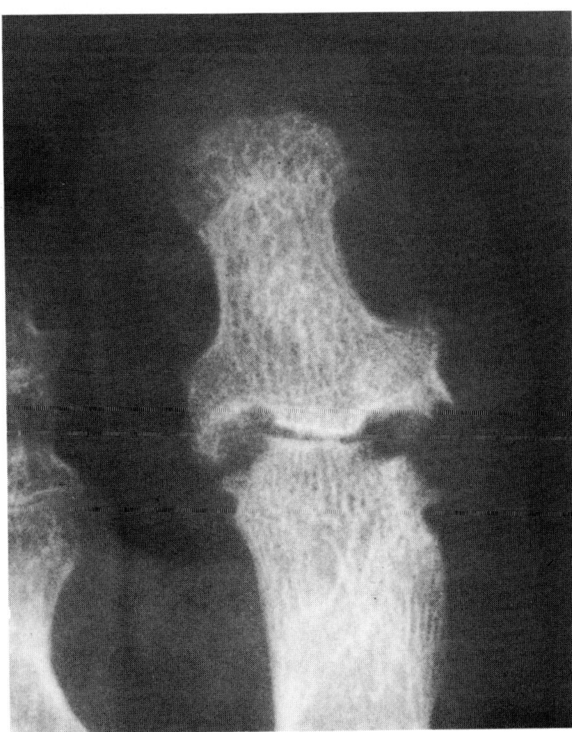

FIGURE 19–9. Psoriatic arthritis involving the interphalangeal joint of the great toe with whiskering and "mouse ear" deformities[9] at the margins of the joint.

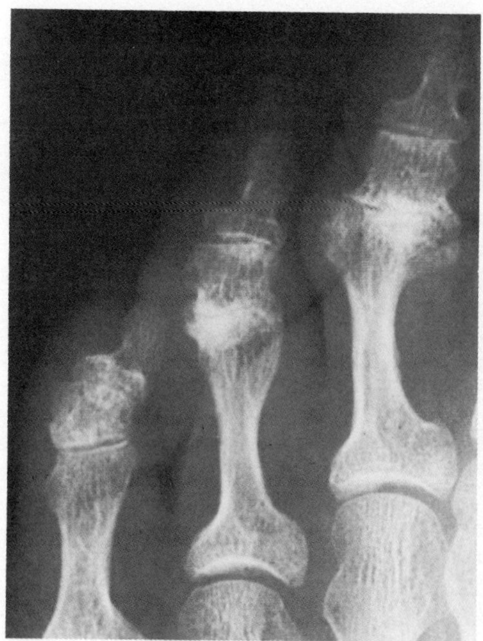

FIGURE 19–10. Psoriatic arthritis involving the proximal interphalangeal joints of the third and fourth digits with joint space narrowing and bony proliferation. (From Stiles RG, Resnick D, and Sartoris DJ: Radiologic manifestations of arthritides involving the foot. Clin Podiatr Med Surg 5:1–16, 1988.)

(Fig. 19–10). Retrocalcaneal bursitis produces soft tissue density that obliterates a portion of the pre-Achilles fat pad. Subjacent bony erosion may occur and can produce the whiskering (enthesitis) that is characteristic of all seronegative diseases. On the plantar calcaneal surface erosions, hyperostosis, and poorly defined enthesophytes may occur. The irregular plantar excrescences of the seronegative diseases may become well defined as the inflammatory process becomes quiescent. During this phase, such outgrowths are indistinguishable from those seen in normal persons or in patients with RA.

Five broad clinical categories of psoriatic arthritis have been recognized:[3] (1) polyarthritis with distal interphalangeal joint involvement; (2) symmetrical seronegative polyarthritis simulating RA; (3) monoarthritis or asymmetrical oligoarthritis; (4) sacroiliitis and spondylitis; and (5) arthritis mutilans. All these patterns can be present in the foot except, of course, sacroiliitis and spondylitis.

DEGENERATIVE DISEASE (OSTEOARTHRITIS)

Degenerative articular disease involving synovial joints is commonly known as *osteoarthritis*. Some authors prefer the term *osteoarthrosis* because inflammation is not thought by them to be a major component of the disease. The process typically does not demonstrate pathologic evidence of inflammation, and hence the morphologic features reflected radiographically are usually distinguishable from those of the synovial inflammatory diseases. The radiographic features of osteoarthritis include joint space loss, subchondral bony eburnation and cysts, osteophytes, and intra-articular bodies (Fig. 19–11). Erosions and soft tissue swelling do not occur in classic osteoarthritis. Osteoarthritis of the first metatarsophalangeal joint is very common and is termed "hallux rigidus." Alterations in the other four metatarsophalangeal joints rarely occur without specific predisposing factors such

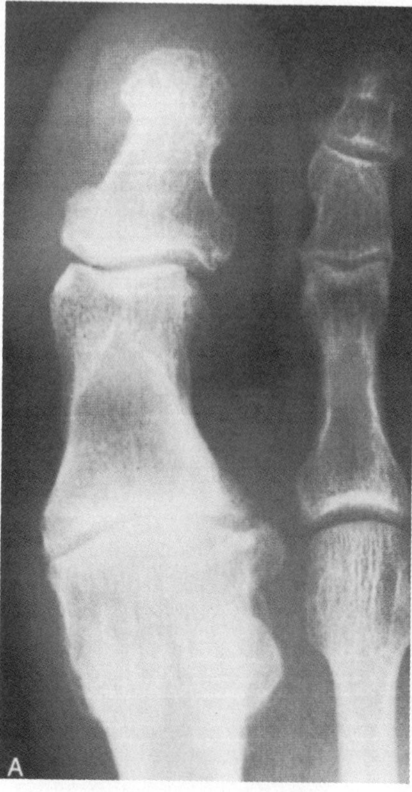
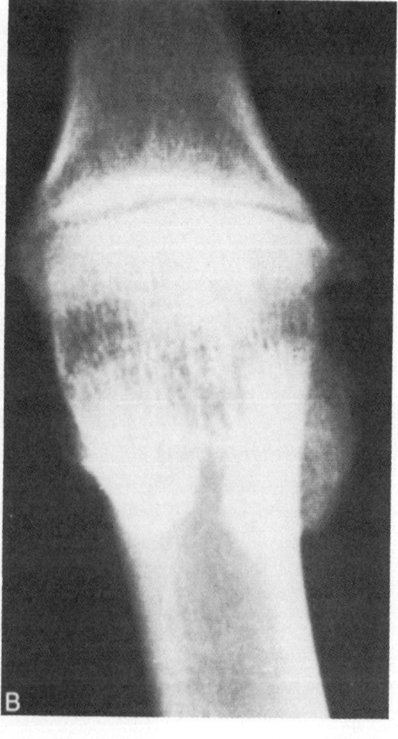

FIGURE 19–11. *A* and *B,* Two examples of hallux rigidus (osteoarthritis) involving the first metatarsophalangeal joint. Compare these examples with Figure 19–14 to observe the difficulty in differentiating osteoarthritis from gout at the first metatarsophalangeal joint. (*A* and *B* from Stiles RG, Resnick D, and Sartoris DJ: Radiologic manifestations of arthritides involving the foot. Clin Podiatr Med Surg 5:1–16, 1988.)

as trauma or osteonecrosis, as in Freiberg's infraction.[2] Interphalangeal joint involvement may occur, but it is usually an incidental, asymptomatic finding. In contrast, hallux rigidus is often symptomatic. Osteoarthritis may be associated with long-standing hallux valgus deformity.

Osteoarthritic involvement of the midfoot and hindfoot is not uncommon. Frequently, a predisposing factor such as talocalcaneal coalition induces degenerative changes in the talonavicular joint. Similarly, prior trauma may predispose to degenerative alterations in the posterior subtalar joint, or any other intertarsal articulation. This is especially common in patients with a calcaneal fracture that violates the posterior facet of the calcaneus.

A variant of osteoarthritis known as *inflammatory* or *erosive osteoarthritis* is usually confined to the joints of the hand and wrist, but occasionally it occurs in the foot.[3] The disease produces changes that simulate those of the previously described inflammatory arthritides, particularly psoriatic arthritis.[2, 3, 19] The radiologic findings are remarkably symmetrical in distribution and include central bony erosions, joint space loss, and osteophytosis. Clinically, this disease exhibits inflammatory manifestations as well.

CRYSTALLINE DEPOSITION DISEASES

As the name implies, the pathogenesis of diseases in crystalline deposition disease is deposition of crystalline material within synovial and parasynovial tissues, where the material incites an inflammatory response. Common diseases in this group include gout (sodium urate crystalline deposition), calcium pyrophosphate dihydrate crystalline deposition disease, and calcium hydroxyapatite crystalline deposition disease. Of these, gout commonly and characteristically involves the foot.

In the past, gout has been known as *podagra*, derived from the Greek words ''pous'' (foot) and ''agra'' (attack).[3, 20] This terminology reflects the strong predilection of gout for the foot, particularly the first metatarsophalangeal joint. Before the advent of chemotherapeutic agents for the treatment of gout, radiographic abnormalities were common. Effective use of these drugs has decreased both the incidence and the severity of radiographically noted changes in the disease, but it has not eliminated them. Although the classic radiographic changes of gout have been well described,[3, 20] the radiographic spectrum of gout is changing because of the effective use of hypouricemic therapy. Recently published reports on gout in two series of patients[21, 22] have demonstrated interesting clinical and radiographic findings. In a prospective analysis of 60 patients using a radiographic survey protocol, Barthelemy and associates[21] found evidence of significant alterations in asymptomatic joints among 24% of patients. This suggests that previous retrospective studies may have underestimated the extent of skeletal manifestations of gout.

The most characteristic site of abnormality in gout is the first metatarsophalangeal joint. Any joint of the foot, however, may be affected. Involvement of the dorsum of the foot[2] may lead to extensive destruction in the tarsometatarsal, intertarsal, and talocalcaneal joints. Soft tissue swelling at involved joints indicates tophaceous deposition of urate crystals. Calcification within tophi is rare unless there is a concomitant abnormality in calcium metabolism, as would occur in gouty nephropathy. Intraosseous tophi also may calcify under similar circumstances.[23]

The erosions caused by gout can be quite extensive and may lie at a significant distance from the adjacent joint (Figs. 19–12 to 19–14). Extensive erosion that is out of proportion to the degree of adjacent joint space narrowing is characteristic. Gouty erosions typically manifest an ''overhanging edge'' of bony cortex that extends around the tophaceous material (see Fig. 21–12). The sign, however, should be used with some caution because overhanging edges may also occur with the osseous lesions of sarcoidosis and psoriatic arthritis.[19] A lacelike pattern has also been described in gouty erosions (see Fig. 21–12).[22] Despite the tendency toward joint space preservation in gout, it should be emphasized that hallux rigidus (osteoarthritis) and gout may be indistinguishable radiographically (see Figs. 19–11 and 19–14).

CONNECTIVE TISSUE DISEASES

Connective tissue diseases are a group of complex disorders for which specific causes are not known. The diseases include systemic lupus erythematosus (SLE), scleroderma, dermatomyositis, and mixed connective tissue diseases (MCTD). The clinical and radiographic spectrum of these disorders is broad. The foot is most likely to be involved in SLE and MCTD. The classic radiographic abnormality in SLE is a nonerosive deforming arthropathy of the hands with easy reducibility of the deformity. Bone and cartilage abnormalities are unusual in SLE, and the arthropathy produces little functional disability. A similar process called *lupus foot* (Fig. 19–15) has been described in the feet of SLE patients.[24, 25] The cases reported in the literature have shown nonerosive deforming arthropathy with passively correctable hallux valgus, widening of the forefoot, subluxation of the metatarsophalangeal joints, and flexion contractures. As in the hands, the deformities of the forefoot are often reducible, but they may show evidence of mechanical dysfunction in the form of calluses and bunions.[24] Despite the evidence of dysfunction, major disability caused by lupus foot has not been reported.[24] MCTD is characterized by clinical and radiographic features that suggest an overlap of SLE, scleroderma, dermatomyositis, and RA. Thus, the radiographs may show deforming, reducible arthropathy as in SLE, but they may also reveal osteoporosis, soft tissue swelling, erosions, and joint space narrowing as in RA. The metatarsophalangeal and interphalangeal joints of the foot are commonly involved in this disorder.

INFECTION AND NEUROPATHIC JOINT DISEASES

Osteomyelitis and septic arthritis relatively commonly affect the foot. Routes of contamination producing infection include hematogenous spread, spread from a contiguous source, direct implantation, and postoperative infection. Typically, direct implantation occurs secondary to puncture wounds as a result of stepping on a contaminated sharp object such as a nail or a thorn. Spread from a contiguous source is typified by nonhealing foot ulcers and cellulitis in a patient with diabetes. Add to this the coexistence of diabetic neuropathic disease of the foot, and an extremely difficult diagnostic situation has developed.[26] This combination of processes represents a frustrating clinical and radiologic dilemma because of the limitations of current diagnostic

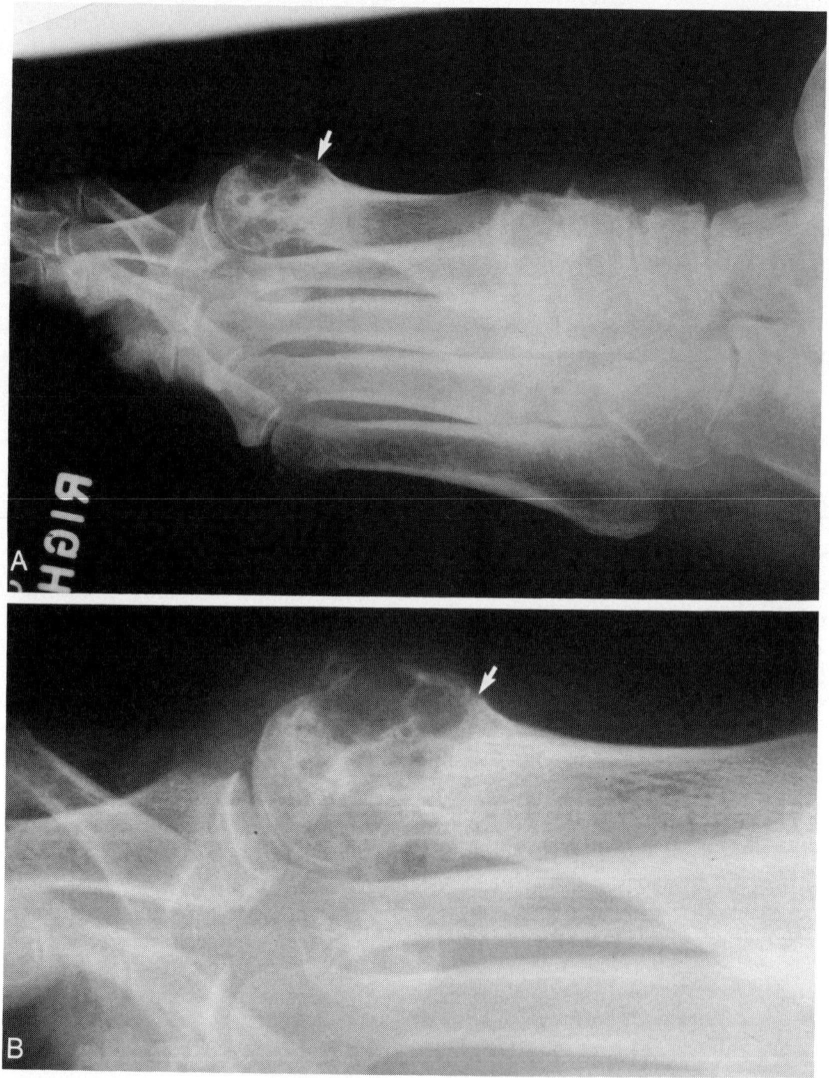

FIGURE 19–12. *A* and *B,* Erosions indicative of gouty arthritis at the first metatarsophalangeal joint and along the dorsum of the foot. Note the overhanging edge *(arrows).* Note also the lacy pattern within the erosions.

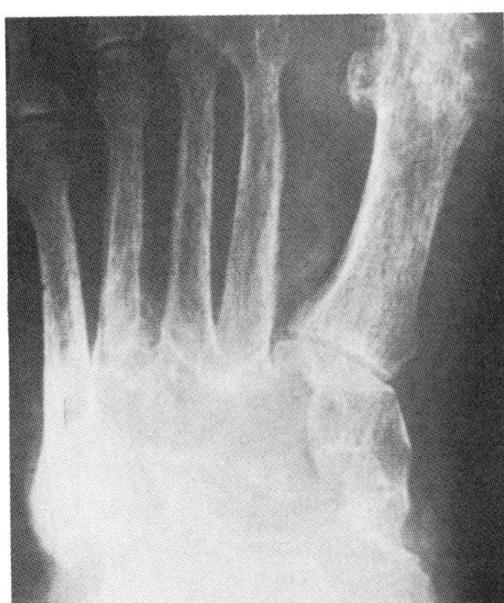

FIGURE 19–13. Extensive erosion of the tarsometatarsal joints from severe tophaceous gout. (Adapted from Stiles RG, Resnick D, and Sartoris DJ: Radiologic manifestations of arthritides involving the foot. Clin Podiatr Med Surg 5:1–16, 1988.)

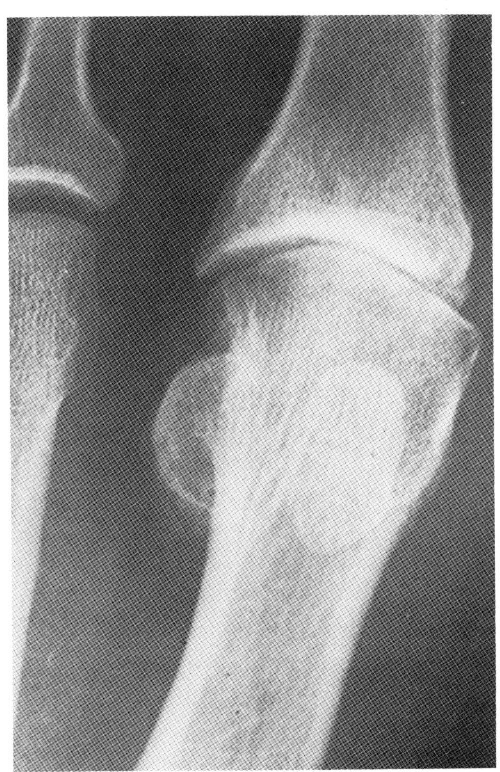

FIGURE 19–14. Gout of the first metatarsophalangeal joint. This stage of gouty arthritis is indistinguishable from osteoarthritis (see Fig. 21–9). (From Stiles RG, Resnick D, and Sartoris DJ: Radiologic manifestations of arthritides involving the foot. Clin Podiatr Med Surg 5:1–16, 1988.)

techniques in evaluating early infection and in differentiating infection from neuropathic disease. Similarly, the presence of any pre-existing articular disorder (such as RA, osteoarthritis, and gout) complicates the ability to clinically and radiographically diagnose septic arthritis and osteomyelitis. Other imaging modalities may be helpful in this situation, however. Radionuclide bone scanning with either bone-seeking agents such as ^{99m}Tc methylene diphosphonate (MDP) or inflammation-seeking agents such as ^{67}Ga citrate and ^{111}In-labeled white blood cells can be utilized to help identify areas of infection. However, the difficulty remains in differentiating neuropathic disease and osteomyelitis with these techniques; neuropathic disease can show characteristics of osteomyelitis, and both of these diseases show increased activity on radionuclide bone scans. Magnetic resonance imaging (MRI) has been applied to this problem as well and does show some promise in demonstrating abnormal marrow replacement in the evaluation of osteomyelitis versus neuro-

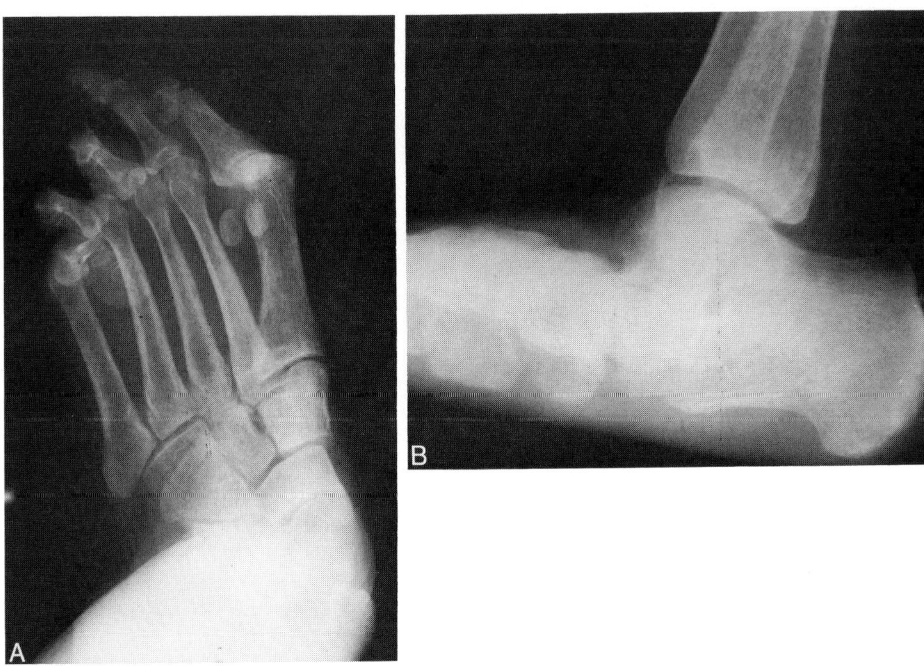

FIGURE 19–15. Lupus foot. *A,* An anteroposterior standing view of the foot demonstrates abduction-pronation deformity with subluxation at the metatarsophalangeal joints. Note the absence of joint space narrowing and erosions consistent with the deforming nonerosive arthropathy of systemic lupus erythematosus. *B,* The lateral view shows midfoot collapse without joint space narrowing or erosive disease characteristic of lupus arthropathy.

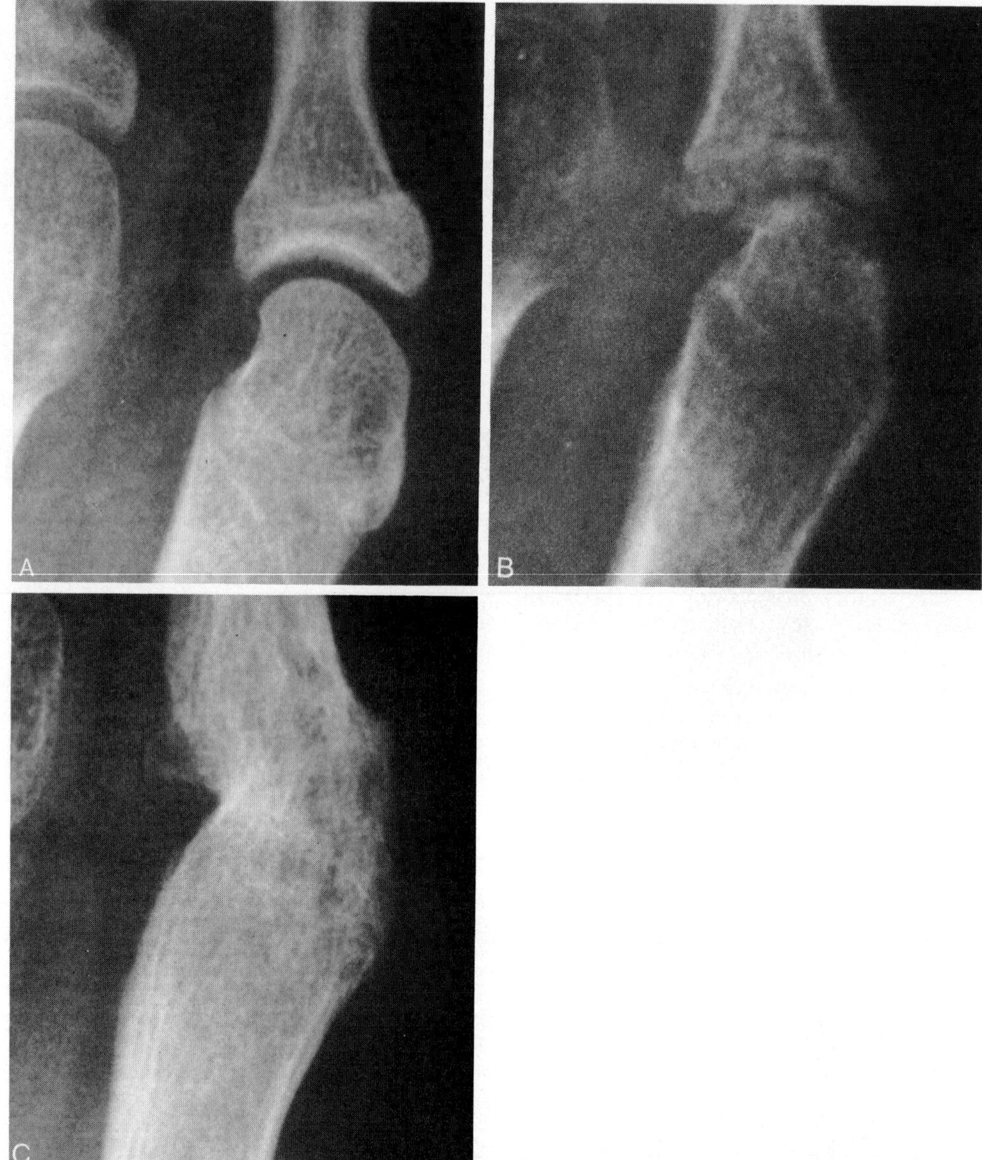

FIGURE 19–16. Progression of septic arthritis of the fifth metatarsophalangeal joint. *A,* At presentation, the radiograph is normal despite clinical signs of septic arthritis. *B,* The infectious process has resulted in loss of cartilage and erosion of articular surfaces. *C,* Chronic phase shows bony ankylosis of the joint.

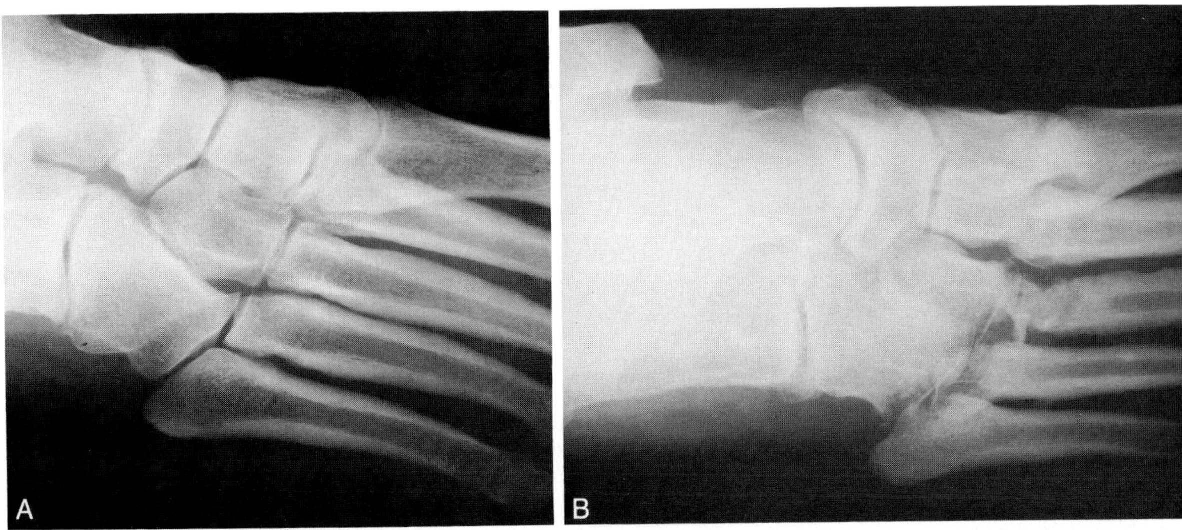

FIGURE 19–17. Neuropathic joint disease. *A,* Oblique view of the foot, approximately 2 years ago, shows a normal Lisfranc's joint. *B,* Radiographic films at the current time demonstrate lateral subluxation and fragmentation, with relative preservation of bone density characteristic of neuropathic joint disease.

pathic disease. Other imaging modalities are discussed in more detail elsewhere in this text.

Septic arthritis implies an infection of the joint itself, including the synovium and cartilage. Infected synovium becomes edematous and hypertrophied, and an exudative joint effusion is produced. With time, the effusion becomes frank pus. This leads to a destructive process involving the articular cartilage and, eventually, the subchondral bone. Early on, then, the radiographic signs of swelling and effusion are nonspecific, and correlation with clinical history is most helpful in making the diagnosis of septic arthritis. Arthrocentesis is required for specific diagnosis. Later, destructive phases are more characteristic, especially when osteolysis and bone destruction occur. The condition of the joint may progress to ankylosis (Fig. 19–16).

Diabetes mellitus has become the most common cause of neuropathic disease in the foot. The process is thought to be secondary to diabetic peripheral neuropathy and probably diabetic vascular disease. Radiographic findings include osseous fragmentation, sclerosis, joint subluxation, and dislo-

cation. At the tarsometatarsal joints, dorsolateral dislocation can occur resembling an acute Lisfranc fracture-dislocation (Fig. 19–17). This leads to a characteristic radiographic appearance of disorganized and destroyed joints. Uncomplicated neuropathic disease in the patient with diabetes is not a difficult radiographic diagnosis. However, vascular insufficiency and neuropathy in diabetes mellitus also predispose to soft tissue infection, which by contiguous spread can produce osteomyelitis and septic arthritis (Fig. 19–18). As mentioned, the superimposition of infection and neuropathic joint disease is a very difficult diagnostic situation. Both of these processes can produce sclerosis and osseous fragmentation. Osteolysis and ill-defined contours of bone are probably the most helpful radiographic clues to the presence of infection superimposed on neuropathy. Magnification radiography can be helpful in defining osteolysis. However, a microfocal spot tube is required, and this is not widely available. Serial radiographs and meticulous comparison with previous films are probably the most helpful methods in this diagnostic situation.

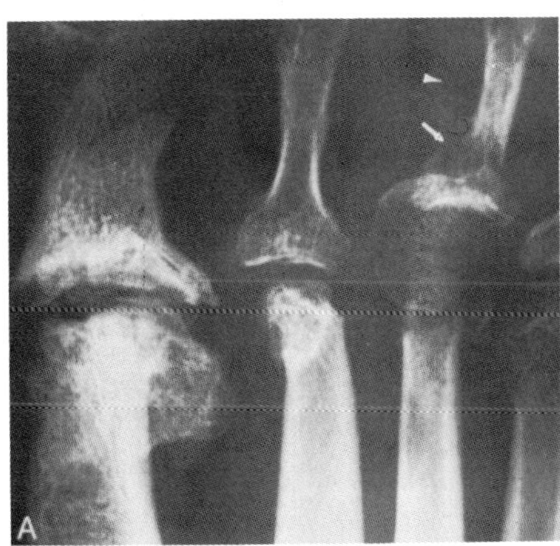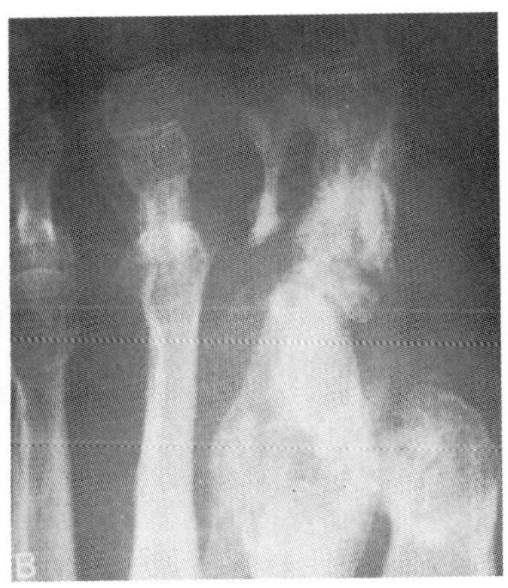

FIGURE 19–18. Neuropathic disease in diabetes mellitus. *A,* Neuropathic disease with soft tissue infection and osteomyelitis. Note the osteolysis of the third proximal phalanx *(arrow)* and the soft tissue gas *(arrowhead). B,* Neuropathic disease involving the fourth ray. Osteomyelitis was also present in this case, but radiographic evidence of infection was difficult to discern. (From Stiles RG, Resnick D, and Sartoris DJ: Radiologic manifestations of arthritides involving the foot. Clin Podiatr Med Surg 5:1–16, 1988.)

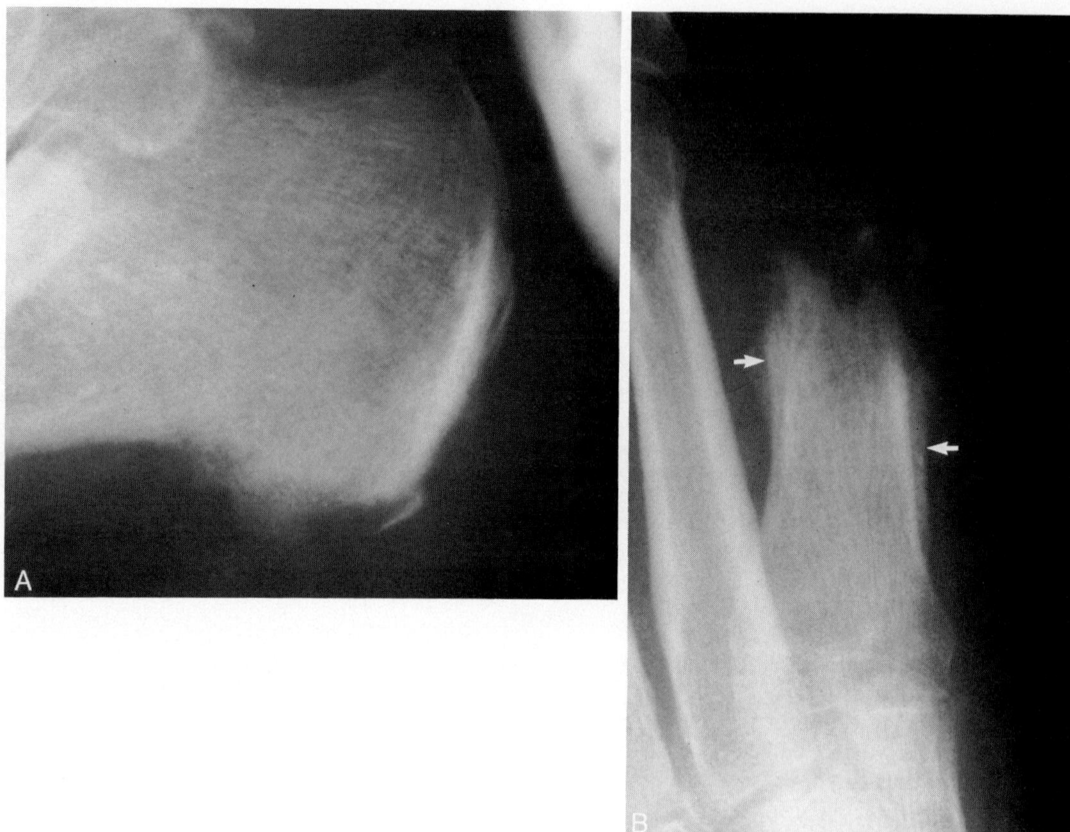

FIGURE 19–19. Acute osteomyelitis. *A,* Acute osteomyelitis of the calcaneus. Cortical margins are indistinct along the plantar surface. *B,* Acute osteomyelitis of the first metatarsal in a diabetic patient after resection of the digit for previous osteomyelitis. Note the acute, immature periosteal new bone formation *(arrows).*

Osteomyelitis produces different radiographic patterns in acute and chronic disease. Acute pyogenic osteomyelitis characteristically demonstrates osteolysis, indistinctness of cortical margins, and immature periosteal bone formation or periostitis (Fig. 19–19). Chronic or nonpyogenic (tuberculous, fungal) osteomyelitis may present with more sclerosis (Fig. 19–20). Although unusual today, occasionally sequestra (dead, infected, and devitalized fragments of bone) sur- rounded by an involucrum (thick, mature periosteal new bone) are demonstrated in chronic osteomyelitis.

DISEASES OF SESAMOID BONES

A brief discussion of sesamoid bones is warranted because they are frequently involved in arthritic disorders, and afflictions of these bones are frequently evaluated and treated by

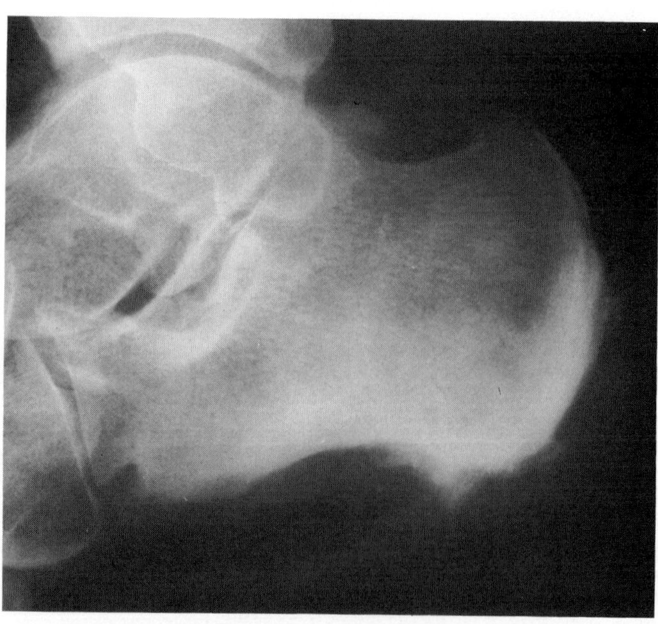

FIGURE 19–20. Chronic osteomyelitis of the calcaneus. Note the sclerosis of the bone.

podiatrists. Sesamoid bones and their relationship to surrounding tissues show all the anatomic features of a synovial joint, with cartilage covering the osseous surfaces and the surrounding synovial lining.[27] As such, sesamoids may be affected by all of the diseases discussed previously. These small bones may show osseous erosion in RA, bony proliferation in seronegative disease, osteophytes in osteoarthritis, and joint space loss and ankylosis with infection. These changes may be present with a normal adjacent first metatarsophalangeal articulation. In these situations, recognition of disease in the sesamoids is important in accurate radiographic diagnosis.[27]

References

1. Kaye JJ: Arthritis: Roles of radiography and other imaging techniques in evaluation. Radiology 177:601, 1990.
2. Martel W: Acute and chronic arthritis of the foot. Semin Roentgenol 5:391, 1970.
3. Resnick D and Niwayama G (eds): Diagnosis of Bone and Joint Disorders, 2nd ed. Philadelphia, WB Saunders, 1988, pp 815–820, 1912–1938.
4. Sartoris DJ and Resnick D: Radiological evaluation of patients with arthritis. PA 86:293, 1986.
5. Winfield J, Young A, Williams P, and Corbett M: Prospective study of the radiological changes in hands, feet and cervical spine in adult rheumatoid arthritis. Ann Rheum Dis 42:613, 1983.
6. Arnett FC, Edworthy SM, Bloch DA, et al: The American Rheumatism Association 1987 revised criteria for the classification of rheumatoid arthritis. Arthritis Rheum 31:315–324, 1988.
7. Kaye JJ, Fuchs HA, Moseley JW, et al: Problems with the Steinbrocker staging system for radiographic assessment of the rheumatoid hand and wrist. Invest Radiol 25:536, 1990.
8. Kaye JJ, Callahan LF, Nance EP, et al: Rheumatoid arthritis: Explanatory power of specific radiographic findings for patient clinical status. Radiology 165:753, 1987.
9. Brower AC: Arthritis in Black and White. Philadelphia, WB Saunders, 1988, p 39.
10. Gold RH and Bassett LW: Radiologic evaluation of the arthritic foot. Foot Ankle 2:332, 1982.
11. Pastershank SP: Midfoot dissociation in rheumatoid arthritis. J Can Assoc Radiol 32:166, 1981.
12. Ang JC, Rubenstein J, and English E: Subtalar dislocation in rheumatoid arthritis. J Rheumatol 9:671, 1982.
13. Spiegel TM and Spiegel JS: Rheumatoid arthritis in the foot and ankle: Diagnosis, pathology, and treatment: The relationship between foot and ankle deformity in disease duration in 50 patients. Foot Ankle 2:318–324, 1982.
14. Downy DJ, Simpkin PA, Mack LA, et al: Tibialis posterior tendon rupture: A cause of rheumatoid flatfoot. Arthritis Rheum 31:441–446, 1988.
15. Resnick D, Feingold MC, Curel J, et al: Calcaneal abnormalities in articular disorders. Radiology 125:355, 1977.
16. Chand Y and Johnson KA: Foot and ankle manifestations of Reiter's syndrome. Foot Ankle 1:167, 1980.
17. Martel W, Stuck KJ, Dworin AM, and Hylland RG: Erosive osteoarthritis and psoriatic arthritis: A radiologic comparison in the hand, wrist, and foot. Am J Roentgenol 134:125, 1980.
18. Resnick DR: Radiologic evaluation of seronegative spondyloarthropathies. Clin Orthop 143:38, 1979.
19. Gold RH, Bassett LW, and Theros EG: Radiologic comparison of erosive polyarthritides with prominent interphalangeal involvement. Skeletal Radiol 8:89, 1982.
20. Resnick D: The radiographic manifestations of gouty arthritis. Crit Rev Diagn Imag 9:265, 1977.
21. Barthelemy CP, Nakayama DA, Carrera GF, et al: Gouty arthritis: A prospective radiologic evaluation of sixty patients. Skeletal Radiol 11:1, 1984.
22. Bloch C, Merman G, and Yu T: A radiologic reevaluation of gout: A study of 2000 patients. Am J Roentgenol 134:781, 1980.
23. Resnick D and Broderick TW. Intraosseous calcification in tophaceous gout. Am J Roentgenol 137:1157, 1981.
24. Mizutani W and Quismorio FP: Lupus foot: Deforming arthropathy of the feet in systemic lupus erythematosus. J Rheumatol 11:80, 1984.
25. Morley KD, Leung A, and Rynes RI: Lupus foot. Br Med J 284:557, 1982.
26. Zlatkin MB, Pathria M, Sartoris DJ, and Resnick D: The diabetic foot. Radiol Clin North Am 25:1095, 1987.
27. Resnick D, Niwayama G, and Feingold M: The sesamoid bones of the hands and feet: Participators in arthritis. Radiology 123:57, 1977.
28. Halla J, Fellahi S, and Hardin JG: Small joint involvement: A systemic roentgenographic study in rheumatoid arthritis. Ann Rheum Dis 45:327, 1986.

CHAPTER 20

Imaging of Musculoskeletal Tumors

Ann Gabrielle Bergman, M.D.

Imaging plays a central role in the evaluation of any abnormality suspected to represent a tumor or tumorlike lesion of the musculoskeletal system. Imaging modalities have increased in number and complexity. Therefore, to select the optimal imaging tests for each type of lesion, it is important to be familiar with the different imaging methods as well as with the radiographic characteristics of the different tumor types.

IMAGING MODALITIES

Conventional radiography remains a cornerstone of tumor imaging. The conventional tomographic technique, however, has been almost entirely replaced by computed tomography (CT), available since the early 1970s. Magnetic resonance (MR) imaging, introduced for clinical use during the mid-1980s, has rapidly become an extremely important modality for evaluation of musculoskeletal tumors. Conventional radiography, CT, and MR imaging all can be used in combination with contrast materials, injected either into a joint or synovial space (e.g., arthrography, tenography, bursography, CT-arthrography, and MR-arthrography) or into a vein or artery (e.g., angiography, contrast-enhanced CT, and contrast-enhanced MR imaging). Nuclear medicine isotope techniques have been available for clinical studies of musculoskeletal structures since the late 1960s and have undergone continued technical improvements. Computerized nuclear medicine methods such as single photon emission computed tomography (SPECT) have also been added. Ultrasonographic Doppler techniques have developed into an excellent noninvasive method of evaluating vascular patency of the extremities, but they are used infrequently in the evaluation of musculoskeletal tumors.

Conventional Radiography

The advantages of conventional radiography include its availability and relatively low cost as well as the excellent contrast detail resolution of imaged bone structures, whereas the disadvantages include the radiation exposure to the patient, the limited ability to evaluate other than osseous structures, and the superimposition of structures on the image.

Computed Tomography

The advantages of CT technique include the ability to image in tomographic sections, thus avoiding structure super-imposition, and cross-sectional imaging in the axial plane. (Sagittal and coronal plane imaging are limited by the difficulties in positioning the patient in the scanner for direct imaging in this plane, but is usually possible for distal extremity joints such as the foot and ankle.) With CT, tissue contrast resolution is better than with conventional radiography but is still inferior to MR imaging, whereas detail resolution is still slightly better with CT than with MR imaging.[1, 2] The technique does involve radiation exposure to the patient, although this is strictly limited to the examined body sections. The cost is relatively high.

Magnetic Resonance Imaging

Major advantages of MR imaging include the excellent contrast resolution of soft tissue structures, including bone marrow, and the absence of ionizing radiation exposure to the patient.[3] The detail resolution is good; however, the cost is still relatively high. Patient acceptance is somewhat limited owing to claustrophobic reaction to the narrow scanner bore in approximately 5% of the population.[4] Intravenous MR contrast has been used but has not markedly increased the ability to separate tumor mass from surrounding edema and is rarely indicated for tumor evaluation.

Isotope Studies

The advantages of isotope studies include the high sensitivity of most scintigraphic techniques and the ability to evaluate the entire skeletal system in one examination. Disadvantages include a poor spatial resolution, limited availability, radiation exposure to the patient, and relatively high cost.

IMAGING CHARACTERISTICS OF MUSCULOSKELETAL TUMORS

General Features

The radiographic features to be evaluated in a lesion suspected to be a tumor of the musculoskeletal system include[5]: (1) matrix type—presence of bone formation or cartilage formation within the tumor tissue; (2) bone destruction type—evaluated at the transition zone between the lesion and surrounding bone; (3) periosteal reaction type; (4) possible extraosseous soft tissue mass; (5) the location of the lesion within the bone in both longitudinal and transverse dimensions; and (6) information regarding the age of the patient.

After reviewing these radiographic features, it becomes important for differential diagnostic considerations to identify the specific tumor types that best fit the particular constellation of radiographic findings.

Before reviewing radiographic features of specific tumor types, the main six features listed earlier are briefly discussed.

Matrix Ossification or Calcification. Most tumor lesions are seen on conventional radiographs as bone destruction without evidence of ossification or calcification. If matrix mineralization is present, it considerably narrows the differential diagnosis to bone-forming or cartilage-forming lesions.

It is sometimes difficult on conventional radiography to separate neoplastic bone formation from the more common reactive bone formation, in which non-neoplastic mesenchymal cells proliferate into osteoblasts as a defense reaction by the host bone against the tumor tissue. Reactive bone formation can be provoked by both malignant and benign lesions. It is most commonly seen around slow-growing benign bone tumors, whereas a more rapidly growing lesion tends to destroy any reactive bone in its way. Reactive bone consists of mature lamellar bone, whereas tumor bone consists of irregular, woven bone. Tumor bone tends to form within the tumor lesion, whereas reactive bone forms at the margin of the lesion as either a sclerotic border or a diffuse increase in bone density around a lesion.

Cartilage formation in a tumor can be identified if characteristic cartilage calcification is present (Fig. 20–1). Owing to the multicentric growth pattern of cartilage, these calcifications are usually seen as curvilinear, circular, spherical, or stippled millimeter-sized densities. Cartilage calcification is homogeneously dense on conventional radiographs, in contrast with ossification that exhibits trabecular structures and a peripheral thin cortical border.

Another type of tumor calcification is due to the presence of calcified necrotic tissue (dystrophic calcification), which is often larger and more irregular than cartilage calcification.

Transition Zone. The character of the border between the

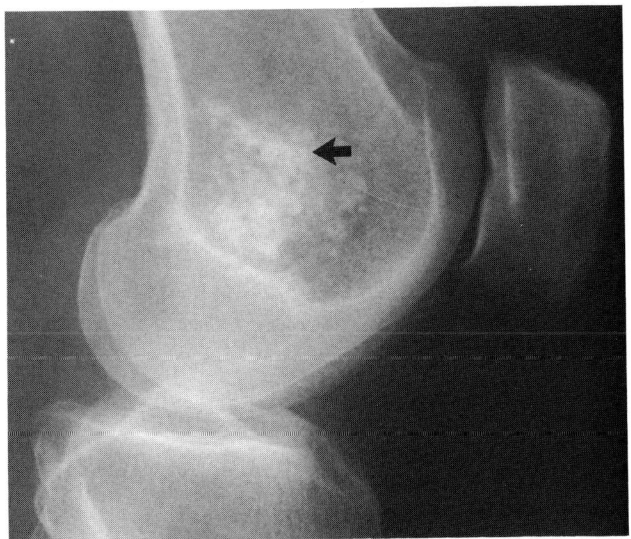

FIGURE 20–1. Characteristic ringlike areas of calcification *(arrow)* in an enchondroma of the distal femur in a 60-year-old woman. The lesion does not have a well-defined sclerotic peripheral margin or a well-defined lytic component.

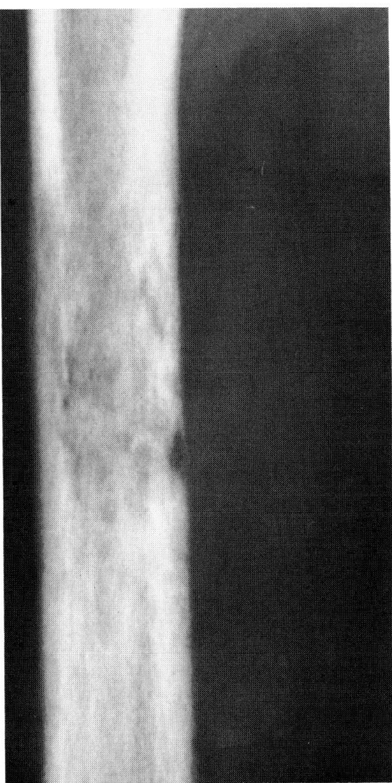

FIGURE 20–2. Ill-defined area of bone destruction involving the femoral diaphysis, illustrating both the moth-eaten (distally) and the permeated (proximally) bone destruction patterns. Lymphoma in an adult.

lesion and the surrounding bone can give information as to whether the lesion is latent or whether it has a more aggressive growth pattern. The transition zone can be classified as narrow or wide, or in Lodwick's classification,[5] as geographic, moth-eaten, or permeative. A narrow transition zone and geographic pattern both indicate a latent lesion, having a sharply delineated border against adjacent normal bone. This border may show a sclerotic line of reactive bone formation or may be sharply delineated but without the presence of a sclerotic line. The moth-eaten pattern indicates more aggressive growth of the lesion, with a transition zone exhibiting focal lytic regions between the lesion and normal bone (Fig. 20–2). The permeative pattern has a wide transition zone with small, poorly defined areas of bone destruction. With the moth-eaten or permeative patterns, the true extent of the tumor is often well beyond that suggested by the conventional radiographs.

Periosteal Reaction. The type of periosteal reaction also adds information regarding latent versus aggressive character of the lesion. Periosteal reactions are classified as benign (solid or single layer), laminated (Fig. 20–3), and spiculated (sunburst or hair-on-end) (Fig. 20–4). The benign type of periosteal reaction is nonspecific as to underlying process and may occur with certain types of benign tumors and also with other pathologic conditions, such as trauma (''callus'') and infection. This type of periosteal reaction is caused by surrounding edema that has elevated the periosteum. The laminated and spiculated periosteal reaction types, however, indicate aggressive growth, and although they are not pathognomonic, they are strongly suggestive of an aggressive and likely malignant tumor. Rarely, laminated or spiculated peri-

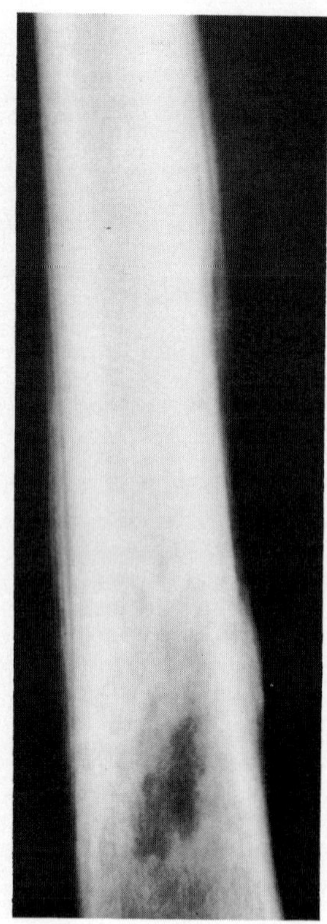

FIGURE 20–3. Laminated periosteal reaction along the femoral diaphysis, associated with an area of cortical destruction. Osteomyelitis in a 14-year-old child.

osteal reactions can occur with a very aggressive form of osteomyelitis. Codman's triangle is a periosteal reaction pattern that occurs when a tumor has broken through the cortical bone and the tumor mass (corresponding to lytic area on the radiograph) starts to destroy the recently formed, solid periosteal reaction. Codman's triangle is therefore always located at the periphery of a tumor.

Periosteal reaction can be identified by MR imaging as well, with a low signal indicating areas of mineralization and an increased signal on T_2-weighted images corresponding with inflammation or tumor.[6]

Extraosseous Soft Tissue Mass. This finding is usually associated with a malignant bone tumor but may also be present in more aggressive benign tumors, such as giant cell tumors. The soft tissue component is rarely identified on conventional radiographs; this usually requires CT or MR imaging. These imaging modalities, especially MR imaging with its increased contrast resolution, can reliably map out the extent of a soft tissue mass and evaluate the compartments that are involved and whether adjacent structures such as vessels, nerves, and joint spaces are displaced, surrounded, or invaded by the mass.

Lesion Location Within the Bone. Most musculoskeletal tumors, benign as well as malignant, are located in the metaphyseal region of a long bone. If the lesion is located in an epiphysis, apophysis, or diaphysis, this leads to strong consideration of certain tumor types. With lesions located in an epiphysis, the adjacent growth plate should be evaluated as to whether it is still open or has closed, and it should also be noted if the lesion reaches the subchondral cortical bone. With lesions located in an epiphysis, it is also important to look for other radiographic signs such as subchondral cysts

or erosions, because inflammatory or degenerative joint disease may sometimes mimic a tumor lesion.

Patient's Age. Primary bone tumors are most common during adolescence, and knowledge of the patient's age is important for generation of the most likely diagnoses when evaluating a musculoskeletal lesion suspected to represent a tumor.

Previous Biopsy or Treatment

Extensive edema hemorrhage or a bone defect from a recent biopsy may be mistaken for a tumor. Tumor imaging should therefore be performed before a biopsy, because both tumor characteristics and tumor extent may be misinterpreted on postbiopsy imaging studies. Previous remote or recent treatment such as radiation therapy should be considered when imaging studies are interpreted.

Staging

Published studies of morphologic tumor appearance as well as true extent of sarcoma in a specimen compared with MR imaging have shown a high correlation, better than with other available imaging methods.[7–9] For pretreatment staging of malignant soft tissue and bone tumors, MR imaging is currently the optimal imaging examination.

CLASSIFICATION OF MUSCULOSKELETAL TUMORS

In 1972, the World Health Organization established an official classification of bone tumors based on histologic cri-

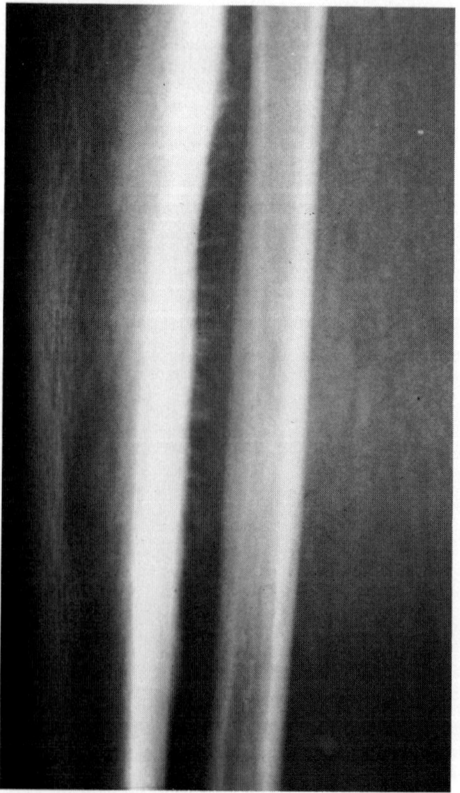

FIGURE 20–4. Spiculated periosteal reaction at the posterior surface of the tibia at the diaphysis proximally. Ewing's sarcoma in a child.

teria.[10] This classification system has also become generally accepted in the radiologic and surgical literature. It consists of the following groups, each with subgroups of benign and malignant varieties: bone-forming tumors, cartilage-forming tumors, giant cell tumors, marrow tumors, vascular tumors, other connective tissue tumors, and other tumors.

SPECIFIC IMAGING CHARACTERISTICS OF MUSCULOSKELETAL TUMOR TYPES

Malignant Bone-Forming Tumors

Osteosarcoma. The conventional type of osteosarcoma is the second most common of malignant bone tumors after multiple myeloma and has a strong predilection for presentation during late teens and early twenties (Fig. 20–5). The other types of osteosarcoma, such as parosteal[11] (Fig. 20–6), periosteal, telangiectatic,[12] and the rare Paget osteosarcoma[13] (Fig. 20–7), may well occur also in patients in their thirties and older, whereas osteosarcomatosis[14] presents in children and adolescents. The most common presentation is a painful mass. Although any bone may be involved, almost half of all cases occur in the femur, another 20% occur in the tibia; and 10% occur in the humerus.

The radiographic findings include periosteal reaction of a type indicating aggressive growth (spiculated, laminated, or Codman's triangle) and evidence of both bone destruction and tumor bone formation.[15] Evaluation of an associated soft tissue mass requires other imaging modalities such as CT or

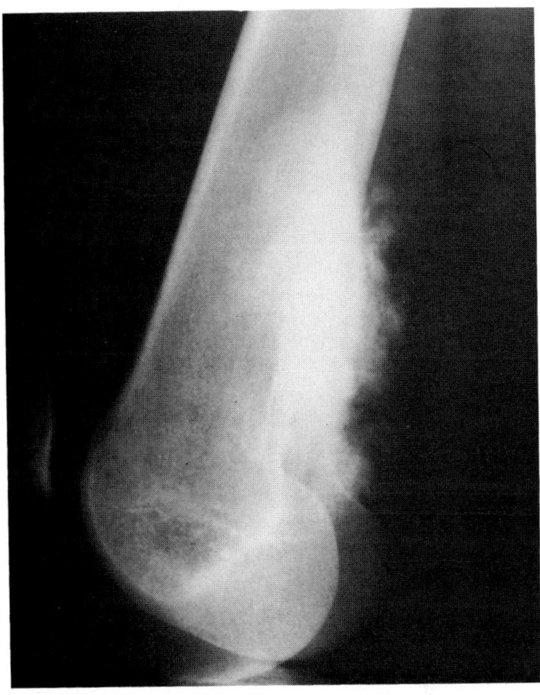

FIGURE 20–6. Parosteal sarcoma of the distal femur, posteriorly, in an adolescent boy. The location is characteristic. The associated soft tissue mass cannot be evaluated.

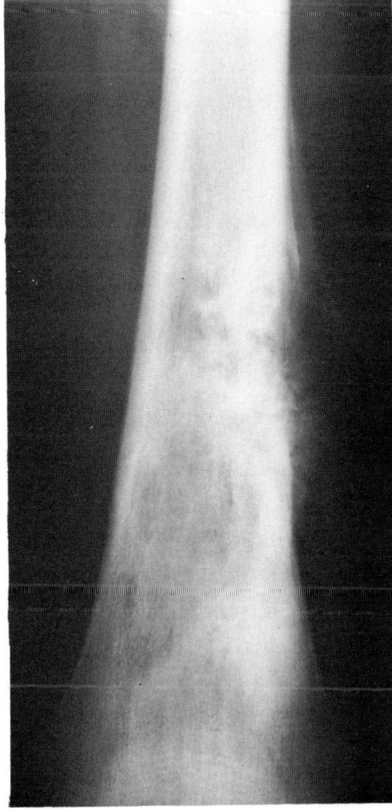

FIGURE 20–5. Dense metaphyseal lesion with cortical destruction and periosteal reaction, indicating an aggressive, bone-forming lesion. Osteosarcoma in the distal femur in a 10-year-old child.

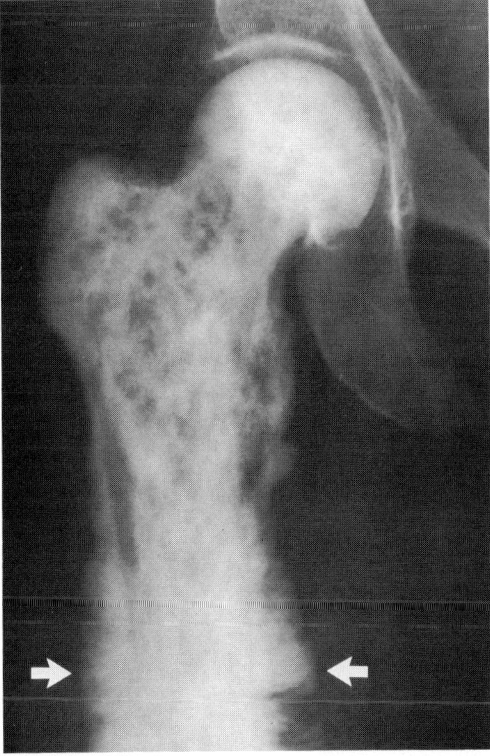

FIGURE 20–7. The aggressive periosteal reaction of spiculated type (*arrows*) involving the proximal femoral diaphysis in this 54-year-old woman indicates the presence of Paget's sarcoma, which is a very aggressive variant of osteosarcoma. The bony sclerosis, expansion, and patchy lucent areas of the proximal femur are characteristic features of Paget's disease.

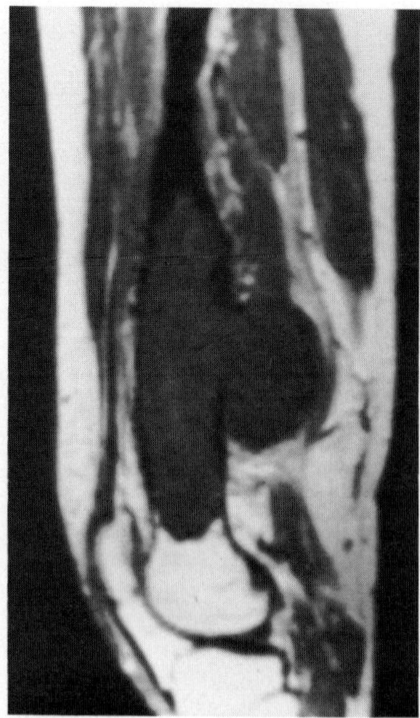

FIGURE 20–8. T_1-weighted magnetic resonance image, sagittal plane, demonstrating osteosarcoma of the distal femur with cortical destruction and an extraosseous soft tissue mass.

preferably MR imaging. The MR imaging findings may range from a homogeneous to a markedly heterogeneous signal intensity, depending on the proportion of mineralized tumor matrix, necrosis, edema, and hemorrhage (Fig. 20–8).[16] The soft tissue components are well visualized on MR imaging, and the possible involvement of adjacent joint spaces and neurovascular structures, as well as skip metastases, can be evaluated.[17]

Benign Bone-Forming Tumors

Osteoid Osteoma. Generally considered a benign bone-forming tumor, this lesion has been suggested to instead represent an inflammatory reaction of unknown etiology.[18] The characteristic clinical presentation is that of regional pain, which is worse at night, with a remarkable response to aspirin. Children, adolescents, and young adults can be affected. The small lesion, by definition smaller than 2 cm in diameter, is usually seen on a radiograph as a lytic area (the "nidus") surrounded by reactive bone sclerosis as well as periosteal bone formation (Fig. 20–9).[19, 20] The nidus, which consists of tortuous vessels and osteoid matrix, often contains areas of bone formation, which if extensive can obscure the identification of the nidus on plain radiographs. To prevent recurrences, the entire nidus has to be removed at surgery, and therefore the preoperative determination of the exact location and extent of the nidus is important. Because of the often extensive surrounding reactive bone formation as well as the frequently associated surrounding tissue edema, and synovial thickening and joint effusion if the lesion is intra-articular, CT is often preferred over MR to identify the small lytic lesion among the reactive bone and soft tissue changes. The location within a bone is often diaphyseal, and the long bones tend to be involved more often than do the small bones of the hands and feet. Radiographic differential diagnosis includes intracortical abscess (Brodie's abscess) and stress fracture or reaction.

Osteoblastoma. Owing to many similar clinical and histologic features, it is not clear if osteoblastoma is a larger version of an osteoid osteoma or a completely separate tumor type. The lytic nidus, which may contain areas of mineralization, is by definition larger than 2 cm in diameter, or the lesion will be called an *osteoid osteoma*. It tends to involve the posterior elements of the spine but can also occur in the diaphysis or metaphysis of long bones. The patients are usually in their teens or twenties. The dramatic response to aspirin that is so characteristic of osteoid osteoma is usually lacking.[21] The radiographic features include a lytic lesion, often expansile, and less frequently areas of mineralization. Differential diagnosis includes osteoid osteoma, enchondroma, and chondromyxoid fibroma.

Osteochondroma. A single osteochondroma is a relatively common benign lesion with a very low incidence of malignant transformation, whereas the familial disorder associated with multiple osteochondromas, hereditary multiple osteochondromatosis, has a more significant risk of secondary malignancy that is estimated at 5% to 10%. Osteochondromas may present during the teens, when the peak skeletal growth occurs, or later owing to symptoms from fracture, mechanical muscle or nerve impingement, overlying bursitis, or development of a malignant mass. Osteochondromas usually originate from the area of a growth plate (epiphyseal or

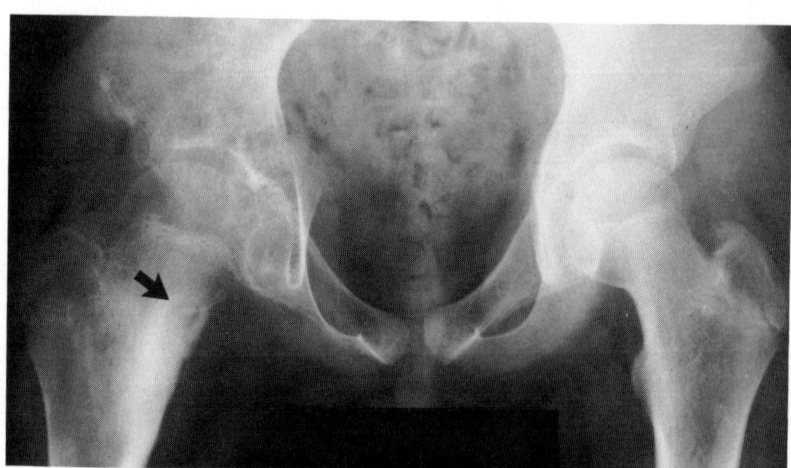

FIGURE 20–9. Osteoid osteoma of the right femoral neck in a 12-year-old boy. The lytic nidus *(arrow)* with a central focal area of mineralization is seen, surrounded by reactive periosteal bone formation. There is extensive osteopenia of both the right femoral neck and the femoral head, and the supra-acetabular portion of the iliac bone, as well as hypertrophy of these areas compared with the normal left hip.

apophyseal) and cease to grow when the adjacent growth plate closes. These tumors may also appear in bony structures that have received prior radiation treatment.[22] The cartilage cap over an osteochondroma is usually a few millimeters in thickness and is the site of potential malignant transformation, usually to a chondrosarcoma. Conventional radiography is usually sufficient for diagnosis of an osteochondroma of the pedunculated (Fig. 20–10) or sessile (broad-based) type (Fig. 20–11). Radiographic features include continuity of the adjacent cortical as well as the trabecular bone into the base of the lesion, and the location is usually at or relatively near a growth plate, with the lesion pointing away from the growth plate. For identification of potential malignancy, however, MR examination is preferable, because the hyaline cartilage cap or mass has a very high signal on T_2-weighted images, and abnormal thickening of the cap or an associated mass is well demonstrated owing to the high contrast against adjacent normal structures such as muscle.[23] Cartilage cap thickness greater than 10 mm has been shown to be associated with an increased incidence of secondary chondrosarcoma. Other signs, such as an associated soft tissue mass and bone destruction of the base of the osteochondroma or adjacent bone structure, also strongly suggest malignant transformation of an osteochondroma. Other possible causes of pain, due to mechanical impingement between an osteochondroma and other musculoskeletal or neurovascular structures, can also be evaluated on MR images. Increased uptake at the site of an osteochondroma on a technetium 99m bone scan is less specific, because it may be caused by a secondary malignancy but also by a fracture or even bone remodeling due to impingement.

Ossifying Fibroma. This disorder is currently thought to be related to fibrous dysplasia. The location in the tibia, particularly the anterior cortex, in the middle third of the

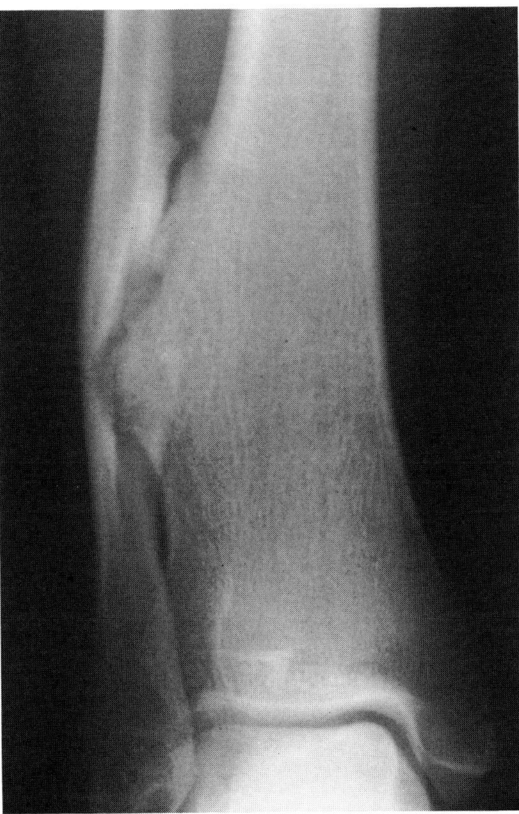

FIGURE 20–11. Sessile osteochondroma of the distal tibia, with a secondary deformity of the adjacent fibula.

diaphysis, is characteristic (Fig. 20–12). Children or teenagers are affected, and enlargement of the lesion can lead to bone deformity with anterior bowing. The lesion may spontaneously regress with age but sometimes progressively enlarges and requires surgical resection.

Radiographically, the lesion is lytic with sclerotic margins, with components of cortical expansion.[24]

Malignant Cartilage-Forming Tumors

Chondrosarcoma. This malignant tumor can be primary (arising de novo) or secondary (arising by malignant transformation in a pre-existing lesion). Development of secondary chondrosarcomas have been reported in single osteochondromas, hereditary osteochondromatosis, single enchondromas, hereditary enchondromatosis (Ollier's disease), Maffucci's syndrome (congenital nonhereditary enchondromatosis and hemangiomatosis), and fibrous dysplasia. A rarely occurring variant of primary chondrosarcoma is the clear-cell chondrosarcoma, which characteristically is located in subchondral bone and early on has a benign radiographic appearance similar to that of a subchondral cyst.[25] Other unusual variants include the dedifferentiated chondrosarcoma, a malignancy with a poor prognosis in which an anaplastic osteosarcoma arises within, but with a well-defined border towards a conventional low-grade chondrosarcoma; and the mesenchymal chondrosarcoma, in 30% to 75% of cases arising within soft tissues and with a poor prognosis owing to high frequency of local recurrences, lymph node involvement, and disseminated metastatic disease.

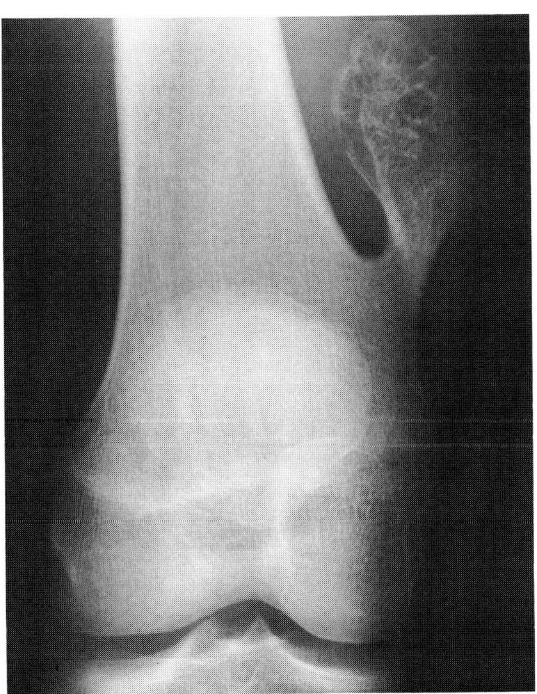

FIGURE 20–10. Pedunculated osteochondroma of the medial aspect of the distal femur in a young adult.

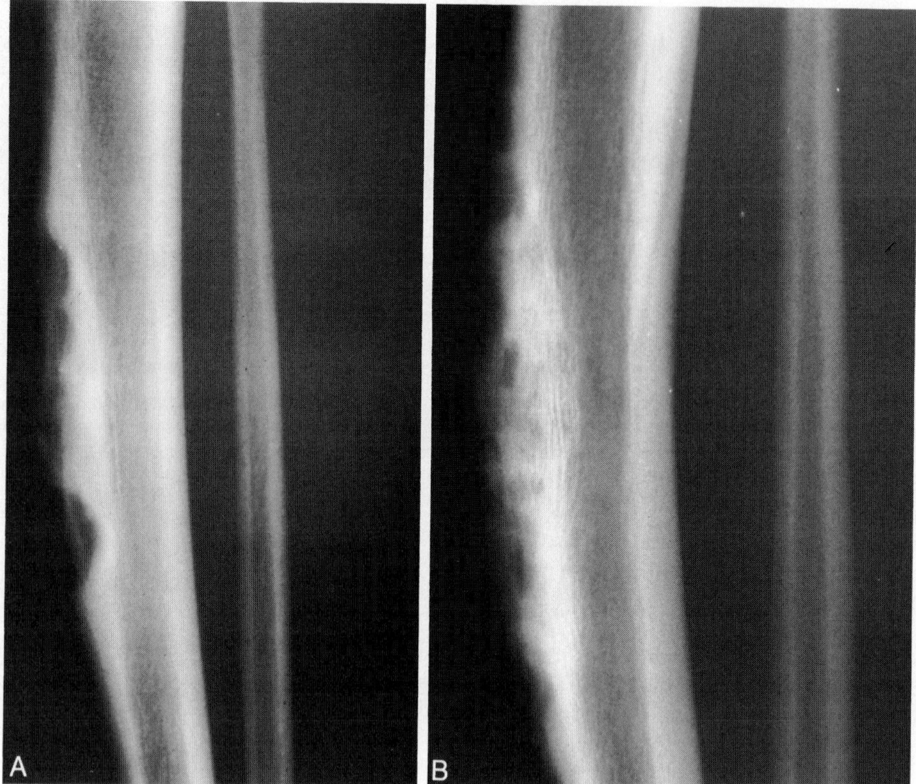

FIGURE 20–12. Multifocal lytic lesions in a thickened anterior tibial cortex in a 5-year-old boy *(A)* were ossifying fibroma on biopsy. Three years later *(B)*, the lytic lesions have become more diffuse and larger, and there is persistence of mild bowing.

Chondrosarcoma tends to affect an older age group than does osteosarcoma, most frequently presenting in adults, although those occurring with multiple osteochondromatosis or with Ollier's disease may present already during childhood or adolescence. The usual presenting symptoms are local pain or a painful mass. Features on conventional radiographs may vary widely and may deceivingly indicate an indolent benign lesion. These usually include a lytic region with central or peripheral location in the involved bone, well to poorly defined transition zone, and periosteal reaction ranging from solid to spiculated (Fig. 20–13).[26, 27] Matrix calcification is seen in as many as two thirds of cases. On MR examination, well-differentiated low-grade chondrosarcomas generally have a homogeneous intermediate signal on T_1-weighted images and a high signal on T_2-weighted images, whereas the more cellular high-grade chondrosarcomas tend to have a heterogeneous signal pattern with an intermediate and high signal on T_1- and T_2-weighted images, respectively.

Benign Cartilage-Forming Tumors

Enchondroma. The most common tumor of the small bones of the hands and feet, this benign lesion consists of hyaline cartilage and is usually seen as a single lytic area. It can present at any age and is usually asymptomatic, although sometimes it may lead to a pathologic fracture. Radiographic features include a lytic lesion, which is often but not always with well-defined sclerotic borders, mild scalloping of the endosteal cortical contour, and frequently with mild expansion of the involved bone.[28] Matrix calcification is present in approximately half of all cases and on close inspection can

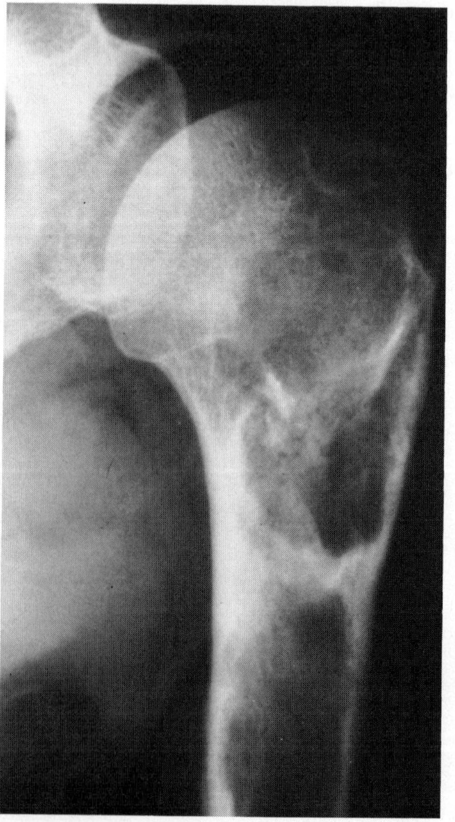

FIGURE 20–13. Chondrosarcoma of the proximal humerus in a 60-year-old man. An ill-defined lytic lesion is seen, with cortical expansion and destruction and coarse calcifications.

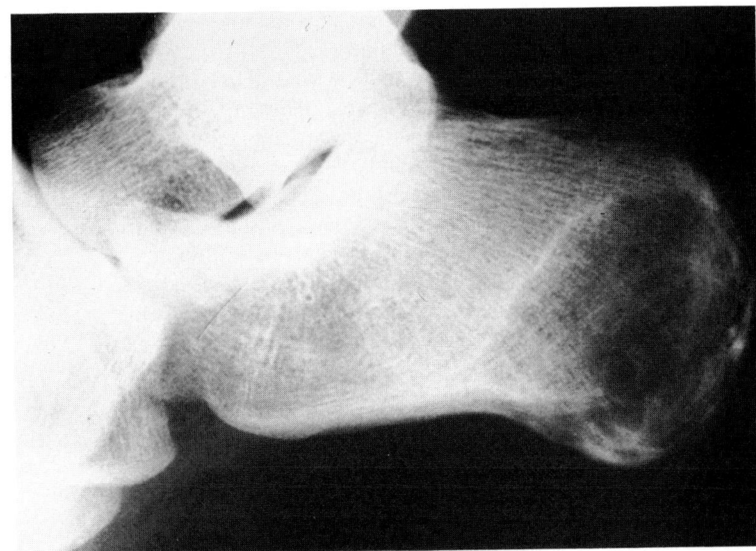

FIGURE 20–14. Chondroblastoma of the calcaneal tuberosity (an apophysis) in a 17-year-old male. Note the faint sclerotic rim and the absence of discrete matrix calcification.

often be seen to have the 2- to 3-mm circular or semicircular configuration, which suggests cartilage matrix (see Fig. 20–1).

Chondroblastoma. This benign bone tumor is almost always located in an epiphysis or apophysis.[29, 30] It contains a component of hyaline cartilage. Chondroblastomas show a strong predilection for people in whom the adjacent growth plate is still open. The lesion can extend across from the epiphysis to the metaphysis (Fig. 20–14).

The radiographic appearance also includes a well-defined margin. Periosteal reaction is frequent. In one third to one half of patients, calcifications can be identified within the lesion.

Chondromyxoid Fibroma. This rare cartilage-forming benign tumor is seen in persons in their second and third decade and may be asymptomatic and noted incidentally or may cause mild pain and local tenderness. Lower extremity involvement is most common, typically in the metaphysis, but may extend into the diaphysis or the epiphysis. The tumor is generally eccentric and radiolucent and is sometimes expansile and contains coarse trabeculations. No or minimal periosteal reaction is seen.[31]

Periosteal Chondroma. A benign hyaline cartilage tumor of the surface of bone, usually associated with long-standing but low-grade pain and swelling, periosteal chondroma occurs in people of any age. Most frequently located in the metaphyseal region, it is seen radiographically only as a mild focal cortical irregularity, which may be due to pressure, erosion, or mild periosteal reaction (Fig. 20–15). Cartilage calcification is frequent and is seen in as many as 50% of periosteal chondromas. The tumor is usually small and may be seen only on MR imaging, where it has intermediate signal on T_1-weighted images and homogeneously bright signal on T_2-weighted images, consistent with its composition of hyaline cartilage. The differential diagnosis includes periosteal chondrosarcoma, periosteal lipoma, and periosteal fibroma.

Giant Cell Tumors of Bone

Giant Cell Tumor. Although many tumors contain giant cells, a specific tumor entity has been named *giant cell tumor*

of bone. These tumors generally have a fairly homogeneous distribution of giant cells throughout the entire lesion, which also contains connective tissue; the cell of origin of this tumor is not known. Giant cell tumors occur in persons after closure of the growth plate, most commonly during the third decade. The presenting symptoms are usually local pain and tenderness. The location of the tumor is characteristically subchondral, most commonly in the distal femur, proximal tibia, or distal radius.

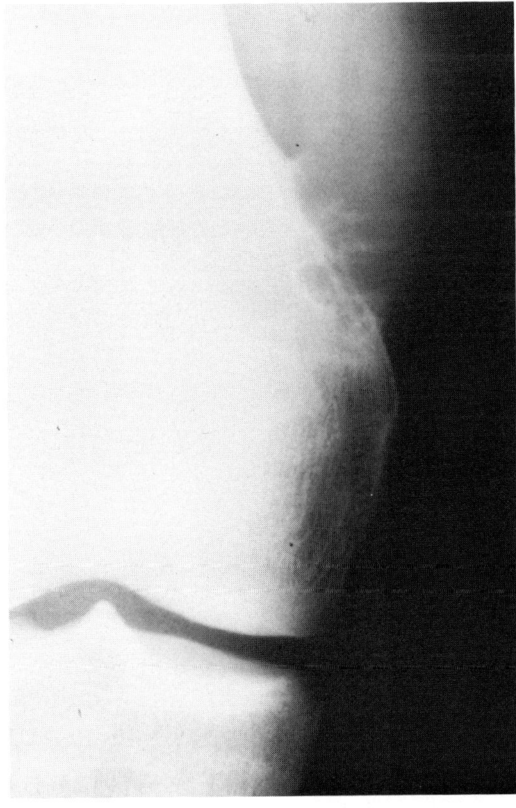

FIGURE 20–15. Periosteal chondroma at the medial metaphysis of the femur in a 21-year-old woman. There is thinning of the cortical bone with periosteal buttressing proximally and several ill-defined areas of calcification with a spiculated appearance located within a soft tissue mass.

Radiographically, the lesion is lytic and sometimes expansile, and may contain thin trabeculae (Fig. 20–16).[32] The transition zone is narrow but may not be well defined. Periosteal reaction is characteristically absent. There is often an extraosseous soft tissue component, best demonstrated by MR imaging, and the tumor usually has an intermediate signal on T_1 and a heterogeneous high signal on T_2. This reflects areas of necrosis or old hemorrhage within the soft tissue mass. MR imaging shows fluid-fluid levels well, which again reflects bleeding into the tumor having resulted in cystic spaces.[33] Tumor size at diagnosis is often relatively large, and sometimes the presentation is due to an intra-articular pathologic fracture. The incidence of local recurrence of the tumor after surgical removal is relatively high, and in rare instances there may also be seeding to the lungs, similar to what may occur in chondroblastomas. This is not considered to be true malignant metastatic disease but tends to occur within a few years of tumor surgery and is thought to be due to passive seeding at the time of surgery. The pulmonary lesions generally remain small and do not grow progressively. The malignant potential of giant cell tumors has been reported following therapeutic radiation to the tumor and is difficult to separate from a radiation-induced sarcoma.

Differential diagnosis of giant cell tumors include chondroblastoma, intraosseous ganglion, and subchondral cysts frequently seen with many inflammatory joint diseases. Brown tumors of hyperparathyroidism can mimic giant cell tumors in radiographic appearance and location and, more rarely, fibrous dysplasia, eosinophilic granuloma, and aneurysmal bone cyst may be considered as well.

Giant Cell Reparative Granuloma. Located mainly in

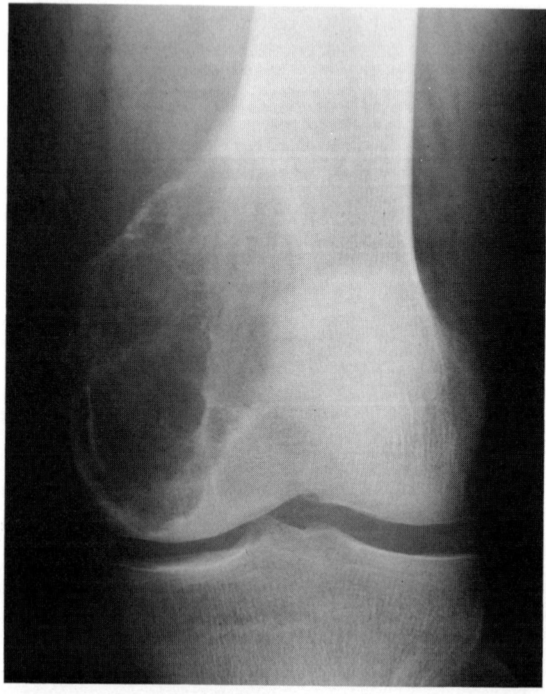

FIGURE 20–16. Giant cell tumor involving the medial femoral condyle, extending into the diametaphysis. The tumor is expansile, and the medial cortex is ill defined. There is no matrix mineralization, but there are a few bony septations. The single most characteristic feature of this tumor is the location, with extension to subarticular bone.

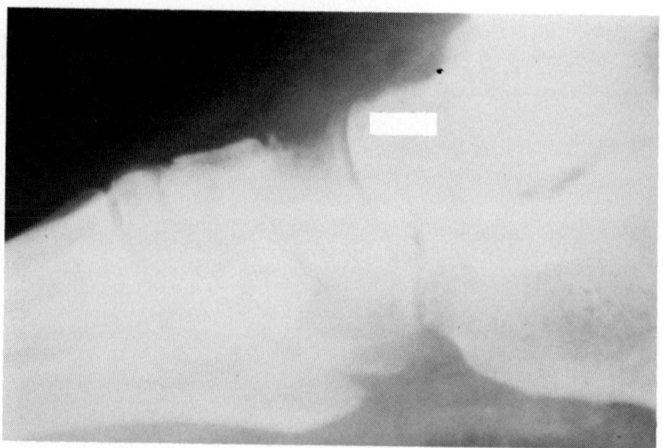

FIGURE 20–17. Giant cell reparative granuloma of the navicular. Note the lytic and expansile lesion. Although not shown in this particular case, the cortex is often intact. (Courtesy of L. M. Oloff, D.P.M.)

the mandible, maxilla, and small bones of the hands and feet in patients of all ages, this lesion is considered different from the giant cell tumor. Symptoms often include pain and swelling, as well as enlargement of the bone. Radiographic changes include a lytic and expansile lesion, usually with intact, although thinned cortex, and without periosteal reaction (Fig. 20–17). The features are similar to those of a giant cell tumor, and other differential diagnostic considerations include enchondroma, brown tumor of hyperparathyroidism, and aneurysmal bone cyst.

Aneurysmal Bone Cyst. A relatively common abnormality found in younger persons, this lesion of unknown etiology may be reactive because it often occurs together with another tumor and has been reported following trauma. Associated tumors include chondroblastoma, osteoblastoma, giant cell tumor, and fibrous dysplasia. Somewhat similar blood-filled cystic spaces also occur with a variant of osteosarcoma, the telangiectatic osteosarcoma. Aneurysmal bone cysts may be located in the diaphysis, metaphysis, and sometimes epiphysis and are most common during the first and second decade. The most frequently involved bones are the tibia, vertebral body, femur, humerus, and iliac bones. Symptoms include pain and swelling. Radiographic characteristics include bone expansion and lysis, and the lesion is often eccentrically located (Fig. 20–18). A small or sometimes quite large extraosseous soft tissue mass may be present, and characteristically a thin rim of periosteal bone formation surrounds the soft tissue mass, indicating that the periosteum has been lifted up by the tumor but has not been breached. Frequently there are thick trabeculas oriented at a right angle to the underlying surface of the bone. MR imaging often demonstrates fluid-fluid levels occupying almost all of the tumor, indicating the presence of multiple loculated spaces containing old hemorrhage (see Fig. 20–18*B* and *C*).[34] The differential diagnosis includes unicameral bone cyst, giant cell tumor, telangiectatic osteosarcoma, brown tumor, chondroblastoma, and fibrous dysplasia.

Marrow Tumors

Multiple Myeloma. Multiple myeloma, also called *plasma cell myeloma* and in its localized form, *plasmocytoma,* is a relatively common malignant disease of bone

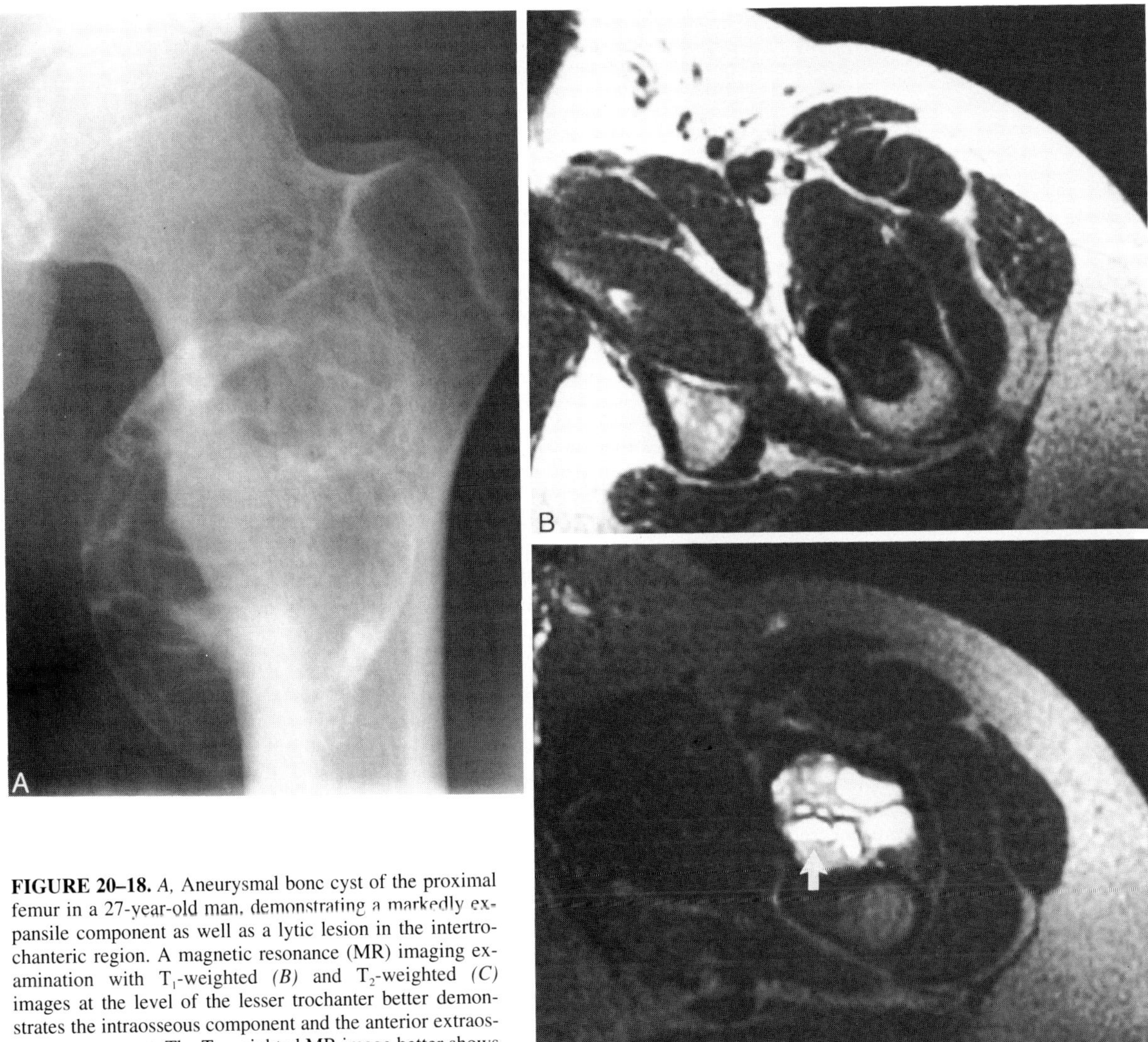

FIGURE 20–18. *A,* Aneurysmal bone cyst of the proximal femur in a 27-year-old man, demonstrating a markedly expansile component as well as a lytic lesion in the intertrochanteric region. A magnetic resonance (MR) imaging examination with T_1-weighted *(B)* and T_2-weighted *(C)* images at the level of the lesser trochanter better demonstrates the intraosseous component and the anterior extraosseous component. The T_2-weighted MR image better shows the presence of fluid-fluid levels *(arrow).*

marrow. The disease is rare during the first four decades. Presenting symptoms are often vague, such as back pain, weight loss, or pain in other bone structures. The sedimentation rate is characteristically elevated, and anemia and sometimes thrombocytopenia are present. As many as half of all patients have hypercalcemia. Associated amyloidosis may lead to renal insufficiency and an increase in serum creatinine levels. Serum electrophoresis typically demonstrates an increase in the serum-globulin fraction, most commonly of immunoglobulin G type.

The most characteristic radiographic finding is bone destruction, usually with ill-defined borders, involving both trabecular and cortical bone. The endosteal aspect of the cortex may show scalloped areas of cortical thinning. Myeloma can sometimes cause bone expansion, particularly if localized as plasmocytoma. Involvement of the vertebral column is most common, and other areas of predilection include the pelvic region, the shoulder region, and the skull. Rib involvement is also relatively frequent, whereas localization of lesions in the distal aspects of the extremities is rare.

Differential diagnosis includes metastasis and lymphoma, as well as osteoporosis, if vertebral compression fractures are the only manifestation.

Plasmocytoma is a localized form of multiple myeloma (Fig. 20–19), and the patients may not have the abnormalities of the serum-globulin fractions present in myeloma to help in diagnosis. It is debated whether plasmocytoma always leads to multiple myeloma or not, and it is known that plasmocytoma may remain a solitary lesion for as long as 20 years. Plasmocytoma tends to occur in a slightly younger age group than does multiple myeloma, and the person's age at presentation is often in the fifth decade. Presenting symptoms are similar, with focal bone pain and sometimes pathologic fracture.

Ewing's Sarcoma. Ewing's sarcoma is the second most common, after osteosarcoma, of malignant bone tumors in children and adolescents. Approximately 90% of patients will be 5 to 30 years of age. It is not clear what the cell origin of this tumor is, but an endothelial origin is suggested. This small round cell tumor has many features in common with both neuroblastoma and primary neuroectodermal tumors of bone. Systemic symptoms may be present, such as fever, weight loss, and anemia. The lower extremities and pelvis are the most common locations, with involvement of tubular bones most frequent in the femur, tibia, humerus, and fibula, and involvement of flat bones most frequent in the ileum, vertebral bodies, and ribs.

Radiographically, the tumor is lytic and has a wide transi-

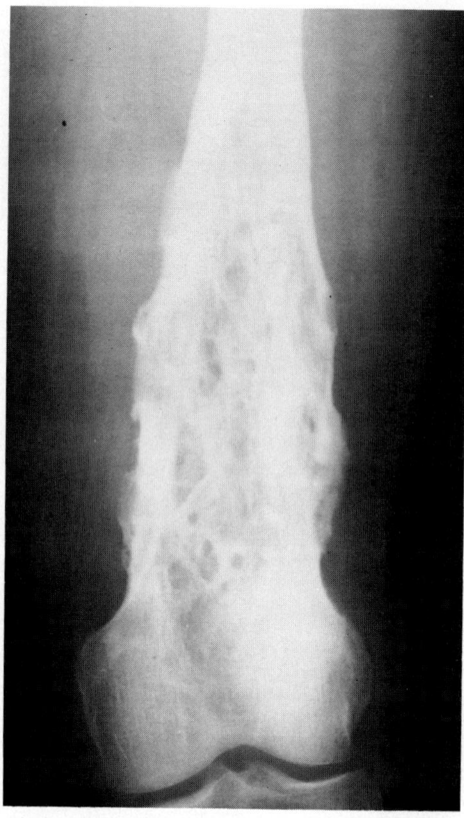

FIGURE 20–19. Plasmocytoma of the distal femoral diaphysis in a 56-year-old woman, with the lytic expansile lesion exhibiting cortical thinning and destruction as well as coarse, randomly oriented bony linear densities.

tion zone (see Fig. 20–20A).[35] A laminated periosteal reaction is strongly suggestive but not diagnostic of Ewing's sarcoma. A radiographic component of increased bone density is frequently seen, owing to a combination of reactive bone formation and superimposition of the laminated periosteal reaction over the lytic diaphyseal or metaphyseal region. Mild bone expansion may also be present.

On MR imaging, the extent of the tumor is better seen and shows a heterogeneous mass with a signal corresponding to tumor tissue, hemorrhage, and necrosis (Fig. 20–20B and C).[36]

Lymphoma. Bone involvement occurs both with non-Hodgkin's lymphoma of different types and with Hodgkin's disease. Lymphoma primary to bone structures is less common but carries a better prognosis than does lymphoma with secondary spread to bone.[37, 38]

In non-Hodgkin's lymphoma, bone involvement is seen in approximately 20% of patients and is usually secondary to involvement of lymph nodes and soft tissues. The bone involvement is most frequently located in the spine, pelvis, ribs, and calvarium. The radiographic changes include ill-defined lytic lesions with destruction of trabecular bone as well as cortical bone (see Fig. 20–2). Periosteal reaction is usually minimal, but variable. Reactive bone formation leading to areas of sclerosis is relatively rare. In Hodgkin's disease, skeletal involvement is somewhat more common than in the non-Hodgkin's lymphoma group and involves as many as 25% of patients in that group. The most frequent sites of involvement are the spine, pelvis, and ribs. The lesions are usually multifocal and lytic with ill-defined borders, whereas the combination of lytic and sclerotic lesions or lesions with only osteosclerotic features is more common. The involvement may be by direct spread from involved lymph nodes or by hematogenous spread to bone.

Vascular Tumors

Hemangioma. A benign tumor that may occur in soft tissues or in bone, hemangiomas are usually asymptomatic during the first decade, and the presenting symptoms include pain, swelling, and sometimes a palpable mass. Intramuscular hemangiomas tend to occur in the extremities, especially in the forearm and the lower leg. Sometimes the overlying skin shows purplish discoloration, whereas pulsations or bruits are relatively rare. Radiographically, a soft tissue mass may be seen to displace the normal fat planes and, in approximately half of the cases, characteristic rounded calcifications (phleboliths) are present within the mass. More rarely there is overgrowth of the adjacent bone and soft tissue structures. The extent of a hemangioma can be evaluated by CT scanning with use of intravenous contrast material, which shows contrast filling of fine-caliber vessels within the mass, but tends to underestimate the lesion size.[39] MR shows an intermediate signal on T_1-weighted images and a high to intermediate signal on T_2-weighted images, and tortuous vascular structures often can be identified.[39, 40]

Glomus Tumor. This rare benign tumor is usually located distally in the extremities, characteristically under the nailbed. The lesion is usually only a few millimeters in diameter but leads to severe tenderness and paroxysmal pain, especially if the mass is exposed to pressure, heat, or cold. The radiographic appearance ranges from cortical scalloping of adjacent bone to no evidence of abnormality.[41]

Lymphangioma. Consisting mainly of cystic spaces filled with lymph, this tumor also has a minor component of lymphoid tissue and relatively poorly defined margins against adjacent normal tissue. These lesions are often superficial and are diagnosed at a young age owing to a mass that is compressible. Radiographs do not demonstrate any abnormalities except for a possible soft tissue mass, and on MR imaging the features are identical to those of hemangiomas.

Other Connective Tissue Tumors

Fibrocortical Defect and Nonossifying Fibroma. These common benign connective tissue tumors are separated mainly by their size, with the former nonossifying fibroma extending from the cortex into the region of trabecular bone.[42, 43] The lesions are rarely symptomatic, but a large nonossifying fibroma may become symptomatic owing to a pathologic fracture. These lesions are seen mainly in children and adolescents and normally spontaneously regress so that they are only rarely found in adults. The cause is unclear, and theories include local trauma to the periosteum, leading to hemorrhage and disturbance of the normal bone formation. The lesions are sometimes multiple within a metaphyseal region of a bone and are less commonly multifocal, involving different bone structures. The distal femur and proximal tibia are most frequently involved, and only rarely is a lesion seen in a diaphysis. The radiographic appearance of a fibrocortical

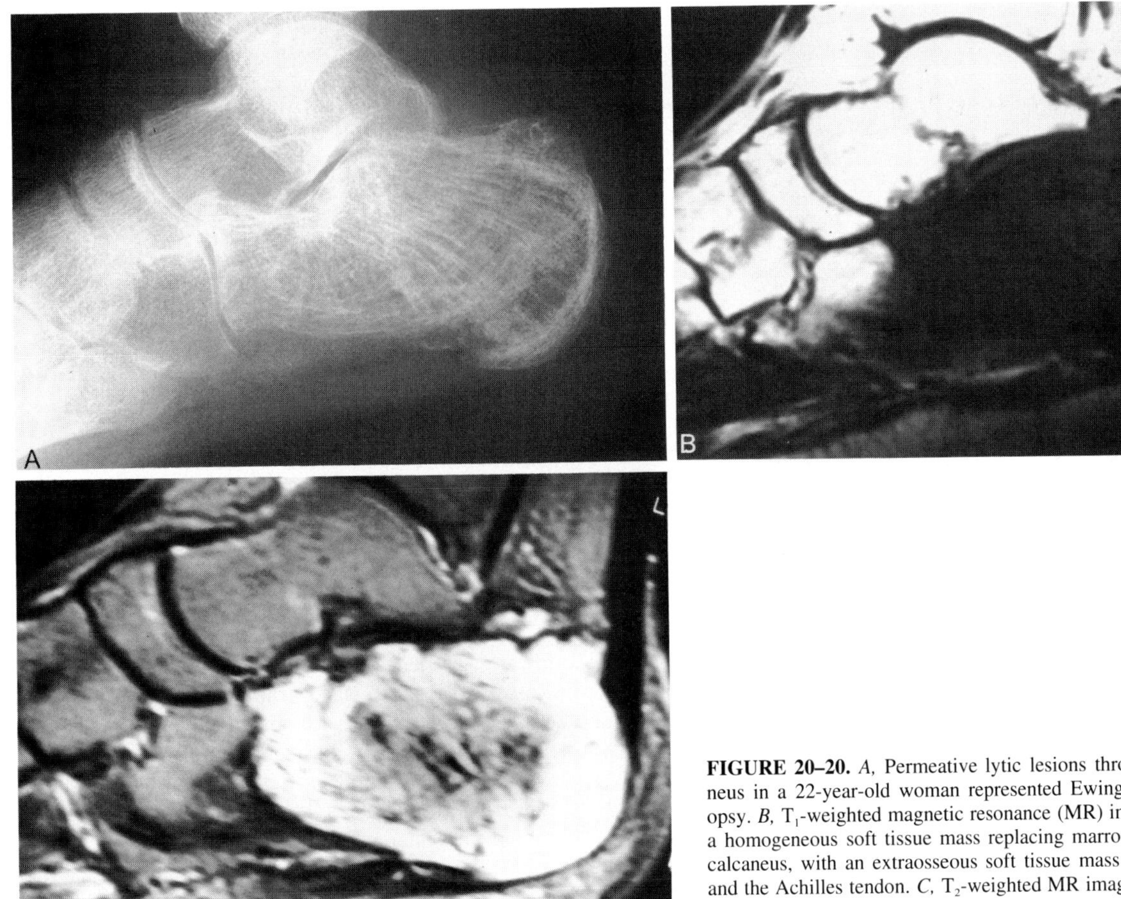

FIGURE 20–20. *A,* Permeative lytic lesions throughout the calcaneus in a 22-year-old woman represented Ewing's sarcoma on biopsy. *B,* T_1-weighted magnetic resonance (MR) image demonstrated a homogeneous soft tissue mass replacing marrow fat in the entire calcaneus, with an extraosseous soft tissue mass between the talus and the Achilles tendon. *C,* T_2-weighted MR image shows increased signal.

defect is that of a radiolucent area within the cortex, often with mild expansion, and with a narrow transition zone against adjacent normal bone. Lesions are characteristically elongated, and the borders may be slightly lobulated, giving a multiloculated impression. The nonossifying fibroma has similar characteristics but is larger.

Epidermoid Cysts. Epidermoid cysts are benign lesions and are thought to result from a penetrating injury that displaces a portion of the epidermis into underlying soft tissues or bone. Location in the fingertips or in the calvarium is most common, and microscopically, squamous epithelium and fibrous tissue surround a cystic structure filled with keratin. If located in bone, the lesion is often asymptomatic, whereas the location in the soft tissues of the fingertip may be symptomatic owing to cyst rupture and a severe inflammatory reaction to the exposed keratin. Radiographically, a lucent, well-defined lesion is seen, often with sclerotic margins and sometimes slightly expansile.[44] Differential diagnosis includes glomus tumor and possibly enchondroma.

Fibrous Dysplasia. This dysplasia involving bone tissue may be limited to a single bone or may be more extensive, involving much of the skeletal structures. The combination of fibrous dysplasia, precocious puberty, and skin pigmentation is termed *McCune-Albright syndrome*; however, it only accounts for a small percentage of the total number of individuals with fibrous dysplasia. The monostotic involvement is most common. The lesions may be asymptomatic or may cause pain, and if they are extensive, the dysplastic lesions lead to insufficiency fracture and bowing.

Radiographic features include progressive bone deformities, which in the proximal femur may lead to a "shepherd's crook" deformity of expansion and bowing. The lesions are lytic, sometimes with a hazy area of mineralization in part of the lesion, called the "ground-glass appearance," which corresponds to metaplastic bone formation within the lytic area.

On MR imaging, fibrous dysplasia may demonstrate an intermediate signal on T_1-weighted images and a low, intermediate, or high signal on T_2-weighted images (Fig. 20–21).[45]

Lipoma. A common benign lesion, lipomas are commonly located in the soft tissues, either in the subcutaneous fat or in muscle. A lipoma's location in bone is less common but has relatively characteristic radiographic findings and is rarely symptomatic.[46] In soft tissues, mature lipocytes are seen microscopically, whereas radiographically the lesion is usually not well demonstrated. Occasionally, it can be seen indirectly because of displacement of other structures, or if it is large, because of its low attenuation. This is better demonstrated by CT or MR imaging, in which a homogeneous lesion with fat attenuation and fat signal, respectively, is shown. A subgroup of lipomas are the angiolipomas, which are benign tumors composed of fat cells as well as abnormal

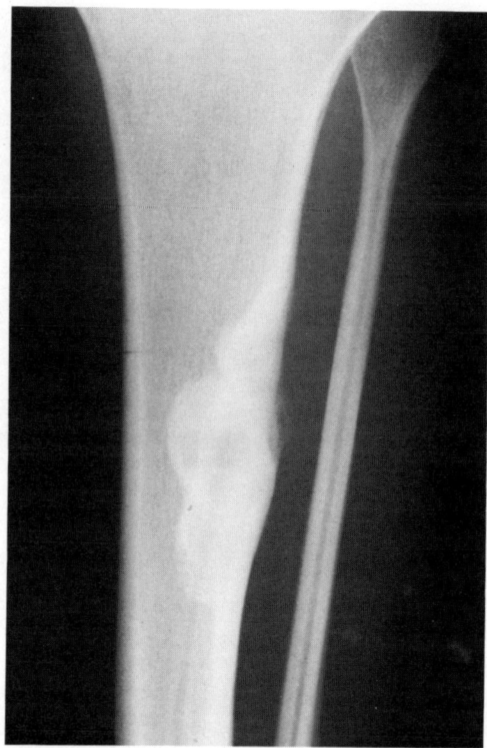

FIGURE 20–21. Fibrous dysplasia of the tibial diaphysis in a 20-year-old woman. This lesion illustrates the homogeneous density with absence of trabecular structures, termed "ground-glass appearance," as well as slight expansion with cortical thinning but sclerotic margins against adjacent bone.

and prominent blood vessels. Intraosseous lipomas are more rare and often asymptomatic but may cause diffuse pain. Radiographic features include a focal lytic lesion, often with sclerotic margin, and central calcification (Fig. 20–22). The calcaneus and the femoral neck are the most common locations. On MR imaging the lesions have a signal similar to that of subcutaneous fat, except for central areas of signal loss if calcification is present.

Liposarcoma. This relatively common malignant tumor usually presents as a painless mass in the lower leg, thigh, or buttock regions. It occurs most frequently in adults and is thought to arise as a primary sarcoma and not as a malignant transformation of a benign lipoma. The radiographic appearance is that of a mass, often relatively large, that may have borders ranging from well-defined to infiltrating adjacent tissues. The fatty component of the tumor may vary greatly, and although the fatty component may occasionally predominate, giving an appearance similar to that of lipoma, most liposarcomas are heterogeneous tumors with no fat or a small component of fat. A prominent myxoid component is frequent in liposarcomas located in the extremities.[47] The CT and MR appearance is usually that of a soft tissue mass with heterogeneous density and signal intensity on both T_1- and T_2-weighted images (Fig. 20–23).[48]

Fibromatosis. A large group of rare fibrous tumors includes several congenital lesions, such as aggressive infantile fibromatosis and congenital, generalized fibromatosis, as well as lesions presenting in adults, such as extra-abdominal desmoid.

Aggressive infantile fibromatosis presents during the first years of life as locally aggressive soft tissue mass tumors that infiltrate adjacent structures. The recurrence rate after surgical removal is high. Radiographically, a soft tissue mass may be seen, sometimes with an adjacent bone deformity with sclerotic margins and an irregular periosteal reaction.[49]

Extra-abdominal desmoid is a benign but aggressively infiltrating fibrous tumor of adults. Plain films are usually normal but sometimes demonstrate bone deformity secondary to the adjacent fibrous tumor. Owing to the high collagen content, these tumors are seen on MR images as having a low signal both on T_1- and T_2-weighted sequences, whereas more cellular tumor foci show an increase in signal on T_2-weighted images (Fig. 20–24).

Other Tumors

Neurofibroma and Neurilemoma. Neurofibromas as well as neurilemomas are benign tumors of peripheral nerves. Neurilemomas are also called *neurinomas* or *benign schwan-*

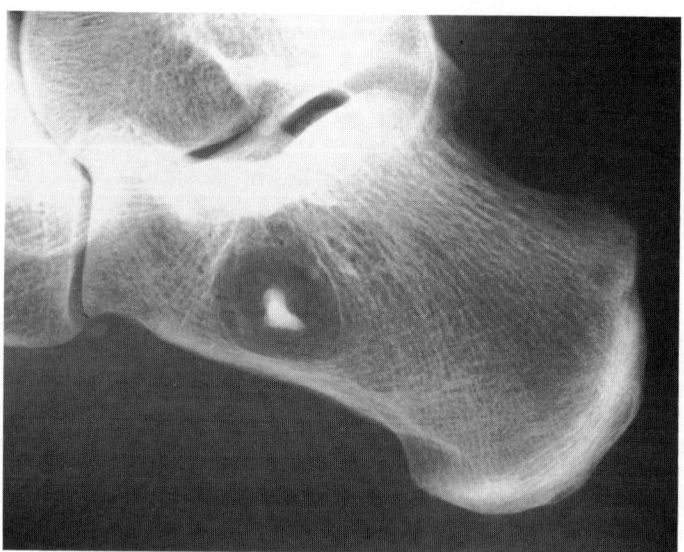

FIGURE 20–22. Intraosseous lipoma of the calcaneus in an adult, manifested by a lytic lesion with sclerotic margins and central dense calcification.

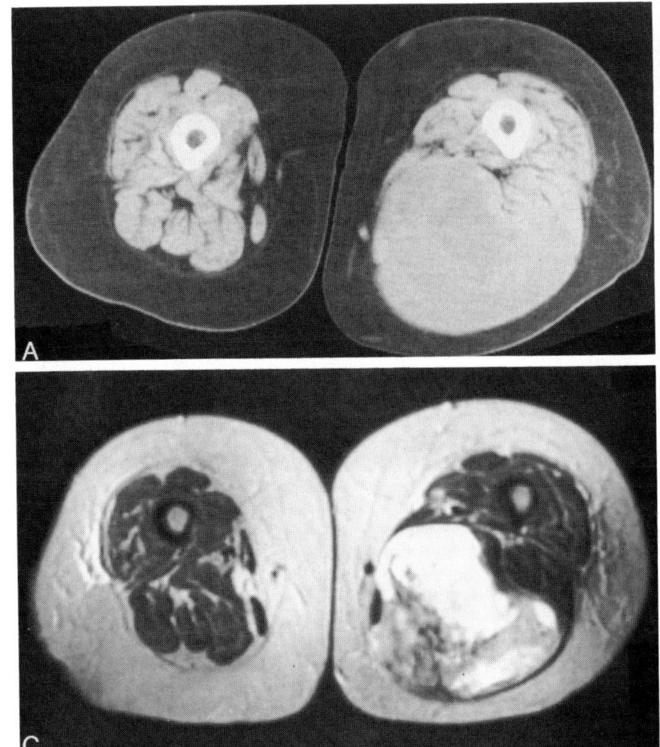

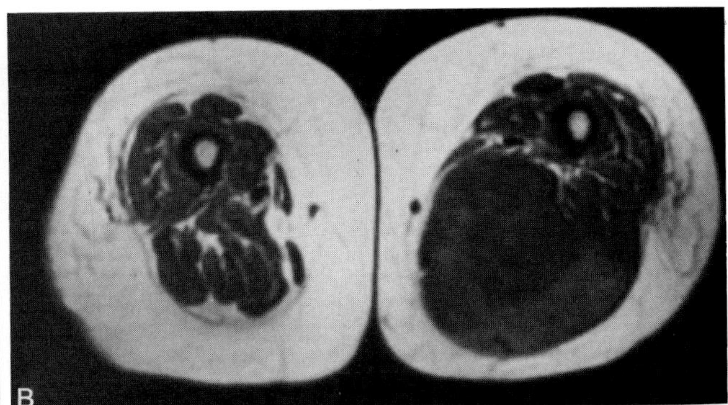

FIGURE 20–23. *A,* Liposarcoma of the left thigh, posterior and medial compartments, in a 61-year-old woman. The computed tomography (CT) scan *(A)* demonstrates the mass, but does not well outline its extent against adjacent muscle structures. The T_1-weighted magnetic resonance (MR) image *(B)* shows a mass with heterogeneous signal and with no component having signal similar to adjacent subcutaneous fat. The T_2-weighted MR image *(C)* also shows the heterogeneity of the mass and best delineates it against adjacent muscle structures. The superficial femoral artery can be well identified.

nomas and are usually solitary lesions that grow slowly and may present as a painful mass. Neurilemomas often arise from spinal nerve roots but may also involve the peroneal or ulnar nerves. Neurilemomas are rarely associated with the syndrome of neurofibromatosis and do not have a tendency to turn malignant.

Neurofibromas are often multifocal as a manifestation of neurofibromatosis but may also occur as a solitary lesion, which is usually located in the subcutaneous tissue.

Radiographic features of neurofibromas or neurilemomas are rare,[50] whereas CT or particularly MR imaging may demonstrate a mass along the distribution of a nerve (Fig. 20–25). The MR imaging features are usually those of an intermediate signal on T_1-weighted images and a high signal on T_2-weighted images, with lobulated, relatively well-defined masses.

Malignant Schwannoma. Occurring as single lesions or in association with neurofibromatosis, the presentation is usually that of a mass that may or may not be painful. Malignant schwannomas are often located in the trunk or in the proximal aspects of the extremities, along major nerve structures. The radiographic features are similar to those of benign neurofibroma or neurilemoma, usually with an absence of findings on conventional radiography but with a mass demonstrated on CT or MR imaging.[51]

Malignant Fibrous Histiocytoma. This malignant tumor arises less frequently in bone structures than in soft tissues. It has also been reported to arise in bone infarcts, in Paget's disease, and in tissue that has received radiation therapy. Presenting symptoms often include pain and tenderness, with a palpable mass that may develop slowly or more rapidly. This tumor may present at any age, with peak presentation in middle-aged and older people. Tumor localization in the lower extremity is most common. Radiographic features include ill-defined bone destruction, usually with an associated soft tissue mass, but an absence of periosteal reaction (Fig. 20–26A). MR imaging often shows a heterogeneous MR signal (Fig. 20–26B and C).[52]

Clinical as well as radiographic features of malignant fibrous histiocytoma are nonspecific, and the differential diagnosis includes bone metastatic disease, fibrosarcoma, lymphoma, myeloma, and osteosarcoma.

Synovial Sarcoma. A malignant tumor usually presenting in young adults, synovial sarcomas show a predilection for involvement of the lower extremity. Despite the name of this

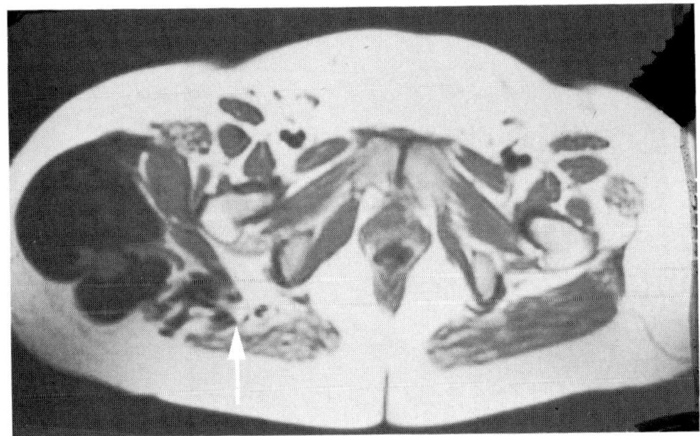

FIGURE 20–24. Aggressive fibromatosis of the right gluteal region in a 29-year-old woman. T_1-weighted magnetic resonance (MR) image shows a large mass laterally with less well-defined, smaller lesions *(arrow)* extending along the deep aspect of the atrophied gluteus maximus muscle. The mass has low signal except for a central portion, suggesting areas of collagen versus more cellular components of the mass.

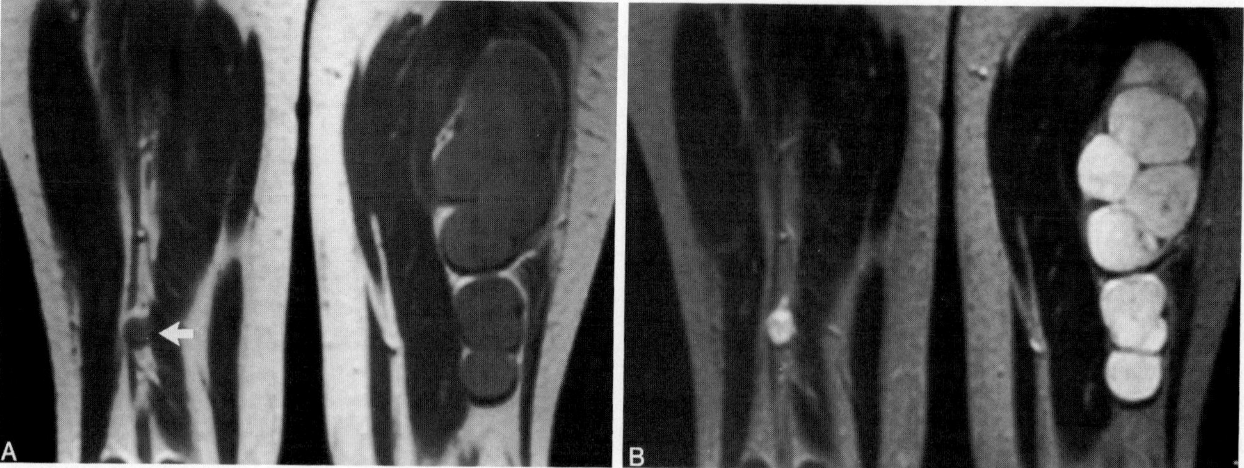

FIGURE 20–25. Neurofibromas shown by magnetic resonance imaging in a 40-year-old woman with neurofibromatosis. The T_1-weighted image *(A)* shows an intermediate signal of a lobulated mass in the left posterior thigh, and the T_2-weighted image *(B)* shows a very bright signal of a lobulated mass with the distribution along the sciatic nerve of the left thigh. A single small mass is seen also in the posterior right thigh *(arrow)*, along the low-signal sciatic nerve structure.

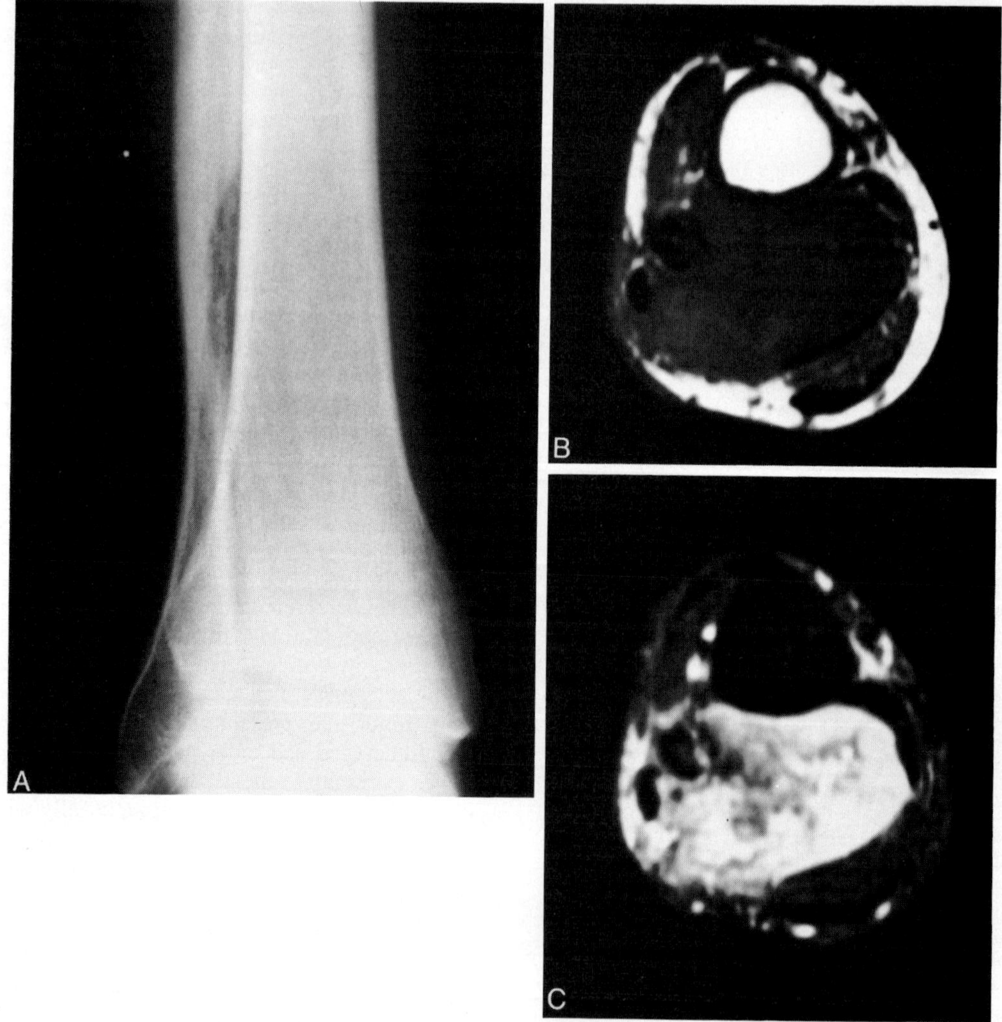

FIGURE 20–26. *A,* Malignant fibrous histiocytoma of the distal fibular diaphysis in a 58-year-old man, presenting on radiograph as a purely lytic lesion without periosteal reaction or matrix mineralization. *B,* Magnetic resonance (MR) examination with T_1-weighted image shows a large soft tissue mass extending posteriorly from the interosseous membrane and absence of marrow fat signal in the fibula. *C,* T_2-weighted MR image better delineates the extent of the soft tissue mass against surrounding muscle tissue.

tumor, it usually arises outside of a joint and not in direct continuity with synovial tissue. The mass may be well defined or ill defined and infiltrating and usually presents as a painful but very slow-growing mass. Conventional radiographs are often normal but may show ill-defined bone destruction or bone remodeling and deformity owing to adjacent tumor. Approximately one third of synovial sarcomas contain areas of calcification, which are often multiple and irregular in size and shape (Fig. 20–27). MR imaging characteristically shows an intermediate signal on T_1-weighted images and a high signal on T_2-weighted images. The signal may be heterogeneous throughout the lesion, or homogeneous,[53] with well-defined lesions mimicking a fluid-filled cyst as to MR extent and signal pattern.

Unicameral Bone Cysts. Likely representing a tumorlike lesion resulting from a disturbance in bone formation at the physis, the unicameral bone cyst is no longer considered to be a true neoplasm. An abnormality in drainage of interstitial fluid with venous obstruction disturbing bone formation is the currently favored hypothesis for the pathogenesis of these lesions. The lesions occur during growth and are located in the metaphysis; they originate at the physis. They may be round or elongated, with the long axis parallel to the long axis of the bone. They can be seen in the diaphysis after the disturbance of bone formation has ceased.[54] The most common location is the proximal end of the humerus, but they may occur in any other long bone as well as in flat bones, especially the iliac bone and the calcaneus. Unicameral bone cysts are usually asymptomatic but may lead to a pathologic fracture if they are large. Treatment often consists of steroid injection into the cyst, which frequently results in progressive

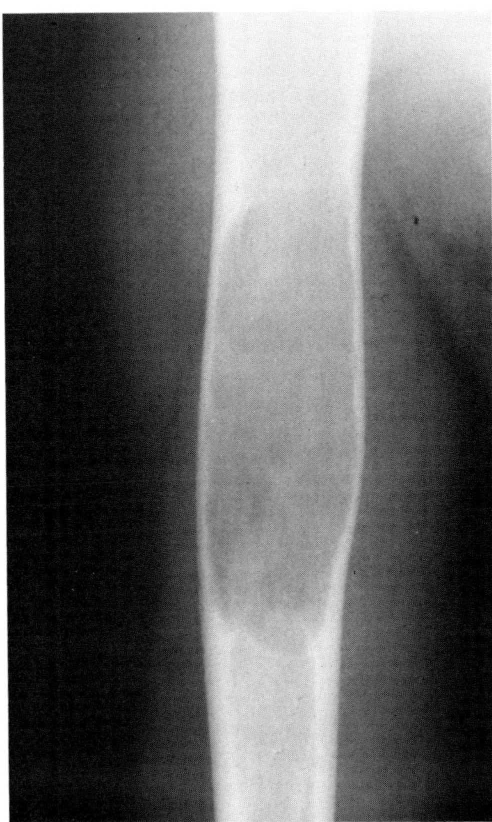

FIGURE 20–28. Unicameral bone cyst in proximal right humerus in a child. The lesion is lytic, has relatively well-defined margins, is expansile with cortical thinning, and does not contain areas of mineralization.

filling-in with bone replacing the cystic space. If resistant to this treatment, surgical curettage followed by packing with bone graft can be performed. Complete bone remodeling and resolution often takes as long as 1 year or more.

Radiographically, the lesion is usually well defined and has a sclerotic margin. There may be mild to moderate bone expansion. The lesion is most often centrally located in the metaphysis (Fig. 20–28). CT or MR imaging shows a homogeneous inner density and signal, respectively, that is consistent with fluid.

Eosinophilic Granuloma. This variant of histiocytosis is currently termed *Langerhans' cell disease* and is usually considered to be non-neoplastic. Eosinophilic granuloma usually presents in adolescence and in young adults and may occur as a single lesion or may be multifocal. Symptoms often include focal pain and tenderness, and sometimes a soft tissue mass is noted. The most common locations include the calvarium, spine, ribs, shoulder girdle, pelvis, and proximal tubular bones of the extremities. In a long bone, a lesion may be epiphyseal, metaphyseal, or diaphyseal in location.

Radiographically, the lesions are lytic and relatively well defined but usually do not have a sclerotic margin.[55] There may be mild bone expansion, as well as a benign type periosteal reaction (Fig. 20–29). Occasionally, a sclerotic focal area is present in the center of the lytic region, simulating the sequestrum of osteomyelitis. Spinal involvement often leads to a loss of vertebral height (vertebra plana), which when affecting a young person may partially or completely

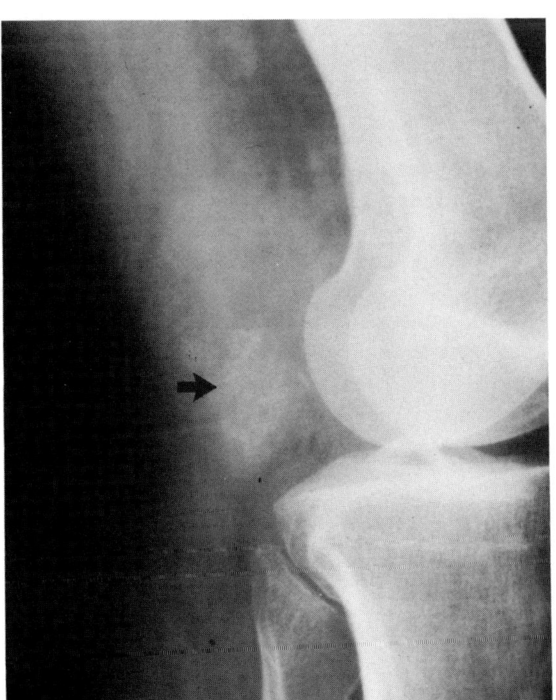

FIGURE 20–27. Synovial sarcoma located in the soft tissues posterior to the knee joint in a 30-year-old man. Soft tissue calcification *(arrow)* is seen, although this conventional radiograph does not allow evaluation of the extent of the soft tissue mass.

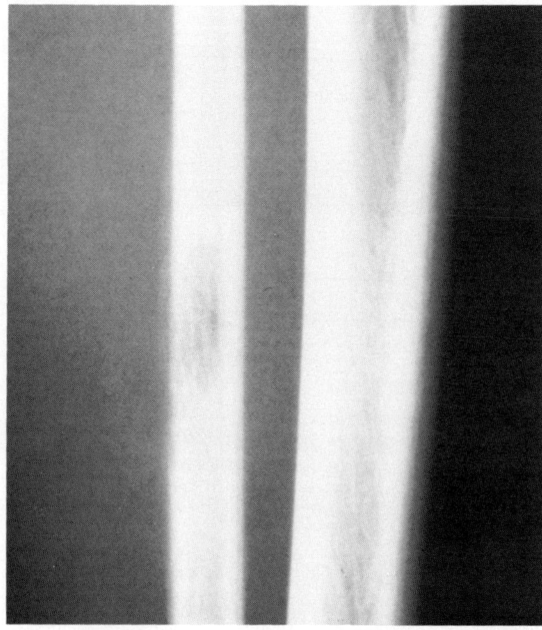

FIGURE 20–29. Eosinophilic granuloma of the fibular diaphysis in a 6-year-old boy. The lesion is lytic, with no evidence of matrix mineralization but with a wide transition zone and a thin layer of solid periosteal reaction.

reconstitute over time. Treatment consists of local radiation, steroid injection, or surgical curettage.

Pigmented Villonodular Synovitis. The cause, reactive or neoplastic, of this synovial proliferation is unclear. It can involve synovial tissue within joints, bursae, or tendon sheaths. The soft tissue masses may involve part or all of the intracapsular joint space. Usually only a single joint is in-volved, and the lesion is characteristically not painful. In the foot, adjacent joints may occasionally be involved (Fig. 20–30).

Radiographically, a soft tissue mass may be seen, and sometimes cortical scalloping peripherally as well, especially in joints that lack communicating bursal structures that may act to decompress pressures from the soft tissue masses. The

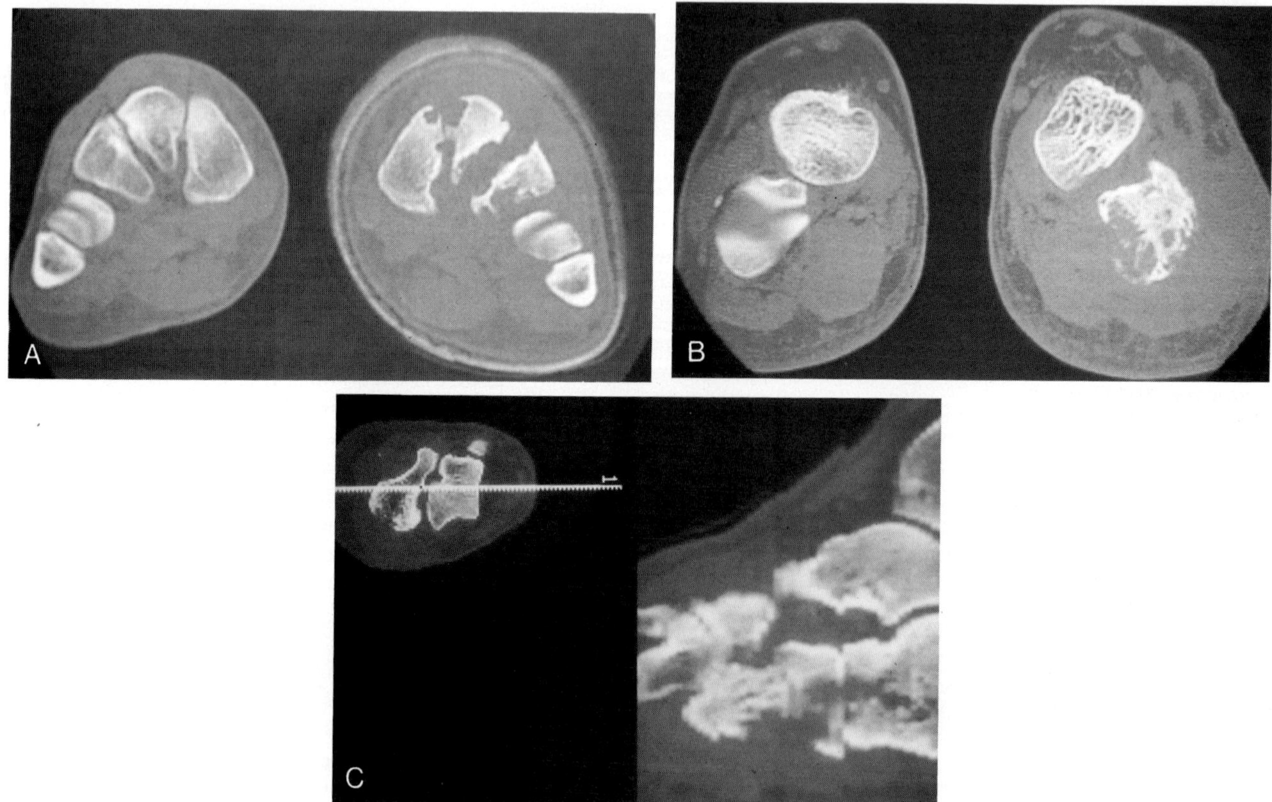

FIGURE 20–30. Pigmented villonodular synovitis may resemble an erosive inflammatory arthritis, such as in the case involving the cuneiforms shown in *A*. Involvement occasionally is more extensive. The cuboid involvement is shown in *B*. The sagittal plane reformation *(C)* illustrates extension into the calcaneus, cuboid, and cuneiforms. (Courtesy of L. M. Oloff, D.P.M.)

synovial hypertrophy often has dark pigmentation and contains hemosiderin deposition, which is seen as foci of signal absence on MR imaging.[56] Joint effusion may be present. The synovial masses do not tend to calcify.

References

1. Zimmer WD, Berquist TH, McLeod RA, et al: Bone tumors: Magnetic resonance imaging versus computed tomography. Radiology 155:709–718, 1985.

2. Sundaram M and McGuire MH: Computed tomography or magnetic resonance for evaluating the solitary tumor or tumor-like lesion of bone? Skeletal Radiol 17(6):393–401, 1988.

3. Frank JA, Ling A, Patronas NJ, et al: Detection of malignant tumors: MR imaging vs scintigraphy. Am J Roentgenol 155:1043–1048, 1990.

4. Erlemann R, Reiser MF, Peters PE, et al: Musculoskeletal neoplasms: Static and dynamic Gd-DTPA-enhanced imaging. Radiology 171:767, 1989.

5. Lodwick GS: A systematic approach to the roentgen diagnosis of bone tumors. *In* Tumors of Bone and Soft Tissues. Chicago, Year Book Medical, 1971.

6. Greenfield GB, Warren DL, and Clark RA: MR imaging of periosteal and cortical changes of bone. Radiographics 11:611–623, 1991.

7. Golfieri R, Baddeley H, Pringle JS, et al: Primary bone tumors: MR morphologic appearance correlated with pathologic examinations. Acta Radiol 32:290–298, 1991.

8. Gillespy T, Manfrini M, Ruggieri P, et al: Staging of intraosseous extent of osteosarcoma: Correlation of preoperative CT and MR imaging with pathologic macroslides. Radiology 167:765, 1988.

9. Bloem JL, Taminiau AHM, Eulderink F, et al: Radiologic staging of primary bone sarcoma: MR imaging, scintigraphy, angiography, and CT correlated with pathologic examination. Radiology 169:805–810, 1988.

10. Schajowicz F, Ackerman LV, and Sissons HA: Histological Typing of Bone Tumors. International Histologic Classification of Tumors, Vol 6. Geneva, World Health Organization, 1972.

11. Lindell MM, Shirkhoda A, Raymond AK, et al: Parosteal osteosarcoma: Radiologic-pathologic correlation with emphasis on CT. Am J Roentgenol 148:323–328, 1987.

12. Vanel D, Tcheng S, Contess G, et al: Radiological appearances of telangiectatic osteosarcoma: Study of 14 cases. Skeletal Radiol 16:196, 1987.

13. Greditzer HG III, McLeod RA, Unni KK, and Beabout JW: Bone sarcomas in Paget disease. Radiology 146:327, 1983.

14. Hopper KD, Moser RP, Haseman DB, et al: Osteosarcomatosis. Radiology 175:233–239, 1990.

15. Ellis JH, Siegel CL, Martel W, et al: Radiologic features of well-differentiated osteosarcoma. Am J Roentgenol 151:739–742, 1988.

16. Sundaram M, McGuire MH, and Herbold DR: Magnetic resonance imaging of osteosarcoma. Skeletal Radiol 16:23, 1987.

17. Seeger LL, Eckardt JJ, and Bassett LW: Cross-sectional imaging in the evaluation of osteogenic sarcoma: MRI and CT. Semin Roentgenol 24:174, 1989.

18. Klein MH and Shankman S: Osteoid osteoma: Radiologic and pathologic correlation. Skeletal Radiol 21:23–31, 1992.

19. Capanna R, Van Horn JR, Ayala A, et al: Osteoid osteoma and osteoblastoma of the talus: A report of 40 cases. Skeletal Radiol 15(5):360–367, 1986.

20. Kransdorf MJ, Stull MA, Gilkey FW, and Moser RP: Osteoid osteoma. Radiographics 11:671–696, 1991.

21. Kroon HM and Schurmans J: Osteoblastoma: Clinical and radiologic findings in 98 new cases. Radiology 175:783–790, 1990.

22. Libshitz HI and Cohen MA: Radiation-induced osteochondromas. Radiology 142:643, 1982.

23. Lee JK, Yao L, and Wirth CR: MR imaging of solitary osteochondromas: Report of eight cases. Am J Roentgenol 149:557–560, 1987.

24. Markel SF: Ossifying fibroma of long bone: Its distinction from fibrous dysplasia and its association with adamantinoma of long bone. Am J Clin Pathol 69:91–97, 1978.

25. Present D, Bacchini P, Pignatti G, et al: Clear cell chondrosarcoma of bone. Skeletal Radiol 20:187–191, 1991.

26. Norman A and Sissons HA: Radiographic hallmarks of peripheral chondrosarcoma. Radiology 151:589, 1984.

27. Rosenthal DI, Schiller AL, and Mankin HJ: Chondrosarcoma: Correlation of radiologic and histological grade. Radiology 150:21, 1984.

28. Resnick D, Kyriakos M, and Greenway GD: Tumors and tumor-like lesions of bone: Imaging and pathology of specific lesions. *In* Resnick D and Niwayama G (eds): Diagnosis of Bone and Joint Disorders, Vol 6. Philadelphia, WB Saunders, 1988, pp 3679–3681.

29. Hudson TM and Hawkins IF Jr: Radiologic evaluation of chrondroblastoma. Radiology 139:1, 1981.

30. Moser RP Jr, Brockmole DM, Vihn TN, et al: Chondroblastoma of the patella. Skeletal Radiol 17(6):413–419, 1988.

31. Schajowicz F: Chondromyxoid fibroma: Report of three cases with predominant cortical involvement. Radiology 164:783–786, 1987.

32. Dahlin DC: Giant cell tumor of bone: Highlights of 407 cases. Am J Roentgenol 144:955–960, 1985.

33. Tsai JC, Dalinka MK, Fallon MD, et al: Fluid-fluid level: A non-specific finding in tumors of bone and soft tissue. Radiology 175:779, 1990.

34. Munk PL, Helms CA, Holt RG, et al: MR imaging of aneurysmal bone cysts. Am J Roentgenol 153:99–101, 1989.

35. Reinus WR and Gilula LA: Radiology of Ewing's's sarcoma: Intergroup Ewing's sarcoma study (IESS). Radiographics 4:927, 1984.

36. Frouge C, Vanel D, Coffre C, et al: The role of magnetic resonance imaging in the evaluation of Ewing's sarcoma: A report of 27 cases. Skeletal Radiol 17(6):387–392, 1988.

37. Phillips WC, Kattapuram SV, Dosoretz DE, et al: Primary lymphoma of bone: Relationship of radiographic appearance and prognosis. Radiology 144:285, 1982.

38. Nghiem HV, Ellis BI, Haggar AM, and Meis JM: Juxta-articular large cell lymphoma. Skeletal Radiol 19:353–357, 1990.

39. Buetow PC, Kransdorf MJ, Moser RP, et al: Radiologic appearance of intramuscular hemangioma with emphasis on MR imaging. Am J Roentgenol 154:563–567, 1990.

40. Cohen EK, Kressel HY, Perosio T, et al: MR imaging of soft tissue hemangiomas: Correlation with pathologic findings. Am J Roentgenol 150:1079–1081, 1988.

41. Enzinger F and Weiss S: Glomus tumor. *In* Soft Tissue Tumors. St Louis, CV Mosby, 1983, pp 450–462.

42. Kransdorf MJ, Utz JA, Gilkey FW, and Berrey BH: MR appearance of fibroxanthoma. J Comp Assist Tomog 12(4):612–615, 1988.

43. Kumar R, Madewell JE, Lindell MM, and Swischuk LE: Fibrous lesions of bones. Radiographics 10:237–256, 1990.

44. Resnick D, Kyriakos M, and Greenway GD: Tumors and tumor-like lesions of bone: Imaging and pathology of specific lesions. *In* Resnick D and Niwayama G (eds): Diagnosis of Bone and Joint Disorders, Vol 6. Philadelphia, WB Saunders, 1988, p 3831.

45. Norris MA, Kaplan P, Pathria M, and Greenway G: Fibrous dysplasia: Magnetic resonance imaging appearance at 1.5 Tesla. Clin Imaging 14:211–215, 1990.

46. Ramos A, Castello I, Sartoris DJ, et al: Osseous lipoma: CT appearance. Radiology 157:615–619, 1985.

47. Vilar JS, Martí-Bonmati L, Poyatos CR, and Ferrer R: General case of the day (myxoid liposarcoma). Radiographics 11:333–335, 1991.

48. London J, Kim EE, Wallace S, et al: MR imaging of liposarcomas: Correlation of MR features and histology. J Comp Assist Tomog 13(5):832–835, 1989.

49. Capusten BM, Azouz EM, and Rosman MA: Fibromatosis of bone in children. Radiology 152:693, 1984.

50. Stull MA, Moser RP, Kransdorf MJ, et al: Magnetic resonance appearance of peripheral nerve sheath tumors. Skeletal Radiol 20:9–14, 1991.

51. Levine E, Huntrakoon M, and Wetzel LH: Malignant nerve-sheath neoplasms in neurofibromatosis: Distinction from benign tumors by using imaging techniques. Am J Roentgenol 149:1059–1064, 1987.

52. Mahajan H, Kim EE, Wallace S, et al: MR imaging of malignant fibrous histiocytoma. Magn Reson Imaging 7:283–288, 1989.

53. Mahajan H, Lorigan JG, and Shirkoda A: Synovial sarcoma: MR imaging. Magn Reson Imaging 7:211–216, 1989.

54. Resnick D, Kyriakos M, and Greenway GD: Tumors and tumor-like lesions of bone: Imaging and pathology of specific lesions. *In* Resnick D and Niwayama G (eds): Diagnosis of Bone and Joint Disorders, Vol 6. Philadelphia, WB Saunders, 1988, p 3820–3831.

55. Resnick D: Lipidoses, histiocytoses, and hyperlipoproteinemias. *In* Resnick D and Niwayama G (eds): Diagnosis of Bone and Joint Disorders, Vol 4. Philadelphia, WB Saunders, 1988, pp 2431–2434.

56. Mandelbaum BD, Grant TT, and Hartzman S: The use of MRI to assist in diagnosis of pigmented villonodular synovitis of the knee joint. Clin Orthop 231:135–139, 1988.

Radiographic Evaluations of Bone and Joint Infections

Allan Bernstein, D.P.M., Gideon Strich, M.D.,
and Mark G. Stein, M.B.B.Ch., B.Sc.

The clinical presentation, subsequent diagnostic imaging, and initiation of medical/surgical therapeutics of an infectious disease involving the bone and joints of the foot and ankle continue to be difficult challenges for the podiatric physician and surgeon. The basic tenets in management of osteomyelitis, regardless of the clinical setting, have remained essentially the same despite explosive advances in medical technology. A high level of suspicion, confirmed by clinical, laboratory, and diagnostic imaging, is the cornerstone of effective treatment for bone and joint infection. Advancement in diagnostic techniques have included radiopharmaceutical imaging, computed tomographic (CT) evaluation, and recently magnetic resonance imaging (MRI). Arthrography, joint aspiration, percutaneous aspiration, and biopsy have also corroborated clinical impressions and have contributed to early diagnosis. The judicious and aggressive utilization of antibiotics and surgery has improved the outcome and treatment of infectious disease of the musculoskeletal system.

The fundamental pathologic process of osteomyelitis in the foot is not dissimilar to that of other locations in the musculoskeletal system; however, certain considerations must be taken into account. Among these are the unique configuration of the bones of the feet, constant exposure of the feet to external trauma, and pathomechanical stresses. Frequent involvement with vascular and metabolic disease makes the diagnostic challenge a more difficult one. It is the intent of this chapter to delineate a practical approach to this difficult diagnostic challenge via an understanding of the physiologic processes and their subsequent radiographic presentations. This will enable the practitioner to direct aggressive and judicious intervention to control this disease process.

PATHOPHYSIOLOGY OF INFECTION

The introduction of the term *osteomyelitis* is attributed to Nelaton in 1844.[1] The interpretation from the French article implies infection of bone and marrow. Although most commonly associated with a bacterial cause, osteomyelitis may be parasitic, viral, or fungal in nature. Infective or suppurative osteitis is indicative of contamination of the bone cortex.

Infective osteitis, although possibly an isolated phenomenon, is usually a concomitant to osteomyelitis. The differentiation, both radiographically and pathologically, of osteitis and osteomyelitis continues to be extremely difficult; however, differentiation is possible and can influence the choice of appropriate medical or surgical therapy. Inflammation of the cortex may be observed in several spondyloarthropathies such as ankylosing spondylitis, Reiter's syndrome, and psoriasis and is not only associated with infection. Infective suppurative periostitis implies contamination of the periosteal cloak surrounding the bone. Subperiosteal accumulation of organisms will frequently lead to infectious osteitis and osteomyelitis because of the interruption of periosteal blood supply to the cortex (Fig. 21–1). This produces necrosis or destruction of the periosteum and accumulation of purulent material in soft tissues. Periostitis may also be associated with metabolic, neoplastic, and traumatic causes.

Osteomyelitis has been classified as acute, subacute, and chronic. Because these may coexist histopathologically, and the clinical presentation may be equivocal because this is a temporal classification with one stage progressing or regressing to another, classification according to pathogenesis appears more reasonable.[2] Hematogenous osteomyelitis accounts for 25% of all cases, and osteomyelitis from a contiguous focus without circulatory disease accounts for approximately 45% of all cases. Adjacent soft tissue infection in patients with associated vascular disorders (diabetes, peripheral vascular disease, and so on) accounts for 35% of clinically documented cases of osteomyelitis.[3, 4] Radiographically, the classification of osteomyelitis has been attempted using the route of contamination, including hematogenous spread, spread from a contiguous infectious source, postoperative infection, and direct implantation.[5] Radiographic findings vary greatly depending on the route of contamination. Hematogenous osteomyelitis originating within the cancellous bone will result in radiographic findings that start inside the bone and eventually work to the cortex of the periosteum. By contrast, direct extension of osteomyelitis will first affect the periosteum, then the cortex, and finally the marrow. Hematogenous spread of infection to the foot is quite uncommon[4–7] and is referred to briefly in this chapter. However, for a complete discourse, one is referred to the text by Resnick and Niwayama.[5]

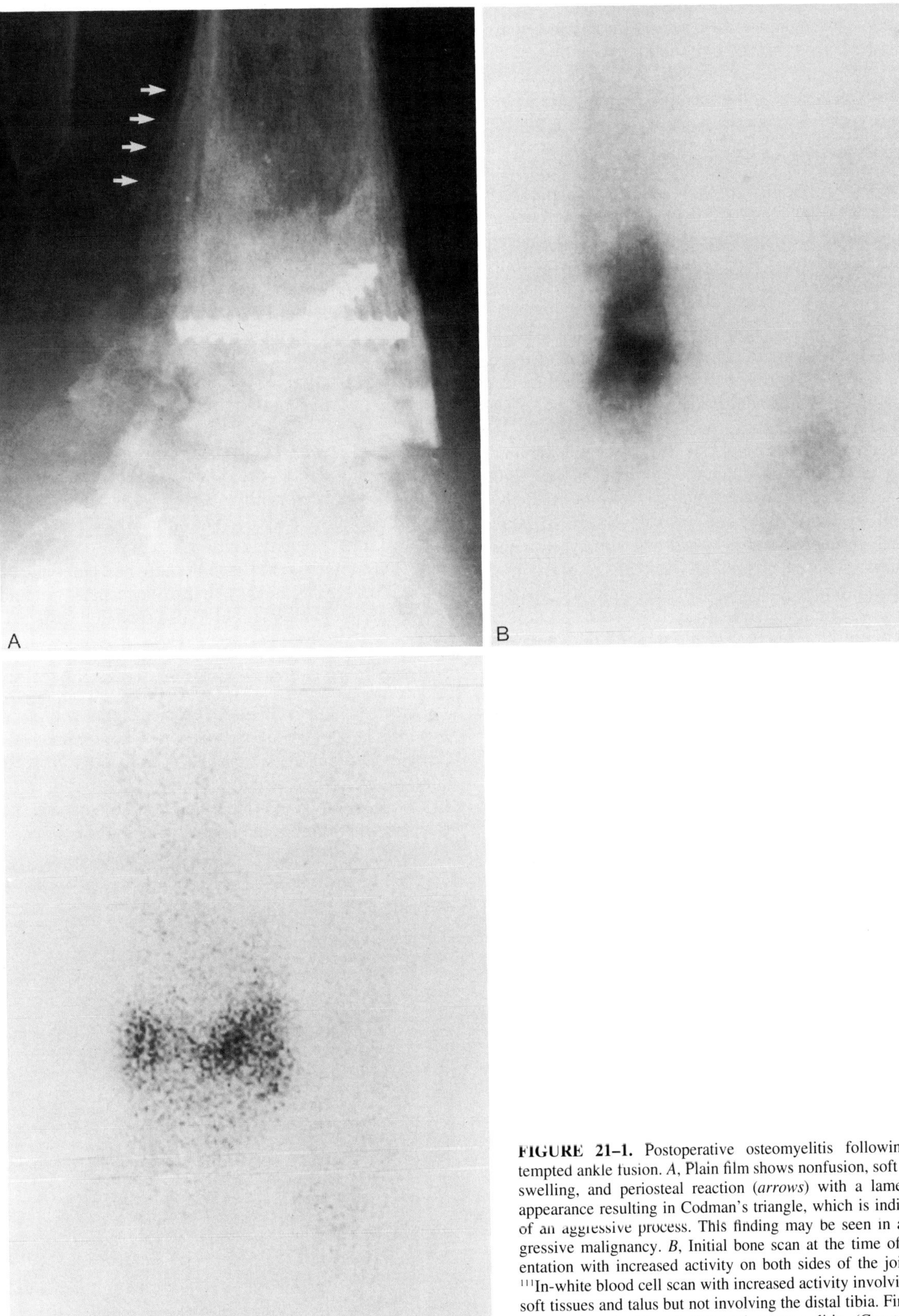

FIGURE 21–1. Postoperative osteomyelitis following attempted ankle fusion. *A,* Plain film shows nonfusion, soft tissue swelling, and periosteal reaction (*arrows*) with a lamellated appearance resulting in Codman's triangle, which is indicative of an aggressive process. This finding may be seen in an aggressive malignancy. *B,* Initial bone scan at the time of presentation with increased activity on both sides of the joint. *C,* ^{111}In-white blood cell scan with increased activity involving the soft tissues and talus but not involving the distal tibia. Findings are consistent with cellulitis and osteomyelitis. (Courtesy of Felix Wang, M.D., Orange, CA.)

CLASSIFICATION OF INFECTION

Hematogenous Spread of Infection

Hematogenously spread osteomyelitis has traditionally been regarded as a disease of childhood, presenting at the ages of 3 to 15 years.[8–17] An increase in the incidence of hematogenous osteomyelitis has recently been noted in older patients, however.[11–23] Neonatal osteomyelitis has also been well delineated. Major clinical and radiographic presentations as well as the course of hematogenous osteomyelitis in infants, children, and adults are well described, particularly because of the vascular anatomy. Blood-borne microorganisms tend to settle in the metaphyseal capillary loops adjacent to the epiphyseal plate. These capillaries and pseudoloops vary greatly in diameter, and their variation in size creates turbulent or sluggish blood flow. The sluggish flow, coupled with poor phagocytic function in bone tissue, leads to an increased likelihood of the establishment of a focus of infection near the epiphysis, with subsequent invasion of the distal metaphysis.[3] In children younger than 1 year, some of the capillaries perforate the epiphyseal plate, and this allows the spread of infection into the epiphysis and joints. Between the age of 1 year and the age at which the epiphysis closes, there is no direct connection between epiphysis and the metaphysis. The capillary loops are therefore end vessels. In adulthood, the growth cartilage is resorbed and epiphyseal anastomosis occurs. Afferent capillaries lack phagocytic lining cells, and the efferent loops contain functionally inactive phagocytic cells. The metaphyseal capillaries are end vessels with stagnation of blood flow. The slow blood flow and lack of phagocytosis make the metaphysis the major focus of hematogenous dissemination of osteomyelitis (Fig. 21–2). In children younger than 1 year, as well as in adults, osteomyelitis may extend into the epiphysis and adjacent joint because of epiphyseal anastomoses.[19] Once bone infection is initiated, organisms reach the periosteum via haversian canals and either occlude nutrient vessels by septic embolization or interrupt nutrient vessel flow by inflammatory elevation of the periosteal membrane.[20–22] Subsequently, leukocytes release osteoclastic activating factors, which initiate bone destruction.[23] Descriptive terminology may now be applied to the pathophysiologic changes that take place depending on the distribution of vascular injury relative to osteoblastic repair. A sequestrum represents a segment of necrotic bone separated from living bone by granulation tissue. Sequestra may be identified in the marrow for protracted periods of time, harboring living organisms that have the capability of evoking acute reactivation of infection. An involucrum may be present, denoting a layer of living bone that is formed around the dead bone (Fig. 21–3). It may surround and eventually merge with the parent bone or may be perforated by tracts or sinuses through which pus may escape. A sinus that leads to the skin surface is termed a *fistula*. Granulation tissue and sequestra may be discharged from the body spontaneously through the fistula channels. Brodie's abscess (a bone abscess) is a sharply delineated focus of infection of variable size occurring at single or multiple locations representing a site of active infection. If it is lined by granulation tissue and surrounded by eburnated bone, it is known as Garré's sclerosing osteomyelitis, a sclerotic, nonpurulent form of osteomyelitis.[24] The descriptive term is associated with intense proliferation of the periosteum, leading to bony deposition in which there is no necrosis or purulent exudate and little granulation tissue.[25] Garré's sclerosing osteomyelitis is extremely rare and typically is due to *Staphylococcus aureus*. It has been most commonly described in the mandible, but it also seen in the distal tibia.[26, 27]

Spread from a Contiguous Focus of Infection

Direct extension of infection in patients without preexisting circulatory disease accounts for approximately 45% of reported osteomyelitis cases.[3] Osteomyelitis derived from a contiguous source usually implies the presence of a soft tissue infection. Contamination from an adjacent site is particularly important in the hands, mandible, skull, and feet.[28–30]

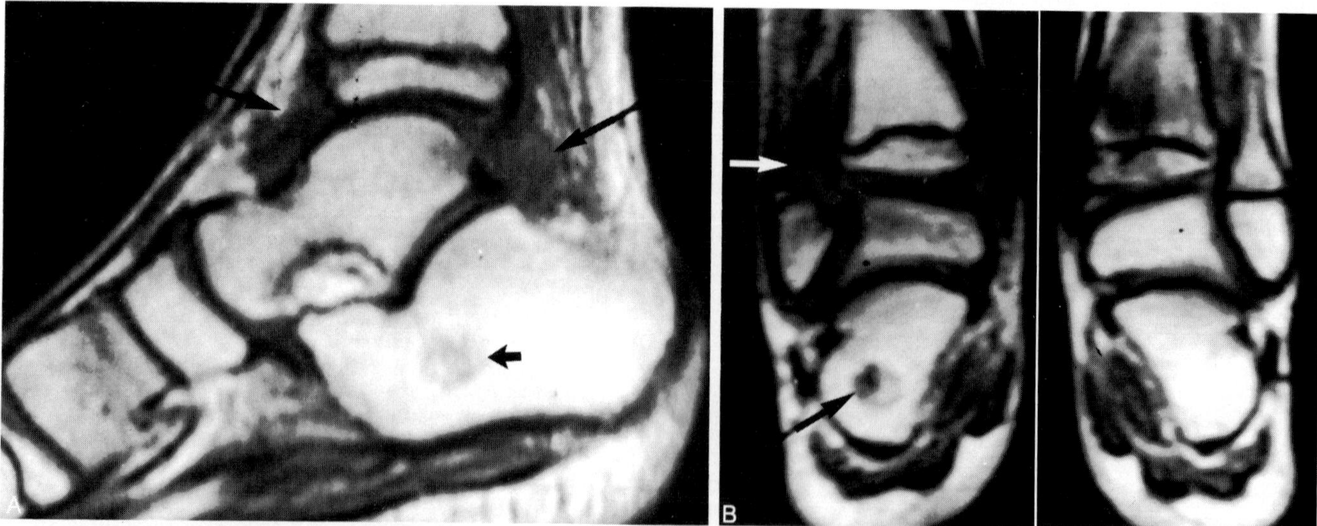

FIGURE 21–2. Blood-borne infection in a child. The plain films had negative findings. *A,* Sagittal T$_1$-weighted magnetic resonance images show the focus of osteomyelitis in the right calcaneus (*short black arrow*) and septic effusion (*long black arrows*). *B,* Coronal T$_1$-weighted images demonstrate additional foci of osteomyelitis in the distal right fibula (*white arrow*) and in the calcaneus, left tibia, crossing the epiphyseal plate (*long black arrows*). (Courtesy of John V. Crues III, M.D., Santa Barbara, CA.)

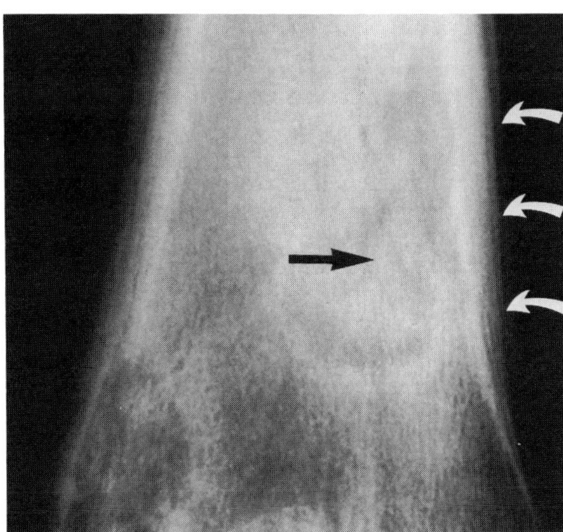

FIGURE 21–3. Chronic osteomyelitis. Anteroposterior view demonstrates typical findings of a sequestrum (*black arrow*), metaphyseal remodeling, and mature periosteal reaction (*curved arrows*). (Courtesy of Joyce Pais, M.D., Orange, CA.)

Soft tissue infection leading to bone and joint contamination frequently involves animal and human bites, puncture wounds, and postoperative infection.[31–39] Koch compared the effect of a contiguous focus of infection of osseous and articular structures to the erosive "action of a turbulent stream of water upon a wall of rock."[40] As previously noted, hematogenously spread osteomyelitis is centrally placed in the marrow and then progresses outward into the soft tissues. The opposite is true of the contiguous spread of osteomyelitis, in which sepsis is spread from the soft tissues inward to the osseous anatomy. Early evidence of soft tissue infection is the rule. Disruption of the soft tissue planes is evident, and abscess formation is common (Fig. 21–4). Extension into the periosteum by initial invasion of its outer, more fibrous portion is noted. Periosteal displacement is more frequent and marked in children because of looser attachment. Resultant periosteal bone formation is commonly the initial radiographic manifestation of osteomyelitis; however, a well-localized loss of bone density, termed *rarefaction*, is generally the earliest finding of this classification of osteomyelitis.[41, 42] As the infectious process ensues, there is gross destruction of bone, termed *osteolysis* (see Fig. 21–7).[42] To complete the lexicon of terminology, we must include the descriptive term *cloaca*. This refers to an opening along the cortex where purulent drainage is noted. A cloaca is seen most commonly in hematogenous infection.[5]

ROLE OF IMAGING MODALITIES IN DIAGNOSIS

Plain Film Screen Radiography

Standard radiography remains the mainstay of diagnostic imaging because of widespread availability, low cost, and rapidity of interpretation. There are, however, significant weaknesses of the plain radiograph in the diagnosis of infection. Often plain radiographs are entirely normal in the pres-

ence of clinically apparent infection.[43] Early findings of soft tissue infection may be subtle soft tissue changes only appreciated using low-KV technique or using a bright light to evaluate the soft tissues on radiographs exposed using bone technique. Findings of soft tissue infections include swelling and loss of the normal fat planes between muscular layers or thickening of fibrous septae within the fat planes. Soft tissue masses may also be seen. Early radiographic findings of septic arthritis are best visualized in the ankle joint as distention of the joint capsule and loss of the normal posterior triangle of fat seen best on the lateral view (Fig. 21–5).

The earliest radiographic appearance of osteomyelitis or bone destruction of cancellous bone is not visible until approximately 50% of the bone mineral is lost.[5, 43] This requires approximately 10 to 14 days depending on the aggressiveness of the infection.[5, 44, 45] Bone loss or destruction in less time suggests other causes (e.g., eosinophilic granuloma). Osteolysis appearing as subtle loss of bone density followed by destruction of the trabecula pattern and cortex may be the first finding in acute hematogenous osteomyelitis (Fig. 21–6; see also Fig. 21–2). Subsequent periosteal reaction and septic or sympathetic joint effusion may occur later.

In osteomyelitis secondary to adjacent soft tissue infection or septic arthritis, the soft tissue changes appear first, followed usually by periosteal reaction and subsequently local bone destruction with a localized decrease in density termed rarefaction. With indolent organisms or chronic infection, the periosteal reaction may be smooth and mature in appearance. With more aggressive infection, there may be marked elevation of the periosteum, with "onion skin" layering of the periosteal new bone and formation of Codman's triangle (see Fig. 21–1) at the ends of the periosteal reaction, a finding that may be suggestive of malignancy, especially in children. Chronic radiographic changes are varied and again depend on the aggressiveness of the organism and whether the infection originates primarily in the soft tissues or the bone. The formation of sequestra, islands of dead bones surrounded by a zone of lucent, osteoporotic bone or active infection, may be seen. Although these findings are more typical of infection with *S. aureus*, this appearance may also be seen in fungal and parasitic infections such as syphilis (see Fig. 21–3). Well-defined zones of sclerosis without central sequestra are typical of a localized bone (Brodie's) abscess, an entity commonly seen in the distal tibial metaphysis (Fig. 21–7).

A permeative, moth-eaten appearance of ill-defined lucency without well-defined sclerotic margins may be seen in cases of very aggressive infection and chronic infection (Fig. 21–8) in which there is mixed osteolysis, periosteal reaction, and reparative changes with replacement of trabecular bone with "woven" bone. This appearance may also simulate malignancy, particularly round-cell tumors such as Ewing's sarcoma in children or metastatic disease in adults.

Chronic periostitis or osteomyelitis may lead to remodeling of the affected bone with widening of the metaphysis and diaphysis as well as increased density radiographically. Occasionally, chronic infection may cause sclerosis only, without significant remodeling, which is termed Garré's sclerosing osteomyelitis, as previously discussed.[24]

Radiographic findings are more complex in patients with previous fractures or with orthopedic hardware or prostheses

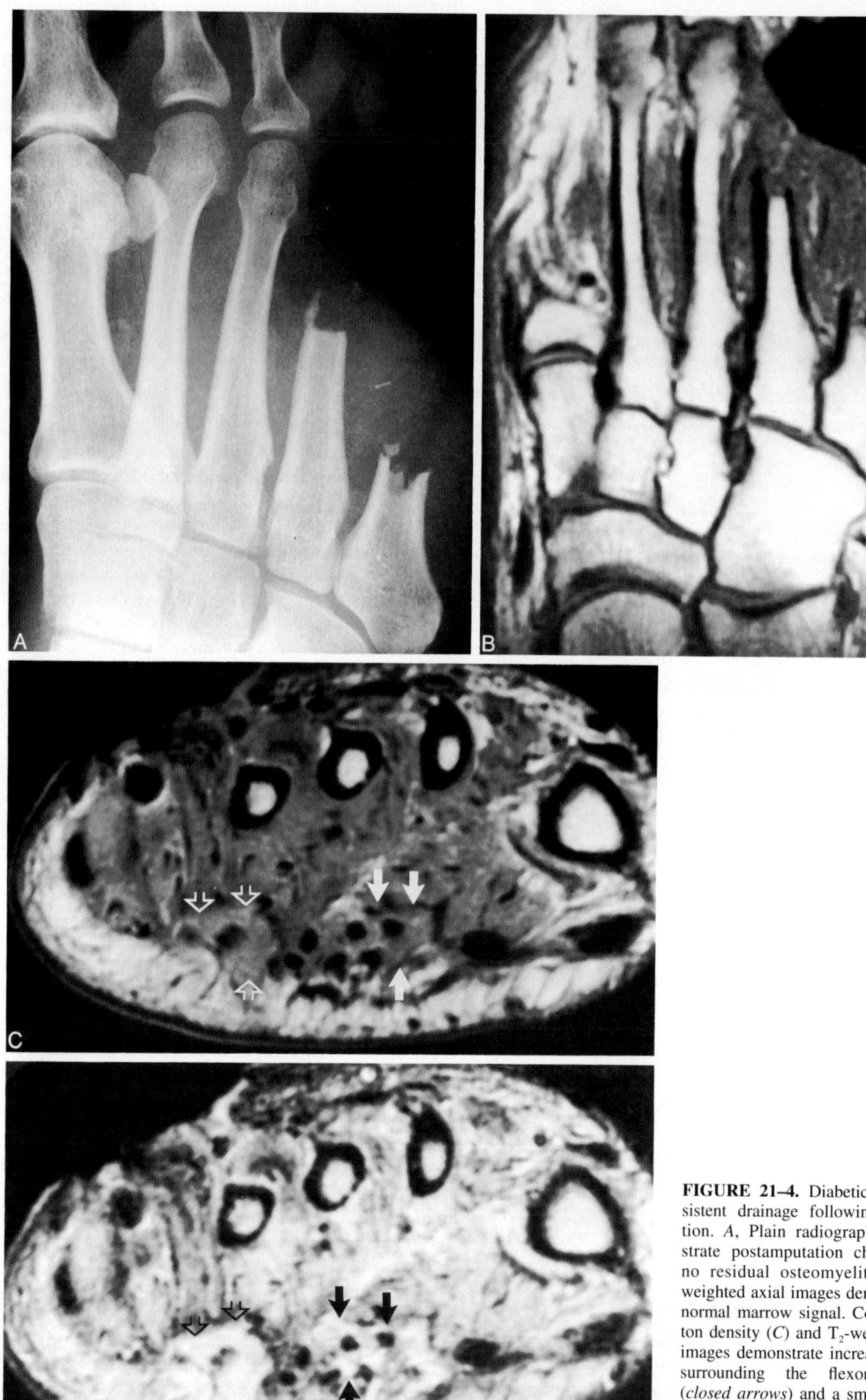

FIGURE 21–4. Diabetic with persistent drainage following amputation. *A*, Plain radiographs demonstrate postamputation changes but no residual osteomyelitis. *B*, T_1-weighted axial images demonstrate a normal marrow signal. Coronal proton density (*C*) and T_2-weighted (*D*) images demonstrate increased signal surrounding the flexor tendons (*closed arrows*) and a small abscess (*open arrows*). Surgical findings were consistent with necrotizing fasciitis but not with osteomyelitis.

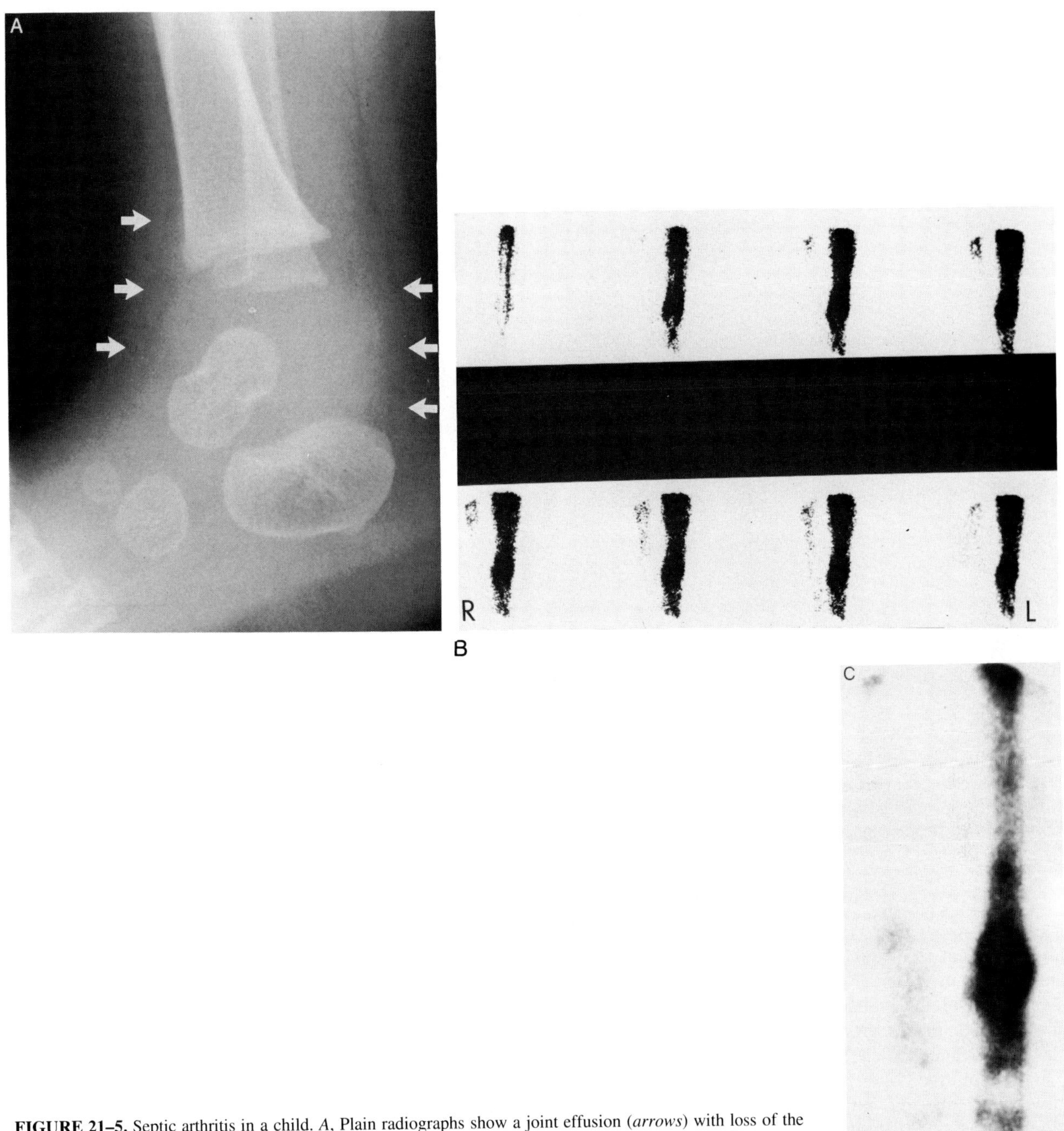

FIGURE 21–5. Septic arthritis in a child. *A*, Plain radiographs show a joint effusion (*arrows*) with loss of the periarticular fat plains. There is no bone destruction. Dynamic (*B*) and delayed (*C*) images from a bone scan with increased flow to the left lower extremity and diffusely increased uptake on both sides of the joint.

(Figs. 21–9 and 21–10). Low-grade chronic infection may result in nonunion at a fracture site, with the radiographic features of osteomyelitis masked by the presence of callus and sclerosis from attempted bone healing. Early osteomyelitis in patients with prostheses or fixation devices often manifests as a zone of lucency surrounding the device, progressing later to frank bone destruction. Unfortunately, the early appearance may be mimicked by simple loosening of the device, causing adjacent osteolysis secondary to motion. In the setting of previous trauma or surgery, radionuclide imaging may have a significant role, as discussed later.

Computed Tomography

The role of CT in the evaluation of disorders of the lower extremity is well established.[46–48] More recently, use of CT in the evaluation of lower extremity infection and the complementary role of CT to plain radiography, radionuclide imaging, and MRI have been described.[49–51]

Typical CT imaging protocols use both direct coronal as well as oblique axial images with the gantry tilted to allow imaging in approximately the same plane as, and perpendicular to, the metatarsals. Slice thicknesses of 3 to 5 mm are

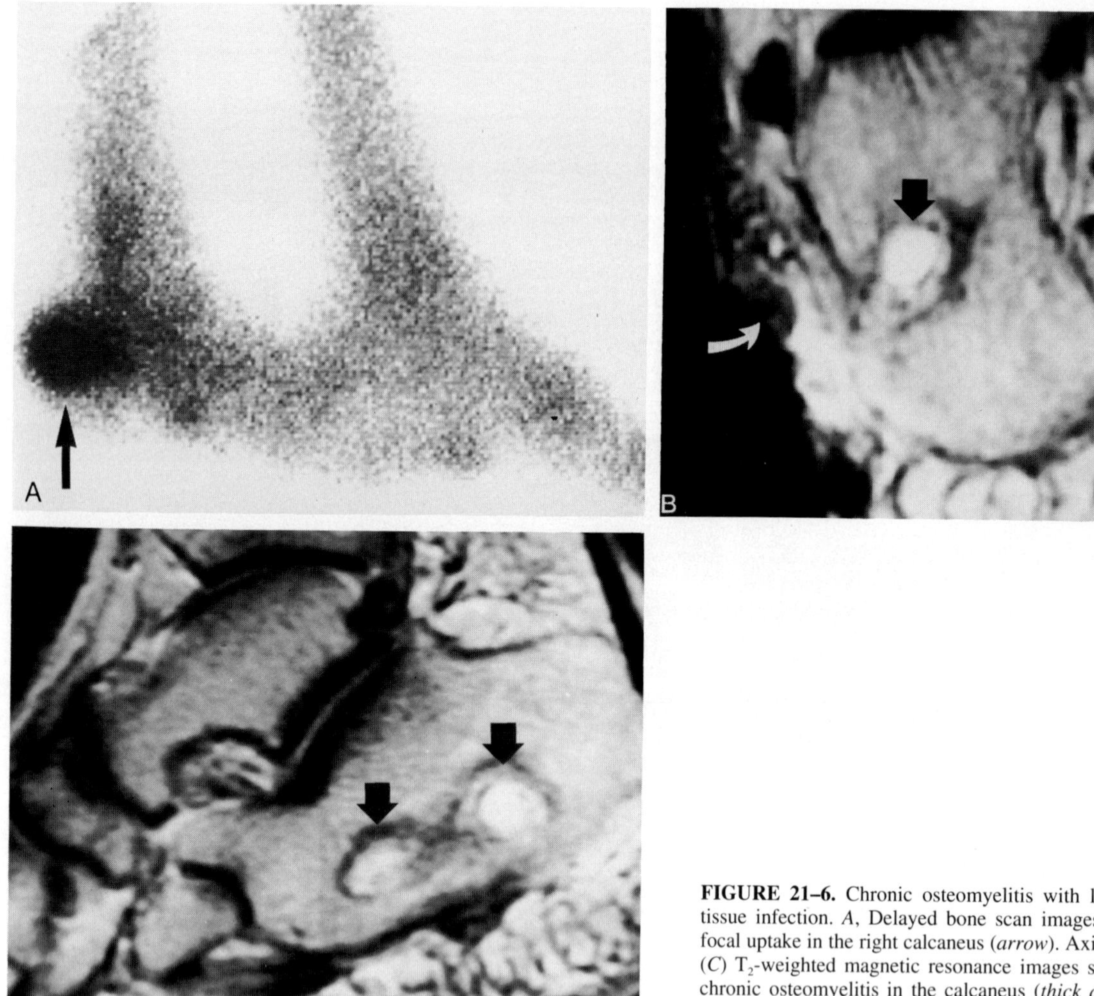

FIGURE 21–6. Chronic osteomyelitis with long-standing soft tissue infection. *A,* Delayed bone scan images demonstrate the focal uptake in the right calcaneus (*arrow*). Axial (*B*) and sagittal (*C*) T$_2$-weighted magnetic resonance images show the focus of chronic osteomyelitis in the calcaneus (*thick arrows*) and demonstrate the extent of soft tissue infection on the plantar surface with associated ulceration (*curved arrows*).

usually sufficient to evaluate the rearfoot and midfoot. Occasionally, 1.5 to 2 mm thick sections are used, especially for evaluation of the metatarsals or digits and when computer-generated images are needed. Generally, two sets of images are obtained for each set of scans performed; one set uses high-resolution bone-reconstruction algorithm and wide windows to display the cortex and trabecular pattern. Wide window widths (2000 to 4000 Hounsfield units [H.U.]) are helpful to demonstrate maximum bony detail and to reduce artifact from metallic devices if any are present. A second set of images using narrower windows (300 to 400 H.U.) demonstrates the extraosseous component of the infection including abscess, edema, and fistula tract formation.

The advantages of CT are due to the tomographic nature of the technique, which allows visualization of abnormalities (e.g., sequestra and fistulas that may be hidden by overlying sclerotic bone). In addition, increased soft tissue contrast resolution allows identification of soft tissue abscesses, fluid collections, and foreign bodies that may otherwise not be seen on plain radiographs (see Fig. 21–8). Tumeh and colleagues found that CT detected virtually all surgically proven sequestra, of which only 33% were visible on plain films.[49]

In cases of extensive bone remodeling, they found a relatively high rate of false-positive findings on the CT compared with the scintigraphy using combined bone and gallium imaging.[50] In comparing CT with MRIs of fungal infections of the foot, Sharif and associates concluded that CT was comparable to MRI in demonstrating soft tissue infection but somewhat more sensitive than MRI in assessing early bone involvement, particularly periosteal and endosteal reaction.[50]

The role of CT is therefore complementary to other imaging modalities. It is particularly good in the preoperative evaluation of patients with known chronic osteomyelitis for localizing abscesses, sequestra, and fistula tracts. CT may complement MRI in defining the extent of bony destruction and adjacent soft tissue abscess collections. CT is more sensitive than MRI in the detection of periostitis and early cortical destruction, particularly in small bones such as the phalanges and metatarsals (see Fig. 21–7). In addition, in postoperative cases in which the presence of metal may produce unacceptable MR images, optimizing CT technique with new state-of-the-art scanners may minimize this problem (see Fig. 21–10).

Text continued on page 351

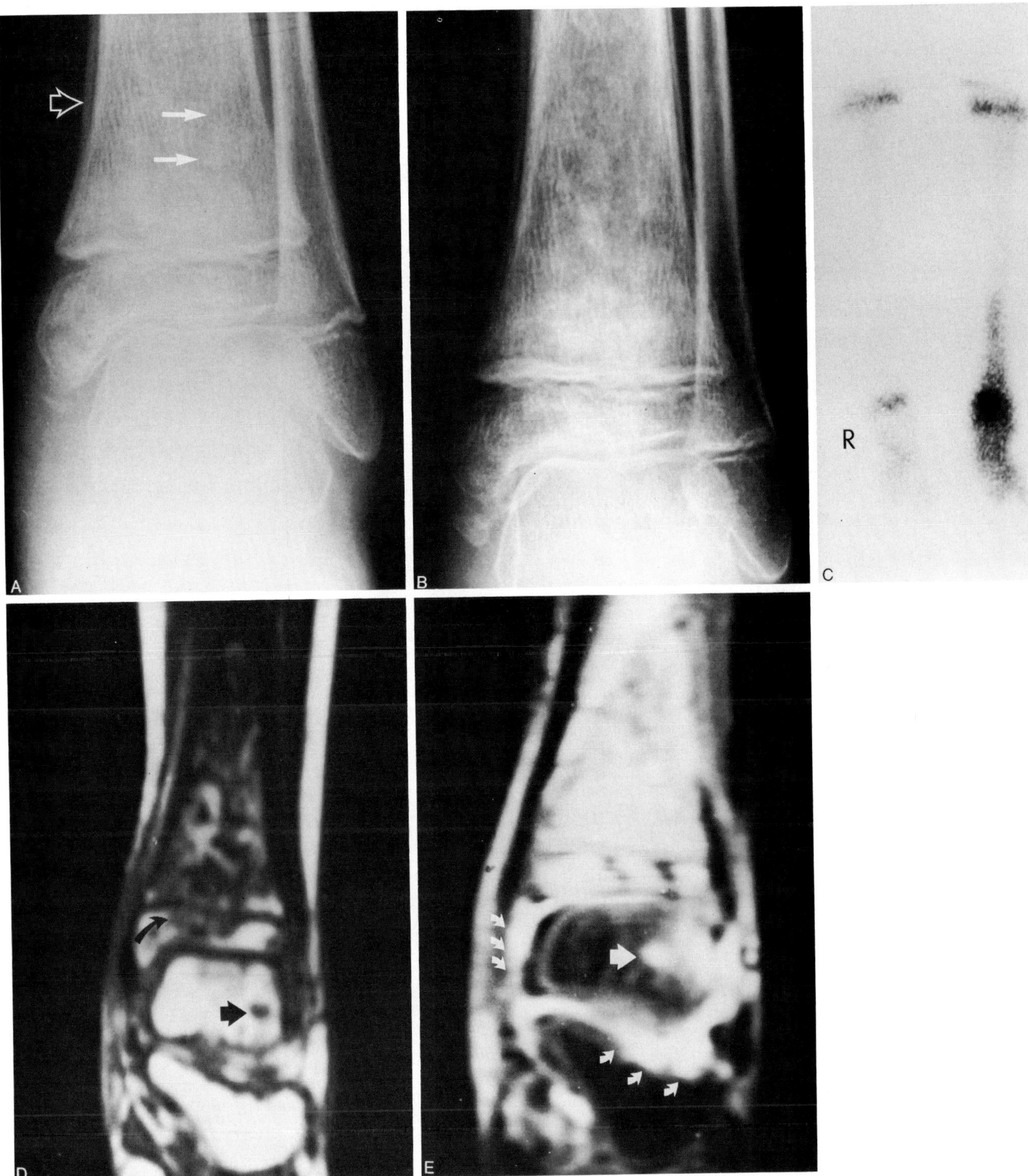

FIGURE 21–7. Osteomyelitis and septic arthritis due to *Staphylococcus aureus*. *A,* Initial plain radiograph shows metaphyseal lucency (*white arrows*) and periosteal reaction (*open arrow*). *B,* Two weeks later, there is progressive destruction despite antibiotic therapy. *C,* A bone scan at the time of initial presentation shows increased activity in the distal left tibial metaphysis. Coronal T$_1$- (*D*) and T$_2$-weighted (*E*) magnetic resonance images demonstrate extensive metaphyseal involvement crossing the epiphyseal plate (*black curved arrow*). Note also the focus of osteomyelitis in the talus (*thick arrows*) and septic joint effusion (*white curved arrows*). (Courtesy of Joyce Pais, M.D., Orange, CA.)

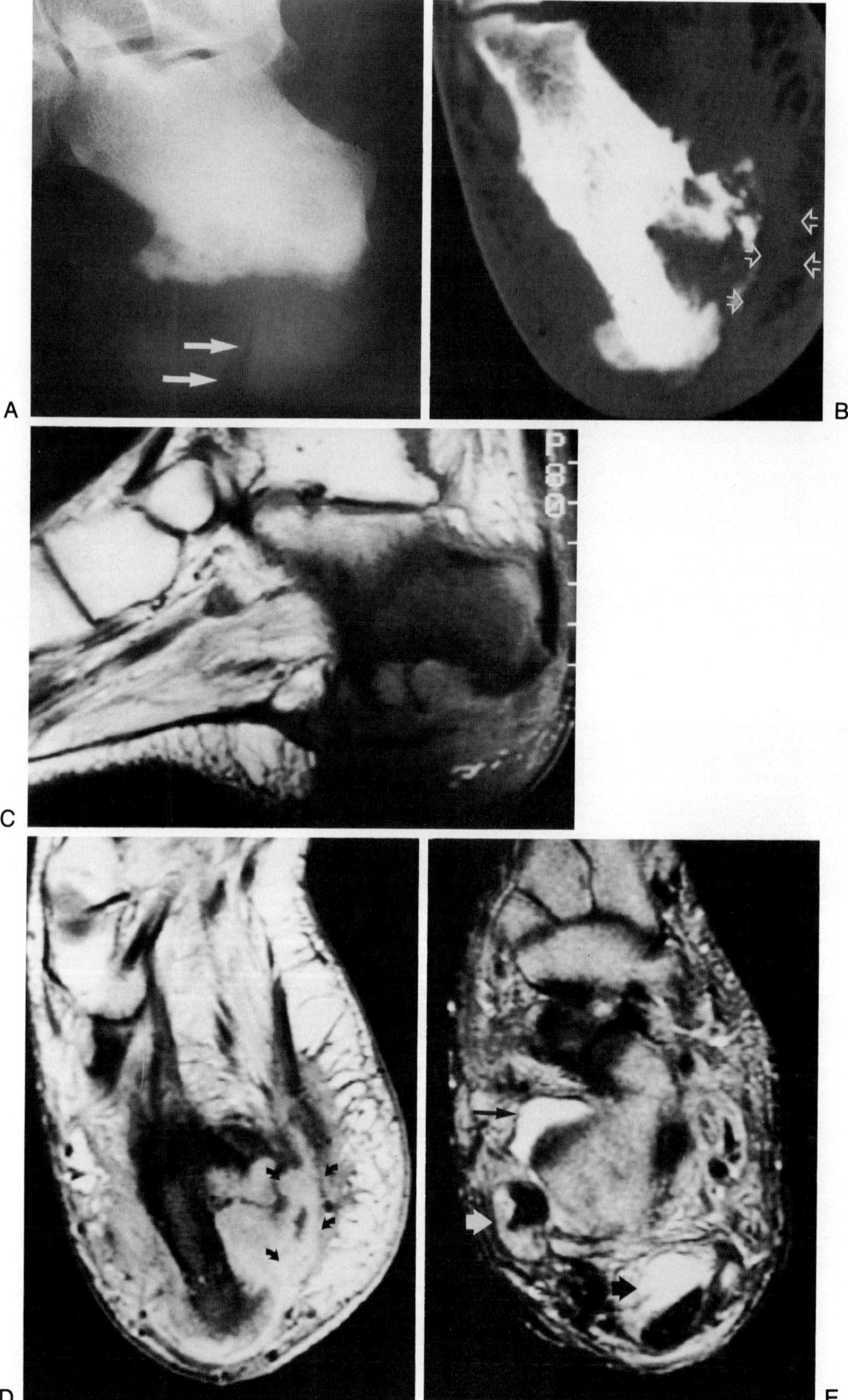

FIGURE 21–8. Patient with chronic osteomyelitis of the calcaneus. *A*, Plain films show bone destruction, soft tissue air (*white arrows*), and distortion of normal soft tissue planes. *B*, Axial CT images demonstrate extensive bone destruction, adjacent sclerosis, and a soft tissue abscess (*open arrowheads*). *C*, Sagittal T₁-weighted magnetic resonance image demonstrating a diminished signal in the calcaneus representing sclerosis and bone marrow edema and the extent of osteomyelitis and soft tissue abscess. *D*, Axial proton density image corresponding with the computed tomography section better delineates the extent of the soft tissue abscess (*curved arrows*). *E*, Axial T₂-weighted (*black arrow*) image obtained superior to *D* demonstrates synovial fluid in the ankle joint (*white arrowhead*), septic tenosynovitis of the peroneal tendons, and an abscess anterior to the Achilles tendon with swelling and edema of the adjacent tendon (*black arrowhead*).

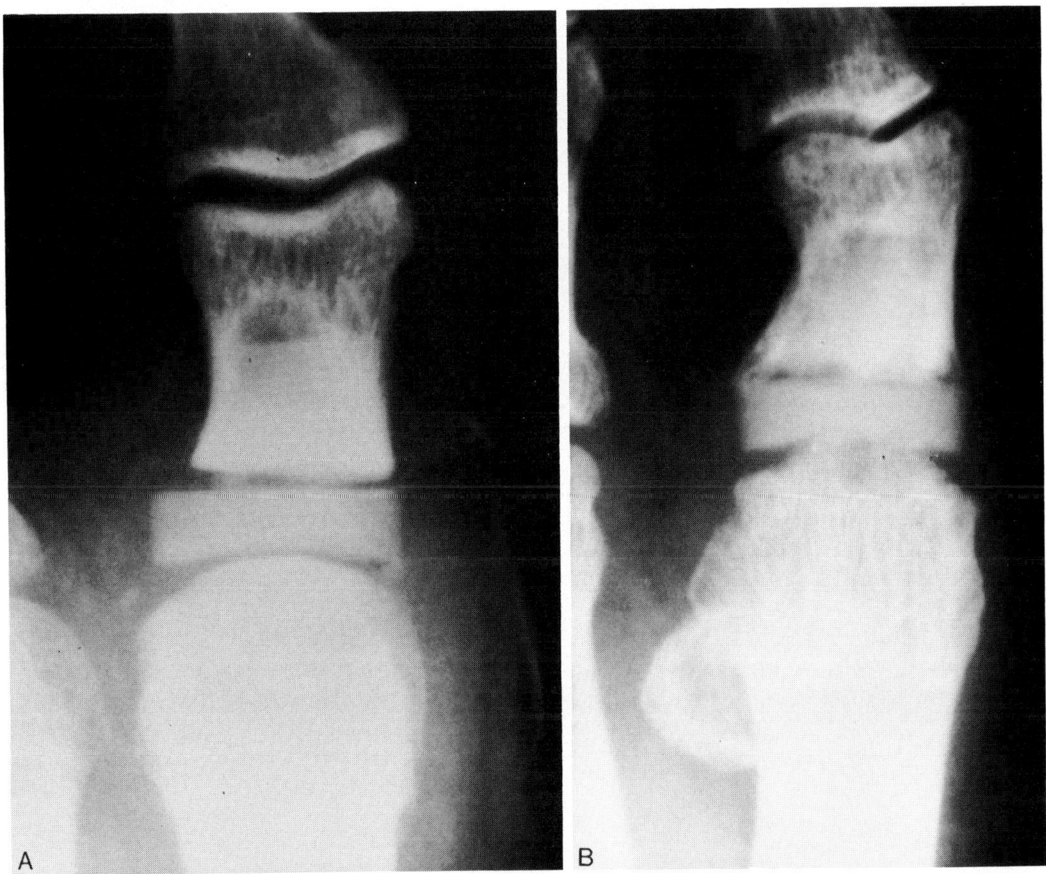

FIGURE 21–9. Osteomyelitis following a joint implant in the left first metatarsophalangeal joint. *A*, The initial postoperative film shows the normal appearance of the implant. *B*, One month later, there is periarticular osteoporosis in the distal first metatarsal and early bone destruction on both sides of the joint implant (surgically confirmed).

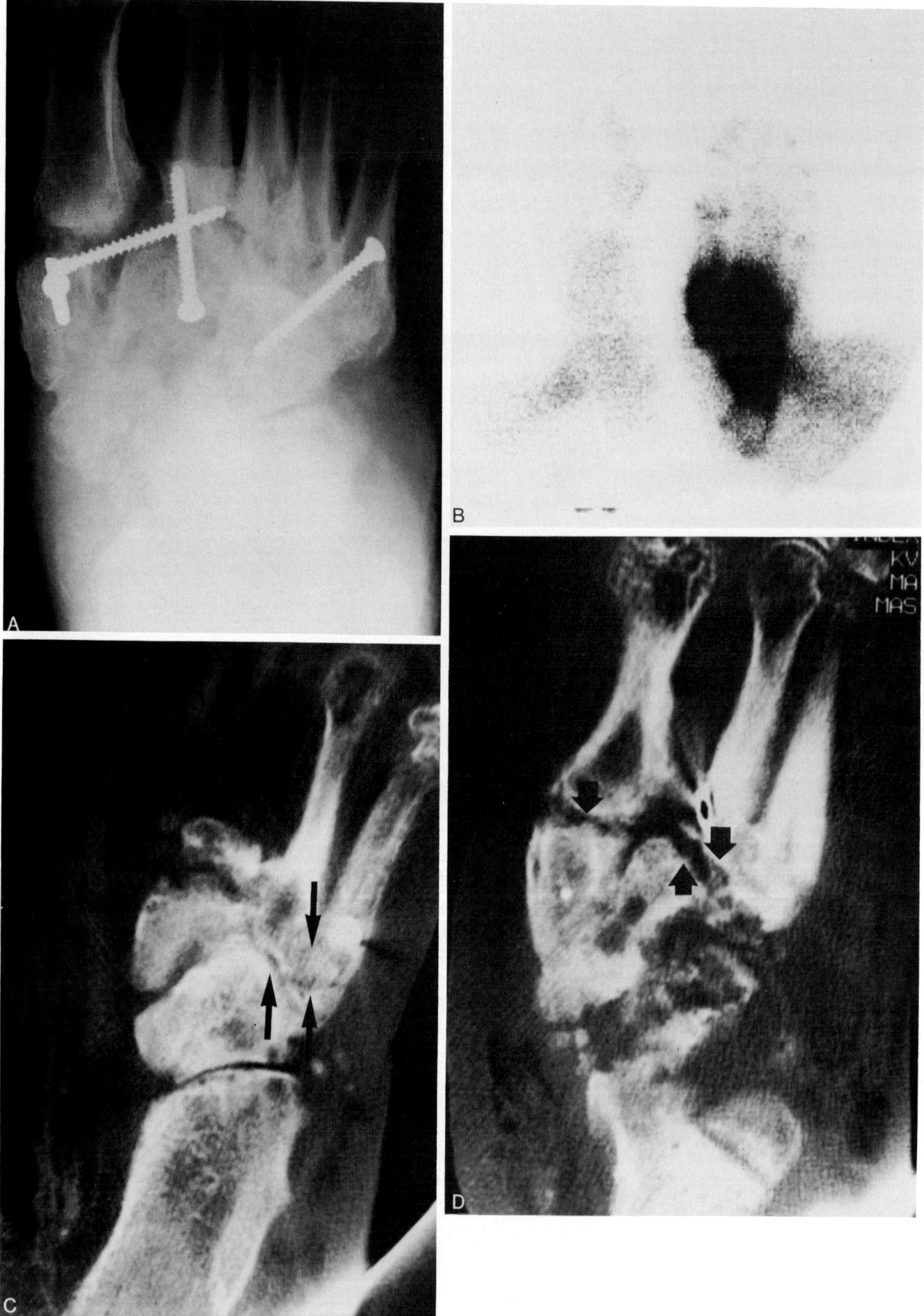

FIGURE 21–10. Postoperative osteomyelitis. *A,* Plain radiograph shows postoperative changes with extensive soft tissue swelling and loss of definition of the bony cortices. *B,* The bone scan shows diffusely increased uptake in the midfoot. *C* and *D,* Computed tomography scans demonstrate areas of intact fusion laterally (*arrows*) and also demonstrate the extent of bone destruction and articular involvement by osteomyelitis in the more medial portion of the midfoot (*thick arrows*).

Radionuclide Imaging

Since the development of the Anger camera made radionuclide imaging of the skeleton feasible, numerous radiopharmaceutical agents have been proposed for imaging pathologic conditions of the bones. These include fluorine (^{18}F), strontium (^{85}Sr), and indium chloride (^{111}InCl^2). These are currently of historic interest only. Currently, radiopharmaceuticals in active use for bone scanning include technetium (^{99m}Tc)-labeled phosphate compounds, gallium (^{67}Ga) citrate, and indium (^{111}In)-labeled white blood cells (WBCs).[52–54]

The first description of technetium-labeled phosphate compounds for bone scanning was described in 1971 by Subramanian and McAfee.[54] Although various phosphate analogues have been used, including pyrophosphate and polyphosphate compounds, the most widely used technetium-labeled bone-scanning pharmaceutical is currently methylene diphosphonate (MDP). Initial uptake of technetium-labeled phosphate compounds into the bone is thought to occur by chemiabsorbtion to the hydroxyapatite crystal matrix in the bone with subsequent integration into the structure of the calcified osteoid.[55, 56] Factors leading to increased uptake in pathologic bone include (1) increased metabolic activity resulting in increased formation of osteoid; (2) increased mineralization of formed osteoid; and (3) increased blood flow to the bone whether mediated by local metabolic factors or regional sympathetic neurologic dysfunction.[57, 58]

^{99m}Tc-MDP is an ideal radiopharmaceutical for imaging. The 6-hour half-life results in low doses to the total body as well as to the critical organs, the kidneys, and bladder, and the 140-KeV photon is ideally suited to currently available Anger cameras. MDP has a rapid rate of soft tissue and blood pool clearance with very high target-to-nontarget ratios 3 hours after intravenous administration. Although imaging may be performed only on a delayed basis, in the setting of inflammatory disease, a two- or three-phase examination is commonly performed. This technique was proposed to be more specific for osteomyelitis by early investigators.[59, 60] The technique involves an injection of 15 to 20 mCi of ^{99m}Tc-MDP as a bolus, during which dynamic images are obtained at 2- to 4-second intervals over the affected extremity, with the unaffected extremity also in the field of view for comparison (dynamic flow phase). The second, or blood pool, phase is obtained approximately 10 minutes after injection (Fig. 21–11). The third, or delayed, phase is generally obtained 3 to 4 hours after injection of the radiopharmaceutical. Whereas the normal bone scan results in symmetrical appearance on all three phases, in the presence of active infection or inflammation, the first, or dynamic, phase will show increased as well as more rapid appearance of activity in the affected extremity. In the presence of cellulitis, there will also be increased activity in the blood pool or the second phase and diffusely increased activity in the bone on the third phase presumably as a result of hyperemia. With osteomyelitis, the appearance is similar to cellulitis except that on the third phase there is focal increased uptake in the affected bone presumably because of abnormal bone turnover superimposed on the generalized increase resulting from increased blood flow. This increased uptake in the third phase is not seen with cellulitis and therefore helps distinguish bone infection from soft tissue infection.

Sensitivity of the three-phase bone scan is generally acknowledged to be quite high (in the range of 90% to 100%).[59–62] A lower range of sensitivity (as low as 70%) has been reported in children and in patients with peripheral vascular disease.[63–65]

More recently, the addition of a 24-hour delayed image (a fourth phase) to the bone scan has been proposed as a way of increasing specificity and therefore diagnostic accuracy.[62–66] Israel and coworkers postulated that the further increase in target-to-nontarget ratio seen on the 24-hour image may be partially due to a further decrease in background activity as well as progressive increased accumulation of ^{99m}Tc-MDP at the site of infection. They postulated that this is caused by the presence of woven bone surrounding the focus of osteomyelitis.[65]

One problem with the ^{99m}Tc-MDP bone scan is lack of specificity. Increased uptake on three or four phases of the bone scan, although typical for osteomyelitis, can also occur in other noninfectious processes such as Paget's disease, vascular disease, primary or metastatic tumors, and even in acute or subacute healing fractures.[60, 66, 67] An additional problem arises in rare cases of osteomyelitis that result in focal areas of decreased activity on the bone scan: "cold" osteomyelitis (Fig. 21–12).[64, 68, 69] The cold appearance is presumably due to decreased blood flow to the infected focus caused by occlusion of the end vessels from spread of infection through the haversian canals, ischemia secondary to increased intramedullary pressure resulting from accumulation of pus within the medullary space, or secondary thrombophlebitis.[69]

In clinical situations in which osteomyelitis or septic arthritis is suspected and radiographs and ^{99m}Tc-MDP bone scan are not diagnostic, imaging with ^{67}Ga citrate may be helpful (Fig. 21–13). Gallium is chemically an iron analogue that has been shown to localize to inflammatory and some neoplastic tissues.[70] The mechanism of localization of gallium to inflammatory lesions is not entirely clear but appears to be multifactorial. Gallium has been shown to bind actively to WBCs, particularly polymorphonuclear neutrophils (PMNs), which then migrate to the site of inflammation.[71] Gallium has also been shown to accumulate actively in some bacteria, particularly *S. aureus*.[72] As an iron analog, gallium binds to iron transport proteins in the serum, particularly transferrin, haptoglobulin, and lactoferrin, compounds that are also found to accumulate at sites of inflammation.[73]

^{67}Ga has a physical half-life of 78 hours and a lengthy biologic half-life, with two thirds of the administered dose being retained in the body for a prolonged period, predominantly in the liver, spleen, bone marrow, salivary, and lacrimal glands. One third of the dose is excreted by the bowel, which is the critical organ. Because of the long biologic and physical half-life and relatively high expense of this cyclotron-produced radiopharmaceutical, the adult dose is approximately 5 mCi. Gallium is not an ideal imaging agent for modern nuclear imaging equipment because of the low dose and multiple energy peaks (93, 184, 296, and 388 KeV), which require use of a high-energy collimator, further decreasing the count rate. Imaging is generally performed 24 and 48 hours after intravenous administration, although delayed images at 72 and even 96 hours may be obtained if further reduction in background tissue activity is desired.

The first articles describing the use of ^{67}Ga imaging for osteomyelitis compared the gallium images with correspond-

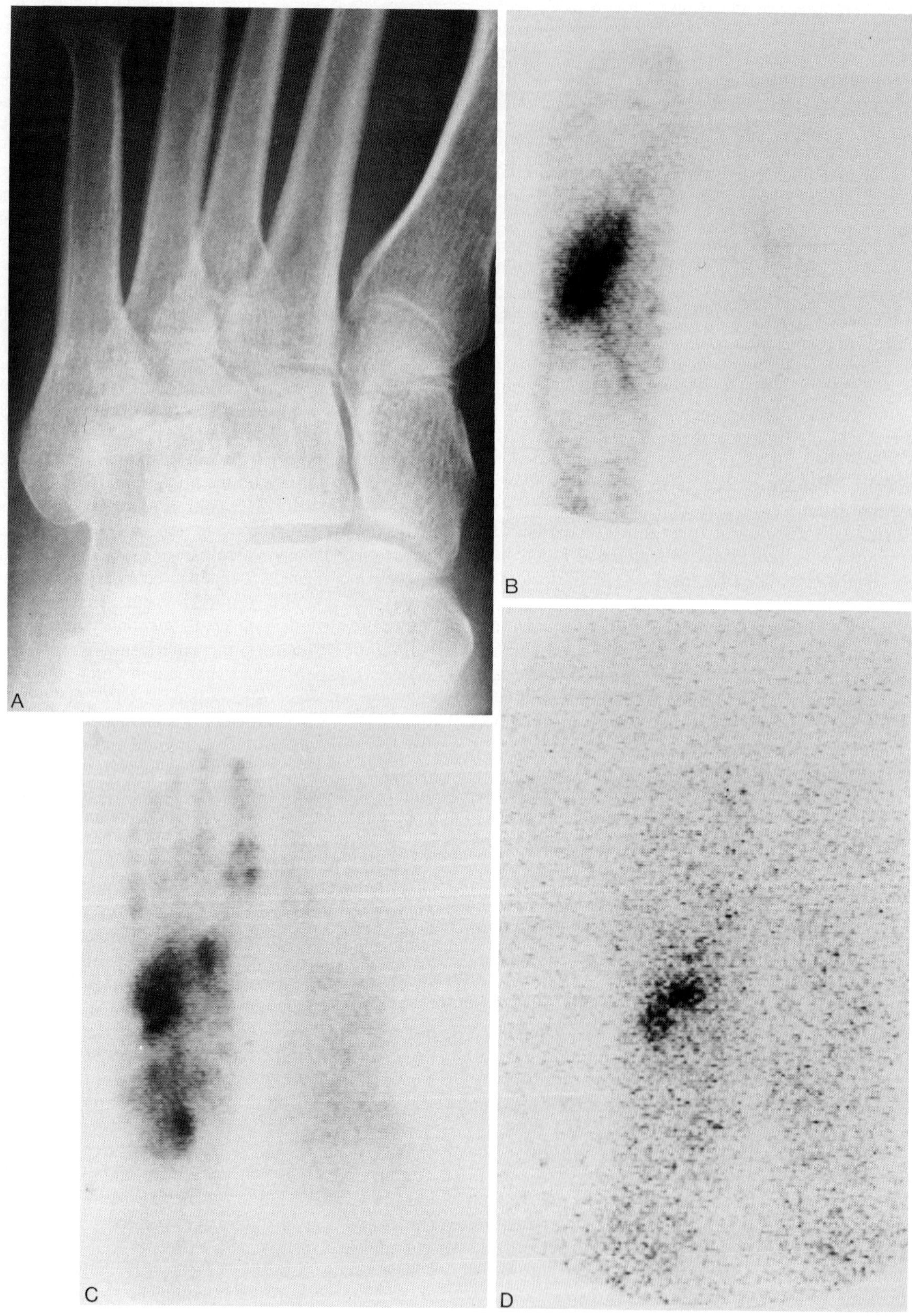

FIGURE 21–11. Osteomyelitis complicating a puncture wound. *A,* The results of plain radiographs are normal. Bone scan blood pool (*B*) and delayed images (*C*) demonstrate focal uptake in the cuboid. *D,* ^{111}In-white blood cell scan confirms osteomyelitis. (Courtesy of Felix Wang, M.D., Orange, CA.)

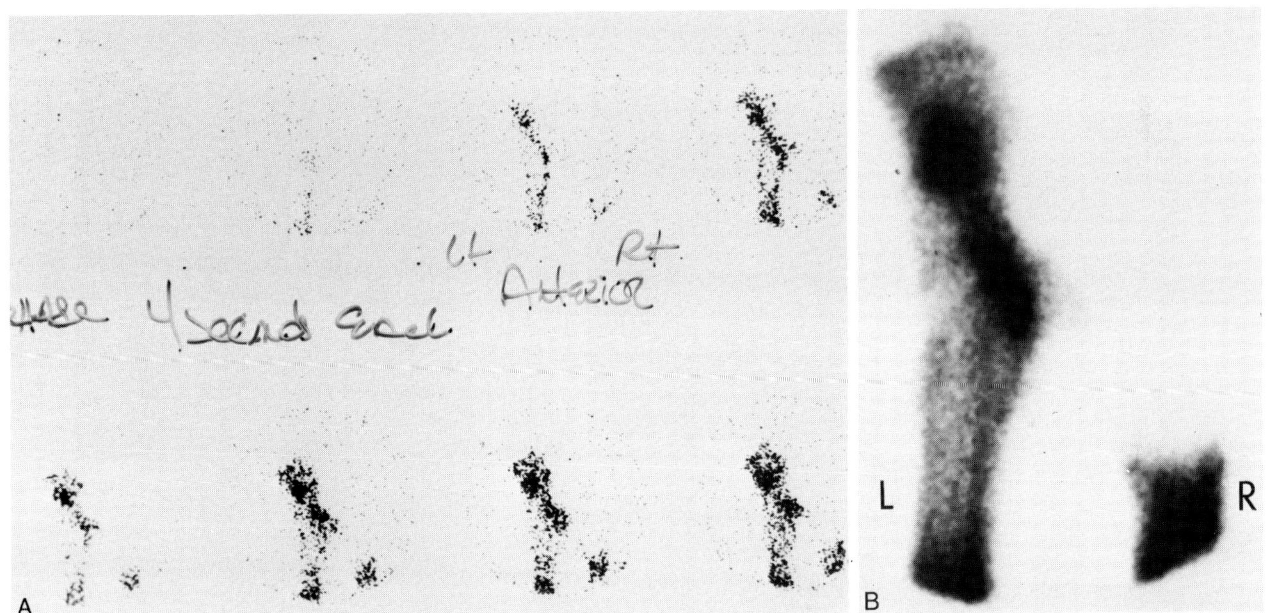

FIGURE 21–12. *A* and *B*, Bone scan images of gangrene of the right foot. Although dynamic (*A*) and delayed (*B*) images appear to show increased flow and uptake in the left foot, clinically, there was cellulitis of the left foot and gangrene of the right foot. An absence of blood flow below the ankle results in a ''cold'' bone scan.

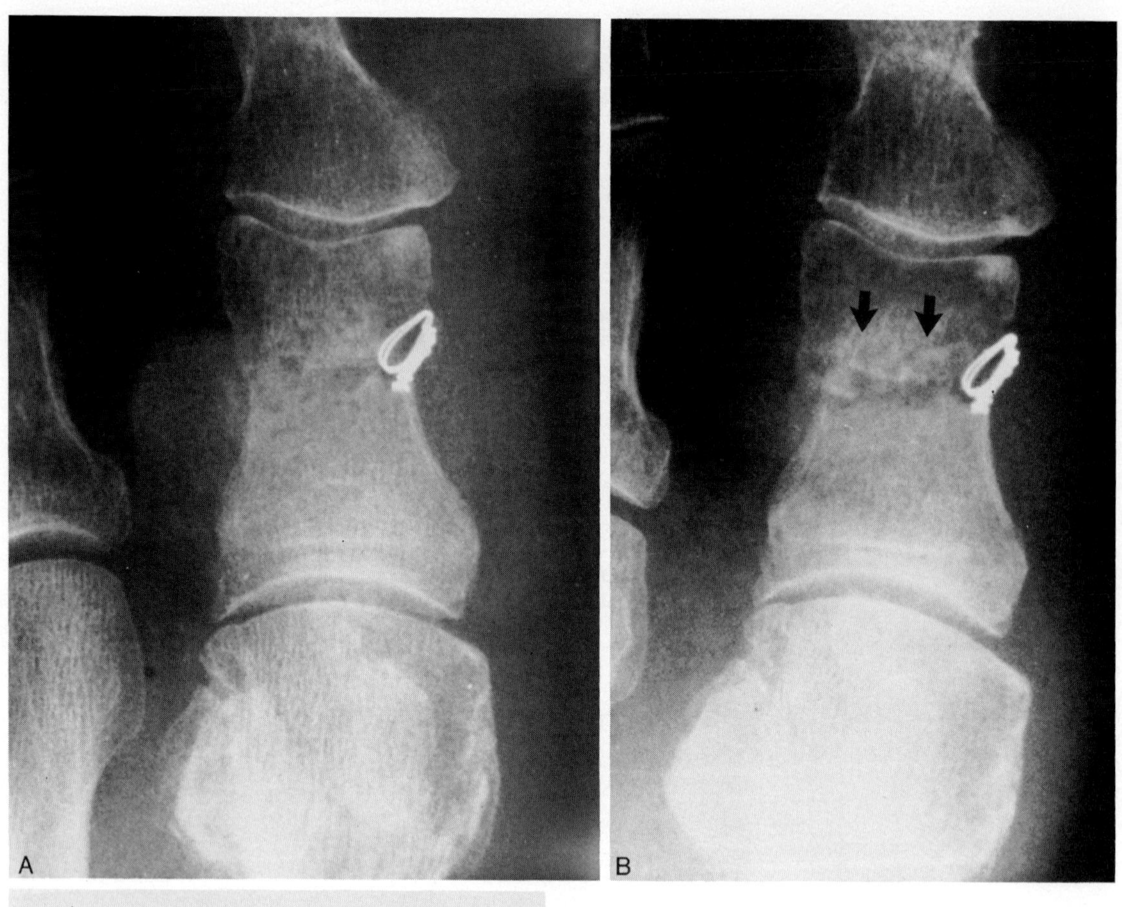

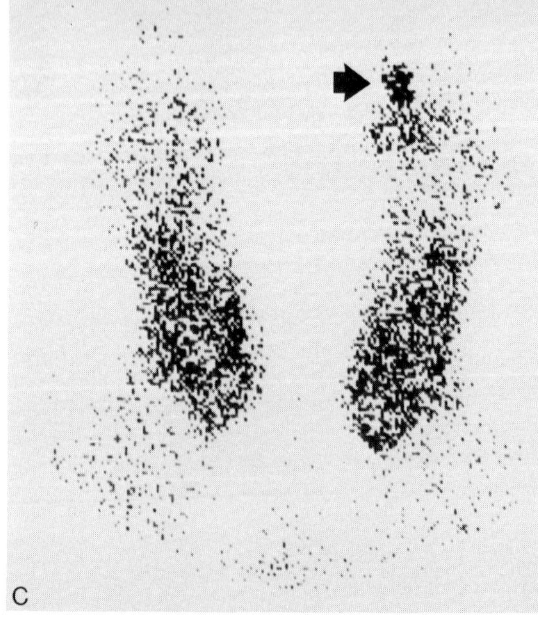

FIGURE 21–13. Postoperative osteomyelitis following osteotomy. *A,* Initial radiograph with early healing of the osteotomy site in the first proximal phalanx. *B,* Two weeks later, there is bone resorption with widening of the osteotomy site and adjacent sclerosis (*arrows*) due to attempted healing. *C,* Gallium scan (*thick arrow*) and subsequent surgery confirmed the osteomyelitis. (Courtesy of Nicholas Grumbine, D.P.M., Fullerton, CA.)

ing ^{99m}Tc-MDP bone scans, a strategy that is still used. Lisbona and Rosenthall[73] studied 40 patients, of whom almost half were children, and described four patterns of radiopharmaceutical uptake, comparing these patterns with the final clinical diagnosis:

1. In patients with negative ^{99m}Tc-MDP and negative ^{67}Ga scan results, there were no cases of active osteomyelitis.
2. Of the patients with a positive result from a gallium scan but without focal accumulation on the MDP bone scan, some had cases of cellulitis and one patient had cellulitis and underlying osteomyelitis.
3. In the group having a focally positive result from an MDP bone scan but a negative gallium scan result, there were no cases of active osteomyelitis.
4. The largest group, having both a focally positive result from an MDP scan and a focally positive gallium scan result, included 16 patients with active osteomyelitis, 6 with septic arthritis, and 3 with unspecified disorders (Fig. 21–14; see also Fig. 21–13).[31]

The same investigators used a similar combined bone scan and gallium scan approach in differentiating infection from loosening in patients with implanted orthopedic devices.[74] Because gallium accumulates to a small extent in normal bone, acting as bone-scanning agent, they introduced the concept of congruence (i.e., for a gallium scan to be considered positive for osteomyelitis, the relative amount of uptake in the abnormal versus normal area should be greater than the relative uptake of bone-scanning agent in the same abnormal versus normal areas). Glynn, however, described a case of marked gallium uptake in a noninfected Charcot's joint.[75] It appears, therefore, that although gallium uptake is somewhat nonspecific, marked gallium uptake must be considered evidence of osteomyelitis until proven otherwise.[76–78] To determine objectively whether there is congruent uptake, some laboratories define regions of interest over normal and abnormal areas using computer-acquired images and calculate a mathematical ratio. In patients with proven osteomyelitis, sequential gallium imaging has been shown to be useful in assessing the success of antibiotic therapy.[78, 79] Decreased gallium uptake is suggestive of successful therapy. The question remains as to whether a return to normal is necessary before antibiotic therapy is discontinued.

Because of the somewhat nonspecific nature of gallium uptake, imaging with radioisotope-labeled WBCs has been suggested as a more specific marker of infection.[80] Although methods have been described for labeling WBCs with technetium,[81, 82] most laboratories prefer the use of ^{111}In with its 67-hour physical half-life. The technique involves withdrawing approximately 50 ml of the patient's own blood into a tube containing anticoagulant, selectively precipitating the erythrocytes and then incubating the leukocyte-rich plasma with ^{111}In-oxime. The isotope diffuses through the cell membranes and binds to intracellular components. The labeled leukocytes are then washed and reinjected into the patient. The entire labeling procedure takes approximately 2 hours. Imaging may be performed at 24 hours, by which time virtually all of the blood pool activity is gone. Physiologic uptake is seen in the spleen, liver, and, to a lesser extent, the bone marrow. Because of the expense of the cyclotron-pro-

bone marrow. Because of the expense of the cyclotron-produced isotope, fairly long physical half-life, and normal accumulation in the spleen, the usual adult dose is in the range of 500 Ci. This low dose, combined with the relatively high energies of the isotope (172 to 247 KeV), results in fairly low count rates in the acquired images. In addition, if a ^{99m}Tc-MDP scan is performed at the same time, there may be some spill over of technetium activity into the indium window because of summation artifact.

Early reports in the use of ^{111}In-WBC for diagnosis of osteomyelitis were encouraging (Fig. 21–15; see also Fig. 21–11). Schauwecker reported a sensitivity of 100% in detection of acute osteomyelitis with a specificity of 96%.[83] They did, however, note a much lower (60%) sensitivity of ^{111}In-WBC in chronic osteomyelitis. Al-sheikh, and colleagues reported a sensitivity of 80% and a specificity of 75%, similar to that reported for gallium.[84] Additional studies confirmed the sensitivity of ^{111}In-WBC scans in the range of 75% to 97%, with a specificity of 56% to 82% for osteomyelitis, which is somewhat better than expected for gallium scanning. These studies also confirmed the lower sensitivity of ^{111}In-WBC scanning in chronic osteomyelitis.[84–88] False-positive results have been reported in noninfected healing fractures, myositis ossificans, heterotopic bone formation, and noninfected bone infarcts, particularly in sickle-cell disease.[89–91] Several authors suggested the addition of bone marrow imaging with ^{99m}Tc-sulfur colloid to improve the specificity of ^{111}In-WBC scans in patients with sickle-cell disease or orthopedic implants.[92–94]

The decision as to which radionuclide imaging technique to use for diagnosis of osteomyelitis or septic arthritis in a patient in whom plain radiographs are negative or nonspecific can be a daunting one. This decision is further complicated by the recent addition of MRI to the armamentarium of the clinician treating the lower extremity.

Magnetic Resonance Imaging

In the last 10 years, MRI has become a mainstay in imaging of the musculoskeletal system.[95–97] Using high-field-strength magnets and specialized orthopedic or surface coils, high-resolution imaging of the lower extremity is routinely feasible with section thicknesses of 3 mm or less, allowing exquisite resolution of small soft tissue and bony structures.[98–100] A full discussion of the physics of MRI is beyond the scope of this chapter. A number of excellent texts are available for a full description of the technique.[101–103] MRI uses no ionizing radiation. Images are generated by the resonation of hydrogen protons within the patient, who is placed into a high-strength magnetic field. Characteristics of the MRI depend on the chemical environment of the hydrogen protons and imaging protocol selected by the operator. Normal bone marrow and subcutaneous fat, which contain large amounts of lipid-bound hydrogen, are bright on T_1-weighted images (T1WI), diminishing in signal intensity on conventional spin echo. On T_2-weighted images (T2WI) with new fast spin echo sequences, fat may remain high in signal intensity on T2WI, and often these sequences are performed using fat saturation to diminish the signal from fat and thereby differentiate fat from fluid or edema. Fluid collections have the opposite characteristic, being of low signal on

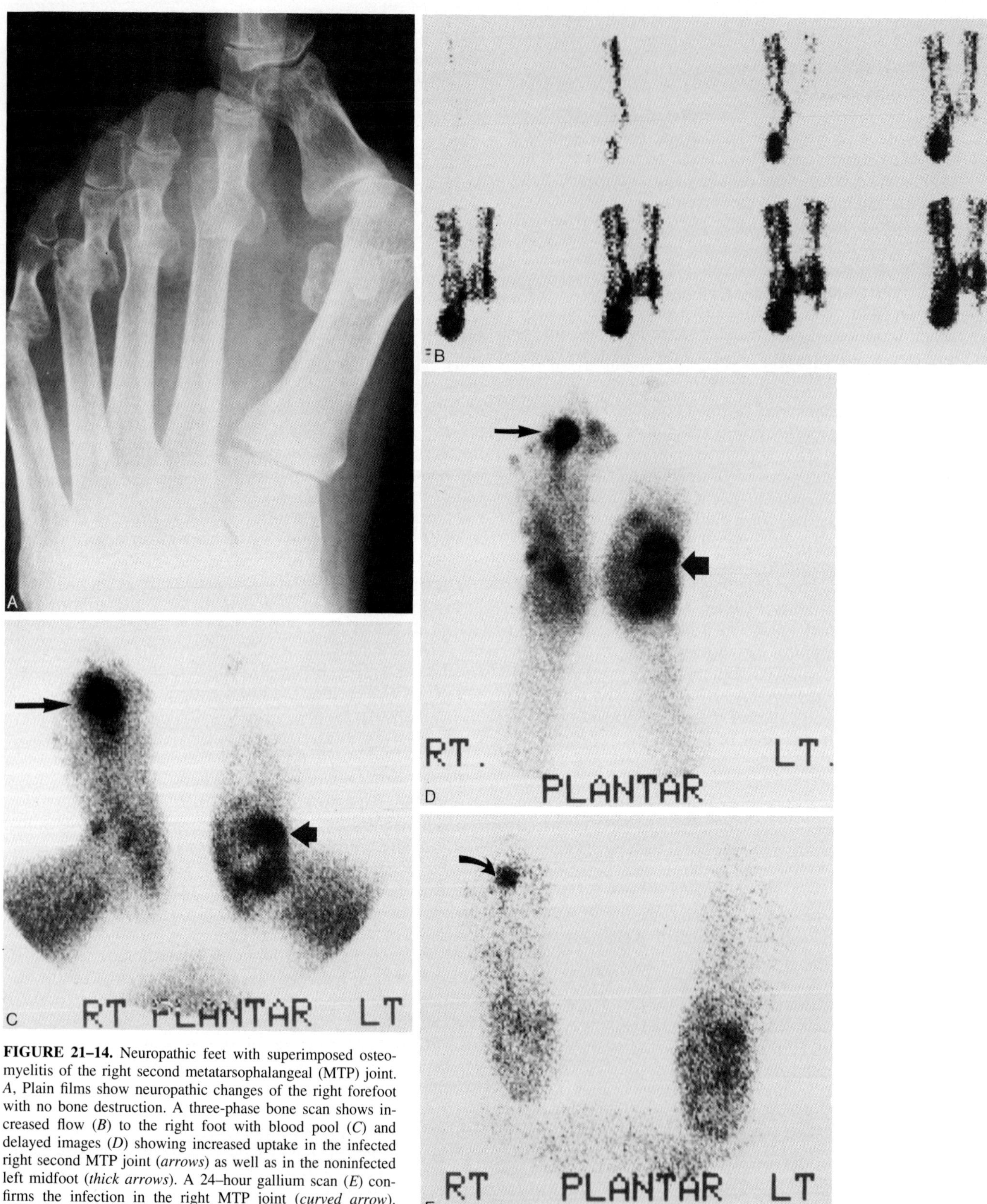

FIGURE 21–14. Neuropathic feet with superimposed osteomyelitis of the right second metatarsophalangeal (MTP) joint. *A,* Plain films show neuropathic changes of the right forefoot with no bone destruction. A three-phase bone scan shows increased flow (*B*) to the right foot with blood pool (*C*) and delayed images (*D*) showing increased uptake in the infected right second MTP joint (*arrows*) as well as in the noninfected left midfoot (*thick arrows*). A 24–hour gallium scan (*E*) confirms the infection in the right MTP joint (*curved arrow*). Mildly increased uptake in the left midfoot is less than would be expected from the bone scan if infection were present and represents the ''bone scanning'' property of gallium.

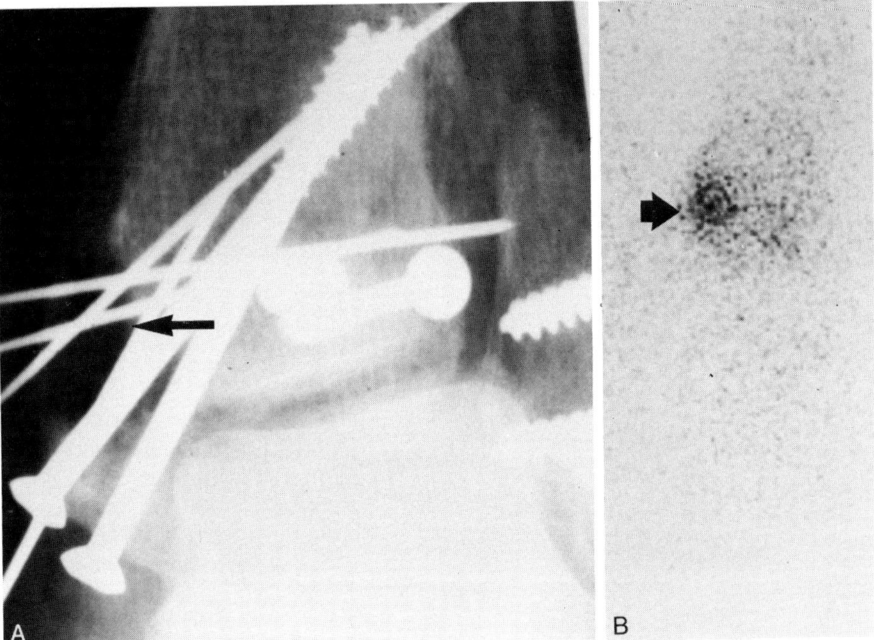

FIGURE 21–15. Postoperative osteomyelitis. *A,* A focal area of lucency at the operative site in the medial malleolus (*arrow*). This area should be checked for osteomyelitis. *B,* ^{111}In-white blood cell scan with increased activity in the medial malleolus (*thick arrow*) confirms osteomyelitis. (Courtesy of Felix Wang, M.D., Orange, CA.)

T1WI and increasing in signal on T2WI. Muscle, proteinaceous fluid, and many soft tissue masses are of intermediate signal intensity on both T1WI and T2WI. Cortical bone, calcification, and dense fibrous tissue, containing very few free hydrogen protons, have a low signal intensity on all pulse sequences. Pathologic conditions including infection and neoplasm often result in increased extracellular water content, causing decreased signal on T1WI and increased signal on T2WI.[104–106] MRI characteristics of infection of the extremities have been described by several authors (see Figs. 21–12 and 21–13).[107–109]

In the case of acute osteomyelitis involving the medullary bone cavity, there is decreased signal in the normally bright bone marrow on T1WI, which then, because of an increase in free extracellular water or edema, increases in brightness on T2 sequences. When there is involvement of the cortex, the normally black cortical bone is interrupted by areas of increased signal. Often the adjacent soft tissue edema is manifested by distortion of the normal anatomy and increased signal on T2WI (see Fig. 21–8).

Chronic osteomyelitis is described in the previously listed sources as being inhomogeneous with zones of both increased and decreased signal intensity. Intraosseous (Brodie's) abscess is of intermediate signal intensity on T1WI, becoming brighter on T2WI consistent with the proteinaceous fluid content. Sequestra, involucra, and sinus tracts are of low to intermediate signal intensity on T1WI, without significant increase on T2WI, consistent with a largely fibrous component. Surgical scars and old fractures are likewise of low signal intensity on all sequences.

Septic arthritis is manifested by distention of the joint capsule, which is filled with fluid (low on T1WI, bright on T2WI). The appearance of infectious tenosynovitis on MRI is of a low-signal-intensity tendon surrounded by a "halo" of fluid that is of low intensity on the T1WI but increases markedly on the T2WI (Fig. 21–16). MRI is not, however, able to differentiate infected from sympathetic, noninfected effusions. In septic arthritis, the signal of the adjacent bone marrow is normal unless there is complicating osteomyelitis. When there is superimposed osteomyelitis, changes in the medullary and cortical bone are present as described previously.

Healing inactive osteomyelitis results in a gradual return of the normal bone marrow signal on both T1WI and T2WI (see Fig. 21–8). Healed septic arthritis often results in marked thinning of the articular cartilage with secondary joint-space narrowing. Often subchondral sclerosis is manifested as a zone of decreased signal in the subchondral bone on T1WI.

Soft tissue abscesses appear as focal, well-marginated fluid collections with increased signal on T2WI, although the degree of increased signal intensity depends on the protein content of the exudate. Septa, debris, or fluid levels may be present (see Fig. 21–8). Cellulitis appears as an ill-defined zone of increased signal intensity on T2WI, infiltrating and distorting normal fat planes and in some cases the muscle planes. When infection or edema extends into the subcutaneous fat, there is a decrease of the normal fat signal on the T1WI.

Caution must be observed in interpreting MRI in patients with other types of marrow-occupying disease such as anemias (e.g., sickle-cell disease), malignancy, or glycogen storage disease such as Gaucher's disease because the bone marrow signal in these diseases may mimic infection.[110]

In the series reported by Unger and associates,[109] of the 35 patients evaluated, 33 also had delayed-phase ^{99m}Tc-MDP bone scans. In the diagnosis of osteomyelitis, the sensitivity and specificity of MRI were 92% and 96%, respectively, with an overall accuracy of 94%. For bone scintigraphy, sensitivity and specificity were 82% and 65%, respectively, with an overall accuracy of 71%. The series by Beltran,[107] and Tang[108] and their coauthors were smaller, with a lower percentage of patients having corresponding bone scans; however, the authors suggested an increased sensitivity and spec-

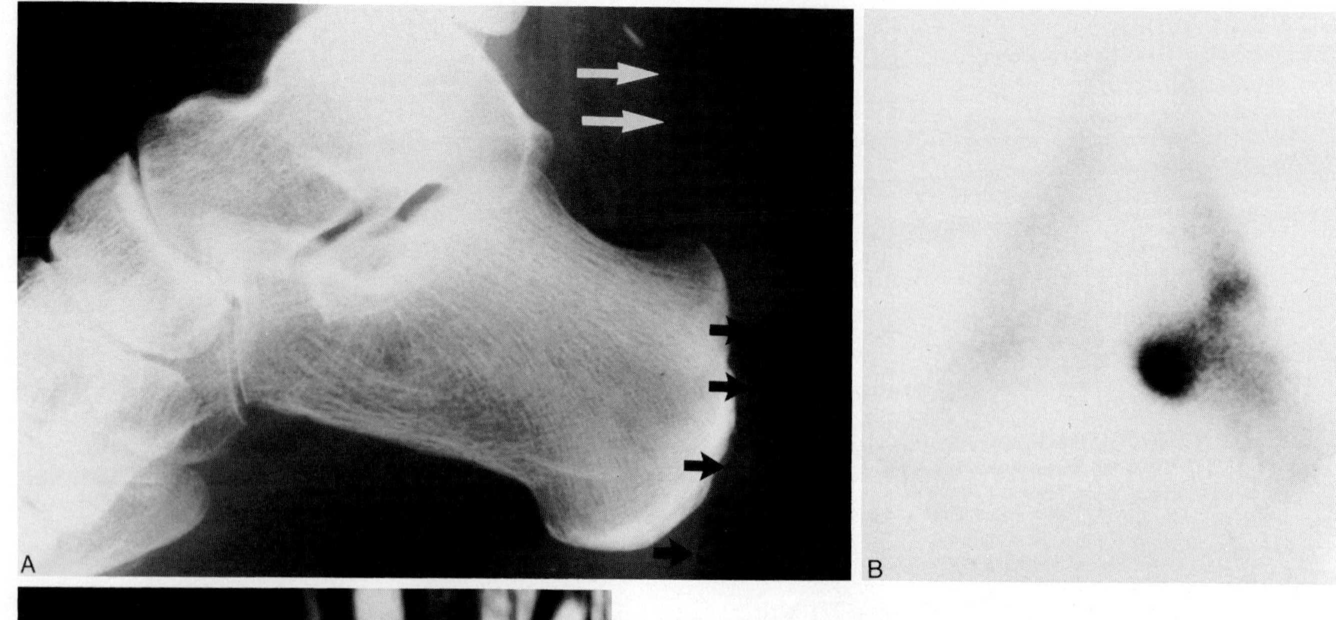

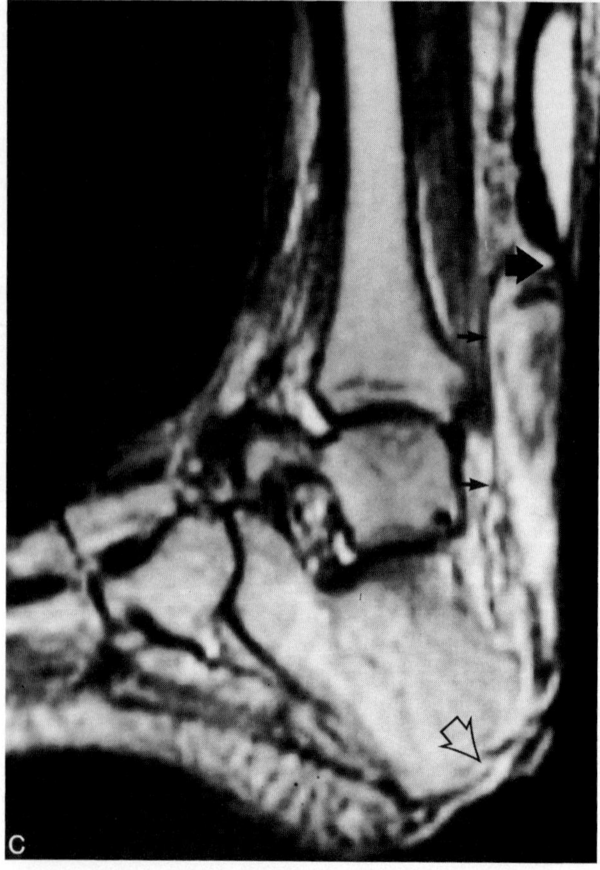

FIGURE 21–16. Diabetic with a soft tissue ulcer. *A,* A plain radiograph shows a large calcaneal ulcer (*black arrows*) and air (*white arrows*) in the soft tissues adjacent to the Achilles tendon. *B,* Bone scan shows focal uptake in the calcaneus. *C,* Sagittal T$_2$-weighted magnetic resonance images show invasion of the calcaneus (*open arrow*) and an extensive soft tissue abscess (*small arrows*) extending up the Achilles tendon with inflammatory rupture of the tendon (*thick arrow*).

ificity of MRI. Experimental work in animals has been performed comparing MRI, three-phase ^{99m}Tc-MDP bone scanning, and ^{67}Ga scintigraphy in acute infection with *S. aureus.*[111] In this series, MRI had a sensitivity of 93% for detection of osteomyelitis, the same as three-phase bone scanning, but overall accuracy of MRI was slightly higher. MRI proved to be more accurate than either bone or gallium scanning in detecting soft tissue infection. Further, MRI proved to be 92% accurate in differentiating drainable abscess from cellulitis in animals with soft tissue infection, a distinction that could not be made at all with radionuclide studies. Two small studies have dealt specifically with MRI of clinical infection in the foot,[112, 113] and one of these[113] specifically deals with the diabetic patient. Although the series were small, the authors suggested a similar sensitivity for MRI compared with combined ^{99m}Tc-MDP and gallium scintigraphy, both of which are markedly more sensitive than plain films and somewhat more sensitive that ^{111}In-WBC scanning. There was a significantly greater number of false-positive diagnoses with radionuclide imaging techniques compared with MRI in these patients, probably as a result of previous infection, trauma, and neuropathic bone disease in this clinical population.

PRACTICAL APPLICATIONS

The Diabetic Foot. It has been estimated that 10% of the 11 million Americans with diabetes will experience podiatric complications (Figs. 21–4, 21–15 to 21–17). More than 20% of all hospitalized diabetic patients are admitted for foot disorders.[114] The pathogenesis of osteomyelitis in the diabetic patient is through a contiguous spread of soft tissue infection. However, clinical and radiographic diagnosis is often complicated by the presence of angiopathy and neuropathy. Soft tissue changes secondary to ulceration may be appreciated radiographically. Gas present in the soft tissues may have dissected through an open ulceration or may be secondary to gas-forming organisms. Both aerobic as well as anaerobic organisms may produce gas. In the face of severe vascular compromise, clostridial organisms may produce gas gangrene with extensive gas formation and subsequent destruction of soft tissue. Interdigital infection may spread through soft tissue planes and sequester within the plantar compartments of the foot, producing a plantar space infection. Osseous demineralization as well as osteosclerosis, cortical thickening, and localized rarefaction are common radiographic findings. However, the distinction between neuroarthropathy and osteomyelitis still remains a diagnostic challenge despite technological advances in diagnostic imaging. MRI and CT are now the diagnostic modalities of choice if the bone scan is equivocal.

Postoperative Infection. After surgical insult to the soft tissues and osseous structures, early recognition of postoperative infection (see Figs. 21–13 and 21–15) is more difficult. Soft tissue swelling and osseous resorption are typical postoperative findings and may obscure the diagnosis and implementation of appropriate therapeutics. Resorptive changes both proximal and distal to the osteotomy site may be the only radiographic clues to an infective process. A high level of suspicion as well as clinical corroboration is most important in determining and differentiating typical postoperative changes from infectious complication. Corroboration of clinical suspicions with more advanced diagnostics (i.e., CT) will allow for appropriate diagnosis and interventional therapy if necessary.

Postoperative Infection After Implant Arthroplasty. Post operative infection with osteoarticular involvement after surgical implant arthroplasty (see Fig. 21–9) is of particular concern to the podiatric surgeon. An infection may occur from direct contamination from adjacent infected tissues or from direct inoculation from surrounding osseous and articular tissues at the time of surgery. Less frequently, these infections may arise from hematogenous spread to an operative site from a distant location.[115–117] A delay in diagnosis is not infrequent because the usual signs of infection are masked by concomitant tissue injury or by the effects of prophylactic antibiotics. Frequently, infective organisms may be of limited or indolent pathogenicity. Osseous and cartilaginous destruction, periostitis, soft tissue swelling, and lucency about the prothesis may be recognized.

Septic Arthritis. Small soft tissue defects, swelling, and gas formation, as well as osteomyelitis with typical meta-physeal destruction originating extraarticularly, may present as general evidence of an infective process (see Fig. 21–5). Joint-space narrowing and marginal as well as central osseous erosion of the metatarsophalangeal joints or interphalangeal joints may be noted. Periostitis, fragmentation, and calcification may as well be observed. Synovial cysts and soft tissue destruction may lead to tendon injury, bony ankylosis, and degenerative bone disease.

Puncture Wounds. Puncture wounds in the plantar aspect of the foot are very common and may lead to osseous infection and septic arthritis (see Fig. 21–11). These injuries are predominantly seen in barefoot children. Infective organisms range among various gram-negative organisms because *Pseudomonas aeruginosa* is a common soil bacteria and is noted to be the most frequently cultured organism from an infection caused by puncture wounds.[118, 119] In addition, the wound must be inspected for the presence of retained foreign bodies as well. Soft tissue swelling, demineralization, and local lytic destruction in the absence of periosteal new bone formation may be evident radiographically.

Granulomatous Infection. This category includes congenital syphilis, tuberculous osteomyelitis, and coccidioidomycosis.

Congenital Syphilis. Transplacental migration of the treponema with subsequent invasion of perichondrium, periosteum, cartilage, bone marrow, and sites of active enchondral ossification, particularly in the metaphyseal region of tubular bone, is indicative of congenital syphilis (Fig. 21–18).[120] Periostitis, irregular destruction of the metaphyses, as well as widening of the epiphyseal plate are common radiographic findings.

Tuberculous Osteomyelitis. Virtually any bone in the foot may be affected by tuberculous osteomyelitis (Fig. 21–19)[121] Radiographically, an initial focus of osteolysis is accompanied by varying amounts of eburnation and periostitis. This focus is typically seen in the epiphysis, with the propensity for geographic cystic destruction. Occasionally, spread to the diaphysis with permeative or moth-eaten appearance is noted. Tuberculous dactylitis is seen in infants in whom multiple small bones of the feet are simultaneously involved, with diffuse soft tissue swelling of the involved digits. These radiographic findings are similar in sickle-cell dactylitis and syphilitic dactylitis.

Coccidioidomycosis. Pulmonary infection secondary to the fungus *Coccidioides immitis* is indigenous to the American Southwest and Mexico. Coccidioidomycosis may also include osseous involvement. Diaphyseal lesions in the feet are common, with a predilection for the calcaneus. Buckley and Barkus noted these lesions to be purely lytic. It is rare for reactive bone to be visualized as periosteal new bone formation or diffuse sclerosis.[122]

Viral Infection. Included in this classification are rubella infection and cytomegalovirus.

Rubella Infection (German Measles). Serious skeletal and nonskeletal alterations in the fetus may occur secondary to a maternal infection within the first trimester of pregnancy (Fig. 21–20). Radiographically, metaphyseal lesions in long bones occur, characterized by symmetrical linear areas of radiolucency as well as increased bone density, producing what has been determined to be a longitudinally oriented striated pattern (celery stalk appearance) with the absence of periostitis.

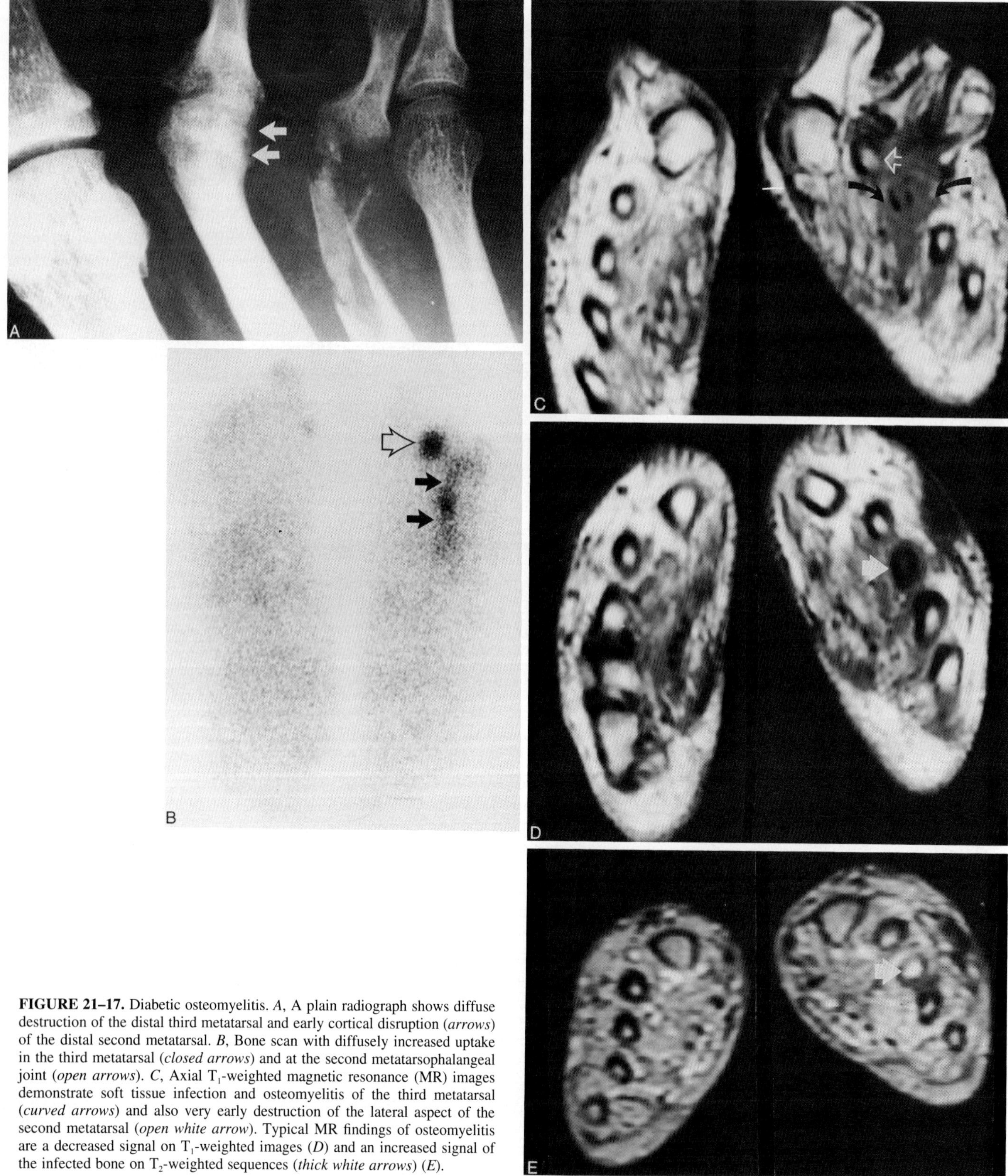

FIGURE 21–17. Diabetic osteomyelitis. *A*, A plain radiograph shows diffuse destruction of the distal third metatarsal and early cortical disruption (*arrows*) of the distal second metatarsal. *B*, Bone scan with diffusely increased uptake in the third metatarsal (*closed arrows*) and at the second metatarsophalangeal joint (*open arrows*). *C*, Axial T_1-weighted magnetic resonance (MR) images demonstrate soft tissue infection and osteomyelitis of the third metatarsal (*curved arrows*) and also very early destruction of the lateral aspect of the second metatarsal (*open white arrow*). Typical MR findings of osteomyelitis are a decreased signal on T_1-weighted images (*D*) and an increased signal of the infected bone on T_2-weighted sequences (*thick white arrows*) (*E*).

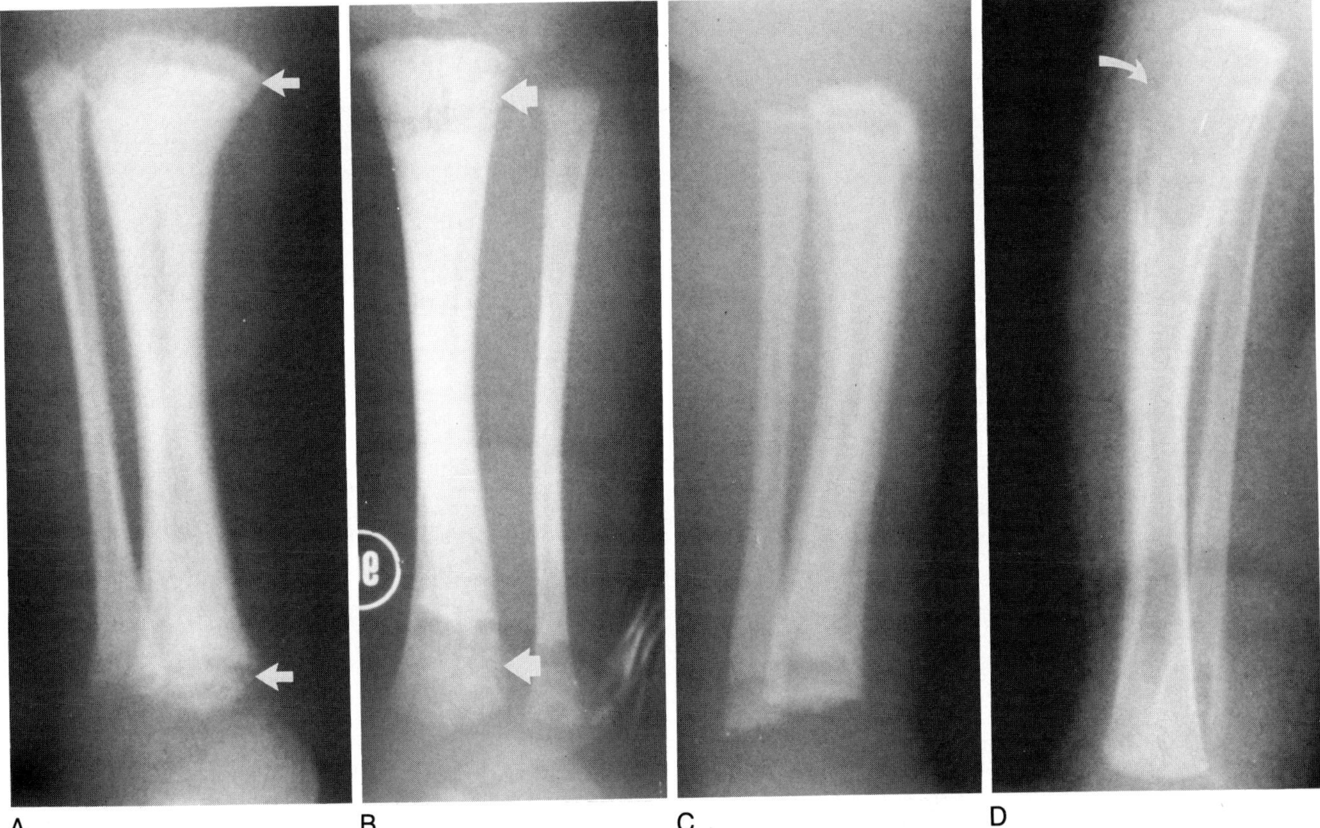

FIGURE 21–18. Variable appearance of congenital syphilis. *A*, Mild involvement with faint periosteal reaction and lucent ''metaphyseal band'' (*arrows*). *B*, Extensive metaphyseal involvement proximally and distally (*thick arrows*). *C*, Extensive periosteal reaction resulting in ''bone within a bone'' appearance. *D*, Corner metaphyseal destruction (Wimburger's sign) (*curved arrows*). (Courtesy of Joyce Pais, M.D., Orange, CA.)

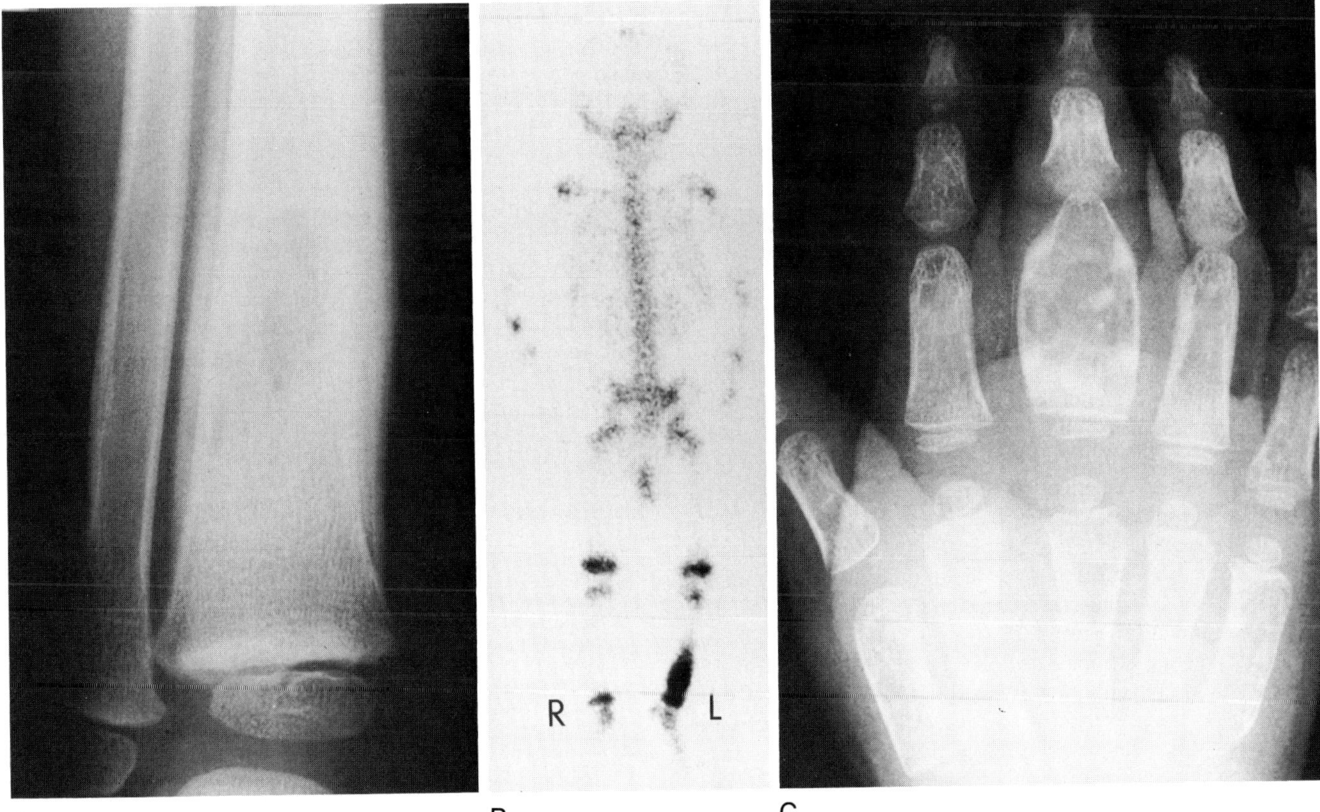

FIGURE 21–19. *A* to *C*, Tuberculous osteomyelitis. *A*, A 2-year-old patient with a 2-month history of a limp. Anteroposterior radiographs of the tibia demonstrate a focal area of destruction, diaphyseal widening, and periosteal reaction consistent with osteomyelitis. *B*, A bone scan obtained at the time of presentation shows an increased uptake of activity in the left tibia. *C*, Typical tuberculous dactylitis of the hand is also seen in this patient. (Courtesy of Scott Rowan, M.D., Orange, CA.)

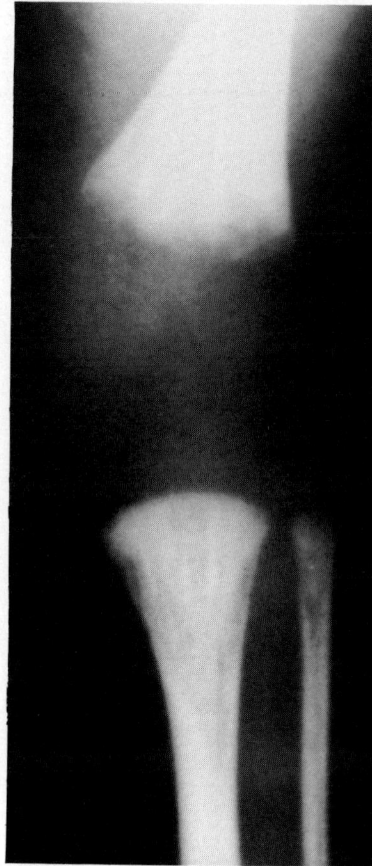

FIGURE 21–20. Congenital rubella. A longitudinal striated pattern is seen in the metaphyses of the femur and tibia.

Cytomegalovirus. Irregularity of the growth plate, a striated pattern parallel to the long axis of the bone similar to that seen with rubella, and metaphyseal osteopenia are associated with this disease. Spontaneous pathologic fractures have also been observed in infants with cytomegalovirus.[123, 124]

SUMMARY

As imaging of musculoskeletal infections of the lower extremity has become more accurate with the advent of multiple radiographic techniques and MRI, it is clear that the critical decision of which imaging modality to use in a given setting has become more difficult. Although plain films remain the mainstay of imaging, they have a fairly low sensitivity and specificity. Various imaging algorithms have been proposed ranging from the simple to complicated (Fig. 21–21).[69, 84, 124–126] Several common factors are present. A negative or nonspecific plain radiograph in the setting of clinically suspected infection should be followed by a three-phase ^{99m}Tc-MDP bone scan. A negative bone scan makes osteomyelitis unlikely, although it does not rule out soft tissue infection. In the presence of soft tissue infection, or if there is a high clinical suspicion of osteomyelitis despite the negative bone scan, correlative gallium scintigraphy or MRI may be suggested. In the presence of a positive bone scan result, gallium or WBC scintigraphy may be helpful in obtaining a specific diagnosis, especially if there are complicating factors

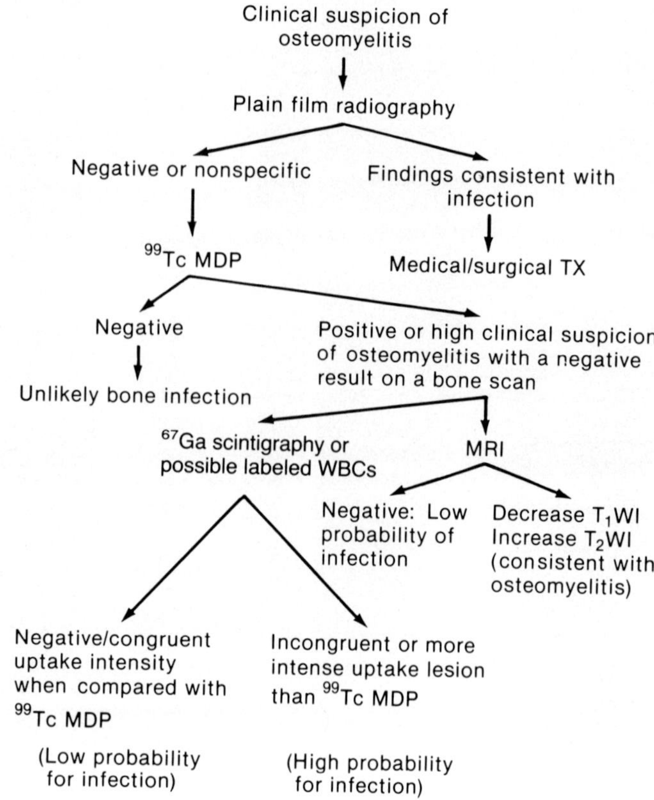

FIGURE 21–21. Proposed algorithm for decision making in diagnostic imaging for musculoskeletal infections of the lower extremity. MDP, methylene diphosphonate; TX, treatment; CT, computed tomography; T$_1$WI, T$_1$-weighted image.

such as previous surgery, trauma, or diabetes. Recently, ^{99m}Tc-labeled WBCs have gained popularity as an imaging modality. Images are obtained much sooner, with better resolution and less radiation exposure to the patient than with indium.[127] Even if the plain radiograph is positive and specific for osteomyelitis, MRI may be very useful in determining the extent of bone involvement before surgery and demonstrating associated cellulitis or drainable soft tissue abscess.

References

1. Elements NA (ed): Pathologie Chiurgical. Paris, Germer-ea. Bailliere, 1844–1859.
2. Hankings CA and Braunstein EM: Osteomyelitis imaging modalities and diagnostic approach. Postgrad Radiol 4:75–92, 1984.
3. Weinstein AJ: Osteomyelitis, microbiology, clinical and therapeutic considerations. J Primary Care 8:557–569, 1981.
4. Ruppert D, Barron BJ, and Madewell JE: Osteomyelitis acute and chronic. Radiol Clin North Am 25(6):1171–1201, 1987.
5. Resnick D and Niwayama G: Diagnosis of Bone and Joint Disorders, 2nd ed. Philadelphia, WB Saunders, 1988.
6. Steinbach HL: Infections of bone. Semin Roentgenol 4(1):337, 1966.
7. Whitehouse WM and Smith WS: Osteomyelitis of the feet. Semin Roentgenol 5(4):367, 1970.
8. Trueta J: The three types of acute hematogenous osteomyelitis: A clinical and vascular study. J Bone Joint Surg 41B:671, 1959.
9. Winters JL and Cahen I: Acute hematogenous osteomyelitis: A review of sixty-six cases. J Bone Joint Surg 42A:691, 1960.

10. Shandling B: Acute hematogenous osteomyelitis: A review of 300 cases treated during 1952–1959. S Afr Med J 34:520, 1960.

11. Waldvogel FA, Medoff G, and Swartz MN: Osteomyelitis: A review of clinical features, therapeutic considerations, and unusual aspects: I. N Engl J Med 282:198, 1970.

12. Mollan RAB and Piggot J: Acute osteomyelitis in children. J Bone Joint Surg 59B:2, 1977.

13. Brill PW, Winchester P, Krauss AN, and Symchych P: Osteomyelitis in a neonatal intensive care unit. Radiology 131:81, 1979.

14. Weissberg ED, Smith AL, and Smith DH: Clinical features of neonatal osteomyelitis. Pediatrics 53:505, 1974.

15. Green WT: Osteomyelitis in infancy. JAMA 105:1835, 1935.

16. Ogden JA and Lister G: The pathology of neonatal osteomyelitis. Pediatrics 55:474, 1975.

17. Dich VQ, Nelson JD, and Haltalin KC: Osteomyelitis in infants and children: A review of 163 cases. Am J Dis Child 129:1273, 1975.

18. Clarke AM: Neonatal osteomyelitis: A disease different from osteomyelitis of older children. Med J Aust 1:237, 1958.

19. Dalinka MK, Yeager BA, Velchik MG, et al: Infectious diseases. In Putman CE (ed): Textbook of Diagnostic Imaging. Philadelphia, WB Saunders, 1988, pp 1453–1474.

20. Garnett ES, Cockshott WP, and Jacobs J: Classical acute osteomyelitis with a negative bone scan. Br J Radiol 50:757–760, 1977.

21. Greenfield G: Radiology of Bone Diseases. Philadelphia, JB Lippincott, 1961, pp 265–279.

22. Murray IP: Photopenia and skeletal scintigraphy of suspected bone and joint infection. Clin Nucl Med 7:13–20, 1982.

23. Rosen RA, Morehouse HT, Karp HJ, and Yu GS: Intracortical fissuring in osteomyelitis. Radiology 141:17–20, 1981.

24. Garré C: Uber Besondere Formen und Folgezustande der akuten infektiosen osteomyelitis. Bruns Beitr Klin Chir 10:241, 1893.

25. Waldvogel FA, Medoff G, and Swartz MN: Osteomyelitis: A review of clinical features: Therapeutic considerations and unusual aspects: I. N Engl J Med 282:198, 1970.

26. Thoma KH and Goldman HM: Oral Pathology, 5th ed. St. Louis, CV Mosby, 1960, p 719.

27. Rabe WC, Angelillo JC, and Leipert DW: Chronic sclerosing osteomyelitis: Treatment consideration in an atypical case. Oral Surg 49:117, 1980.

28. Van Niekerk JP de V: Hand infections: Management and results based on a new classification—a study of more than 1000 cases. S Afr Med J, 40:316, 1966.

29. Kinnman JEG and Lee HS: Chronic osteomyelitis of the mandible: Clinical study of thirteen cases. Oral Surg 26:6, 1968.

30. Blumenfeld RJ and Skolnik EM: Intracranial complications of sinus disease. Trans Am Acad Ophthalmol Otolaryngol 70:899, 1966.

31. Waldvogel FA, Medoff G, and Swartz MN: Osteomyelitis: Review of clinical features, therapeutic considerations, and unusual aspects: II. N Engl J Med 282:260, 1970.

32. Francis DP, Holmes MA, and Brandon G: *Pasteurella multocida* infections after domestic animal bites and scratches. JAMA 233:42, 1975.

33. Hooper G: Tooth fragment in a metacarpophalangeal joint. Hand 10:215, 1978.

34. Lavine LS, Isenberg HD, Rubins W, and Berkman JI: Unusual osteomyelitis following superficial dog bites. Clin Orthop 98:251, 1974.

35. Chusid MJ, Jacobs WM, and Sty JR: *Pseudomonas* arthritis following puncture wounds of the foot. J Pediatr 94:429, 1979.

36. Miller EH and Semian DW: Gram-negative osteomyelitis following puncture wounds of the foot. J Bone Joint Surg 57A:535, 1975.

37. Tscherne H and Trentz O: Gelenkinfektionen nach perforierenden wunden, punktionen und injektioner. Langebecks Arch Cir 334:521, 1973.

38. Brand RA and Black H: *Pseudomonas* osteomyelitis following puncture wounds in children. J Bone Joint Surg 56A:1637, 1974.

39. Swischuk LE, Jorgenson F, Jorgenson A, and Caper D: Wooden splinter–induced "pseudotumors" and "osteomyelitis-like lesions" of the bone and soft tissue. Am J Roentgenol 122:176, 1974.

40. Koch SL: Osteomyelitis of the bones of the hand. Surg Gynecol Obstet 64:1, 1937.

41. Bonakdarpour A and Gaines VD: The radiology of osteomyelitis. Orthop Clin North Am 14(1):21, 1983.

42. Christman RA: Radiographic presentation of osteomyelitis in the foot. Clin Podiatr Med Surg 7(3):433–448, 1990.

43. Butt WP: The radiology of infection. Clin Orthop 96:20–30, 1973.

44. Solomon MA, Gilula LA, Oloff MN, et al: CT scanning of the foot and ankle: 1. Normal anatomy. Am J Roentgenol 146:1192–1203, 1986.

45. Dalinka MK, Lally JF, and Konwer G: The radiology of osseous and articular infection. CRC Radiol Nucl Med 7:1–64, 1975.

46. Solomon MA, Gilula LA, Oloff MN, et al: CT scanning of the foot and ankle: II. Clinical applications and review of the literature. Am J Roentgenol 146:1204–1214, 1986.

47. Sartoris DJ and Resnick D: Computed tomography of podiatric disorders: A review. J Foot Surg 25:394–403, 1986.

48. Wing VW, Jeffrey RB, Federle MP, et al: Chronic osteomyelitis examined by CT. Radiology 154:171–174, 1985.

49. Tumeh SS, Aliabadi P, Seltzer SE, et al: Chronic osteomyelitis: The relative roles of scintigrams, plain radiographs, and transmission computed tomography. J Clin Nucl Med 13:710–715, 1988.

50. Sharif HS, Clark DC, Aabed MY, et al: Mycetoma: Comparison of MR imaging with CT. Radiology 178:865–870, 1990.

51. Blau M, Nagler W, and Bender MA: Fluorine-18: A new isotope for bone scanning. J Nucl Med 3:332–334, 1962.

52. Charkes ND and Sklaroff DM: Early diagnosis of metastatic bone cancer by photo scanning with strontium-85. J Nucl Med 5:168–179, 1964.

53. Gilbert EH, Earle JD, Goris ML, et al: The accuracy of ^{111}In-Cl^3 as a bone marrow scanning agent. Radiology 119:167–168, 1976.

54. Subramanian G and McAfee JG: A new complex of ^{99m}Tc for skeletal imaging. Radiology 99:192–196, 1971.

55. Joans AD, Frances MD, and Davis MA: Bone scanning: Radionuclidic reaction mechanisms. Semin Nucl Med 6:3–18, 1976.

56. Charkes ND: Skeletal blood flow: Implications for bone-scan interpretation. J Nucl Med 21:91–98, 1980.

57. Wagner JW and Dewanjee MK: Drug induced modulation of ^{99m}Tc pyrophosphate tissue distribution: What is involved? J Nucl Med 6:555–559, 1981.

58. Gilday DL, Paul DJ, and Patterson J: Diagnosis of osteomyelitis in children by combined blood pool and bone imaging. Radiology 117:331–335, 1975.

59. Maurer AH, Chien DC, Camargo EE, et al: Utility of three-phase skeletal scintigraphy in suspected osteomyelitis: Concise communication. J Nucl Med 22:941–949, 1981.

60. Duszynski DO, Kuhn JP, Afshani E, et al: Early radionuclide diagnosis of acute osteomyelitis. Radiology 117:337–340, 1975.

61. Alazraki N, Dries D, Datz F, et al: Value of a twenty-four image (four-phase bone scan) in assessing osteomyelitis in patients with peripheral vascular disease. J Nucl Med 26:711–717, 1985.

62. Segall GM, Nino-Murcia M, Jacobs T, et al: The role of bone scan and radiography in the diagnostic evaluation of suspected pedal osteomyelitis. Clin Nucl Med 14:255–260, 1989.

63. Handmaker H: Acute hematogenous osteomyelitis: Has the bone scan betrayed us? Radiology 135:787–789, 1980.

64. Sullivan DC, Rosenfield NS, Ogden J, et al: Problems in the scintigraphic detection of osteomyelitis in children. Radiology 135:731–736, 1980.

65. Israel O, Gips S, Jerushalmi J, et al: Osteomyelitis and soft tissue infection: Differential diagnosis with a twenty-four/four hour ratio of ^{99m}Tc-MDP uptake. Radiology 163:725–726, 1987.

66. Shafer RB and Edeburn GF: Can the three-phase bone scan differentiate osteomyelitis from metabolic or metastatic bone disease? Clin Nucl Med 9:373–377, 1984.

67. Georgen TG, Alazraki NP, Halpern SE, et al: "Cold" bone lesions: A newly recognized phenomenon of bone imaging. J Nucl Med 15:1120–1124, 1974.

68. Barron BJ and Dahekne RD: Cold osteomyelitis: Radionuclide bone scan findings. Clin Nucl Med 9:392–393, 1984.

69. Lavender JP, Lowe J, Barker JR, et al: ^{67}Ga scanning in neoplastic and inflammatory lesions. Br J Radiol 44:361–366, 1971.

70. Tsan MF, Chen WY, Scheffel U, et al: Studies on gallium accumulation in inflammatory lesions: I. Gallium uptake by human polymorphonuclear leukocytes. J Nucl Med 19:36–43, 1978.

71. Menon S, Wagner, HN, and Tsan MF: Studies on gallium accumulation in inflammatory lesions: II. Uptake by *Staphylococcus aureus*: Concise communication. J Nucl Med 19:44–47, 1978.

72. Hayes RL, Nelson B, Swartzendruber DC, et al: Studies of the intracellular deposition of ^{67}Ga [Abstract]. J Nucl Med 12:364, 1971.

73. Lisbona R and Rosenthall L: Observations on the sequential use of ^{99m}Tc phosphate complex and ^{67}Ga imaging in osteomyelitis, cellulitis and septic arthritis. Radiology 123:123–129, 1977.

74. Rosenthall L, Lisbona R, Hernandez M, et al: ^{99m}Tc-PP and Ga imaging following insertion of orthopedic devices. Radiology 133:717–721, 1979.

75. Glynn TP: Marked gallium accumulation in neurogenic arthropathy. J Nucl Med 22:1016–1017, 1981.

76. Tumeh SS, Aliabadi P, Weissman BN, et al: Chronic osteomyelitis: Bone and gallium scan patterns associated with active disease. Radiology 158:685–688, 1986.

77. Lewin JS, Rosenfield NS, Hoffer PB, et al: Acute osteomyelitis in children: Combined ^{99m}Tc and ^{67}Ga imaging. Radiology 158:795–804, 1986.

78. Alazraki N, Fierer J, and Resnick D: Chronic osteomyelitis: Monitoring by ^{99m}Tc and phosphate and ^{67}Ga imaging. Am J Roentgenol 145:767–771, 1985.

79. Behjati K, Boyd CM, Balachandran S, et al: Value of ^{67}Ga SPECT in a patient with "malignant" otitis externa. Clin Nucl Med 12:229–230, 1987.

80. McDougall RL, Baumert JE, and Lantieri RL: Evaluation of ^{111}In leukocyte whole body scanning. Am J Roentgenol 133:849–854, 1979.

81. Guze BH, Hawkins RA, and Marcus CS: ^{99m}Tc white blood cell imaging: False-negative result in *Salmonella* osteomyelitis associated with sickle cell disease. Clin Nucl Med 14:104–106, 1989.

82. McAfee JG and Tacker ML: Survey of radioactive agents for in vitro labeling of phagocytic leukocytes. J Nucl Med 17:488–492, 1976.

83. Schauwecker DS, Park HM, Mock BJ, et al: Evaluation of complicating osteomyelitis with ^{99m}Tc-MDP, ^{111}In granulocytes and ^{67}Ga. J Nucl Med 25:849–853, 1984.

84. Al-sheikh W, Sfakiankis GN, Mnaymneh W, et al: Subacute and chronic bone infections: Diagnosis using ^{111}In, ^{67}Ga, ^{99m}Tc-MDP bone scintigraphy and radiography. Radiology 155:501–506, 1985.

85. Maurer AH, Millmond SH, Knight LC, et al: Infection in diabetic osteoarthropathy: Use of indium-labeled leukocytes for diagnosis. Radiology 161:221–225, 1986.

86. Kim EE, Haynie TP, Podoloff, et al: Radionuclide imaging evaluation of osteomyelitis in septic arthritis. Crit Rev Diagn Imaging 29(3):257, 1989.

87. McCarthy K, Velchik MG, Alavi A, et al: ^{111}In-labeled white blood cells in the detection of osteomyelitis complicated by a preexisting condition. J Nucl Med 29:1015–1021, 1988.

88. Schauwecker DS: Osteomyelitis: Diagnosis with ^{111}In-labeled leukocytes. Radiology 171:141–146, 1989.

89. Seabold JE, Nepola JV, Conrad GR, et al: Detection of osteomyelitis at fracture nonunion sites: Comparison of two scintigraphic methods. Am J Roentgenol 152:1021–1027, 1989.

90. Kim EE, Pjura GA, and Lowry PA: Osteomyelitis complicating fracture: Pitfalls of ^{111}In leukocyte scintigraphy. Am J Roentgenol 148:727–730, 1987.

91. Van Nostrand D, Abreu SH, Callaghan JJ, et al: ^{111}In-labeled white blood cell uptake in noninfected close fracture in humans: Prospective study. Radiology 167:495–498, 1988.

92. Fernandez-Ulloa M, Vasavada PJ, and Black RR: Detection of acute osteomyelitis with ^{111}In-labeled white blood cells in a patient with sickle cell disease. Clin Nucl Med 14:97–100, 1989.

93. Kim HC, Alavi A, Russell MO, et al: Differentiation of bone and bone marrow infarcts from osteomyelitis in sickle cell disorders. Clin Nucl Med 14:249–254, 1989.

94. Palestro CJ, Swyer AJ, Kim CK, et al: Infected knee prostheses: Diagnosis with ^{111}In leukocyte, ^{99m}Tc sulfur colloid and ^{99m}Tc-MDP imaging. Radiology 179:645–648, 1991.

95. Moon KL, Genant HK, Helms CA, et al: Musculoskeletal applications of nuclear magnetic resonance. Radiology 147:161–171, 1983.

96. Berquist TH: Magnetic resonance imaging: Preliminary experience in orthopedic radiology. Magn Reson Imaging 2:41–52, 1984.

97. King CL, Henkelman RM, Poon PY, et al: MR imaging of the normal knee. J Comput Assist Tomogr 8:1147–1154, 1984.

98. Beltran J, Noto AM, Mosure JC, et al: Ankle: Surface coil MR imaging at 1.5 T. Radiology 161:203–209, 1986.

99. Sartoris DJ and Resnick D: Magnetic resonance imaging of the foot: Technical aspects. J Foot Surg 26:351–358, 1987.

100. Ferkel RD, Fannigan BD, and Elkins BS: Magnetic resonance imaging of the foot and ankle: Correlation of normal anatomy with pathologic conditions. Foot Ankle 11:289–305, 1991.

101. Forrester DM, Kricun ME, and Kerr R: Imaging of the Foot and Ankle. Rockville, MD, Aspen, 1988, pp 283–316.

102. Berquist TH: Magnetic resonance imaging of the foot and ankle. Semin Ultrasound, CT and MRI 11(4):327–345, 1990.

103. Bushong SE: Magnetic Resonance Imaging, Physical and Biological Principals. St. Louis, CV Mosby, 1988.

104. Harms SE, Morgan TJ, Yamanashi WS, et al: Principals of nuclear magnetic resonance imaging. Radiographics 4:26–43, 1984.

105. desPlants BG, Falke TH, and denBoer JA: Pulse sequences and contrast in magnetic resonance imaging. Radiographics 4:869–883, 1984.

106. Ehman RL: Interpretation of magnetic resonance images. *In* Berquist TH (ed): MRI of the Musculoskeletal System. New York, Raven Press, 1990, pp 27–51.

107. Beltran J, Noto AM, McGhee RB, et al: Infections of the musculoskeletal system: High field-strength MR imaging. Radiology 164:449–454, 1987.

108. Tang JS, Gold RH, Bassett LW, et al: Musculoskeletal infection of the extremities: Evaluation with MR imaging. Radiology 166:205–209, 1988.

109. Unger E, Moldofsky P, Gatenby R, et al: Diagnosis of osteomyelitis by MR imaging. Am J Roentgenol 150:605–610, 1988.

110. Moore SG, Bissett GS, Siegel MJ, et al: Pediatric musculoskeletal MR imaging. Radiology 179:345–360, 1991.

111. Beltran J, McGhee RB, et al: Experimental infections of the musculoskeletal system: Evaluation with MR imaging and Tc-[99m] MDP and Ga-[67] scintigraphy. Radiology 167:167–172, 1988.

112. Uyuh WT, Corson JD, Baraniewski JM, et al: Osteomyelitis of the foot in diabetic patients: Evaluation with plain films, [99mTc-MDP] bone scintigraphy and MR imaging. Am J Roentgenol 152:795–800, 1989.

113. Mason MD, Zlatkin MB, Esterhai JL, et al: Chronic complicated osteomyelitis of the lower extremity: Evaluation with MR imaging. Radiology 173:355–359, 1989.

114. Staple T: Radiography of the diabetic foot. *In* Levin ME (ed): The Diabetic Foot. St. Louis, CV Mosby, 1983, pp 142–168.

115. Chuinard RG and D'Ambrosia R: Human bite infections of the hand. J Bone Joint Surg 51A:416, 1977.

116. Harris WH: Sinking prostheses. Surg Gynecol Obstet 123:1297, 1966.

117. Gristina A: Musculoskeletal infection, microbial adhesion and antibiotic resistance. Infect Dis Clin North Am 4:391, 1990.

118. Fitzgerald RA Jr and Calland JDE: Puncture wounds of the foot. Orthop Clin North Am 6(4):965–972, 1975.

119. Chisholm CD and Schlesser JF: Planter puncture wounds: Controversies, treatments and recommendations. Ann Emerg Med 18:1352–1357, 1989.

120. Jaffe HL: Metabolic, Degenerative and Inflammatory Diseases of the Bones and Joints. Philadelphia, Lea & Febiger, 1972.

121. O'Connor BT, Steel WN, and Sanders R: Disseminated bone tuberculosis. J Bone Joint Surg 52A:537, 1970.

122. Buckley SL and Barkus JK: Coccidioidomycosis of the first cuneiform: Successful treatment utilizing local débridement and long-term ketoconazole therapy. Foot Ankle 6:300–304, 1986.

123. Kopelman AL, Halsted CC, and Minnefor AB: Osteomalacia and spontaneous fractures and congenital cytomegalic inclusion disease. J Pediatr 81:101, 1972.

124. Smith RF and Specht EE: Osseous lesions and pathologic fractures in congenital cytomegalic inclusion disease: Report of a case. Clin Orthop 144:280, 1979.

125. Berquist TH and Brown ML: Infection. *In* Berquist TH (ed): Radiology of the Foot and Ankle. New York, Raven Press, 1989, pp 277–313.

126. Katz RD and Hawkins RA: A diagnostic algorithm for the systematic evaluation of suspected osteomyelitis. Paper presented at the annual meeting of the Society of Nuclear Medicine, Washington, DC, 1990.

127. Roddie ME, Peters MA, Danpure HJ, et al: Inflammation: Imaging with Tc-99m HMPAO-labeled leukocytes. Radiology 166:767–772, 1988.

CHAPTER 22

Contrast Radiography

Brad L. Naylor, D.P.M.

The use of contrast medium in roentgenographic examination of both acute and chronic disorders and injuries can prove useful for both diagnosis and development or evaluation of treatment plans. Often, when articular disease or injury is evaluated, the contribution and extent of the soft tissue component of the process are difficult to ascertain. This is especially evident in trauma when reactive measures of the body can obscure the actual extent of soft tissue injury and prevent accurate assessment. Use of standard radiographs in the initial evaluation process can be less than optimal for establishing a definitive diagnosis, often leading the clinician to more invasive or costly procedures. The ability to opacify various soft tissue structures can be easily achieved and allows for direct visualization of soft tissue structure, re-evaluation of complex disorders, and initiation of appropriate treatment regimens.

CHARACTERISTICS OF CONTRAST AGENTS

Contrast media available for use are divided into two types: ionic (such as Hypaque, Renografin, and Conray) and nonionic (such as Omnipaque, Amipaque, and Isovue). The ionic group is referred to as the *diatrizoates* and the *iothalamates*, which are also the ionic monoacidic monomers. These agents dissociate in solution at a ratio of 1.5:1 and usually have higher osmolality (in the range of 1200 to 1900 mOsm/kg). The newer nonionic group and a new differing ionic monoacidic dimer, Hexabrix, have also been approved by the Food and Drug Administration for intravascular uses. These agents possess osmolalities between 600 and 900 mOsm/kg. The importance of these newer contrast agents relates to their higher iodine particles per solution and lower systemic toxicities. The nonionic group of agents have been shown to have less central nervous systemic toxicity. Other observations have included less red blood cell rigidity and morphologic changes, including lessened effect on platelets and coagulation time. In addition, fewer electrocardiographic changes and less ventricular irritability and bronchospasm have been observed with the nonionic contrast agents.[1]

Adverse Reactions

Adverse reactions of contrast agents have been well documented[2]; however, this vast data collection study involved injecting large volumes of contrast medium with higher blood volume concentrations than can be reached with small joint or structure studies addressed in this chapter. It has been documented that adverse, even lethal, reactions can be precipitated by very small intravascular and dermal test doses.[3] This should act to reinforce two factors when selection of patients for the studies is considered. First, a complete history should be taken before these materials are administered. This should include specific questioning as to previous sensitivities or allergic reactions to contrast materials, iodine, and seafood. Second, although the procedure itself may be easily employed in an office situation, a degree of caution should be exercised when doing these examinations in that setting. Even though no documented cases of anaphylaxis have appeared in the literature, one must consider that this type of reaction is possible. Thus, a clinician not adequately prepared to handle this situation in an office treatment room might be ill-advised to perform these procedures outside a hospital or properly equipped outpatient facility.

A variety of systemic conditions need to be considered when contrast radiographic studies are contemplated. A history of homozygous sickle cell disease, multiple myeloma, or pheochromocytoma is a contraindication because the contrast agents can displace oxygen and evoke a crisis situation. Other systemic disease states, such as congestive heart failure, hypertension, renal disease, and unstable thyroid conditions, can be exacerbated by increased intravascular or hyperosmolar conditions. Coagulation disorders can predispose to various bleeding diatheses, which may lead to hematoma formation or hemarthroses.

Local factors of the planned examination should also be carefully considered. The presence of infection in the area to be studied is a contraindication, because these examinations should be performed, with the exception of sinograms, in an aseptic manner. The concerns of inducing septic arthritis, suppurative tenosynovitis, and abscesses are inherent potential problems of contrast media studies.

Hypersensitivity reactions may progress in a stepwise fashion and may present initially as nausea, vomiting, flushing, and a lightheaded sensation; fascial edema, bronchospasm, and transient or prolonged hypotension may eventually develop. If left unattended, these situations can continue into circulatory collapse, angina, myocardial infarction, ventricular fibrillation, convulsion, coma, paralysis, and death. Obviously, the risks and benefits of such situations must be carefully assessed. If alternative studies may yield the same information, they need to be considered. The patient with minor sensitivity or allergy represents a gray zone. If contrast examination is likely to provide critical information that may impact the diagnosis and treatment, one may proceed cautiously. Prophylaxis for adult patients with 20 mg of prednisone orally or 100 mg of intravenous hydrocortisone every 6 hours for at least three doses before initiating the contrast study has been shown to be efficacious in preventing reactions in patients at risk.[4]

ARTHROGRAPHY

Most pedal arthrography has been described in relation to the talocrural joint. Evaluations of other lower extremity articulations are possible and can aid in difficult diagnoses, evaluation, and treatment. There are several indications for joint evaluation using radiocontrast materials (Table 22–1). Arthrography is a modality used primarily to rule out or confirm the identity of these structures, which can often be subtle in presentation and as a result be undetected in the initial phases of diagnosis and treatment.

Understanding anatomic dimensions of articulations and communication with extra-articular structures is an important aspect of ankle arthrography. The ability to distinguish normal from abnormal communication is important to appreciate the full value of arthrography. It has been shown that the subtalar articulation, as well as tendons of flexors, extensors, or peroneals coming in close approximation with the talocrural joint capsule, can share synovial fluid.[5] There is some disagreement among authors regarding communication of the peroneals with the talocrural joint as being a normal variant[6, 7] versus traumatic in origin.[8–10] It is generally accepted that this represents an abnormal communication.

Identification and proper treatment of soft tissue injuries can be vital when failure to recognize some of these injuries can result in severe disabling, long-term sequelae.[11] If one can identify the severity of a ''simple sprain'' and proceed to a proper treatment plan, such as casting versus surgical repair, one may prevent development of ligament laxity and later degenerative joint changes.

Normal Ankle Arthrographic Anatomy

Before one can assess abnormal anatomic structure, one must have an understanding of normal anatomy. There are three anatomic recesses in the ankle to remain aware of—normal anatomic recesses can be confusing to the untrained eye. The two recesses that are visible from the lateral projection are the anterior and posterior pouches of the ankle capsule (Fig. 22–1). The third, and often the most confusing, is the interosseous recess, visible on the anteroposterior,

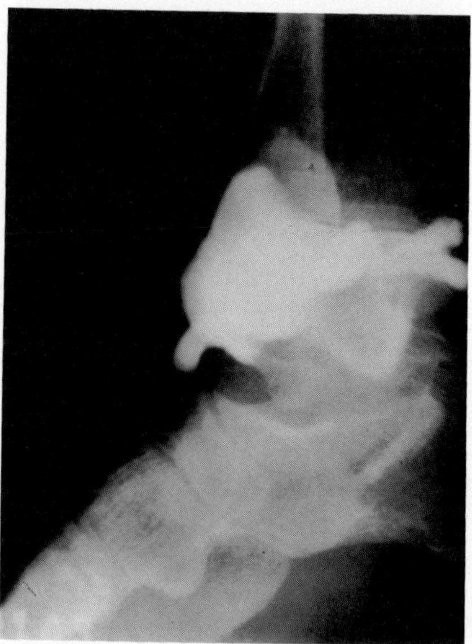

FIGURE 22–1. Normal ankle arthrography. An enlarged anterior recess and a smaller posterior recess are shown.

oblique, or mortise views (Fig. 22–2). This recess projects approximately 1 cm proximally above the most distal tibiofibular articulation. Any leakage of dye proximal to this point is suggestive of a diastasis.[12]

Ankle arthrography is most notable for the assessment of acute ruptures of the collateral ligaments of the ankle (Fig. 22–3). These assessments are based on the observation of contrast material outside the ankle joint, at a point where ligament tears have occurred, allowing contrast material to extravasate extra-articularly. Evaluation of calcaneofibular ligament tears exemplifies these findings. Specifically, assessment of tears of the calcaneofibular ligament is based on the presence of extravasated contrast within the peroneal tendon sheath. The presence of contrast solution from the ankle joint that has made its way into the tendon sheath about

TABLE 22–1

INDICATIONS FOR ARTHROGRAPHY

Ligamentous injuries
Osteochondral/transchondral injury or defects
Intra-articular osseous, cartilagenous, or fibrous bodies
Adhesive capsulitis
Coalitions
Soft tissue impingement

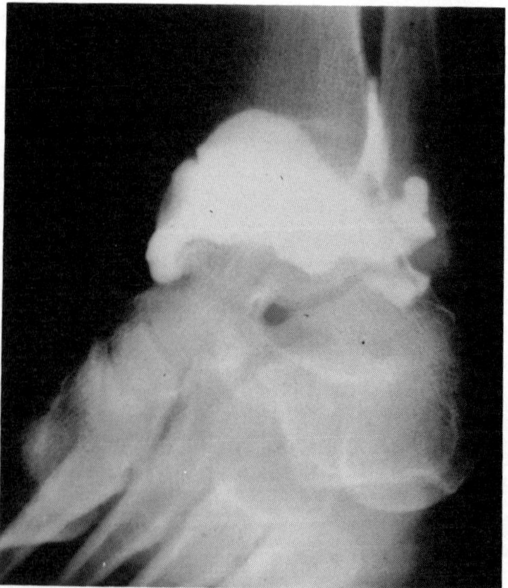

FIGURE 22–2. Normal ankle arthrogram. Oblique view shows the upper limit of the interosseous recess.

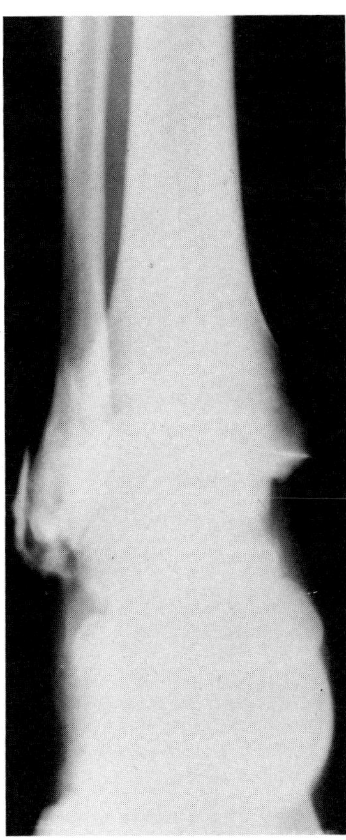

FIGURE 22–3. This ankle joint arthrogram is positive for rupture of the calcaneofibular ligament. Note the leakage of contrast material into the peroneal tendons laterally.

the ankle is not necessarily abnormal. Normal communications do exist on rare occasions and have been documented with cadaveric contrast examinations and dissections.[13] There are limitations also expressed in terms of the time constraints of this study. Capsular repair generally occurs by 1 week after trauma has occurred, at which time the abnormal communication ceases to exist. Studies performed after this period decrease their specificity to tissue damage and can confuse the clinician with false-negative interpretations.[14]

Arthrographic Technique

Arthrography can be employed in either of two typical fashions: a single-contrast or a double-contrast study. Single-contrast arthrography is indicated primarily in the evaluation of soft tissue injury or disease of articular structures. The single-contrast study usually employs an injection of contrast material, alone or diluted for additional diagnostic benefit, with local anesthesia. This is the technique most commonly employed with joint examinations.

Double-contrast technique is identical to that of the single contrast, with the exception that ambient air is added to the syringe. Only small amounts of contrast medium are necessary, and as little as 1 to 2 ml of contrast material is typically used. Double-contrast studies are more advantageous than single studies in profiling osseous or cartilaginous defects. This technique is best applied to the patient who presents with chronic ankle pain following an ankle sprain in whom

standard radiographs are negative and in whom osteochondral defects are included in the differential diagnosis.[12]

Ankle Arthrography. Ankle arthrography is performed with the patient lying supine, the knee flexed, and the ankle in a plantarflexed position. The correct site for introduction of the needle must be carefully chosen. Typically, a 21- or 22-gauge needle and 20-ml syringe are selected. Butterfly needles may be used; an added benefit is that the examiner has a free hand once needle placement is completed. The needle is inserted into an anesthetized area, usually opposite the side of suspected tissue trauma. This is done to decrease the patient's discomfort and to lessen the chance of false-positive studies, such as can occur in acute sprains. In this instance, contrast medium may extravasate in the path of least resistance, which would be the site of capsular injury. The most common site of medial insertion is between the anterior tibialis and the extensor hallucis longus tendons. This avoids the neurovascular bundle, typically located lateral to the extensor hallucis longus tendon. Alternatively, for lateral insertion, topographic identification of the extensor digitorum or peroneus tertius tendons is made, and insertion is made just lateral to these structures. The average entry points are at a level 1 cm proximal to the distal tip of the medial malleolus or 2 cm proximal from the tip of the lateral malleolus. These points of entry can be easily palpated in the nonobese patient, but they must be marked with indelible ink prior to anesthesia.

The ankle is prepared and draped in sterile fashion, and local anesthesia is then infiltrated in the area planned for larger needle insertion. The arthrographic needle is gradually inserted in a slight cephalad orientation, corresponding to the talar trochlear shape. As the needle is gently advanced, resistance is felt at the level of the joint capsule. Confirmation of joint entry is obtained by retrieval of joint fluid. Fluoroscopic or routine lateral radiographs may be obtained to further evaluate needle position. Joint aspiration can be performed and used for analysis, to decrease effusion volumes, and to lavage with sterile saline to rid the joint space of small intraarticular clots or fibrin that could ultimately alter the study interpretation. A 20- or 30-ml syringe is used for slow instillation of contrast material of choice, with or without local anesthesia and ambient air. During instillation, the flow of contrast material is carefully observed to detect any altered flow patterns that suggest blockage by fibrous tissue, meniscoid bodies, or detached articular structures. In addition, close attention should be given to the amount of material accepted without excessive pressure being exerted. Noting this amount can aid in establishing a diagnosis of adhesive capsulitis or chronic effusion states, which are seen in various arthritides. Excessive intracapsular scarring may be the result of various injuries. This fibrosis can lessen the intra-articular volume (Fig. 22–4). Conversely, disease states such as rheumatoid arthritis that produce excessive amounts of synovial fluid can stretch or distend this capsular boundary beyond its normal volume. Normal injection volume of the talocrural joint averages 6 to 10 ml. At the point of firm, yet short of excessive, potentially rupturing pressure, the catheter is removed and range of motion is allowed for a few moments. Radiographic examination in at least two differing planes aids in evaluation and interpretation of the examination.

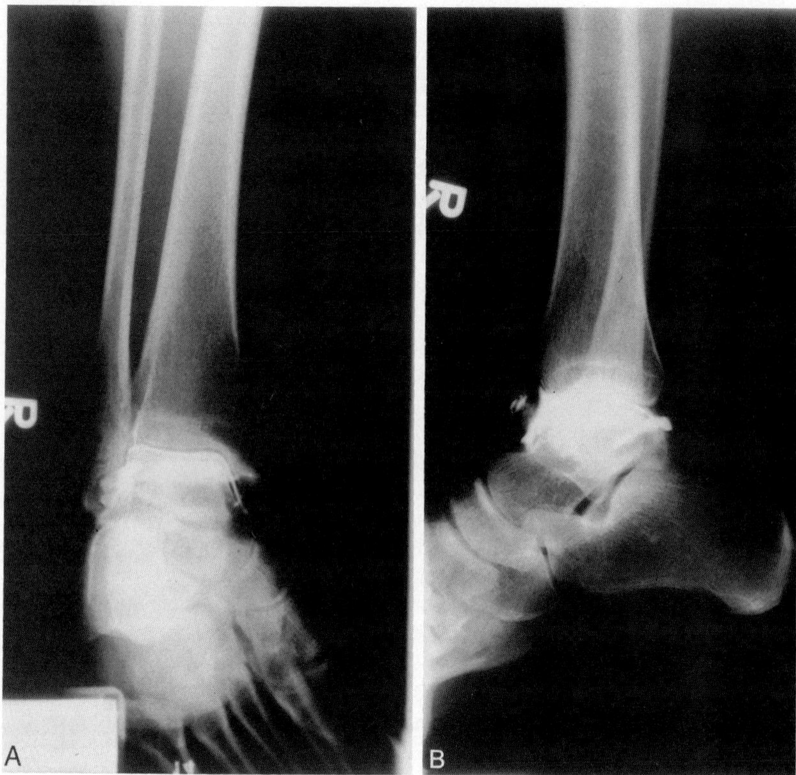

FIGURE 22–4. Adhesive capsulitis. An ankle joint arthrogram showing decreased intra-articular volume. Note the absence of an interosseous recess (*A*) and the reduction of other recesses (*B*).

Posterior Subtalar Joint Arthrography. Two approaches for posterior subtalar arthrography are used: posterolateral and anterolateral. These examinations, as well as more distal pedal arthrograms, are enhanced by fluoroscopic needle placement owing to tight joint accesses. Indications for arthrogram in the hindfoot also include acute or chronic ligamentous damage (Fig. 22–5) and articular evaluation. Sinus tarsi synovitis is another pathologic process in which arthrography may be useful. This condition shows an irregu-

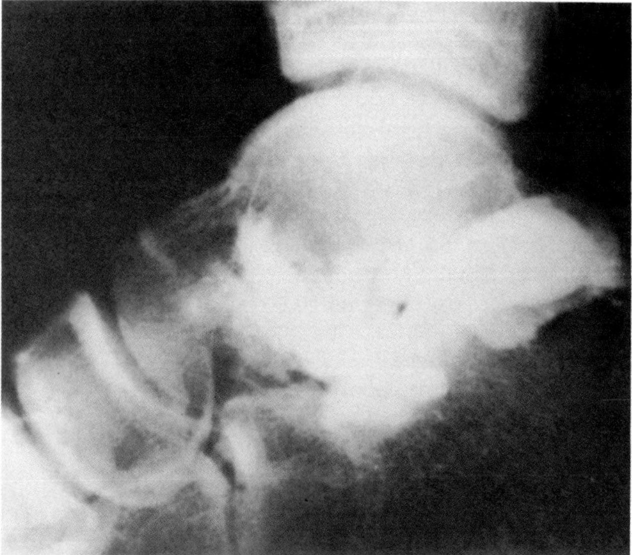

FIGURE 22–5. Abnormal posterior subtalar arthrogram. Contrast is shown traveling dorsally; interosseous ligament rupture is evident. (From Perlman MD: Usage of radiopaque contrast media in the foot and ankle. J Foot Surg 27:3–29, 1988. © by American College of Foot Surgeons, Inc.)

lar, corrugated or obliterated pattern in the talocalcaneal ligamentous space.[15] The posterior subtalar joint normally requires 2 to 4 ml of fluid for examination. Approximately 10% to 20% of the population has a normal communication between the posterior subtalar joint and the ankle joint,[7] in which a larger volume study may be appreciated.

Anteriorly, the subtalar articulation contains the joint spaces of the middle talocalcaneal facet, the anterior talocalcaneal facet, and the talonavicular joints. Also included in this study is the articulation of the distal anteromedial portion of the talar head and the cartilaginous surface of the plantar spring ligament. The middle talocalcaneal joint is a common structure involved in tarsal coalitions (fibrous, cartilaginous, or osseous). An anterior subtalar arthrogram can be an effective evaluation tool in this disorder. Access to the talocalcaneonavicular or the anterior subtalar joint is usually dorsal to the talonavicular capsule. Using a 22- or 25-gauge needle with a slight distal orientation enables the examiner to navigate the needle insertion without producing cartilaginous defects on the concave or convex articulating surfaces. Normal joint volume varies from 2 to 4 ml of synovial fluid. The joint spaces of both the anterior and middle talocalcaneal and the talonavicular are contiguous and evenly defined, which can readily be observed with a normal arthrographic examination (Fig. 22–6). Any variance in these normal findings may be indicative of pathologic changes.

Calcaneocuboid Joint Arthrography. The calcaneocuboid joint can also be examined with the use of contrast arthrography. Acute ligamentous injury can usually be diagnosed using 2 to 4 ml of dye in a single technique (Fig. 22–7).[11] If chronic pain or suspicion of cartilaginous damage or loose bodies is to be evaluated, double-contrast technique using 2 to 3 ml of ambient air can be useful.

Arthrography of Other Small Joints of the Foot. Ar-

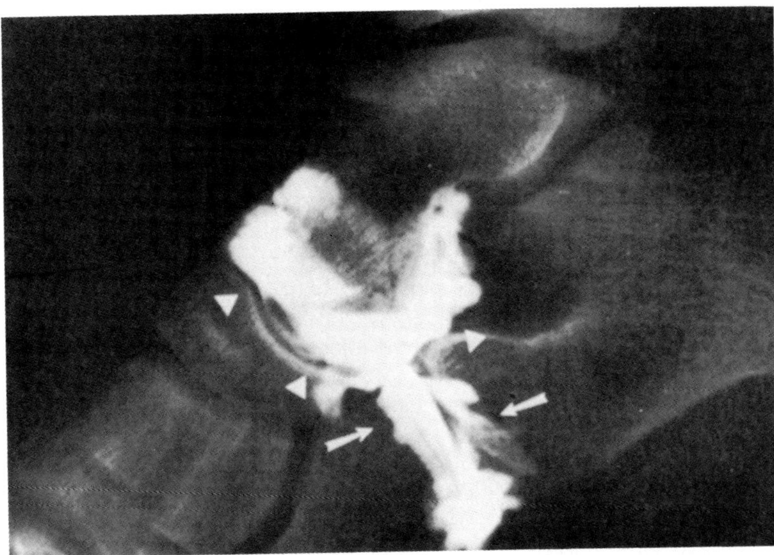

FIGURE 22–6. Normal anterior subtalar (*arrowheads*) and calcaneocuboid (*arrows*) joint arthrography. This examination, visualizing the entire midtarsal joint, requires two separate injections. (From Haller J, Resnick D, and Sartoris D: Arthrography, tenography, and bursography of the ankle and foot. Clin Podiatr Med Surg 5[4]:903, 1988.)

thrography of the joint structures distal to Chopart's joint has been described.[7, 16–18] Contrast radiography of these joints may be useful in evaluating possible coalitions; inflammatory disease involving soft tissue, cartilage, and bone structures; articular or transchondral defects; and acute or chronic capsular/ligamentous ruptures. Of particular interest in podiatry, largely owing to the increased biomechanical stresses and pathologic changes that subsequently develop disease in these joints, are the metatarsophalangeal articulations.

The technique of metatarsophalangeal arthrography starts with sterile preparation and draping. Distal distraction of the corresponding digit produces a characteristic dimple at the joint level.[16] Using local anesthesia, skin is infiltrated with 0.25 to 0.5 ml at this dimple site. A 1-inch, 22- or 25-gauge needle is used at an angle of approximately 15 to 20 degrees from proximal to distal to facilitate capsular puncture and negate the risk of cartilaginous excoriation or laceration. On joint puncture, synovial fluid may be aspirated for analysis. The needle is secured at its hub, and the syringe is twisted off. This is replaced with the contrast mixture of choice. Slow instillation of 1 or 2 ml of fluid is performed to resistance, and the needle is withdrawn from the joint. Radio-

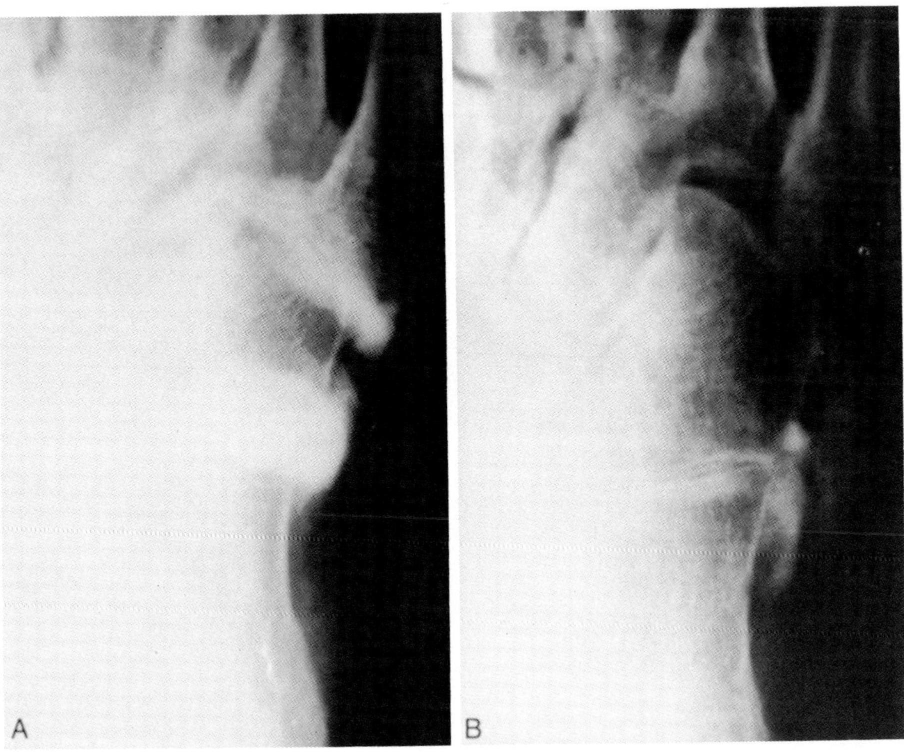

FIGURE 22–7. *A*, Normal calcaneocuboid and cuboid fourth and fifth metatarsal joint arthrogram. *B*, Abnormal calcaneocuboid joint arthrogram. Note the ligamentous rupture laterally. (From Perlman MD: Usage of radiopaque contrast media in the foot and ankle. J Foot Surg 27:3–29, 1988. © by American College of Foot Surgeons, Inc.)

graphic examination using anteroposterior, lateral, and oblique views are then obtained. A plantar axial view can be considered if the sesamoidal apparatus is being evaluated.

Normal examination reveals an even, regular joint space with small recesses, medial and lateral, and larger dorsal and plantar recesses corresponding to the capsular outline. Studies outside these parameters can be viewed as positive findings of injury. It is possible to use contrast material mixed with local anesthetic as a diagnostic block, determining intra-articular versus extra-articular involvement of pain. These principles are exhibited in the patient displayed in Figure 22–8A to C; this patient's pain occurred after bunion surgery. The pain was greatly diminished with the local anesthetic administered in this first metatarsophalangeal arthrographic study. The examination also revealed mild joint space narrowing dorsally (corresponding to the process of plastic deformation) that can occur in certain osteotomies in foot surgery. This examination was used successfully in proposing corrective surgery to derotate the distal metatarsophalangeal head.

TENOGRAPHY

The tendon sheath allows smooth gliding movement around or through fibrous and osseous tunnels. Many tendon disorders involving the tendon sheath structures can be illustrated with the use of radiopaque media. Newer and more costly evaluation of these pathologic conditions may be rendered using technologies such as magnetic resonance imaging (MRI), but tenography offers a dynamic element of flow within the tendon sheath not appreciated by MRI. Perhaps a combination of these studies may bring a better appreciation to some of these disease processes. Treatment of these pathologic processes, whether conservative or surgical in nature, can be aided by this technique.

Etiologic factors are numerous but are usually traumatic in origin. Irritation of tendons by calcaneal spicules following os calcis fractures and tendon and/or tendon sheath fibrosis following ankle sprains have been described and are among the most common post-traumatic sequelae,[11, 21, 22] but other causative factors can produce substantial tendon sheath pathologic changes (Table 22–2). This examination can also be useful in evaluation of a calcaneofibular ligament rupture following an ankle inversion injury. The peroneal tendon's close association with this ligament renders the sheath susceptible for specific involvement after this injury.[11] Knowledge of tendon sheath anatomy is necessary for proper interpretation of these studies.

Tendon and Tendon Sheath Anatomy

The tendon sheath structure consists of a tube of synovial fluid contained by an outer, or parietal, layer and an inner, or visceral, layer that is in close contact with the tendon itself.

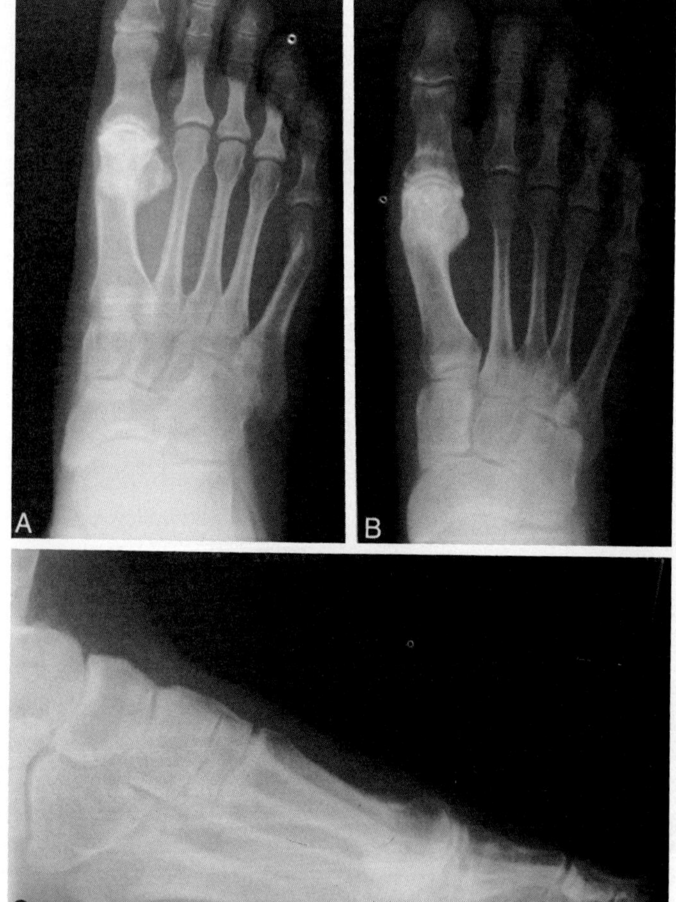

FIGURE 22–8. *A* to *C*, Abnormal first metatarsophalangeal joint arthrogram. Plastic deformation is shown by the metatarsal head position (lateral radiograph) and the thin dorsal capsular contrast filling.

TABLE 22–2

CAUSATIVE FACTORS IN THE DEVELOPMENT OF TENOSYNOVITIS AND OTHER TENDON DISORDERS

Osseous fractures
Soft tissue injury, such as sprains and partial or total tendon ruptures
Inflammatory arthritides
Anatomic anomalies, such as enlarged tubercles and prominences
Static foot and ankle deformities
Repetitive sport- or occupation-related stresses

These two layers connect, typically on the opposite side of greatest tendon pressure, to form a thin membrane, the mesotendineum. This structure is the pathway of vessels, nerves, and lymph channels to and from the tendon.[19] This visceral layer adheres to the epitendineum on the tendon surface, and they, together, move around friction points that usually involve change in tendon direction. These sites are predisposed to either repetitive or acute injury. These types of injuries are not appreciated by standard radiographic techniques.[20]

Three orientations of tendon groups can be evaluated about the ankle joint: lateral, medial, and anterior. The lateral, or peroneal, group consists of a common sheath involving both the peroneal longus and brevis tendons. It extends 2.5 to 3.5 cm above the tip of the lateral malleolus. It then bifurcates at the level of the peroneal tubercle of the calcaneus, proceeding distally with a synovial sac of the brevis, extending as far as 2 cm proximal to the insertion of the fifth metatarsal base. The other sac terminates in the region of the cuboid-peroneal groove on the anteroplantar aspect of the cuboid. In normal peroneal tenography a smooth, confluent sheath is visible in this orientation. Abnormal findings can be found after chronic repetitive or acute traumas (Fig. 22–9). Classically, an extrinsic compression or irregularity,

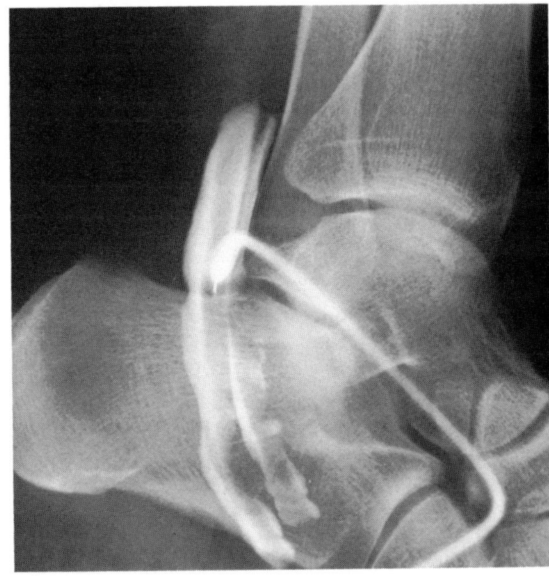

FIGURE 22–10. Peroneal tenogram showing mild corrugation along the peroneus brevis tendon sheath. This patient responded well to conservative treatment, including casting followed by physical therapy.

sometimes referred to as a *corrugated pattern,* is noted on the sheath's outline (Fig. 22–10). Displacement, constriction, or complete obstruction (Fig. 22–11) of the involved tendons can be found.

The medial, or flexor, group of tendons includes the pos-

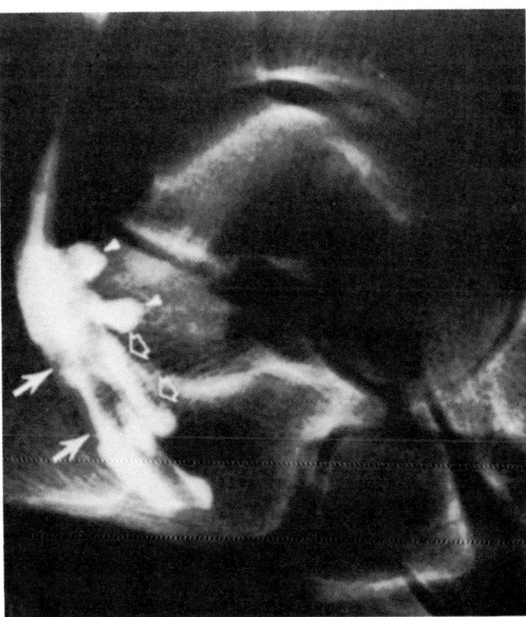

FIGURE 22–9. Abnormal peroneal tenogram with nodular, "pseudodiverticular" changes *(arrowheads)* showing evidence of chronic tenosynovitis. (From Gilula LA, Oloff L, Caputi R, et al: Ankle tenography: A key to unexplained symptomatology: II: Diagnosis of chronic tendon disabilities. Radiology 151:581–587, 1984.)

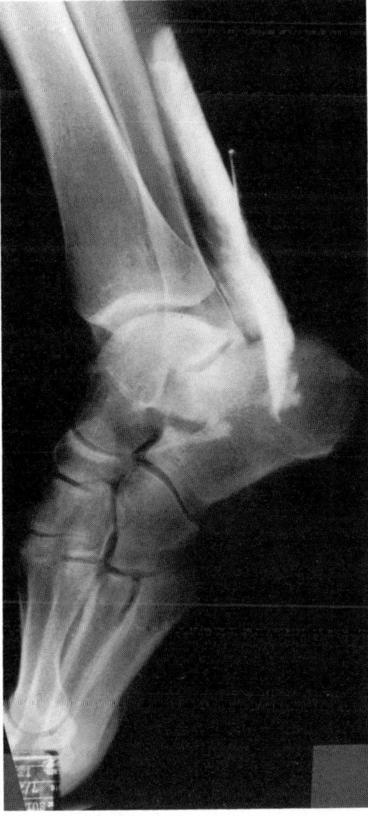

FIGURE 22–11. Abnormal peroneal tenogram. This patient had a history of several severe ankle sprains. Traumatic scarring prevented the flow of contrast material distally past the level of the calcaneofibular ligament.

terior tibialis, the flexor digitorum longus, and the flexor hallucis longus (Fig. 22–12). The posterior tibialis synovial sheath is approximately 7 to 9 cm in length, starting 6 cm proximal to the tip of the medial malleolus; it descends along the tendon in the retromalleolar groove and terminates at the navicular tuberosity. The flexor digitorum longus has two components to its synovial sheath: the malleolar and the digital sections. The malleolar portion starts approximately 1 cm distal to the origin of the posterior tibialis sheath and descends in the retromalleolar groove to end just proximal to or at the cross point with the flexor hallucis longus sheath. This is usually at the level of the talonavicular joint. The digital component envelops the slips of the flexor digitorum longus and brevis tendons of that digit. Originating plantar to the head of the metatarsal, the sheath is closely associated, but not normally communicating, with the plantar pad structure, extending distally and complexly involved with the

vincular system to the insertion at the base of the corresponding distal phalanx.[23]

The flexor group is under great stress as an antigravity muscle group. Tenosynovitis (Fig. 22–13), dislocation, and partial or total rupture are pathologic conditions that can be the result of repetitive microtrauma, altered biomechanics, acute trauma, or various collagen vascular disease. Normal and abnormal interpretations of the flexor are similar to those of the peroneal group.

The anterior, or extensor, group of tendons includes the anterior tibialis, the extensor hallucis longus, and the digitorum longus. The anterior tibialis sheath originates just proximal to the superior extensor retinaculum and reaches distally to or just proximal to the level of the talonavicular joint. The extensor hallucis longus tendon sheath originates at a level lower than that of the anterior tibialis, usually at the interval between the superior and inferior extensor retinaculum. The

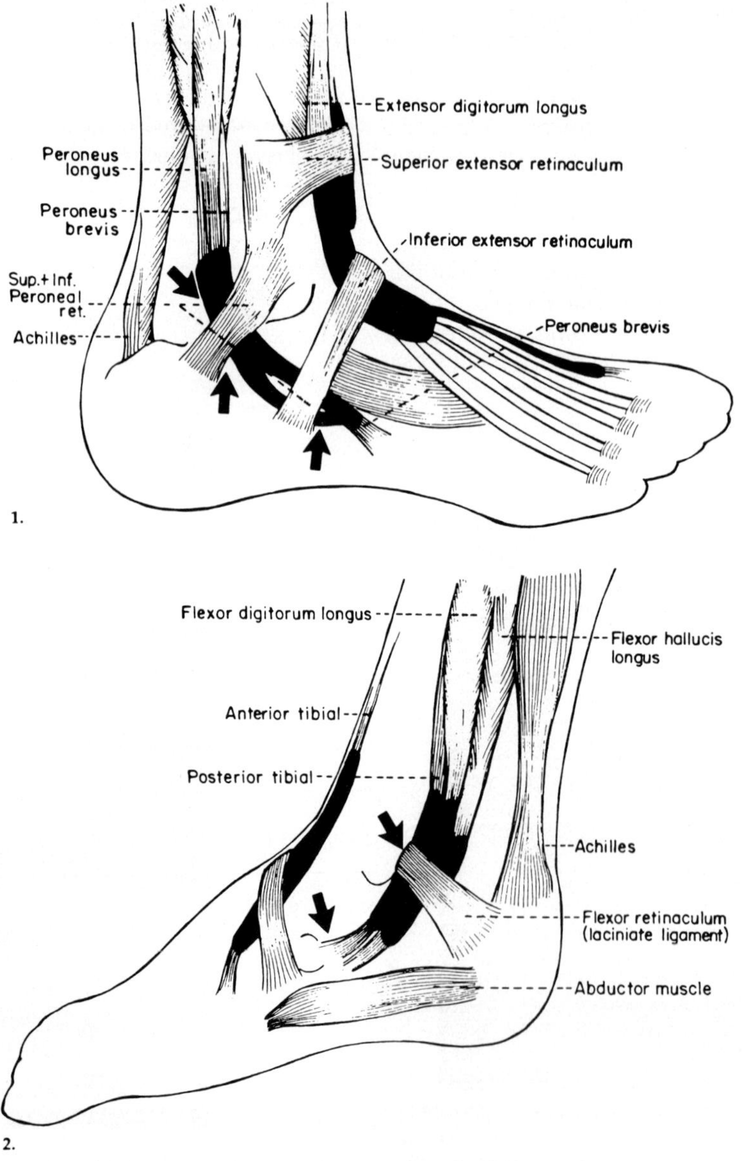

FIGURE 22–12. *1*, Lateral ankle tendons and sheaths. *2*, Medial ankle tendons and sheaths. (From Gilula LA, Oloff L, Caputi R, et al: Ankle tenography: A key to unexplained symptomatology: II. Diagnosis of chronic tendon disabilities. Radiology 151:581–587, 1984.)

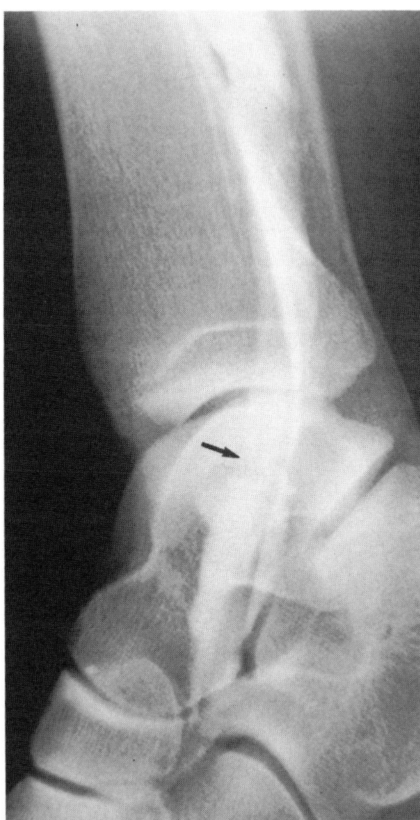

FIGURE 22–13. Posterior tibial tenogram. Note the constricture point on the tendon sheath, marked by the *arrow*.

sheath continues distally to the level that varies between the first metatarsocuneiform joint and the proximal third of the first metatarsal shaft. The sheath of the extensor digitorum longus originates at approximately the same level as the extensor hallucis longus and continues distally in a larger divergent, saclike fashion to envelop the individual slips of the digitorum longus and the peroneus tertius. Distally from this enlarged sac extend small, blunt, saclike projections, approximately 0.5 cm in length, that continue along each individual tendon.[23]

The anterior group of tendon sheaths is subjected to various blunt and mechanical trauma. Certain activities, such as skiing and soccer, and particular shoe gear, such as ski boots, high-top boots, and tennis shoes, are predisposing factors for patients to develop acute and sometimes chronic tendon disorders.

Tenographic Technique

After a review of the anatomic boundaries of the tendon sheath structures to be evaluated, a small amount of local anesthesia is infiltrated in the skin overlying the tendon sheath. This facilitates patient comfort as the needle is manipulated into the sheath structure. A 23- or 25-gauge needle should be introduced into the tendon structure until the tip encounters resistance of the tendon. At this point, either a very slight withdrawal of the needle from the tendon proper or rotation of the needle to open the bevel of the needle toward the sheath structure is performed. After slowly injecting an initial 1 or 2 ml of the radiocontrast material mixture, fluoroscopic or standard radiographs are taken to evaluate the placement of solution into the sheath structure. Placing the fingertips just proximal and distal to the needle insertion can aid in palpating flow into the sheath. Instillation of the remaining fluid to resistance is performed, and the needle is withdrawn.

GANGLIOGRAPHY, HEMANGIOGRAPHY, BURSOGRAPHY, AND SINOGRAPHY

Various soft tissue cavity structures in the body can be visualized to aid in determining the size, shape, and various extensions of these soft tissue cavities. Opacification using contrast media can be employed effectively in this fashion.

One study showed a 24.2% recurrence rate following ganglion excisions.[24] It has been suggested that more preoperative workups using gangliograms might reduce this recurrence rate (Fig. 22–14).[25] The technique commonly used for these examinations involves aspiration of the gelatinous material commonly found in these structures, preceded by a standard sterile preparation as with other contrast studies. The structure is then carefully filled with the contrast me-

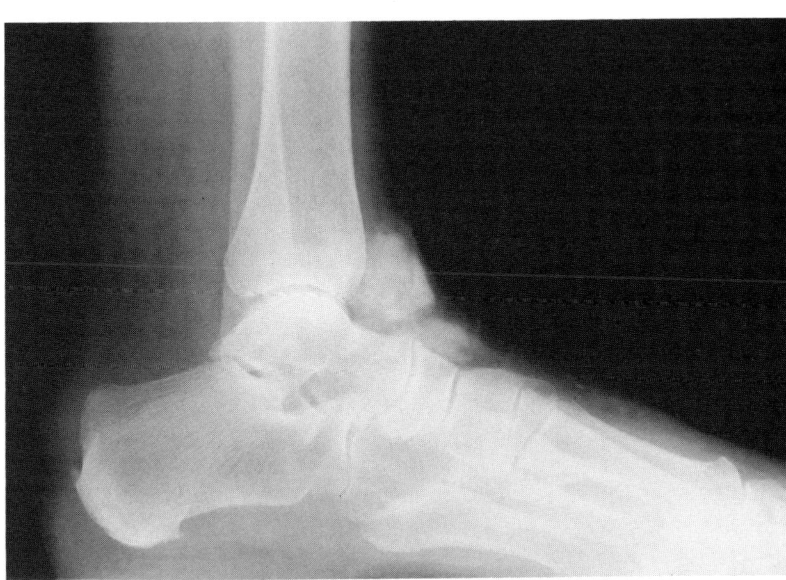

FIGURE 22–14. Preoperative gangliogram. A soft tissue mass in the sinus tarsi area with a gelatinous inner content is present. The mass is identified utilizing contrast demonstrating that this expansile lesion is retained underneath the extensor retinacula.

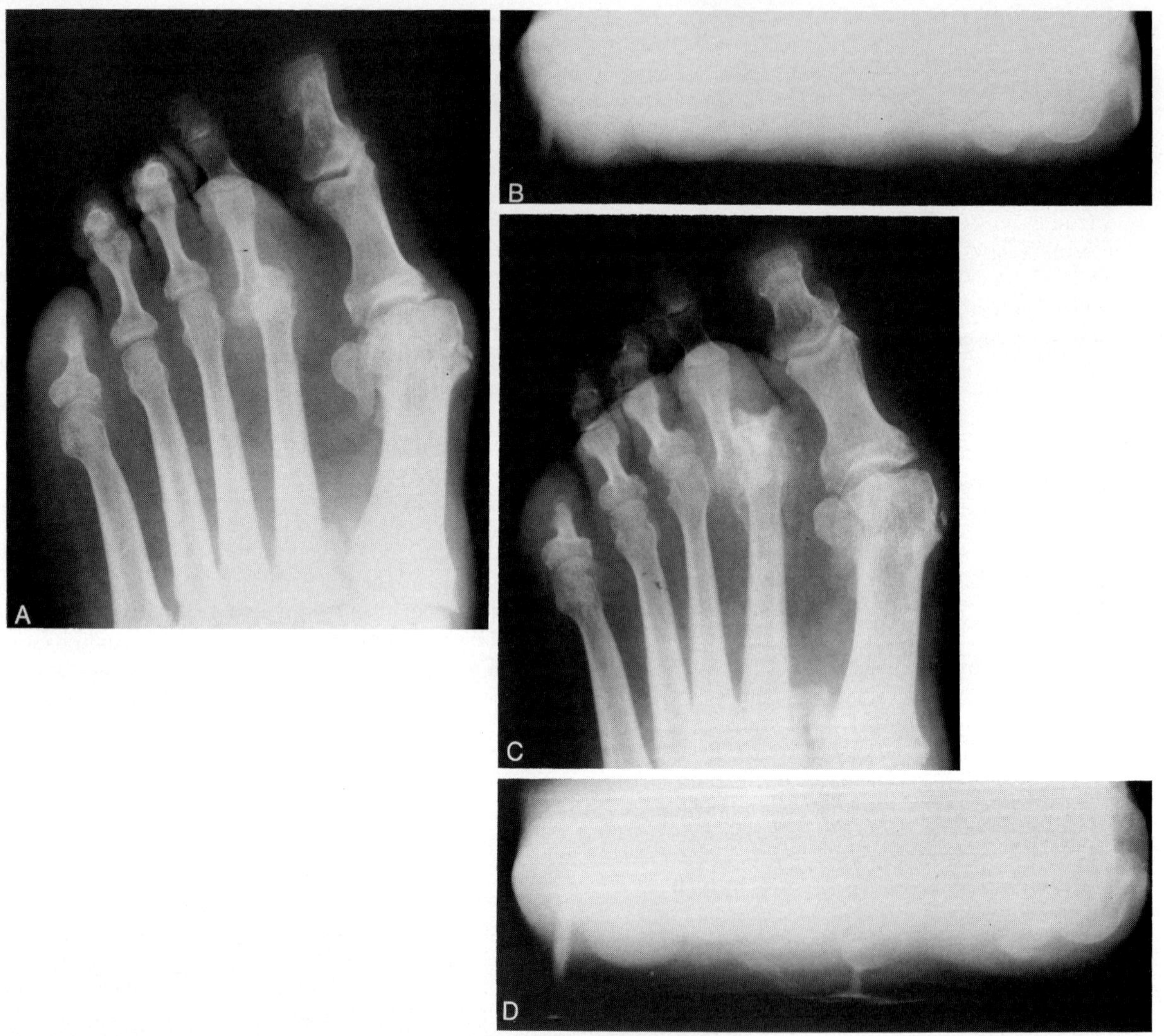

FIGURE 22–15. Anteroposterior (*A*) and plantar axial (*B*) radiographs. The patient presented with chronic draining ulceration on the sub-second metatarsal head. *C* and *D*, Sinograms of this patient. Note the intra-articular involvement in this draining ulceration.

dium until resistance is felt in the syringe. Radiography can then easily detect various extensions, compartments, or pseudopods that are often present and complicate successful excision. The boundaries are thus assessed, allowing for more accurate preoperative planning.

Hemangiomas lend themselves to examination and visualization using contrast medium. The larger cavernous type of hemangiomas often have connections to deep vascular channels that may necessitate arteriography. In evaluation of these larger types of hemangiomas, feeder arteries may be identified for ligation or possible sclerosing purposes.

Bursography can be used when chronic soft tissue masses are suspected to be inflamed anatomic or adventitious bursae. The patient may report that some of these masses exude fluid from time to time. These bursal sac walls can become tenuous, weaken, and even rupture into deeper or more superficial structures or spaces, or they can communicate with the skin and cause chronic draining sinuses. It is this type of lesion that can have extensions into various soft tissues or osseous structures or spaces. The use of radiopaque dye injected into these sinuses can help delineate these extensions. Connections with the external environment can be transcutaneous routes for infectious organisms and ultimately result in complications such as osteomyelitis and pyarthroses. Joint involvement can be documented and treatment customized in these difficult, sometimes confusing cases.

Akin to bursography is the sinogram. Various abscesses, sinus tracts, or other cloacal structures can be outlined effectively with the use of radiopaque study. Patients with neuropathic and chronic bone infection often have sinus tracts of

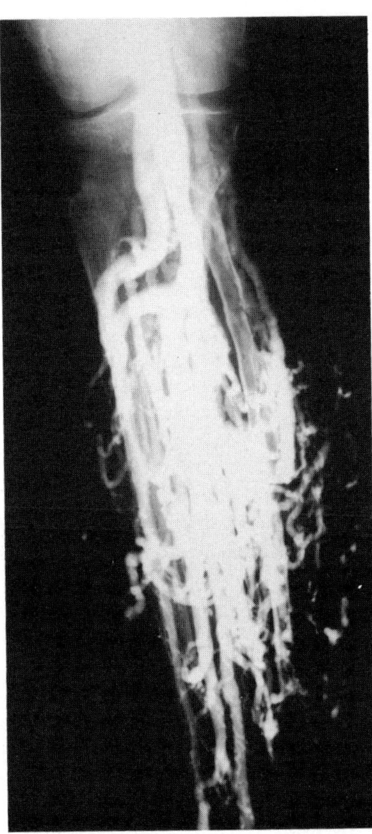

FIGURE 22–17. A venogram demonstrating occlusion of the tributary of the popliteal vein.

various depths and penetrations. Penetrance through deep fascial septa or into joint capsule (Fig. 22–15) or osseous intramedullary spaces can drastically alter treatment intervention. Sinograms have been used in many multidisciplinary centers as an important tool in limb salvage. However, MRI will ultimately surpass this technique in terms of early detection of osteomyelitis when there is an overlying soft tissue defect that communicates with adjoining bone.

Sinographic Technique

A simple plastic catheter can be used with radiopaque dye and syringe to infuse the area of interest. Goldman and associates[26] recommended a 23-gauge Intramedic-Luer stub adapter or French catheter, and they also noted the importance of a snug fit between the catheter and the sinus tract. Care should be taken not to exert excessive pressure, which could be responsible for tenuous cloacal or sinus boundary rupture.

VENOGRAPHIC, ARTERIOGRAPHIC, AND DIGITAL VASCULAR STUDIES

The theory and specific uses of venographic, arteriographic, and digital vascular studies are beyond the scope of this chapter. These studies are used to evaluate the flow and patency of various vascular structures. Various specialists employ them to evaluate occlusion or the possibility for bypass or balloon angioplasty of specific vessels (Figs. 22–16 and 22–17). Another advantageous use of these modalities

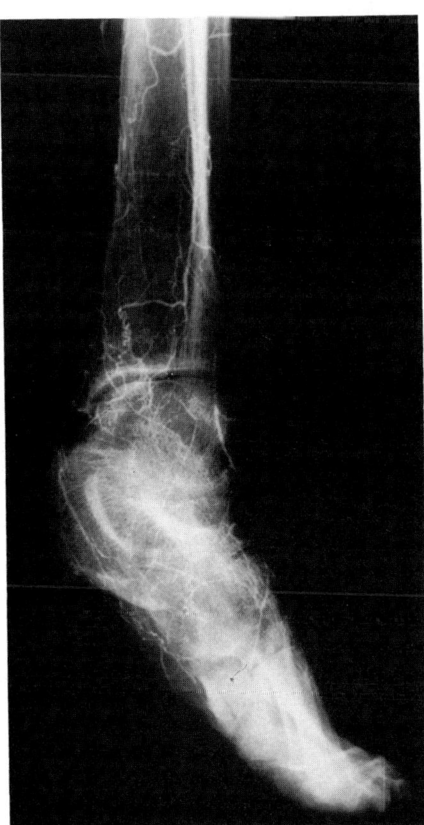

FIGURE 22–16. Arteriogram of the distal leg and foot, demonstrating extensive collateral flow. Posterior, anterior, and peroneal patent vessels are not evident.

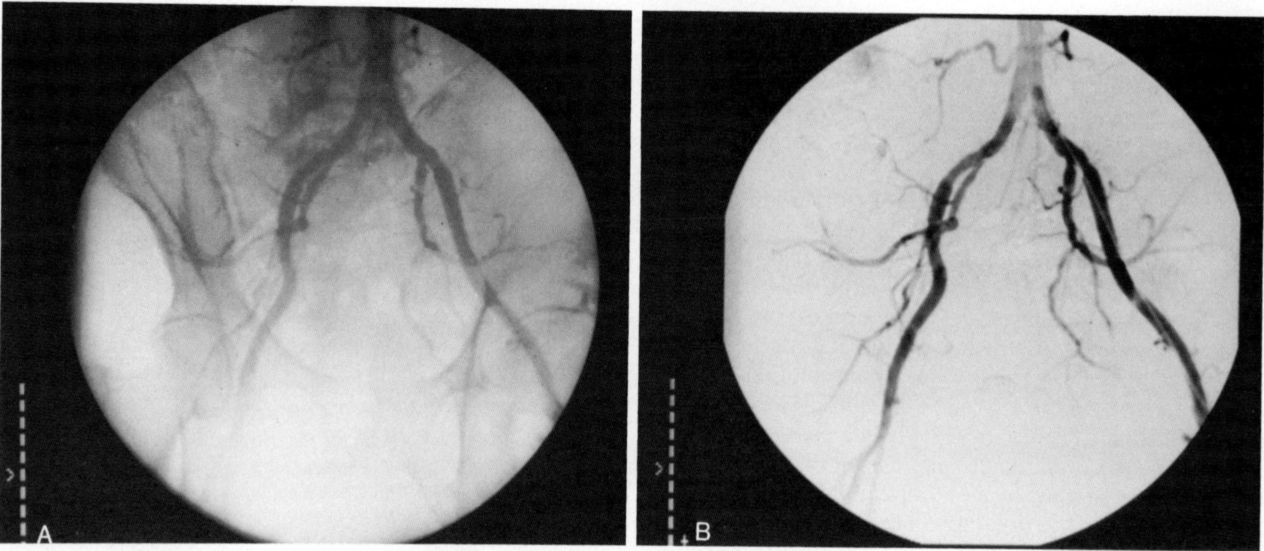

FIGURE 22–18. *A*, An arteriogram of the distal aorta and the iliac branches prior to computed osseous subtraction. *B*, Digital subtraction arteriogram of the same patient.

is the evaluation of blood flow to a specific area being contemplated for vascular-supplied grafts. Figures 22–16 and 22–17 show examples of extensive collateral flow in an arteriogram and occlusion of a tributary distal to the popliteal vein.

Digital subtraction arteriography (DSA) studies, first described in 1935 by Ziedses Des Plantes, has the benefit of providing image enhancement by improving and bringing out detail in areas hidden by overlying bone.[27] Because of the ability of the computer to assist in bringing out this contrast, one can detect extremely low levels of contrast medium not readily apparent in routine arteriography (Fig. 22–18). This might be advantageous in evaluating collateral flow in patients with severe arteriosclerotic disease. It has also been shown that intra-arterial DSA is superior to intravenous DSA in demonstrating the pedal arterial arcades.[28]

CONCLUSION

Contrast radiography is a useful tool for the clinician's armamentarium to decide how a patient will proceed with a diagnostic and treatment plan. It can also be used to evaluate the outcome of treatment. If the results of the study are inconclusive, one still has the opportunity to proceed to more costly and at times more invasive studies.

The author acknowledges and thanks the following people for their contribution to this chapter: Drs. G. Friedland, D. Highsmith, A. Björkengren, L. Oloff, S. Palladino, E. Houtkooper, E. Lang; and Ms. M. Escobar.

References

1. Spataro RF: New and Old Contrast Agents: Pharmacology and Tissue Opacification. Readings from the Society of Uroradiology Meeting, 1988.
2. Shehadi WH and Tonioio G: Adverse reactions to contrast media. Diagn Radiol 137:299–302, 1980.
3. Fischer HW and Doust VL: An evaluation of pretesting in the problem of serious and fatal reactions to excretory urography. Diagn Radiol 103:497–501, 1972.
4. Cohan RH, Dunnick NR, and Bashore TM: Treatment of reactions to radiographic contrast material. Am J Radiol 151:263–270, 1988.
5. Ala-Ketola L, Puranen J, Koivisto E, et al: Arthrography in the diagnosis of ligament injuries and classification of ankle injuries. Radiology 125:63–68, 1977.
6. Brostrom L: Sprained ankles: III. Clinical observations in recent ligament ruptures. Acta Chir Scand 130:560–569, 1965.
7. Resnick D and Niwayamag G (eds): Diagnosis of Bone and Joint Disorders with Emphasis on Articular Abnormalities. Philadelphia: WB Saunders, 1981, pp 596–619.
8. Fordyce AJW and Horn CV: Arthrography in recent injuries of the ligaments of the ankle. J Bone Joint Surg 54B:116–121, 1972.
9. Gordon RB: Arthrography of the ankle joint. J Bone Joint Surg 52A:1623–1631, 1970.
10. Harrington KD: Degenerative arthritis of the ankle secondary to long-standing lateral ligament instability. J Bone Joint Surg 61A:354, 1979.
11. Perlman MD: Usage of radiographic contrast media in the foot and ankle. J Foot Surg 27:3–29, 1988.
12. Kelikian H and Kelikian AS: Disorders of the Ankle. Philadelphia, WB Saunders, 1985, p 141.
13. Arner O, Ekengren K, Hulting B, et al: Arthrography of the talo-crural joint: Anatomic, roentgenographic, and clinical aspects. Acta Chir Scand 113:253–259, 1957.
14. Brostrom L, Liljedahl SO, and Lindvall N: Sprained ankles: II. Arthrographic diagnosis of recent ligament ruptures. Acta Chir Scand 129:485–499, 1965.
15. Meyer JM and Lagier R: Post-traumatic sinus tarsi syndrome: An anatomical and radiological study. Acta Orthop Scand 48:121, 1977.
16. Gerbert J, Spector E, and La Porta G: A preliminary report on arthrography of the first metatarsal-phalangeal joint. Arch Podiatr Med Foot Surg 1:75–84, 1973.
17. Weston WJ: The normal arthrograms of the metacarpo-phalangeal, metatarso-phalangeal and inter-phalangeal joints. Aust Radiol 13:211–218, 1969.
18. Karpman RR and MacCollum MS: Arthrography of the metatarsophalangeal joint. Foot Ankle 9:125–129, 1988.
19. Dykyj D and Jules KT: The clinical anatomy of tendons. J Am Podiatr Med Assoc 81:358–365, 1991.
20. Gilula LA, Oloff L, Caputi R, et al: Ankle tenography: A key to unexplained symptomatology: II. Diagnosis of chronic tendon disabilities. Radiology 151:581–587, 1984.
21. Resnick D and Goergen TG: Peroneal tenography in previous calcaneal fractures. Radiology 115:211, 1975.
22. Deyerle WM: Long-term follow-up of fractures of the os calcis: Diagnostic peroneal synoviogram. Orthop Clin North Am 4:213–227, 1973.
23. Sarrafian SK: Tendon Sheaths and Bursae: Anatomy of the Foot and Ankle. Philadelphia, JB Lippincott, 1983, pp 251–259.
24. Slavitt J, Beheshti F, Lenet M, et al: Ganglions of the foot: A six-year retrospective study and a review of the literature. J Am Podiatr Assoc 70:459, 1980.
25. Reinherz RP: Contrast media in the foot. J Am Podiatr Assoc 72:569–571, 1982.
26. Goldman F, Manzi J, Carver A, et al: Sinography in the diagnosis of foot infections. J Am Podiatr Assoc 71:497–502, 1981.
27. Jeans WD: The development and use of digital subtraction angiography. Br J Radiol 63:161–168, 1990.
28. Hol PK, Heldaas J, and Skjennald A: Demonstration of pedal arterial arcades in occlusive arteriosclerotic disease: Conventional and digital subtraction angiography compared. Acta Radiol 30:61–63, 1989.

CHAPTER 23

Cross-Sectional Imaging

Mark E. Schweitzer, M.D., Juerg Hodler, M.D.,
and David J. Sartoris, M.D.

The human foot may be anatomically subdivided into three parts: hindfoot, midfoot, and forefoot. The hindfoot contains the talus and calcaneus. The midfoot includes the navicular, cuboid, and cuneiforms, although some investigators place the cuboid and navicular in the hindfoot. The metatarsals and phalanges comprise the forefoot.

ANATOMIC STRUCTURES OF THE HINDFOOT

Bones. Osseous structures of the hindfoot include the distal tibia, distal fibula, talus, calcaneus, and inconstant sesamoids. Important landmarks, each of which can be identified on cross-sectional imaging studies, are indicated in Figures 23–1 to 23–4.

Ligaments. The interosseous ligaments of the hindfoot are visualized on cross-sectional imaging studies as thin, soft tissue densities that join adjacent bony surfaces, providing stabilization to the articulations they cover.

Muscles and Tendons. The major musculotendinous units of the hindfoot are indicated in Figures 23–1 to 23–4. They may be classified into two major categories: muscles that originate proximal to the foot and the intrinsic muscles of the foot. Each of these may be further subdivided into dorsal and plantar groups. On cross-sectional imaging studies, muscles are visualized as broad, moderately inhomogeneous soft tissue densities, often with fibrous or fatty septa delineating separate fiber bundles. Tendons are smaller and manifest more uniform, higher computed tomographic (CT) density and lower magnetic resonance imaging (MRI) signal intensity. The musculotendinous transition of a given unit is gradual and may occur over several transaxial images using contiguous 3-mm thick slices. Tendon sheaths can be resolved from the structures they contain by MRI.

Arteries. The major arterial supply to the hindfoot begins with the parent popliteal artery in the calf. Depending on its course relative to the plane of section, this structure is visualized as a curvilinear or round soft tissue density, which may be calcified. Intravenous contrast medium enhances the distinction between arteries and nerves on CT images when the former are not calcified.

Veins. The deep veins of the hindfoot (often paired) accompany their respective arteries, and the combination is generally imaged as a single structure. The two major superficial veins of the hindfoot, the great (long) saphenous and the small (short) saphenous veins, are readily visualized on cross-sectional imaging studies. In addition, various unnamed members of the superficial dorsal and plantar venous networks are seen. Once again, intravenous contrast medium can facilitate indentification of these structures.

Nerves. The innervation of the hindfoot begins with the parent femoral and sciatic nerves. On cross-sectional imaging studies, nerves are visualized as round or curvilinear soft tissue densities that generally course with accompanying vascular structures. Individual muscular branches are difficult to identify with confidence, but cutaneous rami can be resolved.

Fascia. The major fascial structures of the hindfoot are readily visualized on cross-sectional imaging studies. The pedal fascia may be classified as either superficial or deep. The superficial fascia of the hindfoot is best seen in the plantar region, where abundant adjacent fat exists. The retinacula constitute localized, deep fascial thickenings that bind tendons down as they cross the talocrural joint. Major fascial structures, as well as numerous unnamed fibrous strands that traverse the subcutaneous fat, are visualized as thin, linear

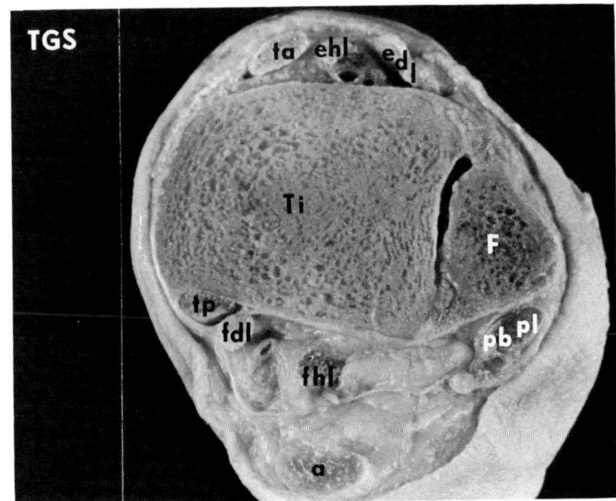

FIGURE 23–1. Axial anatomic section at the level of the syndesmosis. ta, tibialis anterior; ehl, extensor hallucis longus; edl, extensor digitorum longus; Ti, tibia; F, fibula; tp, tibialis posterior; fdl, flexor digitorum longus; fhl, flexor hallucis longus; pb, peroneus brevis; pl, peroneus longus; a, Achilles.

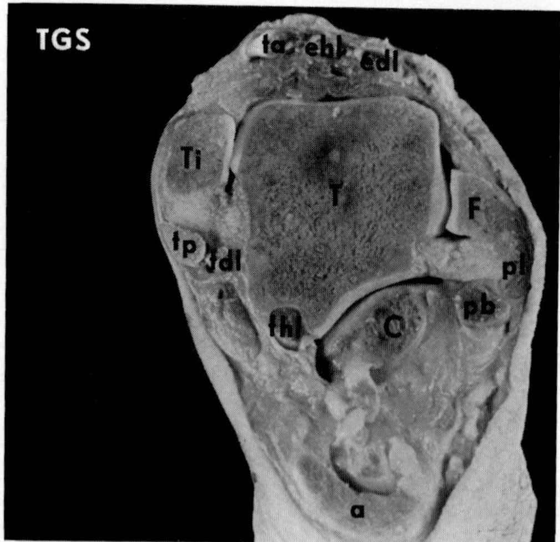

FIGURE 23–2. Axial anatomic section at the level of the talar dome. ta, tibialis anterior; ehl, extensor hallucis longus; edl, extensor digitorum longus; Ti, tibia; T, talus; F, fibula; tp, tibialis posterior; fdl, flexor digitorum longus; fhl, flexor hallucis longus; C, calcaneus; pb, peroneus brevis; pl, peroneus longus; a, Achilles.

bands with density and signal intensity comparable to that of tendons.

Miscellaneous. The lymphatic vessels of the hindfoot are small and unnamed but can be visualized on cross-sectional imaging studies in the plantar region, where low-density subcutaneous fat is plentiful. The medial and lateral superficial channels course, respectively, with the great and small saphenous veins and cannot be resolved from these structures. Soft

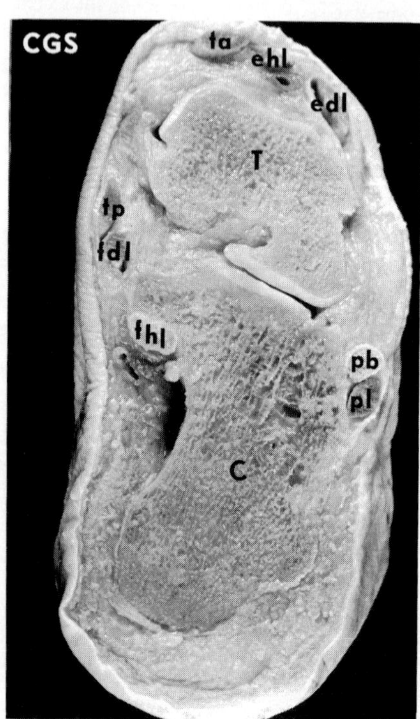

FIGURE 23–3. Axial anatomic section at the level of the subtalar joint. ta, tibialis anterior; ehl, extensor hallucis longus; edl, extensor digitorum longus; T, talus; tp, tibialis posterior; fdl, flexor digitorum longus; fhl, flexor hallucis longus; C, calcaneus; pl, peroneus longus; pb, peroneus brevis.

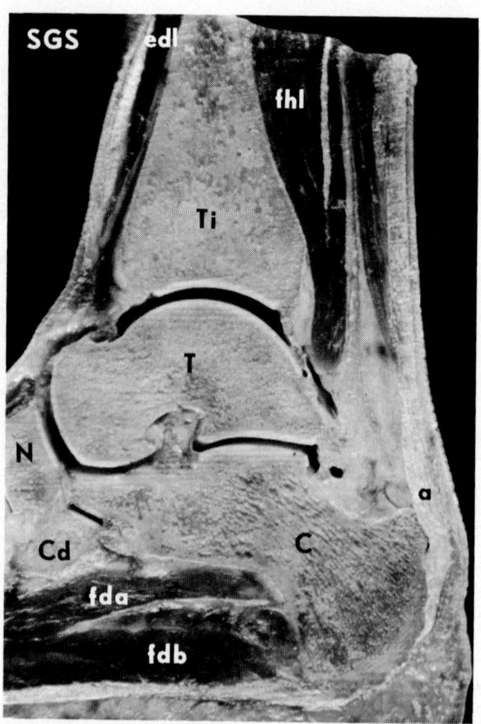

FIGURE 23–4. Midline sagittal anatomic specimen. edl, extensor digitorum longus; fhl, flexor hallucis longus; Ti, tibia; T, talus; N, navicular; Cd, cuboid; C, calcaneus; fda, flexor digitorum accessorius; fdb, flexor digitorum brevis; a, Achilles.

tissue densities between osseous articular facets represent synovium, fluid, cartilage, and fibrous capsule, but individual joint structures can be resolved only by MRI. Skin is recognized between the subcutaneous fat and the surrounding air and is markedly thickened in the weightbearing areas of the sole.

ANATOMIC STRUCTURES OF THE MIDFOOT

Bones. By definition, the midfoot includes the navicular, cuboid, and cuneiform bones, although some investigators place the cuboid and navicular in the hindfoot. The transaxial plane does not respect this strict anatomic division; hence, portions of the talus and calcaneus are included in more proximal images. Similarly, distal images contain the metatarsal bases and proximal shafts laterally.

Important bony structures that can be identified on cross-sectional imaging studies are indicated in Figures 23–5 and 23–6.

Ligaments. The ligaments of the midfoot are generally named for the articulations that they stabilize. On cross-sectional imaging studies, these structures are visualized as flat soft tissue densities of variable size lying immediately superficial to the bones.

Muscles and Tendons. The musculotendinous units of the midfoot are indicated in Figures 23–5 and 23–6. As in the hindfoot, classification into intrinsic/extrinsic and dorsal/plantar groups is possible. On cross-sectional imaging studies, musculotendinous transitions are characterized by a gradual decrease in size and inhomogeneity of density, accompanied by an increase in CT density or a decrease in MRI signal intensity. Intervening subcutaneous fat becomes

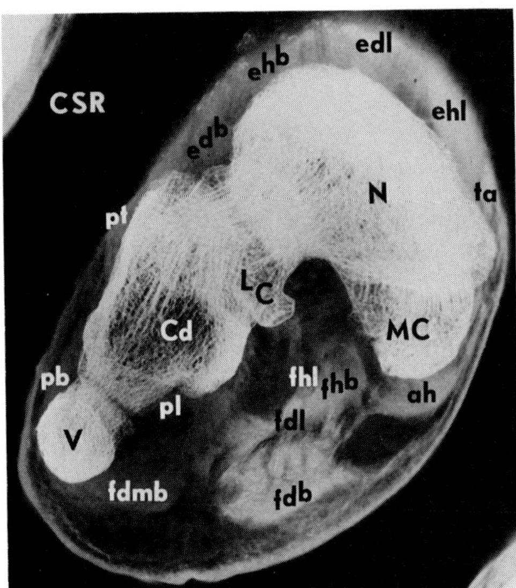

FIGURE 23–5. Specimen radiograph coronal section through the midfoot. pb, peroneus brevis; pt, peroneus tertius; edb, extensor digitorum brevis; ehb, extensor hallucis brevis; edl, extensor digitorum longus; ehl, extensor hallucis longus; ta, tibialis anterior; V, fifth metatarsal; Cd, cuboid; LC, lateral cuneiform; N, navicular; MC, medial cuneiform; pl, peroneus longus; fhl, flexor hallucis longus; fhb, flexor hallucis brevis; fdl, flexor digitorum longus; fdmb, flexor digiti-minimi brevis; fdb, flexor digitorum brevis; ah, abductor hallucis.

sparse in the distal midfoot, resulting in an inability to resolve adjacent muscles as distinct structures.

Arteries. The major arteries of the midfoot are more difficult to visualize on cross-sectional imaging studies than those in the hindfoot because of their progressively diminishing size. Intravenous contrast medium as well as calcification of larger vessels can facilitate their identification.

Veins. As in the hindfoot, the deep veins of the midfoot are generally paired venae comitantes that are not resolved discretely from their respective arteries. The dorsal venous arch, which lies predominantly in the forefoot, continues proximally as the medial and lateral marginal veins. The great saphenous vein is the proximal continuation of the former, whereas the latter becomes the small (short) saphenous vein. In addition to these superficial veins, various unnamed members of the dorsal and plantar venous networks are visualized on cross-sectional imaging studies. Intravenous contrast medium can enhance identification of these structures.

Nerves. Because of their progressively diminishing size, resolution of the major nerves of the midfoot on cross-sectional imaging studies is more difficult than in the hindfoot, particularly in regions of low natural contrast. Their tendency to accompany vascular structures facilitates identification. Cutaneous rami are obscured in areas with thick skin or underlying retinacula, and individual muscular branches cannot be confidently recognized.

Fascia. The major superficial and deep fascial structures of the midfoot are readily visualized on cross-sectional imaging studies. Three retinacula or deep fascial tendon coverings that originate in the hindfoot extend distally into midfoot images. Although all three parts of the plantar aponeurosis become progressively thinner on more distal sections, the central part is obviously thickest at any given level. The lateral and medial vertical intermuscular septa extend from the junctions of the lateral/central and medial/central parts of the plantar aponeurosis, respectively, to the overlying osseous structures and separate the three plantar muscle compartments (Fig. 23–7A to C). Portions of these incomplete structures, as well as the superficial plantar fascia and numerous unnamed fibrous strands, may be identified on cross-sectional imaging studies.

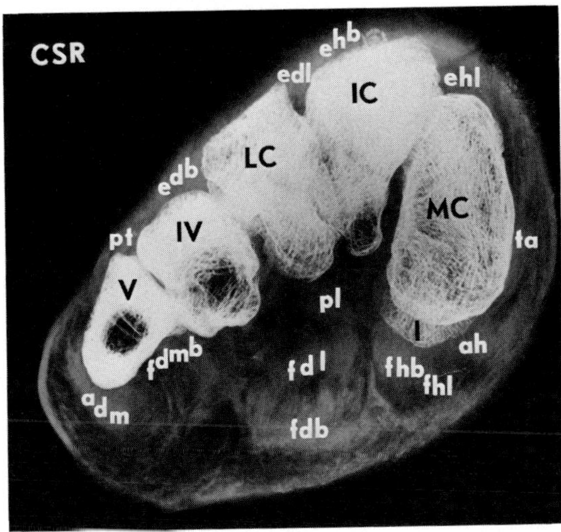

FIGURE 23–6. Specimen radiograph coronal section at the approximate level of Lisfranc's joint. pt, peroneus tertius; edb, extensor digitorum brevis; edl, extensor digitorum longus; ehb, extensor hallucis brevis; ehl, extensor hallucis longus; ta, tibialis anterior; V, fifth metatarsal; IV, fourth metatarsal; LC, lateral cuneiform; IC, intermediate cuneiform; MC, media cuneiform; I, first metatarsal; adm, abductor digiti minimi; fdmb, flexor digiti-minimi brevis; pl, peroneus longus; fdl, flexor digitorum longus; fdb, flexor digitorum brevis; fhb, flexor hallucis brevis; fhl, flexor hallucis longus; ah, abductor hallucis.

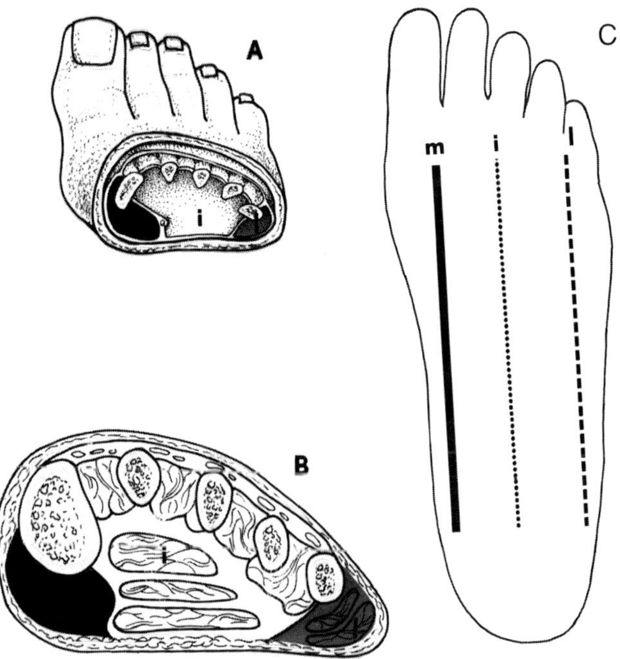

FIGURE 23–7. Compartments of the feet. *A,* Level of metatarsals. *B,* Cross section slightly proximal to *A. C,* Plantar surface of foot with region of compartments labeled. m, medial; i, intermediate; l, lateral.

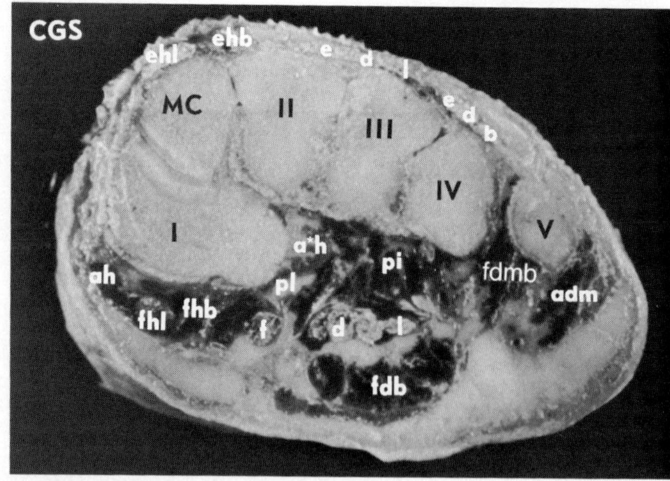

FIGURE 23–8. Coronal anatomic specimen level of Lisfranc's joints. ehl, extensor hallucis longus; ehb, extensor hallucis brevis; edl, extensor digitorum longus; edb, extensor digitorum brevis; MC, medial cuneiform; I, first metatarsal; II, second metatarsal; III, third metatarsal; IV, fourth metatarsal; V, fifth metatarsal; ah, abductor hallucis; fhl, flexor hallucis longus; fhb, flexor hallucis brevis; fdl, flexor digitorum longus; pl, peroneus longus; a*h, abductor hallucis; pi, plantar interossei; fdb, flexor digitorum brevis; fdmb, flexor digiti-minimi brevis; adm, abductor digiti minimi.

Miscellaneous. Midfoot lymphatic vessels are small, unnamed, and generally not confidently distinguished from the vascular structures with which they course. The medial superficial channel travels proximally with the great saphenous vein. As in the hindfoot, intrinsic components of articulations can be resolved only by MRI. Skin thickening in weightbearing areas of the sole is readily apparent on cross-sectional imaging studies.

ANATOMIC STRUCTURES OF THE FOREFOOT

Bones. Osseous structures of the forefoot are indicated in Figures 23–8 to 23–10. Interphalangeal joints that parallel the transaxial plane are not discretely imaged using a slice thickness of 3 mm.

Ligaments. The ligaments of the forefoot are named for their positions relative to the articulations that they stabilize. The collateral and plantar interphalangeal ligaments are not discretely resolved, but their arrangement is comparable to that of the collateral and plantar metatarsophalangeal ligaments.

Muscles and Tendons. The musculotendinous units of the forefoot are indicated in Figures 23–8 to 23–10. As in the hindfoot and midfoot, intrinsic/extrinsic and dorsal/plantar categorizations can be made. Musculotendinous transitions

are gradual and may occur over several transaxial intervals with the use of 3-mm thick contiguous slices. Tendons lying adjacent to each other, such as the flexor digitorum longus and brevis distally, are imaged as a single structure; the fibrous flexor tendon sheaths are not discretely resolved.

Arteries. Visualization of the arteries of the forefoot is more difficult than in the hindfoot and midfoot because of their diminishing size; intravenous contrast medium can facilitate their identification. The arcuate artery, perforating branches of the plantar arch, and distal perforating branches of the plantar metatarsal arteries are not resolved using 3-mm thick coronal slices, because they course relatively parallel to the transaxial plane.

Veins. The deep veins of the forefoot are venae comitantes, which are imaged as single structures with their respective arteries. Superficially, intercommunicating dorsal and plantar digital veins drain proximally into dorsal metatarsal veins and the plantar cutaneous venous arch, respectively. Proximal to the latter, unnamed members of the plantar cutaneous venous network can be identified by cross-sectional imaging studies. The dorsal metatarsal veins unite across the metatarsal bases to form the dorsal venous arch; although the lateral portion of this vein lies at midfoot levels, it is not discretely resolved because of sparse dorsal subcutaneous fat. The dorsal venous network lies proximal to this

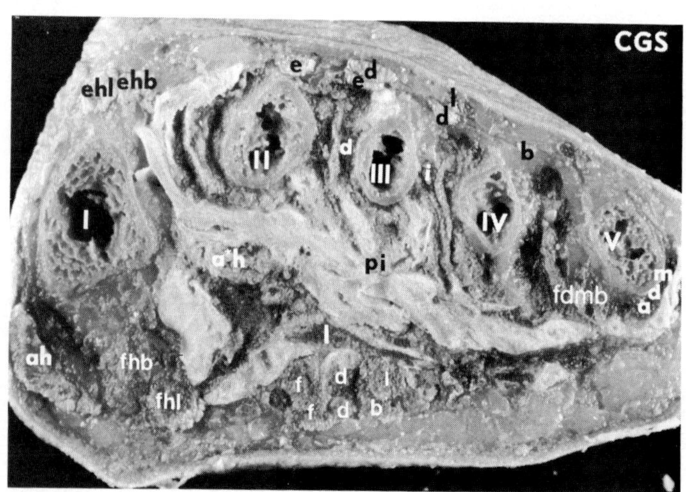

FIGURE 23–9. Coronal anatomic specimen through metatarsals. ehl, extensor hallucis longus; ehb, extensor hallucis brevis; edl, extensor digitorum longus; edb, extensor digitorum brevis; d (white), dorsal; i, interossei; I, first metatarsal; II, second metatarsal; III, third metatarsal; IV, fourth metatarsal; V, fifth metatarsal; ah, abductor hallucis; fhb, flexor hallucis brevis; fhl, flexor hallucis longus; a*h, abductor hallucis; pi, plantar interossei; fdl, flexor digitorum longus; fdb, flexor digitorum brevis; fdmb, flexor digiti-minimi brevis; adm, abductor digiti minimi.

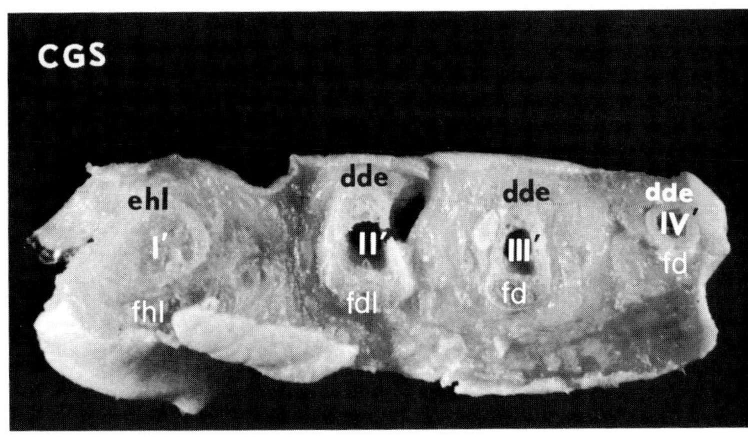

FIGURE 23–10. Coronal anatomic specimen through digits. ehl, extensor hallucis longus; dde, dorsal digital expansion; I', phalanx of the first toe; II', phalanx of the second toe; III', phalanx of the third toe; IV', phalanx of the fourth toe; fhl, flexor hallucis longus; fdl and fd, flexor digitorum longus.

arch, and both drain medially into the medial marginal vein. Intravenous contrast medium can enhance visualization of these structures.

Nerves. Owing to their small size, most forefoot nerves (with the exception of cutaneous rami) cannot be resolved discretely from adjacent structures with confidence. Nevertheless, knowledge of their distribution may be important to the radiologist in the setting of pathologic enlargement (e.g., neurogenic tumors and leprosy) or other clinical situations.

Fascia. The major deep and superficial fascial components of the forefoot are readily visualized on cross-sectional imaging studies. The five digital bands of the plantar aponeurosis (central part) are united by transverse fibers as they diverge plantar to the metatarsal shafts; each has associated retinacula cutis (skin ligaments), paired digital flexor septa, and plantar interdigital (superficial transverse metatarsal) ligaments. The deep fascia on the dorsum of the foot (fascia dorsalis pedis) is continuous proximally with the inferior extensor retinaculum, blends medially and laterally with the plantar aponeurosis, and distally ensheathes the extensor tendons. In addition to these structures, the superficial plantar fascia and numerous unnamed fibrous strands are identifiable. The three plantar muscle compartments (see Fig. 23–7A to C) are less distinctly separated than in the midfoot.

Miscellaneous. Forefoot lymphatic vessels are small, unnamed, and not resolved independent of the vascular structures with which they course. As in the hindfoot and midfoot, individual components of articulations can be distinguished only by MRI. Toenails and skin thickening in the sole are readily identified on cross-sectional imaging studies.

IMAGING TECHNIQUES

Computed Tomography

CT is based on usual radiographic variables, however, computer manipulation of data is performed to obtain cross-sectional images. Because the usual radiographic factors apply, appearance of structures is not dissimilar to that achieved with routine radiography: metal and bone have the greatest density, and air and fat have the least density.

To perform a scan, the patient is placed on a table that passes within a gantry. The gantry contains a ring of x-ray detectors and tubes. A narrow x-ray beam goes from a tube through the patient to the detector on the opposite side of the ring. The process is sequentially performed until the entire 360-degree circle is imaged. This complete arc represents a "slice." The slice is of variable thickness but is usually between 1.5 and 5 mm in the feet. The thicker the slice, the less noise is present, although subtle detail will be lost through tissue volume averaging. Each slice is divided into small units called *voxels*. Each voxel is assigned a number, called the *Hounsfield number,* which is an absolute measure of x-ray attenuation. To create an image, each Hounsfield unit is assigned a shade of gray. These voxels are then called *pixels,* which are filmed. Each pixel makes up a tiny part of the image we see, similar to the dots on a television screen that make up that matrix. The Hounsfield number is absolute and aids in tissue characterization. Numbers close to zero are fluid, small negative numbers represent fat, large negative numbers represent gas or air, and high positive numbers represent calcium or metal. Although the Hounsfield number is absolute, the shade of gray imaged is variable depending on settings called *window* and *level.* By convention, fat and air are dark and bone is white.

The CT scan is performed with both feet symmetrically positioned, which facilitates contralateral comparison. Axial images are performed perpendicular to the long axis of the body. Images in the coronal plane are transverse images of the feet. The patient is positioned supine with knees flexed and soles of the feet flat on the table. True coronal images of the ankle usually require angulation of the gantry. Direct sagittal imaging of the foot is virtually impossible. To acquire sagittal images, computer-assisted reformations are done. The quality of these reformations is dependent on using thin slices on the direct images.

Computed Tomography–Three-Dimensional Reconstruction

Three-dimensional reconstruction usually is based on bone CT images that have good inherent spatial resolution and are of high contrast. Thin, contiguous slices are required. Movements by the patient during the data acquisition have to be avoided because they result in a distorted final image. Typical technical parameters used in the foot are a slice thickness of 2 to 3 mm and no interslice gap. For small bones like the midtarsal bones and toes, overlapping slices may be used. The simplest and most often used reconstruction algorithms are based on a surface reconstruction. The brightness of every pixel is measured and based on a preset value. The computer decides whether this pixel is to be included in the reconstruction. A high preset value is chosen when bone is to be visualized. Soft tissue will be obscured in this instance. This results in a surface reconstruction because internal structures are covered by the dense superficial structures. A simulated light source is used to create the appearance of depth, with bright pixels being closer to the eye (superficial) and darker pixels being farther from the eye (Fig. 23–11). In some programs, the position of this light source can be changed and other program parts of the object can be highlighted. More complicated algorithms may result in simulated transparent images that show both superficial and internal structures. This and more complicated procedures like disarticulations or the demonstration of soft tissue structures with less inherent contrast require more complicated computer hardware and software as well as time-consuming human interaction. Presently, indications for three-dimensional reconstruction in the foot mainly involve CT of trauma, primarily in the calcaneus region.[1] Evolving uses include the perioperative review of complex foot deformities such as clubfoot.

Magnetic Resonance Imaging

In MRI, the influence of a changing magnetic field and radio frequency pulses on hydrogen protons in the body is measured and used to reconstruct cross-sectional images in varying planes. Image intensity depends on a number of different factors. The most important of these are T_1, T_2 proton density, and flow effects. T_1 and T_2 are time constants that describe the reactions of structures to changes in the magnetic field. Depending on how frequently pulses are applied (repetition time [TR]) and on the time when the resultant signal is measured (echo time [TE]), T_1-weighted images or T_2-weighted images result. T_1-weighted images have a short TR (a typical value is 500 ms) and a short TE (a typical value is 20 ms). T_2-weighted images have a long TR (e.g., 2000 ms) and a long TE (e.g., 80 ms). Fat is bright on both T_1- and T_2-weighted images, although it is relatively brighter on T_1-weighted imaging. Free water, as present in cysts but also as occurs in edema in many pathologic processes, is dark (hypointense) on T_1-weighted images and increases in signal on T_2-weighted images. Normal soft tissue–like muscle is gray on both T_1- and T_2-weighted images. Extravascular blood demonstrates different signal behavior depending on the age of the hemorrhage. Fresh blood often appears bright on T_1- and T_2-weighted images, whereas old hemorrhage with hemosiderin formation is dark on both sequences.

The higher the proton density, the higher the image intensity will be. Several soft tissue components have a high density of hydrogen proton (i.e., water, fat) and therefore will usually appear more intense than bone and fibrous tissue, which have smaller amounts of mobile protons and, therefore, appear less intense. Proton density images are acquired with a long TR (e.g., 2000 ms) and a short TE (20 ms). They are routinely acquired together with the T_2-weighted images as a two-echo sequence.

Another important imaging factor is flow: Nonexcited protons may flow into the excited part of the body, resulting in unexpected signal behavior. Rapid flow, as present in arteries, appears hypointense, whereas slow-flowing blood in veins can show variable signal behavior depending on velocity.[2]

The main magnet of the scanner can be used both as emitter and receiver. For smaller regions like the foot, however, surface coils are used that may only receive or both emit and receive signal. Several different types of coils are available: tunnel-like coils, flexible wraparound coils, and flat coils, which are placed underneath the region of interest. These dedicated coils result in improved signal-to-noise ratio and better spatial resolution.

Informing the patient about what to expect from the scan is necessary. The narrow tunnel may cause claustrophobia, and the loud knocking noise caused by moving parts during changes of magnetic fields is disturbing. Moreover, MRI examinations are relatively long (30 to 60 minutes for a foot examination) and must be performed without patient motion. Positioning of the patient and the part to be examined is important to help the patient remain still during the examination. For examinations of the foot, the patient is usually placed supine. The feet are taped together to assist with immobilization. The sole of the foot may be placed against a border to obtain a rectangular position in the ankle joint, or the patient may be scanned prone to further improve immobilization. A typical MRI examination consists of T_1- and T_2-weighted images in the main imaging plane and T_1-weighted images in an additional imaging plane. Sagittal and axial images may be best to depict tarsal bones, their articulations, and related disease as well as the Achilles tendon. Coronal images are more often used for the ankle joint and are helpful for the toes. Slice thickness is 3 to 5 mm with an interslice gap of 1.5 to 2.5 mm in a typical examination.

Contraindications for MRI are cardiac pacemakers, some surgical clips (intracranial clips and most vascular clips) and

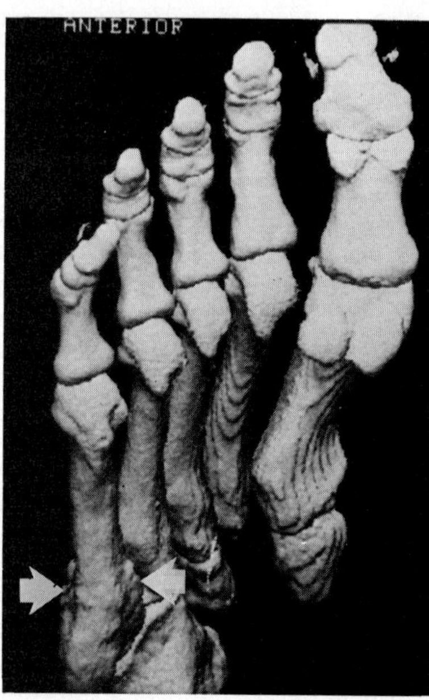

FIGURE 23–11. Three-dimensional reconstruction based on computed tomography (CT) scans with 2-mm slice thickness and 1-mm overlap. View from the plantar, lateral, and anterior. Residual posttraumatic irregularities are at the base of the fifth metatarsal *(arrows)*. Despite the optimal CT technique, a steplike appearance remains, mainly at the first and second metatarsals.

metallic foreign bodies, especially in the eye. Implanted material used for internal bone fixation is usually not dangerous but may degrade the quality of the images. Data are available that describe compatibility of various bioimplants (such as heart, bone, and ear) to decide whether an examination is contraindicated.[3]

Intravenous contrast media are mainly used in the central nervous system and less often in the musculoskeletal system. At present, mainly gadolinium complexes are used. Regions with increased blood flow will appear hyperintense on T_1-weighted images.[4]

Ultrasound Imaging

Ultrasound imaging is based on the differential velocities and reflections of high-frequency sound waves in various types of tissue. Fluid shows nearly no reflection, and the resultant images therefore appear anechoic (dark). Solid tissue reflects acoustic energy depending on its architecture. Very uniform tissue has less reflective surfaces than complex tissue and therefore appears less echoic. Calcifications and bone surfaces are highly reflective to ultrasound waves and appear hyperechoic (bright). Because no energy is transmitted through these structures, objects behind them will be obscured by the resulting acoustic shadow. A contact gel is used to enhance transmission between the transducer and the body surface. Several different types of transducers may be used. For soft tissue evaluation, linear transducers with a frequency of 5 to 7.5 mHz are preferred in most instances. The higher the frequency, the better the spatial resolution. However, these transducers have more limited depth penetration. In addition, structures very close to the transducer are not well visualized. Therefore, the distance between the transducer and the body surface may need to be increased with a standoff gel pad. Its flexibility also helps close gaps between the transducer and the irregular surface of the body that often occur around the foot, and it improves visualization of superficial structures. Ultrasonography of the musculoskeletal system has not become as important as this modality in abdominal or obstetric diagnoses. Ultrasonography has a high-contrast resolution, is inexpensive, is well tolerated by the patient, and is not time consuming. The disadvantages are its limited spatial resolution, operator dependence, and the difficulty in reading images from prints, which result in only limited acceptance of this technique in the musculoskeletal system. Ultrasonography is mainly used to depict soft tissue but not bone because the acoustic waves are entirely reflected at the bone surface, which prevents imaging of the internal structure.[5]

At present, the main indications for ultrasonograms of the foot are the depiction of the Achilles tendon and its surroundings and the differentiation between solid and fluid processes.[6] Ultrasonography may be used to guide fine-needle biopsy of a soft tissue. Real-time control of the needle position is possible and makes the procedure rapid and easy to perform. In addition, ultrasonography may detect early accumulation of subperiosteal fluid and may be helpful in the early diagnosis of osteomyelitis. We believe, however, that MRI is probably more sensitive and specific for the latter.

CLINICAL APPLICATIONS

Neoplasm and Related Disorders

Methods of Imaging

Routine Radiographs. These remain essential in the initial diagnosis of bone tumors because of their high spatial resolution and their depiction of subtle calcifications, bone erosion, and periosteal reaction. They frequently lead to a specific diagnosis on the basis of these findings. Radiographs are not always able, however, to depict correctly the extent of the tumor within bone marrow and adjacent soft tissue. Moreover, the role of plain films is limited in the diagnosis of soft tissue neoplasm because of the limited contrast resolution.

Modern staging systems are designed to plan the optimal surgical intervention.[2, 7] These systems are based on the extent and the aggressiveness of the tumor. Cross-sectional methods are mainly used to assess the extent of the tumor.

Sonography. This has a limited role in the staging of neoplasms because it is operator dependent and shows only the soft tissue regions of the tumor. Only in patients with severe cortical destruction is sonography able to show the intraosseous component of a tumor. Sonography may be the initial examination used to establish the differential diagnosis between a solid tumor and a benign cystic process such as a synovial cyst and a ganglion. The specificity of ultrasonography is limited. Most tumors appear hypoechoic. The surrounding reactive granulation tissue/hemorrhage may be impossible to be differentiated from the tumor itself. Ultrasonography is also limited in the follow-up of tumors because postoperative scars cannot be differentiated from the recurrent tumor itself.

Sonography can be helpful in guiding a needle biopsy in nonpalpable tumors, enabling one to avoid necrotic parts in a solid tumor and avoiding vascular structures.

Computed Tomography. Because MRI is now widely available, CT has a limited role in the staging of tumors. Its main capability is the depiction of cortical bone destruction. CT is also superior in the depiction of calcifications within the tumor, which may be helpful in the differential diagnosis.[8] The main disadvantages of CT are its inherently poor soft tissue contrast resolution and the limited choice of imaging planes. Most tumors cannot be differentiated from surrounding reactive tissue, bleeding, edema, and normal muscle. The injection of intravenous contrast medium can improve this differentiation. Although the role of CT in the local tumor staging is limited mainly to the more exact depiction of cortical bone, it is useful in evaluating visceral metastasis. It is the method of choice with regard to liver and lung metastasis. CT can be used to guide the needle in a percutaneous biopsy of both soft tissue and bone tumors. In the follow-up of tumors after therapy, limitations are expressed in terms of differentiating between scar and tumor.

Magnetic Resonance Imaging. This is the method of choice for the staging of tumors in bone and soft tissue. MRI is very sensitive in depicting tumor extension but is nonspecific.[8] The plain radiograph therefore remains essential. The radiologic evaluation of each patient's bone or soft tissue tumors should be standardized to allow consistent follow-up

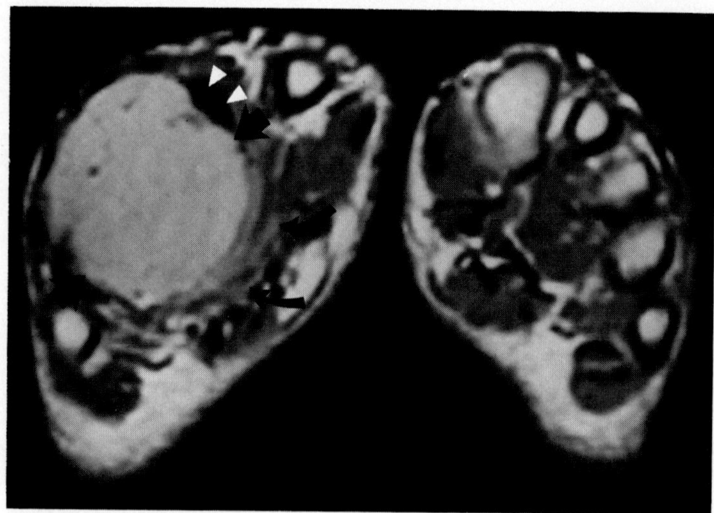

FIGURE 23–12. Chondromyxoid fibroma of the third metatarsal, proton-density coronal image. A large intermediate- to high-signal mass is noted *(black arrowheads)*. Because of the size, it is difficult to ascertain the origin of the mass, although it appears centered at the third metatarsal. Chronic erosion of the second metatarsal is noted with cortical thickening and loss of medullary signal *(white arrowheads).*

and comparison. Most tumors have an intensity similar to muscle on T_1-weighted images and high intensity on T_2-weighted images. Necrotic regions with liquefaction may behave like fluid with low intensity on T_1-weighted images and higher intensity than the rest of the tumor on T_2-weighted images. Large calcifications are visible as signal void. Small areas of calcification are only infrequently noted. Surrounding reactive tissue or even edema may have similar signal behavior as tumor, which may lead to an overestimation of the tumor size (Fig. 23–12). In some instances, however, the surrounding reaction will be less intense on T_2-weighted images than on the tumor itself. Potentially helpful is the use of intravenous gadolinium containing contrast medium, which increases the intensity of vascularized tumor tissue. MRI is superior to the other imaging methods in detecting the infiltration of neighboring soft tissue compartments, vascular structures, and adjacent articulations.

MRI is usually not specific in the characterization of tumors because the signal behavior does not relate to histologic diagnosis in a constant way, with several exceptions.[8–10] A lipoma is relatively characteristic in that it shows the same signal behavior as normal subcutaneous fat. Another tumor with a typical MRI appearance is an osteochondroma, which shows the same characteristic features as on plain films and CT: intact cortical bone continuous with the adjacent normal bone and extension of bone marrow into the tumor. The cartilaginous cap is well shown, and it has been suggested that MRI is the method of choice for follow-up of these tumors to detect malignant degeneration.[11] Neurogenic tumors, tumors containing myxoid tissue, and cartilaginous tumors may have high intensity on T_2-weighted images and may sometimes be confused with fluid collections like a seroma (Fig. 23–13). Cartilaginous tumors tend to be more lobulated. Vascular tumors may show enlarged vessels in and around the tumor. Hemangiomas of soft tissue show a serpiginous pattern and are often hyperintense on T_1-weighted images.[12] Tumors with a high percentage of fibrous tissue or with extensive ossification may be hypointense on both T_1- and T_2-weighted images. Aneurysmal bone cysts can demonstrate a characteristic fluid level, although this finding is described with several other lesions.[13]

The injection of intravenous gadolinium containing contrast medium can depict the degree of vascularity of the tumor and narrow the differential diagnosis. Cartilaginous tumors often show only slight enhancement, whereas other tumors, like the metastasis of a hypernephroma, may be highly vascular and therefore show high signal. The aggressiveness of tumors can be estimated on MRI. The amount of reactive change in the surrounding tissue and the sharpness

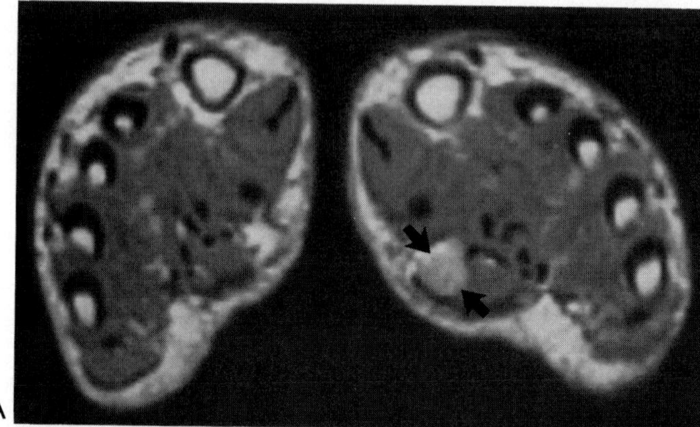

A

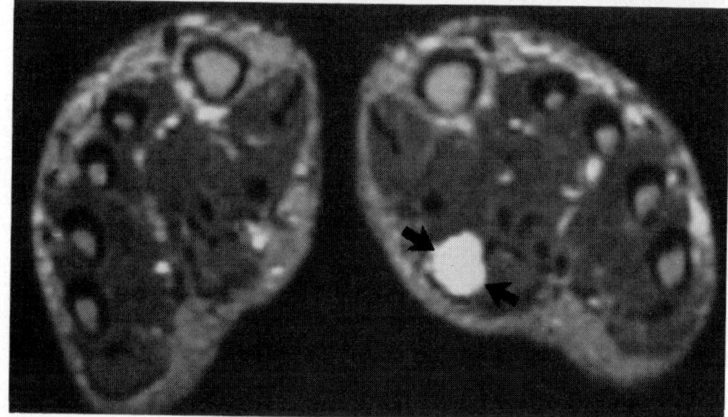

B

FIGURE 23–13. True neuroma. Coronal proton-density image *(A)* at the level of the metatarsals. A well-defined soft tissue mass is seen in the plantar subcutaneous tissue *(arrows)*. This neuroma increases signal significantly on the T_2-weighted image *(B).*

of the tumor border are indirect and limited signs of tumor aggressiveness.

MRI should be performed before biopsy because biopsy will lead to signal changes caused by disruption of tissue with bleeding and reactive reparative tissue.[8] These anatomic changes can imitate tumor invasion into soft tissue or obliterate the borders of the tumor.

MR imaging is useful in the follow-up of tumors treated by chemotherapy. It is able to show indirect signs of therapy response such as diminishing edema[14] and increasing necrosis. The use of MRI has been suggested in the detection of recurrence after resection or radiation therapy as well. There are several limitations. Fibrous tumors may be hard to differentiate from scars. Postoperative and postirradiation changes can persist for a long time. The former will show some signal on T_2-weighted images for several months, and the latter for several years, which makes the differentiation among residual tumor, reactive change, and recurrence difficult. Seromas appear as sharply demarcated structures with high intensity on T_2-weighted images, but a similar appearance is seen with recurrent myxoid or cartilaginous tumors. It is helpful to perform a baseline examination 3 months after the operation or irradiation and then perform follow-up examinations at appropriate clinical intervals. It is not yet clear whether the use of intravenous gadolinium may help in the differentiation of recurrence from postoperative change.

Paget's Disease. Depending on the stage, Paget's disease may appear radiographically mainly as osteolysis or as an increase in bone volume and sclerosis, with coarsened trabeculae. On MRI, Paget's disease has several different appearances. Reactive changes appear hypointense on T1-weighted images and hyperintense on T2-weighted images. Thickened cortex is hypointense on both T1- and T2-weighted images, and regions with fatty marrow appear hyperintense on both T1- and T2-weighted images. Complications like a fracture or malignant degeneration may also be visible on MRI.[15]

Fibrous Dysplasia. Cross-sectional imaging appearance of these lesions is identical to that in plain films. Lesions are expansile, with diaphyseal localization in the tubular bones (in the foot in the tarsal bones), and display sharp borders. Fibrous dysplasia has a very variable MRI appearance. The lesions may be hypointense or hyperintense on T_2-weighted images.[16] The latter is the result of the high cellularity, the complex structure, and the vessels in these lesions. Fractures may occur in fibrous dysplasia. Indirect changes like soft tissue edema and hemorrhage as well as irregular signal within the lesion may be present.

Morton's Neuroma. Morton's neuroma consists of a focal mass of perineural fibrosis involving the plantar digital nerves of the foot, usually located near the metatarsophalangeal joint. Neuromas mainly occur between the second and third or the third and fourth metatarsals, mainly the latter. The diagnosis of Morton's neuroma using ultrasonograms has been described, although it requires a thorough examination by a skilled examiner.[17] Morton's neuroma appears as an ovoid mass with a longitudinal orientation in the typical location for that disease. Experience with MRI is limited. Morton's neuromas appear hypointense on both T_1-weighted images and show only little signal increase on T_2-weighted images (see Fig. 23–13). The surrounding plantar fat helps in the demarcation of the lesion.

Foreign Body

Dense foreign bodies like metal or stones can be detected by plain film. The precise localization may be difficult, especially in the anatomically complicated tarsus. CT is helpful in these cases because it shows the relationship of the foreign body to the surrounding structures.[18] Even if the bodies are not radiodense, CT can help by showing the reaction in the surrounding soft tissue.

Foreign bodies with poor radiodensity, such as wood or fabric particles, may not be visible on plain films or even CT but are visible on ultrasonograms because these objects have high echogenicity.[19] Ultrasonograms also show the extent of the surrounding soft tissue reaction as a hypoechoic rim. MRI has been suggested as a means of detecting foreign bodies. It is superior in depicting the reactive changes that appear hyperintense on T_2-weighted images.[20] The foreign body itself may escape detection because spatial resolution is limited. Some particles, especially if they contain metal, may cause susceptibility artifacts. This occurs because they create a local magnetic field and subsequently distort the main imaging field. The resultant artifact consists of a region of signal void that is larger than the particle itself. It may be accompanied by a hyperintense rim. In postoperative situations, such susceptibility artifacts are a common finding, even in asymptomatic patients. It has been suggested that very small metal particles originating from metallic instruments cause this appearance.

Arthritis

Osteoarthritis. Degenerative changes in the foot and ankle generally do not require cross-sectional imaging because they are readily visible on plain films. One exception is the subtalar joint, which is usually obscured on plain films by overlying structures but can readily be shown on coronal CT images. CT may also be used to show the intertarsal and tarsometatarsal joints. Sonography and MRI do not play a role in the diagnosis of osteoarthritis.

Polyarticular Arthritis. In generalized arthritis, sonography plays a limited role. It depicts joint effusions and secondary synovial cysts (Fig. 23–14). CT is rarely used in these situations. MRI may potentially show effusions and pannus as well as erosions and synovial cysts. The intravenous injection of gadolinium-containing contrast media has been used to differentiate between fluid and pannus.[21] This is not yet routinely performed.

Trauma

Calcaneal Fractures. These fractures may be intra-articular or extra-articular. Because of the complex anatomy of the calcaneus, precise radiographic evaluation is difficult. CT has dramatically enhanced the preoperative assessment of both the osseous component of the injury and the associated soft tissue injuries. CT is usually performed in two complementary planes, most frequently the coronal and axial planes. The latter plane is usually easier to obtain because of less difficulty in patient positioning. In this plane, the calcaneocuboidal joint and the anteroinferior portion of the posterior facet are well visualized. The extent of widening of the calcaneus after fracture is also well seen.

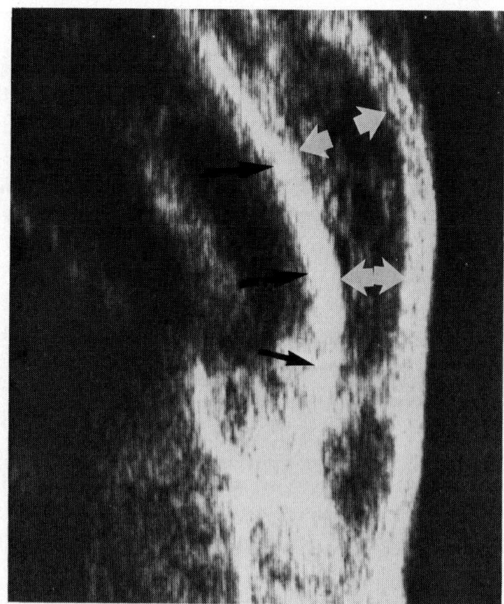

FIGURE 23–14. Synovial cyst of the tibialis posterior tendon sheath, shown by sonography. The transducer is placed over the medial distal tibia and oriented in the long axis of the tibia. The tibial cortical bone appears hyperechoic *(black arrows)*. Overlying the bone, a fluid-filled, hypoechoic cavity is shown *(white arrows)*. Some signal within this cavity probably indicates fibrinous or cellular debris.

When the patient is able to cooperate, coronal scans are useful. In this plane, the patient should be placed with the soles of the feet flat on the table. The plane is difficult to obtain when knee flexion is limited by pain, fracture, or a long leg cast or splint. A compromise scan can occasionally be helpful when knee flexion is limited. For this plane, the patient flexes as much as possible, and the gantry is maximally angulated to obtain modified coronal images. In these planes, the posterior facets and sustentaculum tali are evaluated. Widening or loss of height of the calcaneus, as well as possible impingement of peroneal or flexor hallucis longus tendons, may be demonstrated. This plane also evaluates the integrity of both the medial and lateral walls and assesses for most intra-articular fragments. Occasionally, usually as a sequela to trauma, CT after the intra-articular injection of air may be necessary to determine the precise location of intra-articular bodies.[22]

In summary, CT is optimal for accessing the subtalar and calcaneocuboid joints, the degree of fracture depression, calcaneal widening or shortening, and impingement of adjacent tendons.

Talus Fractures. CT has been less frequently used in evaluating fractures of the talus. Complex fractures of the body of the talus and fractures of the lateral process of the talus may benefit from detailed CT evaluation. In these situations, the degree of displacement and articular involvement of fracture fragments is well seen. In addition, precise localization of the fragments aids in surgical planning. In fractures of the talar head and neck, the degree of displacement or rotation, as well as the status of the talonavicular joint, is well shown. Postreduction scanning visualizes the position of the fracture fragments as well as the integrity of the talonavicular joint. The major utility of MRI after talar injury is in the diagnosis of avascular necrosis (AVN). AVN is characterized by a decrease in the normal high signal of fat on T_1-weighted sequences, with variable behavior on T_2-weighted sequences. The diagnosis of AVN will be made earlier, with higher sensitivity and specificity by MRI than by routine radiography, CT, and bone scintigraphy. MRI, however, is less useful then CT in the evaluation of acute traumatic injury to the talus.

Ankle Fractures. Most ankle fractures are adequately demonstrated on routine radiographs; however, with unusual fractures such as the transitional fractures of adolescence, CT may be beneficial. One such transitional fracture is the triplane fracture, which constitutes 6% to 10% of epiphyseal injuries. This fracture occurs with partial epiphyseal fusion, leaving the anterior lateral physis susceptible to injury. Boys in the 12- to 15-year age group are more frequently affected. The proposed force is controversial, although isolated external rotation, plantar flexion, or a combination of these two may be the cause. This complex consists of fracture lines in three planes: coronal through the metaphysis, horizontal in the physis, and sagittal in the epiphysis. There may be two or three fracture fragments, each with variable geometry. Because of the complexity of the fracture and the necessity for absolute articular congruence to prevent degenerative arthritis, CT is helpful for evaluation. Imaging should be done in the direct axial and coronal planes with sagittal reconstructions.[23]

The pylon fracture is sometimes considered a variant of the triplane fracture. This fracture is more accurately considered a subtype of the trimalleolar fracture because it is not a transitional fracture. The mechanism is an axial compressive force most frequently secondary to a motor vehicle accident. Pylon fractures show severe comminution of the plafond, involvement of the distal tibiofibular joint, and frequent involvement of the talus. Assessment of articular involvement and degree of comminution may be made by CT (Fig. 23–15).[24]

An additional type of transitional fracture is the juvenile Tillaux. This fracture may be classified as a Salter-Harris type III and appears to be a less severe variant of the triplane fracture. CT may occasionally be useful to distinguish these two fractures (Fig. 23–16).

Lisfranc Injuries. Lisfranc fractures are not uncommon injuries among diabetics. The two subtypes are the homolateral type and the divergent type. In the former disorder, dislocation of the second to fifth metatarsals laterally occurs, with rare involvement of the first metatarsal. In the divergent type, the first metatarsal dislocates medially. The injury is often quite subtle on routine radiographs; evaluation is limited by the overlap of structures. CT in the axial plane may demonstrate the metatarsal fractures, the associated additional fractures such as the cuboid, and the metatarsal sublimation. Intra-articular fracture fragments and postreduction articular integrity may be assessed.[25]

Stress Injury. Stress fractures occur secondary to the failure of the skeleton to withstand repeated submaximal forces. These fractures have been divided into two types: insufficiency and fatigue fractures.

Fatigue fractures occur in normal bone in which multiple episodes of unusual stress are placed. Although each episode of stress is insufficient to cause a fracture directly, a cumulative effect occurs. These fractures usually occur after activities such as jogging, marching, and other athletic pursuits,

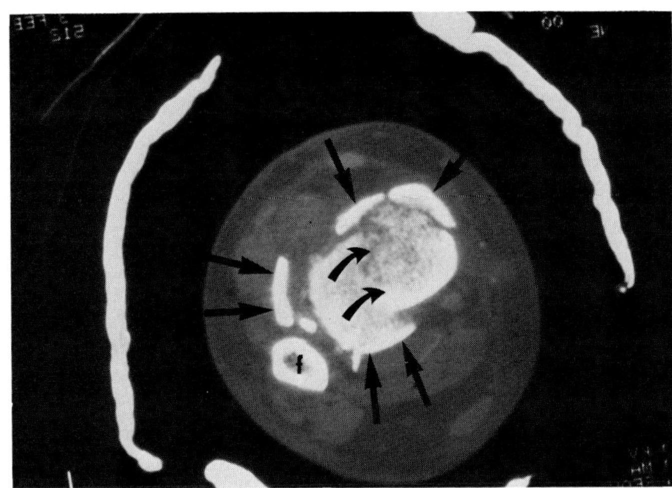

FIGURE 23–15. Pylon fracture. An axial computed tomography (CT) scan through the distal tibia. CT demarcates well several fracture lines *(curved arrows)* and fragments *(arrows)*, as well as the degree of their displacement. f, fibula.

frequently after an episode of activity restriction. In addition, people who undergo surgical procedures have altered biomechanics, leading to abnormal stress. Multiple episodes of stress weaken the bone. This occurs in the early phase of remodeling in reaction to the stress. The bone subsequently has a predisposition to fracture after additional stresses. This has been reported in the metatarsals after forefoot surgery and in the ankle after hip or knee surgery.

Insufficiency fractures are found in patients with deficient bone stock and an abnormal elastic modulus. These occur secondary to disorders such as osteoporosis, osteomalacia, Paget's disease, and fibrous dysplasia. These fractures differ from pathologic fractures in that the bone is diffusely, rather then focally, abnormal. The stresses on these patients are not excessive and, even when cumulative, will not cause an acute fracture.

The diagnosis of some stress fractures may be made on routine radiographs. When no abnormality or only an equivocal finding is noted, scintigraphy remains the most sensitive examination. When the scintigraphic result is nonspecific and a false-negative result is suggested, cross-sectional imaging may be useful. This most commonly occurs with fractures of the navicular and metatarsals. CT best demonstrates bone detail. Although bone scintigraphy is most sensitive to stress fractures, CT more accurately determines restoration of bone continuity, which may help to determine when activity can be resumed. Standard radiographs would be used in this sense for certain structures, whereas CT would be applied to those that are not easily assessed by plain films, such as stress fractures of the navicular. MRI may be more sensitive to subtle changes. Marrow edema with low to intermediate T_1 signal and high T_2 signal may be seen in these patients.

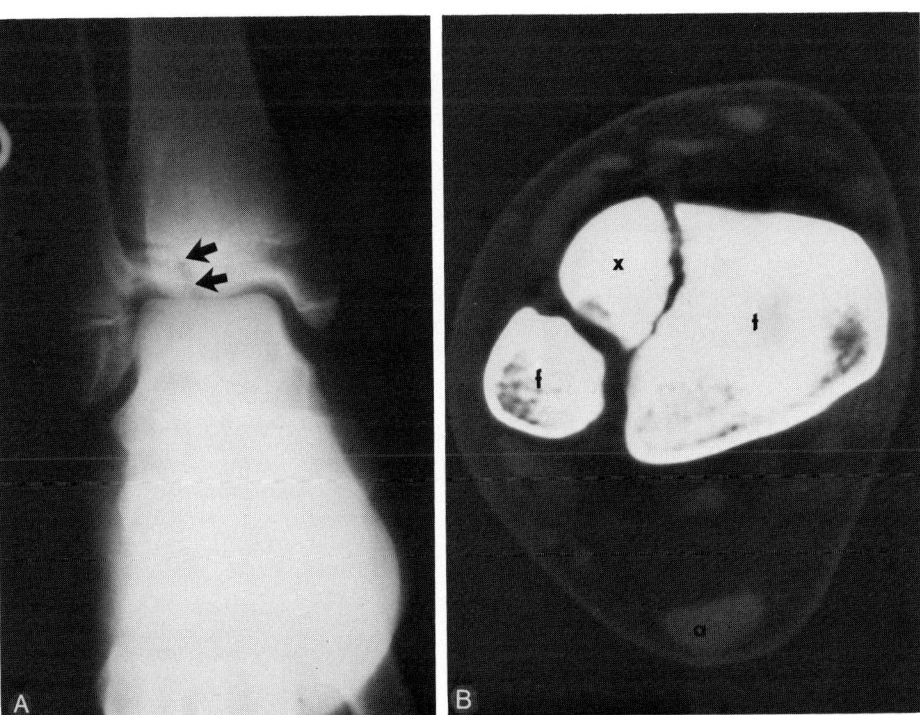

FIGURE 23–16. Juvenile Tillaux fracture. A frontal plane film *(A)* shows the fracture line through the tibial epiphysis *(arrows),* widening of the epiphyseal plate laterally, and partially fused epiphyseal plate medially. *B,* CT more exactly describes the amount of dislocation. t, tibia; x, fragment; f, fibula; a, Achilles tendon.

Two MRI patterns of stress fractures have been described. The globular type presents as an amorphous, poorly defined area of signal loss on T_1-weighted sequences (Fig. 23–17). The periphery will increase in signal on T_2-weighted sequences, with several foci in the center remaining of low signal. The second pattern is more linear (Fig. 23–18), occasionally serpiginous. The region of MRI abnormality may be larger than that initially suspected clinically or on routine radiographs. Abnormalities may be noted in adjacent bones, which may represent adjacent unsuspected fractures or bone contusions.[26] Stress fractures have an appearance on MRI similar to occult intraosseous fractures (Fig. 23–19). However, the latter injury is secondary to a single acute event, not multiple events.

Tendon Abnormalities. Before the advent of cross-sectional imaging, radiographic tendon evaluation was limited. This consisted of routine radiographs and occasionally xeroradiography in evaluating the Achilles tendon. Ultrasonography is emerging as a useful adjunct in tendon evaluation. However, CT and particularly MRI have revolutionized the assessment of tendons in the feet. MRI is able to characterize synovitis, tenosynovitis, tendinitis, tendinosis, and tendon tears by morphologic and signal characteristics. Synovitis of a tendon sheath is manifested as fluid around the tendon. This fluid will be an intermediate signal on T_1-weighted sequences and an increasing signal on T_2-weighted sequences. Tenosynovitis demonstrates similar changes (Fig. 23–20), but, in addition, the body of the tendon will show areas of increased signal on T_2-weighted sequences. Tendinosis is usually manifested as lobular thickening that may be focal or diffuse. In both tendinitis and tendinosis, foci of signal will be seen within the normally black tendon on T_1-weighted sequences. In tendinitis, these areas will remain visible or increase in intensity on T_1-weighted sequences. A partial tear on MRI will appear nearly identical to tendinitis; some retraction of tendon fibers may, however, be infrequently noted. A complete tendon tear will be manifested by discontinuity of the tendon with proximal retraction (Fig. 23–21).

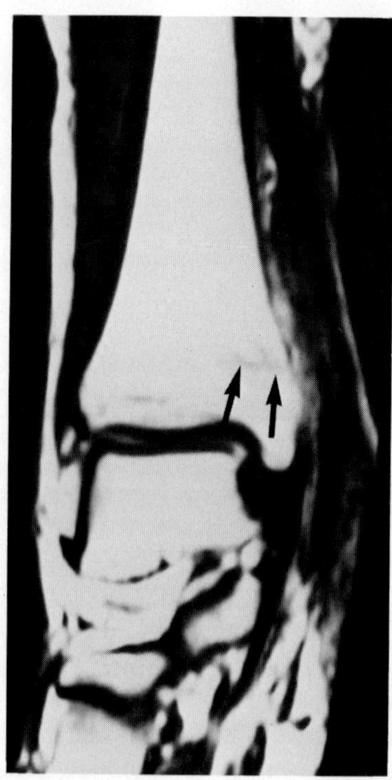

FIGURE 23–18. Stress fracture of the distal tibia. Coronal T_1-weighted magnetic resonance image. More or less linear hypointense fracture line at the level of the medial tibial metaphysis *(arrows)*.

The most commonly injured tendon is the Achilles tendon. This may occur secondary to athletic activities, arthropathies such as rheumatoid arthritis and gout, or corticosteroid use. Most injuries occur 3 to 5 cm proximal to the insertion of the tendon on the calcaneous. The Achilles tendon is best evaluated on axial images, sometimes using the opposite foot for comparison. Sagittal images define the longitudinal extent. Because the Achilles tendon does not have a true syno-

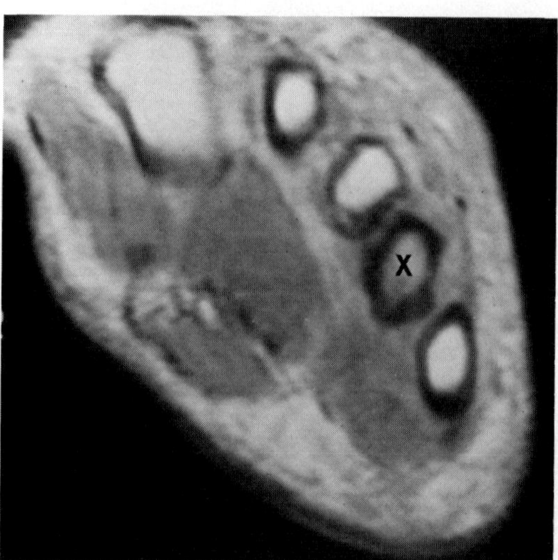

FIGURE 23–17. Stress fracture of the fourth metatarsal. Coronal proton-density magnetic resonance image. The forefoot demonstrates a decreased signal from the fourth metatarsal *(X)* with thickening of the cortex, particularly laterally.

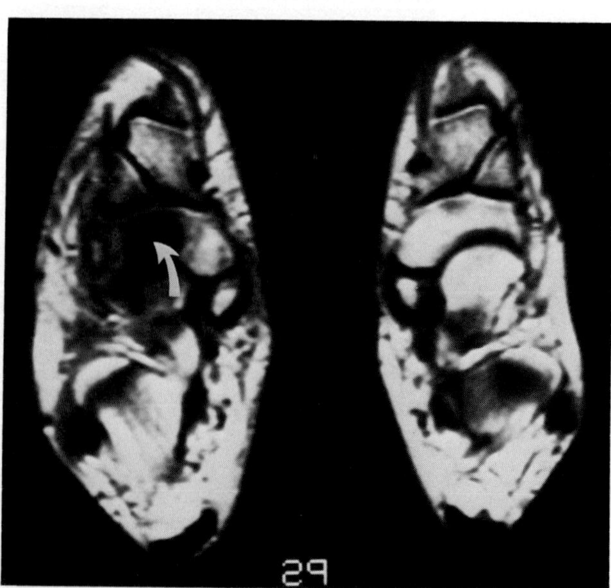

FIGURE 23–19. Fracture of the tarsal navicular. T_1-weighted coronal image. The fracture line is not directly visible on this single image. However, hypointense hematoma and granulation tissue have replaced the lateral fatty marrow *(arrow)*.

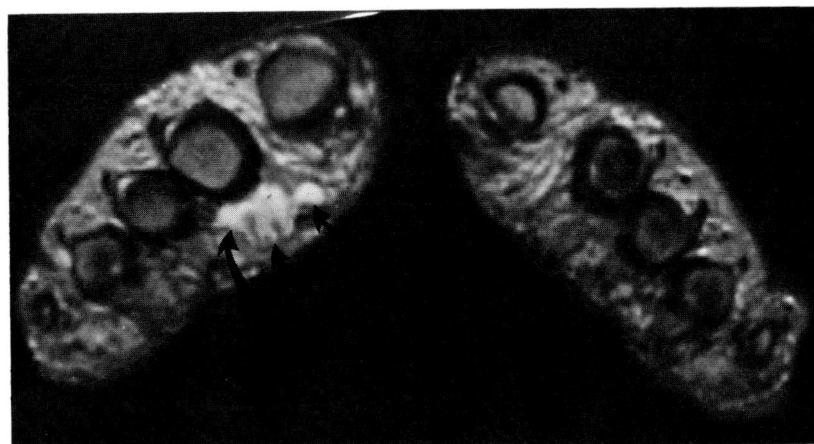

FIGURE 23–20. Plantar tenosynovitis and fasciitis. Coronal T_2-weighted magnetic resonance image. Increased signal in the plantar soft tissues deep to the second metatarsal *(arrows)* is shown.

vial sheath, edema manifests primarily in the loose connective tissue anterior to the tendon (Figs. 23–22 and 23–23).[27]

The posterior tibialis tendon is the second thickest tendon in the foot. It is best visualized on axial images of the ankle and sagittal images of the feet. Three MRI patterns of abnormality have been described. Type I demonstrates a round or linear increase in signal or size and represents a partial tear. Type II also represents a partial tear, but a relative decrease in tendon size is noted at the malleolus secondary to distal hypertrophy. A complete tendon tear is referred to as a type III lesion with a gap noted between bulbous or retracted tendon margins.[28]

Anterior tibial tendon ruptures demonstrate findings similar to those discussed previously. Changes are best demonstrated on axial images.

Ligament Injuries. Injuries to ligaments in the feet are also common and infrequently merit cross-sectional images (Fig. 23–24). Inversion injuries are most common, and these affect the lateral collateral ligament complex, the sinus tarsi, and the tarsal canal.

The lateral complex is made up of the anterior talofibular ligament, the calcaneofibular ligament, and the posterior talofibular ligament. The anterior talofibular ligament has a horizontal orientation and is best seen on axial images. This is the most consistently visualized ankle ligament on MRI. The calcaneofibular ligament has a more vertical course; therefore, the coronal view provides the best image. With the foot placed in a position of plantar flexion, axial images may also demonstrate this ligament. The calcaneofibular ligament is the strongest of the lateral ligaments. This ligament is therefore usually the last one in the complex to tear; isolated tears are rare. When the calcaneofibular ligament tears, associated tears of the peroneal tendon sheath frequently occur.[29]

The cervical ligament lies in the anterior aspect of the sinus tarsi. Because this ligament also limits inversion of the ankle, it may be injured, primarily with the lateral ligamentous complex.[30]

All ligaments are normally low-signal, bandlike structures. Imaging sequences after trauma display edema and hemorrhage within and about the ligaments. This is manifested as high-signal on T_2-weighted sequences. Hemorrhage may be

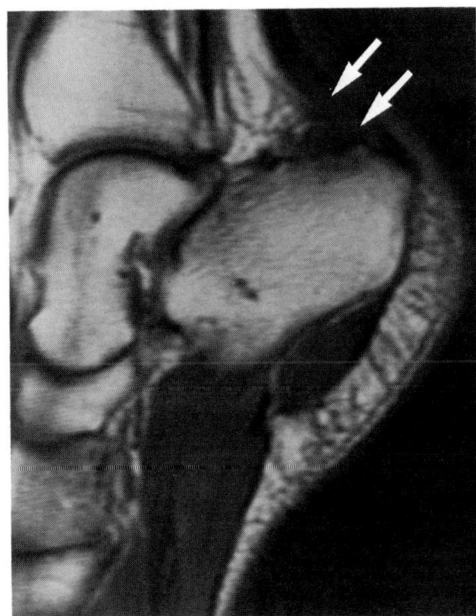

FIGURE 23–21. Tear of the left peroneus brevis tendon. T_2-weighted coronal image. The peroneus brevis tendon in the left foot is slightly enlarged *(arrows)* and contains some signal that is not present in the right foot *(curved arrow).*

FIGURE 23–22. Acute Achilles tendinitis. Sagittal T_1-weighted image. Slight thickening and increased signal within the distal tendon *(arrows).*

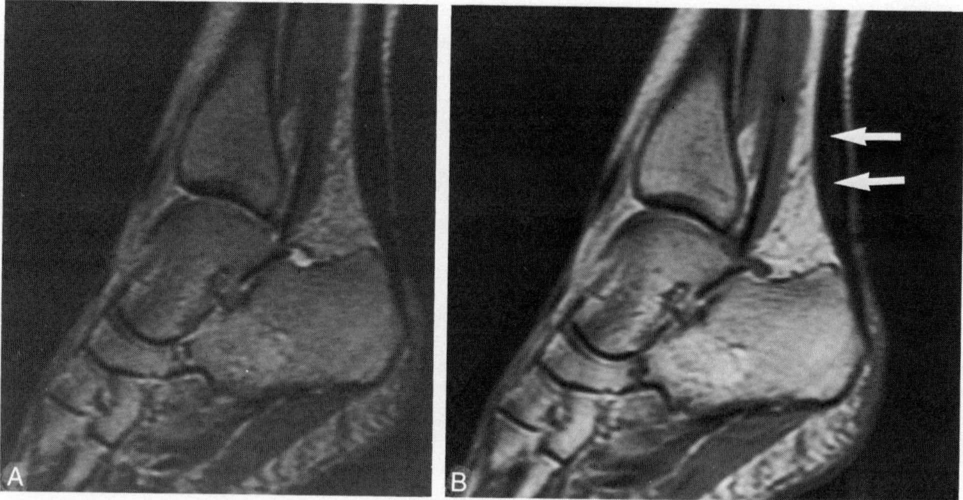

FIGURE 23–23. Chronic Achilles tendinitis. Proton-density *(A)* and T_2-weighted images *(B)*. Thickening of the tendon with internal signal within the normally hypointense tendon *(arrows)*. No signal increase on the T_2-weighted image, and therefore no sign of acute inflammatory changes.

high signal on T_1-weighted sequences as well. Edema in the adjacent soft tissues and subcutaneous fat may also be noted in the acute injuries.

The sinus tarsi is the ovoid space between the talus and the calcaneus. It is continuous with the tarsal tunnel and is located between the posterior and middle facets of the subtalar joint. Within this sinus is fat, the artery of the tarsal canal, a small bursa, several nerve endings, and the talocalcaneal ligaments. These ligaments are seen on all planes as a thin, broad band. With trauma, increased signal within the sinus tarsi is noted on T_2-weighted sequences. Sinus tarsi syndrome has a similar appearance, presumably secondary to edema. Occasionally, fibrous tissue may be seen replacing fat within the sinus tarsi, decreasing the T_1 signal.

Osteochondral Fractures. The clinical management of osteochondral lesions depends largely on the stability, size, and location of the osteochondral fragment (Fig. 23–25). Although routine radiographic signs such as the size of the fragment and the thickness of the sclerotic margins are useful in predicting lesion stability, MRI has been shown to be more accurate. A high-signal interface on T_1-weighted images between the fragment and the underlying bone has a high cor-

relation with instability. The fragment itself, however, shows variable signal characteristics.[31]

Muscle Injuries. Normal skeletal muscle is relatively hypointense on both T_1- and T_2-weighted sequences. Muscle injuries show increased signal on T_1-weighted sequences with often a subtle increase in T_1 signal. These injuries occur in a wide age range and occur with a wide spectrum of severity. Muscle contusions are a milder injury than muscle tears and have a more feathery appearance. Partial tears will have a stellate appearance. Complete muscle tears will demonstrate a gap between the torn ends of the muscle, with more significant hemorrhage and edema than in the milder muscle injuries. Most tears occur within the belly of the muscle and clinically represent a first- or second-degree strain.

Hematomas appearing on MRI have been classically described in the central nervous system. Hematomas in muscles, ligaments, and tendons have different characteristics. Acute hemorrhage has increased signal on T_1-weighted sequences. Acute hemorrhage is isointense to muscle on balanced sequences and hypointense on inversion recovery sequences. With maturation, T_1-weighted and balanced

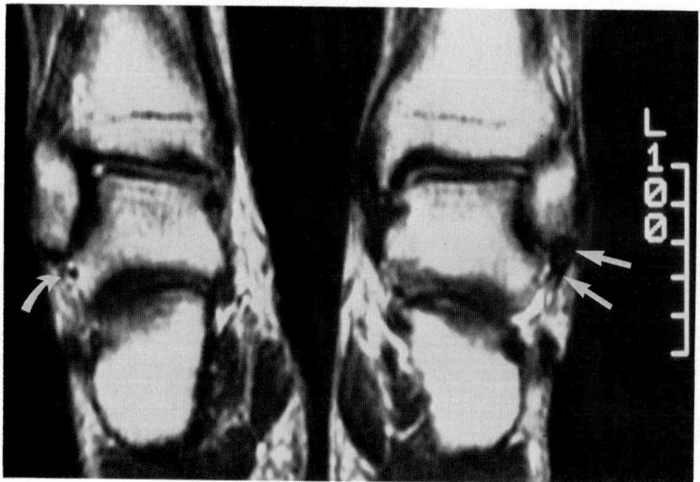

FIGURE 23–24. Tear of the deltoid ligament on the right side. T_2-weighted coronal magnetic resonance image. The normally hypointense deltoid ligament (as shown in the left foot *[arrows]*) is missing in the right foot and is replaced by granulation tissue that demonstrated higher signal intensity than would normal tendon *(curved arrow)*.

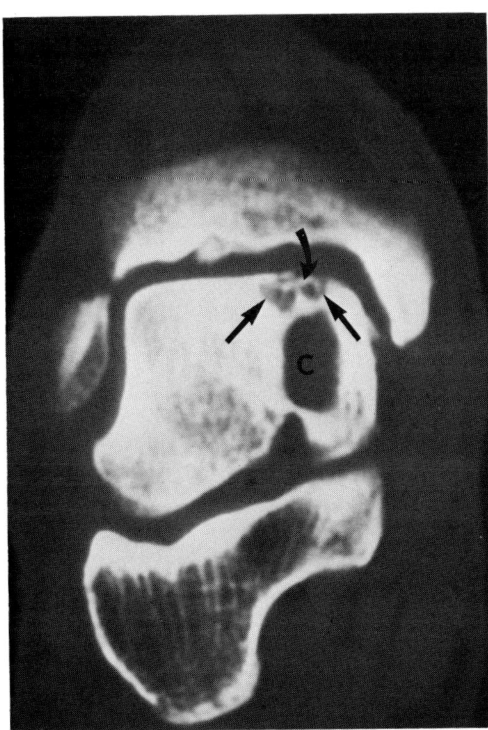

FIGURE 23–25. Osteochondritis dissecans of the right talus. Coronal computed tomography image. Slightly displaced osteochondral fragment *(curved arrow)*. Cystic changes of the underlying bone *(arrows)*. C, calcaneus.

sequences demonstrate signal increase. However, with high-field–strength units (>0.5 Telsa), low signal on T_2-weighted sequences may be seen. With continued maturation and red blood cell lysis, increased T_1 signal is noted at all field strengths.[32]

Atrophy of muscle may be a result of injury or more commonly may occur secondary to a denervation. Sequential imaging reveals a loss of half of the bulk of muscle 12 months after the initiating event. Disuse atrophy also rapidly occurs after immobilization, although the muscle will also quickly recover. After long periods of immobilization (more than 4 months), muscle degeneration is no longer reversible,

and replacement by fat is observed. Preliminary work has demonstrated early changes in skeletal muscle after denervation with alteration of signal characteristics.

Compartment syndrome may occur as a sequela of injury. It is characterized by an increase in pressure within a confined fascial space. This results in decreased capillary profusion below that necessary for tissue viability. Fractures are the most common cause. Although these patients are infrequently imaged, MRI will reveal a unilateral increase in the girth of a compartment with a diffuse, mild increase in the signal intensity.

Tarsal Coalition and Normal Variants

Tarsal coalition is an infrequent condition in which two or more tarsal bones are fused. This occurs as a result of a congenital fibrous union or bony bar. Infrequently, coalition may be acquired as a sequela of trauma or inflammatory arthritis. Symptoms appear after the first decade, usually secondary to a biomechanically induced osteoarthritis. Calcaneonavicular coalitions are most frequently identified on routine radiography. Although calcaneonavicular coalitions are usually appreciated in this sense, CT may be required to assess the subtalar joint for any related osteoarthritic changes. If any changes are present, triple arthrodesis may be indicated versus resection of the calcaneonavicular coalition alone. In contrast, talocalcaneal coalitions, which usually involve the middle facet, may be subtle on plain radiographs. CT may be helpful in these situations. On CT, osseous coalitions are obvious, although imaging of both feet is helpful. Also frequently noted is sclerosis of the adjacent bones when an abnormal articulation is seen. This is believed to represent a cartilaginous or fibrous coalition.[33] MRI may be helpful for differentiation between fibrous and cartilaginous coalitions. On T_1-weighted sequences, fibrous union has a low signal, whereas cartilaginous coalition has an increased T_2 signal.

The most common normal variant of imaging significance is the accessory soleus (Fig. 23–26). This muscle is noted within the pre-Achilles fat in 10% of patients and may be bilateral.

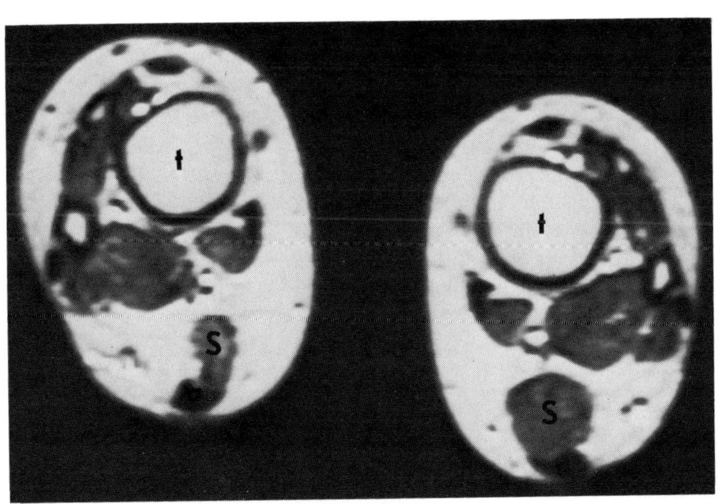

FIGURE 23–26. Bilateral accessory soleus muscle. Axial T_1-weighted magnetic resonance images. t, tibia; a, Achilles tendon; S, accessory soleus muscle.

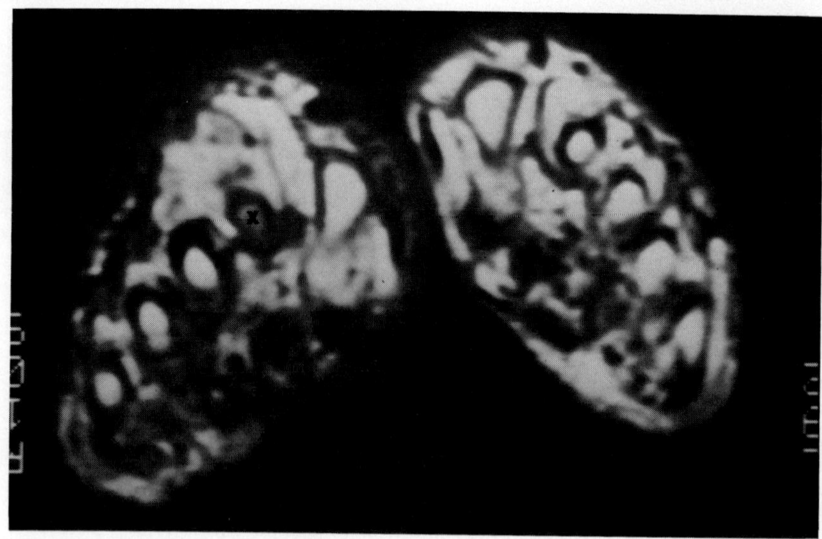

FIGURE 23–27. Osteomyelitis of the right second metatarsal. Coronal T_1-weighted image. Decreased signal from the marrow of the right second metatarsal (x).

Infection

Osteomyelitis in adults has two distinct causes: hematogenous spread or direct spread. The latter cause is most common in the foot and ankle. Routine radiography, although usually quite specific in this diagnosis, has the disadvantage of low sensitivity early in the course of this disorder. Characteristic radiographic changes do not appear until after 7 to 14 days. Initially, these changes consist of deep soft tissue swelling manifested as distortion and loss of visualization of fat planes. Later, focal osteoporosis, periosteal reaction, and eventually bone destruction will be seen. Bone scintigraphy is useful for the early diagnosis of osteomyelitis. Early images show increased blood flow to the involved part, with delayed images demonstrating focal, osseous, radiopharmaceutical uptake. In the diagnosis of osteomyelitis, the technetium bone scan, although highly sensitive, lacks specificity, thus often necessitating either gallium- or indium-labeled white blood cell scanning for more definitive diagnosis. MRI has been shown to have a high sensitivity and specificity for the diagnosis of osteomyelitis. In addition, surgical planning is aided by the improved anatomic resolution and multiplanar capability.

Acute Osteomyelitis. Acute osteomyelitis presents as a decrease in the normal high signal of fatty marrow on T_1-weighted sequences (Fig. 23–27). This signal intensity increases on T_2-weighted sequences and approaches the intensity of water. Short tau inversion recovery (STIR) sequences or other types of fat suppression will show a dramatic increase in the signal intensity of infected marrow. The abnormal marrow will be homogeneous but ill defined on T_1-weighted images. In addition, ill-defined intermediate signal is noted in the adjacent soft tissues and rarely in the cortical bone. These foci increase in signal on T_2-weighted sequences. STIR sequences show the contrast differentiation to greatest advantage. Because the soft tissue and osseous changes have identical morphologic and histologic features, the MRI characteristics are also identical.[34] On CT, an increase in marrow attenuation is noted. Early osteolysis, or periosteal and endosteal bone formation, is readily identified. Rarely intraosseous gas may be seen.

After early treatment, the MRI characteristics are not altered. However, in subacute osteomyelitis with Brodie's abscess formation, both the intraosseous and extraosseous abscesses are of low to intermediate signal on T_1-weighted sequences, increasing in signal intensity on T_2-weighted and STIR sequences. The intraosseous abscess is better defined than in acute osteomyelitis and frequently demonstrates a low-signal rim on all imaging sequences. The low-signal rim is secondary to the sclerotic rim associated with Brodie's abscesses.

Chronic Osteomyelitis. This disorder presents a more confusing picture on MRI. Although the medullary bone is inhomogeneous, the soft tissue margins are better defined then in acute osteomyelitis. In addition, the chronically infected marrow shows a more abrupt demarcation from normal bone than in acute osteomyelitis. The extent of soft tissue abnormality is less prominent than in acute osteomyelitis, but there is greater distortion of soft tissues. Chronic osteomyelitis also more frequently shows cortical involvement.[35] This is seen best on CT, but on MRI may be noted as a thickening of the cortical bone signal void.

Sequestra are isolated fragments of devitalized bone. The signal intensity of these fragments is similar to that of the bone of origin. If the sequestra originate from cortical bone, signal void will be noted; if the origin is cancellous bone, higher signal will be seen. Exudate surrounding the sequestra demonstrates increased signal on T_2-weighted sequences. Because of greater spatial resolution and the confusing signal characteristics, CT or routine tomography may be preferred to evaluate for sequestra.

Involucrum and sinus tracts are seen with CT and MRI. The former is of low signal on T_1-weighted sequences and may infrequently increase in signal on T_2-weighted sequences. The latter more frequently increases in signal on T_2-weighted sequences and may be followed from the skin to the medullary bone.

The diagnosis of an acute exacerbation in a patient with chronic osteomyelitis is difficult radiographically. Foci of increased signal on T_2-weighted sequences are most consistent with this diagnosis; however, this sign may lead to frequent false-negative and false-positive results. This is par-

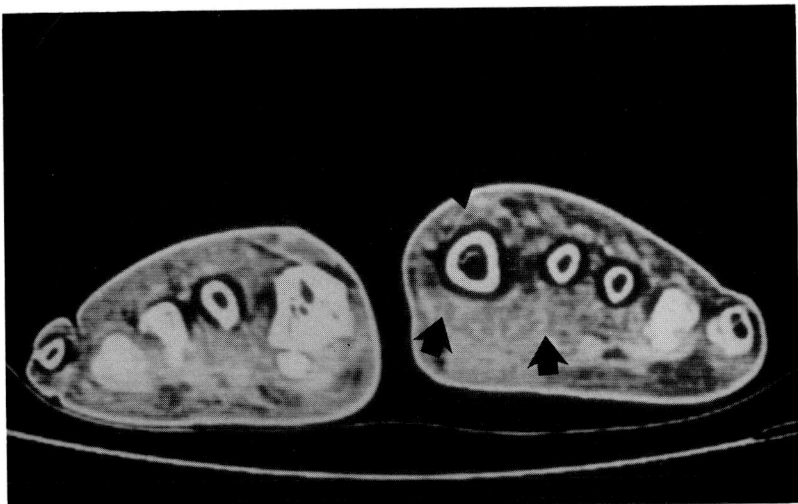

FIGURE 23–28. Bilateral soft tissue infection in diabetes mellitus. Coronal computed tomography image at the level of the metatarsals. Soft tissue infection is evident as an increase in density compared with the normal hypodense surrounding fatty tissue. On the left, the infection is concentrated in the medial compartment *(arrows).* On the right, it is more diffuse.

ticularly noted after surgery, with early fibrosis showing increased T_2 signal. Increased T_2 signal may also be noted in the soft tissues in chronic mature osteomyelitis.[36, 37]

Cellulitis. The differentiation of cellulitis (Fig. 23–28) from osteomyelitis is a common clinical problem. Cellulitis demonstrates MRI characteristics identical to those seen in the soft tissues adjacent to areas of acute osteomyelitis. Ill-defined areas of intermediate T_1 signal, increasing in intensity on T_2-weighted sequences, are seen. When the soft tissue infection involves areas of subcutaneous and deep muscle fat, a decrease in signal intensity of these normally high-signal structures will be noted. Even when the cellulitis extends to the periosteum, unaffected marrow will show normal signal characteristics. This allows ready separation of cellulitis from osteomyelitis.[38]

Soft tissue abscesses (Fig. 23–29) appear as focal, well-defined fluid collections within soft tissue with high signal intensity on T_2 and STIR sequences. These abscesses are convex and lobulated and show a low-signal rim on T_1- and T_2-weighted images. Infrequently, this low-signal rim will be absent.[39]

Periosteal reaction may be difficult to visualize on MRI. When demonstrated, it is immediately adjacent to or slightly separated from the underlying cortex. This area usually increases in signal on T_2-weighted sequences.

Healing of Osteomyelitis. Healing of osteomyelitis shows increased signal intensity on T_1-weighted sequences, with decreased signal on T_2-weighted sequences. This is consistent with fatty infiltration of marrow. This infiltration is also noted after treatment for neoplasms, including radiation therapy and chemotherapy. Alternatively, the marrow may have a low-signal appearance on all imaging sequences from fibrosis or may regain a normal appearance. Abnormal signal intensity may persist for as long as 6 months even in successfully treated patients. The signal intensity should, however, become less pronounced with sequential imaging. In addition, with healing, the soft tissue usually returns to normal. There may be some residual distortion of normal anatomy or residual abnormal signal foci, presumably representing varying manifestations of fibrosis.

Septic Arthritis. In the diagnosis of infectious arthritis, ultrasonography shows increased joint volume. Ultrasonog-

raphy may differentiate between very cellular hyperechoic pus and more liquid, serous hypoechoic fluid. Moreover, sonography can be used for joint aspiration, especially for joints that are not readily accessible. Usually fluoroscopy is the preferred method in these cases, however. Cartilage de-

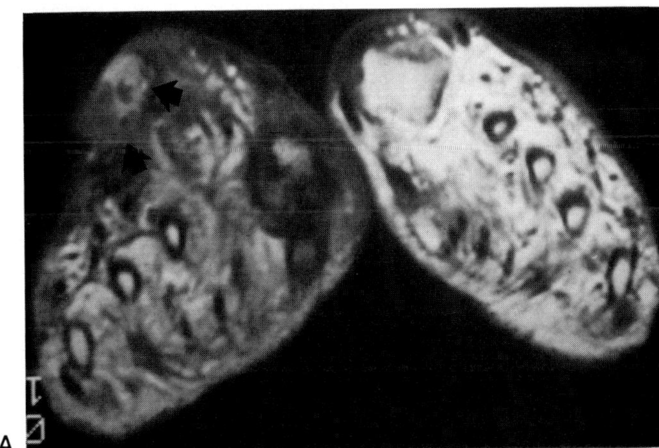

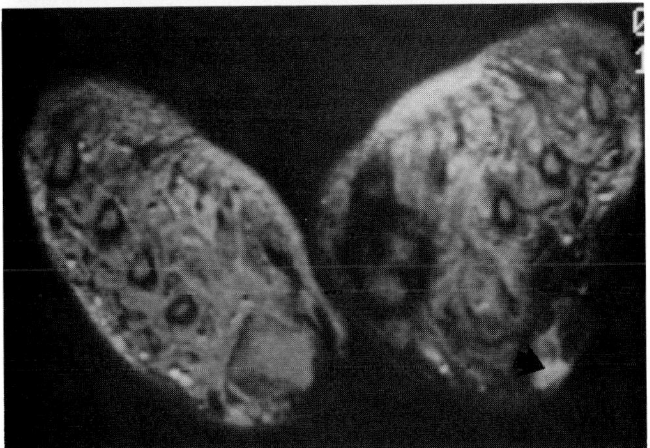

FIGURE 23–29. Soft tissue abscess in diabetes mellitus. Coronal proton-density *(A)* and T_2-weighted *(B)* images. A mass with a complex signal pattern is visible on the dorsal side of the right foot *(arrows in A).* Part of the lesion demonstrates a relative signal increase compared with the surrounding tissue on the T_2-weighted image *(arrow in B).*

struction and erosion are usually not visible on ultrasonograms secondary to the shadowing by bones.

Septic arthritis appears on MRI as homogeneous fluid collection within joint spaces with signal intensity similar to that of water. Although MRI is exquisitely sensitive in detecting effusion, it does not differentiate between noninflammatory, inflammatory, or often even hemorrhagic causes. The periarticular soft tissues frequently demonstrate a high signal on T_2-weighted sequences, presumably representing edema. Destruction of articular cartilage will result in the loss of the normal intermediate signal on this structure. With this cartilage destruction, the joint becomes bordered only by subchondral bone. This will give the appearance on MRI of a more distinct, lower signal joint space. This appearance also occurs in noninfective arthritis. With healing, joint space loss becomes more apparent and there is less signal increase on T_2-weighted sequences.

The Diabetic Foot. The diagnosis of osteomyelitis of the foot in diabetic patients is frequently difficult to establish. The radiographic changes are often subtle or obscured by superimposed neuropathic bone disease. Until recently, bone scintigraphy was the front-line modality used in the evaluation of osteomyelitis in the diabetic foot. A normal bone scan excludes the possibility of infection. A positive bone scan does not differentiate infection from neuropathic changes. The use of concomitant indium-labeled white blood cells and gallium scintigraphy may aid in this differentiation. Preliminary research shows some evidence for the use of MRI in this diagnostic dilemma. The MRI features of osteomyelitis in the diabetic foot are similar to those described previously in nondiabetic patients. False-negative results in MRI in these patients are rare. However, false-positive results occur as in scintigraphy. A significant number of patients with diabetes will show abnormal soft tissue signal and joint effusions without infection. This is thought to be secondary to acute or repetitive trauma and vascular insufficiency. In addition, soft tissue infection may be difficult to separate from osseous infection because of the distorted anatomy. Also, foci of high signal in the soft tissues of diabetic patients are frequently noted in the dorsal subcutaneous and plantar tissue; these are of unknown cause.[40, 41] Therefore, although in the future MRI may be helpful in the diagnosis of infection in diabetic feet, its present use has limitations similar to those of scintigraphy.

Establishing the extent of infection in both diabetic and nondiabetic patients is an application of both MRI and CT. Infection appears to spread in three plantar compartments: medial, lateral, and intermediate. The intermediate compartment is most important because it is the largest and is continuous with the posterior compartment of the calf. Infections with plantar soft tissue involvement spread proximally, with the intermediate septa acting as relative barriers. Although these septa are not directly visualized, indirect assessment of intercompartmental spread and the proximal extent of spread can be established by both MRI and CT.

POSTOPERATIVE ASSESSMENT

Cross-sectional imaging has several uses in the postoperative diagnosis of foot disorders. One significant usage is after fracture reduction in the assessment of residual displacement of fragments. This is most important in intra-articular fractures and in fractures of the hindfoot and midfoot in which, because of the overlap of complex articulations, routine radiographs have limited utility. CT is the preferred modality in detailed osseous evaluation. Metallic fixation, however, creates significant artifacts on CT, particularly in the region adjacent to the fixation device. Although artifacts are less prominent in MRI, they still occur. Less prominent artifacts on MRI occur with titanium and other nonferrous fixation devices. Artifacts are also less impressive near the non-threaded areas of orthopedic screws.

Incorporation of bone graft material and the assessment of the maturity are also indications for cross-sectional imaging. CT shows attachment of graft to adjacent bone, and, with maturity, MRI may show areas of fatty (high T_1 signal) marrow developing in cancellous bone graft material. After surgical arthrosis, CT is an excellent technique for assessing the maturity and extent of the fusion.

A final postoperative use of cross-sectional imaging is to detect postoperative infection. T_1-weighted images show loss of normal marrow signal, although difficulties in interpretation arise when hardware is, or has been, in place. The morphology and extent of signal loss are then helpful discriminating factors. Subtle periosteal reactions and the appearance of the adjacent soft tissues also help discriminate infection from postoperative change. We have found intravenous gadopentetate dimeglumine (Magnevist) helpful, particularly in evaluating possible enhancement of adjacent soft tissue processes and periosteum. Intravenous contrast medium is somewhat less helpful in evaluating medullary bone changes, because enhancement of marrow may occur as a manifestation of postoperative change without infection.

In the assessment of nonunion, both CT and, more important, MRI are useful. Because it is a tomographic technique, CT may demonstrate subtle areas of osseous bridging not demonstrated on routine radiographs. MRI shows crossing medullary bone, albeit at a later stage than is visualized with CT. However, MRI can characterize the interposed tissue at a site of nonunion. MRI may visualize muscle preventing osseous union or may visualize low-signal-intensity fibrous tissue, connoting fibrous nonunion. In addition, the demonstration of high signal intensity at the site of nonunion or T_2-weighted sequences is consistent with pseudarthrosis, often meriting surgical intervention.

References

1. Hirsch BW, Updupa JK, and Roberts D: Three-dimensional reconstruction of the foot from computed tomography scans. J Am Podiatr Med Assoc 79:384–394, 1989.
2. Heare TC, Enneking WF, and Heare MM: Staging techniques and biopsy of bone tumors. Orthop Clin North Am 20:273–285, 1989.
3. Shellock FG: MR imaging of metallic implants and materials. Am J Roentgenol 151:811–814, 1988.
4. Bloem JL, Reiser MF, and Vanel D: Magnetic resonance contrast agents in the evaluation of the musculoskeletal system. Magn Reson Q 6:136–163, 1990.
5. Kremkau FW: Diagnostic Ultrasound. Principles, Instrumentation, and Exercises, 2nd ed. Orlando, FL, Grune & Stratton, 1984.
6. Mathieson JR, Connel DG, and Cooperberg PL, et al: Sonography of the Achilles tendon and adjacent bursae. Am J Roentgenol 151:127–131, 1988.
7. Enneking WF: Staging of musculoskeletal neoplasms. Skeletal Radiol 3:183–194, 1985.
8. Sundaram M and McLeod RA: MR imaging of tumor and tumorlike lesions of bone and soft tissue. Am J Roentgenol 155:817–824, 1990.
9. Keigley BA, Haggar AM, Gaba A, et al: Primary tumors of the foot: MR imaging. Radiology 171:755–759, 1989.
10. Wetzel LH and Levine E: Soft-tissue tumors of the foot: Value of MR imaging for specific diagnosis. Am J Roentgenol 155:1025–1030, 1990.

11. Resnick CS, Levine AM, Aisner SC, et al: Case Report S22. Skeletal Radiol 18:66, 1989.

12. Yuh WTC, Kathol MH, Skein MA, et al: Hemangiomas of skeletal muscle: MR findings in five patients. Am J Roentgenol 149:765–768, 1987.

13. Tsai SC, Dalinka MK, Fallon MD, et al: Fluid-fluid level: A non-specific finding in tumors of bone and soft tissue. Radiology 175:779–780, 1990.

14. Erlemann R, Sciuk J, Bosse A, et al: Response of osteosarcoma and Ewing sarcoma to preoperative chemotherapy: Assessment with dynamic and static MR imaging and skeletal scintigraphy. Radiology 75:791–796, 1990.

15. Roberts MC, Kressel HY, Fallon MD, et al: Paget disease: MR imaging findings. Radiology 173:431–435, 1989.

16. Utz JA, Kransdorf MJ, Jelinek JS, et al: MR appearance of fibrous dysplasia. J Comput Assist Tomogr 13:845–851, 1989.

17. Redd RA, Peters VJ, Emergy SF, et al: Morton's neuroma: Sonographic evaluation. Radiology 171:415–417, 1989.

18. Nyska M, Pomeranz S, and Porat S. The advantage of computed tomography in locating a foreign body in the foot. J Trauma 26:93–95, 1986.

19. Torfing KF, Teisen HG, and Skodt T. Computed tomography, ultrasonography and plain radiography in the detection of foreign bodies in pork muscle tissue. Fortschr Geb Rontgenstr Nuklearmed Erganzungsbd 149:60–62, 1988.

20. Bodne D, Quinn SF, and Cochran CF. Imaging foreign glass and wooden bodies of the extremities with CT and MR. J Comput Assist Tomogr 12:608–611, 1988.

21. Kursunoglu-Brahme S, Riccio T, Weisman MH, et al: Rheumatoid knee: Role of gadopentetate-enhanced MR imaging. Radiology 176:831–835, 1990.

22. Fredrickson BE, Coren AB, and Levinsohn EM: Calcaneal fractures: Clinical and anatomic relevance of computed tomography. Contemp Orthop 14:15–21, 1987.

23. Feldman F, Singson RD, Rosenberg FS, et al: Dohl tibial triplane fractures: Diagnosis with CT. Radiology 164:429–435, 1987.

24. Mainwaring BL, Daffner RH, and Riemer BL: Pylon fractures of the ankle: A distinct clinical and radiologic entity. Radiology 168:215–218, 1988.

25. Goiney RC, Connel DG, and Nichols DM: CT evaluation of tarsometatarsal fracture-dislocation injuries. Am J Roentgenol 144:985–990, 1985.

26. Lee JK and Yao L: Stress fractures: MR imaging. Radiology 169:217–220, 1980.

27. Marus DS, Reicher MA, and Kellerhouse LE: Achilles tendon injuries: The role of MR imaging. J Comput Assist Tomogr 13:480–486, 1989.

28. Rosenberg FS, Cheung Y, Jahss MH, et al: Rupture of posterior tibial tendon: CT and MR imaging with surgical correlation. Radiology 169:229–235, 1980.

29. Daffner RH: Ankle trauma. Radiol Clin North Am 78:395–421, 1990.

30. Erickson SJ, Quinn SF, Kneeland JB, et al: MR imaging of the tarsal tunnel and related spaces: Normal and abnormal findings with anatomic correlation. Am J Roentgenol 155:323–328, 1990.

31. DeSnet AA, Fisher DR, Burnstein MI, et al: Value of MR imaging in staging osteochondral lesions of the talus (osteochondritis dissecans): Results in IU patients. Am J Roentgenol 154:555–558, 1990.

32. Ehmar RL and Berquist TH: Magnetic resonance imaging of musculoskeletal trauma. Radiol Clin North Am 24:291–308, 1986.

33. Sarno RC, Carter BL, Barnkoff MS, and Semire MC. Computed tomography in tarsal coalition. J Comput Assist Tomogr 8:1155–1166, 1984.

34. Modic MT, Pflanze W, Feiglin DHI, and Belhober G: Magnetic resonance imaging of musculoskeletal infections. Radiol Clin North Am 24:247–258, 1986.

35. Tang JSH, Fold RH, Bassett LW, and Seeger LL: Musculoskeletal infection of the extremities: Evaluation with MR imaging. Radiology 166:205–209, 1988.

36. Cohen MD, Cory DA, Kleiman M, et al: Magnetic resonance differentiation of acute and chronic osteomyelitis in children. Clin Radiol 41:53–56, 1990.

37. Movi I, Hekal O, Korhola O, et al: Detector of soft tissue and skeletal infections with ultra low-field (0.2T) MR imaging. Acta Radiol 30:495–499, 1990.

38. Mason MD, Slatkin MB, Esterhai JL, et al: Chronic complicated osteomyelitis of the lower extremity: Evaluation with MR imaging. Radiology 173:355–359, 1989.

39. Beltran J, McGhee RB, Shaffer PB, et al: Experimental infections of the musculoskeletal system: Evaluation with MR imaging and Tc-99m MDP and Ga-67 scintigraphy. Radiology 167:167–172, 1988.

40. Unger E, Modofsky P, Gaterby R, et al: Diagnosis of osteomyelitis by MR imaging. Am J Roentgenol 150:605–616, 1982.

41. Yuh WTC, Corson JD, Barariewski HM, et al: Osteomyelitis of the foot in diabetic patients. Am J Roentgenol 152:795–800, 1989.

Medical Management

CHAPTER 24

Pharmacologic Management of Inflammatory Joint Disease

Thomas J. Kaschak, D.P.M.

DRUGS USED IN THE MANAGEMENT OF INFLAMMATORY JOINT DISEASE

The traditional approach to the treatment of rheumatoid arthritis (RA) and other inflammatory joint diseases (IJDs) has been to attack inflammation itself in the hope of relieving pain and improving mobility. Although symptomatic relief is often realized, the results of therapy on joint structures are not always impressive. Nonsteroidal antiinflammatory drugs (NSAIDs) have been conventionally called on as the first agents to battle joint pain. As of this writing, aspirin retains its status as the prototypical first drug of choice in the management of IJDs. Its status is presently being challenged, especially in RA.

Antirheumatic therapeutic agents have undergone changes in class designation over the years, and a newer classification system was proposed at the 1992 World Health Organization/International League Against Rheumatism Task Force on Rheumatic Diseases. This system places antirheumatic drugs into two broad categories: symptom-modifying antirheumatic drugs (SMARDs), and disease-modifying antirheumatic drugs (DMARDs) (Table 24–1). It is quite likely that all existing drugs will be placed into the SMARD class unless further clinical trials demonstrate prolonged disease-modifying benefit (i.e., effective for 18 months or longer) for the investigated agent.[1]

The older system of classification may be somewhat more cumbersome and less precise. In general, this system recognizes NSAIDs (e.g., ibuprofen, piroxicam, and indomethacin); DMARDs (e.g., antimalarials, gold compounds, D-penicillamine), also known as slow-acting antirheumatic drugs (SAARDs) for their extended onset of action; cytotoxic agents, also known as antimetabolites (e.g., methotrexate [MTX]); immunosuppressive agents (e.g., azathioprine, cy-

clophosphamide, and cyclosporin A); and others. The older classification system is followed throughout this section.

Many rheumatologists are abandoning or at least modifying their traditional therapeutic approach toward IJDs in favor of a more aggressive course of treatment. SAARDs are now being used earlier in the management of RA and other IJDs. With the premise that inflammatory joint changes are irreversible, newer approaches to therapy will focus on preventing joint destruction rather than just relieving pain in a deteriorating joint.

Aspirin and the newer NSAIDs have already established themselves within the drug armamentarium for treating IJD. Their common mode of action is to suppress cyclooxygenase and inhibit the synthesis of prostaglandins. The load of oxygen radicals liberated during the cyclooxygenase pathway is reduced as well, and the tissue damage they cause is averted. Some NSAIDs such as indomethacin and piroxicam have even been shown to scavenge tissue hydrogen peroxide and prevent its production as well.[2, 3] NSAIDs may also suppress inflammatory cell activity.[4]

The SAARDs not only suppress inflammation but may possibly halt or slow the progression of joint destruction. The way in which the SAARDs prevent joint changes is not yet clear.

Corticosteroids are powerful antiinflammatory agents used in the treatment of arthritis. They may be administered either systemically or locally. Their usefulness is limited because of the unacceptable side effects that occur with long-term use.

Nonsteroidal Antiinflammatory Drugs

The NSAIDs are an important group of agents with proven efficacy in the treatment of inflammatory diseases. They in-

TABLE 24–1

WORLD HEALTH ORGANIZATION/INTERNATIONAL LEAGUE AGAINST RHEUMATISM CLASSIFICATION OF ANTIRHEUMATIC DRUGS

Symptom-Modifying Drugs

These drugs improve the symptoms and clinical features of inflammatory synovitis. They include the following:

• Nonsteroidal anti-inflammatory drugs
• Corticosteroids
• Others (e.g., antimalarials, gold, D-penicillamine, antimetabolites, "immunomodulators"); sometimes known as slow-acting antirheumatic drugs

Disease-Modifying Drugs

These drugs modify the course of rheumatoid arthritis, as demonstrated by either or both of the following:

• Prevention or decreased rate of progression of joint erosions
• Sustained improvement in function associated with decreased inflammatory synovitis

Adapted from Paulus HE, Scott DL, and Edmonds JP: Government affairs: Classification of antirheumatic drugs: A new proposal. Arthritis Rheum 35(3):364–366, 1992.

hibit inflammation partly by controlling those mediators liberated through the cyclooxygenase pathway of arachidonic acid metabolism. There have been various reports written on the capacity of NSAIDs to inhibit the enzyme lipoxygenase as well, but these effects are probably minor.

Although it has been generally accepted that NSAIDs reduce inflammation by inhibiting prostaglandin synthesis, this hypothesis does not account for all of the effects of these agents. In many instances, higher doses of NSAIDs are required to suppress inflammation than are necessary to inhibit the synthesis of prostaglandins. On the other hand, clinically effective concentrations of the antiinflammatory agent sodium salicylate are lower than those needed to quell cyclooxygenase activity adequately.[4] These and related issues have challenged the accepted notions about the way NSAIDs work.

Prostaglandins have been shown to exhibit both proinflammatory and antiinflammatory effects depending on the environment and tissue in which they act. They promote inflammation by inhibiting the activity of T suppressor cells; by causing local vasodilatation and increased vascular permeability; and by acting synergistically to promote the effects of C-5a, bradykinin, leukotriene B4, interleukin 1 (IL-1), and other mediators. On the other hand, prostacyclin and prostaglandin E (PGE) have been shown to interfere with the activation of neutrophils, platelets, and mononuclear phagocytes, thus reducing the contribution of these cells to the inflammatory reaction and establishing the antiinflammatory activity of these mediators.[4]

NSAID suppression of prostaglandin antiinflammatory activities may help promote some cellular aspects of inflammation. Also, the NSAIDs can ostensibly shift the direction of arachidonic metabolism toward the lipoxygenase pathway through cyclooxygenase inhibition, paradoxically increasing the contribution of lipoxygenase products to inflammation. Therefore, in some situations, these antiinflammatory agents may themselves be contributing to the chronic disease state.

NSAIDs produce their antiinflammatory effects in a variety of ways. Along with suppressing prostaglandin synthesis, these pharmaceuticals help reduce the contribution of certain immunologic cells to the inflammatory process. For example, cyclic adenosine monophosphate (AMP) has been shown to

stabilize the lysosomal and cell membranes of polymorphonuclear neutrophils (PMNs), preventing the release of inflammatory mediators through the membranes. Indomethacin and a few other NSAIDs inhibit phosphodiesterase, the enzyme responsible for the destruction of cyclic AMP, allowing the intracellular concentration of this nucleotide to increase and thus preventing mediator release.[5]

The structure of the NSAIDs in general enables these agents to exert some of their biologic effects on the inflammatory cells. NSAIDs are planar, anionic molecules that partition into lipid environments. The low pH of the inflamed tissues only increases the drugs' lipophilicity, allowing these agents to insert into the lipid bilayers of the immune cells. This action disrupts a variety of membrane-associated processes, including the generation of superoxide anions by the nicotinamide-adenine dinucleotide phosphate (NADP) oxidase system of PMNs.[4]

Clinical Pharmacology of NSAIDs

All the NSAIDs are well absorbed from the gastrointestinal (GI) tract. Peak plasma levels of most are reached within 2 to 3 hours after oral administration. The rate of GI absorption of these agents varies according to physical factors (e.g., presence of food) or other factors that affect gastric emptying. In the treatment of chronic disorders such as RA, the rate of NSAID absorption is less important than the completeness of absorption, which, for NSAIDs as a class, is virtually whole.[6]

NSAIDs are highly bound to serum proteins; only about 1% of each drug is free to promote pharmacologic activity.[7] The drugs' effectiveness may be partially related to their ability to bind to serum proteins. Because the blood vessels in inflamed areas are highly permeable to high-molecular-weight proteins, the NSAIDs associated with these molecules are effectively delivered in increased concentration to sites of greatest inflammatory activity.[5] Some of the NSAIDs are organic acids with a low pKa, making these agents especially active in the low pH of inflamed tissues.[8]

Many of the NSAIDs contain a chiral center within their structure around which the molecule can exist in either of two configurations, one a mirror image of the other. Although the two enantiomers possess identical chemical properties, their pharmacodynamic and pharmacokinetic characteristics may be quite different. The ability of these stereoisomers to inhibit prostaglandin synthesis lies with the enantiomer of the S configuration, whereas the R stereoisomer is largely inactive. Etodolac, tiaprofenic acid, and all of the propionic acids exist as stereoisomers. Except for naproxen, these agents are administered as racemic mixtures. Some NSAIDs, such as fenoprofen and ibuprofen, can undergo inversion from the inactive R configuration to the active S configuration in vivo.[9]

As with all drugs, NSAIDs must be carefully selected and their use tailored to the condition of the patient. Several pathophysiologic conditions necessitate adjustment in the administration of any medication. Such conditions include cardiac, hepatic, and renal disease and advanced age. Adjustments are made by modifying specific pharmacologic parameters such as drug clearance and drug volume of distribution.[10]

Clearance is the measurement of the body's ability to eliminate a drug by all routes relative to the concentration of the drug in body fluids. The major sites of NSAID elimination are the liver and kidneys. NSAIDs are cleared from the liver by biotransformation of the active drug into inactive metabolites or by elimination of the active drug in the bile. Most of these agents are metabolized by cytochrome P450 oxidation or glucuronide conjugation in the liver. The NSAID-glucuronide linkage can occur as either an ester (aryl) or an ether (phenolic) bond. Significantly, the ester linkage is less stable than the ether linkage. This instability can allow the compound to hydrolyze back to the parent drug spontaneously. Patients with diminished kidney function may then accumulate the drug to dangerous levels. This accumulation has been shown to occur with diflunisal and benoxaprofen, but it is unknown whether this same event occurs with other NSAIDs undergoing aryl conjugation.[9]

The kidneys can eliminate the free drug unchanged, represented as renal clearance, or they may eliminate the drug's metabolites.[10] For most NSAIDs, the kidneys play a lesser role in elimination than does the liver. Overall, clearance of the NSAIDs is quite variable, accounting for the wide range in the elimination half-life of the individual agents.[7]

Prudent use of NSAIDs dictates the use of those eliminated mostly by the liver in patients with renal dysfunction and use of those eliminated primarily by the kidneys in patients with reduced liver function.

Volume of distribution represents the measure of the apparent space in the body that is available to contain the drug. It relates the amount of drug in the body to the concentration of the drug in the blood or plasma. The measurement is not a real measurement in that it indicates the volume of body fluid required to distribute the drug equally throughout all portions of the body, sometimes being reported as a volume much greater than the body itself. This measurement is affected by variables such as plasma and tissue protein binding and by the partition coefficient of the drug in fatty tissues.[10] The volume of distribution of the NSAIDs is small because of the high degree of protein binding of these agents.[7]

NSAID Effects on Renal Function

The eicosanoids are a group of fatty acids that possess diverse pharmacologic actions. In the kidney, these products perform functions primarily related to the control of vascular tone. There appears to be some bias for the site of production of the renal eicosinoids. PGI_2 is produced mainly by the renal afferent arterioles and helps regulate renal blood flow. Both PGE_2 and PGI_2 are produced by the cells of the glomeruli and affect glomerular function. In the medulla, PGE_2 is produced by both the interstitial cells and the cells of the collecting ducts. Here the autacoid helps control the flow of blood to the medulla, and it alters the permeability of the collecting duct cells to water and the duct's responsiveness to antidiuretic hormone.[11]

In general, the actions of PGI_2 and PGE_2 appear vasodilatory; these eicosanoids work to counteract vasoconstrictor stress. Thromboxane A_2 (TXA_2), synthesized by the glomerulus, increases vascular resistance.[12, 13] $PGF_{2\alpha}$, another major eicosanoid product of the kidneys, appears to promote vasoconstriction.[11]

Angiotensin (ANG) II is a potent vasoconstrictor that acts to regulate blood pressure. The pathway to increased ANG-II production begins in the kidneys. When a drop in blood pressure occurs, blood flow through the kidneys is reduced.

The reduced flow stimulates the juxtaglomerular cells within the afferent arterioles to produce and release the enzyme renin. Renin reacts with a plasma protein renin substrate, cleaving the protein to produce ANG-I. Angiotensin-converting enzyme in the lungs further splits ANG-I, forming the active product ANG-II. This hormone raises blood pressure by promoting constriction of the arterioles and, to a lesser extent, the veins.[14]

Arginine vasopressin (AVP), also known as antidiuretic hormone, is another pressure regulatory hormone that promotes long-term pressure control via its effects on the kidneys. A fall in blood pressure provokes the hypothalamus to secrete AVP via the posterior pituitary. AVP produces an immediate rise in blood pressure by increasing peripheral resistance at the level of the arterioles, even more potently than angiotensin. The hormone helps maintain blood volume by reducing renal excretion of water.[14]

The vasodilatory activity of the renal prostaglandins may serve to modulate the vasoconstriction of renal vessels imposed by both ANG-II and AVP. The control of renal function in good health, however, does not rely on basal prostaglandin synthesis. It appears that the effects of the vasoconstrictive hormones are adequately regulated by other means when prostaglandin synthesis is inhibited by NSAIDs in normal persons. However, under pathophysiologic conditions of the cardiovascular, hepatic, or renal systems, prostaglandin suppression can allow a profound suppression of both renal blood flow (RBF) and glomerular filtration rate (GFR) to occur secondary to the vasoconstrictive actions of ANG-II and AVP.[11, 13, 15]

Congestive heart failure, cirrhosis, nephrotic syndrome, and diuretic therapy all lead to a reduction in plasma volume. The reduced plasma volume stimulates the production of both ANG-II and AVP, which, in addition to their effects on peripheral vascular resistance, causes the kidney to produce the regulatory prostaglandins.[15, 16] In these disease states, NSAID therapy can have severe consequences by allowing vascular resistance to be unopposed, further reducing RBF, GFR, and urine output. With sodium retention, a common side effect of most NSAIDs, patients with any condition that produces ineffective circulatory volume are at risk for severe sodium retention and azotemia.[17]

The renal safety profiles of the NSAIDs are reflected in their varying abilities to spare the regulatory prostanoids. When these agents were compared for their effects on the kidneys, indomethacin, phenylbutazone, acetylsalicylic acid (ASA), and fenoprofen were shown to be the most nephrotoxic, whereas the nonacetylated salicylates, piroxicam, and sulindac appeared to possess the least nephrotoxicity.[18, 19] Etodolac was found to produce less renal toxicity than sulindac.[20] A wide array of untoward renal effects have been ascribed to NSAID use, including acute renal failure, acute interstitial nephritis, acute tubular necrosis, acute glomerulitis or vasculitis, chronic renal injury, abnormalities of water metabolism, and abnormalities of sodium and potassium homeostasis.[17, 18, 21]

Patients with heart failure, hypertension, renal insufficiency, diabetes, and cirrhosis, those on diuretic therapy, and those older than sixty years should be observed closely when undergoing NSAID therapy.[17, 18, 22] Blood urea nitrogen (BUN) and creatinine levels should be regularly monitored and routine urine analyses performed. Abnormalities should prompt further renal evaluation and scrutiny of drug use.

Those NSAIDs known for causing fewer side effects on the kidneys should be chosen for use in patients at risk for renal dysfunction.

NSAID Effects on Gastrointestinal Function

The NSAIDs share GI distress as their most common unpleasant side effect. NSAID-induced GI disorders can range from simple irritation to ulcer formation, bleeding, and life-threatening perforations. Two thirds of these GI lesions occur in the antrum and prepyloric regions of the stomach; one third occur in the first segment of the duodenum. Lesions can develop, however, anywhere along the GI tract.[23]

NSAID gastroenteropathy is seen most commonly in the elderly and in women, perhaps reflecting the arthritic diseases commonly occurring in these groups. It is estimated that at least 2600 RA patients treated with NSAIDs experience some form of gastroenteropathy each year. The U.S. Food and Drug Administration (FDA) reported that between 10,000 and 20,000 patients die annually of GI complications during treatment with NSAIDs for any reason. In the elderly, there is a 4.8 times greater likelihood of GI hemorrhage and death compared with a 1.5 times increased risk in younger patients treated with these drugs.[23] Bleeding from peptic ulceration in patients older than 60 years has been strongly linked to NSAID use.[23] The symptoms associated with NSAID-induced gastroenteropathy do not seem to parallel the severity of the damage, and often disease is revealed only when a complete blood count (CBC) or fecal occult blood test (guaiac slide test) reveals hemorrhage.[24]

The integrity of the stomach and duodenal lining is maintained in part by the action of certain prostaglandins, particularly PGE_2 and PGI_2. These eiconsanoids promote cytoprotective activities important to the function of these organs. They improve gastric defensive mechanisms by stimulating mucous production and secretion; by stimulating bicarbonate secretion and inhibiting acid secretion; by inhibiting gastrin secretion; and by enhancing mucosal blood flow.[25–27]

The adherent mucous gel layer is the stomach's first line of defense against the highly acidic fluids that bathe its inner surface. This hydrophobic layer provides a physical barrier against which stomach contents can pass easily with little friction, and it prevents contact of food particles with the mucosa. The mucus itself is strongly resistant to the effects of acid and digestive enzymes.[28] Secretion of bicarbonate, particularly by the duodenum, contributes to the neutralizing capacity of the mucous layer. The production of mucins, mucus, and bicarbonate and the maintenance of hydrophobicity are functions of the mucosal prostaglandins, and these functions are effectively inhibited by the action of most NSAIDs.[26, 29]

Gastric acid aids, but is not essential to, the digestion of proteins.[30] Hydrochloric acid, the acidic portion of gastric secretion, can cause substantial chemical burns to unprotected mucosa. Its production and secretion occur through the activation of one of three receptors. These receptors are activated by acetylcholine, histamine, and gastrin and are effectively inhibited by anticholinergics, histamine-2 (H_2) blockers, and gastrin receptor antagonists, respectively. PGE_2 acts at a common postreceptor site to inhibit the terminal release of acid into the stomach lumen.[26]

Ingestion of food serves as the major physiologic stimulus for gastrin release. This polypeptide hormone is secreted by gastrin cells and is a potent stimulant of gastric acid secretion. Gastric acid, in turn, is an important inhibitor of gastrin secretion, thus establishing a feedback mechanism by which overproduction of either is prevented.[31] The prostaglandins further prevent excess acid secretion through their inhibition of gastrin.

Gastric mucosal blood flow plays an important role in the protection against gastric mucosal injury.[32] When the mucous barrier is disrupted, hydrogen ions can pass into the interstitium, causing inflammation and subsequent increased blood flow. If this flow is sufficient, the acid may be diluted and neutralized by blood buffers, thereby preventing further injury. Poor blood flow would not allow such compensation, and severe damage would result.[33] The vasodilatory effects of the prostaglandins are important in maintaining and augmenting the mucosal blood flow.

NSAIDs can have profound and deleterious effects on the GI mucosa, including (1) direct topical irritation by the ingested agent; (2) systemic inhibition of prostaglandins; and (3) indirect topical contact by drugs undergoing enterohepatic circulation in the bile and possible intestinal reflux into the stomach.[33]

When aspirin or salicylic acid comes into contact with the mucous layer of the stomach, damage occurs to the mucosal barrier as a consequence of the drug being absorbed into the mucosal cells. Aspirin and salicylic acid are soluble in the aqueous milieu of the stomach. In this strongly acidic environment (pH ranging from 1 to 2.5), a considerable amount of aspirin (pKa 3.5) and salicylic acid is present in an unionized form, and as such, these agents can freely diffuse into the mucosal cells. Relatively high concentrations of the drugs can develop within the stomach lining, rendering the cells permeable to hydrogen ions. This allows a back-diffusion of gastric juice from the lumen to the mucosal cells, ultimately causing gastric lesions to develop.[33–35]

The most acidic NSAIDs, such as aspirin, have the greatest effect on the stomach lining, whereas nonacidic drugs, such as nabumetone, cause significantly less injury. Buffering sometimes used in aspirin preparations does not appear sufficient to prevent mucosal damage, but enteric-coated preparations do seem to provide protection at the expense of predictable absorption.[36]

Prodrugs also produce less GI toxicity because they become activated only after they have been metabolized by the liver. Although they suppress GI prostaglandins through their systemic actions, they fail to produce the local changes at the mucosa, which puts the tissue at risk for ulceration. Prodrugs such as sulindac and nabumetone are able to induce direct topical toxicity only when intestinal reflux occurs, placing the now-active agent in direct contact with the stomach mucosa.[33, 37]

The NSAIDs that undergo extensive enterohepatic circulation exert contact toxicity within the duodenum but cause fewer stomach problems.[34] Medications with weaker inhibition of gastric prostaglandin synthesis, such as etodolac and carprofen, have been shown to produce significantly less mucosal injury than other NSAIDs.[38] There is some indication that the nonacetylated salicylates cause less gastric mucosal damage than do acetylated salicylates.[39]

In general, nonaspirin NSAIDs are better tolerated and provide a lower risk for stomach ulceration than aspirin and buffered aspirin products.[38] Highly lipophilic compounds, including ibuprofen, diclofenac, and diflusinal, are not appreciably dissolved in the stomach; therefore, their effects on the stomach are much less than aspirin and salicylic acid.[34]

Any NSAID, whether given orally or parenterally, will cause some amount of gastric mucosal damage. These effects occur principally through the systemic inhibition of GI prostaglandins. The mucosa loses much of its prostaglandin-mediated protection and is easily damaged by the effects of physical or chemical agents.

The GI side effects that accompany NSAID therapy can be minimized by administering these agents in a manner that reduces their local effects. Any NSAID preparation should be taken with food and a full glass of water. The presence of food may delay, but not reduce, absorption of the drug. Pills should not be taken while the patient is in a recumbent position, nor should the medication be swallowed with a short gulp of water, as when a patient takes a last daily dose of medication just before extinguishing the bedside lamp. Such habits could lead to pill-induced esophagitis or frank ulceration attributable to poor esophageal clearance and pill retention. Symptoms of odynophagia, dysphagia, and continuous retrosternal pain have been associated with this disorder and are sometimes confused with symptoms of cardiac or other serious disease.[40] It should be recommended to patients who require a last dose of medication at night to take the pill with a light snack and full glass of water and not sooner than 30 to 60 minutes before retiring.

Cigarette smoking and alcohol abuse are major risk factors for peptic ulcer disease, and use of either substance should be severely restricted or eliminated in patients who must take NSAIDs. Other factors that may increase the risk of NSAID-induced GI lesions include a history of complicated peptic ulcer disease, family history of peptic ulcer disease, age greater than 70 years, use of other NSAIDs or other ulcerogenic drugs,[29] and *Campylobacter pylori* colonization, whose presence in the gut may promote gastric and duodenal ulcers or gastritis.[41]

GI tolerability of NSAIDs can be improved if these drugs are administered with cytoprotective agents. H_2-receptor antagonists, prostaglandin analogues, sucralfate, and other therapeutic agents can be useful in the prevention or treatment of GI disease associated with NSAID use. These and other related medications are destined to find expanded use in the management of IJDs.

H_2-receptor antagonists began to appear on the U.S. drug market in the late 1970s, becoming highly useful in the treatment of gastric mucosal ulcers caused by gastric acid. Stimulation of H_2 receptors causes the stomach parietal cells to produce acid. H_2 antagonists inhibit histamine-induced gastric acid secretion by competing with histamine for the receptor sites. Several marketed and investigational H_2-receptor antagonists have been developed, including cimetidine, the more potent ranitidine, famotidine, nizatidine, roxatidine, and sufotidine.[26, 29, 42, 43] As of this writing, only the first four agents have been approved for use in the United States by the FDA.

Prostaglandins play a favorable role in maintaining the integrity of the GI mucosa, but this protective role is ameliorated by the NSAIDs. By replacing the gut eicosanoids diminished through the use of antiinflammatory agents, the defenses against mucosal damage can be re-established. The PGE_1 analogue misoprostol and the PGE_2 analogues arbaprostil, enprostil, and trimoprostil all have been studied for their usefulness in healing gastric and duodenal ulcers in humans. As of this writing, only misoprostol has been approved for use in the United States. Given in doses smaller than those required for ulcer cure, these analogues have demonstrated cytoprotective properties useful in preventing mucosal damage by injurious substances such as the NSAIDs. The safety of prostaglandin analogues is limited by their potential to induce abortion in pregnant women.[27]

Sucralfate, an aluminum salt of sucrose sulfate, is believed to stimulate endogenous prostaglandin synthesis and release. It also binds to the ulcer base, neutralizing stomach acid locally and absorbing bile salts and pepsin. It is also suggested that sucralfate may display antibacterial effects against *Campylobacter*-like organisms in the GI mucosa.[27, 29] Used along with NSAIDs, this agent may enhance mucosal defenses and afford protection against NSAID-induced GI disease.

Antacid preparations can also provide gastric protection. Aluminum-containing products have demonstrated potent cytoprotective properties not related to their ability to neutralize stomach acid. One such antacid has been shown to strengthen gastric defenses and stimulate prostaglandin release. Other beneficial properties of aluminum-containing antacid preparations include their ability to adsorb pepsin and bile acids, coat the walls of the stomach, and neutralize stomach acid without causing acid rebound.[44]

Still other drugs have been investigated for their effects in healing or preventing damage to the gastric mucosa. Omeprazole is an inhibitor of adenosine triphosphatase, the enzyme that is responsible for hydrogen ion excretion by the gastric mucosal cells. Pirenzepine inhibits vagally mediated acid and gastrin secretion. This anticholinergic agent has effects more selective to the GI system. Colloidal bismuth subcitrate promotes mucous production, provides the stomach with a protective coating, and inhibits pepsin activity. It may also be antibacterial against *C. pylori*.[29]

Various protocols have been proposed for the use of cytoprotective agents with antiinflammatory agents. One such regimen recommends the use of a prostaglandin analogue if the patient has had GI ulceration within the previous 5 years, use of an H_2 blocker in patients with a duodenal ulcer, and use of sucralfate if the patient demonstrates minor GI symptoms when treated with NSAIDs.[24]

NSAID Effects on Platelet Function and the Hematologic System

Platelet function is highly dependent on the activities of certain arachidonic acid metabolites. Those physical processes that initially activate platelet adhesion and aggregation also trigger the release of arachidonic acid from platelet cell membrane phospholipids.

TXA_2, an important product of arachidonic acid metabolism, is a potent vasoconstrictor and is active in stimulating platelet aggregation and release of other vasoactive mediators. Aspirin and the other NSAIDs inhibit the production of TXA_2 by blocking the enzyme cyclooxygenase. Whereas most NSAIDs reversibly inhibit cyclooxygenase, aspirin covalently acetylates the enzyme, causing permanent inactivation. Most cells can synthesize new enzyme, but platelets, lacking a nucleus, cannot recover thromboxane biosynthesis after exposure to aspirin. Thus, platelets are permanently inhibited by aspirin, and restored platelet activity must await the formation of new platelets, a process that may take as long as 10 days. Platelet aggregation is recovered within 1 or 2 days after exposure to nonaspirin NSAIDs.[5, 45]

In most instances, inhibition of platelet activity by the action of NSAIDs is of slight clinical consequence. Patients with coagulation deficits, however, may experience severe bleeding episodes with NSAID-induced platelet torpor. Bleeding time is elevated in patients on NSAID therapy, which may complicate surgical procedures by causing excessive blood loss and postoperative hematoma. In surgical candidates, most NSAIDs should be stopped at least 2 days before surgery, and aspirin should be discontinued for 10 days to 2 weeks before surgery.

Blood dyscrasias remain the leading cause of death attributed to NSAID therapy, although such adverse effects are rare.[46] Agranulocytosis, aplastic anemia, red blood cell aplasia, thrombocytopenia, and hemolytic anemia all have been associated with NSAID use. The pyrazoles, particularly phenylbutazone and oxyphenbutazone, have been associated with a relatively high incidence of fatal blood disease.[47, 48] Benoxaprofen has been linked to severe, nonfatal thrombocytopenia.[49] In general, the later that hematologic symptoms appear after cessation of NSAID therapy, the greater the mortality rate associated with NSAID-induced blood disease. Monitoring the patient for possible late effects of antiinflammatory therapy should continue for several months after the medication is discontinued.

NSAID Effects on the Liver

Most hepatic injuries caused by NSAIDs are idiosyncratic in nature rather than a result of intrinsic toxicity. Injury is usually hepatocellular, but a few of these agents (benoxaprofen and naproxen) cause cholestatic injury. Sulindac can produce both. Fatal liver disease, possibly resulting from reactive metabolites, led to the withdrawal of benoxaprofen from the drug market in 1982.[50, 51] Aspirin and possibly other salicylates are agents with recognized dose-dependent hepatotoxicity, but the salicylate-induced hepatitis is generally mild and reversible with cessation of therapy. Phenylbutazone causes hepatic injury suggestive of hypersensitivity. Phenylbutazone overdosage, however, causes hepatic necrosis, implying hepatotoxicity.[50, 52] Although the incidence of hepatotoxicity resulting from NSAID therapy is low, the pyrazoles, propionic acids, and indole derivatives have shown the greatest propensity for severe toxic liver effects. Those agents with the lowest incidence of liver disease are the fenamates and oxicams.[51]

Almost all the NSAIDs produce a transient increase of liver enzymes, which is probably of no clinical significance. This increase usually reverts to normal despite continued drug use. Regular monitoring of liver function tests should accompany NSAID therapy, including serum aspartate aminotransferase (AST) and alanine aminotransferase (ALT). Persistent elevations greater than three times the normal upper limits should prompt discontinuance of the drug and further evaluation. The physician should also observe for jaundice as an indicator of liver disease.

NSAID Effects on the Cardiovascular System

The effects of NSAIDs on the heart and heart function are not well characterized, and a paucity of information is available in the medical literature. There is probably little direct effect on the tissues of the heart, although prostaglandin inhibition may produce changes in cardiac vascular tone.[53] Leukotriene D_4 can mediate angina and myocardial ischemia through its potent vasoconstricting effects on the coronary arteries.[54] Its production may be enhanced by NSAIDs, which may shunt arachidonic acid metabolism toward the lipoxygenase pathway. In normal doses, indomethacin has been shown to produce a significant rise in mean systolic blood pressure and myocardial oxygen demand, with diminished coronary blood flow when coronary artery disease is present.[53]

NSAID Effects on the Bronchopulmonary System

It is speculated that cyclooxygenase inhibition causes a shift in arachidonic acid production, favoring lipoxygenase pathway products. In patients with chronic bronchopulmonary diseases or allergic diseases affecting the bronchopulmonary system, NSAID-enhanced leukotriene production in the chronically inflamed mucosa may lead to the production of hay fever or asthmatic reactions.[34] Leukotrienes have been shown to be active bronchoconstrictors more potent than histamine.[55] About 10% of asthmatic adults experience bronchoconstriction provoked by aspirin or NSAID use. Most of these patients tend to have nasal polyps.[45]

Whether overproduction of leukotrienes or inhibition of prostaglandin production causes such reactions is not well understood. PGE_2 is a bronchodilator, and it helps stabilize histamine stores in mast cells. Spontaneous degranulation of mast cells may occur when regulatory prostaglandin production is inhibited by aspirin or other NSAIDs in susceptible patients. Release of histamine by these cells in the respiratory tract or skin leads to bronchoconstriction and urticaria.[5]

NSAID Effects on the Skin

Skin reactions generally are not a problem with NSAID use. Still, reactions have occurred with alclofenac, benoxaprofen, and suprofen, all of which are currently withdrawn from the U.S. drug market.[47, 56, 57] Naproxen has been linked to several cases of photo-induced pseudoporphyria.[58] Most reactions caused by NSAIDs are photosensitive, but other side effects include onycholysis, rashes, milia, pruritus, erythema multiforme, Stevens-Johnson syndrome, and toxic epidermolysis.[47, 50] Allergic skin reactions may occur through mast cell release of histamine, allowed by the elimination of stabilizing PGE_2.

NSAID-Induced Allergic Reactions

Although uncommon, NSAIDs can prompt anaphylactoid reactions that can be fatal. Such reactions can occur abruptly, usually within 3 hours of ingesting the drug. Reactions are characterized by dyspnea, flushing, hypotension, chest pain, tachycardia, pruritus, abdominal pain, and diarrhea, most of which are manifestations of systemic mastoid activation. Mast cell activation may occur independent of prostaglandin inhibition because aspirin doses as low as 10 mg have triggered such reactions. At this dose, there is probably no direct inhibition of cyclooxygenase, but shunting arachidonic acid metabolism toward the lipoxygenase pathway may be responsible.[56]

Frank anaphylaxis has occurred with the use of one agent now withdrawn from the drug market. Zomepirac, a pyrrolacetic acid derivative, produced anaphylactic reactions in some patients, usually after uneventful prior exposure. Cross-reactivity has not been shown, but asthma patients sensitive to aspirin were noted to be similarly sensitive to zomepirac.[45]

NSAID Effects on Articular Cartilage

The efficacy of NSAIDs in treating joint inflammation is related to their ability to gain access to the joint synovial fluids through the systemic circulation. Their antiinflammatory activity is directed against those symptoms associated with the ravages of joint disease, but there is evidence suggesting that the therapeutic agents themselves may contribute to joint destruction.[59] Medical literature surveys reveal conflicting information regarding the role of NSAIDs in both preventing and producing cartilage deterioration.

The cellular and humoral mediators of inflammatory arthritis contribute to the degradation of joint structures by provoking cellular, chemical, and enzymatic destruction of cartilage, bone, and supporting soft tissues. Likewise, some of these mediators prevent reparative processes from commencing. By inhibiting prostaglandins and the activation of some inflammatory cell types, NSAIDs can prevent many of the direct and indirect destructive effects of these mediators on joints. In addition, some NSAIDs can scavenge damaging superoxide species and can also prevent the deleterious actions of the lymphokines.[60]

Conversely, NSAIDs have been found to inhibit certain aspects of joint repair itself. Hyaluronic acid and glycosaminoglycans (GAG) are major components of articular cartilage. Therapeutic levels of aspirin and indomethacin have been shown to reduce the synthesis of hyaluronic acid by 32% to 48% in vitro, whereas both fenoprofen and indomethacin were demonstrated to suppress GAG synthesis by 27% and 14%, respectively. The effect on GAG was specific, as witnessed by the fact that general protein synthesis was unaffected.[60] Tiaprofenic acid, however, was found to have no significant effect in organ cultures of normal, osteoarthritic, or atrophic articular cartilage.[61]

Definitive studies comparing the risks and benefits of NSAID use and the effects of these agents on joint structures are lacking as of this writing. It is important for the practitioner to be aware of the possible role NSAIDs play in cartilage destruction, particularly when treating arthralgias, which may be signaling the start of osteoarthritis (OA). Perhaps in this scenario, non-NSAID analgesics such as acetaminophen may be more appropriately recommended for symptomatic relief, and NSAIDs can be administered intermittently for inflammatory flares.

NSAID Effects on the Central Nervous System

NSAIDs have been found to produce side effects within the central nervous system (CNS). These agents are usually dispensed by pharmacists with the notice that the drug may cause drowsiness, a complaint not infrequently encountered. Headaches have been associated with the use of indomethacin in doses higher than 100 mg/day.[5] Dizziness, confusion, disorientation, anxiety, and insomnia have also been associated with NSAID use.[51] Idiosyncratic aseptic meningitis has occurred with use of ibuprofen, and a reversible toxic amblyopia has also been reported with this same agent.[63]

NSAID Effects on the Juvenile Patient

Juvenile patients may be placed on antiinflammatory therapy for any of a variety of reasons. The discomfort associated with musculoskeletal trauma is usually responsive to the analgesic and antiinflammatory effects of the NSAIDs. In this age group, when bumps, bruises, strains, and sprains are sustained with some frequency, NSAIDs are frequently considered for symptomatic relief of pain. Occasional, limited use of these agents probably poses no significant health risks, but the discovery of aspirin's association with Reye's syndrome has tempered the use of most of these agents in children and teenagers. Although Reye's syndrome has not been directly associated with nonaspirin NSAIDs,[63, 64] acetaminophen preparations appear to be a more appropriate choice in relieving symptoms associated with mild to moderate musculoskeletal pain in young patients.

The presence of joint pain in the young age groups may signal the presence of inflammatory disorders such as juvenile RA, ankylosing spondylitis (AS), or rheumatic fever.[65] These patients can face many years of treatment with various antiinflammatory and analgesic agents. Only a few pediatric studies are available at this time from which to cull information regarding the pharmacokinetics, safety, and efficacy of NSAIDs in children.

Generally, the metabolism, activity, and side effects of NSAIDs in healthy children appear to be similar to those in adults. GI symptoms lead the list of adverse effects accompanying NSAID use in the pediatric patient, but children may have greater tolerance or may adapt to NSAID use more readily than do adults.[63] NSAID-induced, minimal-change nephrotic syndrome has been associated with NSAID use in children and teenagers, but most patients have responded favorably when the drug was discontinued.[66]

Aspirin, tolmetin, and naproxen have all been shown to be useful in the treatment of juvenile rheumatic conditions and are the only NSAIDs approved for such use by the FDA.[63] Advances in the development of safe and effective drugs will no doubt expand the list of antiinflammatory agents winning approval for the treatment of arthritis and arthritis-related diseases in the young. Comparative studies of NSAID use in pediatric joint diseases are needed to elucidate the efficacy and safety of these drugs.

NSAID Effects on the Geriatric Patient

The changing physiology of aging patients impacts the effectiveness and safety of many medications, including the NSAIDs. Drug absorption, first-pass elimination by the liver, volume of distribution, extent of protein binding, and renal and hepatic elimination all are compromised in the elderly patient. Some of these physiologic changes influence the pharmacokinetics and pharmacodynamics of the administered drugs, and in many instances, changes must be made in how drugs are used.[67, 68]

Absorption of drugs appears to be little affected by age. Although there may be some delay, it does not appear that absorption in the elderly is incomplete. Once absorbed, the administered drug undergoes extraction by the liver; the remaining active drug is available for therapeutic effect. The agent's bioavailability is therefore determined by the extent to which it survives first-pass elimination. Medications that would normally undergo extensive first-pass elimination may reach relatively high levels in the elderly because of the diminishing capacity of the liver to extract the drug with age. Impaired first-pass elimination in the elderly would thus mandate reduced dosing in this age group.[40, 67] NSAIDs, however, appear to undergo only minor first-pass elimination, resulting in relatively complete bioavailability on absorption.[9]

The liver is less susceptible to the effects of age when compared with other organs, probably because of its ability to regenerate.[69] Still, an age-related decrease in hepatic blood flow can occur, accompanied by a decrease in liver function, whereas liver function tests remain normal.[70] The metabolism and detoxification of chemicals by the liver become increasingly inefficient, depending on the pathway involved. Drug clearance via phase I oxidation by the cytochrome P450 enzyme system deteriorates with age, whereas clearance of drugs through conjugation remains largely unimpaired.[67, 71] Those NSAIDs eliminated through the latter pathway should be considered more closely for use in the elderly arthritis patient.

It is estimated that GFR falls by 10% per decade after the age of 40 years. Further compromise of RBF and GFR by prostaglandin inhibition puts the geriatric patient at risk for renal insufficiency, particularly when other system abnormalities are present, as is often the case in geriatric patients. Serum creatinine measurements generally used to estimate kidney function tend to remain stable, whereas renal creatinine clearance deteriorates. BUN can also be an unreliable indicator of age-related renal impairment because the levels are dependent on dietary intake and metabolic function.[71] Those NSAIDs less dependent on the kidneys for elimination should be considered for use in the elderly patient. Piroxicam and sulindac appear to be the most renal sparing, whereas fenoprofen may have the greatest propensity toward nephrotoxicity.[18] In patients with reduced renal function, oxaprozin, tenoxicam, piroxicam, and nabumetone all appear to be well tolerated and may need no reduction in dosages.[72]

NSAIDs are highly protein bound; about 99% of an individual drug joins with albumin and is unavailable for therapeutic activity. Serum albumin levels decline with age probably as a result of decreased production, changes in metabolism, and changes in dietary habits. With less protein available for binding, normal dosing could permit abnormally high concentrations of free drug to develop, enhancing the drug's pharmacologic and toxicologic actions.[71, 73] With coincidentally diminished drug metabolism and elimination, the elevated levels can persist for quite some time.

Many geriatric patients eventually find themselves under the care of several physicians, all treating one organ system or another. As time passes, patients may find themselves consuming a variety of medications prescribed by each treating physician. A complaint of joint pain may prompt the primary physician to prescribe one NSAID, whereas the patient may already be taking another prescribed by a rheumatologist. In addition, although one prescription may be written generically, another may call for a brand-name drug, causing the patient to ingest the same medication in quantities greater than that recommended. It is easy to envision elderly patients, with poor eyesight and perhaps a diminished capacity for understanding which drug is used for what condition, getting into situations that may put their health at risk rather than help improve it.

It is the physician's responsibility, then, to obtain a complete drug history from each patient before dispensing any drug prescription and to precede treatment with full knowledge of what the patient is already being treated for and by whom. The physician must understand the agent's capacity to interfere with or be interfered by drugs already prescribed. Before committing a patient to potentially long-term therapy with agents that may themselves cause harm, those systems that have been reported challenged by the medication should be thoroughly evaluated by laboratory testing before therapy is initiated and regularly while therapy is continued. This holds true for all patients but particularly the elderly, in whom polypharmacy and poor drug tolerance are the rule.

NSAID Interactions with NSAIDs and Other Medications

NSAIDs are often prescribed for patients who are already taking other medications for a variety of illnesses (Tables 24–2 and 24–3). It is no wonder that many patients will frequently experience adverse reactions to one or more of the medications because of drug conflicts. These conflicts and interactions are particularly dangerous when any of the coadministered agents display a narrow therapeutic index. Slight

TABLE 24–2

PHARMACOKINETIC DRUG–NSAID AND NSAID-NSAID INTERACTIONS

Combination	Effect	Suggested Action
Antacid-NSAID	Reduced absorption rate of some NSAIDs	Not relevant
	Reduced extent of absorption of naproxen, diflunisal, fendosal with certain antacids	Use alternative antacid
Antacid-aspirin	Decreased plasma salicylate concentrations due to increased urine pH	Use alternative NSAID *or* use moderate doses of antacid
Sucralfate-NSAID	Reduced absorption rate of some NSAIDs	Not relevant
Cimetidine-NSAID	Increased plasma concentrations of flurbiprofen, piroxicam	Clinical significance unknown
Probenecid-NSAID	Increased concentrations of NSAIDs forming acyl glucuronides (e.g., naproxen, ketoprofen, carprofen, indomethacin)	Reduce NSAID dose or select alternative NSAID
Cholestyramine-NSAID	Reduced extent of absorption of acidic compounds such as NSAIDs	Separate dosing times of the two medications as much as possible
	Reduced plasma concentrations of certain NSAIDs due to interruption of enterohepatic cycling	Phenomenon not well studied and clinical significance unknown
Corticosteroids-aspirin	Reduced plasma salicylate concentrations	Avoid combination *or* adjust aspirin dose and monitor salicylate concentrations
OCS-NSAID	Increased plasma clearance of salicylate and diflunisal	Clinical significance unknown
Aspirin-NSAID	Decreased plasma concentrations of NSAID	Clinical significance unknown
NSAID-NSAID	Diflunisal increases plasma indomethacin concentrations	Avoid this combination

NSAID, nonsteroidal anti-inflammatory drug; OCS, oral contraceptive steroids.
From Verbeeck RK: Pharmacokinetic drug interactions with nonsteroidal anti-inflammatory drugs. Clin Pharmacokinet 19(1):44–66, 1990.

TABLE 24–3

PHARMACOKINETIC NSAID-DRUG INTERACTIONS

Drug or Class	Effect of NSAID	Suggested Action
Oral anticoagulants	Aspirin enhances hypothrombinemic response	Avoid aspirin
	Pyrazole NSAIDs inhibit metabolism of oral anticoagulants	Avoid phenylbutazone, oxyphenbutazone, azapropazone
	All NSAIDs cause increased risk of bleeding due to inhibition of platelet function and gastric mucosal damage	Other NSAIDs can be used but anticoagulant response should be closely monitored
Oral hypoglycemics	Aspirin (high doses) potentiates hypoglycemic effect	Avoid aspirin, phenylbutazone, oxyphenbutazone, azapropazone; select alternative NSAID
	Pyrazole NSAIDs inhibit metabolism of sulfonylureas	
Anticonvulsants	Pyrazole NSAIDs inhibit metabolism of phenytoin	Use alternative NSAID
	Aspirin displaces phenytoin from plasma protein binding sites	Use alternative NSAID
	Aspirin dsplaces valproic acid from plasma protein binding sites and inhibits its metabolism	Use alternative NSAID
Digoxin	NSAIDs may increase plasma digoxin concentrations (e.g., in the elderly and in reduced kidney function)	Plasma concentrations of digoxin should be more intensively monitored
MTX	NSAIDs (possibly all) reduce the renal clearance of MTX, leading to elevated MTX concentrations and toxicity	Reduce MTX dose and monitor plasma MTX concentrations more intensively
Lithium	NSAIDs (possibly all) reduce the renal excretion of lithium, leading to elevated lithium concentrations and toxicity	Reduce lithium dose and monitor lithium concentration more intensively
Carbonic anhydrase inhibitors	Aspirin decreases plasma protein binding and renal excretion of acetazolamide	Avoid aspirin; select alternative NSAID

NSAIDs, nonsteroidal antiinflammatory drugs; MTX, methotrexate.
From Day RO, Graham GG, Champion GD, et al: Antirheumatic drug interactions. Clin Rheum Dis 10:251–275, 1984.

changes in the kinetics or dynamics of the drug can either eliminate its therapeutic effect or raise its presence to toxic or life-threatening levels. This is especially true for medications such as oral anticoagulants, cardiac glycosides, antiarrhythmics, anticonvulsants, and cytotoxic agents.

Drug interactions are of two basic types: pharmacokinetic, affecting a drug's absorption, distribution, metabolism, and excretion; and, more commonly, pharmacodynamic, causing additive or reductive effects of two or more drugs on the same target organ.[74]

NSAID/NSAID. It is not customary to prescribe more than one NSAID at a time for the control of inflammatory disorders. Occasionally, however, patients may take more than one NSAID preparation unknowingly by combining prescriptions from several different physicians, by adding over-the-counter antiinflammatory agents to prescribed NSAIDs or by combining multiple NSAID prescriptions from one treating physician.

Concurrent use of more than one NSAID provides no increased efficacy but may cause greater toxicity.[6] The potential for problems is especially acute when both agents are metabolized and eliminated by the same route. Some particularly harmful interactions may occur, as witnessed by the twofold to threefold increase in plasma indomethacin concentrations when this drug is coadministered with diflunisal. Eliminated mainly by glucuronide conjugation, diflunisal may inhibit the conjugation elimination of indomethacin.[6] Toxic concentrations of indomethacin may develop through such inhibition.

NSAID/Aspirin. Aspirin is a common medication that patients may consume during NSAID therapy. The drug may be taken reflexively for headache, fever, or other aches or pains that may have been adequately covered by the NSAID anyway. Aspirin, like all NSAIDs, is highly protein bound and competes with the other agents for albumin-binding sites. This competition produces an increase in plasma levels of the displaced NSAID, increasing its clearance and reducing its total plasma concentration. Because the therapeutic and toxic effects of the medication are related to free drug concentration, potentially little change in efficacy or adverse reactions can be expected. Salicylate levels are not usually affected by the coadministered NSAID.[6]

NSAID/Corticosteroid. Oral or intra-articular corticosteroids may be used for IJD in combination with aspirin or other NSAIDs. Corticosteroids administered by any route increase salicylate clearance and reduce its plasma concentration. When the corticosteroid is reduced or withdrawn, salicylate levels rise, potentially causing toxicity, especially in patients being treated with high doses of salicylate. Aspirin/NSAID–corticosteroid combination therapy can also increase the chance of GI side effects.[6]

NSAID/Antacid. Antacids are frequently recommended for patients taking NSAIDs to help relieve or prevent GI discomfort. The potential for drug interactions depends on the antacid preparations and NSAID compounds being used. Aluminum–magnesium hydroxide antacids may increase urine pH, causing enhanced renal excretion of aspirin, but this may not affect the drug's bioavailability. The absorption of aspirin buffered with antacid is accelerated when compared with nonbuffered preparations, but this probably does not affect clinical effectiveness. Oral bioavailability of naproxen and diflunisal both are significantly reduced when administered with aluminum hydroxide alone but to a lesser extent when administered with aluminum–magnesium hydroxide preparations. The oral absorption of fendosal is reduced by 80% after administration of a 30-ml dose of an aluminum–magnesium hydroxide antacid. Ketoprofen bioavailability is slightly reduced when given with aluminum hydroxide alone. With only a few exceptions, NSAID absorption and effectiveness are probably not greatly affected when the drug is taken with an antacid.[6, 75]

NSAID/Cytoprotective Agents. Cytoprotective agents are becoming a popular companion to NSAID therapy, defending the GI mucosa against the ulcerogenic effects of antiinflammatory drugs. The sulfated disaccharide sucralfate does not appear to reduce the absorption of most of the NSAIDs and only slightly reduces that of others. Cimetidine, an H_2-

receptor blocker, binds to cytochrome P450, inhibiting the biotransformation of drugs inactivated by this pathway. Ranitidine binds less avidly to cytochrome P450, therefore affecting this pathway to a lesser extent. These agents do not appear to affect glucuronide conjugation, the favored elimination pathway for most of the NSAIDs.[6] Cytoprotective agents and NSAIDs, therefore, seem to be compatible therapeutic agents, and this combination may allow the arthritis patient who is at risk for GI disease to use NSAIDs with greater tolerance.

NSAID/Probenecid. Probenecid is a uricosuric agent used to decrease uric acid levels in patients with chronic tophaceous gout. Therapeutic doses of the drug inhibit reabsorption of uric acid at the proximal tubules and at a postsecretory site. The overall effect is increased excretion of uric acid and a decrease of the plasma urate pool.[76] The drug is metabolized by the liver through oxidation and glucuronide conjugation, and its metabolites are eliminated by the kidneys. Both the parent drug and its oxidized metabolites bind to serum albumin.[6]

NSAIDs are commonly prescribed for use by gout patients to control inflammatory flares. Renal excretion of these weak organic acids is reduced by the competitive inhibition of probenecid. Probenecid also competes for biliary excretion of the organic acids; it competes for access to enzymes responsible for glucuronidation; finally, it competes with NSAIDs for albumin-binding sites. The overall effect of probenecid on NSAIDs is to increase plasma concentrations of the latter to markedly high levels.[76] Plasma clearance of ibuprofen, a drug eliminated mostly through oxidative metabolism, does not appear to be inhibited by probenecid.[77] The increased NSAID levels caused by coadministration with probenecid are probably tolerable in patients not experiencing GI or renal disease, but for those who do, serious GI or renal toxicity becomes a major concern.

NSAID/Liver Enzyme–Inducing Agents. Certain medications cause the liver to augment the activity of those enzymes responsible for the oxidative and conjugative metabolism of drugs and toxic substances. Phenobarbital, phenytoin, and rifampicin are such enzyme inducers, and coadministration of NSAIDs with these drugs may result in enhanced NSAID metabolism and subtherapeutic drug levels. Oral contraceptive steroids may enhance the metabolism of drugs eliminated through glucuronide conjugation, but it is not clear whether this effect is clinically significant.[6]

NSAID/Anticoagulants. NSAIDs can potentially increase the toxicity of many pharmaceutical agents by altering the plasma levels of the coadministered drugs. The high level of protein binding of the antiinflammatory agents can displace other similarly bound drugs, increasing their free plasma concentration. NSAIDs can also augment the effects of other medications by producing similar therapeutic ends, resulting in dangerously enhanced biologic effects. Both of these actions occur when NSAIDs are administered to patients being treated with oral anticoagulants.

Coumarin anticoagulants are bound to plasma proteins and are readily displaced by NSAIDs. The elevated unbound anticoagulant is then cleared from the plasma, returning free coumarin levels to predisplacement levels.[6] Although the increased levels of anticoagulant are only temporary, the clinician must be aware that such levels may have significant but transient effects, which may put the patient at risk for hemorrhage.

All the NSAIDs and aspirin are potent inhibitors of platelet function. When the coagulation system, already constrained by clotting cascade inhibitors, is further compromised by antiinflammatory-induced platelet restriction, patients are at greater risk for serious bleeding episodes. GI bleeding is of particular concern because of the direct toxicity of aspirin and many other NSAIDs on the gastric mucosa.

Aspirin and the pyrazole-derived NSAIDs have been found to enhance the hypoprothrombinemic response to oral anticoagulants. This same effect can also be seen when sulindac is added to warfarin therapy. No such changes were found when indomethacin, naproxen, tiaprofenic acid, fenbufen, diclofenac, ibuprofen, and oxaprozin were studied. Prolongation of prothrombin time can occur, accompanied by serious hemorrhages, especially in frail, elderly arthritis patients. It is mandatory, then, that prothrombin time be regularly monitored for patients on combined anticoagulant and NSAID therapy, especially during the first few weeks after the NSAID is added or withdrawn.[6]

NSAID/Hypoglycemic Agents. The sulfonylureas are oral hypoglycemic agents used in the management of type II diabetes. These agents are highly bound to plasma proteins and can be displaced from their binding sites by aspirin, temporarily elevating the plasma level of the unbound drug and potentially decreasing plasma glucose to dangerously low levels. Additionally, salicylates themselves have some hypoglycemic effects that can potentiate those of the sulfonylureas or insulin. This same effect may also occur with sulindac.[6, 76]

The pyrazole NSAIDs have been shown to inhibit the metabolism of the sulfonylureas tolbutamide, chlorpropamide, and glyburide, reducing the clearance of the drugs and prolonging their hypoglycemic effects. Many other NSAIDs were studied, including ibuprofen, naproxen, ketoprofen, pirprofen, diclofenac, tolmetin, tenoxicam, and diflunisal, and these agents have shown no significant interaction with the sulfonylureas.[6] Patients being treated with oral hypoglycemic agents should, therefore, not be prescribed aspirin or pyrazole NSAIDs for relief of inflammatory disease, favoring one of the other agents instead.

NSAID/Antihypertensive Agents. Hypertension frequently coexists with arthritis, increasing the probability that patients so affected would be administered both antihypertensive agents and NSAIDs. With the possible exception of sulindac, all NSAIDs can potentially antagonize the effects of antihypertensive drugs. Indomethacin is known to elevate arterial pressure in hypertensive patients being treated with diuretics, β-adrenoreceptor antagonists, or converting-enzyme inhibitors. It interferes with both renal and nonrenal clearance of furosemide, and it impairs the natriuretic effects of the diuretic. Indomethacin, diflunisal, and aspirin have been shown to reduce natriuresis in patients taking spironolactone.[78]

Piroxicam and ibuprofen were found to attenuate the effects of antihypertensive agents, whereas naproxen was found to elevate standing systolic but not diastolic pressure when combined with antihypertensive therapy.[74, 79] Aspirin was noted to decrease plasma protein binding and renal tubular excretion of the carbonic anhydrase inhibitor acetazolamide, but flurbiprofen did not appear to have this effect.[80]

β-blocking agents are commonly used in the treatment of hypertension, but their complete mechanism of action is still incompletely understood. Flurbiprofen and indomethacin have been reported to attenuate the antihypertensive actions of propranolol, whereas sulindac, naproxen, and aspirin lacked this effect.[78]

The possible mechanism by which these drug interferences occur may involve sodium and water retention, suppression of plasma renin, suppression of adrenoreceptors, and impaired prostaglandin synthesis, all produced through NSAID activity.[74, 75, 79, 80] In addition, NSAIDs may themselves have intrinsic pressor activity and may cause fluid retention sufficient to negate the effects of diuretics.[78] Combination therapy using NSAIDs and antihypertensive agents is often overlooked as a cause for poor control of hypertension. Physicians generally respond by altering the antihypertensive drug dose, but eliminating or changing the NSAID may be more appropriate. Patients with such combined therapy should have their blood pressures closely and regularly monitored and should be instructed on the possibility of these drug interactions and their clinical effects.

NSAID/Digoxin. Renal clearance of digoxin is markedly reduced by indomethacin and ibuprofen in the canine model. This inotropic agent is eliminated mostly through renal tubular secretion. Because NSAIDs can have profound effects on renal function, there is a great potential for these drugs to cause increased digoxin levels when the drugs are taken together. Along with indomethacin and ibuprofen, fenbufen, and diclofenac have also been found to increase the serum concentration of coadministered digoxin, whereas ketoprofen and tiaprofenic acid do not affect digoxin levels. With these interactions considered, it is prudent to measure digoxin levels carefully whenever an antiinflammatory agent is added to or discontinued from the digitalized patient.[6]

NSAID/Antiepileptic Agents. The pyrazole NSAIDs have been found to interfere with the metabolism of the anticonvulsant agent phenytoin, producing an increased plasma concentration of the anticonvulsant and a potential for serious drug toxicity. Phenytoin and valproic acid are highly protein bound and may be displaced from their binding sites by aspirin. Total plasma levels of phenytoin may decrease because of aspirin displacement and the subsequent increased drug clearance, but unbound levels of the anticonvulsant return to pretreatment levels within a short period, probably without a change in clinical effect. Aspirin not only displaces valproic acid but also reduces β oxidation of the antiepileptic, promoting an elevation in drug levels and potentially grave toxicity.[6]

NSAID/Lithium. The antipsychotic agent lithium is mostly eliminated through the kidneys, and the clearance of this ion is significantly reduced by the coadministration of NSAIDs. Diclofenac, ibuprofen, indomethacin, and piroxicam all have been shown to increase plasma levels of lithium, probably through their effects on renal prostaglandin synthesis and the diminished renal modulatory activity of these mediators. Because lithium has a narrow therapeutic index, its dosage must be lowered when NSAIDs are also used, and plasma lithium levels should be frequently monitored.[6]

NSAID/Methotrexate. The antineoplastic agent MTX is being used more frequently and earlier in the course of treatment of RA that has failed to respond to NSAID therapy alone. This folic acid antagonist is quite toxic, and its major route of elimination is the kidneys. The diminished RBF caused by NSAIDs can produce elevated MTX levels by reducing the drug's clearance. Serious and sometimes fatal interactions have occurred between MTX and aspirin, phenylbutazone, indomethacin, diclofenac, ketoprofen, naproxen, and azapropazone. It is recommended that NSAIDs be avoided by patients under treatment with intermediate or high doses of MTX and that they be used with caution and with careful monitoring in patients taking low doses of this agent.[6]

NSAID/Aminoglycosides. The aminoglycoside family of antibiotics is disposed of through the kidneys, and their elimination is dependent on the GFR. Indomethacin has been shown to cause a decrease in GFR and urine flow, particularly in preterm infants treated by this NSAID for pharmacologic closure of patent ductus arteriosus. Combined therapy produces elevations in aminoglycoside peak and trough levels, and it is suggested that patients on combined therapy have the dose of antibiotic lowered and readjusted as warranted by regular peak-and-trough measurements.[6, 81]

Laboratory and Clinical Monitoring of Patients Receiving NSAID Therapy

NSAIDs have been shown to potentially interfere with the function of almost every organ system, but this interference does not always produce clinically significant sequelae. In some patients, relatively benign side effects are accompanied by distressing symptoms, whereas some quite serious side effects may remain occult. It is up to the astute practitioner to observe the patient clinically and, through laboratory testing, ensure that the course of NSAID therapy remains safe, effective, and well tolerated by the patient. Observation should continue for several months after therapy is stopped, because some side effects may not surface until well after the last pill was swallowed.

Specific guidelines have not been established for laboratory monitoring during antiinflammatory therapy, but recommendations are regularly published in the medical literature. In general, the function of organ systems most likely affected by prostaglandin inhibition should be monitored throughout the course of therapy and for a period after therapy has stopped. A baseline CBC with hematocrit, and renal and liver function tests should be ordered before therapy is instituted and should be repeated 1 or 2 weeks later. Urinalysis may also be considered. These tests are particularly crucial for patients who are at risk for GI hemorrhage, renal or cardiac failure, or liver disease. If no medically significant changes are noted, the same tests can be repeated 6 weeks and 14 weeks after therapy has begun and then every 3 months thereafter. If abnormalities are noted at any time during therapy, the tests should be repeated every week to 10 days until results are normal or until therapy must be stopped. Significant abnormality on repeat testing should prompt drug withdrawal and further investigation. Patients recuperating from NSAID-induced organ dysfunction should receive regular laboratory monitoring until complete recovery is realized. Patients withdrawn from NSAID therapy for nonurgent reasons should be monitored by laboratory testing at least once more 1 to 3 months after the last pill was taken.

It may be prudent to perform guaiac stool tests for melena during the course of NSAID therapy, especially if the patient has a history of GI ulceration. This test can follow the same time scale described previously. Patients undergoing anticoagulant therapy should have their bleeding time monitored and prothrombin time regularly evaluated. Diabetics need to monitor their glucose levels throughout the day, and patients being treated for hypertension should frequently monitor their blood pressure. Patients who are taking medications with a narrow therapeutic index such as digoxin, lithium, and MTX may experience insufficient drug levels or drug overdosage and serious toxicity if drug interaction occurs when the patient is placed on an NSAID. The levels of therapeutic agents possessing a narrow margin of safety should be measured frequently to ensure patient well-being.

Salicylates

Aspirin, or ASA, is the protypical antiinflammatory agent against which all other NSAIDs are compared. The salicylates have been used for the treatment of rheumatic diseases since the late 1800s, and aspirin continues to be one of the most commonly used antiinflammatory agents.[6, 82, 83]

After oral administration, nonionized ASA is rapidly absorbed in the low pH of the stomach; however, tablet dissolution is greatest in an alkaline environment.[82] On absorption, ASA and nonacetylated salicylates are hydrolyzed by nonspecific liver esterases to salicylic acid. In the tissues and blood, ASA is hydrolyzed to salicylic acid and acetic acid.

Salsalate (salicylsalicylic acid) is a nonacetylated salicylate that is insoluble in the acidic environment of the stomach but dissolves well in the alkaline environment of the duodenum. It is rapidly hydrolyzed after absorption to two molecules of salicylic acid. Both salsalate and aspirin are highly protein bound and widely distributed.[82, 83]

The metabolism of salicylic acid includes glucuronide formation, conjugation with glycine, and oxidation to gentisic acid. The major metabolites of salicylic acid are salicyluric acid and salicyl phenol glucuronide. The pathway to production of these metabolites is saturable, and elimination is dose dependent. With low doses, elimination of the salicylates follows first-order kinetics, resulting in a serum half-life of 2 to 3 hours. Higher doses of the drugs tax the liver's ability to metabolize the agent, and serum half-life can rise to 30 hours or more. Serum salicylate levels reach steady-state in about a week, but this may be delayed because salicylates can induce their own metabolism.[83]

Salicylic acid is eliminated by the kidneys partly unchanged and partly as metabolites. Excretion of free salicylate can be increased with alkalinization of the urine. Concurrent use of antacids such as magnesium hydroxide or sodium bicarbonate increases urine pH, facilitating renal excretion of salicylate. Drugs such as ascorbic acid (vitamin C), commonly used as a dietary supplement, have an opposite effect by acidifying the urine and reducing renal excretion of salicylate, potentially causing elevated plasma salicylate levels.[82]

The pharmacokinetics of salicylates do not appear to differ between the elderly and the young. However, with reduced renal function and a diminished capacity for protein binding, compounded by decreased albumin levels associated with the rheumatic diseases, a higher free fraction of salicylate can develop in elderly arthritic patients, making this group more prone to salicylism.[82]

As many as 1% of the general population can experience anaphylactoid reactions to aspirin and other NSAIDs, sometimes leading to death. In the presence of the dangerous clinical triad of asthma, nasal polyposis, and eosinophilia, anaphylactoid reactions to aspirin and other NSAIDs occur with a frequency 10 times greater than that of the population lacking this clinical triad. The reaction is probably a consequence of prostaglandin inhibition. Nonacetylated salicylates are the only antiinflammatory agents that could possibly be used cautiously in patients with the triad.[83]

Because of weak PGE_2 inhibition, nonacetylated salicylates appear to cause less renal toxicity than do aspirin and some of the other NSAIDs. Along with enteric-coated aspirin, the nonacetylated salicylates may also spare the gastric mucosa from ulceration promoted by most other antiinflammatory agents. They reversibly inhibit platelet function like most nonaspirin NSAIDs, impacting the clotting mechanism to a lesser extent than does aspirin.[83] The nonacetylated salicylates include sodium and potassium salicylate, salsalate, choline magnesium trisalicylate, magnesium salicylate, and diflunisal.

All salicylates have a propensity to produce an annoying tinnitus, which can progress to deafness. Tinnitus can serve as an early warning sign for impending toxicity, and the side effect can be corrected by reducing salicylate dosage.[5] Toxic levels produce metabolic problems, especially in the very young and the elderly. Confusion, mental obfuscation, and symptoms associated with metabolic acidosis accompany salicylate overdose. A reversible elevation of liver transaminase can occur with salicylate use, but it is not always associated with hepatic toxicity. When liver dysfunction occurs, it correlates well with serum salicylate levels. Although liver enzymes may become elevated, they can revert to normal even with continued drug use. When enzymes become markedly or progressively elevated, ASA dosage should be reduced or the drug discontinued.[83] The drug diflunisal has been linked to several cases of photoporphyria.[84]

Drug interactions can occur with the salicylates, and some of these conflicts can be clinically significant. Concurrent use of indomethacin and aspirin results in reduced indomethacin concentrations. The uricosuric effect of probenecid is inhibited by low doses of aspirin. Sulfinpyrazone, a phenylbutazone analogue metabolite, is even more susceptible to aspirin blockade. Aspirin has been found to compete with MTX for renal clearance, increasing the serum concentration of the concurrently administered folic acid antagonist. Clinically important interactions occur with heparin and oral anticoagulants owing to aspirin's effects on platelet function.[82]

The salicylates probably reduce inflammation by inhibiting the prostaglandin-generating enzyme cyclooxygenase, but it is thought that salicylates also protect cartilage from degeneration in inflamed joints by other means. The lysosomal protease cathepsin has been found to be a major factor in the degradation of the articular cartilage matrix. Salicylates were shown to inhibit this reaction by about 20%.[85] Additionally, salicylates may act as scavengers of destructive hydroxyl radicals.[5]

Generally, clinical improvement in the symptoms associated with arthritis is noted when serum salicylate levels reach 20 to 30 mg/dl. Achieving these levels necessitates aspirin doses as high as 3900 mg daily.[52] This requires administration of three 325-mg (5-grain) tablets four times daily. Common doses of the other salicylates are listed in Table 24–4.

All salicylates should be monitored for intrinsic or induced toxic effects when used to treat IJDs, especially in juvenile and elderly patients. Treatment of salicylate overdose includes discontinuance of the drug, alkalinization of the urine, hydration, and cardiopulmonary support.[83]

TABLE 24–4

PHARMACOLOGIC AGENTS USED IN THE MANAGEMENT OF INFLAMMATORY JOINT DISEASE

Drug Class	Agent	Proprietary Name	How Supplied	Usual Daily Dose (No.)	Typical Monthly Patient Cost*
NSAIDs Salicylates		Aspirin†	325-mg tablets	3–4 qid	Less than $10.00
	Enteric-coated ASA	Ecotrin†,[a]	325-mg tablets	3–4 qid	$23.36 (3 qid)
			500-mg tablets	2 qid	$15.00
			325-mg caplets	3–4 qid	$32.45 (3 qid)
			500-mg caplets	2 qid	$32.40
		Generic‡	325-mg tablets	3–4 qid	$7.49
			500-mg tablets	2 qid	$9.90
	Potassium salicylate	Pabalate-SF[b]	300-mg tablets	2 q4h	$32.80
	Sodium salicylate	Pabalate[b]	300-mg tablets	2 q4h	$33.20
	Salsalate	Disalcid [c]	500-mg tablets	3 bid; 2 tid	$74.50
			750-mg tablets	2 bid	$64.45
		Salflex[d]	500-mg tablets	3 bid; 2 tid	$47.41
			750-mg tablets	2 bid	$41.25
		Mono-Gesic[e]	750-mg tablets	2 bid	$36.36
		Generic	500-mg tablets	3 bid; 2 tid	$48.45
			750-mg tablets	2 bid	$41.90
	Choline magnesium trisalicylate	Trilisate[f]	500-mg tablets	3 bid	$92.05
			750-mg tablets	1 tid	$77.65
			1000-mg tablets	3 qd hs; 1 tid	$75.50
			500-mg/tsp liq	3 tsp bid; 4 tsp qd hs	$101.42 (900 ml)
		Generic	500-mg tablets	3 bid	$59.40
			750-mg tablets	1 tid	$36.72
			1000-mg tablets	3 qd hs; 1 tid	$49.14
	Magnesium salicylate	Magsal[g]	600-mg tablets	2 tid	$70.61
		Generic	545-mg tablets	2 tid	$72.27
	Diflunisal	Dolobid[h]	250-mg tablets	1 bid	$59.15
			500-mg tablets	1 bid	$71.25
	Zero-order release ASA	Zorprin[i]	800-mg tablets	2 bid	$36.65
Pyrazoles	Phenylbutazone	Butazolidin[j]	No longer available		
		Generic	100-mg tablets	For gout: 1 qid, discontinue in 1 wk	$20.35
Indoleacetic acids	Indomethacin	Indocin[h]	25-mg capsules	1 bid or tid	$20.35 (tid)
			50-mg capsules	1–2 bid or 1 tid	$77.30 (tid)
			25-mg/5-ml oral suspension (1 tsp = 5 ml)	1–2 tsp bid or 1–2 tsp tid;	$72.80 (480 ml)
			50-mg suppository	1 bid or tid, or 1–2 qd hs	$50.07
		Indocin SR[h]	75-mg capsule	1 qd or bid; 150–200 mg daily maintenance dose divided bid or tid; for gout 50 mg tid until symptoms subside	$122.40 (bid)
		Generic	25-mg capsules	1 bid or tid	$38.70 (tid)
			50-mg capsules	1–2 bid or 1 tid	$50.25 (tid)
			75-mg capsules	1 qd or bid	$79.60 (bid)
	Sulindac	Clinoril[h]	150-mg tablets	1 bid	$59.00
			200-mg tablets	1 bid	$70.05
		Generic	150-mg tablets	1 bid	$35.80
			200-mg tablets	1 bid	$41.70
Pyrrolacetic acids	Tolmetin	Tolectin[k]	200-mg tablets	1–2 tid	$57.10 (1 tid)
			600-mg tablets	1 tid	$100.75
		Tolectin DC[k]	400-mg capsules	1 tid; pediatric 15–30 mg/kg/day divided tid or qid	$84.30

Table continued on following page

TABLE 24–4

PHARMACOLOGIC AGENTS USED IN THE MANAGEMENT OF INFLAMMATORY JOINT DISEASE *Continued*

Drug Class	Agent	Proprietary Name	How Supplied	Usual Daily Dose (No.)	Typical Monthly Patient Cost*
Propionic acids	Ibuprofen	Motrin[l]	300-mg tablets	1 qid	$27.40
			400-mg tablets	1 tid or qid	$21.80 (tid)
			600-mg tablets	1 tid or qid	$28.95 (tid)
			800-mg tablets	1 tid or qid	$38.00 (tid)
		Motrin IB†[l*]	200-mg tablets	1–4 tid or qid	$9.98 (100)
			200-mg caplets	1–4 tid or qid	$9.98 (100)
		Rufen[i]	400-mg tablets	1 tid or qid	$19.24 (tid)
			600-mg tablets	1 tid or qid	$24.17 (tid)
			800-mg tablets	1 tid or qid	$32.46 (tid)
		Advil†,[m]	200-mg tablets	1–4 tid or qid	$10.28 (100)
			200-mg caplets	1–4 tid or qid	$10.28 (100)
		Nuprin†,[n]	200-mg tablets	1–4 tid or qid	$9.61 (100)
			200-mg caplets	1–4 tid or qid	$9.61 (100)
		Medipren†,[o]	200-mg tablets	1–4 tid or qid	$10.52 (100)
			200-mg caplets	1–4 tid or qid	$8.85 (125)
		PediaProfen[o]	100-mg/5-ml oral suspension	3 tsp qid; 4, 6, or 8 tsp tid or qid	$23.61 (480 ml)
	Naproxen	Naprosyn[p]	250-mg tablets	1 bid	$48.80
			375-mg tablets	1 bid	$59.40
			500 mg tablets	1 bid	$70.15
			125-mg/5-ml oral suspension	2 tsp bid	$41.12 (480 ml)
	Naproxen sodium	Anaprox[p]	275-mg tablets	1 bid	$48.70
		Anaprox DS[p]	550-mg tablets	1 bid	$69.45
	Fenoprofen calcium	Nalfon[q]	200-mg pulvules	1–4 tid or qid	$67.65 (1 qid)
			300-mg pulvules	1–2 tid or qid	$77.65 (1 qid)
			600-mg tablets	1 tid or qid	$107.07 (qid)
		Generic	200-mg tablets	1–4 tid or qid	$36.80 (1 qid)
			300-mg tablets	1–2 tid or qid	$42.46 (1 qid)
			600-mg tablets	1 tid or qid	$49.58 (qid)
	Ketoprofen	Orudis[r]	25-mg capsules	1 tid or qid	$86.45 (qid)
			50-mg capsules	1 tid or qid	$124.60 (qid)
			75 mg capsules	1 tid or qid	$138.50 (qid)
	Flurbiprofen	Ansaid[l]	50-mg tablets	1 bid, tid, or qid	$76.65 (tid)
			100-mg tablets	1 bid or tid	$115.55 (tid)
Phenylacetic acids	Diclofenac	Voltaren[j]	25-mg tablets	1 tid or qid	$52.95 (tid)
			50-mg tablets	1 bid, tid, or qid	$93.25 (tid)
			75-mg tablets	1 bid	$111.64 (tid)
Anthranilic acids	Meclofenamate sodium	Meclomen[s]	50-mg capsules	1 qid	$77.53
			100-mg capsules	1 qid	$116.06
		Generic	50-mg capsules	1 qid	$58.20
			100-mg capsules	1 qid	$87.07
Oxicams	Piroxicam	Feldene[t]	10-mg capsules	1 qd or bid	$51.15 (qd)
			20-mg capsules	1 qd	$74.85
Naphthylalkanones	Nabumetone	Relafen[a]	500-mg tablets	1 bid or 2 qd hs	$61.15
Tetrahydroindoles	Etodolac	Lodine[r]	200-mg capsules	1 tid or qid	$102.00 (qid)
			300-mg capsules	1 tid or qid	$115.50 (qid)
DMARDs					
Antimalarials	Hydroxychloroquine sulfate	Plaquenil[u]	200-mg tablets	1 bid	$69.35
Gold salts	Auranofin	Ridaura[v]	3 mg capsules	1 bid or 2 qd	$60.55
	Gold sodium thiomalate	Myochrysine[h]	25-mg/ml solution	1 g total dose	$273.48§
			50-mg/ml solution	1 g total dose	$200.93§
	Aurothioglucose	Solganal[w]	50-mg/ml suspension	1 g total dose	$191.82§
Penicillamines	D-penicillamine	Cuprimine[h]	125-mg capsules	Initial: 125–250 mg qd; maintenance: 500–750 mg qd	$71.40 (500 mg maintenance qd)
			250-mg capsules		
		Depen[x]	250-mg tablets	Initial: 125–250 mg qd; maintenance: 500–750 mg qd	$71.40 (500 mg maintenance qd)

TABLE 24–4

PHARMACOLOGIC AGENTS USED IN THE MANAGEMENT OF INFLAMMATORY JOINT DISEASE *Continued*

Drug Class	Agent	Proprietary Name	How Supplied	Usual Daily Dose (No.)	Typical Monthly Patient Cost*
Antimetabolites	Methotrexate	Rheumatrex[y]	2.5-mg tablet	200 mg total dose given as 5–15 mg once-weekly dose	$226.35 (tablets)
			25-mg/ml injection single-dose vial		$90.20 (assumes wastage of unused vial)
Immunosuppressants	Azathioprine	Imuran[z]	50-mg tablets	1 mg/kg/day as one or two divided doses; may increase to 2.5 mg/kg/day	$67.75 (1 bid)
	Cyclophosphamide	Cytoxan[aa]	4-mg/ml injection		$79.38 (20 ml/vial)
			25-mg tablets	1 bid or tid	$121.90 (1 tid)
			50-mg tablets	1 bid or tid (1.1–1.7 mg/kg/day)	$223.90 (1 tid)
			100-mg injection 200-mg injection 500-mg injection 1.0-g injection 2.0-g injection		
	Cyclosporin A	Sandimmune[bb]	25-mg capsules	5 mg/kg/day‖	$489.72 (420 capsules)
			100-mg capsules	5 mg/kg/day‖	$466.40 (100 capsules)
			100-mg capsules suspension	5 mg/kg/day‖	$466.00 (100 ml)
			50-mg/ml injection	5 mg/kg/day‖	$1,247.76 (2 vials/day)
Others	Sulfasalazine	Azulfidine[cc]	500-mg tablets	2–4 g/day in 2–4 equal doses	$55.05 (2 qid)
		Azulfidine EN[cc]	500-mg enteric-coated tablets	2–4 g/day in 2–4 equal doses	$64.35 (2 qid)
		Generic	500-mg tablets	2–4 g/day in 2–4 equal doses	$35.80 (2 qid)
Antigout Agents Uricosurics	Probenecid	Benemid[h]	500-mg tablets	250 mg bid for 1 week, then 500 mg bid, up to 500 mg qid	$43.40 (1 qid)
		Generic	500-mg tablets	250 mg bid for 1 week, then 500 mg bid, up to 500 mg qid	$28.25 (1 qid)
	Colchicine with probenecid	ColBENEMID[h]	05-mg colchicine with 500-mg probenecid	1 qd first week then 1 bid for maintenance	$25.35 (1 bid)
		Generic	5 mg colchionine with 500-mg probenecid	1 qd first week, then 1 bid for maintenance	$16.50 (1 bid)
	Sulfinpyrazone	Anturane[dd]	100-mg tablets	1–2 bid	$28.65 (1 bid)
			200-mg capsules	1 bid to 2 bid maintenance	$39.95 (1 bid)
		Generic	100-mg tablets	1–2 bid	$16.75 (1 bid)
			200-mg capsules	1 bid to 2 bid maintenance	$21.68 (1 bid)
Xanthine oxidase inhibitors	Allopurinol	Zyloprim[z]	100-mg tablets	200–600 mg/day (if more than 300 mg/day is administered, drug is given in divided doses)	$18.30 (1 bid)
			300-mg tablets		$23.50 (1 qd)
		Generic	100-mg tablets	200–600 mg/day (if more than 300 mg/day is administered, drug is given in divided doses)	$11.90 (1 bid)
			300-mg tablets		$10.60 (1 qd)

Table continued on following page

TABLE 24–4

PHARMACOLOGIC AGENTS USED IN THE MANAGEMENT OF INFLAMMATORY JOINT DISEASE *Continued*

Drug Class	Agent	Proprietary Name	How Supplied	Usual Daily Dose (No.)	Typical Monthly Patient Cost*
Anti-inflammatory agents	Colchicine	Generic	0.6-mg tablets	6.0 mg total dose; see text for usual dosing regimen	Less than $5.00
		Colchicine[ee]	1-mg/2-ml ampules	See text for usual dosing regimen	$22.47 (6 ampules)

*Costs derived from a survey of medical group and hospital pharmacies in the San Francisco Bay area.
†Over-the-counter preparations.
‡Generic prices may vary significantly in different retail chains.
§Expense does not include costs of administering the drug.
‖Assume 70 kg body weight.
[a]Smithkline Beecham Consumer Brands, Pittsburgh, PA 15230.
[b]A.H. Robbins Co., Inc., Richmond, VA 23261-6609.
[c]3M Pharmaceuticals, St. Paul, MN 55144.
[d]Carnrick Laboratories, Inc., Cedar Knolls, NJ 07927.
[e]Central Pharmaceuticals, Inc., Seymour, IN 47274.
[f]Purdue Frederick Company, Norwalk, CT 06856.
[g]Adria Laboratories, Dublin, OH 43017.
[h]Merck Sharp & Dohme, West Point, PA 19486.
[i]Boots Pharmaceuticals, Inc., Lincolnshire, IL 60069-4415.
[j]Geigy Pharmaceuticals, Ardsley, NY 10502.
[k]McNeil Pharmaceutical, Spring House, PA 19477.
[l]Upjohn Company, Kalamazoo, MI 49001.
[m]Whitehall Laboratories, Inc., New York, NY 10017.
[n]Bristol-Myers Products, New York, NY 10154.
[o]McNeil Consumer Products Co., Fort Washington, PA 19034.
[p]Syntex Laboratories, Inc., Palo Alto, CA 94303.
[q]Dista Products Company, Indianapolis, IN 46285.
[r]Wyeth-Ayerst Laboratories, Philadelphia, PA 19101.
[s]Parke-Davis, Morris Plains, NJ 07950.
[t]Pfizer Labs Division, New York, NY 10017.
[u]Winthrop Pharmaceuticals, New York, NY 10016.
[v]Smith Kline & French Laboratories, Philadelphia, PA 19101.
[w]Schering Corporation, Kenilworth, NJ 07033.
[x]Wallace Laboratories, Cranbury, NJ 08512.
[y]Lederle Laboratories, Wayne, NJ 07470.
[z]Burroughs Wellcome Co., Research Triangle Park, NC 27709.
[aa]Bristol-Myers Oncology Division, Evansville, IN 47721-0001.
[bb]Sandoz Pharmaceuticals Corporation, East Hanover, NJ 07936.
[cc]Pharmacia Laboratories, Piscataway, NJ 08855.
[dd]CIBA Pharmaceutical Company, Summit, NJ 07901.
[ee]Eli Lilly and Company, Indianapolis, IN 46285.
ASA, acetylsalicylic acid; NSAIDs, nonsteroidal antiinflammatory drugs; qid, four times daily; q4h, every 4 hours; bid, twice daily; tid, three times daily; qd, every day; hs, bedtime; tsp, teaspoon; liq, liquid; DMARDs, disease-modifying antirheumatic drugs.

Pyrazoles

Phenylbutazone was the first drug referred to as an NSAID. Its major metabolite, oxyphenbutazone, was released as an agent itself several years later, but it has since been taken off the U.S. market because of unacceptable toxicity.[86]

Phenylbutazone is highly protein bound and slowly excreted. The drug increases the renal tubular reabsorption of sodium, which can cause edema and hypertension. The increased volume load can lead to congestive heart failure or pulmonary edema in susceptible patients with cardiovascular disease.[2] Overall, changes in the pharmacokinetics of this drug in the elderly appear to be minor.[67]

Phenylbutazone reduces the renal excretion of tolbutamide and phenytoin, potentiating their pharmacologic effects. It causes an increased prothrombin time in patients receiving warfarin. The metabolism of aminopyrine, digitoxin, and cortisol is enhanced by phenylbutazone, possibly reducing their clinical effectiveness.[87, 88]

Phenylbutazone is a highly effective antiinflammatory agent that has fallen into the disfavor of many clinicians owing to its severe toxicity. There appears to be a high incidence of fatal blood dyscrasias and upper GI bleeding episodes associated with the drug's use. Deaths range from 2.2 to 3.8 in 100,000 patients, depending on patient age.[67, 86] Agranulocytosis, aplastic anemia, and thrombocytopenia all have been reported with the use of this agent.[86]

Although phenylbutazone is effective in the treatment of RA, OA, AS, and other arthritic disorders, it appears to be used mostly in the short-term treatment of acute gout and superficial thrombophlebitis. Because of the severity of its side effects, the use of less toxic and equally effective antiinflammatory drugs is encouraged.

Phenylbutazone is administered at a dose of 100 mg three or four times daily. If the drug is used for more than 5 days, frequent CBCs with differential and urinalyses should be performed.

Indoleacetic Acids

The indoleacetic acids include indomethacin and sulindac, two agents with quite different properties. Sulindac, for example, is quite useful in the treatment of the spondyloarthropathies, whereas indomethacin is much more effective in treating gouty arthritis.[48]

Indomethacin. Orally administered indomethacin is rapidly absorbed and becomes highly protein bound. Its metabolism involves *N*-deacylation, *O*-desmethylation, and glucuronide conjugation. Approximately 65% of administered indomethacin is excreted in the urine and 35% in the stool. There is significant enterohepatic circulation of the glucuronide conjugate; much of the excreted drug is reabsorbed. This may be responsible for the high incidence GI toxicity associated with the drug's use. In elderly patients with decreased renal function, a compensatory increase in GI elimination may occur, making this population particularly prone to GI toxicity.[2, 5, 67]

Headaches occur in half of all patients whose total daily dose of indomethacin exceeds 100 mg. Other CNS symptoms associated with the use of indomethacin include dizziness, confusion, seizures, and syncope. Corneal deposits and retinal toxicity have been reported,[2, 5] along with transient elevations in BUN and serum creatinine levels. Severe azotemia can occur in patients with a diminished GFR secondary to congestive heart failure.[5]

In addition to suppressing cyclooxygenase activity, indomethacin has been found to inhibit the migration of leukocytes to sites of inflammation. It can inhibit phosphodiesterase, thereby increasing intracellular cyclic AMP levels. Cyclic AMP stabilizes the lysosomal enzymes in PMNs and macrophages, thus decreasing the generation of toxic oxygen radicals.[86]

Indomethacin has mostly supplanted phenylbutazone in the treatment of gout and other acute musculoskeletal disorders. For acute gouty attacks, 50 mg of indomethacin is administered three times daily or 75 mg is administered twice daily until symptoms subside. It is then reduced to a maintenance dose of 25 mg twice daily. Indomethacin has also been remarkably useful in treating primary OA of the hip.[5]

Sulindac. This drug resembles indomethacin chemically but is associated with a lower toxicity. It is administered as an inactive sulfoxide, which is rapidly absorbed from the stomach and upper GI tract. Once absorbed, this prodrug is reversibly metabolized to an active sulfide and irreversibly converted to an inactive sulfone. The major sites of these transformations are the liver and the kidney. Metabolites are tightly bound to plasma proteins and eliminated by both the kidneys and the liver. Sulindac sulfoxide and sulindac sulfone are excreted by the kidneys.[2, 19] The parent compound undergoes enterohepatic recirculation, providing a useful drug pool, available for conversion to the active product.[67, 83] The metabolites of the parent drug also appear to undergo hepatic recirculation.[19]

Because sulindac is administered as a prodrug, GI disturbances and occult blood loss are less severe than with other NSAIDs. Constipation is the most common GI complaint associated with its use.[89]

Sulindac does not inhibit cyclooxygenase activity in the kidney because the organ can reoxidize the active sulfide back to its original inactive sulfoxide.[2] This may limit the drug's toxicity in patients experiencing renal compromise. Most studies of sulindac's possible renal-sparing attributes appear to involve patients with minimal renal disease, accounting perhaps for the drug's observed benign action on the kidneys. When patients with higher degrees of renal compromise were studied (i.e., a two-thirds reduction in GFR), the active metabolite sulindac sulfide was found to accumulate to levels high enough to inhibit renal cyclooxy-

genase. With these findings, sulindac's role as a renal-sparing NSAID must be cautiously applied. Although fewer renal side effects occur with sulindac, there is a need for prudent and regular monitoring of patients at risk who are treated with this drug.[19, 20]

In patients using tolbutamide, sulindac was not found to change the 2-hour postprandial blood glucose level. There is little effect on prothrombin time when administered to patients using warfarin. Like indomethacin, sulindac has been shown to inhibit platelet aggregation in vitro.

Overall, sulindac is less potent than indomethacin but has fewer side effects and a longer duration of action. It is effective in the management of RA and OA and may be useful in acute gout. It is less effective than indomethacin in treating AS and OA of the hip. Sulindac is administered at doses of 150 to 200 mg twice daily.

Etodolac. This is the newest indolacetic acid–derived NSAID to be released on the U.S. drug market. It is rapidly absorbed after oral administration, with maximum concentrations reached after 1 hour. The serum half-life of etodolac during chronic therapy was measured at 7.4 hours. Approximately 74% of the administered dose is excreted with the urine and 19% in the stool. Less than 5% of the drug is eliminated unchanged.[56]

Etodolac enjoys improved GI tolerance and a lower incidence of renal side effects than most other NSAIDs.[21, 56] When compared with sulindac and aspirin, etodolac and placebo had significantly lower incidences of drug-induced renal dysfunction. Patients older than 65 years were found to be at no greater risk for renal impairment than were younger patients, and there was no increased risk for renal damage in patients who had abnormal renal values before etodolac therapy was started.[21]

Etodolac is an effective agent for use against RA and OA, and the drug displays favorable efficacy when used to relieve postoperative pain. For treatment of arthritis, etodolac is administered at a dose of 200 mg once or twice daily.[56]

Pyrrolacetic Acids

The pyrrolacetic acids include tolmetin and zomepirac acid. An unusual but important side effect of these drugs is a severe anaphylactoid reaction with bronchospasm and hypotension. This reaction occurs more commonly in patients who are allergic to aspirin, and deaths have occurred.[87] Zomepirac acid, originally introduced as an analgesic, has since been withdrawn from the U.S. drug market.

Although tolmetin is structurally related to the pyrrolacetic acid derivatives, its in vivo behavior resembles that of indomethacin. Tolmetin is rapidly absorbed after oral administration and is highly protein bound. Salicylates can substantially reduce its binding to albumin, and concurrent use provides no additional benefit. The drug is easily metabolized and eliminated as both a conjugate and an inactive oxidant.[87, 89]

Tolmetin is advocated for the management of RA, OA, juvenile RA, and AS. It can also be used for periarticular disorders, but it does not appear effective in the treatment of acute gout.[2] GI side effects are observed in 30% of patients treated with the drug. Symptoms include nausea, vomiting, diarrhea, dyspepsia, and stomatitis. Other side effects encountered with tolmetin use are headache, dizziness, rashes, and edema from sodium retention. This last effect may limit the drug's usefulness when congestive heart failure is present. A false-positive proteinurea test result that would read normal on dipstick may occur with tolmetin use.[87]

Tolmetin is administered in doses of 200 or 400 mg three or four times daily. The drug is approved for use in children, with a recommended pediatric dose of 15 to 30 mg/kg/day.[90]

Propionic Acids

Propionic acids are one of the largest and most commonly used of all the NSAID groups. In 1974, ibuprofen became the first propionic acid–derived NSAID available on the U.S. drug market.

Ibuprofen. When first introduced, ibuprofen was used at a dose of less than 1200 mg per day. Although this dose is adequate for providing analgesia, it succeeds in producing only weak antiinflammatory activity.[89] The drug is now administered at more than twice the originally recommended dose.

More than 90% of ibuprofen is absorbed on oral administration, but absorption is delayed if the drug is taken along with a meal. It is highly protein bound and metabolized by the liver. The drug undergoes hydroxylation and carboxylation, with 12% of the metabolites eliminated by the liver as a glucuronide.[2] Ibuprofen has a half-life of about 2 hours, necessitating frequent dosing.

In general, ibuprofen is well tolerated. Dyspepsia and nausea can develop with the drug's use, but occult blood loss is less than that attributed to aspirin. There have been several cases of idiosyncratic aseptic meningitis reported when ibuprofen was used in patients with systemic lupus erythematosus and mixed connective tissue disease.[2, 88] A reversible toxic amblyopia has also been reported.[89] As with most other NSAIDs, ibuprofen disrupts renal hemostasis through its inhibitory effects on renal prostaglandins.[2]

Distribution of ibuprofen in obese patients was examined.[91] Ibuprofen was found to be distributed 0.44 times as extensively into systems in which actual body weight exceeded ideal body weight. The drug's clearance increases in parallel with the drug's volume of distribution and the patient's total body weight; therefore, to achieve effective plasma concentrations of the drug, the dose of ibuprofen may be increased in obese persons while dosing interval remains unchanged. Further clinical studies are needed to determine whether these findings extend to the other NSAIDs.

Ibuprofen's half-life was found to be longer and total clearance lower in elderly patients compared with that in young men, but the difference was small. The required dosing schedule of three or four times daily is unlikely to cause excessive accumulation of ibuprofen in any person, regardless of age.[92]

Ibuprofen appears to be most useful for the management of OA of the hip, for RA, and, at its highest recommended dose, for acute gout. Other propionic acid derivatives and the salicylates, however, appear to be more effective in the management of RA. Ibuprofen is administered at doses of 300, 400, 600, or 800 mg three or four times daily.[87, 89]

Naproxen. This is one of the most popular NSAIDs available, probably because of its high efficacy, relatively low toxicity, and twice-daily dosing schedule. It is well absorbed from the GI tract and highly bound to albumin. Its rate of absorption is increased when administered with sodium bicarbonate and decreased when administered with food or antacids. Peak plasma concentrations are achieved in 2 hours,

and the drug has a long plasma half-life of 14 hours, allowing twice-daily dosing. Naproxen is excreted in the urine almost entirely as a glucuronide metabolite. Plasma protein binding increases little at doses higher than 500 mg twice daily, which, in combination with rapid renal clearance of free drug, limits plasma levels and subsequent toxicity.[2, 89, 93]

Naproxen causes less GI irritation than does aspirin, but the drug has been associated with several instances of GI hemorrhage. Endoscopic examination showed changes in the gastric mucosa that did not correlate with symptoms. Despite these effects, naproxen can possibly be given safely to patients with a history of peptic ulcer or hiatal hernia if they are monitored closely.[89] Naproxen causes an increased bleeding time, and it displaces warfarin from its albumin-binding sites.[2, 89] Pseudoporphyria, a reversible photo-induced cutaneous bullous disease, has been linked to the use of naproxen.[58] Unusual peripheral neuropathies have also been reported.[94] An atypical distribution of symptoms in patients using this drug should raise suspicion.

There was no increased incidence of side effects noted when naproxen was administered to hypoalbuminemic patients. The hypoalbuminemia commonly associated with RA may prove somewhat beneficial if the drug's efficacy is indeed related to unbound drug concentration.[95, 96] In elderly patients, the mean steady-state plasma unbound concentration of naproxen becomes significantly elevated with usual dosing, suggesting that the prescribed dose should be reduced for this group.[67] Immunoregulatory effects have been attributed to naproxen when it is used to treat RA. Its administration results in a significant enhancement of the in vivo phytohemagglutinin-induced proliferation of leukocytes. The investigator's interpretation suggests that naproxen, and possibly other NSAIDs, used as immunoregulatory agents, may modify the disease process in RA.[97]

Drug interactions have been observed when naproxen was given concurrently with other therapeutic agents. When used with the salicylates, the combination proved to be more toxic than either agent alone and had no greater efficacy.[98] Concurrent administration of naproxen and low-dose MTX (15 mg/day) in patients with RA appears to be a relatively safe regimen, provided patients have normal or only moderately impaired renal function.[99]

Naproxen is useful against all inflammatory diseases and has been found to be as effective as indomethacin in the treatment of RA.[2] The drug was preferred by both patients and physicians compared with aspirin.[100, 101] It appears to be as effective as aspirin when used in the treatment of OA of the hip, and it compares well with phenylbutazone when given as a single 750-mg dose followed by 250 mg twice daily for acute gout.[2] The usual dose for IJDs and musculoskeletal pain is 250, 375, or 500 mg twice daily. A controlled-release tablet using a polymer-matrix formulation designed to release 750 or 1000 mg of naproxen over 24 hours has undergone study.[93] Although unavailable as of this writing, the formulation shows promise that naproxen can be administered once daily with efficacy similar to a conventional twice-daily regimen.

Fenoprofen. Fenoprofen calcium, another propionic acid derivative, is well absorbed after oral administration. Although absorption is impaired when the drug is given with food, the interaction is thought to be clinically insignificant.[89] Concurrent use of magnesium or aluminum hydroxide does not affect absorption. The drug is highly protein bound and undergoes enterohepatic circulation. Metabolites are excreted in the urine as a glucuronide. Fenoprofen is generally better tolerated than aspirin and causes less GI bleeding. Dyspepsia is the most common side effect associated with the drug's use. Fenoprofen appears to be more nephrotoxic than most other NSAIDs. Eosinophilia occurs in 30% of patients using this drug.[18]

Fenoprofen is useful in the treatment of RA, OA, and AS, with the usual dose of 300 to 600 mg three or four times daily. It can be used for acute gout at a dose of 3200 mg daily.

Ketoprofen. Ketoprofen is one of a few antiinflammatory agents whose mode of action includes the inhibition of both the cyclooxygenase and lipoxygenase pathways of arachidonic acid metabolism. This leads to the suppression of both prostaglandin and leukotriene synthesis.

When orally administered, ketoprofen is rapidly absorbed. Food causes a decrease in the rate, but not completeness, of absorption. Ketoprofen is metabolized through hepatic hydroxylation and glucuronidization of the parent compound. Renal insufficiency has only modest effects on serum half-life and does not cause significant accumulation or require dosage adjustment.[2]

Ketoprofen was found to be equivalent to ibuprofen when used for RA but displayed a greater incidence of side effects. It is about as effective as indomethacin for OA of the hip and may be useful in the treatment of AS and gout. Gastric side effects predominate but may be less frequent than with naproxen or indomethacin.[89] CNS disorders can also develop with the drug's use. As with diflunisal and naproxen, ketoprofen has been associated with the infrequent development of pseudoporphyria.[85]

The usual dose of ketoprofen is 50 or 75 mg given three or four times daily.

Suprofen. This drug was found to be more potent as an analgesic than as an antiinflammatory agent despite its potent inhibition of prostaglandin synthesis.

Suprofen is an effective, orally active analgesic used for acute pain of moderate intensity, providing equivalent or superior analgesia to therapeutic doses of aspirin, acetaminophen, dextroproxyphene, codeine, and their combinations. It is rapidly absorbed after oral administration and is eliminated mostly by the kidneys as an acyl glucuronide. Major side effects include mild GI and CNS disturbances. Skin rashes have also been reported.[102] There are several reports of suprofen-related nephrotoxicity manifested as reversible acute renal failure and interstitial nephritis.[103] The drug has been withdrawn from the U.S. market because it produced flank pain probably related to renal toxicity.

Flurbiprofen. This is an effective antiinflammatory agent that exhibits analgesic and antipyretic properties like those of most other NSAIDs. The drug is rapidly absorbed after oral administration and reaches peak blood levels in about 1.5 hours. When the drug is taken with food, its rate of absorption is reduced, but its bioavailability appears unchanged. Once absorbed, about 99% of the drug binds to serum proteins. The elimination half-life of flurbiprofen is about 6.5 hours. The drug is extensively metabolized by conjugation and hydroxylation and is eliminated primarily in the urine.

As with most NSAIDs, flurbiprofen therapy has been associated with GI side effects. GI symptomatology correlates poorly with mucosal erosive changes caused by flurbiprofen use. Gastric irritation from 200 mg of flurbiprofen is similar to that of 2600 mg of aspirin. The drug is better tolerated when administered concomitantly with cimetidine or an antacid, but increased levels of the drug occur with this regimen. A possible drug kinetic interaction may explain the increased levels of flurbiprofen when it is given with the cytoprotective agent, possibly as a result of inhibition of microsomal oxidation by cimetidine.[104, 105]

Overall, genitourinary system effects of flurbiprofen are found to be similar in incidence to those of aspirin. Hemolymphatic system reactions were also infrequent; the most serious was a small decrease in hemoglobin and hematocrit measurements. Peripheral edema occurred in about 2.4% of patients studied, but the edema was not deemed serious. The most common CNS side effect is headache, occurring in about 2.9% of patients using the drug.[106] A severe form of parkinsonian syndrome occurred in a 57-year-old man being treated for a painful knee. The condition developed 1 week after therapy was initiated and was only partially reversed when flurbiprofen was discontinued.[107]

In general, flurbiprofen is a relatively safe, effective, well-tolerated NSAID alternative[106] and is recommended for use in the treatment of RA and OA. It is supplied in 50- and 100-mg tablets. The recommended total daily dose of flurbiprofen is 200 to 300 mg divided into three or four doses. No more than 100 mg should be taken at each dosing.

Benoxaprofen. This NSAID stood out among others by causing only weak inhibition of cyclooxygenase but displaying strong activity against lipoxygenase. Its long half-life permitted once-daily administration. It was removed from the U.S. drug market in 1982 after 2 years of use. Adverse reactions to the drug included cholestatic jaundice and the development of Stevens-Johnson syndrome.[20, 68, 108] The drug was also reported to induce an immediate form of solar urticaria.[109]

Tiaprofenic Acid. A potential drawback of NSAID therapy when used to treat the joint pain of arthritis is for the agent itself to impair the ability of chondrocytes to repair joint cartilage damaged through the disease process. Indomethacin, the salicylates, and the propionic acid derivatives have all been implicated in inhibiting the repair of joint structures.[110–112] Although these agents may not directly produce harmful changes in the cartilage composition, their potential to reduce joint cell activity may, in the long run, extend the effects of the disease process.

Tiaprofenic acid is a propionic acid derivative that lacks the inhibitory effect that others of its class have on proteoglycan synthesis.[113] This major advantage may make the drug useful for the long-term management of RA and OA.

The side effect profile of tiaprofenic acid is similar to that of the other propionic acid derivatives. The drug appears to have a low level of gastrotoxicity, and a sustained-release formulation may provide an even greater degree of gastric tolerance.[113, 114] The incidence of renal side effects also appears comparable to or lower than that of other NSAIDs. It is suggested that tiaprofenic acid may be a suitable NSAID alternate for use in elderly patients who may have renal function impairment.[115] Abnormal liver function was found to occur in about 4% of patients studied as evidenced by an increased ALT and AST. One patient had to be removed from the study, but in all instances, values returned to normal when the drug was withdrawn.[116]

Tiaprofenic acid appears useful for the management of IJDs, particularly RA and OA. The administered drug is rapidly absorbed and eliminated from the plasma; however, synovial fluid concentrations remain constant for at least 8 hours.[117] It is administered at doses of 200 mg three times daily, 300 mg twice daily, or a single 600-mg sustained-release preparation. The drug is not available in the United States as of this writing.

Phenylacetic Acids

Diclofenac is one of the newest of the NSAIDs to be marketed in the United States. Its GI absorption is essentially complete, with peak plasma levels occurring 2 to 3 hours after administration. The drug undergoes extensive first-pass elimination, allowing only 50% of the absorbed drug to be available for clinical effect. More than 99% of the free drug binds to plasma proteins. It appears that diclofenac sequesters into the synovial fluid, extending its duration of clinical efficacy despite a relatively short half-life of 2 hours. Diclofenac is metabolized to glucuronide and sulfate conjugates, and elimination is via the urinary and biliary tracts.[118]

The side effect profile of diclofenac is similar to that of most other nonaspirin NSAIDs. Approximately 5% of patients treated with diclofenac experience an elevation of liver enzymes. It is recommended that liver function be monitored regularly throughout the course of diclofenac therapy, following the ALT in particular, presumably the most sensitive indicator of liver function.[118] Colonic ulceration and bleeding were attributed to diclofenac use in a 67-year-old woman with RA,[119] and abscess formation occurred with one patient in whom the agent was administered intramuscularly during a surgical procedure for control of postoperative pain.[120] GI and renal toxicities are similar to those of other NSAIDs such as ibuprofen, naproxen, and ketoprofen.[118]

Drug interactions are rare with diclofenac. A potentially serious interaction can occur with lithium, which undergoes a decrease in renal clearance and an increase in plasma concentration during concomitant therapy. Serum levels of MTX and digoxin are both elevated when diclofenac is added to the patient's drug regimen, and concomitant use of diclofenac and cyclosporin can increase the nephrotoxicity of the latter.[118]

Diclofenac is useful in the treatment of RA, OA, and AS, and it appears superior to aspirin for the treatment of musculoskeletal injuries.[121] The drug is available in 25-, 50-, and 75-mg enteric-coated tablets and is administered at 150 to 200 mg daily in two or three divided doses for RA and 100 to 150 mg divided two to three times daily for OA. In AS, the drug is given at a dose of 25 mg four times daily, with an additional 25-mg dose at bedtime if needed. For musculoskeletal pain, 75 mg twice daily may be adequate. The drug can be considered as a first-line NSAID for the treatment of those arthritic disorders listed, with only a minor change in dosage needed for elderly patients and patients with mild to moderate renal or hepatic dysfunction.[118] Manipulation of therapeutic regimens is easily performed because the drug is available in several doses.

Anthranilic Acids

The fenamates, meclofenamate sodium and mefenamic acid, are the two currently available representatives of this class of NSAIDs. Because mefenamic acid is an analgesic more useful for the treatment of dysmenorrhea, it is not discussed here.

Meclofenamate sodium is a third-generation fenamate that not only suppresses cyclooxygenase activity but also may inhibit phospholipase A_2 and prostaglandin activity at its binding site. It is rapidly absorbed and highly protein bound. The drug is metabolized; two thirds are excreted in the urine and one third with the feces. Enterohepatic circulation of the drug probably occurs. One of meclofenamate's metabolites, hydroxymethyl meclofenamic acid, possesses antiinflammatory activity.[2]

Like most NSAIDs, meclofenamate can produce GI disturbances. Diarrhea is the side effect most commonly noted. Hemolytic anemia may develop, making regular laboratory monitoring important.[2]

Meclofenamate sodium is useful in the treatment of RA, OA, and AS. In high doses, it is approximately as effective as 150 mg of indomethacin when used for gout. A common dose is 50 or 100 mg given three or four times daily.

Oxicams

As of this writing, piroxicam is the only available agent in this class of NSAIDs. Tenoxicam, a promising new NSAID of the oxicam class, has yet to be released on the U.S. drug market.

Piroxicam. This is easily absorbed after oral administration of a 20-mg dose, with maximum plasma concentration occurring 2 hours later. A second peak is measured 6 to 10 hours after ingestion, suggesting enterohepatic circulation.[122] On absorption, piroxicam is highly metabolized, and about 99% of the drug becomes bound to plasma proteins. The drug's extended plasma half-life of 38 hours allows plasma concentrations to remain stable for 24 to 48 hours, thus permitting once-daily dosing.[123] Steady-state plasma concentration of piroxicam usually occurs within 7 to 12 days of regular daily 20-mg dosing.[124]

Piroxicam is metabolized by hydroxylation; a portion of the hydroxylated product is then conjugated with glucuronic acid. These major metabolites are largely inactive and account for 60% of the daily dose excreted with the urine and feces.[123] There is no increase in plasma levels of the drug in patients with renal failure, nor is there a significantly increased level in elderly patients. This suggests that in elderly patients and those with mild to moderate renal compromise, no dosage adjustment is necessary.[124, 125] As with virtually all NSAIDs, piroxicam can cause a transient elevation of ALT, AST, and BUN levels. The BUN level appears to rise abruptly on initiation of piroxicam therapy, leveling at or just beyond the upper normal limit. Levels promptly return to normal range when the drug is discontinued, regardless of treatment duration.[123] Neither the drug's administered dose nor serum levels correlate well with toxicity or efficacy in any patient group.[123]

During one study,[126] one third of those patients observed were receiving piroxicam concurrently with diuretic therapy. No change in renal function was observed in these patients. Adverse GI effects and discontinuances owing to GI problems were found to be less common with piroxicam than with most other NSAIDs. There appears to be little increase in these problems with age.[127–129] Plasma concentration probably increases with severe liver disorders such as cirrhosis but not with mild liver disease.[122]

Few drug interactions occur with piroxicam, but it may potentiate the anticoagulant effects of warfarin sodium.[122]

Piroxicam is useful in the treatment of RA and AS and is equivalent to naproxen in efficacy and low toxicity when used long term for OA.[130] Compared with sodium salicylate, piroxicam, tiaprofenic acid, and prednisolone sodium phosphate do not appear to exert harmful effects on articular cartilage.[111] Piroxicam is effective in the management of pain from sprains and other musculoskeletal injuries. The convenience of one 20-mg capsule taken daily may be beneficial in the management of arthritic disorders because failures with other agents may be due not to lack of efficacy but rather to lack of compliance.[131] Its long half-life ensures adequate therapeutic levels even if one day's dose is missed. Piroxicam is supplied as 10- or 20-mg capsules, and either is given as a single daily dose.

Some clinicians may be reluctant to administer a drug with a long half-life such as piroxicam to compromised patients or to those who have had previous NSAID side effects. It is thought that if adverse effects occur, the drug could continue to promote such effects for a period after the last dose was taken. In such instances, a drug with a shorter half-life, such as ibuprofen, may be an adequate substitute. Some patients seem to perceive a drug that is given only once daily to be inadequate for relief of their discomfort, particularly when breakthrough pain occurs before steady-state levels of the drug are achieved. In this instance, one may consider giving the patient 10 mg of piroxicam twice daily. Anecdotal evidence shows the drug to be useful in some patients with OA and musculoskeletal pain when 10 or 20 mg is administered as infrequently as once every other day.

Tenoxicam. Tenoxicam is an antiinflammatory agent that shares many pharmacokinetic and metabolic characteristics with piroxicam. The elimination half-life of tenoxicam is 60 to 80 hours, allowing once-daily administration. Its bioavailability is 99%, and the drug is highly bound to plasma proteins after absorption. Clearance of tenoxicam is mainly through oxidative metabolism; less than 1% is excreted unchanged in the urine.[132]

Tenoxicam displays good efficacy and tolerability when the drug is used to treat inflammation associated with rheumatic diseases. It is administered at doses of 20 mg/day. At this writing, tenoxicam remains unavailable on the U.S. drug market.

Lornoxicam. This new oxicam derivative (known also as *chlortenoxicam*) is a powerful inhibitor of cyclooxygenase activity. The drug does not appear to inhibit 5-lipoxygenase activity, nor does it appear to shunt arachidonic acid through this pathway. The potent antiinflammatory and analgesic effects of lornoxicam are supplemented by its ability to suppress bone and joint destruction, as represented by the adjuvant polyarthritic rat model. In such studies, lornoxicam was shown to inhibit PMN migration, inhibit release of superoxide ions from PMNs, inhibit the release of platelet-derived growth factor from platelets, and stimulate the synthesis of cartilage proteoglycans in tissue culture.[133]

Pharmacokinetic studies of lornoxicam show an oral solution of the drug to be rapidly and almost completely absorbed. It becomes highly protein bound and displays a terminal half-life of about 4 to 5 hours. Metabolites of the drug are excreted with the urine and feces, and liver toxicity is low.[134] The elimination half-life of lornoxicam does not appear to increase with age.[135]

There is no evidence of kinetic interaction when lornoxicam is taken with antacids. Lornoxicam has been shown to reduce the clearance and to enhance the hypoprothrombinemic effect of warfarin, similar to other NSAIDs. It leads to an increase in insulin concentrations when administered with the hypoglycemic agent glibenclamide, causing a significant drop in plasma glucose levels. A modest reduction in digoxin clearance occurs when lornoxicam is administered with this drug. Lornoxicam significantly antagonizes the diuretic effect of furosemide.[136]

Lornoxicam has been studied at total daily doses of 4 to 16 mg divided through the day. It is well tolerated, but, as with most other NSAIDs, its primary adverse effects occur in the stomach.[137] GI bleeding was observed less frequently with lornoxicam compared with indomethacin but more frequently compared with placebo. The drug does not appear to alter hemostasis significantly, which may prove useful when other, more hemostatically toxic NSAIDs are contraindicated. Renal toxicity appears to be mild.[138]

As of this writing, lornoxicam is not available on the U.S. drug market.

Naphthylalkanones

The naphthylalkanones represent a novel series of nonacidic antiinflammatory agents potentially useful for the treatment of joint inflammation associated with the arthritides. Nabumetone has undergone extensive testing and shows promise as a favorable alternative to currently available NSAIDs.

The nonacidic prodrug nabumetone is a weak inhibitor of cyclooxygenase. The drug undergoes first-pass metabolism in the liver, where it is converted to 6-methoxy-2-naphthylacetic acid (6-MNA), a potent inhibitor of prostaglandin synthesis. The parent drug is easily absorbed after oral administration and rapidly metabolized to 6-MNA. About 99% of the active metabolite then binds to plasma proteins. Peak levels of 6-MNA occur 3 to 6 hours after ingestion, with a metabolite plasma half-life of 24 hours. Steady-state levels are achieved after 3 to 4 days of daily 1-g doses, with clinically significant levels of 6-MNA detectable in synovial tissues under steady-state conditions.[139–142]

The active molecule 6-MNA is further metabolized through conjugation, *O*-desmethylation, and other pathways. About 80% of the administered nabumetone is excreted as metabolites in the urine and 10% in the feces. Food and milk tend to increase the rate of parent drug absorption but not the extent of drug bioavailability. Antacids have no effect on the coadministered drug.[139, 140]

Studies have shown that nabumetone possesses a remarkably benign GI side effect profile.[143–146] Endoscopic studies in humans show that, at usual therapeutic doses, the drug produces no more GI toxicity than placebo and significantly less toxicity than aspirin and some other NSAIDs, but GI ulceration has been reported. The drug is a weak inhibitor of platelet function compared with other NSAIDs.[139] Nabumetone may provide a margin of safety when used in patients with mild to moderate renal compromise, and dose reduction for these patients is probably not necessary.[139, 147] The bioavailability of nabumetone tends to be reduced in patients with hepatic disease.[139] The rate of elimination of drug metabolites is reduced in the elderly, resulting in a prolonged half-life in this group. It is generally advised that the usual dose of 1 g once daily not be exceeded in the elderly; however, lower dosing may be preferable to avoid possible side effects in the older patient.[139, 148]

Nabumetone offers an acceptable alternative to the other NSAIDs for treatment of IJDs. The drug was found to be comparable to aspirin, indomethacin, naproxen, and sulindac when used to treat such disorders, and it was better tolerated than all except sulindac. In general, nabumetone, administered at a dose of 1000 mg at bedtime, is an effective, well-tolerated agent for use against the inflammation of RA and OA.[139, 149–152] It is also effective against the pain of skin and soft tissue injury when given as a 2000-mg loading dose followed by 1000 mg twice daily.[153]

Indole Carboxamides

Tenidap sodium is an investigative antiinflammatory agent with proported activity against both cyclooxygenase and lipoxygenase.[154, 155] The agent appears to inhibit superoxide production and may help prevent the degradation of tissue collagen—a hallmark of chronic inflammatory disorders—by inhibiting the release of activated neutrophil collagenase.[154]

At this writing, tenidap sodium remains unavailable on the U.S. drug market. It appears to be a unique agent with prompt clinical effect and good tolerance. The agent is administered at a dose of 40 to 120 mg daily.[155]

Final Considerations

The salicylates and nonsalicylate NSAIDs are an important group of pharmacologic agents useful in the management of IJDs. With some exceptions, one drug's usefulness compared with another may be difficult to discern. Ultimately, the drug's cost becomes the deciding factor for use. Table 24–4 compares the formulations, dosages, and costs for most NSAIDs, DMARDs, and other antiarthritic agents available on the U.S. drug market.

The patient will conceivably take these medications for years, so cost becomes an important factor in developing a daily management program. Other factors include drug toxicities, dosing regimens, pre-existing nonrheumatic disease, and other concurrently administered drugs. Effective therapeutic plasma levels of many of these drugs are achieved only after several days on consistent administration. A period of 2 to 4 weeks of uninterrupted therapy may be required before satisfactory clinical results are obtained with any particular agent.

Disease-Modifying Antirheumatic Drugs

NSAIDs are not noted for their ability to alter the disease processes of rheumatic joint disorders. In contrast, disease-modifying agents, as their class designation implies, may provoke a change in disease activity as realized by radiographic improvement in joint architecture. Such claims, however, have not been fully substantiated.

As a group, DMARDs are used primarily for the treatment of RA and are usually reserved for those patients who are found to be refractory to more conservative treatment modalities, such as rest, physical therapy, and NSAIDs, and for patients who have experienced unacceptable toxic or allergic reactions to the NSAIDs. Treatment with the DMARDs usually begins with the less toxic antimalarials or gold compounds and progresses to the more toxic agents.

There has been a general trend toward early use of DMARDs in the course of therapy for arthritic disorders.

This approach is used in the hope of preventing the disease process from irreversibly destroying joint structures. By acting as agents that may alter the pernicious course of RA, DMARDs could possibly help prevent the loss of joint architecture and function or at least delay such loss. Ultimately, these goals may be best achieved by combining modalities such DMARDs, NSAIDs, and physical therapy. Such a multileveled approach would serve to accentuate the beneficial effects and reduce the detrimental effects of each modality.

Antimalarials

The antimalarials have been used for the treatment of IJD since 1951. Their popularity waned when toxic ocular side effects were discovered. Interest has resumed with the observation that these problems are greatly minimized when the drug is administered at reduced doses. Hydroxychloroquine sulfate (HCS) is currently the only antimalarial agent approved by the FDA for use in the management of RA.[2]

HCS is rapidly and completely absorbed when given by mouth and is excreted mostly in the feces and partly in the urine. Acidification of the urine enhances the drug's renal clearance. The drug can be detected in the urine for months after it has been discontinued.[156]

On absorption, the antimalarials become more concentrated in the tissues than in the plasma. They have a predilection for melanin-containing tissues; the most dramatic accumulation occurs in the pigmented retinal structures, perhaps explaining their major ocular toxicity. Chloroquine, another antimalarial agent, has been abandoned in the treatment of RA because of a reputedly higher ocular toxicity.[156]

Ocular toxicity of the antimalarials was first noted when these agents were given at the high dose used for the treatment of parasitic infections. Lowering the doses dramatically reduced the production of retinal lesions. Although there is a direct correlation between serum concentration and side effects, serum levels are not predictive of treatment efficacy.[156]

Like chloroquine, HCS probably interacts with nucleoproteins and double-stranded deoxyribonucleic acid (DNA), inhibiting DNA polymerase. It can stabilize lysosomal membranes and trap free radicals.[156] The lysosomal accumulation may inhibit digestive efficiency of phagolysosomes. Antimalarials have been shown to impair white blood cell chemotaxis and to suppress prostaglandin synthesis. Chloroquine interferes with the generation of immunoglobulin-releasing cells by inhibiting IL-1 from monocytes.[2]

In an effort to develop parameters predictive of response to therapy, investigators evaluated erythrocyte sedimentation rate, proximal interphalangeal joint circumference, number of active joints, duration of morning stiffness, and pretreatment grip strength. HCS was associated with a 63% improvement in several disease parameters, particularly grip strength. Active joint count, erythrocyte sedimentation rate, and hemoglobin levels were found to improve only in those patients showing symptomatic improvement.[157] Controlled studies of 1- to 2-years' duration showed a decline in both rheumatoid factor (RF) and radiologic progression of the disease. Other studies demonstrated no radiologic sparing.[156]

Of the parameters studied, only grip strength showed a statistical difference between those patients responding and those not responding to antimalarial therapy. The importance of this finding is unclear because many factors influence grip strength. What this may suggest is that early disease is more responsive to antimalarial therapy, an observation shared with other disease-modifying agents.[157]

Antimalarial agents may be used as adjunctive therapy along with other disease-modifying agents or in combination with the NSAIDs. Most commonly, HCS is used with the oral gold compound auranofin. Its use with D-penicillamine is questionable.[158]

HCS is usually administered at a dose of 200 mg twice daily or less than 6.5 mg/kg/day. After therapy has been initiated, there is a lag of 6 to 12 weeks before any improvement in clinical parameters can be appreciated.[153, 159] Adverse GI side effects can develop in patients using the drug, with symptoms similar to those in irritable bowel syndrome. Severe diarrhea necessitates discontinuing HCS in about 3% of patients so affected. HCS at therapeutic doses can also produce an irreversible gray discoloration of the skin. A reversible proximal myopathy occurs in 0.1% of patients treated with the drug. Retinal toxicity, the most feared HCS side effect, can possibly be detected on routine ophthalmologic examination. Some authors recommend an initial ophthalmologic evaluation on implementation of therapy, with repeat examinations about every 6 months thereafter.[156, 157, 159] Overall, the incidence and severity of toxic side effects are significantly less with HCS than with the other DMARDs.

Gold Compounds

Gold compounds can be considered the cornerstone of disease-remitting therapy for IJDs. Gold has been used for the management of RA since the 1920s with well-established clinical efficacy. The precise site of action of the gold compounds has not been clearly elucidated; however, multiple targets may be involved.[156, 160]

In vitro studies have shown that gold may interfere with the activity of phagocytes and that it stabilizes lysosomal membranes, inhibits prostaglandin synthesis, and alters humoral and cell-mediated responses to inflammatory stimuli.[161]

Three gold-based compounds are available in the United States as of this writing. These include two injectable compounds, gold sodium thiomalate (GST) and aurothioglucose (ATG), as well as the orally administered auranofin. Both GST and ATG are water soluble, whereas auranofin is primarily lipid soluble. GST is supplied as an aqueous solution and ATG as an oil-based suspension.[160]

The parenterally administered compounds display approximately 95% bioavailability, whereas the orally administered auranofin is only 15% to 25% bioavailable. It can take five to eight doses of weekly administration of injectable gold to reach stable serum concentrations of 3 to 5 mg/l, with concentrations varying greatly from patient to patient and probably from dose to dose for the same patient. Although auranofin produces lower serum concentrations, the levels remain stable at 0.5 to 0.7 mg/l with regular daily dosing.[160]

After administration, intramuscular gold compounds are highly bound to albumin and less well bound to serum globulins. Oral gold seems to be bound less to albumin and more to globulins. All forms of gold bind to the circulating elements of blood[160] and demonstrate wide tissue dispersal. Inflamed synovial membrane may initially show selective uptake of administered gold, after which it is distributed to other organs and tissues. The compounds sequester in areas of chronic inflammation and in tissues rich in reticuloendothelial cells.[156, 160]

More than 70% of parenterally administered gold is slowly excreted in the urine, and the remaining fraction is eliminated erratically in the stool. Eighty percent of orally administered gold is eliminated enterally.[160] The modes of elimination may explain the greater renal toxicity of the injectable gold compounds versus the GI toxicity associated with auranofin.

The action of gold on the cellular elements of the inflammatory response may be crucial to the effectiveness of these drugs. Data suggest that these agents have the capacity to inhibit the differentiation of monocytes into active macrophages and macrophage-like cells. Thus, gold causes a decrease in the synthesis and secretion of C2 complement associated with this cellular transition.[162, 163] On those macrophages that are already present at the site of inflammation or whose differentiation has not been inhibited, GST may significantly inhibit their secretion of collagenase, as demonstrated with cultured macrophages. Gold compounds, then, may be acting on the effector limb of the inflammatory response in erosive joint diseases.[160]

The effect of RF on the pathogenesis of RA is well known. Gold salts have been shown to cause a significant decrease in serum and synovial IgG, IgA, and IgM RFs, suggesting a selective and differential effect of gold salts on RF production.[163, 164]

By convention, the injectable gold compounds are administered at a dose of 10 mg intramuscularly for the first dose; the patient is then monitored during the ensuing week for signs of an idiosyncratic reaction. If the dose is tolerated, 25 mg is administered the second week, 25 to 50 mg the third week, and 50 mg each week thereafter. Doses higher than 50 mg/week do not appear to extend the therapeutic benefits of the drug but may be associated with greater toxicity. In fact, one study demonstrated that weekly doses of 25 mg or less produce the desired effects for responding patients.[165] Therapy continues weekly until toxicity intervenes or until a total of 1 g has been given.[161, 166]

As measured by the effect on several disease parameters, serum and whole blood gold levels do not correlate well with clinical outcome. Also, toxic reactions necessitating removal from therapy cannot be predicted by measuring blood levels. Thus, monitoring serum concentrations of gold during therapy appears unwarranted.[156, 167]

Auranofin, administered at a dose of 3 mg twice daily or as a single 6-mg dose, likewise shows no correlation between serum levels and efficacy or toxicity. Auranofin appears similar to injectable gold in efficacy but is less toxic than either injectable gold or D-penicillamine.[168, 169] This agent may be especially useful alone or in combination with NSAIDs or HCS. Such combination therapy could be used early in the management of RA in an effort not only to achieve prompt suppression of inflammation and pain but also to induce a disease remission before joint destruction can occur.[168, 170]

Toxic side effects of gold therapy can include mucocutaneous and renal disorders, bone marrow suppression, and thrombocytopenia. Neither serum levels nor duration of therapy correlates well with the development of toxicity. Data strongly suggest that patients who show improvement within 6 months may continue chrysotherapy for as long as 3 years with an increasing margin of safety against mucocutaneous and renal toxicity.[171]

In one study, the overall withdrawal from chrysotherapy owing to toxic reactions was found to be about 42%.[171] Of those patients experiencing toxic episodes, rash was the most common, followed by mouth ulcers and proteinuria. The average time of onset for these reactions was 10 months. The mucocutaneous reactions can be surmounted by stopping intramuscular therapy and then reinitiating the therapy at low doses of 5 to 10 mg per week, gradually increasing to tolerance. Proteinuria in excess of 1000 mg every 24 hours requires cessation of chrysotherapy. Proteinuria may continue for many months after the last injection.[156]

Bone marrow suppression is the most serious form of toxicity associated with chrysotherapy. Bone marrow aplasia presenting as pancytopenia has a high fatality rate.[156] Evidence suggests that ATG persists in bone marrow macrophages well after withdrawal from therapy. Aplastic anemia was observed in one such patient, implicating a causative role for gold.[172]

Immunologically mediated, gold-induced thrombocytopenia can occur and may possibly be related to the major histocompatibility complexes (MHCs). In one study, gold-induced thrombocytopenia was found to be associated with the human lymphocyte antigen (HLA)-DR3 alloantigen, a factor that may also correlate with gold-induced nephropathy.[173, 174] The possibility that there is a prognostic value in this alloantigen is speculative. Seventy-nine percent of patients exhibiting toxic reactions were not DR3 positive, and 67% of those with proteinuria lacked the DR3 phenotype.[173] There was a significant positive association with the HLA-Bw35 phenotype and the development of mucocutaneous lesions and a slightly negative correlation in patients carrying the HLA-B27 antigen.[175]

Other toxic side effects observed include bronchiolitis with auranofin[176] and hepatotoxicity associated with the use of AGT.[177] The hepatitis that was observed is self-limiting if gold is discontinued. Liver function tests return to normal usually within 3 months of stopping therapy. Although infrequent, hepatitis should be suspected in any patient experiencing jaundice while on chrysotherapy.

A transient increase in rheumatoid symptoms has been observed after the administration of gold injections. One study described recurring postinjection reactions consisting of transient stiffness, arthralgias, myalgias, and constitutional symptoms, occurring in 15 of 100 patients examined.[178] These reactions were predominantly associated with GST, but similar reactions have been reported with ATG. Still, those experiencing such symptoms with aqueous GST showed a gradual, decremental reduction of reaction severity when switched to the oil-based ATG. It has been suggested that the vehicle for gold compounds may be responsible for some of the side effects linked with parenteral gold therapy, because increased gold toxicity occurs with the aqueous gold preparations.[178]

Drug toxicity and unpredictable response are the two obvious drawbacks to gold therapy. An attempt was made to identify disease parameters that could be associated with a favorable or poor response.[179] Factors found to be unrelated to outcome included patient age at onset of RA treatment, duration of disease, sex, severity of RA, presence of RF, serum globulin levels, antinuclear antibodies, radiographically detectable lesions, and serum gold levels. A composite of six factors related to poor prognosis included a positive RF, two or more swollen upper extremity joints, Raynaud's phenomenon, malaise or weakness at the onset of arthritis, white race, and female gender. The best predictors for a good outcome after 1 years of chrysotherapy were the presence of

HLA-A3 with an absence of HLA-DR4 alloantigens.[179] An improved prognostic edge existed when baseline hemoglobin levels are normal. Further study is needed before the usefulness of such prognostic indicators of response is determined.

Although chrysotherapy has proven efficacy in the treatment of IJD, it is not without the potential for serious toxicity. Still, when administered carefully, such therapy can be relatively safe. Cautious patient selection and judicious monitoring of important systemic functional parameters are essential. Before the initiation of therapy and with each subsequent dose, the patient should have a CBC with differential and a urinalysis performed. Serum electrolytes and liver function tests must also be considered. The patient should be examined for oral and cutaneous lesions, which are not uncommon during chrysotherapy.

D-Penicillamine

D-Penicillamine is a potent antiarthritic agent that chemically resembles the amino acid cysteine. The D-isomer of this compound is used because the L-isomer was found to be too toxic.[156] The drug is rapidly absorbed after oral administration, binds to albumin, and appears to be cleared from the circulation at a rate equal to the clearance of creatinine.[2, 156] Intestinal absorption is significantly decreased when iron preparations, such as those found in dietary vitamin and mineral supplements, are used concurrently. Food also interferes with intestinal absorption of D-penicillamine. Absorption was found to be most effective when the drug was administered several hours before breakfast and much less effective when taken 2 hours after dinner, as is widely practiced.[180]

The occurrence of side effects with D-penicillamine appears to be related to the rapidity with which the dosage is increased. The "go-low, go-slow" dosing regimen has great merit when applied to its use. Using this method, the incidence of toxicity is reduced and therapeutic efficacy is maintained.[156, 181]

D-Penicillamine is quite useful in the management of RA and may be used successfully in patients who have had adverse reactions to gold therapy or in patients who derived no benefit from chrysotherapy.[181] One study demonstrated a 65% improvement in rheumatoid symptoms compared with a 27% improvement noted with placebo.[182] Improvement was assessed by rating favorable physician evaluation of improvement, decline in the rheumatoid activity index, improvement in functional class, decrease in RF, and possible inhibition of erosive change, as noted on radiograph.

The same study demonstrated side effects occurring in 49% of patients treated with D-penicillamine compared with 34% in control groups. Skin eruptions and pruritus were most frequently encountered, but they usually reversed with withdrawal or reduction of therapy. Proteinuria is the most serious complication that can occur. Despite normal renal function, proteinuria may persist for months after therapy has ended.[156, 182] Nephrotic syndrome can occur after 1 year of therapy. Leukopenia and elevation of AST can be avoided with low-dose therapy. Dysgeusia occurs but is usually tolerable and reversible within 1 or 2 months despite continued therapy.[157]

Careful attention to laboratory parameters must be maintained throughout the course of D-penicillamine therapy. Thrombocytopenia can develop, and therapy must be discontinued when the platelet count falls below 100,000/mm³. Therapy can be reinstituted at a lowered dose when the platelet count again rises to 150,000/mm³.[157] Persistently low platelet levels require complete cessation of therapy.[156]

There has been a report of reversible myasthenia gravis developing in a patient receiving alternate therapy with D-penicillamine and chloroquine.[183]

Therapy with D-penicillamine is generally started with a single daily dose of 125 to 250 mg, increasing at 1- to 2-month intervals by the same amount. After 2 to 3 months of treatment at 500 to 750 mg/day, the drug can be increased by 250 mg every 2 to 3 months if no improvement is noticed or until toxicity occurs. If therapy fails after 3 to 4 months at a dose of 1000 to 1500 mg of D-penicillamine daily, the therapy should be discontinued.

Cytotoxic Agents

Cytotoxic and immunosuppressive agents have been used for the treatment of RA since the late 1960s. The main impetus for their use was failure of other available drugs to stop the progression of the disease. These agents are nonspecific, and their potential for systemic toxicity is quite high.[159, 161] Although the cytotoxic agents are generally withheld until all other therapeutic modalities have failed to provide adequate results, some practitioners are now calling the cytotoxic agents into action earlier in the course of the disease, hoping to forestall or prevent irreversible joint destruction.

Methotrexate

MTX is an antimetabolite that binds competitively to the enzyme dihydrofolate reductase, causing an inhibition of the S or DNA synthesis phase of the cell cycle. This effect is most meaningful in diseases characterized by cell proliferation. The drug has been widely used in cancer chemotherapy for diverse conditions such as acute lymphocytic leukemia, non-Hodgkin's lymphoma, osteosarcoma, and breast cancer.[184] It has also become useful in the treatment of psoriasis,[185] and has been found to be beneficial in the treatment of RA intractable to NSAIDs and disease-modifying agents.[186]

The mechanism by which MTX suppresses rheumatic disease activity continues to be debated. The drug has both chemotherapeutic and immunosuppressive effects, but no clear evidence for immunosuppression in RA has been found. MTX produces improvement in disease parameters earlier than most DMARDs and immunosuppressive agents, and termination is usually followed by disease rebound. These observations suggest that the drug may work at least partly as an antiinflammatory agent. Indeed, it has been demonstrated that MTX inhibits IL-1 activity without affecting its production or secretion. A rapid decrease in both erythrocyte sedimentation rate and C-reactive protein levels occurs after a single injection of MTX, supporting the theory of IL-1 inhibition.[187]

MTX may affect lymphocyte function as evidenced by the drug's ability to cause marked decreases in IgM-RF within a day of administration of the first dose. Although low serum concentrations of MTX can inhibit the generation of T suppressor cells and thus stimulate antibody production, higher concentrations directly inhibit B cell proliferation and antibody synthesis independently of T cell activity.[188]

After oral administration of a low dose (5 to 15 mg) of MTX, the drug is rapidly and completely absorbed. Peak plasma concentrations are achieved in 1 to 2 hours, with an elimination half-life of about 8 to 20 hours. The latter value reflects the agent's tissue distribution, renal clearance, and enterohepatic circulation.[184, 189] About 80% to 90% of the dose is excreted unchanged in the urine within 24 hours. More than half of the absorbed dose is bound to serum proteins, particularly albumin. The drug becomes intracellular by simple diffusion and active carrier transport.[184]

Normal glomerular filtration is needed for safe elimination of MTX. Agents with potential renal toxicity such as aminoglycoside antibiotics may increase serum MTX levels. Aspirin, NSAIDs, D-penicillamine, and the sulfonamides compete for tubular excretion, raising MTX plasma concentrations. At low doses of MTX, however, the interaction may be insignificant. The antigout drug probenecid can totally block the renal excretion of MTX, making concomitant therapy rather dangerous.[184]

MTX is quite successful in producing salutary effects against the symptoms and joint destruction associated with RA. The drug is consistently efficacious and well tolerated, with the probability that nearly 50% of patients will still be responding favorably after 6 years of therapy. A large portion of patients, however, become refractory to the drug's effects after 18 to 24 months of therapy.[189] Toxic effects, rather than lack of response, is the main limiting factor for continuing MTX therapy, in contrast with other DMARDs.[186]

Major toxicity is rare at low single doses of MTX. There have been reports of acute, life-threatening pulmonary events occurring when weekly doses have exceeded 20 mg, but pulmonary disease has been noted even with doses of less than 15 mg. Grade III hepatic fibrosis and cirrhosis have been observed in 20% of patients being treated with MTX for long-term psoriasis. In psoriatic patients, however, weekly doses of MTX were much higher than those typically used for RA.[184, 190]

Elevation of liver enzyme levels is the most common adverse event occurring with MTX use. Minor hepatic structural abnormalities are sometimes found in RA patients without the use of MTX. The cause of these abnormalities is probably multifactorial, with previous NSAID, DMARD, and prednisone therapy all taking their toll. Certain changes may be associated with the arthritic disease process itself. Regardless, MTX therapy in RA patients results in worsening of hepatic histologic grade with the development of mild fibrosis. The fibrotic changes appear to correlate well with dose and duration of MTX therapy. These changes may not be of clinical significance,[191] and downward adjustment in MTX dosage may alleviate some of the mild hepatic disturbances.

Increased age is associated with the development of cirrhosis in psoriatic patients. Obesity appears to place the patient at risk for both cirrhosis and hepatic fibrosis. Elevations of AST levels may correlate with worsening of hepatic histologic grade and should be monitored during the course of MTX therapy. Routine pretreatment liver biopsy is probably not warranted unless there is a history of severe liver disease or significant alcohol intake.[191] Biopsy should be considered when a total dose of 1.5 g has been given.[189]

CNS toxicity may develop in patients on low-dose MTX therapy. One study reports subjective neurologic complaints occurring in 5 of 25 patients studied.[192] Most patients experiencing such unpleasant effects were older and had a higher baseline serum creatinine concentration than those without symptoms. It is speculated that impaired renal function may have led to MTX accumulation to toxic levels.

Hematologic toxicity expressed as thrombocytopenia, leukopenia, or pancytopenia occurs rarely during MTX therapy, but the potential for its development warrants routine assessment of hematologic parameters. A CBC with platelet assessment should be performed at least monthly.[184]

Macrocytosis may also be a possible predictor of potential hematologic toxicity resulting from MTX. Severe megaloblastic anemia has been observed during long-term, low-dose MTX therapy, and one study has shown marked macrocytosis to have been present for at least 6 months before the development of this toxic reaction.[193] Patients experiencing an anemic state were more likely to have experienced insufficient diet and a possible folate deficiency before developing the hematologic toxicity. Surveillance of mean corpuscular volume (MCV) is recommended during MTX therapy, and patients should be withdrawn from therapy if the MCV values exceed 106 fl (normal is 80 to 100 fl). Heavy smoking can increase the MCV by at least 3 fl.[194]

Dietary folic acid deficiency or low to normal folic acid status may confer an increased risk for toxicity during MTX therapy. Folic acid supplementation does not appear to compromise MTX efficacy, and adding 1 mg of folate to the daily diet may allow institution of MTX treatment at an earlier stage in the disease process. Such combined therapy may also reduce the toxic effects for those patients already on MTX who have normal pretreatment folate levels. Assaying the C_1 index, a measure of folate-dependent enzyme activity in peripheral blood mononuclear cells, allows the practitioner to monitor the effect of MTX on folic acid metabolism in the RA patient. By measuring the extent of folic acid antagonism, adjustments can be made to the dose of supplementary folate so as to maintain clinical efficacy with reduced toxicity.[195]

One percent to 2% of patients receiving MTX experience herpes zoster infections. The drug is clearly teratogenic and may cause oligospermia in men. MTX has not been shown to be carcinogenic. GI discomfort and skin rash can also develop with its use.[184]

MTX is generally administered at a single, low weekly dose. One study demonstrated that 7.5 mg/week was sufficient to improve symptoms in most patients. Twenty-five milligrams of MTX can be administered per week if given in three divided doses spaced 12 hours apart. However, because toxicity is related to duration of cell exposure to the agent, the single, low-dose schedule is probably safer.[184, 196]

Abrupt withdrawal from MTX after a mean of 40 months of successful therapy was associated with a severe flare of RA symptoms.[191] This suggests that patients can be treated effectively for prolonged periods, but withdrawal from therapy should be gradual.

Low-dose, pulsed MTX therapy has been tested against azathioprine, an immunosuppressive antimetabolite, and has shown similar efficacy. MTX produced a more rapid and complete improvement in disease activity, but overall results were not considered statistically significant.[196] Response to MTX can occur as early as 1 week after initiation of therapy and frequently occurs within the first month. Overall rate of withdrawal from therapy for adverse side effects is between 29% and 32%.[184, 190] Efficacy is reported at 67% to 100% for all patients treated with MTX for RA.[190]

Immunosuppressive Agents

Azathioprine and cyclophosphamide are two immunosuppressive agents that have found use in the treatment of IJDs. Azathioprine is an antimetabolite, and cyclophosphamide is a powerful alkylating agent. The rationale for using such potent agents for the treatment of RA is based on the realization that RA may be an immunologic abnormality.[157] Patients usually begin immunosuppressive therapy when toxic reactions develop with disease-modifying or antimalarial agents or when such therapy fails to produce an adequate response.[197]

Azathioprine. Azathioprine is a structural analogue of adenine and hypoxanthine. On administration, it is well absorbed and quickly converted to 6-mercaptopurine, primarily by the red blood cells. Further metabolism occurs in the liver.[156] The final metabolite, 6-thiouric acid, is excreted in the urine. Xanthine oxidase is responsible for the conversion of 6-mercaptopurine to 6-thiouric acid. It is therefore necessary to reduce the dose of azathioprine if it is to be administered concurrently with the xanthine oxidase inhibitor allopurinol.

Patients who have experienced unsuccessful treatment of RA with gold therapy were found to benefit more from azathioprine therapy than with D-penicillamine, but efficacy was equivalent when tolerance was equal.[198] In clinical trials, azathioprine has been found to be at least as effective as gold, D-penicillamine, MTX, and cyclophosphamide, but because of potentially serious toxicity, azathioprine could not be recommended over gold or the antimalarials for early RA therapy.[198, 199]

GI symptoms are the most common side effects that occur during azathioprine therapy. Nausea occurs with a frequency of 12.4 episodes per 100 patient years of use, and vomiting develops 5.1 times.[197] Severe dose-related hepatotoxicity can occur, which is best monitored with serial alkaline phosphatase measurements, but hepatic fibrosis can develop without laboratory changes.[156] An increase in bilirubin, transaminases, and alkaline phosphatase levels occurs with the use of azathioprine, but these parameters usually revert to normal on cessation of therapy.[200]

Azathioprine is primarily toxic to the bone marrow and can lead to leukopenia, thrombocytopenia, and anemia. Use of the drug has been linked to a risk for neoplasia. Studies of organ transplant patients taking azathioprine demonstrated 300 times increased risk for the development of lymphoproliferative tumors, with a predilection for cerebral localization.[197] There is also a concern for the development of malignancy with the drug's use, but studies do not support such concerns.[156, 197]

A meningitic reaction has been reported with azathioprine use, and restrictive lung disease is a rare complication. In general, the drug has a relatively benign side effect profile when used against RA.[156, 197]

Azathioprine is administered at a dose of 1 to 2 mg/kg/day, increasing to a dose of 2.5 mg/kg/day if tolerated. There appears to be no correlation between laboratory indices and clinical response when the drug is used to treat RA.

When azathioprine therapy is instituted, a CBC, platelet

count, liver function, and renal function tests should be obtained. At least a white blood cell and platelet count, along with liver function tests, should be performed weekly for the first 8 weeks and then every other week thereafter throughout therapy. Renal function should be checked periodically. The drug should be stopped if the white blood cell count falls below 3000/mm³ or other significant abnormalities are uncovered during laboratory monitoring.[200]

Cyclophosphamide. Cyclophosphamide is a cyclic phosphamide mustard metabolized primarily by liver microenzymes to a number of alkylating products, all which are eventually excreted by the kidneys. Alkylating agents such as cyclophosphamide react with nondividing tissue cells but are more toxic to rapidly dividing cells in the S phase of division (i.e., during active DNA synthesis).[2] The agent reacts with DNA by causing intrastrand and interstrand cross-links, inhibiting cell proliferation and the production of antibody.[157, 201]

Cyclophosphamide appears to be superior to both azathioprine and gold for the treatment of RA, but it possesses much greater toxicity than either of these agents. Antiarthritic medications that are this potent are probably useful only in severe RA unresponsive to less toxic treatments. Dosages range from a low of 1.1 mg/kg/day with concurrently administered low-dose prednisone to a high of 1.7 mg/kg/day alone. The former dosing regimen appears to be about as effective but safer than the latter.[157, 201] The drug can be given orally or intravenously, but its dosage must be reduced with renal disease. Its serum half-life is about 5 hours.[201]

Bone marrow depression and predisposition to infection are two major toxicities attributable to cyclophosphamide. A dose-related leukopenia can occur that persists for months after withdrawal from therapy. The metabolites of cyclophosphamide are toxic to the transitional epithelium of the bladder, and cystitis with dysuria and hematuria can occur. In about 50% of those patients in whom cystitis develops, the disorder is asymptomatic. There is also an increased risk for malignancy, which can be reduced by the intake of large volumes of fluid and frequent voiding.[157, 201] Testicular and ovarian functions are affected, with the development of azoospermia in men and amenorrhea in most women within the first year of therapy.[201]

Cyclosporin A. Cyclosporin A is a potent immunosuppressive agent used to inhibit the rejection of allogenic organ transplants. The drug has been investigated for its use in the treatment of RA and may be of benefit in some situations.

On ingestion, cyclosporin A is incompletely absorbed from the GI tract. It is extensively metabolized and eliminated primarily in the bile. Most of the absorbed drug binds to plasma lipoproteins.[202]

Cyclosporin A selectively modulates subpopulations of immunocompetent cells. The immunosuppression is more specific than that of either corticosteroids or alkylating agents. Granulocyte and macrophage migration, phagocytosis, and killing arc unaffected by the drug, and bone marrow production of white blood cells is not suppressed.[203] Cyclosporin A appears to inhibit the capacity for T cells to synthesize and release IL-2. This suppressive action is reversible, suggesting that cyclosporin A is not a lymphotoxic agent.[204]

Trial studies in RA patients using 5 to 6 mg/kg/day did not show remission of the disease but did show a marked improvement in symptoms. No changes in erythrocyte sedimentation rate, RF, or immune complex levels were observed. Major toxicities were noted to include renal dysfunction with significant elevation of BUN and creatinine measures. These effects reversed with withdrawal of the drug. Hypertension related to cyclosporin A responded well to medical therapy.[193]

Other adverse reactions to cyclosporin A include GI intolerance, gingivitis, hypertrichosis, transient paresthesias of the hands and feet, and an erythematous pruritic rash. Thrombocytopenia was also related to the drug's use.[204]

Cyclosporin A appears to be clinically effective in the treatment of refractory RA, but its value is limited because of severe toxicity. The dosage best tolerated appears to be 5 mg/kg/day; higher dosages mainly promote GI intolerance. Patients taking both cyclosporin A and prednisone can generally use a lower dose of prednisone when it is used concurrently with azathioprine.[204]

Cyclosporin A has a tendency to exacerbate hypertension when given to patients who already have this disorder. Thus, use of cyclosporin A in arthritic patients with concurrent hypertension may be contraindicated. The drug was found to be associated with an increased plasma creatinine in patients who were also using cimetidine, suggesting this to be a nephrotoxic drug combination. Because of toxicity, regular laboratory monitoring of renal function is mandatory during cyclosporin A therapy, and a platelet count should be included to detect developing thrombocytopenia.[204]

Other Agents

Corticosteroids. See Chapter 25 for a discussion of the corticosteroids.

Sulfasalazine. Sulfasalazine is beginning to find a place in the management of IJDs. The drug was originally used quite effectively for the short- and long-term treatment of inflammatory bowel disease. It was introduced for the treatment of RA in 1941.[205]

Sulfasalazine is not highly absorbed from the GI tract, and only 2% to 10% of the absorbed drug reaches the systemic circulation. The absorbed drug is highly protein bound and reaches peak serum concentrations in 3 to 5 hours. Metabolism occurs in the liver, producing 5-aminosalicylic acid and sulfapyridine as the major metabolites. The parent drug and its metabolites are eliminated by the kidneys and GI system. The elimination half-life of sulfasalazine is between 5 and 10 hours.[205]

The therapeutic action of sulfasalazine in RA is not entirely clear. The 5-aminosalicyclic acid metabolite is probably not responsible for the suppression of disease, leaving either the parent compound or sulfapyridine as the active agent. Antiinflammatory, antibacterial, and immunomodulatory effects have all been attributed to sulfasalazine, but supporting evidence for any one mode of action is indirect or minimal at best.[206]

Significant improvement in joint tenderness and swelling, morning stiffness, grip strength, and pain were observed when sulfasalazine was compared with placebo for the treatment of RA.[206] Centrally mediated nausea, vomiting, and headaches are the most common side effects, occurring in about 15% of patients using sulfasalazine. The drug can cause reversible azoospermia. Mild neutropenia can also develop, but it is also reversible and is generally mild. Gradual introduction of the enteric-coated preparation reduces the incidence of some adverse effects.[207]

Sulfasalazine therapy may be started at a dose of 500 mg daily with food and increased by 500 mg daily each week until a total daily dose of 2 to 4 g/day divided in three equal doses is reached.[206, 207]

Levamisole. Levamisole is an anthelmintic agent with immunostimulatory properties. The drug can potentiate the immune response by enhancing or inducing T helper, T cytotoxic, and T suppressor cell lymphocyte function.[208]

Levamisole is easily absorbed by the GI tract and metabolized by the liver. The drug is excreted primarily by the kidneys, but some of its metabolites are excreted with the stool.[209]

One controlled study reported significant improvement in grip strength, range of motion, erythrocyte sedimentation rate, C-reactive protein, and reduction of the number of swollen joints with levamisole administered at 100 mg, 4 days per week, for 16 weeks. The drug has been used successfully at doses as high as 150 mg/day for 4 months.[208]

The initial enthusiasm for the use of levamisole in treating RA has been tempered by the frequency of side effects and idiosyncratic reactions. Side effects include alterations of taste, GI disturbances, fatigue, fever, and skin rash. The one side effect that most limits the drug's routine use in RA is granulocytopenia. This reaction occurs with a disproportionatly high frequency in RA patients, especially in those carrying the HLA-B27 alloantigen.[207–209]

Fish Oil Fatty Acid and Olive Oil Diet Supplementation. Two polyunsaturated fatty acids derived from certain fish oils may offer some clinical improvement for patients with RA. Eicosapentaenoic acid (EPA) and docosahexanoic acid (DHA) are classified as omega-3 fatty acids, which competitively inhibit arachidonic acid utilization and the production of prostaglandins and leukotrienes. Ingestion of omega-3 fatty acids leads to the production of TXA_3 and PGI_3, both of which can reduce platelet aggregation.[210] Fish oil supplementation can lead to a decreased production of leukotriene B_4 from the arachidonic acid pathway in favor of leukotriene B_5 derived from EPA as well as a decrease in the production of IL-1.[211]

Leukotriene B_4 is a potent inflammatory and chemotactic compound that has the capacity to modulate immune reactivity. By reducing its production, the lowered levels of leukotriene B_4 should impress a favorable effect on the clinical manifestations of IJDs. IL-1 is an immunomodulating factor that can strongly influence the course of joint inflammation. Its effects on cartilage metabolism and synovial tissue, and the symptoms associated with these effects, may be favorably influenced through the action of dietary fish oil fatty acids. Overall, high doses of fish oil supplement have been reported to reduce the number of swollen joints, decrease duration of morning stiffness, improve grip strength, and improve physician assessment of pain and disease activity in arthritic patients treated for at least 18 to 24 weeks.[211]

Olive oil also appears to offer some relief from the symptoms of joint pain and stiffness when taken regularly in the diet. The monounsaturated fatty acid oleic acid is the component of olive oil most likely to produce the salutary effects.

Olive oil has been observed to induce immune changes and to produce clinical improvement in RA patients consuming the oil in their daily diet. The oil may enhance lymphocyte proliferation but may have less of an effect on leuko-

triene B_4, IL-1, and immunoglobulin G (IgG)-production than does fish oil.[211]

High-dose fish oil supplementation requires the ingestion of the equivalent of 54 mg/kg/day EPA and 36 mg/kg/day DHA, with a caloric load of about 103 kcal. Olive oil is taken at a dose to add about 7 g of oleic acid to the diet while producing a caloric load of 81 kcal. The side effect profile is quite favorable, with ingestion causing only minor GI intolerance and eructation. When taken during aspirin or NSAID therapy, fish oil supplementation was discovered to produce a statistically but not clinically significant increase in bleeding time.[211] One study has shown that omega-3 fatty acid supplementation may produce a decrease in the linoleic, arachidonic acid, and hexosamine content of articular cartilage and may inhibit proteoglycan production in rats.[212] These changes produce cartilage irregularities commonly associated with the development of early OA. Whether such changes are induced in humans remains unknown, but the results do suggest a cautious approach to this seemingly benign therapy when used to enhance the conventional treatment of RA.

Drugs Used in the Treatment of Crystal-Induced Arthropathy

Colchicine. The alkaloid extracts of the autumn crocus, *Colchicum autumnale*, have been known for centuries to alleviate the inflammation of gout. In its pure form, colchicine has been used for this purpose since at least the first half of the nineteenth century.[213]

Colchicine diminishes the inflammation of acute gout through its effect on neutrophils. The drug interacts at a high-affinity binding site with the protein tubulin, a subunit of microtubules. This interaction completely inhibits tubulin polymerization, thereby preventing microtubule assembly and elongation and causing a substantial impairment of leukocytic chemotaxis. Colchicine also alters morphology and pseudopod formation of these cells.[214] As a consequence of preventing the microtubular assembly reaction, release of chemotactic factors, formation of digestive vacuoles, and lysosomal degranulation are reduced. Overall, there is a suppression of migration of PMNs to the site of inflammation and a decrease in metabolic and phagocytic activities of cells already there.[215]

Administered orally, colchicine is almost completely absorbed and reaches peak plasma levels in 30 minutes to 2 hours. It is metabolized and excreted by both the liver and the kidneys and is cleared quickly from the plasma. The drug remains within circulating leukocytes even after plasma clearance and can be detected in granulocytes up to 10 days after a single dose. A scant 10% of the drug is excreted 24 hours after a single intravenous dose.[216]

The major toxic effects of colchicine occur within the GI tract and are manifested by sometimes severe and bloody diarrhea with intestinal cramping. Eighty percent of patients given the full therapeutic dose experience some of these effects. The rapidly proliferating epithelial cells of the intestine, especially those of the jejunum, are most affected by the drug. Because of colchicine's effects on microtubule formation, it presumably disrupts epithelial cell mitosis by preventing aster and spindle cell formation and by inhibiting chromosome distribution and cytokinesis. The drug stimulates adenyl cyclase activity, increases musocal PGE_2 levels, and increases cyclic AMP content, all of which may contribute to the accumulation of intestinal water and diarrhea.[213, 215] Septicemia can develop secondary to intestinal wall damage.[216]

Persistent nausea and weakness secondary to progressive myopathy and neuropathy in patients on chronic therapy suggest acute colchicine intoxication. Electrolyte disturbances may develop by loss through vomiting and diarrhea, and muscle weakness can progress to respiratory failure. Hepatic and muscular necrosis can also occur. Death ensues if therapy is not stopped; however, all manifestations can resolve if the patient survives.[217]

Colchicine overdose can lead to hematologic disorders, of which disseminated intravascular coagulation is the earliest seen. Marrow failure with thrombocytopenia and leukopenia can follow. Agranulocytosis and aplastic anemia have also been observed. Other toxic effects include hepatocellular dysfunction and CNS failure with memory loss, peripheral neuritis, myopathy, alopecia, azoospermia, peripheral neuritis, myopathy, alopecia, burning of the throat and skin, azoospermia, and, rarely, amenorrhea.[213, 218]

In acute podagra, colchicine is administered orally at a dose of 0.6 mg hourly until symptoms cease or the patient experiences nausea, vomiting, or diarrhea or until a total dose of 6 mg has been taken. GI side effects can be decreased by administering the drug intravenously at 2 mg initially, followed by 1 mg every 6 hours until the attack subsides or a total dose of 4 to 5 mg has been delivered. The drug should be diluted with 20 ml of normal saline solution for intravenous administration and should be injected slowly over 10 minutes. Local extravasation of the fluid must be avoided because it can lead to severe local inflammation and necrosis.

Used prophylactically, colchicine can be administered at doses as low as 0.5 mg every other day. Generally, one 0.5-mg tablet is taken once daily for 1 week, followed by one 0.5 mg tablet twice daily thereafter. In recalcitrant cases, the dose can be increased by 0.5 mg every 4 weeks to a total of not more than 2 mg per day in divided doses.[218]

Colchicine dosage by any route should be reduced in the presence of renal or liver dysfunction and in the older patient. The drug should be avoided completely when combined renal and liver disease is present, when there is extrahepatic biliary obstruction, or when creatinine clearance is less than 10 ml/min. Intravenous colchicine is contraindicated in patients with infection or pre-existing depressed bone marrow function. Neither prophylactic oral colchicine nor a second bout of IV therapy should be started within 7 days of completing an initial course of intravenous colchicine because serious toxicity or death can result.[216]

Uricosuric Agents. Uricosuric agents act in part by displacing urate from plasma protein binding sites, thereby increasing the filtered load of free urate. Because only a small portion of free urate is protein bound, this action yields but a small net effect. The predominant action of these agents is to inhibit proximal tubular reabsorption and thus increase renal excretion of uric acid. Several structurally dissimilar drugs have the capacity to induce uricosuria, including probenecid, sulfinpyrazone, high-dose salicylates (more than 3 g per day), several NSAIDs (particularly azapropazone), and other agents. The most commonly used agents are probenecid and sulfinpyrazone.[215, 218, 219]

Uricosuric agents depend on proper renal function to rid the body of excess uric acid effectively. They lose their effectiveness as the GFR drops, and their use is not advised when the GFR falls below 60 ml/min. Uricosurics are not meant for patients who overproduce uric acid or for patients who have the propensity to produce renal stones, because their actions could lead to urolithiasis. They are used most appropriately for normoexcreting or underexcreting patients with tophaceous gout.[218–220]

When uricosuric therapy is started, there is a chance that new attacks of gout will be initiated[219] ostensibly because the mobilized uric acid stimulates a strong immune response. In addition, the hyperuricosuria that develops as a consequence of therapy has the potential for producing pure uric acid stones within the kidneys or uric acid stones containing calcium oxalate.[218, 219] New attacks of gout can be prevented or controlled by combining initial uricosuric therapy with low-dose colchicine or NSAIDs. Renal stone formation can be avoided by instructing the patient to consume large amounts of fluids while undergoing therapy, thus diluting the uric acid and allowing safe excretion. Some patients may require alkalinization of the urine to a pH of 6 to 6.5 to avoid the development of urolithiasis. This can be accomplished by administering acetazolamide, 500 mg, at bedtime.[218] Potassium citrate can also be used to reduce urinary saturation of calcium oxalate by complexing calcium ions. The drug also discourages nucleation and crystal growth while it produces and maintains a urinary pH conducive to uric acid solubility.[219] Sodium bicarbonate, 3 to 7.5 g daily, also adequately maintains urine alkalinity.

Probenecid is readily absorbed from the GI tract and is extensively protein bound. The drug is rapidly metabolized and excreted by the kidney. The well-known effect of blocking excretion of penicillin, thereby increasing plasma levels of the antibiotic, extends to other agents as well, including indomethacin, dapsone, and heparin.[215] Probenecid should thus be used with caution in patients concurrently treated with these agents.

Initially, probenecid can be administered at a low dose of 0.25 g twice daily for a week with adequate hydration. This can be followed by 0.5 g twice daily thereafter. If necessary, the dose can be increased by 0.5 g every 4 weeks to a total dose of 2 g/day divided into two or three doses.

Sulfinpyrazone is completely absorbed from the GI tract and becomes extensively protein bound. Both parent drug and metabolites are excreted by the kidneys. Although it is a derivative of a phenylbutazone metabolite, sulfinpyrazone lacks antiinflammatory properties.

Sulfinpyrazone is administered initially at a dose of 150 to 200 mg twice daily with meals for 3 to 4 days, increasing to a maximum of 800 mg/day or decreased to a low 200 mg/day, given in divided doses.

Neither probenecid nor sulfinpyrazone should be given during an acute attack of gout; however, should an attack occur during their use, either drug may be continued and colchicine or an appropriate NSAID may be added to control the flare. Aspirin should be avoided when either agent is being used because it hinders their uricosuric effect. Toxicity is low with both agents, but GI disturbances and hypersensitivity can occur. These toxic effects are usually controlled by decreasing the drug's dose.

Xanthine Oxidase Inhibitors. Xanthine oxidase inhibitors control serum urate levels by regulating the production of uric acid. The first step in the production of uric acid

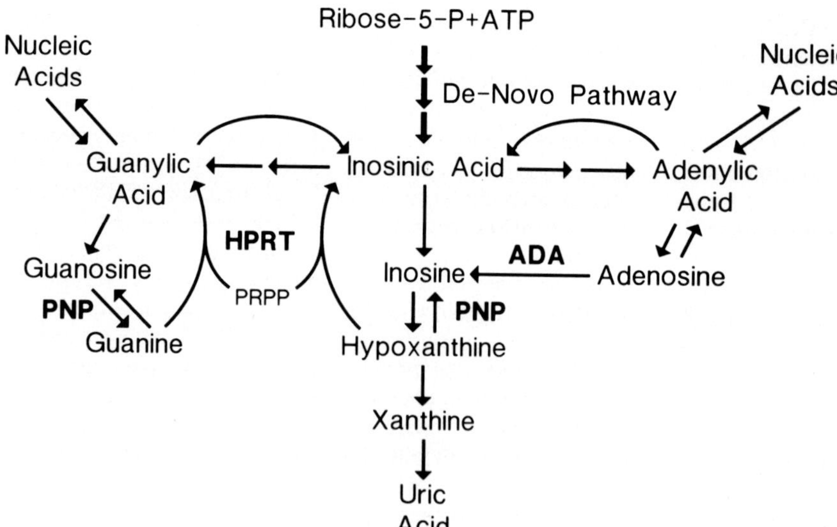

FIGURE 24–1. The metabolic pathways relevant to purine metabolism. Adenosine deaminase (ADA) converts adenosine to inosine. Purine nucleoside phosphorylase (PNP) catalyzes the reversible conversion of guanosine to guanine and inosine to hypoxanthine. Hypoxanthine guanine phosphoribosyl transferase (HPRT) converts guanine to guanylic acid and hypoxanthine to inosinic acid. ATP, adenosine triphosphate. (From Wolff JA and Friedmann T: Approaches to gene therapy in disorders of purine metabolism. Rheum Clin North Am 14(2):460, 1988.)

occurs with the conversion of the purine base hypoxanthine to the intermediate product xanthine; a reaction catalyzed by the enzyme xanthine oxidase. The same enzyme then mediates the conversion of xanthine to the end product uric acid (Fig. 24–1).

Xanthine oxidase can also react with allopurinol, a hypoxanthine analogue, causing its conversion to oxypurinol. Both the parent drug and its metabolite competitively bind to xanthine oxidase, making the enzyme unavailable for the production of uric acid. Although allopurinol has a short half-life (1 hour), oxypurinol has a long half-life of 20 hours. This allows the parent agent to be given only once daily. In addition, allopurinol reduces de novo production of purines by feedback inhibition.[215, 218, 221]

Allopurinol is absorbed well after oral administration, but neither the parent drug nor its metabolite becomes extensively protein bound. Most conversions of allopurinol to oxypurinol occur within the liver and intestinal mucosa; additional conversions occur in capillary endothelial cells. Oxypurinol is excreted through the kidneys. Accumulation of the metabolite can occur during renal dysfunction, necessitating a reduced dosage of the parent drug.[221]

Side effects of allopurinol therapy include GI intolerance, skin rashes, and bone marrow suppression.[221] Hepatotoxicity has also been reported.[222] An allopurinol hypersensitivity syndrome has been recognized, characterized by fever, skin rash, decreased renal function, hepatocellular injury, leukocytosis, and eosinophilia. This immunologic reaction may cause death in 27.5% of patients so affected.[223, 224] The study that defined this statistic has shown that most patients in whom the potentially fatal syndrome had developed did not fulfill the proper indications for receiving the drug (Table 24–5). Hypersensitivity occurs most frequently when allopurinol is given along with diuretics or in patients with renal compromise.

Various drug interactions have been associated with concurrent allopurinol therapy. The purine analogue azathioprine and its metabolite 6-mercaptopurine are both inactivated by xanthine oxidase. The enzyme not only converts the parent drug to its metabolite (itself a chemotherapeutic agent used in the treatment of leukemia) but it further converts 6-mercaptopurine to the inactive end product 6-thiouric acid. By

inhibiting xanthine oxidase activity, levels of 6-mercaptopurine rise, which increases the potential for myelotoxicity. It is, therefore, imperative that the dosage of either azathioprine or 6-mercaptopurine be reduced to one-third or one-fourth normal when administered concurrently with allopurinol.[218, 221]

Allopurinol potentiates the effects of anticoagulants and phenytoin. Unacceptable myelotoxicity precludes the drug's coadministration with cyclophosphamide. Probenecid may increase renal clearance of oxypurinol with uncertain clinical consequences. It has been recognized that renal clearance of allopurinol and oxypurinol is reduced by 28% and 64%, respectively, in patients who ascribe to a low-protein diet. These findings reveal a potential for clinical complication, with patients experiencing protein malnutrition during allopurinol therapy.[221]

Allopurinol therapy is usually started at a low dose of 100 mg daily and is increased weekly at 100-mg increments until favorable uric acid levels are attained. Doses higher than 300 mg should be divided, and the total daily dose should not exceed 800 mg.[218] An acute gout attack may be initiated when allopurinol therapy is introduced. Colchicine can be given prophylactically during the first several months of allopurinol therapy to prevent the acute drug-induced flare.[225, 226]

Allopurinol therapy is not recommended for treating mild to moderate asymptomatic hyperuricemia, uncomplicated

TABLE 24–5

INDICATIONS FOR ALLOPURINOL THERAPY

1. Tophaceous gout
2. Major uric acid overproduction (excretion of more than 900 mg of uric acid per day on a low-purine diet)
3. Frequent gout attacks unresponsive to antigout medications or in patients intolerant to these medications or with renal compromise
4. Recurrent uric acid renal calculi
5. Recurrent calcium oxalate renal calculi when associated with hyperuricosuria
6. Prevention of acute urate nephropathy in patients receiving cytotoxic therapy for malignancy

From Singer JZ and Wallace SL: The allopurinol hypersensitivity syndrome: Unnecessary morbidity and mortality. Arthritis Rheum 29(1):82–87, 1986.

gout, or acute attacks of gout. When strong indications for allopurinol therapy exist in patients showing cutaneous hypersensitivity, cautious desensitization may be feasible and clinically useful.[224]

When faced with the choice of using a uricosuric agent or allopurinol, the less toxic uricosuric agent is preferred. Allopurinol is the drug of choice only for patients who are major excreters of uric acid, who already have renal insufficiency or a urinary stone, or who fit the previously discussed criteria.

Benzbromarone. Benzbromarone is a potent uricosuric agent that is thought to be more effective than other uricosurics when used during renal insufficiency. The drug inhibits tubular reabsorption of urate. Daily doses of 20 to 100 mg have produced significant reductions in serum uric acid levels.[218, 219] As of this writing, benzbromarone is not available in the United States.

Antiinflammatory-Uricosuric Agents. Some NSAIDs have the additional action of promoting uricosuria. Diflunisal and amflutizole are two such drugs, but their usefulness in treating gout seems limited. Azapropazone, on the other hand, appears to show promise for use in chronic gout. Acute attacks of gout caused by uricosuric therapy may be tempered by this agent's double role. As with any uricosuric agent, azapropazone, and possibly diflunisal and amflutizole, should be avoided during an attack of gout and started only after the attack has completely subsided.[218] Both azapropazone and amflutizole are presently unavailable in the United States.

DRUG TREATMENT OF SPECIFIC ARTHRITIC DISORDERS

The pharmacologic management of IJDs, particularly RA, is not completely effective without the concurrent implementation of rest, physical therapy, occupational therapy, patient education, care and protection of the affected joints, and proper nutrition. The maintenance of strength and the protection from disability caused by inactivity are important to the overall success of therapy. The objectives of pharmacologic management of arthritis include relief of pain, reduction or suppression of inflammation, minimization of undesirable side effects, preservation of muscle and joint architecture and function, and a return to productive life.[226]

Rheumatoid Arthritis

RA is a disease of chronic inflammation characterized primarily by the way it affects joint structure and function. The cause of the disease remains unclear, but theories abound. Foreign antigens including Epstein Barr virus, parvovirus, mycoplasma, and several bacteria have been targeted as possible etiologic agents.[227–231] It is known that certain microbes and viruses can cause animal diseases that resemble RA in character, lending some credence to a microbial or viral cause. Human parvovirus B19, in addition to causing childhood exanthem erythema infectiosum, or fifth disease, can cause a chronic arthropathy similar to seronegative RA in adults.[232] Measles virus and parvovirus have been cultured from the joints of a small number of seronegative rheumatoid patients, further supporting this view. Endogenous antigens such as collagen and immunoglobulins have

also been suspected as being responsible for initiating the disease.[228]

Hormonal factors may play a role in the cause and course of RA. It has been observed that women of all ages have a twofold to threefold greater chance than men of acquiring RA. In 80% of arthritic women, the disease appears to be ameliorated during pregnancy, and there is a variation in the severity of the disease in nonpregnant women during menstruation. In one case-controlled study, nulliparity was noted to place women at risk for contracting RA, whereas women who had children and childless women who used oral contraceptive agents were protected from the disease. Of further interest, nulliparous women who had never used oral contraceptives were at a four times greater risk for contracting RA when compared with parous oral contraceptive users.[233, 234] The manner in which hormones influence disease progression is not entirely understood, and perhaps the connection is weaker than suggested by such studies. Still, these observations merit further investigation.

People whose cells express certain class II MHCs, known also as HLAs, appear to have a greater susceptibility to certain rheumatic diseases. Seropositive RA, for example, occurs with greater frequency in people with the HLA-DR4 haplotype; however, only a few people with this genetic constitution acquire the disease.[235, 236] Genetic predisposition to rheumatoid disorders occurs with other class II gene products, including HLA-DQ and DP. Several HLA class I molecules are also associated with augmented susceptibility to disease, the most recognized example being the association of HLA-B27 expression with AS and Reiter's syndrome.[236] Just how immune response surface complexes react with exogenous or endogenous antigens to initiate the course of disease remains to be clarified.

Several theories exist that attempt to explain the relationship between HLA constitution and rheumatic disease susceptibility.[231] One theory postulates that the HLA molecule may be acting as a receptor for the disease-causing antigen. Those patients who display the specific receptor are at a greater risk for acquiring the disease but only if exposed to the etiologic agent. For example, patients who are HLA-B27 positive show an increased risk for contracting AS. When the patient is exposed to the pathogenic antigen (possibly a virus), the antigen is processed and displayed with the HLA molecule. T cell recognition of the complex will then initiate the immune process, leading to illness.

A second hypothesis suggests that only specific HLA molecules possess an antigen-binding groove that is properly configured to accept the processed antigen. Those lacking the correct conformation are unable to display the processed antigen, and no immune response develops.

A third hypothesis puts the onus for antigen recognition on the T cell, which must possess a receptor capable of recognizing the HLA complex. Again, specific HLA type is important because the antigen must be associated with the HLA molecule to react with a properly configured T cell receptor. In this scenario, it is the reaction of the T cell that is responsible for disease pathogenesis.

The fourth hypothesis, known as the *molecular mimicry hypothesis*, postulates that the disease-associated HLA antigen (B27, for example) is immunologically similar to a non–disease-associated HLA antigen that has displayed the processed antigenic agent. That is, when an HLA molecule that is not associated with rheumatic disease susceptibility displays the antigenic particle, it takes on an appearance similar to that of an HLA molecule that is associated with disease expression. This hypothesis allows two alternative explanations for disease development.

The first alternative proposes that the infecting antigen, perhaps a viral particle, is similar in appearance to the disease-associated HLA molecule and is thus recognized as self. This subterfuge allows the antigen to promote the course of the disease without challenge through mechanisms not yet explained. A second alternative again proposes an immunogenic similarity between the antigen and the disease-associated HLA molecule, but in this instance the antigen is recognized as foreign, and a vigorous immune reaction is initiated. The HLA molecule, now recognized as foreign, becomes caught up in the immune melee, and the course toward disease expression is set. This latter scenario lends validity to the hypothesis that certain rheumatic diseases may develop through autoimmune pathways.

It is the T cell receptor that recognizes the HLA complex. Once antigen is processed and displayed by the presenting cell, the T lymphocyte engages the complex, and the immune cascade begins. The intensity of the ensuing response determines whether or not disease occurs. A strong response to an infectious agent would generally prevent disease, but the same intense response to the antigen responsible for RA may be the trigger for the disease process to begin.

RFs are autoantibodies directed against certain epitopes on the Fc fragment of IgG.[237] They have been found among the IgM, IgA, IgE, and IgG classes of immunoglobulins,[238] but IgM-RF is the one most commonly measured.

RF is not specific for RA. It can be found in the sera of patients with other forms of inflammatory diseases. The occurrence of the antibody increases with age, and it is also found in some apparently normal persons.[236, 238]

The B lymphocytes are responsible for producing RF, but the initial immunogenic stimulus for factor production is not yet clear. One theory holds that antigen combining with native IgG causes a structural alteration of the immunoglobulin, revealing antigenic determinants that had been concealed. The new structure is identified as foreign, and an immune response is initiated.[236]

The presence of RF in arthritis is clinically significant. Patients afflicted with RA who are also positive for RF have a more severe form of the disease, with more widespread extra-articular disease manifestations. RFs are associated with a higher frequency of RA-associated vasculitis and subcutaneous nodules. IgM-RF is a potent activator of complement and thus contributes to the progression of the inflammatory process.[237]

The antigens that initiate RA are in all probability arthrotropic.[237] Once established within the joint, these antigens react with locally produced antibodies. However, again, it is quite possible that the antigen itself is a product of resident tissues and not exogenously derived. Potential local antigens include collagen, cartilage, DNA, immunoglobulins, and other such products. Once the immune complexes are formed, they thrust into motion those processes that can eventually cause disease.[236] Clinically, this first stage in the progression of RA produces no observable symptoms.[239]

Early in the course of disease, immune complexes activate complement, increasing vascular flow and permeability within the synovial membrane, whereas complement-derived chemotactic factors summon PMNs to the site. These cells ingest the immune complexes, thereby stimulating the production of additional chemotactic factors, hydrolytic enzymes, oxygen radicals, and other products of inflammation. Eventually, T lymphocytes become activated by antigen-MHC complexes, a process promoted by monocyte/macrophage-derived IL-1. The increased number of T cells prompts the proliferation and differentiation of antibody-producing B cells through the action of cytokines, particularly IL-2. IL-2, interferon, tumor necrosis factor (TNF), arachidonic acid metabolites, and other lymphokines sustain the complex immune reactions. These activities constitute the second and third stages of disease progression, separated by severity and amplitude of inflammation rather than by specific landmark events. Although the architecture remains mostly intact, these stages mark the beginnings of symptomatic arthritis as joints become painful, stiff, and swollen. The presence of certain cytokines, particularly TNF and IL-1, promote the constitutional symptoms of malaise, fatigue, and occasionally fever.[239]

The fourth stage of RA pathophysiology is marked by irreversible structural damage to the joint. The proliferating synovium invades cartilage, tendon, ligaments, and subchondral bone, producing increased discomfort and reduced function.[239] With the fifth stage, the destruction is complete. Joints have been transformed into disfigured banks of rubble, useless for function and a source of chronic agony.

The traditional approach to therapy for RA is to enlist the use of antiinflammatory agents early in the course of the disease. Along with rest, education, and exercise, this combined regimen enjoys a well-established role. It is deemed appropriate to use less benign medications only when the disease passes the NSAID's ability to contain symptoms. This approach minimizes the toxicity of therapy for a disease that may travel a relatively benign and non–life-threatening course (Fig. 24–2).

The treatment pyramid has been challenged since it has been realized that RA not only may pursue an aggressive course toward joint destruction but may also be fatal. The traditional treatment pyramid has revealed many shortcomings and is being replaced with therapeutic plans more suited to the pathomechanics of the disease. The practice of matching drug strength and toxicity with the current severity of disease is being supplanted by an approach that recognizes the potential for modifying the ultimate course of the disease and supplying the necessary therapy at a time that will most favorably affect that course.

A step-down bridge approach[240] has been proposed for RA therapy, combining medications with different mechanisms of action, time to therapeutic onset, and toxicity. The plan calls for the early use of agents that have generally been reserved until late in the course of disease, when former first-line drugs are no longer effective or for drugs that previously have been avoided altogether. Oral corticosteroids, a potent group of antiinflammatory agents generally recognized as being too fraught with dangerous side effects to be useful in standard therapy, enter the treatment regimen at the outset. Although many rheumatologists are reluctant to use large doses of prednisone for treating RA, low doses of the agent (5 to 7.5 mg/day) may benefit patients with minimal risk of toxicity. Mean doses of 6.6 mg/day for a period of 2 years were not found to increase bone loss above that seen in patients with RA without receiving glucocorticoids.[239] A

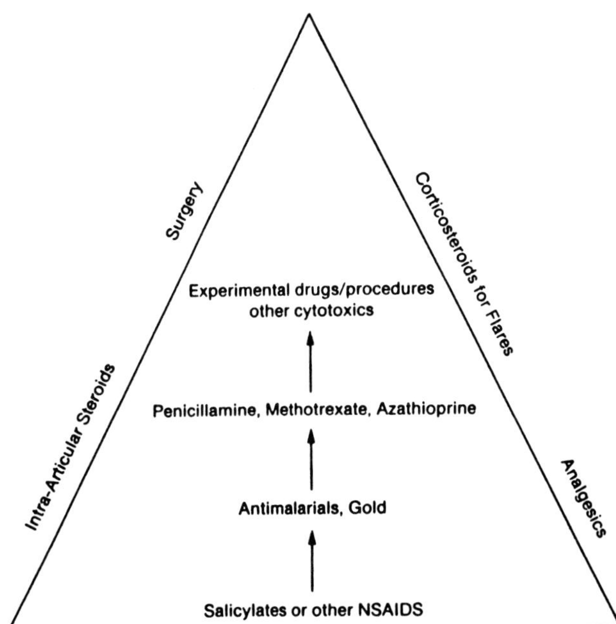

FIGURE 24–2. Treatment pyramid for rheumatic arthritis. (From Schumacher HR, Klippel JH, and Robinson DR [eds]: Rheumatoid arthritis: Epidemiology, etiology, rheumatoid factor, pathology, pathogenesis, treatment. *In* Primer on the Rheumatic Diseases, 9th ed. Copyright 1988. Used by permission of the Arthritis Foundation.)

maintenance dose of 10 mg of prednisone can be used initially, but NSAIDs may also be used at this point if symptoms are mild and responsive to such care. If no relief is achieved after 1 month of therapy, the initial therapeutic agents could be combined with more potent drugs in a stepwise manner rather than using them in sequence, as called for by the treatment pyramid (Fig. 24–3).

MTX is recommended in the next step of RA therapy if the initial antiinflammatory agents fail to quell a persistent synovitis. Under these conditions, the patient faces a high risk of joint destruction; thus, the use of other classes of drugs at this relatively early stage is justified. When used at the low doses established for RA, MTX acts more as an antiinflammatory agent rather than as the cytotoxic or immunosuppressive agent that defined its first use in cancer chemotherapy. Oral and intramuscular gold and HCS can also be added to the prednisone or NSAID regimen along with MTX because lesser combinations fail to render improvement. As the disease is controlled, the toxic agents could be eliminated and the patient maintained on more benign therapeutics agents, such as one antimalarial tablet per day.[240]

With the step-down bridge approach, both prednisone and MTX are used for their early control of the disease process but are discontinued when their job is done. Ideally, prednisone is gradually eliminated after about 3 months of combination therapy, when the full effects of MTX are realized. Six months later, when gold has reached its therapeutic potential, MTX is stopped. Intramuscular gold is used with oral gold to suppress inflammation sooner, and then the intramuscular preparation is discontinued while oral gold maintains control. At any time during the course of therapy, prednisone and MTX could be temporarily introduced to control intermittent flares.[240]

When a therapeutic approach based on the stage of disease is considered, stage 1 RA would require no treatment because no symptoms are produced and the disease is not yet recognized. Stages 2 and 3 produce symptoms, and if treated inadequately, the latter stage can quickly progress to stage 4 when irreversible joint damage develops. Again, NSAIDs, including aspirin, can be used to initiate therapy, but the treating physician must recognize when such care is ineffective and be ready to introduce more potent agents before the stage of destruction begins. The NSAIDs are continued while the other agents are added to suppress those products of inflammation that would otherwise hasten joint destruction.[239]

As with the step-down bridge approach, therapy based on stage of disease calls for the early use of second-line and disease-modifying agents when the disease progresses on antiinflammatory compounds alone. It is recommended that second-line agents such as HCS, sulfasalazine, MTX, aza-

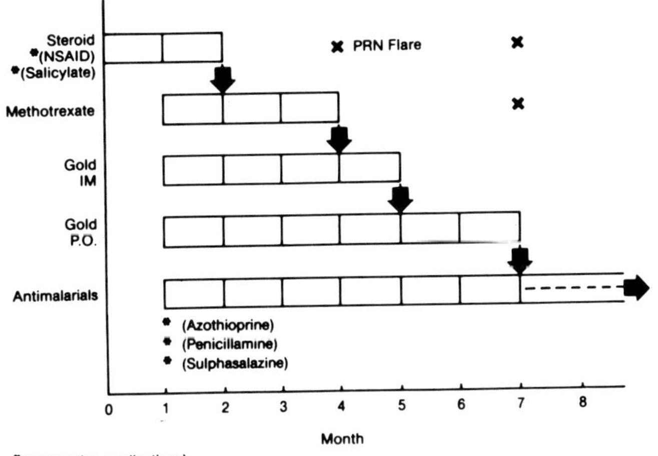

FIGURE 24–3. The step-down bridge. NSAID, nonsteroidal antiinflammatory drug. (From Wilske KR and Healey LA: Remodeling the pyramid—a concept whose time has come. J Rheumatol 16(5):565–567, 1989.)

thioprine, gold salts, or penicillamine be started if the disease remains uncontrolled after 1 month of antiinflammatory therapy.[239] Second-line and disease-modifying agents should be recognized for their toxicity and be used in a manner commensurate with disease severity.

By the time RA enters stage 4, joint structure and function have been irreversibly affected. Advanced therapy should focus on preventing the latter third stage from progressing to the fourth, because therapy during stage 4 would be mostly palliative. Most of the experimental modalities have been used at this stage, but these have shown variable and unclear benefit. Such therapies include high-dose intravenous methylprednisolone, cyclosporin, total lymphoid irradiation, and others. Once the disease has reached stage 5, aggressive therapy is no longer warranted. Control of systemic vasculitis with glucocorticoids or cytotoxic agents may be appropriate, but overtreatment of non–life-threatening disease manifestations with toxic agents should be avoided. Surgical relief of grossly deformed joints using arthroplasties, fusions, and joint prostheses may improve limb function.[239]

The proper management of RA must combine drug therapy with nonpharmaceutical modalities that allow the medications to work most effectively. Educating the patient about the natural history of the disease, particularly concerning the tendency for remissions and flares of disease activity, will do much toward gaining the patient's cooperation and compliance. Rest is important to prevent exacerbation of joint inflammation, and exercises that develop muscle tone without joint stress are important to help maintain joint alignment and function. Activities that overwork inflamed joints may elevate intra-articular pressure, leading to ischemia and additional tissue damage.[239] During flares, the patient should reduce those activities that would potentially hasten joint destruction.

With the revelation that certain dietary components may favorably inhibit some portions of the inflammatory cascade, the physician should encourage arthritis patients to supplement their daily intake with those foods that could possibly curb the course of inflammation. The fish oil fatty acids and particular plant oils described earlier could be substituted for arachidonic acid–containing red meats, which may potentially augment disease expression.

Future strategies for the treatment of RA will most likely focus on the suppression of the immune cascade by regulating the cellular and soluble components of inflammation. The complicated manner in which these components interact to produce inflammation and disease will undoubtedly prove considerably difficult to control because it is the relative concentrations of these elements and their temporal occurrence that determines the harshness of the inflammatory response. Altering any one limb of this elaborate system may do no more than commute reactants along another route that is just as damaging. Successful treatment requires suppression or augmentation of individual components of inflammation by specific agents administered in a timely manner.

Products of recombinant DNA technology may prove useful in interrupting the course of inflammation and tissue proliferation, which causes the disease to be so persistent and ravaging. Cyclic oligosaccharides combined with antiinflammatory steroids can inhibit angiogenesis. Antibodies directed against early-phase components of inflammation may abort the disease process before irreversible destruction can occur. Ferric hydroxide labeled with the isotope dysprosium-165

has been used to destroy proliferating synovium, again stopping the disease at a point at which architecture and function could be preserved.[239]

Certain antibiotics have provoked interest for their use in RA therapy. Minocycline, a member of the tetracycline family of antibiotics, has been observed to chelate calcium, disabling the action of calcium-dependent collagenase. It has also been shown to affect the immune response by upregulating T suppresser-inducer factors.[241]

There is no doubt that new agents will continue to be added to the drug arsenal used to combat this disabling disease, whereas new roles will be discovered for many of the agents currently being used to treat arthritis and others not yet tested against this disease.

RA presents a complicated and ambiguous therapeutic challenge to the treating physician; therefore, the physician must be astute in coordinating all facets of disease management. A thorough familiarity with the therapeutic agents and their toxicities is imperative. Throughout the course of care, the physician must follow those clinical and laboratory parameters that may portend ensuing difficulties. The side effects that accompany the sometimes highly toxic therapy must be recognized early so that mephitic consequences may be averted. Physicians who are not well versed in arthritis care should recognize their limitations and direct the patient to a rheumatologist familiar with symptomatic and remissive therapy. Nonrheumatologist caregivers can play a supportive role by providing additional monitoring of the disease process and by implementing medical or surgical therapy when deemed appropriate. Because RA is a progressive disorder, any surgical therapy rendered should be done properly and with finality so that multiple reconstructive interventions can be avoided. Local anesthetics and systemic analgesics may be used to provide relief during acute flares of joint disease. Intra-articular corticosteroids administered sparingly and judiciously may provide the additional relief necessary to allow arthritis patients to continue a productive life and to maintain those activities deemed most important to them. Throughout the course of arthritis therapy, the treating physicians must pay close attention to each patient's insight and reliability so that proper safety and mutually acceptable results can be realized.

Osteoarthritis

OA, or degenerative joint disease, is the most common of the destructive diseases of the joint. The condition is classified as idiopathic or primary if no direct or obvious cause of joint disease can be identified. The wear and tear of joints that develop with advancing age can thus be classified as primary OA. If joint deterioration develops as a result of previous direct trauma, congenitally or traumatically induced malalignment, previous disease, or any other identifiable condition or event, the disease is classified as secondary.

The clinical characteristics of OA include joint pain, stiffness, crepitus on range of motion, and bony enlargement. The disease usually follows an insidious course, initially producing mild symptoms that are relieved with rest. As the disease progresses, changes in joint architecture develop, causing a further reduction of joint function. Pain becomes a more prominent and persistent feature. The degenerative changes that develop may produce local inflammation, further altering joint integrity.

Although OA is characterized by deterioration and erosion of articular cartilage, this tissue lacks innervation, and local damage produces no pain. The pain that does develop is probably caused in part by the inflamed synovium, which is richly innervated. Additionally, pain may derive from bone microfractures and from the stretching of sensitive soft tissues over enlarged and fragmented bone.

Articular chondrocytes from osteoarthritic joints appear to develop a hypermetabolic state, increasing the rate of synthesis of matrix components. Paradoxically, this increase in production of matrix components, such as proteoglycans, collagen, and hyaluronic acid, is coupled with matrix deterioration.[242] It is apparent that the augmented metabolic state is generalized, so that production of degradative enzymes increases as well. The catabolic action of these enzymes further weakens and fragments cartilage and bone, eventually generating humoral and cellular immune responses.[243] The altered anabolic activity results in proliferation of abnormal joint components.

Treatment of OA consists of reducing those physical activities that stress the joint and cause further deterioration. Strengthening of supporting muscle groups through nonweightbearing exercises may allow better joint tracking, slowing the degenerative processes. Use of supportive devices such as orthoses and braces may also be of benefit.

NSAIDs are useful in relieving much of the pain associated with OA, and, with certain conditions, some agents prove more effective than others. OA of the hip, for example, responds quite well to treatment with agents such as indomethacin, ibuprofen,[8] and ketoprofen.[89] All agents, including the salicylates, however, are useful in treating OA.

Paradoxically, the NSAIDs used to treat the destructive inflammation and pain of OA may in themselves be detrimental. It has been determined that NSAIDs, particularly the salicylates, may suppress proteoglycan synthesis in damaged cartilage tissues.[62] For early OA, when damage to the articular cartilage may still be reparable, use of these agents may actually impede healing. The initial stages of OA, then, may more appropriately be treated with analgesics such as acetaminophen, whereas NSAIDs are reserved to treat acute inflammatory flares. Infrequent and judicious use of short-acting intra-articular steroids may also be used for such flares. Injectible steroids should not be used to treat more than one or two joints concurrently.

In the later stages of OA, when irreversible damage has finally occurred, use of NSAIDs for chronic symptomatic control would probably not be detrimental. Analgesics not related to the NSAIDs may augment relief when antiinflammatory agents alone are not successful. Again, occasional use of intra-articular steroids may be of additional benefit during acute flares. Chronically painful and failed joints may be most successfully treated through surgical intervention.

Gout

Gout is a disease of monosodium urate monohydrate (MSU) crystal deposition. Because of an overproduction or undersecretion of uric acid, or an intolerance to a high dietary purine load, the plasma becomes supersaturated with urate, and the pathologic condition of hyperuricemia develops. This condition in and of itself is usually insufficient to produce the clinical expression of gout,[212] and additional factors including the degree of hyperuricemia, duration of the condition, concomitant disease processes, and diet are generally required to elicit crystal deposition and gout.

Gout is classified as primary, secondary, or idiopathic. *Primary gout* or hyperuricemia is a genetic disorder that directly causes altered uric acid metabolism, yielding chronically elevated uric acid levels and ultimately urate deposition. *Secondary gout* refers to genetic or acquired disorders that indirectly affect uric acid metabolism or excretion, again leading to hyperuricemia. *Idiopathic gout* identifies the gouty condition that cannot be directly attributed to any identifiable systemic cause. Within each class, components of overproduction, undersecretion, or both may be present and contribute to disease expression.[214]

When conditions exist that are favorable for MSU precipitation, crystals of this purine metabolite become deposited predominantly into the connective tissues. Common sites for deposit include the synovial tissue of the small joints of the hands and feet, particularly the first metatarsophalangeal joint, the olecranon bursae, and the pinnae. The MSU deposits can sometimes become concentrated into a large, subcutaneous mass called a *tophus*. These appear as a chronically inflamed red-orange elevation under the skin, again notably on the fingers, toes, elbow, and pinna, sometimes with a white center, which breaks the surface and exudes the tophus material.

Gout is a particularly painful form of arthritis in its acute state. The MSU crystals deposited in the synovial tissues elicit an intense inflammatory response. A common location for the development of acute gout is the first metatarsophalangeal joint, where the condition is called *podagra*. The synovitis that develops is dependent on the influx of neutrophils, a cell line not usually present within the joint space. The crystals are initially taken up by resident activated monocytes, which then produce and release the neutrophil chemotactic factor IL-8. This polypeptide, found in abundance in gouty synovial fluids, not only is responsible for PMN chemotaxis but is also a determinant of PMN degranulation, and it promotes continued ingress and activation of the neutrophils. There is evidence that fibroblasts, vascular endothelium, and urate crystal-stimulated synovial cells can also produce this factor.[245]

Acute gout is often accompanied by the constitutional symptoms of inflammation. Fever, leukocytosis, elevated erythrocyte sedimentation rate, and increased production of the acute phase proteins IL-1 and TNF develop early in the attack. Very high levels of IL-6 have been identified in the synovial fluid of patients with gout and pseudogout. A product of crystal-stimulated monocytes and synoviocytes, IL-6 may be the factor responsible for inducing these systemic effects.[245]

The acute inflammatory response to precipitated MSU crystals is mediated mostly by the neutrophils. Protein-coated MSU crystals are engulfed by these cells, producing urate-filled phagosomes. These phagosomes fuse with the primary lysosomes, creating phagolysosomes. The urate crystals damage the membrane of the phagolysosome, causing it to rupture and spill its contents into the cytoplasm. The injured cell can then lyse, spewing the crystals and digestive enzymes into the joint space. Again, the crystals are phagocytized, and the process is repeated. Throughout, the PMNs put forth additional chemotactic factors, which summon other cellular elements to the site. Superoxide anions are produced by the PMNs along with lysosomal proteases, leukotriene B_4, and a low-molecular-weight polypeptide called *crystal chemotactic factor*.[244, 245]

It is best to act aggressively during an acute attack of gout. Colchicine, administered orally or intravenously, has been the standard therapy for abating the exquisitely painful acute inflammatory episode. If such therapy is delayed longer than 24 to 48 hours, the benefit of colchicine is greatly reduced. Follow-up with an NSAID, particularly indomethacin, is useful over the short term.

Either systemic corticosteroids or adrenocorticotropin can be used to abate an acute attack effectively. It is only when colchicine or NSAIDs fail to produce ablation of a gouty attack that cortisteroids and corticotropin are indicated for the treatment of acute gout. Prednisone, or an equivalent corticosteroid agent, can be administered at a dose of 30 mg/day orally or parenterally. Corticotropin is given as a slow intravenous infusion of 20 USP units or as an intramuscular injection of 40 to 80 USP units daily every 6 to 12 hours over a period of 1 to 3 days. Because about 30% of patients so treated will experience rebound attacks when steroid or corticotropin is withdrawn, prophylactic colchicine (0.6 mg twice daily) should be given during and after therapy has been implemented.[218, 247]

Only a few patients who experience their first attack of acute gout experience relapsing episodes. Follow-up preventive therapy is unnecessary unless the patient suffers three definite attacks within a period of 1 year. Either colchicine or one of the urate-lowering agents can be used depending on specific patient criteria discussed earlier.

Colchicine, when used to treat acute gout, often produces GI symptoms that rival the discomfort of the original condition. In most cases, however, the acute attack can be treated quite effectively without exposing the patient to additional drug-related suffering. A patient presenting with a classic attack of acute podagra can be afforded instantaneous relief with the administration of a fast-acting anesthetic agent such as lidocaine. A 1% or 2% solution of this agent can be injected along the posterior tibial, saphenous, and deep peroneal nerves or just proximal to the area of greatest inflammation. Generally, 10 ml or less provides adequate anesthesia. A long-acting agent like bupivacaine (Marcaine), 0.25% to 0.5%, can be used in addition to or in combination with the faster acting but short-duration anesthetic. This will then ensure quick and long-lasting pain relief.

Once adequate anesthesia is accomplished, the inflamed joint could be entered with a large-bore needle and joint fluid aspirated. The specimen should be sent for crystal identification and for Gram's stain to rule out joint sepsis. If no organisms are seen, the joint could be instilled with a long-acting anesthetic agent and a noncrystalline corticosteroid agent such as dexamethasone phosphate. Usually 1 ml of anesthesia with 4 mg of steroid can be used. The area should be prepared with antiseptic and sterile technique used when the joint is entered so as not to introduce infective organisms into a sterile joint.

The patient should be placed on an antiinflammatory agent such as indomethacin for at least a week to provide continued control of inflammation. Alternatively, a low maintenance dose of colchicine could be used for a short period.

Seronegative Spondyloarthropathies

The seronegative arthritides are characterized by sacroiliac joint inflammation, peripheral arthropathy, enthesopathy, and absence of RF. Disorders include psoriatic arthritis, Reiter's syndrome, AS, and inflammatory bowel disease. Involvement of the eye (uveitis), aortic valve, lung parenchyma, and skin generally occurs.[248, 249]

The seronegative diseases are managed most effectively by treatment of flares rather than by continuous therapy. The patient with psoriatic arthritis can be helped by having the skin manifestations treated when present, which may also relieve the accompanying arthritic process. Again, intra-articular steroids can be used along with NSAIDs, particularly indomethacin. The steroids should be administered with caution despite the success of such therapy. Some patients may have been treated for previous inflammatory attacks in the same manner with favorable results. The tendency to instill the joint automatically with cortisone must be tempered because the patient could be afforded more harm than good when repeated injections are administered by many well-meaning treating physicians. Despite the rapid symptomatic relief of pain provided by steroids for these or any other forms of arthropathy, both the patient and physician must be aware of the inherent dangers of this practice. Hence, a more prudent albeit gradual and effective course of NSAID therapy may provide the greatest overall benefit.

CONCLUSION

The successful pharmacologic management of IJDs requires a full understanding of the underlying disease processes that produce pain, disability, and joint destruction. Knowledge of the mechanism by which each agent controls or modifies the disease is fundamental to choosing the proper course of care. The physician should be aware of the signs and symptoms associated with impending drug toxicity and must be prepared to manage these side effects while successfully maintaining control over the primary disease. Both the treating physician and the patient should realize that drug therapy alone will not be completely effective in treating the disease, and close attention to adjunctive therapeutic modalities is equally important to the overall success or failure of treatment.

I would like to thank my wife, Cissy, and daughter, Shannon, for their support and patience during the preparation of this manuscript.

References

1. Paulus E, Scott DL, and Edmonds JP: Classification of antirheumatic drugs: A new proposal. Arthritis Rheum 35(3):364–365, 1992.
2. McCarty DJ: Arthritis and Allied Conditions. Philadelphia, Lea & Febiger, 1985.
3. Schalkwijk J, Van Den Berg WB, Van De Putte LBA, et al: An experimental model for hydrogen peroxide-induced tissue damage. Arthritis Rheum 29:532–538, 1986.
4. Abramson SB and Weissmann G: The mechanisms of action of nonsteroidal anti-inflammatory drugs. Arthritis Rheum 32(1):1–9, 1989.
5. Simon LE and Mills JA: Nonsteroidal anti-inflammatory drugs: I. N Engl J Med 302:1179–1185, 1980.
6. Verbeeck RK: Pharmacokinetic drug interactions with nonsteroidal anti-inflammatory drugs. Clin Pharmacokinet 19(1):44–66, 1990.
7. Brater D: Clinical pharmacology of NSAIDs. J Clin Pharmacol 28:518–523, 1988.

8. Porter RS: Factors determining efficacy of NSAIDs. Drug Intell Clin Pharm 18:42–51, 1984.

9. Murry MD and Brater DC: Nonsteroidal anti-inflammatory drugs. Clin Geriatr Med 6(2):365–397, 1990.

10. Benet LZ: Pharmacokinetics: I. Absorption, distribution, & excretion. *In* Katzung BG: Basic and Clinical Pharmacology. Los Altos, CA, Lange Medical Publications, 1982, pp 22–33.

11. Dunn M: The role of arachidonic acid metabolites in renal homeostasis. Drugs 33(Suppl 1):56–66, 1987.

12. Henrich WL: Nephrotoxicity of the anti-inflammatory agents. Am J Kidney Dis. 11(4):478–483, 1983.

13. Wilson TW, Kaushal RD, and Dubois M: Prostaglandins, the kidney, and hypertension. West J Med. 153:168–172, 1990.

14. Guyton AC: Hemostasis and blood coagulation. *In* Textbook of Medical Physiology, 5th ed. Philadelphia, WB Saunders, 1981, pp 48–49.

15. Schlondorff D: Renal prostaglandin synthesis. Am J Med 81(Suppl 2B):1–11, 1986.

16. Dunn MJ, Simonson M, Davidson EW, et al: Nonsteroidal anti-inflammatory agents and renal function. J Clin Pharmacol 28:524–529, 1988.

17. Clive DM and Stoff JS: Renal syndromes associated with nonsteroidal antiinflammatory drugs. N Engl J Med 310(9):563–572, 1984.

18. Carmichael J and Shankel SW: Effects of nonsteroidal anti-inflammatory drugs on prostaglandin and renal function. Am J Medicine 78:992–1000, 1986.

19. Klassen DK, Stout RL, Spilman PS, et al: Sulindac kinetics and effects on renal function and prostaglandin excretion in renal insufficiency. J Clin Pharmacol 29:1037–1042, 1989.

20. Whelton A and Hamilton CW: Nonsteroidal anti-inflammatory drugs: Effects on kidney function. J Clin Pharmacol 31:588–598, 1991.

21. Shand DG, Epstein C, Kinberg-Calhoun J, et al: The effect of etodolac administration on renal function in patients with arthritis. J Clin Pharmacol 26:269–274, 1986.

22. Murray MD and Brater DC: Adverse effects of nonsteroidal anti-inflammatory drugs on renal function. Ann Intern Med 112(8):559–560, 1990.

23. Roth SH: NSAID gastropathy. Drugs 40(Suppl 5):25–28, 1990.

24. Zizic TM: The Management of Common Rheumatic Diseases. Lecture, June 27, 1991, San Jose, CA.

25. Carson JL and Strom BL: The gastrointestinal side effects of the nonsteroidal anti-inflammatory drugs. Clin Pharmacol 28:554–559, 1988.

26. Isselbacher KJ: The role of arachidonic acid metabolites in gastrointestinal homeostasis. Drugs 33(Suppl 1):38–46, 1987.

27. Bright-Asare P, Habte T, Yirgou B, and Benjamin J: Prostaglandins, H₂-receptor antagonists and peptic ulcer disease. Drugs 35(Suppl 3):1–9, 1988.

28. Guyton AC: Secretory functions of the alimentary tract. *In* Textbook of Medical Physiology, 6th ed. Philadelphia, WB Saunders, 1981, pp 801–815.

29. Nunes D, Kennedy NP, and Weir DG: Treatment of peptic ulcer disease in the arthritic patient. Drugs 38(3):451–461, 1989.

30. Davenport HW: Digestion and absorption of protein. *In* A Digest of Digestion. Chicago, Year Book Medical, 1978, pp 103–107.

31. Lamers CBHW: The significance of gastrin in the pathogenesis and therapy of peptic ulcer disease. Drugs 35(Suppl 3):10–16, 1988.

32. Cheung LY: Gastric mucosal blood flow: Its measurement and importance in mucosal defense mechanisms. J Surg Res 36:282–288, 1984.

33. Price AH and Fletcher M: Mechanisms of NSAID-induced gastroenteropathy. Drugs 40(Suppl 5):1–11, 1990.

34. Brune K: Is there a rational basis for the different spectra of adverse effects of nonsteroidal anti-inflammatory drugs (NSAIDs)? Drugs 40(Suppl 5):12–15, 1990.

35. Kuwayama H, Matsuo Y, and Eastwood L: Gastroduodenal mucosal injury by nonsteroidal anti-inflammatory drugs. Drug Invest 2(Suppl 1):22–26, 1990.

36. Lanza FL, Royer GL, and Nelson RS: Endoscopic evaluation of the effects of aspirin, buffered aspirin, and enteric-coated aspirin on gastric and duodenal mucosa. N Engl J Med 303(3):136–138, 1980.

37. Lanza FL: Endoscopic studies of gastric and duodenal injury after the use of ibuprofen, aspirin, and other nonsteroidal anti-inflammatory agents. Am J Med 77:19–24, 1984.

38. Lanza FL: A review of gastric ulcer and gastroduodenal injury in normal volunteers receiving aspirin and other non-steroidal anti-inflammatory drugs. Scand J Gastroenterol 24(Suppl 163):24–31, 1989.

39. Kilander A and Dotevall G: Endoscopic evaluation of the comparative effects of acetylsalicylic acid and choline magnesium trisalicylate on human gastric and duodenal mucosa. Br J Rheumatol 22:336–340, 1983.

40. Coates AG, Nostrant TT, Wilson AP, et al: Esophagitis caused by nonsteroidal anti-inflammatory medication: Case reports and review of the literature on pill-induced esophageal injury. South Med J 79(9):1094–1097, 1986.

41. Tytgat GNJ and Rauws EAJ: *Campylobacter pylori* and its role in peptic ulcer disease. Gastroenterol Clin North Am 19(1):183–196, 1990.

42. Sewing K-F, Beil W, and Hannemann H: Comparative pharmacology of histamine H₂-receptor antagonists. Drugs 35(Suppl 3):25–29, 1988.

43. Langman MJS: Antisecretory drugs, safe and effective? Drugs 35(Suppl 3):17–19, 1988.

44. Grim WM: Explaining the cytoprotective properties of an antacid. Drug Invest 2(Suppl 1):59, 1990.

45. Oates JA, FitzGerald GA, Branch RA, et al: Clinical implications of prostaglandin and thromboxane A₂ formation (part 1). N Engl J Med 319:689–698, 1988.

46. Abramowicz M (ed): Toxicity of nonsteroidal anti-inflammatory drugs. Med Lett Drugs Ther 25:15–16, 1983.

47. Hart F and Huskisson EC: Non-steroidal anti-inflammatory drugs: Current status and rational therapeutic use. Drugs 27:232–255, 1984.

48. Jacobs AM, Oloff LM, and Williams GW: Nonsteroidal anti-inflammatory drugs in podiatric medicine and surgery. J Foot Surg 25(3):247–255, 1986.

49. Leen C and Gibb AP: Transient neutropenia and thrombocytopenia due to benoxaprofen. Lancet 1(8284):1302, 1982.

50. Doube A: Hepatitis and non-steroidal anti-inflammatory drugs. Ann Rheum Dis 49:489–490, 1990.

51. Steiner JF: Update on nonsteroidal anti-inflammatory drugs. J Am Acad Physician Assist 3(5):392–400, 1990.

52. Zimmerman HJ: Update of hepatotoxicity due to classes of drugs in common clinical use: Non-steroidal anti-inflammatory drugs, antibiotics, antihypertensives, and cardiac and psychotropic agents. Semin Liver Dis 10(4):322–338, 1990.

53. Duggan DE, Hogans AF, Kwan KC, et al: The metabolism of indomethacin in man. J Pharmacol Exp Ther 181:563, 1972.

54. Michelassi F, Landa L, and Hill RD: Leukotriene D4: A potent coronary artery vasoconstrictor associated with impaired ventricular contraction. Science 217:841–843, 1982.

55. Leitch AG: Leukotrienes and the lung. Clin Sci 67:153–160, 1984.

56. Jacob G, Messina M, Kennedy J, et al: Minimum effective dose of etodolac for the treatment of rheumatoid arthritis. J Clin Pharmacol 26:195–202, 1986.

57. Todd PA and Heel RC: Suprofen: A review of its pharmacodynamic and pharmacokinetic properties, and analgesic efficacy. Drugs 30:514–538, 1985.

58. Suarez SM, Cohen PR, and DeLeo VA: Bullous photosensitivity of naproxen: "Pseudoporphyria." Arthritis Rheum 33(6):903–908, 1990.

59. Palmoski MJ and Brandt KD: Effects of some non-steroidal anti-inflammatory drugs on proteoglycan metabolism and organization in canine articular cartilage. Arthritis Rheum 23:1010–1020, 1980.

60. Furst E: Comments on possible long-term consequences of nonsteroidal anti-inflammatory use. J Clin Pharmacol 28:550–553, 1988.

61. Brandt KD, Albright ME, and Kalasinski LA: Effects of tiaprofenic acid on the concentration and metabolism of proteoglycans in normal and degenerating canine articular cartilage. J Clin Pharmacol 30:808–814, 1990.

62. Collum LMT and Bowen DI: Ocular side-effects of ibuprofen. Br J Ophthalmol 55:472–477, 1971.

63. Mortenson ME and Rennebohm RM: Clinical pharmacology and use of nonsteroidal anti-inflammatory drugs. Pediatr Clin North Am 36(5):1113–1139, 1989.

64. Walson PD and Mortensen ME: Pharmacokinetics of common analgesics, anti-inflammatories, and antipyretics in children. Clin Pharmacokinet 17(Suppl 1):116–137, 1989.

65. Calabro JJ: Optimum management of juvenile chronic polyarthritis. Drugs 26:530–542, 1983.

66. Robinson J, Malleson P, Lirenman D, and Carter J: Nephrotic syndrome associated with nonsteroidal anti-inflammatory drug use in two children. Pediatrics 85(5):844–847, 1990.

67. Woodhouse KW and Wynne H: The pharmacokinetics of non-steroidal anti-inflammatory drugs in the elderly. Clin Pharmacokinet 12:111–122, 1987.

68. Bird HA: Drugs and the elderly. Ann Rheum Dis 49:1021–1024, 1990.

69. Dice JF and Goff SA: Aging and the liver. *In* Arias IM, Jakoby WB, Popper H, et al (eds): The Liver: Biology and Pathobiology, 2nd ed. New York, Raven Press, 1988, p 1246.

70. Beers MH and Ouslander JG: Risk factors in geriatric drug prescribing: A practical guide to avoiding problems. Drugs 37:105–112, 1989.

71. Cusack BJ: Drug metabolism in the elderly. J Clin Pharmacol 28:571–576, 1988.

72. Fillastre J-P and Singlas E: Pharmacokinetics of newer drugs in patients with renal impairment: I. Clin Pharmacokinet 20(4):293–310, 1991.

73. Yuen GJ: Altered pharmacokinetics in the elderly. Clin Geriatr Med 6(2):1990.

74. McInnes GT and Brodie MJ: Drug interactions that matter: A critical appraisal. Drugs 36:83–110, 1988.

75. Gugler R and Allgayer H: Effects of antacids on the clinical pharmacokinetics of drugs: An update. Clin Pharmacokinet 18(3):210–219, 1990.

76. Shearn MA: Nonsteroidal anti-inflammatory agents; nonopiate analgesics; drugs used in gout. *In* Katzung BG (ed): Basic and Clinical Pharmacology. Los Altos, CA, Lange Medical Publications, 1982, pp 369–386.

77. Day RO, Graham GG, Champion GD, and Lee E: Anti-rheumatic drug interactions. Clin Rheum Dis 10:251–275, 1984.

78. Webster J: Interactions of NSAIDs with diuretics and beta-blockers: Mechanisms and clinical implications. Drugs 30:32–41, 1985.

79. Oates JA, FitzGerald GA, Branch RA, et al: Clinical implications of prostaglandin and thromboxane A₂ formation (part 2). N Engl J Med. 319(N 12):761–767, 1988.

80. Sweeney KR, Chapron DJ, Antal EJ, and Kramer PA: Differential effects of flurbiprofen and aspirin on acetazolamide disposition in humans. Br J Clin Pharmacol 27:866–869, 1989.

81. Zarfin Y, Koren G, Maresky D, et al: Possible indomethacin-aminoglycoside interaction in preterm infants. J Pediatr 106:511–513, 1985.

82. Needs CJ and Brooks PM: Clinical pharmacokinetics of the salicylates. Clin Pharmacokinet 10:164–177, 1985.

83. Roth SH: Salicylates revisited. Drugs 36:1–6, 1988.

84. Taylor BJ and Dufill MB: Pseudoporphyria from nonsteroidal anti-inflammatory drugs. N Z Med J 100:322–323, 1987.

85. Van De Putte LBA, Hegt VN, and Overbeek TE: Activators and inhibitors of fibrinolysis in rheumatoid and nonrheumatoid synovial membranes. Arthritis Rheum 20:671–678, 1977.

86. Weiss B and Hait WN: Selective cyclic nucleotide phosphodiesterase inhibitors as potential therapeutic agents. Ann Rev Pharmacol Toxicol 17:441–477, 1977.

87. Hart FD and Huskisson EC: Non-steroidal anti-inflammatory drugs: Current status and rational therapeutic use. Drugs 27:232–255, 1984.

88. Correia MA and Castagnoli N: Pharmacokinetics: II. Drug biotransformation. *In* Katzung BG (ed): Basic and Clinical Pharmacology, Los Altos, CA, Lange Medical Publications, 1982, p 39.

89. Simon LE and Mills JA: Nonsteroidal anti-inflammatory drugs: II. N Engl J Med 302:1237–1243, 1980.

90. Kroop SF and Simon LS: Current pharmacologic therapy of arthritis. Compr Ther 15(1):55–66, 1989.

91. Abernathy DR and Greenblatt DJ: Ibuprofen disposition in obese individuals. Arthritis Rheum 28:1117–1121, 1985.

92. Greenblatt DJ, Abernathy DR, Matlis R, et al: Absorption and disposition of ibuprofen in the elderly. Arthritis Rheum 27:1066–1069, 1984.

93. Ling TL, Yee JP, Cohen A, et al: A multiple-dose pharmacokinetic comparison of naproxen as a once-daily controlled-release tablet and a twice-daily conventional tablet. J Clin Pharmacol 27:325–329, 1987.

94. Rothenberg RJ and Sufit RL: Drug-induced peripheral neuropathy in a patient with psoriatic arthritis. Arthritis Rheum 30:221–224, 1987.

95. Van De Ouweland FA, Franssen MJAM, Van De Putte LBA, et al: Naproxen pharmacokinetics in patients with rheumatoid arthritis during active polyarticular inflammation. Br J Clin Pharmacol 23:189–193, 1987.

96. Van De Ouweland FA, Grabnau FWJ, Tan Y, et al: Hypoalbuminemia and naproxen in a patient with rheumatoid arthritis. Clin Pharmacokinet 11:511–515, 1986.

97. Ceuppens JL, Robaeys G, Verdicdt W, et al: Immunoregulatory effects of treatment with naproxen in patients with rheumatic disease. Arthritis Rheum 29:305–311, 1986.

98. Furst DE, Blocka K, Cassell S, et al: A controlled study of concurrent therapy with a nonacetylated salicylate and naproxen in rheumatoid arthritis. Arthritis Rheum 30:146–154, 1987.

99. Stewart CF, Fleming RA, Arkin CR, et al: Coadministration of naproxen and low-dose methotrexate in patients with rheumatoid arthritis. Clin Pharmacol Ther 47:540–546, 1990.

100. Gall EP, Caperton EM, McComb JE, et al: Clinical comparison of ibuprofen, fenoprofen calcium, naproxen, and tolmetin sodium in rheumatoid arthritis. J Rheumatol 9:402–407, 1982.

101. Wasner C, Britton MC, Kraines RG, et al: Nonsteroidal anti-inflammatory agents in rheumatoid arthritis and ankylosing spondylitis. JAMA 246:2168–2172, 1981.

102. Todd PA and Heel RC: Suprofen: A review of its pharmacodynamic and pharmacokinetic properties, and analgesic efficacy. Drugs 30:514–538, 1985.

103. Hart D, Ward M, Lifschitz MD, et al: Suprofen-related nephrotoxicity. Ann Intern Med 106:235–238, 1987.

104. Friedman H, Seckman CE, Schwartz JH, et al: The effects of flurbiprofen, aspirin, cimetidine, and antacids on the gastric and duodenal mucosa on normal volunteers: An endoscopic and photographic study. J Clin Pharmacol 29:559–562, 1989.

105. Small RE, Cox SR, and Adams WJ: Influence of H_2 receptor antagonists on the disposition of flurbiprofen enantiomers. J Clin Pharmacol 30:660–664, 1990.

106. Brooks CD, Linet OI, Schellenberg D, et al: Clinical safety of flurbiprofen. J Clin Pharmacol 30:342–351, 1990.

107. Enevoldson TP and Wiles CM: Acute parkinsonism associated with flurbiprofen. Br J Med 300(6723):540–541, 1991.

108. Newrick PG and Bainton D: Benoxaprofen—Adverse reactions and monitoring in general practice. Br J Clin Pharmacol 23:195–198, 1987.

109. Webster GR, Kaidley KH, and Kligman AM: Phototoxicity from benoxaprofen: In vivo and in vitro studies. Photochem Photobiol 36:59–64, 1982.

110. Muir H, de Vries SL, and Hall LG: Effects of tiaprofenic acid and other NSAIDs on proteoglycan metabolism in articular cartilage explants. Drugs 35(Suppl 1):15–23, 1988.

111. de Vries BJ, van den Berg WB, Vitters E, et al: Effects of NSAIDs on the metabolism of sulphated glycosaminoglycans in healthy and (post) arthritic murine articular cartilage. Drugs 35(Suppl 1):24–32, 1988.

112. Shinmei M, Kikuchi T, Masuda K, et al: Effects of interleukin-1 and anti-inflammatory drugs on the degradation of human articular cartilage. Drugs 35(Suppl 1):33–41, 1988.

113. Fameay JP: Introductory lecture: Symposium on the therapeutic aspects of tiaprofenic acid. Drugs 35(Suppl 1):1–3, 1988.

114. Warrington SJ, Dana-Haeri J, Horton MA, et al: Comparison on gastrointestinal blood loss in healthy male volunteers during repeated administration of standard and sustained action tiaprofenic acid and sustained release indomethacin. Drugs 35(Suppl 1):90–94, 1988.

115. Ishioka T: Is tiaprofenic acid different from other NSAIDs with regard to effects on renal function in the elderly? Drugs 35(Suppl 1):95–100, 1988.

116. Nagaya T, Niwa S, Harada S, et al: Efficacy and tolerance of tiaprofenic acid during long term administration to rheumatoid arthritis patients. Drugs 35(Suppl 1):101–106, 1988.

117. Nichol FE, Samanta A, and Rose CM: Synovial fluid and plasma kinetics of repeat dose sustained action tiaprofenic acid in patients with rheumatoid arthritis. Drugs 35(Suppl 1):46–51, 1988.

118. Miller LG and Bowman RC: Selective effect of diclofenac in the treatment of osteoarthritis versus dysmenorrhea. J Clin Pharmacol 30:378–379, 1990.

119. Carson J: Colonic ulceration and bleeding during diclofenac therapy [Letter]. N Engl J Med 323(2):135, 1990.

120. Tweedie DG: Unusual reaction to diclofenac [Letter]. Anesthesia 44(11):932, 1989.

121. Duncan JJ and Farr JE: Comparison of diclofenac sodium and aspirin in the treatment of acute sports injuries. Am J Sports Med 16(6):656–659, 1988.

122. Brogden RN, Heel RC, Speight TM, et al: Piroxicam: A reappraisal of its pharmacology and therapeutic efficacy. Drugs 28:292–323, 1984.

123. Wisemam H and Boyle JA: Piroxicam (Feldene). Clin Rheum Dis 6(3):585–613, 1980.

124. Hobbs DC: Piroxicam pharmacokinetics: Recent clinical trials relating kinetics and plasma levels to age, sex, adverse effects. Am J Med 81(Suppl 5B):22–28, 1986.

125. Rugstad HE: The Norway study: Plasma concentrations, efficacy, and adverse events. Am J Med 81(Suppl 5B):11–14, 1986.

126. Zizic TM, Sutton JD, and Stevens MB: A long-term evaluation of the treatment of osteoarthritis. Am J Med 81(Suppl 5B):29–35, 1986.

127. Somerville K, Faulkner G, and Langman M: Non-steroidal anti-inflammatory drugs and bleeding peptic ulcers. Lancet 1:462–464, 1986.

128. Bortnichak EA and Sachs RM: Piroxicam in recent epidemiologic studies. Am J Med 81(Suppl 5B):44–48, 1986.

129. Meisel AD: Clinical benefits and comparative safety of piroxicam: Analysis of worldwide clinical trials data. Am J Med 81(Suppl 5B):15–21, 1986.

130. Husby G: The Norwegian multi-center study. Am J Med 81(Suppl 5B):6–10, 1986.

131. Belcon MC, Haynes RB, and Tugwell P: A critical review of compliance studies in rheumatoid arthritis. Arthritis Rheum 27:1227–1233, 1984.

132. Day RO, Williams KM, Graham S, et al: The pharmacokinetics of total and unbound concentrations of tenoxicam in synovial fluid and plasma. Arthritis Rheum 34(6):751–760, 1991.

133. Pruss TP, Stroßnig H, Radhofer-Welte S, et al: Overview of the pharmacological properties, pharmacokinetics and animal safety assessment of lornoxicam. Postgrad Med J 66(Suppl 4):S18–S21, 1990.

134. Hitzenberger G, Radhofer-Welte S, Takacs F, et al: Pharmacokinetics of lornoxicam in man. Postgrad Med J 66(Suppl 4):S22–S26, 1990.

135. Turner P and Johnston A: Clinical pharmacokinetic studies with lornoxicam. Postgrad Med J 66(Suppl 4):S28–S29, 1990.

136. Ravic M, Johnston A, and Turner P: Clinical pharmacologic studies of some possible interactions of lornoxicam with other drugs. Postgrad Med J 66(Suppl 4):S30–S34, 1990.

137. Berry H and Ollier S: Lornoxicam in clinical practice. Postgrad Med J 66(Suppl 4):S41–S45, 1990.

138. Warrington SJ, Lewis Y, Dawnay A, et al: Renal and gastrointestinal tolerability of lornoxicam, and effects on haemostasis and hepatic microsomal oxidation. Postgrad Med J 66(Suppl 4):S35–S40, 1990.

139. Friedel HA and Todd PA: Nambutone: A preliminary review of its pharmacodynamic and pharmacokinetic properties and therapeutic efficacy in rheumatic diseases. Drugs 35:504–524, 1988.

140. Mangan FR, Flack JD, and Jackson D: Preclinical overview of nambutone: Pharmacology, bioavailability, metabolism, and toxicology. Am J Med 83(Suppl 4B):6–10, 1987.

141. Schrader HW, Buscher G, Dierdorf D, et al: Nambutone—A novel anti-inflammatory drug: Bioavailability after different dosage regimens. Int J Clin Pharmacol 22:672–676, 1984.

142. Miehlke RK, Schneider S, Sorgel F, et al: Penetration of the active metabolite of nambutone into synovial fluid and adherent tissue of patients undergoing knee joint surgery. Drugs 40(Suppl 5):57–61, 1990.

143. Dandona P and Jeremy JY: Nonsteroidal anti-inflammatory drug therapy and gastric side effects. Drugs 40(Suppl 5):16–24, 1990.

144. Lussier A and LeBel E: Radiochromium (chromium-51) evaluation of gastrointestinal blood loss associated with placebo, aspirin, and nambutone. Am J Med 83(Suppl 4B):15–18, 1987.

145. Greb WH, von Schrader HW, Cerlek S, et al: Endoscopic studies of nambutone in patients with rheumatoid arthritis. Am J Med 83(Suppl 4B):19–24, 1987.

146. Roth SH: Endoscopy-controlled study of the safety of nambutone compared with naproxen in arthritis therapy. Am J Med 83(Suppl 4B):25–30, 1987.

147. Boelaert JR, Jonnaert HA, Daneels RF, et al: Nambutone pharmacokinetics in patients with varying degrees of renal impairment. Am J Med 83(Suppl 4B):107–109, 1987.

148. McMahon FG, Vargas R, Ryan JR, et al: Nambutone kinetics in the young and elderly. Am J Med 83(Suppl 4B):92–95, 1987.

149. Lanier BG, Turner RA, Collins RL, et al: Evaluation of nambutone in the treatment of active adult rheumatoid arthritis. Am J Med 83(Suppl 4B):40–43, 1987.

150. Bernhard GC, Appelrouth DJ, Bankhurst AD, et al: Long-term treatment of rheumatoid arthritis comparing nambutone to aspirin. Am J Med 83(Suppl 4B):44–49, 1987.

151. Brobyn RD: Nambutone in the treatment of active adult rheumatoid arthritis. Am J Med 83(Suppl 4B):50–54, 1987.

152. Blechman WJ: Nambutone therapy of osteoarthritis: A six-week placebo-controlled study. Am J Med 83(Suppl 4B):70–73, 1987.

153. Jenner PN: Nambutone in the treatment of skin and soft tissue injury. Am J Med 83(Suppl 4B):101–106, 1987.

154. Blackburn WD, Loose LD, Heck LW, et al: Tenidap, in contrast to several available nonsteroidal anti-inflammatory drugs, potently inhibits the release of activated neutrophil collagenase. Arthritis Rheum 34(2):211–216, 1991.

155. Robinson C: Tenidap sodium. Drugs Future 15(9):898–900, 1990.

156. Bunch TW and O'Duffy JD: Disease-modifying drugs for progressive rheumatoid arthritis. Mayo Clin Proc 55:161–179, 1980.

157. Adams LM, Yocum DE, and Bell CL: Hydroxychloroquine in the treatment of rheumatoid arthritis. Am J Med 75:321–326, 1983.

158. Bunch TW, O'Duffy JD, Tompkins RB, et al: Controlled trial of hydroxychloroquine and D-penicillamine singly and in combination in the treatment of rheumatoid arthritis. Arthritis Rheum 27:267–276, 1984.

159. Wolfe CS and Hughes GRV: The optimum management of arthropathies. Drugs 36:370–381, 1988.

160. Blocka KLN, Paulus HE, and Furst DE: Clinical pharmacokinetics of oral and injectable gold compounds. Clin Pharmacokinet 11:133–143, 1986.

161. Goldenberg DL and Cohen AS: Gold. *In* Goldenberg DL and Cohen AS (eds): Drugs in the Rheumatic Diseases. Orlando, FL, Grune & Stratton, 1986, pp 33–41.

162. Littman BH and Hall RE: Effects of gold sodium thiomalate on functional correlates of human monocyte maturation. Arthritis Rheum 28:1384–1392, 1986.

163. Spalding DM, Darby WL, and Heck LW: Alterations in macrophage secretion induced by gold sodium thiomalate. Arthritis Rheum 29:75–81, 1986.

164. Hanly JG, Hassan J, Whelan A, et al: Effects of gold therapy on the synthesis and quantity of serum and synovial fluid IgM, IgG, and IgA rheumatoid factors in rheumatoid arthritis patients. Arthritis Rheum 29:480–487, 1986.

165. Furst DE, Levine S, Srinivasan R, et al: A double-blind trial of high versus conventional doses of gold salts for rheumatoid arthritis. Arthritis Rheum 20:1473–1480, 1977.

166. Dugowson CE and Gilliand BC: Management of rheumatoid arthritis. DM 32(1):1–74, 1986.

167. Dahl SL, Coleman MI, Williams HJ, et al: Lack of correlation between blood gold concentrations and clinical response in patients with definite or classic rheumatoid arthritis receiving auranofin or gold sodium thiomalate. Arthritis Rheum 28:1211–1218, 1985.

168. Abruzzo JL: Auranofin: A new drug for rheumatoid arthritis. Arthritis Rheum 28:1117–1121, 1986.

169. Hochberg MC: Auranofin or D-penicillamine in the treatment of rheumatoid arthritis. Ann Intern Med 105:528–535, 1986.

170. Bombardier C, Ware J, Russell IJ, et al: Auranofin therapy and the quality of life in patients with rheumatoid arthritis. Am J Med 81:565–578, 1986.

171. Kean WF and Anastassiades TP: Long-term chrysotherapy. Arthritis Rheum 22:495–501, 1979.

172. Cheson BD, Cleeg DO, and Moatamed F: Ultrastructural evidence for persistent gold in the bone marrow of a patient with aplastic anemia. Arthritis Rheum 29:128–132, 1986.

173. Barger BO, Acton RT, Koopman WJ, et al: DR antigens and gold toxicity in white rheumatoid arthritis patients. Arthritis Rheum 27:601–605, 1984.

174. Coblyn JS, Weinblatt M, Holdsworth D, et al: Gold-induced thrombocytopenia. Ann Intern Med 95:178–181, 1981.

175. Nusslein HG, Jahn H, Losch G, et al: Association of HLA-Bw35 with mucocutaneous lesions in rheumatoid arthritis patients undergoing sodium urothiomalate therapy. Arthritis Rheum 27:833–836, 1984.

176. O'Duffy JD, Luthra HS, Unni KK, et al: Bronchiolitis in a rheumatoid arthritis patient receiving auranofin. Arthritis Rheum 29:556–559, 1986.

177. Lowthian PJ, Cleland LG, and Vernon-Roberts B: Hepatotoxicity with aurothioglucose therapy. Arthritis Rheum 27:230–232, 1984.

178. Halla JT, Hardin JG, and Linn JE: Postinjection vasomotor reactions during chrysotherapy. Arthritis Rheum 20:1188–1191, 1977.

179. O'Duffy JD, O'Fallon WM, Hunder GG, et al: An attempt to predict the response to gold therapy in rheumatoid arthritis. Arthritis Rheum 27:1210–1217, 1984.

180. Muijsers AO, Van De Stadt RJ, Henrichs AMA, et al: D-Penicillamine in patients with rheumatoid arthritis. Arthritis Rheum 27:1362–1369, 1984.

181. Tsang IK, Patterson CA, Stein HB, et al: D-Penicillamine in the treatment of rheumatoid arthritis. Arthritis Rheum 20:666–670, 1977.

182. Shiokawa Y, Horiuchi Y, Honma M, et al: Clinical evaluation of D-penicillamine by multicentric double-blind comparative study in chronic rheumatoid arthritis. Arthritis Rheum 20:1464–1472, 1977.

183. Hearn J and Tiliakos NA: Myasthenia gravis caused by penicillamine and chloroquine therapy for rheumatoid arthritis. South Med J 79:1185–1186, 1986.

184. Wilke WS and Mackenzie AH: Methotrexate therapy in rheumatoid arthritis: Current status. Drugs 32:103–113, 1986.

185. Jolivet J, Cowan KH, Curt GA, et al: The pharmacology and clinical use of methotrexate. N Engl J Med 309:1094–1103, 1983.

186. Alarcon GS, Schrohenloher RE, Bartoloucci AA, et al: Suppression of rheumatoid factor production by methotrexate in patients with rheumatoid arthritis. Arthritis Rheum 33(8):1156–1161, 1990.

187. Segal R, Mozes E, Yaron M, et al: The effects of methotrexate on the production and activity of interleukin-1. Arthritis Rheum 32(4):370–377, 1989.

188. Olsen NJ and Murray LM: Antiproliferative effects of methotrexate on peripheral blood mononuclear cells. Arthritis Rheum 32(4):378–385, 1989.

189. Arnold M, Schrieber L, and Brooks P: Immunosuppressive drugs and corticosteroids in the treatment of rheumatoid arthritis. Drugs 36:340–363, 1988.

190. Williams HJ, Willkens RF, Samuelson CO, et al: Comparison of low-dose oral pulse methotrexate and placebo in the treatment of rheumatoid arthritis. Arthritis Rheum 28:721–730, 1985.

191. Kremer JM, Rynes RI, Bartholomew LE: Severe flare of rheumatoid arthritis after discontinuation of long-term methotrexate therapy. Am J Med 82:781–786, 1987.

192. Wernick R and Smith DL: Central nervous system toxicity associated with low-dose methotrexate treatment. Arthritis Rheum 32(6):770–775, 1989.

193. Weinblatt ME, Coblyn JS, Fraser PA, et al: Cyclosporin A treatment of refractory rheumatoid arthritis. Arthritis Rheum 30:11–17, 1987.

194. Ravel R: Clinical Laboratory Medicine, 5th ed. Chicago, Year Book Medical Publishers, 1989, p 10.

195. Morgan SL, Baggott JE, Vaughn WH, et al: The effect of folic acid supplementation on the toxicity of low-dose methotrexate in patients with rheumatoid arthritis. Arthritis Rheum 33(1):9–18, 1990.

196. Hamdy H, McKendry RJR, Mierins E, et al: Low-dose methotrexate compared with azathioprine in the treatment of rheumatoid arthritis. Arthritis Rheum 30:361–368, 1987.

197. Singh G, Fries JF, Spitz P, et al: Toxic effects of azathioprine in rheumatoid arthritis. Arthritis Rheum 32(7):837–843, 1989.

198. Paulus HE, Egger MJ, Ward JR, et al: Analysis of improvement in individual rheumatoid arthritis patients treated with disease-modifying antirheumatic drugs, based on findings in patients treated with placebo. Arthritis Rheum 33(4):477–484, 1990.

199. Dwosh IL, Stein HB, Urowitz MB, et al: Azathioprine in early rheumatoid arthritis. Arthritis Rheum 20:685–692, 1977.

200. Dugowsen CE and Gilliland BC: Management of Rheumatoid Arthritis. Chicago, Year Book Medical Publishers, 1986, p. 48.

201. Baker DG and Rabinowitz JL: Current concepts in the treatment of rheumatoid arthritis. J Clin Pharmacol 26:2–21, 1986.

202. Barnhart ER: Physicians Desk Reference, 41st ed. Oradell, NJ, Medical Economics, 1987.

203. Dougodos M and Amor B: Cyclosporin A in rheumatoid arthritis: Preliminary clinical results of an open trial. Arthritis Rheum 30:83–87, 1987.

204. Gray RG and Gottlieb NL: Intra-articular corticosteroids: An updated assessment. Clin Orthop 177:235–263, 1983.

205. Klotz U: Clinical pharmacokinetics of sulfasalazine, its metabolites and other prodrugs of 5-aminosalacylic acid. Clin Pharmacokinet 10:285–302, 1985.

206. Pinals RS, Kaplan SB, and Lawson JG: Sulfasalazine in rheumatoid arthritis. Arthritis Rheum 29:1427–1434, 1986.

207. Wolfe CS and Hughes GRV: The optimum management of arthropathies. Drugs 36:370–381, 1988.

208. Runge LA, Pinals RS, Lourie SH, et al: Treatment of rheumatoid arthritis with levamisole. Arthritis Rheum 20:1445–1448, 1977.

209. Fauci AS and Young KR Jr: Immunoregulatory agents. *In* Kelley WN, Harris ED, Ruddy S, et al (eds): Textbook of Rheumatology, Vol I, 3rd ed, Philadelphia, WB Saunders, 1989, p. 881.

210. Kremer JM, Jubiz W, Michalek A, et al: Fish-oil fatty acid supplementation in active rheumatoid arthritis. Ann Intern Med 106(4):497–503, 1987.

211. Kremer JM, Lawrence DA, Jubiz W, et al: Dietary fish oil and olive oil supplementation in patients with rheumatoid arthritis. Arthritis Rheum 33(6):810–820, 1990.

212. Lippiello L, Feinhold M, and Grandjean C: Metabolic and ultrastructural changes in articular cartilage of rats fed dietary supplements of omega-3 fatty acids. Arthritis Rheum 33(7):1029–1036, 1990.

213. Malkinson FD: Colchicine: New uses of an old, old drug. Arch Dermatol 118:453–457, 1982.

214. Becker MA: Clinical aspects of monosodium urate monohydrate crystal deposition disease (gout). Rheum Clin North Am 14(2):377–394, 1988.

215. Paulus HE: Nonsteroidal anti-inflammatory drugs. *In* Kelley WN, Harris ED, Ruddy S, et al (eds): Textbook of Rheumatology, Vol I, 3rd ed. Philadelphia, WB Saunders, 1989, p 769.

216. Moreland LW, and Ball GV: Colchicine and gout [Editorial]. Arthritis Rheum 34(6):782–786, 1991.

217. Neuss MN, McCallum RM, Brenckman WD, et al: Long-term colchicine administration leading to colchicine toxicity and death. Arthritis Rheum 29(3):448–449, 1986.

218. Wallace SL and Singer JZ: Therapy in gout. Rheum Dis Clin North Am 14(2):441–457, 1988.

219. Schumacher HR, Klippel JH, and Robinson DR (eds): Mediators of inflammation. *In* Primer on the Rheumatic Diseases, 9th ed. Atlanta, Arthritis Foundation, 1988, p 205.

220. Arie E and Doherty M: Crystal-associated rheumatic disease: Current management considerations. Drugs 37:566–576, 1989.

221. Murrell GAC and Rapeport WG: Clinical pharmacokinetics of allopurinol. Clin Pharmacokinet 11:343–353, 1986.

222. Chawla SK, Patel HD, Parrino GR, et al: Allopurinol hepatotoxicity. Arthritis Rheum 20:1546–1549, 1977.

223. Singer JZ and Wallace SL: The allopurinol hypersensitivity syndrome: Unnecessary morbidity and mortality. Arthritis Rheum 29(1):82–87, 1986.

224. Webster E and Panush RS: Allopurinol hypersensitivity in a patient with severe, chronic, tophaceous gout. Arthritis Rheum 28:707–709, 1985.

225. Kelley WN and Fox I: Antihyperuricemic agents. *In* Kelley WN, Harris ED, Ruddy S, et al: Textbook of Rheumatology. Philadelphia, WB Saunders, 1989, p 898.

226. Webster J: Interactions of NSAIDs with diuretics and beta-blockers: Mechanisms and clinical implications. Drugs 30:32–41, 1985.

227. Harris ED: Pathogenesis of rheumatoid arthritis: A disorder associated with dysfunctional immunoregulation. *In* Gallin JI, Goldstein IM, and Snyderman R (eds): Inflammation: Basic Principles and Clinical Correlates. New York, Raven Press, 1988, pp 753–754.

228. Aire E and Doherty M: Crystal-associated rheumatic disease: Current management considerations. Drugs 37:566–576, 1989.

229. Rook G, Lydyard P, and Stanford J: Mycobacteria and rheumatoid arthritis. Arthritis Rheum 33(3):431–435, 1990.

230. Pope RM, Pahlavani MA, LaCour E, et al: Antigenic specificity of rheumatoid synovial fluid lymphocytes. Arthritis Rheum 32(11):1371–1380, 1989.

231. Schwartz BD: Infectious agents, immunity, and rheumatic diseases. Arthritis Rheum 33(4):457–465, 1990.

232. Naides SJ, Scharoch LL, Foto F, et al: Rheumatologic manifestations of human parvovirus B19 infection in adults. Arthritis Rheum 33(9):1297–1309, 1990.

233. Spector TD, Roman E, and Silman AJ: The pill, parity, and rheumatoid arthritis. Arthritis Rheum 33(6):782–789, 1990.

234. Hernandez-Avila M, Liang MH, Willett WC, et al: Exogenous sex hormones and the risk of rheumatoid arthritis. Arthritis Rheum 33(7):370–377, 1990.

235. McCuster CT, Reid B, Green D, et al: HLA-D antigens in patients with rheumatoid arthritis. Arthritis Rheum 34(2):192–197, 1991.

236. Schumacher HR, Klippel JH, and Robinson DR (eds): Mediators of inflammation. *In* Primer on the Rheumatic Diseases, 9th ed. Atlanta, Arthritis Foundation, 1988, pp 84–85.

237. Harris ED: Pathogenesis of rheumatoid arthritis: A disorder associated with dysfunctional immunoregulation. *In* Gallin JI, Goldstein IM, and Snyderman R (eds): Inflammation: Basic Principles and Clinical Correlates. New York, Raven Press, 1988, pp 755.

238. Carson DA: Rheumatoid factor. *In* Kelley WN, Harris ED, Ruddy S, et al (eds): Textbook of Rheumatology, Vol I, 3rd ed. Philadelphia, WB Saunders, 1989, p. 198.

239. Harris ED: Rheumatoid arthritis: Pathophysiology and implications for therapy. N Engl J Med 322(18):1277–1287, 1990.

240. Healy LA and Wilske KR: Reforming the pyramid: A plan for treating rheumatoid arthritis. Rheum Dis Clin North Am 15(3):615–620, 1989.

241. Breedveld FC, Dijkmans BA, and Mattie H: Minocycline treatment for rheumatoid arthritis: An open dose-finding study. J Rheumatol 17(1):43–46, 1990.

242. Nojima T, Towle CA, Mankin HJ, et al: Secretion of higher levels of active proteoglycanases from human osteoarthritic chondrocytes. Arthritis Rheum 29(2):292–295, 1986.

243. Schumacher HR, Klippel JH, and Robinson DR (eds): Mediators of inflammation. *In* Primer on the Rheumatic Diseases, 9th ed. Atlanta, Arthritis Foundation, 1988, pp 172–173.

244. Terkeltaub R, Zachariae K, Santoro D, et al: Monocyte-derived neutrophil chemotactic factor/interleukin-8 is a potential mediator of crystal-induced inflammation. Arthritis Rheum 34(7):894–903, 1991.

245. Terkeltaub RA and Ginsberg MH: The inflammatory reaction to crystals. Rheum Dis Clin North Am 14(2):353–364, 1988.

246. Guerne P-A, Terkeltaub R, Zuraw B, et al: Inflammatory microcrystals stimulate interleukin-6 production and secretion by human monocytes and synoviocytes. Arthritis Rheum 32(11):1443–1452, 1989.

247. Diamond HS: Control of crystal-induced arthropies. Rheum Dis Clin North Am 15(3):557–567, 1989.

248. Harris ED: The clinical features of rheumatoid arthritis. *In* Kelley WN, Harris ED, Ruddy S, et al (eds): Textbook of rheumatology, V I, 3rd ed. Philadelphia, WB Saunders, 1989, pp 950–951.

249. Schumacher HR, Klippel JH, and Robinson DR (eds): Mediators of inflammation. *In* Primer on the Rheumatic Diseases, 9th ed. Atlanta, Arthritis Foundation, 1988, p 142.

Glucocorticoids: Use in the Management of Rheumatic Disorders

Richard D. Roth, D.P.M.

An adrenal gland sits on top of each of the two kidneys in humans. The clinical syndrome resulting from destruction of these glands, and bearing his name, was initially described by Addison in 1855.[1] Subsequent decades of research have proved that the adrenal glands are essential for the maintenance of human life. In 1932, Cushing published the first clinical description of the syndrome associated with excessive production of adrenocortical agents.[2] By the 1940s, 28 steroid structures had been isolated from the adrenal cortex. Hydrocortisone (cortisol), cortisone, corticosterone, 11-dehydrocorticosterone, and 11-desoxycortisol were five of these agents found to be biologically active.[3]

In the late 1920s, patients with symptomatic rheumatic disorders were noted to have marked clinical improvement during pregnancy or when they became jaundiced.[4] Cortisone became available 20 years later in sufficient quantities to allow for clinical testing. Its initial administration to a patient with rheumatoid arthritis by Hench in 1949 resulted in dramatic relief of clinical signs and symptoms of inflammatory arthritis.[4] The following year, Hench shared the Nobel Prize in medicine for this discovery. Decades of subsequent research have substantiated the dramatic therapeutic benefits that glucocorticoids offer in the management of inflammatory arthritis.

The active glucocorticoids produced by the adrenal cortex are shown in Figure 25–1. Cortisone is the parent compound of this group. Each adrenal gland normally produces about 16 mg/day of cortisone. This can increase from twofold to 15-fold during times of significant physiologic or psychological stress.[5]

The presence of cortisone, and especially of increased amounts of cortisone in the serum during periods of stress, is essential for maintenance of life-sustaining physiologic functions. Cortisone is not biologically active when it is produced by the adrenal cortex. It enters the adrenocortical blood vessels and is transported to the liver. Hydroxylation at the 11-carbon position in the liver creates the biologically active compound hydroxycortisone (see Fig. 25–1).

Decades of efficacious use of glucocorticoids in the management of inflammatory disorders have provided documentation that these agents are among the most beneficial classes of medications known. The issue of whether their use is appropriate in individual instances can be extremely complex. It requires consideration of potential interactions with other agents, physiologic effects, therapeutic limitations, toxicities, and side effects. Dramatic clinical efficacy and widespread use of glucocorticoids in the management of rheumatic disorders requires that any physician treating these disorders be familiar with their use.

SYSTEMIC GLUCOCORTICOID THERAPY

Systemic glucocorticoid therapy is associated with prolonged and profound physiologic alterations, a wide variety of metabolic effects, and numerous potential complications and side effects. Glucocorticoids have widespread influence on carbohydrate, fat, protein, and nucleic acid metabolism. Many of these compounds have significant effects on electrolyte balance and water retention.

Glucocorticoids induce breakdown of protein and fat to produce glucose. The initial administration of these agents to nondiabetic persons is followed by brief and temporary elevations in blood glucose levels that are normalized by compensatory increased insulin production. Administration of these agents to diabetic and prediabetic patients usually results in dramatic increases in serum glucose levels that may require an adjustment in the dosage or choice of oral or parenteral antihyperglycemic medications. In many patients, prolonged administration of glucocorticoids can induce a diabetic state that is usually reversible on their discontinuation.[6, 7]

The presence of glucocorticoids is associated with simultaneously decreased protein synthesis and increased breakdown of proteins in peripheral tissues. Prolonged use of these agents is associated with cutaneous and subcutaneous atrophy, myopathy, osteoporosis, and prolonged wound healing.[8–10] Myopathy and disuse atrophy are seen in most chronic inflammatory arthropathies. Resultant weakness is often compounded by additional loss of muscle strength and mass secondary to therapeutic use of oral glucocorticoids.

Glucose uptake by fat cells is reduced in the presence of glucocorticoids. The combined presence of glucocorticoids

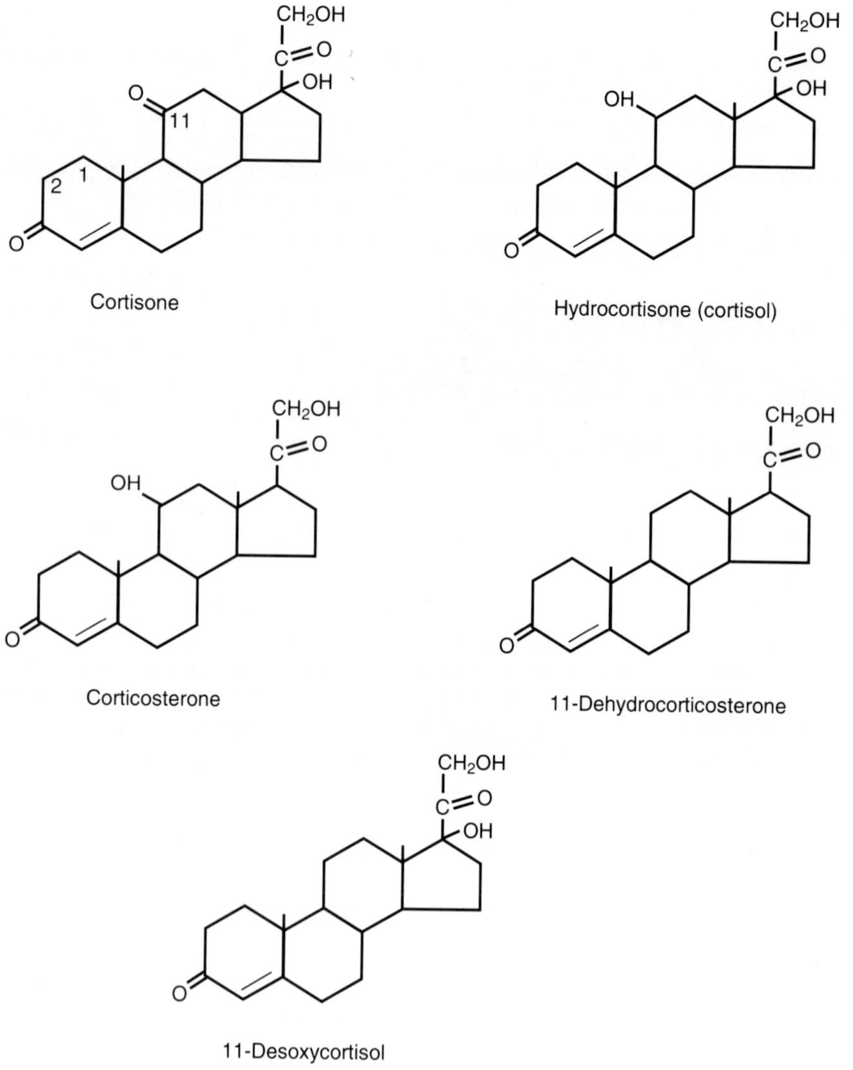

Cortisone

Hydrocortisone (cortisol)

Corticosterone

11-Dehydrocorticosterone

11-Desoxycortisol

FIGURE 25–1. The five natural adrenocortical glucocorticoids: cortisone, hydrocortisone, corticosterone, 11-dehydrocorticosterone, and 11-desoxycortisol.

and catecholamines (epinephrine or norepinephrine) induces breakdown of lipids within fat cells with resultant elevation in serum lipids (hyperlipoproteinemia). In the nondiabetic patient, the presence of insulin counteracts this effect, and significant elevations in serum lipid levels usually are not seen. In the diabetic patient receiving oral glucocorticoids, this effect usually results in dramatic increases in the levels of serum lipids and their byproducts. Glucocorticoids also inhibit production of deoxyribonucleic acid in muscle cells, fibroblasts, and lymphocytes.

The effects of prolonged glucocorticoid administration can also include decreased tensile strength in skin and healing wounds, delayed healing, reduced immunity to infection, and decreased ability to fight infection when it is already present.[11–13] Loss of muscle tissue mass and dramatic weakness may also be associated with their use. These agents also increase retention of sodium with bound water and simultaneously increase excretion of potassium from the kidneys, salivary glands, and sweat glands. Water retention associated with prolonged oral courses of glucocorticoids frequently results in edema that is most apparent in dependent areas.

Increased potassium excretion noted with these agents can be dangerous in patients with compromised cardiac status. This danger is often increased with concurrent use of potas-

sium-depleting antihypertensive medications.[14] It is also increased with vomiting, diarrhea, use of certain antibiotics (gentamicin, carbenicillin, and amphotericin B), and concurrent therapy with insulin or vitamin B_{12}. A patient with concurrent conditions causing potassium depletion who is receiving oral glucocorticoid therapy should be advised of the signs and symptoms of hypokalemia, should have serum potassium closely monitored, and usually should receive potassium supplementation. Signs and symptoms of hypokalemia include bradycardia, cardiac arrhythmia, and weakness or paralysis of striated, smooth, and cardiac muscle.

Because systemic glucocorticoid therapy alters metabolism at the cellular level, all body systems can be affected in its presence. The myriad potential adverse reactions that may be seen with prolonged oral glucocorticoid therapy are reviewed in Table 25–1.

A patient may show any combination of the above findings while on glucocorticoid therapy. The longer such therapy continues, the greater the number and severity of side effects that usually are noted. Many of these complications warrant special consideration of physicians concentrating their efforts in management of rheumatic disorders of the lower extremities. Marked cutaneous atrophy can simultaneously increase the need for protective padding and shielding and increase

TABLE 25–1

**POTENTIAL COMPLICATIONS THAT MAY BE NOTED IN ASSOCIATION WITH
SYSTEMIC GLUCOCORTICOID THERAPY**

Cutaneous
  Acne, facial erythema, cutaneous and subcutaneous atrophy, violaceous striae, petechiae, purpura, ecchymosis, tendency toward excessive bruising, capillary fragility, impaired wound healing, abnormal hairiness (primarily in male-patterned distribution), and subcutaneous panniculitis (potentially noted on steroid withdrawal)
Ophthalmic
  Posterior subcapsular cataracts, glaucoma, exophthalmos, ocular infections
Central nervous system
  Headache, increased intracranial pressure, euphoria, depression, changes in mood and/or personality, psychosis, convulsions
Musculoskeletal
  Growth retardation (children, adolescents), weakness, muscle atrophy, myalgias, osteoporosis, joint instability, pathologic fractures, delayed fracture healing, aseptic necrosis of bone
Gastrointestional
  Abdominal pain, stomach ulcerations, gastrointestinal hemorrhage, pancreatitis, spontaneous viscus hemorrhage
Cardiovascular
  Water retention, dependent edema, hypertension, bradycardia, cardiac arrhythmias, congestive heart failure, capillary fragility, thromboembolism, vasculitis, accelerated arteriosclerosis
Endocrine and metabolic
  Growth retardation or arrest (children, adolescents), impotence, changes in menses (including amenorrhea), hyperglycemia, impaired glucose tolerance, hyperlipoproteinemia, truncal obesity, facial (moon facies), posterior cervical (buffalo hump) and supraclavicular (shoulder pad) fat accumulations, hypokalemia (with cardiac, striated, and smooth muscle weakness or paralysis), diabetes, renal stone formation
Immune
  Increased susceptibility to infections, decreased ability to fight infections once present, decreased inflammatory response, increased peripheral neutrophils, decreased peripheral monocytes and lymphocytes, delayed graft rejections

---

the danger of use of adhesives on thin and friable skin. Skin atrophy, dependent edema, increased risk of infection, and poor dermal healing capacities warrant careful consideration and planning of surgical incisions in the lower extremities of patients receiving these medications. Use of prophylactic antibiotics in perioperative periods and meticulous frequent postoperative wound observation, evaluation, and redressings similarly are warranted.[15] Judicious use and application of adhesive bandages, braces, and casts and use of extra padding, cushioning, and shock-absorptive materials are advisable.

Myopathy and osteoporosis that may be associated with both rheumatic diseases and oral glucocorticoid regimens used in controlling them need to be considered in establishing reasonable and realistic therapeutic goals. These factors can substantially limit the types and rates of rehabilitative measures that can be undertaken safely. The potential for aseptic necrosis of bone mandates meticulous, minimally traumatic surgical tissue handling, limited dissection, and careful planning of any osteotomies in any surgical interventions.[16]

Occasionally, patients on oral glucocorticoid regimens complain of bone pain in the absence of notable trauma, excessive strain, or unusual stress. In such patients, a high index of suspicion should exist with regard to stress fractures, especially in the areas of the central lesser metatarsal heads. Patients on prolonged glucocorticoid therapy have an increased incidence of stress fractures. Occult fractures can be confirmed on triphasic bone scans.

Some patients receiving glucocorticoids may present with vasculitis. Although there is considerable disagreement on this topic in current medical literature, use of chronic glucocorticoid therapy has not been proven to induce or aggravate vasculitis. The presence of vasculitis generally contraindicates elective surgical procedures in the lower extremities. Because treatment of vasculitis customarily involves the use of glucocorticoids, patients already receiving these medications and presenting with clinical evidence of vasculitis usually have severe vascular disease resistant to accepted treatment approaches.

Clinical signs of vasculitis are described in detail in Chapters 7 and 12. They include target lesions, prominent subcutaneous vessels, digital subcutaneous hematomas, periungual hematomas, punctate ulcerations, and gangrene. The increased tendency of patients on oral glucocorticoids to have thromboembolic episodes warrants close postoperative observation for signs and symptoms of phlebitis; ambulation should begin at the earliest reasonable opportunity. Decreased resistance to, and ability to fight, infections warrants use of perioperative prophylactic antibiotics. Bactericidal antibiotics should be used in preference to bacteriostatic antibiotics whenever possible in those receiving oral glucocorticoid therapy.[12, 15]

The present medicolegal climate mandates that informed consent be ensured before any invasive diagnostic or therapeutic procedure is performed. Physicians performing these procedures on patients with inflammatory arthritis controlled with oral glucocorticoid therapy must be acutely aware of the mood and personality alterations, and even psychoses, that may be associated with use of these agents. When possible, family members and other responsible people involved in the patients' lives should be included in the decision-making process preceding these procedures to help ensure that every reasonable effort has been made to obtain such informed consent.[17]

The widespread side effects, toxicities, and complications that are seen with prolonged oral glucocorticoid therapy require that minimal effective doses be used and treatment be confined to the shortest feasible time period. Any patient who has received more than 20 to 30 mg/day of prednisone (or equivalent) for more than 7 days in the previous 12 months must be considered to have adrenal suppression until proved otherwise.[18] A patient continuing to receive a dose in excess of 7.5 mg/day has to be similarly considered.[19] These patients

TABLE 25–2

SIGNS AND SYMPTOMS OF ADRENOCORTICAL (GLUCOCORTICOID) INSUFFICIENCY

Generalized weakness, exhaustion, disinclination toward mental or physical efforts, fever
Anorexia, nausea, vomiting, abdominal pain, weight loss, diarrhea
Hypotension, weak pulses
Irritability, confusion, delusions
Skin discolorations* most prominent at exposed areas (face, neck, arms, hands), points of pressure and friction; freckles; recently formed scars; creases in palms, nipples, and genitalia, appearing as a ''sun tan that doesn't wear off''; coloration may be tinged blue or gray, lips and oral mucosa with spots brown, blue, or gray in color

*Skin and mucosal discoloration are almost exclusively noted in the primary form of adrenocortical insufficiency (Addison's disease).

may be incapable of producing sufficient amounts of adrenocorticoids to meet the physiologic demands posed by significantly increased emotional or physical stress. Similar insufficiency states are noted with excessively rapid reductions in or tapering of oral steroid doses.

Signs and symptoms of adrenocortical insufficiency are shown in Table 25–2. The symptoms of both primary and secondary adrenocortical insufficiency are subtle and nonspecific in the unstressed patient. They include anorexia, nausea, vomiting, diarrhea, and abdominal pain. Hyperpigmentation or a bronze discoloration of skin may be noted in primary insufficiency, but it is rarely seen in the secondary form. In the presence of insufficiency, stress usually causes additive signs of hypotension, weakness, and fever.

Under normal circumstances, mild increases in stress, as seen with minor elective surgeries or influenza, are accompanied by twofold to threefold increases in endogenous adrenal glucocorticoid production, persisting as long as 3 days after the surgery is completed or the infection resolves. Patients receiving oral glucocorticoid therapy who evidence any symptoms of insufficiency with such stress should have their dosages increased to two to three times normal, especially if they have body temperatures in excess of 39°C for 2 to 3 days. Normalization of temperature is an indication to lower the dosage back to normal levels.[20] More severe stress, as is seen with major surgery, can cause normal adrenal glands to increase daily production of cortisol as much as 15 times normal for as long as 3 days after such surgery. Increased oral glucocorticoid coverage should be given beginning shortly before such surgery and extending until at least 3 days following it, with adjustments as necessary for infection or postoperative hemorrhage.[26]

A currently accepted and commonly used regimen for patients undergoing major surgical procedures is 100 mg of hydrocortisone sodium succinate, by intramuscular (IM) or intravenous (IV) route, followed by 100 mg every 8 hours until the patient's condition is stabilized.[20] Many other regimens for coverage have been proposed. Combined physical and emotional stress associated with a specific procedure in a particular patient is variable. Optimal management requires that perioperative glucocorticoid supplementation be individualized. Table 25–3 shows recommended regimens that are commonly employed in lower extremity surgery.[15] Regardless of the specific schedule of supplementation selected, when signs and symptoms of adrenal insufficiency become apparent postoperatively, additional supplementation should be prescribed.

Often, signs of adrenocortical insufficiency are obscured by the side effects anticipated from general anesthetics and injectable narcotic analgesics.[21] Postoperative anorexia, nausea, vomiting, and mild elevations in temperature are not uncommon. Postoperative diarrhea is fairly rare because patients have usually had nothing by mouth for 12 to 24 hours before surgery. Sustained postoperative hypotension, temperature elevation, anorexia, nausea, and vomiting unrelated to narcotic analgesic administration should be considered potential signs of adrenocortical insufficiency. Additional signs of insufficiency may include dramatic systemic flares in inflammatory disease activity, tachycardia, irregularities in cardiac rate and rhythm, and even potential cardiac failure.[22, 23]

Even in the absence of anticipated increases in stress associated with therapeutic measures, signs of insufficiency may be seen during periods of substantially increased physical, occupational, avocational, and familial stress. They are often noted when oral dosages of steroids are being reduced too rapidly. Because the consequences of adrenocortical insufficiency can be serious and even fatal, and because the physician cannot constantly monitor every patient, all patients on oral glucocorticoids should be warned of the signs and symptoms that indicate insufficiency and the need to contact their physician or seek care in an emergency department if such symptoms occur. They should also be advised to carry a medical alert card or wear a bracelet or necklace indicating that they are receiving oral glucocorticoid therapy

TABLE 25–3

RECOMMENDED PERIOPERATIVE SUPPLEMENTAL GLUCOCORTICOID COVERAGE BASED ON SEVERITY OF ASSOCIATED LEVEL OF PHYSICAL AND MENTAL STRESS

Time Dose Given	Level of Stress			
	Minimal	Mild	Moderate	Severe
Day of surgery	M	M	M × 2	M or 50 mg HC
Morning of surgery	M	M	M × 2	100 mg HC
Intraoperatively	—	—	—	— to 100 mg HC/hr
Postoperatively	M	M	M	— to 100 mg HC
First postoperative day	M	M × 2	M × 2	M + 50 mg HC/q 8 hr*
Second postoperative day	M	M × 2	M × 2	M + 50 mg HC/q 12 hr*
Third postoperative day	M	M	M × 2	M*

*May substitute dose of 100 mg HC.
—, no dose given; M, daily maintenance dose; HC, hydrocortisone sodium succinate.
From Roth RD: The rheumatic patient: Medical considerations in foot surgery. *In* McGlamry ED (ed): Fundamentals of Foot Surgery, p 383. © 1987, the Williams & Wilkins Co., Baltimore.

and require supplementation during times of substantially increased stress.

Usually, elective surgical procedures should be postponed when related stress will be superimposed on tapering oral glucocorticoid doses and during times of substantially increased stress in a patient's life. Elective procedures should be undertaken cautiously for as long as 1 year after systemic use of significant amounts of exogenous steroids has been discontinued.[21] It is usually best to individualize additional glucocorticoid supplementation. Individual dosages and regimens should take into consideration the intraoperative physical trauma, the trauma of anticipated rehabilitation, relative psychological stress, amount and frequency of previous glucocorticoid intake, the agent received, signs or symptoms of previous insufficiency, and the stress present and anticipated in the patient's hospital and post-discharge environment. Because there is a period of several hours between the first supplemental dose and its apparent physiologic effects, dosing should begin at least 2 hours preoperatively.

A patient under long-standing control with 7.5 mg/day or less of prednisone who has no significant excessive stress in the home and work environment, has shown no signs of adrenocortical insufficiency, has a calm disposition, and who is anticipating foot surgery under local anesthesia usually needs minimal supplementation. Usually, administration of double the daily maintenance dose on the day of surgery and for 2 to 3 days following surgery provides sufficient supplemental coverage.[18] It is usually best to have a rheumatologist manage postoperative supplementation in patients when high-dose oral glucocorticoids are being used to control severe and disabling inflammatory disease.

Brief courses of oral steroids can be used in managing traumatic and arthritic conditions in the lower extremities. Dose packs are available by prescription to be used for short therapeutic and diagnostic courses. Doses less than 7.5 mg/day of prednisone are usually not associated with significant signs or symptoms of insufficiency during times of increased stress.[19] Most appropriate clinical applications in managing arthritis in the lower extremities involve low doses and brief courses of oral glucocorticoids. Patients should be advised of the anticipated mood elevation and potential for dramatic relief of symptoms before these agents are prescribed. Trials of these agents should be used judiciously in patients with chronic inflammatory arthropathies and those who have become accustomed to tolerating a substantial level of discomfort. Even a short therapeutic trial may provide such dramatic relief that, regardless of risks far outweighing clinical benefits, some patients demand continuation of these agents.

Pharmacists and chemists have created a bewildering number of glucocorticoids that can be clinically efficacious. Most of these agents share the same properties but have differing dosages and scheduling. Forms of cortisone, hydrocortisone (cortisol), betamethasone, dexamethasone, methylprednisolone, paramethasone, prednisolone, prednisone, and triamcinolone are currently available. Table 25–4 lists the relative antiinflammatory potencies of each of these agents when administered orally or parenterally. An arbitrary value of one unit of antiinflammatory activity is assigned to hydrocortisone. Prednisone, prednisolone, and methylprednisolone are approximately four times more potent. Triamcinolone is approximately five times more potent than hydrocortisone, whereas paramethasone is 10 times more potent, and beta-

methasone and dexamethasone are 25 time more potent.[24] Prednisone, prednisolone, and hydrocortisone all cause significant sodium and water retention, whereas betamethasone, dexamethasone, paramethasone, and triamcinolone are not associated with such retention.[30]

Six rules summarize safe guidelines for use of these agents, as listed in Table 25–5. Trial and error are necessary to achieve the appropriate dose for any patient, and that dose requires monitoring through changes in the activity and stages of the disease. A single, large dose of glucocorticoids is virtually without harm. A few days of small to moderate glucocorticoid doses are unlikely to produce any significant harm. However, with prolonged administration cumulative toxicities increase the potential for disabling and potentially lethal effects. Therapy with these agents cannot be viewed as curative but is only palliative control through antiinflammatory and immunosuppressive efficacy. Abrupt withdrawal of glucocorticoid therapy, especially with antecedent high doses, is associated with adrenal insufficiency that may be life threatening. In achieving the smallest possible effective dosage, the goal of therapy with these agents should be to attain tolerable levels of symptoms. In most inflammatory arthropathies involving the lower extremities, complete relief of all symptoms requires unwarranted and dangerously high dose levels. Because of the diurnal nature of endogenous, adrenocortical glucocorticoid production, use of shorter-acting agents administered in the morning hours (as opposed to afternoon or evening) is associated with less adrenocortical suppression. With prolonged use of these agents, alternate-day therapy often proves efficacious and also is associated with less adrenocortical suppression.

TABLE 25–4

RELATIVE ANTIINFLAMMATORY POTENCY OF GLUCOCORTICOIDS

Glucocorticoid	Relative Potency
Hydrocortisone (cortisol)	1
Prednisone	
Prednisolone	4
Methylprednisolone	
Triamcinolone	5
Paramethasone	10
Betamethasone	
Dexamethasone	25

TABLE 25–5

GENERAL RULES APPLICABLE IN USING GLUCOCORTICOID THERAPY

1. Appropriate individual doses are achieved through trial and error and require monitoring through changes in disease stages and activity
2. Any single glucocorticoid dose is virtually without significant harm, and small-to-moderate doses over a few days are unlikely to do harm
3. With prolonged use there is increased risk of encountering dangerous, disabling, and potentially lethal cumulative toxicities
4. Therapy with these agents is only palliative, cannot be viewed as curative, and probably does not alter ultimate disease course and destruction
5. Abrupt withdrawal of therapy or excessively rapid tapering of doses is associated with adrenal insufficiency that may be life threatening
6. In achieving the smallest appropriate dose, the therapeutic goal should be to achieve a tolerable level of symptoms and not a total remission

LOCAL GLUCOCORTICOID THERAPY

The established dramatic antiinflammatory efficacy of glucocorticoids has ensured them a permanent place in the armamentarium of any physician treating rheumatic disorders in the lower extremities. When symptoms are limited to one or a few specific sites, the direct injection of glucocorticoids into these sites can provide dramatic relief, usually without the hazards associated with systemic therapy. Injection therapy has several other advantages. Injection into inflamed bursae, tendon sheaths, and joints also makes synovial fluid available for appropriate examination and for use as a specimen for culture and sensitivity studies. This form of therapy provides an opportunity for immediate removal of excessive amounts of synovial fluid, which often instantly and dramatically relieves pain in previously distended structures. In addition, injection therapy with glucocorticoids involves a relatively simple technique, is accomplished in almost any setting, and is relatively inexpensive. Considering that the primary objective of almost all patients in seeking the care of a physician is pain relief, the instantaneous relief received with this form of treatment is quite beneficial.

Along with these advantages, considerable disadvantages associated with glucocorticoid injection therapy must be considered. Occasionally, this therapeutic approach masks rapidly advancing destructive disease. Such progressive damage can go undetected for considerable periods after injections. Appropriate definitive therapy may be unnecessarily delayed. In the presence of synovitis and inflammation in the lower extremities caused by biomechanical abnormalities, the injections provide only temporary symptomatic relief.

Inadvertent injection of glucocorticoids into a septic joint or infected area may mask or reduce clinical signs and symptoms of infectious processes. Injections also limit the normal inflammatory mechanisms that the body mounts to fight infections, thus delaying appropriate diagnosis and antibiotic therapy. Injections may exacerbate the infectious process and lead to substantially greater tissue destruction than would have otherwise occurred. Prior to injection of any inflamed joint, the synovial fluid should be at least visually examined. If its appearance is cloudy, white to yellow or even brown, and nonviscous, the possibility of infection must be considered. *Glucocorticoids should not be injected under any circumstances into any area that may be infected.*

Inflammatory pain is often a warning and an activity-limiting restraint. It may be the only factor that prevents progressive, potentially disabling tissue destruction. In sprained or strained structures, administration of glucocorticoids to control related symptoms and signs of inflammation can mask the normally restraining pain associated with ongoing application of dangerous levels of stress. In doing so, injections can allow frankly dangerous activity levels to continue and result in substantial additional tissue damage.

The anticipated goals of injection therapy should be discussed with involved patients, especially those with chronically progressive disease activity for which there is no known cure. In many systemic inflammatory arthropathies, the goal of attaining tolerable symptom levels, as opposed to complete pain relief, may need to be stressed prior to initiating injections. The inadvisability of repeated injections into the same area may need to be stressed. Excessive numbers of injections in cases wherein patients have developed dependency on the symptomatic relief or when necessary surgical intervention is unduly delayed should be avoided.

Prior to injection of glucocorticoids, appropriate and realistic assessment of anticipated increases in activity levels should be considered. The physician should ensure that proximal and distal structures are capable of safely handling anticipated increased loads and stresses. Areas with significant risk of injury from such increased stresses should be appropriately protected, cushioned, splinted, or braced.

Injection therapy can be efficacious in a number of applications in managing rheumatic disorders and other conditions in the lower extremities. The antiinflammatory potency of glucocorticoids can substantially decrease postoperative fibrosis, adhesions, inflammation, and pain. The tendency of these agents to atrophy soft tissues can be useful in the treatment of neuromas and nerve entrapments. Keloids and hypertrophic scars can be treated with intradermal injections of these agents. Inflammatory pain in localized structures, whether due to trauma or disease, usually is dramatically relieved with such therapy. These injections can be extremely beneficial in patients with systemic rheumatic diseases that are under good clinical control, especially when inflammatory, disabling pain exists in one or a limited number of joints or other locations.[25]

Use of glucocorticoids combined with local anesthetics can provide substantial relief of associated pain when injected into "trigger point" areas, especially in those patients with fibrositis.[26] Similar injections can be efficacious in reestablishing normal passive range of motion in joints that may have become stiffened or formed adhesions after prolonged periods of casting. Similar efficacy can be attained with inflammatory pain associated with other adhesions or tissue contractures. Caution must be exercised to avoid injecting into areas where osteotomies have recently been performed or where osseous healing may be compromised.

Injection therapy with glucocorticoids is contraindicated in patients with previous hypersensitivity to any of the agents involved, recent or active bacterial or viral infection, bleeding diatheses, or where anticipated levels of use of the involved structure once inflammation has subsided would cause substantial tissue damage. Although this last contraindication is rarely mentioned in the literature, it has special importance in dealing with injection therapy of weightbearing structures. Inflammation associated with a partial tear of the Achilles tendon that is misdiagnosed as synovitis of the paratenon may be completely eradicated by injection therapy, allowing stressful and even athletic use of the involved tendon. This ultimately can lead to an acute and complete rupture. It should be administered to those with myasthenia gravis only with extreme caution. Some patients who report previous allergic reactions to "steroid injections" may be allergic to one or more of the preservatives used. In such instances, the specific agent(s) involved should be determined. Involved preservatives can then be identified. A cutaneous patch test or injection of a diluted agent having different preservatives may indicate that an alternative glucocorticoid preparation can be used without complications.

Degenerative joint disease is the most common form of symptomatic arthritis presenting in the lower extremities. In the absence of antecedent trauma, weightbearing over years on even minor biomechanical imbalances and malalignments is usually the primary etiologic factor causing this type of arthritis. Obesity, vocational demands, and avocational stresses compound the tissue irritation and damage that result from these biomechanical faults. Before significant damage from concentrated internal stresses has occurred, joints tend to form protective osteophytic bone along involved margins that serves to distribute excessive forces over a larger surface area and limit motion within the joint.

With significant tissue damage within involved joints comes further osseous limitation of motion, splinting through increased muscle tone, and guarding of the area, all helping to protect against further damage. Associated painful symptoms cause both disabling discomfort and compensatory protection from further damage and ultimately more intense symptoms. The injection of local anesthetics and glucocorticoids into involved joints provides symptomatic relief and simultaneously eliminates the perceived need for, and use of, well-established protective mechanisms. It can provide symptomatic relief without apparent need for accurate diagnosis and definitive appropriate treatment.

The ultimate result of multiple injections into symptomatic weightbearing joints, following periods of temporary relief, may be marked exacerbation of permanent internal joint damage, associated symptoms, and disability. An appropriate biomechanical assessment of involved joints and related structures should be performed before injection therapy is undertaken. Structural and functional aberrations and related stresses should be identified, evaluated, and minimized. Initial therapy is usually best directed at elimination or optimal control of etiologic and aggravating biomechanical, environmental, and lifestyle factors. Occasionally, this approach proves so successful that there may be no need for injection therapy.

When injection therapy is warranted, previous control of etiologic and aggravating factors ensures that therapy will be optimally efficacious and less dangerous. Each patient should be forewarned that the normal protective mechanisms, which usually produce pain before excessive activity and stress cause damage to involved structures, are masked by the injection. Each should be aware that excessive stress on injected structures may produce permanent and potentially disabling damage in the absence of warning signs or discomfort. Activity levels for 2 to 8 weeks after injection should be no greater than those that would have been reasonably comfortable prior to receiving the injection. The duration of these restrictions depends on the half-life and the amount of specific agent used. When this type of activity reduction cannot

be ensured, either glucocorticoid injection therapy should be withheld or the involved areas should be adequately shielded, strapped, casted, or braced as necessary to guarantee adequate protection. When etiologic biomechanical factors cannot be controlled or occult fractures may be present, or when highly suggestive, neurotic patients without definitive diagnoses are involved, glucocorticoid injection therapy generally should be withheld.

Agents Available for Injection

About 40 years ago, J. L. Hollander was the first physician to inject a glucocorticoid agent into an arthritic joint. In his initial attempts, he injected cortisone and noted no therapeutic benefit.[27] Once it was determined that cortisone had no antiinflammatory activity until it was hydroxylated in the liver, and after the compound hydrocortisone became available in 1951, Hollander injected it into arthritic joints and confirmed its dramatic clinical efficacy in controlling and even eliminating associated pain, swelling, and disability.[28]

Synthetic preparations with substantially increased antiinflammatory efficacy have become available. These agents are generally preferred because small amounts of solution have substantial antiinflammatory efficacy. Currently available agents are shown in Table 25–6. They include prednisolone, methylprednisolone, betamethasone, triamcinolone, and dexamethasone. A number of premixed combinations of agents are commercially available; however, they are significantly more expensive and seem to offer little clinical advantage. Microcrystalline suspensions recently have become available and may offer the benefit of allowing use of smaller diameter needles. Because such needles (27 gauge) are too small to allow for aspiration of most synovial fluid, the advantage of these agents and justification of their increased cost seem questionable.

Table 25–4 lists the relative antiinflammatory potencies of the available injectable glucocorticoids, but the values shown are considered valid only for oral and parenteral use of these agents. Throughout medical literature, reported relative potencies in intra-articular applications have been disputed with regularity. This may be due to the subjective nature of the available reports. Synovial tissues may respond differently to

TABLE 25–6

COMMERCIALLY AVAILABLE GLUCOCORTICOIDS COMMONLY USED IN INJECTION THERAPY OF JOINTS AND SOFT TISSUE STRUCTURES

Generic Name	Trade Name	Salt Type	Concentration (mg/ml)
Hydrocortisone	Hydrocortone, Cortef	Phosphate	50
	Hydrocortone	Acetate	25
Prednisolone	Hydeltrasol	Phosphate	20
	Econopred	Acetate	25, 50, 100
	Hydeltra	Tebutate	20
Methylprednisolone	Depo–Medrol	Acetate	20, 40, 80
	Medrol Acetate		
Triamcinolone	Kenalog	Acetonide	10, 40
	Aristospan	Hexacetonide	5, 20
Betamethasone	Celestone	Phosphate	4
	Celestone Soluspan	Phosphate and acetate	3 of each
Dexamethasone	Decadron, Hexadrol	Phosphate	4
	Decadron-LA	Acetate	8

these agents than do other body tissues. Individual biochemical variations among patients are also factors.

An example of the confusion encountered in trying to determine the relative antiinflammatory potency of these agents is seen with betamethasone. Cameron reported that its relative potency in applications in joints of the feet was 10 to 15 times that of hydrocortisone.[29] Kantor reported that its potency is 30 times that of hydrocortisone.[30] Axelrod reviewed several individual reports and found that the average reported potency was 25 times that of hydrocortisone.[11] In fact, the actual relative potency of this agent may have depended on the manner in which individual injections were given (see later discussion).

Glucocorticoids available for injection are in the form of salts. The glucocorticoid is the cation (positively charged portion). The anions (negatively charged portions) can include phosphate, tebutate, acetate, acetonide, or hexacetonide. Phosphate salts tend to completely dissolve in water and form true solutions. They tend to have rapid onset of antiinflammatory activity (within hours) and fairly limited duration of activity (less than 10 to 14 days). The other salts form crystalline suspensions with longer periods before the onset of their antiinflammatory effects, which are often not noted for 24 to 48 hours or longer. These suspensions have the advantage of prolonged duration of activity, with efficacy often lasting weeks and occasionally months.[31] The phosphate solutions can be instilled with 27- or 30-gauge hypodermic needles, whereas the crystalline suspensions require use of a 25-gauge or larger bore hypodermic needle.

The recommended doses for injection into joints and other soft tissue areas of the lower extremities are quite variable throughout the medical literature.[26, 30–33] Despite considerable variation in the concentration and potency of agents in available solutions, some authors recommend doses by volume of solution used, without specifying any specific solution. Because the antiinflammatory potency of agents ranges from 1 unit to 25 or 30 units, this creates a confusing situation for the physician wishing to follow the basic tenet of using the minimal effective dose to achieve a desired result.

Hollander and colleagues published the most extensive report of glucocorticoid injection therapy available to date, covering more than 100,000 injections.[33] In their paper doses were recommended in milligrams of hydrocortisone, as shown in Table 25–7, for the ankle, tarsal, metatarsal, and interphalangeal joints and for bursae, tendon sheaths, and trigger points. The potential equivalent doses of the other

available injectable glucocorticoids also are shown in Table 25–7 in both milligrams and milliliters. These data are valid only if antiinflammatory potency in intra-articular and soft tissue applications is actually equivalent to that determined to be present in oral and parenteral applications. From this table, it becomes apparent that the increased potency of synthetic agents and their concentration in available solutions may make use of extremely small volumes potentially efficacious when sites in the foot and ankle are injected. It seems that 1 ml of the least concentrated solution of triamcinolone would be more than sufficient in all applications within the foot. Less that 0.2 ml of dexamethasone solution similarly would be efficacious. Excessive amounts of the more potent agents, especially betamethasone and dexamethasone, are used if volume recommendations in many reference texts and research papers are used to determine the amounts of these solutions to be injected at sites in the feet and ankles.

Long-term deposition of undissolved glucocorticoid crystals is occasionally noted in periarticular and other soft tissues. The vast majority of local anesthetics used in daily practice come in multidose vials and contain preservatives such as methylparaben, polyparaben, and phenol. Mixture of local anesthetic agents with these preservatives in the same syringe with glucocorticoid crystalline suspensions can cause flocculation of the steroid crystals, potentially inactivating them. The package insert for Aristospan (triamcinolone hexacetonide) clearly describes this phenomenon and discourages mixture of local anesthetics with preservatives and the triamcinolone hexacetonide contained therein. No similar warning is published in the accompanying literature for any other crystalline suspension of glucocorticoid currently available.[34]

All crystalline suspensions of glucocorticoids should be shaken vigorously immediately before any solution is withdrawn to ensure uniformity of the suspension. Before and after agitation of the suspensions, they should be inspected for any granular appearance or clumps of steroid crystals (agglomeration). Agglomeration can occur after freezing of suspensions or with their excessive aging. Flocculated, agglomerated, and potentially contaminated solutions should be immediately discarded.

Postinjection Flares

Even though local injection therapy with glucocorticoids prevents the complications associated with systemic use of

TABLE 25–7

EQUIVALENT DOSES OF INJECTABLE GLUCOCORTICOIDS IF ESTABLISHED ORAL AND PARENTERAL RELATIVE ANTIINFLAMMATORY POTENCIES ARE CONSIDERED ACCURATE FOR INTRA-ARTICULAR AND OTHER INJECTIONS

Site Injected	Recommended Hydrocortisone		Prednisolone Methylprednisolone		Triamcinolone		Betamethasone Dexamethasone	
	mg	(ml)	mg	(ml)	mg	(ml)	mg	(ml)
Ankle joint	25	(0.5–1.0)	6.3	(0.08–0.31)	5.0	(0.13–1.0)	1.0	(0.12–0.25)
Tarsal joints	15	(0.3–0.6)	3.8	(0.05–0.18)	3.0	(0.08–0.6)	0.6	(0.07–0.15)
Metatarsophalangeal joints	10	(0.2–0.4)	2.5	(0.03–0.12)	2.0	(0.05–0.4)	0.4	(0.05–0.10)
Interphalangeal joints	5.0	(0.1–0.2)	1.3	(0.02–0.06)	1.0	(0.03–0.2)	0.2	(0.03–0.05)
Bursae	25	(0.5–1.0)	6.3	(0.08–0.31)	5.0	(0.13–1.0)	1.0	(0.12–0.25)
Tendon sheaths	12.5	(0.3–0.5)	3.2	(0.04–0.15)	2.5	(0.07–0.5)	0.5	(0.06–0.13)
Trigger points	12.5	(0.3–0.5)	3.2	(0.04–0.15)	2.5	(0.07–0.5)	0.5	(0.06–0.13)

these agents, it does have its own potential hazards. One of the most frequently noted complications in the use of these agents is postinjection flare of synovitis or other inflammation. This phenomenon appears to result from a combination of direct irritation from undissolved crystals and immunologic recognition of such crystals as foreign bodies and subsequent attack by the immune system. Signs and symptoms of postinjection flares are usually noted between 6 and 12 hours after injection.[30] They include increased local temperature, swelling, and pain.[33] Initial symptoms often mimic those of an acute attack of gout but are almost always of significantly less severity and shorter duration.

Patients receiving this type of therapy should be forewarned about the relatively rare possibility of such a flare at the injection site. They should be instructed that if such a flare is noted, the involved area should be rested, elevated, and intermittently massaged with ice. In addition, one to two salicylate, acetaminophen, or ibuprofen pills may be taken every 4 hours as needed for associated discomfort. The self-limiting nature of these attacks should be stressed. Patients should be advised that any such attack should be reported immediately to the physician who administered the injection. Each flare should be followed up at no longer than a 24-hour interval. If symptoms of a flare last longer than 24 hours, clinical suspicion of joint sepsis or other soft tissue sepsis should be entertained. Use of small amounts of rapid-acting phosphate salt solutions of glucocorticoids concurrently with crystalline suspensions usually avert such a flare.

Other Potential Complications Following Injection

Septic arthritis is another potential hazard associated with glucocorticoid injection therapy. Use of strict aseptic technique, avoidance of these injections in immunocompromised patients or in those with active infections, and prevention of placement of the injection through abnormal skin surfaces have made the occurrence of associated septic arthritis exceedingly rare.[33]

Allergic reactions to these agents also are exceedingly rare. Meticulous care should be exercised in administering these injections so as to avoid injury to neurovascular structures. Caution also helps avoid potential intravascular injections, subcutaneous hemorrhage, and nerve damage.

Care also should be taken to avoid use of nonapproved suspensions at subcutaneous sites. Commercially available suspensions of 10 mg/ml of triamcinolone acetonide (Kenalog-10) and 5 mg/ml of triamcinolone hexacetonide (Aristospan) are the only available solutions approved by the Food and Drug Administration (FDA) for subcutaneous administration. The relative potency of suspensions of betamethasone and dexamethasone warrants avoidance of their injection into subcutaneous areas.

Neuropathic arthropathy and *tendon and ligament ruptures* have been reported in association with glucocorticoid injection therapy.[16, 32, 35] Review of these articles has shown that the damage and tissue destruction reported may have been, and most likely was, the result of inadequate protection of injected structures from excessive stresses after the injections had been given. Direct injections of glucocorticoids and local anesthetics into the bodies of tendons or ligaments must be avoided. The density of these tissues provides sufficient resistance to injection so that doing so is quite difficult and often impossible. The necessity of ensuring adequate protection of injected structures from excessive activity, stress, and strain for appropriate durations after any such injection cannot be overemphasized.

Local muscle atrophy and *osteoporosis* also have been reported as potential complications of glucocorticoid injection therapy.[16, 24, 32] It is far more likely that the symptoms requiring these injections and the diseases causing those symptoms caused substantial disuse atrophy of both involved striated muscle and osseous tissue.

Aseptic necrosis of bone reported in the literature may have been due to synovitis resulting in constriction of the blood supply to capital areas of bones, especially at the hip.[16]

Choice of Agent and Dose

Any chances of encountering complications in the administration of injectable glucocorticoids are minimized with use of minimal effective doses. A review of current medical literature reveals that recommended doses for almost all applications of these injections in the feet and ankles, are almost always in excess of 0.25 ml.[14, 17, 25, 31, 33] It seems fairly safe to assume that the relative antiinflammatory potency of the available synthetic glucocorticoids is most likely the same in all body tissues, whether the drug is administered orally, parenterally, or by injection into a joint. If this is true, the dosages listed in Table 25–7 appear to be sufficient for most applications in the distal lower extremities. My clinical experience over the past decade has consistently confirmed the efficacy of these dosages. Effective use of these dosage levels requires meticulous placement of the injected suspensions. When placement is critical, guidance under fluoroscopy may be advisable.

The site to be injected, the condition warranting injection, the potential for patient compliance, and the desired therapeutic goals should be considered in selecting the agent and dosage used in each specific application. When accessibility to the desired site is limited, as with the middle facet of the subtalar joint, when exact placement cannot be ensured, or when atrophy is clinically desirable, use of substantially higher doses may be warranted.

When a condition for which prolonged disease activity is anticipated is being treated, use of longer-acting suspensions should be considered. When patient compliance is in question, initial use of phosphate salts creates less potential danger of self-injury. Once compliance is ensured, longer-acting and more potent agents can be used. Treatment of acute and temporary conditions such as acute gout and lysis of adhesions is often best accomplished with the phosphate salts of these agents.

Patient responses to these agents are often individualized. Similar individualized reactions are frequently seen in the treatment of inflammatory rheumatic disease symptoms with nonsteroidal antiinflammatory agents. Individualized, most likely genetically determined, biomechanical and biochemical variations are probably the cause of variable results in treating similar patients with almost identical disease manifestations with the same oral or injectable antiinflammatory agent. Over the past decade, I have found combinations of agents in the same injection significantly more efficacious than single-agent injections in controlling inflammatory articular manifestations of rheumatic disease. The preferred combination presently includes use of the phosphate salts and suspensions of both betamethasone and dexamethasone.

Techniques of Injection

Safe and efficacious injection therapy with glucocorticoids in the lower extremities requires thorough familiarity with the anatomic structures of involved areas. Damage to vascular, nerve, cartilage, and other soft tissue structures should be minimized. Strict aseptic technique must be employed at all times.

These injections can be given with a minimum of discomfort. Topical refrigerants can be employed to virtually eliminate the initial discomfort of the hypodermic needle piercing the skin surface. Ethyl chloride is readily available, inexpensive, and quite effective for such use. A hypodermic needle with the smallest possible gauge should be used. For example, a 30-gauge hypodermic needle can be used to administer local anesthetics and soluble salt solutions. A 27-gauge hypodermic needle can be used to administer local anesthetics, soluble salt solutions, and some microcrystalline suspensions. A 25-gauge hypodermic needle is usually the smallest bore size that will allow injection of crystalline suspensions. When aspiration of synovial fluid is anticipated or desired, a 22- or even 18-gauge hypodermic needle usually is required, especially for noninflammatory aspirates.

Usually, glucocorticoids and local anesthetic solutions should be loaded into separate syringes. Use of tuberculin syringes for glucocorticoids allows for more precise measurement of administered medications. Single-dose vials of local anesthetic (lidocaine) without preservatives are commercially available. Only when this form of local anesthesia is employed should glucocorticoids be either mixed in the same syringe or injected through the same hypodermic needle.

The best approach to any specific joint in the lower extremity is often individualized. Care should be exercised in avoiding injection through areas of abnormal or inflamed skin. Joints with internal effusions often present subcutaneous bulging at variable sites, and entrance into these areas is often easiest. Before the initiation of any injection into a joint, the exact location where the entrance is planned should be identified. Even with an excellent knowledge of the underlying anatomic structure, it is difficult and often impossible to blindly pierce through the skin and directly enter a desired joint. Direct entrance into desired joints can be facilitated by identification of the joint level and desired site of entrance through palpation of the joint with the index fingernail as the joint is put through a passive range of motion. Once the exact location of the margins of the joint is located, mild to moderate pressure for 10 to 15 seconds applied with the index fingernail leaves a mark that remains a visible guide to the exact entrance site for several minutes.

Some physicians prefer to inject glucocorticoids directly into involved joints and other areas. Even with the area of entrance marked, direct injection of glucocorticoids through the skin and into the joint can be a rather painful experience for the patient. Often, patients describe such injections as the most painful experience that they have ever had. Such discomfort should be avoided and can be eliminated with an appropriate use of local anesthetics.

Once the site of injection has been adequately identified, a *local anesthetic* can be administered. Use of skin refrigerant significantly decreases pain and apprehension associated with these injections. Tensing and stretching skin at the site of entrance decreases the density of pain receptors in the area. The skin usually can be pierced with a minimum of discomfort if the needle is rapidly darted through it in the direction opposite to the tension being applied. If anesthetic solutions without preservatives or other anesthetics combined with only glucocorticoid-soluble solutions are being used, the anesthetic can be injected directly at the proposed site of entrance, down to the level of the joint, bursa, or tendon sheath and even into these structures. If local anesthetics with preservatives are being used concurrently with crystalline glucocorticoid suspensions, injection should be performed sufficiently proximal to the point of entrance to prevent admixture of the local anesthetics and the glucocorticoids. Swabbing the area with alcohol or povidone-iodine where local anesthetic is to be administered is usually sufficient topical antisepsis.

Povidone-iodine or similar antiseptic lavage of any area is mandatory when glucocorticoids are to be injected directly into joints or other underlying structures. Most soft tissues maintain excellent levels of immunocompetence, but the interior of joints and most synovial structures have significantly less immunocompetence, are far more prone to clinical infection with entrance of limited numbers of bacteria, and are sites where it is far more difficult for the body to combat infections. Preparing the skin surface after administration of local anesthetics usually allows sufficient time to ensure adequate anesthesia to the involved area.

Once the area of injection has been properly prepared, a sterile glove should be placed on the physician's nondominant hand and a syringe with the appropriate hypodermic needle and a small amount of sterile saline should be taken up in the dominant hand. Only the hypodermic needle or sterile glove should be allowed to contact the skin at or near the site of entrance. The involved joint should be manipulated so as to distract joint margins at the desired site of entrance. The skin over the area is stretched and the hypodermic needle is inserted with the open side of the bevel facing the interior of the joint. After the skin is pierced, decreased resistance to forward movement is noted unless solid structures such as tendons, bursae, and ligaments are encountered. As the joint capsule is entered, light pressure on the plunger of the syringe is met with similar resistance to injection of the sterile saline that abruptly disappears as the interior of the joint is entered.

Aspiration of synovial fluid should be attempted whenever feasible. Aspirated fluid should be examined for color, clarity, and viscosity. Chalky fluid may indicate urate crystal presence in gout. Purulent fluid is noted with joint sepsis. Viscosity of noninflammatory synovial fluid is quite high; a drop placed on the finger of the sterile glove will tend not to run off. Touching it with another gloved finger and withdrawing that finger reveals a tackiness and produces string-like extensions of the fluid. Inflammatory fluid has substantially lower viscosity and more waterlike qualities. The presence of bright red blood in the aspirate is usually a sign of trauma produced by the injection. Dark red to brown-tinged fluid is usually indicative of previous bleeding within the joint. Fat globules within the fluid may be noted in the presence of intra-articular fracture. If fat globules and previous hemorrhage into an involved joint are noted in the absence of antecedent trauma, intra-articular glucocorticoid injection should be withheld until an occult intra-articular fracture has been ruled out.

Injection should be withheld if there is a significant chance of joint sepsis being present. Under such circumstances, aspirated synovial fluid can be left in the capped syringe and forwarded directly to laboratory facilities for appropriate aerobic and anaerobic culture and sensitivity studies and fungal cultures. These specimens also can be used for Gram's, acid-fast, and fungal staining, microscopic examination, and evaluation for the presence of crystals. All possible synovial fluid should be aspirated to relieve painful distension of capsular structures and allow for injection of glucocorticoids without excessive distension of these structures. Occasionally, the needle tip becomes blocked by soft tissues during aspirations. Slight rotations of the needle, occasional injection of a small amount of aspirate back into the joint, and slow removal of fluid all aid in avoiding such blockages and in clearing them when they do occur.

After aspiration is complete, with care not to move the needle from its site, the first syringe can be removed from the needle and a second syringe with glucocorticoids can be attached to it. The syringe containing glucocorticoids should be vigorously shaken just before its attachment. The glucocorticoids can then be injected directly into the joint. Throughout the injection, the barrel of the syringe should be held horizontally so as to prevent settling of crystals and clogging of the needle. Especially when smaller joints are being injected, an alcohol swab should be held with mild to moderate pressure over the site of needle entrance when the needle is removed to prevent extravasation of glucocorticoids into tissues outside of the joint. Pressure maintained for 1 or 2 minutes after the needle is removed also helps achieve hemostasis. While this pressure is maintained, the injected joint should be passively manipulated to ensure even dispersal of the injected glucocorticoid within it. After removal of the swab, the area should be wiped with povidone-iodine or a similar antiseptic solution and covered with a temporary adhesive bandage.

Generally, injections should be made at the most accessible site that is free of intervening significant vascular or nerve structures. The easiest approach to interphalangeal joints is usually at their dorsal surface. Injection should be made with the needle and syringe held in the frontal plane, slightly oblique to the transverse plane. Entry is made between the dorsomedial or dorsolateral neurovascular bundles and the long extensor tendon. With the bevel of the needle directed plantarly and the toe plantarflexed and distracted, the needle is advanced centrally and slightly plantarly under the long extensor tendon and into the joint. Little if any synovial fluid is available for aspiration in these joints. Care should be exercised to avoid damage to articular cartilage.

The metatarsophalangeal joints are usually best entered with a similar dorsomedial approach, thereby avoiding the short extensor tendons to the toes. Direct dorsal-to-plantar injections along the medial or lateral margins of these joints also can be accomplished. In either instance, the foot should be positioned so that the needle and syringe are held horizontally during injection to prevent settling of glucocorticoid crystalline suspensions into the hub of the needle and subsequently blocking it. As the dorsal intermetatarsal arteries and nerves course and diverge adjacent to these areas, care must

be exercised to avoid injury to them. With a horizontal approach to these joints, plantarflexion of the respective toe aids entrance into the joints. With medial, dorsal-to-plantar injections in these areas, lateral traction on the toe aids in distracting the side of the joint being entered.

Injection of the tarsometatarsal joint requires meticulous identification and marking of the joint margins before any attempts are made to insert a hypodermic needle into them. The subcutaneous positioning of these joints makes dorsal approaches most feasible. Care similarly must be taken to avoid damage to local neurovascular structures. Plantarflexion and abduction of the first metatarsal may allow for significant distraction of the dorsal, and possibly even medial, margin of the first metatarsocuneiform joint. Plantarflexion and adduction of the fifth metatarsal may allow for distraction of its dorsolateral margins. Depending on the flexibility of these joints in the patient, dorsal-to-plantar injections may be preferable to more horizontally oriented injections. The latter type of approach is usually preferable in approaching the central three tarsometatarsal joints.

Similar subcutaneous positioning of most of intertarsal joints makes dorsal approaches to these joints favorable. Familiarity with the anatomic structures in these areas helps prevent injury to neurovascular structures. The calcaneocuboid joint may be somewhat distracted with adduction of the forefoot against a fixed calcaneus, allowing a dorsal-to-plantar approach along the lateral margin of the joint. The talonavicular and navicular-medial cuneiform joints can occasionally be sufficiently distracted by abduction of the forefoot on a fixed calcaneus to allow for dorsal-to-plantar injections along the medial margins of these joints. The dorsomedial-to-plantar lateral angulation of the dorsal surface of the tarsus makes similar approaches in the frontal plane, and slightly oblique to the transverse plane in a lateral-to-medial direction, usually easiest. The naviculocuneiform and talonavicular joints are usually entered in this manner. Intercuneiform, lateral cuneiform-cuboid, and cuboid-navicular articulations are extremely difficult to enter. A direct dorsal-to-plantar approach with slight medial angulation of the needle is usually the best approach for attempting injection of these joints. Attempts to enter the calcaneocuboid joint laterally should be made along the upper margin of this joint to prevent potential injury to the peroneal tendons.

The posterior facet of the subtalar joint is best approached from its lateral aspect. With the calcaneus inverted on a fixed ankle, this joint's lateral margin is found just under the tip of the lateral malleolus. Palpation with the index fingernail of the area just anterior to and beneath the lateral malleolus as the calcaneus is gently inverted and everted often reveals the location of this joint. During this maneuver, the calcaneus should be maintained perpendicular to the leg. Once the precise location of the joint is determined, the calcaneus should be held in full inversion during the actual injection, allowing for slight distraction of the lateral margins of the joint. Occasionally, the anterior and middle facets can be palpated above the sustentaculum tali of the calcaneus. Direct injection of these joints is often quite difficult. Injection of glucocorticoids into the sinus tarsi often allows for sufficient diffusion of the agents into these joints to provide desired clinical benefits. The sinus tarsi is approached from the anterolateral ankle area with the needle directed downward, medially, and posteriorly. The hypodermic needle should be passed plantarly until the floor of the sinus tarsi is encountered before glucocorticoids are injected into this space.

With passive manipulation of the ankle joint into dorsiflexion and plantarflexion and simultaneous palpation with the index finger over its anterior aspect and over the anterior surfaces of the malleoli, the anterior margins of the joint can be identified. The joint is best approached anteriorly, with the needle and syringe in the sagittal plane. Full plantarflexion of the joint facilitates entrance of the hypodermic needle into the dorsomedial or dorsolateral anterior aspects of the joint. Care should be exercised in avoiding injury to any of the anterior tendons, deep peroneal nerve, superficial peroneal nerve, and dorsalis pedis artery.

A medial-to-lateral approach is best used for injections of the plantar fascial insertion and the infracalcaneal bursa, entering the medial side of the heel. Injections directly through the plantar surface may be warranted in specific circumstances but generally should be avoided whenever possible because of the extreme level of discomfort usually associated with them. The retrocalcaneal and retro-Achilles bursae are easily approached from the medial or lateral side of the heel with the syringe and needle held in the transverse plane. Care should be taken to avoid injection directly into the Achilles tendon. The dose and agents chosen should be carefully assessed, as should the reliability of the patient in maintaining satisfactory protection and reduction of activity after these injections.

Rupture of the Achilles tendon and other tendons has been reported after injections of glucocorticoids into or near them.[35] None of these reports documented that the patients provided appropriate activity reduction and protection of involved tendons after their injections. Women who receive injections into the retro-Achilles or retrocalcaneal bursa and who are accustomed to wearing high-heeled shoes for the majority of weightbearing should be advised to avoid the use of unusually low heels or going barefoot for several weeks after any such injection. Even though these patients often note aggravation of initial symptoms with use of lower-than-usual heels prior to injection therapy, with relief of their symptoms they often begin preferentially using low-heeled shoes or going barefoot unless specifically advised against doing so.

The proximal tibiofibular joint is located subcutaneously at the posterolateral aspect of the upper leg. The anterior and superior margins of this joint can be palpated with the index finger, as described earlier. Usually an anterior or anterosuperior approach is preferable. Meticulous care should be taken to avoid the superficial peroneal nerve where it winds around the neck of the fibula. The knee joint is best approached along the palpable subcutaneous margins of the patella. The suprapatellar and infrapatellar synovial reflections of the knee joint capsule are generally easiest to approach along the medial or lateral margins of the patellofemoral joint.

Injecting glucocorticoids into neuromas, chronically inflamed and fibrosed bursae, and areas of adhesions, in addition to providing antiinflammatory effects, provides some atrophy of involved tissues, which is desirable. Care has to be exercised in avoiding undesirable atrophy of adjacent soft tissue structures. Usually, soluble solutions of glucocorticoids induce less atrophy than do crystalline suspensions of these agents. More concentrated crystalline suspensions cause more atrophy than do dilute solutions. Generally, no more than three or possibly four injections should be made into the same site within any 12-month period.

References

1. Addison T: On the Constitutional and Local Effects of Disease of the Suprarenal Capsules. London, Samuel Highley, 1855.
2. Cushing H: The basophil adenomas of the pituitary body and their clinical manifestations. Bull Johns Hopkins Hosp 50:137, 1932.
3. Hartman FA, Brownell KA, and Hartman WE: A further study on the hormone of the adrenal cortex. Am J Physiol 95:670, 1930.
4. Hench PS, Kendall EC, Slocumb CH, and Polley HF: The effect of a hormone on the adrenal cortex (17-hydroxy-11-dehydrocorticosterone, compound E) and of the pituitary adrenocorticotropic hormone on rheumatoid arthritis. Proc Med Staff Mayo Clinic 24:181, 1949.
5. Castles JJ: Clinical pharmacology of glucocorticoids. *In* McCarty D (ed): Arthritis and Allied Conditions, 9th ed. Philadelphia, Lea & Febiger, 1979, p 391.
6. Melby JC: Systemic corticosteroid therapy: Pharmacology and endocrinologic considerations. Ann Intern Med 81:505, 1974.
7. Newman S: Hormone induced diseases. *In* Moser RH (ed): Diseases of Medical Progress: A Study of Iatrogenic Disease. Springfield, IL, Charles C Thomas, 1969, p 361.
8. Ebert RH and Barclay WR: Changes in connective tissue reaction induced by cortisone. Ann Intern Med 37:506, 1952.
9. Ragan C, Howes EL, Plotz CN, et al: The effect of ACTH and cortisone on connective tissue. Bull NY Acad Med 26:251, 1950.
10. Wrenn RN, Goldner JL, and Markee JL: An experimental study of the effect of cortisone on the healing process and tensile strength of tendons. J Bone Joint Surg 36:588, 1954.
11. Axelrod L: Steroids. *In* Kelley WN, Harris ED Jr, Ruddy S, and Sledge CB (eds): Textbook of Rheumatology. Philadelphia, WB Saunders, 1981, p 822.
12. Bale DC and Petersdorf RG: Corticosteroids and infectious disease. *In* Azarnoff DL (ed): Steroid Therapy. Philadelphia, WB Saunders, 1975, p 206.
13. Claman HN: How corticosteroids work. J Allergy Clin Immunol 55:145, 1975.
14. Axelrod L: Glucocorticoids. *In* Kelley WN, Harris ED Jr, Ruddy S, and Sledge CB (eds): Textbook of Rheumatology, 3rd ed. Philadelphia, WB Saunders, 1989, p 845.
15. Roth RD: The rheumatic patient—Medical considerations in foot surgery. *In* McGlamry ED (ed): Fundamentals of Foot Surgery. Baltimore, Williams & Wilkens, 1987, p 383.
16. Fischer DE and Bickel WH: Corticosteroid-induced aseptic necrosis: A clinical study of seventy-five patients. J Bone Joint Surg 53:589, 1971.
17. Roth RD: Steroids in rheumatic disease—A podiatric perspective. Clin Podiatr Med Surg 5:135, 1988.
18. Westerhof L, Van Ditmars MJ, Derkinderen PJ, et al: Recovery of adrenal cortical function during long-term treatment with corticosteroids. Fr Med J 2:195, 1972.
19. Myles AB, Schiller CFB, Glass D, and Daly JR: Single-dose corticosteroid treatment. Ann Rheum Dis 35:73, 1976.
20. Sagel J: Adrenocortical insufficiency. *In* Rakel RE (ed): Conn's Current Therapy—1990. Philadelphia, WB Saunders, 1990, p 560.
21. Good TA, Benton JW, and Kelley VC: Symptomatology resulting from withdrawal of steroid hormone therapy. Arthritis Rheum 2:229, 1959.
22. Salassa RM, Bennett WD, Keating FR, et al: Postoperative adrenal cortical insufficiency: Occurrence in patients previously treated with cortisone. JAMA 152:1509, 1953.
23. Sampson PA, Winsone NF, and Frooke BN: Adrenal function in surgical patients after steroid therapy. Lancet 2:322, 1962.
24. Haynes RC: Adrenocorticotropic hormone: Adrenocortical steroids and their synthetic analogs: Inhibitors of the synthesis of and actions of adrenocortical hormones. *In* Gillman AG, Rall TW, Nies AS, and Taylor P (eds): Goodman and Gilman's the Pharmacological Basis of Therapeutics, 8th ed. New York, Macmillan, 1990, p 1431.
25. Steinbroker O: Management of some non-articular rheumatic disorders. Mod Treatment 1:1254, 1964.
26. Cohen S:Regional corticosteroid therapy. *In* Katz W (ed): Rheumatic Diseases: Diagnosis and Management. Philadelphia, JB Lippincott, 1977, p 910.
27. Hollander JL: Personal communication, 1976.
28. Hollander JL: The local effects of compound F (hydrocortisone) injected into joints. Bull Rheum Dis 11:239, 1951.
29. Cameron DJ: A new rapid and prolonged acting steroid for intraarticular inflammatory disorders. J Am Podiatr Assoc 56:461, 1966.
30. Kantor TG: Anti-inflammatory and analgesic drugs. *In* Katz W (ed): Rheumatic Diseases: Diagnosis and Management. Philadelphia, JB Lippincott, 1977, p 876.
31. Owen DS: Aspiration and injection of joints and soft tissues. *In* Kelley WN, Harris ED Jr, Ruddy S, and Sledge CB (eds): Textbook of Rheumatology. Philadelphia, WB Saunders, 1981, p 553.
32. Fitzgerald RH: Intrasynovial injection of steroids: Uses and abuses. Mayo Clin Proc 51:655, 1976.
33. Hollander JL, Jessar RA, and Brown EM: Intrasynovial corticosteroid therapy: A decade of use. Bull Rheum Dis 11:239, 1961.
34. Physicians' Desk Reference. Oradel, NJ, Medical Economics, 1987, p 1086.
35. Sweetnam R: Corticosteroid arthropathy and tendon rupture. J Bone Joint Surg 51B:397, 1969.

CHAPTER 26

Rehabilitation of the Arthritic Patient

Jon Nordgaard, D.P.M., P.T.

Osteoarthritis affects roughly 37% of the population of the United States, whereas rheumatoid arthritis and less common forms of rheumatic disease affect at least 1% of the population.[1] The toll of these disorders in terms of the patients' pain, deformities, and ultimately their functional abilities is incalculable.

Advances in basic clinical and pharmacologic sciences have allowed us to have more thorough knowledge of these disease processes and methods of treatment. Management of patients with arthritic disease requires knowledge of pharmacologic and surgical methods of treatment. Additionally, clinicians must have a working knowledge of effective techniques in physical medicine and rehabilitation and be capable of appropriate referral.

Given the often life-long and life-changing implications of diagnosed rheumatic disease, it is incumbent on the clinician to educate the arthritic patient. It is essential that patients and their families participate in treatment. This allows for increased awareness and understanding. Patients are given some recourse on a day-to-day basis about the methods they can use to affect symptoms related to their disease. Benefits may be noted on many levels. In addition to the possible physical effects of reduced pain and disability, patients may take a proactive role in maintaining their place as productive, vital members of society. This may act to counterbalance some of the negative psychological implications of a chronic disabling disease. Thorough education can also solidify patients' commitment to the rehabilitation program.

Rehabilitation is a dynamic process designed to assist patients in their attempts to maintain or improve function. Rheumatic disease brings a unique set of problems to those involved in its treatment. These diseases are often chronic, relapsing, and unpredictable and may lead to deformity.[2] This requires that treatment be reassessed and modified frequently. Professionals involved in the care of the rheumatoid patient must be attuned to the changeable nature of these diseases and be prepared to vary treatment goals accordingly.

In our nation's current medical system, a team approach to treatment is often impractical. In the inpatient rehabilitation setting, physiatrists often function as team leaders. They, along with rheumatologists, make appropriate diagnoses and functional assessments, as well as medically manage the patients. These physicians then make referrals within the rehabilitation team. The team often includes physical and occupational therapists, nurses, orthotists, vocational rehabilitation specialists, and in some cases, a representative of social services. Podiatrists can offer unique knowledge to the team regarding the biomechanics of the lower extremity, corrective surgical techniques, shoe gear modification, padding, and orthoses. Decisions regarding surgical consultation may be made most appropriately after a complete functional assessment has been performed.

When a patient is referred to physical or occupational therapy, a prescription is often required. Therapists are not always presented with the tools or the training to allow for specific diagnosis. Radiographs, magnetic resonance imaging (MRI), or bone scan results are often unavailable to the therapists. They rely on the referring physician for pertinent patient information. The fact that a patient has a prosthetic implant or a recent tendon repair is an example of important information the therapist should have. Care should be taken to communicate any specific contraindications. Every prescription should include a diagnosis. The prescription may be detailed as to types of exercise or equipment, or if the referring physician is comfortable with the therapist, specifics of the program may be left to the therapist.

With sophisticated methods now available, definitive diagnoses are made much earlier in the course of articular disease. This creates an opportunity for earlier medical and rehabilitative interventions. Modifications in lifestyle, the use of adaptive aids, methods of nonpharmacologic pain control, and active techniques to minimize deformity can be started early.

Therapeutic care of the arthritic patient melds many of the skills of the rehabilitative team, including therapeutic exercise, physical modalities (heat, cold, electrotherapy, and hydrotherapy), splinting, training in the use of adaptive aids, assistive devices, and modification in activities of daily living. The program should be devised to maintain patient interest, building on strengths while addressing functional weaknesses. Therapy should be thought of not as simply an option to try temporarily but rather as an ongoing process. Optimally, the patient's family should be involved, aiding in their understanding of the disease and ways to help. A strong home program allows for more frequent use of therapeutic techniques, increasing efficacy.

PHYSICAL EXAMINATION

Complete medical evaluation of the patient has typically occurred prior to referral for rehabilitation. This often includes a careful history and physical examination and pertinent laboratory tests. Based on this information, a diagnosis or differential diagnosis is made.

Physical examination in musculoskeletal disorders should include determinations of strength and endurance, range of motion, pain level and location, sensory and motor deficit, and level of function. Specific joint examination should include determinations of tenderness to palpation, warmth, degree of deformity, and quality of range of motion. Motion should be assessed to determine if crepitus is present in a joint. It is important to note whether muscle spasm is limiting motion and to evaluate the "end-feel" of the joint range of motion (e.g., soft or bony). These factors should be quantified when possible and documented for future comparison. With knowledge of the expected course of the disease, the information gleaned from the physical examination helps provide an intelligent approach to designing the rehabilitation program. A program should include appropriate personal, functional, or vocational goals.

Strength Assessment

Muscle strength is frequently affected in rheumatic disease. Strength is the ability of a muscle or body part to produce work or exert force. Power refers to the production of force as related to time, whereas endurance is the body's ability to produce repetitive work efforts or force over time. All are affected in articular or rheumatic disease.[3]

Manual muscle testing techniques have been described and are used to measure strength specifically. Grading systems vary but most use the following scale[4]:

0 *Zero* No muscle contraction palpable.
1 *Trace* Minimal contraction felt in muscle.
2 *Poor* Body part moves through arc of motion with gravity eliminated.
3 *Fair* Body part moves through range of motion, against gravity, but takes no resistance.
4 *Good* Body part has full movement against gravity, tolerates moderate resistance.
5 *Normal* Body part has full movement against gravity, tolerates maximal resistance.

Clearly, other information must be considered when dealing with rheumatic disease patients. Their functional level, pain level, motivation, and degree of deformity are just some of the factors that may influence performance. Positioning and stabilization are important to minimize substitution with other muscle groups. Although less quantifiable, a sense for the patient's specific muscle endurance may be gained by asking the patient to perform repetitive contractions against manual resistance.

Although manual muscle testing remains a relatively simple and useful clinical tool, other methods of determining strength have been devised. Isokinetic equipment has recently been used to measure the peak torque created about a joint. Sophisticated computer algorithms have been created to analyze these measurements objectively. Incremental strength changes can be measured. By evaluating the speed at which torque can be created, indications as to the power of a muscle group can be extrapolated. Similar methods are available to evaluate endurance. These methods can be quite

helpful in evaluation; however, they may be too stressful in the rheumatoid patient.

Range-of-Motion Assessment

Assessment of joint range of motion is inherent to any evaluation of musculoskeletal disorders. Patients with rheumatic disease often lose significant degrees of motion in affected joints. Range of motion can be influenced by a number of factors. Intra-articular or extra-articular edema may limit motion. Pain can reflexly inhibit active motion and cause active resistance to passive motion. Periarticular soft tissue contracture or intra-articular derangement can limit motion. Marginal osteophytes commonly seen in osteoarthritis can cause a bony block to motion. Scleroderma or mixed connective tissue disease can cause skin contractures that may restrict motion. Comparison of available active and passive joint motion should be made of involved joints. Joint crepitus, locking, subluxation, and general quality of movement should be assessed. Abnormal excessive motion should also be noted, because this may lead to joint instability.

Methods for measuring axial skeletal movement have been standardized.[5] Clinicians should have a working knowledge of these techniques as well as a knowledge of normal ranges for joint motion. Both limits and excesses in motion can potentially lead to accelerated joint damage and deformity. Abnormal joint motion can obviously limit function.

Pain Assessment

Because it is largely subjective, pain assessments are notoriously difficult to quantify. The American Rheumatism Association describes a 0 to 4 (0, none; 4, severe) grading scale to help evaluate a joint's pain level.[6] Pain can be rated either at rest, with palpation, or with motion.

Functional Assessment

Functional ability can be simply evaluated as a patient's capacity for ambulation. More subtle levels of function included in activities of daily living are more difficult to assess (Table 26–1). One way to quantify level of function is to assess a patient's independence or need of assistance (minimal, moderate, or maximal) while performing daily activities. This may include the ability to transfer in and out of a bed or chair, climb up and down stairs, perform household tasks or leisure activities, drive, and perform work-related tasks; time able to sit, stand, lie, or walk; and the use of assistive devices and bracing. Functional scales have been developed.[7]

Occupational therapists should be consulted to provide their assessments of patients' functional ability. The ease with which activities of daily living are performed can be improved dramatically with some functional instruction and the use of adaptive aids, splints, and braces.

PHYSICAL MODALITIES IN REHABILITATION

Physical energies, or modalities, are commonly used in the rehabilitative program. Included are the physical modalities of heat (superficial and deep), cold, and electrical stimulation. These are usually adjunctive treatments and should not substitute for sound therapeutic exercise. The various modal-

TABLE 26–1

FUNCTIONAL SCALES FOR RHEUMATIC DISEASES

	MMT	Range of Motion	Pain	Fatigue	Activities of Daily Living	Ambulation	Cognition	Role/Social Interaction
OA		+ +	+ +		+	+ +		
RA	+	+ +	+ +	+ + +	+ +	+ +		+ + + +
Spondyloarthropathies		+ +	+ +		+	+		+
DM-PM	+ +			+ + +	+ +	+ +		+ + + +
PSS		+ +	+ +	+	+ +			+ +
SLE	+			+ + +	+	+	+ +	+ + + +
Gout (crystals)			+ + +			+ +		
Fibrositis			+ + +	+ + +				+ +

+, possibly useful evaluation; + +, recommended evaluation; + + +, strongly recommended evaluation; + + + +, must evaluate.

MMT, manual muscle testing; OA, osteoarthritis; RA, rheumatoid arthritis; DM-PM, dermatomyositis-polymyositis; PSS, progressive systemic sclerosis; SLE, systemic lupus erythematosus.

From DeLisa JA: Rehabilitation Medicine: Principles and Practice. Philadelphia, JB Lippincott, 1988, p 772.

ities may be used in an attempt to mitigate symptoms, thus allowing for participation in therapeutic exercise programs. In extremely acute situations, however, physical therapy in the form of modalities may be all that is tolerated by the patient. The use of these modalities has not been shown to influence the progression of rheumatic disease.[8]

Cold

When musculoskeletal disorders are treated, the use of cold in acute phases has long been considered a most effective form of physical therapy. Cold can have multiple effects. It can increase the pain threshold and reduce muscle spasm.[9] Cold application may inhibit collagenase activity in rheumatic synovium.[10] It may enhance the efficacy of exercise programs, possibly secondary to its analgesic effects.[11]

Cold lowers tissue temperature, resulting in vasoconstriction of inflamed or traumatized vessels. Edema can thus be reduced, particularly in acute phases of injury or inflammation.[12] The ill effects of the application of heat to an acute injury are well recognized. In the acute phase of injury, the combination of cold, compression, and elevation acts to minimize edema, hemorrhage, and pain. This combination is typically used as long as edema or increased warmth exists. In dependent extremities the use of compression is the most maintainable of this combination and possibly the most important approach for control of edema. Frequency of application is determined by the acuteness of the injury and patient motivation. An example is the application of cold every 2 to 4 hours for 20 minutes in the initial acute phase of an injury, progressing to a 20-minute application once a day after activity or therapeutic exercises.

Cold, or cryotherapy, can be provided in a number of methods. Heat is lost by convection and evaporation when air is moved rapidly over skin. Topical refrigerants such as ethylchloride have rapid changes in phase that draw off heat. The more practical and commonly used type of cooling is conduction, which involves the actual application of cold to the part.

Crushed ice is an easily moldable and convenient method of application. Commercially prepared gels are available that hold cold well and are reusable. Care must be taken because some of the gelatinous materials used in some commercial packs frequently remain at temperatures below freezing and as a result this may cause tissue damage. A wet towel should be placed between the body part and the cold pack to protect the skin. Melting ice maintains temperatures at 33°F or higher, offering some protection from frostbite. Immersion ice bath is an effective although often less tolerated technique. Commercial instant ice packs are expensive and do not maintain therapeutic temperatures well. A bag of frozen peas or corn makes an inexpensive, reusable, moldable ice pack. As always when dealing with an insensitive body part, special care must be taken to avoid damaging the tissue.

Contrast baths are a soothing and well tolerated alternate method of application. Used in less acute situations, contrast baths are believed to be an effective method of reducing persistent edema.[11] The alternating vasoconstriction-dilatation effect is thought to help ''pump'' edema from the area. Contrast baths should be combined with gentle active range-of-motion exercises to facilitate venous return.

Patients with systemic lupus erythematosus, Raynaud's phenomenon, diabetes, dermatomyositis, and vasculitis may have vascular and immunologic factors that affect cold sensitivity, which may make the use of cold in these conditions contraindicated. Some arthritis patients claim an intolerance to cryotherapy. Many times it is the mode of application rather than the modality that is the problem.

Heat

Heat has been a soothing modality throughout history. It remains one of the most enduring forms of therapy. Some postulate that this may even be instinctual.[12] Certainly anyone who has experienced the relaxing effects of the sun's rays can understand its attraction. Heat's therapeutic effects have been the subject of much study. There are local, superficial, and deep effects, the most visible of which is hyperemia. As larger body areas are involved, increasing systemic responses are noted.[12] Heat increases threshold responses to pain and can produce sedation.[13] It can also reduce muscle spasm, possibly by its effect on the muscle spindle.[12]

Methods of heating may be divided into superficial or deep. Skin is a poor conductor of heat; therefore, conductive heating techniques produce temperature changes to a depth of only a few millimeters.[12] A paradoxical reduction in intra-articular temperatures has been noted.[15] Deeper forms of heat therapy may be delivered via ultrasonography, short wave or microwave diathermy. Short wave and microwave diathermy are less frequently used in the clinical setting and are less efficacious for deep heating.[12] Ultrasound can reach depths that create increases in intra-articular temperatures, allowing for increased stretch in collagenous structures when placed under tension.[15] This is termed the *viscoelastic effect*, which can be helpful when working to improve joint motion.[15–17]

Heat is most indicated in chronic or subacute situations when attempting to relieve muscle spasm and contracture. Care must be taken in the acutely inflamed joint or in areas of decreased sensation or vascular compromise. Deep forms of heat therapy must be used judiciously in rheumatic disease because increases in intra-articular temperatures can increase collagenase activity and actually accelerate cartilage destruction.[18] The general clinical response to superficial heating that is perceived by patients is relief of joint pain and stiffness. Clearly, this makes heat an important modality in the care of the arthritic patient, particularly as an adjunct to a stretching program. Superficial heat has not been shown to alter the progression of rheumatic disease.[8]

As previously mentioned, heat may be applied either superficially or deeply. Superficial forms of heat may be applied using any number of techniques (Table 26–2). Choice of mode of application should be based on physician and patient preference, convenience, expense, patient tolerance, accessibility of the body part, and treatment goals. Many methods, such as hot water bottles, tub baths, moist heat packs, and heating pads, may be available to the patient for use at home.

Ultrasonography. Since its acceptance by the United States Council on Physical Medicine and Rehabilitation in 1952, ultrasonography has become one of the most used physical modalities. Ultrasound is a high-frequency mechanical vibration produced at frequencies inaudible to the human ear (i.e., frequencies greater than 16,000 to 20,000 cycles/second). Therapeutic ultrasound is produced by converting electrical energy into mechanical energy. High-frequency alternating current applied through a transducer creates mechanical energy in the form of ultrasonic waves. The transducer consists of a crystal capable of producing a piezoelectric effect (e.g., quartz, barium titanate) cemented between two electrodes.[19] The vibrations or ultrasonic waves are adjustable to therapeutic frequencies. The shorter the frequency of sound, the greater the depth of penetration.[17, 20] The optimal frequency band for medical ultrasonography is 800,000 to 1,000,000 Hz. Ultrasonographic energy has been shown to penetrate to greater tissue depths (up to 50% energy at 5 cm) than any other physical agent.[19–21]

Understanding the physiologic effects of ultrasonography enables the clinician to choose appropriate indications for its use. Physiologic effects of ultrasonography are generally recognized to be thermal and nonthermal.[12, 14, 16, 21] Thermal effects result when mechanical energy in the form of sound waves is absorbed by tissue. The amount of absorption depends on tissue density. Tissue with high density or collagen content absorbs most efficiently. Carbohydrates and lipids show the least absorption.[19, 21] Owing to the reflection that occurs at tissues of different densities, increased temperatures are found at interfacing tissues (e.g., muscle and bone).[20] Nervous tissue has been shown to be especially responsive to ultrasonic energy. Changes in nerve conduction velocity are seen in peripheral nerves exposed to standard clinical dosages of ultrasound.[22]

Nonthermal effects of ultrasonography include mechanical and chemical effects. Cell permeability, tissue pressure changes, and local blood flow are all affected at clinical intensities.[23, 24] Effective improvement in joint range of motion can be obtained through changes in tendon extensibility, modification of scar tissue, and relaxation of skeletal muscle, which are shown to be produced by ultrasonography.[16, 19]

The intensity of ultrasound is controlled by the power output divided by the area of the transducer head, measured in W/cm². The intensity and duration of treatment depend on several factors. The clinical diagnosis, the area of the body part to be treated, the acuteness of the injury, and the volume of soft tissue all need to be considered. Proximal limb musculature and the trunk require higher therapeutic intensities in treatment than do the distal extremities. A mild sensation of warmth produced with the sound head moving slowly is a good general guide for appropriate intensity. Of course, patients with sensory deficits require minimum intensities for safety. Pain or burning sensations can indicate too high an intensity or too prolonged a stationary position. Reduced intensity and/or pulsed ultrasound (interrupted sound waves) is indicated when stationary treatment is required.

For effective use of ultrasound, good coupling is necessary between the transducer and the body surface. The coupler should provide reduced friction for application and effective transfer of ultrasound energy to skin. Liquid or viscous materials (e.g., gels, ointments, and creams) are often used. Good coupling is essential because ultrasonic energy is dissipated by air.[20] *Direct coupling* refers to the use of viscous materials interposed directly between the sound head and the skin. *Indirect coupling* refers to the use of ultrasound underwater. This method is especially useful in treating uneven anatomic structures or areas of increased sensitivity.

Some specific indications for ultrasonography use are the following:

- Muscular spasm or strain
- Tendinitis, tenosynovitis
- Capsulitis, sprains, arthritic conditions
- Adhesions, bursitis, calcific deposits
- Neuromas, resolving hematoma
- Limited joint motion
- Application of local medicament

Hydrotherapy. One of the more frequently used heat

TABLE 26–2

HEAT THERAPY: METHODS OF APPLICATION

Superficial	Deep
Solids	
Heating pads	Ultrasound
Hot water bottle	Shortwave diathermy
Peloids (mud, poultices)	Microwave diathermy
Sand	
Liquids	
Water	
Paraffin wax	
Moist heat packs	
Whirlpool	
Wet compress	
Gases	
Dry or moist air	
Fluidotherapy	
Sauna	
Radiant	
Infrared (noncontact dry heat)	

sources is water. Hydrotherapy has many advantages. Gravity can be eliminated, reducing stress to inflamed joints while allowing easy control of temperature. Movement through water can also be used as a low-level form of resistive exercise. Wound care can be performed via the débridement action of air jets or whirlpool. The movement created by these jets also provides a soothing massage effect. Care must be taken to maintain a neutral temperature, particularly because greater percentages of body surface area are exposed to heat (therapeutic range 98° to 105°F).[19]

Paraffin Wax. Paraffin melts at 120°F.[19] The addition of mineral oil lowers the melting point to a more tolerable temperature. Units are available that maintain the wax at therapeutic temperature. This method of heat application particularly lends itself to use in the treatment of hands and feet of arthritic patients. The mineral oil is soothing to the skin while the moist heat prepares stiff, painful joints for motion exercise. Paraffin can be used at home, but caution needs to be taken to ensure the patient maintains proper paraffin temperature. The paraffin can be ''painted'' on, or the body part immersed several times in the wax, then usually wrapped in plastic, and then toweling is used to maintain the heat.

Fluidotherapy. This is a form of dry heat and massage used primarily with the distal extremities. Units use heated cellulose or polypropylene that is rapidly propelled via compressed air. Temperature is readily adjustable. Stimulation is analogous to a whirlpool, but the part is maintained dry.

Infrared Equipment. Infrared equipment provides for application of dry forms of superficial heat. Radiant heat lamps using wavelengths within the electromagnetic spectrum (770 to 12,000 Å) provide comfortable warming.[19] This modality is more commonly used with larger body parts. The lamp must be maintained at the appropriate distance from the body part. Care must be taken to check the skin to avoid burning. The physiologic effects of radiant heat are similar to those of conductive heating methods.

Moist Heat Packs. Commercially prepared silica gel packs or hydrocollator packs are used to provide moist superficial heat. These retain heat for long periods (as long as 1 hour) and can be used at home. They are usually heated to between 140° and 160°F. Appropriate padding (towels or pad covers) and occasional skin checks should be used to avoid burning.

Electrical Stimulation

Interest in the physiologic effects and uses of electricity were first noted when fish producing electrical current were found to produce muscle contraction and relief of pain. Galvani, in the late 1700s, fired the minds of early scientists with his observations of the relationship between muscle contraction and electricity. In the early 1800s, Faraday developed his electromagnetic machine, an early generator. This generator produced current that was found to evoke more sustained muscle contraction.[25, 26] As electrical technology improved, so did clinical applications of electrical stimulation.

Electrical stimulation is often used in the treatment of a variety of neurologic, acute, and chronic musculoskeletal conditions. The excitability of muscle and nerve tissue provides the basic rationale for the use of electrical stimulation in these disorders. Each electrode has been associated with distinct characteristics producing specific therapeutic effects.

The positive pole is generally considered to be the relaxing, or analgesic, electrode, whereas the negative pole is considered the stimulating electrode.

Many claims about the effects of electrical stimulation have been made throughout the years. A person's experience and knowledge of theory, combined with patient presentation and response, dictate the clinician's choice of technique.

Some of the conditions for which electrical stimulation has been used are the following:

- Muscle spasm or strain
- Muscle impaired by surgery, central or peripheral nerve injury
- Atrophied muscle secondary to immobilization
- Acute or chronic inflammation due to sprain, tendinitis, bursitis, or arthritis
- Pain syndromes, postoperative pain
- Biofeedback techniques, muscle re-education
- Edema reduction

The currently popular high-voltage direct-current stimulators (HVDCSs) produce waveforms of very short duration and amplitude.[27] The amplitude of current pulsation appears to be related to the depth of penetration in tissue.[27, 28] The short pulse duration (5 to 75 μsec) seen with the HVDCS seems to be more easily tolerated by the patient than are other forms of electrical stimulation. Chemical and thermal effects often associated with standard galvanic or low-voltage stimulators are not seen. This allows for a longer duration of treatment.

HVDCS units are commonly used to help maintain muscle bulk and strength in immobilized limbs.[29, 30] Because of their short duration of current, they are not used to stimulate denervated muscle. Electrodes may be placed directly over inflamed or edematous body parts. Electrogalvanic stimulation may also be used to reduce muscle spasm.[31] Electrodes are placed parallel to the spasming muscle.

Pain Modulation Using TENS. Transcutaneous electrical nerve stimulation (TENS) has been demonstrated to be effective in increasing patients' tolerance for activity through reduction of pain.[32, 33] Currents have been applied to dermatomes or directly over painful areas. Pain trigger points are abnormally sensitive areas of myofascia that, when treated specifically, can reduce pain and muscle spasm. TENS has specifically been shown to be helpful in controlling pain in patients with rheumatoid arthritis.

Cutaneous electrodes bombard nerves with stimulation, which has been shown to reduce some patients' need for analgesic medication.[34] Theories as to why electrical stimulation reduces pain relate to the neurophysiology of pain transmission. Naturally occurring central nervous system opiates (enkephalins and endorphins) are believed to be secreted as a result of electrical stimulation.[33] The selective stimulation of pain transmitting nerve fibers has been theorized to reduce the overall perception of pain.[32, 33] It remains to be demonstrated whether TENS is helpful on a long-term basis for the treatment of chronic pain due to arthritis. TENS may be considered as a method of pain control particularly in patients who have a poor response to pharmacologic methods of treatment.

THERAPEUTIC EXERCISE

Therapeutic exercise should be the centerpoint to the rehabilitation program and must be designed with many patient

TABLE 26–3

GUIDE TO SELECTION OF THERAPEUTIC EXERCISES FOR PATIENTS WITH RHEUMATIC DISEASES

Disease	Functional Problem	Type of Exercise				Recreational Activities
		Passive (Stretch)	Active Isometric	Active Isotonic	Assistive	
RA						
Acute phase with synovitis	Weakness in specific muscles	−	If involved (quads, rotator cuff, neck retraction)	−	Intrinsic muscles, hands, and feet	−
Subacute/chronic without effusion	Weakness, contracture, fatigue	For contractures	May use isometric or isotonic for weak or atrophic muscles		Intrinsic muscles, hands and feet	+ Swim, walk, bicycle, low-impact aerobics
Systemic lupus (vasculitis)						
Myositis	Weakness and	−	Submaximal	−	−	−
Steroid myopathy	fatigue	−	+	+	−	+ (walk, bicycle)
Polymyositis	Weakness	−	+	Advance to isotonic or isokinetic as enzymes drop	−	None until enzymes are low
Progressive systemic sclerosis	Contractures	+	−	−	+	No restrictions (except when cardiopulmonary system is involved)
	Some weakness		+	+	+	
Ankylosing spondylitis	Limited motion	+	+	−	+	Noncontact sports
Osteoarthritis	Contracture	+	−	−	+	
	Weakness	−	+	+	−	+
	Stamina	−	−	+	−	Encouraged, if no joint effusion (bicycling, walking, swimming preferred)
Crystalline or septic arthritis						
Acute phase		−	+/−	−	−	None
Posteffusion		−	−	+	−	Unrestricted

−, no exercise recommended; +, exercise permitted.
RA, rheumatoid arthritis.
From Kelley WN, Harris ED, Ruddy S, et al: Textbook of Rheumatology, 3rd ed. Philadelphia, WB Saunders, 1989, p 1908.

variables in mind. Although modalities have been discussed extensively, their primary purpose should be to provide relief of symptoms to allow the patient to participate in exercise.

Therapeutic exercise can be designed to maintain or improve range of motion, endurance, and strength. Other less emphasized, although important, components of condition are generalized improvement of function, balance, efficiency of movement, and sense of well-being. In designing a program for any patient, care must be taken to progress the patient appropriately. Initial therapy may be directed at attempting to relieve pain using modalities. Subsequent to this, improvement or maintenance of range of motion may be a goal. Strengthening should begin with less stressful forms of exercise, such as isometrics progressing to isotonic exercise with low resistance. In patients with less severe disease or those seen postoperatively, exercise may progress to isokinetic or isotonic exercise using increased resistance. These last forms of exercise may be inappropriate for the arthritic patient. Generally, with regard to therapy in painful joint disorders, range of motion should be restored first. Strengthening exercise begun too early may worsen symptoms, leading to loss of motion and function.

Rest is an important component of therapy, particularly in the active phases of inflammatory disease; care must be taken not to overtax inflamed joints. Conversely, too much rest can lead to increased fibrosis and decreased cartilage integrity.[35] Also seen are general deconditioning, loss in muscle bulk and strength, diminished range of motion, and reduced kinesthetic awareness. Muscle may lose as much as 30% of its bulk in as little as 1 week of bedrest.[36]

Table 26–3 outlines appropriate therapeutic exercises for patients with rheumatic diseases.

Strengthening Exercise

Isometric exercise is believed to produce the least joint inflammation and least juxta-articular joint destruction.[37] Isometric exercises employ muscle actions with little or no motion of the involved joint and very little fatigue. This form of exercise may be most appropriate for the arthritic patient. It has been shown that repetitive submaximal isometric muscle contractions held for 6 seconds can increase strength and static muscle endurance.[36] These exercises require no equipment but may necessitate demonstration or observation to ensure that the correct muscle group is being contracted. Contractions can be against stationary objects or against a muscle's antagonist. Ideally, contractions are performed at various points in the range of motion, that is, at different muscle lengths.

As joint pain and inflammation diminish and isometric strength increases, isotonic exercise may be initiated. Muscle action is used to move weight through a range of motion. This form of exercise increases strength and dynamic endurance that mimic many functional activities. In general, strength is most rapidly improved by lifting increasing amounts of weight a small number of times (i.e., less than 12). Endurance is improved by moving lesser amounts of weight many times. DeLateur has shown that when carried to the point of fatigue, exercise with low weight and low intensity can build strength.[38] Care should be taken with arthritic patients to avoid dynamic high-resistance exercise because this may exacerbate symptoms.

Isokinetic exercise involves the use of specially designed equipment that maintains a fixed speed of motion but produces a variable resistance. The amount of resistance is equal to the resistance imparted by the patient and may be halted at any moment by the patient. At slower speeds, greater torque or resistance can be created owing to increased time allowed for recruitment of motor units. Because the speed of motion is controlled, exercise can be performed at velocities much higher than those attainable with most weight machines. This should theoretically allow for more functional exercise training. Unfortunately, greater gains in functional performance from isokinetic training have not been documented. Torque measures can be used to determine progress or for comparison to contralateral limbs. This form of exercise may be more appropriate for the athletic patient.

Range-of-Motion Exercise

When patients are in an acute phase of joint inflammation, gentle active-assistive motion performed one or two times a day may be all that the patient will tolerate. Often, splinting is used early to maintain functional positions while resting the body part. As joint inflammation diminishes, increasing degrees of motion may be added within patient tolerance. Exercises should not cause severe pain at the time of exercise, nor should they lead to prolonged residual discomfort. Generally, in inflammatory joint disease, active or active-assistive motions are preferable to passive forms of exercise. The exception is loss of joint motion secondary to trauma, surgery, or immobility. In these instances, passive forms of exercise may accelerate clinical improvements. In distal extremities, passive motions can be performed by the patient or therapist. Active attempts at motion by the patient with passive assist by the therapist allow for reflex inhibition of antagonist musculature, which can facilitate improvements in range.

Mobilization

Techniques for mobilizing joints in nonrheumatic or inflammatory connective disease patients have been the source of much study within the field of physical medicine. Mobilization techniques are outlined for nearly all joints. Accessory motions such as glide, rotation, and joint distraction are used to aid in improvement and maintenance of joint motion. These accessory joint movements are necessary for more classic joint movements to occur. Often, range of motion exercise, performed by the therapist, can begin with small oscillatory motions using accessory joint movement. These are generally well tolerated, even in tender joints, and can greatly improve patients' ability to perform functional motions.

Some definitions are as follows:

- Classic movements: movements that form the more traditional description of movement (e.g., dorsiflexion and plantarflexion)
- Accessory movement: motions that accompany classic movements and are essential for normal full range and painless function (e.g., the glide of the tibia and the fibula on the talus at heel strike)
- Manipulative movement: thrusting, sudden high-velocity, short-amplitude motions that are delivered at the end limit of motion

Mobilizations are performed with the goal of overall improved range of motion and mechanics. These are not considered manipulations, which technically are more sudden, forceful movements. Mobilization can be used to evaluate joint function. An example of this is testing the anteroposterior glide motion available in a first metatarsophalangeal joint. Capsulodesis may limit dorsiflexion and plantarflexion. Anteroposterior glide of the joint also is limited and can be compared with the contralateral limb. By performing oscillating glide motions at the extremes of accessory movement both anteriorly and posteriorly, the capsule may be effectively mobilized in a way that simple classic passive motion may not. These are relatively simple techniques that add tremendously to the clinician's ability to both assess and facilitate improvement in joint motion.

ASSISTIVE DEVICES

The use of assistive devices in patients with articular disease can often present unique challenges. Many factors influence a patient's need for these devices. Deficits in strength, endurance, balance, increased pain, or recent surgery can necessitate the use of assistive devices. Standard assistive devices, such as a cane and crutches, are often appropriate. Quadripod canes of varying sizes can provide a more stable base of support and may be helpful to patients with mild upper extremity involvement. Patients with severe upper extremity involvement, however, may not be able to negotiate with standard axillary crutches or even a pick-up walker. Platform crutches or a platform walker that allows the patient to load weight to the forearms rather than inflamed hands or wrists can be considered. These devices are particularly helpful in postoperative patients who, for reasons related to the surgical procedure, may require a non-weightbearing or partial weightbearing status. A rolling walker may suffice in some instances. A motorized wheelchair or cart can be used to preserve energy and improve endurance.

References

1. Medsger TA and Masi AT: In McCarthy DJ (ed): Epidemiology of Rheumatic Disease: Arthritis and Related Conditions, 10th ed. Philadelphia, Lea & Febiger, 1985.
2. Schumacher HR (ed): Primer on Rheumatic Diseases, 9th ed. Atlanta, Arthritis Foundation, 1988.
3. Spiegel JS, Spiegel TM, Ward NB, et al: Rehabilitation for rheumatoid arthritis patients. Arthritis Rheum 29:628–637, 1986.

4. Kendall HO, Kendall FP, and Wadsworth GE: Muscle Testing and Function, 2nd ed. Baltimore, Williams & Wilkins, 1971.

5. Resnick D and Niwayama G: Diagnosis of Bone and Joint Disorders, 2nd ed. Philadelphia, WB Saunders, 1988.

6. Cooperating Clinics Committee of American Rheumatism Association: A seven-day variability study of 499 patients with peripheral rheumatoid arthritis. Arthritis Rheum 8:302–334, 1965.

7. Jette AM: Functional capacity evaluation: An empirical approach. Arch Phys Med Rehabil 61:85, 1980.

8. Mainard CL, Walter JM, and Spiegal PK: Rheumatoid arthritis: Failure of daily heat therapy to effect progression. Arch Phys Med Rehabil 60:390–392, 1979.

9. Miglietta O: Action of cold on spasticity. Phys Med 52:198, 1973.

10. Harris ED and McCroskery JA: Influence of temperature and fibril stability on degradation of cartilage collagen by rheumatoid synovial collagenase. N Engl J Med 290:1, 1974.

11. Garrick JG and Webb DR: Sports Injuries: Diagnosis and Management. Philadelphia, WB Saunders, 1990.

12. Licht S: Therapeutic Heat and Cold, 2nd ed. Baltimore, Waverly Press, 1965.

13. Lehmann JF, Brunner GD, and Stow RW: Pain threshold measurement after therapeutic application of ultrasound microwaves, and infrared. Arch Phys Med Rehabil 39:560–565, 1958.

14. Hollander JL and Horvath SM: Changes in joint temperature produced by diseases and by physical therapy. Arch Phys Med Rehabil 30:437, 1949.

15. Lehmann JF, Masock AJ, Warren CG, et al: Effect of therapeutic temperatures on tendon extensibility. Arch Phys Med Rehabil 51:481–487, 1970.

16. Gerstein JW: Effect of ultrasound on tendon extensibility. Am J Phys Med 34:362, 1955.

17. Castor CW: Connective tissue activation: Effects of temperature in vitro. Arch Phys Med Rehabil 57:5, 1976.

18. Dorwart BB, Hansell, JR, and Schumacher HR Jr: Effects of cold and heat on urate-induced synovitis in the dog. Arthritis Rheum 17:563, 1974.

19. Griffin JE and Karselis TC: Physical Agents for Physical Therapists, 2nd ed. Springfield, IL, Charles C Thomas, 1982, pp 279–312.

20. Ter Haar G: Basic physics of therapeutic ultrasound. Physiotherapy 64:100–103, 1978.

21. Lehmann JF and Johnson EW: Some factors influencing temperature distribution in thighs exposed to ultrasound. Arch Phys Med Rehabil 39:347–356, 1958.

22. Farmer WC: Effects of intensity of ultrasound on velocity of motor axons. Phys Ther 48:1233, 1968.

23. Helfand A and Bruno J: Therapeutic modalities and procedures: 1. Cold and heat. Clin Podiatr 1:301–313, 1984.

24. Lehmann JF, Warren G, and Scham S: Therapeutic heat and cold. Clin Orthop 99:207–226, 1974.

25. Licht S: Electrodiagnosis and Electromyography, 3rd ed. Baltimore, Waverly Press, 1971, pp 1–23.

26. Benton L, Baker L, Bowman B, and Waters R: Functional Electrical Stimulation: A Practical Guide. Downey, CA, Rancho Los Amigos Rehabilitation Engineering Center, 1980, pp 1–55.

27. Alon G: High-voltage galvanic stimulation. Israel J Physiother 33:1982 [English abstract].

28. Stayodyn Vara/Pulse Operational Manual. Longmont, CO, Stayodyn Inc, 1986.

29. Kramer J and Mendryk S: Electrical stimulation as a strength improvement technique: A review. J Orthop Sports Phys Ther 2:91–98, 1982.

30. Mohr T, Carlson B, and Landry R: Comparison of isometric exercise and high-voltage galvanic stimulation. Phys Ther 65:606–612, 1985.

31. Owens J and Malone T: Treatment parameters of high-frequency electrical stimulation. J Orthop Sports Phys Ther 4:162–168, 1983.

32. Wolfe S: Perspectives on central nervous system response to transcutaneous electrical nerve stimulation. Phys Ther 58:1443–1449, 1978.

33. Bishop B: Pain: Its physiology and rationale for management: 1–III. Phys Ther 60:13–37, 1980.

34. Mannheimer C, Lund S, and Carlsson CA: The effect of transcutaneous electrical nerve stimulation (TENS) on joint pain in patients with rheumatoid arthritis. Scand J Rheumatol 7:13–16, 1978.

35. Woo SL, Matthews JV, Akeson WM, et al: Connective tissue response to immobility. Arthritis Rheum 18:257–264, 1975.

36. Muller EA: Influence of training and activity on muscle strength. Arch Phys Med Rehabil 51:449–462, 1970.

37. Castello BA and El Sallab RA: Physical activity, cystic erosion and osteoporosis in rheumatoid arthritis. Ann Rheum Dis 24:522, 1965.

38. DeLateur B, Lehmann JF, and Fordyce WE: A test of the DeLorme axiom. Arch Phys Med 49:245–248, 1968.

Surgical Management

CHAPTER 27

Perioperative Considerations

Bennett G. Zier, M.D.

Rheumatology has been defined as the area of medicine that deals primarily with disorders of the musculoskeletal system, including all diseases of the joints and periarticular tissues. Rheumatic disorders are among the most common conditions encountered causing pain and loss of physical function and at times may manifest as widespread systemic disease. Many of the rheumatic disorders, such as degenerative joint disease and rheumatoid arthritis, are among the most common diseases encountered in podiatric practice; indeed, there is no other subspecialty of internal medicine that interfaces more closely with podiatry than clinical rheumatology.

This chapter deals with the many clinical issues generated by the arthritic patient who undergoes podiatric medical care or foot and ankle surgery. A number of fundamental clinical concepts are discussed in this context.

GENERAL PREOPERATIVE EVALUATION

The foundation of the preoperative assessment of a patient with an arthritic problem being managed by surgery lies in viewing the patient with a comprehensive medical approach. This is best exemplified by the statement that the foot is connected to the rest of the body. Podiatric pathologic conditions are best approached in the context of whether the foot or ankle problem represents an end manifestation of systemic illness or is the first sign of illness elsewhere in the body. Nowhere is this approach more appropriate than in assessing the patient's medical condition in preparation for podiatric surgery. The podiatrist must perform a thorough preoperative history and physical examination and be able to formulate a perioperative care plan that is dictated by that evaluation.

The ability to define surgical risk is extremely useful for assessing the general medical status of a preoperative patient. Anesthesiologists use a rating scale to correlate a patient's clinical status with a classification of surgical risk (Table 27–1). *Surgical risk* is defined as the probability of morbidity or mortality resulting from an operative procedure. There are five classes of surgical risk, as determined by the American Society of Anesthesiologists (ASA), ranging from class 1 (least risk) to class 5 (most risk). The mortality risk from the same operation obviously increases considerably when comparing a patient with a class 1 risk with a patient with a class 5 risk. Most patients being considered for elective podiatric surgery should fit within a risk class of 1 or 2. If the risk is class 3 or higher, there must be extremely extenuating circumstances that warrant any consideration for elective surgery.

History

Obtaining the patient's medical history is an essential part of a preoperative evaluation. Just as some clinicians believe that 95% of diagnoses can be made through an excellent history, so too can an excellent assessment of the patient's preoperative risk be made through obtaining careful historical information. A preoperative history is specific for surgical risk assessment and need not be as extensive as the type of historical data obtained in an internist's initial comprehensive medical assessment of a patient. The essential elements of a preoperative history are delineated in Table 27–2.

Physical Examination

The physical examination of the preoperative patient is one that mainly emphasizes the cardiopulmonary system because these organ systems contribute most to perioperative morbidity and mortality. Table 27–3 describes the physical examination data that are necessary to evaluate a podiatric surgical patient from a general medical standpoint.

Vital signs are the most important part of the physical examination. Hypertension, hypotension, tachycardia, bradycardia, irregular pulse, fever, tachypnea, obesity, and malnutrition all are readily available information obtained from

TABLE 27–1

AMERICAN SOCIETY OF ANESTHESIOLOGISTS PHYSICAL STATUS MEASURE

P1—Normal and Healthy

There is no physiologic, biochemical, or psychiatric disturbance. The pathologic process for which the operation is to be performed is localized and not conducive to systemic disturbances. Example: A healthy patient with a heel spur.

P2—Mild Systemic Disease

Mild to moderate systemic disturbance caused by the condition to be treated surgically or other pathophysiologic processes. Examples: Presence of mild diabetes, essential hypertension.

P3—Severe Systemic Disease that Is Not Incapacitating

Rather severe systemic disturbance or disorder from whatever cause, even though it may not be possible to define the degree of disability with certainty. Examples: Severe diabetes with vascular complications; moderate to severe degrees of pulmonary insufficiency.

P4—Incapacitating Systemic Disease that Is a Threat to Life

Indicative of a patient with a severe systemic disorder already life threatening and not always correctable by the operative procedure. Examples: Advanced degrees of cardiac, pulmonary, renal, hepatic, or endocrine insufficiency.

P5—Moribund Patient Who Is Not Expected to Live with or without Surgery

Defines the patient who has little chance of survival but is submitted for surgery in desperation. Example: Massive pulmonary embolus.

P6—Emergency Operation (E)

Any patient in one of the classes listed above who is operated on as an emergency is considered to be in somewhat poorer physical condition. The letter E is placed beside the numeric classification.

Data from the Relative Value Guide (copyright 1992) of the American Society of Anesthesiologists, 520 N. Northwest Highway, Park Ridge, IL 60068-2573.

performing vital signs. Because hypertension is often newly discovered on routine preoperative examinations, careful blood pressure recording is an essential task in the preoperative physical examination. Hypertensive disease is not uncommon in a variety of rheumatologic diseases, including systemic lupus erythematosus (SLE), progressive systemic sclerosis, and vasculitis.

An eye examination may reveal evidence of hypertensive or diabetic retinopathy. Podiatrists should be familiar enough with fundoscopic examination to recognize these entities.

A nasal examination should carefully note any nasal obstruction because this is important information when patients are being considered for intubation in general anesthesia. An examination of the neck should denote any presence of carotid bruits, goiter (which may have implications in terms of thyroid disease), and elevated neck veins (which may indicate right-sided congestive heart failure). If patients are to undergo endotracheal intubation, they must have excellent range of motion of their neck. This is of paramount importance when evaluating the rheumatoid patient who may have cervical spine involvement.

A chest and lung examination is extremely important for detecting findings that may indicate congestive heart failure (rales), emphysema (barrel chest, hyperresonant percussion), bronchitis (rhonchi), or asthma (wheezing). An examination of the heart may reveal a heart murmur, a fast or slow apical pulse, or an irregular rate. The presence of a heart murmur may indicate underlying valvular heart disease that may be found in patients with ankylosing spondylitis. Slow, fast, or irregular rates may indicate cardiac rhythm or conduction disturbances.

Abdominal examination must be performed to rule out liver enlargement (acute hepatitis, cancer), splenic enlargement (viral infection, lymphoma, portal hypertension), or abnormal abdominal masses or pulsations (aortic aneurysm). The presence of bowel sounds must be noted both preoperatively and postoperatively because this indicates active bowel function.

Examination of the lower extremities is of obvious importance in podiatry. From a medical viewpoint, podiatrists are most concerned about intact vascular and neurologic systems that would promote excellent wound healing. The musculoskeletal system must be examined because it is helpful in determining the presence of any type of arthritis as well as the existence of any muscular weakness that may indicate an underlying myopathy.

The neurologic examination is of importance in terms of

TABLE 27–2

PREOPERATIVE ASSESSMENT: HISTORY TAKING

I. Introductory statement: name, age, sex, referring physician, planned procedure, primary care physician

II. Patient profile: geographic living situation, support system (husband, wife, significant others, children), line of employment

III. Present medical history: narrative description of the events leading to the decision to undergo planned surgical procedure

IV. Past medical history
  A. Previous operations and complications
  B. Medications: prescribed, over-the-counter, recreational, alcohol, nicotine
  C. Allergies
  D. Nonsurgical hospitalizations
  E. Immunization status (hepatitis, tetanus)
  F. Pertinent review of systems
    1. Head: history of headache, head trauma
    2. Eyes: vision, glasses, contact lenses, glaucoma
    3. Ears: hearing, history of vertigo and dizziness, infection
    4. Nose: nasal stuffiness or obstruction, nose bleeds
    5. Mouth: condition of teeth, bleeding gums; any oral lesions present
    6. Respiratory: cough, sputum production, hemoptysis, asthma, chronic obstructive pulmonary disease, history of pneumonia, tuberculosis screening, last chest radiograph, recent urinary tract infection, function screening
    7. Cardiac: history of shortness of breath, dyspnea, orthopnea, paroxysmal nocturnal dyspnea, chest pain (angina), history of myocardial infarction, edema, palpitations, hypertension, rheumatic fever, heart murmurs, pacemaker, last electrocardiogram
    8. Peripheral vascular: intermittent claudication, history of thrombophlebitis, lower extremity ulcers
    9. Gastrointestinal: heartburn, hematemesis, melena, rectal bleeding, constipation, diarrhea, hepatitis, abdominal pain, jaundice, history of liver disease, diet and nutritional status
    10. Genitourinary/renal: polyuria, nocturia, dysuria, hematuria, incontinence, urinary tract infection, history of renal disease
      a. Male: hernia, discharge from or sores on penis
      b. Female: last menstrual period, possibility of pregnancy
    11. Musculoskeletal: joint pains, arthritis, backache, gout
    12. Neurologic: seizures, fainting, blackouts, paralysis, memory, cognition, burning in feet, dementia, delirium, past or present history of psychiatric problems
    13. Hematology: anemia, easy bruising or bleeding, past blood transfusions; history of thrombocytopenia, postoperative bleeding
    14. Endocrine: thyroid disease, diabetes, history of osteoporosis, any past steroids, history of hyperparathyroidism
    15. Infectious disease: history of acquired immunodeficiency syndrome risk factors, sexually transmitted diseases

V. Family history: occurrence within the family of any significant medical condition, including diabetes, tuberculosis, heart disease, hypertension, stroke, kidney disease, cancer, arthritis, anemia, complications of surgery

TABLE 27–3

PREOPERATIVE ASSESSMENT: PHYSICAL EXAMINATION

I. Introduction, general survey: Succinct paragraph describing patient's general physical appearance
II. Vital signs: height, weight, temperature, blood pressure, pulse, respiratory rate
III. Head and neck
   A. Head: size, shape, trauma
   B. Eyes
      1. Pupillary response to light and accommodation (PERLA)
      2. Extraocular movements (EOM)
      3. Sclera color
      4. Ophthalmoscopic examination (fundi)
   C. Ears: patency of canals, appearance of drum, fundi reflex
   D. Nose: patency of choanae, septal deviation
   E. Mouth: buccal mucosa, state of health of oral structures (teeth, gums, palate, tongue, appearance of pigmentary spots or petechiae)
   F. Throat: presence of obstruction, gag reflex, presence of exudate or erythema
   G. Neck: neck vein distention, tracheal deviation, presence of carotid bruits, presence of goiter, adenopathy, range of motion
IV. Respiratory system: presence of rales, wheezes, rhonchi or pleural rub
V. Heart: rate, regularity, presence or absence of heart murmur
VI. Abdomen: scars, presence of bowel sounds, splenomegaly, hepatomegaly, tenderness, masses
VII. Extremities: presence of clubbing, cyanosis, edema, pulses in all extremities, podiatric pathology
VIII. Skin, nails, hair: erythema, eruptive lesions, rashes (texture, configuration, distribution)
IX. Musculoskeletal system: joints and range of motion, symmetry, tone, deformities
X. Nervous system: mental status (orientation), cranial nerves, sensory, cerebellar, motor reflexes, gait
XI. Lymphatic system: Presence of adenopathy in cervical, axillary, epitrochlear, or inguinal areas

ruling out any involuntary movement disorders, focal deficits, or cognitive problems that may indicate underlying neurologic disease.

The lymphatic system should be examined for the presence of lymphadenopathy, which may represent myriad disorders ranging from acquired immunodeficiency–related complex syndrome to lymphoma to cellulitis.

Podiatrists do not routinely perform genitalia, rectal, and breast examination unless there is some need uncovered in the history or other parts of the physical examination that would necessitate their inclusion.

Laboratory Data

Most textbooks of surgery and anesthesia recommend certain specific laboratory tests for preoperative evaluation. These recommendations often specify a standard complete blood count (CBC), chest radiograph, electrocardiogram on any patient older than 45 years of age, specific blood chemistry determinations, and tests of hemostasis. However, there is little scientific justification for performing these tests. No prospective and few retrospective trials have been carried out to evaluate the necessity of these or any other laboratory tests in the routine preoperative evaluation of otherwise healthy patients. Studies of the value of preoperative chest radiographs and partial thromboplastin times in healthy people show that no significant clinical abnormalities are detected that would not have been apparent from the history or physical examination alone. Suffice it to say that most abnormalities found from laboratory and physiologic data may be predicted from obtaining a careful history and physical examination.

Many patients with rheumatologic disease have systemic illness attributable to their underlying disease. Many of these patients are in an ASA class 2 or 3 risk category because of hypertensive, cardiovascular, pulmonary, or renal manifestations of their disease. Once the history and physical examination data have established a specific rheumatic disease diagnosis, certain laboratory and physiologic tests are appropriate to obtain current information regarding end-organ effects of the primary rheumatologic disease. For instance, if a patient with SLE is a preoperative candidate, a CBC and renal function tests would be necessary to diagnose any anemia or renal dysfunction that is often seen in patients with this disease. Table 27–4 reflects the type of baseline testing

TABLE 27–4

PREOPERATIVE BASELINE TESTING FOR PATIENTS WITH SYSTEMIC ILLNESS

	Connective Tissue Diseases	Vasculitis	Spondylo-arthropathies	Degenerative Joint Diseases	Infectious Arthropathies	Crystal-Induced Arthropathies	Neuro-Arthropathies
Complete blood count	×	×	×	×	×	×	×
Platelet count	×	×			×	×	
Prothrombin time		×					
Partial thromboplastin time		×					
Bleeding time		×					
Serum chemistry panel	×	×	×				×
Uric acid		×				×	
Ca²⁺	×	×				×	
Blood urea nitrogen	×	×			×	×	×
Creatinine	×	×			×	×	×
Arterial blood gases		×					
Urinalysis	×	×				×	×
Electrocardiogram	×	×	×				
Chest radiograph	×	×					
Pulmonary function tests	×						

pertinent to preoperative evaluation in rheumatologic patients. Table 27–4 does not include any rheumatologic laboratory tests because these tests are suited more for disease diagnosis than for general medical preoperative evaluation.

PREOPERATIVE AND POSTOPERATIVE CONSIDERATIONS IN SPECIFIC RHEUMATOLOGIC DISEASE

Connective Tissue Diseases

The last two decades have seen a large increase in the number of joint reconstructive procedures performed in patients with rheumatoid arthritis and osteoarthritis. Certainly, podiatry has played a large role in making available to patients disabled by lower extremity arthritis surgical procedures that correct deformity, restore function, and, most important, relieve pain. As previously discussed, general medical assessment is of utmost importance. Once this is accomplished, the podiatrist should have a reasonable knowledge of the specific rheumatic disease and its manifestations that have made surgery necessary. This knowledge should include any systemic factors expressed by this disease that may have any bearing during the perioperative period. The purpose of this section is to discuss these specific factors by the aforementioned arthritis disease classification.

Rheumatoid Arthritis. It is imperative that the podiatric physician realize that rheumatoid arthritis, in addition to manifesting as a peripheral, symmetrical inflammatory arthritis, may also be a systemic disease affecting other organ systems.

Clinically significant rheumatoid heart disease is uncommon but must be evaluated in all patients with careful cardiac auscultation and electrocardiography. Auscultation may detect pathologic murmurs indicative of valvular incompetence of the mitral or aortic valves. If pathologic heart murmurs are indeed auscultated, echocardiography (cardiac ultrasonography) is indicated to document any possible valvular pathologic changes. Electrocardiography is mandatory in all preoperative patients with rheumatoid arthritis to detect heart blocks or cardiac arrhythmias.

The presence of rheumatoid lung disease, although uncommon, increases in frequency with rheumatoid disease of long duration. Unrelated lung conditions, including pneumonia, emphysema, bronchitis, and bronchiectasis, are more common in rheumatoid patients. Lung function studies often show decreased lung capacity, decreased vital capacity, and arterial hypoxemia. Asymptomatic patients with normal chest radiographs do not require routine pulmonary function studies. If dyspnea is present, or if there are chest radiograph abnormalities, pulmonary function tests are in order, with particular attention to ventilation, diffusing capacity, and arterial oxygen saturation. If these tests confirm pulmonary dysfunction, an internist as well as an anesthesiologist should be consulted regarding the appropriateness of performing certain types of elective reconstructive procedures.

Rheumatoid involvement of the cervical spine is seen in approximately 25% of patients with severe rheumatoid factor–positive disease of long duration. Inflammation of the bursae between the transverse ligament of the atlas and the odontoid process of the axis causes erosion of the bone and ligament, permitting excessive anterior subluxation of the atlas on the axis in cervical spine flexion. Although cervical cord trauma leading to neurologic damage during induction of anesthesia or during a surgical procedure is rare, the surgeon must be aware of the potential problems of an unstable cervical spine in an unconscious patient to avoid unnecessary manipulation of the head or neck. Routine lateral cervical spine radiographs in flexion and extension should be taken in rheumatoid patients with severe disease. The maximum distance between the posterior surface of the anterior arch of the atlas and the odontoid peg in full neck flexion is 2 to 3 mm as measured radiographically in normal subjects. The use of a soft cervical collar for rheumatoid patients being transported to the operating room serves as a reminder to all involved that the patient has a rheumatoid cervical spine. Postoperatively, a soft cervical collar may be recommended as prevention against cord involvement.

A moderate anemia consistent with "anemia of chronic disease" is often seen in patients with active rheumatoid disease. The hematocrit rarely falls below 30 ml/dl. However if this value is lower, other causes of anemia should be sought, such as drug-induced gastrointestinal blood loss. As a rule, transfusions should be avoided in all preoperative patients. It is preferable to treat the primary cause of anemia rather than expose the patient to the multiple risks of transfusion therapy, including infection, volume overload, and transfusion reactions.

Osteoporosis is common in patients with rheumatoid arthritis and becomes worse with progressive deformities and immobility. In addition, corticosteroids used as a treatment modality in rheumatoid patients make generalized osteoporosis worse. Once osteoporosis has been identified by radiographs or bone densitometry, careful handling of these patients by the nursing staff and aides is essential to prevent fractures.

Postoperative infections are not appreciably increased in patients with rheumatoid arthritis who are not receiving corticosteroids. However, if an infection does occur, such as a septic joint, the consequences can be serious. Again it is important to remember that the rheumatoid patient often has multiorgan system involvement; the infectious process as well as the antibiotics used in treatment can compromise rheumatoid-affected organs such as the pulmonary and renal systems. Finally, the possibility of septic arthritis should always be considered in the differential diagnosis of postoperative exacerbation of joint inflammation. Arthrocentesis with synovial fluid culture is essential in these instances.

Pharmacologic Therapy. Pharmacologic therapy of rheumatoid disease poses perioperative problems specific to each drug class. The classic first-line drugs for rheumatoid disease are an aspirin product or one of the nonsteroidal antiinflammatory drugs (NSAIDs). Both of these drugs can cause heartburn, nausea, or epigastric distress. They also exacerbate peptic ulcer disease and worsen gastrointestinal bleeding by interfering with platelet function. Ulcer prophylaxis with histamine blockers or antacids can be given to patients at risk for peptic ulcer disease. NSAIDs reduce renal blood flow in patients with underlying renal disease, congestive heart failure, liver cirrhosis, or hypovolemic conditions and can lead to renal failure, sodium retention, and peripheral edema. Thus, NSAIDs should be used judiciously in these conditions. Aspirin and NSAIDs can produce mild elevations in liver enzyme levels but rarely cause serious liver disease. Salicylates as well as NSAIDs can induce or worsen asthma, especially in those patients with a history of rhinitis, nasal polyps, and asthma. NSAIDs and aspirin also interfere with coagulation. Salicylates bind irreversibly to the platelet membrane and interfere with platelet aggregation and blood clotting. The patient should stop taking aspirin for at least 10 days before elective surgery is performed. NSAIDs also interfere with platelet function, but the effect is reversible within 24 hours of stopping the drug.

Severe exacerbation of arthritis is uncommon following surgery, but increased pain and stiffness can occur following withdrawal of NSAIDs in the postoperative period. In general, antiinflammatory drugs that are part of the patient's treatment program should be restarted as soon after surgery as possible.

Second-line drugs used for rheumatoid arthritis include gold salts, hydroxychloroquine, and penicillamine. Gold is often the first of this group to be used, either in oral or intramuscular form. The most serious gold toxicity is aplastic anemia. A decrease in red blood cell, white blood cell, or platelet counts below normal levels requires termination of gold therapy. Obviously, any preoperative patient receiving gold requires a CBC as well as a platelet count. Gold can also cause a nephrotic syndrome (proteinuria, hypoalbuminemia, edema, and hyperlipidemia), and a urinalysis to detect proteinuria should be obtained on all preoperative patients receiving gold. Hydroxychloroquine, an antimalarial agent, is effective in some patients with rheumatoid arthritis. The drug takes several weeks to months before beneficial effects are observed. The most serious toxicity of antimalarials is retinal damage, which mandates serial ophthalmologic examinations. Perioperatively, the most important concern is that antimalarials may be associated with leukopenia and granulocytopenia. Penicillamine is a disease-modifying agent that is usually given after gold therapy has failed. The most frequent side effect is a rash, which, when extensive, requires stopping the drug. Aplastic anemia, leukopenia, and thrombocytopenia can also develop. Consequently, all preoperative patients on penicillamine require a preoperative CBC and platelet count. Penicillamine has also been associated with a membranous glomerulonephropathy, and a urinalysis to detect proteinuria as well as renal function tests are indicated preoperatively.

Glucocorticoids can be clinically beneficial in some patients with rheumatoid arthritis. In patients with active joint disease who are being started on disease-modifying agents, prednisone gives immediate clinical improvement and allows them to function during the time it takes the disease-modifying drug to become effective. However there are extremely important issues to consider with the use of steroids in any patient being evaluated for surgery. The most common cause of adrenocortical suppression is exogenous long-term steroid use. Supraphysiologic amounts (i.e., doses higher than 7.5 mg/day of prednisone or its equivalent steroid for 3 weeks or longer) of steroids can suppress the pituitary gland's ability to release adrenocorticotropic hormone, a condition that may last as long as 1 year. This has significant implications in terms of how such patients are managed in stress situations such as surgery and infection. It is generally believed that patients who have received supraphysiologic amounts of steroids for 3 weeks or longer should be assumed to have hypothalamic-pituitary-adrenal axis suppression lasting as long as 1 year from the time the prescribed steroid has been stopped. The podiatrist must be able to identify these patients

and to determine if their podiatric surgery will require supplemental steroids. The podiatrist should inquire whether the patient is or has been in the past year receiving steroid therapy. A positive response should be followed with specific questions regarding the type and dosage of the steroid medication, the length of therapy, the frequency and route of administration, and when the last dose was taken. With minor surgical procedures, patients should double their usual steroid dose on the day of treatment. They can then take their normal dose beginning the day after treatment.

A major surgical procedure produces stress, and perioperative administration of steroid is crucial. If the postoperative course is stressful or infection occurs, the rate of tapering is slowed. If there is any question as to whether the patient truly requires steroid coverage, it is far wiser to err on the side of giving steroids. It is always better to administer steroids and taper slowly, because the benefits of allowing the patient to meet stress adequately outweigh any negative effects of transient high-dose steroid therapy. Recommended steroid dosage is mentioned in Chapter 28.

Juvenile Chronic Arthritis (Juvenile Rheumatoid Arthritis). Restriction of cervical spinal motion occurs in nearly 50% of patients with juvenile chronic arthritis. Consequently, careful preoperative evaluation obtained by flexion and extension radiographs of the cervical spine must be obtained before intubation in all children with limited neck motion.

Systemic Lupus Erythematosus. This disease of generalized inflammation is characterized by the presence in the serum of autoantibodies to nuclear constituents and circulating immune complexes. Scheduling a CBC to detect anemia or leukopenia is essential in preoperative patients. Tests of hemostasis are also indicated to uncover any clotting abnormalities. A circulating lupus anticoagulant identified by prolongation of the partial thromboplastin time and slight prolongation of the prothrombin time is present in about 10% of the patients with SLE. The lupus anticoagulant alone is not associated with a bleeding diathesis, and surgery may be performed without risk of hemorrhage. Accelerated platelet destruction from antiplatelet antibodies causes thrombocytopenia in about 33% of patients with SLE, although severe thrombocytopenia with bleeding occurs only in about 5%. Clinical evidence of renal disease is present in more than 50% of patients with SLE and mandates preoperative renal function tests in these patients. Drugs commonly used for first-line therapy in SLE such as aspirin and other NSAIDs may reduce renal function. Complications following surgery in SLE are few, but there is an increased risk of postoperative infection. Many patients with active SLE are treated with corticosteroids, sometimes on prolonged high doses, which will delay wound healing, increase the risk of infection, and mandate perioperative "steroid coverage" because of suppression of the adrenopituitary axis.

Progressive Systemic Sclerosis (Scleroderma). Progressive systemic sclerosis is associated with few perioperative complications. The most important organ in this regard is the pulmonary system. Pulmonary involvement develops in most of the patients. Pulmonary function testing shows reduced diffusing capacity and, later, reduced vital capacity or restrictive lung disease. However, progression is variable, and only a small percentage of patients are significantly incapacitated. If patients do have subjective symptoms of dyspnea, preoperative pulmonary function testing is indicated.

Mixed Connective Tissue Disease. Perioperative concerns are similar to those delineated in the preceding paragraph.

Sjögren's Syndrome. Keratoconjunctivitis sicca occurs in more than 10% of rheumatoid patients and may be accompanied by corneal abrasions and ulcerations. The use of artificial tears every 2 or 3 hours in the immediate postoperative period will avoid potential complications.

Vasculitic Diseases

Vasculitic diseases are characterized by an inflammation of the blood vessels in a number of different organ systems, including the kidney, heart, liver, gastrointestinal tract, and peripheral nerves. Preoperative considerations include knowledge of preoperative renal function (blood urea nitrogen and creatinine levels, urinalysis), cardiovascular status (electrocardiogram, echocardiogram), and liver function (liver chemistry panel). Patients with polymyalgia rheumatica and temporal arteritis who undergo elective surgery should be stabilized in terms of their underlying disease. If they are receiving chronic steroid therapy, they should be administered appropriate steroid coverage. Approximately 20% of patients with polyarteritis nodosa have hepatitis B surface antigen, and it is imperative that this information be known to all health care personnel involved, especially those who have not yet received hepatitis B immunization.

Spondyloarthropathies

Ankylosing spondylitis represents a considerable challenge to the anesthesiologist for reasons of anatomic distortion caused by spine involvement. Endotracheal intubation is particularly difficult in the presence of fixed flexion of the head and neck. An added problem may be the severe restriction in chest wall expansion. Patients with ankylosing spondylitis may also develop pulmonary fibrosis, although rarely does it lead to severe pulmonary insufficiency. Patients with ankylosing spondylitis should have arterial blood gas testing as an initial screening of pulmonary function. Formal pulmonary function tests should be ordered depending on arterial blood gas results. Preoperative electrocardiograms and echocardiograms should be obtained as well in these patients because of spondylitic effects on the heart; either conduction disturbances or aortic insufficiency may be present. If there is evidence of valvular heart disease, endocarditis prophylaxis is warranted.

Similar preoperative issues need to be addressed in the other diseases classified as spondyloarthropathies, such as Reiter's syndrome, psoriatic arthritis, and inflammatory bowel disease–associated arthritis.

Degenerative Joint Disease

Because degenerative joint disease is a local joint disorder, osteoarthritis has no systemic manifestations. The central preoperative issues in this disease are whether the patient is in good enough physical condition to permit surgical intervention and whether the expected gain in function from the procedure outweighs the potential risks common to surgical procedures.

Infectious Arthropathies

Perioperative management of the patient with infectious arthritis presupposes that the invading microorganism has been identified in the synovial fluid. Once this has been accomplished, rapid institution of antimicrobial therapy is imperative. Finally, nowhere in medicine does the time-honored principle of drainage of pus assume more importance than in a joint cavity where a closed-space infection must be opened to complement an effective antibiotic regimen. The podiatric surgeon must also pay strict attention to management of the underlying disease that may have predisposed the patient to joint infection.

The joint cavity maintains a high level of natural protection such that overt joint infection is not a common accompaniment of most septicemic states. Although infection may develop in normal joints, it is likely that the general resistance of the host has been impaired by prior disease (such as tuberculosis, syphilis, Reiter's syndrome, meningococcal septicemia, brucellosis, bacillary dysentery, mycotic diseases, typhoid fever, gonorrhea, and immunocompromised states) or after treatment with drugs that interfere with host-defense mechanisms (such as corticosteroids and immunosuppressive drugs). Sometimes previous damage by trauma or another arthritic disease predisposes a joint to infection.

Crystal-Induced Arthropathies

Gout. Gout is a metabolic disease characterized by increased serum urate levels associated with recurrent attacks of acute arthritis in which monosodium urate crystals are found within the synovial fluid and occasionally deposited in tophi. A perioperative evaluation of the patient with known gouty disease supposes that an acute attack may be precipitated in hyperuricemic or gouty patients by several events, including the use of certain drugs (such as diuretics and aspirin), trauma, starvation, and surgery. The risk of postoperative gout in these patients is high. It is estimated that the risk of developing acute postoperative gout following surgery for removal of tophi exceeds 60% in patients who do not receive prophylactic colchicine.

A gouty attack usually occurs between the third and fifth postoperative day and less commonly thereafter. The diagnosis of acute gout should be suspected in patients who develop monoarticular arthritis or polyarthritis of the lower limb joints in the first few days after surgery. Diagnosis should be confirmed by synovial fluid aspiration and demonstration of negatively birefringent intracellular crystals in synovial fluid white blood cells by compensated polarized light microscopy. Alternatively, if synovial fluid is not obtainable, a trial of oral colchicine may be attempted. A clear-cut response to colchicine is still widely used as confirmatory evidence of gout. Indomethacin is also extremely effective in the treatment of gout and is probably the treatment of choice, assuming there are no contraindications and the diagnosis has been clearly established. An acute attack may also respond to an intra-articular injection of a long-acting steroid preparation. There is occasionally a flare in the intensity of joint pain within 24 hours of such an intra-articular injection, because the material injected is crystalline in nature and may itself induce an inflammatory reaction. Intra-articular injections are contraindicated in the presence of infection or compromised joint access. The effectiveness of other NSAIDs in the management of acute gout is less than that of indomethacin, and they are used only when first-line drugs are contraindicated. Allopurinol and uricosuric agents have no role in management of the acute gouty attack and should never be used until the acute attack has been controlled for at least 2 weeks.

The preoperative approach to the gouty patient should include measurement of plasma urate levels. For patients with a prior history of gouty attacks and those with plasma urate levels higher than 9 mg/dl, colchicine 0.6 mg twice a day, orally, for 3 days before surgery may prevent postoperative gout.

Pseudogout. The presence of microcrystalline deposits of calcium pyrophosphate dihydrate in articular cartilage is associated with self-limited attacks of inflammation in one or, occasionally, two or three joints. Most patients are 60 years of age or older. In contrast with gout, where small peripheral joints in the feet are most affected, pseudogout affects large joints, especially the knees. Surgery and trauma are commonly precipitating factors. The sudden appearance of a warm, effused knee in an elderly postoperative patient may indicate an acute attack of pseudogout. Acute attacks are treated most often by thorough aspiration of the joint followed by intra-articular steroid. The effect of colchicine is unpredictable.

Neuropathic Arthropathies

Neuropathic arthropathies represent a complication of a variety of neurologic disorders, the most common of which are syphilis and diabetes. They are a form of chronic progressive degenerative arthropathy affecting one or more peripheral and vertebral joints that develops owing to a disturbance in normal sensory innervation of the joints. The nature of most of the neurologic diseases responsible for neuropathic arthropathy is such that treatment of these conditions can be expected to have little if any influence on the progression of the joint disease. Immobilization of the affected joint and restriction in weightbearing are basic principles in management. Operative procedures may include amputation or arthrodesis of weightbearing joints. Perioperative concerns should focus most specifically on general medical management of the associated systemic disease. Perioperative management of the diabetic patient entails a comprehensive knowledge of the following issues:

1. The patient's status as a type I or II diabetic.
2. The type of diabetic therapy the patient is receiving (diet, oral agents, insulin).
3. How well controlled the patient's diabetes is.
4. The presence of diabetic complications.

The intraoperative and postoperative management of the diabetic patient is not within the scope of this chapter. The reader is referred to Chapter 28 on anesthesia considerations.

Syphilis, leprosy, and tuberculosis are three infectious diseases that can manifest as neuropathic arthropathy. It is extremely important that the podiatric surgeon be aware of the current status of the patient's disease with specific attention to multiorgan system involvement and history of antibiotic treatment.

CONCLUSION

The success of any surgical procedure has as much to do with careful preoperative appraisal and management as with the technical aspects of the operation itself. The purpose of this chapter has been to provide a functional approach to a working classification of rheumatic diseases commonly encountered by the podiatrist as well as a discussion of general medical factors. Finally, each rheumatologic disease has been addressed in terms of specific perioperative issues. In summary, a reasonable perioperative plan should answer the following questions:

1. What type of rheumatologic disease is this patient manifesting?
2. Is the patient in good enough general medical condition to permit the surgery contemplated?
3. Considering the age of the patient, his or her physical state, and the type of operation indicated, is the expected gain in function from the operation worth the effort?
4. Does the chronic drug therapy that the patient is receiving require specific preoperative management such as ''steroid coverage'' or hemostatic concerns with NSAIDs or aspirin.
5. Does the patient's rheumatologic disease call in question the possibility of widespread systemic illness such as in rheumatoid disease, SLE, ankylosing spondylitis, or vasculitis? What types of preoperative management should address these possibilities?

Whatever surgical decision is ultimately made, effective communication should be established among other disciplines the surgeon decides should be involved in the care of the patient. Internists, anesthesiologists, physical therapists, and nurses all may contribute vital information that ultimately allows the patient to obtain a successful and gratifying outcome.

Bibliography

Harvey AM, et al: The Principles and Practices of Medicine. Norwalk, CT, Appleton & Lange, 1988.

Kammerer W and Gross R: Medical Consultation: The Role of Internist on Surgical, Obstetric, and Psychiatric Services. Baltimore, Williams & Wilkins, 1983.

Larson EB and Ramsey PG: Medical Therapeutics: A Pocket Companion. Philadelphia, WB Saunders, 1989.

Lubin, Walker, and Smith: Medical Management of the Surgical Patient. Boston, Butterworth, 1982.

McCarty DJ: Arthritis and Allied Conditions, 10th ed. Philadelphia, Lea & Febiger, 1984

Molitch ME: Management of Medical Problems in Surgical Patients. Philadelphia, FA Davis, 1982.

Moll JMH: Rheumatic Disorders. New York, Raven Press, 1983.

Rothshild BM: Rheumatology: A Primary Care Approach. New York, Yorke Medical, 1982.

Zier BG: Essentials of Internal Medicine in Clinical Podiatry. Philadelphia, WB Saunders, 1990.

CHAPTER 28

Anesthesia Considerations

Stephen Jackson, M.D., George Lampe, M.D.,
and Donald Silcox, M.D.

THE HEALTHY PATIENT

Anesthesiologists work on the established premise that appropriate preoperative preparations will minimize intraoperative and postoperative complications. A history and physical examination should focus on the patient's general condition and level of physiologic, biochemical, and pharmacologic fitness as well as significant cardiovascular, pulmonary, hepatic, renal, and neurologic dysfunction. Any allergies to medications and the patient's perception of previous anesthetic and surgical procedures should be delineated. Medications, except aspirin, anticoagulants, nonsteroidal antiinflammatory drugs (NSAIDs), monoamine oxidase inhibitors, and certain drugs that may suppress immunity or healing (such as methotrexate), should be continued to the day of operation. Most anesthesiologists even have patients take their medications on the day of the operation with a sip of water, this being the sole exception to the nothing by mouth instructions. The interval of time to the most recent oral intake should be determined. Because the risk of lung injury induced by aspiration is related to gastric content and volume, patients generally are instructed not to eat anything for 7 to 8 hours before scheduled surgery. Pain, narcotics, diabetes, anxiety, obesity, and gastric reflux are additional independent risk factors for aspiration. Recent practice patterns have allowed healthy patients without these known risk factors for aspiration to consume clear liquids until 4 hours before their operation, because this apparently will not increase their gastric volume. Guidelines for children may evolve over even shorter intervals of fasting.[1]

For the healthy patient (American Society of Anesthesiologists class I risk), no preoperative laboratory testing has been shown to be useful in identifying patients whose surgery should be postponed on the basis of clinically significant occult disease. Furthermore, tests have not been useful in identifying patients who are at increased risk for postoperative morbidity. The nonproductive tests that traditionally had been routinely ordered include complete blood counts, urine analysis, chest radiograph, and electrocardiogram (ECG). The Mayo Clinic now proposes that *no* preoperative laboratory tests be performed for healthy ambulatory surgery patients younger than 40 years.[2] Guidelines for suggested tests for older patients or those with significant systemic disease are listed in Table 28–1.[3]

THE PATIENT WITH SYSTEMIC DISEASE

Extra-articular manifestations of the systemic diseases that may lead to podiatric surgery have implications for anesthetic management.[4, 5] Pulmonary, cardiovascular, neurologic, hematopoietic, and renal derangements must be assessed preoperatively (Table 28–1 suggests appropriate laboratory tests), and then must be considered in formulating the anesthetic and postoperative management plans.

Pulmonary Disease

Pulmonary disease is common in patients with rheumatoid arthritis, systemic lupus erythematosus (SLE), and scleroderma and is occasionally associated with ankylosing spondylitis and polymyositis. Diffuse pulmonary fibrosis or multiple pulmonary nodules as well as pleural effusions may be present and cause restrictive functional impairment and impaired gas exchange. Obstructive pulmonary changes are present in bronchiolitis obliterans and occasionally found in rheumatoid arthritis. Ankylosis of the thoracic spine and involvement of the sternomanubrium and sternoclavicular joints also restrict chest (and lung) expansion. In addition, patients with ankylosing spondylitis sometimes contract bilateral pulmonary fibrosis of the upper lobes. Pulmonary fibrosis can also occur with scleroderma. SLE often causes pleural effusions, and pneumonias are not uncommon. Patients with these diseases may not give a history of dyspnea because of the relative inactivity imposed by the underlying disease. Patients with severe or diffuse joint disease should have a chest radiograph and, if deemed appropriate, be evaluated with pulmonary function tests to quantitate the degree of pulmonary functional impairment. Arterial blood gas analysis may detect derangements of oxygen or carbon dioxide exchange and provide a baseline reference for further studies. Continuous pulse oximetry should be extended beyond the operating room at least into the immediate postanesthetic period to ensure early warning of inadequate oxygen stauration values.

Heart Disease

Heart disease is an infrequent manifestation of rheumatologic disorders, although the incidence of asymptomatic disease is significant. Conduction abnormalities, valvular le-

TABLE 28–1

PREOPERATIVE LABORATORY TESTING*

Variable	Hgb	PT/PTT	Plt/BT	Elect	Creat	Bld gluc	LFT	CXR	ECG
Surgery									
With blood loss	X								
Without blood loss									
Age <40 years (healthy)									
Age 40–59 years (healthy)	X								±
Age ≥ 60 years (healthy)	X							±	X
Cardiac disease	X				X			X	X
Digoxin use				X	X				X
Diuretic use				X	X				X
Pulmonary disease	X							X	X
Smoker								X	±
Hepatic disease	X	X					X		
Renal disease	X		X	X	X				
Bleeding history (anticoagulant)		X	X						
Diabetes				X	X	X			X
Steroid use	X			X		X			
Gout					X				X

*Clinical judgment dictates whether this table applies to any given patient. Every woman of child-bearing age should be asked whether there is any chance she is pregnant. For all ''yes'' or ''maybe'' responses, a pregnancy test should be ordered.

X, obtain; ±, maybe; Hgb, hemoglobin; PT, prothrombin time; PTT, partial thromboplastin time; Plt, platelets; BT, bleeding time; Elect, electrolytes (sodium and potassium); Creat, creatinine; Bld gluc, blood glucose; LFT, liver function tests, including aspartate and alanine aminotransferase, alkaline phosphatase, and bilirubin; CXR, chest radiograph; ECG, electrocardiogram.

Modified from Roizen M, Stevens A, and Lampe G: Perioperative management of patients with endocrine disease. *In* Nunn J, Utting J, and Brown B (eds): General Anesthesia, 5th ed. London, Butterworths, 1989, pp 726–740.

sions, and pericardial effusions are occasionally observed. At least 3% of patients with ankylosing spondylitis have aortic valvular insufficiency. This may also occur in Reiter's syndrome as a result of necrosis of the media of the aortic root and dilatation of the aortic annulus. Pericarditis is common in SLE and may cause chest pain and a friction rub; occasionally, a pericardial effusion may cause cardiac tamponade. Myocarditis is less common but can lead to conduction abnormalities or even congestive heart failure. Pulmonary hypertension is not infrequent in scleroderma and lupus variants, and it may progress to right ventricular failure (cor pulmonale). Anticardiolipin antibody syndrome can result in pulmonary emboli. Because the primary disease–imposed inactivity of these patients may conceal symptoms of heart disease, electrocardiograms (ECGs) and chest radiographs should be part of the routine preoperative testing of these patients. Echocardiography also should be considered in patients with abnormal physical findings.

Vasculitis and Vasospasm

Vasculitis may occur as a complication of rheumatoid arthritis and SLE, or it can occur independently such as in Wegener's granulomatosis and polyarteritis nodosa. Although relatively uncommon, the vasculitis can cause serious multiorgan failure. The degree of organ involvement is quite variable, but severe vasculitis may produce significant end-organ disease such as peripheral neuropathy, myocardial ischemia, renal insufficiency, ischemic peripheral vascular disease, and cerebrovascular insufficiency. Raynaud's phenomenon is not a vasculitic but rather a vasospastic condition. Raynaud's phenomenon is common in scleroderma and SLE. Significantly, in these patients the vasospasm can involve the pulmonary circulation and result in right ventricular hyper-

trophy and ultimately require high right-sided filling pressures for normal function. The systemic vascular resistance, in contradistinction to the pulmonary vascular resistance, may be normal because the vasospasm is largely limited to distal extremities. These patients may experience profound hypotension on induction of anesthesia with drugs or techniques that cause vasodilatation, and the cause is thought to be related to decreased right-sided filling pressures. This right-sided heart pathophysiologic state can be detected on physical examination when the second heart sound in the pulmonary artery area is greater than the second heart sound in the aortic area ($P_2 > A_2$). Confirmation of this clinical impression is achieved with ECG and echocardiography. Measurement of blood pressure may be technically difficult when using conventional noninvasive methodology. On the other hand, invasive techniques may further compromise an already tenuous circulation to any extremity. Intra-arterial cannulation should always be preceded by documentation of the adequacy of collateral circulation. Furthermore, these patients may present extreme challenges for peripheral venous access, and on occasion central venous cannulation may become necessary. Patients with scleroderma may be sensitive to the vasoconstrictor effects of the epinephrine in epinephrine-containing local anesthetic solutions. Because the duration of action of these solutions is already markedly prolonged in these patients, epinephrine and phenylephrine should be omitted.

Anemia

Anemia of chronic disease is of the normochromic-normocytic variety and is commonly encountered in rheumatoid arthritis and SLE. At the same time, many of the common drug therapies cause gastrointestinal hemorrhage and secondary anemia from this loss (see later discussion of "therapeutic drugs"). An appropriate medical work-up distinguishes between these two causes; however, the differential diagnosis should consider other causes such as hemolysis, bone marrow depression, and advanced renal dysfunction (decreased production of erythropoietin and erythrocyte survival time). Irrespective of the source of the anemia, it is important to establish whether the anemia is chronic, in which case the patient would likely be homeostatically well adapted from a cardiovascular standpoint. If the anemia is acute, as from recent gastrointestinal hemorrhage, the patient must be stabilized and the bleeding controlled before embarking on elective surgery. The question arises as to what reduced level of hemoglobin concentration (oxygen-carrying capacity) is acceptable for safely proceeding with elective anesthesia and surgery. The answer must be individualized, considering the multifactorial elements influencing this decision: chronicity, condition of cardiovascular system, pulmonary function, risk of corrective transfusion, anticipated surgical blood loss, and ability to collect and reinfuse shed blood. It is clear that in those patients with chronic anemia of chronic renal failure in whom cardiac functional reserve is deemed adequate, hemoglobin concentrations between 8 and 10 g/dl are well tolerated. Severe anemia reduces the blood-gas partition coefficients for the halogenated hydrocarbon anesthetics by 15% to 25%, and this increases the speed of induction and emergence from anesthesia with these agents.

Blood Transfusion Concerns

In the recent past, the hematologic transmission of hepatitis B, non-A, non-B hepatitis, and acquired immunodeficiency syndrome has raised concern in patients and their physicians over the use of blood transfusions for elective surgery. In the highly unlikely event that the podiatric surgery is anticipated to result in the loss of a significant amount of blood, then the use of red blood cell salvaging technology should be considered. In addition, every effort should be made to correct any pre-existing anemia that is amenable to correction such as an iron-deficiency anemia. The use of autologous blood collection and storage should be encouraged if the patient is able to tolerate blood shedding, can be reasonably expected to accelerate erythropoiesis in response to the predeposition, and is anticipated to lose a significant amount of blood.[5a] The preoperative administration of recombinant human erythropoietin (epoetin alfa) to selected patients for the purpose of accelerating erythrocyte production is the newest option to become available to address the issue of blood transfusion in the surgical patient. A permanent, substantial elevation of plasma erythropoietin in response to acute blood loss or chronic small blood losses does not occur until the hematocrit is less than 34%. From a psychological if not medical point of view, designated donors are an acceptable alternative to the general pool of blood donors. Blood banks necessarily carefully screen voluntary donors in great depth with detailed histories and blood testing. Nonetheless, there always remains a small window of time wherein a donor may be carrying an infection early in the disease process when antibody titers have not yet risen to detectable levels. The costs for unnecessary predisposition and intraoperative salvaging are considerable and unacceptable in these days of the poorly controlled and spiraling costs of medical care.

Peripheral Nervous System Disease

Peripheral nervous system disease may be related to compression or entrapment caused by musculoskeletal disease or may be the result of necrotizing vasculitis of the vasonervorum. The clinical manifestations may present as sensorimotor deficits and should be evident on careful history and physical examination. Sympathetic nervous system dysfunction should be ruled out because it can contribute to intra-anesthetic cardiovascular instability. Central nervous system vasculitis can be a manifestation of generalized vasculitis encountered occasionally in SLE. It may manifest as a variable degree of any of a broad spectrum of psychological symptomatology, cerebrovascular insufficiency, or even generalized seizure disorders.

Renal Dysfunction

Renal dysfunction occurs in SLE, vasculitis, and scleroderma. Glomerulonephritis of SLE and vasculitis produces proteinuria, hematuria, cast formation, and hypoalbuminemia, and, in its severest form, renal failure. With the therapeutic effectiveness of allopurinol in patients with gout, it is uncommon to encounter gouty nephropathy (see discussion of therapeutic drugs for gout). Oliguric renal failure accompanies the malignant hypertension of scleroderma. Routine laboratory evaluation of these patients should always include measurement of serum creatinine, albumin, and electrolyte levels as well as routine and microscopic urinalysis. In patients with preexisting renal dysfunction, NSAIDs are more likely to affect further renal dysfunction (see discussion of therapeutic drugs).

Diabetes Mellitus

Diabetes mellitus (DM) affects 5% of the population of Western countries and may be present in an even higher percentage of patients requiring surgery on the foot because of neurovascular injuries associated with the disease. DM is a diverse group of disorders characterized by an absolute or relative lack of insulin, elevated blood glucose concentrations, and characteristic end-organ dysfunction. Anesthesiologists and surgeons frequently are challenged with the demands of caring for these patients, particularly in the preoperative evaluation of associated diseases and in the perioperative control of blood glucose levels.

Clinically, patients are characterized as type I (juvenile-onset or insulin-deficient diabetes) or type II (maturity-onset diabetes). Type I diabetics are chronically treated with insulin in an attempt to maintain euglycemia. They are predisposed to acquire hyperglycemia and ketoacidosis if insulin is withheld, and hypoglycemia may occur if insulin administration is excessive or if inadequate glucose intake occurs perioperatively. Type II DM is characterized by insulin resistance; these patients frequently are overweight and elderly. Their blood glucose usually is regulated by diet or oral hypoglycemic drugs, and they are resistant to ketoacidosis. Type II diabetics also are at risk of hypoglycemia from the residual effects of oral hypoglycemics (most of which have prolonged durations of action) if preoperative, intraoperative, or postoperative glucose intake is inadequate.

Both types I and II DM produce the same organ disease. Suggested preoperative evaluation of these diabetic patients is summarized in Table 28–2, which lists only the conditions associated with DM that may affect surgical outcome and perioperative morbidity.[6, 7] Diabetic patients have an extremely high incidence of coronary artery disease, and they tend to die at an early age from myocardial infarction. Of particular importance is the finding that these patients may have advanced and life-threatening ischemic heart disease that is *asymptomatic*: they may not experience angina. This silent angina occurs as a result of autonomic neuropathy, which also causes delayed gastric emptying (gastroparesis), a pathophysiologic state that places these patients at increased risk for aspiration of gastric contents. Metoclopramide was developed to increase gastric emptying in DM and may decrease the volume of gastric contents if given in a dose of 0.15 mg/kg intravenously at least 10 minutes before induction of anesthesia (or at least 20 minutes if administered orally). Diabetic neuropathy may also lead to sensory nerve deficits, particularly in the feet, which should be carefully documented in the patient's chart before either injecting local anesthetic into the ankle or foot or performing surgery: in this way pre-existing neurologic deficits will not be attributed to the actions of the anesthesiologist or surgeon. Although some studies have found increased mortality in diabetic patients requiring abdominal surgery, others have failed to document either an increase in mortality or complication in diabetic patients undergoing vascular surgery. However, the significant end-organ dysfunction commonly associated with DM (see Table 28–2) must be evaluated, documented, and optimally treated before elective surgery of any type.

Blood Glucose Levels. Both diabetic and normal patients usually increase their levels of blood glucose in response to surgical stress.[8] As part of the "fight or flight" response to surgical pain, the body's sympathetic nervous system mobilizes glucose to meet the anticipated metabolic need. General anesthesia with inhaled anesthetics in combination with intravenous barbiturates, narcotics, benzodiazepines, and other sedative drugs is carefully titrated in an attempt to block these neurohumoral responses to surgical stimulation. However, no form of general anesthesia does, in fact, completely block the hyperglycemic response to surgery. On the other hand, regional anesthesia involving blockade of the sympathetic nervous system (high spinal or epidural anesthesia) can protect the body from these unwanted "stress responses" for the duration of the block. These responses, however, may merely be delayed into the postoperative period until the effects of the local anesthetic wear off. β-adrenergic blocking drugs such as propranolol and the shorter acting esmolol can have a significant antihyperglycemic effect when appropriately deployed, but they are not recommended for this purpose.

It would be wrong, however, to assume that all patients will have normal or high glucose levels intraoperatively and postoperatively. Hypoglycemia may occur because of preoperative fasting aggravated by the residual effects of previously administered oral hypoglycemic drugs or insulin.[9] Most of these preparations have notably long durations of action (Table 28–3). Unquestionably, the single greatest risk to diabetic patients requiring surgery is hypoglycemia. The brain is the organ most susceptible to injury from hypoglycemia because of its absolute dependence on a continuous supply of glucose. The first signs and symptoms of hypoglycemia include light-headedness, hunger, confusion, and drowsiness, these being detectable only in patients in whom regional or local anesthesia allows for an "awake" (or sedated) state. The adrenal medulla responds to hypoglycemia by secreting epinephrine, which causes tachycardia, hypertension, sweating, and pallor. These signs may be blunted or absent in a patient anesthetized with general anesthesia, or they may be misinterpreted as signs of too light a level of general anesthesia. Hypoglycemia may cause seizures, coma, brain damage, and death. A high degree of suspicion for hypoglycemia must be maintained when dealing with diabetic patients, and blood glucose levels must be monitored frequently to prevent its occurrence.[10]

The goal of metabolic control is to avoid marked hyperglycemia or hypoglycemia. Hyperglycemia causes osmotic diuresis, volume depletion, electrolyte abnormalities, acidosis, and ketosis in susceptible type I diabetics. Hyperglycemia may interfere with wound healing and normal host defenses and may exacerbate ischemic brain damage. However, the more "tightly" controlled the blood glucose is, the greater

TABLE 28–3
HYPOGLYCEMIC AGENTS

Agent	Duration of Action (hours)
Genetically Engineered Human Insulin	
Humulin regular	6–8
Humulin NPH	20–24
Humulin Ultralente	24–28
Nonhuman Insulin	
Lente	24–48
Semilente	12–16
Ultralente	More than 36
Oral Hypoglycemics	
Glyburide (Diabeta, Micronase)	24
Chlorpropamide (Diabinese)	36
Tolbutamide (Orinase)	Up to 24
Tolazamide (Tolinase)	10

TABLE 28–2
PREOPERATIVE CONDITIONS, EVALUATION, AND INTERVENTIONS

Hyper- or hypoglycemia	Blood glucose (reflectance meter ideal for immediate and accurate result); electrolytes
Coronary artery disease	Electrocardiogram and history (diabetics frequently have myocardial ischemia without angina, or "silent myocardial ischemia")
Renal insufficiency	Blood urea nitrogen and creatinine (limit total fluids and potassium)
Autonomic neuropathy, gastroparesis	Metoclopramide (Reglan) 10 mg intravenously before the procedure may decrease gastric contents, increase lower esophageal sphincter tone, and perhaps decrease risk of aspiration
Autonomic neuropathy, lower extremity neurologic deficits	Careful preoperative documentation

the risk for catastrophic injury (particularly to the brain) from hypoglycemia.

As a broad recommendation, one should attempt to maintain the blood glucose level between 100 to 200 mg/dl. The regimens in Table 28–4 have been used successfully to control blood glucose levels in fasting diabetic patients; however, the safety and success of any system are related to frequent and accurate blood glucose determinations. All diabetics should have immediate preoperative blood glucose determinations, and then the clinician should be able to predict in which direction the blood glucose is likely to move (e.g., likely increase with general anesthesia; no change or decrease with regional anesthesia; possible decrease in any patient taking insulin or oral hypoglycemic drugs). If insulin is administered, or if a residual hypoglycemic effect is expected, the intravenous fluid should contain 5% glucose (dextrose) and be administered at a rate of about 150 ml/hour (this provides 7.5 g/hour of glucose), which is enough to avoid catabolism. One unit of regular insulin usually lowers serum glucose by 25 to 30 mg/dl in a normal-sized adult. Interventions to treat either high or low blood glucose levels should be followed with another blood glucose determination within 30 minutes.

The common practice of most anesthesiologists has become to administer non–glucose-containing solutions routinely because of the firm data demonstrating a direct relationship between blood glucose levels and the extent of ischemic brain injury under circumstances of circulatory arrest.[11] However, when the potential for hypoglycemia is a concern, the prudent use of glucose solutions is appropriate.

THE PATIENT ON THERAPEUTIC DRUGS

Salicylates

Salicylates commonly produce upper gastrointestinal bleeding ulcerations, with an average blood loss of 3 to 8 ml/day. Salicylates permit back-diffusion of acid into the mucosa and inhibit synthesis of the gastric prostaglandins, which inhibit acid secretion and promote the secretion of cytoprotective mucus. Although gastrointestinal hemorrhage itself can cause an anemia, a primary anemia commonly is encountered in the inflammatory arthritides. An appropriate

---

TABLE 28–4

STRATEGIES FOR BLOOD GLUCOSE MANAGEMENT

Type I Diabetes (Insulin Dependent)

1. No insulin–no glucose is suitable only for brief morning procedures. Once the postoperative oral intake is tolerated for 4 hours, give one third of the usual daily insulin with orders for continued oral glucose intake.
2. Administer one half of the usual insulin dose as intermediate (NPH) insulin after initiating an infusion containing 5% dextrose run at 100 to 150 ml/hour. (Outpatients must tolerate oral intake before discharge.)
3. Administer glucose-insulin-potassium infusion (for inpatients)
   a. Glucose as 5% dextrose at 140 ml/hour (yields 7 g glucose/hour)
   b. Regular insulin 1 unit/hour for blood sugar <150, 2 units/hour if blood sugar >150 (50 units regular insulin in 250 ml of normal saline makes a concentration of 0.2 units/ml)
   c. Potassium should be added up to 40 mEq/L of intravenous fluid

Type II Diabetes (adult onset, noninsulin dependent)

Omit oral hypoglycemic on day of surgery (may be taken postoperatively once oral intake established).

---

medical work-up can distinguish between these two causes and others, including platelet dysfunction and bone marrow depression. The pathophysiologic implications of anemia are discussed later in this chapter.

Salicylate-induced gastrointestinal hyperacidity and bleeding may place these patients at increased risk of lung injury should aspiration of gastric contents occur. Pulmonary aspiration of gastric contents with its subsequent respiratory injury and impaired oxygen and carbon dioxide exchange is a potential complication of (1) general anesthesia and its attendant unconscious state and loss of protective airway reflexes and (2) obtunded states variously characterized as monitored anesthesia care, ''conscious'' sedation, light conscious sedation, and deep sedation, each of which has the potential to compromise protective airway reflexes. The volume of gastric aspirate necessary to produce an acid aspiration and chemical pneumonitis is about 0.4 ml/kg of body weight, but it may be that the pH of the gastric aspirate is the most important factor. A gastric pH greater than 2.5 usually is protective against the acid aspiration syndrome, even when the volume is 1 to 2 ml/kg. Therefore, preanesthetic preparation might include (1) reducing acid secretion during the preoperative fast with histamine$_2$ (H$_2$) blocking drugs and adenosine triphosphate gastric pump inhibitors; (2) nonparticulate antacid ingestion to increase the pH of gastric contents above 2.5; and (3) drug-induced gastric emptying and toning of the gastroesophageal junction with metoclopramide. With these preventive and therapeutic objectives in mind, we recommend the following guidelines:

1. Patients should receive orally 40 mg of famotidine or 300 mg of nizatidine 6 to 18 hours before anticipated surgery. Intravenous ranitidine, famotidine, or cimetidine given immediately before surgery fails to neutralize the gastric acid previously accumulated during the fasting period. Cimetidine and, to a lesser degree, ranitidine are less desirable choices when local anesthetics are used because they inhibit hepatic P-450 microsomal enzyme systems, which metabolize lidocaine and other amino amides, thereby increasing the blood concentrations of these drugs. Metabolism of theophylline, warfarin, and phenytoin is delayed by this same mechanism. Omeprazole is the most recent addition to the pharmacologic armamentarium that suppresses gastric parietal cell acid secretion. It inhibits the hydrogen-potassium ion-adenosine triphosphatase enzyme system, which acts as the acid pump in the gastric mucosa. Published experience with omeprazole in the perioperative setting is sparse, but it appears that a single dose of 20 mg is effective if administered orally 6 to 10 hours before surgery. Because of its potential for interfering with the hepatic cytochrome P-450 system, omeprazole can prolong the duration of action of drugs such as diazepam, phenytoin, and warfarin; no effect on local anesthetics has yet been identified.
2. Thirty milliliters of clear antacid (such as sodium citrate preparation, Bicitra, or Alka-Seltzer Gold) should be ingested 5 to 40 minutes before induction of anesthesia.
3. Metoclopramide administered as a 20-mg dose orally 45 to 60 minutes before anesthesia or a 10-mg dose parenterally at least 10 minutes before induction of anesthesia will relax the pyloric sphincter while tight-

ening the gastroesophageal sphincter, a combination that promotes gastric emptying and may reduce the risk of passive regurgitation.

The use of exogenous prostaglandin supplementation to prevent gastropathy is discussed in the following section of NSAIDs. Sucralfate may have significant beneficial local effects as well.

Another side effect of salicylate therapy is platelet dysfunction as a result of acetylation of platelet cyclooxygenase, which inhibits the biosynthesis of thromboxane A_2 (a potent aggregating agent) and prostaglandins. Platelets are particularly susceptible because they have limited capacity for enzyme biosynthesis. Even a small dose (60 mg) of aspirin will alter platelet function for the 8- to 11-day life of the platelet. Indeed, this effect is best monitored by determining the bleeding time, the most sensitive clinical test for platelet dysfunction. Although salicylate therapy does not affect the platelet count, bleeding times can double. Salicylate-induced platelet dysfunction, even if minimally elevating the bleeding time, is not a contraindication to the use of regional anesthesia or surgery if the patient's coagulation profile is otherwise normal.

High-dose salicylate therapy often causes tinnitus and must enter the differential diagnosis of local anesthetic toxicity because tinnitus is a symptom premonitory to the more serious sequelae of local anesthetic toxicity such as seizures (see discussion of local anesthetic drugs). Full therapeutic doses of salicylates will produce an increased oxygen consumption and carbon dioxide production as a consequence of uncoupling of oxidative phosphorylation. A compensatory increase in alveolar ventilation occurs unless the respiratory response is blunted by opiates, barbiturates, or other respiratory depressant drugs. It is, therefore, more likely that these patients will experience a respiratory acidosis when sedated or on emergence from general anesthesia.

Nonsteroidal Antiinflammatory Drugs

As inhibitors of the cyclooxygenase responsible for the biosynthesis of gastric prostaglandins that play a primary role in maintaining the stomach's mucosal defense mechanisms, NSAIDs can cause toxicity ranging from simple intolerance (dyspepsia) to life-threatening ulcers and bleeding or perforation and peritonitis. Fifteen percent to 35% of NSAID users experience upper gastrointestinal symptoms, but there is little correlation between these symptoms and the more serious NSAID-induced injuries that often remain silent.[12] This upper gastrointestinal injury is distinct from classic peptic ulcer disease in that it primarily involves the stomach and is not necessarily acid dependent. The incidence of substantial upper gastrointestinal bleeding increases considerably in patients with multiple risk factors. These include age greater than 60 years, peptic ulcer disease, alcohol use, cigarette smoking, high-dose and prolonged NSAID use, history of gastrointestinal bleeding, and corticosteroid or anticoagulant treatment. All surgical patients on NSAIDs should have a hemogram and be tested for fecal occult blood loss. Furthermore, NSAIDs alter platelet function and prolong the bleeding time, but unlike aspirin, this effect is rapidly reversible with cessation of drug therapy. NSAID-induced platelet alteration usually will not adversely affect blood clotting;

therefore, regional anesthesia and surgery are not contraindicated on this basis.

The management of patients with upper gastrointestinal hyperacidity was discussed previously with salicylates. NSAID-induced gastric ulcers tend to be only moderately responsive to H_2 blockers and antacids. This reflects the fact that prostaglandin depletion, not hypersecretion of acid, may be responsible for the relative ineffectiveness of conventional antiulcer agents to prevent NSAID-induced gastropathy while proving effective against the much less frequent NSAID-induced duodenal ulceration. Misoprostol, a prostaglandin E_1 analogue, may possess prophylactic efficacy in this respect and, furthermore, may promote healing of NSAID-induced ulcers while the NSAID therapy is continued. Misoprostol will not antagonize the desired analgesia/antiinflammatory effects of the ongoing NSAID treatment.[13, 14] Prostaglandin supplementation will, however, increase visceral motility and produce the dose-related side effects of diarrhea, abdominal cramps, and bloating. A low-dose regimen of 100 µg of misoprostol orally four times a day is more likely to avoid the unpleasant gastrointestinal side effects.

Renal toxicity secondary to NSAIDs is rare in otherwise healthy patients, but the incidence in high-risk patients may approach 20%. These include age greater than 60 years, preexisting renal dysfunction, vascular disease, hypovolemia, and high renin-angiotensin states. Most commonly, renal toxicity is related to reduced renal blood flow caused by NSAIDs' inhibition of renal prostaglandin synthesis. In addition, hyperkalemia and hyponatremia can be induced by NSAIDs. A preoperative determination of the serum electrolytes and creatinine level should be determined for all patients taking these medications. Measurement of blood urea nitrogen (BUN) may not be an accurate reflection of renal function because even small amounts of gastrointestinal bleeding will elevate the BUN. The presence of renal dysfunction is a relative contraindication to anesthesia drugs possessing nephrotoxic potential such as methoxyflurane and enflurane.

All NSAIDs may effect a reversible hepatic dysfunction or even hepatitis, and this mandates preoperative liver function screening for all patients receiving NSAIDs.

Indomethacin not only may cause gastrointestinal blood loss and a resultant anemia, but on rare occasions bone marrow depression with pancytopenia also may be induced. A common (20% to 50%) side effect encountered with chronic indomethacin therapy is cephalalgia (usually frontal), which must be considered when evaluating a patient for a spinal anesthesia or a postsubarachnoid headache. Other common side effects include mental confusion, light-headedness, and vertigo and should be considered during anesthetic emergence and early ambulation after surgery. Patients receiving more than 150 mg/day are likely to experience one or more serious side effects. An intravenous preparation is available to maintain serum levels in a patient unable to ingest indomethacin in the postoperative period. Sulindac, closely related to indomethacin, is a prodrug, and its sulfide metabolite carries the overwhelming majority of its antiinflammatory potency. Its toxicity is less than that of indomethacin. Its rough therapeutic equivalent dose (TED) is 400 mg/day compared with 125 mg/day of indomethacin and 4 g/day of aspirin.

The propionic acid derivatives ibuprofen, naproxen, flurbiprofen, ketoprofen, and fenoprofen are better tolerated by the gastrointestinal system than are the salicylates and indomethacin. However, aseptic meningitis has afflicted normal patients taking ibuprofen, sulindac, or tolmetin, and it is even more likely to occur in patients with SLE or other connective tissue disorders. During the administration of a subarachnoid anesthetic to these patients, it may be prudent to send an aliquot of cerebrospinal fluid for baseline cell count, protein, and glucose determinations. Piroxicam provides an advantage over other NSAIDs with its long biologic half-life, and its single-dose TED is 20 mg/day. Tolmetin may have fewer central nervous system side effects than either aspirin or indomethacin at a TED of 1600 to 1800 mg/day. Diclofenac has a TED of 150 to 200 mg/day, but a small percentage of patients exhibit a marked elevation of hepatic transaminase activity that is reversible with discontinuation of this drug. Diclofenac also may be porphyrinogenic. Flurbiprofen has a TED of 300 mg/day. Etodolac is the first of an entirely new class of NSAIDs. Initial reports suggest significant decreases of gastric toxicity and possibly make it the NSAID drug of choice in the elderly.[15] Nevertheless, the same precautions for gastropathy should be used for all NSAIDs.

All of the NSAIDs except salsalate and trisalicylate can precipitate bronchospasm in patients who are hypersensitive to aspirin. If these patients receive the NSAIDs, they will be more likely to experience increased airway resistance during endotracheal anesthesia. NSAIDs also can cause tinnitus, a premonitory symptom to the more serious sequela of local anesthetic toxicity.

Increasingly, the NSAIDs are being used to provide postoperative analgesia. The considerations favoring NSAIDs over narcotic analgesics have led to the recent widespread acceptance of the parenteral NSAID ketorolac (Toradol), a drug that also possesses significant antipyretic as well as antiinflammatory activity.[16, 17, 17a] The benefits of ketorolac include the following:

1. Good to excellent analgesia in a broad spectrum of postpodiatric surgical pain
2. Apparent lower incidence of nausea and vomiting, because ketorolac is a peripherally acting analgesic and devoid of an opiate receptor effect
3. Designation as a noncontrolled substance
4. No known potential for drug abuse

The recommended initial dose range is 30 to 60 mg intramuscularly 1 hour before the anticipated end of surgery so that therapeutic blood levels are achieved by the end of the procedure. This loading dose is to be followed by half of the initial dose administered every 6 hours with a maximum recommended first-day dose of 150 mg (120 mg on future days). Narcotic analgesics may be used as supplements. The addition of intramuscular ketorolac as a supplemental analgesic to therapeutic doses of narcotics can result in unmasking the respiratory depressant effect of the narcotics. Moreover, ketorolac possesses a mild sedative effect. Ketorolac shares the risks of the other NSAIDs and should not be used in combination with other NSAIDs in which toxic effects become additive. Gastropathy, postoperative hemorrhage, and renal toxicity have been reported even following brief courses of ketorolac therapy postoperatively. It should be clearly understood that any NSAID, when administered in an appropriate manner, will achieve the same therapeutic anal-

gesia goals as will ketorolac. This necessarily would invoke the oral administration of an NSAID before surgery and the continued oral administration postoperatively. An oral preparation of ketorolac is available, and parenteral forms of several oral NSAIDs are likely to make their way into the marketplace. The concomitant administration of low-dose misoprostol with ketorolac or oral NSAIDs postoperatively might prove to be an effective regimen for analgesia without gastropathy. There also may be a role for omeprazole, sucralfate, and H_2 blockers in this modern approach to lowering the morbidity while expanding the indications for NSAIDs in postoperative analgesia.

Gold (Chrysotherapy)

Chrysotherapy is frequently deployed as a disease-remedying drug and commonly is used in combination with NSAIDs. Gold as parenteral aurothioglucose and gold sodium thiomalate or oral auranofin produces cutaneous lesions of the mucous membranes (most frequently of the mouth) in as many as 15% of patients. An exfoliative dermatitis is of concern to the anesthesiologist if the lesions were located in the area to be used for regional anesthesia, intravenous catheter placement, or mask application. Similar concerns apply to the operative site and the area used for a foot block. In the presence of gold-induced inflammatory reactions of the upper airway (stomatitis, glossitis, pharyngitis, laryngitis, or tracheitis), extreme care must be exercised during airway instrumentation and manipulation. These upper airway tissues are prone to traumatic injury, pressure necrosis, and infection. Renal dysfunction such as proteinuria can affect as many as 10% of treated patients. It would be prudent to avoid the potentially nephrotoxic anesthetics as well as the NSAIDs, which decrease renal blood flow (see discussion of NSAIDs). Pancytopenia may occur, and thrombocytopenia is the most prevalent dyscrasia, occurring in about 1% of patients. Therefore, a complete blood count (including platelet count) is indicated, and if thrombocytopenia is found, the patient must be evaluated for the possibility of a clinical coagulopathy. A rare form of gold toxicity is a peripheral neuritis. This may be a concern when a regional anesthetic or peripheral nerve block as well as surgery are contemplated. Detection of such a neuritis should prompt a thorough preoperative neurologic assessment with appropriate documentation. Even though gold only rarely affects hepatic function, liver function tests should be obtained preoperatively. With regard to postoperative use, it is noteworthy that chrysotherapy is devoid of analgesic and antiinflammatory properties.

Immunosuppressive Drugs

Azathioprine and cyclophosphamide are occasionally administered to patients with refractory rheumatoid disease and SLE. These compounds predispose to pancytopenia. Infection may result from the leukopenia, but of greater concern in the perioperative setting should be thrombocytopenia, especially in light of the shorter half-life of platelets. Hepatic biliary stasis is another major concern in patients receiving these drugs. Laboratory evidence of these toxic effects should be screened and addressed preoperatively. Appropriate considerations of the potentially additive toxic effects of anesthetic drugs such as nitrous oxide and halothane are indicated and are addressed later in the discussion of antimetabolites.

Cyclosporine is a recent addition to the drug armamentarium for rheumatoid arthritis. Patients receiving cyclosporine are prone to experiencing hypertension, and chronic nephrotoxicity may occur. At higher doses, lymphomatous lesions within the liver have formed, and airway obstruction can develop related to hypertrophy of the lymphoid components of Waldeyer's ring in children treated with cyclosporine after liver transplantation.[18]

Antimetabolites

Methotrexate in low doses is the most frequently used antimetabolite drug for rheumatoid arthritis patients. It is a folate antagonist that acts as an immunosuppressant. Bone marrow depression is characterized by a pancytopenia and mandates routine monitoring of blood cell counts including platelets. Bone marrow suppression is particularly likely in the setting of renal dysfunction and its associated accumulation of methotrexate in the body.[19] Adherence to a low-dose regimen may avoid hemorrhagic enteritis, but mucosal ulceration of the mouth and rectum as well as nausea and vomiting are commonly encountered. The oral lesions may be worsened by the trauma of intubation on airways, and the vomiting may cause chronic electrolyte abnormalities and dehydration. Because of methotrexate's widespread distribution and its prolonged retention in human tissue, hepatic and renal dysfunction and even nonseptic interstitial pneumonitis may persist for several months after discontinuance of the drug. A preoperative chest radiograph is mandatory in all patients treated with methotrexate within 6 months. Liver disease may become manifest as a slowly progressive fibrosis that may be insidiously associated with normal liver function testing. Even small amounts of ethanol intake markedly accelerates the development of hepatic fibrosis.

Methotrexate may be used in combination with other drugs such as azathioprine and the antimalarials, and potentially additive toxicities must be evaluated before surgery. Methotrexate and antimalarials are especially noteworthy in that methotrexate-induced liver enzyme elevations may be masked by chloroquine or hydroxychloroquine. Concurrent methotrexate and NSAID therapy is particularly dangerous in terms of methotrexate toxicity in the elderly because they are prone to dehydration, may have decreased renal function associated with their age, and then have the synergism of the reduction of renal blood flow caused by NSAIDs. This renal dysfunction reduces the elimination of methotrexate from the body and produces sudden increases in methotrexate blood levels, which, in turn, induce bone marrow depression.

Recent studies suggest that methotrexate may result in increased susceptibility to perioperative infections and may retard tissue healing.[20] The most common route of administration is that of a bolus—orally, intramuscularly, or intravenously—once weekly. It is apparent that the dose scheduled before elective surgery should be eliminated. If other factors predisposing to tissue accumulation are present (renal, circulatory), it might be prudent to discontinue methotrexate 3 weeks before the contemplated surgery. In terms of rheumatoid therapy, the biologic effect of methotrexate lasts for at least a month so that flaring of symptomatology during this window of postoperative recovery is unlikely. The methotrexate may be restarted 1 week after the healing process is deemed adequate. Similar judgment should be applied to all immunosuppressant drugs.

Methotrexate is an analogue of folic acid, a precursor required for deoxyribonucleic acid (DNA) synthesis. There is a close relationship between folic acid and vitamin B_{12}. Nitrous oxide irreversibly oxidizes and inactivates the cobalt atom of cyanocobalamin (B_{12}), a cofactor of the key DNA synthetic enzyme methionine synthetase.[21] Although this blockade of the DNA synthetic pathway is well tolerated in healthy patients undergoing elective surgery, those treated with methotrexate may be extremely sensitive to the B_{12} inhibition, which occurs with even brief (1- to 3-hour) exposures to nitrous oxide.[21–23] Overt clinical toxicity including megaloblastic anemia, pancytopenia, and subacute combined degeneration of the spinal cord may occur in these patients, and it is, therefore, recommended that nitrous oxide not be used to anesthetize or sedate patients currently receiving or recently treated with methotrexate.

D-Penicillamine

A mainstay of therapy for cystinuria and Wilson's disease, D-penicillamine[18, 24] (dimethylcysteine) also is used to treat resistant rheumatoid arthritis. A number of adverse reactions may be encountered with D-penicillamine. During the first week of therapy, one in six patients will experience a hypersensitivity reaction characterized by fever, lymphadenopathy, anorexia, and various urticarial or morbilliform dermatologic lesions. Nonhypersensitivity dermatologic complications including bullous lesions and easy friability also occur. Intraoral lesions may be aggravated by oral airways and endotracheal tubes and require a thorough preanesthetic examination of the oral cavity. Cutaneous lesions may interfere with intravenous catheter placement, mask application, taping, and needle placement for regional anesthesia. Indeed, a small white papule is likely to form at the venous access site. It is prudent to withhold elective surgery until any drug-induced fever subsides, both for patient comfort and because of the serious nature of diagnosing and treating cases of malignant hyperpyrexia. Cessation of drug therapy usually terminates hypersensitivity activity within 1 week.

D-penicillamine may infrequently cause bone marrow depression, toxic hepatitis, and renal dysfunction. Appropriate laboratory screening for these pathologic entities should be done preoperatively, and anesthetic management should protect these organs from further impairment.

A myasthenia gravis–like syndrome can be induced. If general anesthesia with muscle relaxation is planned, it is prudent to administer a small test dose of a nondepolarizing muscle relaxant before induction of anesthesia. Exquisite sensitivity to this class of neuromuscular blocking drugs is characteristic of patients with drug-induced or underlying myasthenic syndromes.

Antimalarial Drugs

An occasional rheumatoid arthritis or SLE patient may receive high doses of antimalarial drugs such as chloroquine and hydroxychloroquine. These drugs must not be administered in doses exceeding 500 mg/day for chloroquine and 400 mg/day for hydroxychloroquine to avoid toxicity. In general, these drugs are well tolerated and have few side effects other than discoloration of the mucous membranes and nail beds. The latter should not interfere with pulse oximetry. Several of the untoward side effects are ophthalmologic and include diplopia and blurred vision. However, the most significant morbidity is that of the deposit of drug and melanin precipitates in the area of the macula and the resultant permanent blind spots within the central visual fields. This, in fact, mandates visual field examinations every 6 months. Detection of these visual symptoms preoperatively can eliminate confusion with similar effects related to muscle relaxants (test doses or residual paresis of incomplete reversal) or corneal injury during administration of anesthesia. A routine preoperative ECG may demonstrate inversion or depression of the T waves and even widening of the QRS complex. Furthermore, cardiomegaly may be detected on physical examination and chest radiograph, but in the absence of clinical findings consistent with cardiac dysfunction, this would not be a contraindication to proceeding with anesthesia. Because antirheumatoid doses can be associated with a peripheral neuropathy, a documented preoperative neurologic assessment of the lower extremities is warranted. The myopathy, cardiomyopathy, and peripheral neuropathy all are reversible with discontinuation of these chloroquinines.

Steroids

Many rheumatoid arthritis patients are receiving steroids[4, 5] or have received them in the past. Steroid therapy causes major effects on the body's ability to maintain homeostasis; therefore, failure to pay meticulous attention to this matter can be life threatening. The adrenal cortex synthesizes corticosteroids, which, in turn, have been categorized as glucocorticoids and mineralocorticoids. The adrenal cortex does not store these biosynthetic products, and corticosteroids have only brief (minutes) plasma half-lives. Table 28–5 lists the relative potencies, equivalent doses, and biologic half-lives of the commonly used steroids.

Cortisol is the standard bearer, or prototype, of the naturally occurring glucocorticoids, which are defined as possessing a high potency to bring about glycogen deposition in the liver but only a weak potency for effecting sodium retention. Aldosterone and deoxycorticosterone are the prototypical mineralocorticoids, which are defined by their strong promotion of sodium retention by the kidney but are virtually devoid of the ability to promote hepatic glycogen deposition. Glucocorticoid activity can, for practical purposes, be equated with an antiinflammatory effect, which, in turn, is loosely coupled with immunosuppressive activity.

Corticotropin (adrenocorticotropic hormone [ACTH]) is produced in the adenohypophysis and stimulates the adrenal cortex to synthesize cortisol, corticosterone, aldosterone, and androgens. The adenohypophysis, in turn, is controlled by both the positive stimulation of the central nervous system and the negative feedback of cortisol and corticosterone. Stimulation of ACTH synthesis and its release into the circulation occurs with stressful states such as surgery, pain, emotional stress, trauma, hemorrhage, hypothermia, and infection. Within minutes, these stress factors will override the normal negative feedback control mechanism. Clearly, the adrenal cortex is a critical organ involved with the ongoing process of homeostasis. The therapeutic use of corticosteroids for several days to as long as 1 month does not result in adrenal insufficiency on discontinuance of therapy. However, more prolonged treatment may cause a suppression of the pituitary's secretion of ACTH, including morphologic changes suggestive of functional impairment. This, in turn, diminishes adrenocortical function and results in atrophy of the adrenal cortex and its inability to produce steroids and release them into the circulation. The adrenal cortex will be unable to respond to endogenous (or even exogenously administered) ACTH if it is atrophied in association with rapid withdrawal from the prolonged administration of steroids in physiologic or supraphysiologic (pharmacologic) doses.

The characteristic withdrawal syndrome for acute, iatrogenically induced adrenal cortical insufficiency may resemble symptoms of rheumatoid arthritis exacerbation: arthralgia, myalgia, malaise, and fever. True adrenocortical insufficiency is life threatening; it results in dehydration, hypotension, hyponatremia, hyperkalemia, hypoglycemia, weakness, and lethargy. Appropriate therapy includes re-

TABLE 28–5

CORTICOSTEROIDS: RELATIVE POTENCIES, EQUIVALENT DOSES, BIOLOGIC HALF-LIVES*

Agent	Antiinflammatory (Glucocorticoid)	Sodium Retention (Mineralocorticoid)	Equivalent Dose (Oral, IV) in Milligrams	Duration of Action (Half-Life) in Hours
Hydrocortisone (Cortisol)	1.0	1.0	20.00	6–8 +
Cortisone	0.8	0.8	25.00	6–8 +
Prednisolone	4.0	0.8	5.00	12–30 +
Prednisone	4.0	0.8	5.00	12–30 +
Methylprednisolone	5.0	0.5	4.00	12–30 +
Triamcinolone	5.0	—	4.00	12–30 +
Betamethasone	25	—	0.75	30–70
Dexamethasone	25	—	0.75	30–70
For reference				
Aldosterone	1.0	3000		
11-Desoxycorticosterone	—	100		
Corticosterone	1.0	15		

*Hydrocortisone (cortisol) has approximately one fourth the antiinflammatory and glucocorticoid potency of prednisone, prednisolone, and methylprednisolone with the same sodium-retaining (mineralocorticoid) potency as each of these drugs. Cortisol and cortisone are essentially equal in glucocorticoid and mineralocorticoid potencies. Dexamethasone, betamethasone, and triamcinolone, although possessing potent glucocorticoid and antiinflammatory properties, do not possess significant mineralocorticoid activity.

IV, intravenous.

placement of intravascular volume with intravenous isotonic sodium chloride solutions containing adequate amounts of glucose and water as well as corticosteroids. The corticosteroid dose should be the equivalent of 100 mg of hydrocortisone and repeated intravenously every 6 hours. This dosage schedule is the rough equivalent of the maximal rate of secretion of cortisol in response to stress by the normal pituitary-adrenal axis. Complete recovery of the pituitary-adrenal axis after prolonged steroid therapy may be as long as 9 to 12 months, and there are patients who are relatively adrenocortical insufficient for as long as 2 years.

Any patient having received several days of consecutive steroid therapy within the previous year must be considered at risk for perioperative adrenal cortical insufficiency. There is no simple, inexpensive test routinely available for measuring the dynamic function of the pituitary-adrenal axis. Therefore, it is mandatory to provide an adequate steroid treatment regimen for every surgical patient who has been treated with steroids within the previous year. This mandate applies even to those patients receiving only local anesthesia with sedation or analgesia (monitored anesthesia care).

Indeed, one of the first case reports of postoperative adrenal cortical insufficiency occurred after an otherwise uncomplicated bunionectomy.[25] The axiom "when in doubt, treat" summarizes our approach. Steroid therapy should be continued throughout the entire perioperative period until patients return to a nonstressful (recovered) physiologic state and tolerate oral ingestion of the appropriate dosage of steroids to which they had previously been accustomed. The dosage of steroid therapeutically deployed for the rheumatoid arthritis patient should never be more than that needed to control the disease process.

The unencumbered adrenal cortex secretes 20 to 30 mg of hydrocortisone each day and generates an average plasma concentration of 10 μg/dl. Diurnal variations result in higher plasma values (16 μg/dl) in the early morning waking hours, a gradual decline during the day, and then a progressive drop to the lowest values usually seen within 2 hours into the sleeping state. The parenteral dose of glucocorticoids in the surgical patient should be at least the generous equivalent of the daily secretion of normal adrenal glands or 30 mg of hydrocortisone.

Recommended regimens for the steroid-dependent patient undergoing podiatric surgery follow.

For *extensive foot surgery* that will result in moderate to severe postoperative physiologic and psychological stress in the form of pain, distress, disability, and multiorgan supranormal demands for as long as 3 days, 100 mg of hydrocortisone or 20 mg of methylprednisolone given intramuscularly every 6 hours is recommended on the operative/anesthesia day. The intramuscular route is preferred because it provides a more steady and reliable blood and tissue concentration of steroid than can be achieved with the intravenous route. The intravenous route is an acceptable alternative only if its uninterrupted function for constant infusion of steroid can be guaranteed until the reinitiation of effective oral intake. The initial dose should be intramuscular 1 to 2 hours preanesthetically. If this initial dose must be administered in the operating room, then the intravenous infusion should be accompanied by an equivalent intramuscular dose. All succeeding 100-mg hydrocortisone or 20-mg methylprednisolone doses are to be intramuscular. The intravenous route is indicated only when the intramuscular depot would be ineffective, as

with circulatory insufficiency or disorders of the muscle system.

On the first postoperative day, 100 mg of hydrocortisone or 20 mg of methylprednisolone should be given intramuscularly or by mouth (if the patient is able) every 12 hours. On the second postoperative day, 100 mg of hydrocortisone or 20 mg of methylprednisolone should be given intramuscularly or orally if this dose is judged to be necessary. This regimen is reduced by 50% each day thereafter until the usual preoperative maintenance dose is reached. Should medical or surgical complications ensue, then a return to a higher dose regimen approximating that of the day of surgery should be instituted.

Steroid-dependent patients subjected to extensive podiatric surgery or physiologic stress should be hospitalized the initial postoperative day to ensure the administration of all medications (including steroids), to guarantee appropriate fluid intake, and to allow for the adequate observation for any medical complications. Regardless of any other circumstances, patients should remain hospitalized until they are able to demonstrate that they can ingest and retain oral steroid preparations.

For *less extensive foot surgery* but which constitutes more than a simple, minimally traumatic or stressful, short podiatric procedure, 100 mg of hydrocortisone or 20 mg of methylprednisolone should be given intramuscularly every 6 hours on the operative/anesthesia day. The initial dose is given 1 to 2 hours preanesthetically. If this must be accomplished in the operating room, the intravenous dose must be accompanied by an equivalent intramuscular dose. Succeeding 100-mg hydrocortisone or 20-mg methylprednisolone doses are to be intramuscular. On the first postoperative day with the patient able to resume oral medications, the resumption of the preoperative daily dose of steroid is appropriate unless the clinical course dictates otherwise.

For *minimally traumatic foot surgery* of short duration and one that can be accomplished with pure local anesthesia or with only minimal supplemental sedation or analgesia (monitored anesthesia care), and after which mild physiologic or psychological stress is anticipated beyond the initial several postoperative hours, 100 mg of hydrocortisone or 20 mg of methylprednisolone should be given intramuscularly before the initiation of anesthesia and at least 1 liter of physiologic salt solution administered intravenously before discharge from the surgical facility. The patient should be able to resume oral medications within 24 hours, and the resumption of the preoperative daily dose of steroid is appropriate unless the clinical course dictates otherwise.

Discharge of the steroid-dependent patient from the hospital or surgical outpatient facility is a medical judgment that is based on (1) actual extent of the podiatric surgery, (2) duration of significant postsurgical stress and physiologic disorder, (3) administration and retention of steroid medications in appropriate doses, and (4) medical clearance for discharge.

Pharmacologic doses of steroids have numerous physiologic effects that may require special management. These include the following:

1. Glucocorticoids effect a diabetic-like state of glucose intolerance. Preanesthetic blood glucose should be measured and then monitored intra-anesthetically and postanesthetically because hyperglycemia is likely in

the milieu of surgical stress (especially with increased catecholamine release), general anesthesia, steroid administration, and infusion of glucose-containing solutions.[8, 10] Hyperglycemia is less likely to occur with regional anesthesia that includes sympathetic nervous system blockade at the spinal cord level and also with administration of β-adrenergic blocking drugs and non–glucose-containing solutions. Should hyperglycemia become significant, such as with values greater than 250 mg/dl, insulin therapy might become necessary.

2. Mineralocorticoids cause sodium retention and expansion of the extracellular fluid volume; an inclination to hypernatremia, hypokalemia, and alkalosis; and a predisposition to hypertension.

3. Glucocorticoids can cause a myopathy in which there is muscle weakness (particularly the proximal musculature of all limbs) and easy fatigability. This may be translated to a sensitivity to muscle relaxants used during anesthesia as well as a hindrance to achieving ambulation.

4. Patients have an elevated hemoglobin concentration and hematocrit.

5. Patients have an increased number of polymorphonuclear leukocytes with a decreased number of lymphocytes, monocytes, and basophils.

6. Patients have an increased susceptibility to infection. This could be a rational basis for the use of prophylactic antibiotics in selected surgical patients.

7. Patients are predisposed to peptic ulcer disease, with the potential for perforation (the signs and symptoms of which can be masked by steroids) and hemorrhage (chronic or acute). In addition, the risk of peptic ulcer disease in patients receiving NSAIDs such as salicylates is increased twofold when the patient is concomitantly receiving steroids. This suggests the prophylactic perioperative use of the H_2 blocking drugs, preferably nizatidine or famotidine, to reduce gastric acid secretion and the likelihood of perforation and bleeding (see Salicylates).

8. Glucocorticoid induction of drug-metabolizing enzymes tends to enhance drug degradation.

9. Behavioral changes may assume any one of numerous abnormal forms, but these may be difficult to distinguish from the anxiety and emotional stress encountered in the preoperative state. Certainly, a manic, euphoric, or hyperactive behavior is more likely to be caused by steroids. Likewise, the differential diagnosis of delirium on emergence from anesthesia must include the possible contributing role of hyperglucocorticoidemia.

10. Predisposition to osteoporosis and the tendency to develop vertebral compression fractures make it imperative to pay meticulous attention to positioning, moving, and transporting these fragile patients.

The anesthetic hypnotic drug etomidate has the potential to cause adrenocortical insufficiency secondary to an inhibition of adrenocortical steroidogenesis.[26] Although this drug is perhaps the most cardiovascular stabilizing of the available anesthesia-inducing drugs, it might be considered relatively contraindicated in the steroid-dependent patient. Nonetheless, one could argue for its use in these situations because appropriate management of these patients already mandates full steroid coverage with ample doses of exogenously administered steroids as discussed previously.

Medications for Gout

Some podiatric surgical patients are afflicted with gout. The most commonly used drugs in the treatment of the hyperuricemia of gout are the xanthine oxidase inhibitor allopurinol and the uricosuric agents probenecid and sulfapyrazole. These drugs are well tolerated and possess minimal side effects, but they are not available in parenteral form. Probenecid infrequently causes cephalalgia, a consideration for the candidate for spinal anesthesia. Probenecid's uricosuric effect is reduced by salicylates administered in low doses; conversely, probenecid may delay the renal excretion of salicylic acid. Probenecid may produce a modest salt and water diuresis, which should be replaced intraoperatively. Hepatic uptake of a number of drugs is reduced by probenecid, including indomethacin, which must be used in lowered dosage, and heparin, whose anticoagulant effect may be increased. The activity of penicillin, ampicillin, nafcillin, and some cephalosporins may be prolonged by probenecid therapy. Furthermore, probenecid increases the plasma half-lives of several NSAIDs, and it reduces the doses of thiopental and ketamine required for induction while increasing their duration of action.

Allopurinol infrequently causes elevations of the alkaline phosphatase, aspartate aminotransferase, and alanine aminotransferase; therefore preoperative liver function screening is indicated. It also has significant interactions with other drugs; among these is an increased incidence of skin rash in patients concomitantly receiving ampicillin, which can present a diagnostic dilemma in an anesthetized patient receiving ampicillin. Allopurinol inhibits the biodegradation of warfarin (anticoagulant), which can result in an elevated prothrombin time that should be measured preoperatively. A reduction (or even cessation) of the dose of warfarin or the administration of vitamin K may be necessary before embarking on surgery or administering a regional anesthetic. Allopurinol also interferes with the metabolism of theophylline and causes an accumulation of methylxanthine (an active metabolite) as well as theophylline. Therefore, the bronchospastic patient receiving theophylline should have blood levels measured, and there will be a heightened concern for the potential for increased ventricular ectopy when such a patient is anesthetized with halothane.

All patients with gout should have BUN and creatinine determinations because of the possibility of uric acid nephropathy. Proteinuria and hypertension are commonly (30%) associated with gout, and each patient scheduled for surgery should have a thorough medical evaluation for the latter.

Patients with hyperuricemia are at risk for gouty arthritis in the postoperative period: This usually occurs between the 3rd and 5th postoperative days but may be as late as the 10th day. It is especially true in those patients who have not had perioperative colchicine or NSAID therapy and also in those in whom some degree of dehydration occurs. NSAIDs control the symptoms of acute gouty arthritis. Oral colchicine still is commonly used, but owing to the significant incidence of gastrointestinal side effects (nausea, vomiting, diarrhea, and abdominal pain), the NSAIDs are the preferred oral agents. Intravenous colchicine circumvents most of the gastrointestinal problems, and in the acute postoperative patient who may not have oral access to drugs, it is a frequently used treatment modality.

Colchicine does potentiate the anesthetic effects of some central nervous system depressant drugs such as the barbiturates and chloral hydrate, and it is synergistic with cyclopropane and nitrous oxide.[28] However, the effect of colchicine on the minimal alveolar concentration of the halogenated hydrocarbon anesthetics remains to be determined.

The administration of colchicine before and after surgery will prevent the occurrence of postoperative acute gouty arthritis. However, such attacks are much less likely to occur in the surgical patient already receiving allopurinol therapy. In fact, with ongoing allopurinol therapy, colchicine need not be administered unless the patient also has been receiving concurrent chronic colchicine therapy (which often is combined with probenecid as well). Acute gouty attacks are more likely to occur in the surgical patient whose oral drug therapy has been withheld (most medications can indeed be safely administered with sips of water even during the traditional preoperative fast) and whose routine oral hydration and self-induced diuresis also have not been maintained via the parenteral route during the fasting period. As the most specific drug therapy for acute gouty attacks, colchicine is given orally, when possible, in 0.5-mg increments every hour until relief is obtained or side effects occur; often between 7 and 10 doses (a maximum of 12 is suggested) are required. Diarrhea frequently is produced by these doses and may necessitate replacement of fluids and electrolytes intravenously. Intravenous colchicine may be necessary if the acute event occurs in the early postoperative period, especially when the patient is unable to tolerate oral medication. If intravenous colchicine is deemed necessary, 1 to 2 mg are diluted in 20 ml of normal saline and administered slowly over 1 hour. Initial amelioration of symptoms usually is noted in 6 to 8 hours, with complete resolution within 24 hours. If relief is not obtained within the 6-hour period after the initial intravenous dose, further colchicine should be administered in 1-mg increments every 6 hours to a maximum total dose of 4 mg in patients not taking colchicine. Extensive tissue necrosis will occur after extravasation of the solution; it behooves the anesthesiologist to use a large-bore, secure intravenous site.

Colchicine has the smallest benefit to toxicity ratio of drugs that are effective in treating acute gouty attacks.[28a] NSAIDs are an effective and appropriate therapeutic alternative. They are most beneficial in doses of 150% to 200% of the usual TED (see earlier section on NSAIDs) during the initial 24 to 48 hours and then must be tapered rapidly to the routine daily TED. Indomethacin and ketorolac are the only currently available parenteral NSAIDs.

If acute monoarticular gout is encountered, arthrocentesis and instillation of corticosteroids are often effective. Triamcinolone hexacetonide, 20 mg—or the more rapidly-acting methylprednisolone acetate suspension in an 80-mg dose—may be aseptically injected into the affected joint. The addition of 1% lidocaine solution to the injectate with a 1:4 ratio of steroid to lidocaine volume is more readily accepted by the patient and offers more immediate relief of symptoms before the steroid's onset of action. In the event of resistance or intolerance to colchicine or NSAIDs, or in the case of

multiple joint involvement, systemic steroid therapy may become indicated. The preferred clinical approach to achieve this goal is the administration of ACTH by slow intravenous infusion in a dose of 20 U, or as an intramuscular dose of 40 to 80 U, every 6 to 12 hours for 1 to 2 days.[28b] ACTH is effective within a few hours, and clinically it has been shown to be more effective than parenteral steroids.

Because both an increased urinary acidity and a decreased excretion of free water increase the urinary concentration of undissociated uric acid—the critical determinant of urinary tract supersaturation and stone formation—the anesthesiologist must guarantee an uninterrupted diuresis and urinary alkalinization (avoidance of inordinate acidity). Unfortunately, the surgical patient normally receives potent antidiuretic stimuli, including the preanesthetic fast (dehydration), the normal decrease in urine flow encountered during preoperative sleep, and the stresses inherent to the preanesthetic intra-anesthetic, and postanesthetic (postoperative) periods. The kidney usually responds homeostatically to these antidiuretic stimuli by decreasing the excretion of water (antidiuresis) and salt. The goal of prophylactic and therapeutic diuresis is achieved by forced fluid intake to greater than 4000 ml/day (proportionately less for children) and administration of alkaline compounds. Hydration is performed preferably by the oral route until the mandatory preanesthetic fasting state begins, at which time one should initiate an intravenous infusion of a *non–lactate*-containing solution with glucose and a pH of approximately 7 at a rate of at least 200 ml/hour. The flow rate should be regulated to guarantee a generous hourly urine output. The presence of glucose in the intravenous solution prevents the generation of lactate and other tubular inhibitory organic acids associated with the fasting state, and the absence of lactate also avoids increasing serum lactate levels, which inhibits renal tubular excretion of urate.

Acetate-containing solutions appear both biochemically and physiologically innocuous for the patient with gout. Once established, this diuresis must be maintained during and after administration of anesthesia and the surgery by appropriate intravenous therapy until the patient is able to resume an oral intake sufficient to sustain the diuresis. The use of the potent diuretic drugs (furosemide and ethacrynic acid) or even mannitol to create or maintain a diuresis in the gouty patient is potentially counterproductive and ultimately may enhance the already pre-existent pathophysiology within the kidney. However, the judicious use of low doses of dopamine to promote a diuresis is justifiable when indicated.

Alkalinization may be effected with oral sodium bicarbonate (3 to 7 g/day) or sodium citrate (Shohl's solution, 30 to 90 ml/day divided into three or four doses and proportionately less in children) before the preanesthetic fast. Bicitra, a stable commercial solution containing sodium citrate and citric acid prepared in a sugar-free base, is the U.S. Pharmacopeia formula for Shohl's solution; it is familiar to anesthesiologists, who use it as a clear antacid for prophylaxis in the patient with a full stomach. Each 5 ml contains 500 mg of sodium citrate as the dihydrate and 334 mg of citric acid as the monohydrate. It usually is diluted twofold or threefold, and flavorings may make it more palatable. Alkalinization of the urine by directly alkalizing the blood is usually unnecessary. Acetazolamide, the potent carbonic anhydrase inhibitor, will bring about both urinary alkalinization (loss of bicarbonate) and promotion of diuresis, but its use in gout is infrequent.

When feasible, the anesthesiologist should ensure continuation of antigout drug therapy throughout the perioperative period. Oral medications with sips of water, therefore, should be continued as an exception to the preoperative fast, and surgical procedures are preferably scheduled at the start of the operative day.

Primary anesthetic considerations for patients afflicted with gout are frequently dictated by other factors. Many patients are elderly and obese and have the usual cardiovascular dysfunction associated with their age and weight. Coronary artery disease and hypertension are particularly common in gout. Because emotional upset may precipitate an acute attack of gouty arthritis and is potentially harmful in the patient with coronary artery disease, a humanistic preanesthetic approach toward establishing a mutually beneficial physician-patient relationship assumes major importance.[29] The patient should be well adapted and adjusted with respect to the total perioperative experience. He or she should arrive in the operating room in an appropriately relaxed state and be handled with an aim to anxiolysis.

No anesthetic agent or technique is clearly superior; however, *methoxyflurane is absolutely contraindicated.*[30] Methoxyflurane is biodegraded to fluoride and oxalate, the former being a potent tubular nephrotoxin when toxic blood fluoride concentrations are achieved. Hyperuricemia and reduced renal clearance of urate are proven potential pathophysiological sequelae of the administration of methoxyflurane. All other currently available potent halogenated hydrocarbon inhalational anesthetics are safe for use in the patient with gout, although enflurane possesses the potential for producing elevated blood fluoride concentrations when given in high concentrations for a prolonged period of time.[31] Although renal dysfunction is less frequently seen with current practice of long-term allopurinol therapy, the elderly patient with long-standing gout may have more renal compromise than his or her nongouty counterpart. The anesthetic considerations for patients with renal disease are similar to those for any patient with a similar degree of renal impairment.[32]

LOCAL ANESTHETIC DRUGS

Podiatric surgery frequently provides the opportunity to choose between various forms of regional anesthesia, a subject that goes beyond the intent of this chapter. The choice of a local anesthetic drug[33] depends on the specific surgical requirements and the distinctive pharmacologic properties of the several local anesthetic drugs currently available.

There are two major chemical groupings of local anesthetics:

1. Amino esters—procaine, chloroprocaine, tetracaine, cocaine, and benzocaine—are hydrolyzed in plasma but have a low, albeit significant, incidence of sensitizing reactions (especially procaine).
2. Amino amides—lidocaine, mepivacaine, bupivacaine, prilocaine, etidocaine, and dibucaine—are biodegraded in the liver and have an extremely low occurrence rate of sensitizing reactions. Most of the alleged allergic reactions to the amino amides might in fact be related

to the preservative methylparaben used in multidose containers.

The pharmacologic properties that dictate clinical utility are as follows:

1. Time of onset of action, this latency interval generally being a function of the pKa
2. Duration of action, largely a function of protein binding
3. Intrinsic anesthetic potency, a function of lipid solubility
4. Toxicity

The following is a general categorical classification of local anesthetic drugs according to their pharmacologic properties:

Short duration of action (30 to 40 minutes), low potency: procaine and chloroprocaine (shortest onset)
Intermediate duration of action (90 to 240 minutes), moderate potency: mepivacaine, lidocaine, and prilocaine
Long duration of action (180 to 600 minutes), high potency: bupivacaine, etidocaine (shortest onset), and tetracaine (longest onset)

The potency of infiltration anesthesia (intradermal or subcutaneous), commonly used in podiatric surgery, parallels the local anesthetic's inherent potency such that:

2% chloroprocaine = 2% procaine = 1% lidocaine = 1% prilocaine = 1% mepivacaine = 0.25% bupivacaine

All of these drugs have a rapid onset of action and have their duration of action significantly lengthened when combined with vasoconstrictor drugs such as epinephrine. This prolongation of effect is achieved by slowing systemic absorption of the local anesthetic, which also reduces the likelihood of rapidly achieving toxic blood concentrations of these drugs. The choice of local anesthetic is determined by the time required for surgery, but the postoperative analgesic potential should be considered as well as in appropriate patients. When larger total volumes of local anesthetics are needed, as in bilateral foot surgery, the potential for toxicity dictates the total doses used and whether the individual foot blocks should be staggered (Table 28–6).

The considerations elaborated for infiltration anesthesia basically apply to all of the peripheral nerve blocks used for the ankle and foot. A common practice to minimize the pain

TABLE 28–6

SUGGESTED MAXIMAL DOSES OF LOCAL ANESTHETICS FOR INFILTRATION OR NERVE BLOCKS

Anesthetic	Dose (mg/kg)
Procaine	15.0
Chloroprocaine	15.0
Lidocaine	5.0 (without epinephrine)
	7.0 (with 1/200,000 epinephrine)
Mepivacaine	5.0 (without epinephrine)
	7.0 (with 1/200,000 epinephrine)
Tetracaine	1.5 (without epinephrine)
	2.8 (with 1/200,000 epinephrine)
Bupivacaine	2.5 (without epinephrine)
	3.2 (with epinephrine)
Prilocaine	7.0

of injection associated with lidocaine is to add 1 mEq of sodium bicarbonate to every 10 ml of lidocaine solution.

Lidocaine and mepivacaine are the gold standards of safe intravenous regional anesthesia in terms of local and systemic toxicity.[34] A double-cuffed tourniquet technique should be used, and exsanguination should be invoked before cuff inflation. On release of the cuff (perhaps most safely accomplished intermittently), lidocaine will generate about 5 to 10 minutes of residual analgesia, whereas mepivacaine may provide twice as much. Larger volumes of more dilute solutions are used for the lower compared with the upper extremities. Procaine (hypersensitivity), chloroprocaine (thrombophlebitis), prilocaine (methemoglobinemia), and bupivacaine (cardiotoxicity) should *not* be used for intravenous regional anesthesia because of their various potential toxicities and the availability of safe and suitable alternative agents.

For a sciatic-femoral nerve block, the onset of action for all the local anesthetics is longer than that noted for peripheral nerve blocks because of the greater temporal requirements for spread along the nerve sheath. Lidocaine and mepivacaine will exhibit a 15-minute onset, and bupivacaine may add as much as another 10 minutes. A longer duration of action accompanies this prolonged onset, with lidocaine and mepivacaine (especially with epinephrine 1/200,000) lasting 2 to 3 hours and bupivacaine (with or without epinephrine) lasting as long as 12 hours. The choice of anesthetic will depend mainly on the desired length of analgesia.

The major toxic effects of the local anesthetic drugs involve the central nervous and cardiovascular systems. Central nervous system toxicity of the various local anesthetic drugs is proportional to their inherent anesthetic potency and is manifest by both excitatory and depressed functions. The earliest symptoms heralding central nervous system toxicity include drowsiness or agitation, tinnitus, disorientation, visual and auditory disturbances, dizziness or presyncopal complaints, and problems with focusing. Muscle twitching, tremors, shivering, and slurred speech may herald generalized convulsions. Seizures should be treated not only with controlled ventilation and oxygenation but also, when appropriate, with drugs that minimize the electrical activity (oxygen consumption) of the brain such as barbiturates, midazolam, or diazepam. Seizures are followed by severe depression of the central respiratory and cardiovascular centers, which must be managed with appropriate supportive measures.

Local anesthetic drugs have direct depressant effects on the heart and peripheral vasculature. Generally, systemic absorption of local anesthetics administered for infiltration anesthesia, nerve blocks, and even central neural blockade will not result in a blood concentration associated with direct cardiovascular depression. However, inadvertent intravascular injection during regional or intravenous regional anesthesia or the use of very large doses of drug for extensive infiltration (e.g., a simultaneous bilateral podiatric procedure) can result in high blood levels of local anesthetic drugs. The consequences include impaired myocardial contractility, various degrees of heart block, and peripheral vascular dilation with ultimate circulatory collapse. Generally, central nervous system toxicity is manifest before cardiovascular depression.

Bupivacaine is unique in its cardiotoxic properties and has been associated with intractable ventricular arrhythmias. As such, extreme care must be taken to limit the total dose of bupivacaine to below a conservative threshold of toxicity doses. Ropivacaine, a new amide local anesthetic under investigation, is similar to bupivacaine in terms of potency, effectiveness, and duration of action but is less cardiotoxic.[35] Prilocaine is unique because methemoglobinemia (reversible with methylene blue) can result from its administration in large doses. Procaine, chloroprocaine, and tetracaine have prolonged durations of action and greater potential for achieving toxic blood levels in the patient with a cholinesterase deficiency. Finally, chloroprocaine has been implicated in rare cases of local neural toxicity. However, the cause may be the sodium bisulfite preservative or the low pH rather than the drug itself. It is prudent to limit the use of chloroprocaine to the newly formulated preservative-free 2% solution.

Table 28–6 presents conservative guidelines that may be used as suggested maximal dosages of local anesthetics for infiltration or nerve blocks in healthy adults. The maximal dose of local anesthetic drugs should be reduced when calculating the value for the extremely obese patient. A safety consideration for bilateral foot surgery under peripheral nerve block or local infiltration is that each foot should be individually anesthetized preceding the actual surgery on that foot. This unilateral approach is inherently safer than simultaneous bilateral blocks before initiation of any surgery because the latter, by doubling the dose of drug given at that time, increases the likelihood of inducing systemic local anesthetic toxicity. Furthermore, unless both feet are operated simultaneously, there is the possibility that the block on the second foot might wear off before the surgery is concluded.

The prophylactic use of diazepam and midazolam to raise the seizure threshold and prevent any such toxic reaction to local anesthetics is a common practice. These benzodiazepines are preferable to the barbiturates because of their minimal cardiovascular depressant effects and their anxiolytic, hypnotic and amnesic properties. The use of epinephrine, usually in a 1/200,000 solution, to retard systemic absorption of the local anesthetics is effective. The epinephrine accompanying local anesthetics also is absorbed into the systemic circulation, and caution must be exercised in the patient with coronary artery disease, arrhythmias, or hypertension.

The halogenated hydrocarbon anesthetics halothane, enflurane, and isoflurane interact with the systemic epinephrine and may sensitize the heart to produce ventricular arrhythmias.[36, 37] The likelihood of ventricular ectopy is greatest with halothane, less so with enflurane, and least likely with isoflurane. The concomitant injection of lidocaine with the epinephrine partially protects against ventricular arrhythmias, thus making lidocaine-containing solutions with epinephrine the most safe in this respect.

The dose of submucosally administered epinephrine required to produce three or more premature ventricular extrasystoles in half of the adequately oxygenated, normocapnic, surgically anesthetized (1.25 × minimal alveolar concentration) patients is as follows:

For isoflurane: 6.7 μg/kg epinephrine
For enflurane: 10.9 μg/kg epinephrine
For halothane: 2.1 μg/kg epinephrine

According to these data, the recommended maximum dose of a 1/200,000 epinephrine-containing solution administered submucosally under halothane anesthesia with normoxia and normocapnia is 20 ml over a 10-minute period or 60 ml over a 60-minute time interval. This would be a conservative figure to carry over to enflurane and isoflurane. The dose-response curve of enflurane is not parallel to those of halothane and isoflurane, and as such, ventricular arrhythmias may occasionally occur during enflurane as well as halothane anesthesia at doses as low as 1 to 2 μg/kg. Therefore, isoflurane produces the greatest freedom from ventricular ectopy. The systemic absorption of any drug from the submucosal area is more rapid and more complete than it would be from local infiltration or peripheral nerve blocks, so that the figures enumerated previously are on the conservative side for nonsubmucosal injections. There are virtually no indications for the use of a 1/100,000 epinephrine solution for local infiltration or peripheral nerve blocks for podiatric surgery.

In those situations in which epinephrine is potentially harmful to a patient's heart, phenylephrine may be substituted as the vasoconstrictor agent. The suggested maximal dose is 10 μg/kg of a solution containing 20 μg/ml of phenylephrine over a 10-minute period or 30 μg/kg over a 60-minute time interval. Phenylephrine is a potent α-adrenergic agonist and can induce significant hypertension in susceptible patients. Its specific antidote is the α-adrenergic blocking drug phentolamine.

AIRWAY MANAGEMENT

The cervical spine may become severely deformed in patients with rheumatoid arthritis, psoriatic arthritis, ankylosing spondylitis, and, less frequently, polyarticular arthritides.[4]

Management of the rheumatoid airway may be especially problematic and associated with morbidity and even mortality.[38–41] Appropriate management begins with a detailed history that includes any past anesthetic experience, a review of old anesthetic records, and an interview of previously involved anesthesiologists if warranted and feasible. Indeed, it is imperative to make the maximal effort to obtain as much specific historic information as possible about previous anesthetic experience before initiating an anesthetic, even if it necessitates postponement of the surgery. One must also be cognizant that the degree of difficulty encountered with airway management of rheumatoid arthritis patients usually increases with time. Potential airway difficulties should be recognized in advance and so allow for detailed planning for optimal management. Accordingly, a thorough preoperative physical examination of the airway should be conducted and should include the mouth, teeth, tongue, hyoid, mandible, uvula, soft palate, tonsillar pillars, larynx, and trachea as well as the cervical spine and neck. The tongue is the largest intraoropharyngeal anatomic structure that influences the accessibility of the laryngeal inlet to direct laryngoscopy.[42]

The normal neck flexes and extends through a range of 90 to 165 degrees, but this decreases about 20% during the third through eighth decades of life.[43] The atlanto-occipital joint provides approximately 35 degrees of range of motion, whereas the lower cervical vertebrae (C3–C7) provide the largest amount of flexion (40 degrees). Atlanto-occipital joint extension and lower cervical vertebral flexion are crucial for achieving the ''sniffing'' position, which facilitates glottic visualization. However, when atlanto-occipital extension is limited, the usual intubation technique of extending this joint may displace the larynx out of the field of view.[44] Indeed, degenerative changes in the cervical spine may cause distortion of the anatomic relationships among the mandible, larynx, and trachea, thereby making endotracheal intubation a

difficult or even impossible task. Some patients with severe rheumatoid arthritis have advanced cervical spine disease that results in displacement of the larynx caudally, deviation or rotation of the larynx to either side, or angulation of the larynx anteriorly. Anterior location of the larynx may be indicated by a thyroid notch to mandibular symphysis distance of less than 3 fingerbreadths. A history of neck pain, occipital headaches, or weakness of the upper extremities points toward cervical spine disease. Physical examination may reveal limited motion of the neck that may even be fixed in a severe flexion deformity, a shortened neck, tracheal deviation, or neurologic deficits caused by cord compression.

Radiographic evaluation begins with standard anteroposterior and lateral (in flexion) projections of the neck and the chest, but more sophisticated studies in the form of computed tomography or magnetic resonance imaging might be necessary to define anatomic structures further. Indeed, cervical spine involvement occurs in as many as 90% of rheumatoid arthritis patients. A triad of radiologic findings is commonly associated with rheumatoid arthritis: atlantoaxial subluxation and instability, which is the most frequent, superior or cephalad migration of the odontoid process, and subaxial subluxation of the mid to lower cervical vertebra.[45] Because of the attendant risk of spinal cord compression during manipulation of the head and neck (especially when the patient is anesthetized), some of these patients may require cervical arthrodesis for stabilization and limitation of neurologic deterioration. Although ankylosing spondylitis primarily affects the lower spine, these patients may have severe neck deformities caused by ankylosis.[46] Cervical subluxation does not occur because the ankylosing cervical spine gradually autoarthrodeses itself into a flexion deformity. However, there is a significant risk of fracture with its neurologic sequelae should the spine be subjected to excessive misguided extrinsic forces.

The importance of a thorough neurologic evaluation in appropriately selected patients for the purpose of documenting a preoperative baseline of sensory and motor function cannot be overemphasized. Appropriate radiographic evaluation would better quantitate clinical suspicions. However, even in the absence of neurologic symptoms or signs, there may be radiographic evidence of severe anatomic changes that would forewarn of difficulties in airway management or the potential for spinal cord injury.

Arthritis of joints other than those of the cervical spine also may complicate airway management. Cricoarytenoid arthritis is a common component of rheumatoid arthritis, but it is rarely observed in patients with other inflammatory arthritides.[47, 48] This condition often is present in the absence of significant symptoms; however, dysphagia, hoarseness, or tenderness or pain to touch of the laryngeal area may be diagnostic aids. Cricoarytenoid arthritis may lead to vocal cord fixation, and this anatomic abnormality increases the likelihood of injury to laryngeal structures during endotracheal intubation. The resultant bleeding and edema can lead to airway obstruction that may even require urgent tracheostomy.[38, 49] In some advanced cases of cricoarytenoiditis, the pre-existing airway compromise may be of such a magnitude that a preanesthetic elective tracheostomy would be prudent. A previous tracheostomy scar is a warning signal of anticipated problems and could be an indication for an elective tracheostomy preanesthetically. Radiologic evaluation of these upper airways is mandatory. An old tracheostomy site might represent the narrowest area of the trachea, which would demand a small-diameter endotracheal tube to avoid tracheal injury.

Involvement of the temporomandibular joint, even unilaterally, can lead to significant restriction of the range of motion and a resultant loss of access to the oropharynx and laryngeal structures. Normal mouth opening generates a space of at least two fingerbreadths. The temporomandibular joint is commonly affected by rheumatoid arthritis, but also has been described in psoriatic arthritis, SLE, ankylosing spondylitis, and gout.[50] Gouty arthritic involvement of the temporomandibular joint is a potential impediment to achieving adequate exposure for direct laryngoscopy and for manipulating the joint for maintenance of an unobstructed airway.[51, 52] Impaired mandibular growth with resultant micrognathia may occur with temporomandibulitis in juvenile rheumatoid arthritis. Preanesthetic evaluation of the range of motion of the mandible (while concomitantly estimating its position relative to the laryngeal structures) should also distinguish between a fixed limitation of motion secondary to the arthritic process and that caused by masseter spasm induced by temporomandibular arthralgia. General anesthesia, especially with muscle relaxants, usually will abolish the masseter spasm.

Selection of a regional anesthetic technique does not obviate concerns for airway management. Indeed, control of the airway may have to be assumed by the anesthesiologist in the patient in whom (1) sedation inadvertently or unexpectedly traverses the continuum of altered states of consciousness into unconsciousness and general anesthesia with attendent loss of protective airway reflexes and hypoventilation, (2) a hypersensitivity drug reaction occurs with accompanying cardiovascular and pulmonary insufficiency, (3) regional anesthesia has failed or becomes inadequate and cannot be re-established, and (4) complications of regional anesthesia are encountered such as toxic reactions to local anesthetic or accompanying vasoactive drugs, cardiovascular insufficiency, as might occur with high sympathetic nervous system blockade, or pulmonary insufficiency relating to high somatic motor nerve blockade. Therefore, contingency plans become essential and should be addressed before any anesthetic intervention.

Some experts argue that, in the case of a patient in whom great difficulty with endotracheal intubation is anticipated, regional anesthetic techniques be postponed until the airway is secured in an elective and controlled manner. Successful exposure of the glottic opening by direct rigid laryngoscopy is benefited by alignment of the oral, pharyngeal, and laryngeal axes, a nonextreme anterior location of the larynx, adequate oral opening, flexible cervical spine, and extensibility of the atlanto-occipital joint. Furthermore, one needs oropharyngeal anatomy that holds enough structural and spatial normality to permit glottic visualization. Intubation in the awake patient who is adequately prepared with topical anesthesia, transtracheal anesthesia, or superior laryngeal nerve block is often the safest approach.[53] Any sedation or anxiolysis to facilitate the intubation must involve doses of drugs that allow spontaneous ventilation and retain patient cooperation. Intubation by direct laryngoscopic vision is probably safer and less traumatic than blind nasal intubation, which has a low incidence of success on first attempt and increases the potential for trauma and bleeding with repeated attempts. Indeed, one must consider that minimal trauma of an already

compromised airway may result in a clinically significant increase of the degree of airway obstruction. Furthermore, bloody secretions from failed blind nasal attempts will worsen the likelihood of successful fiber-optic intubation (see later discussion).

General anesthesia followed by intubation with the patient breathing spontaneously and without the use of muscle relaxants is an alternative approach. However, this method not only encompasses all the difficulties and concerns enumerated previously, but it also adds the encumberment of an unconscious patient unable to assist in maintaining the airway. The use of a muscle relaxant is acceptable only if the patient can be easily ventilated by mask, but even this can be a precarious situation, and only short-acting, readily reversible muscle relaxants should be considered. A preoperative cholinesterase would rule out the possibility of a prolonged reaction to succinyldicholine, the shortest acting relaxant among those currently available. Mivacurium, the shortest-acting nondepolarizing muscle relaxant, also is metabolized by cholinesterase. Fixed intravenous anesthetic drugs for the induction of anesthesia should be short acting. In addition, the initiation of a potent inhalational agent with 100% oxygen provides the most reversible general anesthetic regimen with the greatest margin of safety in terms of oxygenation and reversibility.

An elective tracheostomy with local anesthesia (with or without minimal sedation) has been the classic alternative and ultimate solution to the difficult intubation. This certainly is preferable to an emergency tracheostomy under deteriorating or extreme circumstances. For any case in which the potential for tracheostomy is deemed to be significant, contingency plans should include (1) the availability of tracheostomy instruments and a qualified surgeon and (2) the materials and equipment necessary for performing a large-bore catheter cricothyrostomy and subsequent transtracheal jet ventilation, a procedure that can be accomplished by anesthesiologists. A technique using a wire inserted through the cricothyroid membrane in a retrograde manner through the mouth followed by antegrade endotracheal guidance over this wire has been advocated for both elective and emergent difficult intubations.

Recent advances in flexible fiber-optic laryngoscopy have provided an option to conventional management schemes, and under the right circumstances it may be the method of choice for the controlled management of the difficult airway and tracheal intubation.[54–56] Fiber-optic laryngoscopy is of particular help in the anatomic problems posed by the chronic arthritides. Fiber-optic laryngoscopy requires skill gained through training and experience with proper equipment, and it should not be attempted in a severely deformed patient by inexperienced personnel or under deteriorating, life-threatening situations in which definitive intervention (tracheostomy) is indicated. Proper preparation of the patient is the key to successful fiber-optic laryngoscopy and includes a dry airway, appropriately sedated patient, and complete topical anesthesia. Antisialagogues eliminate the oral secretions that can interfere with airway patency, induce laryngo spasm, and coat the fiber-optic lens. Topical vasoconstrictor drugs will reduce the likelihood of bleeding from a traumatized airway, which can obscure the view. It is entirely appropriate to arrange for two anesthesiologists to manage these high-risk patients, especially if the fiber-optic intubation is attempted under general rather than local anesthesia.

The recently introduced laryngeal mask airway (LMA) is a suitable alternative to the face mask and tracheal intubation in a broad spectrum of clinical situations.[57] As such, the LMA may support airways that are difficult to manage and also may serve to facilitate blind and fiberoptic intubations. However, the LMA is contraindicated in those patients unable to extend their neck or to open their mouth less than 1.5 cm, both of which make LMA advancement into the hypopharynx difficult.

References

1. Cote C: NPO after midnight for children—A reappraisal. Anesthesiology 72:589–592, 1990.
2. Nan B, Hansen T, and Warner M: Preoperative laboratory screening in healthy Mayo patients: Cost effective elimination of the tests and unchanged outcomes. Mayo Clin Proc 66:155–159, 1991.
3. Roizen M: Preoperative patient evaluation. Can J Anaesth 36(3):S13–S19, 1989.
4. Jackson S, Singleton M, Silcox D, et al: Anesthesia and postanesthetic considerations. Clin Pod Med Surg 5:169–192, 1988.
5. Eisele Jr J: Connective tissue diseases. In Katz J, Benumof J, and Kadis L (eds): Anesthesia and Uncommon Diseases, 3rd ed. Philadelphia, WB Saunders, 1990, pp 645–667.
5a. Jackson S: Autologous blood transfusion therapy. West J Med 157:567–568, 1992.
6. Hirsch I, McGill J, Cryer P, et al: Perioperative management of surgical patients with diabetes mellitus. Anesthesiology 74:346–359, 1991.
7. Roizen M, Stevens A, and Lampe G: Perioperative management of patients with endocrine disease. In Nunn J, Utting J, and Brown B (eds): General Anesthesia, 5th ed. London, Butterworths, 1989, pp 726–740.
8. Jackson S: Inborn errors of carbohydrate metabolism. In Katz J, Benumof J, and Kadis L (eds): Anesthesia and Uncommon Diseases, 3rd ed. Philadelphia, WB Saunders, 1990, pp 7–30.
9. Jackson S: Hypoglycemia. In Katz J, Benumof J, and Kadis L (eds): Anesthesia and Uncommon Diseases, 3rd ed. Philadelphia, WB Saunders, 1990, pp 30–43.
10. Jackson S: Blood glucose homeostasis. West J Med 140:441, 1984.
11. Longstreth W and Inui T: High blood glucose level on hospital admission and poor neurological recovery after cardiac arrest. Ann Neurol 15:59–68, 1984.
12. Larkai E, Lacey Smith J, Lidsky M, et al: Gastroduodenal mucosa and dyspeptic symptoms in arthritic patients during chronic nonsteroidal anti-inflammatory drug use. Am J Gastroenterol 82:1153–1158, 1987.
13. Roth S, Fries J, Abadi I, et al: Prophylaxis of nonsteroidal anti-inflammatory drug gastropathy: A clinical opinion. J Rheumatol 18:956–957, 1991.
14. Gabriel S: Is misoprostol prophylaxis indicated for NSAID induced adverse gastrointestinal events? An epidemiologic opinion. J Rheumatol 18:957–961, 1991.
15. Lanza F, Rack M, Lynn M, et al: An endoscopic comparison of the effects of etodolac, indomethacin, ibuprofen, naproxen, and placebo on the gastrointestinal mucosa. J Rheumatol 14:338–341, 1987.
16. Dahl J and Kehlet H: Nonsteroidal antiinflammatory drugs: Rationale for use in severe postoperative pain. Br J Anaesth 66:703–712, 1991.
17. Oosterlinck W, Philip N, Charig C, et al: A double-blind single dose comparison of intramuscular ketorolac tromethamine and pethidine in the treatment of renal colic. J Clin Pharmacol 30:335–341, 1990.
17a. Grass J, Sakima N, Valley M, et al: Assessment of ketorolac as an adjuvant to fentanyl patient-controlled epidural analgesia after radical retropubic prostatectomy. Anesthesiology 78:642–648, 1993.
18. Jackson S and Brill J: Wilson's disease. In Katz J, Benumof J, and Kadis L (eds): Anesthesia and Uncommon Diseases, 3rd ed. Philadelphia, WB Saunders, 1990, pp. 112–127.
19. Mielants H, Veys E, Van Der Streaten C, et al: The efficacy and toxicity of a constant low dose of methotrexate as a treatment for intractable rheumatoid arthritis: An open prospective study. J Rheumatol 18:978–983, 1991.
20. Bridges S, Lopeza-Mendez A, Han K, et al: Should methotrexate be discontinued before elective orthopedic surgery in patients with rheumatoid arthritis? J Rheumatol 18:984–988, 1991.
21. Koblin D, Waskell L, Watson J, et al: Nitrous oxide inactivates methionine synthetase in human liver. Anesth Analg 61:75–78, 1982.
22. Black K and Tephly T: Effects of nitrous oxide and methotrexate administration on hepatic methionine synthetase and dihydrofolate reductase activities, hepatic folate, and formate oxidation in rats. Mol Pharmacol 23:724–730, 1983.
23. O'Sullivan H, Jannings F, Ward K, et al: Human bone marrow biochemical functions and megaloblastic hematopoiesis after nitrous oxide anesthesia. Anesthesiology 55:645–649, 1981.
24. Jackson S: Cystinuria. In Katz J, Benumof J, and Kadis L (eds): Anesthesia and Uncommon Diseases, 3rd ed. Philadelphia, WB Saunders, 1990, pp 54–62.
25. Salassa R, Bennet W, Keating F, et al: Postoperative adrenal cortical insufficiency: Occurrences in patients previously treated with cortisone. JAMA 152:1509–1515, 1953.
26. Fragen R, Weiss H, and Molteni A: The effect of propofol on adrenocortical steroidogenesis: A comparative study with etomidate and thiopental. Anesthesiology 66:839–842, 1987.
27. Jackson S and Silcox D: Gout. In Katz J, Benumof J, and Kadis L (eds): Anesthesia and Uncommon Diseases, 3rd ed. Philadelphia, WB Saunders, 1990, pp 100–112.
28. Jackson S: Anesthetics and cell multiplication. Clin Anesth 11:75–87, 1975.
28a. Roberts W, Liang M, and Stern S: Colchicine in acute gout: Reassessment of risks and benefits. JAMA 257:1920–1922, 1987.
28b. Axelrad D and Preston S: Comparison of parenteral adrenocorticotrophic hormone with oral indomethacin in the treatment of acute gout. Arthritis Rheum 31:303–305, 1988.
29. Jackson S: Humanism and anesthesia safety. Curr Rev Clin Anesth 8:194–199, 1988.
30. Mazze R, Shue G, and Jackson S: Renal dysfunction associated with methoxyflurane anesthesia. JAMA 216:278–288, 1971.
31. Cousins M, Greenstein L, Hitt B, et al: Metabolism and renal effect of enflurane in man. Anesthesiology 44:44–54, 1976.
32. Bastron R: Anesthetic considerations for patients with end-stage renal disease. ASA Refresh Courses Anesthesiol 13:33–41, 1988.
33. Covino B: Clinical pharmacology of local anesthetic drugs. In Cousins M and Bridenbaugh P (eds): Neural Blockade in Clinical Anesthesia and Management of Pain, 2nd ed. Philadelphia, JB Lippincott, 1988, pp 111–144.
34. Holmes C: Intravenous regional neural blockade. In Cousins M and Bridenbaugh P (eds): Neural Blockade in Clinical Anesthesia and Management of Pain, 2nd ed. Philadelphia, JB Lippincott, 1988, pp 443–459.
35. Moller R and Covino B: Effect of progesterone on the cardiac electrophysiologic alterations produced by ropivacaine and bupivacaine. Anesthesiology 77:735–741, 1992.
36. Horrigan R, Eger E II, and Wilson C: Epinephrine-induced arrhythmias during enflurane anesthesia in man: A nonlinear dose-response relationship and dose-dependent protection from lidocaine. Anesth Analg 57:547–550, 1978.
37. Johnston R, Eger E II, and Wilson C: A comparative interaction of epinephrine with enflurane, isoflurane, and halothane in man. Anesth Analg 55:709–712, 1976.
38. Bernstein R and Rosenberg A: Anesthesia for orthopedic surgery. Semin Anesth 6:36–43, 1987.
39. Edelist G: Principles of anesthetic management on rheumatoid arthritic patients. Anesth Analg 43:227–231, 1964.
40. Funk D and Raymon F: Rheumatoid arthritis of the cricoarytenoid joints: An airway hazard. Anesth Analg 54:742–745, 1975.
41. Jenkins L and McGraw R: Anesthetic management of the patient with rheumatoid arthritis. Can Anaesth Soc J 16:407–415, 1969.
42. Mallampati S, Gatt S, Gugino L, et al: A clinical sign to predict difficult tracheal intubation: A prospective study. Can Anaesth Soc J 32:429–434, 1985.
43. Brechner V: Unusual problems in the management of airway: I. Flexion-extension mobility of the cervical vertebrae. Anesth Analg 47:362–372, 1968.
44. Nichol H and Zuck D: Difficult laryngoscopy—The "anterior" larynx and the atlanto-occipital gap. Br J Anaesth 55:141–144, 1983.
45. Keenan M, Stiles C, and Kaufman R: Acquired laryngeal deviation associated with cervical spine diseases in erosive polyarticular arthritis: Use of fiberoptic bronchoscope in rheumatoid disease. Anesthesiology 58:441–449, 1983.
46. Ovassapian A, Land P, Schafer M, et al: Anesthetic management for surgical corrections of severe flexion deformity of the cervical spine. Anesthesiology 58:370–372, 1983.
47. Phelps J: Laryngeal obstruction due to cricoarytenoid arthritis. Anesthesiology 27:518–522, 1966.
48. Grossman A, Martin J, and Root H: Rheumatoid arthritis of the cricoarytenoid joint. Laryngoscope 71:530–544, 1961.
49. Gardner D and Holmes F: Anaesthetic and postoperative hazards in rheumatoid arthritis. Br J Anaesth 33:258–264, 1961.
50. Kovarsky J: Otorhinolaryngologic complications of rheumatoid disease. Semin Arthritis Rheum 14:141–150, 1984.
51. Kleinman H and Ewbank R: Gout of the temporomandibular joint. Oral Surg Oral Med Oral Pathol 27:281–282, 1969.
52. Block C and Brechner V: Unusual problems in airway management: II. The influence of the temporomandibular joint, the mandible, and associated structures on endotracheal intubation. Anesth Analg 50:114–122, 1971.
53. Sinclair J and Mason R: Ankylosing spondylitis: The case for awake intubation. Anaesthesia 39:3–11, 1984.
54. Ovassapian A and Dykes M: The role of fiber-optic endoscopy in airway management. Semin Anesth 6:93–104, 1987.
55. Ovassapian A and Schrader S: Fiber-optic aided bronchial intubation. Semin Anesth 6:133–142, 1987.
56. Marks J and Bainton C: Practical aspects of fiber-optic laryngobronchoscopy. Syllabus for the Annual Meeting of the California Society of Anesthesiologists, 1991.
57. Pennant J and White P: The laryngeal mask airway. Anesthesiology 79:144–163, 1993.

CHAPTER 29

Central Metatarsophalangeal Joint Arthrosis: Evaluation and Surgical Management

William M. Jenkin, D.P.M.

The treatment of end-stage forefoot deformities, wherein multiple metatarsophalangeal (MTP) joints are involved, is for the most part well established. This situation is most often encountered in patients with rheumatoid arthritis. The MTP joints are inflamed with synovitis, unstable, eroded, dislocated, and become malaligned. This malalignment leads to pressure points created by resultant digital deformities and prolapsed metatarsal heads. The soft tissue interface at the new pressure points reacts to the ill effects of abnormal physical forces in several ways, creating the potential for new problems. These range from callous-clavi formation, bursitis, rheumatoid nodules, and nerve entrapments to areas of preulceration, ulceration, sinus tract formation, and eventual infection. In this severe scenario, the treatment goal is to eliminate pain and pressure points. This goal most often is accomplished surgically and is attained at the expense of function and stability. The accepted surgical approach in this instance is panmetatarsal head resection accomplished through various skin incisions along with arthrodesing, resecting, or implanting the first MTP joint and performing appropriate digital procedures.[1-4] In a recent retrospective study of patients who had undergone a panmetatarsal head resection,[4] it was found that the acceptance of the postoperative results of the procedure was highest among those patients who had severe deformities and marked pain preoperatively. Most of these patients also had rheumatoid arthritis. In the same study, those patients who were relatively active preoperatively with fewer disabling symptoms without rheumatoid arthritis tended to be dissatisfied with the postoperative results.[4] It therefore appears that the more functional and propulsive the patient is before surgery, the less likely he or she is to accept the long-term postoperative results of the procedure.

In the rheumatoid patient, the course of the rheumatic disease varies greatly. It may pass through periods of exacerbations and spontaneous remissions; the disease may even arrest completely. Consequently, in both rheumatoid and nonrheumatoid patients, when an isolated arthrosis of an MTP joint occurs, it should be treated. Because the development of symptomatic forefoot deformity and functional impairment does not occur to the same degree in each patient, panmetatarsal head resection should not be used as a panacea for all forefoot symptomatology. This treatment must be individualized, based on the extent of the problem, if applicable, the activity level of the underlying disease, as well as the patient's functional capacity. Should surgical intervention be deemed necessary, the goal of not only eliminating symptoms but also restoring stability and maintaining as much function as possible (restorative surgery) should be kept in mind.

To accomplish these goals one must attain an understanding of the following: pathophysiology of MTP joint arthrosis in both rheumatoid and nonrheumatoid patients; resultant forefoot disorders based on normal forefoot functional anatomic structure; clinical evaluation of isolated forefoot pain (anterior focal metatarsalgia); and procedures available to treat isolated MTP joint arthrosis.

PATHOPHYSIOLOGY

A review of the pathophysiology of arthrosis of the central MTP joints in the rheumatoid and nonrheumatoid patient reveals different inciting events but a sharing of similar outcomes. The outcomes are usually more severe and progress at a more rapid rate in the rheumatoid patient.

As far as the musculoskeletal problems associated with rheumatoid arthritis are concerned, the synovium of synovial-lined structures appears to be the focus of the disease process. In the rheumatoid arthritic patient, through some as yet incompletely understood immunologic defect, the synovium and articular cartilage become the target tissue of pathologic inflammation of an autoimmune nature.[5] An inflammatory joint disorder or primary synovitis develops as a result of the disease process.

In the nonarthritic patient, an idiopathic, nonspecific primary synovitis that is not associated with a systemic disease may develop.[6] This synovitis is most likely secondary to chronic mechanical irritation or stress on the articular and periarticular structures created by faulty biomechanics and skeletal relationships.

Synovitis, whether specific (systemic disease) or nonspecific (idiopathic), in its early phase creates joint distention

TABLE 29–1

PATHOPHYSIOLOGY OF ISOLATED ARTHROSIS

Intra-articular	Extra-articular
Primary synovitis	Muscular imbalance
Joint effusion	Deformity
Synovial hypertrophy	Pressure points
Ligamentous laxity	Mechanically induced lesions
Instability	Bursitis
Articular erosions	Keratosis
Particulate synovitis	Rheumatoid nodules
Secondary synovitis	Ulcerations
Pain and functional impairment	

from synovial hypertrophy that is marked at its junction with articular cartilage. Continued proliferation of synovium leads to pannus formation, which then erodes cartilage and adjoining bone. In its early phases the joint erosions may result in fragments of bone or articular cartilage being lodged into and irritating the synovium, causing a secondary synovitis.[7] This secondary synovitis compounds with the primary synovitis, increasing the likelihood that pain, joint inflammation, and progressive deformity will continue in spite of good medical management.

Initially, the pathologic process results in arthralgia, stiffness, and joint effusion. Eventually, compromise of the integrity of the capsuloligamentous complex with instability of the MTP joint occurs as a result of a laxity or rupture of the joint ligaments and capsule. Joint instability, coupled with an ensuring muscular/supporting structural imbalance, causes partial (subluxation) to complete dislocation of the MTP joint along with secondary functional disorders.

Digital deformities appear in the sagittal, transverse, frontal, or combination planes. Once the deformities are established, secondary changes occur as reactive forces from the ground and shoe result in various degrees of morbidity and functional impairment (Table 29–1).

FUNCTIONAL FOREFOOT ANATOMY

The five metatarsals contribute to the formation of the medial and lateral columns of the foot. The medial column of the foot involves the first, second, and third metatarsals, along with the phalanges, cuneiforms, navicular, and talus. It is flexible and is involved mostly with shock absorption and adaptation to the supporting surface.[8] The fourth and fifth metatarsals, along with the phalanges, cuboid, and calcaneus combine to form the lateral column of the foot. The lateral column of the foot is essentially rigid and functions mostly as a lever for propulsion.[8]

The metatarsal bones are of different lengths. They are curved longitudinally, forming a longitudinal arch, with the central ones extending the farthest distally. This configuration allows for a proximal transverse metatarsal arch corresponding with the arch of the cuneiforms while distally the metatarsals are on one plane.

As long as the entire foot is weightbearing, the metatarsals share a common load. The ratio of weight distribution, however, is 2:1:1:1:1, with the first metatarsal carrying a double load.[9] This common sharing of the load between metatarsal heads comes to an end as soon as the heel leaves the ground because of the different metatarsal lengths.

In most metatarsal length pattern formulas, the second metatarsal is the longest ($2 > 1 > 3 > 4 > 5$ or $2 > 1 = 3 > 4 > 5$). Because of the greatest length of the second metatarsal, there is no common axis for the five MTP joints. However, a transverse axis consists of the first and second MTP joints, and an oblique axis consists of the second through fifth MTP joints.[10] In normal gait, as the heel leaves the ground during push-off, the weight is transferred onto the ball using the oblique MTP joint axis and continues along the transverse axis passing through the first and second metatarsal heads and eventually through the tip of the hallux. It is the body's forward momentum, not muscular contraction, that causes the ultimate push-off. When primarily using the transverse MTP joint axis, the fifth, fourth, and third metatarsal heads are relieved of weight in that order, whereas, when the oblique MTP joint axis is used, the first metatarsal is relieved (Fig. 29–1).[11] Bojsen-Møller and Lamoreux characterized the motion around the oblique axis as low-gear motion such as used in uphill walking with a heavy load and the motion around the transverse axis as being a high-gear motion such as occurs in sprinting.[11] For different demands, it is possible to guide the foot into an appropriate leverage by either adducting the forefoot while internally rotating the leg and thus using the oblique axis of the MTP joint or by

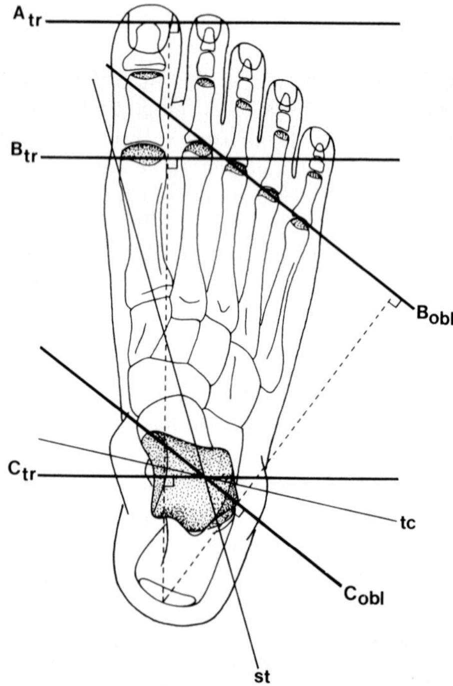

FIGURE 29–1. Axes of the push-off. The push-off is initiated along the oblique axis B_{obl} passing through the metatarsal head 2 to 5 and continuing along the transverse axis B_{tr} passing through the metatarsal heads 1 and 2 and terminating along the distal transverse axis A_{tr} passing through the tip of the big toe. The dorsiflexion of the toes is accompanied by a motion of the ankle complex involving the axes of the talocrural (tc) and subtalar (st) joints, resulting in a secondary axis C_{obl} or C_{tr} that is parallel to the primary axis B_{obl}, B_{tr}, or A_{tr}. The push-off along the oblique axis B_{obl} acts as a low-gear mechanism, whereas the push-off along the transverse axis B_{tr} acts as a high-gear mechanism of take-off. (From Bojsen-Møller F and Lamoreux L: Significance of free dorsiflexion of the toes in walking. Acta Orthop Scand 50:471. © 1979 Munksgaard International Publishers Ltd., Copenhagen, Denmark.)

abducting the forefoot while externally rotating the leg, thereby using the transverse axis.[11]

These same processes may be applied to clinical situations. If the patient has pain in the first MTP joint, such as with hallux limitus or rigidus, and has sufficient internal rotation of the leg available, he or she will often adduct the foot to use the oblique MTP joint axis rather than the transverse axis during the propulsive phase of gait. On the other hand, if the patient experiences pain within the lesser MTP joints, he or she will often externally rotate the leg and abduct the foot, thus using mostly the transverse MTP joint axis. This compensation for forefoot pain often causes secondary symptoms of discomfort in the proximal leg owing to the resultant abnormal biomechanics.

The second or the third MTP joints are the joints that are most often involved when there is an isolated arthrosis of an MTP joint.[6, 12, 13] This is explained by anatomic-biomechanical relationships. The second MTP joint is common to both axes. Therefore, it bears weight regardless of which axis is being used. Additionally, the second and third metatarsals are firmly anchored at their bases such that they cannot dorsiflex.[9] The first and the fifth rays have separate ranges of motion (ROMs) from the central metatarsals. They are able to move independently above and below the central metatarsals. Consequently, any stress that is going to be transferred to the central metatarsals secondary to a biomechanical fault of the first and or the fifth metatarsal is going to be fully borne by the MTP joints. The fourth metatarsal is less firmly anchored at its base and is often able to dorsiflex and thereby avoid the abnormal stress.[14]

The shape or osteochondral form of both the metatarsal head and the corresponding proximal phalangeal base creates the vertical as well as the horizontal axis of each individual joint. The head is quadrilateral and convex. It is covered with articular cartilage that extends further proximally plantarly than dorsally. The capsule encompasses the joint. On its outer surface, it is fibrous and continuous with the periosteum. The capsule is lined by synovium, which secretes fluid, is highly flexible, and helps minimize the volume of the joint space it encloses to allow for a ''better fit.'' The synovial fluid creates an adhesive seal that freely permits a sliding motion between cartilaginous surfaces but resists distracting forces.[15]

The capsule varies in thickness from a thin membrane to a strong fibrous band. The thickened, fibrocartilaginous plantar capsule reinforced by various ligamentous aponeurotic insertions becomes the flexor (plantar) plate.

The flexor plate serves as a checkrein to prevent hyperextension as well as articulates with the plantar condyles to maintain joint congruity and function. On its plantar aspect, it inserts with the flexor tendon sheath.

Within the joint capsule are found the collateral as well as the suspensory ligaments. They are strong, inelastic structures that guide and align the joint throughout flexion and extension and serve as checkreins for the ends of motion. According to Sarrafian, the ligaments are stronger and thicker on the lateral side.[9] The ligaments originate from the epicondyle on each side of the metatarsal head. The suspensory ligaments fan out plantarly, inserting into the flexor plate, whereas the collateral ligaments insert into the plantar sides of the proximal phalanx (Fig. 29–2).

The MTP joints and digits are capable of functioning in-

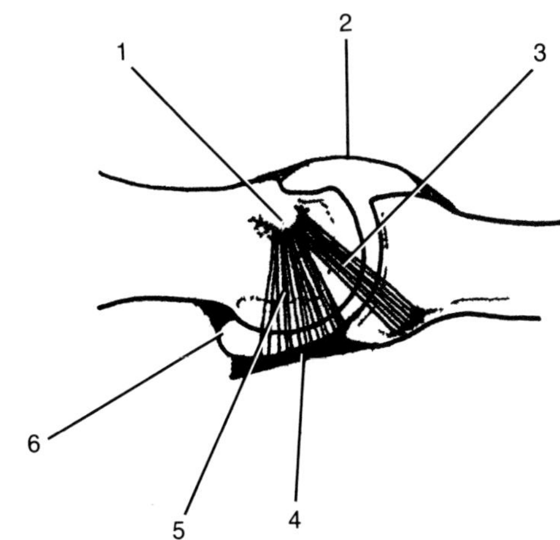

FIGURE 29–2. Intra-articular ligaments. 1, Epicondyle. 2, Joint capsule. 3, Collateral ligament. 4, Flexor plate. 5, Suspensory ligament. 6, Synovial reflection.

dependently yet are bound to each other distally in the transverse plane by the intermetatarsal ligaments, plantar interdigital ligaments, and mooring ligaments, respectively.[16] The deep transverse metatarsal ligament runs as a continuous ligament below the metatarsal heads from the first to the fifth. Below each MTP joint, it incorporates the flexor plate (plantar ligament) and becomes firmly attached to the proximal phalanx.[16] Through collateral ligaments, the deep transverse metatarsal ligament is literally attached from the medial side of the head of the first metatarsal to the lateral side of the head of the fifth metatarsal. The transverse fibers continue distally as transverse lamellae, called the *plantar interdigital ligaments,* which are attached to the sides of the flexor sheaths found in the toes and extend from the medial to lateral margin of the foot.[16] The plantar interdigital ligaments end in a round mooring ligament which arches from one phalanx to the next, securing the transverse stability of the toes while at the same time allowing individual extension of a toe (Fig. 29–3).[16]

The plantar aponeurosis and the flexor plate are critical to forefoot function and stability of the MTP joint. The central slip of the plantar aponeurosis originates from the medial tubercle of the calcaneus and proceeds into the forefoot, where it divides into a superficial and a deep system. The superficial fibers insert into the ball of the forefoot.[16] The deep fibers of the plantar aponeurosis form two marginal and eight intermediate sagittal septa, which pass along the sides of the flexor tendons separating them from the lumbricales, nerves, and vessels to the sides of the fibrous flexor sheath. The fibers now join with the plantar capsule in forming the plantar ligament or flexor plate.[16] Immediately anterior to the septa and below each metatarsal head, vertical fibers form a connective tissue cushion of encapsulated fat. The vertical fibers come from the sides of the flexor tendon sheath and the flexor plate, and insert into the superficial portion of the plantar aponeurosis and through them into the skin (Fig. 29–4).[16] The flexor plates, and through them the plantar aponeurosis, are attached firmly to the bases of the proximal phalanges. Proximally, the flexor plate is connected loosely to the metatarsals by a thin capsule with synovial folds. This configuration allows the flexor plate to glide forward and back-

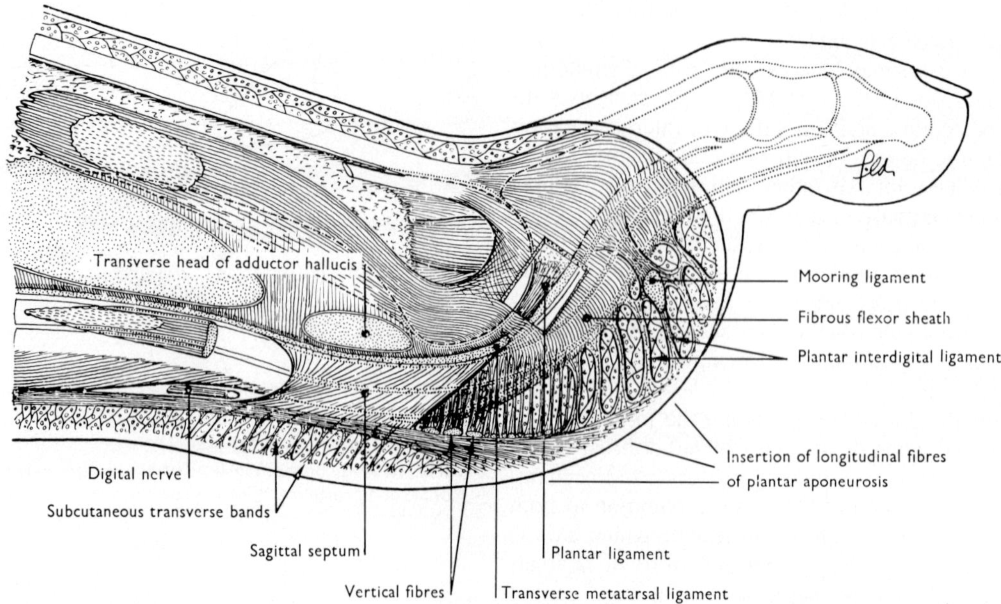

FIGURE 29–3. Architecture of the ball of the foot. Drawing of a sagittal section through the second interstice showing the internal architecture of the three areas of the ball of the foot. The sagittal septum is attached to the proximal phalanx through the transverse metatarsal ligament and the plantar ligament of the joint. The vertical fibers and the lamellae of the plantar interdigital ligament are attached to the proximal phalanx through the fibrous flexor sheath. (From Bojsen-Møller F and Flagstad KE: Plantar aponeurosis and internal architecture of the ball of the foot. J Anat 121:599, 1976; reprinted with permission of Cambridge University Press.)

ward in an unrestricted fashion as the proximal phalanx is dorsiflexed, or plantarflexed.[9] These structures form the capsuloligamentous complex of the MTP joint that, with the proximal phalanx, forms the "phalangeal apparatus," which Sarrafian stated is the main articular unit of the ball of the foot.[9] It is by way of these attachments that the skin of the ball of the foot is tensed and the arch of the foot is raised and shortened while supination occurs as dorsiflexion of the toes exerts a pull on the plantar aponeurosis, thereby plantarflexing the forefoot on the rearfoot, inverting the heel, and causing the leg to externally rotate (Fig. 29–5). This is entitled the "windlass action" of the plantar aponeurosis.[17]

The flexion of the forefoot on the hindfoot occurs at the cuneonavicular and metatarsocuneiform joints. The size of the first metatarsal head as well as inclusion of the sesamoids allows the plantar aponeurosis to have a greater effect on the windlass mechanism of the first ray. The first ray flexes an average of 10 degrees when the plantar aponeurosis is tensed, whereas the central rays flex about 5 degrees.[9] The windlass mechanism is passive and depends entirely on the bony and ligamentous integrity for its function. It is most functional in the medial column, especially the first ray, and is progressively less functional as one proceeds laterally across the foot.[18]

The pull of the tendons passing the MTP joint creates the dynamic stabilization of the MTP joint as well as moves the joint within the restraints of the ligaments. The intrinsic muscles primarily stabilize the MTP joint so that the extrinsic

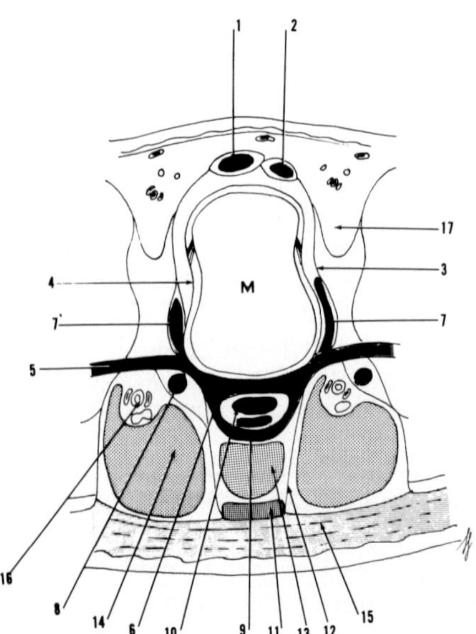

FIGURE 29–4. Cross section of the ball of the foot. M, metatarsal head; 1, extensor digitorum longus tendon; 2, extensor digitorum brevis tendon; 3, transverse lamina of extensor aponeurosis; 4, capsule of metatarsophalangeal joint; 5, deep transverse metatarsal ligament; 6, plantar plate; 7, 7', interossei muscles located in narrow cleft formed by capsule and transverse lamina (7) or incorporated in split of transverse lamina (7'); 8, lumbrical tendon in its own tunnel on tibial side of joint; 9, long flexor tunnel; 10, long flexor tendons; 11, longitudinal band of plantar aponeurosis; 12, vertical thin fibrous band of plantar aponeurosis forming a preflexor tendon space lodging a preflexor adipose cushion (13); 14, fat body on plantar aspect of 5 covering neurovascular bundle (16); 15, transverse component of plantar aponeurosis; 17, triangular adipofascial complex filling intermetatarsal capitular space and carrying superficial nerves and vessels. (From Sarrafian SK: Anatomy of the Foot and Ankle: Descriptive, Topographic, Functional. Philadelphia, JB Lippincott, 1983, p 243.)

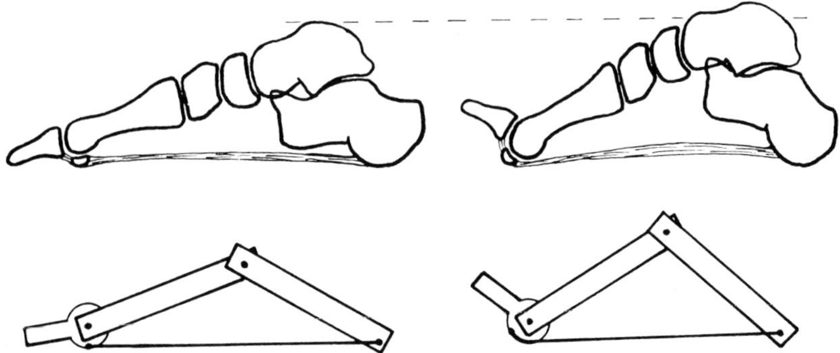

FIGURE 29–5. The ''windlass.'' The drum of the windlass is the head of the metatarsal (including the sesamoid bones). The handle is the proximal phalanx, and the cable wound onto the drum is the plantar aponeurosis through its attachment to the plantar pad of the metatarsophalangeal joint. (From Evans FG [ed]: The Three Weight-Bearing Mechanisms of the Foot in Biomechanical Studies of the MusculoSkeletal System, 1961, p 176. Courtesy of Charles C Thomas, Publisher, Springfield, Illinois.)

muscles may create motion. The extensor system is held in a central location to the MTP joint by the extensor expansion. This fibroaponeurotic band extends from the MTP joint to the proximal interphalangeal joint (Fig. 29–6).[19] The proximal segment of this aponeurosis has transversely oriented fibers originating from the lateral and medial borders of the flat aponeurotic tunnel surrounding the corresponding extensor tendon. The fibers extend around the capsule of the MTP joint and blend on the plantar side with the flexor plate, the deep transverse metatarsal ligament, the flexor tendon sheath, and the base of the proximal phalanx.[19] This slinglike structure (extensor sling) firmly anchors the extensor digitorum longus (EDL) to the plantar aspect of the MTP joint and the proximal phalanx. The EDL actually has no dorsal attachment to the proximal phalanx. Consequently, when the muscle contracts, it lifts the proximal phalanx, which is suspended from the EDL by the extensor sling.[19] The distal segment of the aponeurotic band on each side of the toe is

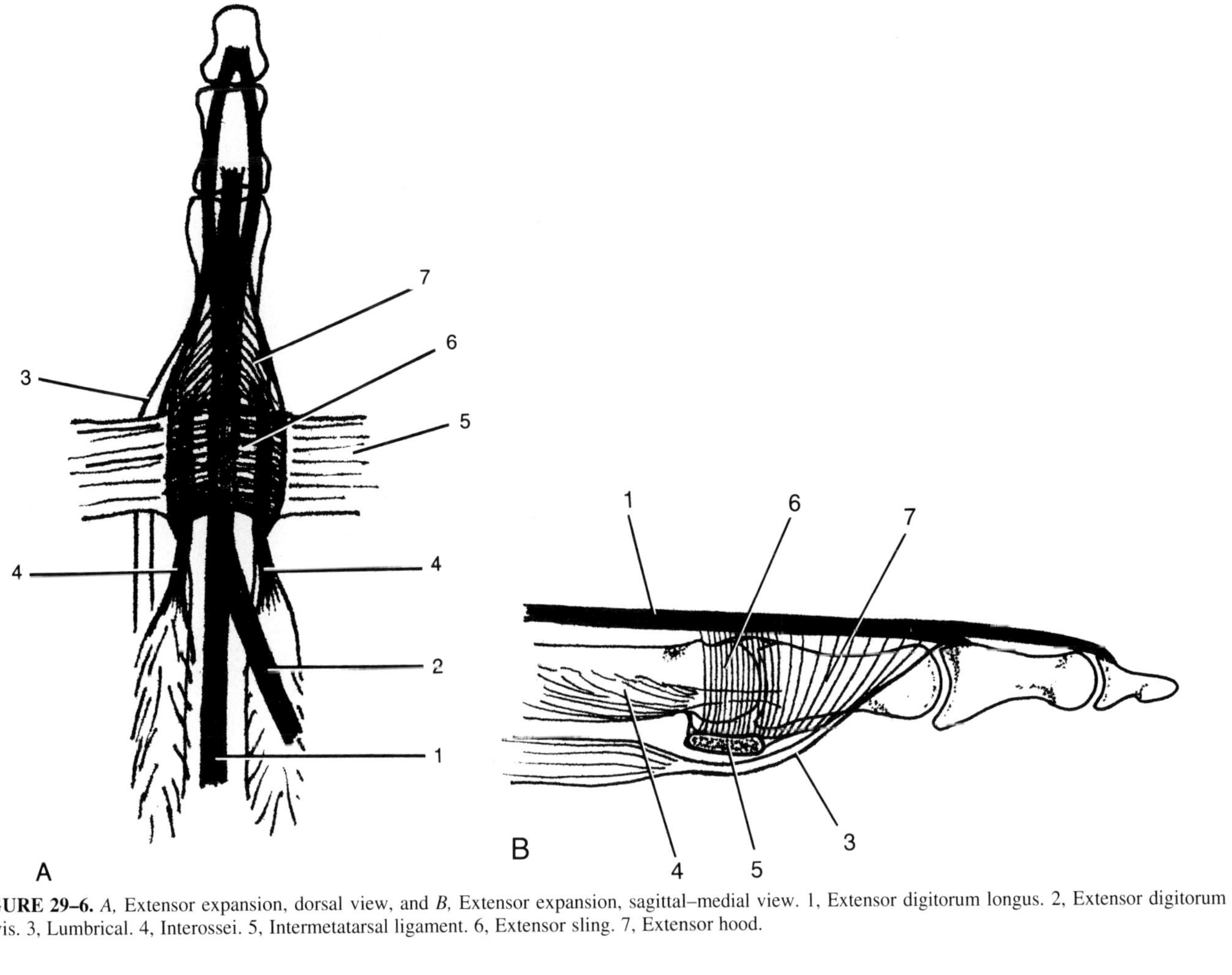

FIGURE 29–6. *A,* Extensor expansion, dorsal view, and *B,* Extensor expansion, sagittal–medial view. 1, Extensor digitorum longus. 2, Extensor digitorum brevis. 3, Lumbrical. 4, Interossei. 5, Intermetatarsal ligament. 6, Extensor sling. 7, Extensor hood.

composed of the obliquely oriented fibers of the extensor wing or hood. This arrangement unites the intrinsic muscles with the trifurcation of the EDL. It enables the tendons of the lumbricales and dorsal and plantar interossei to pass plantar to the axis of motion at the MTP joint and dorsal to the axis of motion at the proximal interphalangeal and distal interphalangeal joints. When contraction of these muscles occurs, it results in flexion at the MTP joint and extension at the proximal interphalangeal and distal interphalangeal joints.[19]

The lumbrical tendon terminates medially into the extensor wing and essentially constitutes the medial portion of the wing. After passing below the intermetatarsal ligament, the lumbricals flex the MTP joint by pulling on the extensor wing in a plantar direction at the same time it extends the interphalangeal joint.[19]

The dorsal and plantar interossei are weak extensors of these joints but strong flexor-pressors of the MTP joint. They have a firm attachment to the flexor plate and proximal phalanx. The dorsal interossei abduct and the plantar interossei adduct the central toes.[9]

The flat tendinous slips of the flexor digitorum longus (FDL) along with the more plantarly placed slips of the flexor digitorum brevis (FDB) tendon pass through an arch formed by the deep septa of the plantar aponeurosis at the level of the transverse head of the adductor hallucis.[9] At the level of the plantar plate, both tendons enter a fibro-osseous tunnel; the FDB is still more plantar to the FDL at this point. The FDB divides into two slips at the level of the base of the proximal phalanx. The tendon of the FDL passes through the bifurcation and continues its distal course now located more plantar to the tendon of the brevis. The FDB inserts into the plantar sides of the intermediate phalanx while the FDL continues distally to insert into the terminal phalanx. Within the fibro-osseous tunnel the flexor tendons are independently surrounded by synovial sheaths extending from the metatarsal heads to the base of the distal phalanx.[9] The FDLs act from their distal insertion. During 30% to 55% of the gait cycle, while the MTP joints are extending, the FDLs are in concentric contraction and act as stabilizers of the toes, invertors of the hindfoot, and plantarflexors of the ankle.[9]

Central MTP joint stability is provided by a combination of factors, some of which are within the joint and some outside the joint. Intrinsic (intra-articular) central MTP joint stability is provided by sufficient cubic content of the metatarsal head, the integrity of the collateral and suspensory ligaments, the flexor plate, the joint capsule, and the adhesive seal of the synovial fluid. Extrinsic central MTP joint stability is provided by the integrity and proper function of the first and fifth MTP joints and their corresponding ray (contiguous stability); the proper length of the metatarsal; the integrity of the plantar aponeurosis; the ability of the intrinsic muscles to plantarflex the MTP joint and stabilize the proximal phalanx onto the metatarsal head; the centralization of the EDL by the extensor expansion dorsally; and the centralization of the flexor plate and FDL plantarly, which is interdependent with the integrity of the intermetatarsal, suspensory, and collateral ligaments.

When the integrity of these structures is compromised, some degree of forefoot or MTP joint instability will occur. This instability is a multifactorial problem. In essence it occurs when the proximal phalanx can no longer be stabi-

lized in its neutral position on the metatarsal head. This instability ultimately results in some degree of forefoot deformity, which often causes pain and dystrophic changes, such as mechanically induced hyperkeratosis, thickened nails, and ulcerations.

The source of the pain varies. It can be secondary to an inflammatory process, such as an adventitious bursitis, tendonitis, and synovitis, as well as nerve entrapments (neuromata) and degenerative joint disease. Because all the MTP joints and digits are directly or indirectly connected, what affects one affects all to some degree. This concept has to be considered in the evaluation process as well as in treatment.

The first MTP joint appears to be one if not the most critical areas as far as forefoot stability is concerned. Once the integrity of the joint is compromised, the entire forefoot appears to follow. When this occurs, the digits often either adduct or abduct depending on which direction the hallux assumes (Fig. 29–7). The next joint of importance appears to be the second MTP joint, then the third MTP joint, with the fourth and fifth joints having less importance in total forefoot stability. In other words, it is the MTP joints of the medial column that appear to be the most significant to forefoot stability, with their importance decreasing from medial to lateral.

The integrity of the first MTP joint can be compromised by disease (rheumatoid arthritis); trauma (either ligamentous or osseous); biomechanical faults; and certain surgical procedures. Each of these, in varying degrees, negates or lessens the effect of the windlass mechanism on the first ray. This results in a loadbearing transference to the central metatarsals

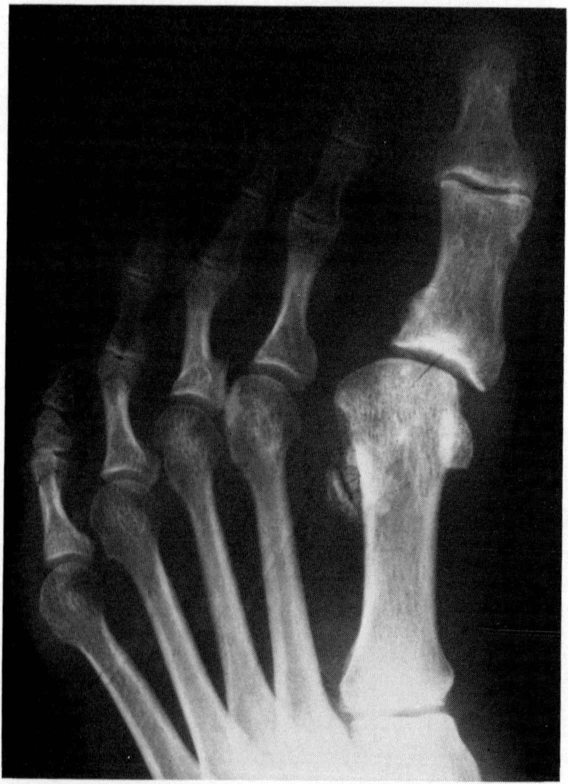

FIGURE 29–7. Importance of the first metatarsophalangeal (MTP) joint on forefoot stability. Dorsoplantar radiograph demonstrating adduction of all digits as a result of hallux varus secondary to intersesamoidal ligament rupture causing intrinsic instability of the first MTP joint.

primarily involving the second MTP joint. This is often found after the Keller procedure, implant arthroplasty, or procedures that cause excessive shortening of the first metatarsal. It is epitomized by amputation of the hallux.

Faulty biomechanics, such as those resulting in hypermobility of the first ray and a first metatarsus elevatus, result in a lateral transference of weight.[14] If present, the consequences of the first ray no longer bearing proper load must be factored into the decision-making during surgical planning for the treatment of isolated arthrosis of the MTP joint. The ability to restore function to the first ray either with orthotic control or through various surgical procedures will improve the prognosis for success of treatment of isolated arthrosis of the second or third MTP joint.

The pathophysiology of instability of the MTP joint essentially involves the loss of integrity of the capsuloligamentous complex of the joint. It occurs insidiously in stages. Sagittal plane stability of the MTP joint is provided mainly by the insertion of the slips of the plantar aponeurosis into the flexor plate as well as the intrinsic muscles that normally pass below the horizontal axis of the MTP joint and insert into the digits and create plantarflexion of the proximal phalanx on the metatarsal head.

According to various sources,[14, 20] when the intrinsic muscles fail to stabilize the proximal phalanx onto the metatarsal head, a hammertoe or claw toe deformity develops. The FDB produces flexion of the proximal interphalangeal joint, resulting in a retrograde force of the intermediate phalanx against the proximal phalanx creating hyperextension of the MTP joint. The long flexor strongly contributes to this action by acting on the terminal phalanx and the interphalangeal joints.

The relationship between the intrinsic musculature, which normally places a plantarflexory stabilizing force on the proximal phalanx, and the toe extensors is disrupted with the result of reinforcing the abnormal proximal phalangeal dorsiflexion by the long and short extensor tendons. As the proximal phalanx dorsiflexes, it plantarflexes the respective metatarsal, which becomes more susceptible to ground-reactive stress.

Additionally, the fifth, fourth, and sometimes third toes in the foot with intrinsic instability as a result of abnormal pronation tend to assume an adductovarus deformity because of the more medially directed pull of the FDL tendon.

In the transverse plane, the centralization of the long extensor tendons relative to the vertical axis passing through the metatarsal head is of prime importance. If the tendon shifts lateral to this axis, it will act as an abductor. If the tendon shifts medially, it will act primarily as an adductor.

With failure of a collateral ligament, the toe initially deviates in an abductory or adductory direction at the MTP joint, creating a space between the adjacent digit.

Accompanying this process, the suspensory ligament also fails, allowing the plantar structures (including the capsule, the flexor plate along with its insertions, and the flexor tendons) to move in the direction of the proximal phalanx. These structures eventually become relocated on the side of the MTP joint and contract along with the capsule. Instead of providing a stabilizing plantarflexory force on the proximal phalanx at the MTP joint, they now exert a deforming adductory or abductory force. With time, secondary to ground-reactive forces and dorsiflexory forces of the extensor tendons, the proximal phalanx hyperextends on the metatar-

sal head, causing the toe to deviate dorsally at the MTP joint, buckle or curl at the interphalangeal joints, and sublux or dislocate at the MTP joint. This allows a retrograde plantarflexory force to occur on the metatarsal, resulting in a prominent plantar metatarsal head.

Additionally, a retrograde abductory or adductory force is placed on the corresponding metatarsal head from the proximal phalanx occasionally resulting in a narrowing of the intermetatarsal angle between this and the adjacent metatarsal, which further aids in the adduction or abduction of the toe.[13]

The plantar structures continue to follow the proximal phalanx and become more anteriorly as well as dorsally located, allowing the plantar capsule to adhere or ''capsulodese'' to the undersurface of the metatarsal head, making the deformity nonreducible.

The dorsal structures, including extensor tendons, extensor expansion, and the capsule, are secondary players in this process. Nevertheless, they do help cause and maintain the deformity. With no plantarflexing stabilizing force on the proximal phalanx, the extensor tendons secondarily contract as the toe moves dorsally.

Additionally, because the dorsal structures also follow the proximal phalanx, the extensor apparatus to the toe becomes relocated to the side of the contraction, resulting in an adductory-abductory force to the toe.

CLINICAL EVALUATION

The purpose of the clinical examination is to define the problem in its entirety. This includes determining the exact source of pain, its cause, as well as the extent of the underlying disease process. The source of pain is determined from the history, the patient's response to the examining hand, and the results of diagnostic procedures. Emphasis is directed in the history as to the existence of inflammatory joint disease. The examination concentrates on determining whether or not the arthrosis is due to a primary synovitis with or without instability or to a secondary synovitis due to joint instability. Furthermore, the presence and extent of erosive joint changes need to be assessed. Once this has been accomplished, the severity and the cause of the process can be established.

The physical examination concentrates on the musculoskeletal system for primary problems and the dermatologic and sometimes the neurologic systems for secondary problems. The examination begins with observation for gross deformity during stance, gait, and non-weightbearing. During stance and non-weightbearing, particular attention is paid to toe purchase, increased toe girth, edema, and dorsal skin contractures.

The gait is further observed for biomechanical faults, noting tendon contracture and their abnormal function such as a premature heel-off (equinus), extensor substitution (equinus), flexor stabilization (pronation), or flexor substitution (triceps surae insufficiency).[21]

Propulsion is noted to see if one MTP joint axis is used over another in a typical antalgic pattern or if, indeed, there is a noticeable limp.

Irritation areas defined by swelling, redness, increased warmth, and mechanically induced hyperkeratosis are noted.

Palpation for areas of forefoot tenderness involves the interspaces, the plantar aspect of the metatarsal head, along the flexor tendons into the toes, dorsal to the MTP joint, and along the extensor tendons.

Determining the patient's response to squeezing the foot from the sides is made (lateral squeeze test).

ROMs along with various stress manipulation studies are performed to further evaluate the MTP joint for painful synovitis, instability, lack of motion (especially in flexion), excessive motion, and arthritis. Pain emanating from the tendons or their sheaths is noted during passive, active, and resistive ROMs.

Pain from synovitis is suspected when there is edema (joint effusion), hyperemia, and pain only at the ends of the ROM when the capsule and ligament are placed on stretch or when the joint is distracted distally. If the synovitis is advanced, pain from the lateral squeeze test will be present.

Pain from both synovitis and erosive arthritis is suspected if, during joint motion, pain is present throughout the entire range and crepitus is felt. The presence of erosive arthritis is further suspected by noting a painful response from compressing the proximal phalanx on the metatarsal head while taking the joint through its ROM.

Instability of the MTP joint is determined by noting toe malalignment or separation, subluxation, or dislocation of the MTP joint in various planes. In the sagittal plane, gross instability is observed by noting any dorsal contracture, subluxation, or dislocation of the MTP joint. Subtle instability is evaluated by performing a test that attempts to dislocate the proximal phalangeal base dorsally out of the MTP joint. This has been called the *modified Lachman test*,[22] but it is more commonly referred to as the *MTP joint luxation test*. It is performed by stabilizing the metatarsal with one hand and placing an upward force on the base of the phalanx with the opposite hand (Fig. 29–8). If the base of the proximal phalanx dislocates when this maneuver is attempted, the test is positive and indicates loss of integrity of the collateral and suspensory ligaments and insufficiency of the flexor

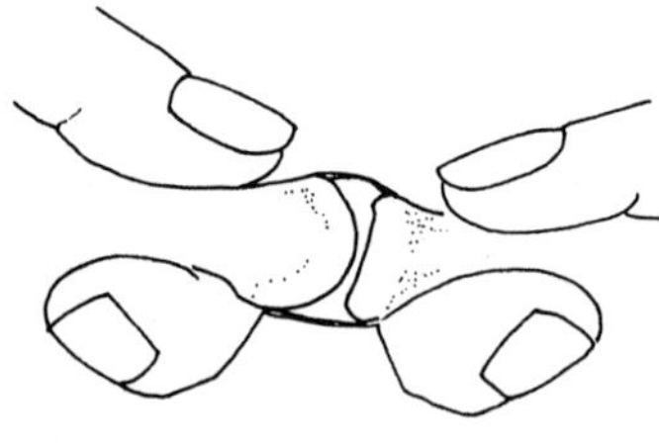

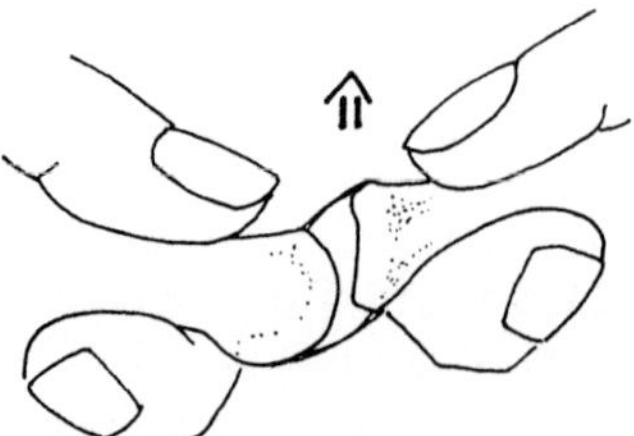

FIGURE 29–8. Metatarsophalangeal (MTP) joint luxation test. Dorsally dislocating the proximal phalangeal base out of the MTP joint is a positive result. It indicates loss of integrity of the "intrinsic ligaments" that results in instability of the MTP joint.

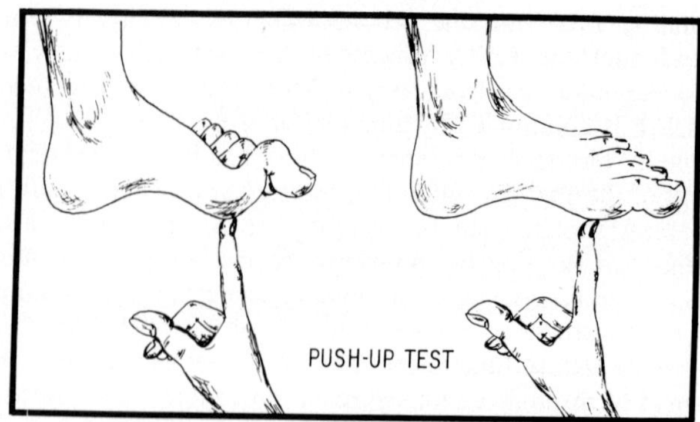

FIGURE 29–9. Kelikian push-up test evaluating the reducibility of the metatarsophalangeal joint. (From Kelikian H: Hallux Valgus and Allied Deformities of the Forefoot and Metatarsalgia. Philadelphia, WB Saunders, 1965, p 314.)

plate.[6, 13, 22] In time this insufficiency will most likely result in subluxation or dislocation of the MTP joint with resultant digital deformity in the form of a hammertoe or an overlapping toe. It is most often seen on the second or third toes.

Transverse plane instability is observed by noting digital splaying, excessive abduction or adduction of the proximal phalanx on the metatarsal head during rest, weightbearing, or while stressing the collateral ligaments of the MTP joint.

Once deformities are developed, a determination as to whether they are reducible, semi-reducible, or nonreducible must be made. Reducibility of the MTP joint in the sagittal plane is determined by performing the Kelikian push-up test. If the toe straightens while a dorsally directed pressure is placed against the plantar aspect of the metatarsal head, the test is negative and indicates reducibility (Fig. 29–9). However, if the proximal phalanx remains contracted at the MTP joint when this manipulation is performed, the test is positive, indicating a nonreducible deformity.[23] This implies that the proximal phalanx is being prevented from properly realigning with the metatarsal head. It occurs because of structural disorders that can be extrinsic as well as intrinsic to the joint. Extrinsic disorders may consist of contracture of the dorsal skin, capsule, and extensor tendons, mainly the extensor digitorum brevis (EDB). Intrinsic disorders consist of contracture of the collateral ligaments; capsulodesis of the capsule to the plantar aspect of the metatarsal head, which accompanies chronic anterior displacement of the flexor plate; and misshapen osteochondral form of the metatarsal head such that no normal articulation of the MTP joint may be obtained. Deformities are further defined as far as the level and extent of joint involvement, whether it be interphalangeal, MTP, or a combination of both. Muscle evaluation is performed to further document tendon contractures as well as strength and atrophy.

Radiographic evaluation is essential to determine mechanical relationships as well as the extent of the disease process, such as joint narrowing, widening, and erosions; bony spurring; subchondral sclerosis; bony fragments (loose bodies); and bone stock. The dorsoplantar view evaluates mechanical relationships in the transverse plane such as metatarsal length, digital alignment, and MTP joint integrity. Elongated metatarsals allow biomechanical forces to have a greater effect on subluxating the MTP joint in the transverse plane. The magnitude of any digital malalignment as well as digital length is noted by comparing its position to the adjacent toes. The longest digit may abut against the tip of the toe box, resulting in the toe buckling with subsequent subluxation of the MTP joint. The integrity of each of the MTP joints is evaluated by noting whether they are congruous, deviated (subluxated), or dislocated. The intermetatarsal angles are noted, especially the first, second, and third as well as the position of the hallux in relationship to the second toe. The first ray is evaluated for hypermobility by noting a metatarsus primus varus, a cuneiform split, or cortical thickening of the second metatarsal diaphysis. Finally, the MTP and interphalangeal joints are evaluated for the presence of osteochondral adaptation as well as for any arthritic changes within the joint, such as subchondral erosions and joint narrowing, arthrodesis, and widening.

The medial-oblique, lateral, and plantar axial views are supportive. The plantar axial view evaluates the soft tissue interface below the metatarsal head as well as any enlargement or erosions of the plantar condyles.

If there is doubt about the source of pain being within the joint, a diagnostic intra-articular injection with local anesthesia alone or mixed with contrast media (arthrogram) can be performed. When completing this test, the clinician should leave the skin sensation intact to evaluate the pain source. Confirmatory information can be gained if contrast media is added to the injection and a radiograph is taken immediately, because the exact location of the injected mixture can be determined and correlated with the clinical response (Fig. 29–10). In other words, when evaluating the radiographs, if all the dye is found to be within the joint capsule and the patient's skin sensation is intact yet the pain has subsided, one can reasonably assume that the pain source is within or associated with the joint. Furthermore, additional information about the integrity of the articular cartilage and joint capsule can be gained from the arthrogram.

At the end of the evaluation process, a working differential diagnosis is established (Table 29–2).

SEVERITY LEVEL CLASSIFICATION

Once the cause and extent of the underlying disease process have been determined, the severity level can be established.

A mild deformity may be defined as one in which there is pain, joint effusion, and edema from synovitis with minimal digital splaying and hyperextension. In its initial phase the associated pain is often attributed to an intermetatarsal neuroma or bursitis. With time the digit begins to deviate subtly in the sagittal or transverse planes as MTP joint instability ensues. The MTP joint luxation test may produce discomfort but is otherwise negative. The digital pulp touches the ground. Digital deformities, if present, are flexible and easily reducible at the MTP joint as well as the interphalangeal joints. The Kelikian push-up test is therefore negative. There are no erosive or other arthritic changes noted on radiograph.

A moderate deformity may be defined as one in which there is pain from synovitis as well as from secondary dystrophic changes. MTP joint instability is more pronounced with digital splaying and hyperextension of the proximal phalanx. The MTP joint luxation test is often positive, especially if the process involves the second MTP joint. The digital pulp may or may not purchase the ground. The Keli-

kian push-up test is positive because the deformity is not entirely reducible at the MTP joint. A reducible hammertoe deformity most often accompanies the problem. There are still no erosive or arthritic changes noted on radiograph.

A severe deformity is one in which the deformity becomes chronic and fixed. The symptoms of discomfort from secondary changes often predominate. The Kelikian push-up and MTP joint luxation tests are strongly positive. MTP joint instability often results in dislocation of the proximal phalanx out of the joint, especially on the second MTP joint where it can become adducted over the hallux (crossover toe). A fixed, nonreducible hammertoe deformity accompanies the problem. Extensor tendon contractures are present. Dorsal skin contracture may or may not accompany the problem, depending on the severity as well as the chronicity of the presentation. Crepitus and pain with ROM of the MTP joint may be present. On radiographic evaluation, osteochondral adaptation as well as erosive changes of the metatarsal head may or may not have occurred.

MANAGEMENT

The treatment of the arthrosis of the central MTP joints varies depending on the severity of the deformity. The mild and moderate deformity is treated medically with one or a combination of antirheumatic drugs, which most often include an appropriate nonsteroidal antiinflammatory drug and injection therapy with local anesthesia and corticosteroids. In addition to pharmacologic therapy, supportive measures are instituted in the form of digital splinting, foot orthosis, footgear modification, and physical therapy. If these measures

---

TABLE 29–2

DIFFERENTIAL DIAGNOSIS OF METATARSALGIA

I. Extra-articular Disorders
- A. Intermetatarsal space-occupying lesions
  1. Neuroma
  2. Bursitis
  3. Ganglion
  4. Synovial cyst
  5. Lipoma
  6. Rheumatoid nodule
- B. Neuritis
- C. Tendonitis and/or tenosynovitis
  1. Flexor
  2. Extensor
- D. Stress fracture
- E. Traumatic dislocation
- F. Referred pain
  1. Tarsal tunnel syndrome
  2. Other entrapment neuropathies: deep peroneal and superficial peroneal nerve
  3. Radiculopathy
- G. Infection

II. Intra-articular Disorders
- A. Nonspecific synovitis (idiopathic)
  1. Metatarsophalangeal joint stress syndrome
  2. Mechanical synovitis
- B. Synovitis of rheumatic disease
- C. Degenerative joint disease
- D. Freiberg's infarction (avascular necrosis)
- E. Gout
- F. Intra-articular fracture
- G. Infection
- H. Dislocation

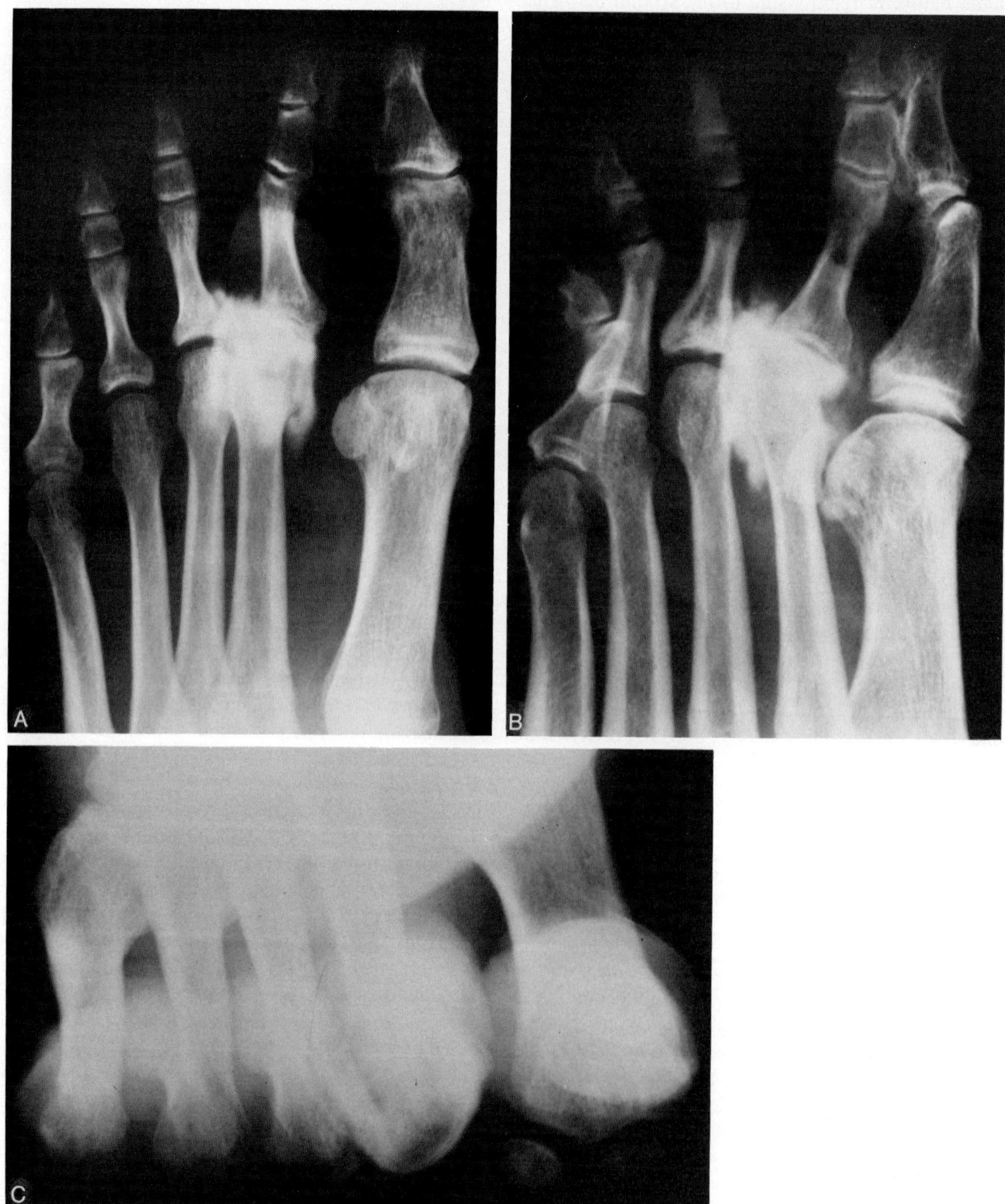

FIGURE 29–10. Radiographs demonstrating diagnostic intra-articular anesthetic block with contrast medium. *A,* Dorsoplantar view. *B,* Medial-oblique view. *C,* Plantar axial view.

are ineffective or if a secondary synovitis, degenerative joint disease, or a more severe deformity is involved, surgical intervention is then an option.

The procedures that are available to treat arthrosis of the central MTP joint are discussed as primary procedures and adjunctive procedures. The primary procedures are those that relieve pain and provide stability. The procedures that are mainly aimed at relieving pain are synovectomy and joint resection, either partial or complete, with or without an implant. The primary procedures that are aimed at providing stability are flexor tendon transfers and, in some instances, arthrodesis of the interphalangeal joints of the involved toe. Adjunctive soft tissue and osseous procedures are performed as necessary to enhance the surgical outcome.

Primary Surgical Procedures

Surgical Synovectomy. The purpose of surgical synovectomy is to remove the inflamed, abnormal synovium that creates pain and leads to joint instability and cartilage destruction. The hypertrophic, hyperplastic, vascularly congested, pink synovium appears as a separate layer from the capsule, which facilitates its removal. An attempt to remove as much abnormal synovium as possible is made without disrupting the ligaments.[21, 22]

Synovectomy as an isolated procedure has been applied mostly to the rheumatoid arthritic patient who has an immunologic defect wherein the synovium appears to be the target tissue. However, Mann and Mizel reported on six nonrheumatoid patients who underwent synovectomy for monarticular synovitis of the MTP joint.[6] Varying degrees of relief are anticipated because the joint is likely denervated by the procedure.[21] The best results of synovectomy seem to be obtained if the procedure is performed early before the signs of crepitus or radiographic changes appear.[15] The main risks or complications of synovectomy include joint instability and excessive joint stiffness.[22]

Flexor Tendon Transfers. The purpose of the flexor tendon transfer is to stabilize the MTP joint mostly in the sagittal plane by enabling the flexor tendon or tendons to assume the function of the intrinsic muscles that normally provide a plantarflexory retrograde force on the MTP joint.

Flexor tendon transfers are accomplished by transferring the plantarflexory power of the FDL and at times the FDB, alone or in combination, to the proximal phalanx. Most often the FDL is transected distal to the proximal interphalangeal joints while leaving the insertion of the FDB intact. It is then transferred to the proximal phalanx by one of the following methods: (1) the transected end is sutured through a buttonhole into the dorsolateral aspect of the extensor expansion[24, 25]; (2) the transected end is split and then the ends are sutured to each other over the neck of the proximal phalanx[26]; and (3) the transected end is passed from plantar to dorsal through a drill hole fashioned in the neck of the proximal phalanx (Fig. 29–11).[27] Another method is simply to leave the insertions of the flexor tendons intact and to suture the FDL to the plantar aspect of the proximal phalanx. Transferring the FDB while leaving the FDL intact has also been described but appears to be less favored.[28, 29] Adjunctive soft tissue procedures are always performed, and osseous procedures are performed as necessary.

Side effects of the procedure consist of a stiff toe, and if the FDL is transferred, loss of the prehensile action of the toe occurs. The toe stiffness actually adds to the success of the procedure, but nevertheless the patient must be advised

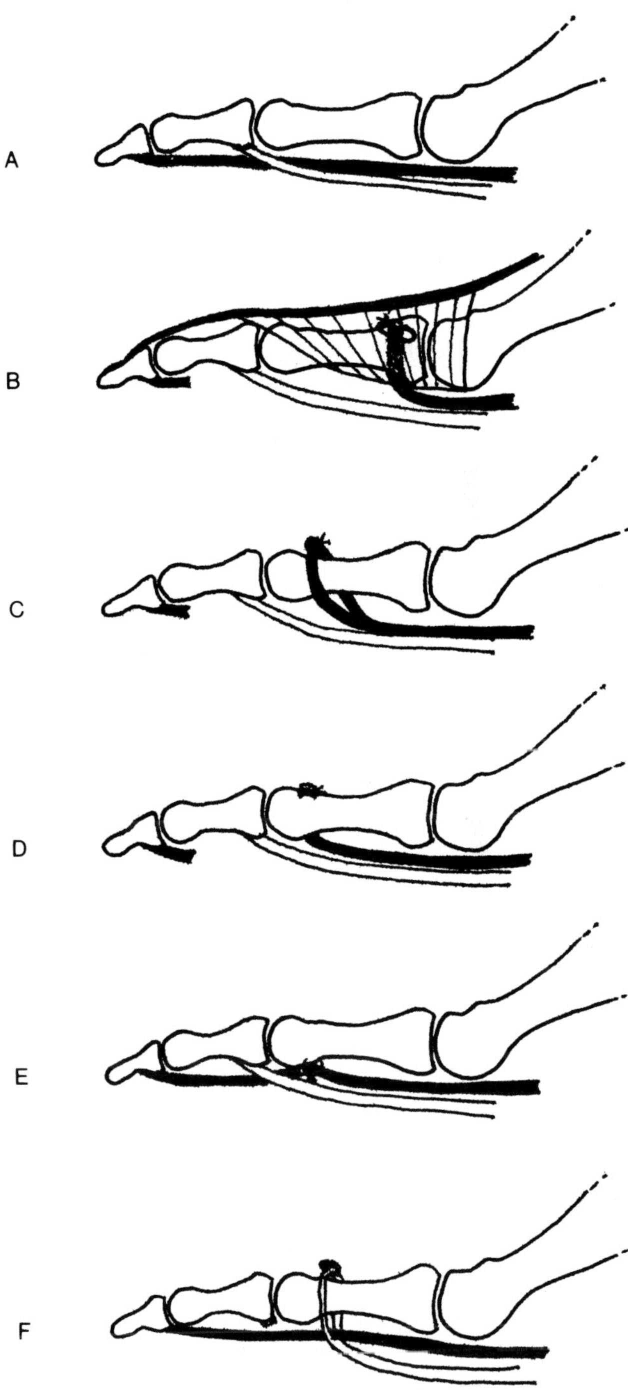

FIGURE 29–11. Methods of flexor tendon transfer. *A*, Normal anatomic relationship. *B*, Transfer of severed flexor digitorum longus (FDL) into extensor expansion while leaving the flexor digitorum brevis (FDB) intact. *C*, Transfer of severed and split FDL around proximal phalanx while leaving the FDB intact. *D*, Transfer of severed FDL through dorsoplantar drill hole in anatomic neck of the proximal phalanx while leaving FDB intact. *E*, Transfer of intact FDL to plantar aspect of the proximal phalanx. *F*, Transfer of severed ends of the FDB around the proximal phalanx while leaving the FDL intact.

of this outcome. Complications include failure, chronic edema, excessive stiffness, lack of toe purchase, and vascular compromise if the tendon is not passed properly.

Simply tenotomizing a flexor tendon releases flexion contractures on the interphalangeal joints but does not help reduce the hyperextended proximal phalanx.[13]

Metatarsophalangeal Joint Arthroplasty. MTP joint arthroplasty is essentially a partial metatarsal head resection. It is performed primarily when there have been erosive changes secondary to an arthritic process or when osteochondral adaptation of the metatarsal head has occurred secondary to chronic subluxation or dislocation. Through a U-shaped dorsal capsulotomy, 3 to 5 mm of the leading aspect of the metatarsal head is resected and rounded so that the proximal phalanx can be relocated. An interpositional capsular flap can be fashioned from the dorsal capsulotomy, which will act as a joint spacer.[30]

If along with the chronic MTP joint dislocation the plantar aspect of the metatarsal head is prominent and associated with a painful intractable keratoma, a plantar condylectomy may be incorporated in the MTP joint arthroplasty. In any event, a 0.045-in. Kirschner wire across the MTP joint is used for approximately 3 to 4 weeks to hold the joint in an overcorrected position while a fibroarthrosis forms (Fig. 29–12).

Metatarsophalangeal Joint Implant Arthroplasty. If more than the leading aspect of the metatarsal head has to be resected owing to severe erosive changes, instability will most likely result because of the loss of internal cubic content as well as intrinsic stability provided by the ligaments. It is here that a double-stemmed lesser MTP joint implant may be used.[31–33] The presently designed lesser MTP joint implants do not duplicate function of the joint but do act as a spacer. Consequently, they provide the intrinsic stability that was lost because of the elimination of collateral ligaments and decrease in the internal cubic content of the joint as a result of resected or eroded bone.

When this procedure is performed, it is imperative to address any extrinsic contractures or contiguous instability because the implant will ultimately fail if external stress is applied.[34] The reader is referred to Chapter 31 on implant arthroplasty for a through discussion of the subject.

Adjunctive Soft Tissue Procedures

The goal of the adjunctive soft tissue procedures is to augment the primary procedures by releasing contractures, thereby relocating the MTP joint, centralizing the long extensor and flexor tendons, and relocating the flexor plate. The success or the failure of the procedure is often predicated on an adequate or inadequate soft tissue release.

Adjunctive soft tissue surgical procedures consist of those that result in an extrinsic as well as an intrinsic MTP joint release. They involve capsulotomies, release of intra-articular ligaments and capsular adhesions, tenotomies, tendon rebalancing techniques, extensor hood recession, and, at times, release of the intermetatarsal ligament. The extrinsic release is performed in two phases. The initial phase is performed before the intrinsic release, and the secondary phase, if necessary, is performed after the intrinsic release.

The initial extrinsic release consists of performing an isolated tenectomy of the EDB tendon at the level of the MTP

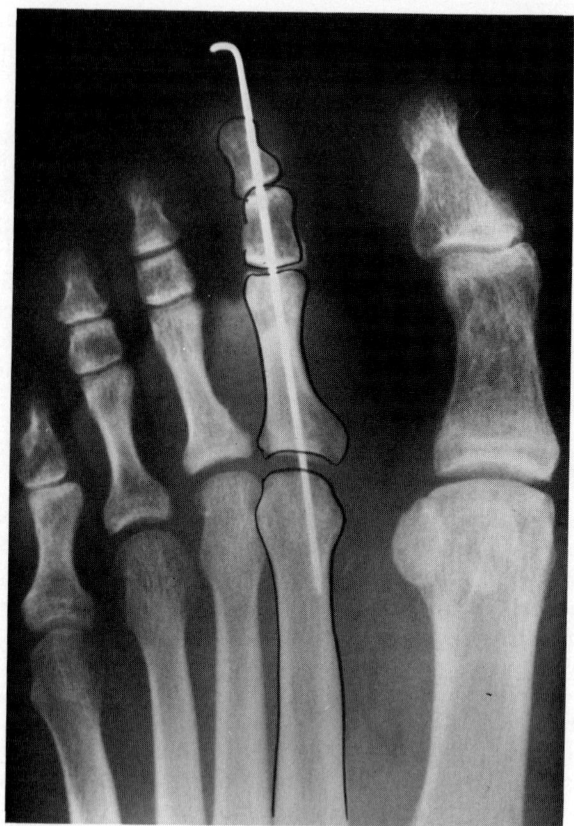

FIGURE 29–12. Dorsoplantar radiograph demonstrating a resectional arthroplasty of the second metatarsophalangeal joint with adjunctive flexor tendon transfer and temporary Kirschner wire stabilization.

joint before it joins with the EDL. The EDB tendon is usually contracted to some degree, causing the extensor expansion to lift the proximal phalanx into a dorsiflexed position. It appears that the muscle with the shortest distance from origin to insertion (i.e., the EDB) proportionally has the most profound effect on causing a dorsal contracture of the proximal phalanx. Most often, once the EDB tendon pull is neutralized and an intrinsic MTP joint release is performed, the dorsal contracture of the proximal phalanx will be reversed, negating the need for a lengthening of the EDL. After an initial extrinsic release is completed, the Kelikian push-up test is performed. If the results are still positive, an intrinsic release of the MTP joint is indicated.

The release is accomplished in a stepwise manner based on preoperative planing and intraoperative evaluation of the reducibility of the MTP joint when the Kelikian push-up test is performed. The intrinsic release begins with a dorsal MTP joint capsulotomy. Once completed, the test is performed again. If the deformity is still incompletely reduced, a release of the collateral and suspensory ligaments from their insertion into the epicondyles is performed. Again, the push-up test is performed, and if the results are still positive, a release of the flexor plate and plantar proximal capsule, which becomes capsulodesed to the underside of the metatarsal head, is performed. This maneuver is best accomplished with a spoon-shaped instrument with a sharp leading edge of appropriate size for the central metatarsal heads (11 mm McGlamry scoop) (Fig. 29–13).

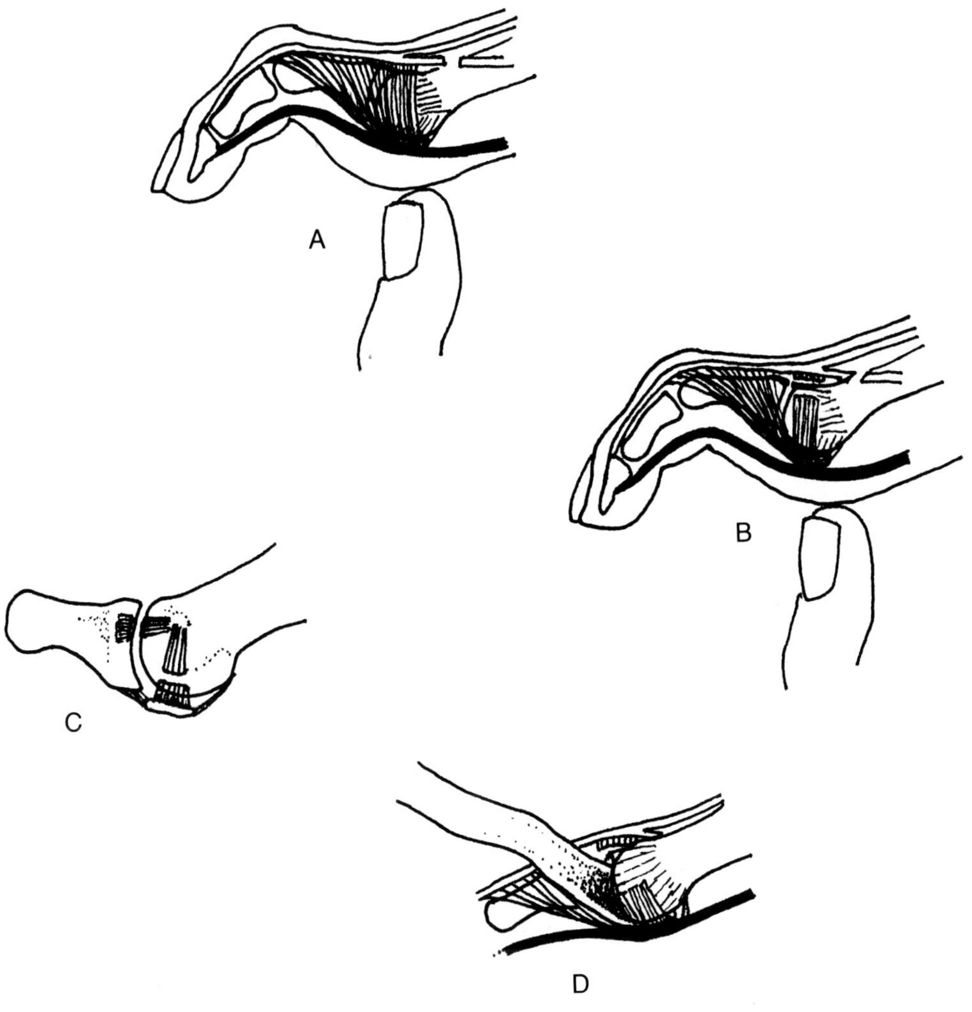

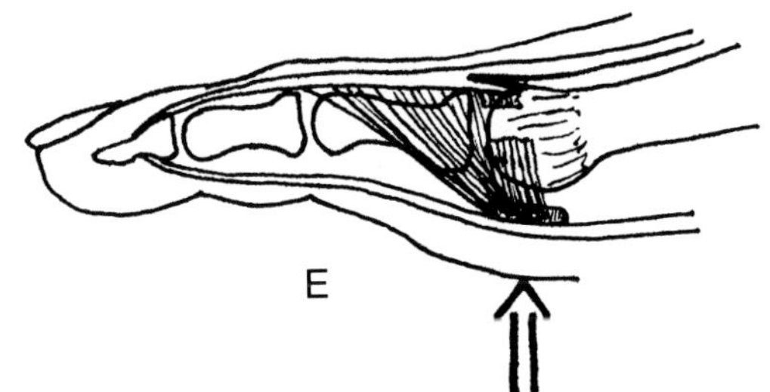

FIGURE 29–13. Sequential metatarsophalangeal (MTP) joint contracture release. *A,* Nonreducible MTP joint even after severance of the extensor digitorum brevis tendon. *B,* Nonreducible MTP joint after partial proximal release of the extensor expansion and dorsal MTP joint capsulotomy. *C,* Nonreducible MTP joint after additional release of intrinsic ligaments indicating plantar capsulodesis. *D,* Freeing of plantar capsular adhesions and relocation of the flexor plate. *E,* Reducible MTP joint after complete intrinsic release.

If all the contractures are released, the Kelikian push-up test will become negative, indicating that the entire phalangeal apparatus, including the flexor plate, has relocated back into a proper alignment. However, if the push-up test is still positive and the proximal phalanx remains dorsiflexed, the secondary phase of the extensor release is performed. This consists of an extensor hood recession (release) and, when necessary, a lengthening of the EDL. The hood recession is performed by freeing the EDL from its attachments to the extensor expansion.[21] If the toe is still dorsally contracted, a Z lengthening of the EDL is performed that virtually frees all the soft tissue structures that could potentially hold the proximal phalanx in dorsiflexion.

The steps just outlined are performed essentially to reverse sagittal plane contractures. If the digit significantly adducts or abducts when the push-up test is performed, instability and contracture in the transverse plane are present. This problem is addressed by centralizing the EDL and FDL tendons above and below the MTP joint. This is accomplished by performing an extensor-flexor ''rebalancing'' procedure that involves releasing the extensor expansion on the contracted side. If necessary, a vertical capsulotomy is performed on the contracted side and tightening or reefing the capsule on the elongated side is done with an appropriately placed suture (Fig. 29–14).

TABLE 29–3

INDICATED PROCEDURES BASED UPON SEVERITY LEVEL OF DEFORMITY

Staged Procedure	Severity Level		
	Mild	*Moderate*	*Severe*
MTP joint			
Capsulotomy	Yes	Yes	Yes
Synovectomy	PRN	PRN	PRN
EDB tenectomy	Yes	Yes	Yes
FLX tendon transfer	PRN	Yes	Yes
MTP joint release			
Ligaments	No	Yes	Yes
FLX plate	No	PRN	Yes
EXT hood recession	No	PRN	Yes
EDL lengthening	No	No	PRN
EXT rebalancing	PRN	PRN	PRN
FLX rebalancing			
IML release	No	PRN	PRN
MTP joint			
Arthroplasty	No	No	PRN
Implant	No	No	PRN
Kirschner wire	Yes	Yes	Yes
Postoperative splint	Yes	Yes	Yes
Z-plasty	No	No	PRN
MET osteotomy			
Transpositional	No	PRN	PRN
Shortening	No	PRN	PRN

MTP, metatarsophalangeal; EDB, extensor digitorum brevis; FLX, flexor; EXT, extensor; EDL, extensor digitorum longus; MET, metatarsal; IML, intermetatarsal ligament.

If the toe still deviates in the transverse plane when the push-up test is performed, a release of the intermetatarsal ligament on the side opposite of the contracture should be performed. This last maneuver should allow the flexor tendon and flexor plate to relocate beneath the metatarsal head.

Adjunctive Osseous Procedures

Adjunctive osseous procedures consist mostly of digital arthroplasties or arthrodeses. They are indicated when the digital deformity is nonreducible secondary to osteochondral adaptation of the interphalangeal joints or when there is excessive digital length.

In rare instances, transpositional metatarsal osteotomies are indicated to better align the MTP joint.[35] Furthermore, shortening osteotomies are indicated if the involved metatarsal is excessively long.[21]

The surgical procedures are performed at one setting but are staged, addressing each component of the deformity as necessary.

For a mild deformity, mostly soft tissue procedures are used because osseous procedures are usually reserved for the moderate or severe deformity (Table 29–3).

Postoperative Management

Postoperative management consists of a 0.045-in. Kirschner wire placed across the MTP joint to maintain the correction obtained by the surgical repair while healing and fibrosis occur. It is removed 3 or 4 weeks after the procedure. The patient is allowed to ambulate in a postoperative shoe that limits propulsion and protects the Kirschner wire.

Once the wire is removed, the toe is splinted for several

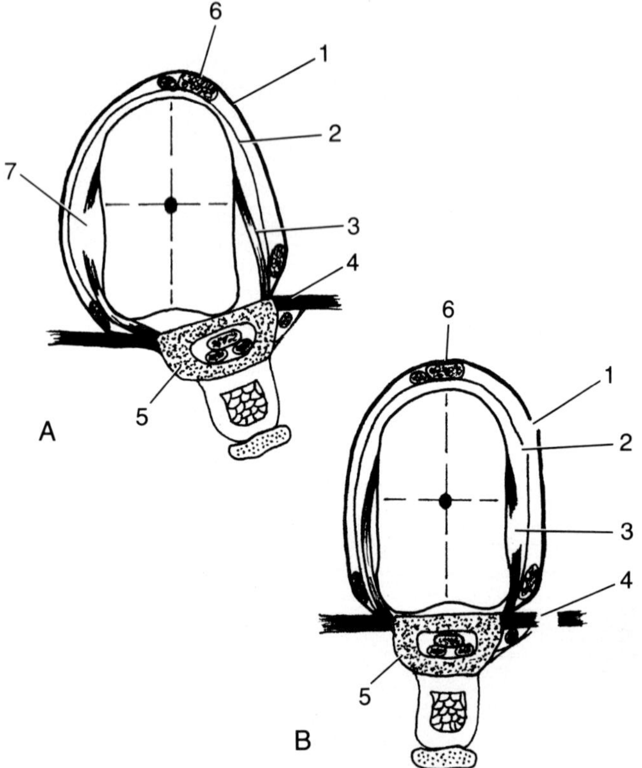

FIGURE 29–14. Extensor-flexor ''rebalancing'' technique. *A,* Medial metatarsophalangeal joint contracture-subluxation of extensor expansion–flexor tendon apparatus. 1, Medial extensor sling contraction. 2, Medial capsule contraction. 3, Medial collateral–suspensory ligament contraction. 4, Medial intermetatarsal ligament contraction. 5, Medially located flexor apparatus. 6, Medially located extensor apparatus. 7, Elongated/ruptured lateral collateral–suspensory ligament. *B,* Relocated extensor expansion–flexor tendon apparatus. 1, Severed medial extensor sling. 2, Severed medial capsule. 3, Severed medial collateral–suspensory ligament. 4, Severed medial intermetatarsal ligament. 5, Relocated flexor apparatus. 6, Relocated extensor expansion apparatus.

months in a plantarflexed position. This can be accomplished with tape or prefabricated splints.

References

1. Gerbert J and Dobbs B: Rheumatoid forefoot. *In* Comprehensive Textbook of Foot Surgery. Vol 1. Baltimore, Williams & Wilkins, 1987, pp 534–543.
2. Gould N: Surgery of the forepart of the foot in rheumatoid arthritis. Foot Ankle 3:173, 1982.
3. Mann RA and Thompson FM: Arthrodesis of the first metatarsophalangeal joint for hallux valgus in rheumatoid arthritis. J Bone Joint Surg 66A:687, 1984.
4. Saltrick KR, Scott AA, and Catanzariti A: Pan metatarsal head resection: Retrospective analysis and literature review. J Foot Surg 28:340, 1989.
5. Cook TD: A scientific basis for surgery in rheumatoid arthritis. Clin Orthop 208:20, 1986.
6. Mann RA and Mizel MA: Monarticular nontraumatic synovitis of the metatarsophalangeal joint: A new diagnosis. Foot Ankle 6:18, 1985.
7. Menninger H, Stiegler A, Mohr W, and Wessinghage D: Detritus synovitis in chronic polyarthritis: A clinical and operation histologic evaluation [Ger]. Z Rheumatol 48:89 [English translation], 1989.
8. Lambrinudi C: Functional aspect: Action of foot muscles. Lancet 2:1480, 1938.
9. Sarrafian SK: Anatomy of the Foot and Ankle: Descriptive, Topographic, Functional. Philadelphia, JB Lippincott, 1983.
10. Bojsen-Møller F: Anatomy of the forefoot: Normal and pathologic. Clin Orthop 142:10, 1979.
11. Bojsen-Møller F and Lamoreux L: Significance of free dorsiflexion of the toes in walking. Acta Orthop Scand 50:471, 1979.
12. DuVires HL: Dislocation of the toe. JAMA 160:728, 1956.
13. Coughlin MJ: Crossover second toe deformity. Foot Ankle 8:29–39, 1987.
14. Root ML, Orien WP, and Weed JH: Normal and abnormal function of the foot. Clin Biomechanics, 2:53, 1977.
15. Schumacher RS Jr (ed): Primer on the Rheumatic Diseases, 9th ed. Atlanta, Arthritis Foundation, 1988.
16. Bojsen-Møller F and Flagstad KE: Plantar aponeurosis and internal architecture of the ball of the foot. J Anat 121:599, 1976.
17. Morton DJ: The Human Foot: Its Evolution, Physiology, and Functional Disorders. New York, Columbia University Press, 1935, p 109.
18. Mann RA and Hagy JL: The function of the toes in walking, jogging, and running. Clin Orthop 142:24, 1979.
19. Sarrafian SK and Topouzian LK: Anatomy and physiology of the extensor apparatus of the toes. J Bone Joint Surg 51A:669, 1969.
20. Jarett BA, Manzi JA, and Green D: Interossei and lumbricales muscles of the foot: An anatomical and functional study. J Am Podiatr Assoc 70:1, 1980.
21. Jimenez AJ, McGlamry ED, and Green DR: Lesser ray deformities. *In* Comprehensive Textbook of Foot Surgery, Vol. 1. Baltimore, Williams & Wilkins, 1987, pp 76–80.
22. Thompson FM and Hamilton WG: Problems of the second metatarsophalangeal joint. Orthopedics 10:83, 1987.
23. Kelikian H: Hallux Valgus and Allied Deformities of the Forefoot and Metatarsalgia. Philadelphia, WB Saunders, 1965, p 314.
24. Girdlestone GR: Physiotherapy for hand and foot. J Chart Soc Physiother 32:167, 1947.
25. Taylor RG: The treatment of claw toes by multiple transfers of flexor into extensor tendons. J Bone Joint Surg 33B:539, 1951.
26. Sgarlato TE: Transplantation of the flexor digitorum longus muscle tendon in hammertoes. J Am Podiatr Assoc 60:383, 1970.
27. Kuwada GT and Dockery GL: Modification of the flexor tendon transfer procedure for the correction of flexible hammertoes. J Foot Surg 19:38, 1980.
28. McCain LR: Transplantation of the flexor digitorum brevis in hammertoe surgery. J Am Podiatr Assoc 48:233, 1958.
29. Parrish TF: Dynamic correction of clawtoes. Orthop Clin North Am 4:97, 1973.
30. Kehr LE: A new surgical technique for the correction of Freiberg's deformity. J Am Podiatr Assoc 72:130, 1982.
31. Sgarlato T: A new implant for the metatarsophalangeal joint. Clin Podiatr Med Surg 1:69, 1984.
32. Cracchiolo A, Kitaoka HB, and Leventen EO: Silicone implant arthroplasty for second metatarsophalangeal joint disorders with and without hallux valgus deformities. Foot Ankle 9:10, 1988.
33. Sgarlato T: Sutter double-stem silicone implant arthroplasty of the lesser metatarsophalangeal joints. J Foot Surg 28:410, 1989.
34. Jenkin WM and Oloff LM: Implant arthroplasty in the rheumatoid arthritic patient. Clin Podiatr Med Surg 5:213, 1988.
35. Johnson JB and Price TW: Crossover second toe deformity: Etiology and treatment. J Foot Surg 28:417, 1989.

CHAPTER 30

Forefoot Arthroplasty

John V. Vanore, D.P.M., and Irving Pikscher, D.P.M.

Rheumatoid arthritis is characterized as a symmetrical polyarthritis, and this symmetry is quite prevalent with regard to the foot deformities (Fig. 30–1). The metatarsophalangeal (MTP) joints are most frequently involved, often all five articulations in both feet. Most striking is the severity of forefoot involvement, commonly with gross dislocation of the joints. Deformities gradually progress from somewhat flexible or semi-reducible to nonreducible and rigid in nature.[1] This rigid deformed forefoot usually makes a comfortable gait or even weightbearing or shoe selection difficult.[2] Clinically, the inflammatory process of the disease may diminish or at some point "burn out." The deformities persist, and symptoms from the markedly altered mechanics dominate the clinical picture.[3, 4] As a result, most surgeons recommend aggressive resection arthroplasties for cosmetic repair and relief of pain. Bunion or hallux valgus deformities with digital and metatarsal dislocations are the concern of this discussion and the pathology addressed in a so-called forefoot arthroplasty.

The problems of rheumatoid arthritis are not new, and surgeons have recommended diverse surgical cures. These have ranged from excision of the metatarsal heads to amputation of each of the toes. Hopefully, with a few ideas from the past combined with our present experiences, a thoughtful surgical approach to the correction of these severe deformities will develop.

Historical Approach to the Surgical Management of Forefoot Deformities

Most authors identify Hoffmann[5] as the initial proponent for the surgical management of the rheumatoid forefoot. Hoffmann did not specifically recognize the condition of rheumatoid arthritis but recommended resection of all the metatarsal heads through a single plantar incision for the severest cases of claw toes with MTP joint dislocations. Clayton[1] attributed most of Hoffmann's patients as having cavus feet as the reason for his use of metatarsal head resection. Probably not until the introduction of the 1958 American Rheumatism Association[6] diagnostic criteria did the use of the term *rheumatoid arthritis* become more prevalent in the literature.

Thompson[7] recognized the contribution of arthritis to the symptoms and severity of the deformities, although he believed that splinting and rest would limit the extent of deformity. He recommended a variety of potential procedures, from the Keller bunionectomy to resection of the entire proximal phalanx to digital amputation. He observed that treatment must be individualized to the patient and presenting deformity.

Key[8] differentiated rheumatoid from degenerative deformities and recommended multiple procedures, possibly 10 or more, to correct the multiplicity of forefoot conditions. He discussed the merits of Keller bunionectomy with or without excision of the sesamoids as well as the potential need for first metatarsal base osteotomy to reduce the intermetatarsal angle. Key recognized the lesser MTP joint dislocations and the requirement for resection of the base of the proximal phalanx and, at times, the metatarsal head as well. He cited the Hoffmann procedure but admitted to performance of limited, partial metatarsal head excisions through a dorsal incision.

Marmon[9] described combining a Keller bunionectomy with lesser metatarsal head excision (Fig. 30–2). This was performed through three incisions: a dorsal longitudinal one over the first ray while the metatarsal heads were excised through web space incisions between the second and third, and fourth and fifth toes, respectively.

The deformities associated with rheumatoid arthritis certainly impressed surgeons attempting to address the patients' suffering. In 1957, Nissen[10] advocated amputation of all the toes with disarticulations of the MTP joints and remodeling of the metatarsal heads to relieve the pain and deformities. Flint and Sweetnam[11] also advised amputation of all the toes in the technique described by Nissen.

Fowler[12] designed his operation for the "severest claw toe deformity when it is impossible to restore the normal anatomy of the MTP joints, and when there is severe pain under the prominent metatarsal heads." His incisional approach was unique, with a dorsal transverse incision over the MTP joints that curves proximally a short distance along the shafts of the first and fifth metatarsals. The osseous resections included the proximal half of the proximal phalanges and remodeling of the metatarsal heads. He described a fairly straight-line parabola from the distal aspect of the first through fifth metatarsal heads with complete excision and remodeling of the plantar condyles. Fowler also recognized the anterior advancement of the plantar fat pad. He recommended excision of a plantar transverse skin wedge proximal to the metatarsal heads to replace this soft tissue pad underneath the metatarsal heads.

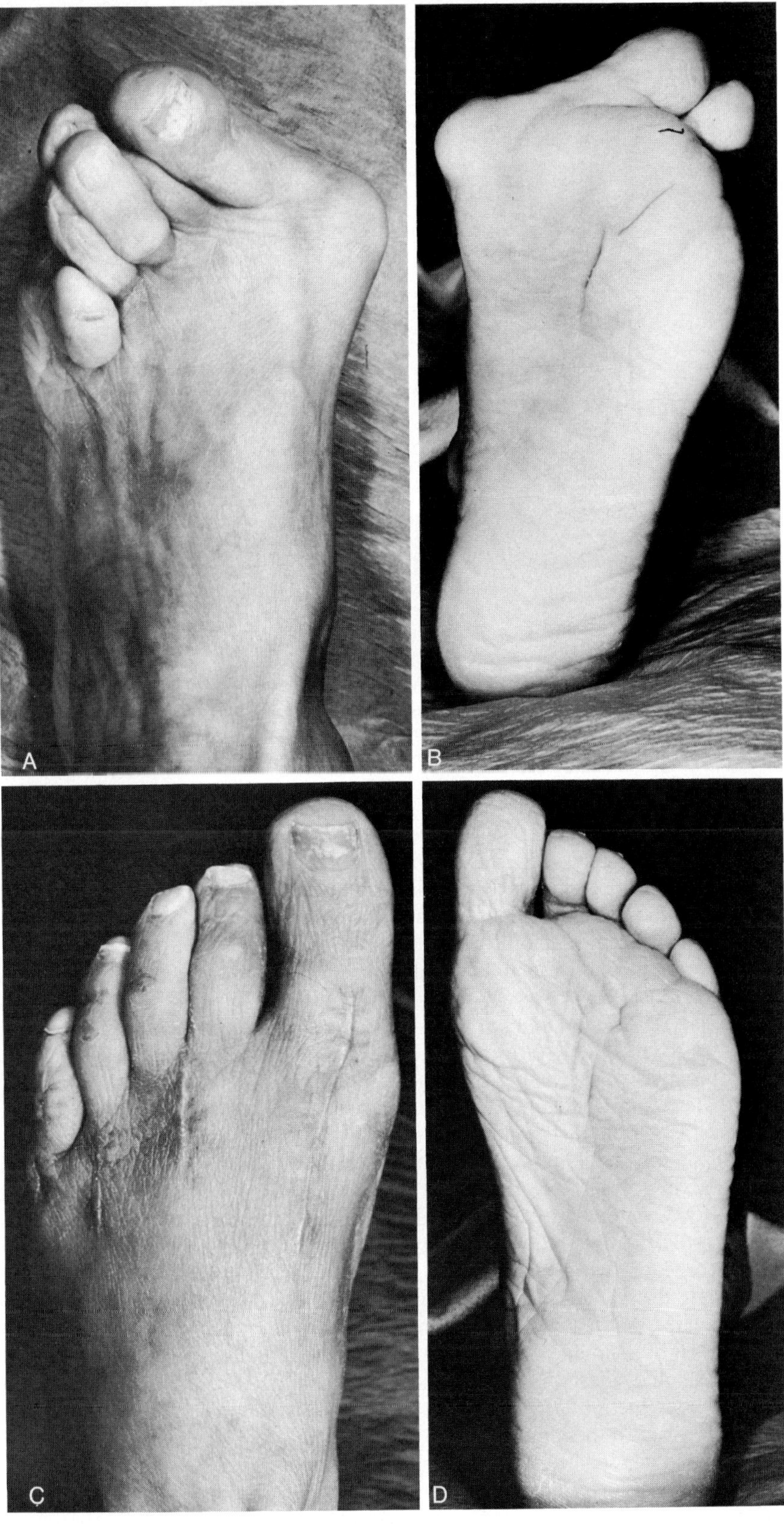

FIGURE 30–1. Clinical result of forefoot arthroplasty. Illustrated are the preoperative deformities that are typically encountered in the rheumatoid forefoot *(A)* and *(B)* and the potential for impressive correction of very severe deformities *(C)* and *(D)*. It is this potential for extraordinary improvements in not only the cosmetic appearance and correction of deformities but also the functional capacity of the foot and the patient that forefoot arthroplasty will allow.

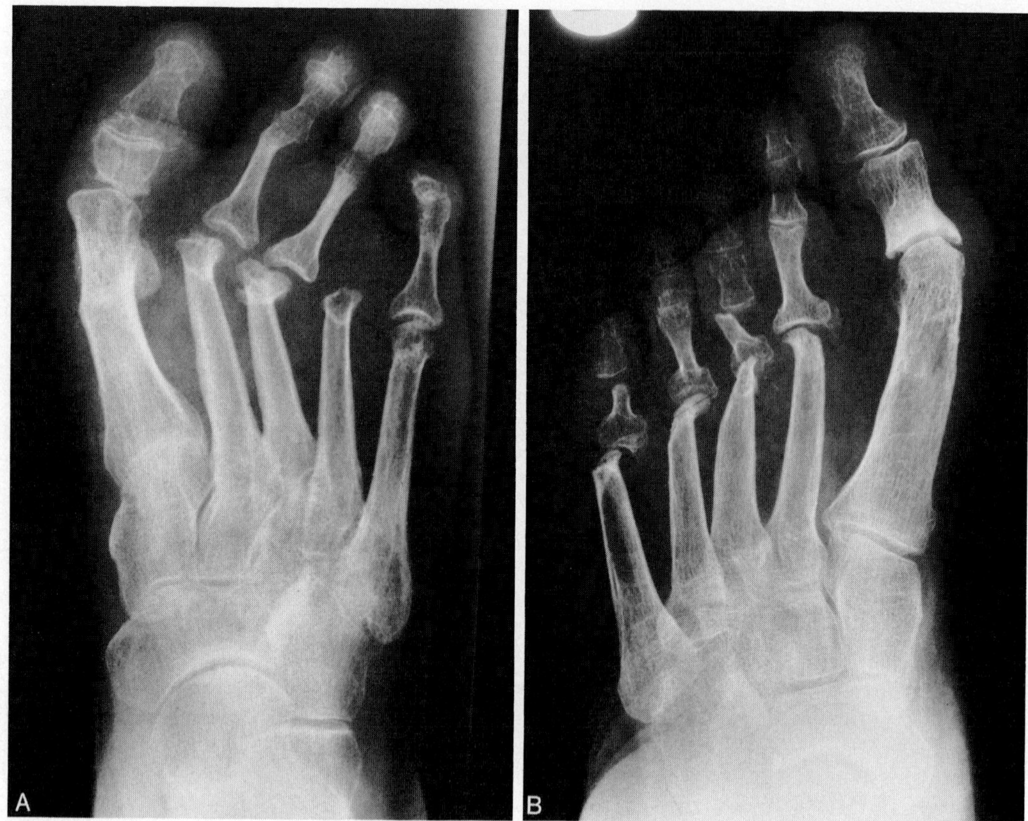

FIGURE 30–2. Variations of the Keller procedure. The Keller arthroplasty has been advocated but, when combined with partial metatarsectomies *(A)* and *(B)*, may leave the foot with a very long first ray and continued transverse plane instability at the first metatarsophalangeal joint.

Clayton[13] described more aggressive osseous resection that included the phalangeal bases as well as the metatarsal heads through a single dorsal transverse incision. He recommended excision of the second phalangeal base, then the third, followed by the fourth. If the fifth toe deformity was insignificant, it was left undisturbed. The hallux could then be approached more easily as a result of the lateral bone resections. This technique then allowed access to the metatarsal heads, and they were excised in the same sequence with a progressive shortening from the second to fifth metatarsals. He recommended that the first and second metatarsal be the same approximate length and that the first metatarsal should possibly be left intact if it was significantly short preoperatively.

In 1963, Clayton[14] further expounded on the forefoot arthroplasty. He admitted to performing excisional arthroplasty only on one or two toes, although he acknowledged that usually all the metatarsal heads require removal. Clayton recommended that if three or more metatarsal heads require excision, all five should be performed. He corrected the distal joints of the toes through manipulation and emphasized adequate bony resection. He also believed that the incisional approach was of minor significance.

Kates and associates[15] described a modification of the Hoffmann and Fowler procedures performed through an excisional skinplasty plantar and proximal to the metatarsal heads. This was planned to accomplish a similar function to the Fowler excision of a plantar skin ellipse. Their osseous resections included the entire metatarsal head in a curved

parabolic manner. The first MTP joint sesamoids were usually excised with the metatarsal head and the arthroplasty stabilized with an axial Kirschner wire.

Raunio and Laine[16] reported good results with MTP joint synovectomies in patients with mild disease. Aho and Halonen[17] also praised synovectomies in patients with joint symptoms unresponsive to medical management or in those with limited deformity.

Lipscomb and associates[18] discussed resection of the phalangeal bases with remodeling of the lesser metatarsal heads and either a Keller arthroplasty or first MTP joint arthrodesis. They used a medial longitudinal incision along the first MTP joint with dorsal linear incisions between the second and third, and fourth and fifth, MTP joints. Following the first ray procedure, the lesser joints were approached. The extensor tendons were divided, and a generous resection of the proximal phalanx was performed. The plantar condyles of the metatarsal heads were resected flush with the metatarsal shafts. They also used 0.045-in. Kirschner wires placed in the toes then retrograded into the metatarsals to maintain the toes in a position of 20 degrees of flexion (they probably meant flexion in relation to the normal degree of 20-degree extension) for 3 weeks. Ambulation in Reese shoes was allowed after 3 or 4 days and continued for 2 or 3 months postoperatively until edema subsided.

DuVries[19] recommended first MTP joint arthrodesis with excision of the proximal phalangeal bases. DuVries rationalized that the stable MTP joint allowed weightbearing by the first ray, yet flexibility was retained through the hallucal interphalangeal and metatarsocuneiform joints. He also recommended leaving the metatarsal heads untouched. He labeled this the *DuVries-Dickson procedure.*

DuVries began with the first MTP joint arthrodesis through a long first web space incision that extended proximally over the medial aspect of the first metatarsal base. Fixation was accomplished with a dorsally placed staple. An adductor release and fibular sesamoidectomy could be performed before the arthrodesis. Through the same incision, the second MTP joint was exposed and the phalangeal base excised. A second incision was then made from the third web space distally and extending proximally over the fourth MTP joint. Through this incision, the bases of the third and fourth toe proximal phalanges were excised, and the fifth, if necessary, was also excised.

Mann and Coughlin[20] recommended a similar approach combining arthrodesis of the first MTP joint with basal resection of the proximal phalanges and variable remodeling of the metatarsal heads. Their report probably still reflects the prevailing orthopedic opinion in the surgical treatment of the forefoot deformities of rheumatoid arthritis.

Podiatric surgeons have for the most part differed from this approach in both the procedures of the first and the lesser MTP joints. Both Hugar and Gucfa[21] and Hodor and Dobbs[22] recommended panmetatarsal head resection, one through five, and both recommended dorsal linear incisions. The earlier report[21] actually described subtotal bone resections of the metatarsal heads at the surgical neck through a three-incision approach, whereas the other authors[22] used five linear dorsal incisions to perform complete metatarsal head resections.

Panmetatarsal head resections or modifications of the Hoffmann-Clayton type procedures have been performed with success in the rheumatoid foot with hallux valgus and lesser MTP luxations. With the advent of silicone implants, the Hoffmann-Clayton procedures were first combined with the Keller and hemi-implant (Fig. 30–3). Many of these procedures failed because of the length discrepancy created between the unaltered first metatarsal and the significantly shortened lesser metatarsals. The hallux was inherently unstable, and lateral dislocation was common.

In the 1980s a modified Hoffmann procedure was performed with resection of the distal portion of the first metatarsal and use of a double-stem hinged implant. This improved the stability of the first MTP joint compared with a Keller arthroplasty or a hemi-implant. The double-stem implants may provide some degree of transverse plane stability, but adequate soft tissue relaxation and correction of the deformity must be accomplished. Recurrence of deformity may occur with frontal plane rotation of the implant within the medullary canals.

Cracchiolo[23] discussed the modifications of various procedures of the forefoot arthroplasty. The first MTP joint may be treated with either excisional arthroplasty of the phalangeal base, metatarsal head, or both, or the joint may be stabilized by fusion or with a double-stem silicone implant. The lesser MTP joint contractures may be addressed with

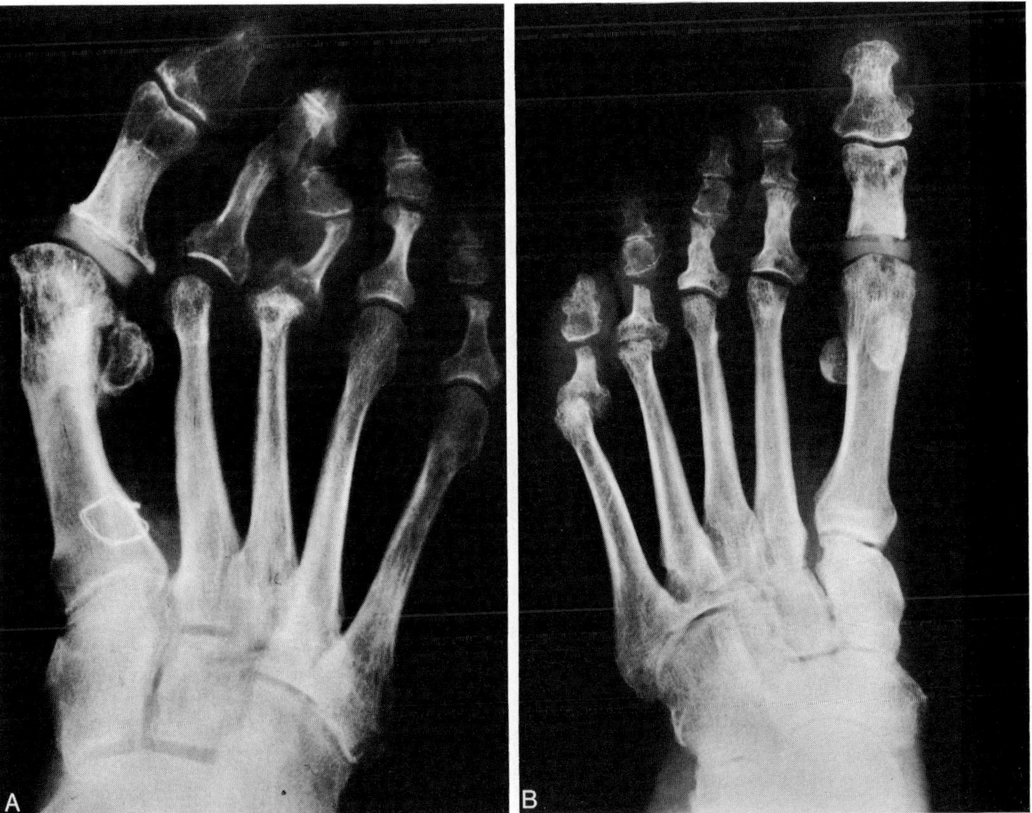

FIGURE 30–3. The role of hemi-implants. Radiographs illustrating the ineffectiveness of the Keller with or without a hemi-implant when combined with panmetatarsectomy. The resultant length discrepancy of the first to lesser metatarsals generally leads to transverse plane instability at the first metatarsophalangeal joint *(A)*. A Keller or hemi-implant is probably best performed in conjunction with resection of the proximal phalangeal bases or simple remodeling of the metatarsal heads *(B)*.

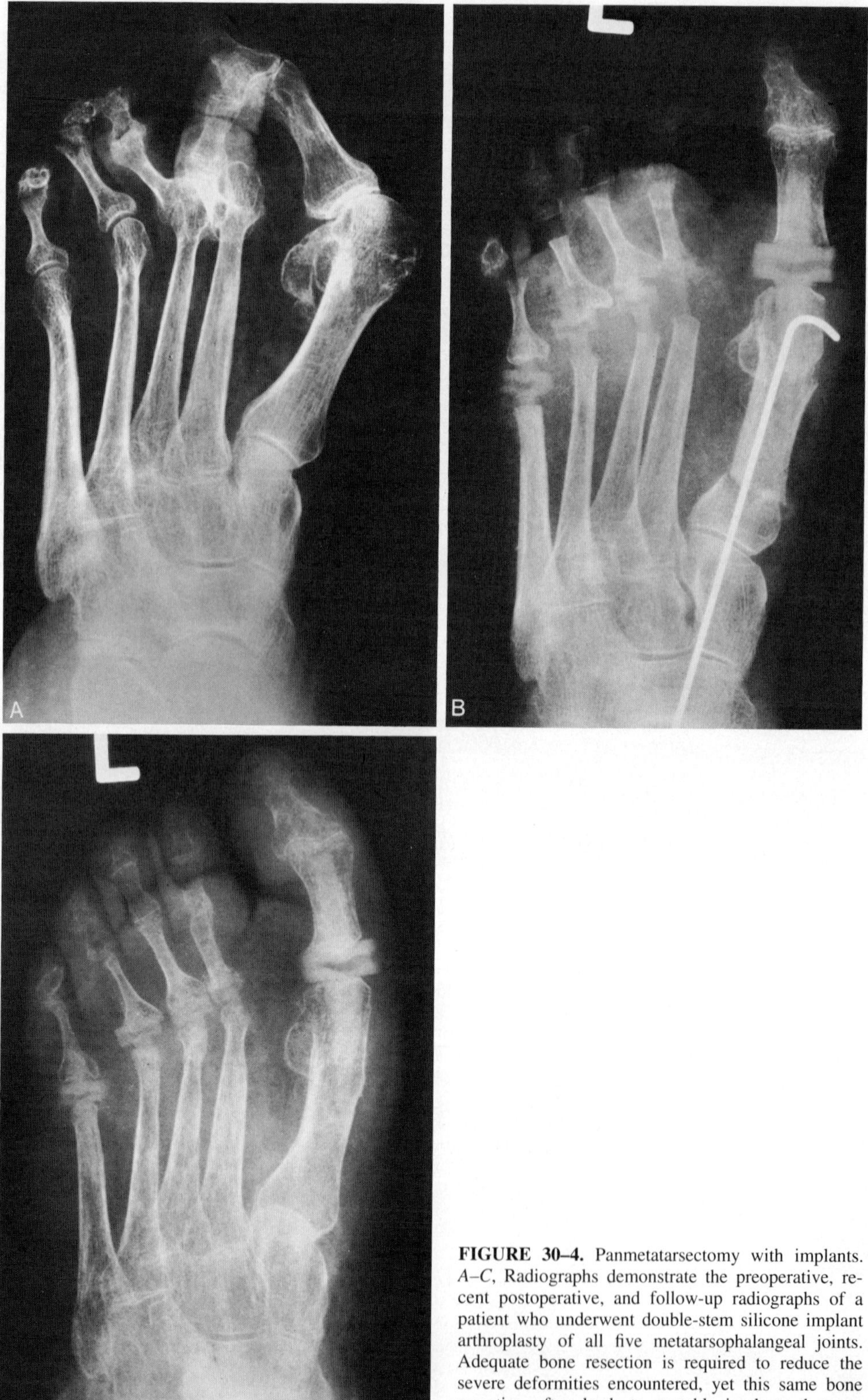

FIGURE 30–4. Panmetatarsectomy with implants. *A–C*, Radiographs demonstrate the preoperative, recent postoperative, and follow-up radiographs of a patient who underwent double-stem silicone implant arthroplasty of all five metatarsophalangeal joints. Adequate bone resection is required to reduce the severe deformities encountered, yet this same bone resection often leads to unstable implants that can easily dislocate postoperatively. There seems to be no advantage to this type of implant.

excision of the metatarsal heads, phalangeal bases, or both as well as the insertion of silicone implants in each (Fig. 30–4). Cracchiolo's plantar approach was through a transverse incision placed just proximal to the metatarsal heads. He believed Hoffmann's incision was too far distal, had a greater likelihood of neurovascular damage, and did not allow for repositioning of the plantar fat pad.

McGlamry and Bernbach[24] discussed forefoot arthroplasty with panmetatarsal head resections and recommended leaving the phalangeal bases and their soft tissue attachments intact. A metatarsal length pattern of $2 > 1 > 3 > 4 > 5$ from longest to shortest was the objective performed through a plantar transverse incision. They used digital fusions of the central three toes and believed that this helped stabilize the lesser MTP joints. Kirschner wire stabilization of the toes across the lesser MTP joints was used. They concluded that the plantar approach was the most practical when severe dorsal contractures of the toes were present.

Vanore and associates[25] discussed forefoot arthroplasty as variations of the Hoffmann procedure: first MTP joint double-stem flexible-hinge silicone arthroplasty with resection of all the lesser metatarsal heads. They recommended all lesser MTP joint resections be stabilized with 0.062-in. Kirschner wires retrograded from the toes deep into the metatarsal bases. They cited poor results with the hemi-silicone implant because of length discrepancies of the first versus the lesser metatarsals (see Fig. 30–3). Other procedures performed but not recommended were double-stem silicone arthroplasty of all the MPJs. This had been considered and performed with both the Swanson-type hinged implant and the Sgarlato lesser MTP joint implants. Problems occurred with dislocation of the stems and difficulty obtaining a properly sized implant as well as one that fit properly within the medullary canals.[26] They concluded that wire stabilization for 4 to 6 weeks relocated the plantar fat pad under the distal metatarsal segments and was more important than the use of lesser MTP joint implants.

More recently, Barouk[27] introduced the concept of a temporary metallic spacer, or "button," that is interposed at the resected MTP joint. He used these in all five MTP joints for forefoot arthroplasty. These "button spacer cups" have a central hole so that a Kirschner wire may be inserted down the long axis of the digital phalangeal and their respective metatarsals. The Kirschner wire may be removed 1 month postoperatively, whereas the buttons are extracted 6 months postoperatively.

Occasionally, proliferative bone at the amputated stumps of the metatarsals has led to plantar keratotic lesions (Fig. 30–5). In an effort to minimize this phenomenon, Zang recommended the use of silicone rubber caps over the lesser metatarsals.[28] These were discontinued due to a relatively frequent finding of bony resorption of the distal metatarsal segment underneath the cap (Personal communication, Kerry Zang, 1992).

McGlamry and Martin[29] acknowledged the success of the Hoffmann procedure in the rheumatoid foot as well as its application in a variety of forefoot derangements, including diabetic ulcerations of the forefoot and the pain and deformity of the iatrogenic foot. They acknowledged the success of the plantar approach in the severely deformed foot but preferred five dorsal longitudinal incisions. These incisions

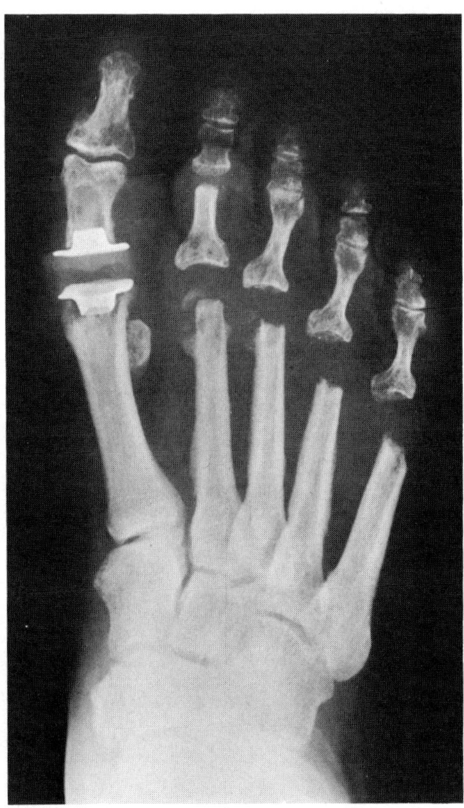

FIGURE 30–5. Heterotopic bone. Heterotopic bone formation at the distal stumps of the lesser metatarsals is not an uncommon radiographic observation. Generally, the degree is not to such an extent that significant symptoms occur or further surgery is warranted. Infrequently, a patient may require additional surgical intervention to simply resect only the proliferative bone.

allow access to both the toes and MTP joints while avoiding the neurovascular structures. Implant arthroplasty was used in the first MTP joint in most situations but avoided in patients with neuropathic disease and prior infection.

In a patient with reasonably good bone stock and particularly in the younger patient, first MTP joint arthrodesis may be the most appropriate procedure combined with panmetatarsal head resections. Stability of the first MTP joint is best accomplished by fusion (Fig. 30–6). The technique has probably been underutilized by podiatric surgeons and with the recent assertions of alternatives to the use of implants, we can expect an increase in its use. Yu and Thornton have suggested that this may be a preferred method of forefoot arthroplasty.[30] The conclusion of Hasselo and associates[31] is that fusion provides a more stable foot for gait and greater likelihood for long-term maintenance of correction in the presence of rheumatoid disease.

THE FOREFOOT ARTHROPLASTY

Obviously, the surgical technique of forefoot arthroplasty varies with the specific approach used and the component procedures included. These require careful preoperative evaluation and planning. The deformities must be assessed, and rational goals of surgery should be formulated by the patient and the surgeon.

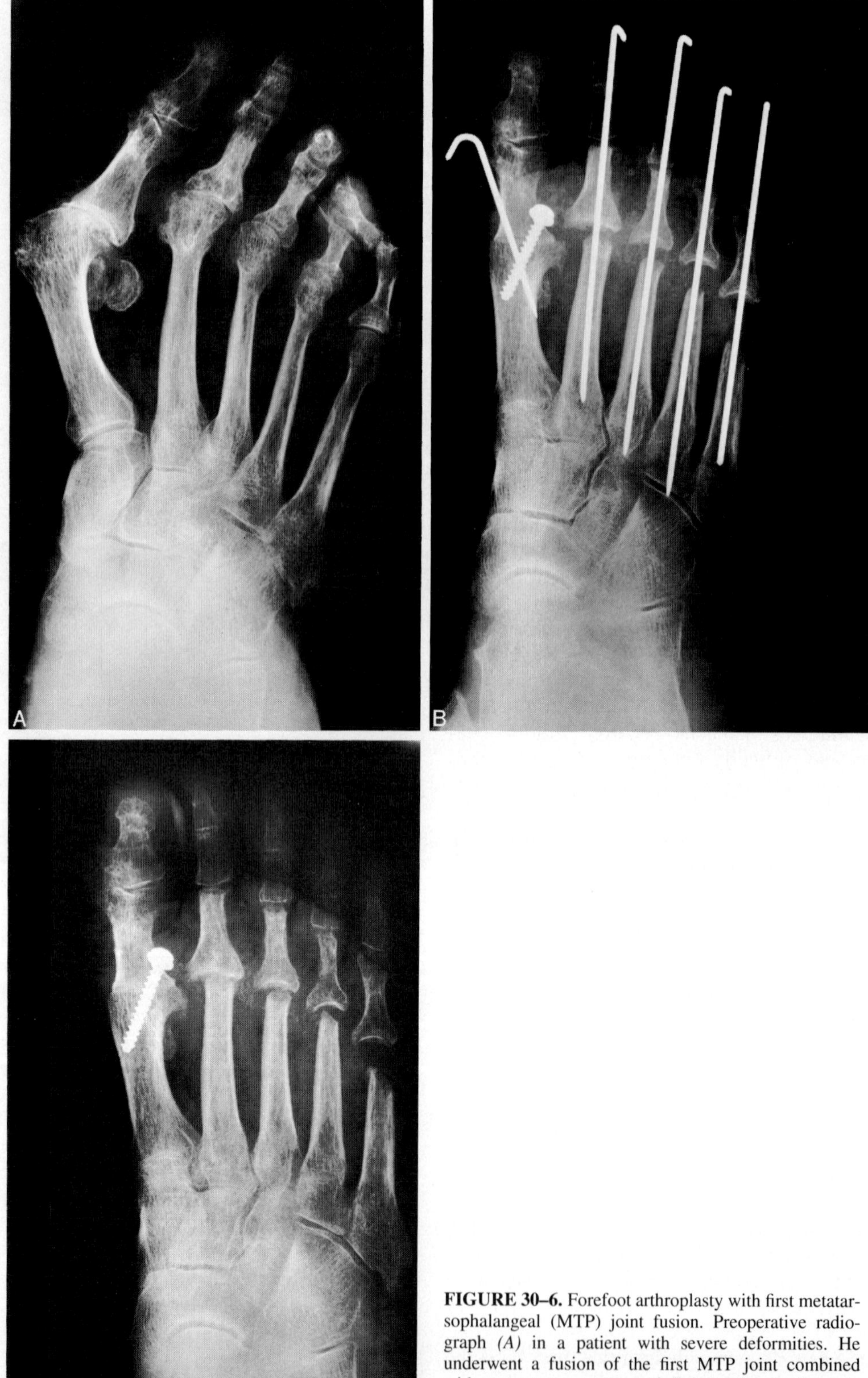

FIGURE 30–6. Forefoot arthroplasty with first metatarsophalangeal (MTP) joint fusion. Preoperative radiograph *(A)* in a patient with severe deformities. He underwent a fusion of the first MTP joint combined with panmetatarsectomy and digital arthroplasties 2 to 5 *(B* and *C)*. First MTP joint fusion provides stability and reduction of the first intermetatarsal angle without a basal osteotomy. *(A* to *C* courtesy of D. Duane Brann, D.P.M., Palos, IL.)

Perioperative Medical Considerations

The medical status of the patient is often the initial area of concern once surgery of some form has been decided on. Whether the patient has rheumatoid disorders or rheumatoid variants, his or her age, activity, and disability as a result of the foot deformities influence the type of procedures performed. Rheumatoid arthritis may affect the greater proportion of synovial joints (Fig. 30–7). Involvement of the tarsus, ankle, knee, or hip as well as spine may influence what deformities are corrected first or which may have a continuing detrimental effect on any surgery.

Age, weight, and quality of the bone influence the decision-making process. Older patients with limited functional demands may do well with some procedures, whereas younger, more active patients may appropriately need other choices. The soft osteopenic bone of rheumatoid arthritis has yielded good results with healing of osteotomies, but their intraoperative fixation and maintenance of stability until union are always tenuous. Questions arise about whether this osteopenic characteristic is one of the disease process or secondary from the administration of corticosteroids and the associated sedentary lifestyle of most patients with significant articular disease.

Immunosuppression as a result of the disease or drug management, including history of steroid use, is important. These patients may require supplemental corticosteroids owing to adrenal suppression, particularly if general anesthesia is anticipated. Careful monitoring perioperatively is important. Overall, most of these types of patients are considered immunocompromised, and the use of preventive antibiotics is a rational choice.

Other ancillary factors are most prevalent with rheumatoid disease and its nonskeletal manifestations, such as a patient still with active disease and the presence of vasculitis. This is probably the leading cause of gangrenous toes after forefoot arthroplasty, not vascular embarrassment due to the surgery. Occasionally, wound healing problems may be encountered but not that commonly. Each patient must be evaluated individually, and cooperation between the surgeon and the internist or rheumatologist is beneficial to the patient.

The optimal timing for surgical intervention is generally when the disease is "burned out," but this is not always practical. Waiting generally results in worsening deformities and the development of concomitant medical problems, both resulting in increased risks from the procedure and greater difficulties in rehabilitation. Thus, timing must be decided on an individual basis, taking all factors into consideration.

Procedural Decision-Making

List the preoperative deformities and develop an operative plan. Generally, a hallux valgus deformity is a prominent aspect of the foot deformity, although hallux varus or even a rectus great toe may be noted. Hallux valgus is the most prevalent deformity, and the severity and aspects of the deformity, such as joint subluxation, intermetatarsal angle, and the presence of an unstable medial column, influence the choice of procedures and the outcomes.

The first MTP joint is worthy of considerable thought. What is the age of the patient? What are the patient's occu-

pation and lifestyle? How severe is the deformity? Is significant metatarsus primus varus present? What is the metatarsal length pattern? It has been our experience that a large degree of deformity, whether hallux abductus or metatarsus primus varus, may be reduced through aggressive resection of the first metatarsal to reduce its length. The length of the first metatarsal should be approximately equal to or slightly less than the second.

In the younger patient, as well as for the more active patient, arthrodesis of the first MTP joint is more a consideration. Arthrodesis is documented to preserve the weight-bearing potential of the forefoot. In addition, arthrodesis helps maintain the corrected position of the lesser toes and may be indicated in patients in whom the disease is not yet in its dormant or burned-out stage.

Should an implant be used in the first MTP joint? Double-stem implants contribute some transverse plane stability, but they should not be relied on to do so. Problems with implants and forefoot arthroplasty have included the surgeon becoming too dependent on the implant for correction. Recurrent or ancillary deformity and adverse reactions may occur.

One of the mistakes in forefoot arthroplasty is the over-zealous resection of the hallucal proximal phalangeal base, as in the Keller arthroplasty. Sometimes more than one half to three fourths may have been resected in attempt to reduce severe deformity and restore a normal digital length pattern. The Keller procedure probably has little indication in the rheumatoid forefoot when resection of the lesser metatarsal heads is performed. It may be appropriate in resection of the phalangeal bases.

Is there deformity or articular disease at the hallucal interphalangeal joint? In the absence of significant articular disease, an arthrodesis of the first MTP joint may be a consideration. Is there deformity of the interphalangeal joint? If there is deformity, an operative procedure may be required at this level. Interphalangeal fusion of the great toe is an option both to correct deformity, be it hallux interphalangeus or hallux malleus, as well as to eliminate erosive disease (Fig. 30–8).

The involvement of the interphalangeal joint of the hallux may influence surgical judgment not to perform a first MTP joint arthrodesis or perform an interphalangeal joint fusion with an implant arthroplasty of the first MTP joint.

The development of hammer or claw toes is usually a part of the lesser MTP joint contracture. Nonreducible lateral and dorsal subluxations lead to severe metatarsalgia, anterior displacement of the fat pad, and production of plantar keratotic lesions. The presence of rheumatoid nodules may lead to sinus formation and the potential for infection. These problems and their severity often dictate both the corrective procedure and its surgical approach. Digital deformities cannot be reduced in the presence of nonreducible MTP joint contractures or subluxations. Occasionally, a capsulotomy and extensor tenotomy or tenectomy may allow reduction, but more often bone resection on either side of the joint is required.

If joint subluxations are present in the absence of metatarsal head lesions, base resections might be a consideration. This is not a common situation. Generally, metatarsal head keratomas are a prominent feature and require resection of the metatarsal heads. It is not usually necessary or recom-

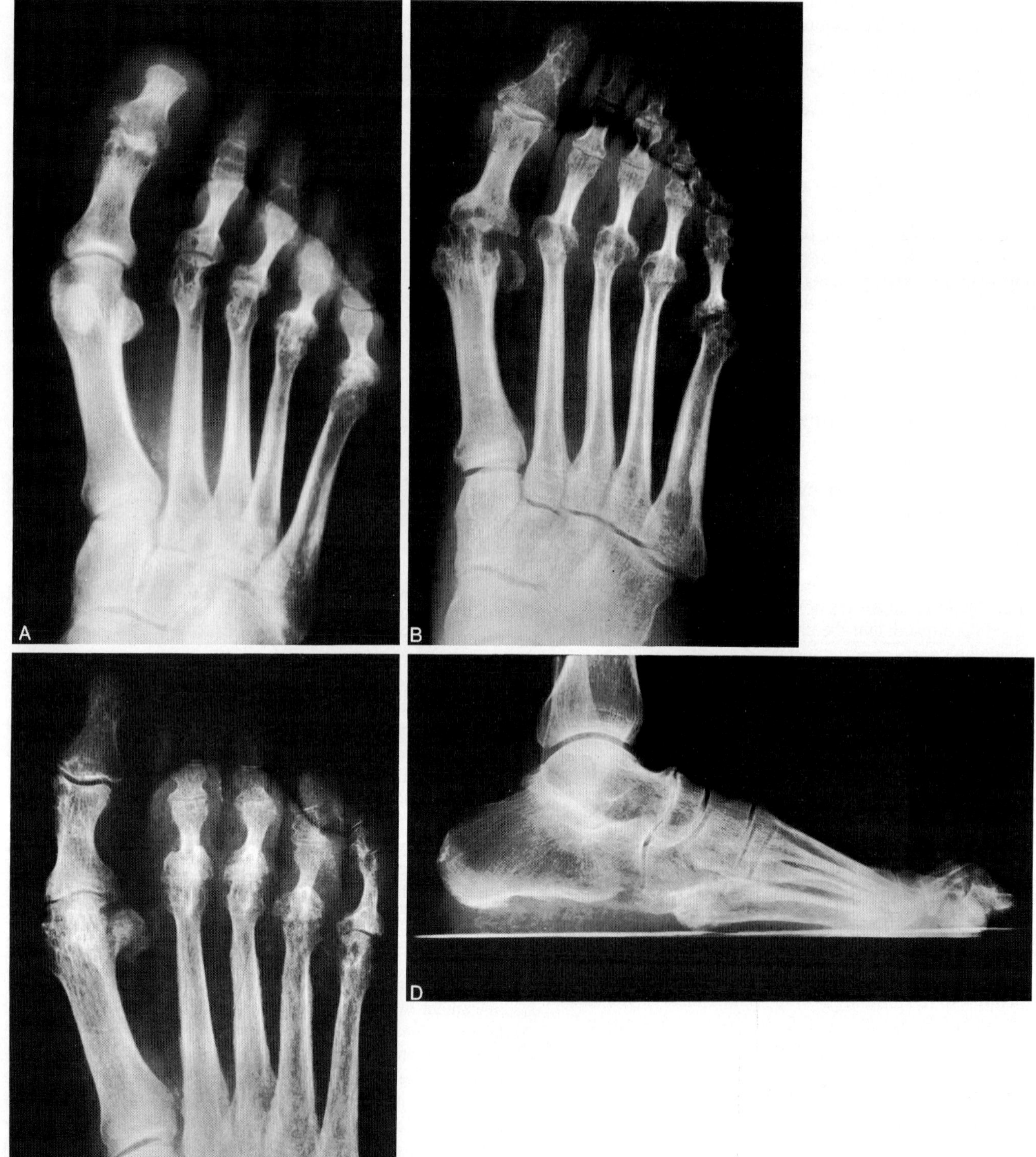

FIGURE 30–7. Erosions of rheumatoid disease. Rheumatoid erosions may begin as marginal lesions in areas of the synovial fold *(A)* but generally progress to lytic or cystic erosions *(B)*. As a result of the synovial disease, joint instability leads to deformity as noted in the forefoot *(C)* or simply in loss of the joint space and ankylosis as seen most commonly in the hindfoot *(D)*.

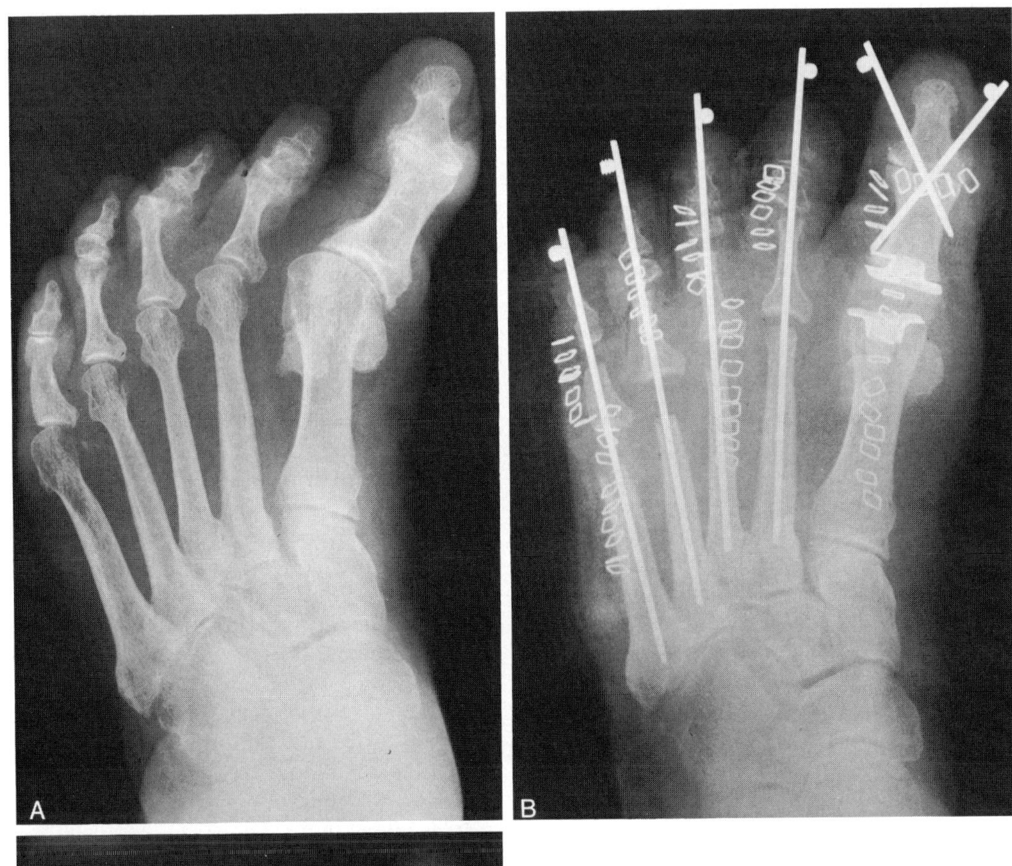

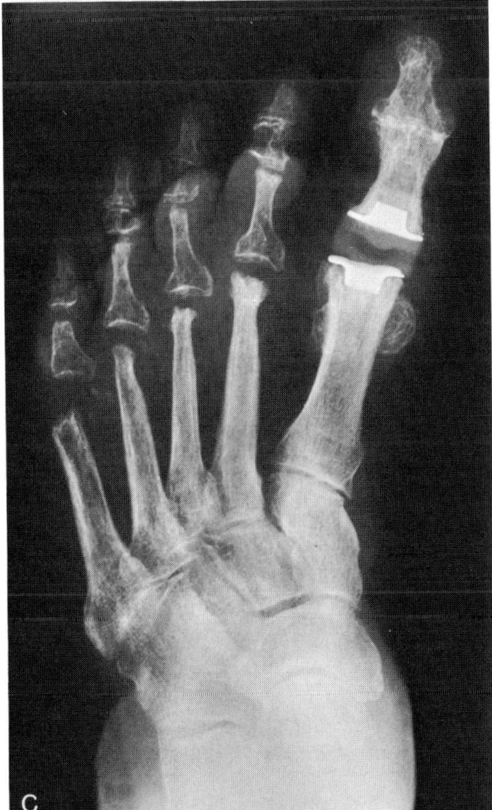

FIGURE 30–8. Rheumatoid deformity with hallux varus. Preoperative radiograph *(A)* of a rheumatoid patient with hallux varus and a hallux malleus who underwent a double-stem first metatarsophalangeal joint implant and hallucal interphalangeal joint fusion with panmetatarsectomy and digital arthroplasties. Intramedullary stabilization of the toes and metatarsals allows reduction of the deformities *(B)*. The follow-up radiograph *(C)* illustrates a good result with these selected procedures.

mended to resect bone from both the metatarsal head and the phalangeal bases. This probably came about because dorsal subluxation of the phalanx is often severe and may limit access from a dorsal approach. Resection of the proximal phalangeal base then allows access to the metatarsal head. Often, only one or two of the lesser MTP joints may present with dislocations. Generally, if the dislocations are severe, or all four of the lesser MPJs are involved, a plantar approach should be considered (Fig. 30–9). If the surgeon elects a dorsal approach, he or she should be adept at dissection and removal of the metatarsal heads because this may be difficult from a dorsal incision. It is our preference to perform pan-metatarsectomies rather than simply to excise one, two, or three of the metatarsal heads.

The digital deformities may be addressed by a variety of techniques. If the deformities are flexible or less severe, resection of the metatarsal heads will allow their reduction. Sometimes, simple manipulation of the toes may allow re-positioning. This is generally performed with Kirschner wire stabilization of the entire ray to maintain position for 4 to 6 weeks. Resection of the phalangeal bases is also a common orthopedic practice and does allow for both reduction of the digital deformity as well as at the MTP joint. Our preference is that of a Post-head arthroplasty or arthrodesis of the proximal interphalangeal joint. Again, Kirschner wires are used to maintain both correction of the digital deformity and maintenance of the MTP joint reduction.

Generally, the disease process alters the biomechanics to the point where little in the way of normal function is present anywhere in the lower extremity. Most of the procedures to be discussed in the following section are ablative in that the synovial joint is sacrificed either to yield a simple resection arthroplasty to allow reduction of deformity or produce stability through fusion of the abnormal joints.

SURGICAL APPROACH

The presence and severity of the involved joints provide the rationale for selection of the component surgical procedures. The need to excise rheumatoid nodules or fixed severe MTP joint dislocations may suggest access via a plantar approach for metatarsal head resections. If the digital deformities are significant, individual arthroplasties or fusions may be combined with a dorsal approach via individual incisions (Fig. 30–10). Performance of partial phalangectomies of the proximal portions of all the phalanges may be accomplished through a dorsal transverse approach if combined with resection of the metatarsal heads; both may be performed through a single dorsal linear incision along the midline of the toe but extended proximal for the metatarsal resection.

The severity of the hallux valgus deformity is usually the governing factor in whether a separate incision will be required for its correction. A fusion or implant arthroplasty of the first MTP joint requires greater exposure than does simple excisional arthroplasty. A plantar transverse approach may be combined with a linear dorsal or medial incision to the great toe.

The dorsal and plantar approaches to forefoot arthroplasty are discussed first, followed by some specific details regarding implant arthroplasty and first MTP joint arthrodesis.

Dorsal Approach: Three to Five Linear Incisions (Pan-metatarsectomy). The dorsal approach to deformities of the

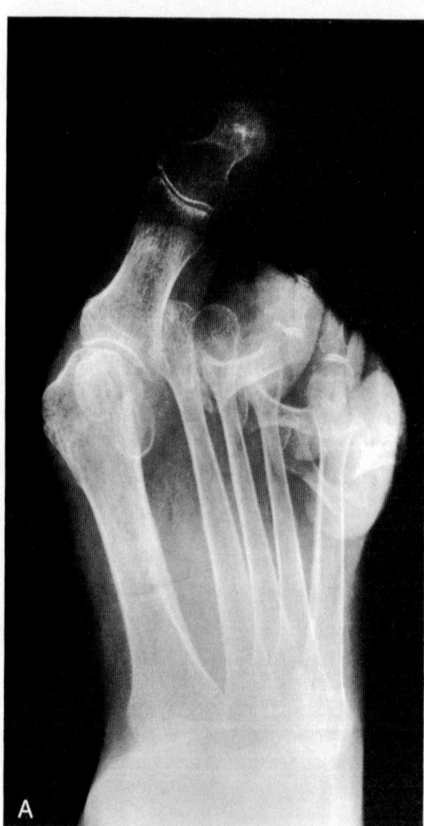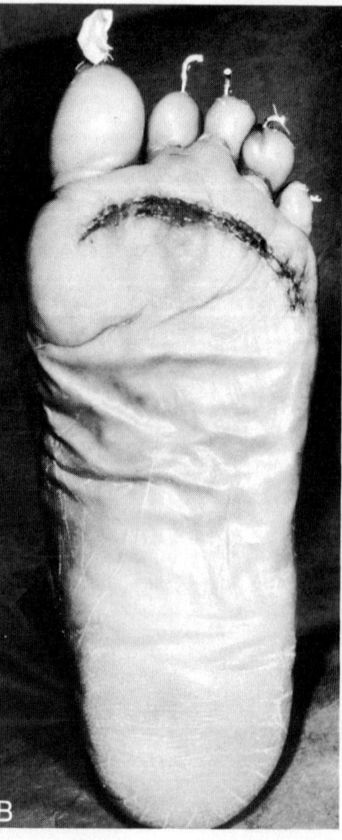

FIGURE 30–9. Rheumatoid arthritis with severe dorsal dislocation. Preoperative radiograph (*A*) of a patient with such severe dorsal luxation of the lesser metatarsophalangeal joints that there is proximal migration of the phalangeal base on their respective metatarsals. It is cases such as this that illustrate the prudence of metatarsal head resections through a plantar approach (*B*).

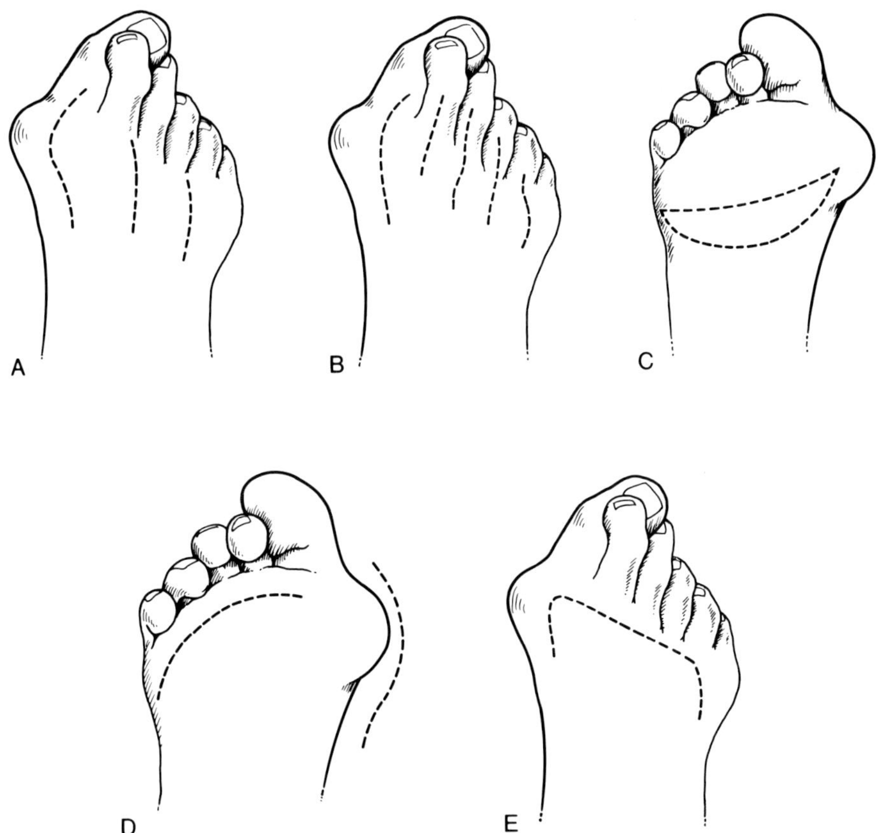

FIGURE 30–10. Forefoot arthroplasty: incisional approaches. *A,* Three linear dorsal incisions: over the first metatarsophalangeal (MTP) joint, between the second and third, and between the fourth and fifth. *B,* Five linear incisions place the incision over each of the toes with proximal extension over the MTP joints. *C,* An elliptical transverse excision wedge skinplasty was advocated to reduce the displaced fat pad. *D,* A transverse planar incision curved with and just distal to the lesser MTP joints may be combined with a medial or dorsomedial incision to the first MTP joint. *E,* A transverse dorsal incision with proximal extensions medial and lateral has been utilized.

forefoot is a practical alternative when the lesser MTP joint contractures are not so severe that access to the metatarsal heads is not significantly impaired.

Variations of this approach usually include a solitary linear incision to expose the first MTP joint. This may be a medial or a dorsal approach and is mainly the preference of the surgeon, although if work at both the MTP and hallucal interphalangeal joints is anticipated, a single medial linear approach is probably best.

For exposure of the MTP joint, the incision extends from the midpoint of the first metatarsal to the midpoint of the hallucal proximal phalanx. This incision affords simple exposure to the MTP joint and access to the articular and periarticular structures that permits adequate bone resection and soft tissue–capsule-tendon balance. Again, this may be performed from a dorsal or a direct medial approach, which has been advocated for its cosmesis. In addition, when multiple linear incisions of the lesser MTP joints are performed, a medial incision provides for a greater separation between skin incisions and may provide less vascular compromise.

The length of the incision may vary depending on the need for basal osteotomy, but its usual length is approximately 7 cm. The dorsomedial approach avoids disruption of the medial proper digital nerve and associated vessels, as does a direct medial or plantomedial incision. Transverse superficial venous tributaries are usually ligated and are small in the

distal portion of the incision. If the incision extends proximally over the base of the first metatarsal, a rather large vein (a component of the dorsal venous arch) will be visualized, and ligation will enhance exposure.

As in most hallux valgus surgery, anatomic dissection of the skin and subcutaneous tissues from the medial joint capsule is recommended if capsular correction is part of the repair. In patients with a rectus toe or hallux varus, only limited underscoring of the medial skin and subcutaneous tissues is necessary.

A linear or lenticular capsular approach between the tendons of the extensor hallucis longus and the extensor hallucis capsularis has proved adequate. If a medial incisional approach is used, a directly medial lenticular capsulotomy is performed.

Alternate capsulotomies include the inverted L, which is usually extended as a T for exposure of the proximal phalanx. The capsular incision begins at the proximal-most aspect of the skin incision and medial to the tendon of the extensor hallucis longus and extends distally over the MTP joint and onto the phalangeal base to an extent required for whatever procedure that is contemplated.

Articular exposure begins with capsular dissection and release of the collateral ligaments from the metatarsal head and the base of the proximal phalanx. Generally, the entire second metatarsal head is resected, and the first should be resected so that it is no longer or even slightly shorter than the second metatarsal. This requires exposure through capsular and subperiosteal dissection of the entire first metatarsal head and all dorsal, medial, lateral, and plantar attachments, whether an implant arthroplasty or a first MTP joint fusion is planned.

The surgical plan is usually to perform the dissection of the first MTP joint and then continue to the lesser MTP joints in sequential order: two, three, four, and then five. Expose each of the lesser MTP joints, then proceed with the joint resections, most typically head resections.

The lesser MTP joints may be approached by adjacent incisions beginning from the web space between the second and third toes and between the fourth and fifth toes. Usually these incisions allow easy access for most deformities. An alternative, particularly when digital arthroplasties are performed, is to use McGlamry's approach of digital longitudinal incisions that extend proximally over their respective MTP joints. In the presence of MTP joint dislocation, this incision offers limited exposure to the metatarsal heads, which allow for easy resection of the base of the proximal phalanx and, subsequently, the metatarsal heads. If the surgical plan is to remove only the metatarsal heads and the proximal phalanx is dislocated dorsally, an alternative approach may be desirable.

Dorsal incisions may be placed over each of the MTP joints or between adjacent joints, or some combination; for example, the second and third MTP joints are easily exposed through an incision between the two, but in severe tailor's bunion, an incision between the fourth and fifth MTP joints may not give adequate exposure for resection of the fifth metatarsal head. Caution with the width of intervening skin island between incisions is necessary because vascular embarrassment is a potential complication.

The initial incision through the skin and subcutaneous tissue should be extended down through the superficial fascia exposing the MTP joint. This is true whether the incision lies between adjacent MTP joints or, in the case of a single incision, directly over the MTP joint. Dorsal venous tributaries may be numerous and require ligation.

Usually, the most prominent finding is that of the bowstrung extensor tendons over their respective MTP joints. In most instances, 1 to 2 cm of the long extensor tendon is excised. Generally, if this is performed at each of the lesser MTP joints, significant relaxation and improved access to the MTP joints are accomplished.

Two techniques of soft tissue dissection are used to expose the lesser MTP joints themselves. In instances wherein no joint dislocation is present, the lesser MPJs are exposed through linear capsular incisions down to bone. Subperiosteal dissection at the anatomical neck allows access for right-angle retractors. With distal traction on the respective toe, the collateral ligaments and joint capsule may then be released through intra-artictular dissection. Neck osteotomy then allows for easy removal of the metatarsal head.

Occasionally, it is necessary to osteotomize the metatarsal before the head is completely dissected free of all soft tissue attachments. This is often the case in complete dorsal luxation with the base of the proximal phalanx sitting on top of the metatarsal head. This second technique is used when significant dorsal contractures or dislocations, or both, are present at the lesser MTP joints.

This also involves a linear approach to the MTP joint, but following exposure of the metatarsal neck, the bone is then osteotomized. Then, with either a Brown or bone forceps, the distal metatarsal fragment is grasped near the osteotomy. With dorsal traction, the metatarsal head will rotate, giving access to the plantar aspect of the MTP joint.

The collateral ligaments and soft tissue attachments may then be severed by placing a No. 15 blade in plantarly and cutting upward to either side.

Partial metatarsectomy with resection at the surgical neck is not recommended owing to the greater likelihood of proliferative bone and subsequent plantar lesion. Resection of the entire metatarsal head at its anatomical neck provides more joint space, and the cut surface of the distal diaphysis usually heals with less bone proliferation. When metatarsal heads are resected, care is taken to ensure maintenance of the metatarsal parabola. This holds greater likelihood of even weight transference (Fig. 30–11).

Once all the metatarsal heads have been resected, the distal stump is rounded with a rotatory bur. We have performed variations of this procedure that included placement of double-stem silicone implants at each of the MTP joints as well as implantation of only the first with use of Kirschner wires to stabilize each of the lesser rays. Generally, once the metatarsal head resections are completed, the toes are then dealt with again in a sequential order from second through fifth.

Digital procedures may include simple manipulation that may be manually reducible once the MTP joint contractures have been released. This reassessment is recommended particularly in patients who do not present with individual keratotic lesions at the proximal or distal interphalangeal joints. Sometimes, only one or two toes must be dealt with, most often the fifth or second toe.

Most of the decision-making process needs to be performed preoperatively because this will influence the planning of skin incisions. If linear incisions were made between adjacent MTP joints, converging transverse semi-elliptical incisions are made across the interphalangeal joints. Either a Post-type digital arthroplasty or a peg-in-hole arthrodesis is our choice of procedure.

The toes are then realigned and stabilized through the use of Kirschner wires. These Kirschner wires are placed in a retrograde technique wherein 0.062-in. smooth wires, in either 6- or 9-in. lengths and pointed at either end, are inserted into the toes from a proximal to distal direction. In a digital arthroplasty, the wire is initially inserted into the base of the middle phalanx. If a digital arthroplasty was not performed, the wire is inserted into the base of the proximal phalanx. The wire is inserted distally into each toe generally from the second to third, fourth, and then the fifth. Once the wire pierces the end of the toe a few inches, the surgeon goes on to the next toe. After all four wires have impaled the digits, the wires are then retrograded across through the proximal phalanges (in digital arthroplasties and otherwise across the MTP joint resections) until the wire is secure within the proximal portion of the metatarsal. No effort is made to deviate from the metatarsal declination during the placement of the Kirschner wires. The toes should be aligned parallel and directly in line with their respective metatarsal (see Fig. 30–11). Wire caps (Jurgan Pin Balls [Jurgan Development & Manufacturing, Madison, Wisconsin] or plastic caps) are placed on the wire at the end of each toe, and the wire is cut short.

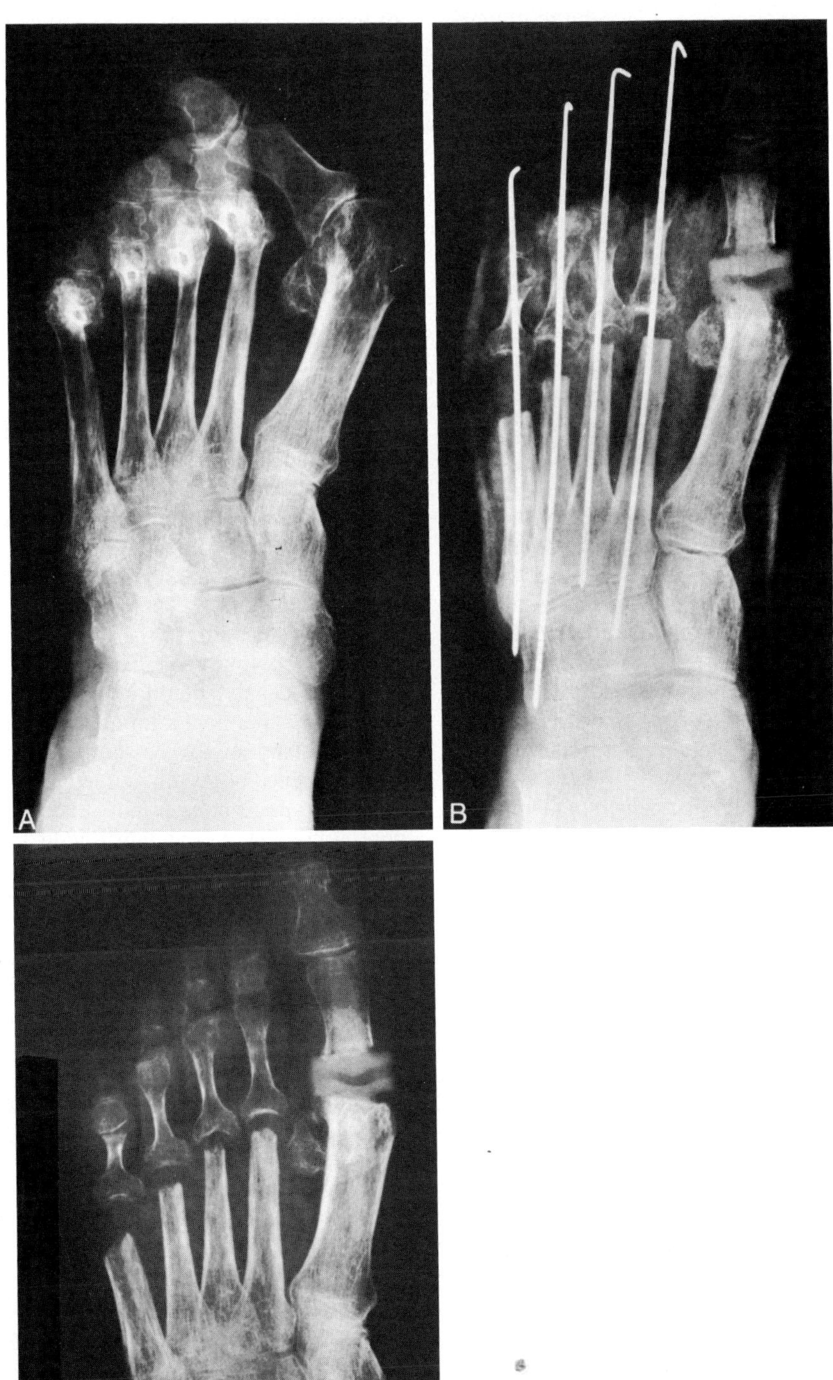

FIGURE 30–11. Forefoot arthroplasty: Kirschner wire stabilization. Preoperative radiograph *(A)* of a patient with severe forefoot deformities. Good reduction was accomplished with panmetatarsectomy, and this was maintained with the use of intramedullary Kirschner wires in the second through fifth rays *(B)*. Follow-up radiograph *(C)* was taken at 3 months postoperatively. Care was taken to maintain the metatarsal parabola.

Once the wires are in place, attention is then redirected to the first MTP joint wherein the implant or arthrodesis may be completed. In an implant arthroplasty, generally all work up to insertion of the actual implant is performed before the insertion of the wires, then the implant is inserted and the wounds are closed. In an arthrodesis, first metatarsal resection is performed following resection of the lesser metatarsals. The Kirschner wires are inserted, and then the proximal phalanx resection is performed so that the hallux will be placed in a position parallel to the second toe, and attempts are made to achieve similar length.

Resection of the first MTP joint should begin on the metatarsal side of the joint. Obviously, the exact manner may vary depending on whether an arthroplasty or a fusion will be performed. Generally, fusions are recommended in younger and more active patients, whereas implants allow early mobilization and weightbearing in older patients. A first MTP joint fusion also maintains the reduction of large, severe deformities.

In implant arthroplasty, following the resection of the first metatarsal head, the base of the proximal phalanx can then be addressed. It is not necessary to excise the entire phalangeal base because resection of the first metatarsal head provides for a good deal of laxity and room to accommodate the implant hinge and its grommets. Assess the overall length of the great toe in relation to the second toe. The hallux should be the same length or just shorter. A long first ray segment often results in first MTP joint instability and recurrent deformity.

The phalangeal osteotomy should just penetrate the plantar cortex. From this point, careful dissection of the soft tissues from the bone helps maintain integrity of the plantar capsule and the aponeurotic insertions of the tendons. Actually after removal of the base, there should be no violation of the plantar tissues; that is, the long flexor should not be exposed.

Resection of the MTP joint provides significant relaxation of the soft tissues, although in patients with long-standing deformity, a fibular sesamoidectomy may also be necessary. This may be performed through the original capsular exposure after the osseous resections. There is generally no need for a secondary approach through the first intermetatarsal space.

Even with the precautions described, instability in the sagittal plane may occasionally lead to a malleus deformity. To avoid this problem, tethering of the long and short flexor tendons to each other usually provides good stability to the first MTP joint. Several authors do describe osseous reattachment of the short flexors through drill holes in the phalangeal base. Generally, the bone is of such poor quality that the least done the better, and simple tethering suture has worked fine.

In a rheumatoid foot or an older patient, the bone density is significantly diminished. The surgeon gets a good idea of the quality of bone both from the preoperative radiographs and during the previously described bone resections. At times following resection of the phalangeal base, the contents of the medullary canal seem to almost pour out. This is another reason to perform a subtotal resection of the phalangeal base, because the cancellous bone can be remodeled and provide greater stability of the implant and grommet.

We recommend the Swanson double-stem silicone implant in situations when the surgeon elects to use an implant. There is no place for the use of a hemi-implant unless phalangeal base resections are performed without concomitant resection of the metatarsal heads. A Keller hemi-implant procedure in combination with metatarsal head resections would create a situation of severe length discrepancy between the first and lesser metatarsals that usually leads to instability of the first MTP joint; valgus deviation of the great toe may be expected as soon as the surgical dressings are removed. In light of the significant bone resections and cortical margins that would otherwise oppose the silicone implant, the use of the titanium grommet as a protective interface prevents insult to the implant. The grommets also seem to decrease the degree of ectopic bone that may encroach on the hinge of the implant and decrease available motion. For these reasons, the Swanson double-stem hinged silicone implant is presently our choice.

The medullary canals in both the first metatarsal and the proximal phalanx are reamed in a tapered fashion. The canals should reflect a negative mold of the implant stem. Implant sizers are used to determine the extent of canal preparation necessary.

Most often a small side-cutting or football bur (e.g., the 4-mm oval side-cutting bur) is used to begin the intramedullary canals. The location of the implant stems within the medullary canals is important. Both within the phalanx and metatarsal, the canals should be placed as dorsal as possible to avoid bony abutment with dorsiflexion. The canal within the metatarsal should also be skewed laterally to avoid overhang or prominence of the hinge medially.

In the type of bone usually encountered during this procedure, following the initial drill hole, the canal is best enlarged to the desired size through the use of intramedullary rasps. If the Dow Corning silicone implants are used, a complete set of rasps for both the proximal and distal stems in each progressive size is available. The shape of the canal is begun with the smallest rasp and then, progressively, a larger one is used until the desired size is obtained. Alternatively, a rasp on the reciprocating saw may be used. Intermittently, the size of the canal is assessed with the use of the implant sizers.

As described earlier, titanium grommets are available for the Swanson double-stem implants. These are recommended because only beneficial consequences can be anticipated. Each size of implant has a corresponding pair of grommets. The grommets are press-fit into the medullary canals of the metatarsal and proximal phalanx. It is not usually necessary to enlarge the medullary canals for fit of the grommet. In most patients undergoing this procedure, the bone is relatively soft, and the grommet can easily be press-fit with hand pressure from the grommet inserter. The inserter improves the surgeon's ability to press-fit the grommet. In dense bone, it may be used as a tamp and tapped with a mallet.

Once the canals are prepared to their exact size, copious irrigation is performed to remove all bone debris that in itself may cause an inflammatory reaction. The correct size of implant is requested and usually placed in saline or antibiotic solution.

The only permissible tampering with the implant is shortening of the stem, and this is really an archaic situation unless the short-stem implants are unavailable. Any other remodeling of the implant must be avoided because early failure of the implant may be precipitated by the introduction of a stress riser.

The implant is then brought to the operative field in a cup of saline or antibiotic solution and placed directly into the wound. The medullary stem of the first metatarsal is inserted first. Plantarflexion of the hallux then allows insertion of the distal stem into the proximal phalanx. Insertion of the implant should be performed without the implant touching the skin. Some surgeons prefer to simply remove the implant from the packaging and place it directly into the wound.

It must be remembered that flexible implant arthroplasty is an adjunct to resection arthroplasty. This type of interpositional arthroplasty is dependent on adequate bone resection and soft tissue release to alleviate the preoperative deformity.

Before capsular closure, the reduction of deformity and the requirements for any adjunctive capsular repair are determined. In most instances, a medial capsular flap is fashioned as a proximally based long U-shaped flap that can then be advanced distally. This capsular flap reinforces the medial side of the joint and acts as a strut to maintain the position of the toe.

Capsular closure is performed with the surgeon's preference of absorbable materials. Our usual choice is 2–0 or 3–0 Dexon or Vicryl sutures, and the medial margin of the extensor hood is also incorporated into the capsular closure. This accomplishes an important function of medializing or maintaining the vector of pull of the tendon of the extensor hallucis longus. Bow-stringing of this tendon laterally may destroy the stability of the joint reconstruction, yielding transverse and frontal plane deformities postoperatively.

Subcutaneous and skin closure is left to the surgeon's preference. Drains are usually not necessary, and a small amount of corticosteroid, usually dexamethasone phosphate, infiltrated periarticularly diminishes postoperative edema and pain. A fluff compression dressing is used postoperatively, splinting the toes in a rectus position and maintaining it in a somewhat plantarflexed position to aid in postoperative toe purchase.

Dorsal Transverse Approach. The dorsal transverse approach described by Fowler[12] and Marmor[9] places an incision over the MTP joints in a medial to lateral fashion. Some authors have extended the incision proximally, laterally, and, in particular, medially to improve exposure of the first MTP joint. Other combinations may include a transverse approach dorsally over the lesser MTP joints combined with a medial lineal approach to the first MTP joint.

The dorsal transverse approach has most often been used for resection arthroplasties of the base of the proximal phalanges, because they may lie superior or dorsal on the lesser metatarsal heads.

Exposure and bone resections must be carefully planned. Usually, chronologic exposure and resection of the second then third, fourth, and fifth MTP joints are performed. Only through the soft tissue laxity created by the resection of the lateral joints can the first MTP joint be exposed with minimal trauma. Alternatively, a separate medial incision to the first MTP joint is made.

The dorsal transverse incision affords good exposure for base resections, although the exposure for resection arthroplasty of the metatarsal alone may be difficult. As described for a Clayton-type procedure, once the base resections are performed, sufficient soft tissue laxity is present, thus allowing for subsequent remodeling of the metatarsal heads if desired. This approach may be advantageous for the timely excision of the digital proximal phalangeal bases and has the obvious advantage of a solitary incision requiring only one closure. Kirschner wire stabilization of the respective rays is easily accomplished. Adequate exposure for MTP joint implantation is also provided. The incidence of wound complications, including skin slough and prolonged edema, may be greater owing to the incision coursing across neurovascular structures.

Plantar Transverse Approach. The plantar transverse approach can be considered analogous to the dorsal transverse approach regarding osseous exposure. The dorsal exposure should be considered when the surgeon desires to resect the phalangeal bases in the presence of severe dorsal subluxations of the MTP joints, whereas a plantar incisional approach is considered more appropriate for the same situation but when the surgeon prefers to resect only the metatarsal heads. A single plantar incision has been adequate, although combining an excisional skinplasty has been advocated to reduce the anterior displacement of the fat pad and the skin. This is often a prominent feature of long-standing deformity.

When resection of plantarly luxated metatarsal heads is planned. The incision is placed distal to the weightbearing surface of the ball of the foot almost in the crest area of the toes. In keeping this transverse incision distal, less damage to the neurovascular structures is seen and, subsequently, less postoperative swelling or vascular complication is noted. Certainly, less effort with less aggressive retraction is usually noted in removal of the metatarsal heads. Working from the bottom of the foot is more difficult for any subsequent remodeling of bone or dorsal capsule and tendon work. Although it is certainly possible, more difficulty is encountered on placement of Kirschner wires, if this is the desire of the surgeon, across the resected joint segments. A retrograde technique as described earlier is recommended, but a capable assistant is mandatory for proper placement.

Usually, the plantar incision is combined with a dorsal or medial lineal incision over the first MTP joint for exposure to that joint. The plantar transverse incision is then used for exposure of the lesser MTP joints.

PROCEDURAL VARIATIONS

First Metatarsophalangeal Joint

Resection Arthroplasty. Resection arthroplasty has the advantage of avoiding many of the complications associated with implanting a foreign material into the human body. Obviously, there can be no host reactions to the implant or need for additional surgery to remove a failed implant. However, there are also a number of problems that can arise related to lack of the stabilizing force that is afforded by some implants. Either a double-stem implant or arthrodesis has been favored for its stabilizing effect on first MTP joint position.

Certainly, a fusion provides for the greatest degree of stability not only in the transverse plane but all planes. Resection arthroplasty is likely as well to result in a progressively shortened toe. Because there is no spacer, the toe will be shorter than would otherwise be the case.

Resection arthroplasty probably has its biggest advantage in that it is a similar procedure to that being performed on the lesser rays. In performing a resection arthroplasty on the first MTP joint, less exposure is generally necessary, and the procedure may performed from the same incision (e.g., dorsal or plantar transverse). The type of resection arthroplasty performed is generally predicated on the procedures performed at the lesser MTP joints. If phalangeal base resections were being performed at the lesser MTP joints, a base resection of the hallucal phalanx would be appropriate. If lesser metatarsal head resections were being performed, osseous resection of the first metatarsal head would be most likely to succeed.

Some surgeons have advocated resecting the base of the proximal phalanx and leaving the first metatarsal full length. However, this results in an uneven metatarsal parabola and is not recommended. If no implant is to be used, the base of the proximal phalanx can be left alone, and the primary resection is done on the first metatarsal. If the lesser metatarsals are to be resected at their anatomical necks, the first metatarsal needs a more generous resection than would be necessary if partial metatarsal head resections are planed laterally.

Regardless of the location of bone resection, generally a capsular flap is interposed and Kirschner wire stabilization is also performed as described for the lesser MTP joints.

Implant Arthroplasty. Single-stem or hemi-implants have been used for the past three decades. However, experience has shown that they are associated with a high complication rate and therefore have fallen into disfavor with many surgeons and should probably be avoided completely. The authors feel strongly that a hemiphalangeal implant has no place whatsoever in forefoot arthroplasty. Nonconstrained and semiconstrained double-stem implants are best for forefoot arthroplasty (see Chapter 31).

Most of the implants manufactured for use in the first MTP joint are now made of a silicone rubber elastomer. Abrasion of the silicone due to its apposition with the resected bone surfaces occurs. To prevent some of these problems, the authors recommend the use of metal grommets that form an interface between the bone and the implant. Currently, titanium grommets are available from Wright Medical Technology, Inc., for use with their short-stem flexible-hinge great toe implants.

The bone resection recommended during the use of a first MTP joint implant should be consistent with that of the lesser joints. The most common procedure is total lesser metatarsal head resections combined with a Swanson double-stem hinged implant. In doing so, most bone resection should occur from the metatarsal head (see prior discussion).

At present little experience is available from the use of the recently available total joint systems, Koenig or Bio-Action, and the possible difficulty in maintaining the position of some of the severe hallux valgus deformities treated by forefoot arthroplasty.

Arthrodesis. In the surgical reconstruction of these complex forefoot deformities, some degree of stability to the forefoot is required. The most important location is at the first MTP joint. Arthrodesis or joint fusion accomplishes several functional objectives for the reconstruction. Weight-bearing through the first ray and hallux generally is maintained. Arthrodesis also provides a significant stabilizing influence to prevent the recurrence of deformity not only at the level of the first MTP joint but also extending to the lesser toes and remainder of the forefoot. It may eliminate or pre-

vent painful weight transfer problems once the patient is restored to a functionally active stage.

The sequence of procedures usually includes planar resection of the first metatarsal at or just less than the length of the second metatarsal following its resection. Generally, the final alignment of the hallux should be determined after the Kirschner wires have been inserted into the lesser rays. The surgeon can then assess the proper transverse plane position and overall length of the great toe and resect a portion of the phalangeal base in an appropriate manner. The hallux is fused in 20 degrees of extension to the long axis of the first metatarsal and parallel to the second toe. The hallux should be just slightly shorter than the second toe. The surgeon must not be misled from the position of the lesser toes with the Kirschner wire stabilization at 180 degrees to its metatarsal. The hallux would therefore appear significantly dorsiflexed compared with the lesser toes.

Lesser Metatarsophalangeal Joints

The surgical plan is usually to perform the dissection and joint resection of the first MTP joint and then to continue to the lesser MTP joints in sequence from medial to lateral. These resection can be accomplished either by severing the collateral ligaments, delivering the metatarsal head into the wound and then resecting it, or by first osteotomizing the bone proximal to the condyles and then dissecting the head free working from proximal to distal. When the joint is severely dislocated, the second method is preferred. When one is doing a partial metatarsal head resection (distal to the anatomical neck), the first method is usually performed. Partial metatarsal head resections are not recommended owing to the greater likelihood of proliferative bone (ectopic bone) developing, which is frequently the cause of subsequent new or recurrent plantar callus. Resection of the entire metatarsal head at its anatomical neck provides more joint space, and the cut surface of distal diaphysis usually heals with less bone proliferation.

If rheumatoid nodules are present, they are most often encountered on the plantar beneath the metatarsal heads and the fifth metatarsal base. Their presence and the plan for excision may dictate the operative approach, generally a plantar transverse incision.

Hallux Interphalangeal Joint

In rheumatoid arthritis, involvement of the hallucal interphalangeal joint is common and may require surgical intervention. When performed in combination with forefoot arthroplasty, interphalangeal joint fusion is the most commonly performed procedure. Both interphalangeal and MTP joint fusions are not performed concomitantly. If hallucal fusion is performed, this is commonly combined with either resection arthroplasty with or without MTP joint implant.

Crossed Kirschner wires across the interphalangeal joint are often used in light of the poor bone density generally encountered. This is probably the best approach if an MTP joint implant is used. An axial cancellous screw is generally not appropriate and does not generally hold well in osteopenic bone. An oblique 2.7- or 3.5-mm screw across the interphalangeal joint has been an approach combined with an implant. This screw placement generally holds more securely owing to its engagement of a cortex. A more recent alternative is to use small power-driven staples (usually two or three 7×7 mm) circumferentially around the fusion site; they will not interfere with the implant stem. The fusion should be fixated after reaming of the medullary canal for the implant, and the sizer may be left in place while the fixation is being applied. Inspection of the medullary canal should be performed before insertion of the implant.

In lieu of arthrodesis, occasionally a simple resection arthroplasty of the proximal phalangeal head may be used to reduce deformity. This may be a reasonable alternative in the patient with extremely poor bone stock.

Postoperative Care

These types of procedures may be performed on an outpatient basis, even in elderly patients. Concomitant medical status may be the determining factor in the patient's hospital stay. Cautious observation of the toes following forefoot arthroplasty is mandatory because digital spasm either secondary to vascular embarrassment, arteritis, or vascular spasm due to the Kirschner wire and applied digital traction is occasionally noted. Dressings should be of a fluff type and nonconstrictive. Postoperative radiographs should be obtained to assess adequate alignment and position of the fixation devices.

The type of surgical procedure generally dictates the patient's limitations postoperatively, specifically whether a first MTP joint arthrodesis or basal first metatarsal osteotomy was performed. These procedures require restricted weightbearing afterward for at least 6 weeks. For a forefoot arthroplasty without either of the above, generally the patient is allowed to ambulate immediately postoperatively with a surgical shoe.

Kirschner wires should be left in place for 6 weeks. During this time, the patient must remember that the toes are at 180 degrees to the metatarsal. This may create a problem with the wires extending beyond the ends of the toes and digging into the toe of the shoe. Breakage of an isolated Kirschner wire may also occur—once two of the four lateral wires have been removed, the remainder should likewise be removed, otherwise the frequency of breakage will increase.

Significant edema is present owing to the extent of the operative procedure. A maturation of the tissues occurs, almost as noted with an amputation and the reduction of edema and maturing of the stump that occur. Whirlpools and various physical therapy modalities may be used to cleanse the wounds and help reduce edema.

Moderation in activity is emphasized early on because edema may be considerable the first month or two. Compression dressings are used for the first 4 to 6 weeks followed by 2 to 4 weeks of above-ankle Unna boots applied at weekly intervals. A Jobst compression device is also a good adjunct to reduce edema, if severe. Coban wraps of the toes minimize digital edema and help maintain digital alignment; these may be reapplied daily by the patient or family during this 1- to 3-month period postoperatively.

Once the edema is sufficiently reduced, placement in a soft leather or gym shoe is possible. At this time the patient should be performing contrast baths at home and using elastic stockings from the tip of the toes to below the knee.

Coban wraps of the toes are also helpful both to reduce edema of the toes and maintain their alignment.

At about 2 months postoperatively, an extra-depth shoe with a Plastizote insole is prescribed. Later, a completely normal off-the-shelf shoe may be possible for most patients, although an in-shoe orthotic is generally prescribed to help support the foot because these patients often present with concomitant tarsal pathologic changes, and the surgeon may anticipate the foot to further pronate postoperatively as a result of the forefoot resections.

The patient is followed postoperatively with serial radiographic examinations at 6 weeks and 3, 6, and 12 months after surgery. If osteotomy or arthrodesis is performed, careful observation is important until bony union is accomplished. Radiographically, the surgeon should inspect the stumps of resected bone for proliferation because this may present as a problem in the future.

RESULTS

Rheumatoid patients present with pain and deformity. Pain may be present at rest or more often during walking. The surgical intervention seeks to correct deformity and thereby eliminate a significant degree of the static and functional symptoms noted as a result of the joint deformity.

Preoperative gait analysis confirms the clinical impression of loss of the normal heel-to-toe gait. The rheumatoid foot is generally placed down flat and then lifted as a whole. The patient often shows a short stride with high-pressure loading at multiple sites in the forefoot. These can often be predicted on the basis of the clinical deformities.

The object of forefoot arthroplasty is to correct deformity and eliminate the adverse forefoot loading pattern. The surgical interventions described eliminate pain, deformity, and loading forces through ablative surgery. Resectional procedures by themselves or as a component of interpositional arthroplasty or fusion perform these functions.

The sine qua non of rheumatoid surgery is adequate bony resection to allow soft tissue relaxation and not only correction of the deformities but maintenance of correction. The U.S. orthopedic community choses to perform most of this resection at the level of the proximal phalanx, whereas podiatric surgeons generally perform total metatarsal head resections. Some form of stabilizing procedure must be performed at the first MTP joint to reduce the likelihood of recurrent valgus deformity and provide a stabilizing influence for the lesser rays. Generally, this has evolved with either double-stem implant arthroplasty or arthrodesis of the first MTP joint combined with lesser MTP joint resections.

Surgeons should attempt to assess the patient and his or her deformities and individualize the surgical intervention based on the presentation. Previous surgeons have had good results with a variety of procedures. This discussion has predominantly addressed the patient with advanced deformities. There have been several surgeons who have advocated synovectomy prior to the development of significant deformity. Synovectomies may be indicated for relief of pain not responsive to conservative or medical measures. Aho and Halonen[17] performed a synovectomy on 84 MTP joints in 25 feet on 18 patients. At a mean of 7 years postoperatively, 50% of the patients were still relieved of pain.

Lipscomb and colleagues[18] operated on 69 patients, and in only 22 of these was there excision of bone from all four lesser MTP joints. Wound healing problems were encountered with the dorsal transverse approach that were not noted after they changed to multiple dorsal linears. The authors believed it was the consensus of U.S. surgeons at the time that plantar elliptical excision of skin was not necessary to reduce the anterior advancement of fat pad. They cited inadequate bone resection as an area of concern and recommended aggressive resection or even complete excision of the proximal phalanx to provide such. Emphasis was placed on maintaining metatarsal length to provide better balance and stance.

Barton[32] reported on 65 arthroplasties in 38 patients. These included variations of (1) the Kates-Kessel-Kay procedure, (2) Fowler's operation, and (3) Clayton's arthroplasty. There were 57 plantar incisions and 32 dorsal incisions with 23 total wound complications; these occurred in almost a 2:1 greater frequency in the plantar. Only two patients rated their procedures as a failure.

MacClean and Silver[33] reported on 36 consecutive procedures on 22 rheumatoid patients. They followed Dwyer's recommendation of arthrodesis of the first MTP joint as well as the lesser toes combined with lateral metatarsal head resections. Their results were good to excellent in 76%, with 12% poor results. This was a restatement of Dwyer's earlier position[34] recommending digital fusions to improve toe function.

Cracchiolo and associates[35] reviewed their use of double-stem silicone arthroplasty with an 18-month to 6-year follow-up. Most patients had rheumatoid arthritis; 133 of 159 feet were included in the study. The authors cited almost uniform relief of pain with improved muscle strength in both flexion and extension at the first MTP joint. They concluded that double-stem arthroplasty does provide maintenance of correction and improved function of the foot.

Beauchamp and coworkers[36] compared the results of forefoot arthroplasty with first MTP joint arthrodesis with those of Keller excisional arthroplasty. The authors noted improved clinical appearance of the foot following arthrodesis versus arthroplasty and that this was definitely reflected radiographically as well. They concluded that the arthrodesis maintained the position of the hallux, whereas in the excisional group there was a tendency toward recurrent valgus. The arthrodesis maintained the position of the lesser toes, whereas fibular deviation also recurred with valgus of the great toe.

Mann and Thompson[37] reported their results of first MTP joint arthrodesis combined with lesser MTP joint arthroplasty (modified Kates-Kessel-Kay procedure) in 12 feet and subtotal forefoot arthroplasty (first MTP joint arthrodesis) in an additional 6 feet. In an average follow-up of 4 years, 14 feet were considered excellent, 2 good, and 2 fair. They were enthusiastic regarding the improved functional stability of arthrodesis compared with either resection arthroplasty with or without an interpositional implant.

Betts and colleagues[38] presented their results of a Kates-type procedure through pedobarographic evaluation of forefoot loading patterns. Preoperatively, 68% of the feet recorded abnormal pressure levels during standing, with the most frequent site occurring centrally. Postoperatively, this complication was eliminated, but the outer rays, first and fifth, showed greater loads, for example, 36% abnormally high pressures under the first metatarsal.

Hughes and associates[39] presented rather troublesome results in their 4-year follow-up review of metatarsal head excision in 38 rheumatoid patients. They compared panmetatarsal head excision (1 through 5) with hallux fusion (first MTP joint arthrodesis) plus metatarsal head excision of the lateral rays. They cited plantar callosities and metatarsalgia as more common with first metatarsal head excision but believed that shoe fitting and maintenance of correction was better in this group. Hughes and coworkers also had difficulty obtaining a satisfactory fusion in more than 30% and included painful pseudarthrosis, malalignment of the fusion site, and recurrent deformity of the great toe and lesser toes. Actually, their results with fusion were quite variable, either quite satisfactory or poor.

Cracchiolo and colleagues[40] reviewed 49 implants in 32 rheumatoid patients. This series included both Cutter (Sutter) implants as well as Swanson silicone implants. At an average follow-up of 68.5 months, these patients underwent both clinical and radiographic evaluation, with an 8% failure rate (four patients). Various ancillary procedures were performed in conjunction with the first MTP joint procedure, including excision of the lateral four metatarsal heads in 34 feet.

DISCUSSION

Forefoot arthroplasty refers to the surgical reconstruction of the entire forefoot usually involving all five ray segments. Since the time of Hoffmann, numerous variations of this reconstruction have been proposed. The general axiom of forefoot arthroplasty is to resect adequate bone to reduce the deformities and eliminate the involved articulation. Recently, there have been some advocates of synovectomy early on in the disease before significant deformity has occurred in an effort to eliminate or at least delay pedal symptoms and deformities.

Some of the long-term studies also reveal that short-term results, less than 4 years postoperative, may not be indicative of long-term maintenance of correction and patient satisfaction. Recurrence of deformity and functional problems is possible. Complications include the proliferation of bone at amputated stumps and the risk for pressure lesions or irritation.

Ablative procedures have dominated the surgical management of pain and deformity of rheumatoid arthritis. Hoffmann[5] advocated excisional arthroplasty of all five metatarsal heads. Later, Keller arthroplasty was combined with metatarsal head excision. Clayton[13] followed with excision of both the phalangeal bases and metatarsal heads but acknowledged that the degree of bone excision should be patient dependent in terms of the degree of deformity. This philosophy of selective arthroplasty is discussed by several authors, although generally all five MTP joints are now addressed.

Long-term maintenance of correction is a problem when the surgical excision creates length abnormalities between the great toe and the lesser MTP joints. This is seen when a Keller arthroplasty with or without the use of a hemi–great toe implant is combined with excision of the lesser metatarsal heads. Because of the length discrepancy, recurrent abductus deformity of the hallux is common. Podiatrists then followed Swanson's lead with double-stem implantation of the first

MTP joint, whereas some orthopedists recommended first MTP joint fusion to maintain hallucal position. Without much discussion, fusion is more likely to restore weightbearing through the entire first ray as well as to provide long-term maintenance of correction.

With regard to the lesser MTP joints and the associated digital deformities, there have been advocates of simply resecting the phalangeal base, which allowed both correction of the MTP joint dislocation and manipulative reduction of the proximal interphalangeal joint deformity. Others have recommended panmetatarsal head resections combined with selective digital arthroplasties, although Dwyer observed the beneficial effect of panmetatarsal head resections and proximal interphalangeal joint fusions to provide better function to the lesser toes.

These procedures have provided dramatic short-term reduction of pain and deformity. Most discussions now need to assess the most appropriate procedures for long-term benefits. These determinations are becoming more sophisticated with the advent of computerized gait analysis and pressure sensors. Notwithstanding these advances, careful postoperative management reduces morbidity and improves the final result.

These patients present with the severest degree of deformities and disability, often with inability to wear shoes comfortably or walk without pain. Aggressive surgical intervention generally is gratifying for both patient and surgeon. The deformities can be reduced, and the patient generally is restored to a more normal gait and shoe.

CONCLUSIONS

A multiplicity of procedures have been recommended as part of the surgical reconstruction of the arthritic forefoot. Determinations as to the requirements must be assessed on a case-by-case or patient-by-patient basis. Variations of the Hoffmann-Clayton procedures are generally performed. Our choice to address the deformity at the first MTP joint is with either a fusion or double-stem hinged silicone implant. The contractures or dislocations of the lesser MTP joints are generally treated with either of two procedures as well: resection of proximal phalangeal bases or metatarsal heads. The former has the advantage of also allowing correction of the often concomitant hammer toe deformities, whereas digital arthroplasty may be required with the latter.

Forefoot arthroplasty is indicated not only for the rheumatoid forefoot but also for any acquired disorder that produces severe disabling deformities of the MTP joints and their toes.

References

1. Clayton ML: Correction of arthritic deformities of the foot and ankle. *In* McCarthy JL (ed): Arthritis and Allied Conditions: A Textbook of Rheumatology. Philadelphia, Lea & Febiger, 1985, pp 785–796.
2. Kuhns JG: The foot in chronic arthritis. Clin Orthop 16:141–151, 1960.
3. D'Amico JC: The pathomechanics of adult rheumatoid arthritis affecting the foot. J Am Podiatr Assoc 66:227–236, 1976.
4. Benson GM and Johnson EW: Management of the foot in rheumatoid arthritis. Orthop Clin North Am 2:733–744, 1971.
5. Hoffmann P: An operation for severe grades of contracted or clawed toes. Am J Orthop Surg 9:441–448, 1911.
6. Rodman GP (ed): Primer on the Rheumatic Diseases, 7th ed. JAMA 224(Suppl):1973.
7. Thompson TC: The management of the painful foot in arthritis. Med Clin North Am 21:1785, 1937.
8. Key JA: Surgical revision of arthritic feet. Am J Surg 79:667, 1950.
9. Marmor L: Resection of the forefoot in rheumatoid arthritis. Clin Orthop 108:223–227, 1975.
10. Nissen KI: The place of amputation of all toes. J Bone Joint Surg 35B:488, 1957.
11. Flint M and Sweetnam R: Amputation of all toes: A review of forty-seven amputations. J Bone Joint Surg 42B:90–96, 1960.
12. Fowler AW: A method of forefoot reconstruction. J Bone Joint Surg 41B:507–513, 1959.
13. Clayton ML: Surgery of the forefoot in rheumatoid arthritis. Clin Orthop 16:136–140, 1960.
14. Clayton ML: Surgical treatment of the lower extremity in rheumatoid arthritis. J Bone Joint Surg 45A:1517–1536, 1963.
15. Kates A, Kessel L, and Kay A: Arthroplasty of the forefoot. J Bone Joint Surg 49B:552–557, 1967.
16. Raunio P and Laine H: Synovectomy of the MTP joints in rheumatoid arthritis. Acta Rheumatol Scand 16:12, 1970.
17. Aho H and Halonen P: Synovectomy of the MTP joints in rheumatoid arthritis [Abstract]. Acta Orthop Scand 62(Suppl 243):1, 1991.
18. Lipscomb PR, Benson GM, and Sones DA: Resection of proximal phalanges and metatarsal condyles for deformities of the forefoot due to rheumatoid arthritis. Clin Orthop 82:24–31, 1972.
19. DuVries HL: Major surgical procedures for disorders of the forefoot. *In* Inman VT (ed): DuVries' Surgery of the Foot. St Louis, CV Mosby, 1973, pp 506–550.
20. Mann RA and Coughlin MJ: The rheumatoid foot: Review of literature and method of treatment. Orthop Rev 8:105–112, 1979.
21. Hugar DW and Gucfa CU: Panmetatarsal head resections: The Hoffmann procedure. J Am Podiatr Assoc 64:983–986, 1974.
22. Hodor L and Dobbs BM: Panmetatarsal head resection: A review and new approach. J Am Podiatr Assoc 73:287–292, 1983.
23. Cracchiolo A: Management of the arthritic forefoot. Foot Ankle 3:17–23, 1982.
24. McGlamry ED and Bernbach M: Panmetatarsal head resections: Plantar approach. *In* McGlamry ED and McGlamry R (eds): Surgery of the Foot and Leg. Atlanta, Doctors Hospital Podiatric Education and Research Institute, 1986, pp 156–160.
25. Vanore JV, O'Keefe RG, and Pikscher I: First metatarsophalangeal joint arthroplasty. *In* McGlamry ED (ed): Comprehensive Textbook of Foot Surgery. Baltimore, Williams & Wilkins, 1987, pp 756–807.
26. Vanore JV and O'Keefe RG: Lesser ray implants and lesser MTP joint implants. *In* McGlamry ED, Banks AS, and Downey MS (eds): Comprehensive Textbook of Foot Surgery. Baltimore, Williams & Wilkins, 1992, pp 392–411.
27. Barouk LS: Forefoot Surgery: A New Approach. Presented at the 49th Annual Meeting of The American College of Foot Surgeons, San Francisco, February 14, 1991.
28. Jenkin W and Oloff L: Implant arthroplasty in the rheumatoid arthritic patient. Clin Podiatr 1:213–226, 1988.
29. McGlamry ED and Martin DE: Panmetatarsal head resection: Indications and uses in forefoot reconstruction. *In* DiNapoli RD (ed): Reconstructive Surgery of the Foot and Leg. Tucker, GA, Podiatry Institute, 1990, pp 37–49.
30. Yu GV and Thornton D: First MTP joint arthrodesis revisited: An update. *In* DiNapoli RD (ed): Reconstructive Surgery of the Foot and Leg. Tucker, GA, Podiatry Institute, 1990, pp 156–162.
31. Hasselo LG, Willkens RF, Toomey HE, et al: Forefoot surgery in rheumatoid arthritis: Subjective assessment of outcome. Foot Ankle 8:148–151, 1987.
32. Barton NJ: Arthroplasty of the forefoot in rheumatoid arthritis. J Bone Joint Surg 55B:126–133, 1973.
33. MacClean C and Silver WA: Dwyer's operation for the rheumatoid forefoot. Orthop Trans 3:349, 1979.
34. Dwyer AF: Correction of severe toe deformities. J Bone Joint Surg 52B:192, 1970.
35. Cracchiolo A, Swanson A, and DeGroot-Swanson G: The arthritic great toe MTP joint: A review of flexible silicone implant arthroplasty from two medical centers. Clin Orthop 157:64–69, 1981.
36. Beauchamp CG, Kirby T, Rudge SR, et al: Clin Orthop 190:249–253, 1984.
37. Mann RA and Thompson FM: Arthrodesis of the first metatarsophalangeal joint for rheumatoid arthritis. J Bone Joint Surg 66A:687–692, 1984.
38. Betts RP, Stockley I, Getty CJ, et al: Foot pressure studies in the assessment of forefoot arthroplasty in the rheumatoid foot. Foot Ankle 8:315–326, 1988.
39. Hughes J, Grace D, Clark P, and Klenerman L: Metatarsal head excision for rheumatoid arthritis. Acta Orthop Scand 62:63–66, 1991.
40. Cracchiolo A, Weltmer JB, Lian G, et al: Arthroplasty of the first metatarsophalangeal joint with a double-stem silicone implant. J Bone Joint Surg 74A:552–563, 1992.

CHAPTER 31

Forefoot Implant Arthroplasty

Albert Burns, D.P.M.

Joint prosthetic replacement has been attempted in numerous joints in the body, with varying degrees of success depending on anatomic location. Because the weightbearing joints of the lower extremity are exposed to stresses that either cause or potentiate joint arthrosis, these have been and are likely to remain the principal areas of joint prosthetic development. The individual joints have different success rates, even though the same materials or combination of materials have been used in each. Knee joint replacement has been immensely successful, whereas ankle joint replacement has been virtually a complete failure. Forefoot implantation, including the first metatarsophalangeal joint, the lesser metatarsophalangeal joints, and joints of the digits, has been partially successful.

The success or failure of joint prosthetic replacement has to be measured against what implantation is ideally trying to accomplish. The primary goals of joint implants are to relieve pain, restore function, allow normal mobility, maintain structural stability, and provide a good cosmetic appearance. These five goals do not necessarily have equal value and may vary from patient to patient. From the physician's prospective, however, the two most important primary goals of joint prosthetic replacement are to relieve .pain and restore function. Knee joint replacement has probably been most successful in these two primary goals and has enjoyed success in the others. Forefoot joint replacement in its current state has been successful in relieving pain and accomplishing the secondary goals, but as it stands now there are no functional forefoot implants. For this reason forefoot prostheses have been only partially successful.

The first metatarsophalangeal joint has had the greatest amount of attention, experimentation, and prosthetic development of all the forefoot joints. The main reason is that its function is far more important than that of the individual lesser metatarsophalangeal joints and the digital joints. Also, this foot joint is most often involved in joint arthrosis from both systemic and local causes. This point is illustrated by many examples. The forefoot is the second most common area of the body affected by rheumatoid arthritis. The first metatarsophalangeal joint is most commonly selectively affected by gouty arthritis involving the forefoot. In other more complex problems such as Sjögren's syndrome and Felty's syndrome, the metatarsophalangeal joints still account for 95% of the rheumatoid arthritis involvement. Although the seronegative spondlyloarthropathies more commonly involve the larger joints of the lower extremity, they are less commonly seen, but one of the most common, psoriatic arthritis, involves the digital and metatarsophalangeal joints. Osteoarthritis is the most predominant arthritic process involving the forefoot, and no joint is more effected by this than the first metatarsophalangeal joint. The abnormal biomechanics of the foot that cause the development of hallux abductovalgus often progress to degenerative joint disease of the first metatarsophalangeal joint. Although the first metatarsophalangeal joint has received the most attention, these same conditions, whether a systemic disease process or biomechanical dysfunction, result in digital contractures, subluxations, dislocations, and arthrosis of the lesser metatarsophalangeal joints and the digital interphalangeal joints.

BIOMATERIAL CONSIDERATIONS

Implantation of the first metatarsophalangeal joint was first reported by Endler in 1951, who used an acrylic to replace the base of the proximal phalanx. Over the years, numerous materials were used for first metatarsophalangeal prostheses, including ivory, glass, acrylic, gold, stainless steel, and other metals. Osteoarthritis was the most common cause of the destruction of this joint, and clinical experience showed articular disease predominantly involved the metatarsal side of the joint. The initial attempts in the late 1960s by both Swanson and Seeburger were thus directed to metatarsal head replacements with metal implants (in 1965, Seeburger implanted a Durallium cap to replace the first metatarsal head). These metal implants failed because they caused osteoporosis, bony resorption around the implant, loosening and dislocation of the implants, and fracturing of the bone.

These early failures illustrate the two most important considerations concerning the composition of the implant material. These are the elastic modulus of the material and the coefficient of friction of the component parts or the component part with anatomic structure. Synovial joints glide easily because of the way that synovial fluid lubricates the articular cartilage of joints. There is, therefore, very little stress passed through the bones as a result of friction. If the prosthesis used to replace a joint has more friction between its components parts or between the implant and bone, then more stress is going to be transmitted through the implant and the bone. If that stress exceeds the tensile strength of the bone or implant, then one or the other, or both, will fracture. The elastic modulus of the implant material refers to the way the material is constructed with standardized dimensions for flexibility. This imparts on the implant the degree of deformation possible and its tensile strength. Ideally, the elastic modulus of the implant should equal the elastic modulus of bone. If the material used is firmer or more rigid than bone, then stresses to the implant site may result in bone resorption or fracturing. If the implant material is more flexible than bone, then stresses passing through it may result in permanent deformation or fracturing of the implant. Besides the appropriate coefficient of friction and elastic modulus, there are other properties that the implant material should possess. The material should be able to withstand contact with tissue enzymes and not deteriorate, not induce a sensitivity reaction, be chemically inert, be incapable of inciting a foreign-body reaction, and be noncarcinogenic. The implants themselves should be capable of resisting deforming forces, returning to their original shape, and being sterilized.

The implant material that has been most universally used in forefoot prostheses almost to the point of being exclusive is silicone. Silicone was first used in 1965. Silicones are polymers of silicone and oxygen, and they are manufactured as resins, elastomers, or fluids. Silicone rubber is manufactured from high-viscosity silicone fluid and a particle size silicone that imparts an effective tensile strength. The silicone rubber is heat stable and may be autoclaved. It is radiopaque and nonadherent to tissues. Silicone rubber has a low-elastic modulus, so when it is subjected to loads within the functional range the implant will deform, but on release the implant will return to its original configuration. The low-elastic modulus also allows the implant to act as a shock absorber. The silicone rubber is considered to be biologically inert, but it has the capability of absorbing cold sterilizing solutions and gases. There is no direct fixation of silicone implants to bone; therefore, the potential for bone resorption and implant loosening is minimized. Because silicone elastomers constitute the vast majority of all forefoot prostheses, there are certain technique considerations that apply to all of them. Silicone tends to develop a static charge, after sterilization, that can attract lint and dust from gauze and powdered gloves. All silicone implants should, therefore, be immersed in sterile solution before implantation. Any tears, flaws, or imperfections in the silicone implant may result in fracturing or other implant failure. Therefore, implants should be handled only with blunt instrumentation, and the only acceptable modification of these implants is shortening the stem.

Implants that are fixed in place cause bone resorption, bone fracturing, implant fracturing, or dislocation, so the implants should be allowed to piston. Pistoning allows for a greater dispersion of forces to pass through the implant, and it increases the available range of motion of the implant. The range of motion is increased because pistoning allows greater bending in the stem. Pistoning, however, does increase the abrasion between the stems and the bone, thus increasing the microfragmentation of the silicone implant and the likelihood of reactive synovitis. The amount of motion in an implant made of silicone is inversely proportional to the size of the implant. The smallest possible implant should be used, therefore, but it must be large enough to bridge the resected cortices to prevent it from telescoping into the bone. Steroids should not be used adjunctively with implants. The introduction of any foreign body decreases the number of organisms necessary to cause an infection from 10^5 to 10^2/g of tissue, and anything that would further reduce the patient's immunologic response would be inappropriate.

Conversely, the introduction of an implant does not mandate the use of prophylactic antibiotics. Follow-up studies on surgeries involving a single implant have shown infection rates to be less than 1%. Because it reduces the number of organisms necessary to cause an infection, however, the insertion of an implant is a risk factor that requires consideration of antibiotic prophylaxis. The potential risk is weighed in relation to any other existing risk factors. Other complicating factors that warrant the consideration of antibiotic prophylaxis are an operating time that exceeds 2 hours, procedures that require excessive dissection, procedures that result in tissue having a diminished blood supply, procedures that result in the creation of a large dead space or hematoma, procedures on patients who have an existing infection distant from the operative site, incisions through cicatrical tissue, any breaks in sterility during surgery, and any medical condition that increases the risk of infection. Diabetes is a classic example of a systemic process that reduces a patient's immunologic response. The atrophic skin and minimal subcutaneous tissue seen in rheumatoid arthritis can also be a serious impediment to wound healing and resistance to infection. If the risk of infection is adequate to warrant the use of prophylactic antibiotics, then the choice of antibiotic is based on the most likely pathogen, the current antibiotic profile in the local hospital or community, and the risk of adverse side effects. The most common cause of intraoperative contamination in extremity surgery is *Staphylococcus aureus*. Because the incidence of penicillinase producing *S. aureus* is so high, penicillin is not used. First-generation cephalosporins have become the drug of choice for prophylaxis in these cases. For those patients with documented allergy to cephalosporins, vancomycin is a current alternative. The antibiotic should be administered parenterally at the time of surgery and on a short-term basis, never exceeding 24 hours.

FIRST METATARSOPHALANGEAL JOINT IMPLANTS

Hemi-Implants

The specific criteria for the hemi-implants have virtually precluded their use. The joint arthrosis of the first metatarsophalangeal joint must be restricted to involve only the base of the proximal phalanx. Because the implant is going to be articulating with the head of the first metatarsal, degenerative changes in the first metatarsal head will dramatically increase the coefficient of friction and ensure failure. There must be an adequate range of motion of the first metatarsophalangeal joint, and the presence of a hallux rigidus or limitus contraindicates their use. Limited range of motion will cause jamming of the implant, which would impart undue stress through the implant and bone. This limited range of motion applies to both structural and functional hallux limitus. Hypermobility of the first ray will create a metarsus primus elevatus with weightbearing, which, in turn, will cause a hallux limitus and jamming of the joint. This will cause a failure of the implant. The hemi-implants are, therefore, the one implant design that is contraindicated by uncontrollable pronatory forces, even if all the other criteria are met. To use

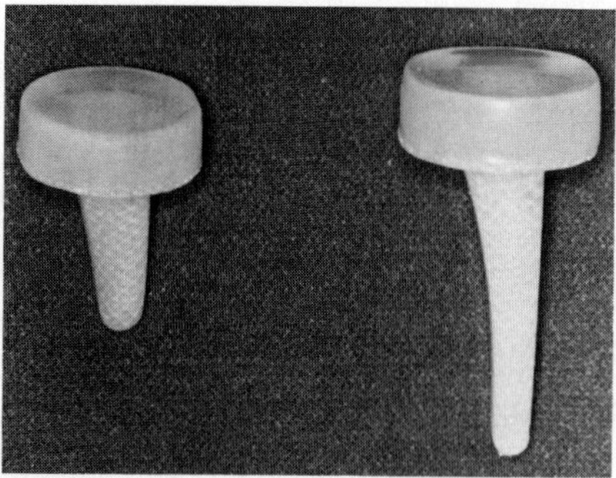

FIGURE 31–1. The standard hemi-implant produced by Dow Corning Wright and Sutter has two stem lengths available. The stems are rectangular, with one concave curved side that is intended to be the plantar aspect of the stem.

these implants, there must be a normal intermetatarsal angle unless it is corrected by an osteotomy procedure. There must also be a normal proximal articular set angle unless it is corrected by an osteotomy or a hemi-angled implant is used.

There are two standard designs for the hemi-implants: the standard Swanson and Weil angled. The implants are designed to supplement resection arthroplasty of the first metatarsophalangeal joint by replacing the resected base of the proximal phalanx with the implant. The Swanson design is a cylinder that has a concave surface for articulation with the head of the first metatarsal, and there is a rectangular stem designed for insertion into the medullary canal of the proximal phalanx (Fig. 31–1). The stem has a concave curvature on one side, which should be plantar at the time of insertion. The implant is available in five sizes, with the choice of two stem sizes: regular and short. There is a sizing set for the implant, and either a silicone or a titanium implant is available. All can be used interchangeably in the right foot and left foot. The titanium implants are available with the short stems only, and the stems are square, lacking the plantar curvature in the standard models (Fig. 31–2). The Weil angled hemi-implant has the additional modification of a 15-degree angulation of the cylindrical base in the transverse plane (Fig. 31–3). The thicker side of the angled implant is placed to the lateral aspect of the metatarsal head. To make the implant interchangeable for both the right and left feet, the rectangular stems have no curvature. The implant is available in three anatomic sizes, and it has only the regular stem size. There is a sizing set for the implant, and it is available only in silicone.

Serious questions have to be raised about the use of these implants. The coefficient of friction of either silicone or tita-

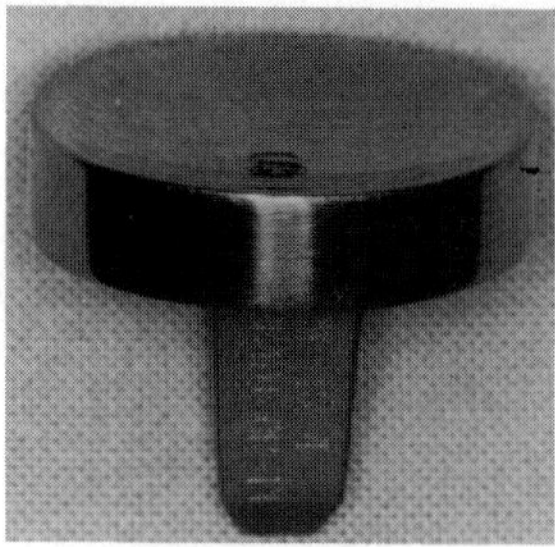

FIGURE 31–2. The standard hemi-implant is also available in titanium produced by Dow Corning Wright.

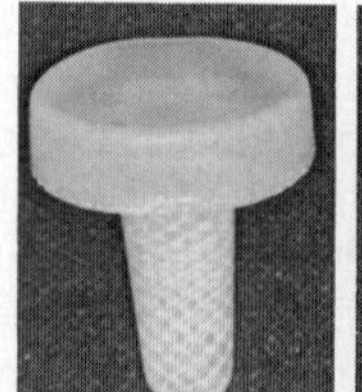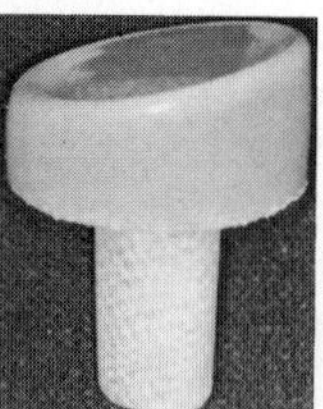

FIGURE 31–3. The hemi-angled implant is shown in comparison with the standard short-stemmed hemi-implant. The hemi-angled implant is only available with the short stem, and there is no concave curvature. The buildup for the lateral side of the base is at a 15-degree angle in the transverse plane.

nium articulating with a metatarsal head will far exceed that of a synovial joint. That, coupled especially with the titanium model, in which the elastic modulus is extremely more rigid than bone, raises the question of whether this implant is ever indicated. Additionally, because almost all patients with joint arthrosis have some limited motion and involvement of the first metatarsal head, its use seems to be precluded in all instances.

The operative technique for these implants is a modification of the Keller bunionectomy technique. One modification is to perform a capsulotomy that can be used for positional corrections. The base of the proximal phalanx is resected with power instrumentation perpendicular in both the transverse and sagittal planes. This will usually involve anywhere from one fourth to one third of the proximal phalanx, depending on the size of the implant. After removal of the base of the proximal phalanx, the sesamoids are examined to make sure there are no adhesions and that they have retracted. A stem hole is fashioned in the remaining proximal phalanx, using either burs or broaches, or a combination of the two. The stem hole is fashioned as dorsally as possible to avoid exiting through the concave plantar cortex of the phalanx and to help ensure hallux purchase postoperatively. When inserting the implant, it should neither be handled with the gloved hand nor touch the patient's skin.

This is an ambulatory procedure unless a concomitant base osteotomy was performed. The patient may ambulate in a postoperative shoe, and passive and active range-of-motion exercises are started immediately. Sutures are removed at 2 weeks, and the patient may start progressing back to normal shoe gear at that time. Compressive wraps and physical therapy are used as warranted.

Total Hinged Implants

Joint arthrosis of the first metatarsophalangeal joint that involves the head of the first metatarsal or the base of the proximal phalanx is the primary indication for these implants. Hallux limitus or rigidus secondary to joint arthrosis or any other problem is also an indication for these implants. Uncontrollable pronatory forces do not contraindicate their use, and a normal intermetatarsal angle should be present unless it is corrected by an additional procedure. There are currently four total implant types available, all of which are made of silicone: the Swanson flexible toe implant (Dow Corning Wright), the La Porta and Lawrence total implants (Sutter Biomedical, Inc.), and the GAIT (great toe arthroplasty implant technique; Sgarlato Labs, Inc.).

The Swanson flexible toe implant is a double-stemmed flexible hinge implant in which the midsection of the implant

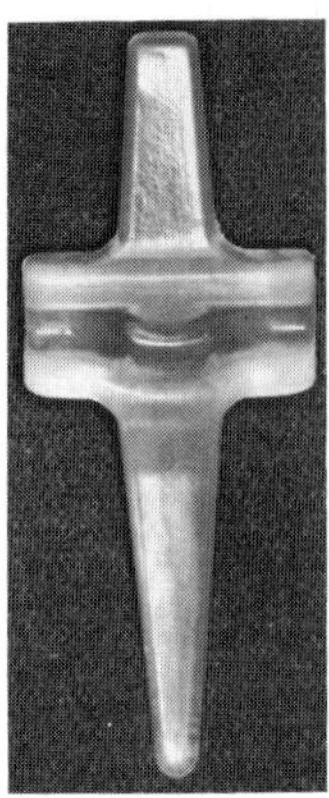

FIGURE 31–4. The Swanson Flexible Toe Implant has a horseshoe-shaped hinge. Both stems are perpendicular to the hinge in both the transverse and sagittal planes.

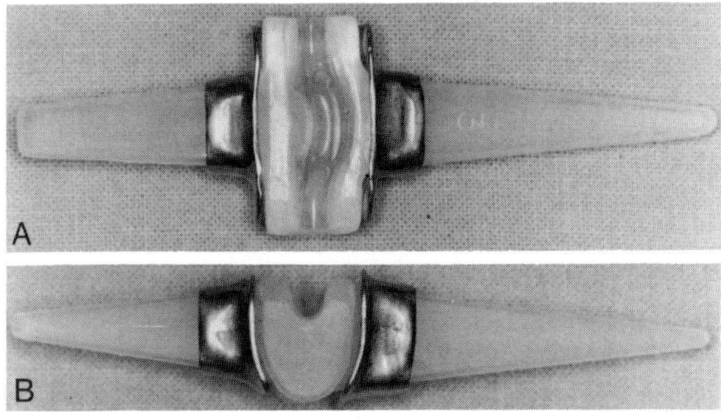

FIGURE 31–5. The Swanson Flexible Toe implant *(A)* with its grommets *(B)*. The grommets are marked with their size and either **P** or **D** for proximal and distal. The grommets are made of titanium, and the sizes correspond to the size of the implant. The implant should be used with either the same size or the next larger size grommet.

is U-shaped and the two stems are perpendicular to this hinge in both the transverse and sagittal planes (Fig. 31–4). The proximal stem is the longest of the two stems, and it fits into the medullary canal of the first metatarsal, whereas the shorter distal stem fits into the proximal phalanx.

The stems are rectangular in cross-section and taper from the hinge out. Their implant is available in two stem sizes, standard and small, and there are eight sizes to choose from. There is a sizing set for this implant. In 1986, Dow Corning Wright introduced the Swanson flexible hinge toe grommet (Fig. 31–5A and 5B). This is a thin, titanium shield contoured to conform to the shape of the midsection of the flexible implant and the base of both stems. The grommet is intended to protect the implant from the biomechanical shearing forces of sharp bone edges during joint motion. The grommets are marked with the size implant that they are intended for as well as with the letters **P** or **D**, indicating whether it is a proximal or distal grommet. Neither the implant nor the grommet requires fixation to bone.

The La Porta implant has a hinge with a broad collar on both sides of the hinge. This design feature is suppose to prevent or retard osteophyte development. The literature states that another design feature is a 10-degree angulation of the metatarsal stem in the transverse plane. This transverse angulation in the metatarsal stem is designed to accommodate for the natural hallux abductus position. This is some-

what misleading, however, because the lateral edge of the proximal stem is perpendicular to the implant hinge, as is the long axis of the distal stem. Therefore, if the bone cuts on the metatarsal and the proximal phalanx are made perpendicular to their long axes, the hallux is going to rest in a straight line with the metatarsal with proper implant seating. There is no intrinsic abduction in the implant itself. To obtain the abduction, the bone must be cut on the metatarsal head; that is, the resected surface of the metatarsal head is abducted or laterally deviated to the long axis of the first metatarsal. Because the medial side of the proximal implant stem is tapered at a 10-degree angle, the metatarsal head bone cut can be angled up to 10 degrees abducted to the long axis of the metatarsal before the medial side of the stem becomes parallel to the medial cortex of the first metatarsal (Fig. 31–6A). Another design feature that is optional is a 15-degree angulation of the metatarsal stem in the sagittal plane (Fig. 31–6B). This angulation is designed to accommodate for the normal metatarsal declination, so the implant can be inserted without losing any of its range of motion with simple weight-bearing. Those implants that have both the transverse and sagittal angulations in the metatarsal stem can be used only in one foot, so they are designated as right and left. The implant that has only the transverse plane angulation may be used in either foot by simply rotating it 180 degrees in the frontal plane, so it is designated as the neutral design. The

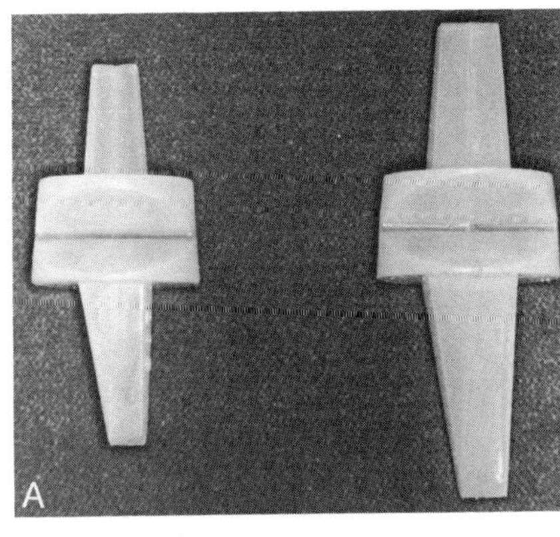

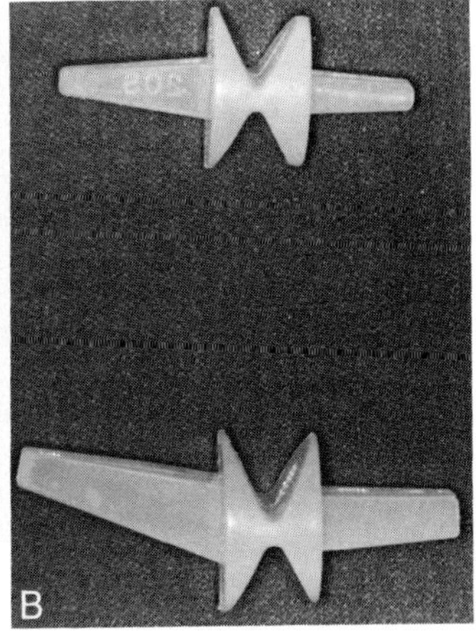

FIGURE 31 6. *A,* The LaPorta total implant illustrating a smaller size neutral and a larger size right. The 10-degree transverse plane angulation of the metatarsal stem that is a standard feature of all the LaPorta implants is illustrated. *B,* The same two LaPorta implants in the sagittal view. The neutral implant has both stems perpendicular to the hinge in the sagittal plane and should be used in patients with a low metatarsal declination angle. The right or left LaPorta implant has the optional 15-degree declination of the metatarsal stem and should be used in patients with a normal metatarsal declination angle.

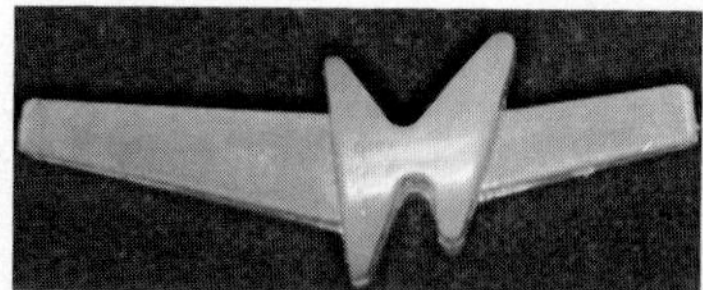

FIGURE 31–7. The sagittal view of the Lawrence implant. The metatarsal stem has a 15-degree declination, and the dorsal angulation of the hinge is 85 degrees. The phalangeal stem is perpendicular to the proximal hinge, and the distal hinge is angled 30 degrees from the proximal hinge so that the bone cuts will preserve the attachment of the flexor hallucis brevis.

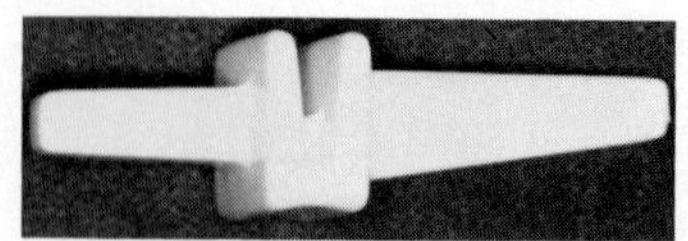

FIGURE 31–9. A sagittal view of the GAIT implant. The implant is similar in design to the Swanson total implant, in that there is a U-shaped hinge and both stems are perpendicular to the hinge in the transverse and sagittal planes. It is similar in design to the Sutter implants in that the hinge has a broader collar to presumably reduce ectopic bone formation.

neutral design is indicated when there is a low metatarsal declination angle. There are four sizes of the implant available and a set of yellow silicone sizers for all three implant configurations. The stems are rectangular in cross-section and taper from the hinge out, and there are broaches that work on a reciprocating saw for fashioning the stem holes in the bone. The hinge is designed with a 60-degree angulation.

The Lawrence total implant also has a hinge with a broad collar on both sides of the hinge, and the hinge is designed with an 85-degree dorsal angle. This implant is designed specifically to preserve the insertion of the flexor hallucis brevis tendon to the proximal phalanx. This is accomplished by angling the distal collar 30 degrees from the proximal collar in a plantar proximal to dorsal distal direction. The distal stem is perpendicular to the proximal collar. The proximal stem is angled 15 degrees in the sagittal plane to accommodate for the first metatarsal declination angle (Fig. 31–7). The stems are rectangular in cross-section and taper from the hinge out. Five sizes are available, and there is an accompanying sizer set. There is also a template instrument used to determine the angulation of the cuts on the proximal phalanx and first metatarsal (Fig. 31–8). The preservation of the insertion of the flexor hallucis brevis by the way the bone cut is made on the proximal phalanx implies the preservation of the weightbearing capacity of the first metatarsal, because the sesamoids do not retract. It also implies, however, that this implant would be restricted to only those patients who have no degenerative process involving the sesamoids, unless the flexor hallucis brevis tendons are resected on purpose. It is rare that any patient with first metatarsophalangeal joint arthrosis would not have involvement of the sesamoids. Additionally, although a normal foot type has a metatarsal declination, patients with painful first metatarsophalangeal joint arthrosis usually have a pronated or laterally deviated foot

type with little or no first metatarsal declination. The use of any implant with sagittal plane declination would be contraindicated because it would cause a hallux elevatus. The usual involvement of the sesamoids in the arthrosis and typical foot type of these patients, coupled with the more difficult bone cuts, have limited the use of this implant.

The last and most recently introduced total hinge implant is the GAIT (Fig. 31–9). The design is somewhat similar to the Swanson total implant. There is a U-shaped hinge, except that the hinge is larger and broader, akin to the two Sutter implants. The proximal collar is larger than the distal collar. The two stems are perpendicular to the hinge in both the transverse and sagittal planes, and the metatarsal stem is larger than the phalangeal stem. The stems are rectangular in cross-section and tapered from the hinge out. Three sizes of the implant are available, and there is an accompanying sizer set.

Surgical Technique. The operative technique for all four total hinge implants is essentially the same; the only difference is in the way the bone cuts are made and how the implant is inserted. The approach is through a dorsomedial bunion incision. An extensor hallucis brevis tenotomy or tenectomy is usually performed. Because there is no positional correction to be achieved and hallux stability is dependent on the implant, the joint is exposed through dorsolinear capsulotomy. The capsule and periosteum are reflected off the base of the proximal phalanx and the head of the first metatarsal. If there is a bunion, it is resected at this time. The base of the proximal phalanx is then resected using power instrumentation. For the Swanson, La Porta, and GAIT implants, the resection is made perpendicular to the bone in both the transverse and sagittal planes, removing one fourth to one third of the phalanx, depending on the intended size of implant to be used. For the Lawrence implant, the tem-

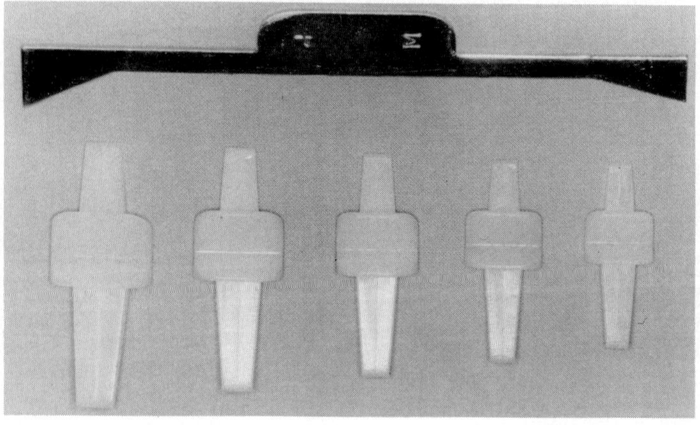

FIGURE 31–8. A transverse view of the five sizes of the Lawrence implant and the template instrument. The template is marked M and P for metatarsal and phalanx, and each end has a scored line that is supposed to be aligned with the long axis of the corresponding bone in the sagittal plane. The angled part of the template then indicates the direction of the bone cut.

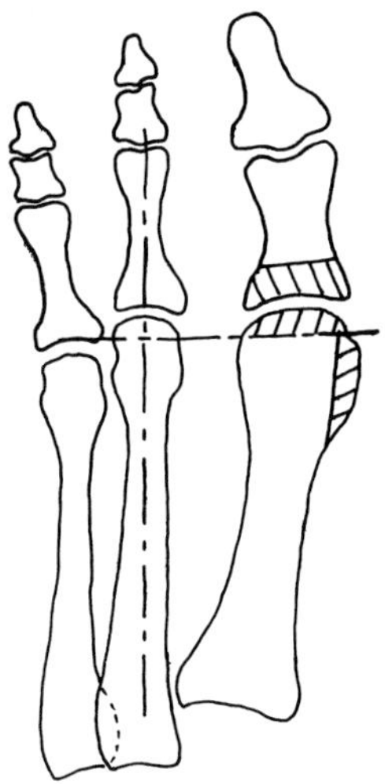

FIGURE 31–10. The transverse plane bone cuts for the Swanson Flexible Hinge Implant are illustrated. The resection on the proximal phalanx is perpendicular to the long axis of the phalanx, removing one fourth to one third of the bone. The resection on the head of the metatarsal is approximately perpendicular to the long axis of the second metatarsal. This will vary slightly to allow the hallux to lie parallel with the second digit.

plate device is placed medial to the phalanx, and the scored line is aligned with the long axis of the bone. This gives the angle of the cut, which is 30 degrees from the perpendicular to the weightbearing surface running from plantar proximal to dorsal distal.

The resection of the metatarsal head is then completed, and this varies for each implant. For the Swanson implant, the cut in the transverse plane should be perpendicular to the long axis of the second metatarsal (Fig. 31–10). Obviously, to do this, the intermetatarsal angle has to be normal or close to normal or reduced with a base wedge osteotomy to get the stem into the metatarsal. In the sagittal plane, the cut should be somewhere between the perpendicular to the long axis of the first metatarsal and the perpendicular to the weightbearing surface. There is some available implant motion lost with dorsiflexion of the hallux with simple weightbearing, but keeping the cut between these two perpendiculars keeps that loss to a minimum. In the excessively pronated foot with loss of metatarsal declination, these two perpendiculars virtually become one and the same.

For the La Porta implant, the metatarsal cut is also perpendicular to the long axis of the second metatarsal in the transverse plane. There is more stem latitude to work with than in the Swanson implant before it becomes necessary to perform an osteotomy to reduce the intermetatarsal angle (Fig. 31–11). In the sagittal plane, the cut is always perpendicular to the weightbearing surface. Indication for the neutral implant is a pronated foot that has little to no metatarsal declination, so the perpendicular to the weightbearing surface is virtually the same as the perpendicular to the long axis of the first metatarsal. For the right and left designated implants, the patient should have a relatively normal first metatarsal declination. This way, the cut perpendicular to the weightbearing surface will allow the stem to go up the metatarsal and the collar to be flush with the resected bone.

The metatarsal cut for the Lawrence implant is made with the template. This assumes a first metatarsal declination angle of 15 degrees, however, which will result in a cut perpendicular to the weightbearing surface. The template is laid on the medial aspect of the first metatarsal, and the scored line is aligned with the long axis of the bone. Obviously, if the metatarsal declination is less than 15 degrees and the template is used, it will result in a cut that is angled dorsally,

and the implant will then act to hold the hallux in an extensus.

For the GAIT implant, there is no cut on the metatarsal head, and the metatarsal stem hole is fashioned directly through the cartilage. For the stem holes in all the implants, they should be as dorsal as possible in the phalanx and as plantar as possible in the metatarsal head. This helps ensure hallux purchase. Additionally, it avoids passing through the plantar cortex of the phalanx, which is significantly concave in shape. All of these implants have broach systems for fashioning the stem holes, and their use is recommended to prevent slippage and malposition of the implant. After the stem holes are fashioned, the grommets for the Swanson implant may be inserted simply by doing a press fit. The

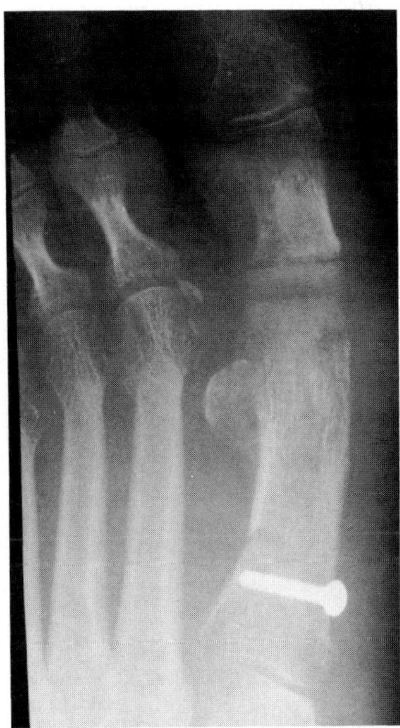

FIGURE 31–11. LaPorta implant done concomitantly with a closing abductory wedge osteotomy. Even with the transverse plane modification of the metatarsal stem, the intermetatarsal angle may still need to be reduced to have the hallux in proper position.

sizers are then used to ensure proper fit, pistoning, and range of motion.

The surgical site is flushed and the implant immersed in fluid before insertion, taking care to make sure that the implant does not touch the patient's skin during insertion. The LaPorta and Lawrence implants can be inserted only one way, as determined by the stems. The Swanson and the GAIT implants may be inserted with either the hinge facing dorsally or plantarly. With encapsulation of the implant, the concavity will be filled with fibrous tissue, and that part of dorsiflexion that would occur with the hinge closing would be blocked. With the hinge facing plantarly, the hinge would open with dorsiflexion instead of closing. Closure is achieved in the usual manner, and the patient is allowed to ambulate in a postoperative shoe, assuming no osteotomies were performed. Postoperative x-rays are taken within 24 hours. Assuming nothing untoward occurs, sutures are removed at 2 weeks, and the patient may start progressing to normal shoe gear. Range-of-motion exercises and physical therapy are performed to keep fibrosis to a minimum.

Two-Component Implants

The latest development in first metatarsophalangeal joint implants is the introduction of two-component implants. There is the Biomet Total Toe System (Biomet, Inc.); the Bio-Action Great Toe Implant (Orthopaedic Biosystems); and the Acumed Great Toe System (Acumed, Inc.). Although each has its own design characteristics, there are common features shared by each. All of the systems have a polyethylene phalangeal component that articulates with a metal alloy metatarsal component. All three of the implants are designed to preserve the attachment of the flexor hallucis brevis, and all are promoted as maintaining the full weight-bearing capacity of the first ray, yet none claim to be a functional prosthesis. They all stress that they maintain the normal anatomic shape of the great toe and that they are engineered to follow the anatomic radii of the first metatarsal, even in extremes of dorsiflexion and plantarflexion. The relevance here is that the anatomic radii change with motion of

the first metatarsophalangeal joint, and the axis of motion is dynamic and moves within the head. The implication is that greater motion can be achieved with a dynamic axis of motion as opposed to a static axis of motion. This has always been one of the criticisms of the total hinged implants. Not only is their axis of motion static but it is located in an anatomically incorrect position. It is in the center of the joint instead of in the center of the metatarsal head.

The Biomet Total Toe System has a metatarsal component that is made of a titanium alloy, which has been implanted with nitrogen ions for improved wear characteristics (Fig. 31–12). It replaces the entire articular surface of the metatarsal, and it is designed to have the sesamoids articulate with the implant. The phalangeal component is available either as a total polyethylene component or as a metal-backed polyethylene component. There are three sizes of metatarsal components and three sizes of phalangeal components. The system is modular so that any metatarsal component may be used with any size phalangeal component. There is a guide that is secured with two .035-inch Kirschner wires that is used to make the cuts on the metatarsal head to accept the implant. A second metatarsal guide is placed over the resected metatarsal head to check the exactness of the cuts, and a pilot hole for the metatarsal component stem is drilled through a center hole in the guide. The stem hole is completed with a broach. The base of the proximal phalanx is resected in the usual manner, and a pilot hole for the phalangeal component stem is made using the phalangeal template. The stem hole is completed with broaches, and the components are then inserted.

The Bio-Action Great Toe Implant is constructed of cobalt chrome and polyethylene (Fig. 31–13). The metatarsal implant is cobalt chrome and condylar in shape. The phalangeal component is backed with cobalt chrome and has a concave polyethylene component that articulates with the metatarsal component. The metatarsal components are available in small and large sizes as well as right, left, and neutral geometry. Phalangeal components are available in various sizes for use in complete resection of the phalangeal base and modified design for use in notched resection to preserve completely

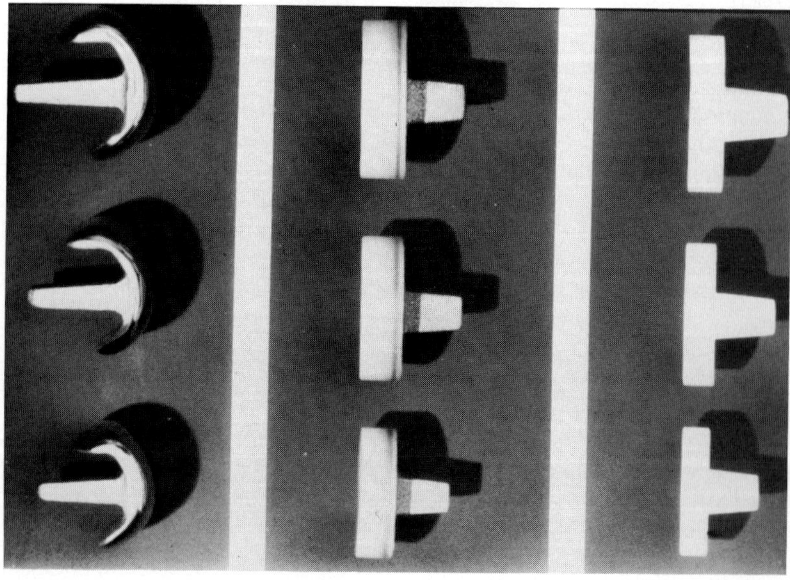

FIGURE 31–12. The Biomet Total Toe System has three sizes in the metatarsal component made of titanium *(right column)*. The plantar curvature is designed to articulate with the sesamoids. There are three sizes of the phalangeal component made either solely of polyethylene or polyethylene backed with titanium. All phalangeal components articulate with all metatarsal components.

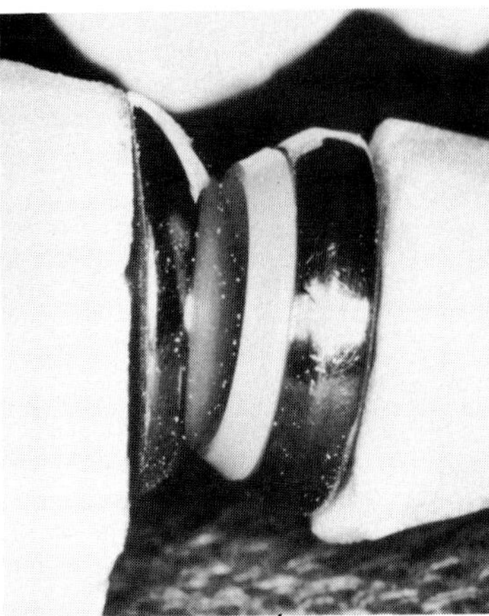

FIGURE 31–13. The Bio-Action Great Toe Implant is demonstrated in sawbones. The metatarsal component is a condylar cap with a stem that is made of cobalt chrome. The phalangeal component is polyethylene backed by cobalt chrome. The polyethylene articulates with the metatarsal cap.

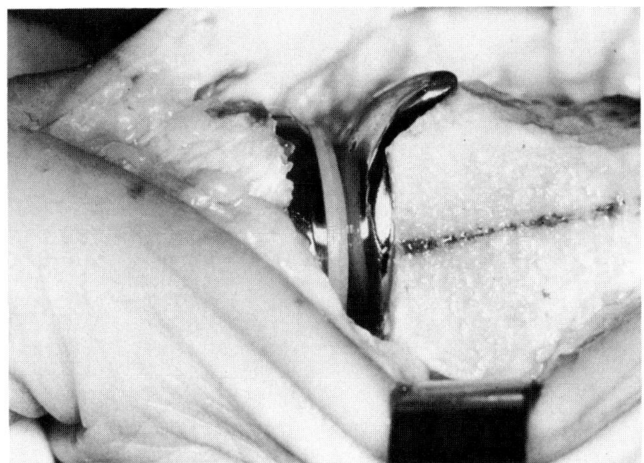

FIGURE 31–14. Intraoperative view of the Acumed Great Toe System inserted.

the attachment of the flexor hallucis brevis. The metatarsal head and proximal phalanx are resected with a power saw, making straight cuts. Broaches are used to make stem holes, and sizers are available.

The Acumed Great Toe System has a metatarsal component made of cobalt chromium and a phalangeal component made of polyethylene that is backed with titanium (Fig. 31–14). There are three metatarsal component sizes and two phalangeal sizes with two available thicknesses. The metatarsal component is designed as a condylar component with an extended dorsal curvature (Fig. 31–15A and B). A saw jig guides the cuts on both the metatarsal and phalanx, ensures that both cuts are vertical, and removes a precise amount of bone. A chamfer guide makes the second cut on the metatarsal head to accommodate the dorsal extension. Metatarsal and phalangeal drill guides and stem burrs fashion the stem holes. Sizers are used to check the fit before inserting the implant components. The system is modular so that any metatarsal component can be used with any phalangeal component.

For all of the two-component implants, there are questions

that need to be answered. All of these implants are approved by the U.S. Food and Drug Administration only if they are cemented in. The more than occasional disastrous past results of cemented implants have led some surgeons to simply press fit the implants. However, this approach has not yet gained Food and Drug Administration approval. By preserving the attachment of the flexor hallucis brevis and weightbearing capacity of the first metatarsal, increased stress will be passed through the implants. Experience has shown that implants that are rigid or that have an increased elastic modulus cause bone resorption, bone fracturing, and implant loosening with this type of stress. Although the intrinsic coefficient of friction of these implants is minimal, what will be the long-term effect with implantation and possible increased stress? In addition to these general questions, there are specific questions based on the individual design characteristics of each implant. The Biomet system allows for articulation with the sesamoids. The increased friction with movement and weightbearing makes very little sense. With the Bio-Action implant, the phalangeal component articulates with the dorsal bone of the first metatarsal with maximal dorsiflexion (Fig. 31–16). The Acumed design appears to be the most logical, but the cuts and stem hole for the metatarsal component are

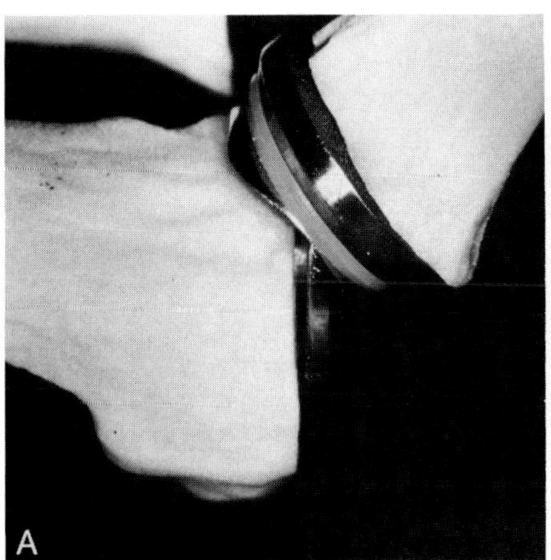
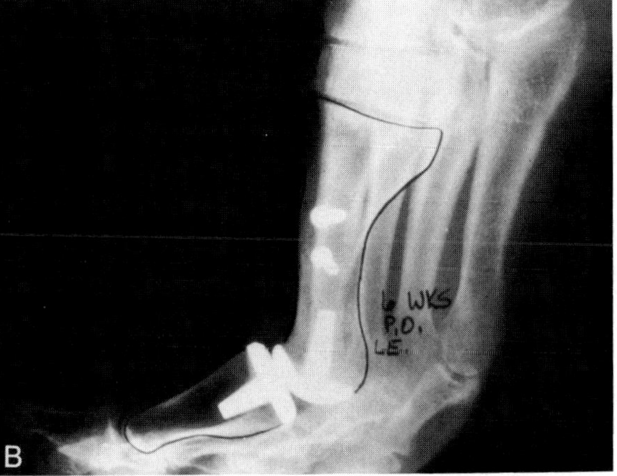

FIGURE 31–15. A, Acumed Great Toe System inserted into a sawbones model. This demonstrates how the phalangeal component articulates with the dorsal metatarsal component extension with dorsiflexion of the hallux. B, This radiograph demonstrates maximal dorsiflexion of the hallux, and it shows how the phalangeal component articulates with the dorsal metatarsal component extension.

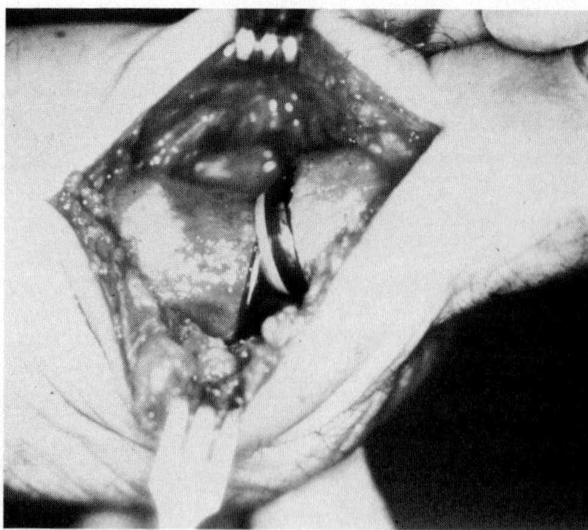

FIGURE 31–16. Intraoperative picture of an inserted Bio-Action implant with the hallux dorsiflexed. It can be observed that the phalangeal component is articulating with the dorsal bone of the metatarsal with dorsiflexion of the hallux.

based on the smallest component. If the medium or large metatarsal component is used, there will be no bone backing the most dorsal aspect of this component, and pressure from the phalangeal component on this part of the metatarsal component will cause increased stress.

LESSER METATARSOPHALANGEAL IMPLANTS

The first lesser metatarsophalangeal prosthetic replacement was attempted by Seeburger in 1962. The procedure was used to treat plantar keratomas. The initial implants were metal and in a convex condylar shape with a stem for replacement of the metatarsal head. Neither the implant nor the criteria were appropriate, and both have changed over time. Lesser metatarsophalangeal implants are indicated primarily

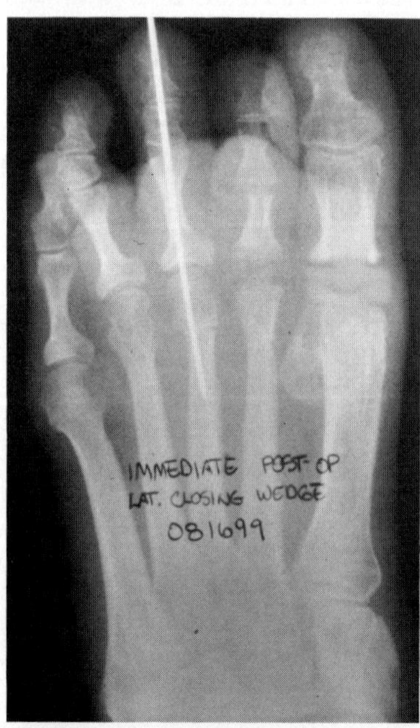

FIGURE 31–17. Radiograph demonstrating use of the Swanson total implant in both the first and second metatarsophalangeal joints. It is recommended that in both instances the implant be inserted with the open hinge facing plantar.

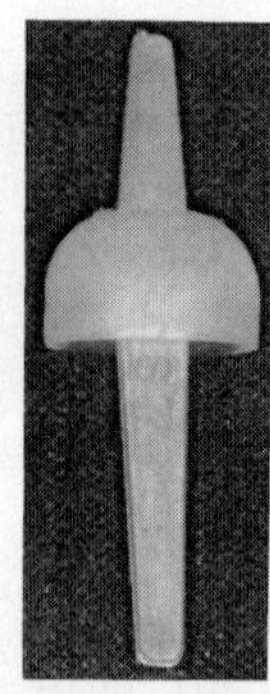

FIGURE 31–18. The Sgarlato lesser metatarsophalangeal joint implant produced by Sutter. The hinge is half a sphere with the flat surface resting against the resected metatarsal head. All of the motion in this implant comes from bending of the stems.

for articular disease, when primary joint reconstruction fails to provide a satisfactory result. They are also used for the treatment of brachymetatarsia, Freiberg's disease, and flail toes secondary to previous base resection of the phalanx or head resection of the metatarsal. The primary objectives of this implant arthroplasty are to provide pain relief, provide digital stability, and maintain the normal length of the digit.

On the basis of the size of the bones alone, lesser metatarsophalangeal implantation was more susceptible to the pitfalls of stresses than the first metatarsophalangeal implantation, and all of the early implants that were made of high-elastic modulus materials failed. Currently, therefore, the lesser metatarsophalangeal implants available are all made of silicone. There are three implants, including the Swanson double-stemmed hinge implant (Dow Corning Wright); the Sgarlato double-stemmed implant (Sutter Biomedical, Inc.); and the Lesser Metatarsal Cap (Zang design) (Sutter Biomedical, Inc.).

The Swanson double-stemmed hinge implant is identical in design to the first metatarsophalangeal implant but smaller (Fig. 31–17). There is a U-shaped hinge with two stems, both of which are perpendicular to the hinge in both the transverse and sagittal planes. There are six sizes available with only one stem size. The implant is detailed to be used with the hinge opening facing plantar.

The Sgarlato implant is also a double-stemmed implant that is available in three sizes (Fig. 31–18). There is no hinge to this implant; instead, there is a half sphere with the flat part designed to rest against the resected metatarsal head. This implant relies solely on the flexibility of the stems and pistoning for its motion.

The last of the lesser metatarsophalangeal implants is the Lesser Metatarsal Cap designed by Zang (Fig. 31–19). This

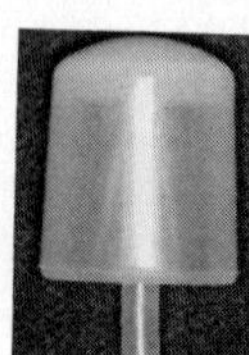

FIGURE 31–19. The Lesser Metatarsal Cap (Zang design) is a hollow cylinder that is closed at one end and has a stem running through the middle of it. The closed end has a buildup to replace the resected bone of the metatarsal head, and it is convex in shape to articulate with the base of the proximal phalanx. This same design without the stem was once used for digital implantation, but it has been abandoned.

is a cup-shaped implant that is thickened at its closed end. There is a single stem passing through the center of the cup. The stem is designed to be placed into the distal metatarsal shaft after metatarsal head resection. There are two holes in the cup part of the implant to suture it in place. The distal end of the implant is designed to articulate with the base of the proximal phalanx. Five sizes of this implant are available. The extension of the cap proximally is promoted to prevent hyperostosis, but experience has shown, however, that a large amount of hyperostosis occurs at the proximal end of the implant and that the bone underneath the implant resorbs. This implant has other troublesome features also. The addition of holes with which to suture the implant was added because the implant is readily dislocated otherwise. This fixes the implant, and there are inherent problems associated with all fixed implants. Having the implant articulate with the proximal phalanx causes increased stress because of the increased coefficient of friction.

The operative technique is essentially the same for all three of the implants. A serpentine incision is used over the joint because of the high digital contracture potential. Any soft tissue contractures must be released, and the metatarsal head is exposed through a linear capsulotomy. A partial metatarsal head resection is performed with a power saw. All of the classic protocols describe resection of the base of the proximal phalanx at this point. This has been fraught with problems, however, because of the fragility of this bone. Stress passing distally has routinely resulted in fracturing and resorption of the proximal phalanx. Instead, it is recommended that all the bone necessary to accommodate the implant be resected off the head of the metatarsal, and the phalangeal stem hole bc fashioned directly through the intact cartilage of the phalangeal base. The stem hole in the metatarsal for all three implants is fashioned with a side-cutting bur or an equivalent instrument. The stem hole in the phalanx for the Swanson and the Sgarlato implants is also fashioned with a side-cutting bur. After adequate irrigation, sizers are used to ensure proper fit and digit position. The implant is inserted using all the previously described precautions. The Zang cap is sutured to the metatarsal at this time. Closure is achieved in the usual manner, and the foot is dressed with a compressive dressing. The patient is allowed to ambulate in a postoperative shoe, with suture removal at 2 weeks and return to normal shoe gear at 3 to 4 weeks. It must be understood that the insertion of any of the implants does not restore the weightbearing function of the metatarsal and that transfer lesions are very common. Although a panmetatarsal head resection seems to be an indication for these implants, it is not. The increased risk of infection, the additional trauma and dissection, and multiplication of inherent implant complications contraindicate their use. The one implant indicated for the panmetatarsal head resection is a total implant for the first metatarsophalangeal joint to give the hallux stability and prevent drift of the lesser toes.

DIGITAL IMPLANTS

Digital implants were developed and have been modified because of the dissatisfaction of the results with digital arthroplasty and arthrodesis procedures. Digital implants are designed to provide either motion or stability to toes. Digital implantation is restricted to the proximal interphalangeal joint of digits two, three, and four. Although some have stated they are indicated for the fifth digit, the restoration of motion and stability are not needed as they are in the other digits and, more importantly, the predictability of failure and problems far outweigh any possible improvement. Other goals of digital prostheses are to maintain digital length, alignment, and purchase of the ground. The primary indication for digital implants is joint arthrosis of the proximal interphalangeal joint of the second, third, and fourth digits. There are numerous contraindications to these implants that will cause their failure. Inadequate bone stock or bone size will result in bone fracturing. The size of the intermediate phalanx is especially important: It must be large enough to accept the implant stem. Inadequate skin covering or vascular status, the presence of infection, and history of previous implant material intolerance contraindicate their use.

Two functional considerations preclude the use of these implants: nonreducible contractures at the corresponding metatarsophalangeal joint and a pes cavus foot type. An implant cannot achieve the same degree of stability that is needed and gained with a digital arthrodesis in a cavus foot, and the likelihood of implant dislocation is significant.

Three digital implant designs are available, all of which are made of silicone: the Swanson flexible hinge toe implant and the Weil design hammertoe implant (Dow Corning Wright) and the Sgarlato design hammertoe implant (Sutter Biomedical, Inc.) (Fig. 31–20). The Swanson flexible toe implant is simply a smaller version of the first metatarsophalangeal implant, and it is available in six sizes with only one stem size. The Weil design implant has a cylindrical collar instead of a hinge and two stems of equal size. The stems are also cylindrical and perpendicular to the collar. This implant is available in seven sizes with two stem sizes, six collar lengths, and two collar diameters. The Sgarlato implant is also a double-stemmed hinge implant available in four sizes. The stems are rectangular and tapered, and they are perpendicular to the hinge. The implant is impregnated with a Dacron mesh throughout its length. All three implants have sizer sets and are radiopaque on radiograph.

The operative technique limits the ellipse of any skin lesions to maintain adequate skin closure. The extensor digitorum longus tendon may be split longitudinally or transected transversely and dissected proximally or distally for exposure of the joint. It is recommended that any bony resection be performed with power instrumentation rather than cutting forceps to avoid microfracturing.

In the past, it was recommended to resect both the head of

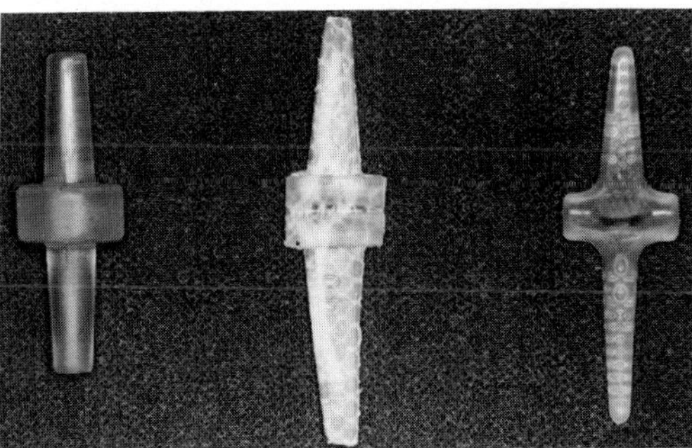

FIGURE 31–20. The available implants for digital implantation. From left to right are the Weil design hammertoe implant, the Sgarlato design hammertoe implant, and the Swanson flexible hinge toe implant.

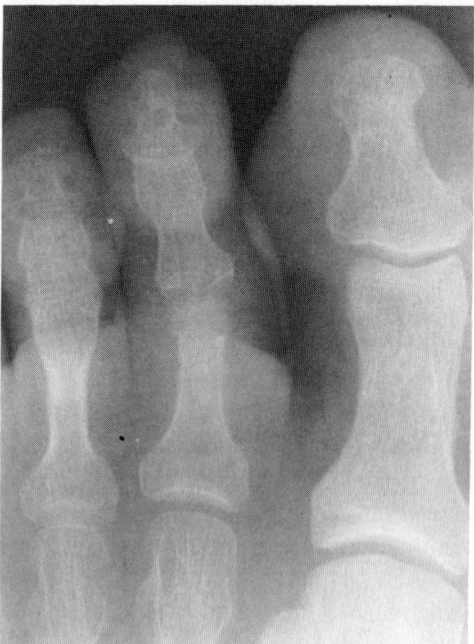

FIGURE 31–21. Radiograph demonstrating the implantation of a Weil hammertoe implant used in the proximal interphalangeal joint of the second digit. Note that the implant bridges the resected cortex of the proximal phalanx and the stem hole in the intermediate phalanx is fashioned directly through the cartilage.

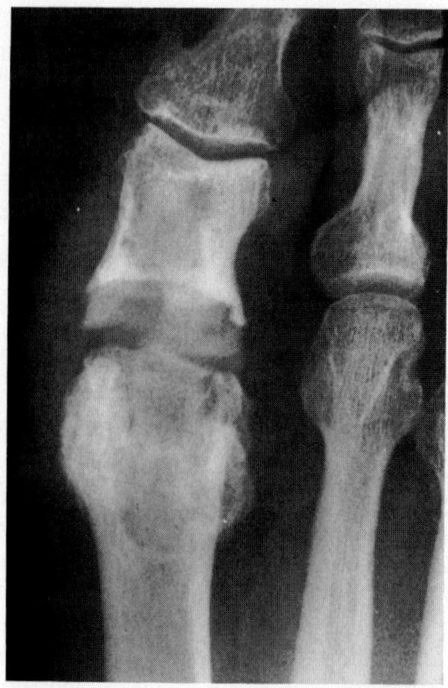

FIGURE 31–22. Radiograph revealing fracturing and fragmentation of a LaPorta implant. This implant was exposed to stresses that exceeded its design characteristics.

the proximal phalanx and the base of the intermediate phalanx, but this has resulted in the same problem associated with the lesser metatarsophalangeal implants, namely, fracturing of the distal segment. Therefore, it is recommended to resect the head of the proximal phalanx only, and fashion the stem holes through the resected end of the proximal phalanx and through the cartilage of the intermediate phalanx (Fig. 31–21). The sizing sets are used to determine the proper size, utilizing all the generic parameters previously described. The surgical site is irrigated adequately; the implant is inserted, using the previously described precautions; the extensor digitorum longus tendon is reapproximated; and skin closure is achieved in the usual manner. The procedure is ambulatory, and the sutures are removed in 2 weeks. A compressive wrap is maintained for as long as 6 weeks to reduce the amount of postoperative fibrosis, and the patient may start to progress to normal shoes as early as 2 weeks postoperatively.

IMPLANT COMPLICATIONS

The insertion of any prosthetic device has the potential for complication. There are inherent possible complications with the devices themselves, or there may be surgical technique problems. As described earlier, the possibility of infection is increased with the insertion of any foreign body, because the level of contamination necessary to cause an infection is reduced. If an infection does develop, one must determine whether it is superficial or a deep-space infection. A superficial infection can be treated with antibiotics and local wound care, but a deep-space infection requires implant removal. A deep-space infection is feared because of the possible development of osteomyelitis. The development of a deep-space infection or osteomyelitis does not, however, preclude ever using an implant again. Reimplantation, if seen to be of adequate benefit to the patient, may be accomplished 6

months to 1 year after the initial implant removal, provided the infection was eradicated.

Implant fracturing or deformation may occur any time an implant is exposed to forces that exceed its design characteristics (Fig. 31–22). Anything that can cut or create flaws in the implant can potentiate this possibility. The examples of using a hemi-implant when a hallux limitus exists or traumatically handling an implant have been discussed. Removal

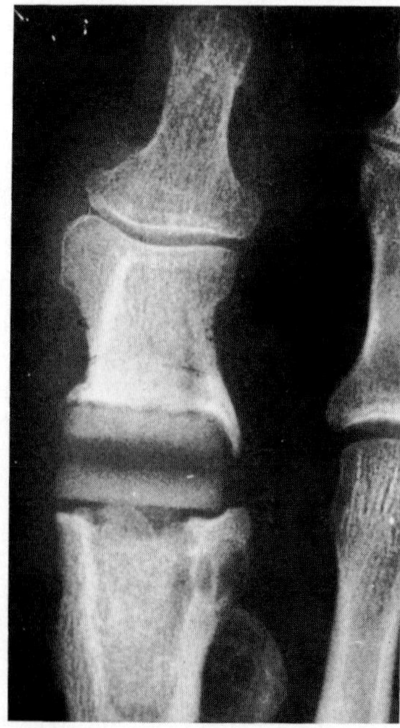

FIGURE 31–23. Radiograph showing ectopic bone formation around a LaPorta implant. Even with the proper size implant and using the broader collar implants, this is still a common finding. It is only a problem if it limits motion or becomes large enough to be irritated by shoegear.

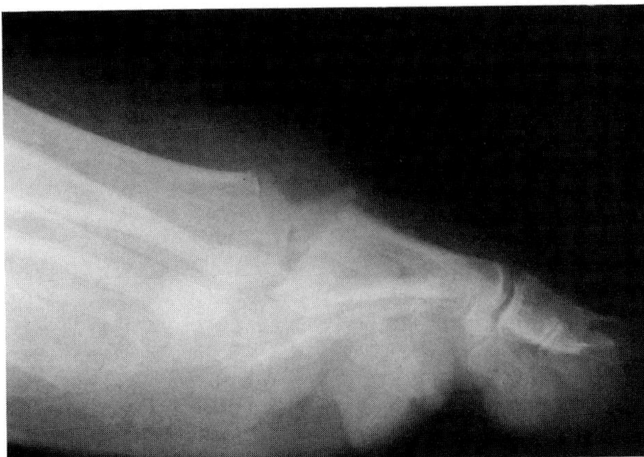

FIGURE 31–24. Radiograph revealing two errors in surgical technique in using the Lawrence implant. First, an inadequate amount of bone was resected, causing jamming of the implant. Second, the metatarsal cut is angled improperly in a dorsal direction. If this cut had been done properly, it should appear perpendicular to the weightbearing surface.

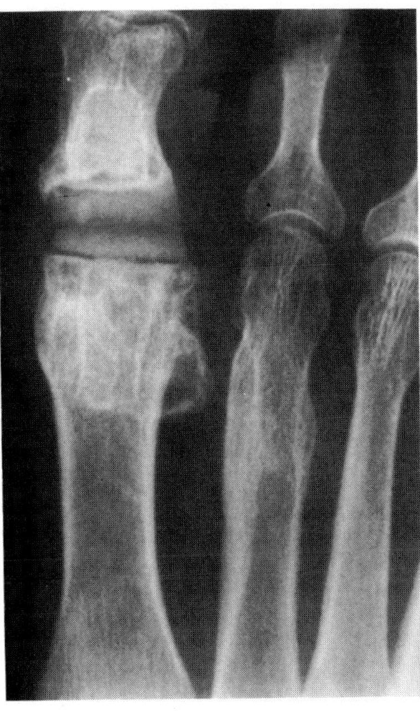

FIGURE 31–26. Radiograph showing a healed fracture of the second metatarsal that occurred following the first metatarsophalangeal joint implantation procedure. The elimination of the weightbearing capacity of the first ray in implantation procedures shifts the weight to the lesser metatarsals. This will lead to the inherent problems of metatarsalgia, metatarsophalangeal capsulitis, transfer lesions, and stress fractures.

of the implant in these instances depends on whether the implant was symptomatic for the patient or not. There can be reaction to the implants, which will require their removal. A foreign-body reaction occurs in only 0.01% of the population, but it occurs early and requires immediate implant removal. Reactive synovitis is a foreign-body, giant-cell inflammatory reaction to particulate matter of silicone. This is a byproduct of anything that causes implant abrasion, such as implant pistoning, and requires implant removal and synovectomy to improve the symptoms. Ectopic bone formation may limit motion enough to become symptomatic (Fig. 31–23). Whether this is a biological response of the bone to the implant material or a mechanical response to the motion of

the implant becomes irrelevant once symptoms develop because implant removal is required to relieve the symptoms.

Inappropriate techniques such as overzealous soft tissue releases, excessive bone resection, inaccurate angulation of bone cuts, remodeling of the implant, or failure to release or to structurally correct deforming forces may cause several problems (Fig. 31–24). Complications that result from these technique errors include implant dislocation, implant malposition, limited range of motion, digits that fail to purchase the ground, aseptic necrosis of the bone, fracturing of the bone, telescoping of the implant into the bone, and abducted or adducted digits (Figs. 31–25 and 31–26). Implant removal depends on whether the complication is symptomatic to the patient. Reimplantation depends on whether the cause of the complication could be identified and neutralized and whether reimplantation would be beneficial. A unique problem to the digital implants is prolonged edema, resulting in an enlarged digit that is often stiff, elevated, and painful.

In conclusion, it must be repeated that there exists no forefoot prosthesis that is functional. The most that can be expected from prosthesis use is relief from pain, mobility at the joint, some stability, and improved cosmetic appearance. Prosthesis use must always be weighed against the possible detriment, and one must be prepared to deal with the potential problems.

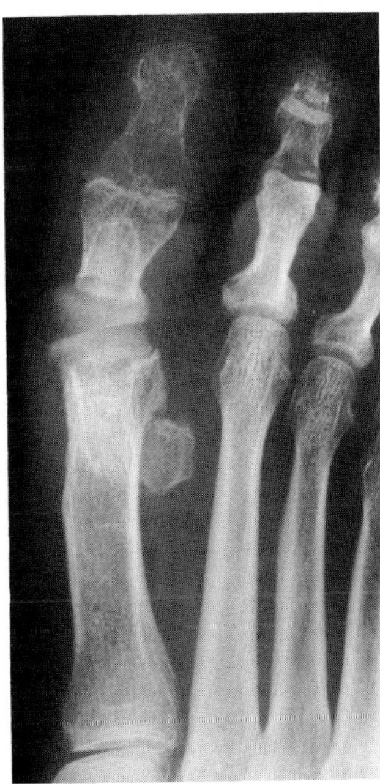

FIGURE 31–25. Radiograph revealing malposition of a LaPorta implant, which has rotated 90 degrees in the frontal plane. This is most commonly due to excessive reaming of the stem holes. This rotation can occur only in the early postoperative period, because once fibrosis around the implant occurs, it will not shift.

Bibliography

1. Acumed, Inc: Acumed great toe system. Commercial Prospectus. Beaverton, OR, Acumed, Inc., 1992
2. Arenson DJ: The angled great toe implant (Swanson design/Weil modification) in the surgical reconstruction of the first metatarsophalangeal joint. Clin Podiatr 1:89–102, 1984.
3. Arenson DJ and Wil LS: Aseptic necrosis: An unusual cause of Silastic (Swanson) implant failure, a case report. J Am Podiatr Assoc 69:616–620, 1979.

4. Biomet, Inc: Total toe system. Commercial Prospectus. Warsaw, IN, Biomet, Inc., 1990.

5. Burns A: Implant procedures. *In* Gerbert J (ed): Textbook of Bunion Surgery. Mt. Kisco, NY, Futura, 1991, pp 269–312.

6. Burns A: Implant complications. *In* Gerbert J (ed): Textbook of Bunion Surgery. Mt. Kisco, NY, Futura, 1991, pp 525–542.

7. Clark JR: Implant procedures. *In* Gerbert J (ed): Textbook of Bunion Surgery. Mt. Kisco, NY, Futura, 1981, pp 199–225

8. Cracchiolo A, Swanson A, and Swanson GD: The arthritic great toe metatarsophalangeal joint: A review of flexible silicone implant arthroplasty form two medical centers. Clin Orthop 157:64–70, 1981.

9. Davis JA: Rheumatology. *In* Zier B (ed): Essentials of Internal Medicine in Clinical Podiatry. Philadelphia, WB Saunders, 1990, pp 135–177.

10. Dobbs B: Implants in foot surgery. Clin Podiatr 1:79–88, 1984.

11. Dobbs B: LaPorta® great toe implant: Long term study of its efficacy. J Am Podiatr Med Assoc 80:379, 1990.

12. Dow Corning Wright: Silastic® orthopaedic implants H.P. for the foot. Commercial Prospectus, Arlington, TN, 1984.

13. Dow Corning Wright: Swanson titanium great toe implant. Commercial Prospectus. 1987.

14. Dow Corning Wright: Silastic® HP100 Swanson flexible hinge toe implant. Commercial Prospectus. 1986.

15. Dow Corning Wright: Silastic® HP100 Swanson flexible hinge toe implant and Swanson flexible hinge toe joint grommet. Commercial Prospectus. 1986.

16. Edlich R: Modern concepts of treatment of traumatic wounds. Adv Surg 13:169–197, 1979.

17. Farnworth C, Haggard S, Nahmias M, et al: LaPorta® great toe implant: A preliminary study of its efficacy. J Am Podiatr Med Assoc 76:625–630, 1986.

18. Fox I and Pro A: Lesser metatarsophalangeal joint implants. J Foot Surg 26:159–163, 1987.

19. Frisch EE: Biomaterials in foot surgery. Clin Podiatr 1:11–28, 1984.

20. Gerbert J and Benedetti L: Swanson design finger joint implant utilized in the proximal interphalangeal joints of the foot: A preliminary study. J Foot Surg 22:60–65, 1983.

21. Gerbert J: Digital implantation. Clin Podiatr Med Surg 3:95–102, 1986.

22. Gerbert J and Dobbs B: Forefoot derangement. Part I: Rheumatoid forefoot. *In* McGlamry ED (ed): Comprehensive Textbook of Foot Surgery. Baltimore, Williams & Wilkins, 1987, pp 534–543.

23. Granberry W, Noble PC, Bishop JO, and Tullos HS: Use of a hinged silicone prosthesis for replacement arthroplasty of the first metatarsophalangeal joint. J Bone Joint Surg 73A:1453–1459, 1991.

24. Groman AD, Solomon MG, and Ketai NH: Repair of cocked hallux secondary to Keller procedure using silicone rubber implant. J Am Podiatr Assoc 66:181–189, 1976.

25. Hunter WN and Borovoy M: Prophylactic antibiotics: Control of implant contamination. J Am Podiatr Assoc 74:284–290, 1984.

26. Jacobs A and Oloff L: Implants. *In* Marcus A (ed): Complications in Foot Surgery, 2nd ed. Baltimore, Williams & Wilkins, 1983, pp 274–308.

27. Jarvis B, Moats D, Burns A, et al: Lawrence® design first metatarsophalangeal joint prothesis. J Am Podiatr Med Assoc 76:617–624, 1986.

28. Joseph J: Range of movement of the great toe in men. J Bone Joint Surg 36B:84–88, 1954.

29. Kampner SL: Total joint prosthetic arthroplasty of the great toe—A 12 year experience. Foot Ankle 4:249–261, 1984.

30. Kaplan E, Kaplan G, Kaplan D, et al: History of implants. Clin Podiatr 1:3–10, 1984.

31. Landry J, Lowhorn M, Black A, et al: Antibiotic prophylaxis in Silastic joint implantation—A retrospective study. J Am Podiatr Med Assoc 77:177–181, 1987.

32. Lanham RH: Digital implant arthroplasty. Clin Podiatr 1:47–68, 1984.

33. LaPorta GA, Piloa P, and Rickter KP: Keller implant procedure. J Am Podiatr Assoc 66:126–147, 1976.

34. Lauf E, McLaughlin B, and McLaughlin E: Swanson great toe flexible hinge endoprosthesis—Design, flexibility, and function. J Am Podiatr Med Assoc 75:393–400, 1985.

35. Lemon RA, Engber WD, and McBeath AA: A complication of Silastic hemiarthroplasty in bunion surgery. Foot Ankle 4:262–266, 1984.

36. Mann RA and Thompson EM: Arthrodesis of the first metatarsophalangeal joint for hallux valgus in rheumatoid arthritis. J Bone Joint Surg 66A:687–692, 1984.

37. McCarthy DJ, Kershisnik W, and O'Donnell E: The histopathology of silicone elastomer implant failure in podiatric surgery. J Am Podiatr Med Assoc 76:247–265, 1986.

38. McDonald RJ, Griffin JM, and Edleman RO: Consecutive bilateral failures of first metatarsophalangeal joint prosthesis. J Foot Surg 25:226–233, 1986.

39. McGlamry ED and Ruch J: Status of implant arthroplasty for the lesser metatarsophalangeal joints. J Am Podiatr Assoc 66:155–164, 1976.

40. Mednick D, Norgaard J, Hallwhich D, et al: Comparison of total hinged and total nonhinged implants for the lesser digits. J Foot Surg 24:215–218, 1985.

41. Mondul M, Jacobs PM, Caneva RG, et al: Implant arthroplasty of the first metatarsophalangeal joint: A 12 year retrospective study. J Foot Surg 24:275–279, 1985.

42. Orien WP: Biomechanics of implanted joints of the foot. Clin Podiatr 1:29–45, 1984.

43. Orthopedic Biosystems: Bio-Action great toe implant. Commercial Prospectus. Scottsdale, AZ, Orthopedic Biosystems, 1991.

44. Rude CC, Karlin JM, Scurran BL, et al: Implant arthroplasty of the first metatarsophalangeal joint: A follow up study. J Am Podiatr Med Assoc 75:279–287, 1985.

45. Sbarbaro J: Surgery on the rheumatoid foot and ankle. *In* Evarts C (ed): Surgery of the Musculoskeletal System. New York, Churchill Livingstone, 1983, pp 191–202.

46. Schilero J: The implications of silicone implant surgery. J Foot Surg 23:66–69, 1984.

47. Sgarlato T: A new implant for the metatarsophalangeal joint. Clin Podiatr 1:69–78, 1984.

48. Sollitto RJ and Shonkwiler W: Silicone shard formation: A product of implant arthroplasty. J Foot Surg 23:362–365, 1984.

49. Sollitto RJ and Werner MS: A preliminary report on the status of implants for the lesser toes. J Foot Surg 24:453–455, 1985.

50. Sutter Biomedical, Inc: The Sutter hinged great toe metatarsophalangeal joint implant (Lawrence design). Commercial Prospectus. San Diego, CA, Sutter Biomedical, Inc., 1982.

51. Sutter Biomedical, Inc: The Sutter hinged great toe joint implant (LaPorta design). Commercial Prospectus. San Diego, CA, Sutter Biomedical, Inc., 1983.

52. Swanson R, Meester W, Swanson G, et al: Durability of silicone implants: An in vivo study. Orthop Clin North Am 4:1097–1112, 1973.

53. Teich L, Frankel J, and Lipsman S: Silicone hinge replacement arthroplasty. J Am Podiatr Assoc 71:266–272, 1981.

54. Vanore J, O'Keefe R, and Pikscher I: First metatarsophalangeal joint implant arthroplasty. *In* McGlamry ED (ed): Comprehensive Textbook of Foot Surgery. Baltimore, Williams & Wilkins, 1987, pp 756–807.

55. Vanore J, O'Keefe R, and Pikscher I: Complications of silicone implants in foot surgery. Clin Podiatr 1:175–198, 1984.

56. Vanore J, O'Keefe R, and Pikscher I: Silastic® implant arthroplasty—Complications and their classification. J Am Podiatr Assoc 74:423–433, 1984.

57. Vanore J, O'Keefe R, and Pikscher I: Lesser metatarsophalangeal joint. *In* McGlamry ED (ed): Comprehensive Textbook of Foot Surgery. Baltimore, Williams & Wilkins, 1987, pp 808–820.

58. Weil LS, Pollak RA, and Goller WL: Total first joint replacement in hallux valgus and hallux rigidis: Long term results in 484 cases. Clin Podiatr 1:103–129, 1984.

59. Weinstock RE, Bass SJ, Wolfson SF, et al: Osseous engulfment of a silicone prothesis with foreign body reaction. J Am Podiatr Assoc 74:80–88, 1984.

60. Zeichner AM: Component first metatarsophalangeal joint replacement—A new approach. J Am Podiatr Assoc 75:254–257, 1985.

CHAPTER 32

Joint Preservation Techniques in Hallux Limitus/Rigidus Repair

Kieran T. Mahan, M.S., D.P.M.

Hallux limitus/rigidus is a common condition in the foot. Cotterill coined the term *hallux rigidus* in 1888.[1] The terms *hallux limitus* and *hallux rigidus* are often used interchangeably. However, hallux limitus is best used to describe a decrease in the range of motion beyond normal. Hallux rigidus is best used to describe the absence of motion at the first metatarsophalangeal (MTP) joint. Each of these terms describes a point along a continuum of limitation of motion, with each step along the continuum having some degree of hallux equinus. A variety of surgical treatments have been described for the management of hallux limitus/rigidus. These techniques include the Keller bunionectomy, first MTP joint fusions, and implant arthroplasty. Each of these joint-destructive procedures has significant functional limitations that it imposes on the foot. It is because of these limitations and other problems associated with these procedures that great attention has been paid toward developing reconstructive techniques for salvageable joints. The focus of this chapter is the surgical management of the reconstructible first MTP joint by joint-preserving techniques.

ANATOMY AND MECHANICS OF NORMAL FIRST METATARSOPHALANGEAL MOTION

The normal functioning of the first MTP joint is critical for normal gait. Under most circumstances, 65 to 75 degrees of dorsiflexion of the hallux on the first metatarsal is required for normal gait. These values are based on the angulation of the tibia and foot to the ground at toe-off. In order for the hallux to function properly in propulsion, the hallux must dorsiflex at least 65 degrees on the first metatarsal to keep the hallux on the ground.[2]

The first MTP joint is a ginglymoarthrodial joint. In normal function, the motion about the first MTP joint occurs primarily in the sagittal plane. The motion of the first MTP joint is interesting for two reasons: (1) The axis of the first MTP joint is not static but dynamic, changing position as the hallux changes position with respect to the first metatarsal (Fig. 32–1) and (2) the motion of the first MTP joint is ultimately dependent on the stability and position of the more proximal structures. For example, first-ray plantarflexion (which is dependent on a stable lateral column and functional peroneus longus) increases the available dorsiflexion at the

first MTP joint. On the other hand, dorsiflexion of the first ray reduces the available dorsiflexion at the first MTP joint. In order for the first MTP joint to function properly during gait, the first metatarsal must stabilize and plantarflex as the hallux becomes stable along the supporting surface.

There are some key elements necessary to allow for adequate dorsiflexion of the hallux on the first metatarsal. The first metatarsal must be structurally and dynamically stable, there must be adequate joint function without mechanical blockade, there must be adequate joint lubrication (in which the dorsal synovial fold at the end of the dorsal articular cartilage plays a critical role), and the sesamoids must glide unrestricted along the plantar aspect of the first metatarsal head (Fig. 32–2). Interference with any of these aspects of normal MTP joint motion creates a pathologic condition.

As is clear from the previous discussion, the position and function of the first metatarsal and proximal joints are primary considerations in determining the available range of motion of the first MTP joint. The first ray, in turn, is affected by the stability of the subtalar and midtarsal joints and by the pull of the peroneus longus. In order for the peroneus longus to function properly, the lateral column must be rigid.

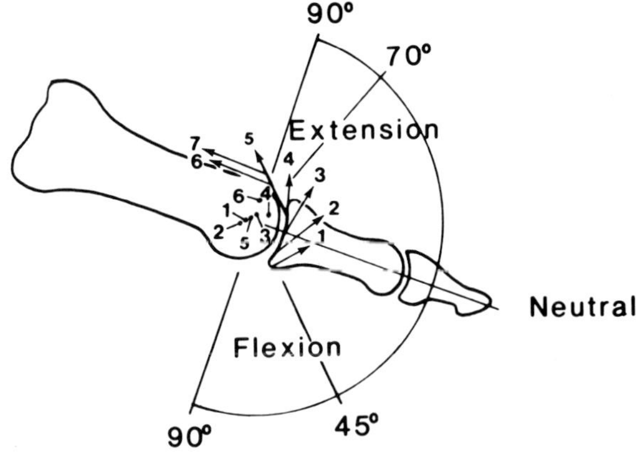

FIGURE 32–1. Diagram illustrating the rotation of the first metatarsophalangeal joint axis of motion as the hallux dorsiflexes on the first metatarsal. (From Smith T, Malay DS, and Ruch JA: Hallux limitus and rigidus. *In* McGlamry ED [ed]: Comprehensive Textbook of Foot Surgery, Vol 1, p 240. © 1987, the Williams & Wilkins Co., Baltimore.)

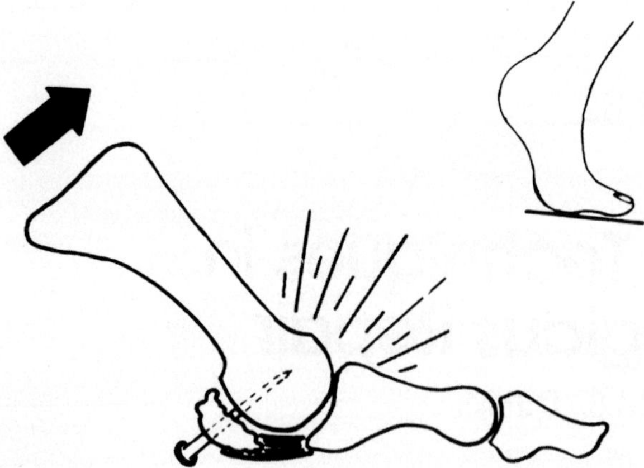

FIGURE 32–2. Diagram illustrating the effect of frozen sesamoids on first metatarsophalangeal joint dorsiflexion. (From Smith T, Malay DS, and Ruch JA: Hallux limitus and rigidus. *In* McGlamry ED [ed]: Comprehensive Textbook of Foot Surgery, Vol 1, p 243. © 1987, the Williams & Wilkins Co., Baltimore.)

Without the plantarflexion that occurs in the first ray during propulsion, only 25 to 30 degrees of MTP joint dorsiflexion will occur before the base of the proximal phalanx compresses into the metatarsal head. However, as the first metatarsal plantarflexes, the distal aspect of the first metatarsal head articulates more and more with the sesamoids. The sesamoids function as a pulley for the intrinsic muscles, stabilizing the hallux against the ground. Once the articular cartilage of the metatarsal head contacts the sesamoids, it continues to rotate plantarly and proximally, allowing a passive migration of the proximal phalanx over the dorsal aspect of the first metatarsal. As the joint reaches its end range of motion, the proximal phalanx will start to compress against the metatarsal head in a hinge-like manner. It is the premature hinge motion created by a lack of adequate dorsiflexion that creates the dorsal flag effect commonly seen in hallux limitus.

MEASUREMENT OF THE FIRST METATARSOPHALANGEAL JOINT MOTION

Because the functional aspects of the first MTP joint motion are so critical, measurement of first MTP joint motion must take into account what occurs during the normal gait cycle. A variety of techniques have been described for measurement of first MTP joint range of motion. The lack of a consistent, reproducible technique has hindered comparison among various studies concerned with management of the first MTP joint. Buell and colleagues proposed a series of measurements to evaluate first MTP joint range of motion:[3] (1) the relaxed hanging position of the hallux, (2) the straight line position of the hallux, (3) unassisted dorsiflexion of the hallux, (4) assisted dorsiflexion of the hallux, and (5) assisted plantarflexion of the hallux (Fig. 32–3).

Dorsiflexion of the hallux is measured from the straight-line position of the hallux. Straight-line position of the hallux refers to moving the hallux into a position in which the proximal phalanx is parallel to the longitudinal bisection of the first metatarsal. For measurement of assisted dorsiflexion, the examiner exerts pressure on the proximal phalanx of the

hallux in a dorsiflexory direction. This creates a retrograde plantarflexion of the first metatarsal. In their study, Buell and colleagues found unassisted dorsiflexion of 77 degrees in the normal group and 51.4 degrees in the first-ray pathology group.[3] Assisted dorsiflexion was 82 degrees in the normal group and only 55 degrees in the first-ray pathology group.[3] The measurement and terminology system proposed by Buell and coworkers provide a significant basis for the standardization of measurement of the first MTP joint. It should allow for more accurate comparison among retrospective surgical studies.

ETIOLOGY OF HALLUX LIMITUS/RIGIDUS

A large number of causes have been described for hallux limitus. Nilsonne[4] classified hallux rigidus/limitus into primary and secondary forms. He described the primary hallux rigidus form as typically having an onset in adolescence with the appearance of localized degenerative changes. He described secondary hallux rigidus as a degenerative osteoarthritis of long-standing duration.

Further refinement of this categorization was advanced by the hypothesis that the primary hallux limitus in adolescent patients may be associated with a long first metatarsal bone.[5] The long first metatarsal bone, in turn, could be related to the presence of a distal first metatarsal epiphysis, adding to the length of the bone. The presence of dorsal lesions in and above the joint led some authors to speculate that osteochondritis dissecans might be related to the cause of primary hallux limitus. McMaster described the cause as acute or chronic trauma resulting in a characteristic head lesion.[6]

Metatarsal head shape may also be related to hallux limitus. Brahm[7] demonstrated that the degree of hallux abductus

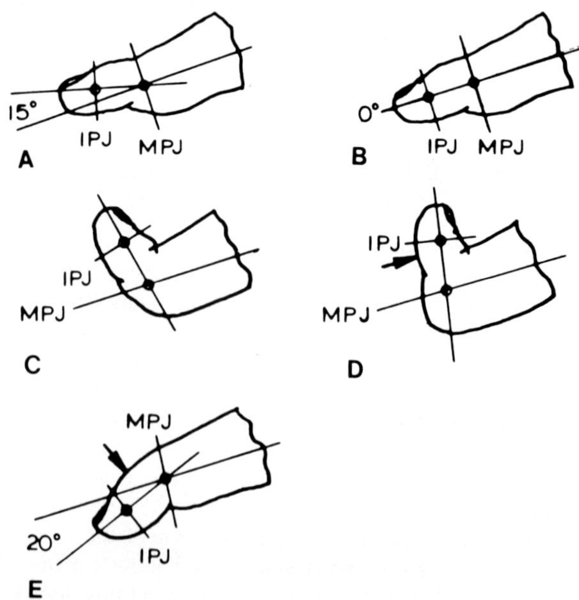

FIGURE 32–3. Diagrams illustrating measurements described by Buell and associates.[3] *A,* The relaxed hanging position of the hallux. *B,* The straight line position of the hallux. *C,* Unassisted dorsiflexion of the hallux. *D,* Assisted dorsiflexion of the hallux. *E,* Assisted plantarflexion of the hallux. (From Buell T, Green DR, and Risser J: Measurements of the first metatarsophalangeal joint range of motion. J Am Podiatr Med Assoc 78:439–448, 1988.)

is related to the radius of curvature of the first metatarsal head. Similarly, a more square head may be more likely to develop hallux limitus.

Bingold and Collins[8] noted a high correlation between unilateral hallux rigidus and the patient's footedness.

In the classical description of secondary hallux limitus, a variety of causes are hypothesized for the onset of degenerative joint disease. These include hallux valgus and other deformities, trauma to the joint (particularly blunt trauma to the dorsal aspect of the first metatarsal head), infection, systemic arthritides, and primary osteoarthritis.

Although there are no good data for support, it appears that the most common form of hallux limitus is the primary form. This is associated with a variety of structural and functional causes, including a long first ray or a long hallux creating jamming at the first MTP joint; hypermobility of the first ray secondary to proximal hyperpronation, creating distal instability; neuromuscular disorders affecting the ability of the peroneus longus to pull down on the first ray; lack of available range of motion of the first ray as a result of degenerative joint disease; and structural first metatarsal elevatus. All of these structural and functional disorders create a functional gait disorder because of a lack of normal hallux dorsiflexion. When repetitive jamming and premature hinge motion of the first MTP joint occurs, synovitis of the first MTP joint will develop, followed by fibrillation of cartilage, erosion, and the development of subchondral cysts. Long-term changes include the development of hypertrophic bone formation on the dorsal aspect of the joint from repetitive jamming. Eventually, this dorsal spur formation creates a mechanical blockade that, if left untreated, may lead to ankylosis of the first MTP joint.

Although a variety of other causes have been described for hallux limitus, it is the structural and functional cause that bears the greatest impact on the discussion of surgical management. It is particularly crucial to understand the primacy of first-ray plantarflexion as the determining element in the dorsiflexion of the hallux on the first ray.[9] If the first metatarsal is too long or too elevated to allow the hallux to glide over the first metatarsal head, then jamming will occur. If the sesamoids do not have a functional articular cartilage to allow the first metatarsal head to glide, then premature hinge motion will occur at the joint, with a resultant repetitive jamming and hypertrophic bone formation. Kessel and Bonney[10] noted that their evidence ''suggests that hyperextension of the first metatarsal is the primary cause of hallux rigidus,'' and indeed much of the hallux limitus we repair results from first metatarsal dorsiflexion.

The proof of these concepts of first MTP joint motion can clearly be seen in the causes for iatrogenic hallux limitus. Iatrogenic hallux limitus most frequently occurs when the first metatarsal head is excessively dorsiflexed surgically in comparison to the second metatarsal.[11] Other causes include the failure to address all deforming forces in a hallux valgus repair, resulting in continued abductory range of motion of the first MTP joint. This abduction range of motion can result in a dorsal lateral jamming of the first MTP joint with hypertrophic bone formation. Although excessive dorsiflexion of the first metatarsal is the most common mechanism for the creation of an iatrogenic hallux limitus, inappropriate lengthening of the first metatarsal can also create jamming of the first MTP joint. Failure to provide for free articular motion

of the sesamoids can also result in hallux limitus deformity. Excessive tightening of soft tissue structures, or prolonged joint immobilization, can also create hallux limitus. The former commonly occurs when plantar soft tissue structures adaptively shorten in long-standing cases of hallux limitus.

CLINICAL FINDINGS AND EVALUATION

The patient with hallux limitus/rigidus usually presents with a gradual onset of pain and loss of motion in the first MTP joint. The hallux is usually in some element of plantarflexion with respect to the first metatarsal. There may be a hyperextension deformity at the interphalangeal joint of the hallux as compensation for the loss of motion about the first MTP joint. There is frequently a bony prominence on the dorsal and lateral aspects of the first metatarsal head. Dorsiflexion range of motion is restricted and may demonstrate crepitus. Plantarflexion range of motion may be normal and will often have no element of crepitus. There is usually pain to direct palpation of the first MTP joint. In the later stages, there may also be spasms about the extensor hallucis longus. The first metatarsal is usually in an elevatus position, which may represent either a primary deformity or a secondary adaptation.

It is important to assess motion with the foot loaded as well as in a relaxed non-weightbearing position. The more subtle functional cases of hallux limitus may only be detected by the former method. Of equal importance in the clinical evaluation are findings about the foot in areas other than the first MTP joint. Because of the lack of motion at the first MTP joint, the patient will generally redirect motion to the lateral side of the foot. Depending on the patient's foot type and the available range of motion of the first ray, this may present as either a lesion beneath the second metatarsal or lesions on the lateral border of the foot (Fig. 32–4). There may be severe metatarsalgia. In fact, the metatarsalgia pain may greatly exceed that of the pain around the first MTP joint and may be the presenting complaint.

A variety of other pathologies directly or indirectly related to inadequate hallux motion may be present, including plan-

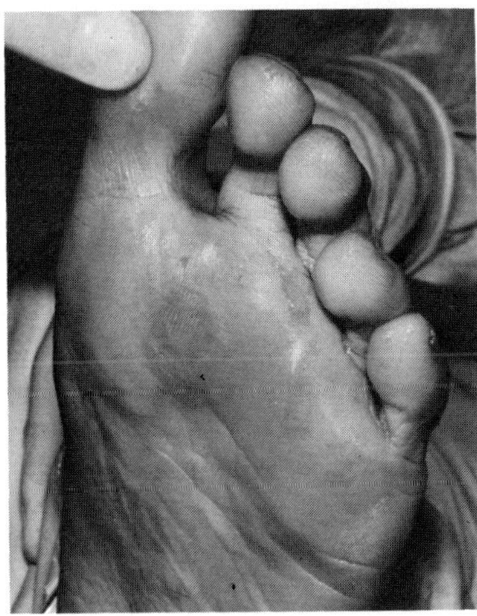

FIGURE 32–4. Preoperative photograph of hallux limitus. Note the absence of dorsiflexion of the first metatarsophalangeal joint and the presence of a keratotic lesion beneath the second metatarsal from lateral shifting of weight.

tar keratosis beneath the hallux interphalangeal joint associated with the presence of interphalangeal sesamoids, subungual exostosis of the hallux, onycholysis and paronychia of the hallux, and ulceration.[12] Dananberg and colleagues described the effects of functional hallux limitus on aspects of the superstructural skeleton.[13] They emphasized that a full range of motion may be present in the first MTP joint during non-weightbearing examination. However, if functional hallux limitus is present, heel lift can be delayed or restricted, making the deformity difficult to evaluate with the naked eye during the gait cycle. Dananberg and coauthors documented primary complaints of cephalgia, lower back pain, hip pain, knee pain, and leg pain caused by functional hallux limitus and alleviated by orthotic control of the functional hallux limitus.[13] The use of sophisticated clinical gait instrumentation has made it easier to observe the magnitude of the effects of functional hallux limitus on the human foot (Fig. 32–5). As this type of instrumentation becomes more commonly used, it will also allow earlier diagnosis of functional hallux limitus and perhaps result in a decrease in the number of patients requiring surgical management of the condition.

IMAGING FINDINGS

When hallux limitus has been present for some time, a variety of classic radiographic findings will be present: flattening of the first metatarsal head, narrowing of the first MTP joint, dorsal hypertrophic bone formation, subchondral bone cysts, particularly on the lateral side of the first metatarsal head, osteophytic proliferation on the base of the proximal phalanx, occasional loose bodies within the first MTP joint, and subchondral sclerosis. It is important to note that the width of the first MTP joint space can be particularly misleading. There are occasions when the hypertrophic bone formation serves to prop open the joint, making the radiographic appearance of the joint seem normal. After debridement of the hypertrophic bone formation, the joint drops back into a collapsed position, and it becomes clear that there is very little functional cartilage left. This misleading aspect of the radiologic appearance of hallux limitus/rigidus is a significant problem to the operating surgeon.

Radiographic appearance should be used as simply one tool to correlate with the clinical evaluation, including the available quantity and quality of the motion of the first MTP joint and the direction in which that motion is present. Meyer and coauthors demonstrated that lateral radiographic evidence of structural elevatus may not be significant.[14] Other imaging studies can also be useful, including computed tomographic scans for examination of the relationship of the sesamoids to the plantar aspect of the first metatarsal head (Fig. 32–6) and magnetic resonance imaging, which can be particularly useful for determining the extent of synovitis and cartilage destruction. As arthroscopic instrumentation and techniques improve, it may become more common to use arthroscopic techniques both diagnostically and therapeutically in the management of mild to moderate hallux limitus deformities.

CLASSIFICATION

No universally accepted classification system yet exists for hallux limitus and rigidus. Regnauld[15] classified hallux limitus as follows: Grade one, mild and functional; grade two, moderate and structural; and grade three, severe and exten-

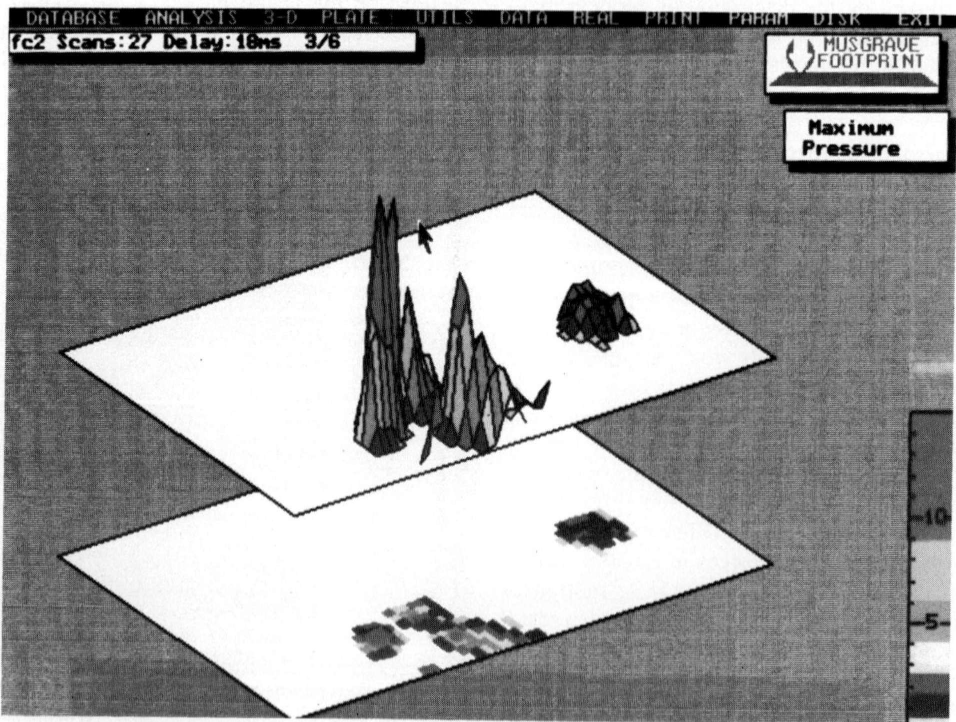

FIGURE 32–5. One type of output from the Musgrave Footprint. This patient presented with 0 degrees range of motion of the first metatarsophalangeal joint. The plantar pressures are greatest at the hallux and the third metatarsal head. The three-dimensional footprint depicts the relative magnitudes of pressures in height and are color coded. (Musgrave Footprint from Preston Communications, Llangollen, Wales, UK.)

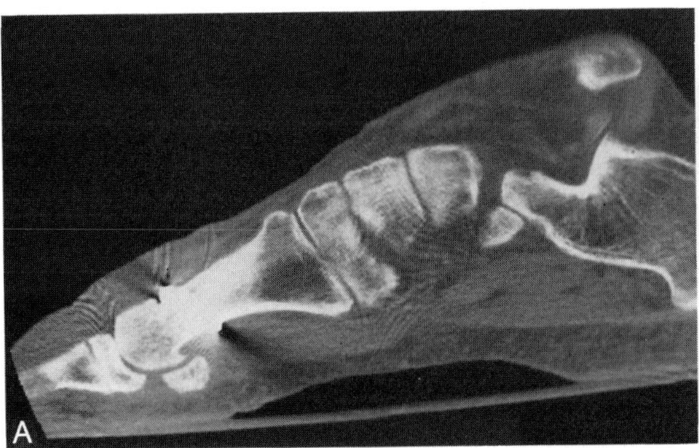
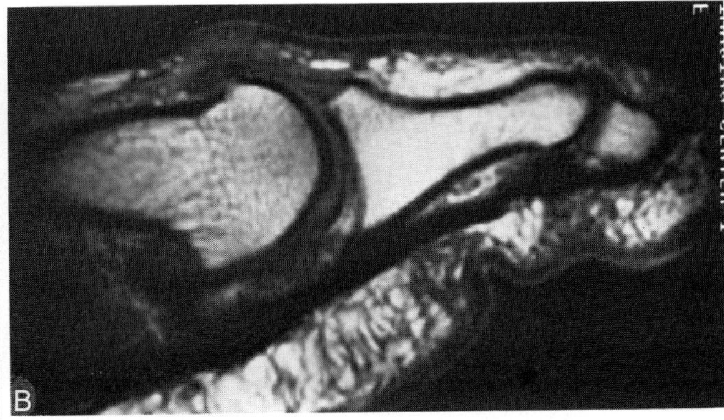

FIGURE 32–6. *A,* Computed tomography scan of the medial column. Note the narrowing of superior aspect of first metatarsophalangeal joint. Artifact at the distal shaft head junction represents a screw from prior surgery. An incompletely healed Akin is also noted. *B,* Magnetic resonance imaging scan of first metatarsophalangeal joint. Note the thickened dorsal synovial fold.

sive. Regnauld's grade one consists of functional limitation of motion with mild dorsal spurring and without structural disease (Fig. 32–7). Regnauld's grade two is demonstrated by a broad and flat metatarsal head, narrowing of the joint space, structural elevatus, hypertrophy of the sesamoids, and osteochondral defects in the metatarsal head (Fig. 32–8). Regnauld's grade three demonstrates severe loss of joint space with extensive periarticular spurs. There is extensive first metatarsal sesamoid disease and both osteochondral defects and joint mice (Fig. 32–9).

Drago and associates in 1984 proposed a four-step classification system.[16] In their scheme, grade one is a prehallux limitus with significant metatarsus primus elevatus, plantar subluxation of the proximal phalanx of the first metatarsal head, and significant pronatory changes in the rearfoot. The grade one deformity is functional in nature with minimal adaptive changes. Drago and associates' grade two demonstrates some flattening of the first metatarsal head, occasionally with osteochondral defects. Clinically, there is pain on end range of motion as in grade one, but structural adaptation may also have occurred. Passive range of motion is also limited. Plantar cartilage is in good condition with dorsal degeneration of cartilage and a dorsal exostosis. Drago and colleagues' grade three demonstrates more severe flattening of the metatarsal with greater hypertrophic bone formation, including a large dorsal exostosis on both the proximal phalanx and the first metatarsal head. The joint is narrowed with crepitus and pain on full range of motion. During surgical exploration, degeneration of articular artilage is found. Drago and colleagues' grade four is more severe than grade three, with total obliteration of the joint space, loose bodies within the joint capsule, and less than 10 degrees of total MTP joint motion. It is a subtotal ankylosis condition and may also progress to total ankylosis.[16] Rzonca and colleagues[17] also proposed a hallux equinus staging classification. They described three stages: stage one, young patients, functional limitus, with no osseous disease; stage two, moderate limitus, osseous disease, age variable; stage three, age variable, osseous disease at end stage, no motion.

As indicated previously, the usefulness of these classification systems is somewhat compromised by the misleading radiographic appearance that may be present. Nonetheless,

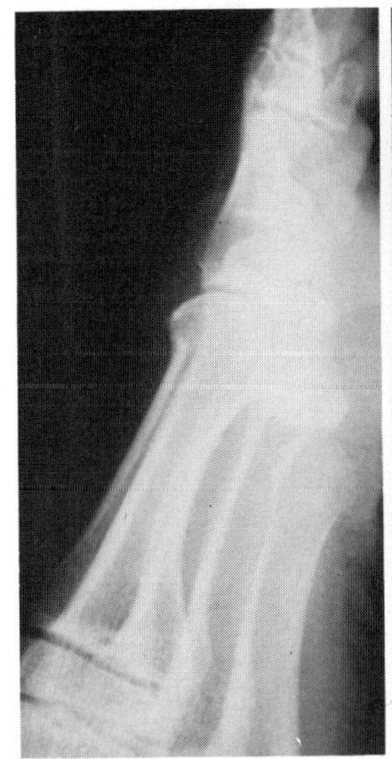
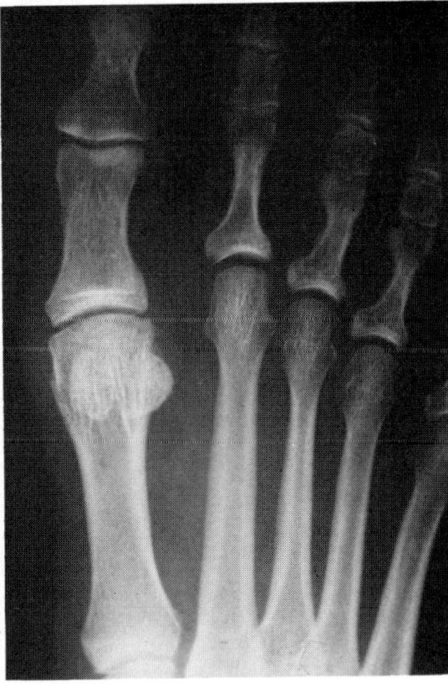

FIGURE 32–7. Radiographs *(A* and *B)* of a patient with symptomatic hallux limitus consistent with Regnauld grade I. Note the increased soft tissue density and very early dorsal spur. Small subchondral cysts are present in the first metatarsal head.

A   B

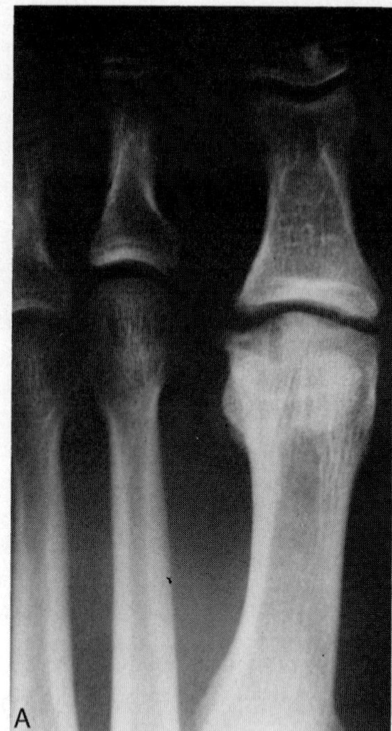
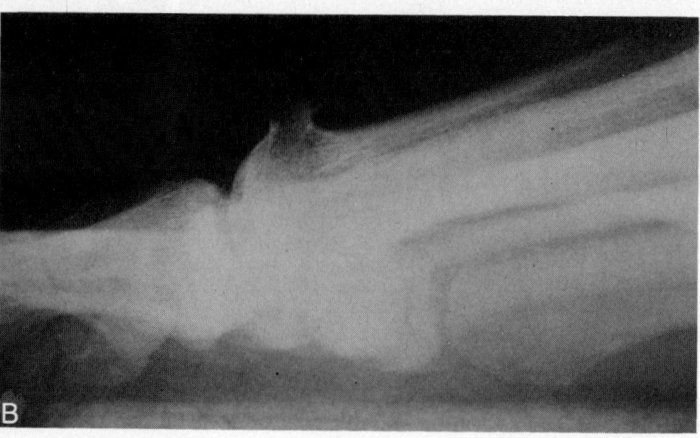

FIGURE 32–8. Radiographs of a typical hallux limitus consistent with Regnauld grade II. *A,* Dorsoplantar view demonstrating lateral hypertrophic bone and subchondral cysts. *B,* Lateral view demonstrating a dorsal flag of hypertrophic bone.

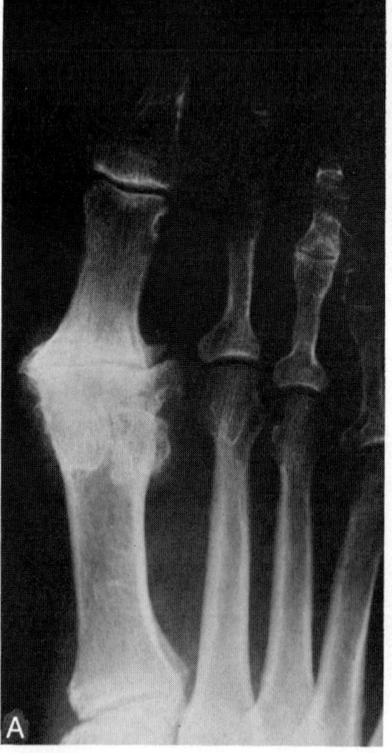
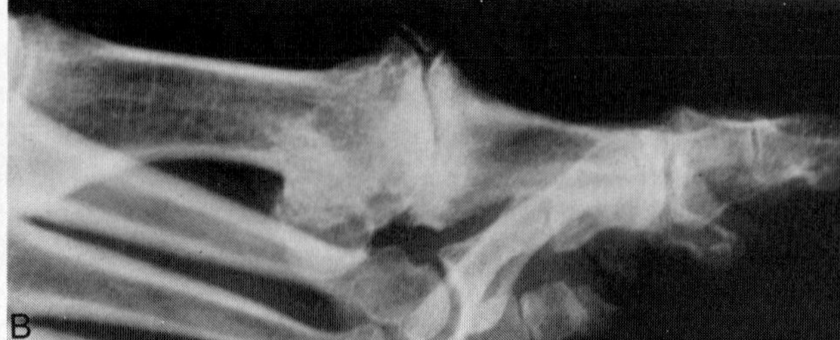

FIGURE 32–9. Radiographs of a patient with hallux rigidus consistent with Regnauld grade III. *A,* Dorsoplantar view demonstrates loss of joint space and large lateral exostoses. *B,* Oblique view demonstrates dorsal loose body and severe joint narrowing.

such classification systems are helpful in discussing treatment options. Clearly, there is a wide range of disease present in hallux limitus. The surgical management within this continuum varies quite significantly, from simple cheilectomy and perhaps synovectomy on one end and fusion or implant arthroplasty on the other end.

TREATMENT OF HALLUX LIMITUS

Conservative Modalities

There are a variety of nonsurgical modalities for the treatment of hallux limitus. Nonsteroidal antiinflammatory drugs, corticosteroid injections, and various physical therapy modalities can all be used to treat the symptoms of a painful or inflamed hallux limitus. Biomechanical treatment of the disorder is based on two principles: (1) to reduce the necessity for first MTP joint dorsiflexion and (2) to increase the available dorsiflexion range of motion by stabilizing the medial column and dropping the first metatarsal in a sagittal plane. These treatment modalities can be very effective for a functional hallux limitus without significant secondary changes. They can also be effective for patients in whom secondary changes have developed but who have limited functional demands. Patients with secondary changes and significant functional demands will generally not respond to these types of conservative modalities in the long run. It is also important to recognize that functional stabilization of the foot is an important component of the surgical repair. Following the variety of reconstructive techniques available, maintenance of the stability of the foot is ensured by the continued utilization of orthotic devices. Regardless of the sophistication of the surgical reconstruction of the foot, patients usually will benefit from postoperative functional stabilization by means of orthotic devices.

Joint-Destructive Procedures

To discuss the development of joint-reconstructive procedures fully, it is important to consider the implications of joint-destructive procedures. Procedures such as the Keller bunionectomy, the various implant arthroplasties, and first MTP joint fusion have a significant place in the management of hallux rigidus.[18] In a patient with more limited functional demands and significant secondary joint changes, some form of joint-destructive procedure may be the only alternative.

It is important to recognize that these procedures do have some significant disadvantages. Stutz and colleagues, in their review of 36 Keller arthroplasties, demonstrated shortening of the hallux in 73% of the cases, poor hallux purchase in 40%, malposition of the hallux in 70%, decreased range of motion in 81%, and reduced hallux purchase power in 73%.[19] Nonetheless, patients did report an 84% satisfaction rate. A variety of modifications have been described for the Keller bunionectomy, including those described by Ganley and colleagues in 1986.[20] Ganley and others reported a revision rate of 5% in Keller bunionectomies.[20] In apropulsive patients, the Keller bunionectomy has some significant advantages, including a relatively rapid recovery time and little postoperative morbidity. For patients with poor bone stock, the Keller bunionectomy may be the only alternative. On the other hand, for patients with good bone stock and high functional demand, the Keller bunionectomy has some significant functional disadvantages. O'Doherty and associates, in their 2-year follow-up study, reviewed a series of 81 patients in whom they compared Keller arthroplasty versus arthrodesis of the first MTP joint.[21] Their study was for both hallux valgus and hallux rigidus in the older patient. They reported a 44% incidence of nonunion in their first MTP joint fusions, although in retrospect they believed that perhaps their fixation technique was less than adequate. There was significant postoperative metatarsalgia after both the fusion and the arthroplasty procedures. Ultimately, they concluded that a Keller arthroplasty may be the treatment of choice in the older patient.[21]

First MTP joint prostheses have had considerable popularity in the treatment of hallux limitus and rigidus. However, in 1984, a significant article by Vanore, O'Keefe, and Pikscher enumerated and categorized the types of complications that can result from silicone implant arthroplasties.[22] This article very graphically demonstrated intrinsic implant failures such as deformation and fatigue fracture as well as microfragmentation. Others reported on implant complications. Verhaar and colleagues[23] reported on the presence of foreign-body, giant-cell reactions to silicone and on the pervasiveness of osteolysis. Only 25% of the patients in their series were free of cysts; 75% of the metatarsal heads and 59% of the proximal phalanges were cystic.[23] Verhaar and others noted an increase in shortening of the toe over time.[24] The overall increasing incidence of these problems led many surgeons to begin reviewing alternatives to implant arthroplasties. Additional problems with adjacent bones, such as aseptic necrosis, bone detritus, bone cysts, and ectopic bone formation further served to raise concern among foot and ankle surgeons.[25–28] The publication of Vanore and coworkers' article served to crystallize surgical thought regarding the limitations of silicone implant arthroplasties.[22] It particularly became clear that the hemi-implant arthroplasty should be restricted to those situations in which there is not significant double-sided degenerative joint disease. In addition, significant functional load increases the likelihood of the development of some of these complications. Resection of an adequate amount of bone is critical to prevent excessive compression of the implant device on the metatarsal head. First MTP joint prostheses still have a place in reconstructive foot surgery. New materials and designs continue to be developed in response to some of the limitations of current procedures.

Regnauld[15] described a procedure that avoids silicone endoprostheses but accomplishes intracapsular shortening to relieve tension on the joint (Fig. 32–10). The procedure has limitations but may occasionally be useful.

First MTP joint fusion is a time-honored procedure.[29] It has been used particularly in the orthopedic community and in the military for the treatment of painful hallux rigidus and limitus. A variety of technical modifications are available to increase the likelihood of success after first MTP joint fusion. These include techniques to preserve the contour of the metatarsal head and base of the proximal phalanx and superior internal fixation techniques. These have raised the union rate after first MTP joint arthrodesis. There continue to be limitations with the procedure, particularly for individuals who wish to wear a variety of different heel heights. Increased lateral loading on the forefoot after arthrodesis can create

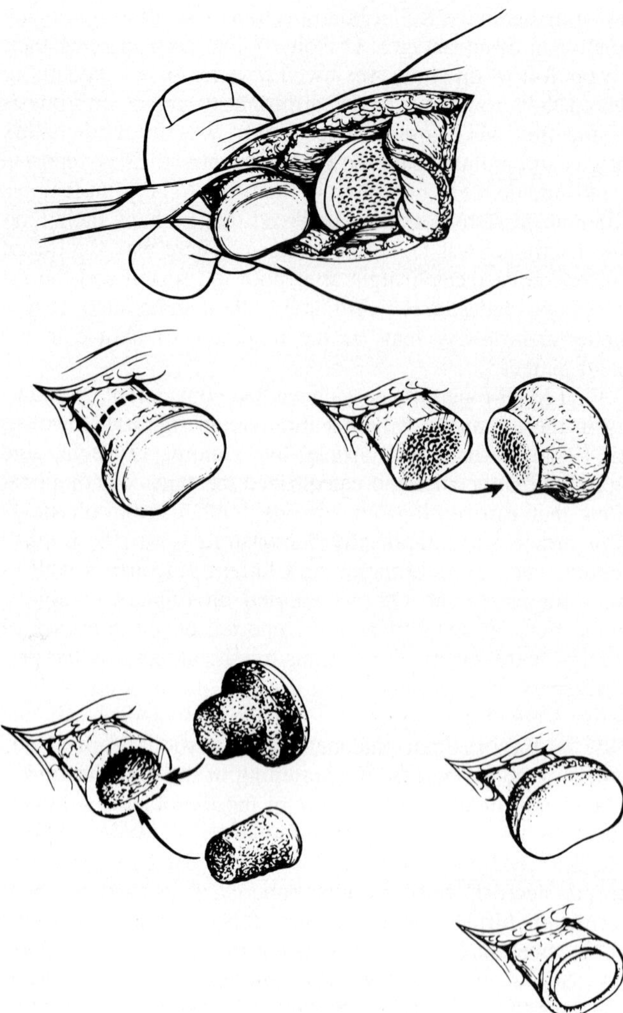

FIGURE 32–10. Diagram illustrating the Regnauld procedure. The procedure creates an autogenous osteocartilaginous graft out of the base of the proximal phalanx and shortens the hallux. (From Jahss M: Disorders of the Foot, Vol 2, 2nd ed, Philadelphia, WB Saunders, 1991, p 1038.)

significant gait disturbances. For patients with severe degenerative joint disease who have significant functional demands, arthrodesis is an acceptable treatment alternative. It provides stability within the medial column and avoids the risks associated with silicone devices. It can be particularly successful in middle-aged and older men with severe degenerative joint disease for whom reconstructive surgery is not an option.

RECONSTRUCTIVE TECHNIQUES FOR REPAIR OF HALLUX LIMITUS/RIGIDUS

A variety of techniques are available for repairing the joint with hallux limitus/rigidus.[30] Most of these procedures can be grouped under one or more of the following concepts: (1) plantarflexion of the first-ray segment to increase dorsiflexory reciprocal motion; (2) stabilization of the medial column again to allow greater reciprocal plantarflexion of the first ray; (3) decompression of the joint by intracapsular shortening; (4) extra-articular shortening to decrease the digital length pattern of the hallux; (5) removal of the mechanical

blockade; (6) rearrangement of the effective articular cartilage to provide more dorsiflexion; and (7) stimulation of new cartilage. There are also some miscellaneous procedures that partially fall into one or more of these categories. The philosophy behind reconstruction of the first MTP joint involves the following criteria: (1) The joint must be reconstructible to an acceptable quantity and quality of motion; (2) the cause of the hallux limitus must be addressed surgically or postoperatively by orthotic control; and (3) postoperative rehabilitation must begin very soon after surgery to allow for maximum preservation of the increase in range of motion obtained during surgical correction.

CHEILECTOMY

Reduction of the mechanical blockade of hallux limitus is an important element in most types of hallux limitus repair. It is routinely performed in association with a variety of other hallux limitus reconstruction procedures. It can also be performed as an isolated procedure in certain instances. Mann, Coughlin, and DuVries described the use of the cheilectomy procedure for hallux rigidus in a series of 20 patients observed for more than 5½ years.[31] In these patients, cheilectomy was the only procedure performed. The average age of the patients was 56.8 years. Mann and colleagues found that patients were satisfied with the procedure and that an increase in motion occurred.[31, 32]

In our own experience, cheilectomy is most often used as an adjunctive procedure, as described previously. However, there are instances in which cheilectomy is performed as an isolated procedure. In cases of traumatic hallux limitus in which the removal of one or more fragments is the principal surgical objective, cheilectomy is often the only procedure required. In some older patients with insignificant functional demands, cheilectomy may produce a significant reduction in symptoms, even when motion is not significantly increased. However, there is also another side to the removal of the mechanical blockade. Without treatment of the initial cause, many younger patients will have an exacerbation of the symptoms caused by the increase in available range of motion on a poor articular surface. These patients respond to cheilectomy with an increase in symptoms caused by an increase in local synovitis.

The technique for cheilectomy involves a dorsal medial incision similar to that used for hallux valgus repair. Capsule is incised in a linear manner and reflected medially and laterally. The joint is inspected and hypertrophic and inflamed synovium is removed (Fig. 32–11). The synovectomy portion of this procedure can be an important adjunct in the reduction of symptoms. If there is any question about the appearance of the synovium, a synovial biopsy is obtained. The dorsal flag on the first metatarsal head is then removed with either power or hand instrumentation. The lateral side of the metatarsal head is also inspected for hypertrophic bone formation. The dorsal and lateral sides of the base of the proximal phalanx are also inspected, and a rongeur is used to debride any hypertrophic bone. The articular surface is carefully inspected on the base of the proximal phalanx and the head of the metatarsal (Fig. 32–12). The sesamoids are inspected and evaluated for range of motion. After remodeling the metatarsal head with a hand rasp or power bur, a significant cancellous area may be exposed. This may be

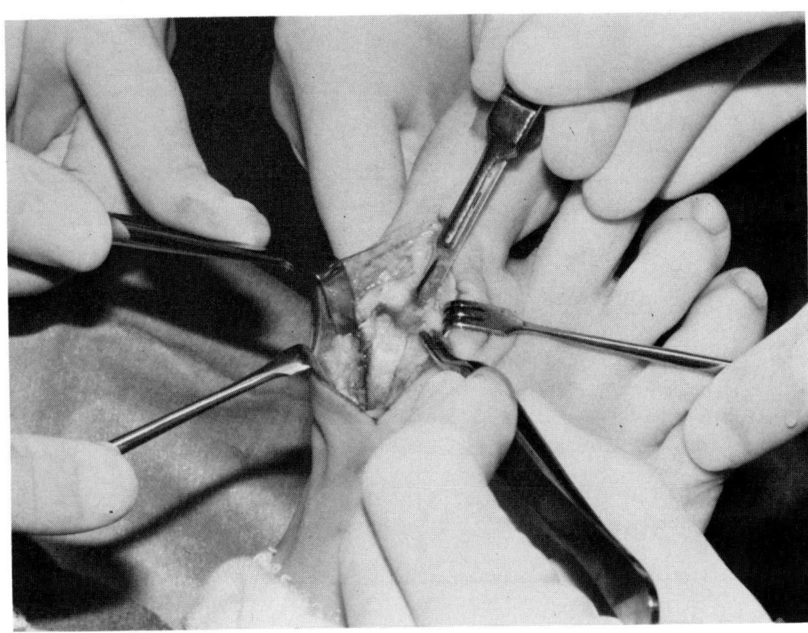

FIGURE 32–11. Excision of a hypertrophic inflamed synovium.

treated with bone wax or topical thrombin to reduce bleeding. Careful hemostasis is critical during this procedure. Excessive bleeding into the joint space will result in hematoma, fibrosis, and the early return of stiffness and mechanical blockade. When cheilectomy is performed as an isolated procedure, a minimum of 45 degrees of dorsiflexion should be obtained on the table after removal of the mechanical blockade.

SHORTENING PROCEDURES

A long first ray or hallux has often been associated with the development of hallux limitus. With a long medial column, jamming of the joint occurs prematurely, resulting in the development of a dorsal flag and subsequent mechanical blockade. Shortening can be achieved in a variety of ways.

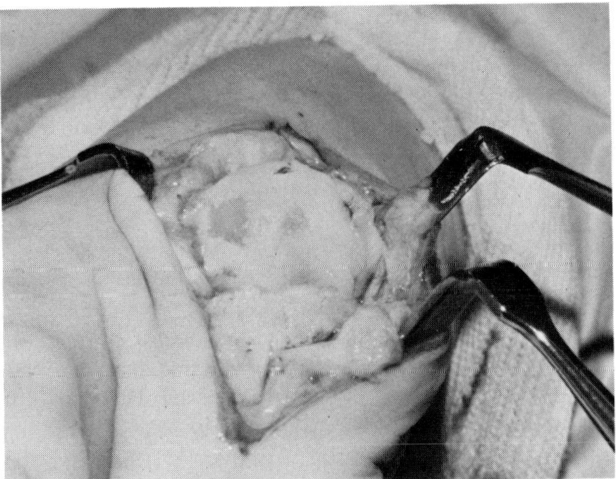

FIGURE 32–12. Intraoperative view of the metatarsal head in a Regnauld grade II hallux limitus. The two dorsal cartilage defects flank an area of chondromalacia. Abrasion chondroplasty and continuous passive motion may allow resurfacing of these defects.

If the cause of the deformity is a long hallux, then a cylindrical Akin-type procedure can be performed at the base of the proximal phalanx. In my own experience, this is not a common manifestation of the problem. More commonly, shortening is required in the metatarsal head region. This can be performed either as a secondary objective, such as with a Watermann procedure, in which the primary objective is to redirect the cartilage dorsally, or it can be achieved as the primary objective. Shortening of the first metatarsal at the head can be accomplished by segmental shortening of the bone, such as with a true Chevron-type procedure, or it can be achieved by means of the hinge-axis concept. The axis technique of the Austin osteotomy is modified to achieve shortening (Fig. 32–13). For this objective, the osteotomy axis is directed from medial distal to lateral proximal. This creates shortening of the first-ray segment as the metatarsal head is displaced in a lateral direction. The utilization of the axis concept can be limited in situations in which the metatarsal is very narrow or the intermetatarsal angle is low, creating little opportunity for lateral displacement of the metatarsal head. In most situations, there is adequate metatarsal width and intermetatarsal space to create adequate shortening. The shortening procedure itself creates less jamming at the joint and also serves to relax the surrounding tissue structures.

PLANTARFLEXION PROCEDURES

Most commonly, surgical shortening of the first-ray segment is combined with plantarflexion. To have a functional first MTP joint, the first metatarsal must be in a position to allow reciprocal motion of the hallux over a plantarflexing first metatarsal. Just as the axis of the Austin osteotomy can be modified to create shortening, so can the axis be modified to create plantarflexion. When the axis is raised dorsal medial to plantar lateral, the capital fragment will displace in a plantar direction as it displaces laterally (Fig. 32–14). Again, there is a limitation to this technique based on the width of

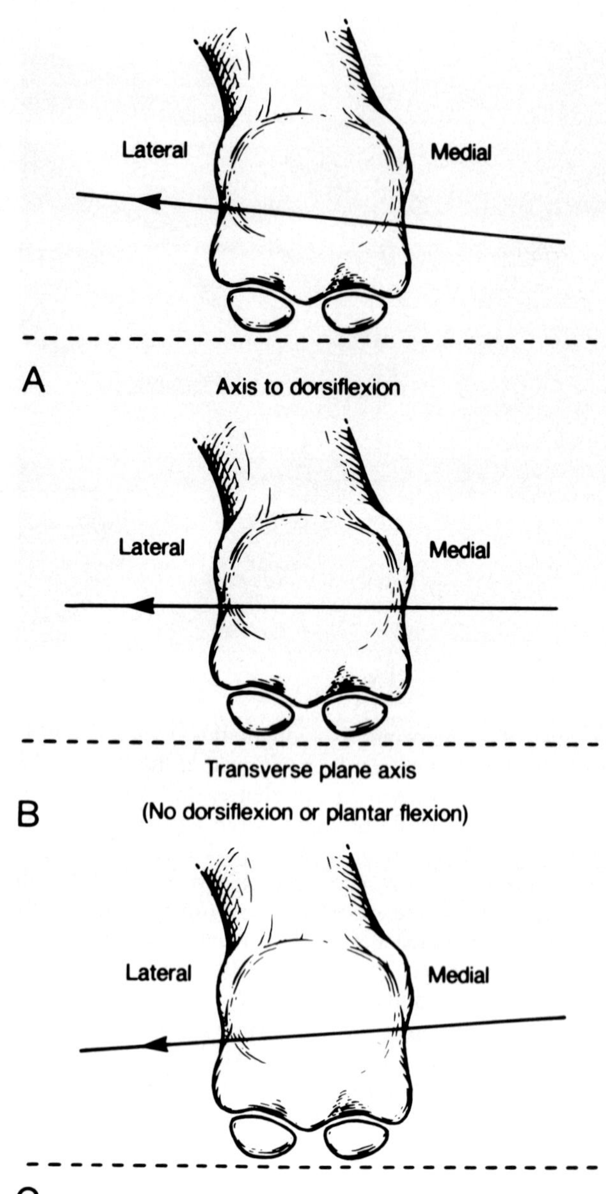

FIGURE 32–13. Diagram illustrating the axis concept and the technique for altering the sagittal plane position of the metatarsal head during a transposition osteotomy. (From Boberg J, Ruch J, and Banks A: Distal metaphyseal osteotomies in hallux abducto valgus surgery. *In* McGlamry ED [ed]: Comprehensive Textbook of Foot Surgery, Vol 1, p 179. © 1987, the Williams & Wilkins Co., Baltimore.)

the metatarsal and the intermetatarsal separation. Nonetheless, a very significant amount of plantarflexion can be created using this technique. In fact, overplantarflexion is a hazard that must be carefully avoided. Use of the Kirschner wire as an axis guide, rather than simple "eyeballing" of the axis, is the most effective way to ensure accurate positioning of the metatarsal head.

The Youngswick modification of the Austin osteotomy can also be used in hallux limitus repair.[33] This modification involves another bone cut parallel to the plantar component of the traditional Austin cuts. This serves to shorten and plantarflex the first ray. The Mitchell and Hohman procedures also can be used to create plantarflexion. Both of these osteotomies are distal transverse osteotomies that allow the metatarsal head to be shifted plantarly and laterally. Each one creates some significant shortening of the first metatarsal as well. Metatarsalgia has been reported to be a common complication after these types of osteotomies. This may most

often be attributed to early weightbearing or inadequate fixation. These osteotomies are often the cause of iatrogenic hallux limitus, but with proper technique they can be used for plantarflexion.

CARTILAGE REARRANGEMENT

In hallux limitus deformity, there is often good functional articular cartilage on the plantar aspect of the metatarsal head with more eroded cartilage dorsally. The Watermann-type osteotomy has been described for rearrangement of functional articular cartilage to improve the cartilage in a dorsal direction.[34] Essentially, the osteotomy is a dorsiflexory osteotomy of the articular cartilage of the first metatarsal. The procedure was originally described as the removal of a trapezoidal wedge of bone, with the wider side of the wedge being dorsal. Removal of the wedge of bone creates a less stable osteotomy but increases the amount of shortening of

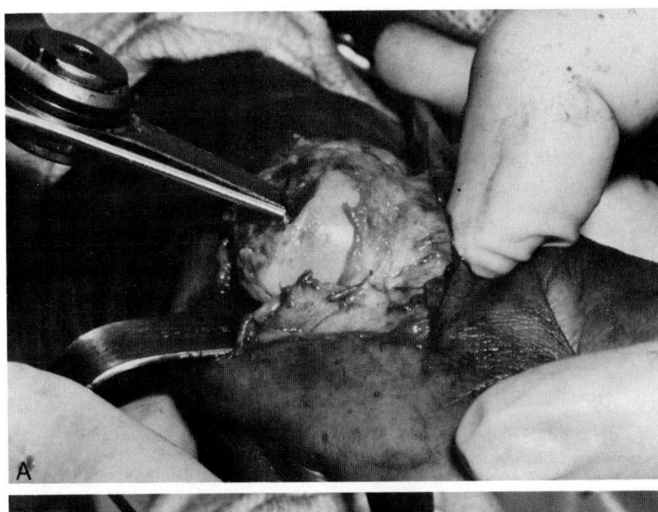
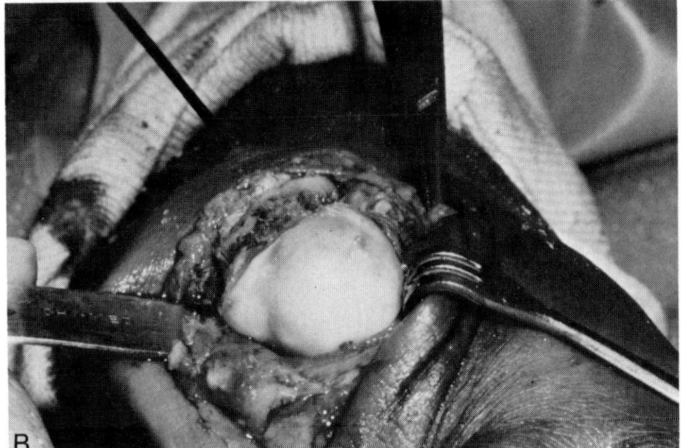

FIGURE 32–14. *A,* Intraoperative view demonstrating the application of the axis concept to achieve plantarflexion during an Austin osteotomy. A saw-blade is placed parallel to the guide wire. *B,* Intraoperative view demonstrating plantarflexion of the first metatarsal head after lateral transposition.

the segment (Fig. 32–15). Most commonly, the osteotomy is performed with an intact plantar hinge (Fig. 32–16). The procedure can be performed either very distally, just behind the articular cartilage, or more proximally, at the junction between the neck and head. The advantage of performing the procedure more distally is that it creates less disturbance over the sesamoids.[35] Malay (Personal communication, 1992) demonstrated that these types of very distal osteotomies may have a greater incidence of avascular necrosis. More proximal placement of the Watermann-type osteotomy may reduce the incidence of avascular necrosis and may allow for more secure fixation.

Another modification of the procedure is the Watermann-Green technique. This procedure is similar to a distal L or Reverdin Green osteotomy, in which a plantar cut is made parallel to the supporting surface, exiting proximal to the sesamoid apparatus. In the Green-Reverdin procedure, a wedge osteotomy is then performed on the dorsal cut to correct the proximal set angle. With the Watermann-Green procedure, the wedge is resected with the base of the wedge dorsal and the apex at the midpoint of the metatarsal head.[35] This allows for dorsiflexion of the functional articular cartilage without interruption of the sesamoid apparatus. The Watermann osteotomy, in combination with a cheilectomy, can be a useful procedure in middle-aged patients with less stressful functional demands.

Because stability of these osteotomies allows earlier mo-

bilization of the joint, fixation should be ensured. A variety of techniques can be used, but internal fixation is preferred to avoid interfering with dorsal skin excursion. Suture, buried Kirschner wires, small staples, absorbable pins, and stainless steel or titanium screws can all be used. So long as the fixation is secure and internal, early motion can begin. Kessel and Bonney[10] described a dorsiflexory osteotomy at the base of the proximal phalanx. Their series included just 10 procedures on nine patients, but the technique developed some degree of acceptance as a way to transfer good range of plantarflexion to a functionally useful dorsiflexory range. Excessive dorsiflexion can create nail disease, but the procedure has some limited use for moderate limitus deformities in patients with limited functional demands.

ABRASION CHONDROPLASTY

A great deal of attention of has been paid to the healing of cartilage defects. Cartilage itself comes in three basic forms: (1) fibrocartilage, containing a high proportion of collagen; (2) elastic cartilage, containing a high number of elastin fibers; and (3) articular cartilage, which is of greatest concern in joint reconstruction. Articular cartilage is made of both collagen fibers and a hydrated glycoprotein gel. The collagen fibers are oriented in a structural pattern reflecting stresses applied to that particular joint. It is the properties created by the combination of the collagen network and the proteogly-

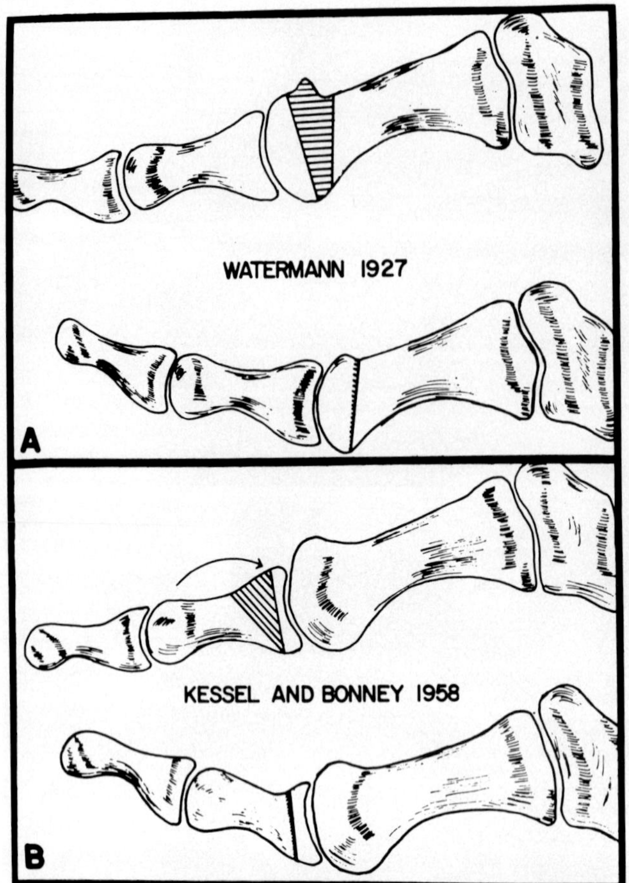

FIGURE 32–15. Diagrammatic representation of original Watermann and Kessel and Bonney procedures. Note that the Watermann osteotomy shortens the first metatarsal as well as dorsiflexes the articular cartilage. The Kessel and Bonney procedure acts by reducing the amount of dorsiflexory motion necessary during propulsion. (From Kelikian H: Hallux Valgus, Allied Deformities of the Forefoot and Metatarsalgia. Philadelphia, WB Saunders, 1965, p 280.)

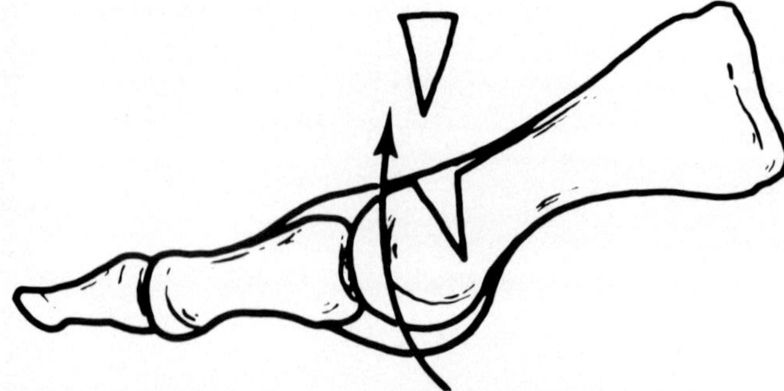

FIGURE 32–16. Diagram illustrating a Watermann procedure variation with wedge osteotomy to rotate effective plantar cartilage dorsally. (From Smith T, Malay DS, and Ruch JA: Hallux limitus and rigidus. *In* McGlamry ED [ed]: Comprehensive Textbook of Foot Surgery, Vol 1, p 245. © 1987, the Williams & Wilkins Co., Baltimore.)

The principles behind this technique have been extensively studied by Salter.[36] The technique is useful only if patient rehabilitation begins immediately postoperatively with either continuous passive range-of-motion or frequent passive range-of-motion exercises on a daily basis. Akeson and colleagues[37] noted that stress deprivation from immobilization produces an increase in fibrofatty connective tissue within the joint, ulceration at points of cartilage—cartilage contact, atrophy of cartilage, adhesions between synovial folds, and a collagen mass decrease of 10%. Figure 32–17 demonstrates resurfacing of a previously drilled defect in the first metatarsal head.

COMBINATION PROCEDURES

The reconstruction of a hallux limitus joint frequently necessitates a variety of procedures on any given patient. These usually include cheilectomy, partial synovectomy, abrasion chondroplasty, and osteotomy reconstruction either in the form of capital osteotomies or base osteotomies (Fig. 32–18).

In patients with significant elevatus deformities, a plantar-flexory base osteotomy is performed. This is usually fixed with two screws, with the cortical hinge left intact. Most frequently, this procedure is performed with the apex and

can gel that allows articular cartilage to function. Articular cartilage must provide for two properties: (1) adequate slipperiness and resilience and (2) significant durability despite severe loading. Although articular cartilage appears smooth macroscopically, it is actually made up of small undulations on the surface of the cartilage, which help to entrap synovial fluid. This mechanism facilitates lubrication of the joint.

The technique for abrasion chondroplasty involves multiple fine drill holes into areas of devitalized cartilage. Drilling is performed down onto subchondral bone. A fine drill bit or a .035 or .045 Kirschner wire is used to make the drill hole depending on the size of the defect and the size of the metatarsal head. The drill holes must not be placed so close together that the holes will collapse on each other, making one large defect. In addition, because making the drill holes will increase the possibility of intracapsular bleeding, drill holes should be limited strictly to those areas where it is vital to have functioning cartilage. The technique is not performed until final positioning of the metatarsal head has occurred. The principle of abrasion chondroplasty is to allow healthy fibrocartilage to migrate into areas of chondromalacia or fibrosis within the joint. This technique has been successfully used after removal of osteochondral fractures of the talus.

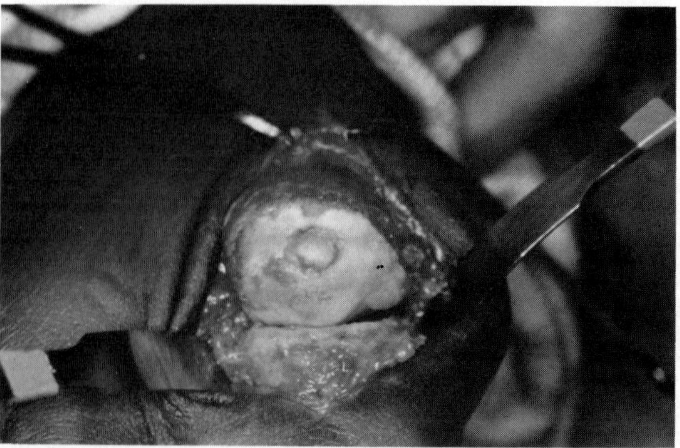

FIGURE 32–17. Intraoperative photograph demonstrating resurfacing of a central defect 1 year after subchondral drilling. (Courtesy of Raymond Cavaliere, D.P.M.)

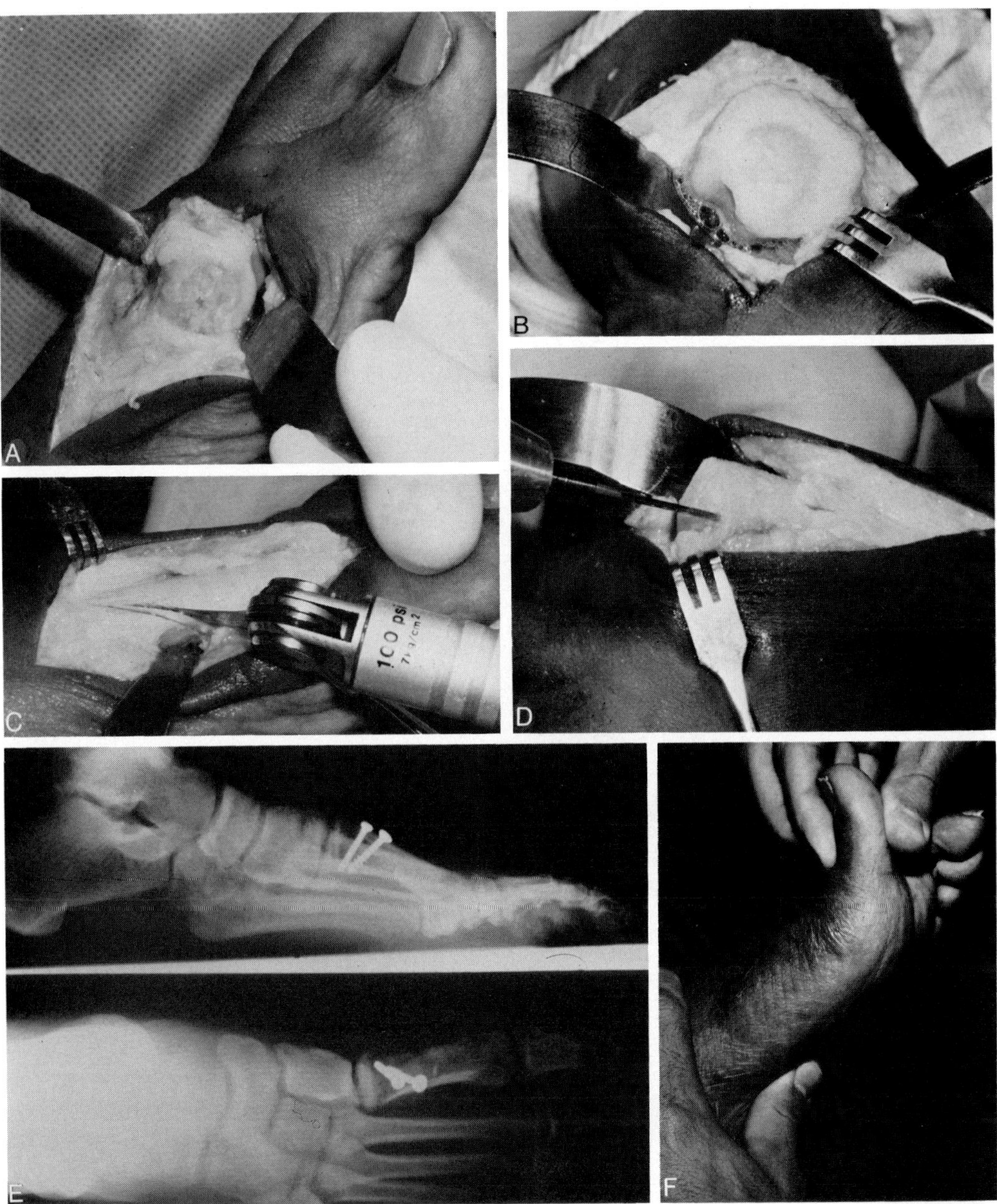

FIGURE 32–18. Hallux limitus in a 35-year-old soldier (preoperative radiographs are seen in Fig. 32–8). *A,* Intraoperative lateral view demonstrating a dorsal spur. *B,* Intraoperative view of the metatarsal head demonstrates severe chondromalacia and thick synovial fluid. *C,* Plantarflexory base osteotomy. *D,* Subchondral drilling of the first metatarsal head. *E,* Postoperative radiographs at 2 months. Note the lucency of the first metatarsal head indicating revascularization following subchondral drilling. *F,* Photograph demonstrating a dorsiflexory range of motion at 3 months postoperatively.

hinge of the osteotomy located in a dorsoproximal direction to maximize the amount of plantarflexion that occurs. The base osteotomy is performed after the cheilectomy and synovectomy. After completion of the plantarflexory osteotomy, the joint is once again inspected. Plantarflexory osteotomies may actually exaggerate the angulation deformity in a joint in which articular cartilage is located only on the plantar aspect of the metatarsal head. In these patients, it is particularly important to inspect the joint once again after completion of the plantarflexory osteotomy. Frequently, it will be clear that a Watermann-type osteotomy is necessary. Although double osteotomies may increase the possibility of avascular necrosis (Malay DS, Personal communication,

1992), it is also clear that reconstruction of the arthritic first MTP joint frequently requires the combination of these two osteotomies. In order for this combination of procedures to be successful, stable internal fixation is required for both osteotomies. This is most commonly performed with screw fixation for the base osteotomy and buried Kirschner wire or absorbable pin fixation for the capital osteotomy. The combination of the plantarflexory osteotomy and Watermann osteotomy is usually performed on younger patients and on those patients with greater functional demands (Fig. 32–19).

Middle-aged patients and those with somewhat less significant functional demands most commonly require a cheilectomy, partial synovectomy, and capital osteotomy. The capi-

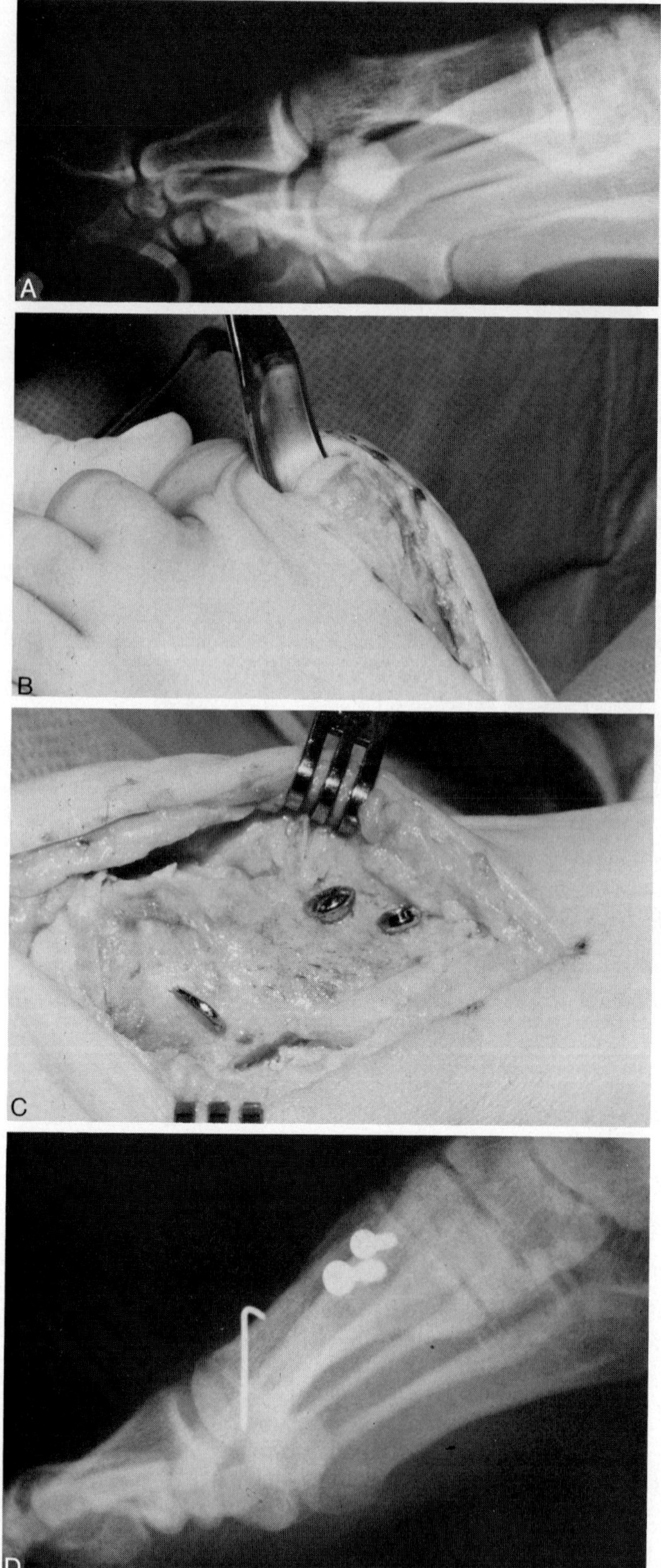

FIGURE 32–19. Iatrogenic hallux limitus following a Mitchell bunionectomy. *A*, Lateral radiograph demonstrates elevation of the distal first metatarsal segment. *B*, Use of the McGlamry elevator is critical for stripping adhered soft tissues in revisional surgery. *C*, View of buried fixation: Kirschner wire for Watermann osteotomy, screw fixation for sagittal closing wedge–plantarflexory osteotomy. *D*, Lateral radiograph demonstrating fixation placement and osteotomy position.

tal osteotomy is most commonly involved in correction of the angulation of the cartilage or the creation of plantarflexion or shortening.

POSTOPERATIVE CARE

Although postoperative care is important in every procedure performed, it is imperative that the patient actively participate in the postoperative care after hallux limitus reconstruction. Patients selected for the procedures listed previously should be willing to engage in the immediate and vigorous rehabilitation of the joint. Failure to begin immediate rehabilitation will result in fibrosis, readhesion of soft tissues, and joint stiffness.

The typical rehabilitation of a patient with a plantarflexory base osteotomy, Watermann procedure, and cheilectomy begins with a below-knee cast applied at the time of surgery. Two days postoperatively, the cast is given a bivalve, and a dressing change is performed. Assuming that there is no significant edema or sign of infection, passive range of motion of the joint is demonstrated to the patient. A dry, sterile dressing is then placed on the osteotomy site, and the bivalved cast is reapplied. The patient is instructed to begin range-of-motion exercises twice daily; movement of the hallux is performed with full reciprocal motion. That is, as the hallux is dorsiflexed, the first metatarsal is plantarflexed passively. Full available excursion is performed 10 times in each direction and held each time for 10 seconds. At 12 to 14 days postoperatively, the bandages are removed, and the patient is placed into an elastic stocking and bunion splint, followed by reapplication of the bivalved cast. With the absence of the dry, sterile dressing, the patient is now able to begin more vigorous range-of-motion exercises. Because of the use of internal fixation, the patient is also able to bathe the foot. Patients are instructed to bathe the foot in warm water before the range-of-motion exercises and to continue with exercises two to three times daily. Should the joint become inflamed or painful, it is important to treat the symptoms quickly to keep the patient from becoming discouraged and discontinuing the exercises. The use of ice after the exercises is encouraged and the use of nonsteroidal antiinflammatory drugs is also encouraged on an as-needed basis. The patient is not allowed to bear weight on the cast until approximately 5 to 6 weeks postoperatively. Serial x-rays are performed at 2 weeks and 6 weeks postoperatively. Assuming adequate consolidation, the patient is able to wear a running shoe with an elastic sock. If the patient has previously worn orthotics, he or she may wear the orthotics on a short-term basis until recasting of the foot can occur with the fabrication of new devices that will accommodate the change in foot position.

Because patient cooperation is so important, the frequency of office visits must be determined by the anticipated cooperation of the patient. If at 2 weeks postoperatively it is clear that the patient has performed very little range-of-motion exercises, then the patient may need to be seen weekly or be seen by a physical therapist to ensure compliance. In my own experience, most patients do not require a therapist for these types of exercises. However, a physical therapist and the use of physical therapy modalities may be very helpful in some patients. The recent development of a first MTP joint continuous passive motion device will change the postoperative care and allow for more significant joint motion exercises earlier (Fig. 32–20).

For patients who have only a capital osteotomy performed, the rehabilitation is somewhat different. The patient is placed in a wooden-soled postoperative shoe and is kept nonweightbearing for 2 weeks. The schedule of range-of-motion exercises is otherwise the same. Partial weightbearing is performed weeks 2 through 4 followed by full weightbearing after week 4. This is entirely dependent on the type of capital osteotomy performed, the security of the fixation, and the adequacy of the bone stock.

The use of postoperative orthoses is helpful for most of these patients for at least 1 year after the surgery. Depending on the extent of full structural correction, some will require continuing orthotic control.

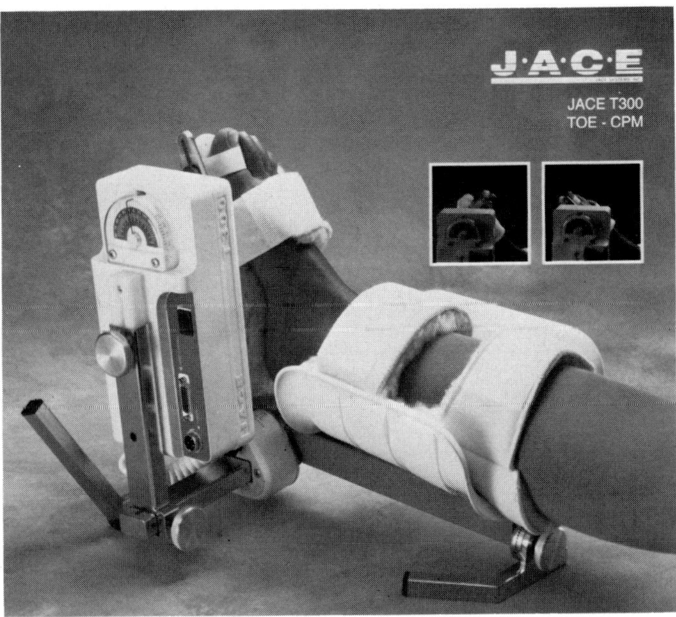

FIGURE 32–20. First metatarsophalangeal joint continuous passive motion device. (Courtesy of JACE Systems, Inc., and Thera Kinetics, Mt. Laurel, NJ.)

COMPLICATIONS

This type of reconstructive surgical intervention on the first MTP joint is meticulous surgery requiring both finesse in the execution of the soft tissue dissection and accuracy in the placement of osteotomies. The lack of patient cooperation can result in continued stiffness of the joint by failure to move the joint sufficiently during the initial postoperative period. Hematoma or excessive edema can also significantly delay early range of motion and result in compromising the final postoperative result.

Depending on the availability of good cartilage, an adequate Watermann procedure may take away some plantarflexory purchase power of the hallux. Placement of the osteotomies can also create complications through overplantarflexion or inadequate correction. Excessive plantarflexion can occur both with a base osteotomy and with capital osteotomies. Most frequently, this occurs in the patient with a flexible or semirigid forefoot valgus-type deformity. Although these patients do end up compensating through subtalar joint pronation, the plantarflexed first metatarsal can create tibial sesamoiditis in these patients. Because the available range of motion often allows excessive dorsiflexion of the first ray, it is tempting to plantarflex these patients significantly. Some plantarflexion is usually required, but the remainder of the correction needs to occur through postoperative orthotic control.

Early range of motion can also create problems of osteotomy stability if the osteotomies are not fixated properly. Usually the postoperative care can be tailored to the degree of stability present at the osteotomy site. Early weightbearing on a less stable capital or base osteotomy can create loss of correction.

Most importantly, it is necessary to review with the patient preoperatively the surgeon's expectations and the patient's expectations for the surgery. It is important to give the patient realistic expectations, depending on the degree of arthrosis, the bone quality, and the patient's age. The most important goals are a decrease in pain and restoration of adequate, if not normal, function to the first MTP joint. Using the combinations of procedures described previously, it is usually possible to give the patient accurate expectations regarding the degree of pain relief and the degree of increase in range of motion to be expected.

References

1. Cotterill J: Stiffness of the great toe in adolescents. Br Med J 1:1158, 1888.
2. Root M, Orien W, and Weed J: Normal and abnormal function of the foot. Clin Biomechanics 3:358, 1977.
3. Buell T, Green DR, and Risser J: Measurement of the first metatarsophalangeal joint range of motion. J Am Podiatr Med Assoc 78:439–448, 1988.
4. Nilsonne H: Hallux rigidus and its treatment. Acta Orthop Scand 1:295–303, 1930.
5. Malay DS: Etiology of hallux limitus and hallux rigidus. *In* McGlamry ED (ed): Categoric Foot Rehabilitation. Doctors Hospital Fourteenth Annual Surgical Seminar Text. Tucker, GA, Podiatry Institute, 1985, p 182.
6. McMaster MJ: The pathogenesis of hallux rigidus. J Bone Joint Surg 60B:82–87, 1978.
7. Brahm S: Shape of the first metatarsal head in hallux rigidus and hallux valgus. J Am Podiatr Med Assoc 78:300–304, 1988.
8. Bingold A and Collins D: Hallux rigidus. J Bone Joint Surg 32B:214–222, 1950.
9. Jack EA: The aetiology of hallux rigidus. Br J Surg 27:492–497, 1940.
10. Kessel L and Bonney G: Hallux rigidus in the adolescent. J Bone Joint Surg 40B:668–673, 1958.
11. Mahan KT: Repair of iatrogenic hallux limitus. *In* DiNapoli DR (ed): Reconstructive Surgery of the Foot and Leg: Update '90. Tucker, GA, Podiatry Institute, 1990, pp 144–148.
12. Daniels E: Neuropathic foot ulcer prevention in diabetic American Indians with hallux limitus. J Am Podiatr Med Assoc 79:447–450, 1989.
13. Dananberg H, Lawton M, and DiNapoli DR: Hallux limitus and nonspecific gait related bodily trauma. *In* DiNapoli DR (ed): Reconstructive Surgery of the Foot and Leg: Update '90. Tucker, GA, Podiatry Associates, 1990, pp 52–59.
14. Meyer J, Nishon L, Weiss L, and Docks G: Metatarsus primus elevatus and the etiology of hallux rigidus. J Foot Surg 26:237–241, 1987.
15. Regnauld B: The Foot: Pathology, Aetiology, Seminology, Clinical Investigation and Treatment, edited and translated by Elson R: Berlin, Springer-Verlag, 1986, pp 335–350.
16. Drago J, Oloff L, and Jacobs A: A comprehensive review of hallux limitus. J Foot Surg 23:213–220, 1984.
17. Rzonca E, Levitz S, and Lue B: Hallux equinus: The stages of hallux limitus and rigidus. J Am Podiatr Med Assoc 74:390–393, 1984.
18. Pontell D and Gudas C: Restrospective analysis of surgical treatment of hallux rigidus/limitus. J Foot Surg 27:503–510, 1988.
19. Stutz J, Druse-Edelman I, and Green D: The Keller bunionectomy. *In* DiNapoli DR (ed): Reconstructive Surgery of the Foot and Leg: Update '90. Tucker, GA, Podiatry Institute, 1990, pp 152–155.
20. Ganley J, Lynch F, and Darrigan R: Keller bunionectomy with fascia and tendon graft. J Am Podiatr Med Assoc 76:602–610, 1986.
21. O'Doherty D, Lowrie I, Magnussen P, and Gregg P: The management of the painful first metatarsophalangeal joint in the older patient. J Bone Joint Surg 72B:839–842, 1990.
22. Vanore J, O'Keefe R, and Pikscher I: Silastic implant arthroplasty. J Am Podiatr Med Assoc 74:423–433, 1984.
23. Verhaar J, Vermeulen A, Bulstra S, and Walenkamp G: Bone reaction to silicone metatarsophalangeal joint hemiprosthesis. Clin Orthop 245:228–232, 1989.
24. Verhaar J, Bulstra S, and Walenkamp G: Silicone arthroplasty for hallux rigidus: Implant wear and osteolysis. Acta Orthop Scand 60:30–33, 1989.
25. Beverly M, Horan F, and Hutton W: Load cell analysis following silastic arthroplasty of the hallux. Int Orthop 9:101–104, 1985.
26. Schneider H, Weiss M, and Stern P: Silicone-induced erosive arthritis: Radiologic features in seven cases. Am J Roentgenol 148:923–925, 1987.
27. Rogers L, Longtine J, Garnick M, and Pinkus G: Silicone lymphadenopathy in a long distance runner: Complication of a Silastic prosthesis. Hum Pathol 19:1237–1239, 1988.
28. McCarthy D, Kershisnik W, and O'Donnell E: The histopathology of silicone elastomer implant failure in podiatric surgery. J Am Podiatr Med Assoc 76:247–265, 1986.
29. McKeever DC: Arthrodesis of the first metatarsophalangeal joint for hallux valgus, hallux rigidus, and metatarsus primus varus. J Bone Joint Surg 34A:129–134, 1952.
30. Smith TF: Hallux rigidus treatment. *In* McGlamry ED (ed): Categoric Foot Rehabilitation, Doctors Hospital Fourteenth Annual Surgical Seminar Text. Tucker, GA, Podiatry Institute, 1985, pp 91–96.
31. Mann R, Coughlin M, and DuVries H: Hallux rigidus: A review of the literature and a method of treatment. Clin Orthop 142:57–63, 1979.
32. Mann RA: Hallux rigidus: Treatment by cheilectomy. J Bone Joint Surg 70A:400–406, 1988.
33. Youngswick FD: Modifications of the Austin bunionectomy for treatment of metatarsus primus elevatus associated with hallux limitus. J Foot Surg 21:114, 1982.
34. Cavolo DJ, Cavallaro DC, and Arrington LE: The Watermann osteotomy for hallux limitus. J Am Podiatr Med Assoc 69:52–59, 1979.
35. Phillips A and McGlamry ED: Hallux limitus: Technique. *In* McGlamry ED (ed): Reconstructive Surgery of the Foot and Leg: Update '89. Tucker, GA, Podiatry Associates, 1989, pp 34–41.
36. Salter RB: The biologic concept of continuous passive motion of synovial joints. Clin Orthop Rel Res 242:12–25, 1989.
37. Akeson W, Amiel D, Dip I, et al: Effects of immobilization on joints. Clin Orthop 219:28–37, 1987.

CHAPTER 33

First Metatarsophalangeal Joint Arthrodesis

John V. Vanore, D.P.M.

Joint fusion, or surgical arthrodesis, is a time-honored orthopedic method used to eliminate joint pain, reduce periarticular deformities, and provide stability in the face of neuromuscular imbalances or contractures.[1]

Arthrodesis of the first metatarsophalangeal (MTP) joint has been advocated since 1941 with Duncan McKeever's fortuitous ankylosis of an infected bunionectomy. McKeever noted that from a cosmetic and functional standpoint, the result was better in the foot with the surgical complication as compared with the contralateral foot that had undergone a similar bunionectomy.[2] He also stressed that success is judged by a satisfactory fusion position and not the surgical technique used to produce it.

Arthrodesis eliminates first MTP joint motion yet provides for a stable medial column and weightbearing through the hallux.[3, 4] Consistent with McKeever's subjective evaluation, most of the studies reveal reduction of metatarsalgia and high patient satisfaction.[5–7] This discussion emphasizes the indications and the benefits of the operation.

RATIONALE

Some significant deformities and arthritic conditions occur involving the first MTP joint and first ray. In most patients, joint preservation procedures should be the prime objective of the surgeon[8]; therefore, arthrodesis should be considered when other procedures are less likely to produce a successful outcome. Arthrodesis is one of several joint-destructive procedures of the first MTP joint that also include resection arthroplasty with or without an interpositional implant and total joint replacement.

There are patients who undergo revision surgery for a previous unsuccessful result. Often, these patients present with degenerative arthritis, recurrent deformity, previous infection or osteomyelitis, and functional imbalances of the forefoot. Dealing with this diverse group of problems in a patient population with a similarly diverse age and functional demands requires thoughtful surgical planning. Careful evaluation and planning for the needs of a particular patient are the hallmarks of an experienced surgeon.

Biomechanically, the cause of most foot deformities, particularly those involving the first MTP joint, is related to musculoskeletal imbalances. Specifically, subtalar pronator syndromes that are responsible for first ray hypermobility must be considered when dealing with pathologic changes in the first MTP joint.

Some biomechanists suggest that the recurrence of deformity seen after bunion surgery is the result of not controlling these forces postoperatively. In addition, the patient may present with ancillary forefoot symptoms of metatarsalgia and plantar keratotic lesions. Instability of the medial column exacerbates symptoms in these patients. Joint reconstruction should address the patient's functional problem as well as the static deformity.

Resection arthroplasty was and still is performed frequently. With the advent of interpositional implant arthroplasty, early reports were promising,[9–13] and the functional and cosmetic inadequacies of resection arthroplasty were supposed to be solved. However, first MTP joint implants were overused, the indications were much too broad, and there was little appreciation of the potential adverse effects. Subsequently, patients experienced symptoms related to functional limitations and tissue reactions to the biomaterials.[14] Surgeons have now narrowed their indications, and first MTP joint implant arthroplasty is more predictable than it was in the late 1970s.

Today, there is a stigma associated with arthrodesis not only of the first MTP joint but of almost any joint. Over the last two decades, orthopedic practitioners have emphasized joint arthroplasty in combination with the introduction of artificial materials in an attempt to maintain or provide joint motion. Analogous procedures and materials have been used in the first MTP joint, although with limited success. Clinical trials by surgeon-inventors did not warrant their continued use.[15–19] Interpositional arthroplasty with a number of biomaterials, such as silicone and titanium, has been somewhat successful.

The focus is to broaden the surgical armamentarium of foot surgeons to include joint arthrodesis. Various surgeons, including Scranton[20] and Mann and Oates,[21] have advocated arthrodesis of the first MTP joint not only to achieve reduction of complex deformities but also to relieve the metatarsalgia that often accompanies the pathologic changes of hallux valgus and hallux rigidus.

Although there is no longer movement at the first MTP joint, fusion offers stability of the medial column and efficient weight transfer through the medial portion of the foot. A study performed by Henry and Waugh[6] concluded that the surgical plan should not destroy but attempt to restore the ability of the great toe to bear weight. Moynihan[5] identified the ability of the hallux to bear its share of weight as a reason for the reduction of metatarsalgia following fusion. Stokes and associates[4] identified the need for a stable medial column for patient satisfaction after bunion surgery. Beauchamp and coworkers[22] used the pedobarograph to illustrate the improved stability of the medial column following arthrodesis.

Why should arthrodesis be viewed enthusiastically, and what does it offer the patient? Arthrodesis offers longevity and durability, once bony consolidation is complete. It does not wear out, and recurrence of arthrosis is not possible. Although arthrodesis of the first MTP joint eliminates motion at that joint, it does allow for a functional foot. A young person may have a more functional foot following an arthrodesis compared with a foot plagued with persistent medial column instability that may accompany osteotomy or resection arthroplasty with or without an interpositional implant.

INDICATIONS

End-Stage Hallux Valgus or Hallux Rigidus

The indications for first MTP joint arthrodesis (Table 33–1) include the common conditions of hallux valgus and hallux rigidus in situations when joint deterioration has progressed to the point that a joint preservation procedure is unlikely to yield a pain-free reconstruction.[23–25]

First MTP joint arthrodesis performed for late stages III and IV hallux rigidus eliminates the movement that results in joint symptoms. In hallux valgus, first MTP joint arthrodesis additionally helps maintain reduction of metatarsus primus varus and provide stability with first ray hypermobility. This is important in the patient with associated metatarsalgia and plantar keratoses.

Revision Surgery

Revision surgery must often deal with a variety of conditions; often, revision attempts to give some finality or provide a durable reconstruction. Surgical complications of first ray surgery can result in postsurgical arthritis, recurrent deformity, and persistent medial column inadequacies. Implant arthroplasty does not address functional problems of hypermobility or metatarsus primus elevatus. Arthrodesis is a valuable alternative for revision of failed or prior unsatisfactory surgery of the first MTP joint.[26, 27]

Rheumatoid and Other Inflammatory Arthritides

Rheumatoid deformities and the arthritides that cause inflammatory synoviopathies of the forefoot should be a consideration for fusion. Arthrodesis eliminates symptoms through resection of the joint and restores stability. In rheumatoid arthritis, fusion of the first MTP joint helps maintain correction and is effective when combined with panmetatarsal head resections.[28–33]

Patients with these inflammatory arthropathies often present with osteopenia either secondary to the disease or their medications. As a result, maintenance of an implant within the confines of bone may not be relied on. Arthrodesis in osteoporotic bone is usually successful. The literature supports the use of arthrodesis in both the elderly and rheumatoid populations.

Synoviopathies such as gout are also a good indication for arthrodesis because the procedure eliminates the synovial articulation. Acute gouty arthritis may still occur after silicone implant arthroplasty; therefore, arthrodesis may be the joint-destructive procedure of choice.

Previous Infection

Arthrodesis is a useful procedure for the reconstruction of the joint destroyed by pyarthrosis or osteomyelitis. In these instances, significant osseous defects and functional alterations may be addressed through fusion with or without bone grafting.

CONTRAINDICATIONS

There are few contraindications to the implementation of first MTP joint arthrodesis. Hallucal interphalangeal (IP) joint degenerative disease has been cited as a relative contraindication to MTP joint fusion by Coughlin[34] and others.[35]

Active infection and severe osteoporosis are also contraindications. As with any surgical procedure, adequate neurovascular and general medical status are required.

THE SURGICAL PROCEDURE

The goals of surgery, regardless of the preoperative condition, remain fairly uniform and include the following:

- Permanent correction of the deformity
- Stable first ray
- Comfortable gait pattern

A successful surgical result is dependent on proper alignment of the arthrodesis and osseous consolidation of the arthrodesis site.

Position of Fusion

In determining the proper position of arthrodesis (Fig. 33–1), normal alignment of the first MTP joint in static stance must be considered. In the sagittal plane, the first metatarsal

---

TABLE 33–1

INDICATIONS FOR FIRST METATARSOPHALANGEAL JOINT–FUSION

Hallux Valgus
Rheumatoid arthritis
Unstable due to neuromuscular imbalance
Severe endstage deformity in younger patient
End-stage with secondary arthrosis

Hallux Rigidus—late Stages III and IV

Osteoarthrosis
Secondary to previous surgery, trauma

Prior Infection

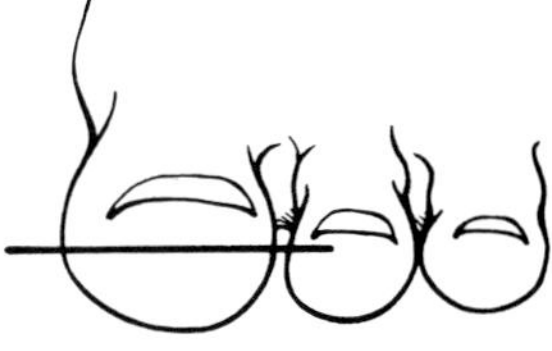

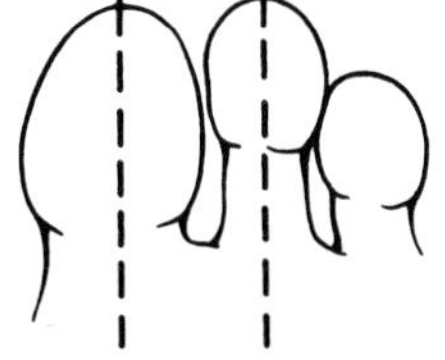

FIGURE 33–1. Position of the first metatarsophalangeal joint arthrodesis.
Sagittal plane
20 to 30 degrees of extension (males lower limit; females upper limit)
Transverse plane
Place the hallux parallel to the second toe
The degree of abduction varies with each patient
Frontal plane
Neutral—no varus or valgus rotation
Hallucal length
The great toe should be a little shorter than or approximately the same length as the second toe.

is in a position of 15 to 20 degrees of declination with the hallux lying flat on the ground supporting surface. In the transverse plane, the hallux is abducted 0 to 15 degrees. In the frontal plane, generally there is no axial rotation of the hallux.

To delineate the correct position of fusion and correlate the results of other authors, a standard nomenclature must be understood. The position of the great toe is referenced to the long axis of the first metatarsal. This means that a position of the great toe at 180 degrees from the metatarsal is one of 0 degrees extension and 0 degrees flexion. A position of 20 degrees of extension means that the great toe is angulated 20 degrees dorsal to the long axis of the metatarsal.

Proponents of arthrodesis acknowledge that the resection and fixation techniques are less a consideration than the actual position of the fusion. The sagittal plane position is based on the normal declination of the first metatarsal. Most authors recommend 15 to 25 degrees of extension (Table 33–2). The transverse plane position of the hallux should be parallel to the lesser toes.

To reduce any metatarsus primus varus, McKeever recommended pressing the first metatarsal close to the second, then aligning the first and second toes side by side. This usually results in a position of 10 to 15 degrees of abduction at the MTP joint. Generally, reduction of the intermetatarsal angle is believed to accompany the reduction at the first MTP joint with arthrodesis.[2, 3, 24, 36, 37]

Techniques of Joint Resection

Although a description of surgical techniques follows, this discussion also focuses on the potential advantages and the implementation of arthrodesis as a valuable alternative procedure for destructive arthropathies of the first MTP joint. Although fusion position must be emphasized, the preoperative anatomy and pathology may dictate the most appropriate technique. Methodologies of joint resection and the techniques of fixation are discussed.

Techniques of joint resection may include simple denuda-

tion of the articular surfaces, planar resections, crescentic resection, and resection with hand or power reamers. Some of these techniques demand that the position of fusion in one or more planes be determined prior to osteotomy, whereas others allow variable adjustment of position after joint resection (Table 33–3).

Maximal bone preservation and maintenance of bone length are best attained through denuding the articular surfaces. The cartilage can be removed with a rongeur and the surface abraded with a bur. In patients with degenerative joint disease with dense subchondral bone, perforating the surface with multiple drill holes is recommended (Fig. 33–2). This allows for vascularization and subsequent osseous remodeling across the fragments. Following simple denudation of the joint surfaces, a certain degree of latitude is present regarding the position of fusion. Preliminary fixation may be applied and intraoperative position assessed with or without the use of an intraoperative radiograph. The position and bony apposition may then be determined prior to definitive fixation of choice.

TABLE 33–2
RECOMMENDED POSITIONS OF FUSION*

Author	Position	
	Plane	*Angle*
McKeever[2]	Sagittal	15–20 degrees in males
		15–25 degrees in females wearing medium heels
		Up to 35 degrees in females wearing high heels
	Transverse	Place hallux parallel to second toe
Mann and	Sagittal	20–30 degrees
Thompson[32]	Transverse	20 degrees (abduction)
Coughlin[34]	Sagittal	20 degrees in males (may vary in females)
	Transverse	15–20 degrees (abduction)

*See also Figure 33–1.

TABLE 33–3

COMPARISON OF METHODS OF JOINT RESECTION

Method	Degree of Shortening*	Position and Adjustment After Osteotomy
Simple denudation	+	Allows adjustment in all three planes after joint resection
Planar resection†	+ + to + + + +	Frontal plane freely variable
		Must reosteotomize to adjust transverse or sagittal plane position
Crescentic resection	+ + to + + +	Allows adjustment/reposition in the sagittal plane
Wilson hand reamers	+ + + +	No adjustment
Coughlin reamers	+ +	Allows for minor degrees of positional change in all three planes
Truncated cone reamer	+ + + +	No adjustment

* +, minimal; + + + +, maximal.

†Varies with surgeon's discretion.

Planar resections necessitate careful planning of the osteotomies of joint resection prior to their performance (Fig. 33–3). Once the cut is made, the position of fusion is now determined unless recutting is done. If the surgeon is not satisfied with the position of fusion once preliminary fixation is applied, further modification of the osteotomies is necessary. Planar resections often involve more bone removal compared with denudation of the surfaces. This may be a useful technique in the rheumatoid foot to reduce first metatarsal length when combined with panmetatarsal head resections (Fig. 33–4).

Resection of the first MTP joint with a crescentic blade is performed from the medial aspect so that the resection may correspond to the anatomic concavity of the phalangeal base and the convexity of the metatarsal head (Fig. 33–5). It requires that the transverse and frontal plane positions be

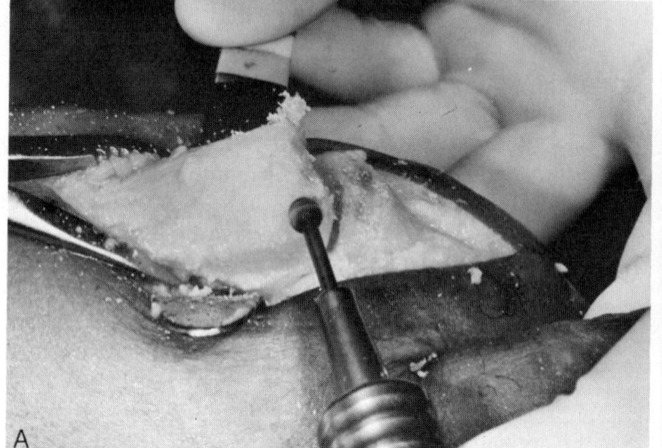

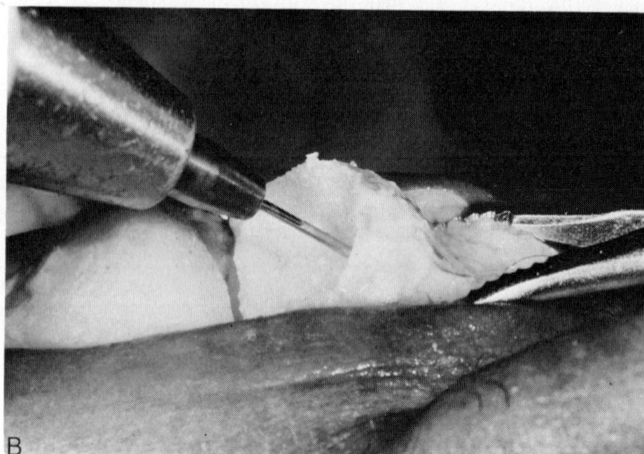

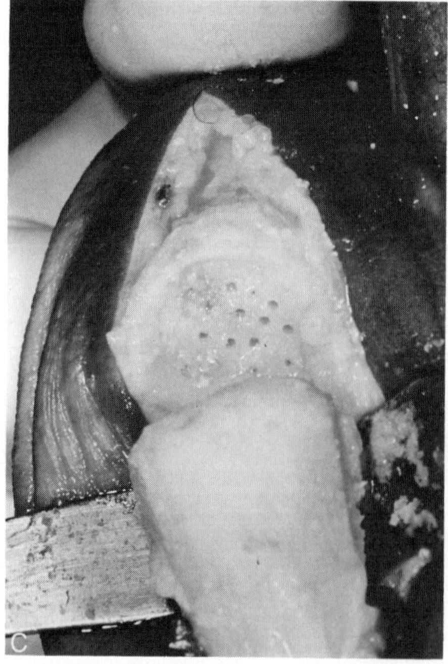

FIGURE 33–2. Joint resection: denuding surfaces with a rongeur and a bur followed by fenestration of subchondral bone. McKeever initially described simply denuding the articular surfaces to accomplish arthrodesis (*A* and *B*). Generally, a 6- or 8-mm round side-cutting bur is used to débride the articular surface of the phalanx *(A)* and metatarsal *(B)* surfaces. This is followed by fenestration of the subchondral bone *(C)* on both sides of the joint with a Kirschner wire to encourage revascularization and bony union.

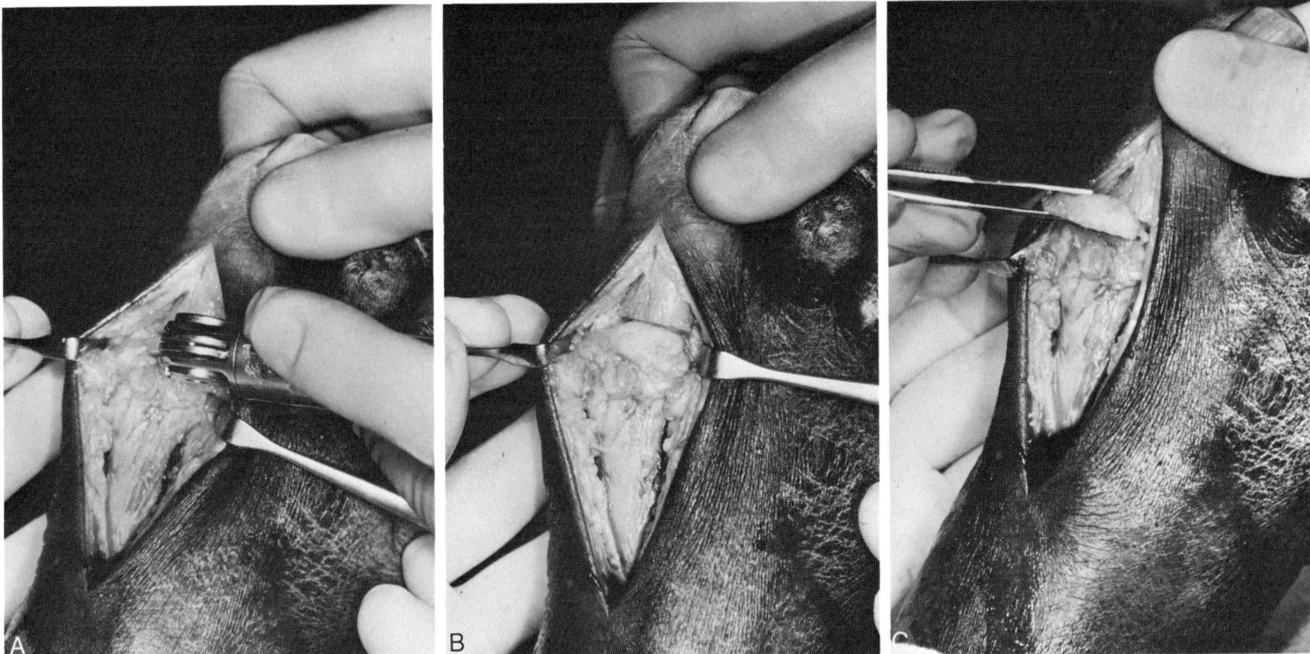

FIGURE 33–3. Joint resection: planar resections. A simple planar joint resection may seem the most straightforward, but the surgeon must determine the proper sagittal and transverse plane positions before performing the osteotomies. Generally, the proximal phalangeal osteotomy *(A and B)* is performed first, followed by that of the first metatarsal *(C)*. Planar osteotomies allow greater variability with respect to shortening of the first ray, for example in the case of reconstruction of a rheumatoid foot, but mandates that proper angles of resection for fusion alignment be achieved with the osteotomy.

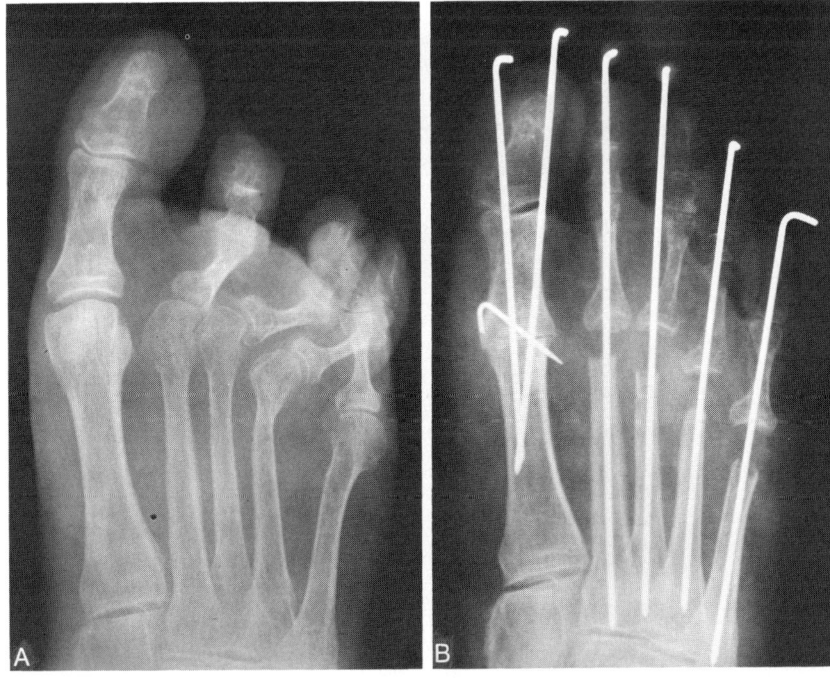

FIGURE 33–4. Planar arthrodesis in combination with forefoot arthroplasty. Preoperative radiographs *(A and B)* of a patient who underwent arthrodesis in conjunction with panmetatarsal head resections for repair of rheumatoid forefoot deformities. The arthrodesis site was fixated with the use of two 0.062-in. Kirschner wires retrograded across the fusion site with the addition of a third wire placed obliquely to increase stability.

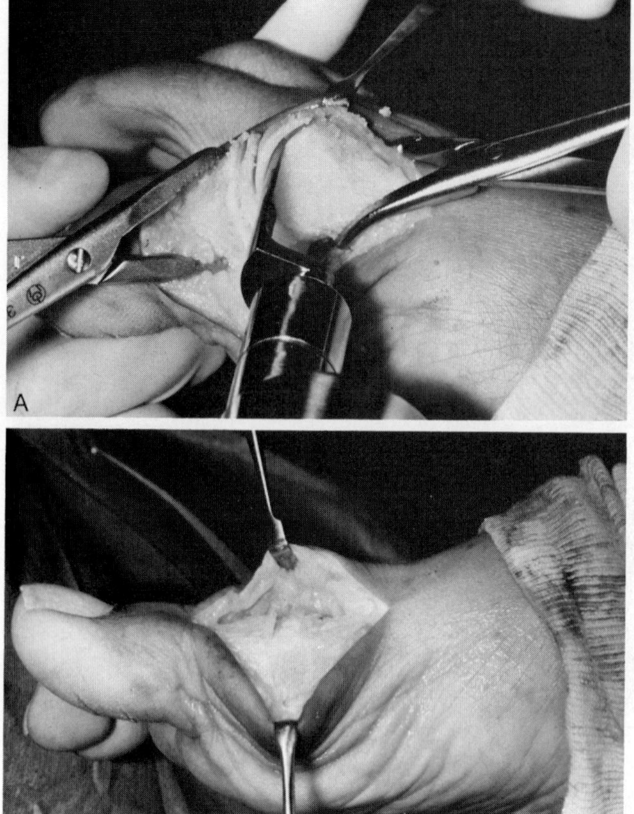

FIGURE 33–5. Joint resection: crescentic resections. Use of a crescentic blade that allows resection of the adjacent joints *(A)* in a corresponding concave-convex configuration allows for excellent bone-to-bone contact area *(B)* and adjustment in the sagittal plane even after performance of the osteotomies.

predetermined prior to osteotomy. The toe may then be positioned in a variable degree of extension prior to fixation (Fig. 33–6).

Reamer systems, consisting of corresponding concave and convex instruments, have evolved over the years. Some of the simplest hand reamers, such as those used by Moynihan,[5] create a peg-and-hole interlock (Fig. 33–7). This provides a greater degree of stability than does simple articular denuda-

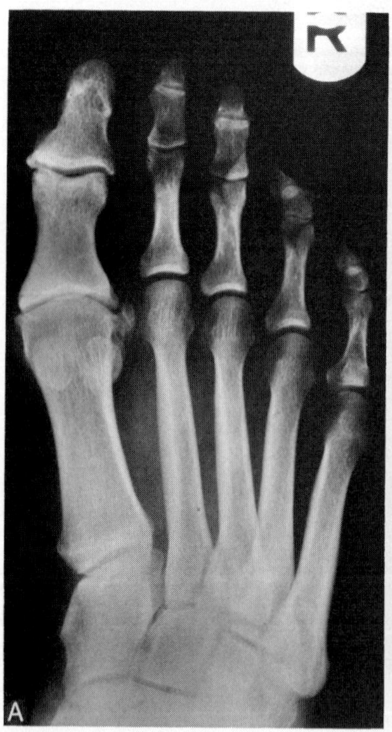

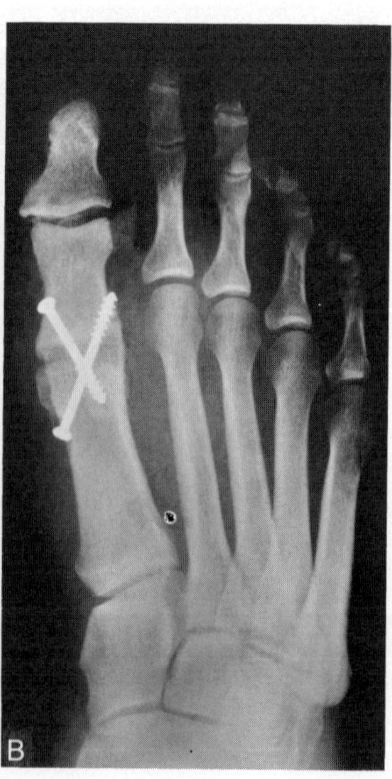

FIGURE 33–6. Crescentic resection arthrodesis. Preoperative radiographs *(A)* of a patient who underwent arthrodesis due to osteoarthrosis with grade IV hallux rigidus. Two crossed, partially threaded cancellous screws were used for intrafragmentary compression of the fragments *(B)*.

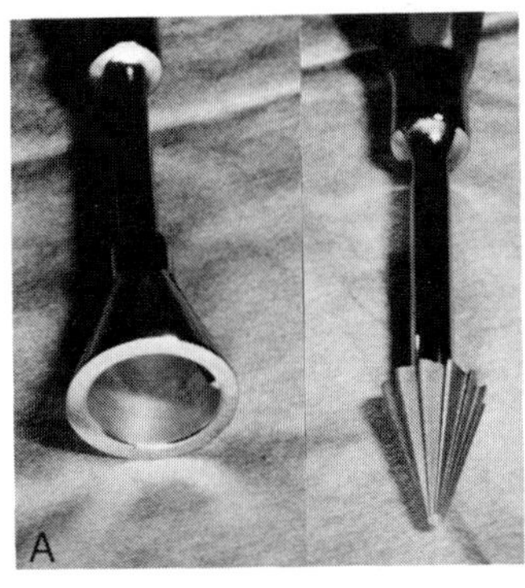

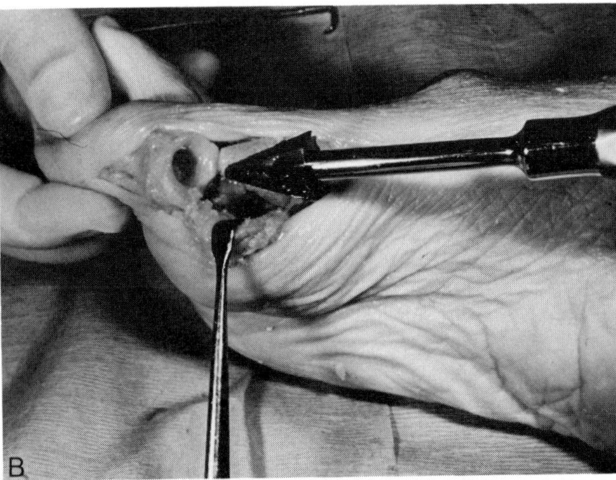

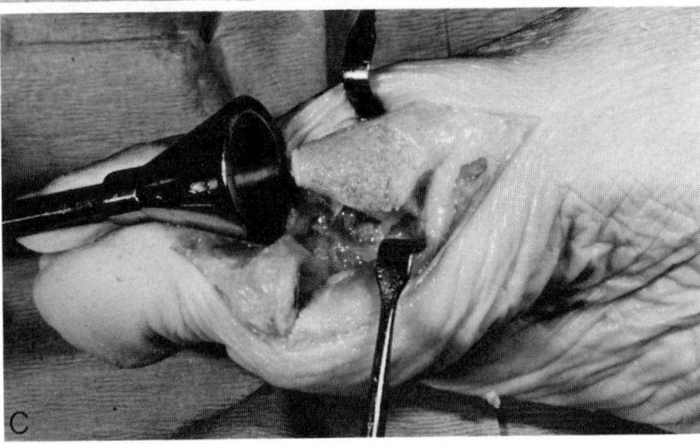

FIGURE 33–7. Joint resection: hand reamers. The Wilson hand reamers are corresponding concave-convex peg-in-hole–type reamers *(A)* that provide good stability as the result of the interlocking bone configuration *(B)* and *(C)* but do so at the expense of significant bone loss. Also, no adjustment in the position of fusion is possible after the peg and canal are formed.

tion or planar resection but requires significant bone removal from the distal third of the metatarsal resulting in substantial length reduction.

Another system described by Coughlin[7, 34] uses a concave and convex reamer that creates a peg-and-hole configuration with a gentle radius (Fig. 33–8). In contrast with the previous hand reamers,[38, 39] this device is used with power instrumentation. Some variation in the position of fusion in all three planes is possible owing to the hemispheric configuration of the reamers. To expedite the process, these instruments are

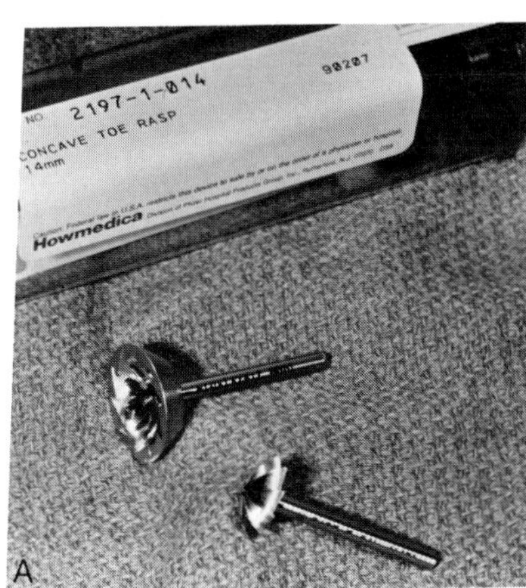

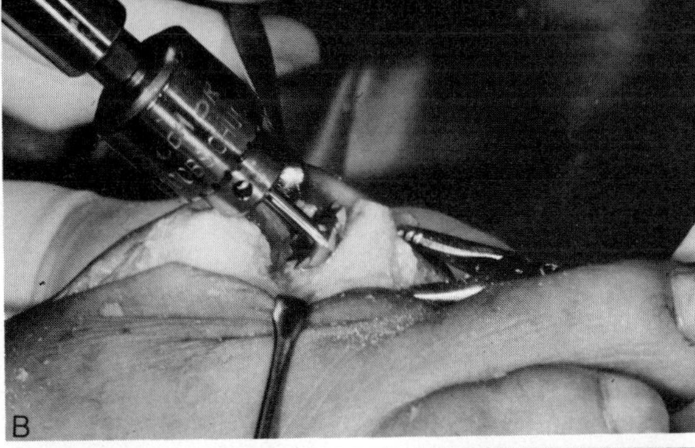

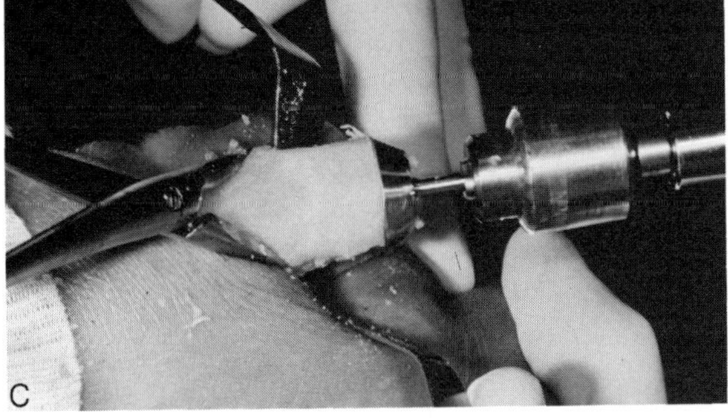

FIGURE 33–8. Joint resection: Howmedica reamers. Corresponding concave and convex reamers *(A)* have been advocated by Johnson[15] to fashion an arthrodesis with good bone contact yet allow for minor positional variations after the sites have been prepared. These power reamers create a 14-mm oval concavity in the phalangeal base *(B)* and mirror image convexity to the first metatarsal head *(C)*.

cannulated to allow the axis of resection and the position of fusion to be estimated. In addition, before the reamers are used, a third instrument called a *hole saw* is employed to reduce the girth of the metatarsal head.

The truncated cone reamer is a system for peg-in-hole–type fusion performed with a series of instruments.[40] It attempts to allow precise predetermination of the position of fusion with templates and a goniometer (Fig. 33–9). Osseous stability is enhanced by the final configuration of resected bone. This is a complex system that removes a significant amount of bone, particularly from the first metatarsal. Problems are encountered if the position of fusion is unacceptable after the creation of the peg and hole. The technique is not forgiving, and careful study of the instrumentation before its use is judicious and considered mandatory.

These various techniques each have their advantages and disadvantages, and the surgeon should choose a technique that is most appropriate for a given patient or pathologic condition (see Table 33–3). Generally, the potential for (or requirements to avoid) length reduction to the first metatarsal and first ray are determinant factors in the type of resection employed. Earlier, the example of fusion combined with forefoot arthroplasty was cited as a reason to shorten the first metatarsal. This is easily accomplished with planar osteotomies. In hallux rigidus with an index plus, shortening of the first metatarsal is desirable. Significant shortening occurs with most of the described resection techniques, and it is important to determine the limits.

Often, surgical revision of a failed Keller arthroplasty is required because of a short hallux and lateral metatarsalgia. Secondary fusion with a bone graft may restore cosmetic length and weight transfer through the great toe (Fig. 33–10). Proximal phalangeal stumps, shorter than one third the original length, with recurrent deformity or pain may be salvaged with grafting.

Fixation

Fixation may be as variable as the techniques of joint resection for first MTP joint fusions. The goal is timely consolidation of the arthrodesis. The fixation device usually dictates the postoperative course regarding external immobilization and length of non-weightbearing.

The fixation applied ranges from a simple design such as a single Kirschner wire to complex screw-and-plate configurations. Rigid internal fixation is a fundamental goal, and this is usually best accomplished with either a single-screw or dual-screw technique. Clinical situations may dictate the fixation device and technique of application. Kirschner wire techniques are appropriate for use in osteopenic bone and in instances when the bone shape may preclude other techniques. Many satisfactory fusions have been accomplished with much less than the absolute stability of rigid internal fixation.

Kirschner wires or Steinmann pins, generally two, are sufficient to provide stability and union as documented in a number of studies. A single wire may allow rotational instability; therefore, at least two are recommended. Because of the extended period required for union of most fusions, the wires may be cut and buried subcutaneously. Wire fixation is often used in conjunction with forefoot arthroplasty in the management of the rheumatoid forefoot (see Fig. 33–4).

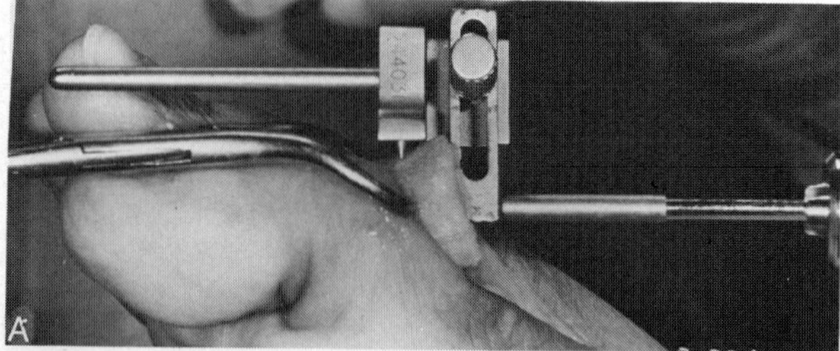
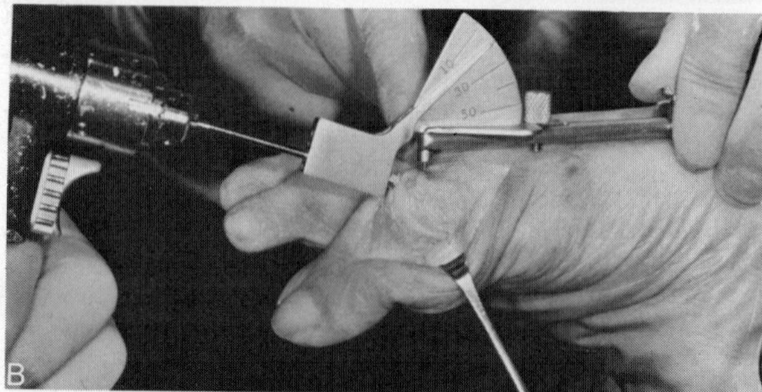
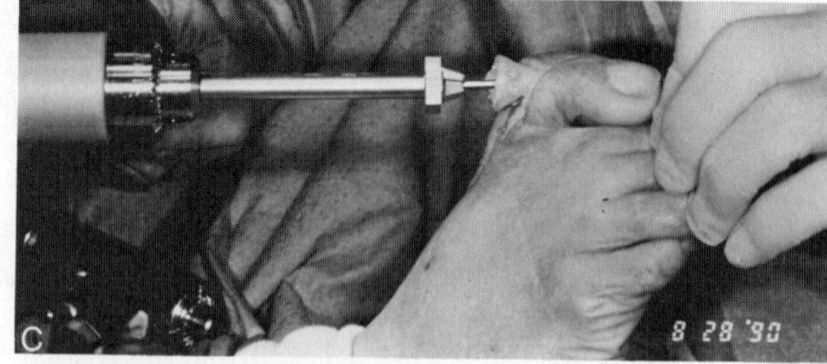
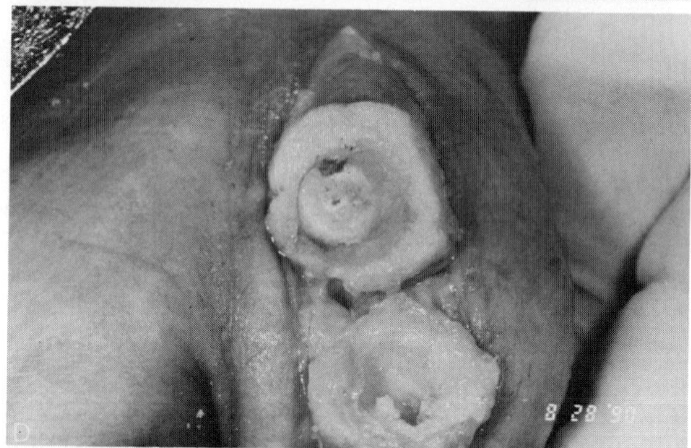
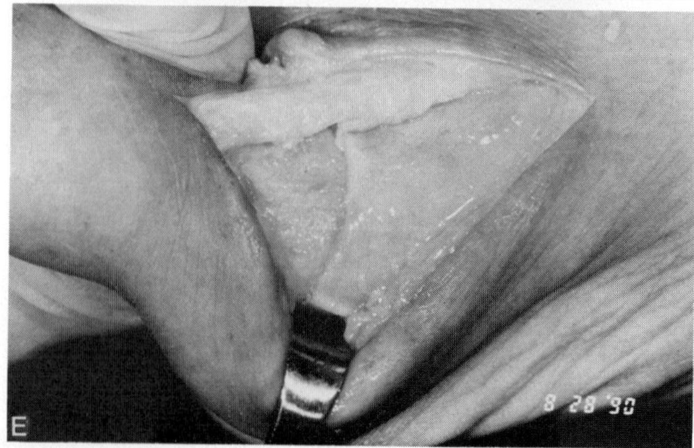

FIGURE 33–9. Joint resection: truncated cone reamers. This complex set of instrumentation uses a variety of jigs *(A)* to ascertain the proper placement of guide wires *(B)*, whereupon cannulated reamers *(C)* are placed. The result is a peg-and-hole configuration *(D)* to the respective ends of the metatarsal and phalanx that should provide precise interlock *(E)* and position. (Courtesy of Irving Pikscher, D.P.M., Chicago, IL.)

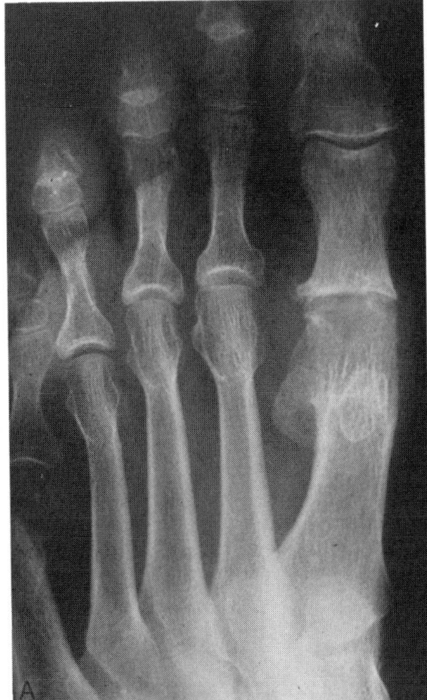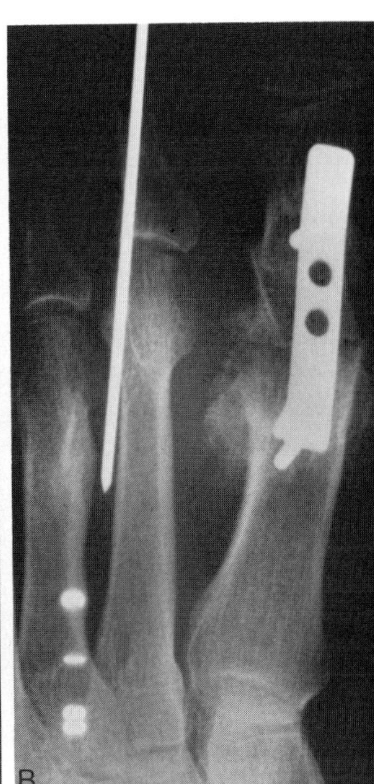

FIGURE 33–10. Planar arthrodesis for revision fusion of Keller with bone graft. Preoperative *(A)* and postoperative dorsoplantar *(B)* radiographs of a patient with a failed Keller procedure revised to a fusion using a bone graft and a tubular plate. Grafts are considered in such cases when the arthrodesis would yield an objectionable shortening to the first ray and a plate would provide stability to the fixation of the three fragments. The planar resection allows for easy fitting of an interpositional bone graft. (Courtesy of Jack Schuberth, D.P.M., San Francisco, CA.)

McKeever described use of a large Woodruff screw canted plantarly placed down the greater length of the first metatarsal. With the AO (Arbeitsgemeinschaft für Osteosynthesefragen) influence, interfragmentary compression is the objective to provide rigid screw fixation.[41] The result is primary bone union where the union is precise without resorption or callus formation. One screw may not provide sufficient stability (Fig. 33–11) and may be augmented with one of numerous devices, including a Kirschner wire, monofilament wire, or a second screw. A technique that combines an interfragmentary screw and tension band is one of the most physiologic and may be used even in osteoporotic bone (Fig. 33–12). Using two crossed screws has been a successful technique to achieve timely fusion. Either partially (Fig. 33–13) or fully threaded screws (Fig. 33–14) can be used for interfragmentary compression and rigid internal fixation.

Coughlin[34] has advocated plate fixation for the arthrodesis. Because the plate is usually placed on the dorsal surface, bending the plate in the desired degree of extension is required (Fig. 33–15). Owing to its placement of the compression surface, the plate may require additional fixation implants plantarly to resist tensile forces that may distract the osseous surfaces (see Fig. 33–15). Personal experience has not shown plate fixation to be advantageous except in interpositional bone grafting. The plate must then span the length of the graft as well as adjoin the segments of the phalanx and metatarsal. A minimum of a four-hole plate with purchase of four cortices in the first metatarsal is recommended. This may require later removal owing to its subcutaneous placement and potential for irritation.

An external fixator may be configured to provide good stability and maintenance of position but is generally not the technique of choice unless osteomyelitis or an open wound or one with a skin defect is present.

Results

The literature verifies the good results that can be expected with first MTP joint fusions. Orthopedic practitioners perform these procedures regularly, yet because a fusion eliminates motion at the first MTP joint, the procedure is looked on with disdain by podiatrists. No one is recommending that all Coughlin's results are good and bear out the ability of first MTP joint fusion to correct deformity, provide a stable foot, and most important, relieve pain on a long-term basis. Fusions do not usually deteriorate but may subject adjacent joints to increased stress. Coughlin noted that IP joint arthritis is usually minimal until 3 years postoperatively. He used Fitzgerald's rating scale to assess this.[35]

Coughlin[7] agreed with Fitzgerald[35] that a comfortable gait pattern is possible after first MTP joint arthrodesis, reporting only 1 patient in 63 having a poor result. Along with Mann,[32] these authors noted a gait with an early heel lift. Both the transverse plane and sagittal plane positions of the first MTP joint are important. IP joint arthritis is correlated with the hallux being too straight versus any relation to first MTP joint extension. Fitzgerald found that first MTP joint fusion with the toe in less than 20 degrees of abductus tripled the incidence of IP joint arthritis, although this was predominantly a radiographic abnormality. Their findings of radiographic arthritis at the IP joint did not correlate with clinical symptoms reported by the patients. Mann and Thompson[32] concurred in that 65% of the feet showed abnormal IP joints on radiographs, yet none were symptomatic.

In patients with hallux valgus, 20 degrees of abduction is reasonable, but in patients with a rectus toe, such as hallux rigidus, the second toe may be used for positioning. In men, first MTP joint fusion appears to be a good salvage procedure for MTP joint arthritis. Extension of less than 10 degrees

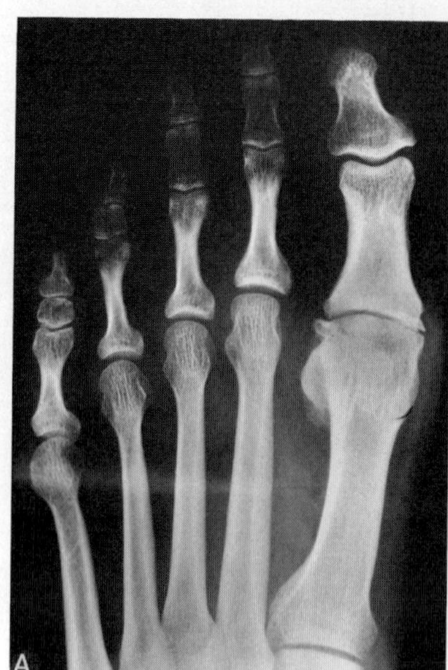

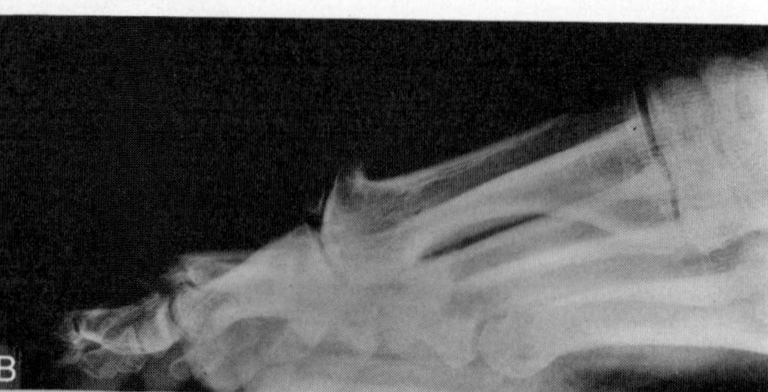

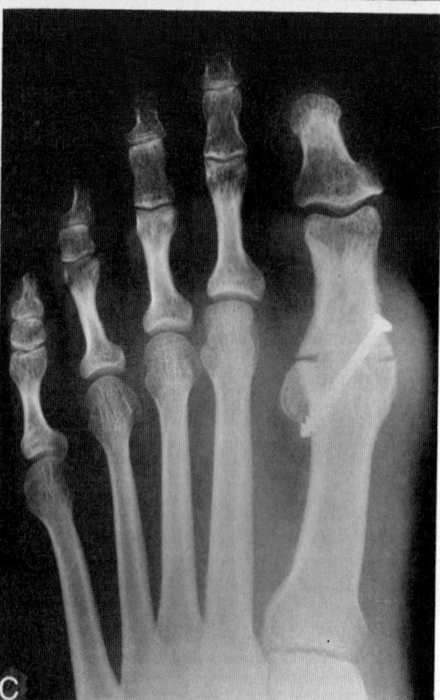

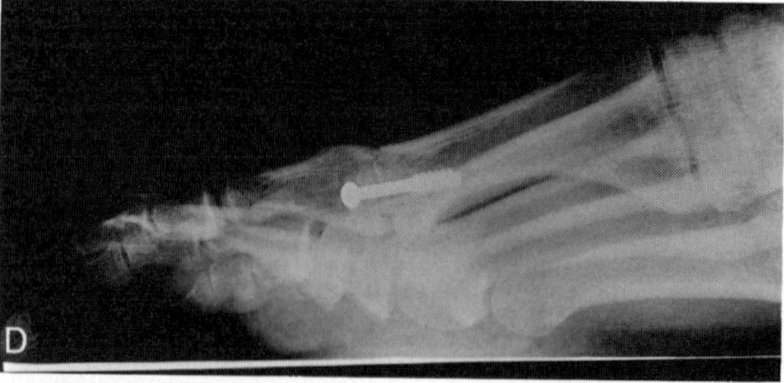

FIGURE 33–11. Fixation: single interfragmentary partially threaded cancellous screw. Preoperative radiographs *(A)* and *(B)* of a patient who underwent arthrodesis due to osteoarthrosis with grade III hallux rigidus. The arthrodesis site has a certain degree of intrinsic stability, and only one interfragmentary screw was used for osteosynthesis *(C)* and *(D)*. Placement of the screw using the plantar medial portion of the base of the proximal phalanx as a buttress is usually the easiest and most reliable approach. This is preceded by preliminary fixation of the arthrodesis site in the desired alignment with a Kirschner wire. (Courtesy of William Noorlag, D.P.M., Westmont, IL.)

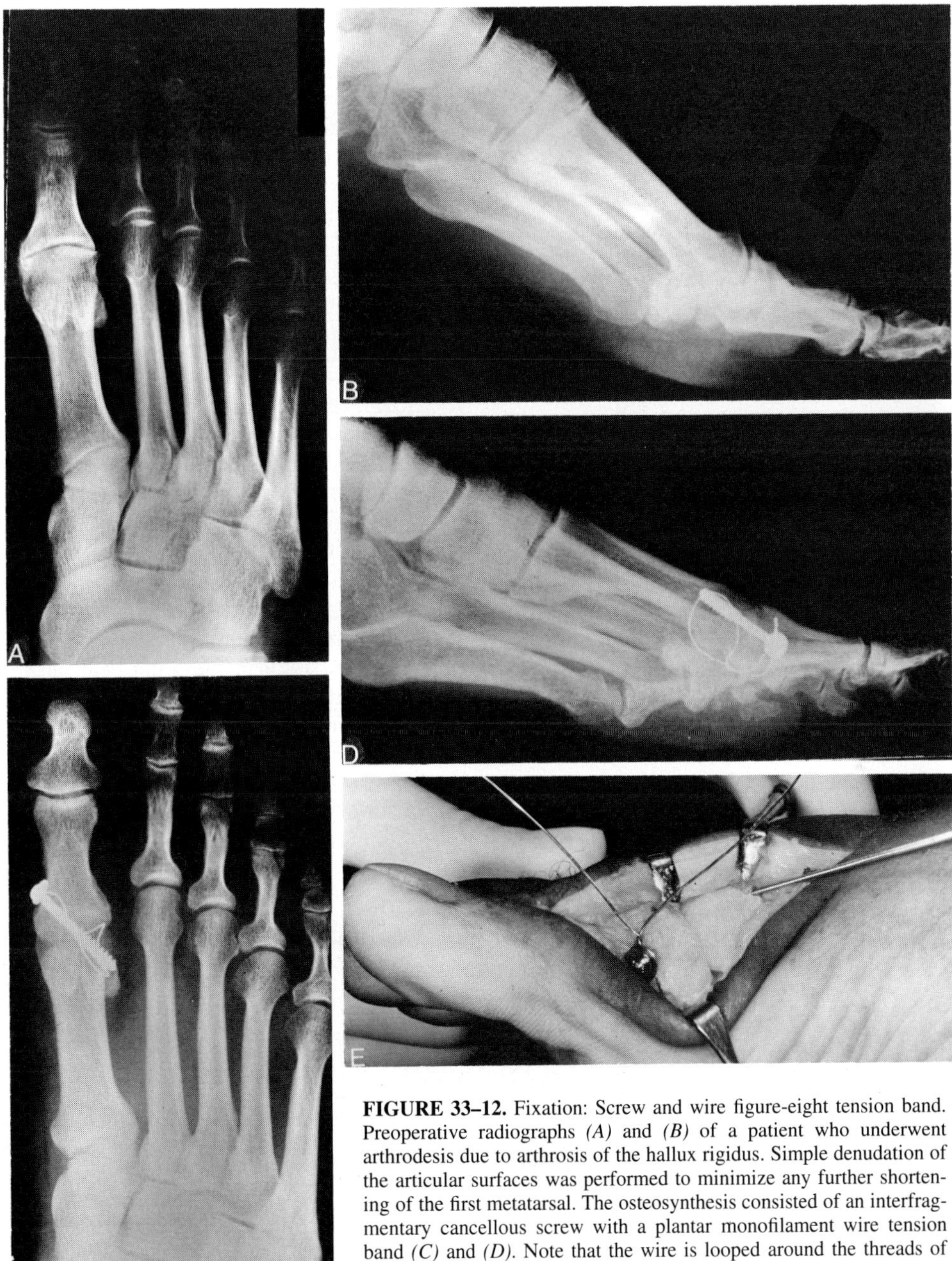

FIGURE 33–12. Fixation: Screw and wire figure-eight tension band. Preoperative radiographs *(A)* and *(B)* of a patient who underwent arthrodesis due to arthrosis of the hallux rigidus. Simple denudation of the articular surfaces was performed to minimize any further shortening of the first metatarsal. The osteosynthesis consisted of an interfragmentary cancellous screw with a plantar monofilament wire tension band *(C)* and *(D)*. Note that the wire is looped around the threads of the screw laterally and the head of the screw with a washer medially *(E)*.

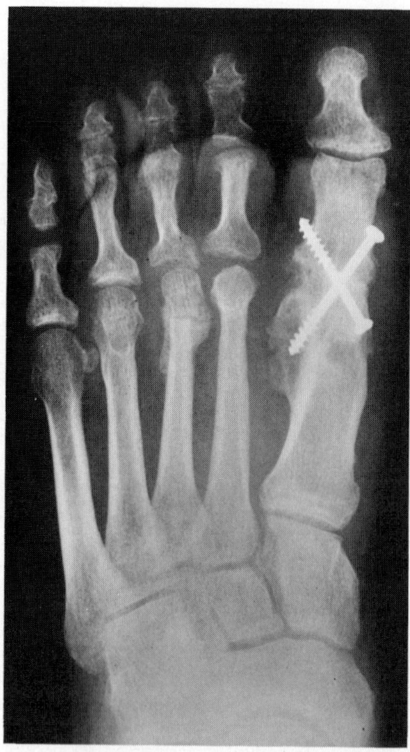

FIGURE 33–13. Fixation: dual partially threaded cancellous screws. In a patient who underwent arthrodesis as a salvage procedure for arthrosis secondary to prior surgery, the arthrodesis site was fixated with two crossed partially threaded cancellous screws to provide interfragmentary compression.

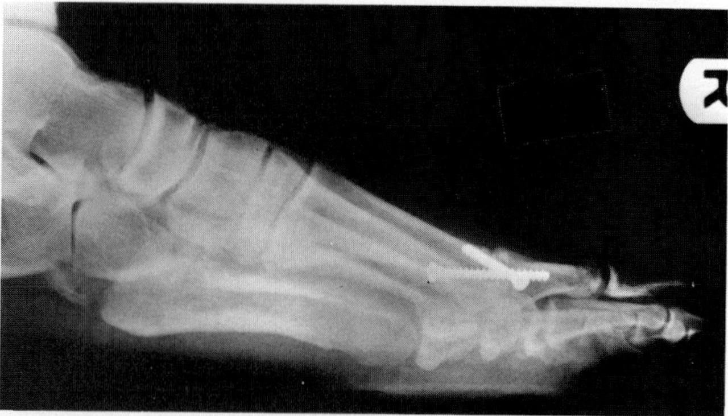

FIGURE 33–14. Fixation: dual fully threaded cancellous screws. In a patient who underwent arthrodesis due to osteoarthrosis with grade IV hallux rigidus, the joint resection was accomplished using the Howmedica power reamers and was fixated with two crossed fully threaded interfragmentary screws.

may lead to irritation at the tip of the hallux, whereas more than 40 degrees is associated with increased pressure under the first MTP joint. Owing to the variability in heel height in women's shoes, a compromise position of first MTP joint extension must be decided on. Coughlin[7] also noted that in women, the position of fusion in extension may need to be greater because of the demands of their shoe preferences.

McKeever[2] was among the first proponents of first MTP joint fusion. Bonney and MacNab[42] acknowledged their less than ideal results with resection arthroplasty in hallux rigidus and recommended arthrodesis except in patients with metatarsus primus elevatus without significant joint arthritis. They concluded that functional results are the major objective, not necessarily any cosmetic one. They specifically mentioned the resistance of women to undergo the procedure and their uniform success in adult men; however, the long-term results of Riggs and Johnson[36] did not bear out a sex-related dissatisfaction with the procedure.

Others, including Bingold,[43] Lipscomb,[25] Mann and others,[21, 32, 37] Fitzgerald,[35] Harrison and Harvey,[23] and Coughlin,[7, 34] have recommended arthrodesis for hallux rigidus. Most authors state that the technique of obtaining the arthrodesis is less a consideration than the actual position of the

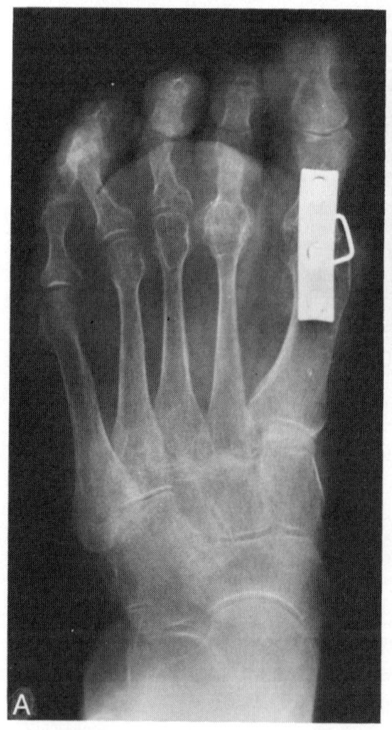

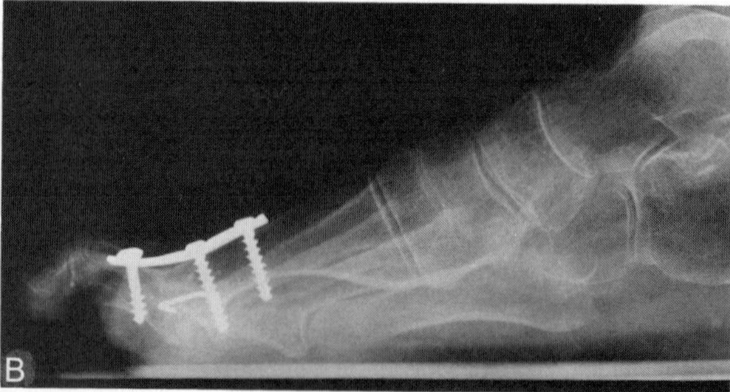

FIGURE 33–15. Fixation: plate and staple. *A* and *B,* The radiographs of this fusion illustrate some of the difficulties encountered with the use of plate fixation. The plate placed on the dorsal surface must be bent in the proper degree of extension and yet avoid gapping of the plantar area. A staple was inserted to resist these tensile forces. Generally bicortical screw fixation is preferred, particularly with any degree of osteopenia. (Courtesy of Robert G. O'Keefe, D.P.M., Chicago, IL.)

fusion. The sagittal plane position is based on the normal declination of the first metatarsal—most authors recommend 15 to 25 degrees. The transverse plane position is usually reflected to that of the lesser toes. McKeever[2] recommended pressing the first metatarsal close to the second, more a consideration with hallux valgus than with hallux rigidus, then aligning the first and second toes side by side. This is usually a position of 10 to 15 degrees of abduction.

As discussed in the section on fixation, McKeever[2] used a type of peg-and-hole resection and screw fixation. This involved remodeling of the first metatarsal head "down to a blunt point" approximately 0.375 in. in diameter. He would then begin with a 0.25-in. drill hole in the phalangeal base and ream it out to a conical shape, corresponding to the remodeled metatarsal head. In this manner, he could position the fusion in the desired manner after the joint resection.

Regarding fixation, McKeever used a long screw and washer from the plantar flare of the phalangeal base down the entire first metatarsal to provide secure, rigid fixation. Lipscomb[25] followed the basic technique of McKeever except that he inserted the screw from a plantar medial point on the phalangeal base without a washer, which he cited as being irritative in his experience. He also revealed that casts and prolonged non-weightbearing were discontinued because successful fusion was accomplished just as well with the use of wooden surgical shoes.

Mann and Thompson[32] used simple planar resection of both the metatarsal head and the phalangeal base in 18 feet. They placed the hallux (proximal phalanx) in 15 degrees of abduction and 15 degrees of dorsiflexion, *or about 30 degrees of extension from the long axis of the first metatarsal.* The arthrodesis was fixated with two heavy Steinmann pins (3.2 and 3.6 mm). The pins were retrograded from the fusion distal out the tip of the hallux and then back across the first MTP joint, and they were cut just under the skin and left in place until radiographic consolidation of the arthrodesis site was noted. Wooden surgical shoes were worn until this point. The Steinmann pins were removed between 60 and 210 days postoperatively (an average of 111 days), and consolidation occurred at an average of 97.5 days.

The cone arthrodesis of Wilson[39] was an attempt to provide increased bone-to-bone contact and some degree of stability by way of the configuration of the osteotomy. The male and female hand reamers were difficult to use, and the resultant resections did not allow for adjustment of position. Moynihan[5] described the use of these reamers as well.

Coughlin[7] acknowledged the potential difficulty of alignment of the hallux in all three planes with simple resection. He described a technique of conical reamers that allows adjustment after the joint resection and before the internal fixation. These also minimize the shortening that often accompanies joint resection arthrodeses. Mann and Thompson[32] recommended that the hallux protrude no more than 5 mm beyond the second toe. This is usually not a problem, because most toes are shortened significantly following arthrodesis.

Lipscomb[25] is another author who was convinced of the superiority of arthrodesis. He believed that the most satisfied patients following bunion surgery were those who underwent a first MTP joint fusion. He quoted an unpublished study at the Mayo Clinic wherein 95% of the patients who underwent fusion were satisfied with their surgical result.

As concluded by Henry and Waugh,[6] reconstruction of the first MTP joint should restore the ability of the great toe to bear weight. Others, including Moynihan,[5] verify the improvement in metatarsalgia following fusion. In his series of 35 patients with metatarsalgia, Moynihan found that 63% were relieved of their preoperative symptoms. Beauchamp and associates[22] used the pedobarograph to illustrate the stability of the medial column that resulted from arthrodesis.

Arthrodesis may eliminate first MTP joint motion, but it maintains the weightbearing capacity of the great toe. There has been concern for postfusion IP arthritis, but radiographic features may not correlate well with the patient's clinical or subjective feelings. Often, grafting must be considered to eliminate a preoperative osseous abnormality or defect.

Discussion

In planar resections, a greater amount of bone is usually removed, and it is difficult to give perfect alignment in both the transverse and sagittal planes without some recutting. Generally, either crescentic resection or the use of simple reamers provides adequate articular resection with more intrinsic stability than planar resection. Simple abrasion of the surfaces with a bur allows the formation of a cup or concave-convex surfaces while it minimizes bone resection. Each of these techniques may allow for a variable degree of repositioning following the osteotomy.

The truncated cone reamer provides the greatest degree of intrinsic stability at a significant cost. This involves not only purchase of the system but also the complexity of the procedure. If the position is not ideal, modification may be difficult. This system allows for precise resection and positioning of the arthrodesis; however, these are entirely dependent on the surgeon's placement of guide wires, which is an estimate at best.

The end-stage condition of hallux rigidus involves ankylosis of the first MTP joint. Usually, once the patients have progressed to this point where the joint can no longer move, they become asymptomatic. Therefore, arthrodesis seems to be a logical alternative in patients with hallux rigidus with a non-salvageable joint. This is particularly true for younger patients who must labor on their feet and require a stable foot that offers durability and longevity. Yet, somehow, resistance to fusion is apparent from both patients and clinicians.

References

1. Stewart M: Arthrodesis. *In* Edmonson AS and Crenshaw AH (eds): Campbell's Operative Orthopaedics, 6th ed. St Louis, CV Mosby, 1980, pp 1100–1141.
2. McKeever DC: Arthrodesis of the first metatarsophalangeal joint for hallux valgus and hallux rigidus and metatarsus primus varus. J Bone Joint Surg 34A:129–134, 1952.
3. Raymakers R and Waugh W: The treatment of metatarsalgia with hallux valgus. J Bone Joint Surg 53B.684–687, 1971.
4. Stokes IAF, Hutton WC, Mech MI, et al: Forces under the hallux valgus foot before and after surgery. Clin Orthop 142:64–72, 1979.
5. Moynihan FJ: Arthrodesis of the metatarsophalangeal joint of the great toe. J Bone Joint Surg 49B:544–551, 1967.
6. Henry APT and Waugh W: The use of footprints in assessing the results for hallux valgus. J Bone Joint Surg 57B:478, 1975.
7. Coughlin MJ: Arthrodesis of the first metatarsophalangeal joint. Orthop Rev 19:177–186, 1990.
8. Vanore JV, O'Keefe RG, Bidny MA, and Pikscher I: Hallux limitus and rigidus. *In* Marcinko DE (ed): Medical and Surgical Therapeutics of the Foot and Ankle. Baltimore, Williams & Wilkins, 1992.

9. Swanson AB: Implant arthroplasty for the great toe. Clin Orthop 85:75, 1972.
10. Swanson AB, Lumsden RM, and Swanson GD: Silicone implant arthroplasty of the great toe: A review of single-stem and flexible-hinge implants. Clin Orthop 142:30–43, 1979.
11. Albin RL and Weil LS: Flexible implant arthroplasty of the great toe: An evaluation. J Am Podiatr Assoc 64:967–975, 1974.
12. LaPorta GA, Pilla P, and Richter KP: Keller implant procedure: A report of 536 procedures using a Silastic intra-medullary stemmed implant. J Am Podiatr Assoc 66:126–146, 1976.
13. Kalish SR and McGlamry ED: The modified Keller hallux valgus repair utilizing Silastic implants. J Am Podiatr Assoc 64:761–773, 1974.
14. Vanore JV, O'Keefe RG, and Pikscher I: Silastic implant arthroplasty: Complications and their classification. J Am Podiatr Assoc 74:423–433, 1984.
15. Johnson KA and Buck PG: Total replacement arthroplasty of the first metatarsophalangeal joint. Foot Ankle 1:307–314, 1981.
16. Kampner SL: Pyrolytic carbon: An alternative implant material in orthopaedic surgery. Contemp Orthop 10:13–29, 1985.
17. Weil LS, Pollak RA, and Goller WL: Total first metatarsophalangeal joint in hallux valgus and hallux rigidus. Clin Podiatr 1:103–129, 1984.
18. Merkle PF and Sculco TP: Prosthetic replacement of the first metatarsophalangeal joint. Foot Ankle 9:267–271, 1989.
19. Koenig R: Koenig total great toe implant: A preliminary report. J Am Podiatr Med Assoc 80:462–468, 1990.
20. Scranton PC: Metatarsalgia: Diagnosis and treatment. J Bone Joint Surg 62A:723–732, 1980.
21. Mann RA and Oates JC: Arthrodesis of the first metatarsophalangeal joint. Foot Ankle 1:159–166, 1980.
22. Beauchamp CG, Kirby T, Ridge SR, et al: Fusion of the first metatarsophalangeal joint in forefoot arthroplasty. Clin Orthop 190:249–253, 1984.
23. Harrison MHM and Harvey FJ: Arthrodesis of the first metatarsophalangeal joint for hallux valgus and rigidus. J Bone Joint Surg 45A:471–480, 1963.
24. Humbert JL, Bourbonnière C, and Laurin CA: Metatarsophalangeal fusion for hallux valgus: Indication and effect on the first metatarsal ray. Can Med Assoc J 120:937–941, 956, 1979.
25. Lipscomb PR: Arthrodesis of the first metatarsophalangeal joint for severe bunions and hallux rigidus. Clin Orthop 142:48–54, 1979.
26. Vanore JV, O'Keefe R, and Pikscher I: Complications of silicone implants in foot surgery. Clin Podiatr 1:175–198, 1984.
27. Coughlin MJ and Mann RA: Arthrodesis of the first metatarsophalangeal joint as salvage for the failed Keller procedure. J Bone Joint Surg 69A:68–75, 1987.
28. Benson GM and Johnson EW: Management of the foot in rheumatoid arthritis. Orthop Clin North Am 2:733–744, 1971.
29. Clayton ML: Surgery of the forefoot in rheumatoid arthritis. Clin Orthop 16:136–140, 1960.
30. Gould N: Surgery of the forepart of the foot in rheumatoid arthritis. Foot Ankle 3:173–180, 1982.
31. Mann RA and Coughlin MJ: The rheumatoid foot: Review of the literature and method of treatment. Orthop Rev 8:105–112, 1979.
32. Mann RA and Thompson FM: Arthrodesis of the first metatarsophalangeal joint for rheumatoid arthritis. J Bone Joint Surg 66A:687–692, 1984.
33. Yu GV and Thornton D: First metatarsophalangeal arthrodesis revisited: An update. In DiNapoli DR (ed): Reconstructive Surgery of the Foot and Leg, Update '90. Tucker, GA, Podiatry Institute, 1990, pp 156–162.
34. Coughlin MJ: Arthrodesis of the first metatarsophalangeal joint with mini-fragment plate fixation. Orthopaedics 13:1037–1044, 1990.
35. Fitzgerald JAW: A review of long-term results of arthrodesis of the first metatarsophalangeal joint. J Bone Joint Surg 51B:488–493, 1969.
36. Riggs SA and Johnson EW: McKeever arthrodesis for the painful hallux. Foot Ankle 3:248–253, 1983.
37. Mann RA and Katcherian DA: Relationship of metatarsophalangeal joint fusion on the intermetatarsal angle. Foot Ankle 10:8–11, 1989.
38. Johansson JE and Barrington TW: Cone arthrodesis of the first metatarsophalangeal joint. Foot Ankle 4:244–248, 1984.
39. Wilson JN: Cone arthrodesis of the first metatarsophalangeal joint. J Bone Joint Surg 49B:98–101, 1967.
40. Alexander IJ and Kotschi H: Truncated cone reamer system for first MTP joint arthrodesis: Surgical technique. Biomet product literature YBMT-170/0022890. Warsaw, IN, Biomet, Inc., 1990.
41. Turan I and Lindgren U: Compression screw arthrodesis of the first metatarsophalangeal joint of the foot. Clin Orthop 221:292–295, 1987.
42. Bonney G and MacNab I: Hallux valgus and hallux rigidus: A critical survey of operative results. J Bone Joint Surg 34B:366–385, 1952.
43. Bingold AC: Arthrodesis of the great toe. Proc R Soc Med 51:435–437, 1958.

CHAPTER 34

Fusions in the Arthritic Patient*

John M. Schuberth, D.P.M.

In the past, surgical procedures in the rheumatoid patient have been labeled as radical treatment. However, despite aggressive medical therapy, severe pain and deformity may progress relentlessly. It is becoming clear, then, that the insistence on conservative therapy may be a radical departure from the optimal form of treatment. The patient and the primary caregiver may have significant reservations about any surgical therapy for a variety of reasons. This may range from a patient's natural fear of any surgical treatment to the primary physician's unfamiliarity with the results of carefully planned, well-performed surgical procedures. Last, the memory of other rheumatoid patients with poor surgical results will dampen the enthusiasm of both well-intended primary care physicians and patients alike.

Nevertheless, rheumatoid surgical patients must be chosen carefully. The surgeon who operates on such patients must be fully aware of the pathologic and physiologic differences between rheumatoid and osteoarthritic joints. The management of these patients demands a thorough understanding of the pathophysiologic and psychological aspects of the disease as well as the special technical considerations applied to the surgery. Last, the perioperative management of these patients requires a higher level of care than that for the otherwise healthy patient who presents for elective foot surgery. This includes a consideration of the effect of the disease on other joints of the body. These clinical situations may inhibit the patients' ability not only to be mobile but also to perform activities of daily living postoperatively. Surgery on the foot or ankle can impart significant limitations to the patient during convalesence that must be anticipated well in advance.

There are three primary indications for fusion in the rheumatoid patient: pain, instability, and deformity. Patients may have more than one of these conditions, and it may be difficult to distinguish one from the other. There may be significant overlap or a cause-and-effect relationship of any of these factors. Nevertheless, patients who exhibit enough symptomatology for any reason should be considered for surgical treatment.

The most common indication for arthrodesis in the rheumatoid foot and ankle is pain in the presence of aggressive yet failed medical therapy. The underlying pathologic processes that mediate the pain include instability, secondary degenerative arthritis, synovitis, ankylosis, and an asymptomatic proximal or distal defect that unduly stresses the symptomatic joint. Even though the common denominator of these conditions is pain, it is incorrect to assume that a universally performed fusion will yield uniform results if the underlying pathologic process is not addressed. For example, a painful subtalar joint as a result of synovitis in the absence of deformity will require only an in situ fusion, whereas a painful subtalar joint secondary to excessive pes planovalgus demands selective wedging to improve the position of the foot and thereby eliminate the deforming forces.

The second indication for arthrodesis is deformity that interferes with function. There may be a direct correlation between deformity and pain but not in all cases. Severe valgus of the heel or abduction of the forefoot can result in a painless but apropulsive gait. Even though the local disease process may be burned out, the increased oxygen demands incumbent on these patients' cardiorespiratory systems may make arthrodesis a reasonable option even in the absence of pain (Fig. 34–1). In addition, the altered gait mechanics may unduly stress the joints distal or proximal to the deformed joint, which may cause significant pain in the distant location.

Deformity is somewhat more common in patients in whom rheumatoid arthritis develops later in life in contrast to those in whom the disease develops earlier in life.[1] In these younger patients, the joints are usually stiffer and less likely to experience severe deformity, particularly if braced appropriately. It is also unlikely for patients with juvenile rheumatoid arthritis to exhibit the clinical features of the adult form of rheumatoid arthritis. Therefore, deformities either attained or prevented in the juvenile form of the disease are usually quite stable with regard to deformity; however, the degree of pain or degenerative change may increase.

Instability of a pedal joint without pain or deformity is uncommon in the rheumatoid patient but will be observed on occasion in isolation. The most obvious example is the patient who has suffered a ruptured posterior tibial tendon in the early stages. Initially, there is usually minimal deformity, but the patient will relate a feeling of instability or weakness. As the condition goes untreated, there will be progressive flattening of the longitudinal arch and eventually deformity and progressive dysfunction.

The final indication for fusion is failed total joint replacement arthroplasty or interpositional arthroplasty. Surgeons

---

*Adapted from Schuberth JM: Pedal fusions in the rheumatoid patient. Clin Podiatr Med Surg 5:227–247, 1988.

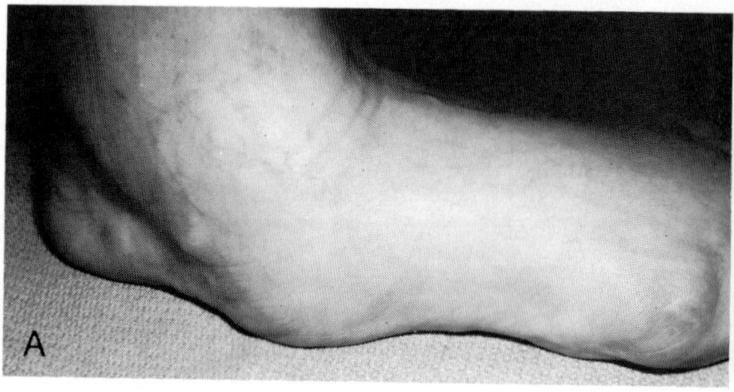

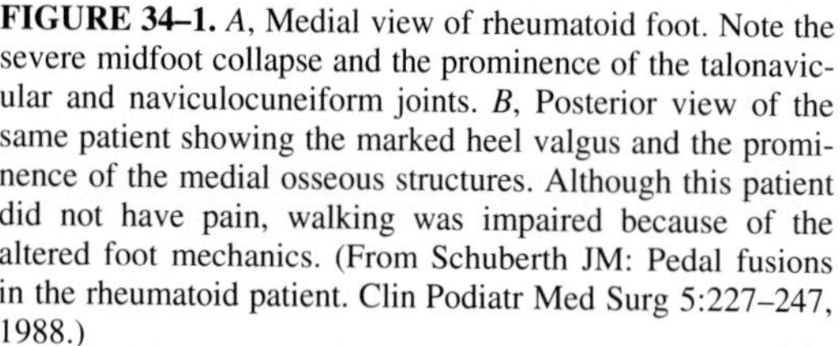

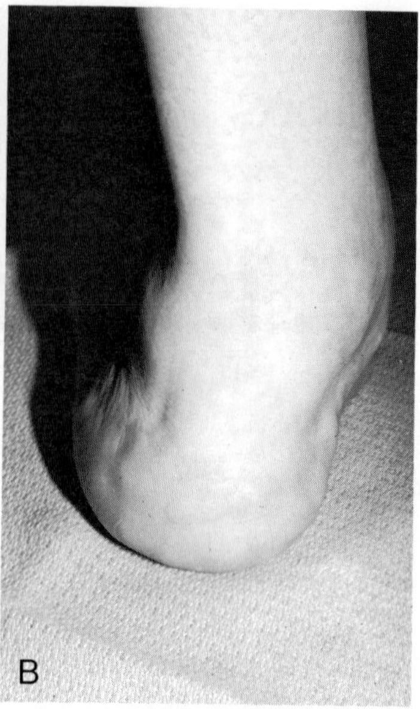

FIGURE 34–1. *A*, Medial view of rheumatoid foot. Note the severe midfoot collapse and the prominence of the talonavicular and naviculocuneiform joints. *B*, Posterior view of the same patient showing the marked heel valgus and the prominence of the medial osseous structures. Although this patient did not have pain, walking was impaired because of the altered foot mechanics. (From Schuberth JM: Pedal fusions in the rheumatoid patient. Clin Podiatr Med Surg 5:227–247, 1988.)

realize that total joint replacement in rheumatoid patients is often necessary much earlier than in a random group of patients with osteoarthritis. Therefore, patients should be informed that fusion procedures are often necessary after failed replacement arthroplasty if either revision or implant removal is not an alternative. Both the ankle[2, 3–4] and the first metatarsophalangeal joint[5] have been treated with these joint replacement procedures over the years in rheumatoid patients. Other joints have had limited short clinical trials[6, 7]; however, dismal results have all but eliminated replacement arthroplasty in other locations.

Even though forefoot problems have been addressed with modest success by replacement or resectional arthroplasties, there is a general trend toward more stringent use of these implants in the first metatarsophalangeal joint. This is due, in part, to the recognition of more frequent complications associated with the use of these devices.[8–16] Silicone-implant arthroplasty, in particular, has become much less popular because of the discovery of these complications. Although patients who have had a failed silicone or other implant can often be treated with simple removal of the implant, fusion of the first metatarsophalangeal joint may be desirable when a higher functional demand is anticipated.[17] Even though the same logic can seemingly be applied to the lesser metatarsophalangeal joints, fusion of these joints makes ambulation more difficult, and failed implant arthroplasty is better treated with simple resection.

Although total ankle replacement is hardly considered the standard of care in the management of the rheumatoid ankle, the best results to date are in the rheumatoid patient.[2–4] Many patients have benefited from the insertion of these devices. Nevertheless, the problems of cement disease, loosening, and subsidence are still causes of failure in the rheumatoid patient. Simple removal of the device is obviously not a viable alternative in these patients. Therefore, fusion is the procedure of choice in the presence of a failed total ankle arthroplasty unless revisional surgery has a high probability for success.

Subtalar joint arthroereisis has been used experimentally in the management of the valgus hindfoot, but it has not passed the all-important test of time.[6, 7] Until the usual problems of implantation of the pedal joints can be solved, any and all implants of the foot and ankle will often fail with time. Salvage procedures such as arthrodesis are often the most predictable in terms of the restoration of some function and the relief of pain.

GENERAL PRINCIPLES OF FUSION

When fusion or any surgical procedure is contemplated for the rheumatoid patient, one must remember that the goals of surgery, and therefore the results, must not be compared with those of patients with unrelated or relatively static conditions. Surgical or functional results that may be inadequate for the nonrheumatoid patient may be considered excellent by the rheumatoid patient. Outcome parameters should be based on realistic surgical goals but more importantly functional goals because levels of acceptable function differ widely between the rheumatoid patient and the nonrheumatoid patient. Care should be taken when evaluating the clinical studies of surgical procedures when there is little or no similarity between the patient populations.

Similarly, patients' expectations may be drastically different between these two groups. Major therapeutic gain in the overall rehabilitation of the rheumatoid patient may be realized with the performance of a procedure with seemingly trivial benefit. It is my impression that rheumatoid patients learn early in life to cope with pain and disability and often are quite grateful for any enhancement of lifestyle or level of independence that may be gained from surgical treatment. Many patients submit to surgery with the expectation that there is likely to be some improvement regardless of the amount. Barring a disasterous complication, they are seldom worse off after surgery. This mode of rationalization helps many rheumatoid patients make decisions relative to the appropriateness of surgical treatment.

The frequent involvement of multiple joints in the rheumatoid patient may complicate the surgical decision-making process. First, one must decide when in the scheme of the overall surgical plan for the patient the pedal procedure should be performed. This holds true in the relation of both the forefoot to the rearfoot and the foot/ankle to other anatomic areas. When reconstruction of both the forefoot and hindfoot is necessary, it is probably advisable to perform the forefoot procedure first and then observe the effect during ambulation. Often more proximal pedal symptoms will wane as the patient is able to bear more weight on the forefoot. This relief of pain may make the hindfoot procedure unnecessary. Second, compensation of overall forefoot alignments can be accounted for during the hindfoot arthrodesis procedure,[18] but the converse is seldom possible. Although malposition in any fusion procedure is usually poorly tolerated in any situation, subtle adjustments can be made during the forefoot procedure to compensate for the malpositioned hindfoot.

If total hip or total knee arthroplasty is indicated, it is usually performed after the forefoot reconstruction but before the hindfoot fusion because the hip or knee procedure may have a profound effect on pedal alignment. If the pedal procedure is done first, the plantigrade position attained during surgery might be lost when suprastructural frontal, sagittal, or transverse plane alignments are corrected. A common example is the correction of genu varum or valgum with a total knee procedure, which will obviously alter the position of the foot to the ground.

The forefoot should be reconstructed first to allow for pain-free ambulation in the recovery period after total hip or knee arthroplasty, which most orthopedic surgeons consider essential to the overall success of the procedure and expedient to ambulation and recovery.[19]

One of the most difficult decisions regarding the rheumatoid patient with regard to arthrodesis procedures is the determination of which joints need to be fused. This situation is unduly complicated by the often widespread articular disease seen on conventional radiographs (Fig. 34–2). Patients' subjective complaints either may be localized to a more finite area or may be unable to be localized at all. Correlation of radiographic and clinical findings is then quite difficult.

I believe that it is paramount to the long-term success of the procedure to be able to predict where the majority of the symptomatology is originating. In my hands, this is accomplished best with sequential local anesthetic blocks into the suspected joints. If one is concerned with multiple joint involvement, then 0.25% bupivacaine should be injected into the joint that is most likely causing the symptoms. I like to wait 15 to 20 minutes after the injection before asking the patient to walk. The subjective relief of pain as a result of the injection will usually help the surgeon determine whether there are multiple locations that contribute to the pain. If the patient reports 100% relief of pain from a monoarticular injection, then isolated fusion of that joint is often all that is necessary. If the patient reports less than significant pain relief, either he or she will be able to localize a secondary and contributing source of pain or the surgeon will be able to exclude the more likely source from the list of possibilities. A common clinical situation that often masquerades as hindfoot pain is the painful rheumatoid ankle joint with lateral talofibular impingement and resultant pain. The patient may complain of lateral hindfoot pain where, in effect, the pain is emanating from the ankle joint. Injection into the ankle joint will often eliminate the pain. Regardless of the clinical scenario, several visits to the office and thoughtful sequences of local injections may be necessary to localize the painful areas accurately.

Well-established compensatory mechanisms from a surgically ankylosed joint will often incite symptoms in a previously benign joint. Triple arthrodesis, for example, will usually increase the functional load-bearing demands of the ankle joint. Fusion of the ankle will often place excessive stresses on the talonavicular joint, particularly in the presence of any residual plantar flexion. As with any fusion, the compensation required of adjacent joints is increased with malposition of the joints being fused. Symptoms are more likely to be incited if the compensation necessary is more than

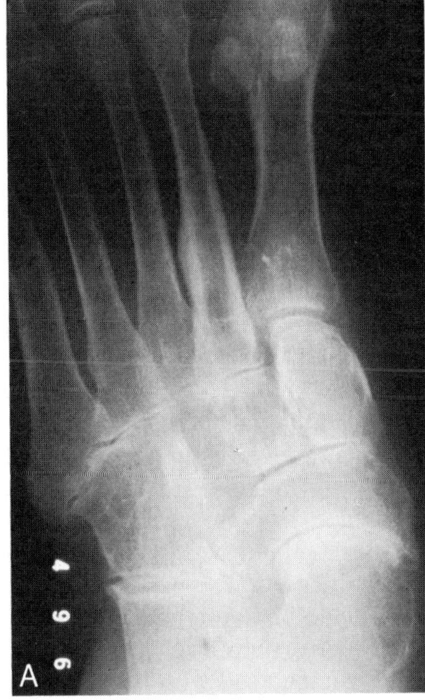
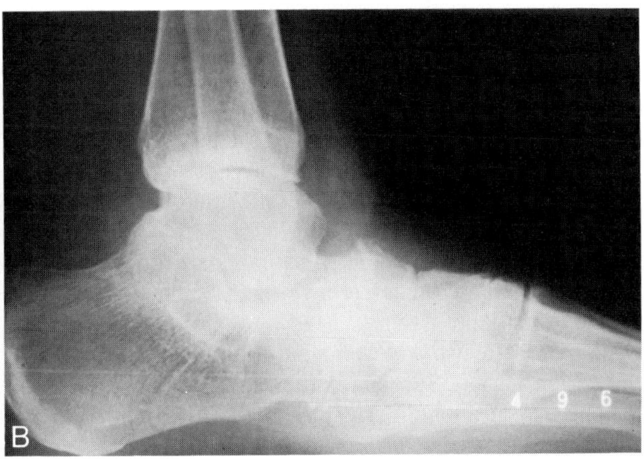

FIGURE 34–2. *A,* Anteroposterior view of middle-aged woman with panarticular involvement of her feet. There is narrowing at the talonavicular, calcaneocuboid, naviculocuneiform, and tarsometatarsal joints. Isolation of symptoms to any or all of these joints is often difficult. *B,* Lateral view of the same patient demonstrating involvement of the subtalar joint as well.

would have occurred with an optimally positioned fusion. Examples of this phenomenon are quite prevalent in the rheumatoid foot.

However, an anatomic study demonstrated that the commonly accepted compensatory mechanisms may not play as significant a role as once thought. Gellman and associates[20] showed a lower-than-expected reduction of the range of motion in adjacent joints after simulated arthrodesis of major tarsal joints. The most illustrative and striking examples are included in the discussion of the individual procedures.

In spite of the attainment of an excellent position of fusion to reduce unnecessary compensatory mechanisms, it is still difficult to predict which joints will become symptomatic after a distant joint is surgically fused. One of the determining factors is the amount of motion that is eliminated from the fused joint. In rheumatoid patients, it is common to fuse joints that exhibit minimal motion in the first place as a consequence of the disease process. In those cases, subsequent symptomatology in distant joints may be less common because the loss of motion is minimal, and compensatory mechanisms may have already been established.

Because of the lower demands on the pedal joints, rheumatoid patients with some radiographic evidence of deterioration in the compensatory joints may be better served by concomitant fusion of the compensatory joint. This is the opposite philosophy exhibited when dealing with nonrheumatoid patients, in whom the preservation of motion is usually the dominant philosophy. Certainly, the converse argument can apply. When there is little but pain-free motion in a joint distant to one to be fused, it is wise to spare that joint because a little motion is better than none at all. Regardless of one's thinking, each patient should be evaluated individually. When fusions are performed, patients need to be aware that subsequent fusions of adjacent joints may prove necessary.

Many conventionally performed hindfoot and midfoot fusions demand a period of non-weightbearing in the postoperative course. This is often difficult in view of the frequent involvement of the upper extremity in the disease. Integrity of the wrists, metacarpophalangeal joints, elbows, and shoulders, as well as sufficient upper body strength, is integral to the use of conventional three-point crutch or walker ambulation. Second, suprastructural deformity or flexion contractures of the lower extremity may also preclude use of conventional ambulatory aids. Patients should be evaluated for the ability to be non-weightbearing well in advance of the fusion operation. Therapists well versed in the rheumatoid patient and modalities should be employed.

Numerous options exist for the patient who cannot use conventional crutches. Platform crutches relieve most of the weight borne by the wrist and transfer it to the elbow. Second, patients may need to use a wheelchair for the required non-weightbearing period. Surgical compromise may also be necessary. The use of an alternative method of fixation may enable some weightbearing with or without weight-relieving casting techniques. Infrequently, wrist fusion may be indicated well before the proposed lower extremity fusion to enable crutch ambulation. Thoughtful preparation for the postoperative course is of the utmost importance in the arthritic patient population and should be done well in advance.

If arthrodesis of a joint is indicated, the only absolute contraindication relative to the temporal performance of the procedure is an acute exacerbation of the involved joint. Acute flares of the joint usually dictate a period of disease quiescence to maximize the perioperative conditions, which can impact on the immediate or long-term result. Even the most astute clinician will have difficulty predicting the period of time that the disease will be active. Therefore, a period of immobilization or other conservative modalities aimed at abatement of the acute process is indicated. On the other hand, waiting for disease abatement or burnout may only allow for progression of the deformity and complication of the surgical procedure. Prevention of the progression of existing deformities via bracing, immobilization, or unweighting of the part may be necessary during acute flares of the joint.

SURGICAL CONSIDERATIONS

There are several conditions in the rheumatoid patient that may cause some alteration in procedure selection, technique, or postoperative management. The density of bone in the rheumatoid patient is often quite different from that in the nonrheumatoid patient. Osteoporosis is quite common in the rheumatoid patient for several reasons. First, the higher incidence of the disease in women naturally inflates the incidence of osteoporosis resulting from hormonal influences. Second, there is a percentage of patients who have been managed with systemic corticosteroids, which in itself contributes to osteopenia. Third, the juxta-articular osteopenia, which results from the inflammatory joint disease, may accentuate the global osteopenia. Last, the decreased activity level and subsequent decrease in the physiologic stress to the lower extremity will further contribute to the lack of bone mass.[21]

Regardless of the cause, decreased bone stock may necessitate alternative methods of fixation other than those the surgeon is accustomed to using. Rigid internal fixation is often difficult if not unattainable. This is most evident when the screw threads must be placed in the cancellous bone. To optimize the chance of success when using screws, the surgeon should try to engage cortical bone with the threads of the screw if the geometry of the procedure allows. The density gradient between cancellous and cortical bone may allow for rigid fixation if one of the cortices can be captured with the threads of the screw. When screw fixation is used, it is usually ill advised to countersink the head of the screw unless it is in relatively dense bone. Particularly vulnerable locations include the distal phalanx and the neck of the talus (Fig. 34–3).

When screw fixation fails to provide rigid fixation intraoperatively, the device should be abandoned and replaced with axially oriented Kirschner wires or Steinmann pins (Fig. 34–4). Threaded pins may be necessary to prevent migration when the bone density is insufficient to provide adequate friction or when additional stability is desired.

The lack of compression in these procedures does not threaten healing as long as the caliber of the alternative device is large enough to prevent bending or failure. Kirschner wires, if used, should be 0.062 inch or larger. External fixators can also be used. The pins should be placed perpendicular to the vector of compression and in cortical bone whenever possible to minimize the chance of migration or pullout. Staples can be used with the same precautions.

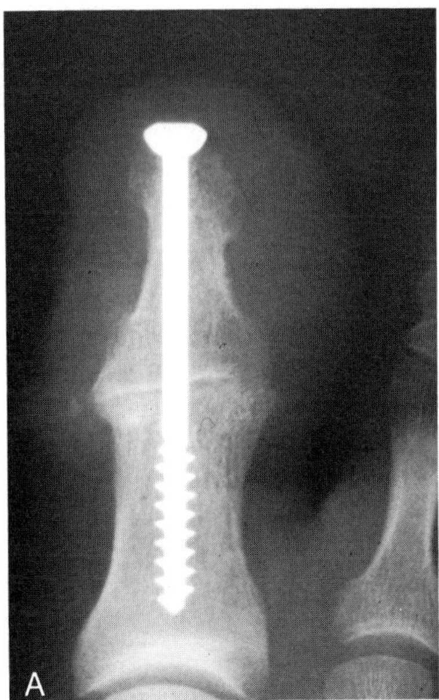
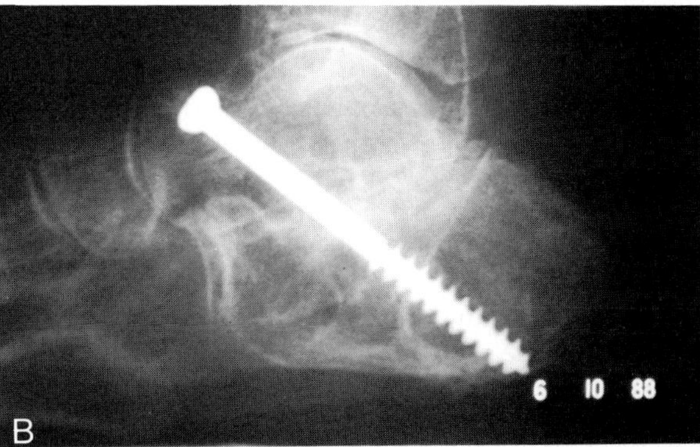

FIGURE 34–3. *A,* Anteroposterior view of an interphalangeal joint fusion where the screw head has been countersunk at the distal phalangeal tuft. This patient had sufficient bone density to allow for a recessed seating of the screw. *B,* Lateral view of a subtalar fusion in an elderly rheumatoid patient with advanced osteoporosis. The head of the screw was not countersunk, but the soft bone consistency allowed for a flush seating of the screw head on the neck of the talus. (From Schuberth JM: Pedal fusions in the rheumatoid patient. Clin Podiatr Med Surg 5:227–247, 1988.)

BONE GRAFTING

Bone grafting may, on occasion, be necessary in the treatment of the rheumatoid foot or ankle. Bone grafting applied to fusion procedures is done primarily to correct large deformities. The most striking example of the latter is the rheumatoid hindfoot that exhibits severe valgus deformity of the subtalar joint (discussed later).

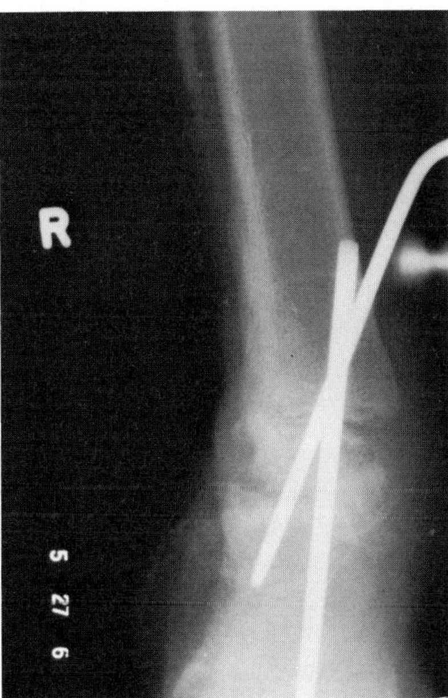

FIGURE 34–4. Anteroposterior radiograph of a compression distraction arthrodesis in a 9-year-old girl. The axially oriented Steinmann pin crosses the physis but maintains alignment. The lateral portion of the physeal plate has been destroyed secondary to trauma.

Autogenous bone is clearly the material of choice in the rheumatoid patient regardless of the anatomic site involved because it will reduce the time required for fusion. This is important in the overall rehabilitation of these patients. There is no substitute for autogenous bone with regard to its osteogenic potential.[22] Excellent sources of cancellous bone are the distal and proximal tibia and calcaneus when small portions are needed and the iliac crest when larger quantities are necessary or when corticocancellous grafts are needed.

Allogeneic bone is rarely indicated in these patients because its primary advantage of strength is seldom realized in the rheumatoid patient. Although allogeneic bone does not require an additional surgical procedure to procure, the longer incorporation time outweighs any advantage, because the postoperative rehabilitative process may be protracted. If allograft is desired, there are numerous sources of material and multiple anatomic parts that can be used depending on the needs of the procedure.

ARTHRODESIS OF SPECIFIC JOINTS

Hallux Interphalangeal Joint

The need for fusion of the hallux interphalangeal joint is infrequent in the rheumatoid patient. Although many rheumatoid patients will have significant radiographic findings with regard to deterioration, few of them have complaints specific to this joint.[23] Occasionally, a patient will have severe lateral deviation at the interphalangeal joint, which will place undue stress on the lateral digits. This may make shoe fitting a problem, thereby indicating fusion. Second, the presence of lateral deviation may necessitate surgical fusion when other reconstructive procedures are performed because the overall alignment of the digit attained from adjacent or more proximal procedures would be compromised (Fig. 34–

5). Finally, patients who have had Keller procedures or resectional arthroplasty may have hallux flexus deformities as late complications. If the contractures are severe, surgical fusion may be indicated (Fig. 34–6).

The osteoporotic environment of the hallucal phalanges frequently precludes the use of compression screws. Seldom is there sufficient cancellous bone in the medullary canal of the proximal phalanx for satisfactory compression. Preoperative evaluation should include thorough radiographic assessment of the distribution of cancellous bone to determine the modifications in fixation that are necessary. If enough metaphyseal bone appears to be present, one should be aware that it is likely to be soft and may preclude compression in spite of ensuring that the threads of the screw are situated in that area. If screws are used, the distal phalangeal tip should not be countersunk except in patients with more dense bone (Fig. 34–7).

Instead of the traditional axially oriented screw in the interphalangeal joint fusion, one may also use the obliquely oriented screw technique. This configuration takes advantage of the denser cortical bone and allows for hardware that does not protrude through the skin. Care should be taken to ensure that the alignment is maintained by temporary fixation of the fusion site so that lateral migration of the distal phalanx does not occur as the screw is tightened.

One should be prepared to use another fixation device if the apparent radiographic density is not supported by the intraoperative findings or it is determined that the bone is inadequate. The most reliable form of fixation in osteoporotic bone is crossed Kirschner wires placed obliquely across the fusion site. Large-caliber wires should be used to prevent bending during the ambulatory stages of postoperative care. In extremely osteoporotic bone, threaded Kirschner wires may be indicated to reduce pin migration. Care should be taken not to remove too much of the metaphyseal components because this will result in excessive loss of cancellous bone. If this occurs or there is insufficient bone in the first place, cancellous bone grafting is indicated. Because of the small quantity of bone needed, it is easily procured from the calcaneus.

The optimal position of fusion should be biased toward

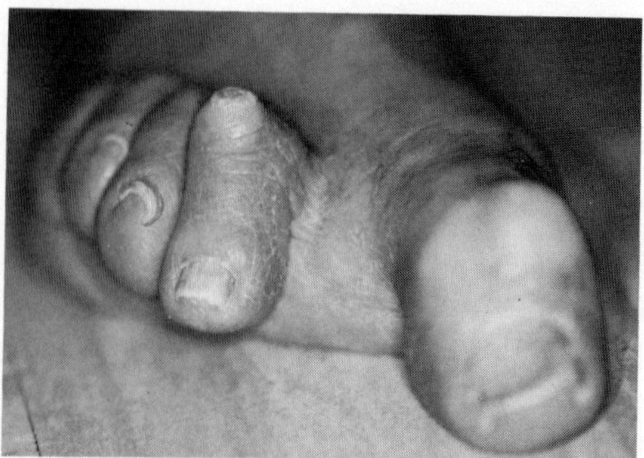

FIGURE 34–6. Male patient who underwent resection of all five metatarsal heads with excessive shortening of the metatarsals. Gradual and progressive hammering of all of the toes ensued, creating a significant shoe-fitting problem.

abduction and dorsiflexion. This will facilitate ambulation and shoe fitting. Neutral positioning in all three body planes is also acceptable and is not likely to cause problems. Varus or valgus rotation is usually complicated by irritation of the remaining plantar condyle and should be avoided. Care should also be taken to avoid plantar displacement of the distal phalangeal base because this can be a significant irritant (Fig. 34–8).

First Metatarsophalangeal Joint

Options abound for the surgeon addressing the rheumatoid first metatarsophalangeal joint. These include the Keller procedure, Keller procedure with implant, and arthrodesis. Proponents of arthrodesis contend that the fusion of this joint reestablishes a normal weight-bearing pattern, protects the lesser toes from valgus stress, and prevents recurrence of the deformity.[23] Although these observations may be valid, fusion has not gained widespread acceptance in the podiatric literature. Perhaps this is because the techniques and materi-

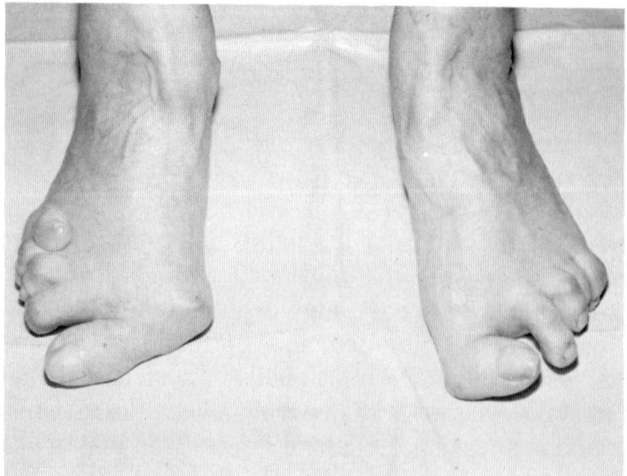

FIGURE 34–5. Dorsal plantar view of a middle-aged woman with asymmetric yet advanced forefoot deformities. Fusion of the left interphalangeal joint is indicated because of the plantar medial digital callosity and the severe lateral deviation of the digit at this level. (From Schuberth JM: Pedal fusions in the rheumatoid patient. Clin Podiatr Med Surg 5:227–247, 1988.)

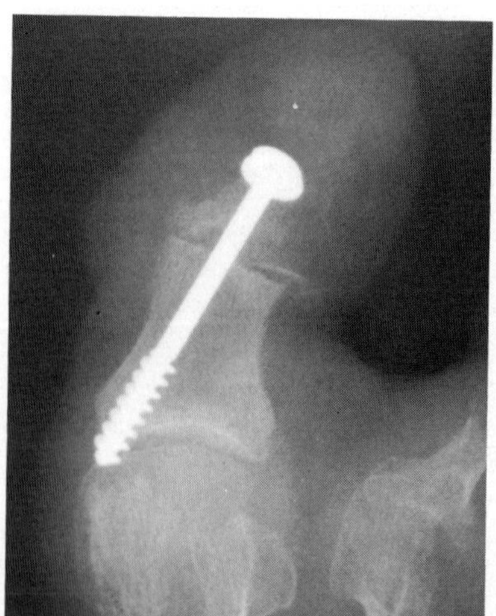

FIGURE 34–7. Intraoperative radiograph in a rhematoid patient with severe osteoporosis. Despite the use of a washer, the distal tuft density was insufficient to prevent intraosseous migration of the screw head. This situation necessitated screw removal and fixation with crossed Kirschner wires. (From Schuberth JM: Pedal fusions in the rheumatoid patient. Clin Podiatr Med Surg 5:227–247, 1988.)

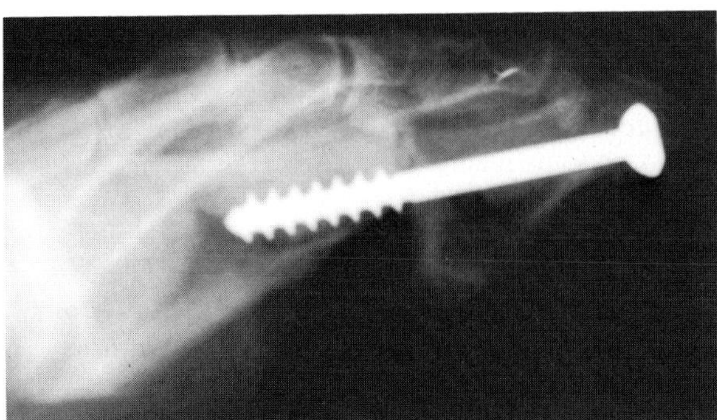

FIGURE 34–8. Lateral view of the hallux showing the plantarly displaced distal phalangeal base on the proximal phalanx. The excessive overhang of the phalangeal base was quite symptomatic to the patient.

als of implant arthroplasty have been refined, thus offsetting the disadvantages that the advocates of fusion profess.[5, 24–26] However, recognition of the complications of Silastic implant arthroplasty may tip the scales in the other direction. Many of the complications resulting from implant arthroplasty have been from inappropriate selection of patients and improper technique.[8–16] Although it may be tempting to place an implant into a first metatarsophalangeal joint in a patient who has a high intermetatarsal angle, it usually predisposes the implant to failure because of the residual forces that abound. Correction of the intermetatarsal angle usually requires a proximal osteotomy, which is undesirable for many surgeons and patients alike. The difficult postoperative course and the complexity of the procedure in the rheumatoid patient often convince the surgeon and patient alike to seek other alternative procedures.

Fusion of the first metatarsophalangeal joint remains a useful procedure in the patient for whom implant arthroplasty is contraindicated or as a salvage for a failed implant or Keller procedure. In the latter example, it is often useful to re-establish the weightbearing capabilities of the first metatarsophalangeal joint, especially when the original Keller procedure was performed with excessive bony resection and shortening.[27] First metatarsophalangeal joint fusion is slowly becoming the primary procedure of choice for painful arthrosis or for correction of malalignments at this joint. The advantages of the procedure are that it allows for a stable and propulsive gait, there is little chance for migration or change with time, and it has a high success rate for the resolution of pain. It also has been shown to impede dorsal migration of the lesser toes and the occurrence of lateral metatarsalgia after panmetatarsal head resection because of the stability the procedure imparts to the forefoot.[23] The procedure provides protection and stabilization of the lesser digits, particularly if the lesser metatarsophalangeal joints have been resected.[23]

Re-establishment of digital length may necessitate bone grafting or other length-attaining maneuvers, but care should be taken to prevent establishment of the fulcrum in a position that is too distal, which will impede proper pushoff. Although it has been reported that the interphalangeal joint of the hallux undergoes some radiographic deterioration,[23, 27] it is seldom a clinically significant entity.

Many patients are likely to be skeptical about the benefits of fusion because they equate it with stiffness and loss of flexibility. This is its primary disadvantage. Even though there is stiffness, the actual loss of flexibility is often less than the preoperative perception. Although the fusion is considered to be ''reversible'' with takedown and insertion of an implant, as a practical matter this simply does not work well.

Arthrodesis of this joint requires considerable preoperative planning. The heel height and style of shoe that the patient prefers to wear should be ascertained preoperatively. This will indicate the preferential angle of sagittal plane position of the hallux. However, in the majority of rheumatoid patients, heel height and shoe style choices are foregone conclusions. Most patients with significant disease are grateful to be wearing conventional shoe gear in comfort so that their choice is usually one of reason.

The position of the hallux in the fusion operation is somewhat variable depending on several factors. The hallux should probably not be fused in neutral position because this situation tends to limit the propulsive phase of gait. Some degree of dorsal angulation is most desirable, particularly in female patients. Excessive dorsiflexion is bound to be complicated with shoe-wear difficulties, particularly in male patients. Toenail problems are quite common because of the excessive pressure from the top of the shoe on the unyielding hallux.

Several authors noted that arthrodesis in 20 to 30 degrees of lateral deviation afforded optimal results.[23, 28, 29] This position enables normal shoe fitting and protects the hallux and interphalangeal joint from stress from the shoe in a lateral direction.

Care should also be taken with regard to proper orientation on the frontal plane. Just as in fusion of the interphalangeal joint, neutral rotation is probably best to avoid irritation to the medial or lateral condyles of the interphalangeal joint.

The same basic tenets of technique should be applied to fusion of the first metatarsophalangeal joint as are applied to the arthrodesis of the hallux with regard to osteoporosis, fixation, and bone grafting (Fig. 34–9). Mann and associates described the technique in both rheumatoid and nonrheumatoid patients.[23, 30] The actual techniques are addressed in Chapter 33.

Tarsometatarsal Junction

Radiographic evidence of disease at the tarsometatarsal level is common. Surprisingly, it correlates little with symptoms (Fig. 34–10). In fact, the overwhelming majority of patients with radiographic disease at this level are not symptomatic at this articulation. Perhaps the lack of correlation of these changes with symptoms is due to the relative lack of motion at this level or the decreased demands placed on this joint in this group of patients. The requirement for fusion at this level in the rheumatoid patient is an infrequent event.

It is extremely rare to encounter the patient who has symptomatic panarticular disease at this level to a point at which arthrodesis of all of the tarsometatarsal joints would require fusion. When a patient presents with symptoms at this level, it is important, again, to localize the joints responsible for the majority of the pain. This also can be accomplished with strategically placed injections of local anesthesia. In most cases, patients with symptoms at this level will find relief with injection of the medial two rays and, on rare occasion,

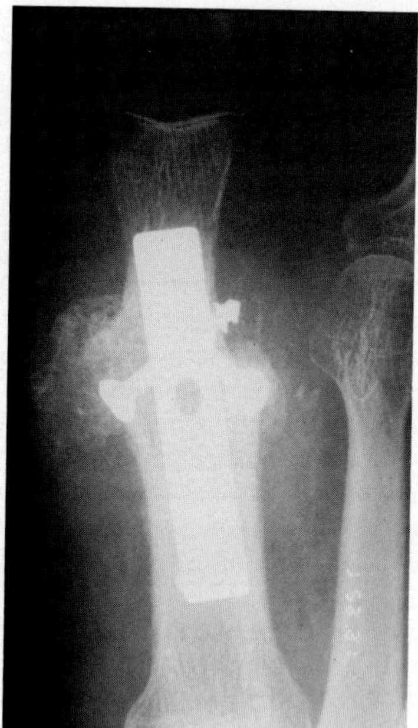

FIGURE 34–9. Anteroposterior radiograph of a first metatarsophalangeal joint fusion with crossed screw fixation. In this case the bone stock was satisfactory, but a supplemental plate was applied to stabilize the construct.

the third tarsometatarsal joint. This is probably due to the increased stress on the medial column with any pronatory attitude of the foot. Symptomatic involvement of the lateral two rays is extremely rare.

If surgery is deemed necessary, limited local arthrodesis is the procedure of choice. Fusion of the first metatarsocuneiform joint is a well-established procedure for the correction of hallux abductovalgus in the nonrheumatoid patient.[31–34] The same principles and techniques are applicable to the rheumatoid patient. However, the situations described previously may complicate the performance of the procedure and make internal fixation a bit more difficult.

If the first metatarsocuneiform joint is fused in conjunction with hallux abductovalgus, correction of choice is performed first at the metatarsal head. A separate incision or proximal extension of the primary incision will provide exposure. Once the joint is exposed, resection is best accomplished with power instrumentation from either the dorsal or medial approach. It is critical to place a wide retractor just against the lateral surface of the metatarsal base to protect the deep plantar vessels that course between the first and second metatarsals. The advantage of the dorsal approach is that the amount of necessary correction can be easily gauged. However, the depth of the base of the bone requires that a long saw blade be used to resect the plantar aspect of the bone. With a longer saw blade, the amount of wobble increases, which may reflect the accuracy of resection. There is a tendency to remove less bone on the plantar aspect of the joint, which would create a dorsiflexion of the first metatarsal. This situation is avoided by the more medial approach, but it is more difficult to remove the amount of bone that was calculated to correct the deformity.

I find it easier to cut both the base of the metatarsal and the distal aspect of the first cuneiform from the medial aspect before removing the articular surfaces. Cuts perpendicular to

the long axis of the respective bones provide excellent alignment of the first ray. It is easier to remove the entire joint than piecemeal resection of the respective joint surfaces. The only difficult part is severance of the peroneus longus tendon insertion from the plantar lateral aspect of the first metatarsal base.

Once the bony resections have taken place, the surfaces are opposed and the fixation is introduced. In the rheumatoid patient, the bone is usually of insufficient density to accept compression screws, particularly the cannulated variety. This is because the currently available cannulated screws have shallow pitches, which lessens the hold in softer bone. Conventional cancellous screws have deeper pitches and may suffice. Crossed Kirschner wires or Steinmann pins provide reliable fixation in most cases.

Fusion of the lesser articulations is less well documented but is usually accomplished without significant difficulty. When more than one metatarsal is fused to the respective tarsal bone, care should be taken to ensure that all of the involved metatarsal heads end up on the same plane so that there is no iatrogenic deformity. The best way to prevent sagittal plane malalignment is to resect minimal but adequate bone from the metatarsal base and the distal aspect of the cuneiform joint. Even though the dorsal approach is the only one possible, these joints are not as deep as the first metatarsocuneiform joint; therefore, fusion is not as technically difficult.

The options of fixation are essentially the same as for the first metatarsocuneiform joint, except that single-point fixation is often adequate for the central three metatarsals because of the support from the adjacent metatarsal bases. If dual-point fixation can be done easily, it is inherently more stable than a single device.

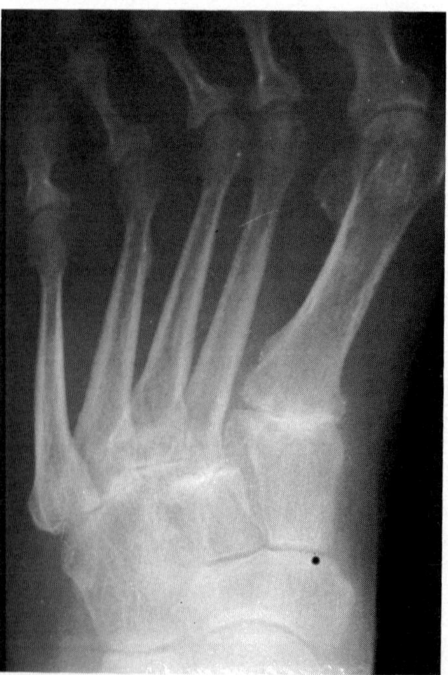

FIGURE 34–10. Anteroposterior radiograph showing advanced narrowing of the tarsometatarsal joint in this seronegative rheumatoid arthritic patient. There is significant loss of joint space and subchondral sclerosis.

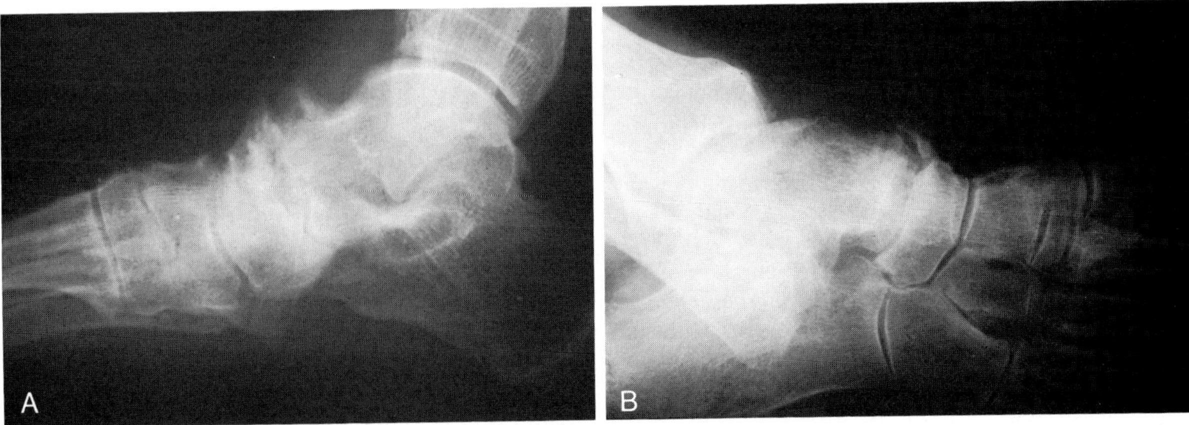

FIGURE 34–11. *A*, Lateral radiograph of a woman with rheumatoid arthritis showing severe narrowing and osseous proliferation of the talonavicular joint. Note the relatively unaffected subtalar joint. *B*, Oblique radiograph of the same patient showing preservation of the calcaneocuboid joint.

Talonavicular Joint

The talonavicular joint shows the earliest signs of joint space narrowing when compared with the other joints of the hindfoot complex (Fig. 34–11). According to the classic study by Vahvanen,[35] talonavicular narrowing and collapse of the midfoot occurs within 3 years from establishment of the diagnosis. Similarly, this joint has been shown to be severely narrowed most frequently when compared with the ankle, the talocalcaneal joint, and the calcaneocuboid joint. Even though it usually exhibits the earliest narrowing, progression does not correlate with the disease process in contrast with the calcaneocuboid and talocalcaneal joints. Many authors believe that this joint is most responsible for sagittal and transverse plane collapse, leading to the pes planovalgus deformity.[1, 36] According to Vainino,[37] the naviculocuneiform sagittal breach is most commonly responsible for midfoot collapse (Fig. 34–12). Nevertheless, the talonavicular joint is often found to be arthritic and narrowed.

Isolated fusion of the talonavicular joint in the rheumatoid patient has definite but limited application. Elboar and colleagues evaluated 35 isolated talonavicular fusions and reported complete relief of pain in 75% after a minimum follow-up of 1 year.[38] They contended that the radiographic presence of subtalar disease does not contraindicate solitary talonavicular fusion. In addition, they found no significant progression of degenerative changes with time as a result of the procedure. Although the statistical analyses presented are inadequate, these procedures seem to have been performed early in the course of symptoms. When one considers the early onset of collapse of this joint, perhaps it is then tenable that its fusion would eliminate the need for fusion of the subtalar joint. Because of the integrated motion of the hindfoot complex, stoppage of one joint could prevent excessive motion in the others.[39] In addition, they also found a decrease in the amount of plantarflexion available in the forefoot after talonavicular fusion in a group of nonrheumatoid patients. This resultant loss of propelling action during swing phase led to a decrease in step length and velocity. In rheumatoid patients, particularly those with multiarticular involvement, this is probably not significant and probably will not adversely alter gait capabilities at all.

It is important, however, to scrutinize the patients' symptoms and location of pain. Although patients may exhibit minimal, if any, radiographic evidence of change in the subtalar joint, they may complain of lateral symptoms that seem to emanate from the sinus tarsi or posterior aspect of the subtalar joint. Even though fusion of the talonavicular joint

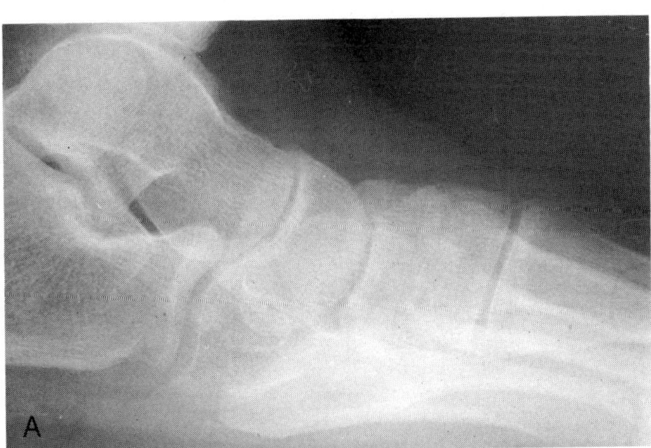
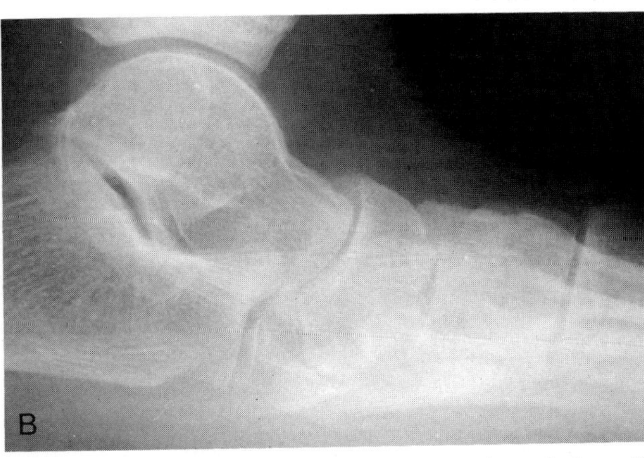

FIGURE 34–12. *A*, Lateral view of a 31-year-old woman with rheumatoid arthritis. There is significant collapse and narrowing at the naviculocuneiform joint but sparing of the more proximal articulations. *B*, Lateral view of a different patient with collapse of the talonavicular and naviculocuneiform joints. (From Schuberth JM: Pedal fusions in the rheumatoid patient. Clin Podiatr Med Surg 5:227–247, 1988.)

may be performed in a manner to "unweight" the lateral aspect of the foot, patients' lateral symptoms often do not abate postoperatively. Although the reasons for this remain obscure, patients with lateral symptoms in addition to the medial column disease should be considered for triple arthrodesis.

Technical considerations of isolated talonavicular fusion relate primarily to the attainment of adequate bone-to-bone apposition and satisfactory position. The latter is often difficult because of the ball-and-socket-like configuration of the joint and the often abundant but necessary bone resection of the concave portion of the navicular bone. The surgeon should thus be prepared to pack the interstices with autogenous bone graft or, less preferably, allogeneic bone (Fig. 34–13). The need for bone graft can occasionally be obviated when careful denuding of just the articular cartilage and subchondral bone is performed. This is somewhat technically difficult, however, because of the limited exposure afforded by monoarticular fusion. Care must be taken not to place the other articulations at risk by unduly stressing the other joints of the hindfoot complex at the expense of attaining bone-to-bone apposition.

Stiff or ankylosed calcaneocuboid or subtalar joints may prevent significant mobility for bone surface approximation even if cartilage is kept to a minimum. Care must be taken not to create a forefoot adductus by aggressive manipulation. I believe that when fusion of this joint alone is done in the presence of even marginal subtalar disease, every effort should be made to prevent excessive stress on the subtalar joint, which may be caused by overzealous intraoperative mobilization. Therefore, an interposition bone graft should be considered to facilitate bony apposition without redirecting adjacent joints.

Fixation is usually best accomplished with compression screws of 4.0 or 6.5 mm in diameter. The relatively new 4.5-mm cannulated cancellous bone screw is ideal in this procedure. Alternatives include staples, Kirschner wires, and Steinmann pins (Fig. 34–14). Onlay or inlay graft techniques are also acceptable.[40]

Subtalar Joint

The subtalar joint is clearly the most frequently involved joint of the hindfoot complex in the rheumatoid foot[35, 36] and

is often a source of considerable disability. Although solitary fusion of the subtalar joint has had minimal exposure in the early[41] literature, it is a useful technique when significant subtalar arthrosis is present in the absence of ankle and midtarsal disease. The potential for adaptability of the foot for uneven terrain is significantly maintained if the midtarsal joint is able to be spared. However, this notion may not hold entirely true if there is stiffness or other arthrosis in the midtarsal joint preoperatively. Range of motion of the midtarsal joint should be assessed about both of its axes to determine the adaptability potential of these joints when the subtalar joint undergoes arthrodesis. Frequently, these articulations have already undergone moderate adaptation, particularly when there is some subtalar or, more commonly, ankle stiffness or deformity. If any existing frontal plane deformity of the subtalar joint is going to be corrected, the midtarsal range of motion should be assessed, with the subtalar joint held in the desired position of fusion if possible.

Although it is generally believed that subtalar arthrodesis will place additional stresses on the ankle joint, it is seldom a problem in the rheumatoid patient when one considers the progression of ankle arthritis.[35, 36] The development of ankle joint arthritis is a very slow process and may be more related to the progression of the disease itself rather than being induced by the subtalar arthrodesis. Conceivably, the sparing effect on the ankle can be attributed to the small component of sagittal plane motion that is lost as a result of the subtalar fusion. This small amount of compensatory motion may not be needed by the sedentary rheumatoid patient; therefore, there is no additional sagittal plane motion requirement for gait to occur.

Increases in frontal plane talar tilt have been observed in the rheumatoid ankle after subtalar arthrodesis.[35] This is most likely caused by the increase in the lever arm of the talocalcaneal apparatus and not from damage to the lateral ligamentous complex from the surgical procedure. Any inversion stress applied to the calcaneus is no longer dampened by an intact subtalar joint. The increase in talar tilt is not as evident when ankle joint space narrowing is present preoperatively because of the partially ankylosed condition of the ankle itself.

If subtalar fusion is indicated, the general principles of fusion of this joint should be followed. Several technical considerations warrant discussion. Because of the often se-

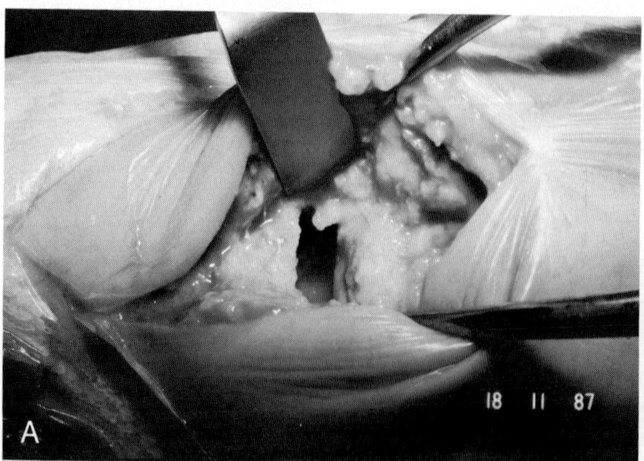
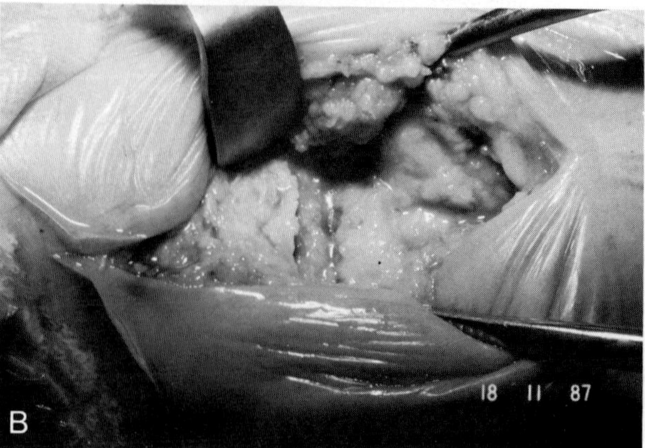

FIGURE 34–13. *A,* Intraoperative view of a talonavicular fusion after appropriate resection of the articular surfaces. A large void is between the talus and the navicular. *B,* Autogenous iliac crest bone is packed into the void to prevent shortening of the medial column.

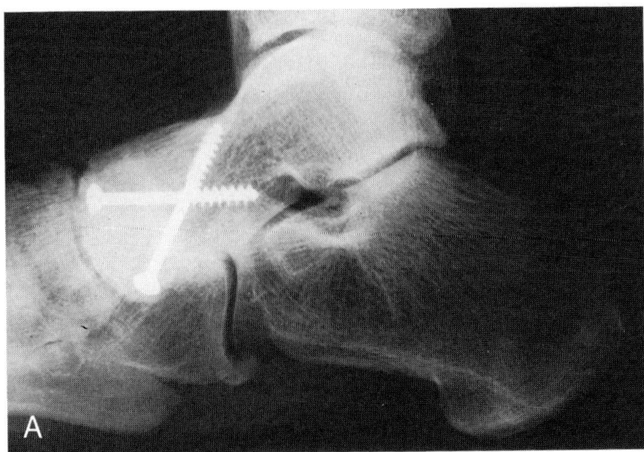
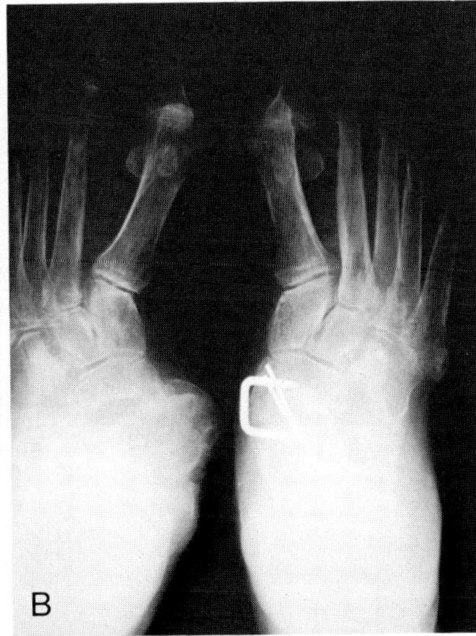

FIGURE 34–14. *A*, Lateral view of an isolated talonavicular fusion showing crossed cannulated screw technique for fixation. *B*, Anteroposterior view of a patient with bilateral dislocation of talonavicular joint secondary to rheumatoid arthritis. In this patient, the right foot underwent talonavicular fusion with wire and staple fixation owing to the soft bone.

vere valgus position of the heel preoperatively, one should be careful not to create excessive heel eversion. This is often inadvertent if one uses the conventional lateral approach. The intact sustentaculum tali and the middle talar articular facet serve as a hinge in which the joint is booked open for preparation of the fusion surfaces. As the articular surfaces are denuded of cartilage, there is a natural tendency to create additional valgus because of the normal limitations of access to the medial joint structures from this approach. In fact, wider resection of the more lateral cartilaginous tissue may be done to improve exposure and access to the medial aspect of the joint. This problem is compounded if subchondral bone is removed. However, complete removal of subchondral bone is recommended to enhance the fusion rate. It has been my observation that a higher incidence of nonunion of the subtalar joint occurs when the subchondral bone is left intact. Some surgeons elect to obviate this problem by drilling holes into the subchondral plate to promote vascular ingrowth across the fusion site. In most cases, this is inadequate because the relatively sclerotic bone has a poorer potential for fusion than raw cancellous bone.

It is also difficult to reduce heel valgus with selective wedging from the lateral approach. Even with the direct approach of McGlamry and associates,[42] the varus-producing maneuver is difficult. This technique is best accomplished with a power saw. One must be aware of the juxtaposition of the medial aspect of the talus and the neurovascular bundle when cutting through the medial aspect of the talus and calcaneus during the wedging process. Large, spoon-shaped retractors should be optimally placed to avoid damage to these structures. In spite of an accomplished technique, the resultant shortening of the height of the foot may create other problems of limb-length inequality or, more likely, impingement of the peroneal tendons between the fibula and calcaneus on the lateral side of the foot.

Therefore, bone grafting is often desirable to reduce or prevent worsening of the valgus heel position and will help preserve foot height. This is best accomplished by a tricorti-

cal or bicortical iliac crest bone graft. The graft should be situated with the superior surface of the iliac crest in a lateral position at the base of the wedge (Fig. 34–15). This will help prevent collapse of the graft with resultant loss of position. Precise positioning of the subtalar joint is thereby possible by refining the thickness of the wedge. The cortical surfaces of the thinner part of the wedge should be removed so that vascular cancellous bone is exposed to the respective denuded surfaces of the talus and calcaneus. As with standard subtalar fusions, some residual valgus is the optimal position.

Fixation of the subtalar fusion is not particularly difficult in the rheumatoid patient. The calcaneus will usually hold large compression screws placed from the neck of the talus. If it does not hold in the cancellous portions of the body, the screw can be oriented more laterally to engage the lateral cortical wall of the calcaneus (Fig. 34–16). Countersinking in this area is seldom necessary, but if so, it should be done with caution. Occasionally, bone density dictates use of a washer (Fig. 34–17). Another option includes reversal of the

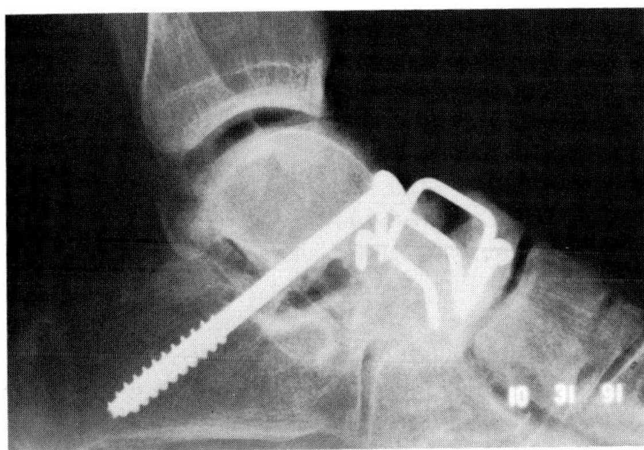

FIGURE 34–15. Lateral view of a patient who underwent a talonavicular and subtalar fusion with severe preoperative valgus position. The tricortical iliac crest wedge has been placed into the subtalar joint to reduce the valgus position.

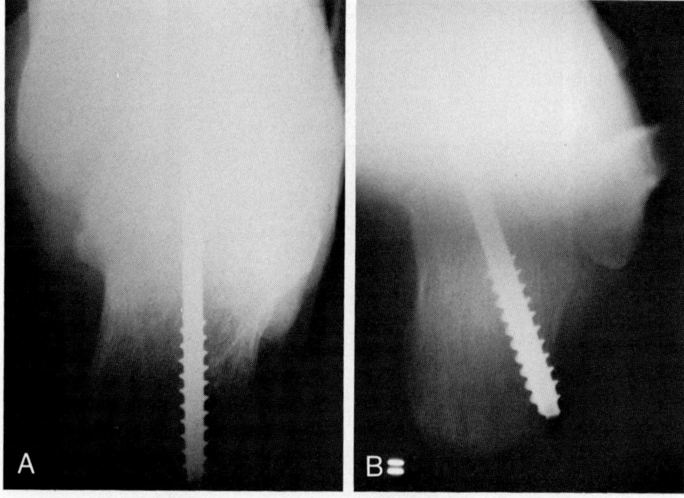

FIGURE 34–16. *A,* Axial view of an isolated subtalar fusion indicating the optimal placement of the compression screw into the cancellous bone of the tuber. *B,* Axial view of an isolated subtalar fusion showing the screw engaging the lateral wall of the calcaneus to enhance purchase in this osteoporotic patient.

direction of the screw by placing it from the calcaneus into the talus from a posterior inferior approach. The talus is usually a bit more dense than the calcaneus, and this approach can be considered as a back-up technique or a primary method. A third alternative is the use of threaded or nonthreaded Steinmann pins placed across the subtalar joint. Last, staples have been used with some success in some of the reports in the literature.[43]

Extra-articular fusion procedures are not recommended for several reasons.[44] First, diseased articular cartilage is still present in a weightbearing attitude and can account for residual pain even in the alleged absence of motion. In addition, if synovitis is activated or pannus formed, the intact articular cartilage serves as an excellent substrate for the process. Therefore, elimination of as much of the articular cartilage as possible should minimize the chances of reactivation of the joint symptoms. Second, even if the procedure is performed correctly, the absolute absence of motion is not ensured, particularly with small bridges of bone that are expected to limit motion of the involved joint completely.

TRIPLE ARTHRODESIS

Triple arthrodesis is indicated when the patient requires ultimate stabilization of the hindfoot or relief of symptoms stemming from multiple joint involvement. Again, pain, deformity, and instability may be present in variable degrees. One must carefully assess the condition of both the proximal and distal joints to determine whether additional fusion should take place at these levels. Joints distal to the midtarsal joint are often spared and are seldom the site of postoperative arthrosis regardless of their preoperative condition.

Although arthropathy in the ankle joint has been cited as a complication after triple arthrodesis, I believe that this is a rare occurrence and a very slow process. Wilson and colleagues[45] did not mention this complication after 301 cases of triple arthrodesis, and Vainino[37] reported only 4 of 209 feet with significant worsening of the ankle joint arthrosis in the rheumatoid patient. Radiologic changes are more common, but it is difficult to say whether these changes are due to the natural progression of the rheumatic disease process or are mediated by the triple arthrodesis. Gellman and associ-

ates[20] reported only a 15% loss of plantarflexion and 12.5% loss of dorsiflexion of the entire foot after triple arthrodesis. Only 50% of total foot inversion and eversion was lost after triple arthrodesis, and 60% of total hindfoot motion was lost. This suggests that there may be some inherent protective mechanism that spares deterioration of the ankle joint after triple arthrodesis. This supports the work cited previously and confirms personal clinical impressions.

The principles of triple arthrodesis do not differ appreciably between rheumatoid and nonrheumatoid patients except as already mentioned. Excessive frontal plane deviations are to be avoided because suprastructural adapting mechanisms may be dampened by stiffness, total joint replacement, or both. The preferred technique is that popularized by McGlamry and associates.[42] Modifications of this technique as described previously will yield satisfactory results in most cases.

ANKLE FUSION

The rheumatoid ankle exhibits some innate if not surprising properties that reduce the need for ankle fusion. Although this joint is commonly affected by rheumatoid disease, relatively few ankle fusions are indicated in this patient popula-

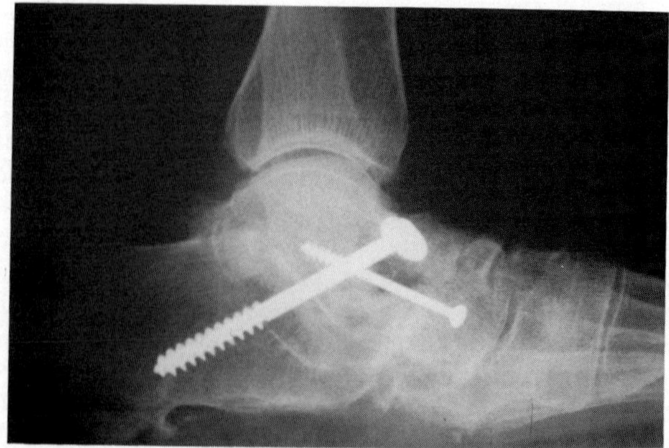

FIGURE 34–17. Lateral view of a triple arthrodesis using a washer at the talar neck to prevent migration of the screw into the talus. Most of the fixation of the calcaneocuboid and talonavicular joints has been removed.

tion.[46] The most striking characteristic is the relatively poor correlation between pain and the radiologic findings. Patients may complain of pain in the hindfoot that is localized to the subtalar complex by astute clinical examination and yet have radiographs that demonstrate advanced ankle joint disease and a relatively benign subtalar joint. The converse situation of hindfoot pain later localized to the ankle is observed less frequently. It is also interesting that spontaneous fusion in the ankle joint is quite uncommon in the osteoarthritic joint but occurs more commonly in the rheumatoid ankle. Fibrous ankylosis occurs more often than true bony ankylosis (Fig. 34–18). When fibrous or bony ankylosis does occur, pain will be sparse. It has been stated that the ankle is resistant to

rheumatoid arthritis.[37] Our experience at Kaiser Foundation Hospital confirms this. In a review of 261 patients with rheumatoid arthritis requiring a major lower extremity joint procedure, only 4 required a talocrural arthrodesis. From 1983 to 1992, 55 ankle fusions have been performed here, and 4 were in the true rheumatoid category. Four total ankle replacements have been performed during the same period on rheumatoid patients. Two of these required secondary arthrodesis because of prosthesis loosening.

The indication for arthrodesis is almost invariably pain. Because of the tendency for symmetric joint space narrowing, deformity at the talocrural joint is uncommon. However, in the presence of severe varus or pes planovalgus deformity,

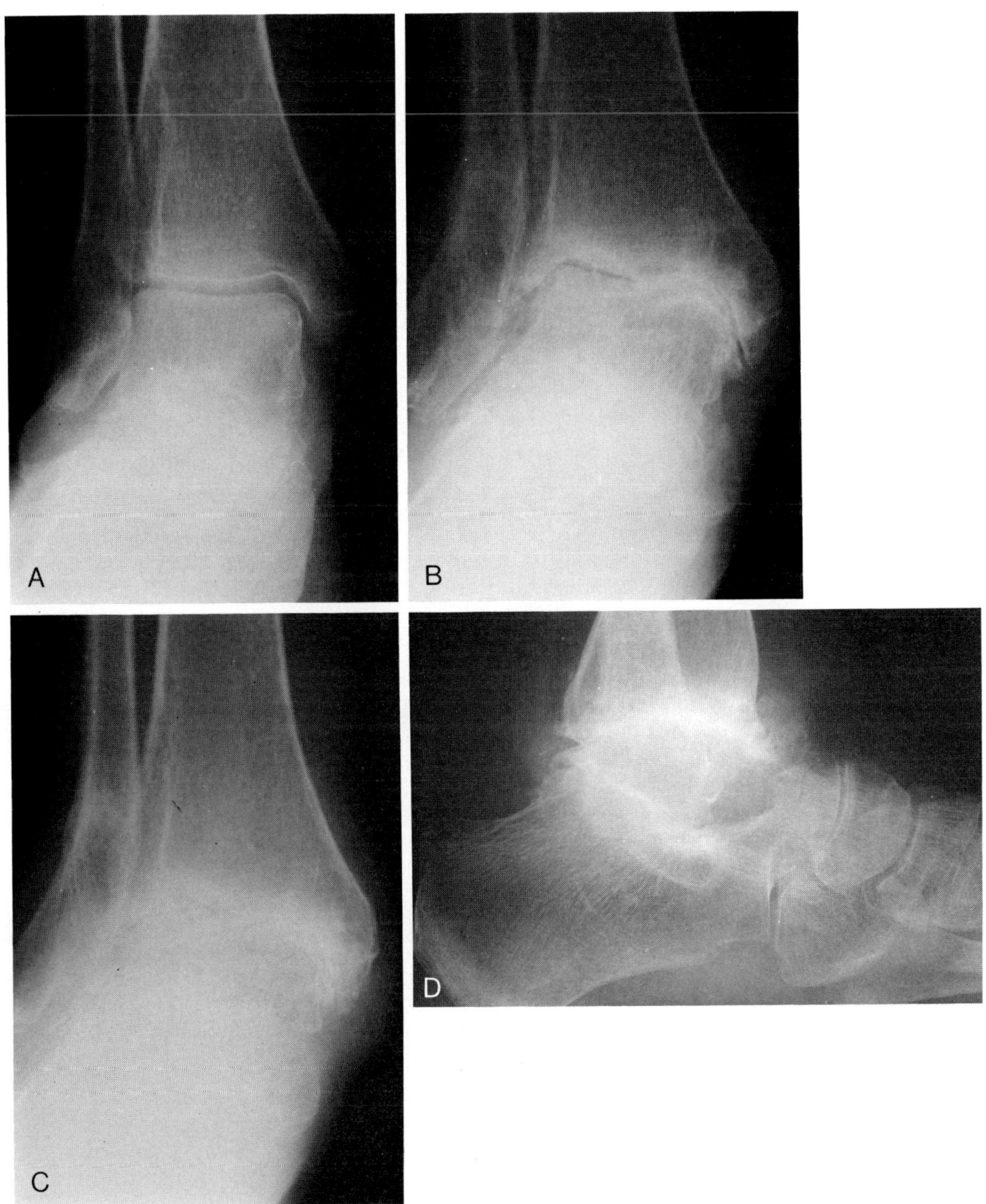

FIGURE 34–18. *A*, Anteroposterior view of the ankle of a woman taken at the onset of the disease. Minimal articular changes are noted. *B*, Anteroposterior view of the same ankle taken 2 years later showing the progressive erosive changes with joint space narrowing. The fibula exhibits an old healed stress fracture. *C*, Anteroposterior view taken 4 years after onset of disease showing the spontaneous fusion that has occurred. There was no perceptible motion at this articulation. *D*, Lateral view of the same patient, confirming the completion of radiographic union. (From Schuberth JM: Pedal fusions in the rheumatoid patient. Clin Podiatr Med Surg 5:227–247, 1988.)

weightbearing radiographs of the ankle should be taken to determine to what degree true ankle varus or valgus contributes to the condition. Some gradual collapse and adaptation of the tibial plafond may occur, particularly in the presence of severe hindfoot valgus. Ankle varus is extremely rare in the rheumatoid patient, as is instability of the talocrural joint.

A painful rheumatoid ankle requires attention to the joints distal to the ankle. Although typically there is a considerable decrease in the range of motion at the ankle preoperatively, the loss of additional sagittal plane motion may unduly stress the joints distally. The midtarsal joint is the major compensatory mechanism in the foot for decreased ankle joint dorsiflexion. Although traditional teaching and prior published reports[47–50] suggest that midtarsal range of motion increases after ankle arthrodesis, Gellman and associates[20] showed that 51% of dorsiflexion of the foot remains after ankle arthrodesis. They pointed out that isolated motion of this joint in the plane of compensation has not been adequately studied in the nonarthrodesed foot. Perhaps those who have studied this range of motion after fusion had erroneously assumed that the motion had increased when, in fact, it had been present before the fusion operation. The work by Jackson and Glasgow[51] further supports this notion. They also noted that degenerative changes about the midtarsal joint developed in 33% of patients undergoing ankle fusion and that midtarsal hypermobility was not a common observation after fusion. These findings, however, were not able to be correlated with clinical results.

Even though the studies cited previously involved primarily patients without rheumatoid disease, they raise the question of whether or not one should be more or less aggressive in deciding whether to spare or fuse the midtarsal joint. In view of these works, perhaps pantalar fusion should be performed more sparingly. On the other hand, in the face of significant midfoot or hindfoot arthritis, pantalar arthrodesis should be considered if ankle fusion is performed. If there are additional symptoms at the subtalar joint or midtarsal complex, then the decision for pantalar arthrodesis is simplified.

Another option is total ankle arthroplasty, which preserves the limited motion and spares the involved midfoot joints from additional stress (Fig. 34–19). Long-term follow-up is lacking,[2, 4] and even though the best results to date are in the low-demand rheumatoid patient, the ultimate efficiency of total ankle arthroplasty is uncertain. As follow-up increases, more unsatisfactory results may emerge.[52]

The principles of fusion in the rheumatoid ankle do not deviate from those in the post-traumatic or osteoarthritic ankle. Juxta-articular softening of the osseous structures does not seem to be a problem when compared with other rheumatoid pedal joints. Loss of cartilage from the talofibular and talotibial articulations is common as a result of the erosive processes but is seldom clinically relevant.

The favored technique is the transfibular approach, as described by Mahan.[53] This allows for excellent visualization of the entire joint and facilitates posterior displacement of

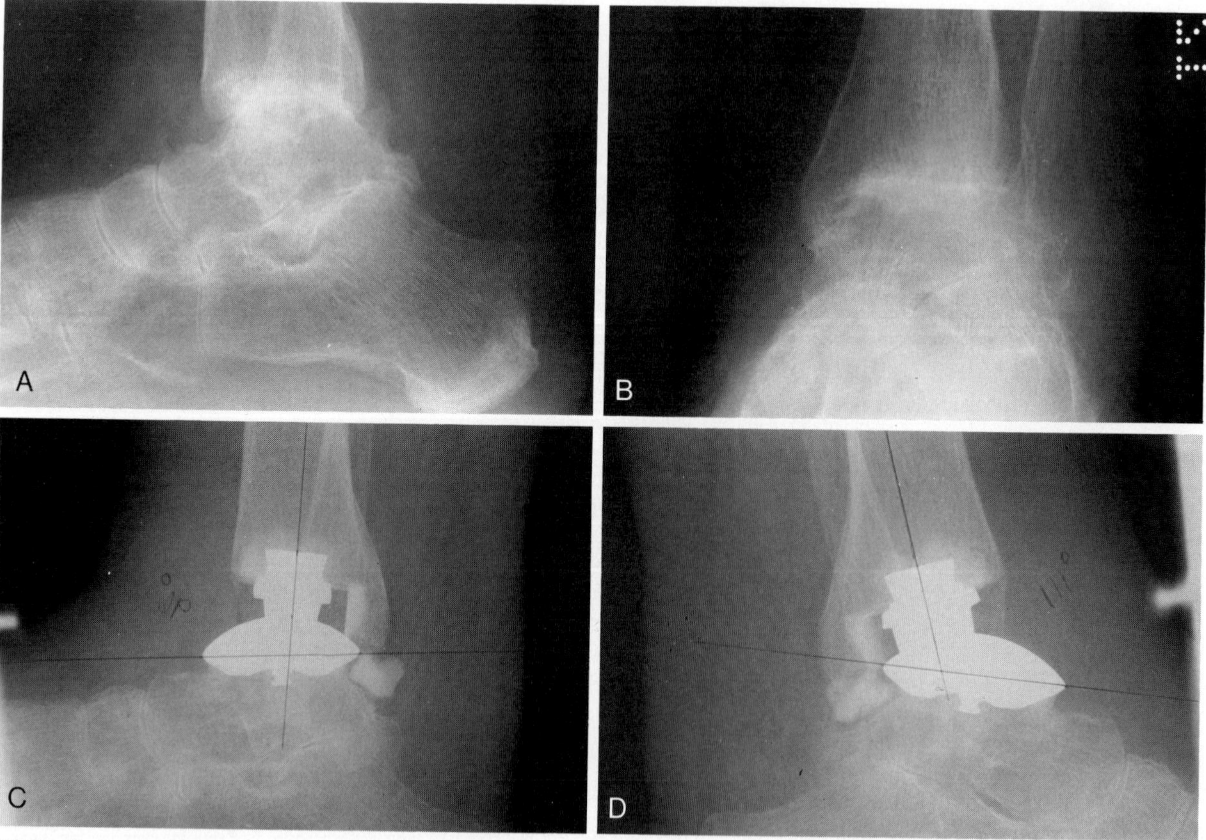

FIGURE 34–19. *A* and *B*, Preoperative radiographs of a 67-year-old rheumatoid patient with a markedly painful ankle. There was 10 degrees of painful motion in the ankle joint. There is moderate narrowing of the subtalar and midtarsal joint. *C* and *D*, Stress films of a cemented total ankle arthroplasty 3 months postoperative demonstrating 15 degrees of motion. This is postulated to spare additional stress at the talonavicular joint. Observe the degree of motion available at the talonavicular articulation. Had an ankle arthrodesis been performed, the demand for motion at the talonavicular joint could have stressed this joint excessively. (From Schuberth JM: Pedal fusions in the rheumatoid patient. Clin Podiatr Med Surg 5:227–247, 1988.)

the talus on the tibia. The more posterior position allows for the effective elongation of the lever arm of the Achilles tendon, which aids in propulsion during the heel-off phase of gait. In patients with presumably weaker muscle groups, this mechanical property may be advantageous in reducing the energy needed for efficient gait.

The ankle joint is exposed through a midfibular incision, which is carried to the tip of the lateral malleolus and then curved slightly anterior. The superficial peroneal nerve is reflected with the skin and subcutaneous tissue and the fibula is exposed. Subperiosteal dissection of the entire distal fibula is performed. The fibula is cut transversely just above the level of the syndesmosis. As much of the soft tissue attachments as possible is transected, with attention directed to the syndesmotic ligaments. The fibula can be removed completely or can be hinged out of the way on its inferior hinge of the calcaneofibular ligament. I prefer to remove it completely to improve access to the ankle. The tibiotalar joint is now completely visible to the surgeon. The soft tissues on the anterior and posterior aspect of the distal tibia are reflected and then protected with wide, flat retractors. It is important to expose the entire distal tibia so that careful monitoring of the position of power instrumentation can occur at all times. This is especially true for the posterior tibial neurovascular bundle. It must be adequately protected from the lateral incision.

Next, attention is directed to the medial side of the ankle joint, where a second incision is made over the medial gutter of the ankle. This is usually just anterior to the saphenous neurovascular bundle. These structures are also reflected with the skin and subcutaneous layer, and dissection is carried to the level of the capsule. The joint is opened with a vertical arthrotomy, and the medial talotibial articulation is identified. Care should be taken to preserve the deltoid if possible because it carries one of the crucial blood supplies to the talar body. A saw cut is made in the distal tibia, which parallels the orientation of the medial tibiotalar articulation. The cartilage from the lateral surface of the medial malleolus is thus removed. The blade is detached from the saw and left in place, thus serving as a stopper to prevent overzealous resection of the medial aspect of the distal tibial bone.

Attention is now redirected to the lateral side. The cartilage and the subchondral bone on the distal aspect of the tibia are now removed. It is easiest to use a large sagittal or oscillating power saw from lateral to medial. If there are any angulatory deformities, they should be corrected with this cut because one strives to preserve as much of the talar bone stock as possible. The saw is carried as far medial as the previously placed saw blade will allow. With some final adjustments in the saw cuts, the distal aspect of the tibial plafond should now be completely detached from the rest of the tibia.

The cartilage from the medial and lateral sides of the talus is now removed. The final cut involves the removal of articular cartilage from the talus. The optimal position of the ankle joint is first determined by dorsiflexing and plantarflexing the talus against the prepared tibial surface. When the desired position of fusion is obtained, the talus is prepared by removing its articular surface in a manner parallel to the distal tibial surface. The talus and tibia have now been prepared in what should resemble two table top surfaces with an intact medial corner or mortise. The talus should be posteriorly displaced on the tibia. Refinement of the cut surfaces

should ensure maximal bone-to-bone apposition and optimal positioning of the osseous segments. The medial corner of the talus should fit securely into the denuded medial corner of the tibia.

The optimal position of fusion in the rheumatoid patient is neutral. A few degrees of equinus or calcaneus are tolerated, but excesses should be avoided at all costs. Equinus is tolerated less by rheumatoid patients because their shoe requirements are often more confined than those of nonrheumatoid patients and they cannot substitute shoes of varying heel heights for malposition. Therefore, midfoot compensation for an equinus ankle should be minimized by a more neutral position of fusion. An excessive calcaneal attitude will further enhance the development of knee contractures and make ambulation extremely difficult.

Rotational or transverse plane positioning of the fusion is often difficult. Because of the often abducted forefeet in these patients, there may be confusion as to where the true line of progression lies. The rule of thumb is to align the foot with the axis of the second metatarsal joint positioned in line with or very slightly external to the long axis of the tibia. This will facilitate a relatively smooth gait pattern. Iatrogenic internal rotation should be avoided at all costs.

The frontal plane position of fusion should be neutral or biased slightly toward a valgus attitude. Varus is always contraindicated.

Frontal plane deviations at the level of the ankle are less common, but if they are encountered, some correction is advisable. In most cases in which there is frontal plane deviation, it is usually valgus. This is particularly true in the patient who has had long-standing disease and valgus deformity of the foot and in the juvenile rheumatoid arthritic. The longevity of the disease in the former and the long-term effects of abnormal loading in the latter will predispose the patient to a valgus ankle. This usually occurs at the expense of asymmetric talotibial joint narrowing in the adult patient and remodeling in the pediatric patient.[37] In either case, the talus must be medialized to place it under the strong and intact medial column of the tibia. Varus deformity of the ankle joint in the rheumatoid patient is rare but should be eliminated if present.

Temporary fixation should now be introduced and intraoperative radiographs should be taken. The radiographs are important not so much to attain position of the ankle joint but rather to serve as a checkpoint for the position of the temporary and thus final fixation devices. I believe that careful visual assessment of the position of the foot relative to the leg is more useful than radiographic assessment. However, intraoperative radiographs can assist the surgeon in attaining optimal position. If one is compelled to use radiographic images for attainment of optimal position, then 14 × 17–inch plates should be used. This will allow for better visualization of the long axis of the tibia so that accurate position can be attained.

In most routine cases of ankle arthrodesis, I favor the use of cannulated 7.0-mm screws placed across the fusion site. In the rheumatoid patient, this is still the favored technique if bone stock is sufficient. The first guide pin for screw placement is best inserted at the medial aspect of the tibia so that the screw traverses the corner formed by the medial malleolus and the remaining portion of the tibia (Fig. 34–20). When the screw is tightened, the talus will be drawn into the mortise-like configuration. The second screw is

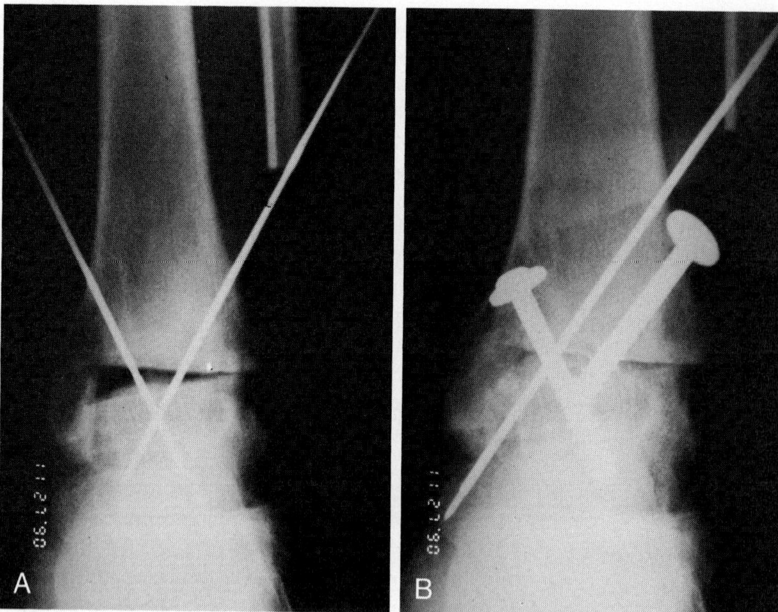

FIGURE 34–20. *A*, Intraoperative radiograph showing the position of the guide wires for screw placement across the fusion site. Ideally, there is less gapping at the medial corner prior to screw placement. *B*, Appearance of the fusion site after the screws have been placed. Note the reduction of the gap and the excellent apposition of the bony surfaces. A third guide pin was also placed for added stability.

placed at the anterolateral aspect of the tibia and directed distal and medially. A third screw can be added from antero-proximal to posterorinferior, if necessary.

Once the talotibial joint is fixated, the fibula is decorticated and then replaced to augment the fusion mass. The medial cortical surface or medial one third of the bony fragment is removed with a power saw to expose the cancellous bone of the malleolus and distal metaphysis. It is usually fixated to the tibia only with 4.5-mm cortical screws placed from lateral to medial (Fig. 34–21). The drill holes in the fibular component are overdrilled to allow for some compression, but care is taken not to overtighten the screws because the fibula will often fracture.

Intraoperative assessment of the position of the replaced fibula is important if there is significant eversion of the calcaneus. With the fibula displaced medially as a result of medial decortication, the distal tip of the bone may be impinged by the calcaneus as it everts through the subtalar joint. It is, therefore, important to slide the fibula superiorly a sufficient distance to prevent this complication. If if will not pass easily under the proximal aspect of the intact fibula, the distal fragment can be shortened a bit to allow for the necessary proximal placement. This entire maneuver is unnecessary if the subtalar joint is surgically stabilized.

If there is significant damage to the lateral aspect of the tibial plafond because of collapse from the valgus orientation of the ankle joint, then it is preferable to medialize the talus rather that attempt to fixate the talus to softer and damaged lateral bone. However, this requires resection of the medial malleolus and sacrifice of the deltoid ligament. The talus is displaced medially so that the medial edge of the talus lines up with the medial edge of the tibia. Internal fixation is similar to the previous example, but three screws are preferable because the absence of the intact medial corner causes some rotatory instability.

Screw fixation can usually be accomplished in most cases of ankle fusion, but, as Mahan pointed out,[53] there is certainly no universal technique for ankle fusion. This is particularly true in the rheumatoid patient because of the problems with

decreased bone density. Alternative fixation devices should be procured and available if the primary method proves unsatisfactory. We usually have the external fixator available as an option. A series comparing use of the external fixator with internal screw compression showed no significant difference between fusion rate or the time to fusion.[46] Because of the increased technical difficulty with external fixation, it is preferable to attempt internal screw fixation at first. If there is insufficient compression or outright failure of the technique, then one should resort to external fixation for optimal compression. Although the infection rate is probably a bit higher in the external fixation group,[54] the primary objective is a

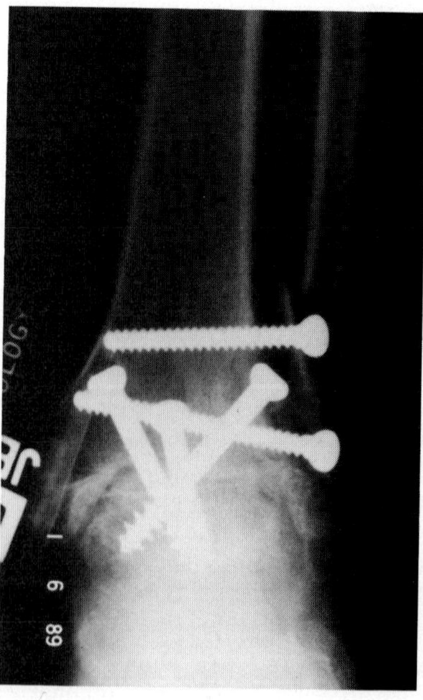

FIGURE 34–21. Anteroposterior radiograph showing the completed fusion with placement of all hardware. This patient is 3 months postoperative. Note the lateral contact of the talofibular fusion site, which serves to stabilize the construct.

solid fusion. In view of the higher percentage of patients with osteoporotic bone, external fixation will provide the most stable construct when all else fails.

PANTALAR ARTHRODESIS

The need for pantalar arthrodesis is infrequent. The patient with a painful arthrosis in all of the peritalar articulations is rare. As discussed before, it is extremely difficult to determine which of the joints are responsible for the most disabling symptoms and which joints are likely to cause symptoms later. Radiographic appearance of the joint may be contradictory to the level of symptoms produced. The converse can also be true. However, because of the significant morbidity associated with both the rigidity of the foot and the surgical procedure itself, the procedure should be used sparingly. One must weigh the alternatives of a potentially staged pantalar arthrodesis versus a one-stage operation. Although this philosophical question has many facets, I believe that if pantalar arthrodesis is not absolutely indicated, then a more limited arthrodesis should be performed instead. The patient should be informed that a secondary procedure may be indicated if there is evolution of new symptoms or unmasking of pre-existing ones.

Absolute indications for pantalar fusion in the rheumatoid patient include severe degeneration and pain in the ankle joint coupled with a grossly deformed and relatively rigid hindfoot. Even though there is a paucity of symptoms in the hindfoot, the severe deformity can make attainment of a plantigrade foot difficult or impossible without a concomitant triple arthrodesis.

The key articulations are the midtarsal (particularly the talonavicular) joint and the ankle joint. If fusion of either one of these joints is indicated in the presence of advanced degenerative changes or symptomatology of the other, pantalar arthrodesis should be considered. The subtalar joint plays a much lesser role in the decision-making process because its plane of compensation is more suited to frontal plane devia-

tions. The principles of fusion for each of the individual joints should be followed. Excessive planar deviations are poorly tolerated, and meticulous care should be taken to obtain a plantigrade foot.

POSTOPERATIVE IMMOBILIZATION

As with all rearfoot fusions in the rheumatoid patient, longer periods of non-weightbearing and immobilization are often required. The osteoporotic condition does not hinder bone healing itself, but it does not tolerate compression or weightbearing well until secondary stress trabeculae develop. Valgus deformity with premature weightbearing may ensue, particularly at the subtalar and ankle joints. The union rate is clearly affected by the patient who is taking relatively high doses of prednisone or other corticosteroids. A higher nonunion rate is expected in those steroid-dependent patients because of the negative effect of the steroid on osteogenesis.

JUVENILE RHEUMATOID ARTHRITIS

Arthrodesis procedures in the juvenile rheumatoid arthritic patient are seldom indicated. Because these patients are much more prone to joint stiffness than to joint laxity, joint instability is seldom observed. Similarly, successful fusion of a painful joint depends on the painless integrity of those joints proximal and distal to the fused joint. This is rarely observed in the juvenile rheumatoid patient in whom multiple joint involvement is common.

Joint stiffness may progress to the point of fibrous or even bony ankylosis. This phenomenon is much more common in the juvenile patient than in the adult rheumatoid patient. Therefore, appropriate splinting or soft tissue release may allow for a solid spontaneous fusion in a physiologically acceptable position. This principle is best illustrated in the juvenile rheumatoid ankle joint (Fig. 34–22). A plantigrade foot with the ankle ankylosed at 90 degrees is the optimal result.

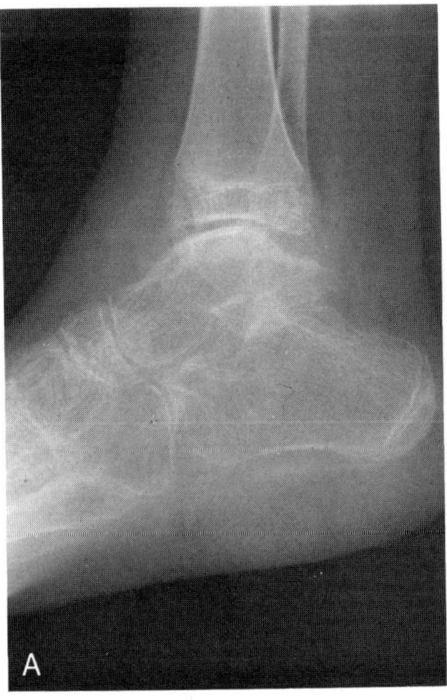
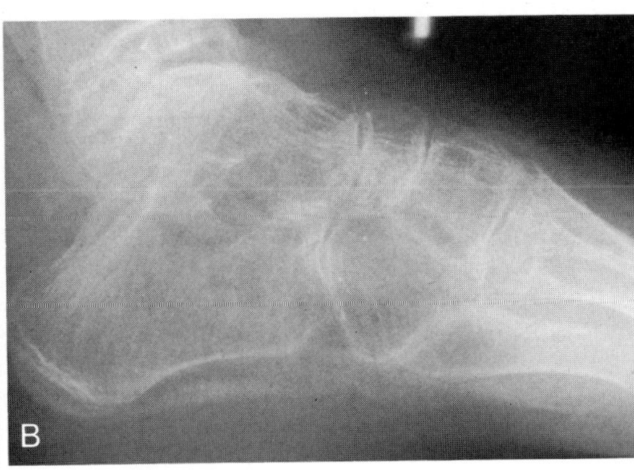

FIGURE 34–22. *A*, Lateral radiograph of a juvenile rheumatoid arthritic patient with ankylosis of the ankle joint. This child has been braced throughout the progression of the disease process, and a plantigrade foot has resulted. *B*, The opposite ankle has ankylosed into equinus in spite of the same bracing protocol. (From Schuberth JM: Pedal fusions in the rheumatoid patient. Clin Podiatr Med Surg 5:227–247, 1988.)

When fusion is indeed indicated, one must remember that stiffness is the predominant feature in the neighboring joints, and an increase in the compensatory joint's range of motion is seldom realized.

References

1. Clayton ML: Surgical treatment of the rheumatoid foot. *In* Giannestras NJ (ed): Foot Disorders: Medical and Surgical Management. Philadelphia, Lea & Febiger, 1967, pp 319–340.
2. Lachiewicz PF, Inglis AE, and Ranawat CS: Total ankle replacement in rheumatoid arthitis. J Bone Joint Surg 66A:340, 1984.
3. Newton SE III: Total ankle arthroplasy. Clinical study of 50 cases. J Bone Joint Surg 64A:104, 1982
4. Stauffer RM and Segal NM: Total ankle arthroplasty. Four years' experience. Clin Orthop 160:217, 1981.
5. Cracchiolo A, Swanson A, and Swanson GD: The arthritic great toe metatarsophalangeal joint: A review of flexible silicone implant arthroplasties from two medical centers. Clin Orthop 157:64, 1981.
6. Samuelson KM, Tuke MA, and Freeman MAR: A new reconstructive procedure to correct hindfoot valgus. Orthop Trans 3:149, 1978.
7. Samuelson KM, Tuke MA, and Freeman MAR: A study of hindfoot mechanics with relation to valgus deformity. J Bone Joint Surg 60B:282, 1978.
8. Vanore JV, O'Keefe RG, and Pikscher I: Silastic implant arthroplasty: Complications and their classification. J Am Podiatr Med Assoc 74:423, 1984.
9. Lim WT, Landrum K, and Weinberger B: Silicone lymphadenitis secondary to implant degeneration. J Foot Surg 22:243, 1983.
10. Gordon M, and Bullough PG: Synovial and osseous inflammation in failed silicone rubber prosthesis. J Bone Joint Surg 64A:574, 1983.
11. Lemon RA, Engber WD, and McBeath AA: A complication of Silastic hemiarthroplasty in bunion surgery. Foot Ankle 4:262, 1984.
12. Sethu A, D'Netto DC, and Ramakrishna B: Swanson's Silastic implants in great toes. J Bone Joint Surg 62B:83, 1980.
13. Bass SJ, Gastwirth CM, Green R, et al: Phagocytosis of Silastic material following Silastic great toe implant. J Foot Surg 17:70, 1978.
14. Shereff MJ and Jahss MH: Complications of Silastic implant arthroplasty in the hallux. Foot Ankle 1:95, 1980.
15. Glod D and Frykberg RG: Foreign body reaction in a Dacron-meshed hemiimplant. J Foot Surg 29:250, 1990.
16. Worsing RA, Engber WD, and Lange TA: Reactive synovitis from particulate Silastic. J Bone Joint Surg 64A:581, 1982.
17. Coughlin MJ and Mann RA: Arthodesis of the first metatarsal phalangeal joint as a salvage for the failed Keller procedure. J Bone Joint Surg 69:68, 1987.
18. Betts RP, Stockley MB, and Getty CJM: Foot pressure studies in the assessment of forefoot arthroplasty in the rheumatoid foot. Foot Ankle 8:315, 1988.
19. Rana NA: Rheumatoid arthritis, other collagen diseases and psoriasis of the foot. *In* Jahss MH (ed): Disorders of the Foot. Philadelphia, WB Saunders, 1982, pp 1027–1039.
20. Gellman H, Lenihan M, Halikis N, et al: Selective tarsal arthrodesis: An in vitro analysis on foot motion. Foot Ankle 8:127, 1987.
21. Saville PD and Kharmosh O: Osteoporosis of rheumatoid arthritis: Influence of age, sex, and corticosteroids. Arthritis Rheum 10:423, 1967.
22. Mahan KT: Bonegrafting. In McGlamry ED (ed): Comprehensive Textbook of Foot Surgery. Baltimore, Williams & Wilkins, 1987, p 646.
23. Mann RA and Thompson FM: Arthrodesis of the first metatarsophalangeal joint for hallux valgus in rheumatoid arthritis. J Bone Joint Surg 66A:687, 1984.
24. Gerbert J and Dobbs B: Forefoot derangement: Rheumatoid forefoot. *In* McGlamry ED (ed): Comprehensive Textbook of Foot Surgery. Baltimore, Williams & Wilkins, 1987, p 534.
25. Rude CC, Karlin JM, and Scurran BL: Implant arthroplasty of the first metatarsophalangeal joint. A follow-up. J Am Podiatr Assoc 75:279, 1985.
26. Weil LS, Pollak RA, and Goller WL: Total joint replacement in hallux valgus and hallux rigidus: Long term results in 484 cases. Clin Podiatr 1:103, 1984.
27. Henry APJ and Waugh W: The use of footprints in assessing the results of operations for hallux valgus: A comparison of Keller's operation and arthrodesis. J Bone Joint Surg 57B:478, 1975.
28. Fitzgerald JAW: A review of long-term results of arthrodesis of the first metatarsophalangeal joint. J Bone Joint Surg 51B:488, 1969.
29. Raymakers R and Waugh P: The treatment of metatarsalgia with hallux valgus. J Bone Joint Surg 53B:684, 1971.
30. Coughlin MJ and Mann RA: Arthrodesis of the first metatarsophalangeal joint as salvage for the failed Keller procedure. J Bone Joint Surg 69A:68, 1987.
31. Lapidus PW: Operative correction of the metatarsus primus varus in hallux valgus. Surg Gynecol Obstet 58:183, 1934.
32. Hernandez A, Hernandez PA, and Hernandez WA: Lapidus: When and why? Clin Podiatr Med Surg 6:1, 1989.
33. Lapidus PW: Author's bunion operation from 1931 to 1959. Clin Orthop 16:119, 1960.
34. Rutherford RL: The Lapidus procedure for primus metatarsus adductus. J Am Podiatr Med Assoc 64:8, 1974.
35. Vahvanen VAJ: Rheumatoid arthritis in the pantalar joints: A follow-up study of triple arthrodesis on 292 adult feet. Acta Orthop Scand Suppl 107:3, 1967.
36. Vahvanen VA: Arthrodesis of the talocalcaneal or pantalar joints in rheumatoid arthritis. Acta Orthop Scand 40:642, 1969.
37. Vainino K: The rheumatoid foot: A clinical study with pathologic and roentgenological comments. Ann Chir Gynaecol 45(Suppl):1, 1956.
38. Elboar JE, Thomas WH, and Weinfield MS: Talonavicular arthrodesis for rheumatoid arthritis of the hindfoot. Orthop Clin North Am 7:821, 1976.
39. Fogel GR, Katoh Y, Rand J, et al: Talonavicular arthrodesis for isolated arthrosis. 9.5-year results and gait analysis. Foot Ankle 3:105, 1982.
40. Potter TA: Talonavicular fusion with bone graft for spastic arthritic flatfoot. Surg Clin North Am 49:883, 1969.
41. Mann RA and Baumgarten M: Subtalar fusion for isolated subtalar disorders. Preliminary report. Clin Orthop 226:260, 1988.
42. McGlamry ED, Ruch JA, and Mahan KT: Triple arthrodesis. *In* McGlamry ED (ed): Reconstructive Surgery of the Foot and Leg—Update, Tucker, GA, Podiatry Institute Publishing, 1987, pp 126–153.
43. Bennett GL, Graham MD, and Maudlin DM: Triple arthrodesis in adults. Foot Ankle 12:138, 1991.
44. Jones WN: Treatment of rheumatoid arthritis of the foot and ankle. *In* Cruess RL and Mitchell NS (eds): Surgery of Rheumatoid Arthritis, Philadelphia, JB Lippincott, 1971, pp 87–92.
45. Wilson FC, Lamotte P, and Williams JC: Triple arthrodesis. J Bone Joint Surg 47A:340, 1965.
46. Cracchiolo A III, Cimino WR, and Lian G: Arthrodesis of the ankle in patients who have had rheumatoid arthritis. J Bone Joint Surg 74A:903, 1992.
47. Kimberly AG: Malunited fractures affecting the ankle joint. Surg Gynecol Obstet 62:19, 1960.
48. Kennedy JC: Arthrodesis of the ankle with particular reference to the Gallie procedure. J Bone Joint Surg 42A:1308, 1960.
49. Said E, Hunka L, and Siller TN: Where ankle fusion stands today. J Bone Joint Surg 60B:211, 1978.
50. Colton CL: Injuries of the ankle. *In* Wilson JN (ed): Watson-Jones Fractures and Joint Injuries, 5th ed. Edinburgh, Churchill Livingstone, 1976, pp 1091-1156.
51. Jackson A and Glasgow M: Tarsal hypermobility after ankle fusion—Fact or fiction? J Bone Joint Surg 61B:470, 1979.
52. Unger AS, Inglis AE, Mow CS, et al: Total ankle arthroplasty in rheumatoid arthritis: A long term follow-up study. Foot Ankle 8:173, 1988.
53. Mahan KT: Ankle and pantalar fusion. *In* McGlamry ED (ed): Comprehensive Textbook of Foot Surgery. Baltimore, Williams & Wilkins, 1987, pp 519–533.
54. Rothacker GW and Cabanela ME: External fixation for arthrodesis of the knee and ankle. Clin Orthop 180:101, 1983.

CHAPTER 35

Tendon Dysfunction

Lawrence M. Oloff, D.P.M.

Tendon injuries of the foot and ankle may be manifest in many ways. They may present as acute or chronic problems. The acute manifestations are often associated with a traumatic event. Acute injuries have received considerable attention over the years. These type of injuries are best exemplified by Achilles tendon ruptures, and the vast array of literature devoted to the management of these injuries is testimony to the focus on acute problems. Although chronic tendon defects are far more common, only recently has attention been directed to these conditions. The foot serves as a specific target site for tendon injuries presumably because of a combination of factors, including the prevalence of foot dysfunction, anatomic predispositions of the foot, and the repetitive loads to tendinous structures under weightbearing conditions.[1–4] Although the causes of these tendon conditions are discussed in more detail during the course of this chapter, it should be briefly mentioned that systemic disease influence is significant in the foot and ankle, as it is elsewhere in the body. Prominent among systemic diseases are those that target synovial tissues and hence are likely to affect tendons in areas where tendon sheaths exist.[5–8]

This chapter discusses some of the more common tendon diseases encountered in practice. Attention is focused on chronic conditions because I believe that these are far more common.

TENDON STRUCTURE AND FUNCTION

Tendons are a specialized connective tissue whose function is to anchor muscles to bone to enable motion of the part. Tendons are composed primarily of collagen, whose basic repeating molecule is tropocollagen. Strong cross-linking is witnessed between molecules, which results in significant strength to this basic repeating unit of tendons.[9] The tropocollagen is arranged in fibrils, which are, in turn, arranged in fibers. Specialized connective tissue coverings separate component parts: the endotenon, which surrounds the fibrils, and the epitenon, which surrounds the aggregates of fibers.[10] These connective tissue encasements serve specialized functions in terms of the reparative processes of tendons and are dealt with in greater detail in the discussion of tendon healing. The insertion of tendon into bone occurs via so-called Sharpey's fibers. The endotenon becomes continuous with the periosteum at the point of attachment. There are gradual zones of transition where tendons attach: starting

with tendon, then fibrocartilage, mineralized cartilage, and eventually the bone itself. This has been theorized as allowing for a gradual release of forces at this site.[11]

Tendon fibers are arranged longitudinally. The longitudinal orientation coincides with the line of tension, which, in addition to the cross-linkage, imparts significant strength to tendons. The high end of tensile strength of tendons has been related as being four times the isometric strength of the associated muscle.[12]

The blood supply to tendons is arranged via internal and external systems.[13] The internal system occurs primarily through longitudinal vessels that traverse within the endotenon. The external system is derived from the muscular branches on one end and the periosteal blood supply on the opposing insertional end. These supply the proximal one third and distal one third, respectively.[14] The paratenon also contains vessels that provide nourishment, supplying the middle one third. Interfascicular branches serve as the network to connect the vessels in the endotenon to the paratenon, muscular branches, and perosteal vessels. A significant vascular contribution is brought in via the mesotenon.

Tendon motion or glide is an important aspect of tendon function. There are specialized structures that help to facilitate this process, namely the tendon sheath and the paratenon.[15] The sheath represents a specialized structure that is located in areas where tendons alter position or change direction.[16] These directional changes serve as pulleys to add efficiency to the system. In these areas, the tendon is typically kept restrained in place by an overlying retinaculum, under which is located a synovium-lined tendon sheath. The latter serves to lubricate the tendon and facilitates necessary motion, as previously mentioned. The sheath has two layers: a visceral layer that covers the tendon and a parietal layer that lines the osseofascial tunnel.[17] The two layers conjoin to form the mesotenon, through which a significant vascular supply passes to the tendon. In contrast, the paratenon is a loose, areolar tissue located around tendons that do not appreciably change their direction: The Achilles tendon is one example. The high sialic acid content of the paratenon facilitates its gliding function.[18]

Tendon healing is a subject of relatively recent interest and debate. It is believed that healing is achieved by contribution from the tendon directly or the surrounding tissues.[19, 20] In the case of the former, or so-called intrinsic repair, specialized cells called tenocytes are believed to participate directly in the necessary fibroplasia.[19, 21] In regards to the latter, or so-called extrinsic repair, the surrounding tissue invests the area and contributes to the repair.[22] The intrinsic pathway seems to be preferred because there is less tendency to adhesion formation that might potentially restrict tendon motion. This intrinsic pathway is encouraged when there is less tissue damage.[20] It also seems to be encouraged when passive motion is incrementally started during the healing period.[23]

Many of the chronic problems that occur with tendons do so on the basis that injured tendons become welded to surrounding tissues during the reparative process.[24] This can occur as a result of either an acute injury to the tendon or chronic low-grade repetitive trauma. With an acute tendon injury, tissue injury evokes an intense inflammatory condition. The torn tissues may become part of the surrounding tissues in the healing process and may serve as irritation points. With chronic trauma, unabated repetitive trauma will evoke a prolonged inflammatory reaction that will gradually weaken the tendon apparatus and eventually lead to tendon rupture. Acute injuries can thus lead to chronic processes, and chronic injuries can lead to an acute process. Both types of injuries are discussed in detail.

TENDINITIS

One of the most commonly encountered groups of tendon injury is tendinitis. These injuries are manifest in different ways. They occur most commonly as localized inflammation about the tendon or tendon sheath apparatus, giving rise to the terms *tendinitis* or *tenosynovitis*. When there is no tendon sheath, the term *paratenonitis* is sometimes substituted, such as might occur with the Achilles tendon.[25–27] The terminology used reflects the specific tissue type involved. In reality, it may be quite difficult to discern this subtle difference between contiguous tissue. In addition, even if the inflammatory reaction was specific to the tendon, one would suspect that adjacent tissues would eventually be involved in the resulting inflammatory reaction.

As previously mentioned, tendinitis may be precipitated by trauma or repetitive strain.[3, 4, 28, 29] Tendinitis usually evokes images of a rather innocuous condition that follows a very benign course without sequelae, and this, fortunately, is usually the case. However, in certain instances, the functional components of the tendon apparatus are irreparably damaged. In these more severe instances, tendon replacement by graft or transfer or removal of the functional need for that tendon muscle unit by arthrodesis may be necessitated. This should serve to emphasize the potential morbidity of these types of injuries. It, therefore, becomes important to recognize that tendinitis is progressive to varying degrees, and if the cause is not reversed or the inflammation is not abated, then permanent changes will eventually occur.

Etiology

There are many causes of tendinitis, and the differential diagnosis poses a challenge to the examining physician. The causes of tendinitis may be conveniently divided into local causes, systemic causes, and anatomic predispositions.[2, 4, 30]

The two most common local causes for tendinitis include trauma and abnormal function. Traumatic causes include injuries that directly or indirectly affect the tendon apparatus. Direct injuries occur when the tendon is either contused or partially or totally torn. Total ruptures initiate a perpetual inflammatory response and cause the torn ends to adhere to surrounding tissues. There is obvious alteration in function. This injury is covered in greater detail in the discussion on tendon dysfunction. Partial tears and contusions are more subtle injuries and often go undetected. A case in point is a peroneus brevis tendon defect after an inversion ankle sprain.[31] Little is said about the occurrence of these lesions, and confirmation of this injury is often incidental, more often detected after the fact in those patients undergoing ankle stabilization or primary ligament repair. Indirect injuries include those traumatic cases in which tendon function is altered by injury to adjacent structures, such as would occur with injury to retinaculum. When retinacula are disturbed, the tendon may be predisposed to subluxation and resultant chronic irritation.[32–35] There are also those cases in which tendon subluxation is due to congenital abnormalities, such as a shallow retromalleolar groove that predisposes either the posterior tibial tendon or peroneal tendons to chronic subluxation.[2, 36]

When one considers trauma, it is also important to consider the secondary effects of altered osseous anatomy. For example, the more severe calcaneal fractures are associated with widening of the body of the calcaneus. These injuries potentially result in a blowout fracture of the lateral calcaneal wall. While these injuries are healing, there may be incorporation of the peroneal tendons into the healing bone callus or fibrosis, thereby interfering with peroneal tendon function.[37] Once healed and as a late development, there may be impingement of the peroneal tendons by the altered lateral calcaneal anatomy. When these injuries become the focus of chronic complaints several months later, they prove to be diagnostic challenges because one needs to discern between post-traumatic subtalar joint arthritis and peroneal tendon impingement as the cause of the complaints. Diagnostic anesthetic blocks and diagnostic imaging studies prove valuable in making this distinction. In the case of the former, one should first anesthetize the tendon to see whether there is relief of complaint. If not, one can assume that the source of the patient's complaint is intra-articular, and this can be confirmed by the administration of local anesthetic into the subtalar joint.

One of the unique aspects of the foot and ankle is the causative relationship of foot function to a variety of disorders. Foot dysfunction plays a prominent role as one of the more common local causes of the development of tendinitis. The most characteristic example of this is the relationship of flexible flatfoot deformity and posterior tibial tendinitis.[38–40] It is generally accepted that various muscles work in an overtime posture with flatfoot deformity.[41, 42] Such is the case with the tibialis posterior muscle/tendon unit, in which this overuse ultimately leads to tenosynovitis. Further support of this association comes from the observation that patients with recalcitrant tibialis posterior tenosynovitis typically display significant equinus and forefoot varus deformities.[43] This observation supports taking a proactive stance and instituting strict biomechanical control in all such cases with such symptoms to prevent permanent damage to the tendon. A similar presentation is also observed in tendons that perform some repetitive action that overworks the tendon muscle unit. Flexor hallucis tendinitis that occurs as the result of excessive plantarflexion during pointe work in ballet dancers illustrates this type of disorder.[44–46] Tendons have been demonstrated to withstand so many repetitive motions before injury occurs. One study supports this viewpoint by observing that tendons withstand up to approximately 1500 to 2000 repetitions per hour before injury occurs.[47] The removal of the inciting factor is the key to improving symptoms in such patients.

When one considers local causes, anatomic predispositions need to be taken into account.[4, 43, 48] The prominent role of these contributing factors is appreciated when one considers that tendinitis of the foot and ankle typically occurs in the same location time and time again, usually the tendon sheath area, where the tendon alters direction.[49] It seems that these sites represent vulnerable points for tendon injury. The tendon seems to tether against the pulley mechanisms that normally help to increase the efficiency of the tendon/muscle units in question.[43] The medial malleolus thus becomes a common site of occurrence for tibialis posterior tendinitis, the lateral malleolus and plantar cuboid groove for peroneus longus tendinitis, and the lateral malleolus and peroneal tubercle for peroneus brevis tendinitis. A further contributing factor seems to be the retinaculum and ligaments that restrain the tendons. The fibro-osseous tunnels and spaces beneath these structures are limiting. The spaces can be further compromised when accessory tendons exist or tendons are dimensionally enlarged. Cases of tendinitis resulting from the presence of accessory tendons has been described.[50] Furthermore, local masses such as ganglionic cysts may take up space and irritate contiguous structures such as tendons.

Another local factor that needs to be considered is the vascular supply inherent to specific tendons. In a case model of the upper extremity, the supraspinatus tendon ruptures at the point of poorest vascular supply.[51] Similar situations are witnessed in the lower extremities. Microangiographic studies indicated that the poorest vascular supply to the Achilles tendon occurs 2 to 6 cm proximal to the calcaneal insertion.[52] This seems to be the area that most frequently ruptures.[53] More recently, a similar zone of hypovascularity has been described within the posterior tibial tendon.[54] In the case of the posterior tibial tendon, the zone is located approximately 20 cm proximal to the navicular tuberosity. As with the Achilles tendon, this area does represent a common site for rupture of the posterior tibial tendon.

In terms of systemic factors, one needs to remember that tendon sheaths are lined with synovial tissues. Any systemic disease that focuses on synovial tissues will affect tendon sheaths as well as joints. Rheumatoid arthritis and other synovium-based disorders, therefore, can manifest themselves clinically as tendinitis.[5, 6] Although this presentation may be focal, systemic disorders usually manifest themselves at multiple sites. Besides rheumatoid arthritis, seronegative inflammatory disease may affect tendon sheaths. Unlike rheumatoid arthritis, the seronegative disorders are less likely to be confined to synovial tissues. The points of attachment of tendons and ligaments also may be target sites.[7, 55, 56] These sites of attachment are referred to as enthesis, and hence the clinical manifestations at these sites are referred to as enthesopathy. The examiner should check the patient for other musculoskeletal manifestations, particularly low back pain, as well as for the presence of urethritis, conjunctivitis, papulosquamous skin eruptions, oral ulcers, and the many other manifestations of these disorders. The reader is encouraged to refer to the chapters on the seronegative disorders for detailed discussion of the characteristics of these disorders.

Although inflammatory arthritis is directly contributory to tendon involvement, degenerative arthritis is indirectly so. Degenerative arthritis does not cause any significant inflammation of the tendon sheath, but the formation of degenerative spurs at joint margins may irritate juxtapositional tendons. Besides the arthritides, infectious causes may show up in the synovial tissues of tendon sheaths as well as joints. Multifocal presentation may occur in this case as well. Last but not least is the aging process. The vascularity of tendons has been demonstrated to decrease with age. Because there does seem to be a correlation of rupture sites with vascularity to these sites, any further compromise to vascularity by aging seems to play some role in the genesis of gradual tendon deterioration.[54]

Classification

The key to initiating proper treatment and prognosticating different types of tendon disorders lies in the ability to label and define more accurately the different types of tendon injuries. It is generally accepted that there are three distinct types of tendon injuries: *peritendinitis crepitans, chronic tenosynovitis,* and *stenosing tenosynovitis.*[2, 4, 29, 47, 48, 57] The first two are rather benign entities that usually respond to traditional treatment programs that combine basic principles such as removal of inciting factors, antiinflammatory-directed therapy of some type, and limitation of activity. Stenosing tenosynovitis usually requires surgery, so that the distinction of this entity from the other types is most important.[4, 30]

Peritendinitis crepitans is a tendon lesion that occurs at the musculotendinous junction.[58] Swelling localized to these areas helps to differentiate this injury from the other types. These injuries are usually the result of repetitive strain. Although not always present, the finding of crepitus by auscultation is pathognomonic. Pain is usually elicited with resisted motion of the muscle unit in question or by stretching the muscle/tendon unit. As mentioned, peritendinitis crepitus is a benign tendon problem that usually resolves with cessation of the inciting event and institution of conservative measures.[4, 37]

Chronic tenosynovitis also represents a type of tendinitis that follows a benign course. It occurs in and about the tendon sheath that is involved. Fusiform swelling at this location is the typical finding. Clinical findings again include pain on both resisted motion and passive stretch of the muscle/tendon unit in question. The presence of multiple sites should alert the examiner to one of the previously cited systemic causes of this disorder. Traditional conservative care is usually successful in improving symptoms, although cases that are systemic in origin are likely to recur until the specific disease that is causing the inflammation is arrested or brought under control.[4, 37]

Stenosing tenosynovitis (STS) is the type of tendinitis that is most refractile to conservative care. This fact was first appreciated in the upper extremities when it was noted how poorly de Quervain's disease of the thumb responds to conservative care.[59] It was subsequently recognized in the lower extremities and has since been noted in most of the tendinous structures about the foot and ankle.[2, 4, 29, 30] The genesis of this particular disorder is believed to be the result of either an acute injury or conversion of one of the more benign tendinitis presentations previously discussed. In the case of an acute injury, extensive scarring renders the tendon immobile. In regards to the more benign cases of tendinitis, some contend that chronic tenosynovitis and peritendinitis, if left untreated or ineffectively treated, will progress to STS.[4, 48] This occurs on the simple premise that chronic inflammation will eventually lead to fibrosis. This fibrosis can exist in various locations. STS can involve adhesions between the tendon and tendon sheath or between the entire tendon apparatus and surrounding structures. In either case, the tendon is prevented from gliding freely, being bound down at some point along its course. The tendon undergoes varying stages of deterioration from mild to more severe. When severe, eventual tendon deterioration and rupture can occur. Protracted trials of conservative care are usually futile in resolving this condition. Early diagnosis will prevent unnecessary protracted periods of unsuccessful conservative care.[4, 48]

Diagnosis

Diagnosis of the type and extent of tendon injury is often difficult on the basis of the clinical examination alone. The clinical examination seems best suited to acute injuries, especially in regards to complete tendon ruptures. The presence of a palpable gap within the substance of a tendon, the inability of the traumatized muscle/tendon unit to move the part, and the presence of a recently acquired deformity that is the result of either lack of support or overpowering by opposing muscles all indicate that a complete disruption of a tendon has occurred. Not all acute injuries are this clear. Unlike complete tendon ruptures, partial tendon tears may defy detection because the findings outlined previously may not be present. This is the case with chronic injuries such as the various types of tendinitis. In these cases, the clinical picture may be the same. There may be subtle differences in location, such as the more proximal location for peritendinitis. However, for the most part, all of the chronic injuries display varying degrees of swelling, pain, and loss of function.

The diagnosis of tendon injuries often requires sophisticated diagnostic imaging techniques because tendons are not adequately appreciated on plain radiographs. The special techniques that may be used to visualize tendons directly include soft tissue radiography, tenography, ultrasonography, computed tomography (CT), and magnetic resonance imaging (MRI).[4, 37, 60–64] Selection of the most appropriate technique is made on the basis of a variety of factors including whether the problem is acute or chronic, the specific type of disease, whether the suspected problem is intratendinous or extratendinous, the availability of the particular technology, and cost, to mention a few. Some mention of each visualization technique is warranted.

Soft tissue radiography is inexpensive and generally accessible. It provides indirect evidence of acute and chronic problems by detecting changes in the girth of the tendon. These findings are unfortunately nonspecific for tendon swelling is seen after complete and incomplete ruptures as well as in cases of chronic tendinitis.

Tenography provides valuable information in regards to extratendinous defects. When performing tenography, contrast is injected into the tendon sheath proximal to the area of symptoms. In the case of STS, contrast flow is interrupted,

whereas in the other types of tendinitis, it is continuous along the course of the tendon sheath (Fig. 35–1).[4] It provides a dynamic study when the contrast is injected under fluoroscopic control because it very accurately detects areas of tendon/tendon sheath adhesions that restrict flow and displays where these adhesions may be most severe. Tenography is also useful in differentiating pain caused by peroneal tendon entrapment after calcaneal fracture with that resulting from post-traumatic arthritis.[37] These cases often require both CT and a tenography examination, the former to assess the status of the subtalar joint and the latter to determine the status of the tendon.[4, 62] Tenography provides indirect evidence of old tendon tears and tendinopathy, the latter representing progressive tendon degeneration. It does so in a manner similar to soft tissue radiography, namely by detecting tendon enlargement. It will also detect whether a tendon is displaced, such as might occur as a result of an adjacent mass. It provides little direct information as to the internal status of the tendon; this is one of the major limitations of tenography. It also seems to be of limited value in diagnosing acute tendon tears.[65] One advantage unique to tenography is that the examination can potentially prove to be therapeutic as well as diagnostic. In selected patients, the introduction of the local anesthetic and contrast mixture has an adhesiolytic effect. This occurs by injecting a large volume of fluid under pressure into a confined space. This essentially is the principle followed with treatment of adhesive capsulitis of a joint. On the other hand, one must consider that tenography is an invasive study with attendent infection risks.

Ultrasonography has advantages in terms of cost, availability, dynamic potentials of the examination, and use of nonionizing radiation.[66] Ultrasonography has shown value in diagnosing partial tendon tears and total rupture that may have defied detection.[67] Unfortunately, it is limited in its ability to assess deeper structures and does not allow for concurrent osseous evaluation.[63] As the medical field continues its cost-containment focus, this test holds potential for greater utilization.

CT serves several useful purposes. First and foremost, CT is the best technique for detailing osseous structures. As a result, its best application in these clinical settings is in the evaluation of any contiguous exostosis or other bony deformities that may be irritating tendons.[64] This is most important in the hindfoot, where such osseous deformities may not be disclosed by plain films because of the complex anatomy. This is also exemplified in cases of post-traumatic deformi-

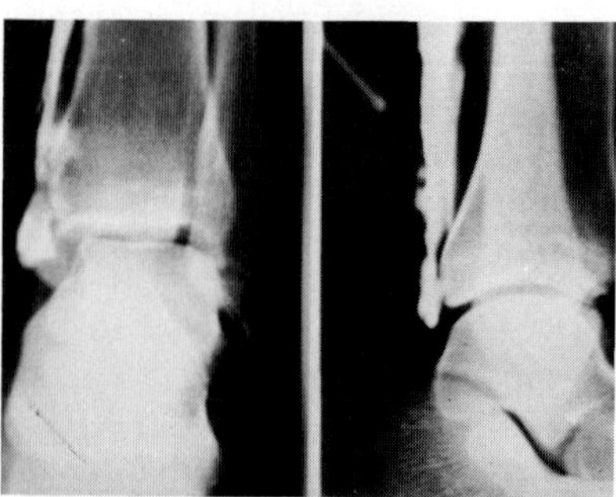

FIGURE 35–1. Abnormal tenogram demonstrating attenuation and eventual interrupted contrast flow of the posterior tibial tendon due to stenosing tenosynovitis. The point at which contrast stops usually corresponds to the site of maximal point tenderness.

ties. Furthermore, CT can be calibrated for a soft tissue window, allowing for greater detail of soft tissue structures, including tendons.[62] Through this imaging technique, tendons can be assessed for increased diameter, suggesting whether intratendinous defects exist. It does not reflect the extent of tendon defect present. One limitation of CT is that it does not allow for direct sagittal imaging. A computer-generated image can be used, but it lacks the detail of direct studies.

MRI is the gold standard at present for assessment of tendon injuries.[63, 64] It offers the best soft tissue contrast of all the imaging techniques discussed, without using ionizing radiation, and is useful for a variety of tendon diseases. Unlike CT, MRI allows for direct multiplanar imaging. This study is useful for both acute and chronic injuries. MRI allows for accurate intratendinous evaluation, unlike many of the other studies already mentioned. In the case of acute injuries, complete tears will appear as areas of discontinuity.[68] Partial tears reflect a high signal within the tendon at the site of the tear. Chronic injuries appear as a diffuse thickening that may be accompanied by increased signal, the presence and degree of which are indicative of the amount of associated tendon degeneration.[63] Tendon degeneration is an important aspect of chronic injuries. First, it indicates the severity of tendon defect, and it enables one to prognosticate these injuries. Tendon degeneration is often a precursor to tendon rupture, such as is observed with tibialis posterior dysfunction. MRI does have some limitations in regards to STS. It will detect fluid within the tendon sheath, displayed as low-signal accumulations around tendons on short TR/short TE sequences.[63] The effusions are seen with greater detail on long TR/long TE sequences.[63] Low-signal areas around an enlarged tendon suggest the presence of STS. One limitation at present is that collagen essentially appears as collagen, so that although fibrosis is displayed it is not qualified. With cases of STS, the diagnosis may be made with MRI, but if surgical release is contemplated, additional information and potential therapeutic advantage may be obtained with tenography.

Treatment

The choice and success of treatment of chronic tendon injuries are ultimately based on the specific diagnosis. The treating physician should suspect that the condition of a patient diagnosed with STS by one of the aforementioned methods is unlikely to improve with conservative care alone.[4, 30] Nonetheless, each patient seems to be deserving of some form of conservative care because there are rare exceptions to most rules in medicine. Also, fundamental to treatment protocols is that conservative care needs to be started promptly to avoid excessive scarring brought on by protracted inflammation. Unnecessary delays potentially allow one of the more benign tendinitis conditions to progress to one that requires surgery.[4]

The key to ameliorating peritendinitis and chronic tenosynovitis is to remove the inciting cause.[37, 38] In those cases in which some activity, work or recreational, is an initiating or aggravating event, a modification or cessation of the activity is necessary.[69] Immobilization may also be considered, but one needs to recognize that this approach has both a risk and a benefit potential. Although immobilization has to be used at times, complete immobilization may predispose the

patient to further scarring. Immobilization favors the production of restrictive rather than nonrestrictive adhesions.[19] This premise holds true in both the conservative and surgical treatment groups, so one needs to take this into consideration in the postoperative care of those patients who eventually undergo surgery. As a result, a removable immobilization device is used so that a physical therapy program that encourages motion can be initiated. Passive motion is initially used to protect the injured or inflamed tendon. Active-resistance programs are gradually phased in. Simultaneously, some form of antiinflammatory drug program is initiated. This may require use of nonsteroidal antiinflammatory drugs. Readers are encouraged to refer to Chapter 24, which discusses these medications in detail. If there is a systemic cause, the associated inflammation needs to be controlled, and appropriate consultation is thus sought out to accomplish this. In regards to steroid injections, caution is exercised because of the risk of intratendinous steroids precipitating tendon rupture.[2] If a tenogram is contemplated, steroids can be administered at the time the needle is in the tendon sheath, thus ensuring accurate placement. If steroids are used, short-acting preparations are preferred to limit the risks associated with the use of these drugs. Once the acute aspects of this disorder are over, one should consider the use of orthotic devices, primarily in those cases in which foot dysfunction has played a prominent role in the cause.

Surgery has a limited role in cases of chronic tenosynovitis or peritendinitis. Surgery is usually reserved for those patients who experience repetitive episodes of tenosynovitis that can be attributed to some specific cause and in whom conservative care is not effective in preventing frequent occurrences; for example, an exostosis that was produced by trauma and now serves to irritate an adjacent tendon. In this instance, exostosectomy is considered. The other extreme may be a case of flatfoot deformity that cannot be controlled by orthotics. In such cases, consideration may be given to improving foot structure so that soft tissue structures are not stressed. STS often requires surgery, as previously mentioned. The goal of surgery is to restore the gliding capacity to an immobilized tendon apparatus. The simplest method of restoring tendon function is by what might be best labeled a tenolysis. In this procedure, the tendon sheath is opened, and the tendon is freed from all adhesions until motion is restored.[2, 4, 29, 48, 70] What is done beyond this point varies considerably and is best dictated by the diagnostic studies previously mentioned and may ultimately depend on the intraoperative findings. A case in point is the tendon itself. If circumferentially enlarged, it may prove necessary to perform a tenoplasty, whereby the tendon is reduced dimensionally to facilitate its passage beneath the retinaculum and fibro-osseous channels (Fig. 35–2). One may remove longitudinal sections of the tendon, carefully placing the incision in a location that is unlikely to be subject to friction in the channels. It is important to assess for intratendinous changes. Removal of focal areas of degeneration has been advocated by some.[71] I have personally found this useful in selected patients, particularly in regards to the Achilles tendon and posterior tibial tendon. The pulley mechanisms also need to be assessed. Sometimes they are fibrotic, calcified, or attenuated. They likewise may need to undergo syndesmoplasty to help facilitate tendon motion.[4] If the tendon is significantly destroyed, consideration is given to reconstruction of the soft

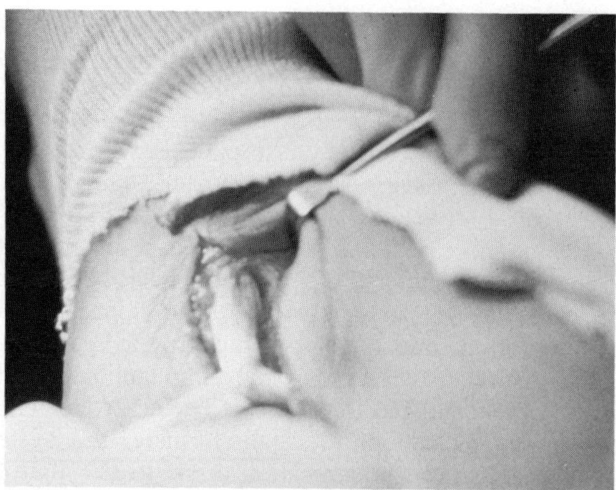

FIGURE 35–2. The goal of surgery for cases of stenosing tenosynovitis is to restore tendon mobility. The tibialis posterior tendon has been released. The tendon is significantly enlarged in the area between the retractors. To facilitate motion of the tendon, tenoplasty is sometimes performed.

tissue portions of the pulleys by borrowing the parietal side of adjacent retinaculum.[4] Any adjacent exostosis or post-traumatic osseous deformity may be reduced concurrently. However, resection of hypertrophic bone adjacent to tendon can potentially produce raw, bleeding bone, which may encourage hematoma and fibrosis at the site, leading to restenosis. Bone wax is considered to deter this. In addition, careful surgical planning may limit the amount of fibrosis. For example, exostoses that are adjacent to tendons may be approached surgically by raising periosteal flaps distant to the exostoses and tunneling under the periosteal tissues until the exostoses in question are reached. Bleeding directly into the area of the tendon is thus minimized. Use of drainage systems is also advised when hematoma is imminent.

The postoperative follow-up care is as critical as the procedure itself. Mobilizing the tendon as quickly as possible to discourage adhesions should be emphasized. Tenolysis alone allows for immediate mobilization. The use of continuous passive motion devices helps to facilitate this process. The patient may be dispensed a unit for home utilization. Greater caution needs to be exercised in those cases in which early motion may jeopardize repair sites, such as when the pulley mechanisms have been restored, tendon graft has been used, or new points of tendon attachment have been established. Each case needs to be individually assessed in this regard.

TENDON DYSFUNCTION

Tendon dysfunction is the term often applied to describe the series of stages through which a tendon passes when subject to repetitive injury, which ultimately culminates in rupture of the tendon and results in associated foot deformities.[72] The end result is a foot that has lost its ability to provide a basis of support and is severely compromised in function. The terminology is most commonly applied to the tibialis posterior tendon (TPT), although any tendon can be affected. For the sake of this discussion, emphasis is directed to the TPT because this is the tendon that has received the most attention.

It has been suggested that a normal TPT is unlikely to rupture and, when witnessed, it is generally assumed that the tendon has previously undergone some degeneration.[43, 73] There is often predisposing local or systemic disease that has weakened the TPT unit and has predisposed it to eventual rupture. This distinction is important because it helps to clarify further that the term TPT dysfunction (TPTD) is best applied to the patient in whom a unilateral flatfoot deformity develops as a result of a compromised TPT resulting from repetitive irritation or stress on either a normal or abnormal tendon and not from an acute injury per se.[43] This is not meant to imply that the onset may not be acute, but rather it was a long time in development before the actual rupture occurred. The previous discussions on tendinitis are pertinent to a discussion of TPTD because, many times, tendinitis was the antecedent condition or event that weakened the tendon and predisposed it to rupture. Finally, it is likely that, as a clearer understanding of the pathogenesis of this disorder evolves, there will be greater appreciation that this condition is not uncommon and may actually represent a greater number of patients than originally thought. Designation of many of the cases as traumatic in origin was likely incorrect. One only needs to question the patient with a traumatic rupture to realize that there was often a history of tendon symptoms and that the traumatic event described by the patient seemed too trivial in nature to produce such a severe injury.[2, 43, 74]

Spontaneous tendon ruptures have been noticed for some time and have been described in a variety of locations. The TPT and the Achilles tendon have received the most attention; however, just about every tendon has been described at some time.[60, 74, 75] Emphasis is directed to the TPT because the pathogenesis of this particular disorder seems best understood at this point in time.

Etiology

One needs to be familiar with all of the causes cited in the discussion of tendinitis because tendon dysfunction may represent one end of a continuum of the same developmental process. Therefore, the local and systemic causes previously cited are considered.

There are numerous systemic causes for tendon degeneration and rupture. The literature is full of reports of such occurrences and include such disorders as synovial-based disease such as rheumatoid arthritis, seronegative spondyloarthropathies, systemic lupus erythematosus, hyperparathyroidism, and chronic acidosis from lead toxicity.[5, 6, 7, 76–78] Myerson, Solomon, and Shereff suggested that there are two groups in whom TPTD develops and that distinctive findings arise for these two groups.[7] Myerson and colleagues observed that those patients with TPTD with possibly a systemic cause were generally younger than those with TPTD without systemic influence. This younger group displayed multiple manifestations of enthesopathy, a strong family history of ligament and tendon inflammation, and a higher incidence of positive human lymphocyte antigen typing. The older group had no such findings, suggesting that this group had TPTD associated with a mechanical traumatic cause.

STS emphasizes those processes that encourage the formation of adhesions, whereas tendon dysfunction emphasizes those processes that result in internal degeneration of the tendon itself. Although unabated tendinitis or STS may represent the singularly most important contributing factor, as previously stated, one also needs to consider those processes that encourage tendon alteration. In this regard, the vasculature is important. The areas of hypovascularity may serve as an explanation as to why tendon dysfunction and rupture are most often witnessed in the TPT and Achilles tendons, these two tendons in particular having recognized areas of avascularity that correspond to rupture sites.[52, 54] Iatrogenic causes should also be considered and are easily ascertained from the patient history. Injudicious steroid injections, either by excessive repetitive injections or injections directly into the tendon itself, may either cause degeneration or weaken an already injured part and predispose to rupture.

The area of pathomechanics has been touched on previously. It seems that biomechanical factors play a prominent role in TPTD.[42, 43] The more advanced cases of TPTD have an exaggerated flatfoot appearance; in fact, a unilateral severe flatfoot is the hallmark presentation of this disorder. However, many have noted that the contralateral foot often displays a less severe and less symptomatic flexible flatfoot deformity as well in most patients with this disorder. Funk, Cass, and Johnson described the development of similar symptoms on the contralateral side years after surgical repair.[79] Henceroth and Deyerle noted the presence of osteoarthrosis at the cuneiform-first metatarsal joint in those patients who experienced foot collapse.[80] Banks and McGlamry further refined these findings by noting the prevalence of forefoot varus and ankle equinus, and they further commented on how the changes that Henceroth and Deyerle noted are radiographic changes often witnessed with severe ankle equinus.[43] In any case, functional overload of the TPT/muscle unit is commonly witnessed in a flatfoot deformity. The exact mechanism for TPT/muscle unit overuse can vary and may have a variety of contributing factors. Basmajian and Stecko noted that muscles are not called on to maintain the arch unless the foot is significantly pronated.[41] Any structural or functional abnormality that causes a pronated foot can theoretically contribute to this phenomenon. Once uncontrolled inflammation occurs, tendon degeneration eventually results. Mueller described in detail the pathoanatomic findings that are observed, which would perpetuate some of the associated deformities.[65] The tendon will eventually undergo functional or spontaneous rupture. Once lengthened, the resting length of the tendon increases, which adversely affects the contractile force. The midfoot becomes unstable and begins to abduct. The initial deformity occurs at the talonavicular and calcaneocuboid joints. As the midtarsal and subtalar joints are functionally integrated, subtalar joint instability ensues. Further complicating the process is the fact that the tendon often becomes enlarged, serving as a source for further irritation of the tendon as the enlarged tendon rubs against the restraining retinaculum.

Diagnosis

The presenting history and physical findings vary depending on the disease present. In its earlier stages, the presentation is relatively quiescent; patients realize that they have a problem but are not yet incapacitated.[43] As the problem progresses, and if the tendon is intact and rupture has not yet occurred, tenosynovitis symptoms predominate. The course is more gradual, and the description by the patients is usually of a vague medial arch/ankle discomfort that is accompanied by swelling along the course of the involved tendon. There

are varying degrees of increased warmth and tenderness from the medial malleolus to the navicular bone.

The diagnosis is often clinically apparent once rupture has occurred. The rupture may have been gradual or the result of an acute spontaneous event, and it may be complete or incomplete. Incomplete in situ tears are sometimes referred to as functional tears.[81] The patient sometimes tries to relate a specific traumatic event but is usually unable to do so. The typical presentation in either case is a patient with an accentuated flatfoot deformity on one side, although the asymptomatic side, as previously mentioned, displays varying degrees of less severe flexible flatfoot deformity. The hindfoot is everted and the forefoot abducted. The patient ambulates with an apropulsive and abducted gait that is antalgic. The tibialis anterior and digital flexor muscles may be hyperactive. The patient displays those characteristic findings described by Johnson and others: too many toe signs, inability to rise on the heel of affected side, and local signs of inflammation.[72, 79] There is some distinction between the actual clinical presentation and the chronicity of the rupture. Early on, the deformity is flexible, and medial tendon and arch symptoms predominate. With time, sinus tarsi and lateral tarsal complaints begin. This is a poor prognostic sign and usually indicates a more rigid adapted deformity that displays varying degrees of tarsal arthrosis.

Plain film radiography, soft tissue radiographic techniques, ultrasonography, tenography, CT, and MRI may be used to evaluate tendon defects.[4, 62–64] Each test has its own specific advantages and disadvantages. Standard radiographs help to support the clinical findings of a severe flatfoot deformity. Ultrasonography is a relatively safe and inexpensive method of diagnosing acute tears. More sophisticated diagnostic techniques prove useful for filling in some of the details regarding the presence of tendon adhesions, presence and extent of tendon degeneration, and presence of any secondary arthrosis of the subtalar joint. It is important to consider these factors before embarking on surgical solutions. Tenography will not prove useful for diagnosing a tendon rupture, but it will determine the presence of any tendon/tendon sheath adhesions and will therefore support the diagnosis of STS, as previously mentioned. This can prove useful when deciding whether early surgical intervention is warranted to avert more severe and advanced stages of dysfunction.[4] CT, when calibrated for soft tissue evaluation, can determine whether the tendon is enlarged or not.[62] It does not address whether this enlargement is due to imminent rupture or reflects a functional tear. CT is the procedure of choice for evaluating whether there is any secondary arthrosis of the subtalar or midfoot articulations. MRI provides a vital function in the evaluation of tendon dysfunction, namely the status of the tendon. MRI provides the best soft tissue contrast of studies mentioned, and spatial resolution has been enhanced by the use of extremity coils, reduced-field-of-view imaging, and decreased scanning time.[63] An additional advantage is MRI's capability of direct multiplanar imaging. It determines whether the tendon is thickened, whether the tendon is ruptured, and the degree of tendon degeneration, if any. Fluid collections are best visualized on long TR/long TE sequences (Fig. 35–3).[63]

Treatment

The most appropriate treatment for TPTD depends on the stage of the disorder.[65, 82] The success of conservative meas-

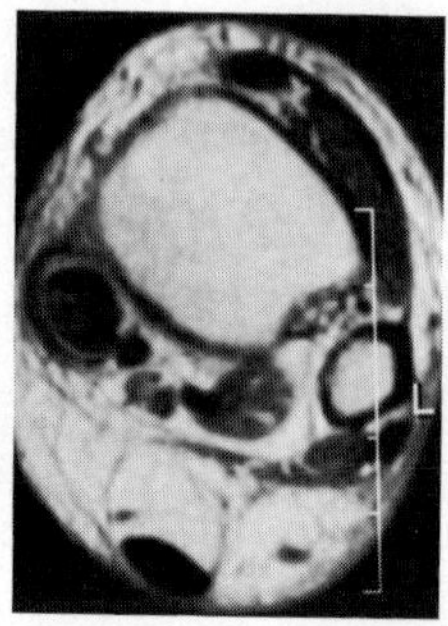

FIGURE 35–3. Magnetic resonance imaging scan demonstrating thickening of the tibialis posterior tendon. There is increased signal circumferentially, suggesting a tendon sheath effusion. The intratendinous signal is increased, suggesting tendonopathy. Advancement of the tendon is usually ill advised when tendon degeneration exists, unless the areas of degeneration can be dealt with concomitantly.

ures is directly linked to the status of the tendon itself as well as any accompanying changes in the architecture of the foot. If the tendon is intact and there is no change in the position of the foot, then removal of inciting causes, symptom-oriented antiinflammatory measures, and improved positioning of the foot through appropriate orthosis and shoe modification should be attempted. Clearly, those patients on the opposite end of the continuum, namely those who have undergone frank rupture followed by the development of a severe flatfoot, experience an unrelenting course of problems that are usually unresponsive to conservative therapy. Those patients in the middle of the continuum follow varying degrees of limited short-term success with conservative means. If the tendon has ruptured, either completely or as an in situ tear, then conservative measures usually produce less than desirable results.[40, 65, 79, 82] However, not every patient is a surgical candidate, and other considerations need to be taken into account. In the nonoperative candidate, stabilization and unweighting the extremity become considerations. Stabilization is often difficult with a compromised tendon/muscle unit; however, use of the University of California Biomechanics Laboratory (UCBL) device is sometimes effective in the TPTD patient. Unweighting can be achieved by various bracing devices that shift weightbearing more proximally, such as an ischial or patellar weightbearing brace.

Much of the basis for surgical repair has resulted from staging of TPTD by various authors who have taken many factors into consideration. Funk, Cass, and Johnson[79] identified four types of TPT lesions at surgery: TPT avulsion at the insertion, midsubstance rupture, incontinuity tear, and no tear with tenosynovitis. Treatment was individualized on the basis of these findings.[79] The avulsion group was treated by reattachment, the midsubstance ruptures by transfer of the flexor digitorum longus, and the incontinuity tear and tenosynovitis groups by synovectomy. The study group was admittedly small, and consideration focused mostly on the appearance of the tendon. The avulsion group seemed to fare the worst of all the groups. The remaining groups did reasonably well. One interesting finding was that the appearance of the foot did not appreciably change postoperatively in any of the patient groups. A later study by Johnson and Strom[82] expanded the staging process and considered the functional development of TPTD. Staging emphasized whether the tendon was elongated, degree of tendon degeneration, position of the foot, and status of the joints (Table 35–1). This staging is most interesting because it reflects on the clinical aspects of the foot and how this translates into the observed defect. It is becoming increasingly clear that the surgical approach to the patient with TPTD is complicated but is facilitated by careful consideration of multiple factors, including status of the tendon, presence of any associated foot deformities from the ensuing muscle imbalance, presence of any associated degenerative joint disease, and whether control of the foot is feasible or not. Each of these considerations is discussed in greater detail.

The status of the tendon is an important consideration in determining the most appropriate procedure. One prime consideration is whether tendon length has been maintained and whether frank rupture or functional in situ tears have occurred that have resulted in increased tendon length. Alteration of tendon length is usually appreciated by the clinical examination because a typical flatfoot presentation develops, as previously discussed. If the tendon length is suspected as being near normal, then tenolysis with synovectomy is a consideration in the patient with unrelenting discomfort.[79, 82] If tendon length has changed, attempts may be made to restore origin to insertion resting muscle length to restore or improve muscle function to near-preinjury status. This may occur through either a repair of a frankly torn tendon or

TABLE 35–1

CHANGES ASSOCIATED WITH VARIOUS STAGES OF TIBIALIS POSTERIOR TENDON DYSFUNCTION

Factor	Stage 1	Stage 2	Stage 3
TPT condition	Peritendinitis and/or tendon degeneration	Elongation	Elongation
Hindfoot	Mobile, normal alignment	Mobile, valgus position	Fixed, valgus position
Pain	Medial: focal, mild to moderate	Medial: along TPT, moderate	Medial: possibly lateral, moderate
Single-heel-rise test	Mild weakness	Marked weakness	Marked weakness
"Too-many-toes" sign with forefoot abduction	Normal	Positive	Positive
Pathology	Synovial proliferation, degeneration	Marked degeneration	Marked degeneration
Treatment	Conservative, 3 months; surgical, 3 months with synovectomy, tendon débridement, rest	Transfer FDL for TPT	Subtalar arthrodesis

FDL, flexor digitorum longus; TPT, tibialis posterior tendon.
From Johnson KA and Stram DE: Tibialis posterior tendon function. Clin Orthop 239:196–206, 1989.

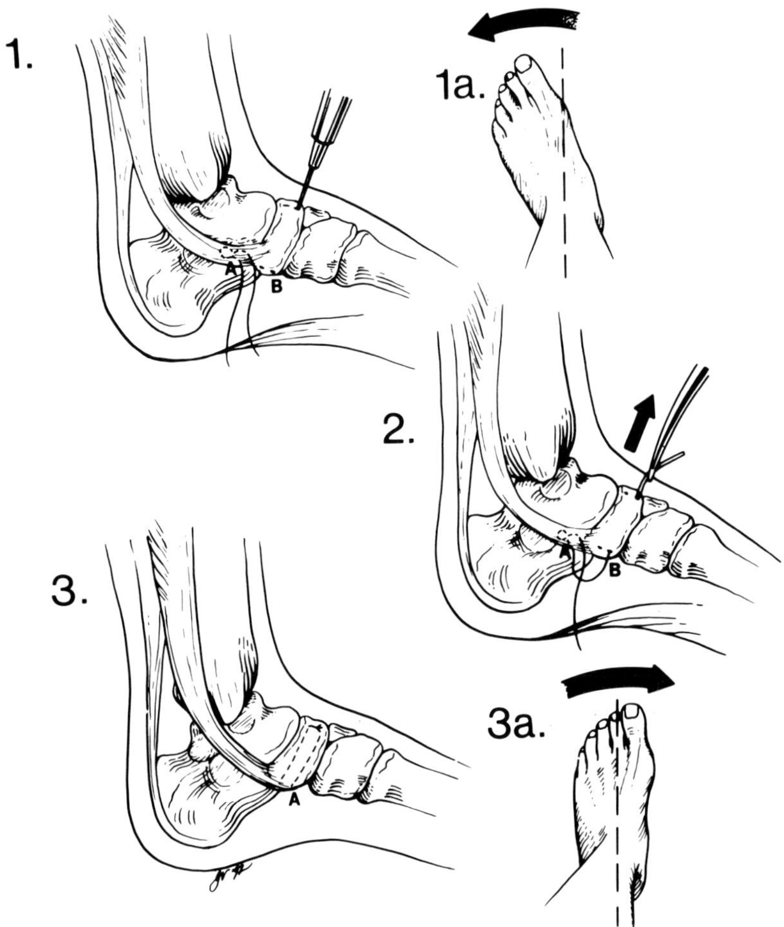

FIGURE 35–4. *1,* The tibialis posterior is being prepared to be advanced. The tendon is threaded with a nonabsorbable suture, with the sutures exiting the tendon at the point of the proposed new primary attachment site (A). Two drill holes are being placed dorsal to plantar through the navicular to eventually receive the tendon sutures. *1a,* The position of the foot prior to advancement, demonstrating significant abduction. *2,* The tendon sutures are being passed through the drill holes in the navicular. *3,* The suture is tied dorsally on the navicular, dragging the tendon forward. Point A has been repositioned to what was point B. *3a,* With greater tension on the tendon, the foot is brought into improved alignment on the transverse plane.

advancement of an intact tendon that has undergone lengthening as a result of a previous partial tear.

One additional consideration exists for those patients in whom tendon advancement is considered. If a tendon has suffered any cystic changes or any form of degeneration as a result of chronic irritation/trauma, then any attempt to restore resting length will likely fail because the altered tendon will be unable to sustain normal functional loads and will be subject to increased risk for rerupture. Advancement of the tibialis posterior tendon in the presence of advanced cystic changes is akin to stretching out a frayed rubber band. These cases are best determined by MRI before any surgical intervention. By carefully assessing tendons by this method, the clinician should be able to appreciate whether there is internal tendon derangement.[63, 64] This is reflected on MRI as increased signal on those studies that emphasize fluid, namely the T_2-weighted images, gradient echo, and short tau inversion recovery (STIR) sequences. When severely compromised, use of the injured tendon alone to restore function should be avoided; another tendon unit via tendon transfer is preferred.

Although there are no satisfactory long-range studies at this time, some consideration should be given to the benefit of excising areas of tendon degeneration, when limited, thereby lessening the risks of further degeneration and future rupture.[2, 71, 82] Some success has been seen in the Achilles tendon, but, as mentioned, additional work is needed to determine whether this same philosophy can be applied to other

tendons. I have noticed some short-term benefits to this approach, but, again, further research is warranted. The excision of wedges of abnormally enlarged tendons, in essence debulking tendons, also benefits the passage of the tendons within the confined spaces beneath the retinaculum.

Careful consideration also needs to be given to the position of the foot. When the TPT becomes lengthened, a flatfoot develops. Initially, the flatfoot is flexible and reducible. With time, it becomes more rigid and fixed. Once it reaches the latter stages of development, there is associated arthrosis of the hindfoot and later the midfoot articulations.[65, 82] This can usually be determined by the nature of the patient's symptoms. All through the course of development, symptoms predominate medially, mostly along the course of the TPT. Desmopathy then may be seen, with medial arch strain symptoms. When symptoms progress laterally, about the lateral tarsal and sinus tarsi, usually arthrosis has started. When in the earlier, more flexible stages, consideration exists for restitution of the TPT as previously mentioned either through tendon advancement or tendon transfer. Advancement is carried out, much like the Kidner procedure in which the TPT is advanced forward and a new attachment point is developed on the undersurface of the navicular bone (Fig. 35–4). A relatively good tendon is a necessary prerequisite for this procedure, as previously mentioned. If the TPT is compromised, then tendon transfer is preferred usually using the flexor digitorum longus tendon (Fig. 35–5).[79, 82, 83] The tendon transfer has not been observed to produce any appreciable

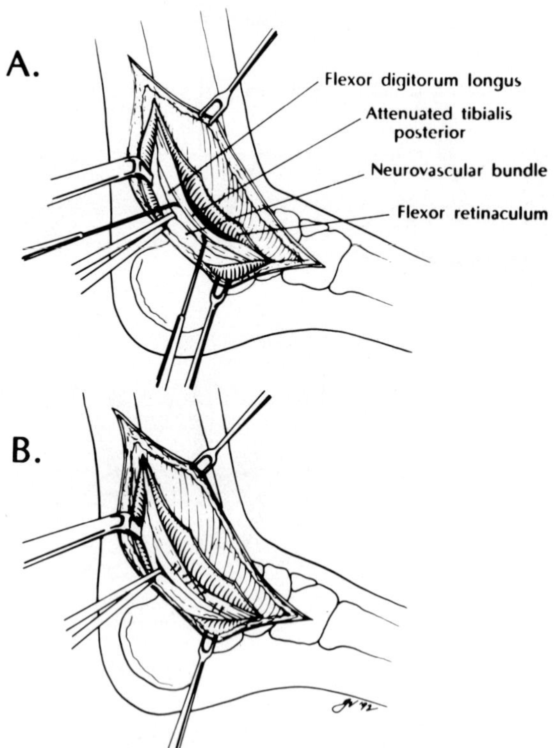

FIGURE 35–5. *A,* When the tendon is severely compromised, tendon transfer is considered. *B,* Use of the flexor digitorum longus is usually preferred in such instances. If there is accompanying arthrosis, fusion procedures of the hindfoot are preferred.

improvement in the appearance of the foot.[79] For that matter, neither does the advancement produce any significant changes in position. Both procedures do seem to effect a significant improvement in symptoms. Either tendon advancement or tendon transfer will be less than completely successful in situations in which functional control of the foot cannot be achieved postoperatively. In such instances, the transferred or advanced tendon will potentially be placed under inordinate stress, predisposing to recurrence of the tendon defect.

Special consideration should also be given to more rigid deformities and to those cases in which joint symptoms are manifest. As previously mentioned, the symptoms often shift laterally when the patient progresses to this stage. CT can confirm the joint symptoms as well. These situations are best managed by arthrodesis. Differing opinions exist regarding which joints should undergo arthrodesis.[82, 83] The time-honored tradition has been triple arthrodesis, although some investigators have argued for limited arthrodesis, such as the talocalcaneal joint alone.[82] This question may be more accurately addressed by careful assessment of the components of the flatfoot deformity. The flatfoot deformity with TPTD has been characterized as displaying significant hindfoot valgus in combination with marked forefoot abduction. Although the symptoms are predominantly talocalcaneal in location, the forefoot abduction also often becomes fixed in those deformities that are of greater duration. In these instances, talocalcaneal arthrodesis alone may not be sufficient, and considerations might best indicate triple arthrodesis.

References

1. Andrews JR: Overuse syndromes of the lower extremity. Clin Sports Med 2:137–148, 1983.
2. Trevino S, Gould N, and Korson R: Surgical treatment of stenosing tenosynovitis at the ankle. Foot Ankle 2:37–45, 1981.
3. Jackson MA and Gudas CJ: Peroneus longus tendinitis: A possible biomechanical etiology. J Foot Surg 21:344–348, 1982.
4. Gilula LA, Oloff L, Caputi R, et al: Ankle tenography: A key to unexplained symptomatology: Part 2. Radiology 151:581–587, 1984.
5. Cruickshank B: Lesions of joints and tendon sheaths in systemic lupus erythematosus. Ann Rheum Dis 18:111–119, 1959.
6. Downey DJ, Simkin PA, Mack LA, et al: Tibialis posterior tendon rupture: A cause of rheumatoid flatfoot. Arthritis Rheum 31:441–446, 1988.
7. Myerson M, Solomon G, and Shereff M: Posterior tibial tendon dysfunction: Its association with seronegative inflammatory disease. Foot Ankle 9:219–225, 1989.
8. Guerra J and Resnick D: Arthritidis affecting the foot: Radiographic-pathologic correlation. Foot Ankle 2:325–331, 1982.
9. Piez KA: Cross-linking of collagen and elastin. Annu Rev Biochem 37:547–570, 1968.
10. Hurst LN: The healing of tendon. *In* Kerahan DS and Vistnes LM (eds): Biological Aspects of Reconstructive Surgery. Boston, Little, Brown, 1977, pp 383–389.
11. Cooper RR and Misol S: Tendon and ligament insertion. J Bone Joint Surg 52A:1–20, 1970.
12. Harkness RD: Mechanical properties of collagenous tissues. *In* Gould BS (ed): Treatise on Collagen. Orlando, FL, Academic Press, 1968.
13. Mayer L: The physiological methods of tendon transplantation. Surg Gynecol Obstet 22:182–197, 1916.
14. Peacock EE: Research in tendon healing. *In* Tubiana R (ed): The Hand. Philadelphia, WB Saunders, 1981.
15. Miller SJ: Principles of muscle tendon surgery and tendon transfers. *In* McGlamry ED (ed): Comprehensive Textbook of Foot Surgery. Baltimore, Williams & Wilkins, 1987.
16. Semple C: The design of tendons and their sheaths. *In* Owen R, Goodfellow J, and Bullough P (eds): Scientific Foundations of Orthopedics and Traumatology. Philadelphia, WB Saunders, 1980.
17. Sheinberg R and Bayne O: General concepts in the management of tendon trauma to the foot and ankle. *In* Scurran B (ed): Foot and Ankle Trauma. New York, Churchill Livingstone, 1989.
18. Peacock EE Jr and Van Winkle W Jr: Wound Repair, 2nd ed. Philadelphia, WB Saunders, 1976.
19. Matthews P and Richards H: The repair potential of digital flexor tendons. J Bone Joint Surg 56B:618–624, 1974.
20. Strickland JW: Flexor tendon injuries. I. Anatomy, physiology, biomechanics, healing, adhesion formation around a repaired tendon. Orthop Rev 15:632–645, 1986.
21. Manske PR, Gelberman RH, VandeBerg JS, and Lesker PA: Flexor tendon intrinsic repair: A morphological study in vitro. J Bone Joint Surg 66A:385–396, 1984.
22. Lindsay WK and Birch JR: The fibroblast in flexor tendon healing. Plast Reconstr Surg 34:223–232, 1964.
23. Gelberman RH and Manske PR: Factors influencing flexor tendon adhesions. Hand Clin 1:35–42, 1985.
24. Peacock EE Jr: Biological principles in the healing of long tendons. Surg Clin North Am 45:461–476, 1965.
25. Klein SN, Oloff L, and Jacobs AM: Functional and surgical anatomy of the lateral ankle. J Foot Surg 20:170–176, 1981.
26. Sarrafian SK: Tendon sheaths and bursae. *In* Sarrafian SK (ed): Anatomy of the Foot and Ankle. Philadelphia, JB Lippincott, 1983, pp 251–259.
27. Hartman A: The tendon sheaths and synovial bursa of the foot. Foot Ankle 1:247–269, 1981. (Original published 1896.)
28. Fitzgerald RH Jr and Coventry MB: Post-traumatic peroneal tendinitis. *In* Bateman JE and Trott AW (eds): The Foot and Ankle. New York: Thieme-Stratton, 1980, pp 103–109.
29. Parvin RW and Ford LT: Stenosing tenosynovitis of the common peroneal tendon sheath. J Bone Joint Surg 38:1352–1357, 1956.
30. Gould N: Stenosing tenosynovitis of the flexor hallucis longus tendon at the great toe. Foot Ankle 2:46–49, 1981.
31. Sammarco GJ and DiRaimondo CV: Chronic peroneus brevis tendon lesions. Foot Ankle 9:163–170, 1989.
32. Zoellner GZ and Clancy W Jr: Recurrent dislocation of the peroneal tendon. J Bone Joint Surg 61A:292–294, 1979.
33. Stein RE: Reconstruction of the superior retinaculum using a portion of the peroneus brevis tendon. J Bone Joint Surg 69A:298–299, 1987.
34. Lowy A, Kruman N, and Kanat IO: Subluxating peroneal tendons. Treatment with the use of an autogenous sliding bone graft. J Foot Surg 75:249–253, 1985.
35. Perlman MD, Wertheimer SJ, and Leveille DW: Traumatic dislocations of the tibialis posterior tendon: A review of the literature and two case reports. J Foot Surg 29:253–259, 1990.
36. Edwards ME: The relations of the peroneal tendons of the fibula, calcaneus and cuboideum. Am J Anat 42:213–253, 1928.
37. Resnick D and Goergen TG: Peroneal tenography in previous calcaneal fractures. Radiology 115:211–213, 1975.
38. Jacobs AM and Oloff LM: Surgical management of forefoot supinatus in flexible flatfoot deformity. J Foot Surg 23:410–419, 1984.
39. Kidner FC: The pre-hallux (accessory) scaphoid in relation to flatfoot. J Bone Joint Surg 11:831–839, 1929.

40. Cozen L: Posterior tibial tenosynovitis secondary to foot strain. Clin Orthop 42:101–102, 1965.
41. Basmajian JV and Stecko G: The role of muscles in arch support of the foot. An electromyographic study. J Bone Joint Surg 45A:1184–1190, 1963.
42. Mueller TJ: Ruptures and lacerations of the tibialis posterior tendon. J Am Podiatr Assoc 74:109–119, 1984.
43. Banks AS and McGlamry ED: Tibialis posterior tendon rupture. J Am Podiatr Assoc 77:170–176, 1987.
44. Fond D: Flexor hallucis longus tendinitis—A case of mistaken identity and posterior impingement syndrome in dancers: Evaluation and management. J Orthop Sports Phys Ther 5:204–206, 1984.
45. Hamilton WG: Stenosing tenosynovitis of the flexor hallucis longus tendon and posterior impingement upon the os trigonum in ballet dancers. Foot Ankle 3:74–80, 1982.
46. Reinherz RP: Management of flexor hallucis longus tendon injuries. J Foot Surg 23:366–369, 1984.
47. Lipscomb PR: Nonsuppurative tenosynovitis and paratendinitis. Am Acad Instruct Course Lec 7:254–261, 1950.
48. Burman M: Stenosing tendovaginitis of the foot and ankle. Arch Surg 67:686–689, 1953.
49. Jagerink TA: Uber zei noch nicht beschriebne Formen von Tendovaginitis Stenosans. Z Orthop 50:703–705, 1929.
50. Ghormley RK and Spear IM: Anomalies of the posterior tibial tendon. Arch Surg 66:512–516, 1953.
51. Rathbun JB and McNab I: The microvascular pattern of the rotator cuff. J Bone Joint Surg 52B:540–553, 1970.
52. Lagergren C and Lindholm A: Vascular distribution in the Achilles tendon—An angiographic and microangiographic study. Acta Chir Scand 116:491–495, 1958/1959.
53. Ralston EL and Schmidt ER: Repair of the ruptured Achilles tendon. J Trauma 11:15–21, 1979.
54. Frey C, Shereff M, and Greenidge N: Vascularity of the posterior tibial tendon. J Bone Joint Surg 72A:884–888, 1990.
55. Bluestone R: Collagen diseases affecting the foot. Foot Ankle 2:311–317, 1982.
56. Jacobs J: Sponyloarthropathies and enthesopathy: Current concepts in rheumatology. Arch Intern Med 143:103–107, 1983.
57. Lapidus PW and Seidenstein H: Chronic non-specific tenosynovitis with effusion about the ankle. J Bone Joint Surg 32A:175–179, 1950.
58. Howard NJ: A new concept of tenosynovitis and the pathology and physiologic effort. Am J Surg 42:723–730, 1938.
59. Engel J, Luboshitz S, Israeli A, and Ganel A: Tenography in DeQuervain's disease. Hand 2:142–146, 1981.
60. Bruce RK, Hale TL, and Gilbert SK: Ultrasonography evaluation for ruptured Achilles tendon. J Am Podiatr Assoc 72:15–17, 1982.
61. Weinstabl R, Stiskal M, Neuhold A, et al: Classifying calcaneal tendon injury according to MRI findings. J Bone Joint Surg 73B:683–685, 1991.
62. Solomon MA, Gilula LA, Oloff L, and Oloff J: CT scanning of the foot and ankle: 2. Clinical applications and review of the literature. Am J Roentgenol 146:1204–1214, 1986.
63. Sartoris DJ and Resnick D: Magnetic resonance imaging of tendons in the foot and ankle. J Foot Surg 28:370–377, 1989.
64. Rosenberg ZS, Cheung Y, Jahss MH, et al: Rupture of posterior tibial tendon: CT and MR imaging with surgical correlation. Radiology 169:229–235, 1988.
65. Mueller TJ: Acquired flatfoot secondary to tibialis posterior dysfunction: Biomechanical aspects. J Foot Surg 30:2–11, 1991.
66. Kalebo P, Goksor L-A, Sward L, and Peterson L: Soft-tissue radiography, computed tomography, and ultrasonography of partial Achilles tendon ruptures. Acta Radiol 31:565–570, 1990.
67. Blei LC, Nirschl RP, and Grant EG: Achilles tendon: US diagnosis of pathological conditions. Radiology 159:765–767, 1986.
68. Daffner RH, Reimer BL, Lupetin ARE, and Dash N: Magnetic resonance imaging in acute tendon ruptures. Skeletal Radiol 15:619–621, 1986.
69. Clement DB, Taunton JE, and Smart GW: Achilles tendinitis and peritendinitis: Etiology and treatment. Am J Sports Med 12:179–184, 1984.
70. Tudisco C and Puddo G: Stenosing tenosynovitis of the flexor hallucis longus tendon in a classical ballet dancer. Am J Sports Med 12:403–404, 1984.
71. Leach RE, James S, and Wasilewski S: Achilles tendinitis. Am J Sports Med 9:93–98, 1981.
72. Johnson KA and Strom DE: Tibialis posterior tendon dysfunction. Clin Orthop 239:196–206, 1989.
73. McMaster P: Tendon and muscle ruptures. J Bone Joint Surg 15:705–722, 1933.
74. Jahss MH: Spontaneous rupture of the tibialis posterior tendon: Clinical findings, tenographic studies, and a new technique of repair. Foot Ankle 3:158–166, 1982.
75. Kashyap S and Prince R: Spontaneous rupture of the tibialis anterior tendon. Clin Orthop 216:159–161, 1987.
76. Werner JA and Shein AJ: Simultaneous bilateral rupture of the patellar tendon and quadriceps expansion in systemic lupus erythematosus: A case report. J Bone Joint Surg 56A:823, 1974.
77. Murphy KJ and McPhee I: Tears of major tendons in chronic acidosis with elastosis. J Bone Joint Surg 47A:1253, 1965.
78. Cirincione RJ and Baker EB: Tendon ruptures with secondary hyperparathyroidism: A case report. J Bone Joint Surg 57A:852, 1975.
79. Funk DA, Cass JR, and Johnson KA: Acquired adult flat foot secondary to posterior tibial-tendon pathology. J Bone Joint Surg 68A:95–102, 1986.
80. Henceroth WD II and Deyerle WM: The acquired unilateral flatfoot in the adult: Some causative factors. Foot Ankle 2:304, 1982.
81. Mueller T: Tibialis posterior dysfunction. In Jay R (ed): Current Therapy in Podiatric Surgery. St. Louis, CV Mosby, 1989, pp 99–107.
82. Johnson KA and Strom DE: Tibialis posterior tendon dysfunction. Clin Orthop 239:196–206, 1989.
83. Mann RA and Thompson FM: Rupture of the posterior tibial tendon causing flat foot. J Bone Joint Surg 67A:556, 1985.

CHAPTER 36

Tendon Transfers

John M. Schuberth, D.P.M.

Tendon transfers of the foot and leg are valuable procedures that lower extremity surgeons should have at their disposal. The ability to alter locomotor mechanics is essential in providing for patients with neuromuscular disease states or dynamic gait aberrations. These patients present with muscular imbalances that are usually poorly compensated for by the musculoskeletal system. The application of tendon transfer surgery can make a substantial difference in that particular patient's ability to ambulate, which may in turn elevate the functional capacity and quality of life.

Tendon transfers can be defined as the relocation of all or part of a tendon insertion to another location to alter the function of that tendon-muscle unit. Although there are other subcategories of procedures such as tendosuspension, they are discussed in this chapter only if there are direct applications to the field of foot and ankle surgery. *Tendosuspension,* often referred to as *tenosuspension,* is defined as the transfer of a tendon or portion of a tendon to another bony location. The proposed mechanism of action is to ''suspend,'' or support, the bony structure rather than move it through a specific range of motion.

Four types of patients may benefit from tendon transfer surgery. The first category is the patient with a known neuromuscular disease. This includes a wide array of diseases ranging from polio to Charcot-Marie-Tooth disease. This group comprises patients who have either spastic or flaccid muscular activity. Although many of these diseases are uncommon, the underlying neurologic lesions that are produced generally fit into reproducible patterns that are amenable to classification. On the other hand, there are seldom two patients who are alike in actual clinical presentation even though they have the same disease. This is because of the variable involvement of either the peripheral or the central nervous system.

Until the polio vaccine was discovered in 1954, poliomyelitis was responsible for tremendous numbers of patients with lower extremity locomotor imbalances. Poliomyelitis is the disease that alone accounted for large series of clinical cases from which we are able to draw on the experiences of those surgeons who treated this epidemic disease. Although polio is largely eradicated throughout the modern world, there are still some patients living in the United States who have the disease. It is especially prevalent on the West Coast, which has a higher proportion of immigrants from Mexico and the Philippines, where the vaccine may not be readily available. Most of the vast clinical experience of the 1930s,

1940s, and 1950s can be applied to the neuromuscular patient of today.

The second category of patients who may benefit from tendon transfer surgery is the group without a true neuromuscular disease but with a significant gait disturbance caused by faulty biomechanics. This includes patients with overt muscular imbalances and those with subtle mechanical aberrations that lead to significant symptoms when allowed to persist. As the study of biomechanics becomes more scientific and parameters are easier to quantify, the indications and applications of tendon transfers continue to expand.

The third type of patient who may benefit from tendon transfer surgery is the group with a traumatic nerve injury. These injuries may have occurred at the root level during excision of a tumor, for example, or they may be the result of gunshot wounds or traction injuries to the common peroneal, femoral, and sciatic nerve or their branches.

Acquired neurologic conditions such as cerebral vascular accidents, head injury, or other centrally mediated conditions constitute the last group of patients that may benefit from tendon transfer surgery. Although patients in this category typically present with spastic activity, the principles and procedures discussed here can be applied in many instances.

Regardless of the specific clinical situation, tendon transfers can generally be relied on to either restore function, prevent future or worsening deformity, or facilitate rehabilitative efforts. This chapter discusses the principles of tendon transfers in general and presents some of the techniques used in the performance of these procedures. Musculoskeletal conditions that would benefit from tendon transfers and the more commonly used lower extremity tendon transfers are also disscussed.

GENERAL PRINCIPLES

Although most of the procedures discussed in this chapter require a certain skill level and advanced training, it is absolutely imperative for anyone who performs these procedures to be well versed in the principles of tendon transfer. This includes a thorough understanding of the principles of physics involved, the local anatomic factors, and the specific disease processes. Misapplication of any of the principles of physics or surgery often compromises the desired result. Failure to consider the natural course of the disease may temporize the surgical result but end in ultimate failure.

The surgeon must understand the goal of the proposed transfer. One must understand whether or not the proposed new function is physiologically or anatomically possible. Tendon transfers cannot be relied on to correct fixed or bony deformities regardless of the strength of the transferred tendon. In addition, the tendon transfer functions best if the excursion of the transferred tendon can be along a straight line. It should also be designed to work perpendicular to a joint axis of motion to be optimally effective. Performing transfers that function obliquely to a joint axis of motion is akin to expecting a door to swing freely if one of the hinges is twisted or damaged. Additionally, the chosen tendon-muscle unit should be about the same size and have a similar length of excursion as the tendon it is replacing. This ensures that the strength of the transferred tendon will be sufficient to perform the proposed action.

Phasic transfer, or transfer of a tendon that functions in the same phase of gait as the tendon it is replacing, is preferable to out-of-phase transfer. However, when phasic transfer is not possible, out-of-phase transfers can work effectively when the principles of tendon transfer surgery are followed. When more than one choice of out-of-phase transfer is available, the tendon with the higher probability of phasic conversion is most desirable.

Once the tendon is transferred, the antagonist may still be working. If so, new deformities can be created that may be worse than the original problem. There is also some evidence to suggest that antagonists may actually function better postoperatively when the agonist is weakened or lengthened and one can gain additional benefits from the tendon transfer surgery.[1] However, this concept was founded on the results of Achilles tendon lengthening for equinus deformities in patients with spastic cerebral palsy.[2] In addition, the new action of the transferred tendon may then overpower existing muscle antagonists at its new location, and a new deformity may result.

Many of the patients who are candidates for tendon transfer surgery have some neuromuscular disease. The surgeon must be acutely aware of the natural course of the disease process to accurately and effectively treat the condition. According to a seemingly simple tenet, neuromuscular diseases do not improve with time—these disease states often get worse in terms of function. Therefore, the procedure selected should be able to withstand the test of time. In some instances, delay of any surgical procedure for a period may be prudent to observe the patient's response to the disease. We can benefit from the experiences of those clinicians who treated patients with polio. Although there is some concern for the so-called post-polio syndrome, it is so uncommon that it is probably not prudent to deny these patients useful surgical procedures on the chance that increasing weakness may occur many years after the disease process has supposedly stabilized. Similarly, delay of procedures in other conditions is unnecessary if the surgeon is reasonably certain that the neurologic deterioration has stabilized or there are no other alternatives at the time of evaluation.

Other conditions such as spasticity also are unrelenting unless the underlying cause of the spasticity is treated or the hyperactivity is controlled with medication or surgery. Patients with nonprogressive diseases should be observed carefully because the amount of spasticity often may vary from day to day. Those patients who acquire neuromuscular imbalances after cerebrovascular accidents should not have any

surgical procedure until at least 6 months after the event because it is possible for complete or partial neurologic recovery to occur.[3] Stabilization of the neurologic sequelae should be allowed to occur if at all possible. If the patient has such a severe disability that ambulation is impossible without surgery, earlier surgery would be appropriate in selected cases. Nevertheless, spastic conditions are difficult to treat with tendon transfers owing to the marked uncertainty of the disease course and are often a contraindication to tendon transfer. However, there are few situations in which transfer or release of a spastic tendon may be appropriate. In these instances, the patient should be fully aware of the goals and the long-term prognosis of the operation. Miller[4] has provided guidelines that indicate the appropriate timing for the performance of tendon transfer surgery.

It is usually preferable to perform stabilizing procedures of the foot prior to performance of a tendon transfer. Often, the apparent need for tendon transfer disappears when proper foot position is achieved via stabilizing operations such as arthrodesis procedures. If the malfunctioning joints or motions are eliminated, the pathologic forces acting on those joints are significantly dampened to the point of having little or no detrimental effects on foot function. In fact, the tendon may have positive effects on foot function now that the pathologic motions have been eliminated. An example of this is the patient with a dynamic varus deformity that has some fixed structural components of the forefoot. If a triple arthrodesis is performed, correction of the forefoot varus could and should be done via derotation of the forefoot, thereby possibly obviating the need for a tendon transfer. However, this philosophy does not hold true when dealing with a pediatric patient. In this patient population it is often preferable to perform early tendon transfer to prevent further deformity and even reverse existing postural components before the onset of fixed structural changes. If an arthrodesis is performed early, especially in the hindfoot, the growth of that portion of the foot will usually cease, which is undesirable in most patients. However, in a few instances, the foot size may stabilize well before physical maturity. In this situation it is permissible to perform an early arthrodesis. The surgeon should be acutely aware of the long-term effects of the existing tendon imbalance even with a stabilized hindfoot complex. The tibialis posterior tendon can still cause unremitting cavovarus-deforming forces on the forefoot even in the face of a well-positioned triple arthrodesis. This occurs through the multiple insertions of the tendon distal to the transverse tarsal joint.

When at all possible, a tendon should be passed within an existing tendon sheath.[5] This necessitates passing the tendon under the extensor retinaculum, which increases the mechanical advantage of the transfer by increasing the lever arm mechanics. If it is not passed within a tendon sheath, the tendon should be passed superior to the retinaculum at the cost of a significant mechanical advantage. This is because the excursion of the transposed tendon is less likely to be affected if passed in the subcutaneous fat. If it is passed beneath the retinaculum but not in a sheath, the chance of adhesion of the tendon to the adjacent structures is significantly increased.

Even when one recognizes and understands the principles of tendon transfers, each successful transfer can be expected to lose at least one grade in muscle strength. This expectant loss of power occurs even with a technically perfect operation. Therefore, only a good or normal muscle should be used for tendon transfer. Slight imperfections in the performance of the procedure or misapplications of the principles can allow for the loss of more than one grade of muscle function, which will translate into a less desirable result in most instances.

Axes of Motion: Muscle and Joint Mechanics

Regardless of the muscles that act on a particular joint, motion can occur about that joint only in a direction that is perpendicular to the axis of motion. One cannot expect a joint to function in a different plane regardless of the efficiency or strength of the tendon transfer. Although most of the joints in the foot are composed of complex multiplanar facets, major movement can be thought to occur primarily about a relatively stationary axis.

The arrangement of muscle fibers is dependent on the required length of excursion, the strength required of the particular action, the mechanical advantage of the system, and the speed of action necessary for powerful or efficient movement. Regardless of the arrangement of the fibers of the particular muscle belly, the ultimate action on the tendon usually results in a force that is in line with the long axis of the tendon. Although the final action of the tendon may be altered by a system of pulleys, the force generated causes the tendon to be pulled directly toward the muscle belly itself.

Efficient and powerful excursions of muscle action are mediated through the proper length of the muscle when contraction is initiated. The length-tension curve of Blix[6] conveniently explains the fact that any muscle functions with the most power when contraction is initiated with the muscle at its resting length (Fig. 36–1). Maximal tension can be realized when this condition is met. As the muscle is shortened or lengthened, the amount of potential tension decreases accordingly. Transferred muscles should be anchored with this concept in mind. Attainment of the optimal resting length requires experience, analysis of the excursion of the transferred muscle, and careful attention to detail. Any deviation

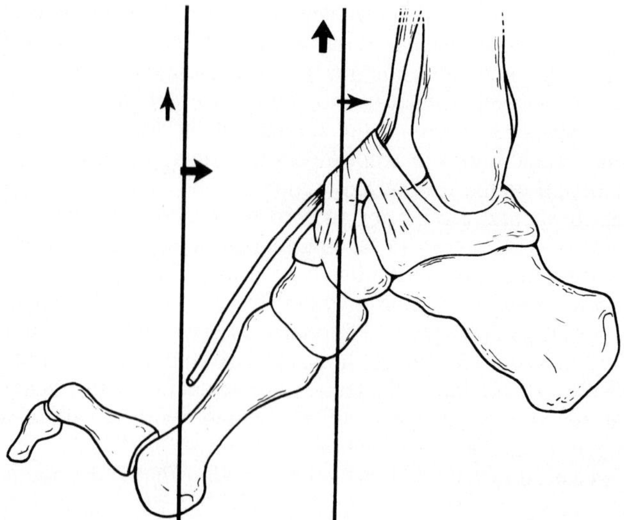

FIGURE 36–2. Diagram depicting the dual function of the extensor digitorum longus tendon. At the metatarsophalangeal joint, the tendon has the primary function of moving the digit through its range of motion. At the midtarsal joint, the direction of force stabilizes the midtarsal joint. (From McGlamry ED, Butlin WE, and Ruch JA: Treatment of forefoot equinus by tendon transpositions. J Am Podiatry Assoc 65:872–888, 1975.)

from the resting length will likely result in loss of power of the transferred tendon.

As mentioned, the resultant pull of the muscle may be along a line that is different from one that is parallel to the long axis of the muscle. This is accomplished by an efficient system of pulleys in the foot and ankle. The various retinacula of the ankle allow for transmission of muscle action to more distal articulations without a significant loss of mechanical advantage.

The foot-ankle unit also has an inherent system of level arms that dictate particular function of specific muscles. By virtue of the class of level that is created, some tendons serve to stabilize a particular joint that they cross, whereas others serve to move the joint through a range of motion. This is usually dependent on the direction and distance from a specific joint that a tendon crosses or inserts into the bone. A tendon that crosses a joint but does not actually move the articulation through a range of motion functions as a shunt muscle. It usually inserts some distance away from the joint. A tendon that moves a joint through a range of motion functions as a spurt muscle. Here, the tendon usually inserts in close proximity to the axis of motion. The extensor digitorum longus (EDL) muscle serves both as a spurt and a shunt muscle. The tendon serves as a spurt muscle at the lesser metatarsophalangeal (MTP) joint and as a shunt muscle at the midtarsal joint (Fig. 36–2). The Hibbs tenosuspension makes use of an alteration in level arm mechanics by converting the action of the EDL tendon from a shunt muscle to a spurt muscle at the midtarsal joint.

Phasic Conversion

It is well known that the cyclical action of walking is mediated in the central nervous system. This central control dictates the phasic activity of each of the muscles used for locomotion. The walking response is learned at an early age and becomes more or less ''reflexive.'' For this reason it is

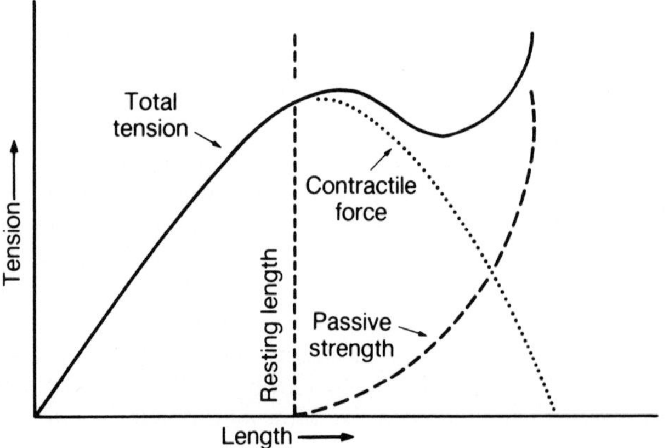

FIGURE 36–1. Length-tension curve of Blix[6] showing that the maximal tension that can be generated by a muscle is at 120% of its resting length. If the length of the muscle is shorter or longer, the resultant tension decreases proportionately. (From Bechtol CO: Muscle physiology. Am Assoc Orthopedic Surgeons Instructional Course Lectures 5:181, 1948.)

difficult for muscles to convert phase when out-of-phase transfers are performed. Close and Todd[7] have shown that most of the time the transferred muscle retains its preoperative phasic activity, regardless of its new location or desired function. There are a few factors that seem to influence the capability of a muscle to convert phases. Intensive perioperative training by a physical therapist skilled in this technique is essential, particularly when either of the tibialis muscles is involved. However, it seems that certain muscles have a predetermined ability or inability to convert phase, regardless of the intensity of perioperative training. Peroneus brevis seems to convert from stance phase to swing phase automatically, whereas peroneus longus conversion seems to be random. This is predicated on the assumption that the transferred muscle is essentially normal and is substituting for a diseased or absent muscle.

There are some instances when phasic conversion is desirable. However, if it does not occur, it does not necessarily signify a failure of the operation. The transferred tendon may provide enough support to the joints by its tenodesis effect so that the surgical goal is partially attained. For example, one may be able to rely on the intact stretch reflex in some cases of posterior tendon transfer.[8] As Miller[4] has suggested, some patients are able to discard their ankle-foot orthoses (AFOs) following surgery in which a tendon has been only partially successful in phasic conversion. Biofeedback is another modality that can aid in the conversion of phasic activity. Voluntary activity can also help in attaining the desired function. It is important that this training be initiated preoperatively and by a therapist who is skilled and trained in the techniques.

PREOPERATIVE EVALUATION

The preoperative evaluation is absolutely critical to the successful application of the procedures discussed in this section. A complete diagnostic work-up is required to accurately assess the pathologic mechanisms that are acting on the foot and the leg in almost all instances. Although some of the procedures discussed are not technically demanding, the value of clinical experience in the preoperative assessment of these types of patients cannot be overemphasized.

Historical Factors

Probably the most critical determination in the preoperative assessment is the expectation of the patient who faces a reconstructive surgical procedure. The surgeon should be careful not to convey a sense of euphoria or a miraculous cure for the patient's disease or locomotor discrepancy. This is especially true in the patient with an acquired neuromuscular disease. Most of the patients are reasonably educated with regard to their disease process as well as to the ultimate prognosis and the effect the disease has on their ability to ambulate. Patients should be interviewed extensively with regard to present limitations, course of the disease, genetic variants if applicable, and what they would like to be able to do if surgery were performed. Patient expectations may range from being able to walk ''normally'' to being able to ambulate without a brace or walking aid. Patients who are not independent ambulators may still be candidates for tendon transfer surgery if simple tasks such as standing and transfer-

ring from wheelchair to bed are difficult. Patients who are wheelchair dependent may require tendon-balancing procedures just to be able to sit in their wheelchairs in a balanced posture (Fig. 36–3).

It is critical to be familiar with any neuromuscular disease, with special attention to the natural course of the problem. The patient should be questioned regarding the impact of the disease on the activities of daily living. Modifications in the perioperative program may need to be made for successful attainment of the goal. The practitioner should also ascertain whether other joints of the lower or even upper extremity are affected or weakened. If the condition affects both lower extremities, some modifications to the patient's shoes, braces, or ambulatory aids may be in order so that the patient can comply with the postoperative regimen. Patients may also have significant upper extremity problems that preclude the use of crutches if a period of non-weightbearing is required.

Although most of the patients who present for these techniques do not have disease states that pose additional anesthetic risk, there are certain situations in which early preoperative evaluation of the patient by an anesthesiologist or pulmonary specialist may be in order. These include diseases such as multiple sclerosis and amyotrophic lateral sclerosis, which can alter pulmonary function. Evaluation by a physical or occupational therapist may also be appropriate to anticipate postoperative needs.

Patients without significant neuromuscular disease but who have functional aberrations causing some problem with comfortable ambulation should also be questioned carefully. Many patients' perceptions of the problem are several orders of magnitude lower than what most surgeons would consider serious enough for extensive reconstructive surgery. Nevertheless, many patients with relatively minor imbalances can be helped with carefully applied tendon transfer surgical procedures if it is deemed that the cumulative effect of the problem is likely the cause of significant symptoms or potential problems.

Physical Examination

A complete examination of the lower extremities is necessary for accurate diagnosis and appropriate selection of the

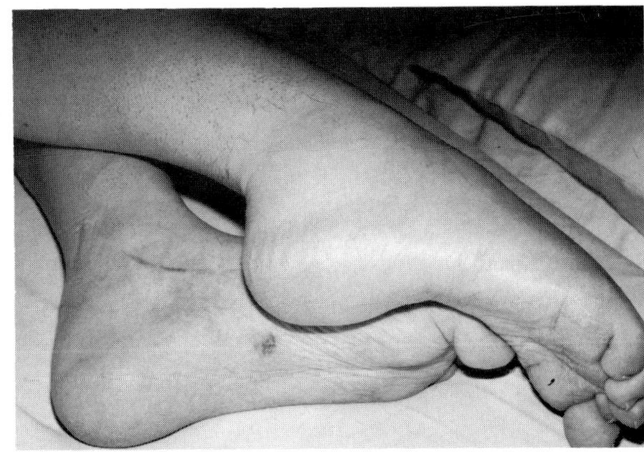

FIGURE 36–3. A nonambulatory wheelchair-bound patient with multiple sclerosis who had difficulty in maintaining balance in the wheelchair due to spastic equinus deformity. The patient had recurrent ischial tuberosity ulcerations. The right extremity is preoperative, and the left leg has had an extensive posterior release and transfer of the posterior tibial tendon to the dorsum of the foot. Note the difference in the resting posture between the two extremities. After surgery on both legs, the patient was able to balance in the wheelchair without additional ischial tuberosity ulcerations.

surgical procedure. This includes a determination of the range of motion of the major joints of the lower extremities, muscle testing of all muscles, and a detailed neurologic examination. A neurology consultation may be indicated in some instances when the neurologic status or condition is complex.

Manual muscle testing techniques are well known to most practitioners and can be found in the standard textbooks. However, each individual muscle must be isolated so that the effect of synergistic muscle action will be eliminated. This information, combined with gait analysis, should be processed so that realistic expectations of each particular muscle and muscle group can be ascertained. Whatever scheme of muscle grading is chosen, it is important to specify the system of evaluation in the medical record so that consistency throughout time is ensured. It will also help the practitioner to provide meaningful comparisons of function from time to time.

It is essential that the patient be examined during gait for an extended period. If there is a particular time of day that the patient has more difficulty, that is the time to conduct the examination. If available, videotaped gait analysis with slow motion capacity may aid the practitioner in detecting subtle discrepancies to further refine the surgical plan. The patient should be dressed in running shorts or the equivalent to assess the entire lower extremity during walking. If the patient normally uses a walking aid such as a brace, cane, and other device but can walk without it, gait analysis should be conducted with and without the device. Finally, the patient should be observed for postural tendencies that may require surgical attention to enhance the result.

The evaluator must remember that there is extreme variation from patient to patient with the same disease. There may also be significant variation in the same patient when examined on different days.[9] Usual techniques of muscle testing are seldom appropriate in patients with any neuromuscular dysfunction. This is especially true in those patients with spastic components to their specific problem. Differences in muscle control are likely to be manifested as inconsistent responses to the specific task that is requested by the examiner. Manual muscle grading is dependent on both the patient's ability to selectively activate the chosen muscle and relax the antagonists. The consistency of response is predicated on muscles that are indifferent to the rate of active and passive stretch. These two conditions are not necessarily present in the patient with a centrally located cause of paralysis.[9] This explains the inconsistency and abnormal responses that are seen in these patients.

In the normal person, walking is a habitual response. The hemiplegic patient has lost the ability to walk as a patterned response. However, the functional loss may be incomplete, and the patient may have difficulty attaining fine motor control even though he or she may perform reasonably well during manual muscle testing. This phenomenon may not be manifested until the patient is asked to ambulate when there is more tendency to exhibit gross limb motion. The loss of selective control and an inaccurate habitual performance make the gait pattern erratic, even though the simpler task of firing a single muscle appears to be intact.[9]

Electrodiagnostic Testing

Electrodiagnostic testing is also an integral part of the preoperative assessment in most instances. The surgeon may use this type of information in a variety of ways, ranging from the confirmation of findings observed during clinical examination to more elaborate analysis of patients with the more complex neurologic status. In patients with spastic conditions, it is often difficult to determine which muscles of a particular group are involved in the spasticity. Often, the resultant deformity masks subtle differences in the muscle activity. This is particularly evident in the patient with acquired spastic disease processes such as multiple sclerosis, cerebral vascular accidents, and head trauma. The particular dynamics of the neuromuscular activity are not consistent, and electrodiagnostic testing helps clarify the electrical activity of each muscle.

The diagnostician can also electrically determine the recruitment availability of a particular muscle. In some instances, the recruitment potential can be far more promising than the clinical examination indicates. However, the surgeon is cautioned against betrayal of clinical impressions. It is prudent to trust clinical findings more than electrical findings when the patient stands to suffer from an idiosyncratic response. In other words, if a muscle tests poorly on clinical examination but tests better from an electrical perspective, the practitioner should assume that the muscle will function poorly rather than as the electrical testing indicates. On the contrary, one should make sure that the patient is able to override the difficulties in isolated firing of the involved muscle. The electrical response may in fact be the more accurate reflection of muscle capability during gait.

If available, dynamic electromyography is invaluable in determining the phasic action of muscles, particularly in the spastic conditions. It is helpful in determining the temporal relationship of the muscle activity as well as the duration of the gait cycle that a particular muscle fires. Lastly, it may also clarify if a particular muscle is firing in a phase other than one it was destined for. This testing maneuver requires sophisticated equipment and is subject to expert interpretation. It also helps sort out the discrepancy between the clinical impression and static electrodiagnostic findings.

Force plate analysis may also be useful in the determination of the temporal relationships of muscle activity. It would be particularly useful to integrate force plate measurements with those obtained from wire electrodes. Discrepancies in the slopes of the respective curves might signify abnormal joint mechanics or other osseous obstructions to normal excursions. Practically, this notion will require significant research.

Radiographic Evaluation

Radiographic examination is also mandatory prior to surgical intervention. Although routine radiographs seldom impact the ultimate surgical plan, they are extremely helpful for a number of reasons. First, they help determine whether there are any bony causes for lack of motion. This is especially critical in assessment of ankle joint motion. In many instances, there is a bony equinus that would prevent ankle dorsiflexion regardless of the success of the tendon transfer. On the other hand, it is my experience that in some instances the radiographic determination is misleading with regard to the amount of available dorsiflexion at the ankle. The stress dorsiflexion lateral radiograph may indicate the presence of a bony equinus. However, it is more important to correlate this finding with the clinical examination. If the end point of motion appears soft or spongy, it is probable that there is more dorsiflexion than the radiographic picture would indicate. If the end point of motion is firm or abrupt, the radiographic findings are probably quite accurate (Fig. 36–4). The discrepancy between the radiographic and the clinical examination can often be explained by the radiographic positioning technique. Second, the surgeon can assess bone density, which would indicate the feasibility of stable fixation in fusion procedures or attachment of tendon to bone. Third, the surgeon can decide if the bony anatomy can support the proposed surgical plan.

Routine radiographs should be taken in a weightbearing attitude in all instances. In some situations it may be necessary to take non-weightbearing films to see if there is any change in osseous architecture or the configuration of the medial arch from the weightbearing profile. Degenerative changes should be searched for to make sure the joint would not be predisposed to early arthrosis with the new functional demands or positions of the joints.

CONDITIONS AMENABLE TO TENDON TRANSFER TECHNIQUES

There are several categories of dysfunctional conditions that are amenable to tendon transfer techniques. However, it is important to evaluate each patient individually so that the functional limitations may be determined with the patient's individual needs in mind. The surgeon should direct the examination and the surgical plan with a goal of solving the problem for the patient. It is inappropriate to address the deformity alone without weighing both the risks and benefits to each particular patient. A simple example of this concept can be a patient with a drop foot with anterior tibial paralysis who also presents with a symptomatic cock-up hallux deformity. It may not be appropriate to perform a dorsiflexion attainment procedure if the patient is content wearing an AFO. The relatively simple correction of the cock-up hallux deformity may be all that is necessary to correct the patient's main complaint. On the other hand, patients should be presented with all the surgical and nonsurgical options so that an informed decision can be made.

Although no two patients present exactly alike, similar patterns can be discussed together with the preceding concepts in mind. Careful clinical evaluation segregates those patients requiring similar yet different combinations of surgical procedures.

Extensor Insufficiency

Extensor insufficiency is one of the more common conditions for which tendon transfer techniques can be applied. Most of the patients present with some degree of anterior group paralysis that translates into a lack of power in swing-phase ankle joint dorsiflexion. The gait pattern that is manifested depends on the specific deficit, but the functional loss will be along the continuum of a complete drop foot to a mild loss of power in dorsiflexion. Lack of activity in isolated muscles is uncommon but can be seen in traumatically induced situations. In addition, incomplete penetrance of some disease states may produce these unique and focal losses.

Although these isolated losses are easily discovered and treated, most of the patients with a clinically detectable drop foot have some weakness of the tibialis anterior muscle. This is the most powerful and thus most important muscle for dorsiflexion of the foot at the ankle. Loss of the extensor hallucis longus (EHL) and EDL alone or in combination leaves most patients with enough dorsiflexion power to ambulate without a perceptible slapfoot gait. On the contrary, most patients have sufficient power of dorsiflexion with an intact tibialis anterior. If the tibialis anterior is intact and the remaining muscles are not, there is likely to be a dynamic varus deformity that manifests during swing phase. Lateral column overload, lateral ankle or subtalar instability, and symptoms from lack of shock absorption are likely presenting complaints (Fig. 36–5).

Isolated weakness of the tibialis anterior muscle often results in a clinically detectable drop foot. However, additional presentations may complicate the surgical plan. Overpowering by the peroneus longus results in a plantar flexed first ray. This results in a forefoot cavovarus posture, with possible calcaneal varus deformity. In addition, the attempt of the other two long extensors to assist in dorsiflexion, the so-called extensor substitution phenomenon, results in digital deformities. Claw toes and hallux hammertoe are common deformities seen with tibialis anterior insufficiency. Each condition can become rigid if left unattended for a prolonged period.

Isolated weakness of the EHL is uncommon but usually manifests as a hallux flexus deformity at the interphalangeal joint. There is usually little deformity of the first MTP joint due to the lack of long extensor power. However, there may be some retrograde force of the mallet toe resulting in some degree of extension at the MTP joint.

It is extremely rare to observe a patient with an isolated weakness or absence of EDL activity. I have seen only one

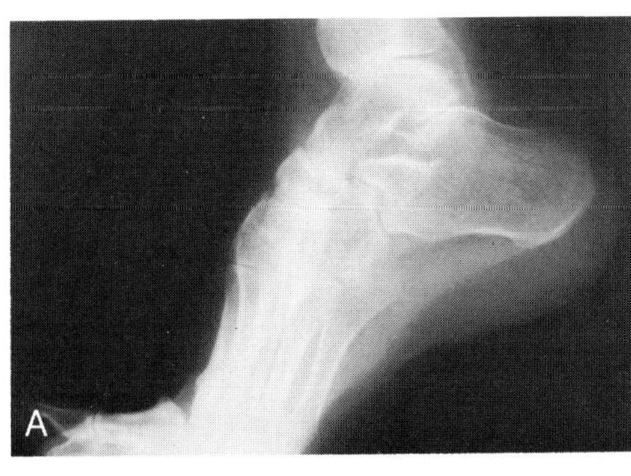
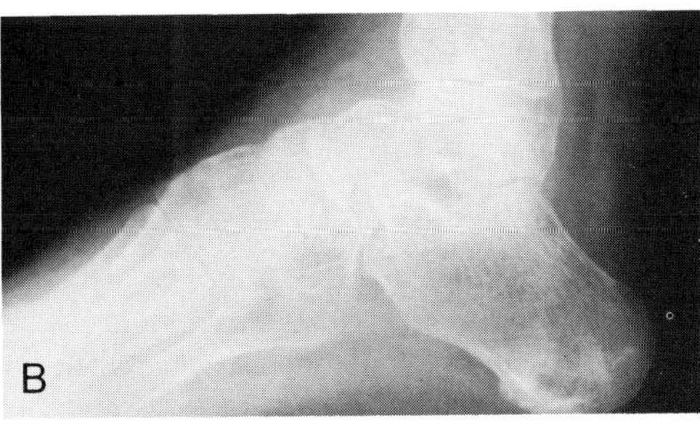

FIGURE 36–4. *A,* Preoperative stress lateral radiograph of a patient with severe equinus. Note the apparent lack of dorsiflexion owing to bone block equinus. *B,* Postoperative radiograph showing the amount of dorsiflexion after a soft tissue release of the triceps surae.

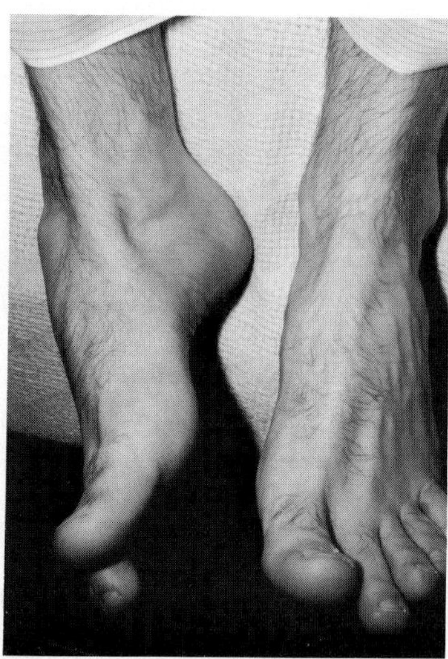

FIGURE 36–5. A 37-year-old male patient with an L5 nerve root deficit secondary to deliberate sacrifice during excision of a spinal cord tumor 10 years ago. Note the hypertrophy of the tibialis anterior on the involved side. There is resultant dynamic swing phase varus deformity with lateral symptomatology.

patient with an isolated EDL insufficiency, which was the result of a gunshot wound to the common peroneal nerve area. This patient had slow development of mallet toes, which was easily addressed. If followed for a long period, patients with similar lesions would be expected to develop some mild degree of cavovarus.

There are a few surgical alternatives for the patient who has a paralytic drop foot. However, because of the degree of force necessary to resist the moment arm of force created by heel strike, few of the posterior muscles are suitable for sufficient dorsiflexion power because of the size of the remaining tendons. The most commonly employed procedure is transfer of the posterior tibial tendon through the interosseous membrane. This is the most desirable because the posterior tibial tendon is generally regarded as the third strongest muscle below the knee, preceded only by the gastrocnemius and the soleus.[10] The second tendon transfer that is used when the posterior tibial tendon is insufficient is the hemigastrocnemius-soleus transfer to the anterior aspect of the leg.[11, 12] I have had little practical experience with this procedure. However, it should probably be reserved for those patients who have an insufficient posterior tibial muscle and who refuse to wear a brace.

The peroneus longus has been used for the correction of drop foot.[13, 14] However, its relatively small girth makes it a last choice for the correction of a severe drop foot. It is useful when there is a need for more power in dorsiflexion or there is no other suitable alternative.

Peroneal Insufficiency

Although isolated peroneal muscle insufficiency is uncommon, there are certain conditions that can result in paresis isolated to either the peroneus longus or the peroneus brevis, or both. Gunshot wounds or fractures that involve the lateral proximal aspect of the leg may injure the common peroneal or superficial peroneal nerve. If either of these muscles is injured alone or in combination, a severe varus deformity

will develop by way of an intact and untethered tibialis posterior–tibialis anterior tendon unit.

Peroneus longus weakness or paralysis can result in a significant first metatarsal elevatus. If hallux limitus is the presenting complaint, the practitioner may not recognize early peroneus longus insufficiency as the etiologic factor. If it is recognized early, a peroneal stop procedure can be performed to assist in plantar stabilization of the first metatarsal. This involves anastomosis of the intact peroneus brevis to the tendon of the weak peroneus longus. When the peroneus brevis contracts, it will serve to plantarflex the first metatarsal by virtue of the conjoined tendons. Second, a lateral transfer of the tibialis anterior can be performed. The primary purpose is to remove the deforming force from the first metatarsal. If the deformity is long-standing and irreducible, bony procedures may be necessary to plantarflex the first metatarsal at the base (Fig. 36–6).

If the peroneus brevis muscle or nerve is injured or weakened, a progressive varus deformity of the forefoot and later the hindfoot will develop. With the EDL and EHL as the only active everters of the foot, the tibialis posterior will eventually overpower and create the varus deformity. In this situation, several surgical options are available. An anastomosis of the peroneus longus to the peroneus brevis can be performed above the level of the lateral malleolus. Because the phasic activity of both peroneal muscles is approximately the same, the effect of the peroneus longus can be used to power the peroneus brevis. The tibialis anterior can be split and transferred to the lateral aspect of the foot, or the tibialis posterior can be weakened. The latter approach is preferable if the tibialis posterior muscle is spastic throughout swing and stance phases.[15]

Tibialis Posterior Insufficiency

Paresis or dysfunction of the tibialis posterior has predictable consequences, including a progressive flatfoot and an apropulsive gait. This condition has a presentation that is quite similar to one in those patients with a rupture of the tibialis posterior tendon. However, there may be crossover paresis into the other deep posterior muscles that may complicate the clinical picture. The reader is referred to Chapter 35, which discusses attritional posterior tibial dysfunction.

Transfer of the flexor digitorum longus (FDL) into the navicular tuberosity has been reported as an effective procedure to restore inversion function,[16, 17] but it is useful only if there is an absence of fixed compensatory deformities. In addition, if there is additional weakness of the adjacent muscles, soft tissue supplementation transfers will be insufficient. If there is fixed deformity, bony stabilization procedures will be necessary.

Triceps Insufficiency

Although triceps insufficiency is uncommon, it presents a difficult problem for the surgeon and the patient. The resultant cavus deformity is difficult to reverse without bony correction. The lack of propulsion in stance phase also makes for an inefficient gait. The primary problem in addressing this deficit surgically is the obvious mismatch between the size of the Achilles tendon and the tendons available for transfer. The triceps surae is four times stronger than any of the other tendons, so it is unlikely that a single transfer will be sufficient for adequate plantar flexory power. To transfer

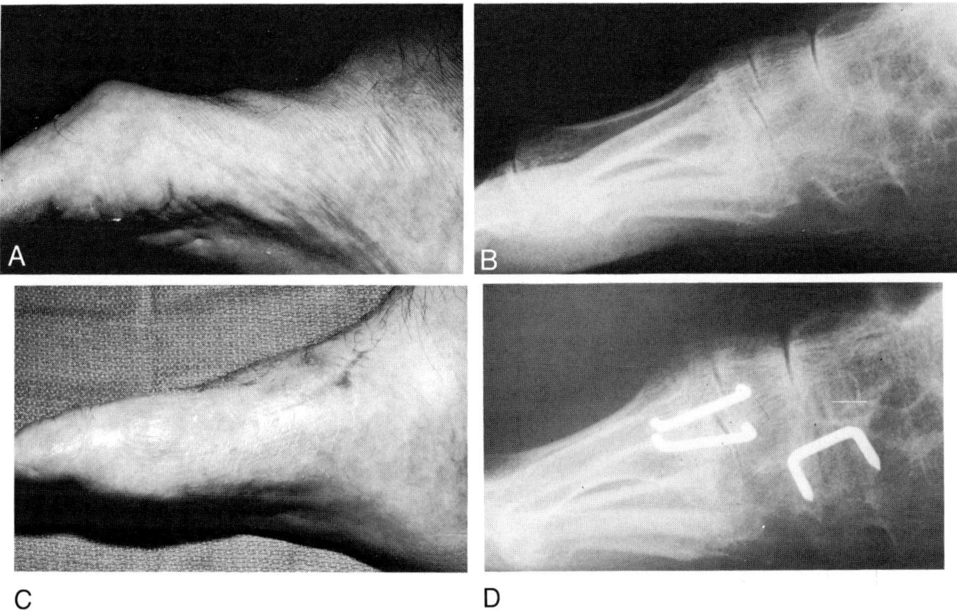

FIGURE 36–6. *A,* Preoperative photograph showing severe metatarsus primus elevatus in a patient with a spinal cord injury. Manual muscle testing showed only a complete absence of the peroneus longus, which was confirmed electromyographically. The deformity was irreducible. *B,* Preoperative lateral radiograph confirming the first metatarsal primus elevatus. *C,* Postoperative photograph showing the result after split tibialis anterior tendon transfer, cuboid osteotomy, and fusion of the first cuneometatarsal joint. *D,* Postoperative lateral radiograph showing the reduction of the bony deformity.

a stance-phase muscle, one must use either of the peroneals, the tibialis posterior, or one or both of the long digital flexors. These can be used alone or in combination; however, the discrepancy in the caliber of these muscles would necessitate the use of more than one. As Miller[4] suggested, it would be prudent to preserve the tibialis posterior and peroneus brevis to avoid development of frontal plane deformity. Both the great toe flexors and the peroneus longus can be used in combination. The appropriate digital procedures may need to be performed to prevent extensus deformity, especially of the hallux. In the great toe, either an interphalangeal joint fusion or an anastomosis of the long and short extensors is required. Surgical intervention is probably unnecessary when the lesser digital long flexors are sacrificed.

For out-of-phase transfers, the choices are more limited and less desirable from a conceptual standpoint. However, the tibialis anterior muscle is a prudent choice if a single muscle transfer is desirable or all of the posterior muscles are paretic. Close and Todd[7] have shown a tendency for the tibialis anterior to transfer phase, particularly if it is the only tendon transferred. Its advantage is that it may be sufficient to provide adequate plantar flexion because of its girth and resultant strength. The technique is more difficult to perform.

The peroneus brevis has also been used for weakness of the gastrocnemius after Achilles tendon rupture.[18] I am unaware of any significant number of procedures that have been performed for paralytic conditions of the gastrocnemius or soleus.

Regardless of the technique or muscles chosen for transfer, restoration of normal strength cannot be attained. However, even modest plantar flexor strength is beneficial in the push-off phase of gait.

Extensor Substitution

The phenomenon of extensor substitution occurs when the anterior muscle group must work harder to make the heel strike the ground first in the weight-acceptance phase of gait. This occurs primarily if there is some condition or anatomic abnormality that predisposes to an ankle equinus. In a superimposed equinus, the Achilles tendon or triceps surae acts as a tether, and the anterior group acts longer and pulls harder to make heel contact more prominent. Although any of the tendons of the anterior group can cause an imbalance, it is most common to see the effects of the substitution at the level of the EDL. This usually causes a retrograde plantar flexion of the metatarsal heads and resultant metatarsalgia. The EDL and EHL are most likely to display the effect of extensor substitution because of the laws of physics. These two tendons act on the toes at the MTP joint, whereas the tibialis anterior acts on the entire first ray at the less mobile first metatarsal cuneiform joint. The lateral digits are a much lesser mass than the first metatarsal, and the design of the joints facilitates dorsiflexion of the digits more so than the first ray.

Spastic Conditions

Spastic conditions of the lower leg are less amenable to traditional tendon transfer because of several factors. First, the spastic muscle is sometimes present in disease states that are quite variable and unpredictable with regard to long-term prognosis. Therefore, muscle function may change in time with a concomitant change in the power, effect, or mechanical advantage of the tendon.[15] Second, the effect of clonus tends to induce dampening of the effect of the transfer because the tendon shortens with time. Because the clonus is irreversible, the exaggerated stretch reflex will continually be active, and adaptive shortening will ensue. However, if one can transfer the tendon where the reflex will not be triggered by virtue of the new position, the long-term action of the muscle may be uniform.

Spastic equinovarus deformity is one of the more common

conditions seen in the patient with hyperactive muscular activity. Most commonly, this phenomenon is a result of either a cerebral vascular accident or cerebral palsy. The unpredictable behavior of any spastic muscle complicates the choices of appropriate surgical procedures. The most distinguishing factor in these patients is that there is usually overpowering of the spastic muscles over the remaining muscles. In most instances, the tibialis posterior–gastrocnemius-soleus complex constitutes the spastic components, particularly in patients with cerebral palsy.[19] In those patients who have had a cerebral vascular accident, the anterior and lateral compartment muscles may not function normally. Various procedures and combinations of procedures have been described to restore motor balance to the foot. These include posterior tibial tenotomy,[20] tibialis posterior tendon transfer,[21–23] and split transfer of the tibialis posterior.[24, 25] There is usually no clear indication of one procedure over another.

Combinations of the split tibialis anterior tendon transfer and weakening of the tibialis posterior tendon have been shown to be efficacious in patients who have spastic equinovarus of the foot due to cerebral palsy.[19]

SURGICAL TECHNIQUES USEFUL IN TENDON TRANSFERS

Several surgical techniques are helpful in the performance of tendon transfer procedures. Most of the procedures presented in this chapter require the use of one or more of these techniques. The most important technique is the ability to anchor the tendon to the new insertion point so that the attachment site is stable during the postoperative phase. The new insertion should be strong and should not pull off its bony or soft tissue attachment.

The trephine technique[26] involves the excavation of a solid cylinder of bone at the new insertion point. The tendon to be transferred is then threaded into the trephine cavity, and the bone plug is then replaced. The advantage of this technique is that it is usually quite stable and promotes a direct tendon-to-bone anastomosis. The trephines come in various sizes and are used on an oscillating power handpiece.

The disadvantages of this technique are numerous enough, in my opinion, to preclude its routine use. Although the concept is sound, it is difficult to consistently replace the plug into the cavity without breaking it into pieces. The loss of adequate space, which is necessitated by the transposed tendon, makes it difficult to complete the reinsertion. The harvesting of the plug also generates a great deal of heat, which can be dampened by copious flushing of the surgical site during procurement of the plug. I have observed several plugs that appeared to dissolve during the postoperative period (Fig. 36–7). This might be the result of thermal necrosis of the bone or lack of adequate blood supply to the plug by virtue of the tendon stump partially surrounding the graft. However, in most instances, the integrity of the anastomosis was not compromised due to the early mechanical stability of the dowel. There was usually ample time for the tendon to attach to bone before dissolution of the plug.[27]

The tunnel technique involves the fashioning of a bony tunnel and passing the tendon through the passage. It is useful when there is abundant tendon available for transfer so that the tendon can be sewn back on itself. The advantage of the technique is that the tension of the tendon can be

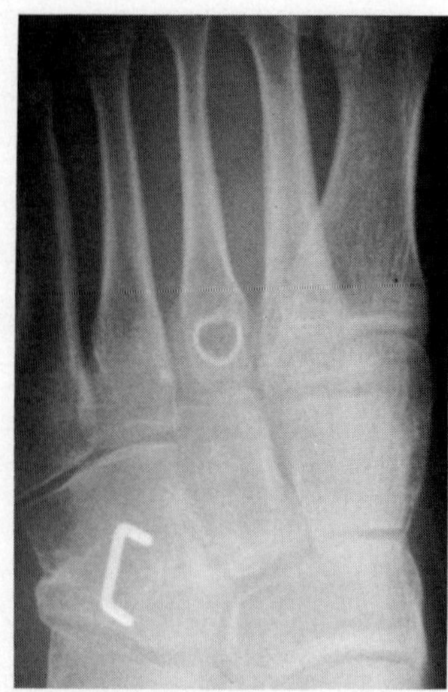

FIGURE 36–7. Postoperative radiograph of a patient who had a Hibbs tenosuspension performed 6 months earlier. Note the absence of the bone plug that was replaced into the trephine hole in the third metatarsal. The plug had necrosed during the postoperative period, but the transferred tendon was firmly anchored into the bone.

adjusted easily just by the amount of tendon that is pulled through the tunnel. It is performed by drilling two converging holes while leaving a roof of cortical bone. The drill caliber should be chosen on the basis of the size of the tendon that is to be inserted into the tunnel. The tunnel technique has limited applicability in the foot because of the lack of large surface areas. It is best used at the base or neck of the first metatarsal for the Jones tenosuspension. It can also be used on the dorsolateral surface of the cuboid.

The three-hole technique is useful in the lesser metatarsals because it does not require a lot of bony surface area. It involves a larger single hole to accommodate the tendon and two smaller drill holes to anchor the Bunnell-type suture that is placed in the tendon (Fig. 36–8). This technique is helpful

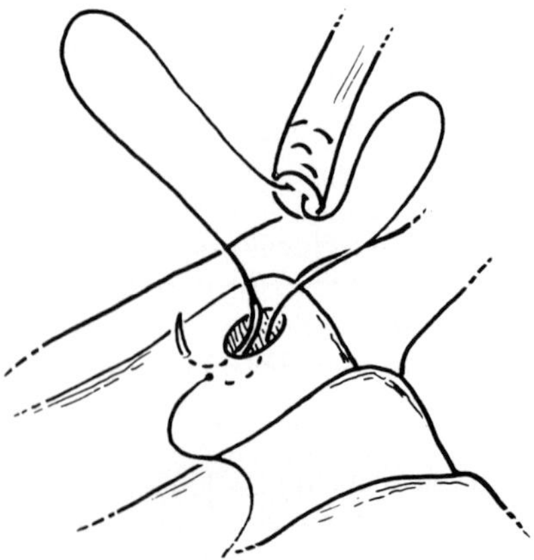

FIGURE 36–8. The three-hole technique for anchoring a tendon to bone is shown. Note the Bunnell-type stitch in the tendon that is threaded through the two smaller holes distal (or proximal) to the larger hole that contains the transferred tendon. (From McGlamry ED, Butlin WE, and Ruch JA: Treatment of forefoot equinus by tendon transpositions. J Am Podiatry Assoc 65:872–888, 1975.)

when there is a short tendon stump that would often preclude other techniques. The tendon needs to be only long enough to just approximate the bone in which it is to be transferred. On the other hand, it is difficult to adjust tension on the tendon intraoperatively unless the Bunnell-type stitch and the tendon are both shortened.

The most widely used technique is where the tendon is passed through a through-and-through drill hole in the bone. The suture in the tendon is then tied to a button on the bottom of the foot. This is best applied when the posterior tibial tendon transfer or the Hibbs tenosuspension is performed. These two tendons' stumps are quite large, and a large hole is required. There are several technical disadvantages to this technique. First, the drill hole must often be placed in the midfoot. Because of the complex bony anatomy, it is easy to violate the intertarsal articulations with the passage of the drill. Even with a properly oriented drill hole, the threading of the sutures through the drill hole must pass through all the plantar layers of the foot. The neurovascular bundles can be injured with the Keith needles as they are passed to the bottom of the foot. One might anticipate aneurysm formation if the vessel is violated or traumatic neuromas if the nerve is injured. However, I have not recognized any complications from this maneuver in approximately 60 cases.

In those instances when the tendon stump is too wide to pass through the hole in the bone easily, one can employ the technique of Krackow and Cohn,[28] which uses the principles of the Chinese finger trap. Two nonabsorbable sutures of the surgeon's preference are wrapped around the tendon from proximal to distal and are tied at the end of the tendon. It is important to wrap the sutures out of phase so that as the suture is pulled through the bone, the tendon is not allowed to expand or become frayed (Fig. 36–9).

Although tendon washers are excellent devices to anchor tendon to bone, the application in the foot is limited because of the bulky nature of the instrument. Even with recession of the washer below the cortical surface, the prominence of the device in a subcutaneous position makes the application quite limited.

The advent of two new devices to anchor tendon into bone may have significant impact on the ability to secure tendon to osseous structures. Both innovations involve the insertion of a small metallic device directly into bone. There are sutures attached to the device that are then tied to the tendon. The Statak device is inserted by actually drilling it into the cortical bone by means of a screw-type mechanism. It is placed subcortically, and the suture is anchored below the cortical surface. The biggest disadvantage to this device is that the caliber of the suture is No. 2-0, which is quite large for many of the smaller tendons in the foot.

The Mitek device involves a springlike mechanism similar to a Molly bolt in which the device is placed subcortically through a previously placed drill hole. The spring-loaded arm on the anchor expands after insertion, thereby preventing extrusion from the bone (Fig. 36–10). Variable suture calibers and types are able to be attached to the anchor, which makes this device somewhat more versatile. The use of both devices greatly reduces operative time and eliminates the complications that result from drilling entirely through the midfoot.

Direct tendon-to-tendon anastomosis can be used to anchor the transferred tendon. Side-to-side attachment is the easiest

and most reliable technique, but any alternative tendon suture technique can be employed to complete the anastomosis. Regardless of the technique, it is recommended that a nonabsorbable suture be used.

SPECIFIC TENDON TRANSFERS

Split Tibialis Anterior Tendon Transfer

The *split tibialis anterior tendon transfer* is defined as a transfer that takes the lateral one half of the tibialis anterior tendon and moves it to a more lateral location on the dorsum of the foot. It was designed to balance out the dorsiflexion force of the anterior group of muscles. Although this procedure was usually performed in stroke patients for spastic equinovarus secondary to the cerebral vascular infarction, the procedure has been expanded to a variety of indications ranging from spasticity to dynamic biomechanically induced imbalances. It became popular in the treatment of cerebral palsy after studies in the laboratory of Hoffer and colleagues[29] showed that much of the deforming force causing equinovarus was attributed to the tibialis anterior. Other causes of imbalance are often created from an overactive or overpowering tibialis anterior muscle. This situation may be created by a weak or absent peroneus longus due to peroneal nerve injury or disease or an overactive tibialis anterior in the face of extensor substitution. As the anterior tibial muscle tries to overcome a shortened posterior group, it pulls more vigorously against the unyielding tether in the back of the leg; the result is a dynamic varus deformity that occurs during swing phase. Lateral metatarsal lesions, ankle instability, and lateral column overload are the resultant symptoms.

Indications. The indications for performance of a split tibialis anterior tendon transfer are usually an excessive supinatory force to the forefoot. In most instances, this involves excessive rotation about the longitudinal midtarsal joint axis and the subtalar joint axis. There may be an insufficiency of the lateral-most dorsiflexors, such as the EDL and EHL. Often, this imbalance is the result of trauma to the anterior compartment of the leg. Because the tibialis anterior is innervated much higher in the leg than are the latter two muscles, the tibialis anterior is often spared with injury to the lateral compartment. Open tibiofibular fractures are often responsible for the trauma.

Loss of peroneus longus and brevis strength or power can also result in an overpowering of the tibialis anterior. A rigid or flexible dorsiflexed first ray can accompany this imbalance. If the deformity is rigid, a plantar flexory procedure of the first metatarsal should also be performed.

Technique. The technique of the tibialis anterior tendon transfer is performed with the patient in the supine position. If a heel cord lengthening or posterior release procedure is needed, it should be performed before the tendon transfer. If possible, one should evaluate for the presence of a peroneus tertius preoperatively, which is present most of the time— this will serve as a convenient lateral anchoring point for the lateral slip of the tibialis anterior. Tourniquet control is preferred, but the procedure can be performed safely without hemostasis.

The first stage of the procedure is the harvesting of the tibialis anterior tendon at its insertion. A curvilinear incision is made along the course of the insertion of the tendon at the

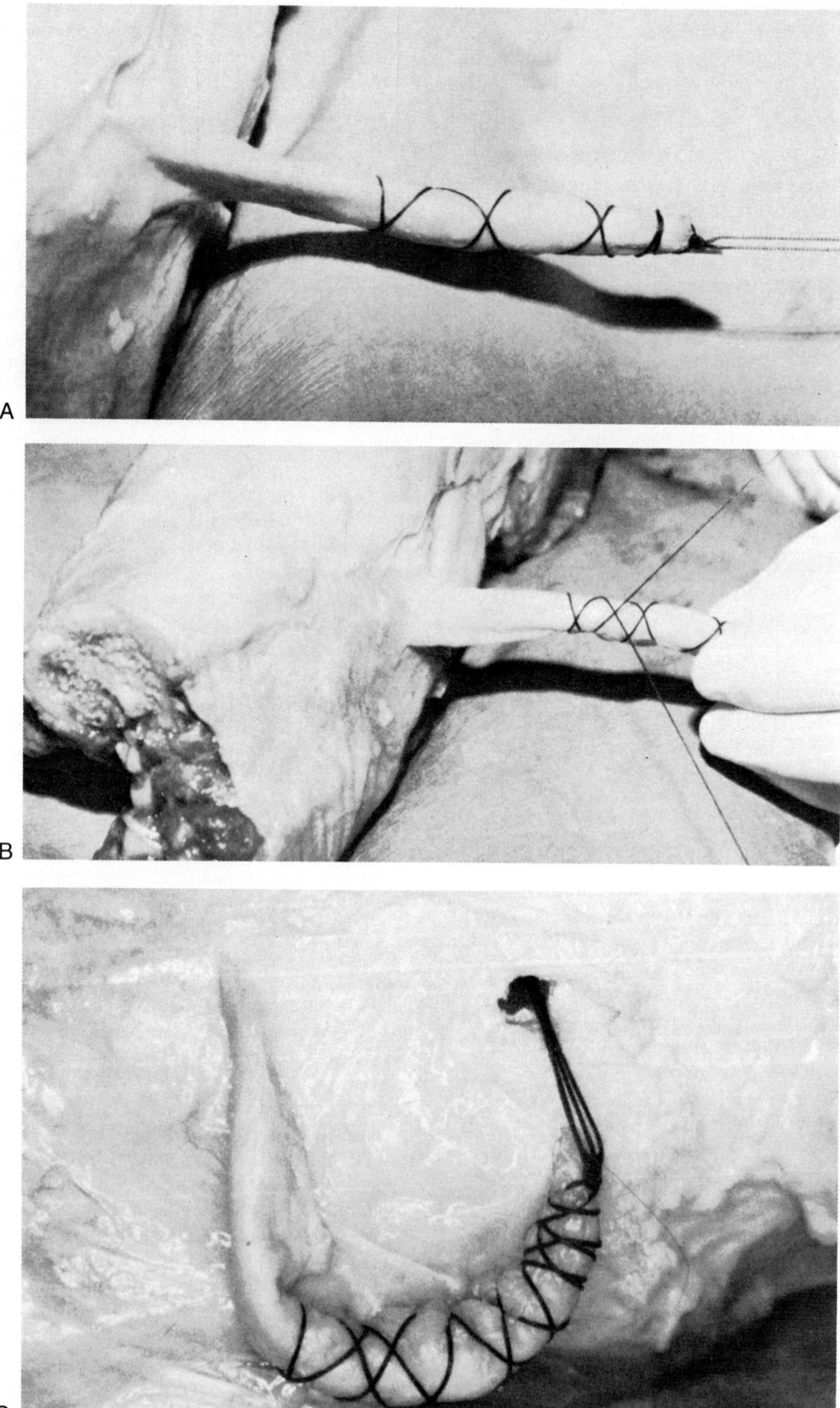

FIGURE 36–9. The technique for wrapping the tendon that is to be passed through a bone tunnel in the manner of the Chinese finger trap. *A,* Suture is wrapped about the distal end of the tendon and tied, leaving the ends long. *B,* A second suture is wrapped in a similar fashion but out of phase with the first. *C,* The Chinese finger trap suture in place. (From Krakow KA and Cohn BT: A new technique for passing tendon through bone. J Bone Joint Surg Am 69(6):922, 1987.)

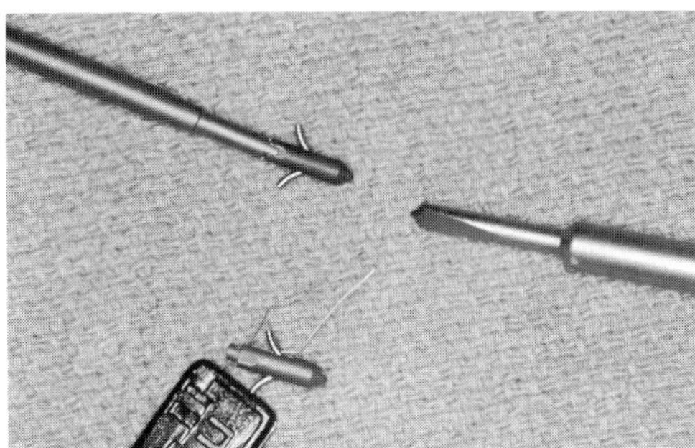

FIGURE 36–10. Mitek device. (Courtesy of Mitek Surgical Products, Inc., Norwood, MA.)

first metatarsal cuneiform joint. The tendon sheath is identified and split longitudinally. The tendon is captured by placing a hemostat clamp under the tendon (Fig. 36–11*A*). The tendon is then freed to the most distal part of its insertion. A Penrose drain or umbilical tape is placed around the tendon and then wrapped in a saline-moistened sponge.

The second stage of the procedure is the splitting of the tendon into medial and lateral portions. This is done approximately 2 or 3 cm above the level of the ankle joint directly over the tibialis anterior tendon. A linear incision is made over the tendon, and the synovial sheath is then incised. The tendon is retrieved with a clamp and delivered into the wound. Care must be taken not to twist the tendon abnormally while it is taken out of the sheath. I prefer to split the tendon from a proximal to distal direction to better ensure that the sections of tendon are of equal diameter. To accom-

plish this, a sharp scalpel blade is then used to divide the tendon into a medial and a lateral half with a stab incision. Two 10- to 12-cm lengths of umbilical tape are placed around the lateral portion of the tibialis anterior tendon (Fig. 36–11*B*). The tendon is split by placing a long uterine-packing forceps from distal to proximal from the distal wound. It is critical to place the forceps directly into the sheath of the tendon so that the tip of the packing forceps is visualized in the tendon sheath in the most proximal wound. The jaws are opened, and the ends of one of the slips of the umbilical tape are placed into the forceps. The forceps is then withdrawn from the distal wound, thereby pulling one of the umbilical tapes into the distal wound. The tape is grasped manually, and a strong, steady pull directly along the line of the tendon is performed. If the tape has not violated the boundaries of the tendon sheath by virtue of improper passage of the forceps, this maneuver should be accomplished without difficulty.

Other techniques, such as stainless steel wire or suture, can be used to split the tendon; however, I have found the umbilical tape method to be the most consistent and reproducible. Proximal-to-distal splitting is an important concept because it is the proximal end of the tendon that actually does the work of the transfer. If the tendon is split disproportionately, the resultant forces can be expected to be disproportionate. On the contrary, if the distal ends of the tendon are unequal, local or distant tissue grafts can be used to supplement the disparity.

Once the tendon is split, the lateral slip is dissected as far distal as possible. If any of the periosteum can be included in the lateral half of the tendon, it should be incorporated.

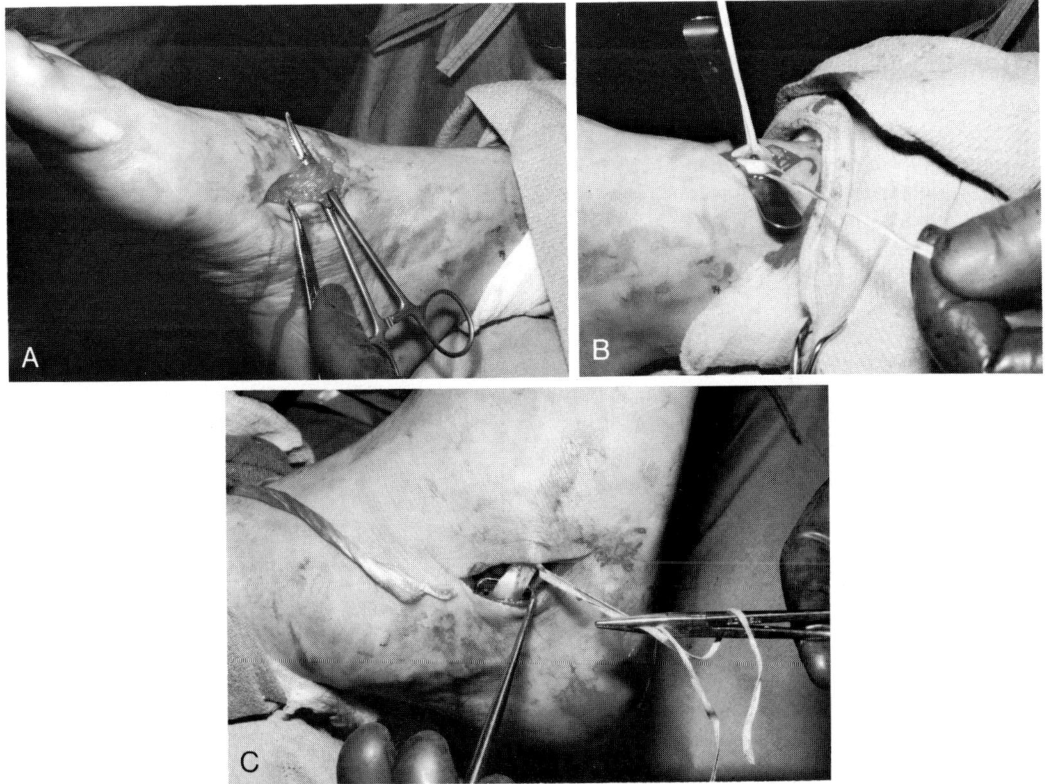

FIGURE 36–11. *A,* Intraoperative photograph showing the capture of the tibialis anterior tendon at its insertion. *B,* Intraoperative photograph showing the splitting of the tibialis anterior above the level of the ankle joint. *C,* The tendon is placed across the dorsum of the foot in the proposed line of action. In this case there is not enough length, thus the peroneus brevis is being prepared for acceptance of the lateral portion of the tendon.

The lateral tendon is then detached as far distal as possible. The tendon is then retrieved from the proximal wound by withdrawing the second remaining umbilical tape. The tendon portion is then checked for length by placing it on the skin in the line of the proposed path of action (Fig. 36–11C). It is usually aimed at the insertion of the peroneus tertius and the fifth metatarsal base. If there seems to be sufficient length, the anchoring point is prepared. The tendon half is wrapped in a saline-soaked sponge.

A third incision is made over the cuboid along the course of the peroneus tertius in a longitudinal fashion. The common tendon sheath of the peroneus tertius and EDL is then entered with a vertical incision. The same uterine-packing forceps are delivered into this sheath and directed proximal and aimed at the tibialis anterior tendon at the site where it was split proximally. It is essential to the success of the transfer to pass the tendon deep to the superior retinaculum. One should palpate the forceps under the retinaculum before passage of the tendon.

Although the EDL and tibialis anterior are adjacent to one another in the leg, the lateral aspect of the EDL sheath must be punctured to allow for passage of the lateral slip of the tibialis anterior tendon to the lateral side of the foot. It is essential that the forceps be passed to the level of the tibialis anterior within the sheath of the EDL. Once the tibialis anterior sheath is entered, the lateral slip is grasped and pulled into the distal lateral wound. If there is appropriate length of the tendon, it is anchored into the previously determined location. In most instances, it is sutured to the peroneus tertius if present. If there is no peroneus brevis, it can be anchored to the cuboid. Any technique can be used, but it is imperative to position the foot in the proper degree of pronation before attachment of the tendon slip. Neutrality is the desired attitude in most instances.

The concept of passing the tendon under the retinaculum in this procedure is credited to McGlamry and coworkers.[30] Their technique uses fundamental lever arm mechanics and is preferable to the subcutaneous technique described by Hoffer and colleagues.[29] In the latter technique, there is obvious bowstringing of the tendon in the subcutaneous tissue.

If there is not enough length to anchor the tendon to the cuboid or the peroneus tertius, a split graft of the insertion of the peroneus brevis is used (Fig. 36–11C). The sheath is opened, and the tendon is located and split with a scalpel. The most medial half is then detached proximally and anastomosed to the lateral half of the tibialis anterior. This effectively anchors the tibialis anterior to the fifth metatarsal base.

The sheaths are closed with a minimum of fine nonabsorbable suture. This decreases the amount of inflammatory response, which will hopefully reduce the tendency for postoperative adhesions. The rest of the closure is in routine fashion.

Postoperative Care. For the first several days after the surgical procedure, the patient is ambulating on crutches in a splint or cast that has been positioned in the pronated attitude.

Postoperative protocol then calls for a short-leg cast in which the patient can ambulate if there are no other procedures that would preclude this activity. Cast immobilization is then employed for a minimum of 6 weeks. One may elect to initiate gentle passive range-of-motion exercises at 4 weeks. To do this, a removable external immobilization device may be employed. However, if this latter approach is

chosen, the patient should be told that active contractions to the tibialis anterior are to be avoided at all costs for fear of destroying or compromising the transfer site. If the suture or anastomosis technique is tenuous, it may be pulled away and the effective muscle-tendon length relationship and the mechanical advantage of the transfer will be lost. In most instances, a supervised physical therapy program is necessary to avoid this event.

Complications. Aside from the usual complications of any surgery, there are several problems that are indigenous to this procedure. The most significant complication is failure for the transfer to function owing to iatrogenic passage of the tendon above the superior retinaculum. The transfer will function poorly because the lateral slip will adhere to the other structures. Revision surgery is possible, but the scarring in the area and on the tendon itself compromises the natural gliding excursion even if placed in the sheath properly the second time.

Damage to the peripheral nerves is also possible, especially near the lateral incision.[31] Although this is relatively rare, it is difficult to treat because of the repetitive trauma on the nerve from the tendon excursion.

Undercorrection of the varus is also a possible complication. It is usually seen when the surgeon has not recognized a fixed varus attitude in the preoperative evaluation. In that instance, the tendon transfer would be insufficient in overcoming the fixed bony deformity. The other cause of undercorrection is sewing the transferred slip under inadequate tension to the lateral structures.

Hibbs Tenosuspension

The Hibbs tenosuspension procedure redirects the effect of the EDL tendons from the lesser digits to the midfoot. The procedure is indicated for a well-defined set of clinical criteria.

Indications. Patients benefit from the Hibbs tenosuspension when there is extensor substitution during the swing phase of gait. There is usually a concomitant gastrocnemius or a gastrocnemius-soleus equinus that is addressed at the same time. Because of the effect of the extensor substitution, there are usually flexible hammertoes or mallet toes of the lesser digits and a reducible contracture at the lesser MTP joint. In addition, a flexible anterior cavus deformity is observed with the apex at the midtarsal joint. When the foot is loaded, the contractures reduce almost completely and return when the foot is non-weightbearing (Fig. 36–12). The deleterious effects of this imbalance then become manifest during the swing phase of gait as the patient actively overcontracts the EDL tendon, which causes buckling of the digits. The resultant pressure on the top of the shoe produces the clavi. As the foot becomes plantigrade, the digits have now caused a retrograde plantarflexion of the forefoot around the oblique axis of the midtarsal joint and the typical plantar metatarsalgia occurs.

This group of biomechanical aberrations is fairly consistent in presentation, with some minor variations. The clavus can be observed at either the distal or the proximal interphalangeal joint. The former is a more common occurrence. When plantar callosities are present, they almost always occur under the third metatarsal head, but careful clinical examination will not yield a true plantarflexed third metatarsal.

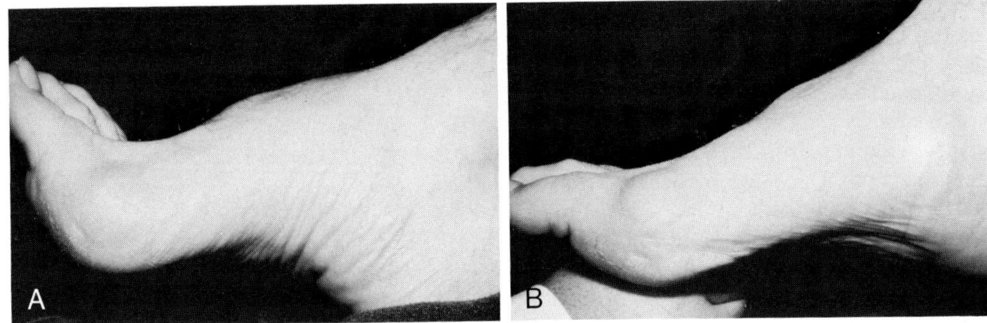

FIGURE 36–12. *A,* Foot with a flexible anterior cavus deformity in the nonloaded attitude. Note the contracture of the digits, and the relative cavus architecture. The apex of the deformity is at the midtarsal joint. *B,* Foot in the loaded attitude. Note the reduction of the digital and metatarsophalangeal joint contractures as well as the height of the arch.

Patients who have all or part of this clinical scenario are candidates for the Hibbs tenosuspension. The design of the procedure is such that it addresses all the destructive forces that occur. As mentioned earlier, the success of the procedure is heightened by eliminating the equinus deformity, usually with operative methods. Digital fusion procedures may also be necessary if some of the digital contractures have become fixed.

Technique. The technique of the Hibbs tenosuspension involves a curvilinear incision commencing at the base of the third and fourth toes that is concave medially. It courses over the fourth ray and ends at the fourth metatarsal cuboid joint (Fig. 36–13*A*). The incision is deepened through the subcu-

taneous tissue to the deep fascia. However, it is likely that the surgeon will encounter multiple nerve branches from the superficial peroneal nerve, especially the intermediate dorsal cutaneous component. Although it is preferable to spare these branches, it is often necessary to sacrifice them to obtain exposure. The skin and subcutaneous tissue are reflected off the underlying fascial layer, thereby exposing the EDL and brevis tendons. Starting from the second extensor tendon apparatus, the longus and brevis tendons are anastomosed together. However, it is critical to fully extend the respective digit to preserve some extensor capacity of the digit through the action of the short extensor on the extensor hood. The MTP joint should also be held in neutral before the anasto-

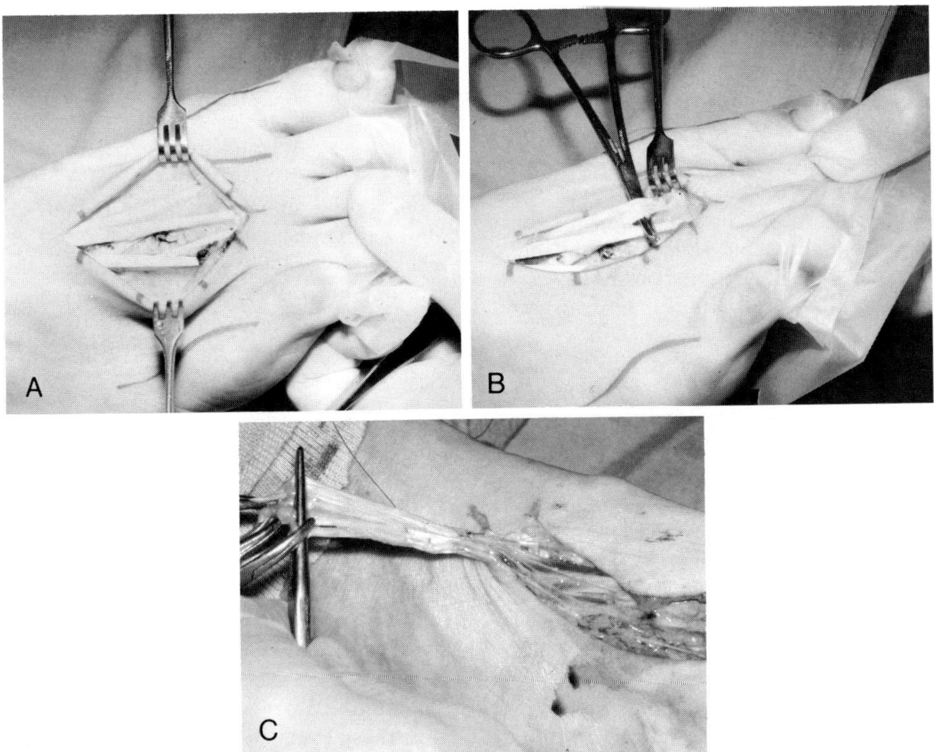

FIGURE 36–13. *A,* Intraoperative photograph showing the placement of the incision for the Hibbs tenosuspension. The skin and subcutaneous layer have been reflected off the tendons as a single layer. *B,* Both the long and short extensor tendons to the second toe have been isolated and are ready to be clamped together for anastomosis. Note that the interphalangeal joints are fully extended, and the metatarsophalangeal joint is held in neutral position before the two tendons are attached together. *C,* The four common extensors are being sewn from side to side to facilitate insertion into the midfoot. This is a different patient from the patient shown in *A* and *B*.

mosis is performed (Fig. 36–13*B*). A nonabsorbable or absorbable suture should be used to secure the longus to the brevis at or distal to the level of the MTP joint. It may be helpful to rough up the surfaces that are to be in contact to increase the chance of fibrosis and to secure attachment. This is easily accomplished with an Adson-Brown forceps or any instrument with multiple teeth. Once accomplished, the long extensor is severed just proximal to the point of attachment and retracted proximally. It is often necessary to use a scalpel or scissors to free up the tendon from the underlying sheath.

This process is repeated for the third and fourth tendon and digital structures, with each tendon being retracted to the proximal level of the incision. Each tendon is tagged with a clamp, alternating between curved and straight hemostats so that the correct order of the tendons can be determined later. Alternative methods of labeling the tendons can be used.

The fifth tendon is identified at the level of the fifth MTP joint and transected at this level. It is then delivered to the other tendons by sharp dissection. This tendon lies in a somewhat deeper plane and is slightly more difficult to isolate. Because it does not have a short extensor component, it is retracted without anastomosis. Loss of active extension of the fifth digit is of no significance from a functional standpoint.

The four long extensor stumps are then dissected proximally to at least the level of the third cuneiform and placed adjacent to one another in order of occurrence. A straight clamp is then placed across all the tendons, and they are sewn together in the form of a sheath by using a straight Keith needle. A stout suture is used from side to side. Once the suture is tightened, the four tendon stumps will roll into a common tubular or rod-shaped structure (Fig. 36–13*C*). Additional peripheral sutures may be placed to assist in maintaining the extensor tendons in a tubular shape. It is then wrapped in a saline-soaked sponge for later transfer into the midfoot. An alternative technique is use of the modified Chinese finger trap suture.[28]

The third cuneiform is exposed by reflecting the extensor digitorum brevis muscle to the medial or lateral side. Care must be taken to isolate all the bony boundaries of the third cuneiform. This will prevent iatrogenic violation of the intercuneiform joints, the cuneometatarsal joints, or the naviculo-cuneiform joint during drilling of the hole into which the tendons will be passed.

Once the cuneiform and its boundaries have been isolated, a ¼- or ⅜-in. drill is used to drill a hole completely through the cuneiform from dorsal to plantar. Because the cuneiform is oriented in an oblique fashion, the drill should be oriented in a similar manner to facilitate through-and-through drilling of the bone. Although there is negligible movement between the intertarsal joints, iatrogenic violation of the articular surfaces should be avoided if at all possible (Fig. 36–14). The tendon is then passed plantarly through the midfoot and secured either to a button on the plantar aspect of the foot or to the midfoot through some other suitable method.

Postoperative Care. Postoperative care involves a short-leg walking cast for 6 weeks unless additional procedures preclude weightbearing. Physical therapy may be instituted after the period of immobilization.

Complications. Complications from the Hibbs procedure are uncommon but predictable. In the earlier stages of performing this procedure, the incision was curved to a much higher degree than is now described. A higher incidence of

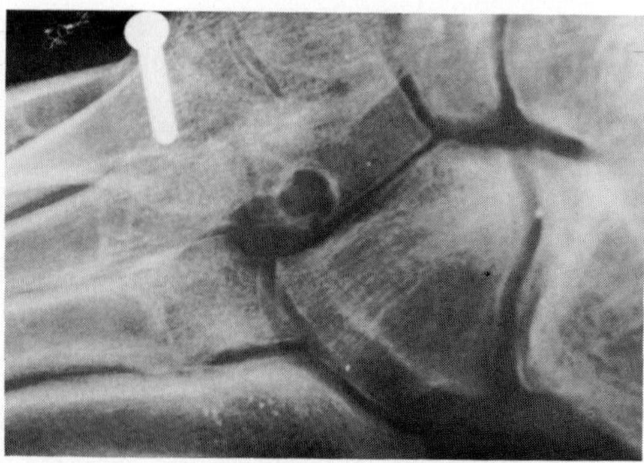

FIGURE 36–14. Postoperative radiograph in which the drill hole has been placed too close to the lateral cortex. Note the cortical break in the cuneiform. This patient had no symptoms relative to this finding.

central wound sloughs was observed that usually resolved with local wound care. One can also minimize wound complications by careful elevation of the skin flaps with a thick layer of subcutaneous tissue. Prolonged use of self-retaining retractors on this delicate skin layer must be avoided.

Gradual development of mallet toes may ensue in some patients for several reasons. If the gastrocnemius equinus has been released, there may be a period of posterior group weakness that would result in flexor substitution. This can also occur if the Achilles tendon was overlengthened. This imbalance, coupled with a weakened extensor complex, can predispose to mallet toe formation. This complication may be slightly more prevalent in those patients who have had concomitant digital fusions of the proximal interphalangeal joint because the mechanical advantage of the FDL is increased by virtue of the longer lever arm. Mallet toes are best prevented by proper maintenance of the digit in extension before anastomosis of the long and short digital extensors. When they occur, early treatment with flexor tenotomy may prevent the deformity from becoming rigid.

Limitation of plantar flexion of the foot at the ankle may occur if the transferred EDL complex is attached to the midfoot in a shortened attitude. Careful attention to establishment of physiologic tension minimizes this tendency.

Violation of the intertarsal articulations is also a possible complication. However, it is usually not a clinically significant event owing to the relative lack of motion available at these joints.

Posterior Tibial Transfer

The posterior tibial tendon transfer is a useful technique in most patients who have a paralytic drop foot or a dynamic equinovarus foot. It is most commonly employed for the treatment of the paralytic drop foot deformity when there is little or poor function of the anterior group muscles. The technique was first published by Watkins and associates[32] in 1954, but there are now several variations, depending on the specific functional needs and the condition being treated.[33–35]

In most instances, the posterior tibial tendon transfer involves the conversion of the muscle-tendon unit from a stance-phase supinator of the foot to a stance-phase dorsi-flexor of the foot. The passage of the tendon is usually through the interosseous membrane, although it can be passed to the front of the leg by going around the anterior crest of the tibia. In other well-defined situations, the tendon can be split to weaken the force of the tendon on the navicular tuberosity. In those instances, the split tendon is usually rerouted around the back of the leg to the lateral side of the foot.

Indications. As mentioned earlier, there are two clinical situations when consideration for transfer of the tibialis posterior tendon is appropriate. The most common is the patient who presents with a deficit in ankle dorsiflexion for any reason. The deficit may range from a mild slapfoot gait to that of a profound paralytic drop foot. Owing to the wide variability of involvement of most neurologic diseases, patients usually present somewhere along the continuum described.

The second indication for posterior tibial tendon transfer is spastic equinovarus due to the hyperactive muscle. Similarly, many diseases can present with focal or more widespread spastic states that adversely impact normal gait. This is usually mediated by overpowering of the antagonist muscles by the spastic muscle. Even though there is a dynamic imbalance, the antagonist muscles may be neurologically and physiologically normal. The principle of tibialis posterior transfer, then, is to redirect the forces of the spastic muscle so that it will provide movement of the osseous segments that facilitate rather than hinder normal gait mechanics.

Technique. The technique that I most favor is the transfer through the interosseous membrane. This procedure gives the transferred tendon the most direct line of pull to the midfoot to assist in dorsiflexion. Maximization of the mechanical advantage of the tendon transfer enhances both the long-term and short-term results. It is critical when the transferred tendon is going to be the only muscle to supply dorsiflexion power to the foot. I have little experience with the technique of passing the tendon around the anterior crest of the tibia.[13] However, it is difficult to conceive how this arrangement would be able to establish clinically useful dorsiflexion in the face of a weak anterior compartment. The only advantage of this method is the relative ease in performing the procedure compared with the following method.

The procedure is performed in the supine position after any posterior lengthening procedures have been carried out. Because Achilles tendon lengthening and posterior release are often necessary, I find it much easier and safer to initiate the operation with the patient in the prone position where the appropriate components of the triceps surae, ankle, and subtalar joints are released or lengthened. The wound should be closed, and a temporary dressing is applied. The patient is then repositioned in the supine attitude and prepared and draped again.

The procedure begins with a curvilinear incision over the insertion of the tibialis posterior at the navicular. The convexity is superiorly based. The tendon is retracted from the wound with an umbilical tape and followed to the navicular tuberosity. A scalpel is used to make an osteoperiosteal flap off the navicular to ensure maximal length of the tendon end (Fig. 36–15). It is freed sharply from the navicular. The most distal attachments of the tibialis posterior should not be disturbed.

A second incision 10 cm in length is then made over the medial aspect of the leg just anterior to the saphenous neurovascular bundle at the junction of the middle and distal one third of the leg. The deep fascia is exposed by retracting the saphenous vein and nerve posteriorly in its protective subcutaneous layer (Fig. 36–15B). The gastrocnemius and soleus are retracted posteriorly. The deep fascia is incised longitudinally, and the deep posterior compartment is then entered (Fig. 36–15C).

The tibialis posterior is located between the flexor hallucis longus (FHL) and the FDL. Careful isolation of the FDL from the tibialis posterior muscle belly exposes the tibialis posterior tendon. A blunt instrument is then used to encircle and secure the tendon of the tibialis posterior. The surgeon's index finger or a 0.75-in. Penrose drain is then placed around the tendon, and firm but gentle traction is placed on the tendon (Fig. 36–15D). Gradual force is applied to the tendon to pull it from its deep location. Caution should be exercised owing to the close proximity of the posterior tibial neurovascular bundle and the peroneal artery that lie just lateral to the tibialis posterior tendon and muscle.

In most instances, the vast origin of the muscle from the lower portions of the interosseous membrane and the tibia gives rise to multiple muscular processes. This may complicate the retrieval of the tendon from the distal part of the leg. Excessive trauma to the muscle belly can be avoided by gentle separation of the distal attachments from their origins. It may also be necessary to free up the distal end of the tendon if the tendon cannot be retracted easily from the wound. It is easily accomplished by passing Metzenbaum scissors into the posterior tendon sheath from below. If retrieval is still not possible, it is necessary to extend either the proximal or distal wound to detach any remaining adherent areas. Once the tendon can be retrieved out of the leg, it is wrapped in a saline-soaked sponge (Fig. 36–15E).

Next, the approach for passage of the tendon to the anterior compartment of the leg is done. A third incision is made over the anterior compartment approximately 8 cm in length, slightly inferior to the incision over the posterior compartment. It is made just lateral to the belly of the tibialis anterior, centering the incision over the EDL. The deep fascia is exposed and then incised longitudinally. The interval between the EHL and the EDL is developed and deepened to the interosseous membrane. The anterior tibial artery should be retracted medially with the EHL tendon. The surgeon then places an index finger on the interosseous membrane from the anterior compartment approach and the opposite index finger on the interosseous membrane from the posterior approach so that only the interosseous membrane is palpated. The passageway for the transferred tendon is created by using blunt-tipped scissors from either wound and directing it at the opposite finger. Once penetration of the membrane is accomplished, the scissor tips are spread and the window is created. It becomes readily apparent that creation of the window to pass the tendon to the front of the leg is shaped more like a slit in the membrane rather than a large opening. Nevertheless, the muscle and tendon have ample room to function if the procedure is performed properly.

A clamp is then placed through the window from front to back, and the tendon is grasped and pulled through the interosseous membrane. It is important to ensure that muscle fibers are in direct contact with the opening of the membrane. If not, the tendon is likely to adhere to the interosseous membrane and hinder the tendinous excursion.[32, 36] The tendon is then pulled through the interval between the EHL and the EDL. It should be wrapped in a saline-soaked sponge for later use (Fig. 36–15F).

A fourth incision is made over the site where the tendon

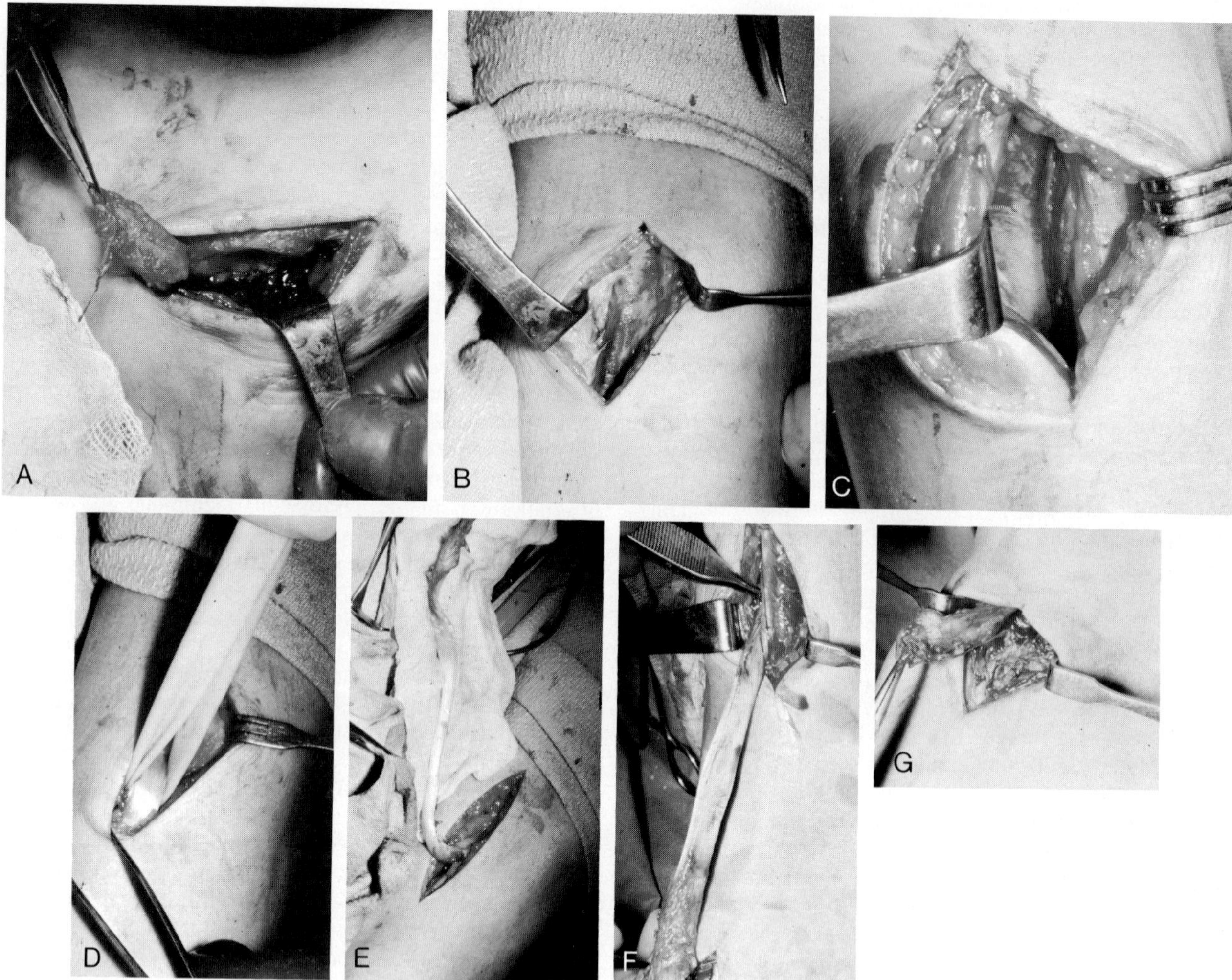

FIGURE 36–15. *A,* Intraoperative photograph of the posterior tibial tendon after it has been harvested from the navicular tuberosity. As much length as possible has been preserved. *B,* The saphenous neurovascular bundle in the subcutaneous layer. *C,* The saphenous neurovascular bundle has been retracted posteriorly, and the deep fascial compartment has been entered. The gastrocnemius and soleus are being retracted off the posterior compartment. *D,* The Penrose drain is now encircling the posterior tibial tendon ready for retrieval. Alternate manipulations of the distal and proximal wounds will aid in mobilization of the tendon. *E,* The tendon is now retrieved from the distal wound into the proximal wound ready for transfer through the interosseous membrane. *F,* The tendon has been passed from the posterior aspect of the leg to the anterior compartment. The tendon is bound by the extensor digitorum longus and by the extensor hallucis longus muscle bellies. *G,* The tendon is now located at the third cuneiform area after being rerouted along the tendon sheath of the extensor digitorum longus. It is now ready for attachment into the bone.

will be anchored. It is usually preferable to transfer the tendon to the third cuneiform, because this is considered to be the center of the foot. It is also an appropriate location to obtain eversion around both the longitudinal and the oblique axes of the midtarsal joint. This necessitates a longitudinal incision over the extensor hallucis brevis muscle belly. Once the muscle belly is identified, it is retracted to one side, depending on the orientation of the fibers. Sharp elevation may be necessary to visualize the third cuneiform. Adequate dissection needs to be performed to visualize the entire boundary of the third cuneiform. This is similar to the technique that is used for the Hibbs tenosuspension.

The sheath of the EDL tendons is located. A uterine-packing forceps is then inserted into the distal aspect of the sheath and passed superior to the ankle joint. One should make certain that the forceps is passed under the superior retinaculum. The tips of the forceps should exit the superior wound at the level that the tendon passes to the front of the leg. It then passes laterally to puncture the septum between

the EDL and the EHL. The free end of the tibialis posterior tendon is grasped and pulled into the sheath of the EDL. The tendon is then transferred to the dorsum of the foot by exiting below the ankle joint and into the area of the third cuneiform (Fig. 36–15*G*).

A ¼- or ⅜-in. drill is used to fashion a channel for insertion of the tibialis posterior to the midfoot. The tendon is attached under physiologic tension and tied to a button on the bottom of the foot. If tourniquet control was used, the cuff is released to assess any iatrogenic damage to the major vascular structures and to control any residual bleeding. The wounds are closed in layers, and a short-leg cast is applied in the operating room, with the foot at 90 degrees of dorsiflexion at the ankle.

Although several authors[33–35] have described modifications to the technique to prevent the creation of a varus or valgus deformity, I have found it unnecessary to split the tendon to balance the foot as long as there is no other predominant, albeit weakened, muscle that supplies dorsiflexor power. In those instances, the tendon may be split or moved medially or laterally to compensate for any other muscular activity. Anchoring of the tendon into the third cuneiform takes advantage of the oblique axis of the midtarsal joint and serves to dorsiflex the foot by locking first at the midtarsal joint and then at the ankle.

Postoperative Care. The patient is immobilized with a short-leg cast for approximately 6 to 8 weeks. If concomitant procedures do not preclude weightbearing, progressive weightbearing is allowed after a few weeks of non-weightbearing. Gentle passive range of motion exercises are initiated at 2 to 3 weeks postoperatively. This can be facilitated with a removable short-leg cast.

At 6 weeks postoperatively, the patient can be started on phasic transfer exercises, which may be quite extensive. These exercises should be supervised by a therapist specifically trained in these techniques.

Complications. Significant complications can result from the performance of the tibialis posterior tendon transfer. The most devastating is damage to either of the neurovascular bundles that are encountered during the procedure. Although injury to the vessels is usually detected intraoperatively, injury to the nerve may be a latent discovery. Although the diagnosis of neural damage may be relatively easy, the treatment may present some difficulty because of the limited accessibility and the potential need for reoperation.

Failure of the transfer to function as expected may be due to a number of reasons. First, the tendon may not function during its desired swing phase of gait in spite of aggressive preoperative and postoperative rehabilitation. In this situation, the best that can be hoped for is a functional tenodesis that may provide some passive dorsiflexion. However, this is quite uncommon in the patient who has a spastic neurologic component. One must be sure that the reason for failure is physiologic problems and not technical mistakes. These can include passage of the tendon outside existing tendon sheaths, damage to the branches of the nerve supplying the muscle, or restriction of the excursion of the tendon at the site of passage from the posterior to the anterior compartment.

Lack of plantarflexion may also be realized when the tendon is anchored under excessive tension. This is usually not a significant problem with regard to ambulation, but it is often disconcerting to the patient.

Inadequate correction is seldom observed but is usually due to performance of the procedure in the face of irreducible bony deformities.

In the more mobile foot, gradual collapse of the midfoot may be a consequence of the loss of the tibialis posterior tendon stabilizing force on the talonavicular joint. This is akin to the acute or attritional rupture of the tibialis posterior tendon and is best remedied with an orthotic device in most instances. In the more symptomatic patients, talonavicular fusion or another hindfoot stabilization procedure is indicated.

Of those patients in whom the procedure was done for correction of spastic or flaccid equinus, a significant percentage will develop digital deformities, assuming the equinus deformity was addressed. Keenan and colleagues[37] reported a 78% incidence of new digital deformities in 41 feet corrected for spastic equinovarus deformities. With the new dorsiflexed attitude of the foot, the flexor tendons are now placed on stretch. This often results in flexion deformities of the digits at the interphalangeal level. This situation may be further complicated in the spastic patient by concomitant spasticity of the FDL, the FHL, or intrinsic musculature (Fig. 36–16).

Split Tibialis Posterior Tendon Transfer

Indications. The split tibialis posterior tendon transfer is indicated in the patient with cerebral palsy who has spastic activity of the tibialis posterior tendon.[38] The typical equinovarus gait is observed with activity of the posterior tibial during both swing and stance phases of gait. The lateral aspect of the forefoot is usually observed to strike the ground first during weight acceptance. There is also lateral instability of the entire stance phase of gait.

If there are no adaptive bony changes, this procedure is preferred in lieu of a formal tibialis posterior tendon transfer or a posterior tibial tendon lengthening. The problem of the unpredictability with transfer of entire spastic muscle is circumvented by this technique. In addition, recurrence of the deformity is much less likely with the split transfer than with simple lengthening of the tendon. The basic premise of the procedure is the application of the spastic condition of the muscle to balance the hindfoot. Most of the patients who are candidates for this procedure also require triceps surae lengthening procedures.

Technique. The basic procedure differs from the transfer of the entire muscle in that it does not pass anterior to the ankle joint axis. The tendon is prepared for splitting by making a curvilinear incision along the course of the tibialis posterior tendon from distal to the medial malleolus to the navicular. The sheath is opened and the tendon identified. A second incision 4 to 5 cm in length is made just posterior to the medial tibial crest, commencing 4 cm superior to the medial malleolus. The deep fascia is opened, and the tibialis posterior tendon is retrieved. The tendon is divided into a posterior and an anterior portion using a stab incision in the

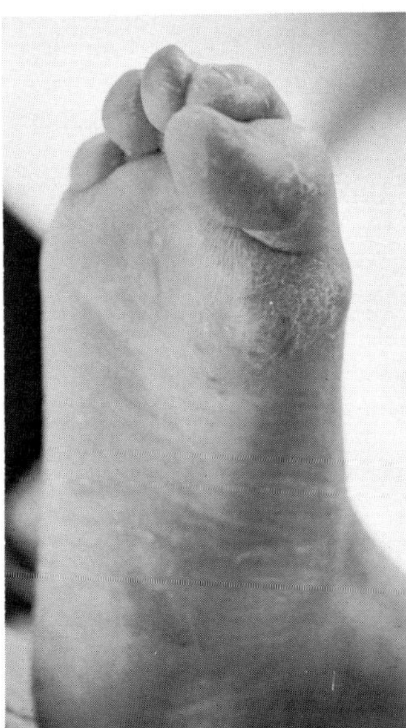

FIGURE 36–16. Plantar view in a patient who underwent tibialis posterior tendon transfer for spastic cerebral palsy. Note the development of new digital deformities of the toes and the hallux.

proximal wound. The stab incision should be made just distal to the myotendinous junction so that maximal length of the tendon can be transferred and the line of pull can be initiated from the most proximal point. Umbilical tape is placed around the posterior portion. The tendon is split by passing uterine-packing forceps or other long instruments from the distal to the proximal wound along the course of the tendon sheath. The umbilical tape is grasped, and the uterine-packing forceps is withdrawn, thereby splitting the tendon into the posterior and the anterior halves. The posterior stump is detached sharply from the navicula and is then pulled out of the proximal wound.

The third incision is made over the peroneal sheath superior to the lateral malleolus for a distance of 4 or 5 cm. The sheath is opened, and the peroneus brevis tendon is found. A tunnel is made directly behind the tibia and fibula that is anterior to the soft tissues. The posterior half of the tibialis posterior tendon is passed to the lateral side of the foot via this tunnel. The tendon slip is grasped and then sewn to the peroneus brevis tendon. Although two prior discussions[24, 25] on this technique describe anchorage of the tibialis posterior tendon to the peroneus brevis distal to the fibula, it is usually not necessary to perform the anastomosis at this level. I favor the modification proposed by Median and coworkers,[39] which involves the attachment of the tendon to the peroneus brevis well proximal to the fibular malleolus. This modification prevents another incision and avoids crowding of the peroneal groove and the tendon sheath. The most important aspect of this maneuver is to make sure that the transferred end of the tibialis posterior is running in a direct line to its distal target. This is best accomplished by splitting the tendon all the way up to its superior extent.

Regardless of the technique chosen, the tendon is sewn under the appropriate tension with the foot in a neutral or slightly overcorrected attitude.

An alternative surgical approach has been described using a Cincinnati-type incision.[40] I have not tried this approach, but the authors stated that the intraoperative vision is improved and the scar is more cosmetically acceptable.

Postoperative Care. A short-leg cast is applied with the foot in the overcorrected position and left in place for 6 weeks. After the cast is removed, the patient is allowed to bear weight as tolerated. Most of the patients in the reported series in the literature obtained good results.[21, 22] Most of the poor or fair results were consequences of technical error. Two groups of investigators[20, 21] found that the electromyographic patterns of the tibialis posterior did not change after the operation. This would be expected in the spastic muscle that is simply split and transferred. However, this procedure takes advantage of this property by converting the hyperactivity to a corrective balancing force rather than a destructive one.

Anterior Advancement of the Achilles Tendon

The anterior advancement of the Achilles tendon, the so-called Murphy procedure, was first described in the English literature by Pierrot and Murphy in 1974.[41] (Murphy had been performing the procedure since 1959.) However, Esteve[42] first published a description of this procedure in 1936. The procedure evolved through a realization of a certain failure rate following Achilles tendon lengthening procedures in children with cerebral palsy. It is well established that spastic conditions that are treated with tendon lengthenings are often helped on a temporary basis and are subject to recurrence of the deformity. This can be mediated by growth of the extremity when the triceps surae crosses the three epiphyseal plates of the lower extremity. The Murphy procedure alters the mechanical advantage of the triceps surae complex without changing the length of the Achilles tendon. By transferring the insertion of the Achilles tendon forward or more anterior, the muscle serves as a shunt muscle more than as a spurt muscle. The problem of recurrence is lessened because the lever arm is lessened, and the tendon substance itself is undisturbed. In addition, if one realizes that spasticity is accompanied by a lack of inhibition of the stretch reflex, the alteration of the lever arm will also diminish the tendency to set off the hyperactive stretch reflex that precipitates recurrence.

Indications. The indications for use of the anterior advancement of the Achilles tendon have been broadened since the inception of the procedure. Pierrot and Murphy[41] applied the procedure to children with spastic equinus from cerebral palsy for reasons discussed earlier. The indications currently also include any other fixed spastic neurologic deficit from other diseases or injuries in the pediatric population. Although the problem of open epiphyseal plates contributes to the possibility of recurrence in the younger age group, it is not a problem in the skeletally mature group. The procedure has a limited, but definite, place in the management of spastic equinus in the adult patient. The most opportune situation to use the procedure in adults is in the stroke patient who has developed spastic equinus. Although many of these patients are best managed with AFO, there are some patients who are not braceable due to the existence of insurmountable equinus caused by a lack of postinfarction bracing or prolonged convalescence. In many of these patients, the ability to ambulate efficiently is compromised by the persistence of equinus. Balance is affected because of the toe-toe gait, and the ambulatory capacity is lessened. Restoration of a plantigrade foot with damping of the hyperactive stretch reflex can be quite effective in the establishment of a slow but stable gait.

The patient should be examined for any fixed compensatory deformities, especially if he or she has ambulated with a spastic equinus for a long period before surgery. Sagittal and frontal plane compensations may be well tolerated by the patient preoperatively. Advancement of the heel cord allows for a plantigrade foot, but the patient may tolerate this poorly due to the fixed suprastructural conditions. The most obvious example is the compensation that occurs from a long-standing equinus at the level of the spinal column. By effectively shortening the surgical leg, the patient may have acute symptoms due to the abrupt correction of the compensatory limb-length discrepancy. Other compensatory mechanisms are equally at risk for acute exacerbation after reduction of the functional limb-length unequally.

Technique. The procedure is performed with the patient in the prone position with the foot free over the end of the operating table. Tourniquet control is optional but preferred. A longitudinal incision is placed along the medial border of the Achilles tendon, which then curves slightly anterior at its distal end. Thick flaps are developed that include the skin and subcutaneous tissue in a single layer. They are reflected off the underlying Achilles tendon and the paratenon. The

41. Pierrot AH and Murphy OB: Heel cord advancement: A new approach to the spastic equinus deformity. Orthop Clin North Am 5:117, 1974.
42. Esteve R: Un procede d'equilibration des pieds spastidae. La Vie Medicale 1:51, 1936.
43. Throop FB, DeRosa GP, Reeck C, and Waterman S: Correction of equinus in cerebral palsy by the Murphy procedure of tendo calcaneus advancement: A preliminary communication. Dev Med Child Neurol 17:182, 1975.
44. Downey MS: Ankle equinus. *In* McGlamry ED (ed): Comprehensive Textbook of Foot Surgery. Baltimore, Williams & Wilkins, 1987, p 392.
45. Sharrard WJW and Bernstein S: Equinus deformity in cerebral palsy. J Bone Joint Surg 54B:272, 1972.
46. Jones R: Arthrodesis and tendon transplantation. Br Med J 1:728, 1908.
47. Jones R: The soldier's foot and the treatment of common deformities of the foot. Br Med J 1:749, 1916.
48. McGlamry ED: Unfavorable long-term results in the Jones metatarsal suspension. J Am Podiatr Med Assoc 65:479, 1975.
49. Green WT and Grice DS: The management of calcaneus deformity. Am Acad Orthop Surg Instructional Course Lectures 13:135–149, 1956.
50. Bickel WH and Moe JH: Translocation of the peroneus longus tendon for paralytic calcaneus deformity of the foot. Surg Gynecol Obstet 78:627, 1944.
51. Makin M and Vossipovitch A: Translocation of the peroneus longus in the treatment of paralytic pes calcaneus: A follow-up study of thirty-three cases. J Bone Joint Surg 48A:1541, 1966.
52. White RK and Kraynick BM: Surgical uses of the peroneus brevis tendon. Surg Gynecol Obstet 108, 117, 1959.
53. Schuberth JM: Management of Achilles tendon trauma. *In* Scurran BL (Ed): Foot and Ankle Trauma. New York, Churchill Livingstone, 1989, pp 214–215.

Bibliography

Chick LR and Walton RL: A history of tendon operations. Surg Gyncol Obstet 168:183, 1989.
Fulford GE, Veldman HJ, and Stewart K: Dynamic inversion of the forefoot and dorsiflexion of the big toe treated by transfer of extensor hallucis longus. J Bone Joint Surg 71B:21, 1989.
Johnson WL and Lester WL: Transposition of the posterior tibial tendon. Clin Orthop 245:223, 1989.
Jones JR, Smibert JG, McCullough CH, et al: Tendon implantation into bone: An experimental study. J Hand Surg [Br] 12:306, 1987.
Kaufman KR, An KN, and Chao EY: Incorporation of muscle architecture into the muscle length-tension relationship. J Biomech 22:943, 1989.
Lagast J, Mylle J, and Fabry G: Posterior tibial transfer in spastic equinovarus. Arch Orthop Trauma Surg 108:100, 1989.
Loitz BJ, Zernicke RJ, Vailas AC, et al: Effects of short-term immobilization versus continuous passive motion on the biomechanical and biochemical properties of the rabbit tendon. Clin Orthop 244:265, 1989.
Pandey AK, Pandey S, and Prasad V: Calcaneal osteotomy and tendon sling for the management of calcaneus deformity. J Bone Joint Surg 71:1192, 1989.
Pinzur MS, Kett N, and Trilla M: Combined anteroposterior tibial tendon transfer in post-traumatic peroneal palsy. Foot Ankle 8:229, 1988.
Richard BM: Interosseous transfer of tibialis posterior for common peroneal nerve palsy. J Bone Joint Surg 71B:834, 1989.
Roper BA: The orthopedic management of the stroke patient. Clin Orthop 219:78, 1987.
Roper BA and Tibrewal SB: Soft tissue surgery in Charcot-Marie-Tooth disease. J Bone Joint Surg 71B:17–20, 1989.
Wijesinha SS and Menalaus MB: Operation for calcaneus deformity after surgery of club foot. J Bone Joint Surg 71B:234, 1989.

CHAPTER 37

Role of Arthroscopy in the Treatment of Arthritic Ankle Disorders

Richard O. Lundeen, D.P.M.

ANATOMY OF THE ANKLE

Cartilage

Cartilage is a unique, specialized tissue responsible for the primary functions of the joint: motion and shock absorption. Articular cartilage has no blood supply, nerves, or blood vessels. It receives nourishment mainly from the synovial fluid and, to some extent, from the underlying subchondral bone on which it rests. Because it has no nerves, damage to cartilage goes highly undetected unless or until the surrounding bone, capsule, synovium, or ligaments are involved.

Hyaline cartilage consists mainly of type II collagen fibers between which is ground substance or matrix. Chondrocytes are sparsely interspersed within the matrix. New cartilage is formed by chondrocytes, which are more numerous in the deeper layers of cartilage. In the adult, the mitotic ability of the chondrocyte is retained but, because of their sparsity within the matrix and dependence on synovial fluid for nourishment, the ability of cartilage to heal is poor, especially in the presence of an ongoing disease process. Response to injury depends on the level at which cartilage is damaged. Superficial lesions that do not extend to the subchondral bone do not heal because of the acellularity of cartilage and subsequent lack of inflammatory response. It is only the deeper layers that involve the subchondral bone plate that will heal, because, in these instances, good vascularity is present, allowing for fibrin clot formation.

The resistive, elastic properties of hyaline cartilage are due to the combination of proteoglycan aggregates and type II collagen fibers that are contained within a sponge-like network. A proteoglycan molecule is able to bind large amounts of water. With compression, the proteoglycan molecule, which exists as a long chain, compresses. Opposing links of this proteoglycan chain consist of anionic molecules, which, when compressed, oppose one another, thereby resisting the force. This gives cartilage its elastic properties.

The resistive properties of cartilage come from the arrangement of collagen fibrils. These exist as large loops of type II collagen anchored in subchondral bone just below the zone of calcified cartilage. This zone, also known as the tidemark because of its basophilic staining properties, is also the level at which vascularity exists. At the upper surface of cartilage, the collagen loops intertwine, forming a tangential layer above the deeper vertical layer. At the surface of cartilage, a closely packed, horizontal layer protects the structure. It is these three layers of cartilage that make up its unique properties. Any disorganization can be termed *arthritis*.

Subchondral Bone

The main supporting structure of hyaline articular cartilage is the subchondral bone. It provides the anchor into which the deep vertical fibers of collagen attach and is the closest source of vascularization for nourishment of the chondrocyte and source of repair for cartilage. Any change in the subchondral bone will affect the cartilage by altering its ability to bear loads or by decreasing its nourishment. Also, any change in the cartilage can affect the subchondral bone by altered load-bearing characteristics, inducing sclerosis or exposure to enzymatic degradation. In either event, any change in the subchondral bone plate will elicit pain because this is the point at which the nerves terminate before the cartilaginous zones.

Capsule

The joint capsule completely surrounds but does not isolate the joint as a separate body cavity. The capsule is continuous with the periosteum covering bone and consists largely of fibrous tissue with some elastic fibers contained within it. Its vascularity comes from the adjacent bone and forms an arterial circle around the joint. Nerves are present and consist of both sensory and autonomic fibers. Small sensory fibers are responsible for forming pain endings, whereas larger sensory fibers form proprioceptive endings responsible for detecting motion and position.

Because the ligaments that support the ankle joint are usually vested or in close association with the capsule, they share similar nerve and vascular arrangements.

The combined fibrous and somewhat elastic nature of the capsule makes it extremely resistant to stretching and tearing. Because of the abundance of sensory nerve endings contained within it, the capsule is important because any alteration in its structure or function will produce sensation that is perceived as pain.

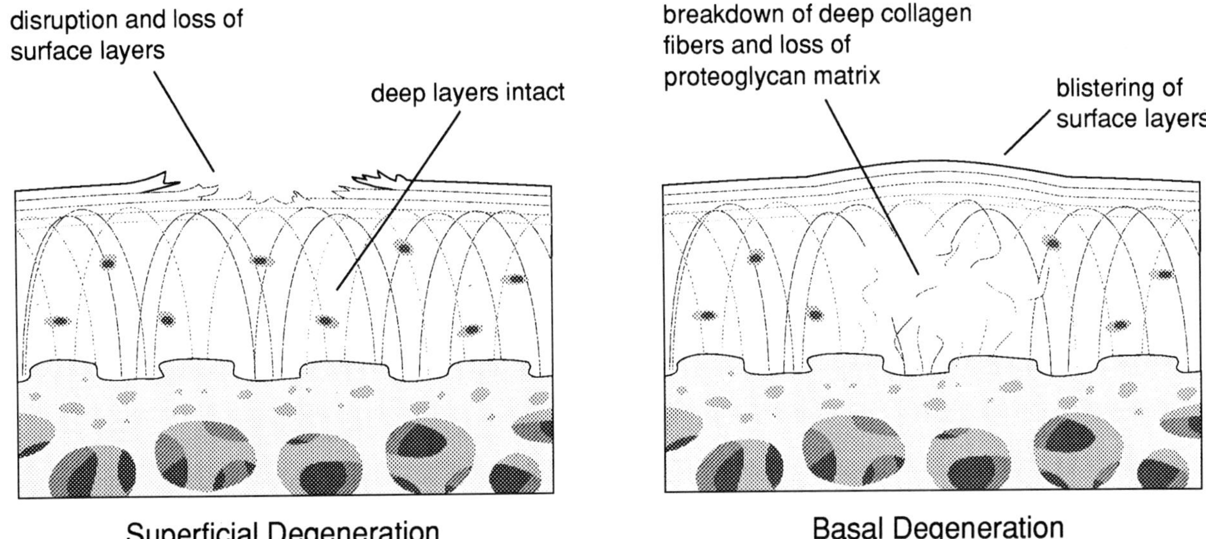

FIGURE 37–1. Types of degeneration of cartilage, based on Goodfellow's classification of chondromalacia. Disruption of the upper layer begins superficial degeneration, whereas disruption of the tangential and deep layers leaving the superficial layer intact initiates basal degeneration.

Synovium

Lining the interior of the capsule is a continuation of the cambium layer of periosteum, termed the *synovium*. A highly vascular tissue, it lines the capsule and intra-articular ligaments. It does not cover the cartilage. Specialized synovial cells control fluid and colloid transport into and out of the joint, lubrication, and phagocytosis for joint débridement. Cells close to the surface may be one or more layers thick and appear as a smooth surface or form villi or even holes. Tissue deep to the surface may be fatty, fibrous, or areolar. Besides being vascular, synovium is also rich in lymphatic vessels and contains some nerve fibers. Substances can, therefore, exit or enter the joint or be absorbed from the joint by the circulating blood. The lymphatic vessels are responsible for removing most matter from the subsynovial tissue; larger particles are removed after phagocytosis.

Synovial Fluid

Synovial fluid is responsible for lubrication and nourishment of the articular cartilage. A distillate of plasma and mucin, it is 95% water and contains hyaluronic acid, which gives it the ability to bind large amounts of water, forming a viscous solution. It is normally clear to pale yellow in color, and only small amounts can be aspirated from the ankle in noninflammatory conditions. Any process that increases the amount of water in the joint, such as effusion, will dilute the hyaluronic acid, decreasing the viscosity of the solution and leading to increased wear of the cartilage.

ARTHRITIC PROCESS IN THE ANKLE

As knowledge of different disease processes increases, the generalized term arthritis takes on new meaning as it is further subdivided into separate entities. Arthroscopy allows surgeons to microscopically evaluate the joint in its in situ environment. As a result, the arthritic process can be broken down into chondral, osteochondral, and soft tissue compo-

nents. This forms the diagnostic basis for the evaluation of the arthritic disease process.

Chondral Lesions

Chondral lesions affect only the cartilage. Late changes may affect subchondral bone by sclerosis or osteophytic lipping, and soft tissue changes often occur secondary to the inflammatory process.

Chondral lesions have been described in numerous ways with different classifications. Three classifications seem to fit most circumstances. These are based on the gross or macroscopic changes of cartilage, microscopic changes of the histologic components of cartilage, and the appearance of degenerated cartilage arthroscopically.

Macroscopic classification of cartilaginous changes grades these lesions into four types.[1] Grade I presents with a softening of the cartilage, progressing then to grade II, which is represented by fibrillation of its superficial layers. Grade III is recognized by the development of fissures through the cartilage, progressing to grade IV, in which there is exposure of subchondral bone.

A microscopic description of cartilaginous degeneration designates such changes on the basis of the layer in which the degeneration originally occurs.[2] This forms two types: superficial and deep degeneration (Fig. 37–1). Each type of degeneration can be broken down into four stages depending on the progression of the disease process.

Superficial lesions begin by disruption of the superficial horizontal layer of cartilage appearing as fibrillation (stage I). With deeper involvement of the tangential and deep vertical layers, more matrix is exposed and fissures form (stage II). Eventually, small areas of subchondral bone (stage III), and then larger areas, are exposed, often with small cartilaginous islands (stage IV).

Deep degeneration begins with the initial disruption of the deep collagen layer, with a characteristic "blister" formation of the tangential and superficial collagen layers (stage I). With progression, the superficial layer erupts, leaving a fibrillated area of exposed matrix with loss of ground substance (stage II). Progression results in fissuring with exposed subchondral bone (stage III) and eventual crater formation with exposure of larger areas of subchondral bone (stage IV).

Classification of cartilaginous lesions as they appear arthroscopically categorizes the disease process into six types (Fig. 37–2A–C). Types I through IV are traumatic in origin, whereas types V and VI result from degenerative processes. Type I lesion appears as a linear crack in cartilage, type II is a stellate-appearing lesion, type III is a cartilaginous flap, and type IV is a crater with exposed subchondral bone. Type V lesions appear fibrillated, whereas type VI lesions appear fibrillated with exposed subchondral bone. The primary trauma creating types I through IV lesions are impaction and excessive rotational forces. Degenerative lesions, as represented by types V and VI, are due to enzymatic degradation or excessive wear.

It is obvious in studying these classifications that similarities in the appearance of chondral lesions exist. The most important feature of these classifications is the understanding of the different types of degeneration and how they occur. Ultimately, the end result is the same: loss of cartilage integrity with exposure of matrix and loss of ground substance with altered loadbearing characteristics and potential destruction of the joint.

Chondral lesions can occur anywhere in the joint where there is hyaline cartilage. This includes the direct articular surfaces and also the peripheral areas of hyaline cartilage such as portions of the tibia and fibula that are adjacent to the articular surface of the talus. In the anterior aspect of the ankle, peripheral lesions occur on the anterior tibial lip or the front of the medial and lateral malleoli and are usually degenerative, occurring secondary to hypertrophic synovium that accumulates at the margins of the joint. Enzymatic degradation by the synovium will induce degeneration of the cartilage. It can also pile up and cover the adjacent cartilage, preventing synovial fluid from washing the cartilage, effectively preventing the nourishment of the chondrocytes, and resulting in degeneration.

Osteochondral Lesions

Osteochondral lesions involve both the cartilage and underlying subchondral bone. They are primarily traumatic, being secondary to impaction or rotational forces, but may be degenerative in nature because of loss of the integrity of the subchondral bone plate. Probing the involved area can easily differentiate a chondral lesion from an osteochondral lesion.

These lesions are classified in the same manner as chondral lesions, depending on their arthroscopic appearance (see Fig. 37–2A–C). As with chondral lesions, types I through IV are traumatic in origin, whereas types V and VI result from the degenerative process. Type I lesions appear as linear cracks through the cartilage and subchondral bone. Type II lesions appear as stellate fractures through the subchondral bone, and type III lesions appear as osteochondral flaps. Type IV lesions give the appearance of a crater-shaped defect, exposing underlying cancellous bone. Type V lesions consist of cartilaginous fibrillation with subchondral softening, and type VI lesions appear fibrillated, with exposed cancellous bone and fragmented subchondral bone.

Osteochondral lesions are important in that they are more reactive than chondral lesions, often being covered with hemorrhagic fibrous tissue. Loss of the subchondral bone plate significantly alters the load-bearing characteristics of the joint to a much greater extent than the loss of its overlying cartilage.

Osteochondral lesions can appear anywhere within the joint but are common on the anterior tibial lip and are termed *subchondral erosions.* They are also important clinically on the anterior border of the fibula directly adjacent to the anterior talofibular ligament.

Synovial and Related Soft Tissue Disorders

In the arthritic process, synovium can be either the mediator of inflammation or the primary tissue affected by the presence of an inflammatory process. In general, acute exudative inflammatory synovitis can be manifested clinically by joint swelling, heat, effusion, and redness. Chronic synovitis is predominantly proliferative in nature; as the synovial villi hypertrophy, synovium piles up and accumulates within the joint. In injuries in which there is no disruption of the capsule, the synovium is the first tissue to respond. The synovial villi proliferate and enlarge almost immediately, a process that will continue as long as the irritation persists. As the villi proliferate, a fibrin exudate is produced. These small particles can often be seen initially when first entering the joint arthroscopically. The acutely inflamed villi are transparent with a visible, red central vessel indicative of acute inflammation (Fig. 37–3). With age, the villi lose transparency, taking on an opaque appearance, and the central ''injected'' vessel is not apparent. Next, the villus tips necrose and appear frayed. Eventually, the entire villus structure degenerates, resulting in whitish, frayed elements that have been described as having a ''crab meat'' appearance (Fig. 37–4).

In cases of prolonged stimulation, the villi can hypertrophy, filling large areas of the joint pouch. With motion, the capsule is impinged against the joint surface (i.e., with plantarflexion of the foot on the leg), and the hypertrophic synovium is caught in between. Such compression of the synovium compacts or hyalinizes it, thereby allowing for the formation of a distinct mass shaped to the joint contour. This lesion is termed a *meniscoid body* and most commonly appears in the lateral gutter of the anterolateral aspect of the ankle (Fig. 37–5).

The fibrin exudate that is produced by the proliferating villi is also important because these particles can become hyalinized and aggregate within the joint, leading to the formation of fibrous bands and perhaps the creation of osteochondral bodies.

Immune responses can initiate trauma to the synovium also, as seen in rheumatoid arthritis. Lymphocytic, plasma cell, and macrophage infiltration along with proliferation of fibroblasts in the hypertrophic synovium can combine to form the characteristic granulation tissue indicative of rheumatoid arthritis that is responsible for much of the joint destruction seen in this disease.

In instances of trauma in which the capsule is injured, a chronic inflammatory condition can result if normal healing does not occur. Adhesive capsulitis forms when there is an

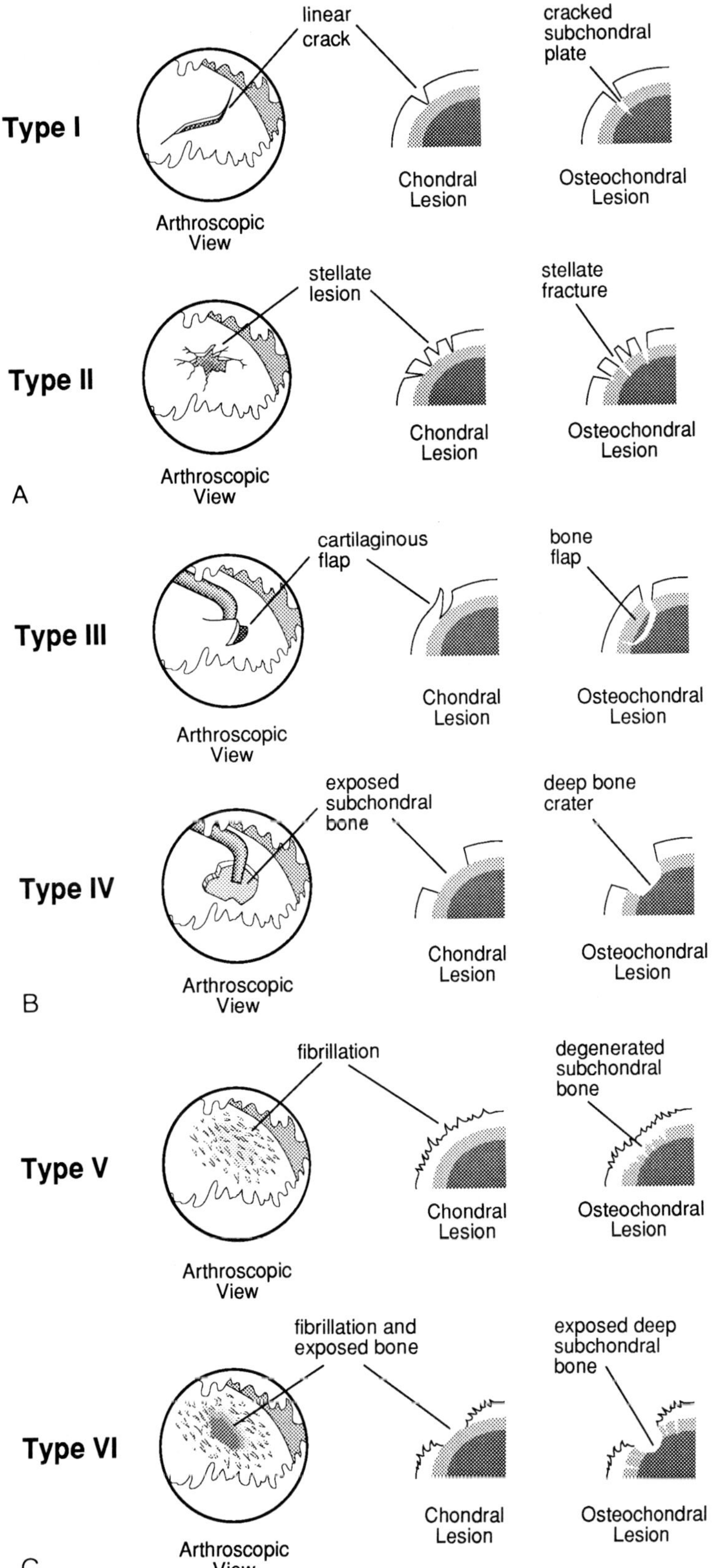

FIGURE 37–2. *A* to *C.* Classification of chondral and osteochondral lesions.

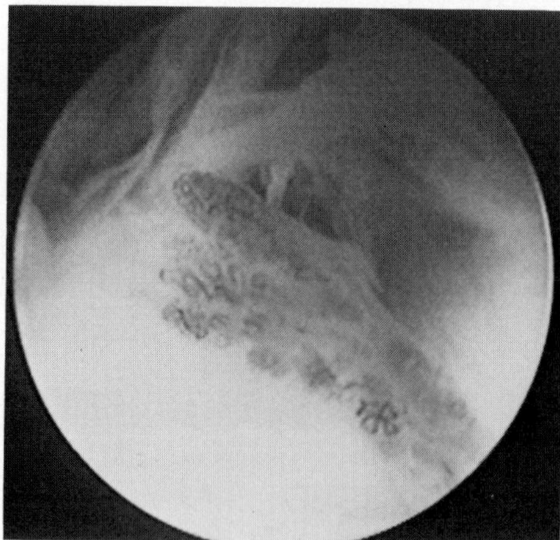

FIGURE 37–3. Acute synovitis. The villi become long and slender with a central, visible, injected vessel.

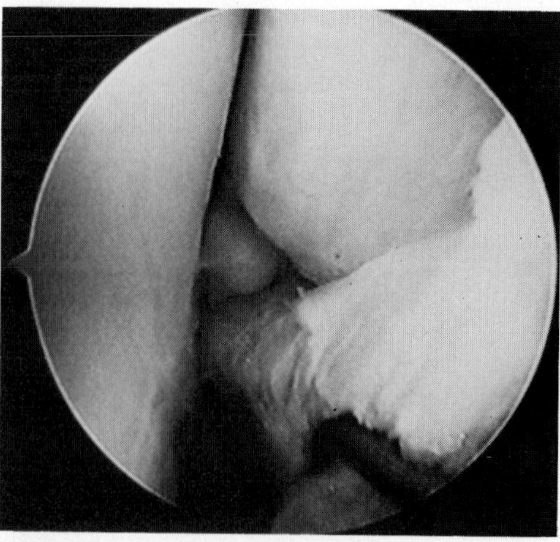

FIGURE 37–5. A small meniscoid lesion can be seen deep in the lateral gutter. The probe is reflecting the anterior talofibular ligament.

increased fibroblastic response to the injury, causing thickening and loss of flexibility of the capsule when the joint is moved (Fig. 37–6). This can initiate a hypertrophic response of the synovium, causing even more thickening. When entering this type of joint arthroscopically, the joint pouch is almost obliterated, thus making entry difficult but not impossible. The lateral gutter of the joint is most commonly affected because of the predominance of lateral ankle injuries, but it can be present in any portion or all of the joint capsule. Although the term *adhesive capsulitis* may infer that the capsule actually adheres to the joint surface, in actuality it does not. There invariably is a small space adjacent to the cartilage where there is some joint pouch. It is not uncommon, however, for adhesed capsule to form in areas where osteochondral erosions occur at the margins of the joint such as the medial and lateral malleolus or anterior tibial lip. Here, it can firmly adhere to the exposed subchondral or cancellous bone.

ANKLE ARTHROSCOPY TECHNIQUE

When approaching the arthritic patient, the basic guidelines for performing arthroscopic surgery are the same as for any other individual. Because of the nature of the disease, patient ages can vary from as young as 4 years up to the 80s. Normal precautions for each age group should apply. Typically, in the younger patients, arthroscopic treatment is for the diagnosis of inflammatory conditions. In the elderly patient, it is primarily for treatment of the byproducts of inflammation mediated by the degenerated joint. Individuals who do not have significant degenerative changes apparent in the joint or ankylosis are treated by resecting the synovium as well as by removing the byproducts of inflammation that the disease process has produced. Special emphasis should be placed on obtaining a good history, especially of medications, because precautions need to be taken, especially when treating patients on prednisone or aspirin therapy.

In approaching the arthritic ankle arthroscopically, the surgery is usually performed on an outpatient basis. If a type of arthritic condition is expected but has not previously been diagnosed and a diagnosis cannot be made from laboratory tests or by diagnostic imaging, care must be taken to preserve all synovial shavings and to perform a thorough synovial fluid analysis by obtaining adequate samples for the laboratory.

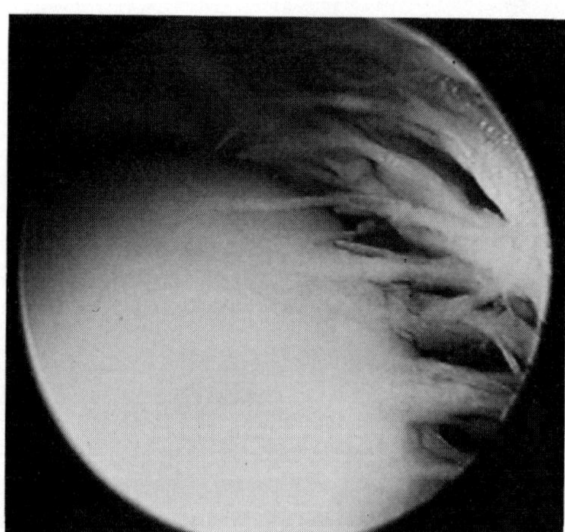

FIGURE 37–4. Chronic synovitis. The villi become opaque with frayed tips, indicating degeneration.

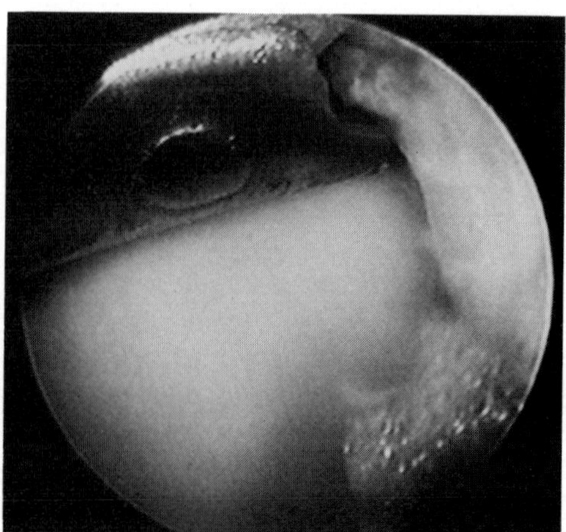

FIGURE 37–6. Adhesive capsulitis is best resected with a punch because it is thick and usually hyalinized. Note that it is not adhered to the underlying talar dome.

General or local anesthetic may be used. When using a local anesthetic, conscious sedation is used in conjunction with it. Anesthetizing the ankle with a local anesthetic can be easily and painlessly performed as follows: Ten cc of 2% lidocaine with epinephrine is drawn in the usual manner and a wheal of the solution is placed into each desired portal. A small amount of anesthetic is placed under the wheal to the level of the joint. Through one of the anticipated portals, the joint is distended with the remaining 5 to 6 cc of the anesthetizing solution. Because the synovium rapidly takes up the anesthetic, the arthroscopic procedure can begin immediately after the injection.

After anesthesia or analgesia, a tourniquet may be applied for hemostasis. The reason for using epinephrine in the local anesthetic is that when an ankle tourniquet must be used, if the tourniquet leaks or needs to be deflated, the hemostasis provided by the epinephrine usually allows for adequate completion of the surgical procedure. Thigh tourniquets provide better hemostasis than do ankle tourniquets but are usually reserved for cases performed under general or spinal anesthesia.

After application of a tourniquet, a leg holder is applied to the leg and angled caudally. When an ankle tourniquet is used, the leg holder is placed just above it. When using a thigh tourniquet, the leg holder is placed just distal to the head of the fibula to prevent compression of the common peroneal nerve. The foot is then secured in its desired position within the frontal plane, the foot and ankle are prepared in the usual manner, and routine arthroscopic drapes are applied.

The anterior aspect of the joint is palpated and a cut-down incision is made over the extensor digitorum longus tendon at the level of the joint. A second incision is made medially along the joint line at the level of the medial shoulder of the talus. The 4.0-mm and 2.7-mm arthroscopes are well suited for use in the ankle. The appropriate arthroscopic cannula is placed centrally, and an egress cannula is placed medially. On initial entry into the joint, the inflow is turned on and fluid is allowed to ingress into the joint, allowing for distension through the arthroscopic cannula. A power insufflator should be used to help maintain joint distension. Suction is not needed to evacuate fluid from the joint. A small cannula, using gravity flow, works well for this. Once the joint is distended, and with the arthroscope in the joint, a diagnostic arthroscopy is performed to identify any defects. If entry into the joint is difficult, adhesive capsulitis, severe hypertrophic synovitis, or ankylosis of the joint is likely present. In these instances, the surgeon must make sure that the tip of the arthroscope is on the joint margins and then blindly introduce a shaver to the tip of the arthroscope. Using a shaver such as a 3.5-mm full radius, a rent can be made in the capsule, allowing visualization of the articular surface. Once the joint surface can be seen, the remainder of the soft tissue is resected to the point at which the joint space has been re-established.

On entry into the joint, the various abnormal entities are identified and prioritized for treatment. Invariably, hypertrophic synovium is present, and a synovectomy is first performed. This is accomplished initially through the medial portal and then, once the medial gutter and anteromedial aspect of the joint are free of abnormal synovium, the arthroscope is directed laterally. On visualizing the lateral talar shoulder, the skin is transilluminated. A cut-down incision is

then made, establishing an anterolateral portal. A blunt obturator is used to make a channel into the joint through which a 3.5-mm shaver is placed into the joint, and the synovectomy is completed in the anterolateral aspect of the joint and lateral gutter.

If a synovectomy of the posterior aspect of the joint needs to be performed, an ankle distractor can be used or the patient is turned to a prone position and posteromedial and posterolateral portals are made to access the joint. If the joint is lax, the arthroscope can sometimes be placed into the posterior pouch through the sagittal groove of the talus with manual distraction of the joint using an anterocentral portal. A posterior transtendo-Achilles portal has also been described but adds to the potential risk of complication, as does the use of an ankle distractor. Some noninvasive ankle distractors are available that may prove useful.

After synovectomy, abnormal chondral or osteochondral lesions are identified and appropriately addressed. Once the arthroscopic procedure has been performed, all arthroscopic equipment is removed, and the joint is flushed with a 20-cc solution containing 18 cc of bupivacaine plain and 2 cc of dexamethasone phosphate. Excess fluid is then exsanguinated manually from the joint. The use of an additional 2 cc of synthetic morphine sulfate (Duramorph), administered into the joint concurrently with the bupivacaine and dexamethasone phosphate, appears to enhance the analgesic effect of the injection postoperatively, thereby greatly decreasing pain in the postoperative period.

The arthroscopic portals can then be sutured, leaving at least one portal open for postoperative drainage to prevent hemarthrosis. A compression dressing is applied from the base of the toes to an area well above the ankle. If an extensive synovectomy or an abrasion arthroplasty has been performed, a cast brace can be used postoperatively. Continuous passive motion (CPM) can be instituted at the surgeon's discretion. Animal studies have shown that CPM is effective in promoting a more mature fibrous filling of an abraded osteochondral defect and aiding chondroneogenesis.[4] Some surgeons use CPM as a physical therapy modality to increase ankle range of motion. I use it only in an attempt to resurface large, abraded defects or in therapy the first 2 weeks after an arthroscopy. Here it is used three times a week, one-half hour per session. In either event, no significant advantage has been demonstrated over standard techniques and procedures.

Patients are re-examined 3 to 5 days after surgery, and a fresh compression dressing is applied. Regular arthritic medications can be restarted after arthroscopic surgery, or nonsteroidal antiinflammatory drugs can be prescribed. Immobilization is usually continued for 3 to 4 weeks, followed by a physical therapy program for an additional 2 to 3 weeks at the surgeon's discretion if one is believed to be advantageous over routine home therapy.

ARTHROSCOPIC MANAGEMENT

A review of the arthroscopic literature shows that various joints of the human body have undergone arthroscopy for both localized joint defects as well as systemic medical conditions. In discussing the arthroscopic management of arthritic conditions, emphasis is limited to those one can anticipate seeing in private clinical practice. Arthritis, in general, can be broken down into three types of disease processes: degenerative or noninflammatory, inflammatory, and septic.

Degenerative or noninflammatory disease processes are a direct result of the poor healing response of cartilage to injury. Here, the breakdown of cartilage exceeds the ability of cartilage to repair itself; therefore, a pathologic condition is produced.

Inflammatory disease processes can be primarily proliferative when there is an initial increased amount of synovial fluid or joint effusion or primarily exudative when the initial response is synovial villus hypertrophy. A combination of these two types of inflammatory processes can also occur.

Septic disease processes, the third category, occur from a joint that has become infected. They can be the result of either a primary infection within the joint or hematogenous spread of an infection originating elsewhere.

Each of these disease processes are discussed separately. Emphasis is placed on any unique features of the disease and how to approach each disease process arthroscopically.

Degenerative Arthritides

Degenerative types of arthritis revolve primarily around the presence of osteoarthritis, post-traumatic arthritis, arthritis secondary to ankle instability, and the neuropathic joint.

Osteoarthritis. Much discussion exists as to whether osteoarthritis is an actual disease process or secondary to wear and tear and primarily age related. For this discussion, osteoarthritis is considered an age-related condition and, therefore, exists in the presence of a negative history for trauma to the ankle joint. Osteoarthritis occurs primarily in weight-bearing joints or in those joints that are subjected to large degrees of shearing forces. A wearing away of the cartilage can occur by the simple inability of cartilage to repair itself from repetitive joint motions over long periods of time or from microtrauma that may exist from one's occupation, angle and base of gait, weight, or other environmental, job related, or extra-articular conditions. As the cartilage degenerates, one can arthroscopically document the presence of chondral lesions (early type V and type VI lesions). More commonly, one will see chondral lesions that result from superficial and deep types of degeneration within the cartilage. This can be visualized as stage I superficial lesions consisting of fibrillation of the surface of the cartilage or stage I deep degenerative lesions as evidenced by softening and blistering of the cartilage.

As the wear and tear to the affected joint continues, progression of the type of chondral lesion ensues. The superficial lesions further degenerate into fissuring and exposure of subchondral bone while the deep lesions degenerate, with the opening of the blistered areas of cartilage and exposure of matrix, fissuring, and eventual exposure of the subchondral bone plate. As these disease processes progress, the load-bearing characteristics of the joint rapidly change, as evidenced by the presence of sclerosis of the subchondral bone. Here we see a proliferation of bone in the subchondral area with increased density of the bony structures under the cartilage. The subchondral bone plate becomes more dense, hardened, and eburnated. With progression, this can even degenerate with cystic lesions and very large amounts of sclerosis of adjacent areas of bone.

In conjunction with the later stages of subchondral sclero-

sis, osteophytes can be seen at the margin of the joint. These develop at the periphery of the articular cartilage where the latter blends with the periosteum. These osteophytes may extend into the joint cavity, or they may develop within the capsule and ligamentous attachments of the joint margins. In general, these osteophytic lesions grow in the direction governed by the lines of mechanical force. After cartilage degeneration, subchondral sclerosis, and osteophytic lipping, narrowing of the joint margins gradually occurs, and, radiographically, geometric changes in the joint are visualized.

When approaching osteoarthritis arthroscopically, the surgeon must be aware of the presence of any secondary factors that contribute to the formation of osteoarthritis such as a foot that is not biomechanically stable. In these cases, the effect of a significant pes cavovarus, pes planovalgus, or other biomechanical abnormality must be controlled postoperatively to reduce external forces acting on the joint. At times, surgical intervention for a predisposing foot type is necessary to reduce abnormal stress on the ankle joint and prevent further degeneration.

When approaching the osteoarthritic joint, the degree of deformity must be assessed. Osteophytic lipping must be differentiated from an impingement exostosis. An impingement exostosis is a primary abnormality of the joint in which there is a definite impingement of the tibia or talus on one another. These respond well to resection arthroscopically or by open arthrotomy. Osteophytic lipping is degenerative in nature. It often accompanies geometric changes of the joint and is an early sign of ankylosis. When large areas of osteophytic lipping are resected, the joint can be significantly mobilized, further aggravating the arthritic condition that is present. This creates a dilemma in arthroscopy as to how aggressive the surgeon should be in treating these arthritic joints. Experience dictates that resection of osteophytic lesions that impinge on the joint surface is necessary. Abrasion arthroplasty of large chondral or osteochondral defects should be avoided and attention placed primarily on débriding the synovial lesions and extracting the inflammatory byproducts from the joint.

On initial entry into the osteoarthritic joint, a thorough diagnostic arthroscopy should be performed. This includes recognition of synovial defects such as hypertrophic synovitis. Acute hemorrhagic synovitis indicates an active area of the disease process, and, once resected, the adjacent areas must be thoroughly probed to identify additional bony or cartilaginous defects to ensure that it is effectively treated. Areas of chronic synovitis as represented by opaque, frayed white synovium need to be thoroughly resected and adjacent degenerative areas thoroughly débrided.

A complete synovectomy should be performed first to visualize the entire joint adequately. Once the synovectomy is complete, other pathologic lesions are addressed in the cartilaginous or bony structures. Cartilaginous lesions should be staged and a chondroplasty or gentle débridement performed. Aggressive curettage or abrasion arthroplasty may be necessary in some instances but, generally, should be avoided unless a specific lesion exists such as a large chondral or osteochondral flap or regeneration of damaged chondral areas is being attempted. Areas of fibrillated cartilage should be gently débrided or left alone. Blistered areas of cartilage can be débrided if they appear loose or are spongy on probing. Large fissures or exposed subchondral bone should be only gently débrided of any fibrous tissue covering. Areas of osteochondral degeneration in which there is distinct erosion through the subchondral bone plate should be gently débrided and resected of fibrous tissue, but care must be exercised not to resect underlying cancellous bone excessively and further weaken its osseous structure. Osteochondral erosions on the anterior aspect of the tibia should be débrided if covered with a reactive fibrous tissue. These lesions are invariably secondary to synovial pileup and do not represent a pathologic entity unless they eroded through the subchondral bone plate or are covered with a reactive fibrous tissue. Osteochondral lesions on the anterior border of the fibula need to be resected accordingly. Once all lesions have been addressed, the joint is thoroughly flushed and the patient is maintained in a compressive wrapping. Immobilization in a cast brace is useful if further bracing is needed. Because the treatment of the osteoarthritic joint often leaves exposed cancellous or subchondral bone and involves the resection of abnormal synovial changes, postoperative hemarthrosis is the greatest threat to the surgical procedure. Therefore, ice, elevation, compressive dressings, and rest need to be maintained a minimum of 48 hours after surgery. If hemarthrosis does occur, aggressive débridement and flushing of the joint should be instituted if regular conservative measures fail to reduce the condition.

Post-Traumatic Arthritis. Perhaps the most common reason for performing arthroscopy on the ankle is for persistent pain after traumatic injuries. In this patient population, a careful history must be taken to ascertain when and how many times injury has occurred, what specifically was injured, and what was done after diagnosis. Radiographs taken at the time of examination should be compared with those taken at the time of injury to get a feel for the progression of the disease process. In cases in which there has been a fracture with shortening of the fibula when anatomic reduction was not achieved (with or without surgery), arthritis will gradually develop in the joint anywhere from 1 to 10 years after injury depending on how poor the reduction was. Avulsion fractures are also present many times after post-traumatic injury to the ankle and frequently are diagnosed as ''calcifications.'' Often small fragments are left unattended, and chronic inflammation and irritation will produce degenerative joint changes or chronic pain in the ankle. Commonly associated with ankle fractures are transchondral fractures, which may present as stage I lesions that are not able to be imaged at the time of the initial injury. These lesions are degenerative in nature and present themselves only with time. Here, a compressive force will form a contusion in the cartilage and subchondral bone, cutting off vital circulation. The resultant necrosis of bone, sclerosis, and cystic degeneration will show up in subsequent radiographs when the patient continues to complain of pain. CT scans are invaluable in evaluating these lesions. Incomplete (stage II) and complete (stage III) fractures usually show up at the time of injury but are treated conservatively. These must be addressed after the injury if conservative care fails to render the joint asymptomatic. In these instances, CT scanning is also very valuable.

Complete fractures that are displaced (stage IV) are usually diagnosed at the time of injury and are treated surgically by fixation of the avulsed fragment or by resection of the fragment if it is small. If not diagnosed on initial injury, these lesions are treated arthroscopically when diagnosed. Avulsed fragments in stage IV lesions are commonly appar-

ent on initial entry into the joint but, at times, are elusive and need to be aggressively sought after. When found, they can be extracted from the joint with a grasper, and the base of the lesion from which the fragment originated either is abraded or undergoes curettage to restore vascularity to the defect to promote healing.

Because of the importance of treating the fractured fibula, other fractures in the ankle can, at times, be overlooked. This includes not recognizing the importance of a syndesmotic injury, a fracture of the anterior or posterior tibial lip, and small avulsion fractures. Also, attempts should be made on initial injury to reduce any medial malleolar fragment anatomically. Follow-up must be provided after the injury to ensure that all fractures that are open or closed-reduced heal, because nonunion of these fragments is a common cause of chronic ankle pain.

Accurate preoperative assessment of the joint is mandatory when approaching post-traumatic pain. This involves a thorough knowledge of the actual injury and the ability to image the type of lesion present. In the presence of an avulsion fracture, a transchondral fracture, or nonunion without significant joint changes, the pathologic entity can be treated on an isolated basis. On entering the joint for any of these conditions, a thorough synovectomy is first performed. Other synovial elements such as meniscoid bodies or fibrous bands need to be addressed at this time. Unless the joint is free of abnormal synovial tissue, assessment of any osseous lesion is difficult. Avulsion fractures commonly treated arthroscopically are off the tibial insertion of the anterior tibiotalar ligament, the fibular insertion of the anterior talofibular ligament, tibial or fibular insertion of the anterior tibiofibular ligament, and, less commonly, the fibular insertion of the posterior talofibular or tibiotalar ligaments. Small anterior tibial lip fractures can occasionally be identified off the anterior tibial tubercle or anterior tibial lip.

Once visualized arthroscopically, avulsion fractures can be loosened with a synovial shaver or grabbed with a grasper and cut free with an arthroscopic knife before evacuation from the joint. When large, these fragments can be sectioned into pieces, reduced to morsels, and removed. After resection of the fragment, the areas around it should be thoroughly probed and débrided with a synovial resector to prevent inadvertently leaving any osseous fragments.

Most avulsion fractures can be resected without concurrent detrimental effect on the function of the joint. The exception is the inadvertent creation of an unstable ankle after the resection of an avulsion fracture off the fibular insertion of the anterior talofibular ligament. In these cases, once the avulsed fragment has been resected, the ankle should be stressed and if excessive talar tilt or significant widening of the lateral gutter is present, an appropriate stabilization procedure is concurrently performed. An arthroscopic stapling of the anterior talofibular ligament into the fibula or the trochlear surface of the talus is usually performed, but an open procedure would suffice.

Transchondral fractures are treated by resection of the involved area of talus. Besides resecting the lesion, a secondary goal of revascularizing the defect also needs to be achieved. Stage I transchondral fractures are resected by probing the softened area and performing curettage on the defect. An abrader may also be used, but, because a significant amount of sclerosis is usually associated with these lesions, an angled curette is invaluable in resecting its deeper portions. Stages II, III, and IV lesions are resected in a similar manner. It should be noted that the arthroscopic appearance of transchondral fractures does not follow the usual classification. Several authors proposed different arthroscopic classifications, but, unless the lesions are acute, they do not appear as classically described. Radiographically, or on computed tomographic scanning, the old transchondral fracture may appear to fit within a definite classification, but, on direct visualization arthroscopically, the lesion will appear as an opaque, whitish area that is not easily discernible from the surrounding cartilage, or it may be raised above the surface of the adjacent cartilage. Other lesions can appear as a crater, which will, most likely, represent an old stage IV lesion.

As a result of these three different appearances of transchondral fractures seen on arthroscopy, nonacute transchondral fractures can be classified by their appearance: softening of the cartilage and subchondral bone or contusion (type I), a raised flap of cartilage, soft tissue, or subchondral bone (type II), and depression or crater (type III). Types I and II lesions are soft, the contents of the defect can be pried loose with a probe or a curette, and the base of the lesion is usually sclerotic or cystic. These areas must undergo curettage or abrasion to be resected and revascularized. Resection should continue to the level of normal cancellous bone. If sclerosis is deep and unable to be fully resected with a curette or abrader, drilling with a 0.45-in. Kirschner wire is required. Type III lesions are usually not soft and do not contain small areas of reactive or nonreactive fibrous tissue. Sclerotic areas of the lesion are evident on probing. Because these are representative of old stage IV lesions, they are usually found on the anterolateral border of the talus. Therefore, by nature, they are shallow lesions and easily undergo curettage or abrasion.

It must be noted that, whether transchondral fractures are classified as acute or by their appearance in chronic cases, they all occur on distinct anatomic areas of the talus. Laterally, lesions appear on or near the shoulder of the talus anteriorly and medially on or near the talar shoulder from the middle to the posterior aspect of the talus. In addition, posteromedial lesions are typically cup shaped and deep, whereas anterolateral lesions are shallow and wafer-like. Because of the compression between the articular surfaces of the tibial plafond and the talar shoulder, stage IV lesions are rare posteromedially and primarily occur from injuries to the anterolateral aspect of the talus.

Posteromedial transchondral fractures are associated with medial impingement lesions. These are areas on the tibial plafond and anterior tibial lip that have been compressed from the posteromedial talar shoulder being driven into the adjacent surface of the tibial plafond, with the foot plantarflexed and inverted at the time of the original injury. The resultant impactional rotation creates the transchondral fracture and causes a concurrent injury to the tibial plafond whereby the subchondral bone is violated and loses its vascularity, resulting in softening and degeneration in a characteristic triangular manner.[5] These lesions are 6.0 to 8.0 mm in width at the level of the anterior tibial lip directly in the medial bend and extend posteriorly onto the tibial plafond, where they assume a triangular appearance. In the apex of the triangle is a characteristic apical fibrous plug, which, when resected, will determine the most posterior progression of the lesion. Treatment of these lesions is by curettage or

abrasion through the softened fibrous areas to the normal adjacent subchondral or cancellous bone. Once the lesion has been abraded, the obliquity of the arthroscope can be turned downward onto the talar surface, where, with the foot plantarflexed, the transchondral fracture will be located.

Delayed union, nonunion, and malunion also contribute to degenerative arthritis and cause chronic ankle pain. Small, nonunited fragments can easily be resected arthroscopically, but larger fragments need to be stabilized by appropriate open reduction and internal fixation. Nonunions that have failed to heal 1 year after injury need to be resected when small and open-reduced and internally fixated or bone grafted when large. Avulsion fractures, even if large, can usually be resected unless they affect the primary stability of the ankle. This includes the resection of larger bony fragments off the posterior tibial lip (involving less than one third of its articular surface), tibial tubercle, and medial malleolus. In all instances, maintenance of the length of the fibula must be attempted. Therefore, resection of large fibular avulsion fractures or portions of the fibula that will result in any shortening must be avoided.

Malunion of an ankle fracture presents a special problem in that the fragment has healed and cannot simply be fixated or resected. More common malunions involve a medial malleolar fragment, anterior tibial tubercle, and transverse or spiral fractures of the fibula. When associated with degenerative arthritis, these ankles are treated in a similar manner as osteoarthritis. When malunion of the fibula is present and there is a visible medial clear space, this will appear arthroscopically as a fibrous plug between the medial malleolus and the talus. This tissue needs to be resected sparingly inasmuch as overaggressive removal from the medial gutter can result in an increased amount of talar instability in the ankle, resulting in persistent ankle pain. Gentle débridement and re-establishment of the anterior joint pouch is the rule when approaching these types of ankles.

When approaching these ankles arthroscopically, one area requires special mention. This is in an ankle in which there is fibular shortening and a posterior displacement of the fibula as seen in a supination/external rotation stage III injury. On the fibular fracture line at the level of the joint, there is often a spike of bone off the proximal fibula around which the distal fragment of the fibula has rotated superiorly, posteriorly, and laterally (Fig. 37–7). When this area is freed of abnormal soft tissue, the adjacent shoulder of the lateral talus will contain a chondral or osteochondral defect if there is impingement of the fibular spike on the talus. Here the fibular spike needs to undergo abrasion or curettage to prevent further damage to the talus. If a talar lesion is intact and there is no reactive fibrous tissue or exposure of subchondral bone, resection of the fibular spike is adequate in treating this lesion, and any cartilaginous defects can be left untreated.

In summary, post-traumatic ankle arthritis can be treated by either resection of the offending lesion or generalized joint débridement. Lesions responsive to resection include avulsion fractures, transchondral fractures, and some nonunions and malunions. In these instances, the associated soft tissue changes or degenerative chondral and osseous lesions are treated simultaneously. Care must be exercised so as not to create instability in removing lesions that involve the fibula or anterior talofibular ligament.

Joints that require generalized débridement are those in which the arthritic process has caused significant change in

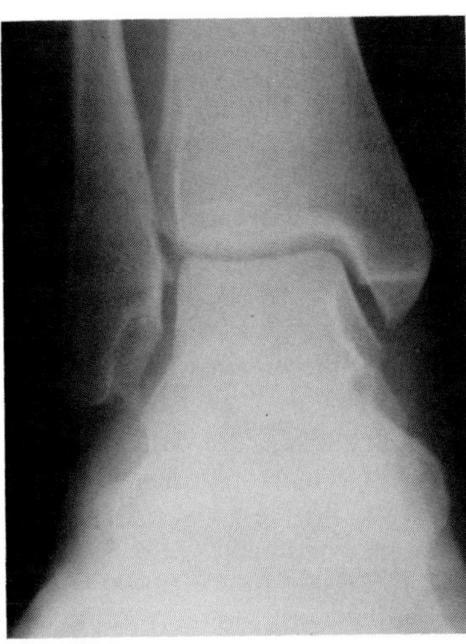

FIGURE 37–7. Residual ''spike'' resulting from a supination external rotation injury to the fibula. The fibula is displaced posteriorly and caudally, leaving the proximal fracture line prominent in the lateral interval.

the joint as indicated by geometric changes of the joint on radiograph as well as subchondral sclerosis, cystic changes, osteophytic lipping, and generalized ankylosis of the joint. These cases are treated in a similar manner for the progressive stages of osteoarthritis by generalized débridement of the joint, resection of hypertrophic and hemorrhagic synovium, resection of loose bodies, chondroplasty, and abrasion arthroplasty. In general, the goal in the arthroscopic treatment of the end stages of this disease is to recreate the joint space and resect abnormal soft tissue, chondral, and osseous lesions, being careful not to overaggressively mobilize the joint or create additional lesions and trauma, thereby causing persistent and progressive ankle pain.

In joints in which significant degeneration occurs, arthroscopy may be effective, if only temporarily, in relieving the pain. It is not uncommon that many of these joints may need to undergo repeat arthroscopy every 1 to 3 years depending on how long the procedure remains effective. If the procedure is not effective and symptoms persist, appropriate measures need to be taken, including the possibility of ankle fusion. When evaluating for fusion, the geometry of the joint and ankylosis, if present, must be considered. If the joint architecture is fairly well preserved, a fusion can be attempted arthroscopically. If significant changes in the shape of the joint are present, then open means of ankle fusion will be necessary.

Ankle Arthritis Secondary to Instability. Ankle instability has been implicated as a cause of degenerative arthrosis.[6] Excess motion and the resultant incongruity of the joint can be as notorious as a loose avulsion fracture within the joint in causing inflammatory changes and joint degeneration. Instability must be detected initially by patient history and then by appropriate radiographs to ascertain its effect on the overall condition of the ankle. This is particularly true if the patient complains of multiple sprains or strains of the ankle or a feeling of instability when stepping off a curb or down a stair and when an avulsion fracture of the fibular attachment of the anterior talofibular ligament exists. In these cases, stress radiographs should be taken before surgery and confirmed with diagnostic arthroscopy by stressing the ankle during the surgical procedure.

On entering an unstable joint, a thorough diagnostic arthroscopy is first performed followed by a synovectomy. Special attention should be given to the lateral aspect of the ankle because the lateral gutter and areas around the anterior talofibular ligament are what tend to be primarily affected. The ligament should be identified and inspected as to its laxity and the presence of scar tissue. Once the lateral gutter is visualized, the ankle is stressed with visualization of the posterior talofibular ligament as a good indication that a significant amount of instability is present. The ankle can then be stressed, looking at the anterior aspect of the joint, with instability being expressed as full visualization of the tibial plafond and the tibiofibular synovial recess and fringe. The lateral aspect of the ankle (lateral interval) may open up enough on varus stress to enable the passage of a 4.0-mm arthroscope into the posterior ankle pouch.

In most cases, the unstable ankle can be stabilized through an arthroscopic stapling procedure whereby the anterior talofibular ligament is plicated into the anterior tibial border or into the lateral trochlear surface of the talus. If the ligament is too frayed or the deformity too great, a traditional open arthrotomy with peroneus brevis tenoplasty is performed.

Medial impingement lesions are, many times, associated with ankle instability. These lesions are identified on visualization and probing of the medial bend of the anterior aspect of the tibia. A softened area of subchondral bone with reactive or nonreactive fibrous covering is indicative of this lesion. These lesions need to undergo curettage or abrasion to ensure that they are thoroughly resected.

A type IV, V, or VI osteochondral lesion is often present on the anterior border of the fibula adjacent to the insertion of the anterior talofibular ligament. These lesions are important because they are reactive in nature and represent a pathologic entity that requires treatment. This consists of débridement with a full radius shaver, curette, or abrader. The significance of this type lesion is that it affects the integrity of the insertion of the anterior talofibular ligament, precipitating pain from altered function much as a sprain does. In addition, when the lesion is reactive, it is associated with hypertrophic and hemorrhagic synovitis and can be associated with meniscoid bodies and fibrous bands. Often, under anesthesia, a moderate amount of instability is evident, yet gross instability is not obvious. In these cases, when an osteochondral fibular lesion is identified with some laxity and scarring of the anterior tibiofibular ligament present, a stabilization should be performed if the patient attests to a feeling of an unstable ankle in the presence of normal stress radiographs. The osteochondral defect is resected and an arthroscopic staple placed into the anterior talofibular ligament. The staple tines and ligament are then plicated into the débrided portion of the osteochondral defect, restoring the insertion and reefing up the ligament, thereby effecting a stabilization.

Neuropathic Joint. The insensitive joint is an important clinical entity and can be present in diabetes, syringomyelia, spinal cord lesions, or pernicious anemia. Usually only one joint is involved, such as the hip, knee, or ankle. The neuropathy in the joint prevents any proprioceptive response from its protective reflexes, subjecting the joint to repetitive injury. In addition, the supporting structures are relaxed in the absence of pain, which leads to potential joint destruction.

Symptomatic neuropathic joints are treated arthroscopically in the same manner as discussed when approaching the osteo- or post-traumatic arthritic patient.

Inflammatory Arthritis

Inflammatory disease process can be characterized as being primarily exudative or proliferative or a combination of both.

Exudative inflammation includes the classic manifestations of pain, redness, swelling, and heat. These correlate with the impairment of the microcirculation of the synovial tissues and are mediated by a variety of agents and mechanisms not well understood. With alterations in the microcirculation and impaired synovial function, there is a concurrent increased vascular permeability. Because the lymphatic and vascular supply to the joint is predominantly in the synovium or just below it, it is this tissue that is primarily involved and initially affected with inflammation in the joint.

Exudate inflammation is initially present with acute synovitis. Along with the classic signs of inflammation, such as redness, warmth, pain, and swelling, there is an increased amount of synovial fluid produced that distends the joint capsule. Along with the increased synovial fluid, there is an increased amount of inflammatory cells present, usually polymorphonuclear neutrophils (PMNs). The synovium enlarges as it and the subsynovial tissues become infiltrated to varying degrees with inflammatory cells. Acute rheumatic fever is an example of exudative inflammation but is self-limited and subsides without residual joint damage.

Proliferative arthritis is actually a continuation of the exudative process. In the more chronic forms of arthritis, the proliferative phase of inflammation develops and may dominate the pathologic and clinical features of the disease. A prototype for this form of inflammation is rheumatoid arthritis, which actually is a combined exudative and proliferative inflammatory process.

A primarily proliferative inflammatory process can be seen in joints that are chronically inflamed. Here, because of the build-up of the proliferative intra-articular soft tissue structures, the exudative phase is not apparent. These patients complain of pain on activity and after-rest pain, present with no significant joint effusion, and usually do not complain of joint swelling. Examination reveals pain around the joint margins on palpation. Radiographic and laboratory studies may be negative.

Along with alteration of the permeability of the synovial and subsynovial tissue, changes can be seen in the joint fluid as well. Water, electrolytes, and protein easily diffuse into the joint, along with other colloids. Fibrinogen, immune globulins, and leukocytes can also be found. The increased diffusion of water also decreases the viscosity of the synovial fluid, affecting the nourishment and the fluid mechanics of the joint.

Evaluation of the synovial fluid extracted from the joint before an arthroscopic procedure can aid in differentiating inflammatory from noninflammatory synovial effusions. Effusions in traumatic and degenerative joint disease are relatively clear and may present with increased red blood cells and a moderate increase in white blood cells. Viscosity in these joints is well maintained. Inflammatory synovial fluids are turbid and, because of the presence of fibrinogen, may clot on standing and present with large numbers of leuko-

cytes, most of which are PMNs. The viscosity of the fluid in these joints is also altered in varying degrees. In septic joints, the synovial fluid can be purulent or turbid with an extremely high number of leukocytes, most of which again are PMNs, and the infectious microorganism may be able to be cultured directly from the synovial fluid.

Laboratory examination of the synovial fluid is extremely important in differentiating inflammatory from noninflammatory arthritic conditions and even, at times, in differentiating between septic conditions. This is especially true in younger patients or patients who have not been previously diagnosed as having a type of arthritis and in whom the disease process is limited to a single joint. In these instances, the synovial fluid can be subjected to laboratory tests such as antinuclear antibody, rheumatoid factor, lupus erythematosus preparation, and refractive light microscopy for the differentiation of crystalline arthritis. The other more common tests on synovial fluid can also be performed such as clotting time, white blood cell count, glucose, and so on.

Inflammatory arthritis can manifest itself in the form of different disease processes. The prototype of this inflammatory process is rheumatoid arthritis. Also classified as inflammatory is crystalline arthritis as evidenced by gout and pseudogout. Other inflammatory conditions include that seen in hemophilia, ochronosis, systemic lupus erythematosus, and psoriasis.

Rheumatoid Arthritis. The synovitis with subsequent destruction of articular cartilage in rheumatoid arthritis results from an antigenic stimulus that induces an inflammatory process. An immune response is triggered by these exogenous or endogenous antigens to a variable degree in a susceptible individual. Antigen is presented to synovial T lymphocytes, which, in turn, activate B lymphocytes, which produce antibodies that react with the antigen activating the complement system. This, along with other mediators, increases the vascular permeability of the synovial and subsynovial cells, attracting PMNs into the synovial fluid. Chemotactic factors attract the PMNs to ingest the antigen/antibody complexes, releasing lysosomal enzymes. As these enzymes accumulate, they saturate the capacity of their inhibitors to deactivate them within the synovial fluid, leading to the initiation of the exudative inflammatory process. The synovial villi elongate with concurrent injection of the central vessel. The acuteness of the reaction often perpetuates hemorrhagic synovitis, which denotes the extent to which the tissue becomes inflamed. The synovial villi replicate and enlarge, accumulating within the joint pouch. The increased permeability allows diffusion of plasma cells and macrophages and T lymphocytes. These all may appear in a follicle-like arrangement on histologic examination. As the proliferative phase of inflammation ensues and continues, the angioblastic proliferation and fibroblastic proliferation of the synovial villi and related structures form granulation tissue, which replaces the synovium and invades the joint capsule and periarticular structures.

Because of the acellularity of cartilage and lack of adequate inhibitors to stop the lysosomal enzymes from the antigen/antibody complexes, granulation tissue is actually able to invade the matrix and destroy the physical properties of hyaline cartilage. In early stages of the disease or in the early acute phases, the antigen/antibody complexes are also able to enter the matrix, releasing lysosomal enzymes and causing degradation of the cartilage before pannus formation.

This can be seen arthroscopically by subchondral erosions at the periphery of the joint where the synovium tends to accumulate.

In understanding the natural course of rheumatoid arthritis, it is obvious that the earlier the disease process is arrested, the better the prognosis for long-term results when considering arthroscopic treatment. Because the rheumatoid disease process is mediated in the synovial and subsynovial tissues, it stands to reason that the treatment of choice to arrest the process is to resect the synovium. Synovectomy has long been discussed as a treatment for the disease, but previous open arthrotomy has required hospitalization along with the risk of complication in terms of the adjacent tendinous structures around the joint and neurologic and vascular structures as well. Excess amounts of scar tissue can also inhibit range of motion after surgery and, even though the synovium has been resected, it does have a good capacity for regeneration, allowing for the procedure to be potentially performed every 1 to 3 years.

With the advent of arthroscopy, the traumatic nature of synovectomy and associated complications has been greatly reduced. The therapeutic results of merely flushing the joint of noxious substances, especially in diseases such as rheumatoid arthritis, have recently become known. When performing arthroscopy on ankles before the advent of power equipment, a dramatic relief of symptomatology was found merely by performing a diagnostic procedure to identify the defect and thoroughly irrigating the joint.[7] With the advent of power instrumentation, the added effect of synovectomy has greatly enhanced the therapeutic value of the arthroscopic procedure, making it an important tool for the early diagnosis and treatment of inflammatory arthritic processes.

After the soft tissue changes, the invasion of cartilage with granulation tissue, and the breakdown of cartilage from lysosomal enzymes, secondary effects on the rheumatoid joint are seen such as subchondral sclerosis, osteophytic lipping at the joint margins, changes in the geometry of the joint, and restrictions of range of motion. A build-up of inflammatory tissue and debris along with the rheumatoid disease process accounts for exacerbations and remissions in pain and disability suffered by the patient. In addition, intervention by medical means often decreases the inflammatory process, placing the disease in remission.

Many inflammatory arthritides are diagnosed with arthroscopy. In cases in which a diagnosis has not been made despite standard history and physical examination along with appropriate diagnostic testing, arthroscopy of the painful ankle may be the only means of effectively diagnosing and treating an inflammatory disease process. This is particularly true in juvenile rheumatoid arthritis, in which one sees a chronic nonsuppurative arthritis often involving only one joint. Joint tap reveals an increased amount of synovial fluid with a high number of PMNs, which is often associated with a low sedimentation rate and is misdiagnosed as a suppurative arthritis. Early diagnosis and treatment of these patients are particularly important: The sooner it can be diagnosed and a synovectomy performed, the greater the possibility of total arrest of the disease.

The arthroscopic appearance of the rheumatoid joint varies with the progression of the disease process. In early cases or in juvenile rheumatoid arthritis, one sees the classic signs of exudative inflammation consisting of increased amounts of synovial fluid, warmth, redness, and pain associated intra-

articularly with enlargement of the synovial villi and injection of the central vessel. Because of the intense synovial reaction, the synovitis is usually hemorrhagic but not necessarily in all parts of the joint. Fibrin is produced along with the hypertrophy of the villus structures often clouding the joint. The unique aspect of synovial villus hyperplasia in the rheumatoid patient is the size to which the villi hypertrophy. These are often cigar shaped in appearance, are very large, like a long grain of rice, and have been termed ''rice bodies.'' As the synovial reaction continues, the hypertrophic villus structures pile up in the various recesses of the joint. In older patients in whom there have been remissions and exacerbations, it is not uncommon to see acute hemorrhagic hypertrophic synovitis associated with chronic hypertrophic synovitis characterized by frayed, whitish accumulations of synovial tissue. In treating these joints, the most important portion of synovium to resect initially is that which is hemorrhagic, because this is more acute in nature and can be associated with other defects in the cartilage or subchondral bone. Once that synovial tissue has been resected, the more chronic hypertrophic synovium can be addressed. The goal is to re-establish the joint pouch of the ankle in its anterior or posterior aspects. Aggressive synovectomy must be undertaken but not to the extent at which the capsule is violated, causing extravasation of fluid or perpetuating the postoperative risk of adhesive capsulitis. Once a thorough synovectomy has been performed, cartilaginous and osseous lesions can be addressed. In most cases of rheumatoid arthritis without obvious geometric changes in the joint preoperatively, a synovectomy is adequate. If cartilaginous defects exist, they can be gently débrided or abraded if large. Care must be exercised to prevent overaggressive treatment of cartilaginous or osseous lesions because these are secondary in nature. Resection of the synovium is primary because it is this tissue that is the mediator of the rheumatoid disease process. As in dealing with degenerative arthritic processes, the same tenets of treatment are followed: Cleanse the joint of its byproducts of inflammation and abnormal hypertrophic soft tissues, gently débride the chondral and osseous elements, and get out of the joint.

In more chronic rheumatoid ankles, granulation tissue, if present, must be resected off the cartilage and a chondroplasty performed simultaneously. If the granulation tissue is fibrosed, it must be resected with a shaver or a punch to re-establish the joint space. In ankles in which secondary osseous changes have occurred such as marginal osteophytic lipping and bony ankylosis, the same tenets of treatment exist as for the other arthritic joints of severe nature, as previously discussed.

In approaching the painful rheumatoid ankle, it is important to identify the location of the pain. The majority of complaints revolve around pain at the anterior aspect of the joint compared with the painful posterior joint pouch. I do not advocate routine synovectomy of the anterior and posterior joint pouches if only one of the joint pouches is symptomatic. It is not common for the posterior joint to be symptomatic; therefore, the majority of defects will occur anteriorly. In these instances, only the anterior joint pouch is treated.

Postoperative treatment involves the application of a mild compression dressing, with rest, ice, and elevation of the affected joint for 48 hours. Because of the large amount of synovial tissue resected, all attempts are made to reduce postoperative hemarthrosis. Medications for the rheumatoid arthritis are continued the day after surgery, and the patient is followed weekly with dressing changes until the fourth week, at which time the ankle is maintained in an elastic wrap. Physical therapy can be instituted at the surgeon's discretion as needed.

Because synovium will regenerate, repeat arthroscopies may need to be performed occasionally. Before repeating an arthroscopic procedure, it is highly recommended that the occasional use of a nonrepository steroid such as dexamethasone phosphate with a local anesthetic be injected into the joint when symptoms recur to break the inflammatory process. In addition, control of abnormal foot mechanics with the use of a functional foot orthosis is advocated if other joints of the foot are involved or on recurrence of symptoms. An ankle/foot orthosis is sometimes used, especially when ankylosis is apparent. If symptoms of the rheumatoid ankle appear shortly after arthroscopic procedure and are only partially helped by bracing and injection therapy, an option to arthroscopy is articular pumping. Here the joint is anesthetized in a manner similar to performing an arthroscopic procedure. Through an anteromedial and anterolateral portal, an 18-gauge needle is introduced into the joint and a 1-liter bag of lactated Ringer's solution is attached to one needle in its respective portal. Fluid is then allowed to run through the joint to cleanse it, along with manual palpation of the joint to disperse the fluid. Nonrepository steroids, local anesthetics, and synthetic morphine can also be flushed through the joint as is routinely done after an arthroscopic procedure to enhance postprocedure relief of pain. This can be done in the office setting and can easily be performed with minimal risk and cost to the patient.

Crystalline Arthritis. The two most common types of crystalline arthritis result from the systemic effect of gout and pseudogout. In both disease processes, it is virtually impossible to distinguish one from the other arthroscopically. It is necessary, if particulate matter is visible on initial diagnostic arthroscopy, to send the synovial fluid for analysis so that any crystalline matter can be examined microscopically. Microscopic examination is the only way to differentiate between the two conditions. When initially performing arthroscopy on an ankle, at times, crystalline-type aggregates can be identified in the periarticular structures. These are usually soft and embedded in synovium but not attached to cartilage. This probably represents a previous injection with a repository corticosteroid such as betamethasone phosphate or dexamethasone acetate. These deposits can be probed and, if loosely attached to the synovium, can be easily débrided with a synovial shaver. If hard, they represent crystalline deposits and can be sent to the laboratory for identification if a diagnosis has not previously been determined. Such crystalline deposits also should be resected when seen arthroscopically.

The deposition of crystalline matter into the joint differs when comparing gout and pseudogout. Gouty infiltrate is a precipitate of uric acid that crystallizes into the joint from the synovium. These crystals then propagate an inflammatory process as evidenced by hypertrophic synovitis. Prolonged irritation by the uric acid crystals can cause synovial accumulation in the various recesses about the joint and can lead to the formation of synovial pileup and meniscoid bodies. Enzymatic degradation from the chronic synovitis can evoke degenerative changes in the cartilage as can alteration in the mechanical properties of the joint because of the crystalline deposition into expired matrix.

Pseudogout or chondrocalcinosis is a disease in which calcium pyrophosphate dihydrate is deposited within a joint. Although this crystal can be deposited in synovium and capsule, it can also precipitate into hyaline cartilage because of its metabolic disturbance of chondroitin sulfate. Secondary alterations can result in the covering of the cartilage with a thin layer of pannus, which, rather than being granulation tissue from fibroblastic proliferation, is actually a dense mucoprotein layer.[8]

Treatment of gout and pseudogout is identical. A synovial fluid analysis consisting of refractive microscopic examination should be performed if the disease has not been diagnosed. Arthroscopically, a thorough synovectomy of the synovial and subsynovial tissue to the capsular layer is imperative. Secondary effects on the cartilage and osseous structures can then be undertaken initially by resection of crystalline deposits by chondroplasty. Aggressive arthroplasty should be avoided.

Other Inflammatory Arthropathies. Other inflammatory arthropathies can be seen that might require arthroscopic treatment, including the painful joint in patients with hemophilia, ochronosis, systemic lupus erythematosus, and psoriatic arthritis. In these instances, the medical management of the overall condition is primary, and arthroscopic treatment is reserved as a final procedure when medical treatment fails or is not adequately effective in rendering the joint asymptomatic. The diagnosis is not made arthroscopically but rather has already been made by an internist or rheumatologist. The usual conservative care before arthroscopy is carried out, and when this fails, arthroscopic assessment and treatment of the joint are rendered. Usually, the primary pathologic process is the hypertrophic synovitis and associated impingement syndrome that results. Again, the synovium and subsynovial tissues are the mediators of the disease, and effective treatment revolves around adequate resection of those tissues. Secondary débridement of the joint by chondroplasty or, if indicated, abrasion arthroplasty can be performed after synovectomy.

Septic Arthritis

The basic foundations of arthroscopy were formed on the treatment of the infected knee. As a means to rid a tuberculosis-infected knee of its pain, enabling the patient to kneel respectfully again, Kenji Takagi first conceptualized the method to invade the joint minimally.[9] When this became effective, other applications for the procedure were found and so grew the field of arthroscopy. Because of this, treatment of septic joints is one of the primary indications for arthroscopy. Any type of organism can affect joint tissue. Rarely, infection is by laceration or extension from a contiguous area. The primary mechanism of joint infection is through the blood stream. Organisms known to primarily infect joints are *Staphylococcus, Streptococcus, Gonococcus, Meningococcus,* and *Pneumococcus.* Usually, only one joint is involved, but multiple joints may be affected, especially with *Gonococcus* and *Meningococcus.*

When approaching a septic joint arthroscopically, it is important to classify the infection as acute or chronic in nature. With acute infections, the primary goal is to culture the synovial fluid and flush the joint. Concurrent synovectomy can be performed if indicated. Usually, secondary changes to the cartilaginous and osseous structures are not evident.

In cases suspected of being septic, a synovial analysis is also performed to rule out the presence of an inflammatory arthropathy and is cultured to isolate any organisms. Acute changes in the joint result from exudative inflammation. The longer the condition persists, the more proliferative changes that occur within the joint, which need to be treated appropriately.

Chronic septic arthritis such as that with gonococcal infections will lead to significant joint degeneration consisting of impingement syndrome not only from hypertrophic synovial tissue but also from cartilaginous and osseous degeneration. Often marginal lipping, subchondral sclerosis, and geometric changes of the joint can be seen. In approaching these ankles, a thorough synovectomy with resection of any impinged and hypertrophic synovial tissue is first performed. Further evaluation of the joint will determine the extent of osseous and cartilaginous defect. As in the severe osteoarthritic joint, these joints should be gently débrided and flushed of all inflammatory exudate. Chondroplasty should be performed on appropriate cartilaginous lesions, with curettage or abrasion arthroplasty conservatively used at the surgeon's discretion. Caution is again urged to débride the joint gently after complete and thorough resection of hypertrophic synovial and subsynovial tissues, being careful not to violate the normal capsular structures.

References

1. Collins DH: The Pathology of Articular and Spinal Diseases. London, Edward Arnold Publishing, 1949, p 74.
2. Goodfellow J, Hungerford DS, and Woods C: Patello-femoral joint mechanics and pathology: Part 2. Chondromalacia patella. J Bone Joint Surg 58B:291, 1976.
3. Bauer M and Jackson RW: Chondral lesions at the femoral condyles: A system of arthroscopic classification. Arthroscopy 4:99, 1988.
4. Salter RB, Simmons DF, Malcolm BW, et al: The biological effect of continuous passive motion on the healing of full thickness defects in articular cartilage. J Bone Joint Surg 62A:1232–1251, 1980.
5. Lundeen RO: Medial impingement lesions of the tibial plafond. J Am Podiatr Med Assoc 26:37, 1987.
6. Harrington KB: Degenerative arthritis of the ankle secondary to longstanding lateral ligamentous instability. J Bone Joint Surg 61A:354, 1979.
7. Watanabe M, Takeda S, and Ikeuchi H: Atlas of Arthroscopy. Tokyo, Igaku-Shoin, 1979, p 52.
8. Zitnan D and Sitaj S: Chondrocalcinosis articularis. Ann Rheum Dis 22:142, 1963.
9. Lundeen GW: Historical perspectives of ankle arthroscopy. J Foot Surg 26:3, 1987.

CHAPTER 38

Surgical Management of Soft Tissue Tumors

Robert G. O'Keefe, D.P.M.

Soft tissue neoplasms of connective tissue can occur anywhere in the body; they are found in the head and neck (10%), upper extremities (20%), trunk and retroperitoneum (30%), and lower extremities (40%).[1] It is not unusual to expect a variety of tumors to affect the nonosseous tissues of the foot. These tumors make up a vast and heterogeneous group of benign and malignant lesions that develop in connective tissue other than bone; that is, fibrous tissue, tendon, fat, muscle, and neurovascular tissue. These lesions are more common than bone tumors and may form a benign mass or its malignant counterpart. Soft tissue tumors of the foot are generally more apparent on physical examination than on routine radiography.[2]

With magnetic resonance imaging (MRI), a more accurate preoperative evaluation of the extent of the lesion can be performed. MRI establishes exceptional soft tissue contrast of these lesions and is capable of direct multiplanar imaging in the extremities. Although MRI has not proven useful in predicting tumor histology, it has aided greatly in understanding benign and malignant behavior and in staging musculoskeletal neoplasms. Accurate identification of lesions and determination of the extent of bone and soft tissue involvement can be established with a high degree of reliability with MRI.[3]

A reliable system of staging musculoskeletal neoplasms has been developed by Enneking and colleagues over the past 12 years.[4] This system applies only to benign and malignant lesions of connective tissue histogenesis and not to primary lesions of round-cell origin (leukemias, lymphomas, myelomas, and so on) or metastatic lesions.

STAGING OF SOFT TISSUE TUMORS

Benign

Benign tumors may appear aggressive but should not metastasize. They are usually slow growing and have an intact capsule or fibrous tissue pseudocapsule surrounded by a narrow zone of reactive or inflammatory tissue. Benign neoplasms may be inactive, active, or aggressive in behavior (Table 38–1).

Inactive Benign Tumors (Static, Latent). These tumors are enclosed by a capsule of mature fibrous tissue. These lesions remain localized and rarely deform or expand overlying soft tissues. The reactive zone is minimal, and histologic characteristics are benign. These processes are usually asymptomatic.

Active Benign Tumors. These tumors remain encapsulated with a mature fibrous tissue. They continue to grow and may deform overlying tissues. A narrow reactive zone develops around the tumor with irregularity of the intracapsular structure. The tumor may appear septate or loculated. Active benign tumors may be symptomatic and cause anatomic dysfunction.

Aggressive Benign Tumors. These lesions appear locally invasive and behave like low-grade malignant tumors. Tumors will penetrate adjacent tissue, forming a pseudocapsule of reactive tissue around the expanding lesion. These neoplasms may penetrate adjacent anatomic compartments and may involve neurovascular structures. The histologic characteristics demonstrate impressive pleomorphism or mitoses, but these cytologic features may not correlate with their clinical aggression. These processes are often symptomatic and can be associated with significant anatomic dysfunction and neurovascular complications.

Malignant

Malignant tumors usually grow rapidly and possess the ability to create metastatic disease to remote anatomic sites, most commonly the lung. Other remote anatomic sites may be the lymphatics, liver, or the rest of the skeletal system. The only soft tissue sarcomas with significant risk of primary metastatic lymph node involvement are synovial sarcoma and rhabdomyosarcoma. The rapid growth of malignant tumors results in less distinct tissue borders and a wider inflammatory reactive zone. The biologic behavior of sarcomas varies considerably, from indolent local growth with few metastases to aggressive local growth and a high incidence of metastases. The histologic grade of the tumor will be the most accurate indicator of the prognosis rather than the histologic type. These neoplasms may be described as low-grade or high-grade sarcomas.

Low-Grade Sarcomas. These are malignant lesions that slowly invade local tissue with a low risk of metastasis. An interrupted capsule is observed with an inflammatory reactive

TABLE 38–1

STAGES OF SOFT TISSUE TUMORS*

Benign
1. Inactive (stage I)
2. Active (stage II)
3. Aggressive (stage III)

Malignant
1. Low grade without metastasis (stage I)
   Intracompartmental
   Extracompartmental
2. High grade without metastasis (stage II)
   Intracompartmental
   Extracompartmental
3. Low/high grade with metastasis (stage III)
   Intracompartmental
   Extracompartmental

*Some tumors of the extremities are not located in distinct anatomic compartments such as the ankle and may require radical en-bloc resection.

Adapted from Enneking WF: A system of staging musculoskeletal neoplasms. Clin Orthop 204:9–24, 1986.

zone and pseudocapsule around the lesions. Tumor nodules may be found in but not remote to the reactive tissue zone. Low-grade sarcomas will gradually erode natural anatomic barriers such as fascia and bone. The histologic characteristics demonstrate malignant cytologic features. Low-grade malignant tumors by virtue of their nonaggressive growth rate appear as slow-growing masses. Malignant, aggressive induction may occur in late stages of development.

High-Grade Sarcomas. Uninhibited by anatomic barriers, these lesions overgrow a wide reactive zone and appear to have little or no pseudocapsulation. They extend into regional and extracompartment tissue by destroying contiguous tissues. "Skip" metastases are observed beyond satellite nodules in the reactive tissue. The histologic features of these lesions include poor cellular differentiation and, especially, tumor necrosis.

Tumor Characteristics: Staging

Significant progressive changes in the biologic behavior of soft tissue neoplasms may be progressive and can be categorized as (1) localized, inactive, benign; (2) localized, active, benign; (3) aggressive, invasive, benign; (4) indolent, invasive, malignant, low risk of metastasis; (5) rapid growing, destructive, malignant, and high risk of metastasis; and (6) regional and distal metastatic disease.[5]

The biologic behavior of the neoplasm involves evaluating the histologic grade of the tumor (G), the extent of involvement at the primary site (T), and the presence or absence of distant metastases (M). The Enneking staging system for lesions of connective tissue histogenesis recognizes three histologic grades, one benign and two malignant. Thus, the biologic activity of a primary tumor is graded as follows: G_0, benign; G_1, low-grade malignant; G_2, high-grade malignant.[6]

The anatomic site of the tumor indicates whether the lesion is contained by its capsule (intracapsular) or has breached it (extracapsular) and whether the tumor remains enclosed within its anatomic compartment of origin (intracompartmental). Tumors that have penetrated their anatomic compartment are considered extracompartmental. The emphasis on anatomic compartmentalization is best suited for well-documented neoplasms arising in the extremities. Ankle tumors are extracompartmental as are lesions in extrafascial planes or spaces of the midfoot and hindfoot. Lesions of intrafascial compartments or rays of the foot are regarded as intracompartmental.

T_0 denotes a tumor that is both intracapsular and intracompartmental; T_1, extracapsular but intracompartmental; and T_2, extracapsular and extracompartmental.

The presence of metastatic disease (M) from the neoplasm is the third parameter in the staging system. Tumors with regional or distal metastasis have a similar outcome.[4–11]

MORPHOLOGIC FEATURES OF SOFT TISSUE NEOPLASMS ON MRI EXAMINATION

Evaluation of soft tissue lesions may be quite difficult with routine radiographs and even xeroradiography. Until recently, computed tomography (CT) has been the technique of choice for evaluating bone and soft tissue neoplasms. As experience has increased, MRI has become the ideal technique for detecting and determining the extent of involvement of soft tissue tumors.[12]

MRI is highly sensitive in establishing soft tissue detail but lacks high specificity in establishing significant differentiation between benign and malignant lesions and in predicting their histologic features. The relaxation times of benign and malignant lesions overlap too greatly to be of diagnostic value alone. Despite the apparent lack of tissue specificity, MRI establishes certain features that can be useful in differentiating neoplasms. The morphologic features noted on MRI examination such as homogeneity, margination of the lesion,

TABLE 38–2

APPEARANCE OF SOFT TISSUE TUMORS ON MAGNETIC RESONANCE IMAGING

Lesion	Homogeneous	Marginated	Neurovascular Encasement	Signal Intensity
Cyst	+	+	−	$\downarrow T_1$; $\uparrow T_2$
Lipoma	+	+	−	$\uparrow T_1$; $\uparrow T_2$
Fibroma	+	+	−	Intermediate T_1 and T_2
Desmoid	−	Variable	Occasional	Slight T_1 and T_2
Hemangioma	−	−	Numerous vessels	$\downarrow T_1$; $\uparrow T_2$ (occasionally mixed)
Malignant	−	− (partial margins)	+	Mixed T_1 and T_2

+, positive; −, negative; $\downarrow$, lower; $\uparrow$, higher.

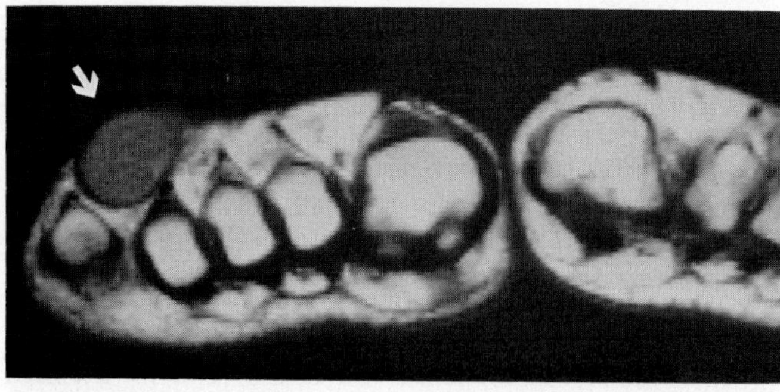

FIGURE 38–1. Leiomyoma of the foot. T_1-weighted magnetic resonance image of the right foot. Note the homogenicity of the lesion with clear margination of borders (encapsulation). (Courtesy of M. A. Solomon, M.D., Redwood MRI, Redwood City, CA.)

neurovascular encasement, and signal intensity differentiate malignant processes from most of their benign counterparts (Table 38–2). Even though T_1 and T_2 relaxation times of benign lesions overlap considerably with malignant lesions, morphologic characteristics are of more value in the relationship of tumor margins, uniformity, and aggressive behavior.[13]

Benign soft tissue masses are usually well marginated, have homogeneous signal intensity, and do not encase neurovascular structures or invade bone (Fig. 38–1). Malignant soft tissue lesions are poorly marginated, are inhomogeneous, encase neurovascular structures, and usually invade bone.

Lipomas are homogeneous on MRI examination with a high signal intensity on both the T_1- and T_2-weighted sequences. They are well marginated and may contain clearly defined fibrous septae. Larger lipomas may appear irregular with adjacent soft tissue distortion of the mass such as a muscle group. This lesion is clearly separated from adjacent tissue with a distinct margin or capsule. Liposarcomas should be considered when there are areas of inhomogeneity or when significant irregularity of the tumor margins is noted. Mixed signal intensity of the T_1- and T_2-weighted sequences may be demonstrated. Atypical lipomas in the extremities may be difficult to differentiate from low-grade liposarcomas.

Benign cysts have high signal intensity on T_2-weighted sequences and homogeneous low signal intensity on T_1-weighted images. These lesions are very distinct and well marginated. Cystic lesions, such as ganglia, are typically associated with tendons and joints. Signal intensity of communicating articular cysts and ganglia do not differ significantly. Soft tissue ganglion cysts usually occur in periarticular locations or along tendon sheaths. The fluid in the cyst will usually demonstrate a high T_2 signal intensity, but if mucoid degeneration and necrosis have occurred, the T_2-weighted sequence will appear somewhat decreased (Fig. 38–2).

Giant-cell tumors of tendon sheath are noncollagenous lesions that arise from histiocytes with a prominent giant-cell component. These are well-marginated lesions with decreased signal intensity on T_2-weighted sequences. The signal intensity may vary depending on the size of the lesion and deposition of hemosiderin.

Most other benign lesions excluding lipomas are also well marginated and homogeneous with increased signal intensity on T_2-weighted sequences and decreased signal intensity on T_1-weighted sequences. There are two notable exceptions to the morphologic appearance of benign lesions: hemangiomas and vascular malformations. These lesions are observed with mixed signal intensity on MRI and may be very extensive. Hemangiomas may vary from capillary-like vessels to cavernous lesions with large sinusoids. The cavernous variety is common in the muscles of the peripheral extremities. Numerous serpiginous vessels may be observed with increased signal intensity on both T_1- and T_2-weighted sequences. These

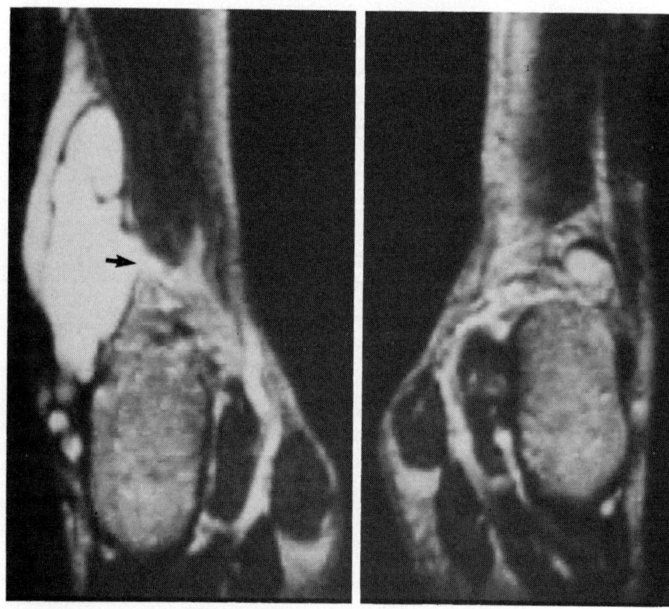

FIGURE 38–2. Ganglion cyst of right ankle. T_2-weighted magnetic resonance image of the ankle demonstrates a mass of high signal intensity *(arrow)*. A thin, low signal intensity capsule is identified. Note the anatomic association with the ankle joint. (Courtesy of M. A. Solomon, M.D., Redwood MRI, Redwood City, CA.)

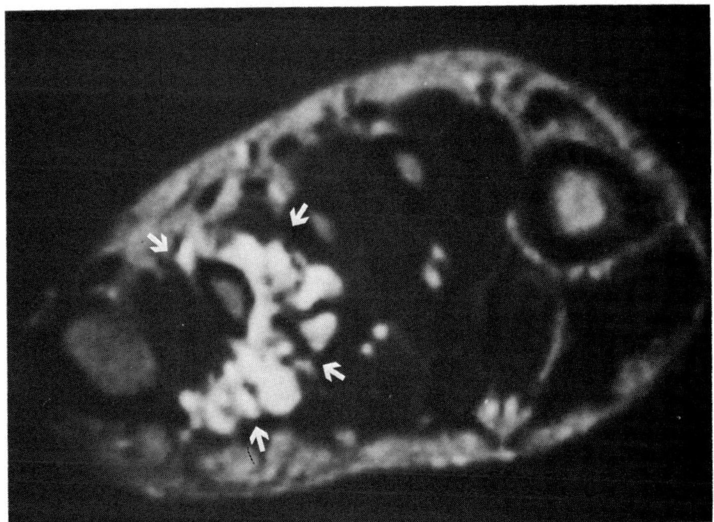

FIGURE 38–3. Hemangioma of the foot, T_2-weighted magnetic resonance image. Although benign, these lesions *(arrows)* appear aggressive with inhomogenicity and lacking clear margins. Mixed signal intensity may be observed. (Courtesy of M. A. Solomon, M.D., Redwood City MRI, Redwood City, CA.)

lesions may not appear homogeneous or well marginated. Apparent aggressive vascularity may be extensive with irregularity and mixed signal intensity (Fig. 38–3). Selective angiography may still be necessary to identify feeding arteries and draining veins in arteriovenous malformations.

Fibromas may be well-demarcated lesions of fibroblast origin found in subcutaneous tissues. These lesions are benign and may vary in size. They are homogeneous and well marginated and do not invade neurovascular structures. Fibromas are observed with an intermediate signal intensity in both T_1- and T_2-weighted images (Fig. 38–4).

Extra-abdominal desmoid tumors are locally aggressive fibrous tissue lesions of aponeurotic or fascial origin. These aggressive hypocellular lesions are poorly marginated with partial encapsulation and pseudoencapsulation. These tumors are inhomogeneous and poorly marginated and occasionally

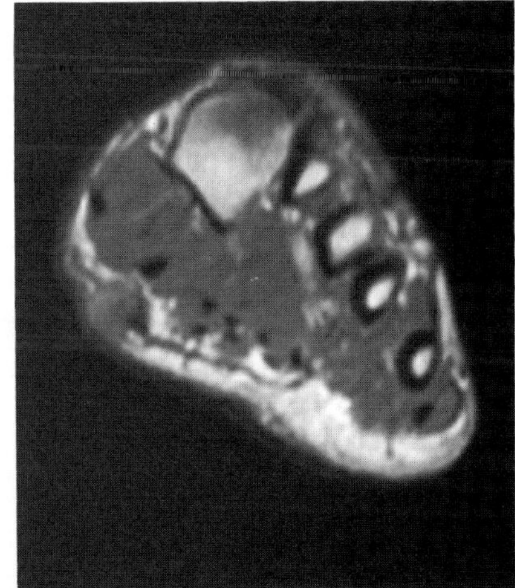

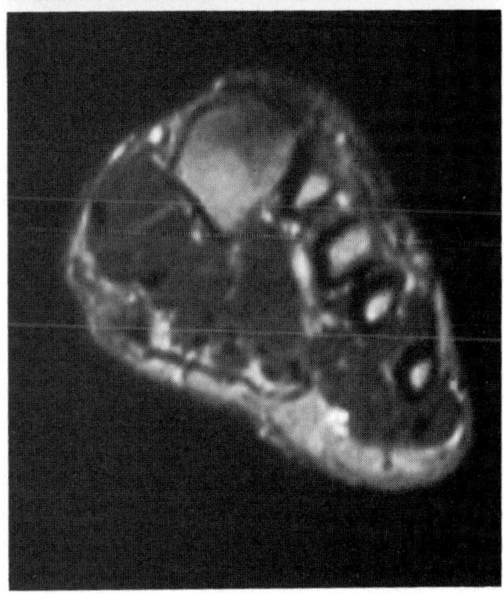

FIGURE 38–4. Plantar fibromatosis of the left foot. T_2-weighted image with intermediate signal intensity. The lesion is well marginated and homogeneous.

involve neurovascular structures. The signal intensity with MRI is absent or low on both T_1- and T_2-weighted sequences. Marginal irregularity and inhomogeneity with significant scar tissue is typical in recurrent desmoid tumors.

Malignant soft tissue neoplasms are irregular along a portion of their margins. There may be increased signal intensity surrounding lesions on the T_2-weighted sequence. This is not specific for malignant neoplasms because it may be observed with infection and hemorrhage. The signal intensity is inhomogeneous on both T_1- and T_2-weighted sequences but most appreciated on the T_2-weighted sequence. Neurovascular encasement is common along with local bony involvement (neoplastic infiltration with primary destruction of bone).[14–16]

The MRI characteristics of benign and malignant soft tissue masses have been described in much detail.[17] Such characteristics can be used as reasonable criteria for accurately identifying benign and malignant tendencies. Malignant lesions were accurately identified 91% of the time with a negative prediction value of 94.5% by Berquist and coworkers.[18] MRI has become a valuable tool for the physician in determining appropriate biopsy and surgical margin technique.

SURGICAL CONSIDERATIONS

Not all soft tissue lesions require surgical biopsy. The low incidence of malignant lesions supports this promise. Benign soft tissue tumors outnumber their counterparts by a margin of approximately 100:1. The annual incidence is about 300 per 100,000 population.[1] The incidence of benign tumors in the general population may even be higher on the basis of the probability that many lesions go unnoticed. Soft tissue sarcomas are relatively rare and may account for 1% of all cancers. The incidence of malignant tumors is probably better appreciated because they ultimately come to medical attention.

Certain characteristics indicate a need for biopsy. If a lesion is clinically active with demonstrated aggressive tendencies on MRI, surgical biopsy is indicated. If the tumor is malignant, the biopsy findings form the basis of histopathologic diagnosis and tumor grade. Once obtained, appropriate surgical staging and adjunctive therapy can be instituted. An open incisional biopsy is preferred, providing an adequate tissue sample with little probability of exfoliation of tumor cells. In contrast, an excisional biopsy removes most of the tumor. Contamination of the surrounding tissue is certain if the tumor is aggressive or malignant. Excisional biopsy may be used for benign tumors less than 3 cm in diameter. These lesions should not demonstrate aggressive tendencies on MRI and should be well marginated.[8, 9, 19]

Intracapsular excision of a neoplasm should be avoided. Remnants of neoplasm with capsular or pseudocapsular tissue invariably remain. Aggressive benign and malignant lesions most certainly will recur. Marginal local excisions are by definition performed extracapsularly through the marginal reactive zone, sequestering the tumor in the specimen. Appropriate excisional biopsy may be considered a marginal excision, but this type of ''shell-out'' procedure is recommended for latent and moderately aggressive benign neoplasms with excellent margination and no pseudocapsule. Wide-excision or en-bloc local excisions are performed through normal tissue beyond the pseudocapsule or reactive zone of more aggressive benign lesions and less aggressive malignant neoplasms but within the compartment of origin. Local recurrence is likely if microsatellite tumors and skip lesions are observed on microscopic examination. Abnormal microscopic tissue borders assume incomplete surgical ablation of the neoplasm. Radical excision requires removal of the anatomic compartment of origin. This is usually beneficial in the treatment of sarcomas that are not extracompartmental. Aggressive benign lesions such as recurrent pigmented villonodular synovitis, extra-abdominal desmoid, and nodular fibromatosis may require radical en-bloc resection. Most benign lesions are treated with marginal and occasional wide-excision techniques. In the foot and ankle, anatomic compartments may not be sufficiently distinct and may require radical en-bloc resection of poorly marginated malignant lesions. Radical local or amputative procedures have

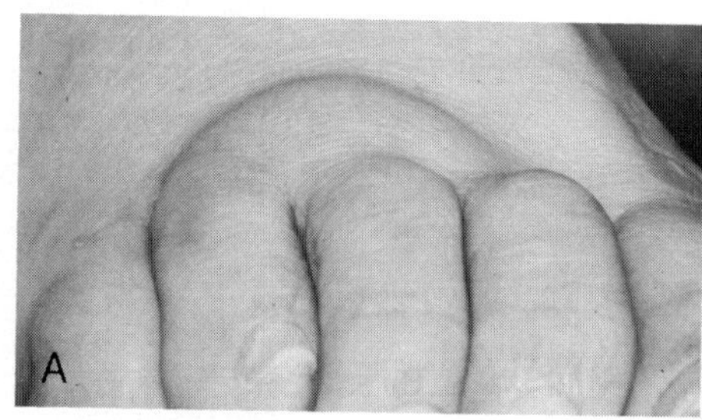
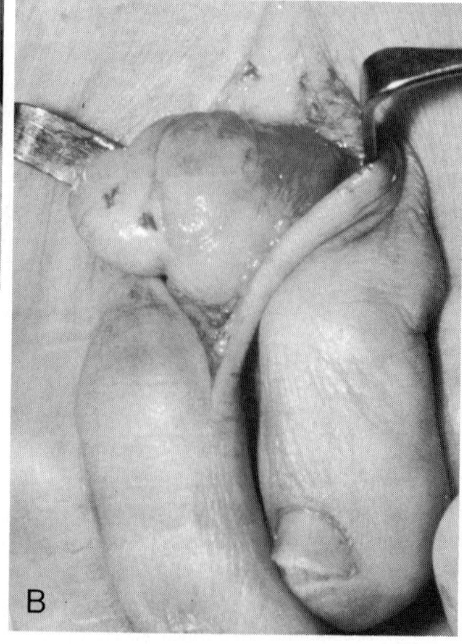

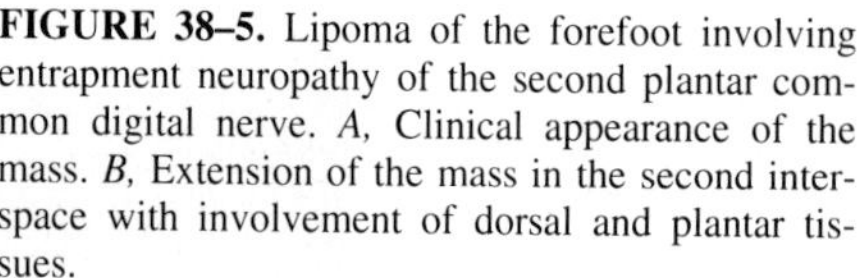
FIGURE 38–5. Lipoma of the forefoot involving entrapment neuropathy of the second plantar common digital nerve. *A,* Clinical appearance of the mass. *B,* Extension of the mass in the second interspace with involvement of dorsal and plantar tissues.

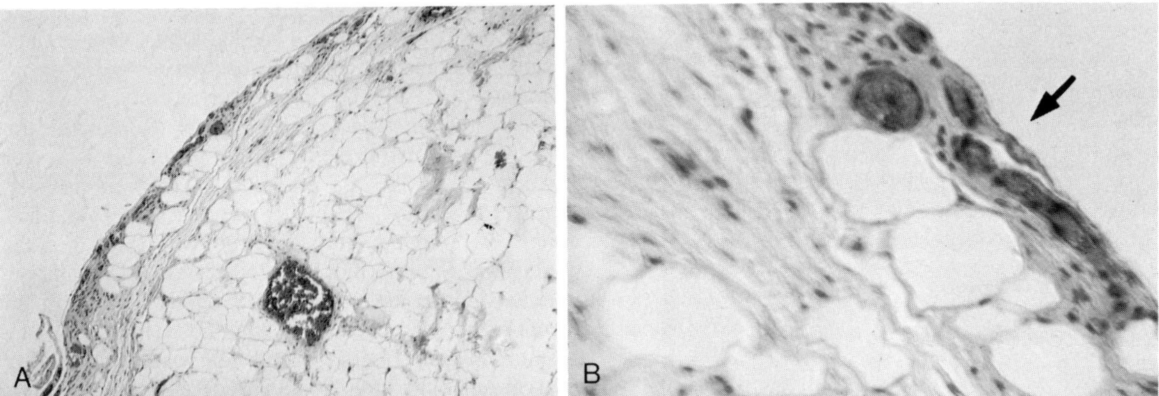

FIGURE 38–6. *A,* Lipoma showing sharp circumscription with typical fat cells; fibrous connective tissue is observed. *B,* Angiolipoma showing prominent fatty tissue with perivascular channels in the subcapsular tissues.

yielded the lowest local recurrence rates for highly aggressive or malignant lesions. The histologic grade, anatomic site, and presence or absence of metastatic disease will influence both surgical and medical management.

LIPOMA

Lipoma is a well-encapsulated, benign neoplastic proliferation of adipose tissue that is composed of mature fat and represents, by far, the most common mesenchymal tumor. Although uncommon in the distal extremities, this tumor varies in size and is usually observed as a superficial solitary mass. Lipomas usually appear as asymptomatic inactive or latent lesions (stage I). They rarely exhibit rapid growth changes. However, some lipomas may present as active lesions (stage II) involving deep structures as a space-occupying lesion, which may evoke neurovascular complication (Fig. 38–5).

Variants of lipoma are uncommon in the extremities and rare in the foot. Angiolipoma may occur in the foot as a subcutaneous palpable tender lesion. Unlike the typical asymptomatic lipoma, this neoplasm is painful in the initial growth period (stage II). These lesions are located in subcutaneous tissue and present as an encapsulated yellow nodular mass with perivascular tissue. The vascularity is usually prominent in the subcapsular areas (Fig. 38–6). Late forms of this tumor usually undergo perivascular and interstitial fibrosis. I have confirmed the presence of angiolipoma in two patients.

Most locally occurring lipomas are less than 5 cm, are usually inactive or latent (stage I), and, because of their proximity, can be surgically removed without the need for establishing staging characteristics via MRI. Only large lipomas greater than 5 cm need to be staged via MRI (Fig. 38–7). These lesions may encroach on adjacent anatomy and may make surgical excision difficult if appropriate surgical exposure has not been determined. MRI is useful not only in staging large neoplasms but also in determining appropriate surgical exposure (Fig. 38–8). Large lipomas that are compartmentalized or extend along distinct anatomic compartments can be visualized with MRI to determine their characteristics and association with adjacent tissue structure (Fig. 38–9). Using axial views as an aid in marginal excision of large lipomas is helpful in determining anatomic structures that may be adjacent to the mass. Injury to neurovascular structures can be avoided. A variety of incisional approaches to large plantar masses can be made such as the Curtin incision,[20] simple serpentine incision, or Z-incisional approach. It must be emphasized that marginal excision requires adequate extensive exposure to avoid damaging intimate neurovascular structures. Complete marginal excision of lipomas is usually successful; recurrence is uncommon.[1, 21]

PLANTAR FIBROMATOSIS

Plantar fibromatosis is part of a group of non-neoplastic growths that demonstrate a varying degree of infiltrative behavior. Nodular aponeurotic lesions from the plantar fascia

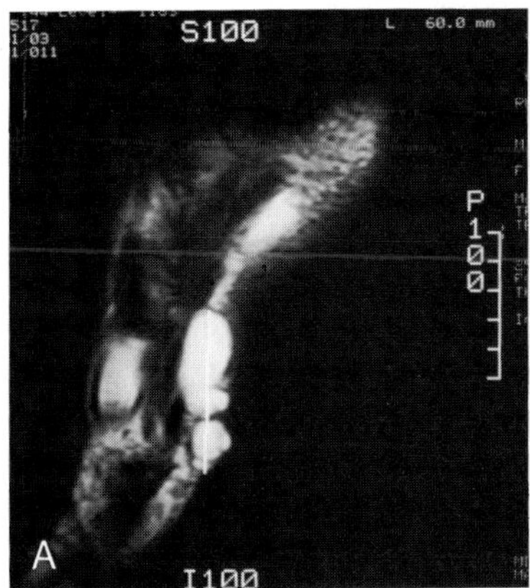
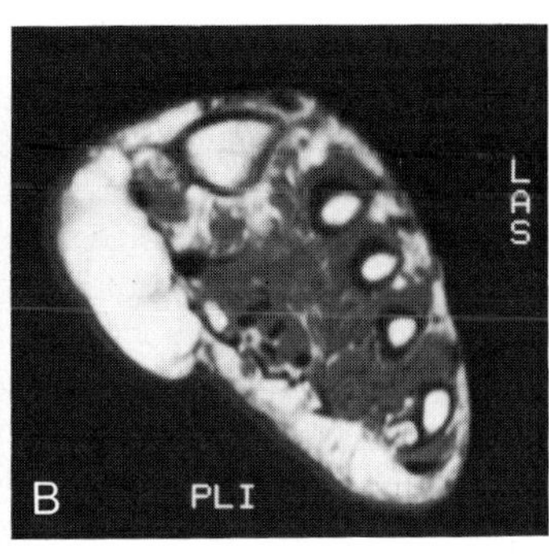

FIGURE 38–7. Lipoma. *A,* Sagittal T$_1$-weighted image. *B,* Axial view of T$_1$-weighted image. This is a distinctive, well-marginated lesion with increased signal intensity that is homogeneous and separate from adjacent tissue.

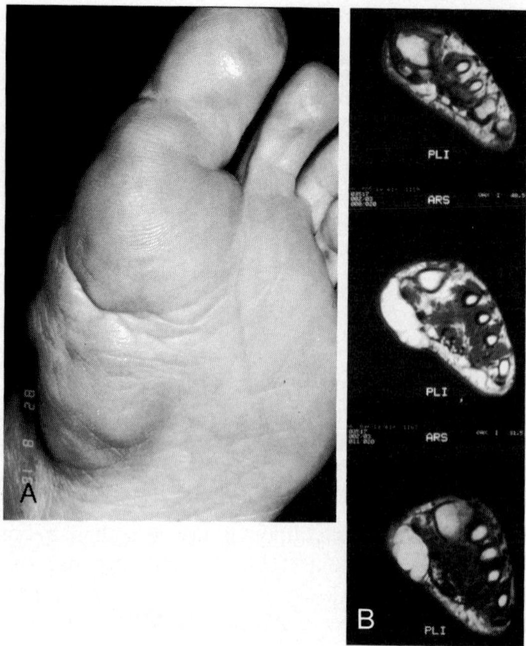

FIGURE 38–8. Lipoma. *A,* Lipoma of the foot approximately 9 cm in length. *B,* Magnetic resonance image of lesion with T$_1$-weighted image in the axial view.

may demonstrate local infiltration along intimate fascial tissues, primarily the medial septum and medial border of the central band of the plantar aponeurosis (see Fig. 38–4). Aggressive behavior of plantar fibromatosis can vary from simple local involvement to more infiltrative nodular activity. The classic plantar fibromatosis is usually multinodular and can occur along the medial aspect of the central aponeurosis. This lesion is usually locally aggressive (stage II), and subtle infiltration to surrounding fibrous septae and fascia planes is not usually observed (Fig. 38–10). Nodular fasciitis is clinically more aggressive than plantar fibromatosis (stage III). This lesion may appear to expand beyond the plantar aponeurosis and infiltrate myofascial tissues. Although benign, this lesion has been mistaken for sarcoma because of rapid growth, clinically aggressive behavior, rich cellularity, and mitotic activity. The terms *pseudosarcomatous fibromatosis, infiltrative fasciitis, proliferative fasciitis,* and *pseudosarcomatous fasciitis* have been ascribed to nodular fasciitis. Although seldom encountered in the lower extremities, nodular fasciitis should be appreciated as an aggressive variant of plantar fibromatosis. This nodular fibrous proliferation arising within the plantar aponeurosis may appear as a large eccentric mass with less well-circumscribed borders than the typical plantar fibromatosis (Fig. 38–11).

Plantar fibromatosis is best visualized by axial MRI. Large, multinodular fibromatosis should be staged and tissue margins established before excision. MRI will demonstrate the extent of soft tissue involvement and neurovascular margins. Nodular fibromatosis may involve deep tissue compartments, with infiltration along myofascial planes (stage III). Fibromatosis is by definition an aggressive, benign lesion, and simple marginal excision is not recommended. Simple resection of the nodular lesion underestimates typical local infiltration of normal-appearing fascia. These attempts at simple excision fail. These lesions should be treated aggres-

sively with wide-margin excision requiring at least a radical fasciectomy. Usually the medial septal border and central band of the plantar aponeurosis are removed. However, wide excision may include portions of the medial and lateral expansion of the aponeurosis. If local nodular infiltration has occurred involving the flexor digitorum brevis muscle, wide excision may include partial myectomy. If nodular lesions adhere to the hypodermal tissue and skin, the attached cutis may be removed. Surgical approaches vary but the Curtin incision[20] is preferred, involving a medial plantar serpentine incision along the margin of the lesion. This approach allows exposure to the medial septal border, central band, and lateral septal border. Deep compartment exposure may require a large Z incisional approach. Wide excision with removal of the lesion with normal tissue borders should be attempted. Local recurrence may further compromise regional tissue including neurovascular structures. Radical fasciectomy should be included in the wide-excision technique. Neurovascular complication is usually one of surgical error. The medial plantar neurovascular complex courses along the medial septum, under the flexor digitorum brevis, and through the distal fascial and tendinous expansion. Error in margin resection may lead to damage of vital anatomy.[21, 22]

GANGLION

A ganglion is not a true neoplasm but develops from myxoid degeneration of connective tissue involving joint capsule, synovial membrane, or tendon sheath. It presents as a soft, tumor-like mass in the foot and ankle regions. Ganglia or synovial cysts are usually inactive lesions that lack aggressive behavior (stage I). Ganglion cysts are firm, nodular masses fixed to a tendon sheath or joint capsule. Aspiration of ganglia usually demonstrates mucinous fluid if mucoid degeneration and necrosis have not occurred. Sophisticated staging studies are rarely needed for diagnosis. The cyst may appear unilocular or multilocular, with firm encapsulation with synovial lining and clear gelatinous fluid. Marginal excision of this stage I lesion with removal of ligamentous tissue around the base of the cyst is usually adequate (Fig. 38–12).[11, 21]

PIGMENTED VILLONODULAR SYNOVITIS

Pigmented villonodular synovitis (PVNS) is a benign tumor of synovial origin. This lesion may be diffuse or nodular in clinical presentation. The diffuse variety encompasses 75% of PVNSs and involves synovial joints. Nodular lesions involve the synovial lining of tendon and are termed giant-cell tumors of tendon sheath. The diffuse type usually has a more difficult and protracted course. PVNS is a locally aggressive benign lesion (stage III). It is locally destructive and will penetrate adjacent tissue, including bone. Erosive bone changes will resemble an aggressive intraosseous tumor (Fig. 38–13). PVNS extends initially as a hypertrophic hemorrhagic synovitis, creating capsular synovitis distension and periarticular erosion. There is no disorganization of the joint space because the articular cartilage is not directly affected. The disease process will extend beyond the joint and involve periarticular structures. Chronic joint effusion, pain, and hemarthrosis are common. Aspiration of the joint may reveal bloody, brown, or serosanguineous fluid. The aggressive be-

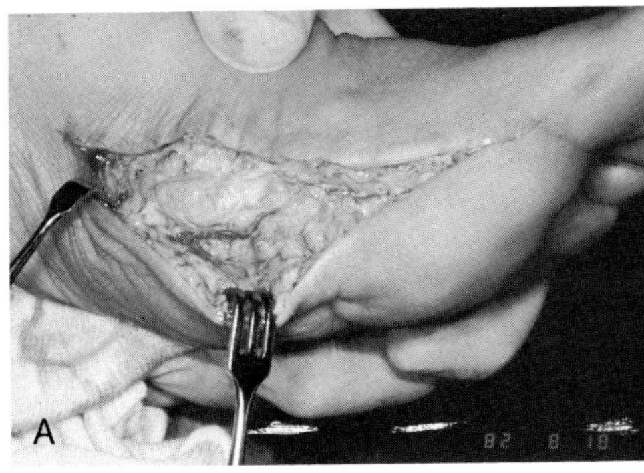
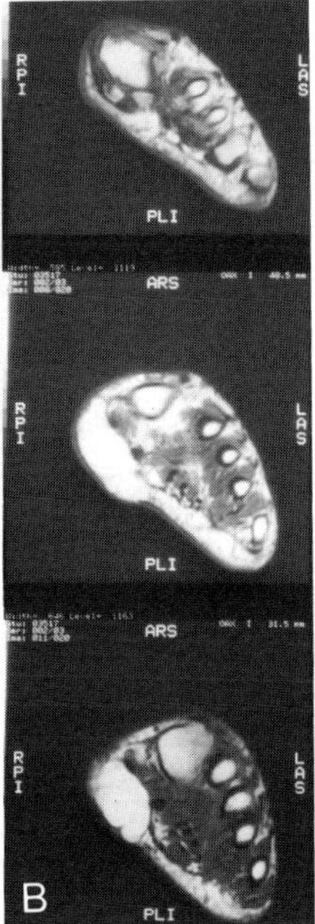

FIGURE 38–9. Lipoma. *A*, Surgical approach. *B*, Three-stage axial view to aid in surgical excision of a large lipoma.

havior of PVNS may mimic severe rheumatoid arthropathy or synovial sarcoma.

Radiographs demonstrate joint effusion, thickened synovium, and periarticular bony erosions. MRI will demonstrate extensive synovitis and joint distension. Focal areas of decreased signal intensity on T_2-weighted images are observed (hemosiderin deposition). Soft tissue characteristics will show margination of the lesion with extension beyond the involved joint. Because of the aggressive appearance of PVNS, a biopsy should be performed to rule out malignancy.

Wide-margin excision is the treatment of choice. Periarticular tissue involvement will make surgical intervention diffi-cult. Local wide-margin or en-bloc resection is recommended with advanced diffuse lesions with periarticular involvement. Local recurrence after excision may require adjunctive radiation therapy.[11, 23]

DESMOID TUMOR

Extra-abdominal desmoid tumor is an infiltrative fibrous lesion of musculoaponeurotic or fascial origin. It may be observed as a partially encapsulated or pseudoencapsulated lesion. The biological behavior of desmoid tumor is very aggressive, with rapid growth and infiltration into adjacent tissue such as muscle and bone. Although this is a stage III aggressive benign neoplasm, it differs from well-differentiated fibrosarcoma only in its inability to metastasize. Anatomic dysfunction and neurovascular complication may arise depending on the location of the desmoid tumor. Desmoid tumors can be palpated but are usually not well demarcated.

Radiographs demonstrate local bony erosion if the lesion is adjacent to skeletal tissue. MRI will demonstrate an inhomogeneous lesion with variable margination that may encase neurovascular structures. Indistinct margination on MRI indicates the infiltrative behavior of this neoplasm. Wide-margin excision is recommended to avoid local recurrence. If the infiltrative fibrous tumor involves pedal digits, adequate surgical ablation may require local amputation (Fig. 38–14).[24]

HEMANGIOMA

Hemangioma is a benign vascular tumor that may involve capillaries, veins, or arteries. Most of these lesions involve more than one vessel type, although one may predominate. Hemangioma is found more commonly in the lower extremity and may involve the foot. This neoplasm may appear as a solitary tumor that may be diffuse and infiltrative or well circumscribed. Infiltrative types may encroach muscle and intimate neurovascular structures, resulting in anatomic dysfunction. Cavernous hemangioma is an example of an ag-

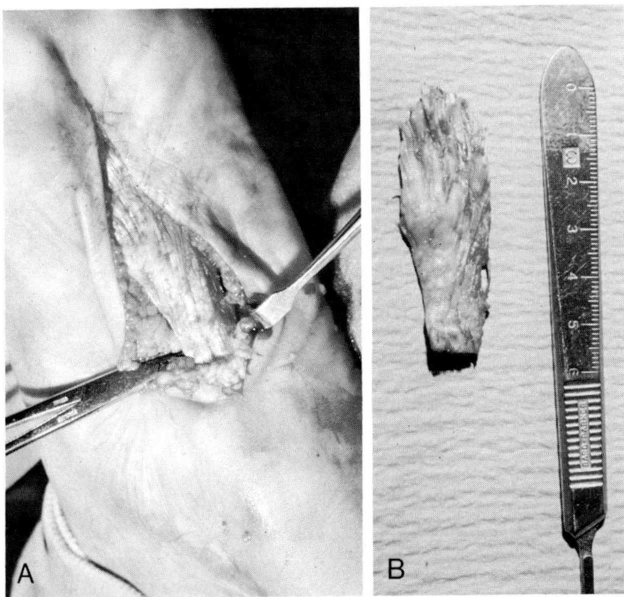

FIGURE 38–10. Plantar fibromatosis. *A*, Serpentine surgical approach exposing the central division of the plantar aponeurosis. *B*, Specimen with infiltrating fibromatosis along the fascia.

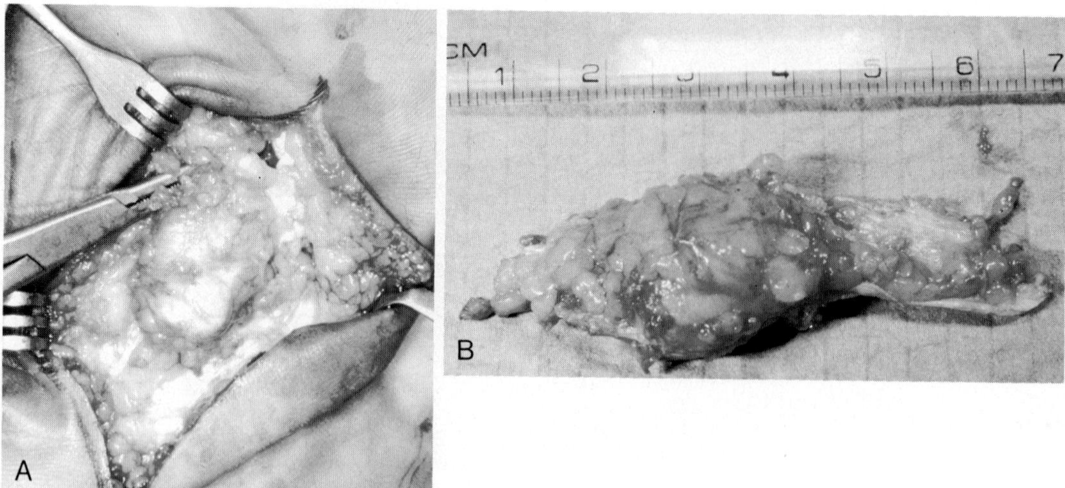

FIGURE 38–11. Nodular fibromatosis. *A,* Serpentine surgical approach exposing less well-defined fibromatosis. *B,* Specimen with aggressive nodular fibromatosis obliterating the plantar fascia. (Courtesy of John V. Vanore, D.P.M., Chicago, IL.)

gressive benign stage III lesion that is locally invasive. MRI will demonstrate an intermediate or increased signal intensity on T_1-weighted images and increased signal intensity on T_2-weighted images (see Fig. 38–3). A serpiginous pattern may be observed as well as the precise anatomic extent of the hemangioma. It will appear as a mixed infiltrative-like tumor composed of both large and small vessels. In contrast, well-circumscribed hemangiomas are small vessel and capillary types and are not invasive. Capillary hemangiomas are more cellular than cavernous lesions. Intravenous phleboliths may be observed with cavernous hemangioma via radiographs and contrast-enhanced CT. Angiography will identify feeding arteries and draining veins in the cavernous hemangioma. Angiography is helpful in determining vascular implications to surrounding structures and aid in establishing hemostasis during surgical removal.

Aggressive stage III mixed cavernous hemangioma requires wide-margin excision or en-bloc resection to establish safe tissue margins. Inadequate marginal resection along the border of this neoplasm may precipitate a recurrence rate as high as 30%. Intramuscular hemangiomas are more easily resected because wide-margin excision is consistently obtainable. Unlike angioendothelial neoplasm, hemangiomas do not metastasize or undergo malignant transformation.[25]

LEIOMYOMA

Leiomyomas are benign smooth muscle tumors that parallel the distribution of smooth muscle tissue in the body. They are commonly found in the genitourinary and gastrointestinal tracts. Leiomyomas are less frequently found in skin and are uncommon in deep soft tissue. Soft tissue leiomyomas can arise from pilar arrector muscles of the skin (cutaneous leiomyomas), superficial vessels (vascular leiomyomas), and deep tissue smooth muscle elements presumed to be vascular in origin (leiomyomas of deep soft tissue).

Cutaneous leiomyomas are usually nodular and multiple and are associated with pain. Vascular leiomyomas are pain-

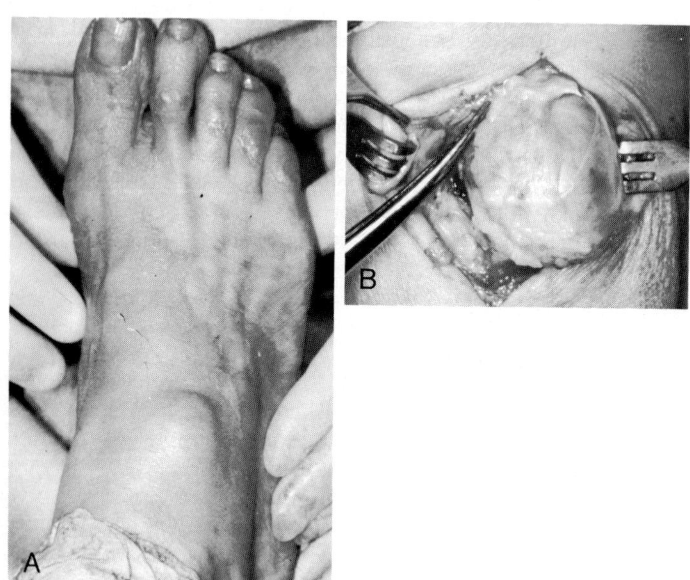

FIGURE 38–12. Ganglion of the ankle. *A,* Clinical appearance of the ganglion on the anterior aspect of the ankle. *B,* Surgical exposure of the cyst with intact fibrous capsule.

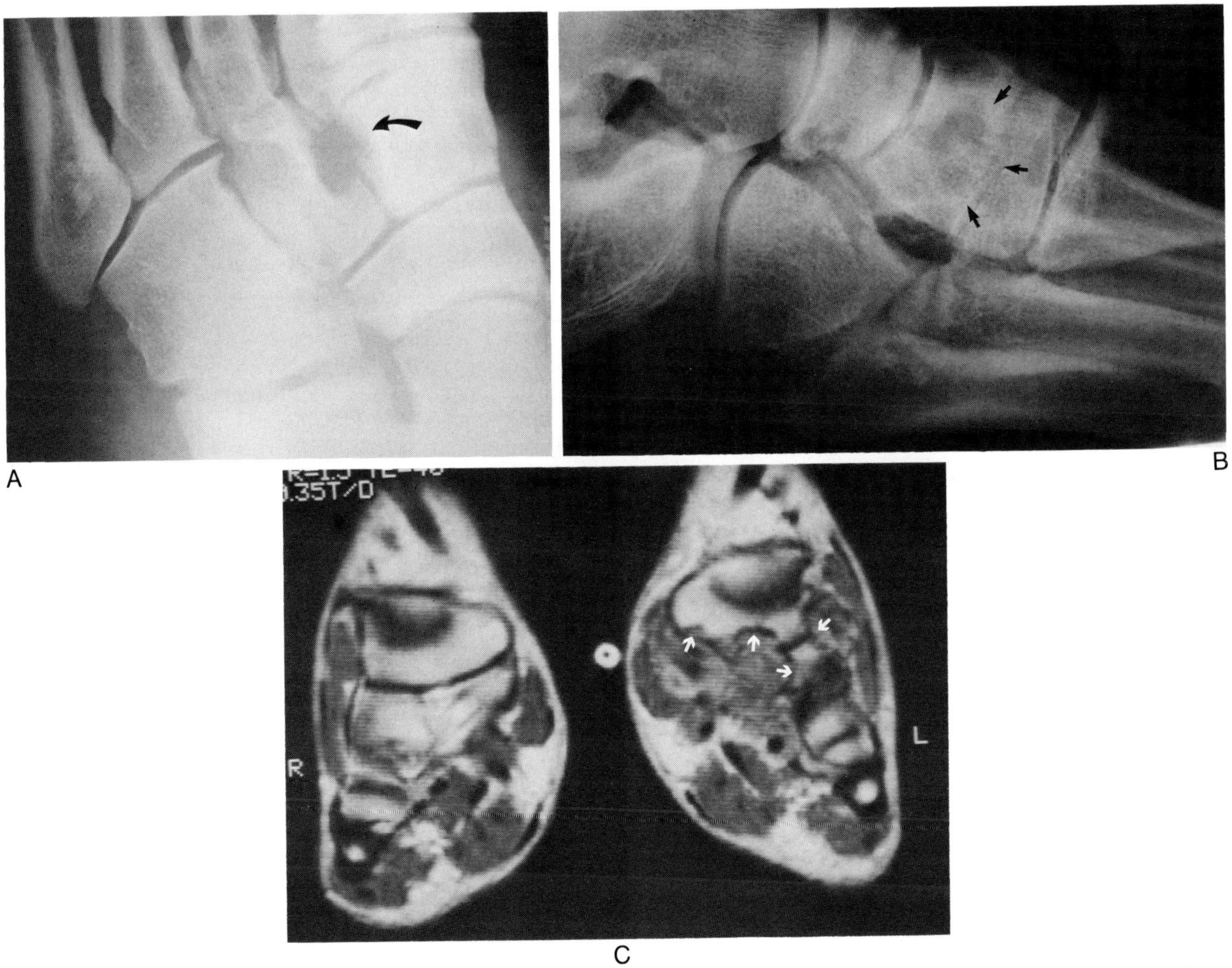

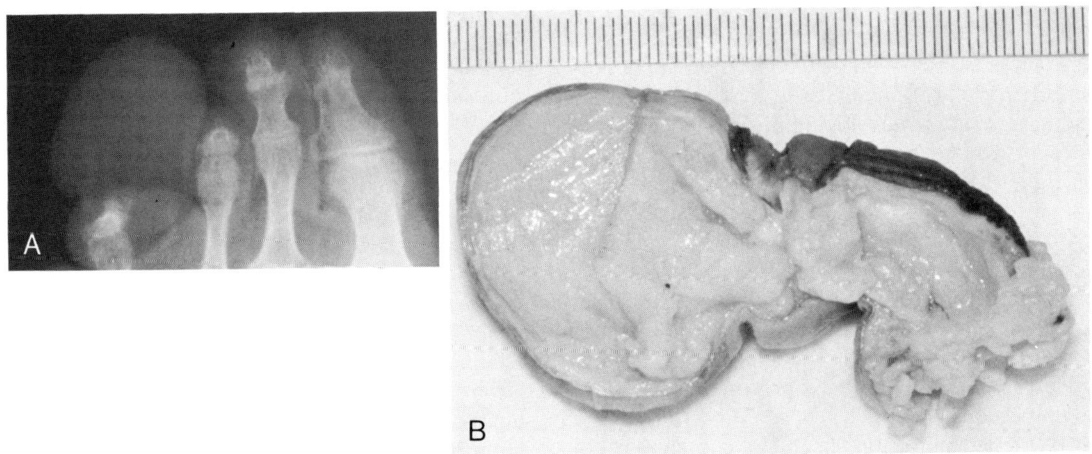

FIGURE 38–13. Pigmented villonodular synovitis. *A*, Radiograph of bony erosion between the second and third cuneiform *(arrow)*. *B*, Lateral view demonstrating apparent ''punchout'' lesions in the cuneiform area *(arrows)*. *C*, Magnetic resonance image proton-density image enhancing soft tissue periarticular involvement and bony destruction, which appear more extensive *(arrows)*. This lesion required en bloc resection, bone graft, and myocutaneous vascular graft. (Courtesy of L. Oloff, D.P.M., San Francisco, CA.)

FIGURE 38–14. Extraabdominal desmoid of digit. *A*, Radiograph demonstrates desmoid tumor with extension of soft tissue. *B*, Sagittal section of tumor specimen with aggressive fibrous infiltration in the confines of the digit without distinct margins.

ful subcutaneous tumors composed of thick-walled vessels associated with smooth muscle tissue. They are common in the lower extremities, reaching a size of approximately 2 cm. Simple excision of superficial leiomyomas is adequate therapy.

Leiomyomas of deep tissue are uncommon but have occurred in the lower extremities (see Fig. 38–1). Most are located in the deep muscle of the extremities. They are usually larger than cutaneous and subcutaneous lesions. Grossly, they are well-circumscribed, gray-white lesions (stage I). Marginal excision of these benign soft tissue lesions is usually curative. Because of the association of leiomyosarcoma in deep tissue, biopsy must be performed to rule out malignancy from pleomorphic leiomyoma.[11]

NEURILEMOMA (SCHWANNOMA)

Neurilemoma (schwannoma) is a benign neoplastic tumor that arises from Schwann's cells that form the sheaths around myelinated nerves. The collagenous type of neurilemoma may develop well-demarcated lesions surrounded by a true capsule consisting of the epineurium. Tumors of small nerves may resemble neurofibromas by virtue of their fusiform shape and usually obliterate the nerve of origin. In larger nerves, the tumor will present as an eccentric mass with adjacent splayed nerve fibers.

Neurofibromas are well-demarcated, small, round, or fusiform lesions that have been identified in the foot and ankle. A solitary neurofibroma is usually found. Multiple lesions are usually associated with neurofibromatosis. Plexiform neuromas may be observed with a multinodular pattern and clinically appear similar to a neuroma (stage I).[26]

Excisional biopsy is curative. Normal perilesional borders should be attempted to ensure complete removal of the tumor. Occasionally, neurilemomas of the collagenous variety can undergo malignant transformation.

LIPOSARCOMA

Liposarcoma constitutes the most common lower extremity sarcoma in adults. The tissues of origin are primitive mesenchymal cells rather than mature adipose tissue. This implies that various histologic subtypes of liposarcoma exist. They range from well-differentiated lipoma-like and myxoid tumors (stage I) to extremely cellular or pleomorphic tumors (stages II and III). Well-differentiated lesions are low-grade sarcomas and have a risk of developing distinct metastasis of less than 25%. They are nonaggressive and slow-growing lesions. The round-cell and pleomorphic subtypes are very aggressive, high-grade sarcomas that produce metastatic disease in many cases via microvascular invasion.[11]

Liposarcomas are localized primarily in the extremities and retroperitoneum. These lesions arise from deep structures such as intramuscular fascial planes or similar deep-seated and richly vascular structures. The neoplasm may be presented as a deep nodular bulging mass or symptomatic, deep space-occupying lesion.

MRI may vary depending on the histologic subtype of liposarcoma. Well-differentiated types may appear well marginated, and pleomorphic types may appear highly aggressive with poor margination. Regardless of subtype, inhomogeneous characteristics will appear, especially on the T_2-weighted image. MRI aids in staging liposarcoma and its relationship with regional anatomy. Better definition of the tumor extent and histologic grade (frozen section) will assist in combination therapy, varying from radical surgical extrication to chemotherapy and irradiation. Surgical intervention will vary from local amputation to wide-margin excision of this neoplasm. Combination therapy including chemotherapy and regional irradiation will be predicated on the extent of the lesion and metastatic disease, if present. Long-term follow-up is necessary to monitor recurrence or occult metastatic disease.[27]

FIBROSARCOMA

Like other sarcomas, fibrosarcoma causes no early characteristic symptoms and is difficult to diagnose clinically. This neoplasm is slow growing and may reach a large size before causing pain. The tumor is common in the region of the thigh and knee and distal portions of the extremities but is rare in the foot. Fibrosarcoma usually involves deeper structures originating from intramuscular fibrous tissue, fascia, aponeurotic tissues, and tendon.

The tumor is usually solitary, soft to firm, rounded or lobulated, gray-white to tan-yellow, and poorly defined. Small lesions may appear well circumscribed and partially or completely encapsulated (pseudocapsule). Fibrosarcoma appears aggressive with eventual extension of multiple processes into surrounding tissues. This lesion may grow in a more typical diffuse invasive or destructive manner. Pseudoencapsulation is usually incomplete, with extension of the tumor into adjacent and remote tissue sites.

Fibrosarcoma is a high-grade malignant neoplasm whose features are appreciated on MRI. The lesion will appear inhomogeneous and partially marginated (pseudocapsule) and will demonstrate neurovascular encasement and mixed signal intensity on T_1- and T_2-weighted images.

Once the diagnosis of fibrosarcoma is established by incisional biopsy, wide-margin or en-bloc resection may be attempted in well-differentiated lesions (stage II). Anaplastic tumors with poorly differentiated fibroblasts and minimum collagen formation are best treated with local amputation. Excisional biopsy and margin resection should be avoided. Metastatic disease should be investigated, especially to the lungs and bone (stage III). Adjunctive systemic chemotherapy and radiotherapy are beneficial in the treatment of fibrosarcoma.[28, 29]

SYNOVIAL SARCOMA

Synovial sarcoma is prevalent in adolescents and young adults. It occurs primarily in periarticular areas in close association with tendon sheaths, bursae, and joint capsules. It is found in joint cavities approximately 5% of the time. This neoplasm's resemblance to normal synovium has been well recognized, but its origin from preformed synovial tissue has never been substantiated. This sarcoma is regarded as a highly malignant, metastatic tumor with synovial tissue features arising from mesenchymal cells.

Several basic and closely interrelated types of synovial sarcoma are recognized: the classic biplasic type with distinct spindle-cell and epithelial-cell components, the monoplasic fibrous type, a fibrosarcoma-like neoplasm without epithelial component, the monoplasic epithelial type, and poorly differentiated synovial sarcoma. It may be difficult to draw a sharp distinction between well-differentiated and poorly differentiated synovial sarcomas. Poorly differentiated lesions behave very aggressively and metastasize in a greater percentage of cases. Although this sarcoma usually metastasizes hematogenously, anaplastic types have a 15% to 25% incidence of lymph node metastasis. Lymphangiogram is valuable in assessing metastatic disease in patients with synovial sarcoma.

This sarcoma occurs predominantly in the extremities, with a predilection for periarticular tissues of large joints, especially the knee region. The region of the ankle and foot accounts for 13% of synovial sarcoma reviewed by Armed Forces Institute of Pathology between 1970 and 1979.[11] The tumor generally grows slowly and insidiously and may be wrongly diagnosed initially as synovitis, bursitis, or arthritis. A palpable, deep-seated swelling or mass may be associated with pain or tenderness. Limitation of motion and severe functional disturbances are uncommon.

The majority of synovial sarcomas present radiographically as round or oval to lobulated swellings or masses of moderate density located in close proximity to a large joint. Periosteal reaction, superficial bone erosion, or invasion is observed in 20% of the cases. If remarkable bony destruction is demonstrated, a poorly differentiated synovial sarcoma of long duration is usually encountered. In approximately one third of all cases, the presence of multiple spotty radiopacities from focal calcification can be observed. The appearance of synovial sarcoma on MRI varies. Slow-growing lesions tend to be sharply circumscribed and round to multilobular with a pseudocapsule. Cyst formation may be prominent, and the neoplasm can be confused with ganglion features. This sarcoma can be well marginated and cystic, mimicking a benign lesion.

Synovial sarcoma is treated with radical or wide-margin excision. Low-grade variants occurring in the hands and feet may be adequately controlled by clean margin excision (stage I). High-grade synovial sarcomas are best treated with local wide resection or regional amputation (stage II). The incidence of both regional and pulmonary metastases is high with synovial sarcoma. Lymph node examination and pulmonary evaluation should be assessed before surgery to rule out early metastatic disease (stage III). Adjunctive therapy involving chemotherapy and radiation therapy is beneficial.[30]

LEIOMYOSARCOMA

Leiomyosarcoma is regarded as a high-grade sarcoma (stage II) arising from smooth muscle elements of the cutis, blood vessels, or visceral walls. This neoplasm is divided into three geographic groups presenting certain clinical and biological differences: retroperitoneal, superficial, and deep vascular types.

Extremity involvement of leiomyosarcoma includes the superficial and deep varieties. Superficial cutaneous leiomyosarcomas may appear as solitary lesions averaging less than 2 cm in size. Surface changes include discoloration and ulceration. Subcutaneous tumors are more organized and grow to a large size without cutaneous involvement. Deep lesions are usually located in deep muscle structures capable of growing more than 10 cm in size and are locally invasive.

Tumors confined to the dermis rarely metastasize; however, subcutaneous lesions may metastasize one third of the time. Metastatic disease in deep tissue leiomyosarcoma is common, with spread typically occurring hematogenously to the lung. Regional lymph node involvement may be observed.

MRI characteristics are variable for subcutaneous and deep lesions. Subcutaneous lesions may appear well organized with some margination. There will be mixed signal intensity on T_1- and T_2-weighted images and inhomogeneity noted primarily on the T_2-weighted images. Deep leiomyosarcomas appear poorly marginated and demonstrate neurovascular encasement as well as inhomogeneity on T_2-weighted images. Angiography is appropriate, especially for deep lesions when compartment resection is anticipated.

Superficial forms of leiomyosarcoma have a better prognosis than infiltrative deep lesions. Staging and biopsy may be difficult, especially with deep neoplasms. To avoid exfoliation in deep leiomyosarcoma, needle biopsy or intraoperative frozen section is recommended.[31, 32]

Local surgical management includes wide-margin excision with normal histologic borders. If the lesion is regionally infiltrative and extracompartmental, amputation is recommended. Patients with leiomyosarcoma must be evaluated for metastatic disease. Combination therapy including chemotherapy and radiation is recommended.

NEUROSARCOMA (MALIGNANT SCHWANNOMA)

Neurosarcoma is the primary sarcoma of peripheral nerves. It arises from mesenchymal elements of peripheral nerve sheath and Schwann's cell. This lesion has also been termed neurofibrosarcoma and fibrosarcoma of nerve sheath. Neurosarcoma is a high-grade sarcoma (stage II) with metastatic disease (stage III).

This neoplasm may involve primary induction of an isolated lesion or secondary malignant transformation of longstanding neurofibromatosis (von Recklinghausen's disease). Primary lesions are well demarcated, but lesser differentiated neoplasms arising from neurofibromatosis may be more difficult to determine histologically. The lesion is locally aggressive with the potential for metastatic disease. The patient may exhibit paresthesia and other motor and sensory abnormalities and occasionally pain. A fusiform mass can occasionally be palpable.[33]

MRI is helpful in delineating the size of the lesion and its relationship with other anatomic structures. Partial margination is observed as well as inhomogeneity, mixed signal intensity, and neurovascular invasion. Margins of the lesion along the proximal course of the nerve are difficult to delineate with MRI. Tumor extension and local infiltration are typical events with this neoplasm.

Wide-margin excision/resection or amputation is recommended in the surgical management of neurosarcoma. Adequate margins may be complicated by difficulty in differentiating long-standing neurofibromatosis from neurosarcoma. Primary solitary lesions of neurosarcoma are usually better defined. Proximal tumor resection must be microscopically clear of tumor cells. Prognosis is less satisfactory for patients with undifferentiated lesions. Adjunctive chemotherapy and radiation therapy are recommended.[11, 21]

References

1. Rydholm G and Berg N: Size, site, and clinical incidence of lipoma. Factors in the differential diagnosis of lipoma and sarcoma. Acta Orthop Scand 54:929, 1983.
2. Seale KS, Lange TA, Monson D, and Hackbarth DA: Soft tissue tumors of the foot and ankle. Foot Ankle 9:19–27, 1988.
3. Petterson H, Gillespy T, Hamlin DJ, et al: Primary musculoskeletal tumors: Examination with MRI imaging compared with conventional modalities. Radiology 164:237–241, 1987.
4. Enneking WF, Spanier SS, and Goodman MA: A system for the surgical staging of musculoskeletal sarcomas. Clin Orthop 153:106, 1980.
5. Enneking WF: Staging of musculoskeletal neoplasms. *In* Current Concepts of Diagnosis and Treatment of Bone and Soft Tissue Tumors. Heidelberg, Germany, Springer-Verlag, 1984.
6. Enneking WF: A system of staging musculoskeletal neoplasms. Clin Orthop 204:9, 1986.
7. Enneking WF, Spanier SS, and Malawer MM: The effort of the anatomic setting with results of surgical procedures for soft parts sarcomas of the thigh. Cancer 47:1005–1022, 1981.
8. Enneking WF: The issue of the biopsy [Editorial]. J Bone Joint Surg 64A:1119–1120, 1982.
9. Enneking WF: Musculoskeletal Tumor Surgery. New York, Churchill Livingstone, 1983.
10. Enneking WF: Staging of musculoskeletal neoplasms, from Musculoskeletal Tumor Society. Skeletal Radiol 13:183–194, 1985.
11. Enzinger FM and Weiss SW: Soft Tissue Tumors, 2nd ed. St. Louis, CV Mosby, 1988.
12. Weekes RB, Bergguist TH, McLeod RA, and Zimmer WD: Magnetic resonance imaging of soft tissue tumors: Comparison with computed tomography. Magn Reson Imaging 3:345–352, 1985.
13. Petterson H, Slone RM, Spanier S, et al: Musculoskeletal tumors: T_1 and T_2 relaxation times. Radiology 167:783–785, 1988.
14. Aisen AM, Braunstein EM, McMillin KI, et al: Magnetic resonance imaging and computed tomography: Evaluation of primary bone and soft tissue tumors. Am J Roentgenol 146:749–756, 1986.
15. Kirby EJ, Shereff MJ, and Lewis MM: Soft tissue tumors and tumor like lesions of the foot. J Bone Joint Surg 71A:621, 1989.
16. Richardson ML, Kilcoyne RF, and Gillespy T: Magnetic resonance imaging of musculoskeletal neoplasms. Radiol Clin North Am 24:259–265, 1986.
17. Totty WG, Murphy WA, and Lee JKJ: Soft-tissue tumors: MR imaging. Radiology 160:135–141, 1986.
18. Berquist TH, Ehman RL, King BF, et al: Value of MR imaging in differentiating benign from malignant soft-tissue masses: Study of 95 lesions. Am J Roentgenol 155:1251–1255, 1990.
19. Simon MA: Biopsy of musculoskeletal tumors. J Bone Joint Surg 64A:1253–1257, 1982.
20. Curtin JW: Fibromatosis of the plantar fascia. J Bone Joint Surg 47A:1605, 1965.
21. Hajdu SI: Pathology of soft tissue tumors. Philadelphia, Lea & Febiger, 1987.
22. Haedicke GJ and Sturim H: Plantar fibromatosis: An isolated disease. Plast Reconstr Surg 83:296–300, 1988.
23. Rao AS and Vigorita BJ: Pigmented villonodular synovitis (giant cell tumor of tendon sheath and synovial membrane). J Bone Joint Surg 66A:76–94, 1984.
24. Rock MG, Pritchard DJ, Reiman HM, et al: Extra-abdominal desmoid tumors. J Bone Joint Surg 66A:1369–1374, 1984.
25. Kaplan PA and Williams SM: Mucocutaneus and peripheral soft-tissue hemangiomas: MR imaging. Radiology 163:163–166, 1987.
26. White NB: Neurilemomas of the extremities. J Bone Joint Surg 49A:1605–1610, 1967.
27. Kelly PC and Shramowiat M: Liposarcoma of the foot. A case report. J Foot Surg 17:27–31, 1978.
28. VanWerf-Messing B and Unnik JAM: Fibrosarcoma of the soft tissues—A clinicopathologic study. Cancer 18:1113, 1965.
29. Wu KK: Tumor review: Fibrosarcoma of the foot. J Foot Surg 26:535, 1987.
30. Cadman NL, Souk EH, and Kelly PJ: Synovial sarcoma. An analysis of 134 tumors. Cancer 18:613, 1965.
31. Bernardone JJ and Scarlet JJ: Leiomyosarcoma: A case report and literature review. J Am Podiatr Med Assoc 78:183, 1988.
32. Wu KK: Leiomyosarcoma of the foot. J Foot Surg 27:362, 1988.
33. Giannestras NJ and Bronson JL: Malignant schwannoma of the medial plantar branch of the posterior tibial nerve. J Bone Joint Surg 57A:701–703, 1975.

CHAPTER 39

Avascular Necrosis of Bone

Jeffrey C. Page, D.P.M.

Avascular necrosis describes the process of osseous necrosis that results from causes other than infection. Synonyms and other overlapping labels include aseptic necrosis, osteonecrosis, osteochondrosis, osteochondritis dissecans, and ischemic necrosis. The label of aseptic necrosis indicates that microorganisms are not recoverable from the affected site. Osteonecrosis is a nonspecific term applied to osseous destruction. The term ischemic necrosis aptly describes the dysvascular component of the necrotic changes.

The osteochondroses are a set of idiopathic conditions appearing in children or adolescents that are characterized by disorderly endochondral ossification. They are discussed separately in this chapter. Osteochondritis dissecans is a distinct entity typified by osteochondral injury. The cause, diagnosis, and treatment are reviewed.

Avascular necrosis may be classified according to cause as postoperative, traumatic, secondary to systemic disease, or idiopathic. Each of these subsets is presented.

The common link between all of these entities is that at some point in the progression of the avascular necrosis a dysvascular phase is reached with relative ischemia of all or part of the affected bone. Avascular necrosis may affect any bone in the body but has a predilection for weightbearing structures such as the femur, tibia, and talus. Weightbearing joints are three times more commonly affected than those of the upper limb, and some lesions in the upper limb may be clinically silent.[1]

ETIOLOGY

A long list of potential causes of avascular necrosis and associated disorders has been reported (Table 39–1).[2-19] The disease has been documented in association with trauma,[2, 3, 20–26] connective tissue diseases,[4, 5, 27–32] blood dyscrasias,[6–9, 3–37] metabolic disorders,[9, 19] transplantation,[10, 11] neuropathy,[12] Caisson disease,[13] steroid use,[16, 38] and many others.[14, 15, 17–19, 39–43] Some of the factors are considered to be directly contributory, whereas others are simply reported, associated factors.

Trauma is the most common cause of avascular necrosis. Fractures, dislocation, overuse injuries, and surgical trauma are all etiologic. Of the connective tissue disorders, systemic lupus erythematosus has the highest reported incidence of avascular necrosis.[44] Avascular necrosis is also seen in rheumatoid arthritis, osteoarthritis, hyperuricemia,[4] and several other inflammatory diseases.

Avascular necrosis is a serious complication of organ transplant surgery and is seen in patients on immunosuppressive therapy. Renal transplant patients are particularly susceptible.[45, 46]

A history of significant alcohol intake has been reported in 10% to 39% of patients with avascular necrosis.[9] Standardizing the diagnosis of alcoholism is difficult. The daily amount of alcohol that a patient will admit to consuming is, at best, unreliable. A history of alcoholism was found in 74% of patients in one study, a figure much higher than that found in similar studies.[47] It is not known why alcoholics are susceptible to osseous necrosis; however, it has been suggested that showers of systemic fat emboli may be released into the

TABLE 39–1

ETIOLOGY OF AVASCULAR NECROSIS*

Trauma	Transplantation
Fracture/dislocation	Renal
Overuse	Cardiac
Surgical	
Fat embolization	**Neuropathy**
	Diabetes
Connective Tissue Diseases	Myelomeningocele
Systemic lupus erythematosus	
Rheumatoid arthritis	**Caisson Disease (Dysbaric)**
Osteoarthritis	
Gout	**Thermal Injuries**
Vasculitis	Burns
Osteoporosis	Electrical
Polymyositis/dermatomyositis	Frostbite
Ankylosing spondylitis	
Scleroderma/Raynaud's	**Miscellaneous**
phenomenon	Allergic dermatitis
	Asthma
Blood Dyscrasias	Cocaine abuse
Immune thrombocytopenic purpura	Inflammatory bowel disease
Hemoglobinopathies	Radiation
Leukemia	Obesity
Sickle cell	
Autoimmune granulocytopenia	**Steroid Use**
Coagulopathy	Intravenous
Hodgkin's disease	Oral
Gaucher's disease	
	Idiopathic
Metabolic	
Alcoholism	
Pancreatitis	
Cushing's syndrome	
Hyperlipidemia	

*This list includes disorders that have been reported concurrent with the onset of avascular necrosis. Steroids are commonly used to treat many of these disorders.

circulation when alcoholism is severe enough to induce fatty infiltration of the liver.[48] Alcohol abuse may lead to peripheral neuropathy, which is a known associated factor for avascular necrosis. A rare report of avascular necrosis of the head of the talus was linked to alcohol abuse.[18]

Myelomeningocele and diabetes mellitus also cause neuropathy and have been associated with avascular necrosis. Glucose tolerance tests were performed on 34 patients with idiopathic femoral head necrosis and on a matched control group. Elevated levels of blood glucose were found in 41% of the abnormal patients, whereas only 4% to 5% of the general population had elevated glucose levels.[49] The relationship has not been explained. Charcot's disease affects the feet of many diabetic patients with radiographic changes that in some ways resemble those of avascular necrosis. However, Charcot's disease occurs only in relatively well-vascularized patients and presumably does not pass through an ischemic phase.

Gaucher's disease is characterized by the accumulation of glucocerebroside in macrophages.[8] These lipid-containing cells deposit throughout the body but particularly in the liver, spleen, and bone marrow. When Gaucher's cells deposit in bone, the result is osseous necrosis. Several other blood dyscrasias have been cited in association with avascular necrosis, including hemophilia, sickle cell, and leukemia.[7] It is likely that intraosseous thrombosis is the cause of osseous necrosis in the case of coagulopathy.

Caisson disease, or dysbaric osteonecrosis, is a form of avascular necrosis that develops in deep-sea divers, those working at depths such as mine workers, and those working in an environment of compressed air such as tunnel workers. The pathologic and radiologic features are similar to those found in traumatic avascular necrosis.[13, 50] It is, therefore, assumed that there is a vascular obstruction of the affected bone, but the cause is not clearly understood. Arterial obstruction could result from the impaction of emboli, vascular thrombosis, or extravascular obstruction. It is known that bone death results after only 6 to 12 hours of ischemia.[51] Bubbles are present in the arterial system with both severe and safe decompressions, which could potentially occlude the lumen of small vessels.[52] Furthermore, platelet aggregation may occur at the liquid/gas interface, resulting in microemboli.[53] The bones most commonly affected are the femur and the humerus.

Steroid use is a common finding in many cases of avascular necrosis. Many of the disorders known to be associated with avascular necrosis are treated with corticosteroids. Patients treated with corticosteroids constitute the largest group of individuals with nontraumatic avascular necrosis.[4] The evidence that corticosteroids produce avascular necrosis of bone, although overwhelming, is largely circumstantial. It is not possible to differentiate the contribution of corticosteroids from the underlying disease in the case of connective tissue disorders. Avascular necrosis is not an unexpected complication of other steroid-treated disorders such as dermatologic disease, asthma, ulcerative colitis, or renal transplantation. There are no characteristic histologic features unique to steroid-induced avascular necrosis, however, some patients show evidence of fatty infiltration of the bone marrow on biopsy. The appearance of avascular necrosis is closely related to the total daily dose and to the length of therapy.[1] The frequency with which avascular necrosis develops in steroid-treated patients is not known; however, it is clear that the majority of patients undergoing corticosteroid therapy do not acquire radiologically detectable necrosis.

Intra-articular and periarticular injection of corticosteroid is widely used in clinical practice. Three large studies reported no avascular necrosis after intra-articular cortisone injection.[55–57] However, there are also reports of unexpectedly rapid deterioration of joints after intra-articular injection.[58, 59] The radiologic appearance is often indistinguishable from neuropathic arthropathy. Evidence seems to indicate that avascular necrosis does not follow single or isolated intra-articular injection, and it is more likely to occur in patients with rheumatoid disease. Patients requiring intra-articular steroid therapy should be carefully reviewed after the first few injections for early signs of arthropathy.

Three local mechanisms are believed to play a role in the pathogenesis of avascular necrosis: (1) compromise of vessel wall integrity (e.g., trauma or vasculitis), (2) intraosseous venous congestion (e.g., increased marrow contents or pressure), and (3) intravascular occlusion (e.g., thrombus or embolus).[60] These factors may act independently or in concert to cause ischemia and death of osteocytes. Increased bone marrow pressure is often present in preradiologic and preclinical disease and may be a final common pathway in the development of avascular necrosis.[61] Patients who have any of the disorders listed in Table 39–1 or who are receiving corticosteroid therapy for any reason are more likely to acquire avascular necrosis.

DIAGNOSIS

The differential diagnosis of unexplained osseous or articular pain should include avascular necrosis. Avascular necrosis has been misdiagnosed as reflex sympathetic dystrophy, arthritis, bone cysts, and bone tumor. Symptoms usually precede radiographic changes; therefore, a high index of suspicion will aid in the early diagnosis of ischemic necrosis of bone.

Patients with avascular necrosis of bone in the lower extremity most often present with a history of gradual onset of pain, stiffness, and swelling. Pain on active motion is almost invariably present. Weightbearing and physical activity aggravate the symptoms, and rest and antiinflammatory medication make the patient feel better. Clinical examination may reveal pain with palpation, painful range of motion (and crepitus in later stages), limitation of motion, warmth, edema, and erythema. Clinical presentation can mimic that of an infectious process, which should be ruled out.

Zizic, Hungerford, and Stevens pioneered the use of hemodynamic studies in the early diagnosis of avascular necrosis, particularly for idiopathic cases appearing in childhood.[61] These studies include bone marrow pressure, the saline stress test, and intraosseous venography. Increased bone marrow pressure or decreased venous flow are present in patients with avascular necrosis regardless of the radiologic stage of the disease. These tests are accomplished using a rigid needle inserted percutaneously through the cortex and connected to saline-filled cannulas. A pressure transducer records the intraosseous bone marrow pressure. Saline is then injected intraosseously. A new pressure reading is taken 5 minutes after the injection. After pressure readings are concluded, a soluble contrast medium is injected through the needle, and radiographs are taken for intraosseous venography. Hemodynamic studies are reliable measures of disease but are not widely available. They are, therefore, not a practical clinical tool but are of value in the research laboratory.

Routine radiographs may appear normal in the early stages of avascular necrosis. However, progression of the disease causes patchy, increasing osteopenia and sclerosis, subcortical lucency, joint narrowing, cystic changes, fragmentation, and shortening or collapse. A classification scheme based on radiographic appearance was developed by Arlet and Ficat for necrosis of the femoral head.[62] However, the scheme is applicable to other joints of the lower extremity as well.[19] They described four stages:

Stage I: Minimal osteoporosis
Stage II: Significant osteoporosis and osteosclerosis
Stage III: Translucent subcortical band, ''the crescent sign,'' and partial collapse
Stage IV: Discrete discontinuity, ''joint step,'' and joint-space narrowing

Stage I is the preradiologic stage often characterized by the absence of radiologic signs and the presence of clinical signs and symptoms. Despite the absence of radiologic signs, diagnosis can be accomplished through hemodynamic, isotopic, or histopathologic testing. Stage II is characterized by the radiologic evidence of bony remodeling but without overall change in the shape of the bone or the associated joint space. Several types of bone reaction can be distinguished: osteoporotic, sclerotic, cystic, or mixed. Osteoporosis may be diffuse or patchy and may be interspersed with areas of sclerosis or cysts. The sclerosing type of stage II avascular necrosis is most often homogeneous in appearance. The appearance of a subcortical radiolucent line, the crescent sign, represents a transition from stage II to stage III. Cortical continuity is disrupted in stage III, with depression or partial collapse that constitutes irreversible structural damage. The changes in this stage result in progressive deterioration. Stage IV is characterized by progressive secondary deterioration of the cartilage revealed by joint-space narrowing and osteophyte formation.

Radionuclide scintigraphy can help diagnose avascular necrosis at an early stage.[63] It has been used for this purpose since 1953 with sensitivity of up to 89%. Radiography, by comparison, was found to be only 41% sensitive in detecting avascular necrosis.[64] Bone marrow scintigraphy, a variation of conventional skeletal scintigraphy using a radionuclide of very small particle size, was found to be even more sensitive. Although highly sensitive, scintigraphy is limited by poor specificity and poor anatomic resolution. In cases in which avascular necrosis is likely to be bilateral (e.g., systemic lupus erythematosus, steroid therapy), bone scans are unlikely to be helpful. A photon deficiency of one hip in comparison with normal uptake in the opposite hip indicates the possibility of avascular necrosis. Strömqvist showed that most cases of avascular necrosis of the femoral head can be seen on scintigraphy 2 to 14 days after fracture.[65] The first metatarsal head probably acts in the same way.[26] In hospitals without easy access to magnetic resonance imaging, scintigraphy remains the most practical and sensitive method of diagnosing avascular necrosis.

Computed tomography can be very useful in elucidating structural changes of avascular necrosis. Although not as sensitive to marrow changes, computed tomography clearly shows collapse or fragmentation of cortical bone, which may be difficult to visualize on standard radiographs. It is particularly useful in cases of osteochondritis dissecans of the knee or ankle. Computed tomography is useful for assessing late osseous destruction and for planning preoperative care, but it is less useful as an early diagnostic tool than scintigraphy or magnetic resonance.

Magnetic resonance imaging is believed to be more sensitive than scintigraphy for early lesions[66, 67] and has an overall sensitivity approaching 100%.[68, 69] Some authors found that magnetic resonance imaging may miss some early lesions because the signal is not significantly altered until fat cells die.[70, 71] Nonetheless, magnetic resonance is the imaging technique most sensitive to marrow-based pathologic changes. It provides intrinsically high soft tissue contrast, and has the ability to image in multiple planes and to manipulate tissue contrast.

Four patterns of abnormality on magnetic resonance scans have been described for the femoral head:[67]

1. Homogeneous pattern: a well-defined, homogeneous area of low signal intensity limited to the subarticular region
2. Inhomogeneous pattern: larger irregular areas of inhomogeneously decreased signal intensity that may extend into the femoral neck
3. Band pattern: a band of decreased intensity that extends across the femoral neck
4. Ring pattern: a ring of decreased intensity surrounding an area of relatively normal intensity

The significance of these patterns is unclear. The hallmark of avascular necrosis on magnetic resonance imaging appears to be a focal region of decreased signal intensity in a subarticular location.[69] This pattern is expected in other joints as well as the hip. Other diagnostic possibilities should be included in the differential inasmuch as almost any process that invades or displaces marrow can cause focal regions of decreased intensity. The list of possibilities might include metastatic disease, primary bone tumors, leukemia, and subchondral cysts. Spin shift or chemical shift techniques enhance the specificity of the magnetic resonance examination. In addition to its use in diagnosis of avascular necrosis, magnetic resonance imaging may be important in planning surgical procedures and in evaluating the effectiveness of therapy.

OSTEOCHONDROSES

The osteochondroses are idiopathic conditions characterized by disorderliness of endochondral ossification that develops in a previously normal site of growth. These idiopathic syndromes usually bear eponymic titles and present during childhood or adolescence. Osteochondrosis develops most often in children who are active in sports and who are actively growing. It is a self-limiting disorder that has a generally predictable outcome. Osteochondrosis does not continue past the age of osseous maturity. However, alterations in the vascular supply to bone as a result of known systemic causes (see Table 39–1) may result in the development of avascular necrosis at the same anatomic locations at any age. Only a small percentage of patients with osteochon-

TABLE 39–2

OSTEOCHONDROSES OF THE LOWER EXTREMITY

Articular Osteochondroses

Primary Involvement of Articular and Epiphyseal Cartilage
Metatarsal head (Freiberg's infraction)

Secondary Involvement of Articular and Epiphyseal Cartilage
Hip (Legg-Calvé-Perthes disease)
Osteochondritis
Navicular (Köhler's disease)
Talus (Mouchet's disease)

Nonarticular Osteochondroses

At Tendon Attachments
Tibial tuberosity (Osgood-Schlatter disease)
Trochanteric (Mandl disease)
Patella (Sinding-Larsen disease)
Fifth metatarsal base (Iselin's apophysitis)

At Ligament Attachments
Femoral condyles (Ahlback's disease)
Ankle malleoli

At Impact Sites
Calcaneus (Sever's syndrome)
Sesamoids (Treve's disease)

Physeal Osteochondroses

Tibia (Blount's disease)

---

drosis present with a history of significant trauma.[72] Familial associations have been reported. The pathomechanics of osteochondrosis in the foot often involve excessive pronation secondary to pes planus and equinus deformities.[73] Trauma in the form of compression on articular surfaces or tension on nonarticular surfaces may be the common final pathway of all of the osteochondroses.[74]

Siffert offered a clinically useful classification of the osteochondroses that divides them into articular, nonarticular, and physical osteochondroses.[75] On the basis of this scheme, Table 39–2 lists some of the osteochondroses presenting in the lower extremity. The most common sites for the development of osteochondrosis are the hip, tibial tuberosity, calcaneus, navicular, and metatarsal heads.

Typically, rest and protection will control the symptoms of osteochondrosis and prompt a resolution of the process. Residual deformity and continued pain are best avoided by early recognition and intervention.

Legg-Calvé-Perthes Disease

One of the earliest reports of osteochondrosis was by Georg Perthes (Germany), who, in 1910, described arthritis deformans juvenilis of the hip.[76] Articles describing coxa plana by Legg (United States) and Calvé (France) appeared almost simultaneously.[77, 78] The disease presents between 4 and 8 years of age, predominantly in boys. Avascular necrosis of bone is the hallmark of Legg-Calvé-Perthes disease. However, the exact cause remains unclear.

The natural history of Legg-Calvé-Perthes disease can be divided into four stages. The first stage, lasting 1 to 3 weeks, is the incipient or synovitis stage. Synovial membrane and capsule are edematous and hyperemic. The aseptic necrotic or avascular stage lasts 6 to 12 months and includes death of the ossific nucleus. Increased homogeneous sclerosis is noted on x-ray at this stage. The regenerative or fragmentation stage begins with revascularization and "creeping substitution." The femoral head is flattened and fragmented (Fig. 39–1). This stage may last 1 to 3 years. The fourth stage is the residual stage. It corresponds to the disappearance of lucency and sclerosis on x-ray and to the development of normal trabecular bone. This progression through four stages also occurs in the foot. However, the duration of each stage varies with the bone involved.

Treatment for Legg-Calvé-Perthes disease may be either conservative or surgical and depends on the age of onset, extent of disease, stage, and adequacy of previous treatment. The goals of treatment for Legg-Calvé-Perthes disease are to preserve normal congruity and range of motion of the hip, provide a painless, weightbearing joint, and prevent prolonged confinement. Treatment approaches may be divided into recumbent, ambulatory, and operative classes. Recumbent therapy relies on bed rest, traction, casting, and abduction bracing to rest the hip joint. Recumbent therapy is appropriate for very young children and for initiation of therapy but is not used as the sole treatment approach. The ambulatory approach allows for the use of crutches for unilateral cases. Long-leg cylinder spica walking casts or ischial ring

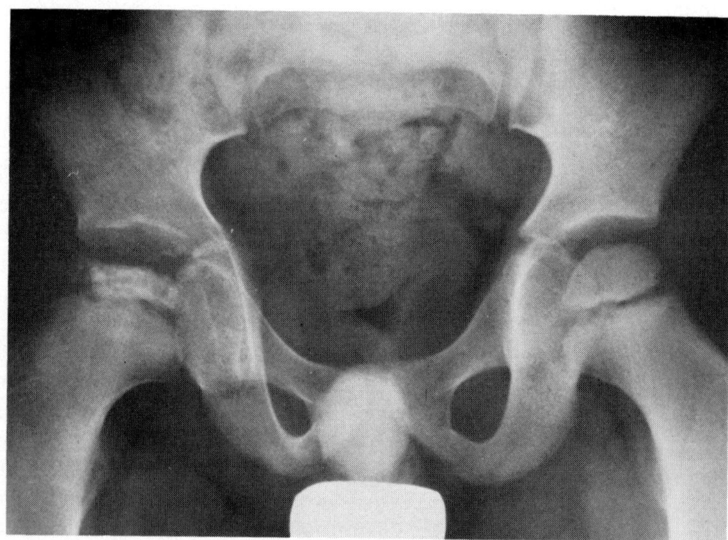

FIGURE 39–1. This 5½-year-old boy has reached the fragmentation stage in the progression of Legg-Calvé-Perthes disease.

leg braces allow the patients to ambulate. Only in cases of severe, permanent deformity is the operative approach considered. Procedures that have been used successfully include drilling, grafting, ostectomy, osteotomy, and obturator neurectomy.

Osgood-Schlatter Disease

Osgood-Schlatter disease is characterized by tenderness and edema of the patellar tendon and enlargement of the tibial tubercle. It was first described independently by Osgood[79] and Schlatter[80] in 1903. Presenting in adolescence, it has its onset most often between the ages of 11 and 15 years. Participation in sports and rapid growth are often a part of the history. Running, jumping, and climbing stairs are often difficult. Although this disease is more common in boys, its incidence in girls is increasing.

The cause of Osgood-Schlatter disease is traumatic, but there is disagreement as to the primary mechanism. Most likely, it is the repeated stress on the patellar tendon, which causes tendinitis and subsequent heterotopic bone formation at the tendinous insertion. Osgood-Schlatter disease is not a true osteochondrosis inasmuch as avascular necrosis does not occur at any stage of the disease.

Soft tissue swelling is the only radiographic indication of active disease. Irregularity and fragmentation of the ossification center of the proximal tibial tubercle are normal variations and are not diagnostic of Osgood-Schlatter disease.

The disease is self-limiting, resolving when the tibial tubercle fuses to the diaphysis. Enlargement of the tibial tuberosity may persist. The type of treatment depends on the severity of the disease. Simple restriction of physical activity is sufficient for mild cases. More severe cases may require long-leg casting from 4 to 6 weeks. Surgical intervention is indicated only for excision of the persistent enlarged tubercle.

Köhler's Disease

Avascular necrosis of the navicular bone in children was first described by Köhler in 1908. In some cases, it presents with clinical manifestations that include pain and tenderness localized to the navicular bone. Physical activity aggravates the symptoms. Mild edema and a flat foot may be present. Antalgic gait may result. The midtarsal and subtalar joints have a full range of motion. Radiographic appearance is characterized by flattening, sclerosis, and irregular rarefaction of the navicular bone (Fig. 39–2). The anteroposterior diameter is narrowed on the lateral view. Ossification of the navicular bone occurs later in boys than in girls; hence, the symptoms of avascular necrosis present later and more often in boys than in girls.[81] Irregular ossification results from compression of the bony nucleus at a critical phase of growth. These compressive forces occlude the vessels in the cancellous bone and produce avascular necrosis of bone.

Treatment varies with the severity of the condition. Limited activity, strapping, and arch supports may be all that is required in moderate cases. More severe cases will require casting for 6 to 8 weeks and non-weightbearing with crutches. The prognosis is excellent in Köhler's disease, resolving without residual deformity or disability.

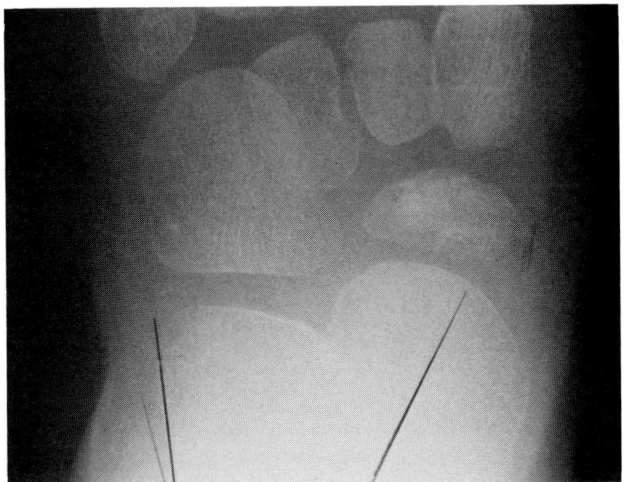

FIGURE 39–2. Flattening, sclerosis, and irregular areas of lucency in the navicular of this 8-year-old child typify the changes of Köhler's disease.

Sever's Disease

Haglund first described calcaneal apophysitis and likened it to osteochondrosis of the tibial tuberosity.[82] The syndrome derives its eponym from Sever, who published a comprehensive article on the subject in 1912.[83] The symptoms may appear as early as age 8 and may extend well into adolescence. The disease most often occurs in active children who participate in sports.[24]

A number of possible causes for Sever's disease have been proposed, but the definitive cause has yet to be established. There is a definite link between equinus deformity and Sever's disease.[73] Obesity, acute and chronic trauma, infection, heredity, and other factors have been implicated.[84–86] Direct pressure may play an etiologic role, but the most likely cause is tension created by the pull of the plantar fascia and the Achilles tendon.

The center of secondary ossification (apophysis) of the calcaneus appears earlier in girls (4 to 6 years old) than in boys (7 to 8 years old). It develops into a crescent-shaped osseous structure at the posteroinferior aspect of the calcaneus. The Achilles tendon inserts into the apophysis, and the plantar aponeurosis originates from it. There may be deep clefts dividing the apophysis into a bi- or tripartite structure (Fig. 39–3). Fusion of the apophysis to the primary ossification center occurs as early as age 12 in girls and age 15 in boys.

Patients with Sever's disease usually relate an increase in pain with activity. Poststatic dyskinesia is not a feature with this syndrome as it is with plantar fasciitis or Achilles tendinitis. Parents may have noticed a recurrent limp. Swelling and redness are not usually seen; however, the posterior heel will be distinctly tender to palpation.

Treatment for calcaneal apophysitis should always be conservative. Reduction of activity, heel lifts, and strapping are usually sufficient. Resistant cases may require oral antiinflammatories or casting. Orthotics are often used for follow-up. Steroid injections must be avoided. Even without treatment, Sever's disease is a self-limiting process. Symptoms resolve as the apophysis fuses with the body of the calcaneus.

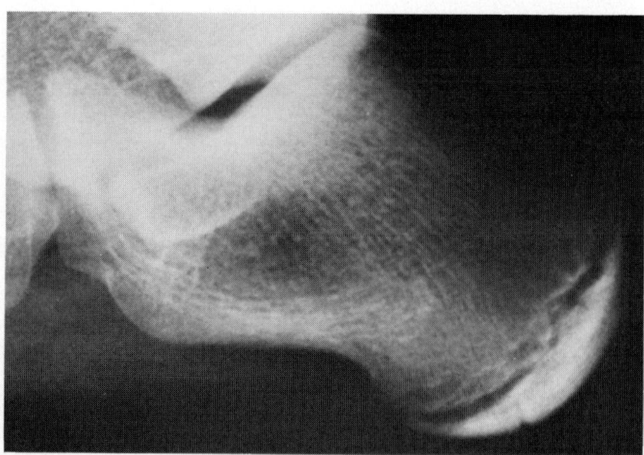

FIGURE 39–3. A deep cleft divides the apophysis of this 12-year-old boy with Sever's disease.

TABLE 39–3

CLASSIFICATION AND TREATMENT OF FREIBERG'S DISEASE

Type	Description	Treatment
I	No degenerative joint disease; articular cartilage intact	Non-weightbearing with metatarsal pad; low-heel shoe; cessation of sports; orthotics; NSAIDs
II	Periarticular spurs; articular cartilage intact; metatarsal head flattening	Cheilectomy; all of the conservative measures for type I
III	Severe degenerative joint disease; loss of articular cartilage	Arthroplasty/metatarsal head resection, with or without soft tissue interposition or implantation
IV	Epiphyseal dysplasia; multiple head involvement	Same as indicated for types I, II, and III

NSAIDs, nonsteroidal antiinflammatory drugs.

Freiberg's Disease

Freiberg was the first to describe an infraction of the second metatarsal bone in which the metatarsal head had a "crushed in" appearance.[87, 88] Avascular necrosis of the lesser metatarsal heads is also sometimes referred to as Köhler's second disease. The disease appears in adolescence after 13 years of age. Seventy-five percent of all cases occur in girls. The second metatarsal head is the most commonly involved site; however, other metatarsals may be affected.

The precise cause of the avascular necrosis that occurs in Freiberg's disease is uncertain. It may be the result of a single traumatic event or the cumulative result of chronic minor trauma. The clinical presentation of pain under the second metatarsal head is often accompanied by swelling, limitation of motion, and pain or crepitus with motion. Radiographs show flattening, irregularity, and sclerosis of the involved metatarsal head along with marginal osteophytes. Radiographic appearance varies with the stage of the disease.

A staging scheme was developed by Thompson and Hamilton, which helps to correlate radiographic appearance with treatment. The four types are summarized in Table 39–3 with my treatment recommendations. Type I is not often recognized in practice. It is typified by mild symptoms that can be self-limiting. A transient lesion appears, but there is no joint-space narrowing or osteophytic degeneration (Fig. 39–4). Surgery is not indicated, but the patient should reduce activity, wear an accommodative pad, and wear lower heels. Short-term nonsteroidal antiinflammatory drugs help relieve symptoms. Steroids may interfere with the reparative process. Type II is the result of significant bony ischemia, which leads to marginal osteophytes and synovitis. The joint is usually not subluxable at this stage, and articular cartilage is preserved. Surgical treatment may be limited to synovectomy and excision of the degenerative osteophytes. However, casting or orthotics may relieve the symptoms and should be attempted with cartilage damage and cortical disruption. For type III Freiberg's disease, complete arthroplasty is usually required with débridement or metatarsal head resection (Fig. 39–5). Soft tissue interposition or double-stemmed implant can help maintain digit length but provides no weightbearing support. Type IV is quite rare because it involves multiple metatarsal heads. It may represent a form of epiphyseal dysplasia. Treatment is selected according to the stage of each metatarsal head.

OSTEOCHONDRITIS DISSECANS

Osteochondritis (osteochondrosis) dissecans is the development of an osteochondral injury through the articular cartilage of a diarthrodial joint. The injury is produced by a force transmitted from the articular surface of a contiguous bone across the joint and through the articular cartilage to the subchondral trabeculae of the damaged bone. Two physical types of fracture may result: (1) The injury may result in a small area of compressed trabeculae, with or without demonstrable damage to the overlying cartilage, or (2) the in-

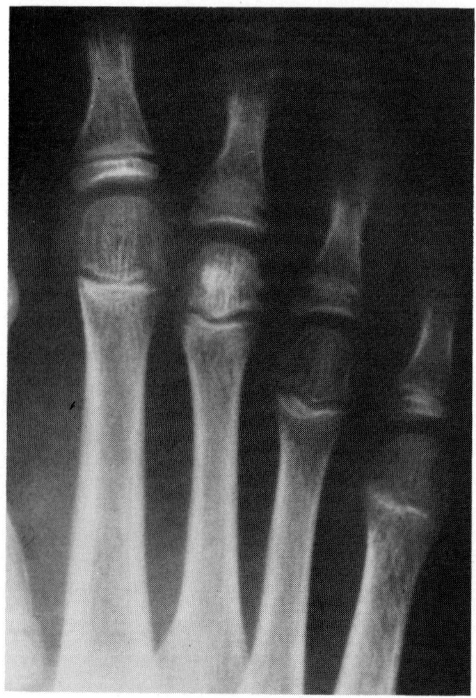

FIGURE 39–4. An uncommon example of type I Freiberg's infraction displays a transient sclerosis of the third metatarsal head. (Courtesy of Paul Scherer, D.P.M., San Francisco, CA.)

jury may produce an osteochondral fragment. The fragment may remain in situ, incompletely detached, and free to move within the joint. The compressed or avulsed fragment of bone has no soft tissue attachments, has poor blood supply, and is susceptible to avascular necrosis.

In 1888 König described loose bodies in joints other than the ankle.[89] He decided that they could not have been caused by any known disease, tumor, or trauma and concluded that they must have been produced by a process of spontaneous necrosis. He termed this hypothetical process *osteochondritis dissecans*. Although the term *osteochondritis* has been used for many years to indicate the presumed role of inflammation in the cause, the belief that the disease is primarily inflammatory has not been substantiated.[90]

The first use of the term osteochondritis dissecans to apply to the ankle was made by Kappis in 1922.[91] Thereafter, it became the accepted term. As subsequent studies were developed, different terms were proposed for this entity. Osteochondrosis dissecans, transchondral fracture, and osteochondral fracture may be preferable terms. Trauma has been identified as an apparent etiologic factor in more than 50% of reported cases; however, the cause is likely to be multifactorial.[92–94]

The clinical presentation of osteochondritis dissecans is one of joint pain and swelling. The transchondral injury may result from significant trauma or from an injury so trivial as to pass unnoticed. The presence of transchondral injury may be masked by adjacent soft tissue injuries. Instability, joint locking, and articular degeneration may develop. The most commonly affected joints are the knee, ankle, elbow, and hip. It is most common in young males. It may be misdiagnosed as a sprain or as arthritis.

Radiographs may reveal crescent-shaped lucent areas in subchondral bone or loose ossicles in the joint space (Fig. 39–6). However, in many cases of osteochondral injury, the radiographs are normal in appearance. This is usually due to the small size of the fragment and its location adjacent to or "behind" other cortical surfaces. Double constant arthrography is useful in both the knee and the ankle in delineating both the intra-articular fragment and the degree of separation

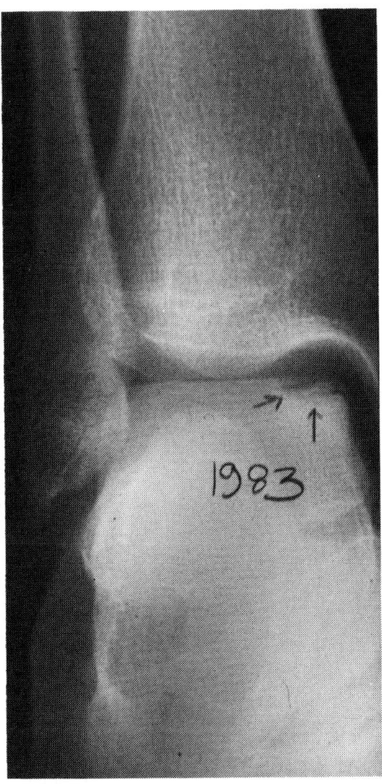

FIGURE 39–6. Standard radiographs may reveal crescent-shaped intra-articular bodies, as demonstrated by this ankle view of a patient with an osteochondral fracture.

from the talus.[95] Computed tomography is most helpful in determining the presence, size, and location of the osteochondral fragment (Fig. 39–7). The slices must be small, and sagittal reconstructions are useful. Bone scanning is a useful screening tool when the diagnosis is obscure and usually demonstrates an area of increased uptake. Magnetic resonance imaging is the best available tool to evaluate the condition of the overlying cartilage but is not often necessary.

Histopathologically, the primary changes occur in the bone, whereas secondary changes follow in the cartilage. Avascular necrosis is evident in the subchondral bone as

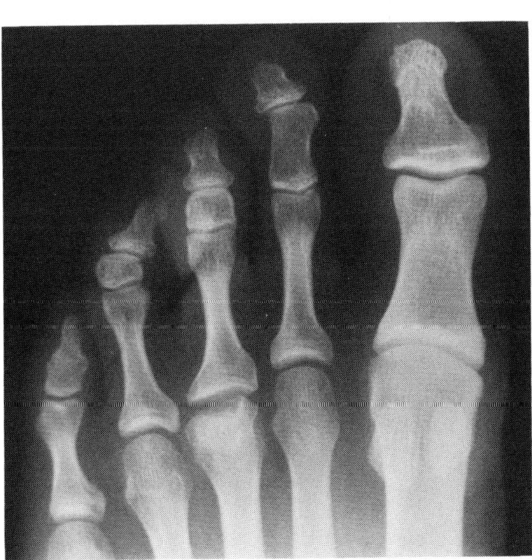

FIGURE 39–5. Flattening and marginal osteophytes are seen in cases of type III Freiberg's infraction.

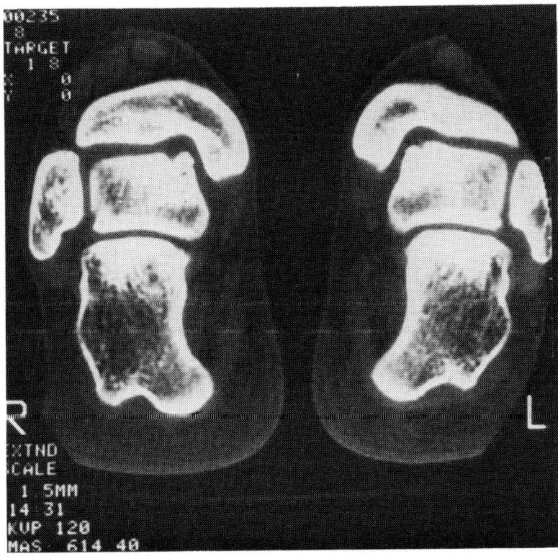

FIGURE 39–7. Computed tomography scan clearly reveals the size and displacement of an osteochondral talar dome fracture. Note the bilateral distribution in this patient.

either a loose fragment or a compressed area. A zone of fibrocartilaginous tissue often develops between the fragment and its bony bed.

In the landmark article by Berndt and Harty, a staging scheme was proposed[94] (Fig. 39–8). Stage I consists of impaction of the talus on the fibula or tibia with compression of the subchondral bone. Stage II consists of an incompletely detached osteochondral fragment. The lesion is considered a stage III lesion if the fragment is completely detached but remains in its bed. Stage IV is achieved when the osteochondral fragment is both completely detached and displaced from its original site. The value of the Berndt and Harty classification lies in guiding therapeutic choices.

Lateral lesions are most often shallow osteochondral "flakes" that lie in the central portion of the dome of the talus. Medial lesions are more often deep fragments that lie in the central to posterior area of the talar dome.

The objectives of treatment for osteochondritis dissecans are to eliminate pain and prevent articular degeneration from a free osteochondral fragment. Children up to the age of 11 (girls) or 13 (boys) years usually do well with conservative care, including activity modification and immobilization. Between the ages of 12 (girls) or 14 (boys) and 20 years, youths are becoming skeletally mature. Stage I and II lesions may achieve good results with the use of rest and protective devices.[96] Stages III and IV lesions and patients older than 20 years will most often require surgery. Small fragments should be excised with saucerization and drilling of the defect. Softened, compressed areas should likewise be débrided, saucerized, and drilled. Larger fragments may be fixed using metallic or absorbable pins. Arthroscopy is useful both diagnostically and therapeutically in many cases of osteochondritis dissecans.[97] When a talar fragment is difficult to reach by arthrotomy, osteotomy of the medial malleolus may be necessary. This is most often necessary with posterior medial fragments.

POSTOPERATIVE AVASCULAR NECROSIS

Speculation about the causes of avascular necrosis in the postoperative patient centers on the role of disruption of medullary circulation, overzealous stripping of soft tissue attachments, and excessive motion of an osteotomy. Aggressive dissection and vigorous reaming of the medullary canal may contribute. Interruption of blood supply, either intraosseous or extraosseous, is the primary cause of aseptic necrosis after foot surgery.

The incidence of avascular necrosis after foot surgery, particularly bunion surgery, is a matter of some disagreement in the literature. Avascular necrosis has been documented in lesser metatarsals after forefoot surgery.[24] Increased pressure with weightbearing on the involved metatarsals appeared to be the cause. Arenson reported a case of avascular necrosis after implant arthroplasty.[98] The incidence of avascular necrosis after first metatarsal osteotomy was reported to be unacceptably high in a letter by Mann.[99] Jahss stated that transmetatarsal head osteotomy invariably results in avascular necrosis.[100] Meier and Kenzora also reported a significant incidence of avascular necrosis after first metatarsal osteotomy.[26]

Surgeons in Great Britain reviewed the incidence of avascular necrosis after chevron distal metatarsal osteotomy. Avascular necrosis did not develop in any of the 64 feet studied.[101] A 4% incidence of avascular necrosis after 54 first metatarsal osteotomies was also reported by Meisenhelder and colleagues.[102] A Swedish study of 41 feet that had undergone chevron osteotomy revealed no cases of avascular necrosis despite the fact that all patients were monitored with bone scans and no internal fixation was used.[103] Boberg and associates put the incidence of avascular necrosis after forefoot surgery in perspective, saying "only one case of avascular necrosis in several thousand distal procedures performed at Doctors Hospital [occurred] over the past thirty years."[104]

There is little consensus on the ideal treatment modalities for postoperative avascular necrosis except that the best results are derived from the earliest possible intervention. If the condition remains untreated once radiographic changes have occurred, the involved bone will collapse, resulting in severe dysfunction. Furthermore, once radiographic changes have occurred, the results of nonoperative management alone are often not satisfactory (Fig. 39–9A–D).

Conservative management of postoperative avascular necrosis always includes rest of the affected part and the elimination of any weightbearing stress. Crutches, patellar tendon bearing brace, wheelchair, or a modified postoperative shoe

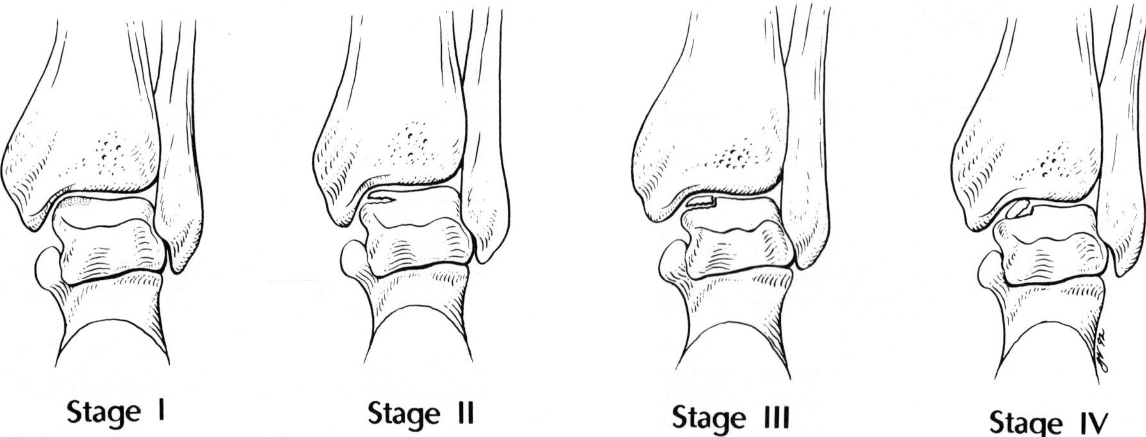

FIGURE 39–8. Berndt and Harty classification. Stage I—compression of subchondral bone; Stage II—incompletely detached osteochondral fragment. Stage III—completely detached osteochondral fragment remaining in its bed. Stage IV—completely detached and displaced osteochondral fragment.

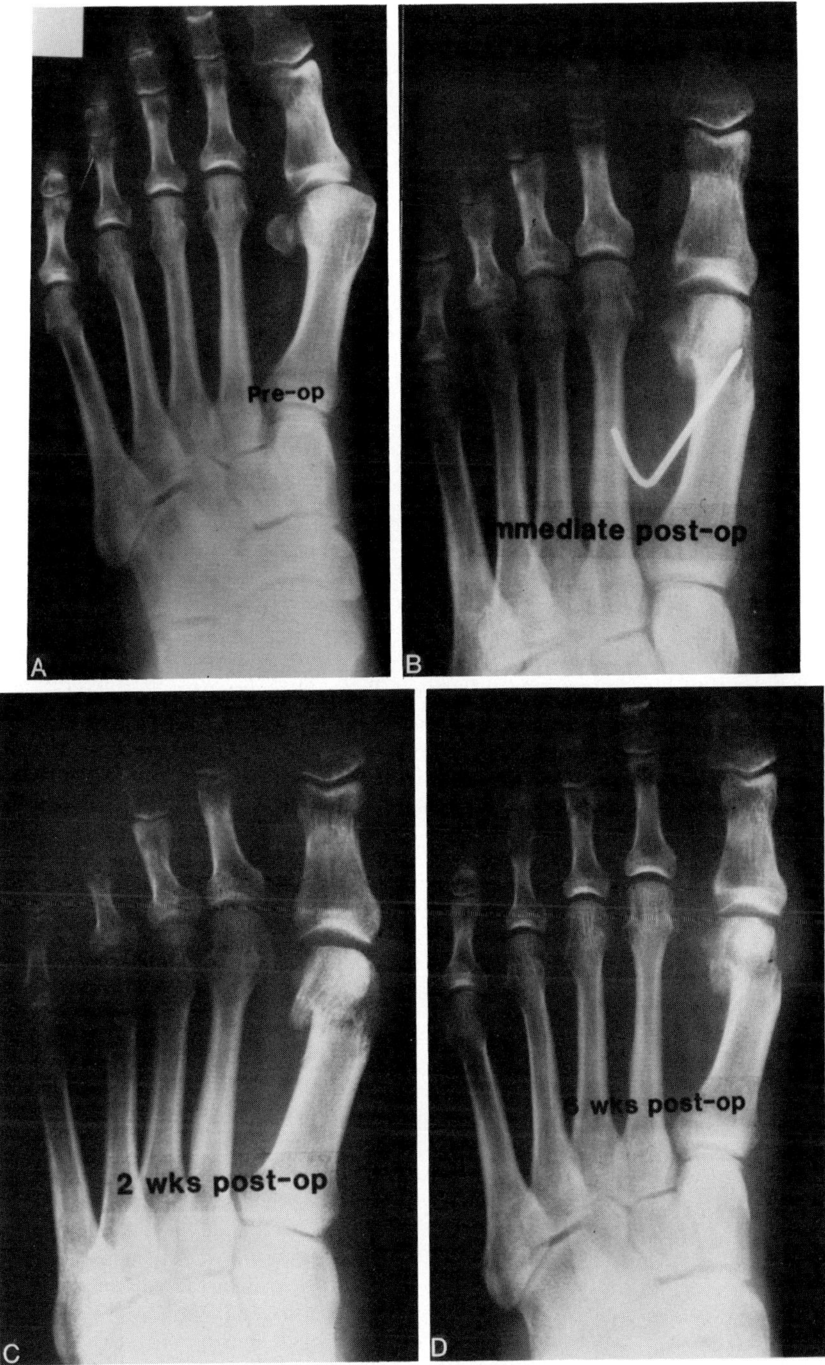

FIGURE 39–9. *A*, Preoperative radiograph of a bunion deformity. *B*, Immediate postoperative radiograph following an Austin bunionectomy. *C*, Postoperative radiograph taken 2 weeks after bunionectomy. Note the increased sclerosis, patchy lucency, and the beginning of the collapse of the capital fragment. *D*, Postoperative radiograph taken 6 weeks after bunionectomy. Note the shortening of the metatarsal, increased sclerosis and erosion of the metatarsal head.

may be used to off-load avascular bones in the foot. Casting or splinting is often advisable. Corticosteroid injections are contraindicated during the active phase because of the potential for impairment of the reparative process. Nonsteroidal antiinflammatory medication may give some symptomatic relief. When avascular necrosis has run its full course and the patient has been allowed to return to full weightbearing, concern must be given to alteration of weight distribution, particularly in the forefoot. Avascular necrosis of the metatarsals may result in shortening and elevation, causing meta-

tarsalgia of adjacent metatarsals, which share a disproportionate load. Avascular necrosis of the talus can result in varus or valgus position of the foot in relation to the leg. Functional or accommodative orthotics are often necessary. Shoe modifications such as varus wedges or rocker soles may be helpful.

When conservative, nonoperative management of avascular necrosis gives unsatisfactory results, operative intervention must be a consideration. Remodeling of a joint with the removal of exostoses and loose ossicles may be sufficient in mild cases. The saucerization and fenestration of articular defects serve to decompress and promote fibrocartilage formation. Realignment may be accomplished through osteotomy. Severe cases of arthrosis will require arthrodesis or implantation. Lyophilized allograft, autograft, and demineralized bone paste have all proven to be effective adjuncts to joint fusion. Joint implants can be used in the foot to maintain length and restore some motion in selected cases. Double-stemmed or two-component implants function best in the forefoot, but the ideal implant has yet to be designed. Successful revascularization has been accomplished through the use of vascularized bone grafts.

TRAUMA

When avascular necrosis of bone develops after trauma, it usually does so at sites with few arterial anastomoses. The most common of these are the humeral head, the carpal scaphoid, the femoral head, and the body of the talus. The similarity of these sites is that they are all intra-articular with limited soft tissue attachments and arterial supply.

Traumatic avascular necrosis is seen most frequently in the femoral head after fracture of the femoral neck.[40] The incidence of avascular necrosis after hip trauma ranges from 15% to 45%. Avascular necrosis is common in cases of displaced or malaligned fractures and occurs more frequently in women than in men.[54] The incidence of avascular necrosis is much higher in fracture dislocations of the hip that remain unreduced for longer than 12 hours.[105] If diagnosed early, avascular necrosis of the hip can be successfully treated to preserve the joint. The hip must be rested and protected from weightbearing. Surgical decompression, rotational osteotomy, and grafting have been used successfully to achieve revascularization. If diagnosis and treatment are instituted before the subchondral bone has collapsed (stage III), the potential for painless ambulation is good. If structural damage has already occurred before treatment is begun, the likelihood of arthrosis and worsening pain with ambulation is high. Joint replacement may be the only alternative.

Fracture of the talar neck is the most dangerous talar fracture. Avascular necrosis of the talus is the most serious complication with a generally poor prognosis. The talus is a primarily cancellous articular bone with no muscular attachments, and three fifths of its surface are covered with cartilage.

The talus has an extraosseous blood supply that depends solely on the fragile periosteal vascular network formed by the anastomoses of the dorsalis pedis, posterior tibial, and peroneal arteries. The vascular supply is retrograde from three main sources: through the neck of the talus, through the sinus tarsi and tarsal canal, and through foramina on the medial side of the body. The most important arterial supply to the talus, and to the talar body in particular, is the intraosseous anastomosing network of the sinus tarsi and the tarsal canal arteries. Other important vessels include the lateral talar artery, the medial recurrent tarsal artery, and the posterior recurrent branch of the lateral tarsal artery.

Forced supination or pronation can result in fracture/dislocation or complete dislocation of the intact talus. Avascular necrosis of the body of the talus has been widely reported after fractures and dislocations of the talar neck. Avascular necrosis of the talar head after talar neck fractures

is rare.[20] Most modern talar neck fractures result from motor vehicle accidents and, less commonly, falls from heights or direct blows to the dorsum of the foot.

The most widely accepted classification of talar neck fractures was proposed by Hawkins,[106] who categorized talar neck fractures into three distinct groups: type I, nondisplaced vertical fracture of the talar neck; type II, displaced vertical neck fracture with subluxation or dislocation of the subtalar joint; and type III, displaced vertical neck fracture with subluxation or dislocation of the subtalar and ankle joint. This classification scheme did not include subluxation and dislocation of the talonavicular joint. Of the 71 talar neck fractures studied by Canale and Kelly, 4% had accompanying dislocation of the talar head from the talonavicular articulation.[107] Bodamer and coauthors proposed the addition of a fourth group that includes displaced vertical fractures of the talar neck with subtalar and ankle subluxation and subluxation or dislocation of the talar head from the talonavicular joint.[21]

Avascular necrosis is a rare complication of type I fractures of the talar neck. However, the incidence of avascular necrosis has been reported to be as high as 50% with Hawkins' type II talar fractures and ranges from 75% to 100% with Hawkins' type III fracture dislocations.[18] Only the talar body is at risk for avascular necrosis in types I to III. The talar head may develop necrosis as well in type IV injuries. Avascular necrosis after total dislocation of the talus occurs very often.[108] However, Ritsema demonstrated that talectomy can be avoided and the incidence of avascular necrosis minimized with rapid, open reduction after total dislocation of the talus.[23] Avascular necrosis can also occur in cases of apparently minor trauma in which no fracture or dislocation has occurred.[2]

The first radiographic sign of avascular necrosis after talar trauma can be observed anywhere between 4 weeks and 6 months after trauma. An apparent increase in radiodensity of the talus may actually be the result of increasing osteopenia in the surrounding bones (Fig. 39–10). A decrease of relative sclerosis and the appearance of subchondral lucency (Hawkins' sign) herald the beginning of revascularization. Hawkins' sign is a simple, reliable, early (it usually appears within the first 8 weeks after injury) indicator of viability after fracture of the talus. So reliable is Hawkins' sign that the pathognomonic sign of osteonecrosis in post-traumatic avascular necrosis of the talus is the absence of the normal, early resorption of subchondral bone from the dome of the talus.[109]

Because marrow necrosis is an early part of avascular necrosis, magnetic resonance imaging is an excellent tool for early detection of osseous necrosis in many bones, including the talus. It is more sensitive than plain radiographs, computed tomography, and radionuclide bone scanning. However, false-negative magnetic resonance scans have been reported in the hip, wrist, and talus.

When avascular necrosis has been diagnosed, weightbearing must be avoided until revascularization is complete. Some authors advocated talectomy followed by tibiocalcaneal arthrodesis.[110, 111] Tibiocalcaneal arthrodesis can give only fair results and causes a disabling shortening of the extremity. Revascularization of a partially necrotic talus has been accomplished through the use of a vascularized bone graft.[112]

Avascular necrosis has also developed in bones of the foot other than the talus after trauma. Mullen and Kashuk reported

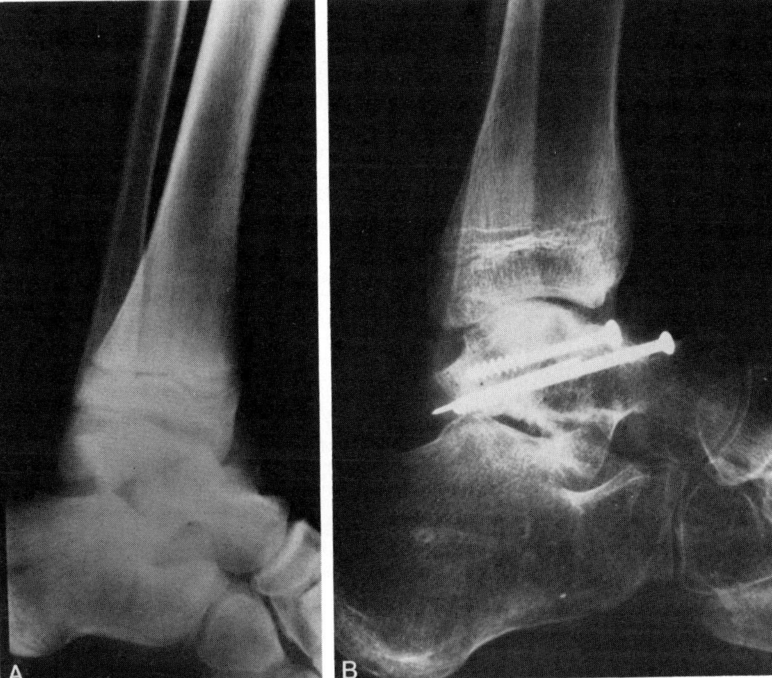

FIGURE 39–10. *A*, Fracture of the talar neck of this 14-year-old boy resulted from a rock-climbing accident. *B*, Increased sclerosis of the talar body was emphasized by relative osteopenia of surrounding bones.

a case of avascular necrosis in the distal phalanges of the halluces in a dancer.[113] The apparent mechanism of injury was through a bony infarct created by compression ischemia. Avascular necrosis of the first metatarsal sesamoid was described in 1972 and has become more common with the popularity of aerobic dance.[114, 115] This painful condition most often affects the fibular sesamoid. Avascular necrosis may also develop in the accessory sesamoids beneath the lesser metatarsal heads in response to local trauma.[116] Radiographs reveal mottling, irregularity, fragmentation, and abnormal density. If pain from the traumatized sesamoid does not respond to conservative measures such as padding, strapping, orthoses, and rest, surgical excision must be considered.

IDIOPATHIC AVASCULAR NECROSIS

When primary avascular necrosis of the tarsonavicular bone occurs in adults, it may be termed Mueller-Weiss syndrome.[17, 117] This must not be confused with Köhler's disease (osteochondrosis of the navicular bone in children). Although no clear cause has been defined for spontaneous avascular necrosis of the navicular bone, repetitive trauma, chronic stress, and obesity have been implicated. Pes planus and rearfoot valgus are associated as well. Avascular necrosis of the navicular bone is also known to occur in patients with an underlying systemic disease who are receiving steroid treatment. Radiographic findings are characteristic, with increased density, fragmentation, medial and dorsal protrusion, and a comma-shaped configuration. Magnetic resonance imaging most often displays homogeneous loss of signal intensity on T_1-weighted images, whereas T_2-weighted images show a less impressive focal loss of intensity. Initial treatment of avascular necrosis of the navicular bone is conservative with non-weightbearing and casting. Unremitting pain may require surgical reconstruction with grafting.

Bilateral avascular necrosis of the first metatarsal heads was reported in a 12-year-old girl; surgical intervention was required. No apparent cause could be discovered, and the patient was reportedly doing well.[118]

Four cases of histologically confirmed avascular necrosis of the first metatarsal sesamoid were reported in 1986.[119] None of the patients were athletes, and none recalled noticeable trauma or stress. No foot deformities or joint malalignments were found. Excision of the affected sesamoid achieved excellent results.

Spontaneous avascular necrosis can also occur in the knee, in either the femur or the tibial plateau.[120] Because of the relatively normal radiographic appearance in the early stages, the differential diagnosis of a painful knee may be shortened with the use of triphasic bone scanning or magnetic resonance imaging.

Idiopathic punctate necrosis has been reported in the phalanges of the feet.[121] Small areas of discrete radiolucency surrounded by well-defined margins of sclerosis were incidental, asymptomatic findings. The cause was not proven, but musculoskeletal stress was suspected.

The author gratefully acknowledges the invaluable assistance of Sherry Heldens and John Griffith in the preparation of this chapter.

References

1. Park WM: Spontaneous and drug-induced necrosis. *In* Davidson JK (ed): Aseptic Necrosis of Bone. Amsterdam, Excerpta Medica, 1976, pp 213–270.
2. Feller JA, Hart JA, and Doig SJ: Avascular necrosis of the talus following apparently minor ankle injury: A case report. Injury 19:213, 1988.
3. Binek R, Levinsohn EM, Bersani F, and Rubenstein H: Freiberg disease complicating unrelated trauma. Orthopedics 11:753, 1988.
4. Giacomello A, Zoppini A, Sorgi ML, et al: Hyperuricemia, gout and idiopathic aseptic necrosis of bone. Adv Exp Med Biol 253A:211, 1989.
5. Feldman JL, Alcalay M, Queinnec JY, and de Bray JM: Spinal cord compression related to vertebral osteonecrosis. Clin Exp Rheumatol 6:297, 1988.
6. Smith RE, Chelmowski MK, and Anderson T: Osteonecrosis in a patient with immune thrombocytopenic purpura. Am J Hematol 26:97, 1987.

7. Hanada T, Horigome Y, Inudoh M, and Takita H: Osteonecrosis of vertebrae in a child with acute lymphocytic leukaemia during L-asparaginase therapy. Eur J Pediatr 149:162, 1989.

8. Wounlund J and Lohmann M: Aseptic necrosis of the capitate secondary to Gaucher's disease: A case report. J Hand Surg 14:336, 1989.

9. Hungerford DS, and Zizic TM: Alcohol associated ischemic necrosis of the femoral head. Clin Orthop 130:144, 1978.

10. Patton PR and Pfaff WW: Aseptic bone necrosis after renal transplantation. Surgery 103:63, 1988.

11. Isono SS, Woolson ST, and Schurman DJ: Total joint arthroplasty for steroid-induced osteonecrosis in cardiac transplant patients. Clin Orthop 217:201, 1987.

12. Kjaerulff H and Hejgaard N: Neuropathic osteonecrosis of the knee in childhood. Two cases of myelomeningocele. Acta Orthop Scand 58:436, 1987.

13. Williams ES, Khreisat S, Ell PJ, and King JD: Bone imaging and skeletal radiology in dysbaric osteonecrosis. Clin Radiol 38:589, 1987.

14. Amano M, Ohsawa S, Saito M, and Ueno R: Multiple osteonecrosis associated with allergic dermatitis. Arch Orthop Trauma Surg 109:170, 1990.

15. Kuriloff DB and Kimmelman CP: Osteocartilaginous necrosis of the sinonasal tract following cocaine abuse. Laryngoscope 99:918, 1989.

16. Bomelburg T, von Lengerke HJ, and Ritter J: Aseptic osteonecroses in the treatment of childhood acute leukaemias. Eur J Pediatr 149:20, 1989.

17. Haller J, Sartoris DJ, Resnick D, et al: Spontaneous osteonecrosis of the tarsal navicular in adults: Imaging findings. Am J Roentgenol 151:355, 1988.

18. Schmidt DM and Romash MM: Atraumatic avascular necrosis of the head of the talus: A case report. Foot Ankle 8:208, 1988.

19. Ficat P and Arlet J: Necrosis of the femoral head. In Hungerford DS (ed): Ischemia and Necrosis of Bone. Baltimore, Williams & Wilkins, 1980, pp 53–74.

20. Larson B, Light TR, and Ogden JA: Fracture and ischemic necrosis of the immature scaphoid. J Hand Surg 12:122, 1987.

21. Bodamer WJ, Torre RJ, Cotch MT, and Goldman FD: Avascular necrosis of the talar head. A complication of group 4 fracture of the talar neck. J Am Podiatr Med Assoc 77:217, 1987.

22. Simkin PA and Downey DJ: Hypothesis: Retrograde embolization of marrow fat may cause osteonecrosis. J Rheumatol 14:870, 1987.

23. Ritsema GH: Total talar dislocation. J Trauma 28:692, 1988.

24. Wirtz PD, Vito GR, and Long DH: Calcaneal apophysitis (Sever's disease) associated with tae kwon do injuries. J Am Podiatr Med Assoc 78:474, 1988.

25. Bayliss NC and Klenerman L: Avascular necrosis of lesser metatarsal heads following forefoot surgery. Foot Ankle 10:124, 1989.

26. Meier PJ and Kenzora JE: The risks and benefits of distal first metatarsal osteotomy. Foot Ankle 6:7, 1985.

27. Outwater E, Oates E, and Sarno RC: Bilateral distal tibial osteonecrosis in systemic lupus erythematosus. Am J Roentgenol 152:895, 1989.

28. Nagasawa K, Ishii V, Mayumi T, et al: Avascular necrosis of bone in systemic lupus erythematosus: Possible role of haemostatic abnormalities. Ann Rheum Dis 48:672, 1988.

29. Fishel B, Caspi D, Eventor I, et al: Multiple osteonecrotic lesions in systemic lupus erythematosus. J Rheumatol 14:601, 1987.

30. Wang TY, Avlonitis EG, and Relkin R: Systemic necrotizing vasculitis causing bone necrosis. Am J Med 84:1085, 1988.

31. Vakil N and Sparberg M: Steroid-related osteonecrosis in inflammatory bowel disease. Gastroenterology 96:62, 1989.

32. Jones JG: Avascular necrosis and pulsed methylprednisolone in rheumatoid arthritis. Br J Rheumatol 27:497, 1988.

33. Murphy RG and Greenberg ML: Osteonecrosis in pediatric patients with acute lymphoblastic leukemia. Cancer 65:1717, 1990.

34. el-Sabbagh AM and Kamel M: Avascular necrosis of temporomandibular joint in sickle cell disease. Clin Rheumatol 8:393, 1989.

35. van Leeuwen HJ, Witkamp D, Verdonck LF, et al: Multiple sites of ischemic necrosis of bone following long term corticosteroid treatment in a patient with auto-immune granulocytopenia. Clin Rheumatol 8:103, 1989.

36. McGill NW, Warburton P, Kronenberg H, et al: Ischaemic necrosis of the ilium complicating haemolytic anaemia due to an unstable haemoglobin. Ann Rheum Dis 47:957, 1988.

37. Smith RE, Chelmowski MK, and Anderson T: Osteonecrosis in a patient with immune thrombocytopenic purpura. Am J Hematol 26:97, 1987.

38. Perlman MD, Gold ML, and Schor AD: Usage of long-term steroid therapy. J Foot Surg 26:233, 1987.

39. Xue HL: Dysbaric osteonecrosis and its radiographic classification in China. Undersea Biomed Res 15:389, 1988.

40. Davidson JK: Aseptic necrosis of bone—An introduction. In Davidson JD (ed): Aseptic Necrosis of Bone. Amsterdam, Excerpta Medica, 1976, pp 1–2.

41. Yamaguchi H, Masuda T, Sasaki T, and Nojima T: Steroid-induced osteonecrosis of the patella. Clin Orthop 229:201, 1988.

42. Felson DT and Anderson JJ: Across-study evaluation of association between steroid dose and bolus steroids and avascular necrosis of bone. Lancet 1(8538):902, 1987.

43. Havel PE, Ebraheim NA, and Jackson WT: Steroid-induced bilateral avascular necrosis of the lateral femoral condyles. Clin Orthop 243:166, 1989.

44. Zizic TM, Marcoux C, Hungerford DS, et al: Corticosteroid therapy associated with ischemic necrosis of bone in systemic lupus erythematosus, Am J Med 79:596, 1985.

45. Zizic TM and Hungerford DS: Avascular necrosis of bone. In Kelley WN, Harris ED, Ruddy S, and Sledge CB (eds): Textbook of Rheumatology, 2nd ed. Philadelphia, WB Saunders, 1985, pp 1689–1910.

46. Resnick D: Osteonecrosis of metacarpal and metatarsal heads following renal transplantation [letter]. Br J Radiol 55:463, 1982.

47. Boettger WG, Bonfiglio M, Hamilton HH, et al: Nontraumatic necrosis of the femoral head. J Bone Joint Surg 52A:312, 1970.

48. Jones JP, Jameson RM, and Engleman EP: Alcoholism, fat embolism, and avascular necrosis. J Bone Joint Surg 50A:1065, 1968.

49. Hartmann G: The possible role of fat metabolism in idiopathic ischemic necrosis of the femoral head. In Zinn W (ed): Idiopathic Ischaemic Necrosis of the Femoral Head in Adults. Baltimore, University Park Press, 1971, pp 140–144.

50. Nellen JR and Kindwall EP: Aseptic necrosis of bone secondary to occupational exposure to compressed air: Radiological findings in forty-one cases. Am J Roentgenol 95:512, 1972.

51. Woodhouse CF: Dynamic influences of vascular occlusion affecting aseptic necrosis of the femoral head. Clin Orthop 32:119, 1964.

52. Walder DN, Evans A, and Hempleman HV: Ultrasonic monitoring of decompression. Lancet 1:897, 1968.

53. Philp RB, Inwood MJ, and Warren BA: Interactions between gas bubbles and components of the blood. Aerospace Med 43:946, 1972.

54. Zizic TM: Osteonecrosis. In Schumacher HR (ed): Primer on Rheumatic Diseases, Atlanta, Arthritis Foundation, 1988, pp 253–257.

55. Hollander JL: Intraarticular hydrocortisone in the treatment of arthritis. Ann Intern Med 39:735, 1953.

56. Kendall PH: Untoward effects following local hydrocortisone injection. Ann Phys Med 4:170, 1958.

57. Keagy RD and Keim HA: Intraarticular steroid therapy: Repeated use in patients with chronic arthritis. Am J Med Sci 81:45, 1967.

58. Bentley G and Goodfellow JW: Disorganization of the knees following intraarticular hydrocortisone injection. J Bone Joint Surg 51B:498, 1969.

59. Steinberg CL, Duthie RB, and Piva AE: Charcot-like arthropathy following intra-articular hydrocortisone. JAMA 181:851, 1962.

60. Sweet DE and Madewell JE: Pathogenesis of osteonecrosis. In Resnick D and Niwayama G (eds): Diagnosis of Bone and Joint Disorders. Philadelphia, WB Saunders, 1981, pp 2780–2831.

61. Zizic TM, Hungerford DS, and Stevens MB: The early diagnosis of ischemic necrosis of bone. Arthritis Rheum 29:1177, 1986.

62. Arlet J and Ficat P: Biopsy drilling as a means of early diagnosis. In Zinn W (ed): Idiopathic Ischemic Necrosis of the Femoral Head in Adults. Baltimore, University Park Press, 1971, pp 74–80.

63. Tawn DJ and Watt I: Bone marrow scintigraphy in the diagnosis of post-traumatic avascular necrosis of bone. Br J Radiol 62:790, 1989.

64. Conklin JJ, Alderson PO, Zizic TM, et al: Comparison of bone scan and radiograph sensitivity in the detection of steroid-induced ischemic necrosis of bone. Radiology 147:221, 1983.

65. Strömqvist B: Femoral head vitality after intracapsular hip fracture. Acta Orthop Scand 54(Suppl 200):25, 1983.

66. Mitchell DG, Rao VM, Dalinka MK, et al: Femoral head avascular necrosis: Correlation of magnetic resonance imaging, radiographic staging, radionuclide imaging, and clinical findings. Radiology 162:709, 1987.

67. Totty WG, Murphy WA, Ganz WI, et al: Magnetic resonance imaging of the normal and ischemic femoral head. Am J Roentgenol 143:1273, 1984.

68. Markisz JA, Knowles RJR, Altchek DW, et al: Segmental patterns of avascular necrosis of the femoral head: Early detection with MR imaging. Radiology 162:717, 1987.

69. Gillespy T, Genant HK, and Helms CA: Magnetic resonance imaging of osteonecrosis. Radiol Clin North Am 24:193, 1986.

70. Beltman J, Herman LJ, Burk JM, et al: Femoral head avascular necrosis: MR imaging with clinicopathologic and radionuclide correlation. Radiology 166:215, 1988.

71. Ehman RL, Berquist TH, and McLeod RA: MR imaging of the musculoskeletal system. Radiology 166:313, 1988.

72. Wynne-Davies R and Gormley J: The etiology of Perthes' disease. J Bone Joint Surg 60B:6, 1978.

73. Szames SE, Forman WM, Oster J, et al: Sever's disease and its relationship to equinus: A statistical analysis. Clin Podiatr Med Surg 7:377, 1990.

74. Douglas G and Rang M: The role of trauma in the pathogenesis of the osteochondroses. Clin Orthop 158:28, 1981.

75. Siffert RS: Classification of the osteochondroses. Clin Orthop 158:10–18, 1981.

76. Perthes GC: Über Arthritis Deformans Juvenilis. Deutsch Z Chir 107:111, 1910.

77. Calve J: Sur une forme particuliere de coxalgie greffeé: Sur des deformations caracteristique de l'extremité superieure du femur. Rev Chir 42:54, 1910.

78. Legg AT: An obscure affection of the hip joint. Boston Med Surg J 162:202, 1910.

79. Osgood RB: Lesions of the tibial tubercle occurring during adolescence. Boston Med Surg J 148:114, 1903.

80. Schlatter C: Verletzungen des Schnabel Formigen Forsätzes der Oberen Tibiaepiphyse. Beitr Klin Chir 38:874, 1903.

81. Waugh W: The ossification and vascularization of the tarsal navicular and their relation to Kohler disease. J Bone Joint Surg 40B:765, 1958.

82. Haglund P: Über Fraktur des Epiphysenkerns des Calcaneus, Nebst all Gemeinen Bemerkung en über Einige Ahnliche Juvenile Knochenkern Verletzungen. Arch Klin Chir 83:922, 1907.

83. Sever JW: Apophysitis of the os calcis. N Y Med J 95:1025, 1912.

84. Krantz MK: Calcaneal apophysitis: A clinical and roentgenologic study. J Am Podiatr Assoc 55:801, 1965.

85. Meyerding HW and Stuck W: Painful heels among children (apophysitis). JAMA 102:1658, 1934.

86. Stess RM: Persistent calcaneal apophysitis: A case report. J Am Podiatr Assoc 63:147, 1973.

87. Freiberg AH: Infraction of the second metatarsal bone: A typical injury. Surg Gynecol Obstet 19:191, 1914.

88. Freiberg AH: The so-called infraction of the second metatarsal bone. J Bone Joint Surg 8:257, 1926.

89. König F: Ueber freie Körper in den Gelenken. Deutsche Z Chir 27:90, 1888.

90. Pappas AM: Osteochondrosis dissecans. Clin Orthop 158:59, 1981.

91. Kappis M: Weitere Beiträge zur Traumatischmechanischen Entstehung der ''Spontanen'' Knorpelablösungen (sogen. Osteochnodritis Dissecans). Deutsch Z Chir 171:13, 1922.

92. Stougaard J: Familial occurrence of osteochondritis dissecans. J Bone Joint Surg 46B:542, 1964.

93. Ribbing S: The hereditary multiple epiphyseal disturbance and its consequences for the etiogenesis of local malacias, particularly the osteochondritis dissecans. Acta Orthop Scand 14:286, 1955.

94. Berndt AL, and Harty M: Transchondral fractures (osteochondritis dissecans) of the talus. J Bone Joint Surg 41A:996, 1959.

95. Wershba M, Dalina MK, Coren GS, and Cotler J: Double constant knee arthrography in the evaluation of osteochondritis dissecans. Clin Orthop 107:81, 1975.

96. Canale ST and Belding RH: Osteochondral lesions of the talus. J Bone Joint Surg 62A:97, 1980.

97. Silvani S: Injuries to the talus. Clin Podiatr 2:287, 1985.

98. Arenson DJ and Weil LS: Aseptic necrosis: An unusual cause of Silastic (Swanson) implant failure. J Am Podiatr Assoc 69:616, 1979.

99. Mann RA: [Letter]. In Jahss MH: Editorial. Foot Ankle 3:125, 1982.

100. Jahss MH: Hallux valgus: Further considerations—The first metatarsal head. Foot Ankle 2:1, 1981.

101. Williams WW, Barrett DS, and Copeland SA: Avascular necrosis following Chevron distal metatarsal osteotomy: A significant risk? J Foot Surg 28:414, 1989.

102. Meisenhelder DA, Harkless LB, and Patterson JW: Avascular necrosis after first metatarsal osteotomy. J Foot Surg 23:429, 1984.

103. Resch S, Stenström A, and Gustofson T: Circulatory disturbance of the first metatarsal head after Chevron osteotomy as shown by bone scintigraphy. Foot Ankle 13:137, 1992.

104. Boberg J, Ruch JA, and Banks AS: Distal metaphyseal osteotomies in hallux valgus surgery. In McGlamry ED (ed): Comprehensive Textbook of Foot Surgery. Baltimore, Williams & Wilkins, 1987, pp 177–184.

105. Brav EA: Traumatic dislocations of the hip. J Bone Joint Surg 44A:1115, 1962.

106. Hawkins LG: Fractures of the neck of the talus. J Bone Joint Surg 52A:991, 1970.

107. Canale ST and Kelly FB Jr: Fractures of the neck of the talus: Long-term evaluation of seventy-one cases. J Bone Joint Surg 60A:143, 1978.

108. Pennal GF: Fractures of the talus. Clin Orthop 30:53, 1963.

109. Henderson RC: Posttraumatic necrosis of the talus: The Hawkins sign versus magnetic resonance imaging. J Orthop Trauma 5:96, 1991.

110. Pennal GF: Fractures of the talus. Clin Orthop 30:53, 1963.

111. Detenbeck C and Kelley PJ: Total dislocation of the talus. J Bone Joint Surg 51A:283, 1969.

112. Hussl H, Sailer R, Daniaux H, and Pechlaner S: Revascularization of a partially necrotic talus with a vascularized bone graft from the iliac crest. Arch Orthop Trauma Surg 108:27, 1989.

113. Mullen BR and Kashuk KB: Primary avascular necrosis of the halluces in a ballet dancer. J Am Podiatr Med Assoc 76:544, 1986.

114. Ilfeld FW and Rosen V: Osteochondritis of the first metatarsal sesamoid. Clin Orthop 85:38, 1972.

115. Golding C: Sesamoids of the hallux. J Bone Joint Surg 42B:840, 1960.

116. Keating S, Fisher D, and Keating D: Avascular necrosis of an accessory sesamoid of the foot. J Am Podiatr Med Assoc 77:612, 1987.

117. Viladot A, Rochera R, and Viladot A Jr: Necrosis of the navicular bone. Bull Hosp Jt Dis Orthop Inst 47:285, 1987.

118. Fu FH and Gomez W: Bilateral avascular necrosis of the first metatarsal head in adolescence. Clin Orthop 246:282, 1989.

119. Ogata K, Sugioka Y, Urano Y, and Chikama H: Idiopathic osteonecrosis of the first metatarsal sesamoid. Skeletal Radiol 15:141, 1986.

120. Traflet R, Desai A, and Park C: Spontaneous osteonecrosis of the knee. Scintigraphic findings. Clin Nucl Med 12:525, 1987.

121. Keats TE, Johnson RR, and Fechner RE: Idiopathic punctate necrosis of the phalanges of the feet. Skeletal Radiol 18:25, 1989.

CHAPTER 40

Congenital Deformities

Richard M. Jay, D.P.M.

One of the keys in treating children with congenital deformities is redirecting the forces of growth and development into an accepted normal position. It is also understood that if an abnormal force is applied to any growing child, a deformity will result.[1] Wolff's law[2] describes the reaction of bone to forces acting on it: "Every change in the form and function of bones or their function alone is followed by certain definite changes in their normal internal structure and equally definite changes in their external configuration in accordance with mathematical laws." Forces of weightbearing and the action of muscles reshape and remodel the bone, gradually correcting the deformity. Bone can thus change its architecture in response to altered mechanical loads.

CALCANEOVALGUS

Clinical Signs

In calcaneovalgus, the foot is in an up-and-out position relative to the leg (Fig. 40–1). This dorsiflexed and abducted position leaves the foot in a calcaneal position. There exists a limitation of motion in plantarflexion, inversion, and an increase in dorsiflexion, eversion. The ranges of these motions vary, and all are dependent on the degree of the deformity. With calcaneovalgus deformity, the dorsum of the foot lies in close proximity to the anterior aspect of the tibia. If the leg is held and the foot is rapidly shaken and then released, the foot will still assume a dorsiflexed everted position relative to the leg. The normal foot assumes a plantarflexed or at least a right-angle attitude to the leg. Increased skin folds are common along the lateral border of the foot in the area of the sinus tarsi. When present, these folds blanch when the foot is plantarflexed and inverted.

Etiology

Intrinsic and extrinsic factors that affect the position of the calcaneovalgus foot can be attributed to and aggravated by the following (in degree of severity):

1. Small uterus
2. Tight amniotic membranes
3. Breech or transverse-lying fetus
4. Large child
5. Sitting and sleeping positions that force the foot outward. Sleeping in a prone position with the feet outward and in a reverse tailor sitting position with the feet forced outward will maintain the deformity.
6. Muscular imbalances. In the calcaneovalgus foot type, the anterior tibial tendon becomes shorter because its origin and insertion are brought closer together. This maintains dorsiflexion and pulls the flexible forefoot into supination. The peroneus longus muscle is greatly overstretched and is essentially functionless. The heel cord and the tibialis posterior muscle are also elongated. The peroneus brevis muscle becomes active at about the fourth to sixth week of age and pulls the heel

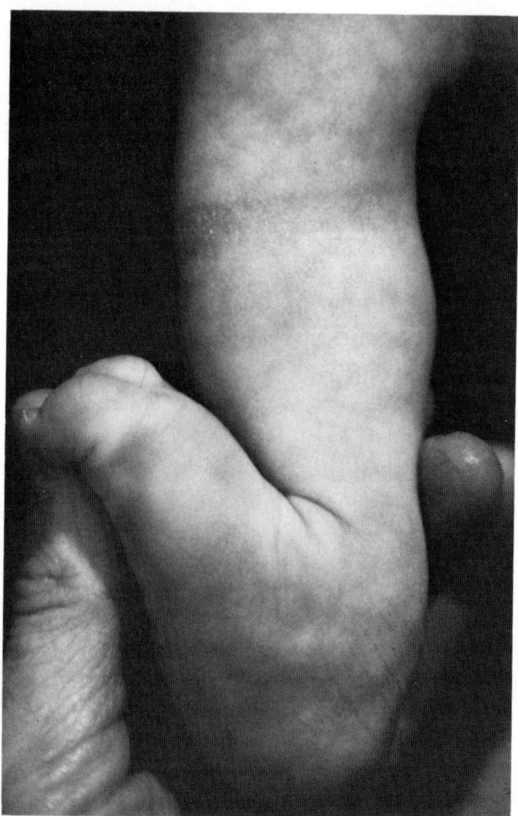

FIGURE 40–1. Three-month-old child with calcaneovalgus. The right foot is maximally dorsiflexed, leaving the heel in a calcaneal position. The foot easily rolls into an abducted and dorsiflexed position. The dorsum of the foot rests against the anterior aspect of the leg.

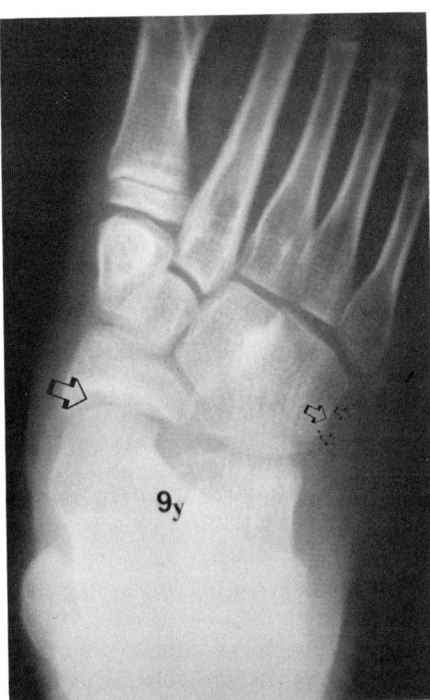

FIGURE 40–2. Right foot of a 9-year-old girl with calcaneovalgus. The talar head flattens as the navicular drifts laterally along with the cuboid. The medial surfacer loses its articular covering, creating a more rigid, nonreducible, cone-shaped head.

into marked eversion and abduction secondary to the position of the calcaneovalgus foot.

7. Weak ligaments. These allow bone structures to follow a course of least resistance. If an abnormal force is applied to a loose joint, the bone will deform in the direction of the applied force. In the presence of joint laxity (in Ehlers-Danlos syndrome, Marfan's syndrome, hypertonia, or children with trisomy 21), the joints are going to respond to extrinsic pronatory factors. In time, the muscles acting around the joints begin to change the bone positions further, and the bones themselves will change their shapes (Fig. 40–2).

Radiologic Evaluation

One must be aware that calcaneovalgus at an early age is determined clinically and not radiographically. However, if the condition is severe and warrants casting or surgery, then a radiograph can be beneficial in determining the degree of the deformity. With a young child, the bones are not fully matured, and interpreting navicular position on the head of the talus will be impossible because the primary ossification center of the navicular bone does not appear until at least 2 years of age. One can, however, on a lateral radiograph determine the bisection of the talus through the upper segment of the cuboid (Fig. 40–3). This is performed by moving the child's foot into a weightbearing position on the x-ray table. In the calcaneovalgus foot, holding the same position in a lateral view, the talus is plantarflexed and the line bisecting the talus extends far below that of the plantar surface of the cuboid. What is also noticed is the overlapping of the head of the talus on the anterosuperior surface of the calcaneus. Also, the talus itself appears to be smaller because of the plantar medial position of the head on the calcaneus, thus giving the visual appearance of a shortened talar neck. The bone itself is not shortened but is only a radiographic finding. Because the navicular bone is locked toward the calcaneus by the spring ligament, the navicular bone now lies lateral to the talar head. This is seen by the increase in the talocalcaneal angle on the anteroposterior view of the foot.

Conservative Treatment

Casting Technique. The assistant holds the child's toes with one hand and stabilizes the thigh with the other hand. If a concomitant external tibial torsion is present, the cast will be applied from the toes to the proximal segment of the thigh. If an isolated calcaneovalgus is present, then only a below-the-knee cast is necessary.

The technique for casting should completely reverse the component deformities. One should keep in mind the position of the foot and the tendons and ligaments that maintain the deformity. With the foot up and out, the peroneus brevis and lateral ankle ligaments are tight. In addition, the dorsiflexed position is maintained by the tightened anterior tibial

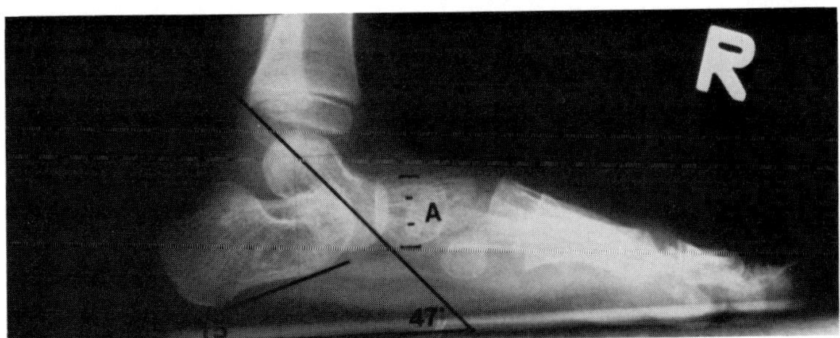

FIGURE 40–3. Bisection of talus forms a 47-degree angle to the supporting surface. The bisection lies below the lower ⅓ trisection of the cuboid (A). The normal bisection should pass through the upper third. The cartilaginous surface develops on the superior aspect of the talar head. As the distal head completely develops with maturity, the bisection of the talus changes. The gradual decrease in the head and neck bisection to the supporting surface makes trisecting the cuboid unnecessary. This occurs at approximately 10 years of age.

tendon and the anterior ankle ligaments. The anterior ankle is stretched out by plantarflexing the foot at the ankle. The tight peroneus brevis is further lengthened by inverting the calcaneus and adducting the forefoot. The tibialis anterior is stretched by plantarflexion of the ankle. Plantarflexing the first ray isolates this tendon, and an increase in length can be attained. The cast is molded into these positions to maintain correction. The soft tissue and osseous structures will adapt to a correct position over a 4- to 12-week period of casting (Fig. 40–4).

Because of varying degrees of deformity, the cast should be changed until the foot is brought to the desired position. It is recommended that the cast be worn an extra week or two beyond the time that correction is noted to overcorrect slightly. This is advised because the foot has a tendency to draw back to its original position. According to Giannestras, after the foot has gained its position of correction, the foot alone is casted in the desired position and then gently dorsiflexed on the leg and casted in that attitude. Giannestras indicated that prolonged casting in a plantarflexed position induces an equinus. By maintaining the foot in this position of correction, one can stretch out the heel cord and prevent any of the pronatory effects of the equinus on the foot.[3] This correction may take up to 12 weeks.

Bebax Shoe. The Bebax shoe is used as an adjunct to the application of casts in children with metatarsus adductus, talipes equinovarus, and calcaneovalgus (see Table 40–1 for information on this and other manufacturers). The construction of the shoe allows a multidirectional change through the universal joints placed underneath the forefoot and hindfoot shoe compartments. The Bebax shoe allows motion on all three planes and can maintain any of these deformities. It is recommended to be worn from birth to approximately 9 months of age. The shoe is to be worn at all times because it is simulating the cast application.

For use with calcaneovalgus, the forefoot is adducted, plantarflexed, and everted in relation to the hindfoot. The medial column of the forefoot shoe is also translated plantarly.

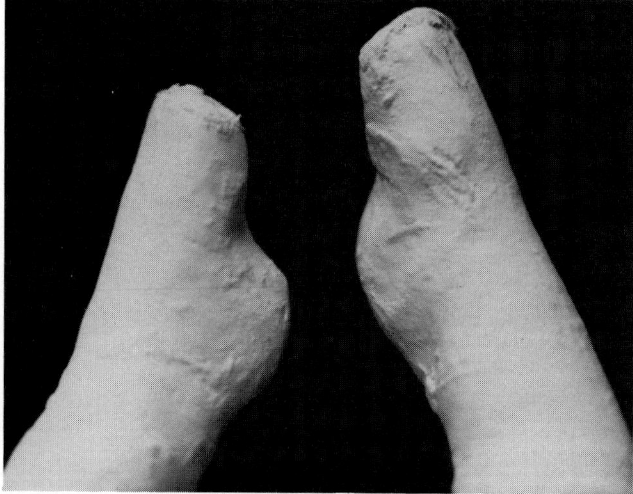

FIGURE 40–4. Correct cast position of the calcaneovalgus foot: plantarflexed ankle; inverted hindfoot; plantarflexed first ray on hindfoot; and adducted forefoot on hindfoot. The cast should extend past the toes but open distally for inspection. The cast should be well molded to capture and maintain correction.

Ganley Splint. Now that the deformity is reduced, it must be maintained in a corrected position. The most accurate device to accomplish the desired position is the Ganley splint (see Table 40–1). The purpose of the Ganley splint is to maintain the correction in the foot and leg of young children. Adjustments are made by rotating and torquing the shanks and bars. It is intended for the reduction and correction of tibial torsion, calcaneovalgus, metatarsus adductus, and talipes equinovarus.

The splint is placed directly on a pair of leather-bottom oxford shoes. The plate of the shoe, as well as the medial and lateral vamps, are cut along the transverse plane of the shoe to allow for motion of the forefoot against the hindfoot. Each shoe on the torsion bar is set apart a length equal to that of the distance between the anterior iliac spines. This length in a young child is usually between 6 to 8 inches. For calcaneovalgus, the torsion bar is bent to create an internal or medial rotation of the foot relative to the long axis of the body. External tibial torsion is usually seen secondary to calcaneovalgus because the foot is malpositioned on the transverse plane in an up and out position. The torsional bar is set internally to maintain an internal alignment rather than maintaining an external rotatory force through the foot. The shank bar is then also bent inward to adduct the forefoot on the hindfoot. At the same time, the rear heel plate is inverted to maintain a subtalar neutral position. With the inverted position of the hindfoot to the forefoot, in effect what is created is a plantar flexion of the first ray on the hindfoot (Fig. 40–5).

When initially applying the splint to the child, it is a good idea to torque the bars and shanks gradually, rather than placing the splint into its full correction. The device should not be cranked any further than resistance because it will become uncomfortable, and the child will not tolerate the device. The device is intended to be used during times of sleep only and is not intended for use when walking or sitting during the day.

Counter Rotational System. The Counter Rotational System (CRS) is a dynamic orthosis that can replace the use of the rigid Fillauer or Denis Browne Bar (see Table 40–1). This system is a flexible parallelogram that allows rotation on the transverse plane and allows motion and freedom to

TABLE 40–1

PRODUCTS AND MANUFACTURERS

Bebax: Inter Axial France, Sallanches, France
CRS: Langer Laboratories, Deer Park, NY
Denis Browne: Durr-Flower Medical Inc., Orthopedic Division, Chattanooga, TN
Dexon: Davis and Geck, Pearl River, NY
EBI: EBI, Parsippany, NJ
Fillauer: Durr-Flower Medical Inc., Orthopedic Division, Chattanooga, TN
Ganley Splint: J. Ganley, Norristown, PA
IPOS: Ipos USA, Niagara Falls, NY
K-Wire: Micro-Aire, Valencia, CA
Plastizote: BXL Plastics, Ltd., Croydon, England
PPT: Langer Laboratories, Deer Park, NY
Richard's Buck Plug: Richards, Memphis, TN
Scotchrap: 3M Health Care Products, St. Paul, MN
STA-Peg: Dow Corning Medical Products, Midland, MI
Unibar: Spectra Industries Corp., Yeadon, PA
Webril: Johnson and Johnson Orthopedics, Raynham, MA
Wheaton Brace: Wheaton Brace Co., Carol Stream, IL

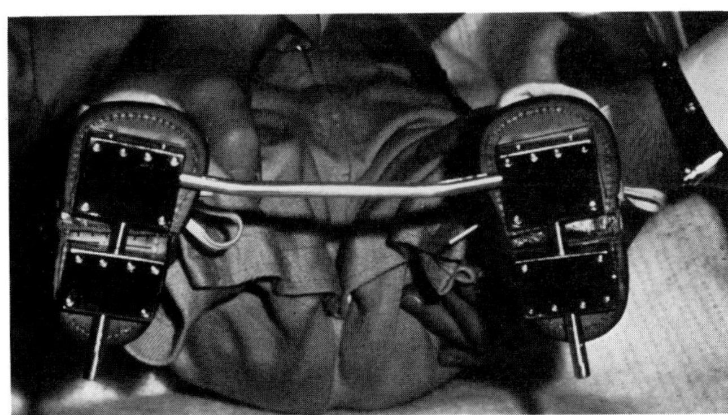

FIGURE 40–5. Ganley splint maintaining correction of a calcaneovalgus foot. The hindfoot plate is inverted in position to the forefoot plate along the longitudinal bar. The longitudinal bar can be bent with bending irons to increase the forefoot adduction. The transverse bar is bent to an internal position.

occur within the leg, hip, and knee. With calcaneovalgus, the foot plate should be set approximately 10 degrees internally. Because this device allows for more dynamic motion and does stimulate normal muscle development to allow movement during the night and day, the child can be in the splint a greater amount of time than the conventional rigid devices (Fig. 40–6).

Fillauer and Denis Browne Bar. These two bars also maintain transverse plane position of the foot relative to the axial segment. They do not address calcaneovalgus directly. Care must also be taken with the use of any of these splints and devices. As seen with children sitting in a reverse tailor position, an actual internal rotation will occur at the hip while the leg is being maintained externally. If the child presents with an internal hip deformity, this will only increase with the use of these splints and bars. Again, these splints are to be used only when sleeping. The devices are not intended for correction of any of these deformities; they are intended only to maintain correction and prevent further increases in malposition.

Orthotics. A Roberts plate, calcaneal brace, or rigid, molded acrylic orthosis to stabilize the hindfoot is essential in the treatment of the child with calcaneovalgus with or without prior casting. The use of an orthosis with a lateral extension is needed to stabilize the rearfoot in an approximate 5-degree inverted position. The lateral flange prevents the abductory transverse plane deformity that is seen in calcaneovalgus foot types. The medial flange at the same time is supporting the medial column and preventing the midtarsal and subtalar joint breakdown. The child should be placed into this orthosis as early as possible, usually at 24 months of age. This orthosis can be placed directly into a running sneaker. Replacement of this orthosis is usually necessary when an increase of approximately two shoe sizes occurs. When the child becomes older and there is less fat around the heel and arch area, it may be necessary to continue this deep-seated heel cup with the addition of a Plastizote or SBR flange (see Table 40–1) to protect irritations on the medial talar bulge. As the child continues to grow, at approximately 7 or 8 years of age, the child will not tolerate this very deep, flanged orthosis and will need to have one constructed that eliminates the far lateral flange and stops just short of the fifth metatarsal base. The younger child can tolerate the flange extending as far distally as the fifth metatarsal head because of the extra fat that is present. With the older child, it will be necessary to decrease the depth of the heel seat.

Dynamic Stabilizing Insole System. The design concept of the dynamic stabilizing insole system incorporates a deep offset heel seat that will be able to cup the calcaneus and maintain it in a correct alignment relative to the ground, which has been predetermined to be approximately 5 degrees of varus. This inverted position is accomplished by a unique design. All other orthotic devices try to invert the heel from the plantar aspect of the insert itself or the shoe. This new design concept of offsetting the calcaneus within the interior of the cup will give direct contact control.

The deep heel seat is offset to maintain the calcaneus in an inverted position but to allow normal pronation. The lateral and medial flanges of the present device extend to the

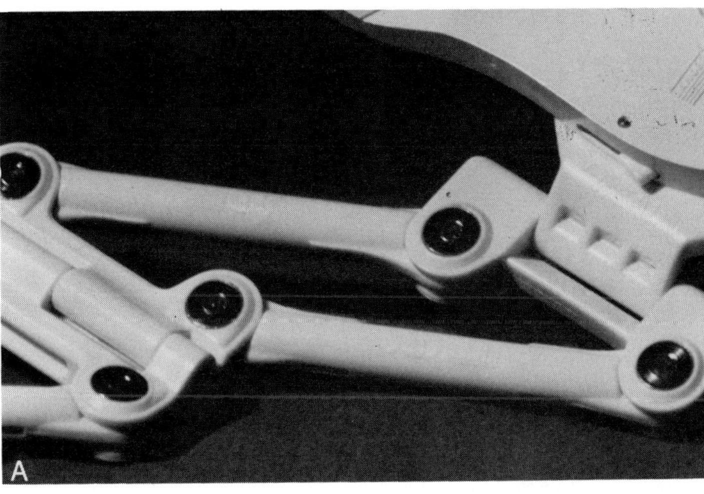

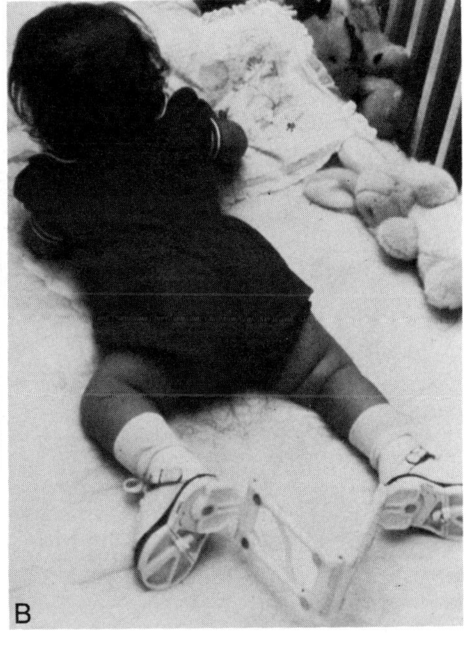

FIGURE 40–6. *A*, Counter Rotational System (CRS). A double-flexible parallelogram allows motion and maintains the desired transverse, fixed plane position. *B*, A CRS with a flexible parallelogram design allows the child full mobility while it maintains an external position to the limb.

neck of the first and fifth metatarsals and function in a different capacity. The stiff lateral counter, which extends high in the present device from the cup of the heel seat and continues along the entire lateral border, is designed to prevent a lateral shifting of the entire foot, which occurs in conjunction with the medial shift with rotation of the talus. In pronation, the talus plantarflexes and adducts, whereas the calcaneus, the midtarsus, and the forefoot abduct. There is a component of eversion of the calcaneus with pronation, and this is controlled by the offset inverted heel cup of the dynamic stabilizing insole system. Transverse plane function is maintained by the medial flange and the offset varus heel as it controls the adduction of the talus while the lateral flange controls the abduction of the forefoot (Figs. 40–7 and 40–8).[4–13]

Surgical Treatment

Subtalar Arthroereisis. Arthroereisis is based on the premise that abnormal subtalar motion may be limited by insertion of an implant into the sinus tarsi. This procedure is indicated in the calcaneovalgus flatfoot, with a forefoot supinatus deformity. With realignment of the subtalar joint to neutral and an increase in the range of dorsiflexion of the ankle joint, the peroneus longus can function under a stable cuboid. Plantar flexion of the first ray can then occur, thereby reducing the supinatus. Usually present with this deformity is a primary or secondary gastrocnemius equinus deformity (described in the discussion of equinus), which may have to be addressed when the arthroereisis procedure is performed.

The procedure limits pronation by the insertion of a Silastic or polyethylene plug into the lateral sinus tarsi. Various techniques have been described with the insertion and the type of plug used (Sta-peg, high-density silicone, or Richard's Buck plug) (see Table 40–1).[14–18] The procedure seems best applied to the skeletally immature foot, thereby allowing for functional adaptation to a more normal position. Calcaneovalgus is one type of pronation disorder for which this procedure may be applied.

Surgical Anatomy. The canal of the sinus tarsi is cone shaped with the apex positioned medially. The internal ligaments guard against excessive inversion and eversion, thus stabilizing the subtalar joint. In the flexible flatfoot, the interosseous ligament, which limits eversion, is not doing its job and allows the deforming forces to take their toll on the subtalar joint. The cervical ligament, which limits inversion of the subtalar joint, begins to be taut and further limits

inversion.[19] Some authors performed the procedure by severing the interosseous and cervical ligaments. The main advantage of this approach is that one is able to open the sinus tarsi floor with greater ease. However, by incising the interosseus ligament, eversion is left unchecked. The cervical ligament alone should be isolated to gain inversion of the subtalar joint and allow entrance into the canal.

I personally use this technique with the insertion of the Richard's Buck plug. The implant has two rings of polyethylene that become incorporated with fibrous tissue within the sinus tarsi. This has an advantage in terms of limiting the possibility of implant extrusion (Figs. 40–9 and 40–10).

The procedure is sound in the young child but is not advised in the older, mature child because irritation to the surrounding tissue can occur, creating a synovitis of the sinus tarsi. This eventually necessitates removal of the plug. The synovitis reduces immediately on removal with no permanent changes to the osseous surface.

Evan's Calcaneal Osteotomy

Indications. The indications for Evan's procedure is a flexible flatfoot with excessive transverse plan motion as exhibited by the abducted excursion of the midtarsal joint. This type of flatfoot is observed when the oblique axis of the midtarsal joint is more vertically oriented. This is fairly visible on the anteroposterior radiograph, which demonstrates a prominently abducted lateral border witnessed with an increased talocalcaneal angle. It is important that the lateral and medial columns be equal in length. If the lateral column is significantly shortened, as seen on the anteroposterior view, the cuboid will not rotate properly in an adducted manner and will jam into the talus (Fig. 40–11). It will be necessary to lengthen and equalize the lateral column to ensure that the proper adductory rotation will occur and to reduce the abducted forefoot.

Procedure. The procedure entails an osteotomy of the calcaneus, with insertion of a bone graft into the site. Placement of the bone graft encourages the forefoot into adduction. The placement of the wedge should be 1 cm proximal to the calcaneocuboid joint. If the osteotomy is placed too far anteriorly, avascular necrosis will potentially develop on the distal surface of the calcaneus. Placing the graft too far proximally will invade the medial subtalar joint facet and will invite arthritic changes (Fig. 40–12).

The graft should be composed of either cortical or corticocancellous bone. The graft can be fenestrated to encourage

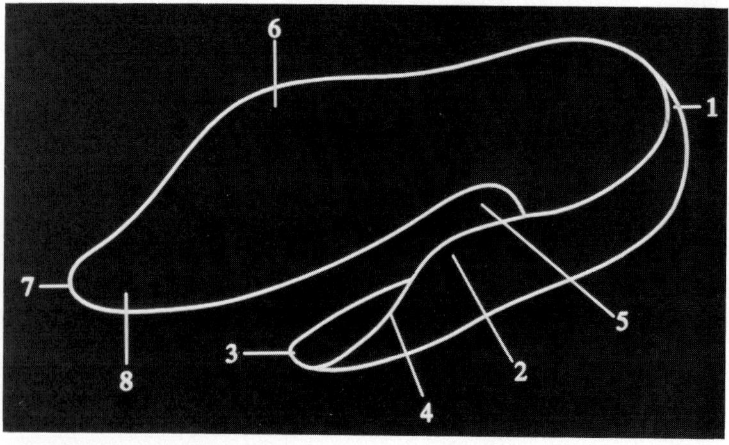

FIGURE 40–7. Dynamic stabilizing insole system (DSIS). An orthographic view of one preferred embodiment of the DSIS showing a molded structure comprising the deep-offset inverted heel cup (1) with the lateral flange (2). This flange continues distally to just proximal to the fifth metatarsal head (3 and 4). There is a cutout in the deep heel seat that creates a plantar support both medially and laterally (5). The high medial flange (6) rests adjacent to the talonavicular and cuneonavicular articulation. The distal end of the medial flange ends proximally to the first metatarsal head (7), and the plantar medial flange ends proximally to the sesamoid apparatus (8).

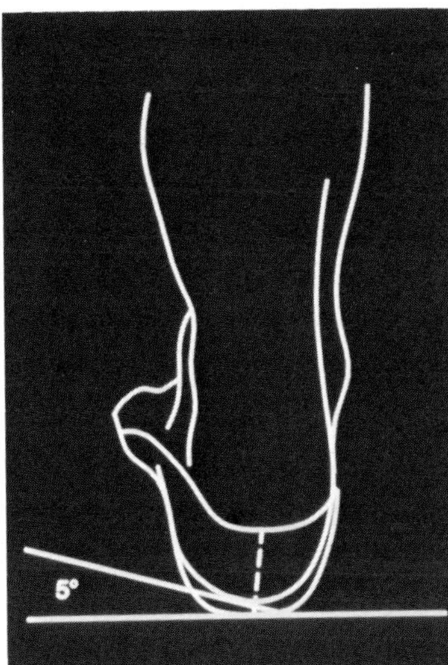

FIGURE 40–8. Dynamic stabilizing insole system (DSIS). Normally, the vertical axis of the calcaneus is perpendicular to the ground. By application of the DSIS, the axis of the calcaneus is tilted with 5 degrees of varus. This tilt prevents displacement between the calcaneus and the overlying talus. Stabilization of the hindfoot and midtarsal joint is maintained. Transverse drift of the forefoot is prevented by the locking mechanism and the inherent stability of the DSIS flanges, medially and laterally.

vascular ingrowth and promote osteogenesis. With creeping substitution, the graft will be incorporated into the surgical site. The cortical portion of the bone graft provides a strong strut that keeps the cut surfaces apart and maintains the adducted alignment.[20] The use of allografts is an acceptable approach.

Strict attention is given to the cast application because the position of the foot is critical. The foot must be maintained in a neutral position; however, the foot should not be actively dorsiflexed above its neutral position or the graft will slip. The foot should also not be inverted and plantar flexed, or the graft will become loose and will dislodge. After 3 to 4 weeks, the cast is changed to a walking cast and kept in position for another 5 to 6 weeks.

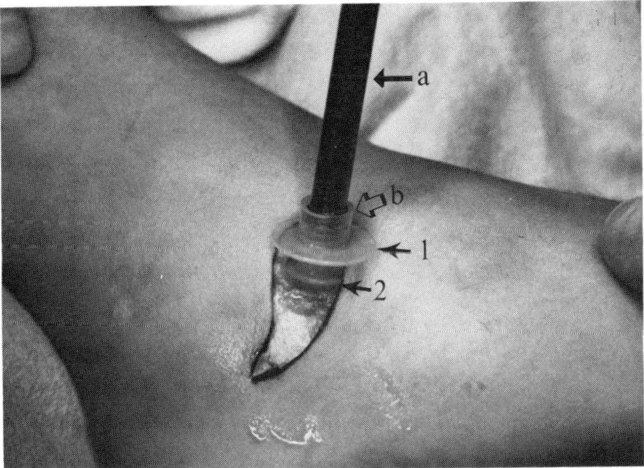

FIGURE 40–9. Impactor rod (a) attached to Richard's plug. Rings (1 and 2) can be cut depending on the diameter of the sinus tarsi. The neck (b) can also be cut back if the depth of the sinus tarsi is short. This surface is kept flushed below the ligament and prevents a sinus tarsi bulge.

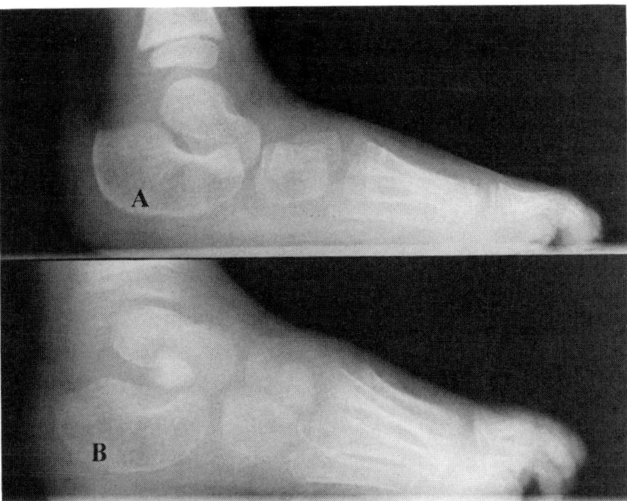

FIGURE 40–10. *A*, Preoperative calcaneovalgus foot. The talar bisection plantarflexed below lower third of cuboid trisection. *B*, Postoperative sagittal plane corrected as noted by talar bisection rises above upper third of the cuboid trisection.

METATARSUS ADDUCTUS

Metatarsus adductus can be described as an osseous transverse plane deformity that occurs at the tarsometatarsal articulation (Lisfranc's joint). It has been described as a skew foot or serpentine foot. Kite used the term *metatarsus adductus* to describe one third of a clubfoot deformity;[21] however, this is not exactly accurate. In metatarsus adductus, the navicular rides laterally to the talar head, whereas in clubfoot deformity, the navicular rides medially to the talar head. The

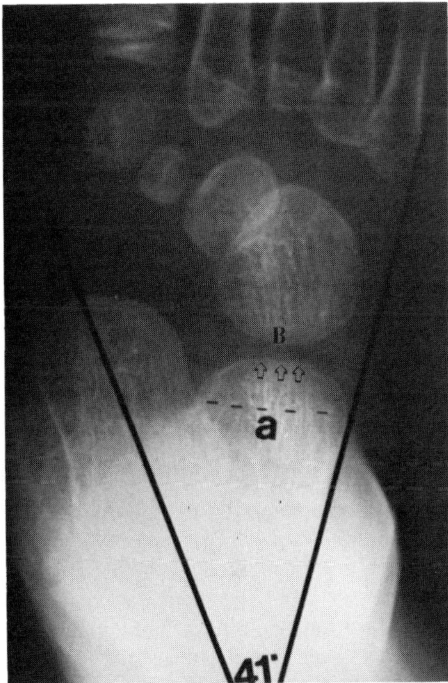

FIGURE 40–11. Evan's preoperative cut (a) 1 cm proximal to calcaneocuboid joint. This distal fragment must be advanced anteriorly to equalize the calcaneocuboid joint (B) to the talonavicular joint if forefoot adduction is to occur.

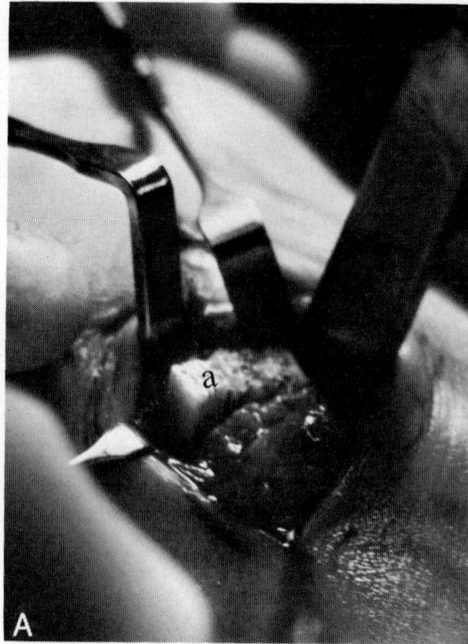
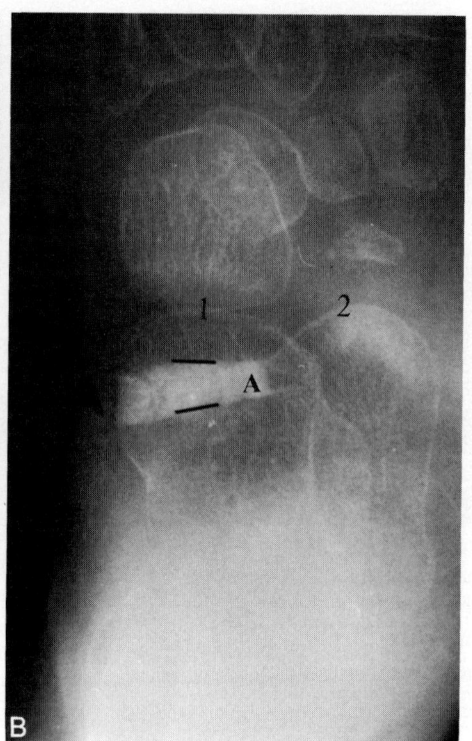

FIGURE 40–12. *A*, Graft insertion (a). *B*, Evan's postoperative cut with a trapezoidal wedge (A). This shape anteriorly advances and adducts the distal fragment. The calcaneocuboid and talonavicular joints become equalized (1 and 2).

cause of metatarsus adductus is not fully understood at this point, but it is possibly a result of excessive intrauterine forces. It is also possible that the malpositioning of the fetus and lack of ontogeny have a deforming effect on the metatarsals. With this resultant malpositioning, certain muscles gain a mechanical advantage and become more powerful. Possibly, the abductor hallucis can become overactive, maintaining a metatarsus adductus deformity. In addition, with weak peroneal muscles, the tibialis anterior and tibialis posterior muscles can gain a mechanical advantage to supinate and adduct the forefoot.

One must remember that the diagnosis of metatarsus adductus is predominantly a clinical diagnosis. The following five criteria can be observed in the weightbearing or nonweightbearing position.

1. The foot maintains an inward position when you stroke the lateral border; it may twist outward for a moment but returns to the original adducted position.
2. A medial concave border and a lateral convex border develops in the foot, with a prominent base of the fifth metatarsal. The prominence of the fifth metatarsal base becomes more evident after the foot loses some of its fat and the metatarsal bases becomes ossified.
3. The metatarsus adductus foot may appear with a high arch. The foot appears as though it were in a cavus position in the infant.
4. One can observe a marked separation of the great toe from the lesser toes. The great toe can remain in this adducted position, yielding a hallux varus and a high first metatarsal adductus angle. In the presence of a tight heel cord, the foot will pronate, and eventually the adducted hallux will drift laterally. If the first ray is adducted, as in a metatarsus primus adductus, a hallux valgus will develop.

5. When you view the metatarsus adductus foot in a nonweightbearing attitude, look at the plantar aspect of the foot and construct two imaginary lines. One line should bisect the heel longitudinally, and the other line should bisect the forefoot area longitudinally. In a metatarsus adductus foot, these two lines will intersect and create an angle greater than 25 degrees.

Radiographic Evaluation

Radiographs are not needed to establish a diagnosis because metatarsus adductus is a clinical diagnosis. They are, however, used to establish the criteria for the surgical procedure and to monitor treatment postoperatively or after casting. The normal angle of metatarsus adductus as seen on radiographs should be less than 22 degrees. Anything greater than 22 to 23 degrees is considered to be an adduction of the metatarsals. It should not be considered a pathologic entity unless the metatarsus adductus angle is greater than 25 degrees.

Three types of metatarsus adductus can be demonstrated:

1. Total metatarsus adductus. The first to fifth metatarsals are adducted relative to the lesser tarsus with a mild to moderate degree of pronation at the subtalar and midtarsal joints.
2. Atavistic form or metatarsus primus adductus. The first ray is adducted so that the intermetatarsal angle is increased greater than 15 degrees. The hallux stays in a varus attitude or stays in line with the metatarsal, and the lesser metatarsal remains normal or slightly adducted.
3. Serpentine, S-shaped foot. This is a severe metatarsus adductus, with all five metatarsals being adducted and compensated for by an increased amount of subtalar

and midtarsal joint pronation. Also noted is that the hallux goes into a valgus deformity because of the pronatory effect of the rearfoot. An uncontrolled, long-standing total metatarsus adductus can develop into this type of metatarsus adductus deformity.

Metatarsus adductus is frequent in children, but whether it will correct spontaneously or whether early treatment is necessary is somewhat controversial. In a study performed by Berg[22] of the Alfred I. DuPont Institute in Wilmington, Delaware, 84 patients with metatarsus adductus were examined. Fifty boys and 34 girls, and a total of 124 feet, were evaluated. Patients' ages ranged from 5½ months to 2½ years. Dorsiplantar and lateral weightbearing radiographs were taken.

More than 43% of the children with simple metatarsus adductus (i.e., the midfoot and hindfoot were in normal alignment) required no treatment. This compared with 24% of children with metatarsus adductus and the midfoot also being laterally translated. Children with a severe complex flattening of the rearfoot and an adducted deformity of the forefoot required cast treatment twice as long as those with simple metatarsus adductus. When presenting with a severe breakdown at the midtarsal or subtalar regions, more aggressive therapy is needed. Prolonged cast therapy with the possibility of surgical intervention, to include hindfoot stabilization with or without tendo-Achillis lengthening, needs to be considered.

The dorsoplantar view allows measurement of the adductus deformity and localization of the deformity at the tarsometatarsal joint, the midtarsal joint, or both. The metatarsus adductus angle is the angular relation between the line representing the bisection of the second metatarsal and a line representing the lesser tarsus abductus angle (Fig. 40–13). A normal metatarsus adductus angle is approximately 22 degrees. A significant metatarsus adductus angle is greater than 25 to 30 degrees with a normal midtarsal joint position.[23]

The calcaneocuboid relation is also studied to determine the presence or absence of a forefoot adductus. *Forefoot adductus* is defined as a soft tissue deformity produced by midtarsal joint oblique axis supination, resulting in plantar flexion, adduction, and inversion of the forefoot. In the presence of abduction of the cuboid (i.e., midtarsal joint pronation), a metatarsus adductus deformity will need to be addressed more radically and aggressively.

The position of the navicular on the talar head must also be considered because it reflects existing foot deformity. A lateral position of the navicular will demonstrate subtalar pronation, whereas the medial position of the navicular on the talar head is seen with talipes equinovarus and cavus foot deformities. That type of supinatory position has to be addressed separately and is usually seen with a forefoot adductus deformity.

Radiographically, on the dorsiplantar view, the metatarsal position needs to be assessed as to whether the first to fifth metatarsals are adducted as a group or whether the first metatarsal is adducted individually. Adduction of the first metatarsal alone is an atavistic type of metatarsus adductus in which the hallux is usually directly in line with the first metatarsal, yielding a hallux varus deformity. If left untreated, this type of early intermetatarsal primus adductus angle will result in a juvenile hallux valgus deformity. It is usually complicated further by the midtarsal and subtalar joint pronation that occurs.

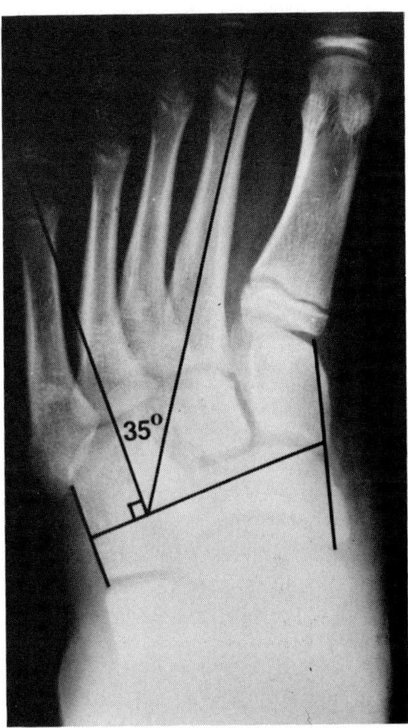

FIGURE 40–13. Metatarsus adductus angle determination in mature child's foot. This angle cannot be determined in a child younger than 6 years of age, because the joint margins of the talonavicular joint, calcaneocuboid joint, fifth metatarsal cuboid, and first cuneometatarsal joint articulations are not mature, and placing points are too variable.

Conservative Treatment

Casting Technique. Cast application started before the age of ambulation will respond favorably because the weightbearing factors have a direct effect in the pronatory direction of the midtarsal and subtalar joints. For this reason, care must be taken when casting children after the age of ambulation because the foot is maturing and the bases of the metatarsals are becoming more rigid.[24] If a transverse force is applied to this weightbearing foot, it is not Lisfranc's articulation that is affected but rather the more proximal articulations, namely the midtarsal and subtalar joints. The entire foot will abduct except the originally deformed adducted metatarsals. The result will be a maximally pronated, iatrogenically induced flatfoot. An increase in shifting the transverse torque to the midtarsal joint occurs with an increase in age. Straightening of the foot is obtained at the cost of pronating the foot at the subtalar and midtarsal joints. I personally cease casting within 2 months after the age of ambulation.

The infant's foot is manipulated by the assistant for approximately 5 to 10 minutes before the casting procedure. Initiating reduction is more successful with this preparatory method. The ligaments become loose, and the child becomes more relaxed during this hands-on method. Place the heel between your thumb and index finger, and lock it to prevent motion. With the opposite hand, grasp the forefoot and apply an abductory motion. Be sure that the motion is applied at the first metatarsal head, with counterpressure on the base of the fifth metatarsal. Hold the transverse motion to resistance for approximately 15 seconds and then release. Repeat this maneuver for 5 to 10 minutes. You will eventually notice that the stiff deformity becomes easily reducible. At this point, the cast can be applied. If the deformity in the foot is still stiff or the infant is unmanageable, have the parent continue this manipulation for another week. Make sure that the parent does not allow the heel to unlock and force the foot into a pronatory position.

As stated previously, the reduction must be precise. It is recommended that plaster cast material be used in the reduction rather than flexible fiber glass because plaster is more easily molded. While the plaster is setting, the hands are positioned about the foot, ready to reduce the deformity. One hand is held on the calcaneus; the position of the heel should be slightly inverted to the leg and prevented from everting when the forefoot pressures are applied. Be sure that the fifth metatarsocuboid joint is stabilized with the same hand as it extends distally on the lateral border of the foot. In the infant's foot, this is simply performed with the thumb and index finger; positioning the opposite hand or fingers is a little trickier. It has been described that counterpressure on the first metatarsal head is enough to reduce the metatarsus adductus deformity. To reduce the metatarsus adductus deformity completely, the metatarsals must be abducted as a unit. Place the first metatarsal head in the sulcus between the index finger and thumb. The remainder of the metatarsals are then grasped by the thumb and index fingers of the same hand. While stabilizing the rearfoot and applying a counterpressure on the fifth metatarsal base, an abductory force is applied on the forefoot. This provides reduction on the first metatarsal head and a sequential abductory reduction on the lesser metatarsals. The fingers and hands should be continually smoothing the plaster while maintaining correction. This will eliminate pressure point mark on the cast.

Modified Furlong Casting Procedure. A short-legged cast is applied to the foot, with the foot maintained in a neutral position; the hindfoot is maintained in the stable neutral position as described previously. A window is then cut out of the dorsolateral aspect of the cast, and this wedge window is removed. The cast is cut out to allow the forefoot, and only the forefoot, to abduct at Lisfranc's articulation, and the hindfoot is held locked in an inverted stable neutral position. A wedge felt piece is then placed between the medial aspect of the cast and the great toe joint. The foot is then wrapped in an Ace bandage to avoid window edema. Each week the wedge felt is increased in size. By placing the wedge, an abductory force is created about Lisfranc's articulation. One must be cautious when attempting this procedure because, as the forefoot abducts, it has a tendency to abduct at the midtarsal joint rather than at Lisfranc's articulation. It is imperative that the rearfoot be locked and stable in as neutral a position as possible to prevent midtarsal and subtalar joint breakdown. It is also important that the cast be cut so that the dorsolateral piece that is removed extends no further proximally than the fifth metatarsal base. The casting procedure is continued until the desired abduction is maintained, and then the final position is maintained in a below-the-knee closed cast (Fig. 40–14).[25]

After-Cast Maintenance. Now that the deformity has been reduced with casting, the correction must be maintained. The question arises as to how long the position must be maintained. Consider casting the child for 3 weeks to 3 months before the age of ambulation and follow with a Ganley splint (see Table 40–1) for an additional 3 to 6 months.

Ganley Splint. The technique of application follows the

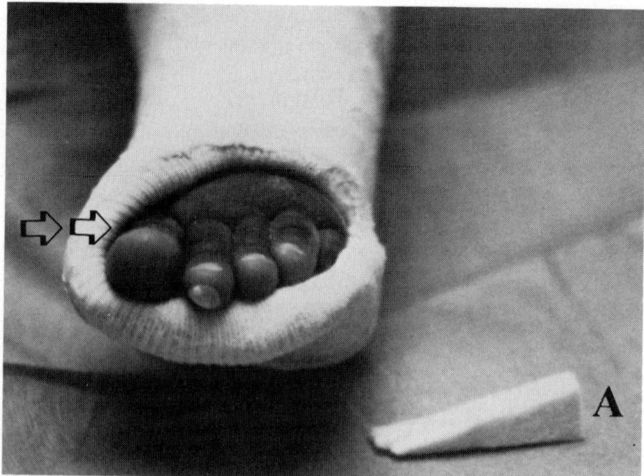

FIGURE 40–14. Furlong cast wedge (A) is placed along the medial surface of the first metatarsal *(arrows)* on the cast. The wedge is placed deeper into the cast each week. The size is also increased with progression of correction. It is important to completely lock the hindfoot to prevent unlocking of the midtarsal joint.

same directions as described for calcaneovalgus except the position of the longitudinal bar is bent by the bending irons to create an abducted forefoot position. With the treatment of metatarsus adductus, the torsion bar is bent to allow the foot to be externally or laterally rotated with reference to the leg. As is commonly seen with metatarsus adductus, a concomitant internal tibial torsion is present, and the external rotation of this bar will maintain an abductory position rather than allow the foot to rotate inward. The shank bar is bent outward to allow the forefoot to abduct on the hindfoot, and at the same time the heel plate is placed in varus. It is important to maintain hindfoot inversion with the abduction of this shank to prevent severe pronatory changes that can be driven through the entire hindfoot and midfoot joints. The hindfoot is still maintained in approximately 5-degree varus.

Bebax Shoe. As with calcaneovalgus, the Bebax shoe is recommended for use in the child with metatarsus adductus from birth to approximately 9 months of age (Fig. 40–15). It is used at all times and is taken off only when bathing the child. The device can also be used after casting, but if the child is ambulatory it must only be used at nap and sleep times.

The Wheaton Brace. This device is an orthosis made of polypropylene (see Table 40–1). The orthosis features the corrective aspects of casting without the disadvantages of the casting technique. It is molded to conform to the inner border of the foot in the overcorrected position and uses three-point fixation to correct the deformity as seen in metatarsus adductus. The hindfoot is held securely by the heel portion of the orthosis to prevent hindfoot pronation with the abductory force on the forefoot. The amount of correction obtained can be altered by adjusting the tightness of the straps. The device is relatively inexpensive, but correction is individually adjusted. The device is intended as an alternative to serial casting. Serial casting itself has the advantage of providing an exact mold and positioning of the foot. The Wheaton brace is manufactured and does not mold to the exact shape of the foot. With the application of the brace and its three-point pressures to reduce the deformity, little control is af-

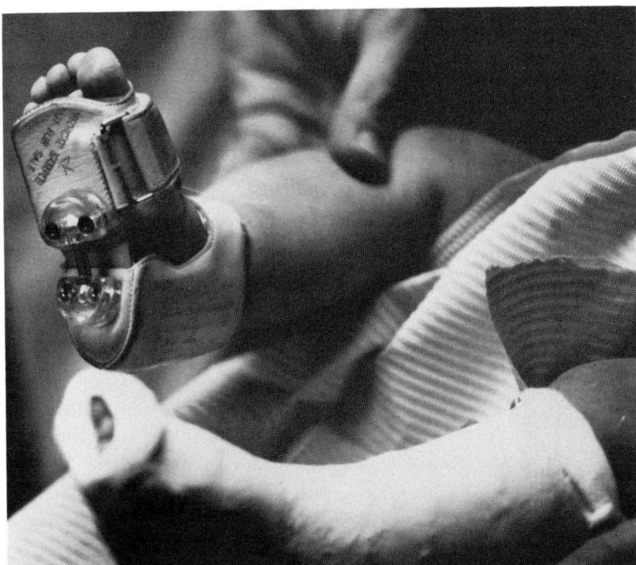

FIGURE 40–15. Bebax shoes securely holding a foot in a corrected position for the maintenance of a metatarsus adductus deformity. The forefoot is adducted on the hindfoot at the distal universal joint in the area of Lisfranc's. The hindfoot is held tightly in a neutral position.

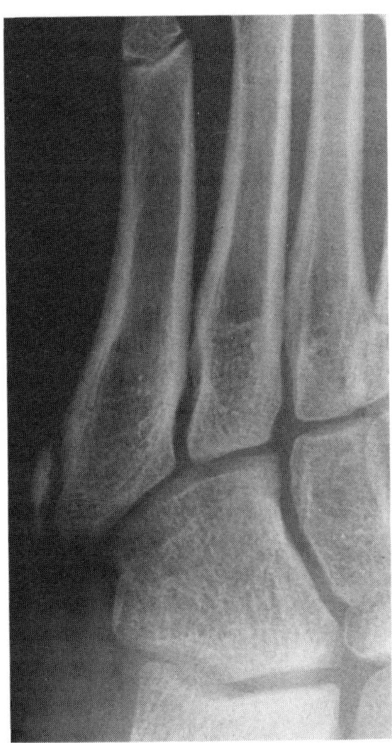

FIGURE 40–16. Fifth metatarsal apophysis with metatarsus adductus. The apophysis can be irritated owing to an increase at the vertex of Lisfranc's articulation, and an apophysitis can develop.

forded to the rearfoot. With no or only minimal control to the hindfoot, the midtarsal joint will abduct and the desired correction at Lisfranc's articulation will not occur. This may result in a pronated, straight foot. The device is a good adjunct in the treatment of metatarsus adductus after casting has been initiated.

Orthotic Device Control. The child who presents with compensated metatarsus adductus who is ambulating needs to be controlled with an orthosis. This orthotic device will visually increase the apparent toe-in position and at the same time prevent the foot from pronating. Because the foot is maturing, a device needs to be constructed that will control hindfoot pronation and also prevent the transverse drift of the forefoot that is commonly seen in the compensated metatarsus adductus deformity.

If a concomitant internal axial deviation (internal tibial torsion, internal femoral position) occurs at the same time as the metatarsus adductus, the result is an internal positioned foot (i.e., controlled). It is imperative to explain to the parent the purpose of control with the orthosis as well as the visual effect of intoe.

The child with a metatarsus adductus is prone to Iselin's apophysitis because of the lateral prominence, with an increase in pressure and irritation (Fig. 40–16). An effective approach to decrease this pressure is with use of a rigid, molded acrylic orthosis. This orthosis is a modified version of a Roberts plate; the flanges are kept low but with a deep heel seat. The lateral flange is cut proximally to the fifth metatarsal base. The orthotic device manages to control pronation and removes the direct pressure on the base. With a healthy, young fat pad, this cutout is not necessary. The flange should be extended distally to just proximal to the fifth metatarsal head (Fig. 40–17).[26]

Shoes. Reverse last shoes are contraindicated because they maximally pronate the foot at the midtarsal and subtalar joints. In the toddler, a straight last shoe with a scaphoid pad can be used before the construction of an orthosis. The straight last shoe will maintain the foot in a rectus position, and the scaphoid pad will prevent some of the midtarsal joint abduction.

Surgical Treatment

Indications. The decision to perform surgery on the metatarsus adductus foot is based on cosmesis. The child should present with one or more of the following: difficulty in finding shoe gear that is comfortably worn, tripping, or pain on the various pressure points of the foot (i.e., first metatarsal head, fifth metatarsal base). Surgery all too often addresses the cosmetic appearance rather than the cause and compensatory findings.

Closing Base Wedge Osteotomies. Steytler and Van der Walt,[27] in their procedure originally reported in 1966, described osteotomies using connecting drill holes. This was accomplished in a wide V fashion, and the metatarsals were then forced into a corrected abducted position. The procedure was later modified using a crescentic osteotomy that allowed rotation along the long axis of the metatarsal to occur.

The apex of base wedge osteotomies is located on the proximal medial aspect of each metatarsal and is distal to the articular facet on the second to fifth metatarsals. On the first metatarsal, it must be held further proximally to avoid the epiphysis at the base of the first metatarsal. The various techniques that are used to fix the osteotomies can include use of external Kirschner wire fixation, which provides a uniplanar stability on the osteotomy site. Alternatively, internal monofilament wire fixation can be used along the lateral aspect to close down the osteotomy site but only when the medial cortex is still intact. Screw fixation is another alternative; however, a larger base is needed to allow the insertion of the smallest 2.7-mm cortical screw.

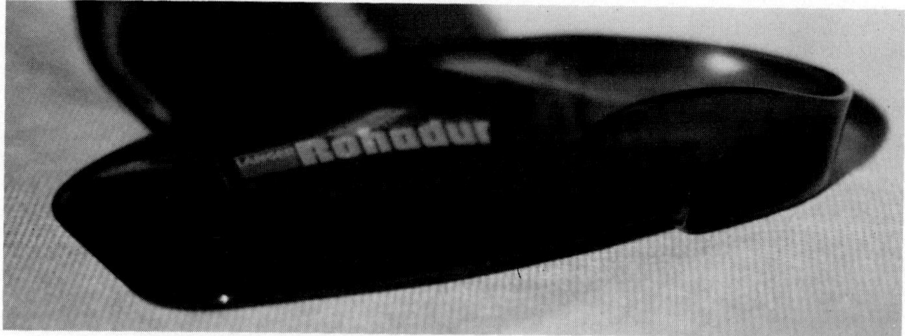

FIGURE 40–17. Deep heel seat orthosis with flange cut proximal to fifth metatarsal base. Flange decreases pressure at fifth metatarsal base by acting as a barrier.

Crescentic Osteotomies. The development of the crescentic osteotomy to correct metatarsus adductus was the result of the inability to apply the closing and opening wedge osteotomies to all cases. Specifically, the closing wedge osteotomy was an acceptable procedure when the first metatarsal was not too short or when the second metatarsal was not too long. In those instances in which an absolute or relative shortening of the first metatarsal was a consideration, the opening wedge osteotomy could reduce the intermetatarsal angle while preserving a functionally acceptable metatarsal length.

The modification of the crescentic osteotomy is technically simple. The osteotomy is made with the crescentic blade angulated and rotated medially. One of the most important effects of the angulated crescentic osteotomy is that an intrinsic bolstering effect is produced by the high medial lip on the medial side of the base created by the angulated cut. This bolster, or lip, of bone acts as a significant counterforce to any medially directed forces at the osteotomy site (Figs. 40–18 and 40–19).[28]

When performing crescentic osteotomies on the metatarsals for the correction of metatarsus adductus, two methods of fixation are commonly used: transverse pin fixation and cross-pinning of the first and fifth metatarsals. A large Kirschner wire (see Table 40–1) is placed across the metatarsals distally, and the pin is secured in a plaster cast, which maintains alignment. This provides adequate maintenance of the fracture sites, but if a proper sequence of pin fixation is not followed, complications of delayed union, malunion, or nonunion may result. Care must be taken to avoid the distal growth plates of the second to fifth metatarsals. If one enters from the lateral side of the fifth metatarsal, and the pin is placed just proximal to the neck, one will avoid damaging the plates because the fifth growth plate is the most proximal. Another advantage of the lateral entrance is the ease in guiding the pin from the thin fifth metatarsal to the thicker first metatarsal shaft.

The crescentic cut metatarsals rotate at the longitudinal axis of each individual metatarsal and do not rotate as a group. Therefore, reduction of the osteotomies and proper alignment before pin placement of each individual metatarsal

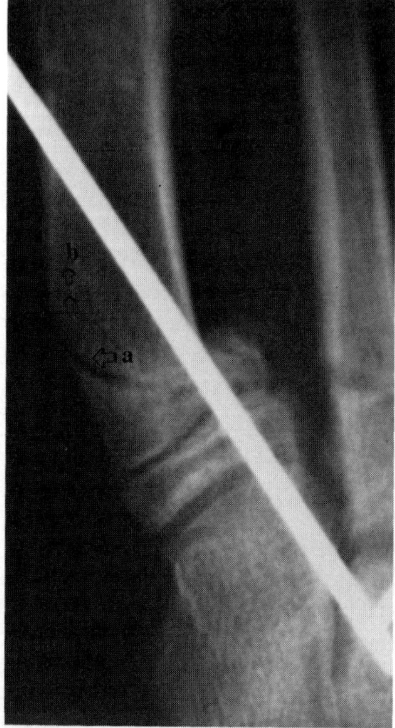

FIGURE 40–18. Crescentic osteotomy, with medial high buttress inhibiting proximal metatarsal shaft from shifting medially (a). Angle of osteotomy allows greater surface contact as well as increasing the length of metatarsal (b). This accommodates for loss of length from the thickness of a saw cut.

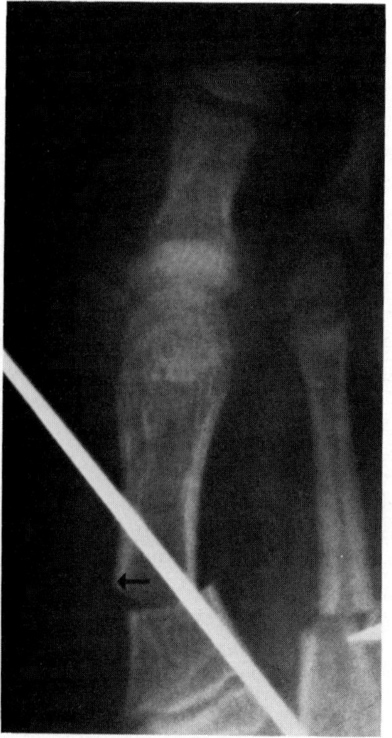

FIGURE 40–19. Crescentic osteotomy without angle. With no medial buttress, the metatarsal can shift medially *(arrow)*.

are necessary. The transverse pin is incorporated within the cast. The foot is still maintained in correction with the hindfoot in the neutral position, and the first to fifth metatarsals are abducted as a unit. The position during cast application is of paramount importance because this is when complications are most likely.

An alternative in the fixation of the metatarsals is to drive two Kirschner wires, one fixing the first metatarsal to the middle cuneiform and the other fixing the fifth metatarsal to the medial portion of the cuboid. It is most important that the metatarsals be properly aligned.

Heymen-Herndon Tarsometatarsal Capsulotomy. Tarsometatarsal capsulotomies have received mixed reviews. The procedure seems to have merit in that the procedure can be performed in younger children, 3 to 8 years of age, thereby avoiding osseous procedures. Despite being a soft tissue procedure, 3 months of casting is required, actually in excess of what is recommended for panmetatarsal osteotomies. Mixed postoperative results have led some to believe that it is better to forgo soft tissue release and wait for the child to mature further in order to become a candidate for metatarsal osteotomy.

In a study performed by Stark and associates[29] at the Gillette Children's Hospital in St. Paul, Minnesota, 37 children with metatarsus adductus—for a total of 56 feet—underwent a capsulotomy as described by Heymen-Herndon and Strong after conservative treatment had failed. A 41% failure rate was present with this tarsometatarsal capsulotomy release with no true overcorrection occurring, raising the question of whether this procedure deals with the actual defect as presented.

The high failure rate in this study of capsule releases of the metatarsal bases shows that care must certainly be taken in the release of these cartilaginous surfaces. Joint damage and future degenerative changes have been recorded and, with this study, significantly so.[29]

Open Wedge Osteotomy of the First Cuneiform. Resistant metatarsus adductus deformities were reviewed by Kling and coworkers[30] at Indiana University. They noted a severe varus first metatarsal cuneiform joint angle in these patients and elected to perform an opening wedge osteotomy of the first cuneiform to correct this angulation.

All records and radiographs of 32 feet in 22 patients who had an opening wedge first cuneiform osteotomy with two to four metatarsal osteotomies were reviewed. The mean age at osteotomy was 11 years (range, 3.5 to 21 years), and the mean length of follow-up was 2 years (range, 1 to 5.5 years). All patients and parents rated the foot as good or excellent in appearance; shoe fitting was easy; and none had pain or limited activity postoperatively. Radiographically, correction of the adduction deformity was 13 degrees (64%) as measured by the talar-first metatarsal angle. Patients with greater adduction deformities preoperatively had the largest adduction deformities postoperatively. This suggests that there is a limit to the amount of correction possible with this procedure.

MEDIAL TIBIAL TORSION

The most common cause of intoe in children is internal or medial tibial torsion. During development of the fetus, the lower limb buds rotate externally along the axial plane. Tibial torsion at birth has been estimated at 0 degrees. During the child's development, the tibia normally torques laterally to approximately 23 degrees external. This gradual unwinding of the bone in a lateral direction takes place over the course of 18 years, with an increase in external torque of 1 to 1.5 degrees per year.[31]

Various studies of this outward growth of the tibia have been performed.[32–35] Arkin[36] demonstrated a plasticity of the bone under direct perpendicular stress to the epiphyseal plate that always allows an outward or inward spiraling effect to occur. This stress causes newly formed bone to change its position either internally or externally. Many of these studies on the hip, femoral, and leg segments substantiated the original premise by Heuter[37] and Volkmann[38] in 1862—otherwise known as the Heuter-Volkmann law—that increased pressure inhibits growth and decreased pressure accelerates growth at the epiphyseal growth center.

These findings substantiated the cause of medial tibial torsion. A rapidly growing fetus can be subject to extrinsic constraining forces that will mold the fetal tissues into certain positions according to the laws of bone growth. This is more likely seen with first-born infants when the mother has tight uterine musculature, with a large fetus, or with multiple fetuses. In the presence of uterine fibroids or a paucity of amniotic fluid, the fetus cannot develop or continue through a normal ontogeny. Constrained by these underlying problems, extrauterine compressions can prevent normal lateral unwinding of the tibial segment. A tight abdominal muscle with a small pelvis or prominent lumbar spine can also inhibit the natural lateral twisting of the tibial segment. The vertex position maximizes uterine space and allows the fetus to go through its normal stretch and rotation of the limb buds. The breach position, or a transverse lie, further creates a constraint and prevents normal ontogeny.

Diagnosis

The diagnosis of tibial torsion is simple to make. In a clinical assessment, the child is placed in a seated position with the legs dangling over the table top and the knees parallel to the frontal plane. In younger children, this can become difficult in that the femoral segment is also going through an external position and the hip is normally in an abducted position; with this child, the hips are drawn together and adducted while the child is in the seated position. This brings the legs closer together and the knees then parallel the frontal plane; the malleoli are examined. When the foot and leg are in a normal position in the developing child, the tibial malleolus should face forward and the lateral malleolus lies posterior to the medial malleolus. Jakob,[39] in 1980, determined a relation between tibial torsion and the trans malleolar axis. This transmalleolar axis is the angle made between the distal tips of the tibial and fibula malleolus in the frontal plane. Jakob computed that a line drawn from the tip of the medial malleolus to the tip of the lateral malleolus on the frontal plane should be approximately 27 degrees in the adult. Jakob's values, determined by computed tomography, showed that the transmalleolar axis is normally 5 to 7 degrees greater than the tibial torsion angle. In earlier studies, La Damany[31] and Elftman[40] noted normal tibial torsion at birth of 0 degrees. Thus, a newborn should have no tibial torsion and a 5- to 7-degree lateral transmalleolar axis. With a normal unwinding of the tibial segment throughout growth, the transmalleolar axis increases 1 to 1.5 degrees per year. It is a simple matter, then, to compute the appropriate normal axis for a given age. A child of 10 years, for example, should have a transmalleolar axis of approximately 15 degrees. Keeping in mind that tibial torsion is normally 5 degrees less than the transmalleolar axis, we can extrapolate normal tibial torsion angle by subtracting 5 degrees from the transmalleolar axis.

The tensile and compressive forces that act on immature, rapidly growing bone will eventually become permanently fixed. For this reason, early diagnosis and treatment are of paramount concern. Unfortunately, a child is not usually brought into the physician's office for this complaint until it is too late. Certain sequelae will occur, including apparent bowing of the lower leg or increased tripping as the foot becomes locked in the ankle joint and positioned inward. An unlocking mechanism can occur in which the leg is twisted and driven internally, and the foot is locked and positioned on the ground and, through the reactive force of gravity, starts to abduct at the subtalar joint. The midtarsal joint, along the transverse plane, also abducts, dorsiflexes, and pronates. The result is a flatfoot deformity secondary to the reaction of the internal drive of the tibia. As this child develops, the intoe appears to reduce. The leg unscrews the talus downward and the midtarsal joint unlocks, giving the appearance of an externally positioned foot at the cost of an abduction and pronation position of the foot. When seen by the parent or the untrained eye, the answer is simple: The child outgrew the deformity. Unfortunately, the child did not actually outgrow the deformity; rather, a new flatfoot deformity has replaced the intoe.[41]

Treatment

Consider the younger child between the ages of 6 months and 1 year who has just started to stand. It is at this age that parents will notice that the legs are bent and the feet turned inward. We physicians who are fortunate enough to see children at this age can undo constraining factors and use, to our advantage, the laws that promote outward bone growth. Understanding that the tibia will normally go through an external torque, and taking away all the constraining internal factors, we can promote external rotation of the tibia. This can be done simply by placing the child in an outward position and maintaining the child in that position for a period of time. However, there remains much disagreement over whether to treat medial tibial torsion or not.

One method of treatment is with a long-leg, externally torqued cast that is generally maintained for a period of 3 to 4 weeks and longer in more recalcitrant cases. Casting is recommended before the child is ambulatory, and one need not dorsiflex the foot. If the older child is ambulating, the foot must be dorsiflexed and held in a neutral position. With the knee flexed approximately 25 degrees, the foot must also be flexed; otherwise, the child will not be able to stand flat on the cast and walk. Plantar flexion of the cast needs to be avoided in this ambulating child because pressure sores (blisters) will develop on the dorsal surface of the toes (Fig. 40–20).

After the removal of the cast, the foot and leg must be maintained in their new laterally torqued position. If they are

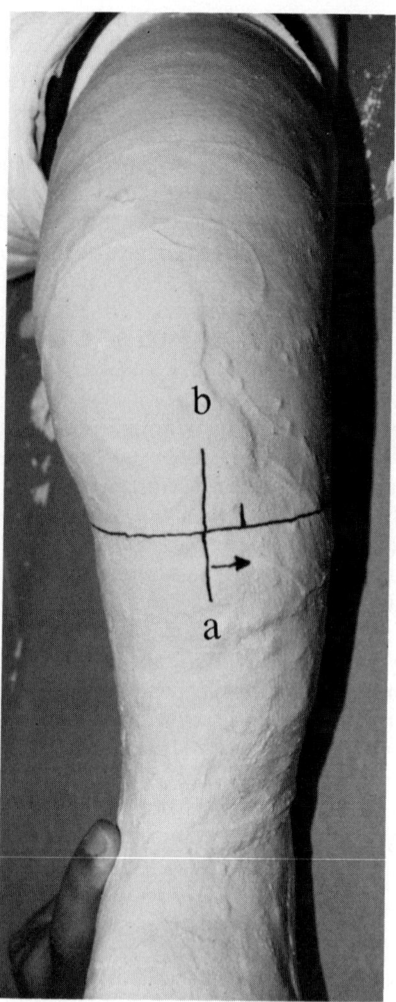

FIGURE 40–20. Cast application for medial tibial torsion. Segment a is rotated externally at weekly intervals (3 weeks maximum). The proximal segment b stabilizes the thigh and knee. Approximately 2 cm is available at each torque session and should not be forced into further medial rotation.

not, the deformity may recur. Arkin[36] described that a torque in the long bone will produce a spiraling of the growth cells in the direction of the applied torque. However, it was also noted that when the torque was released, the spiraling effect returned to the original columnar position. Applying these principles of bone growth, an externally placed splint or bracing system should be applied. The use of a CRS is recommended because this not only allows for an external position to the transverse plane of the leg but also allows the child to go through his or her normal muscular development and allows motion within the knee and hip. It must be noted that bars, splints, and braces do not obtain correction of any torque or rotatory changes in the bone. They do, however, maintain the desired position and eliminate any extrinsic, internally directed forces. When using a CRS, Fillauer, Denis Browne Bar, Unibar, and so on, the position should not exceed 15 to 25 degrees external, and the hindfoot must be maintained in approximately 5- to 7-degree varus. Excessive external position of the shoe plates will not have the desired effect on the leg; rather, it will force the foot to abduct and pronate the talocalcaneal joint. The talocalcaneal joint will increase as the talus unlocks in the ankle mortise. The result is that the foot (calcaneus) will abduct under the talus.

For children older than 18 months, casting for the intoe deformity is quite difficult. These children are more active; there is more motion in the lower extremity and more awareness of being constrained by a cast. Placing a cast on these children makes it more difficult for them to crawl, stand, and walk. For these children, it is especially important to remove the constraining factors that continually inhibit the leg from correcting itself. Children may not go through their normal external rotation in the axial segment of the leg because of either sitting or sleeping positions that gently torque and maintain the leg inwardly. These are seen in children who sit in a reverse tailor position or who sleep with their legs tucked up to their chests. Removing constraining positions and maintaining an external attitude at this stage requires a bar, splint, or other system that maintains correction. Again, it must be stressed that these devices should be used only to maintain position and not to obtain correction.

For children 6 years of age or older who still possess an inward tibial torsion, the deformity probably will not decrease, and the sequelae of a flatfoot will increase. Flatfoot secondary to suprapedal transverse plane abnormalities can become a fixed, rigid flatfoot. A simple orthosis is recommended for these children. By maintaining the hindfoot in a subtalar neutral position, one can prevent the internal driving forces through the midtarsal and subtalar joints that encourage development of a flatfoot. The question that is often asked is, ''Because we are supporting the subtalar and midtarsal joint in a supinated position, will the toeing-in be accentuated?'' It will, but the support is needed to maintain a corrected position of the foot so as not to create another problem as the child grows older. The child is still encouraged to remove all the internal medial forces that are torquing the leg.

Operative correction of tibial torsion is considered for more severe cases and should be delayed until after 9 years of age, when tibial torsion has been stabilized and posthealing changes are unlikely. Rotational tibial osteotomies can be performed safely at either the proximal level or distal level, but fewer serious complications occur with distal osteotomies.

EQUINUS FLATFOOT

Equinus is a limitation of dorsiflexion of the foot on the leg. By definition, for normal foot function, it is necessary to have 10 degrees of dorsiflexion of the foot on the leg with the knee joint fully extended and the subtalar joint in its neutral position with the midtarsal joint maximally pronated and locked.

With a limitation of dorsiflexion at the ankle, when the knee joint is extended, the foot must compensate by dorsiflexing. This is accomplished somewhat at the subtalar joint, but, more importantly and more significantly, it is accomplished at the midtarsal joint. With the midtarsal joint using its oblique axis, a compensation for the deformity occurs and causes significant changes around the midtarsal joint. An equinus deformity is considered a midstance pronator (Fig. 40–21).[42] Equinus may be defined by the degree of compensation.

The uncompensated equinus presents with no dorsiflexion at the ankle, midtarsal, or subtalar joints. These children appear to walk on the metatarsal heads with the toes maxi-

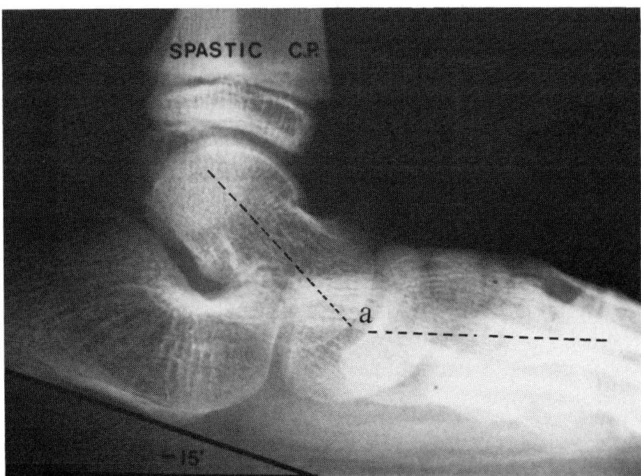

FIGURE 40–21. Compensated equinus with resultant flatfoot. Decrease in calcaneal inclination with dorsiflexion occurring at talonavicular joint (a).

mally dorsiflexed at the metatarsophalangeal joints. No heel contact is made during the gait or stance cycle (Fig. 40–22).

The partially compensated equinus allows the heel to approach the ground by the midtarsal and subtalar joints with some pronation taking place. These children have a bouncing gait and early heel-off. Calcaneal apophysitis is a common finding in these children.

The fully compensated equinus with complete and abnormal subtalar and midtarsal joint pronation the foot attains the necessary 10 degrees of dorsiflexion to the leg. This is a severe, deforming force to foot function (see Fig. 40–21).

A variant is noted in the young healthy child who toewalks out of habit rather than any overt tightness of the posterior group muscles. The child's foot is in equinus at stance, and if the child is allowed to stand still, the heel will eventually drop. If the same child is told to run, the heel will immediately rise. The deep tendon reflexes are usually intact, and the foot can be actively dorsiflexed to a right angle. This should be considered a normal variation of gait. It is advisable for these children to wear a serial cast over a 6-week period with the possibility of reapplying the cast over the

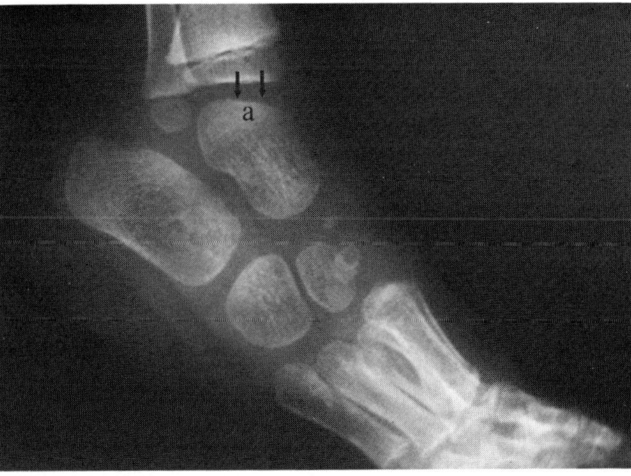

FIGURE 40–22. Uncompensated equinus. Plantar flexion at ankle with decrease in endochondral bone growth on the talus. A flat top talus is developing (a).

next few months to ensure the dorsiflexed position. These habitual toe walkers have normal orthopedic and neurologic findings, and the condition reduces without surgery. On occasion, heel-cord lengthening is needed but is reserved for resistant cases that have failed conservative therapy.[43, 44]

The child will display a markedly abducted foot on stance with an obvious break in the direction of abduction along the calcaneocuboid joint. The forefoot will demonstrate a high degree of soft tissue varus deformity, otherwise known as a forefoot supinatus. The supinatus is secondary to midtarsal joint oblique axis pronation; this occurs as the midtarsal joint unlocks because of the lack of dorsiflexion at the ankle joint. With a gastrocnemius equinus, the posterior calf loses its definition and the muscle appears to run directly into the distal leg. Normally, one can visually define the gastrocnemius heads proximally. The non-weightbearing foot shows no arch formation, with no apparent plantar flexion of the first ray.

Clinical Diagnosis

The child is placed in a prone position with the leg extended and the toes hanging over the edge of the examination table. Place your hand under the leg distally, and raise it slightly to bring the leg parallel to the table surface. Grasp the forefoot with the opposite hand and visualize the lateral border of the calcaneus as it runs just proximal to the fifth metatarsal base and cuboid. The foot is dorsiflexed at the ankle. The forefoot is neither abducted nor adducted relative to the tibia. With abducting the foot (pronating), dorsiflexion is appeared to be increased. This is midtarsal joint oblique axis dorsiflexion and not ankle joint dorsiflexion. An angle is then observed between the leg and the lateral calcaneal border. Repeat the dorsiflexion of the foot with the knee flexed; the angle should increase as the gastrocnemius muscle becomes lax. A gastrocnemius equinus can now be distinguished from a gastrocsoleus equinus. If dorsiflexion is inadequate but does increase with knee flexion, the gastrocnemius muscle alone is considered to be contracted. If dorsiflexion is inadequate with the knee flexed or extended, the gastrocnemius and soleus muscles are both held accountable. An osseous limitation of dorsiflexion may also be considered in the latter case. Lateral radiographs of the foot with the knee flexed will usually discern cases that are osseous in origin.

Conservative Treatment

With control of equinus by an orthotic device, one must be cautious. Because the dorsiflexory component of gait is taken up at the midtarsal joint, the foot will pronate with great impact into the medial part of the orthosis, causing discomfort. If there is no dorsiflexion available at midstance, the orthosis will probably fail, and the child will most likely be a candidate for a lengthening procedure. If, however, at least 5 degrees of dorsiflexion is available at the ankle joint, then an orthosis is likely to be effective. The orthosis could be casted with the child's foot in a slightly pronated position to eliminate the possibility of medial arch fatigue and to allow the foot to pronate through gait but blocking end-range pronation. This allows dorsiflexion to occur at the midtarsal joint. When a child is wearing a fully posted orthosis (hind-foot and forefoot post), stretching exercises should be encouraged. The subtalar and midtarsal joints remain in neutral position. The cuboid remains stable and will allow the peroneus longus tendon to plantarflex the first ray. When this occurs, the forefoot posting will have to be reduced gradually. It is easier to reduce extrinsic posts rather than intrinsically repositioning the forefoot in varus. Every month, the forefoot post is ground down approximately 1 to 2 degrees. If this posting is not reduced, the creation of a first-ray elevatus develops. Some believe it is necessary to recast the child completely at 2-month intervals to capture the changing forefoot design. If cost is no factor, this is the best approach. Otherwise, gradual reduction of the forefoot extrinsic post is usually sufficient.

When controlling the equinus foot, and if concern exists over the midtarsal joint breakdown creating pain from the orthosis medially, the addition of compressible posts will also allow some give into the orthotic in the direction of pronation.

Surgical Treatment

Equinus is a severe pronatory force, especially when it is of a primary or congenital nature. The equinus now creates a compensatory pronated foot that is most difficult to control, and surgical attention is required. All too often with the compensated equinus foot, a standard Achilles tendon lengthening is performed when in fact the deformity does not lie in the gastrosoleus complex but rather is isolated to the gastrocnemius muscle. The result is an instability at the knee joint with the possibility of recurvatum because of lost stability about the knee. In addition, because we have increased the amount of dorsiflexion at the expense of power for propulsion, an apropulsive gait results and is easily demonstrated by the child's inability to stand on the toes. The isolated gastrocnemius recession or lengthening allows an increase in dorsiflexion at 50% to 60% of the midstance in the gait cycle and reduces the resultant and compensated dorsiflexion at the midtarsal joint.[42, 45] The power to plantarflex at this segment of gait is not reduced, and propulsion is not reduced as it is with the complete Achilles tendon lengthening.

Modified Gastrocnemius Lengthening

In performing a modified gastrocnemius lengthening,[44] a linear incision about 5 cm in length is made over the lower to middle thirds of the leg. The short saphenous vein and sural nerve need to be avoided. The peritenon and fascia are incised, and the hemostat is placed from the lateral to the medial borders. The hemostat allows the separation between the myotendinous junction of the gastrocnemius tendon and the soleus fibers. The hemostat is gently opened, separating these two bodies. Incisions in the tendon are made medial to lateral at the proximal end of the incision and lateral to medial in the distal segment of the incision. Both of the cuts should run just past the midline. This allows all of the fibers to be cut and is essential to allow the tendon to glide on itself. What is being accomplished is a Z lengthening of the tendon to the gastrocnemius muscle. Once these cuts have been made, the foot is actively dorsiflexed, ensuring that the knee is held in full extension. Approximately 1 to 1.5 cm of length will be noted in both the distal and proximal segments (Fig. 40–23).

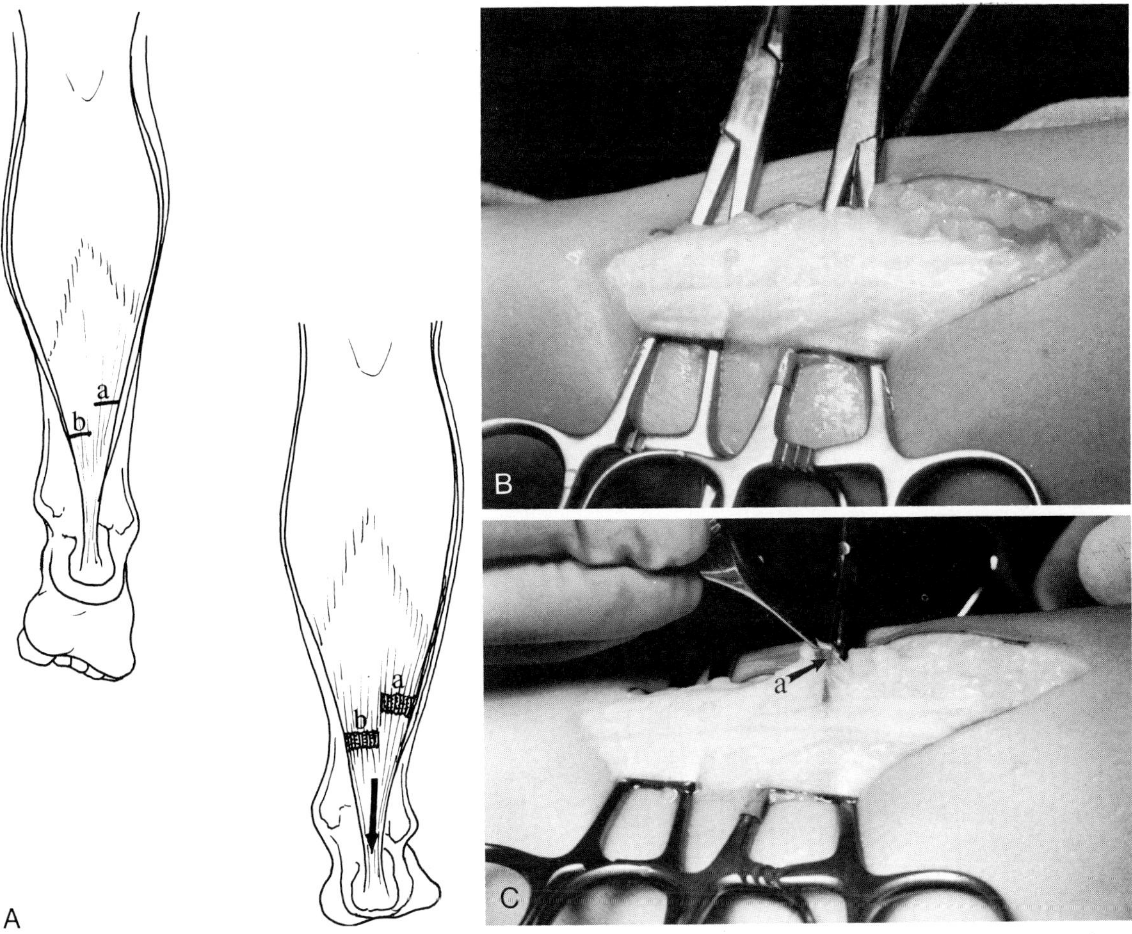

FIGURE 40–23. *A*, Cuts a and b are in the myotendinous junction of the gastrocnemius muscle. With dorsiflexion of the foot, a gap is created; the peritenon remains intact over this separated gap area. *B*, Hemostats shown placed under the gastrocnemius tendon and separating it from the soleal fiber. The peritenon remains complete. *C*, Gastrocnemius lengthening. The peritenon (a) is carefully retracted and No. 11 blade cuts the tendon of the gastrocnemius muscle.

The child is placed in a below-the-knee cast with the foot held in a neutral position. If this is a bilateral procedure, the child can be placed in this cast and allowed to ambulate. After 3 to 4 weeks, the child is removed from the cast and immediately placed into an orthosis that had been constructed before the surgery. This orthotic is the same as described earlier with a gradual reduction of the forefoot posting. In addition, the postoperative orthotic can also have included a one-eighth inch heel raise to allow the hindfoot to attain a more supinated position. This too is gradually reduced over a period of 3 months.

SPASTIC EQUINUS DEFORMITY

Spastic equinus deformity may be caused by either of the following: The gastrocsoleus complex can be partially or entirely spastic, or weakness of the anterior muscles can result in relative overpowering by the posterior muscles.

The gastrocsoleus complex is spastic throughout the gait cycle. The gait is no longer that of a heel-toe; the pattern becomes one of a toe-toe, with the spastic condition of the triceps surae being so tight that not even the child's weight can force the hindfoot down. If the triceps spasticity is of a lesser quality, the heel may come down after the toe touches or the entire foot may strike in a plantargrade manner.

In many patients with spastic equinus, preventing compensation via pronation is paramount to achieving adequate functional gait. Spastic equinus occurs when the triceps surae is cerebrospastic and performs in a panphasic manner during the swing and stance phases of gait. This spasm creates a strong deforming force to the foot.

Midtarsal instability results from subtalar malposition and promotes increased subtalar pronation to compensate for the lack of dorsiflexion necessary for adequate propulsion. This pronation subsequently creates a flexible flatfoot deformity.

Conservative Treatment

The conventional medial column support, the Whitman plate, and Roberts plate provide hard, nonconforming braces for calcaneal stability, which can cause medial blistering and callus formation. A more appropriate support is in the use of a custom, heat-molded support attached to an orthotic. This device supports the calcaneus as conventional supports do; however, it is lightweight, soft, and moldable. When used in conjunction with a high-top sneaker, it prevents the calcaneus from abducting or everting and maintains the subtalar joint in a neutral or slightly supinated position.

Constructed from an inner lining of one-eighth inch PPT and one-fourth inch Plastizote (black firm) on the exterior (see Table 40–1), the support maintains high medial and lateral flanges, which extend just below the malleoli and taper as the orthotic extends more distally. A deep-seated heel cup is advised to give the maximum support (Fig. 40–24).[46]

Surgical Treatment

When conservative measures fail to address the deformity adequately, surgical considerations exist. Traditional lengthening procedures of the Achilles tendon are considered. In addition, Achilles tendon advancement anteriorly on the calcaneus is advised. This procedure shortens the lever arm to the ankle joint more significantly than it affects the distance to the metatarsophalangeal joint. The net effect is a reduction of equinus in stance without significant effect on gastrocnemius muscle strength during propulsion.

CAVUS DEFORMITY

It has been well documented that many forms of cavus deformity are associated with neuromuscular disease, and the incidence of association has been stated to be as high as 65%. When cavus foot is associated with an established neurologic disease process, it is observed that the cavus foot deformity is progressive in that the structure of the foot changes with time. Even when the cause is not progressive, position may secondarily change over time but in a less dramatic manner. Although the young child with a cavus foot still has a fairly flexible foot type, it is not uncommon that these feet develop into rigid, stiff foot types in adulthood. The gait is awkward in that lesions start to develop on the plantar aspects of the metatarsals and on the dorsally contracted digits. This is typically a late finding in children; however, in more severe cases, these lesions can be present as early as 4 and 5 years of age. The heel becomes inverted, and the plantar fascia starts to tighten. With the changing shape of the cavus deformity, the foot is prone to ankle sprains. There is also an increase in the plantarflexion of the first metatarsal, which induces a greater amount of inversion to the rearfoot. Excessive wear is noted on the lateral aspect of the heel of the shoe.

The osseous alignment is ever changing in cavus foot deformity. Mechanical advantages are gained by the increased angle of the calcaneus and the supinated appearance. The peroneus longus increases its mechanical advantage and further plantarflexes the first ray. This, in effect, brings the plantar fascia closer and aids in the contracture of this plantar structure. With a strong peroneus longus and the new position of the plantarflexion deformity, the anterior tibialis becomes a weakened structure, and the deformity continues to be progressive. This will be present whether we are dealing with spasticity, hyperinnervation, or a relation of one weak muscle over a stronger muscle secondary to mechanical advantage.

A cycle develops to produce an increase in the cavus foot. The intrinsic muscles plantarflex the forefoot on the hindfoot. This in turn causes an altered function of the anterior extensors of the forefoot with a loss of dorsiflexory power to the metatarsals. The stabilizing force on the metatarsophalangeal joints is lost, and the digits are further contracted by these extensors. As the ankle dorsiflexes in an attempt to bring the forefoot up, the toes contract again, creating dorsal excrescences. With the plantarflexion of the forefoot, the plantar fascia begins to contract. The primary origin to insertion is on the medial aspect of the calcaneus to the medial first metatarsal, and as weightbearing increases and the child's weight increases, the deformity of the calcaneus changes in the direction of a prominent medial tubercle, with an increase in varus deformity. The tightened medially inserted Achilles tendon further throws the calcaneus into its inverted and heel varus attitude. Continuing to the lateral side, the lateral column becomes more and more stable with this heel varus, yielding a stronger peroneus longus and further plantarflexing the first ray.

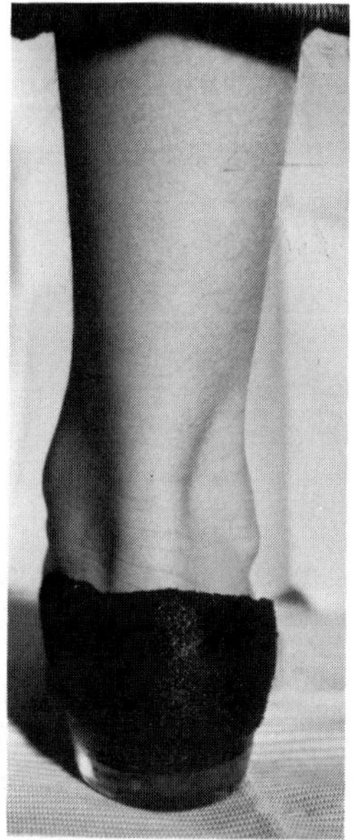

FIGURE 40–24. Deep-seated orthotic device constructed of Plastizote outer shell and PPT intersurface. The materials sandwich deep acrylic orthoses.

Area of Deformity

The classification as to which portion of the foot is involved is determined with reference to the three body planes.

Sagittal Plane. The cavus foot may present with a sagittal plane deformity, referred to as an *anterior* or *posterior cavus deformity*. The anterior cavus foot presents with a forefoot that has become plantar flexed on the hindfoot either at Chopart's joint or Lisfranc's joint. There are two types of anterior cavus. When the first ray is involved alone, it is termed an anterior local cavus. If all of the metatarsals are plantar flexed at Chopart's or Lisfranc's joint, or both, this is considered a global deformity. The sagittal plane posterior cavus relates to the angle of inclination of the calcaneus. An inclination increase of more than 35 degrees when measuring the plantar surface of the calcaneus to the supporting surface indicates a posterior cavus. It is not unusual for both deformities, anterior and posterior, to be present in one foot. This is considered to be the combined cavus foot type.

Frontal Plane. In addition to the sagittal plane deformity, the foot can also present with a deformity on the frontal plane. The calcaneus can be in either varus or valgus. The cavovarus foot with its subtalar varus and heel varus position has greater ankle instability and usually a greater degree of sagittal plane deformity when combined.

Transverse Plane. Finally, the cavoadductus foot is the most significant defect noted in the child with a cavus deformity. This is a rare finding and is usually seen in cases of long-standing rigid deformities. As stated earlier, most foot types of children with cavus deformities are flexible. The transverse plane deformity does not usually present itself until marked osseous changes have developed over a number of years as a result of the inverted and plantar flexed position of the forefoot.

Degree of Deformity

The degree of deformity of the cavus foot in a young child is classified into three categories: flexible, which is a mild deformity; semiflexible, which is a moderate deformity; and rigid, which is the most severe.

Flexible Deformity. This deformity may be difficult to differentiate from the normal foot. On weightbearing, the flexible deformity presents with plantar flexion of the first ray and slight inversion of the hindfoot. When the child is in a weightbearing position, the medial arch is usually compressed, and all of the digital contractures can be reduced.

Flexible deformity is significant in that it is usually overlooked by the physician and may very well be non-neurologic. However, in the presence of a mild cavus deformity that is flexible, one must rule out neurologic etiology.

Semiflexible Deformity. This moderate deformity presents itself on weightbearing because the deformity does not completely reduce. The contracted digits are also present and are not reducible. At this point, plantar keratomas as well as digital contractures with overlying heloma dura start to appear. Usually noted on the great toe interphalangeal joint, a cock-up hallux is starting to appear and beginning to become more rigid than flexible. Soft tissues are increased in their contractures at all of the joints in the forefoot. On radiographic appearance, osseous changes start to develop with mild jamming of joints and with lipping on the dorsal surfaces.

Rigid Deformity. This is the most severe of all of the cavus deformities and usually is not present in children until the later adolescence/early adulthood period. Feet with rigid deformities do not change on or off weightbearing. Joint motion is usually subluxed to rigid with no motion available. The gait is awkward with an increase in lateral ankle instability. All of the digits are flexed and contracted with large bony prominences on the plantar aspects of the metatarsals depending on whether the anterior deformity is global or local. Shoe gear is most difficult to find for these young people because the foot is so arched and inverted that it is rolling off of the shoe and creating maximal wear on the lateral surface in the heel area.

Conservative Treatment

The conservative management of cavus deformities has been a perplexing problem for as long as the deformity has been recognized. It has been well documented that many forms of cavus deformity are associated with neuromuscular disease, and the incidence of association may be as high as 60% to 70%[47] and could be as high as 95% if our methods of neurologic evaluation could be refined. Associated with or without established neurologic disease, cavus deformity is often progressive and the structure of the foot and its functions significantly change with time. Therefore, when considering orthotic control, we must realize that periodic changes in the device are advised.

In the past, conservative treatment of rigid forefoot valgus included balanced padding, semirigid orthoses, metatarsal bars, and lateral Dutchmen's wedges as well as numerous shoe modifications. Many practitioners have questioned the use of rigid orthoses with these foot types, and many have shied away from using them.

The common misconception in using a rigid orthosis with a rigid foot type is that the orthosis is rigid and the foot is rigid, and, therefore, it will not be tolerated. Briefly, a functional orthosis is intended to allow normal function of the foot and to eliminate abnormal compensatory movements. One might even go so far as to say that a rigid orthosis may be the best form of control regarding certain symptoms. Using ankle sprains associated with the supinatory rock of the contact phase as an example, after a biomechanical examination and neutral position casting, one is faced usually with a forefoot valgus and hindfoot varus deformity. The question arises as to what deformity to post and how much. If the patient has a total forefoot valgus, the forefoot should be posted in valgus according to the number of degrees measured. Additionally, the hindfoot should be posted the number of degrees measured. However, this should not exceed 7 degrees, or contact-phase instability may lead to ankle sprains. Commonly, the amount of hindfoot varus is equal to the amount of forefoot valgus. This type of control eliminates the rapid subtalar resupination after the forefoot hits the ground because of its equalizing of the weight across all of the metatarsals. In addition, the retro-Achilles irritation will also be eliminated. In the forefoot, by distributing weight across all metatarsal heads, the concentrated pressure below the first to fifth metatarsals will be diminished.

The plantarflexed first ray is probably the most common type of forefoot valgus and is associated usually with uncompensated or partially compensated hindfoot varus or compensated or partially compensated forefoot varus. With the latter, the relation of the second to fifth metatarsals to the calcaneus is a position of varus, but the first to fifth metatarsals demonstrate a perpendicular relation. It is proposed that the first ray has plantarflexed because of an increased pull by the peroneus longus, which has an increased force because of a stable cuboid. In the management of this foot type, a hindfoot post is used to control the hindfoot varus, and a forefoot post is used beneath the second to fifth metatarsals in the amount of degrees of the forefoot to hindfoot. The first ray is not posted in the medial border. The orthosis is in the first intermetatarsal space and is intended not to support the first ray but to allow it to use its own range of motion.

It should be mentioned, at this point, that the first ray should not be casted out, as had been proposed a few years ago. The reason simply is that, by dorsiflexing the first ray, the longitudinal axis of the midtarsal joint may be inverted as well, and this is undesirable. Furthermore, by dorsiflexing the first ray, a functional hallux limitus will be created, which may lead to structural abnormalities. This type of forefoot valgus can also be posted if the plane beneath the first and fifth metatarsals relative to the hindfoot is in valgus.

In flexible forefoot valgus, which on weightbearing flat-

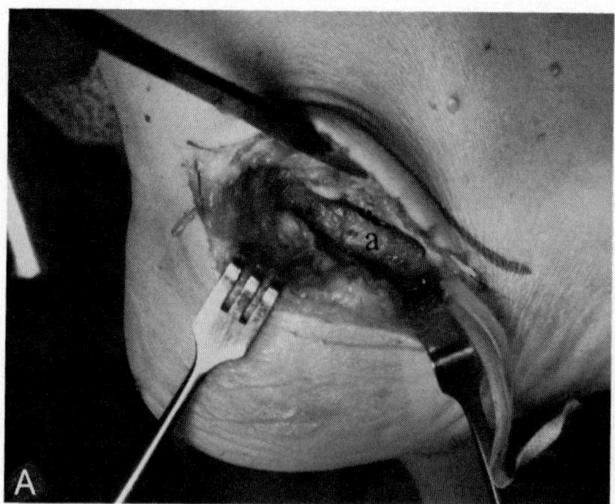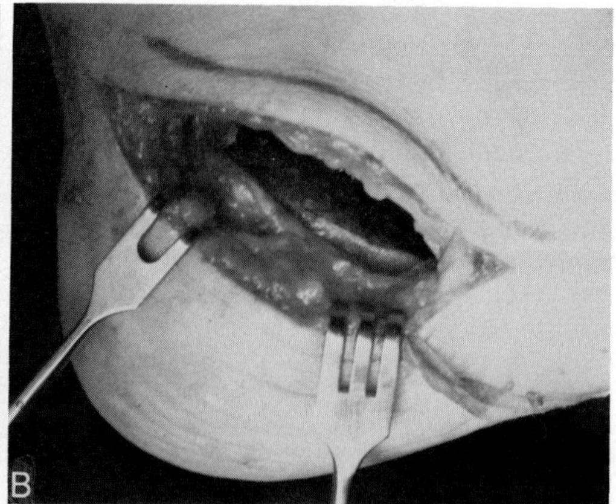

FIGURE 40–25. *A*, Osteotomy is made parallel to peroneal tendons. *B*, A sizeable wedge (a) of bone is removed.

tens significantly, the foot is very unstable and significant forefoot symptomatology develops, including severe hallux abductovalgus and submetatarsal lesion patterns in various combinations. The non-weightbearing attitude, the structural forefoot to hindfoot relationship, is one of valgus, but when weight is superimposed, the forefoot collapses. In gait the forefoot is not locked against the hindfoot; therefore, instability exists. The primary role of the rigid orthosis in such situations is to stabilize the hindfoot and maintain the forefoot in an everted position and to lock the midtarsal joint in a pronatory direction. This is necessary for stable propulsion. Therefore, the neutral position orthosis is used with a hindfoot varus post and a total forefoot valgus post for the first to fifth metatarsals. With this type of device, the forefoot symptomatology is greatly reduced. Earlier recognition of this foot type is necessary to prevent severe hallux abductus and bunion deformity.

The key in the conservative treatment of congenital cavus is stabilization of the hindfoot and maintenance of the everted forefoot. With the midtarsal joint locked, stable propulsion is guaranteed. If a child presents with forefoot lesions, an extension can be incorporated into the orthosis. This is rare in the young child because lesion patterns usually do not develop until the deformity is rigid and long-standing. Flexible sport orthotics are recommended with compressible posts. If a rigid orthosis is used, compressible posts are recommended to aid in shock absorption to this heel under tension from the Achilles tendon and the plantar fascia. No matter what type of orthosis is used, one should maintain the heel in a deep heel seat because this will provide the best control.[48]

Surgical Treatment

Hindfoot. Of prime importance in the consideration of surgery for the cavus foot is the location of the deformity. When the deformity is present in the early stages of a child's development, the calcaneus will start to change its frontal plane alignment. The insertion of the Achilles tendon has its pull on the medial side of the posterior surface, and the predominate origin of the plantar fascia is also on the medial inferior surface. The net effect is a continual deforming force on the calcaneus, creating a heel varus. When the decision is made to osteotomize the calcaneus to reduce the heel varus,

correct placement of the osteotomy is essential. The osteotomy must be parallel to the peroneals if complete reduction is to occur (Fig. 40–25*A* and *B*). Often the cuts are made too perpendicular to the supporting surface, providing no change to the frontal plane deformity but rather rotating the posterior surface along the transverse plane. Fixation is required, and bone contact must be complete. The osteotomy is only made to and not made through the lateral cortex. The foot should be slowly dorsiflexed on the leg because the tension from the Achilles tendon will help close the osteotomy site. A Kirschner wire can be driven from the plantar aspect proximally while the osteotomy is held closed. Pin fixation should not enter the subtalar or ankle joint. Staple fixation provides firm fixation; however, care must be taken not to strike the staples too hard because the medial cortex could fracture.

With a cavovarus foot type, a triplane calcaneal osteotomy may be indicated. The approach is as previously described. The distinction lies in the wedge being directed from the lateral side to the medial side but is modified so that it passes from the dorsolateral aspect to the medial plantar aspect. There is a change of position in all three body planes as this osteotomy site is closed. Again, depending on the degree and location of the deformity, the osteotomy can be modified to address a specific plane.

Other osteotomies are indicated for the reduction of the hindfoot component in a cavus foot type, including an opening wedge osteotomy with the insertion of a bone graft. This serves the same purpose as a closing wedge; however, the intricacies are greater when using a medial approach to insert a bone graft. However, heel length is preserved with this approach should this be a concern.

Forefoot

With regard to the location in the forefoot, the deformity will usually be present at the metatarsal-tarsal joint. The metatarsals, predominantly the first, second, and third, will be plantar flexed in relation to the lesser tarsus. Usually, as noted on a lateral view, the first to fifth metatarsals appear in a plantar flexed position; however, the fourth and fifth metatarsals are essentially dorsiflexed in relation to the midfoot and hindfoot. When addressing this deformity, the metatarsals affected are dorsiflexed by performing an osteotomy at the base to raise the metatarsal declination. One can note this visually on a child because there is a dorsal prominence

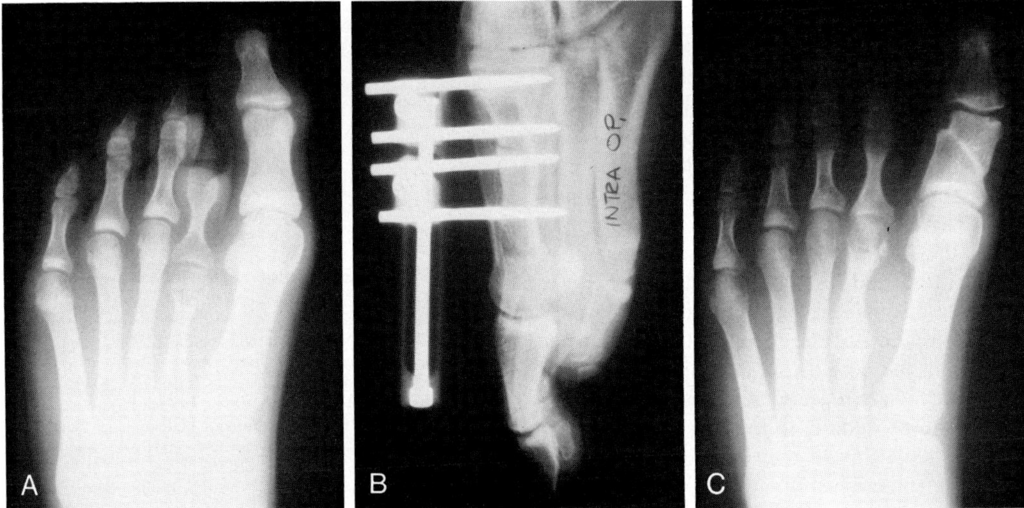

FIGURE 40–26. *A,* This patient presented with a congenitally short fourth metatarsal. Her concerns were cosmetic and her symptoms mostly related to metatarsal transfer complaints. *B,* The external fixator is in place. The device created distraction of the metatarsal. *C,* The metatarsal is displayed approximately 4 months after the procedure and is healed and lengthened. (Courtesy of Dr. William Jenkins, San Francisco, CA.)

noted at the area of the first metatarsal cuneiform. The first metatarsal is dorsiflexed to a position that will lie perpendicular to the bisected calcaneal inversion axis. If a calcaneal varus deformity is present, then a Dwyer osteotomy will be necessary to rotate this axis perpendicular to the supporting surface. In doing so, this will also bring the forefoot parallel to this surface as well. With no calcaneal varus, it will not be necessary to perform any osteotomy in the hindfoot.

BRACHYMETATARSIA (CONGENITAL SHORT METATARSAL)

The hypoplasia of the metatarsal is commonly seen in the fourth metatarsal bilaterally. However, any metatarsal can be affected and can present unilaterally. A shortened fourth metatarsal does not present with any functional disturbance in the child. It is, however, a concern with regard to cosmesis. Most parents are more concerned about the cosmesis than future functional problems. The cosmetic concern is an acceptable reason for surgery; however, the surgeon should be aware that if brachymetatarsia is left untreated, an increase in pressure results on the adjacent metatarsals. This sequela is not usually observed until the child loses the supple fat pad plantarly. Calluses develop, and the toes begin to override and start to contract; at this point, surgery is indicated for this functional deformity (Fig. 40–26).

Surgical Treatment

With an understanding of the future sequelae of the short metatarsal, the physician's goal is proper function first and then cosmesis. The selected procedure should maintain length and joint motion.

Grafts. Bone grafts from adjacent metatarsals are placed in the distal cut shafts of the shortened metatarsal.[49, 50] The cylindrical graft is held by a longitudinally placed Kirschner wire (see Table 40–1). I personally use a mini external fixator to maintain bone length and graft compression. Two screws are placed distally and proximally to the graft site. With a

compressor adjusted in place, the set screw is torqued gently with enough compression to hold the graft without slipping. One full turn is applied in a counterclockwise direction; this equals approximately 8 to 12 pounds of torque.

An alternative to the cylindrical bone graft is autogenous bank bone. Cancellous and cortical bone is placed in the osteotomy site, creating the desired separation without shortening of the adjacent metatarsal. Keep in mind that a dermal Z plasty and a Z lengthening of the tendon may be necessary.

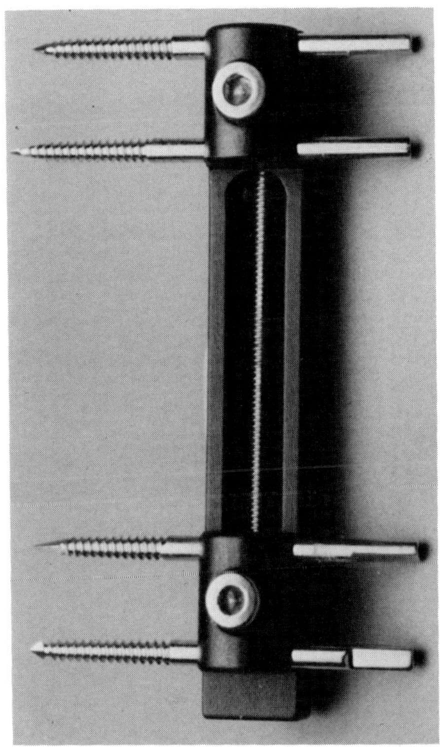

FIGURE 40–27. EBI mini-bone fixator used to compress or distract bone fragments.

Callotasis

Surgery intended to lengthen the metatarsal rather than shorten the healthy normal bones seems to be more efficacious. Callotasis[18] (callus distraction) is another method of lengthening a bone. After an osteotomy has been performed on the diaphysis of the metatarsal, an early callus is gradually elongated with the aid of an external bone fixator. A mini-bone fixator is placed over the osteotomy site, and the screws are placed on both sides of the osteotomy. The periosteum is incised dorsally and reflected around the entire shaft. The transverse cut is made through the entire shaft, and the periosteum is closed. Distraction of the metatarsal is performed gradually by separating the new callus at a rate of approximately 0.25 mm per day. Care must be taken with distraction, as with any lengthening procedure, to prevent neurovascular compromise. Periodic cleansing of the pin sites is important to minimize the risk of infection (Fig. 40–27).[51–54]

References

1. Jay RM: Don't worry, your child will outgrow it . . . [Editorial]. J Foot Surg 29:412, 1990.
2. Wolff J: Das Gesetz der Transformation der Knochen. Berlin, Hirschwald, 1892.
3. Giannestras NI: Foot Disorders. Philadelphia, Lea and Febiger, 1973.
4. Otman S: Energy cost of walking with flatfeet. Prosthet Orthot Int December:73–76, 1988.
5. Wickstrom J: Shoe corrections and orthopedic foot supports. Clin Orthop 70:30, 1970.
6. Cowell H: Shoes and shoe corrections. Pediatr Clin North Am 24(4):791, 1977.
7. Gould N: The development of the toddler arch. Foot Ankle 9(5):241, 1989.
8. Gould N: Shoes versus sneakers in toddlers. Foot Ankle 6(2):105, 1985.
9. Menkveld SR: Analysis of gait patterns in normal school-aged children. J Pediatr Orthop 8(3):263–267, 1988.
10. Doxey GE: Clinical use and fabrication of molded thermoplastic, foot orthotic devices: Suggestions from the field. Phys Ther 65:1679–1682, 1985.
11. Smith LS: The effects of soft and semi-rigid orthoses upon rearfoot movement in running. J Am Podiatr Med Assoc 76:227–233, 1986.
12. Minns RJ: A study of foot shape, underfoot pressure patterns, lower limb rotations and gait of children. Chiropodist March:89–99, 1986.
13. Johnson GR: The effectiveness of shock-absorbing insoles during normal walking. Prosthet Orthot Int 12:91–95, 1988.
14. Smith RD and Rappaport MJ: Subtalar arthroereisis: A four-year follow-up study. J Am Podiatr Med Assoc 73:356–361, 1983.
15. Lelievre J: Current concepts and correction in the valgus foot. Clin Orthop 70:43, 1970.
16. Kuwada GT and Dockery GL: Complications following traumatic incidents with sta-peg procedure. J Foot Surg 27:236–239, 1988.
17. Subotnick S: The subtalar joint lateral extra-articular arthroereisis. J Am Podiatr Med Assoc 67:3, 1977.
18. Lanham RH: Indications and complications of arthroereisis in hypermobile flatfoot. J Am Podiatr Assoc 69:178–185, 1979.
19. Schmidt HM: Shape and fixation of band systems in the human sinus and canalis tarsi. Acta Anat 102:184, 1978.
20. Jay RM: Current therapy in podiatric surgery. *In* Ganley JV (ed): Flatfoot: Evans Procedure. Toronto, B. C. Decker, 1989, pp. 251–253.
21. Kite JH: Errors and complications in treating foot conditions in children. Clin Orthop 53:31–38, 1967.
22. Berg EE: Reappraisal of metatarsus adductus and skewfoot. J Bone Joint Surg 68A:1185–1196, 1986.
23. Sgarlato TE: A Compendium of Podiatric Biomechanics. California College of Podiatric Medicine, San Francisco, CA 1971, p 31.
24. Jay RM and Johnson M: Recurrent metatarsus adductus. Curr Podiatr Med 33:33–42, 1984.
25. Bestard EA: A modified Furlong procedure for the correction of metatarsus adductus. Contemp Orthop 8:19–23, 1984.
26. Schwartz B, Jay RM, and Schoenhaus HD: Apophysitis of the fifth metatarsal base: Iselin's disease. J Am Podiatr Med Assoc 81:128–130, 1991.
27. Steytler JCS and Van der Walt ID: Correction of resistant adduction of the forefoot in congenital clubfoot and congenital metatarsus varus by metatarsal osteotomy. Br J Surg 53:558, 1966.
28. Jay RM, Schoenhaus HD, and Donohue CM: A modified crescentic osteotomy in children. J Foot Surg 29:417–420, 1990.
29. Stark JG, Johanson JJ, and Winter RB: The Heyman-Herndon tarsometatarsal capsulotomy for metatarsus adductus. J Pediatr Orthop 7:305–310, 1987.
30. Kling TF, Schmidt TL, and Conklin MJ: Open wedge osteotomy of the first cuneiform for metatarsus adductus. J Bone Joint Surg 15B:331, 1991.
31. LaDamany P: La torsion du tibia. J L'Anat Physiol 45:598–615, 1909.
32. Wilkinson JA: Femoral anteversion in the rabbit. J Bone Joint Surg 44B:386, 1962.
33. Salter R: The present state of innominate osteotomy in congenital dislocation of the hip. J Bone Joint Surg 48B:853, 1966.
34. Brookes M and Wardle EN: Muscle action and the shape of the femur. J Bone Joint Surg 44B:398, 1962.
35. Moreland MS: Morphological effects of torsion applied to growing bone. J Bone Joint Surg 62B(2):230–237, 1980.
36. Arkin AM: The effects of pressure on epiphyseal growth: The mechanism of plasticity of growing bone. J Bone Surg Joint Surg 38A:1056–1076, 1956.
37. Heuter C: Anatomische Studien an den Extremita Tengelenhen Neugeborener und Erwach Sener. Virchows Arch 25:572, 1862.
38. Volkmann R: Chirurgische Erfahrungan uber Knochenverbiegurgen. Arch Pathol Anat 24:512, 1862.
39. Jakob RP: Tibial torsion calculated by computerized tomography and compared to other methods of measurement. J Bone Joint Surg 62B:238–242, 1980.
40. Elftman H: Torsion of lower extremity. Am J Physiol Anthropol 3:255–265, 1945.
41. Jay RM: In-toe secondary to medial tibial torsion. Curr Podiatr Med 39:9–13, 1990.
42. Schoenhaus HD and Jay RM: Modified gastrocnemius lengthening. J Am Podiatr Med Assoc 68:31–37, 1978.
43. Griffin PP, Wheelhouse W, Shiavi R, and Bass W: Treatment of toewalking, habitual toewalkers. J Bone Joint Surg 59A:97–101, 1977.
44. Illingworth RS: General articles on toewalking of unknown etiology. *In* Common Symptoms of Disease in Childhood. Oxford, England, Blackwell Scientific, 1979, pp 237–238.
45. Kalen V and Breecher A: Relationship between adolescent bunions and flatfoot. Foot Ankle 8:331–336, 1988.
46. Jay RM: Orthoses for cerebral palsy patients. Curr Podiatr Med 38(1):26–27, 1989.
47. Dwyer FC: The present status of the problem of pes cavus. Clin Orthop 106:254, 1975.
48. Jay RM and Schoenhaus HD: Cavus deformity—Conservative management. J Am Podiatr Med Assoc 70(5):235–238, 1980.
49. Marcinko DE and Rappaport MJ: Post-traumatic brachymetatarsia. J Foot Surg 23:451–453, 1984.
50. Kaplan EG and Kaplan G: Metatarsal lengthening by use of autogenous bone graft and internal wire compression fixation: A preliminary report. J Foot Surg 17:2, 1978.
51. Kojimoto H and Yasui N: Bone lengthening in rabbits by callus distraction. J Bone Joint Surg 70B:543–549, 1988.
52. Aldegheri R: The callotasis method of limb lengthening. Clin Orthop 241:137–145, 1989.
53. De Bastiani G, Aldegheri R, Renzi-Brivio L, and Trivella G: Limb lengthening by distraction of the epiphyseal plate: A comparison of two techniques in the rabbit. J Bone Joint Surg 68B:545–549, 1986.
54. De Bastiani G, Aldegheri R, Renzi-Brivio L, and Trivella G: Limb lengthening by callus distraction (callotasis). J Pediatr Orthop 7:129–134, 1987.

Chronic Pain Syndromes

CHAPTER 41

Physiology of Pain

Pamela K. Westfahl, Ph.D.

Pain is a perception that involves not only noxious sensation but the emotions and experiences that accompany this sensation. The perception of pain is different for each individual because we each have our own expectations and memories, which are integrated with nociceptive input to provide the experience we call pain. For example, one individual may report that a specific stimulus is moderately painful, but a second individual may say it is severely painful even though the stimulus is the same. Nociception is the sensation that results from activation of specific sensory receptors by modalities that can cause tissue injury. These modalities include pressure, heat, and chemicals. Activation of nociceptors and transfer of this information along nociceptive pathways to the brain elicit specific behaviors and reflexes that tend to protect the individual from further damage. These reflexes include somatic and autonomic responses such as withdrawal reflexes, increased heart rate, and sweating.

Nociceptive input can arise from viscera, skeletal muscle, joints, bones, and cutaneous tissue. Pain may be acute, such as a pinprick, and last only as long as the stimulus is present. Perhaps of more clinical importance is chronic pain, which may persist even after damaged tissue has healed and the stimulus is no longer present. Sometimes pain in deep somatic or visceral tissue results in spasm of neighboring skeletal muscle. The muscle spasm provokes ischemia and muscle pain, thus exacerbating the nociceptive input. The severe abdominal pain associated with appendicitis is an example of this reflex.

Chronic pain may involve long-term changes in behavior such as disrupted sleep and inability to perform one's work or daily activities. Thus, unrelieved chronic pain may significantly decrease an individual's quality of life. An understanding of the mechanisms that underlie persistent changes in nociceptive responses may lead to the development of ways to alleviate chronic pain.

To understand noxious reflexes better, physiologic studies of the component parts of these reflexes have been con-ducted. Much information has been learned about the receptors that detect noxious stimuli and the afferent fibers that carry this information into the central nervous system. Interactions between noxious and innocuous input at the level of the spinal cord and the ascending pathways carrying noxious information to the brain have also been described. Data indicating the presence of endogenous control over the transmission of nociceptive information in the central nervous system have also been collected. Intensive investigation of this area has been carried out because of its clinical relevance to pain control. Therefore, in this chapter, the following areas are discussed: nociceptors, peripheral afferents, spinal cord interactions, ascending pathways in the central nervous system, and endogenous control of pain.

RECEPTORS

Sensory receptors are characterized by the form of energy or modality to which they respond, the minimum stimulus necessary to evoke a response (called the threshold), the relationship between stimulus strength and the firing rate of the receptor, and how quickly the receptor adapts to continued stimulation. Most of the physiologic research on peripheral aspects of nociception has been conducted on cutaneous tissue because of the accessibility of sensory receptors and afferents, but the deep somatic and visceral nociceptors that have been studied seem to have similar characteristics.

Nociceptors are sensory receptors that specifically respond to stimuli that are damaging or potentially damaging to tissues. Free (unencapsulated) nerve endings have been identified as nociceptors in cutaneous tissue[1] and are probably the nociceptors in deep somatic and visceral tissue as well. Nociceptors are abundant in cutaneous tissue and some deep somatic and visceral tissue.[2] Some nociceptors respond only to extremes of pressure and are called mechanical nociceptors. Other nociceptors respond only to extremes of heat (greater than 45°C) and are identified as thermal nociceptors.

Chemical nociceptors respond to certain chemicals released by damaged or inflamed tissues. These chemicals include kinins, histamine, potassium ion, prostaglandins, and serotonin.[3] Polymodal nociceptors respond to two or more of these modalities. Deep somatic and visceral nociceptors respond to mechanical distention, thermal stimuli, and chemicals released by inflammation or ischemia.

Other cutaneous sensory receptors respond to sensory modalities that are similar to those that activate nociceptors. For example, the pacinian corpuscle responds to pressure. The characteristic that distinguishes nociceptors from innocuous receptors is the high threshold of nociceptors. Under normal circumstances, nociceptors respond only to intense stimulation,[3] much greater than that required to elicit a response from non-noxious receptors. Nociceptors do not exhibit spontaneous activity and do not respond to innocuous mechanical or thermal stimuli because the intensity of these stimuli is not sufficient to reach threshold for nociceptors.

The firing frequency of nociceptors increases in direct proportion to the intensity of the stimulus.[4] A similar relationship is true for all sensory receptors. Nociceptors adapt slowly, which means that they maintain activity in the presence of continued stimulation.[4] This characteristic is unlike that of sensory receptors such as the pacinian corpuscle, which adapts rapidly and only signals a change in the stimulus. The functional significance of slowly adapting nociceptors is that the individual continues to receive input about a noxious stimulus. However, in the presence of sustained intense stimulation, some nociceptors can become less responsive.[3]

Some nociceptors become sensitized when repetitively stimulated[5] or when previously exposed to noxious stimuli.[3] A sensitized nociceptor exhibits an increase in firing frequency, a lower threshold, a shorter latency to response, and the appearance of spontaneous activity. Thus, it is easier to evoke a response in a sensitized receptor. Tissue injury or inflammation can also decrease the threshold for nociceptors at or near the site of injury, resulting in hyperalgesia (i.e., excessive sensitivity to pain).[6] The affected area sometimes becomes so sensitive that even an innocuous stimulus such as light touch may elicit a response from the nociceptor and be perceived as painful. Administration of aspirin or nonsteroidal antiinflammatory drugs often relieves hyperalgesia. These compounds inhibit the synthesis of eicosanoids such as prostaglandins, prostacyclins, and thromboxanes.[7] This observation suggests that local release of eicosanoids by injured or inflamed tissues causes the hyperalgesia. Prostaglandin E_2 and prostacyclin lower the threshold for mechanical nociception in the rat hind paw.[6] Other metabolites of arachidonic acid were not effective in this situation, but that does not mean that other types of nociceptors are unaffected by these metabolites. Leukotrienes may also affect the responsiveness of nociceptors,[3] but cyclooxygenase inhibitors such as aspirin do not inhibit the production of leukotrienes. McMahon and Koltzenburg[8] suggested that there is a separate group of nociceptors specifically recruited by inflammatory agents. They suggested that these nociceptors are not stimulated by acute injury but participate in the chronic pain associated with inflammation. This may explain some of the differences in the response to acute and chronic pain.

Causalgia is a severe, burning pain that can develop after peripheral nerve injury. The mechanisms underlying the development of this phenomenon are not clearly understood.

One hypothesis suggests that spinal cord neurons, which receive input from nociceptive afferents, are sensitized and thus fire more than usual. This results in an increase in activity along the central pain pathways. In a small proportion of patients with causalgia, the pain is accompanied by localized sympathetic effects and is relieved by transection of sympathetic nerves innervating the damaged area. Therefore, this response has been termed sympathetic maintained pain.[9] A hypothesis to explain the symptoms associated with the latter form of causalgia is that sympathetic input onto sensory nociceptive afferents maintains and reinforces transmission along nociceptive pathways. Normal nociceptors do not respond to norepinephrine or sympathetic stimulation, but Sato and Perl[10] demonstrated that peripheral nerve injury induces changes in nociceptors that make them responsive to norepinephrine. One of the changes is an increase in the number of α_2-adrenergic receptors on sensory nerve terminals. Thus, a circuit could be established whereby the stress that accompanies pain activates the sympathetic nervous system, which increases the sensitivity of peripheral nociceptors and results in sustained activation of these receptors and chronic pain.

PERIPHERAL AFFERENTS

Nociceptors are innervated by Aδ or C afferent neurons. Non-nociceptive receptors, which detect crude touch and innocuous temperatures, are also innervated by Aδ and C afferent fibers.[2] Aδ fibers are small-diameter (2 to 5 μm), myelinated fibers with a conduction velocity in the range of 5 to 30 m/second. C fibers are smaller (0.4 to 1.2 μm), unmyelinated neurons with a slower conduction velocity (0.5 to 2 m/second). The difference in conduction velocities between these two groups of fibers may explain the distinction between "fast" (first) pain and "slow" (second) pain. Fast pain is described as sharp and localized, such as a pinprick, and is perceived immediately after application of the stimulus. Slow pain is dull, diffuse, and burning and takes longer to reach consciousness. C fibers mediate the chronic, unpleasant sensations associated with pain. The cell bodies of sensory afferents lie in the dorsal root ganglia, and their processes extend peripherally to the receptor and centrally into the spinal cord. Most Aδ and C fibers enter the spinal cord through the dorsal root; however, some C fibers also enter through the ventral root.[3]

Substance P is believed to be one of the neurotransmitters released by nociceptive afferents.[11] This 11–amino acid peptide is present in afferent C fibers and is released when the fibers are activated by natural noxious stimuli or high-intensity electrical stimulation.[12, 13] Substance P produces slow, excitatory postsynaptic potentials in dorsal horn neurons, which brings them closer to their firing threshold.[11] Other peptides such as somatostatin, vasoactive inhibitory polypeptide, bombesin, and calcitonin gene-related peptide are also present in small-diameter afferent fibers and may coexist with substance P[14]. The conditions affecting the secretion of these neuropeptides and their effects are not well understood, but they may also participate in nociceptive signal transmission.

In addition to serving as a neurotransmitter mediating pain transmission, substance P may also participate in the development of inflammation associated with noxious stimuli. The triple response is a frequently observed result of mechanical irritation of the skin. The response consists of a reddening of the skin at the site of irritation followed a few minutes later by localized swelling and diffuse redness radiating away from the site of irritation. The latter response (the flare) is believed to be due to the release of substance P from a branch of the peripheral afferent fiber that innervates tissue near the site of stimulation. Substance P either directly dilates cutaneous blood vessels or stimulates the secretion of histamine by mast cells,[15] which induces vasodilation and causes the flare. The other peptides found in small-diameter sensory fibers may also participate in the local inflammatory response.[15] A hypothesis concerning a potential role for substance P in the cause of rheumatoid arthritis has been forwarded by Levine and others.[16] They correlated the severity of arthritis with the amount of substance P present in a joint and suggested that substance P may mediate the inflammatory response associated with rheumatoid arthritis.

SPINAL CORD INTERACTIONS

Aδ and C fiber afferents enter the spinal cord, ascend or descend for a few segments in the tract of Lissauer, and then synapse on neurons in the dorsal horn gray matter of the spinal cord. Fine-diameter afferent fibers terminate on neurons in Rexed's laminae I, II, and V. Lamina I, or the marginal layer, is the most superficial of the gray matter layers in the dorsal horn. Most of the cells in lamina I are nociceptive specific; that is, they are excited by noxious thermal and mechanical stimuli but are unaffected by touch or hair movement (innocuous stimuli). Lamina V is located in the medial portion of the gray matter. Lamina V cells receive input from Aβ collaterals as well as Aδ and C fibers and are stimulated by innocuous stimuli such as touch, vibration, and hair movement as well as by noxious stimuli. Therefore, lamina V cells are called wide-dynamic-range neurons.[17] The distinction between noxious and innocuous stimuli is coded for by the firing frequency of wide-dynamic-range neurons.[3] Nociceptive input onto the lamina V cells results in a greater frequency of action potentials in the lamina V neurons than does innocuous input. This difference in frequency allows the central nervous system to distinguish between noxious and non-noxious input.

The synapses between peripheral nociceptive afferents (first-order neurons) and dorsal horn cells in laminae I and V (second-order neurons) provide locations for summation of information and modification of transmission. Temporal and spatial summation of sensory input onto dorsal horn cells may explain the afterdischarge phenomenon observed in many of these cells. Afterdischarge is the sustained activity of dorsal horn neurons that persists longer than the firing of nociceptors.[3] Thus, the nociceptive pathway continues to be active after peripheral stimulation has ceased. Modification of transmission between first-order and second-order neurons has also been observed in the nociceptive pathway. Peripheral injury can result in prolonged sensitization of dorsal horn neurons.[18] Sensitization of the second-order neurons facilitates the transmission of nociceptive information because not as much input is needed to cause firing of the second-order neuron. Sensitization of dorsal horn cells has also been suggested as a mechanism of causalgia because the nociceptive

pathway is easier to activate at the level of the second-order neuron.[9]

Referred pain is a phenomenon in which stimulation of visceral or deep somatic nociceptors is perceived as pain in a superficial structure. The pain in the left shoulder and arm associated with angina pectoris is an example of referred pain. Usually the superficial structure is derived from the same dermatome as the deeper structure. There are two hypotheses to account for this phenomenon. One is that superficial and visceral pain afferents synapse on the same spinal cord neuron in either lamina I or lamina V.[19] However, because this input usually originates from superficial sources, stimulation of the dorsal horn cell by visceral afferents is perceived as arising from superficial sources. The second hypothesis is that branches of the same afferent fiber innervate cutaneous and visceral areas.[20] Therefore, activation of either branch results in the same input onto the second-order neuron.

There are interactions within the spinal cord that may control the transmission of nociceptive information. Interneurons originating in Rexed's lamina II (substantia gelatinosa) also receive C fiber input. These interneurons terminate in lamina V and are believed to be inhibitory in nature.[21] Gamma-amino butyric acid and enkephalins have been proposed as dorsal horn neurotransmitters that mediate this inhibition.[11] Both substances are present in the dorsal horn, and application of them to the dorsal horn inhibits nociceptive reflexes. There is evidence that the inhibitory neurotransmitter hyperpolarizes the membrane of the lamina V neuron and thus suppresses its activation.[3] This action is termed postsynaptic inhibition because the inhibition acts on the postsynaptic cell. There is also evidence that the inhibition is mediated by a decrease in the amount of neurotransmitter released by the C fiber.[3] This is an example of presynaptic inhibition because the action is exerted on the presynaptic cell.

ASCENDING PATHWAYS

Axons of most second-order nociceptive neurons cross over the midline of the spinal cord at their segment of origin and ascend in the anterolateral quadrant of the contralateral spinal cord, forming the spinothalamic tract. This tract is not nociceptive specific because it also carries non-nociceptive information from thermal receptors and crude touch receptors, which synapse on lamina V second-order neurons.[2] Identification of the anterolateral pathway as a carrier of nociceptive information led to the development of techniques for transection of the pathway as a means of relieving chronic pain in patients. Anterolateral cordotomy is effective in many instances, but there are patients who still have pain after this procedure.[2]

Dennis and Melzack,[22] among others, divided the spinothalamic tract into a lateral portion, which mediates specific, localized nociceptive transmission, and a medial portion, which carries burning, diffuse, unpleasant pain. The lateral spinothalamic tract terminates in the ventrobasal complex of the thalamus (posteromedial and posterolateral thalamic nuclei), and third-order neurons carry information from the thalamus to the somatosensory areas of the cerebral cortex. The thalamic and cortical projections of the lateral spinothalamic tract are similar to those of the dorsal column–medial lemniscal pathway, which carries touch and vibration sensations.[2] Simultaneous input from innocuous mechanoreceptors onto the somatosensory cortex via the dorsal column–medial lemniscal pathway may facilitate the localization of acute, painful stimuli.

The medial portion of the spinothalamic tract also ascends in the anterolateral quadrant of the spinal cord but is more accurately termed the spinoreticulothalamic tract because of its terminations.[17] This tract sends information into the brain stem reticular formation with projections onto the intralaminar and midline nuclei of the thalamus. The spinoreticulothalamic tract carries the "slow" component of nociception, and the diffuse nature of this component may result from the spread of activity into the reticular formation, diencephalon, and various forebrain regions. Input from the spinoreticulothalamic tract onto the reticular formation also mediates the increased level of cortical arousal associated with nociception.[2] This is probably the mechanism underlying the adage about pinching yourself to stay awake.

Although the contralateral anterolateral system is the major ascending pathway for nociceptive information, other ascending nociceptive pathways exist. These include a small ipsilateral component of the anterolateral spinothalamic tract, a dorsolateral spinothalamic tract, a spinocervical tract, and a postsynaptic dorsal column pathway.[23] None of these pathways carry only nociceptive information. The failure of anterolateral cordotomy to relieve pain in all patients[2] may be explained by the presence of the secondary pathways. The presence of more than one nociceptive tract implies that surgical transection of "the" nociceptive pathway as a means of relieving chronic pain in all patients is an unrealistic goal.

The role of the cerebral cortex in pain perception has not been well defined because of the difficulty in finding a significant number of cortical neurons that respond to painful stimuli and the problems with interpreting data from patients with lesions in cortical areas. However, Talbot and coworkers[24] used a combination of subtractive positron emission tomography and magnetic resonance imaging to identify cortical areas in human subjects that preferentially responded to painful thermal cutaneous stimuli as opposed to innocuous stimuli. These investigators found three areas of increased neuronal activity in the cortex that were specifically associated with noxious thermal stimulation: the contralateral anterior cingulate, the secondary somatosensory cortex, and the primary somatosensory cortex. Whether the same areas respond to other noxious modalities or to deep somatic and visceral pain remains to be determined.

Branches of the ascending nociceptive pathways also terminate in the periaqueductal gray of the midbrain and the nucleus raphe magnus of the medulla oblongata.[25] These brain stem areas are involved in the descending control of nociceptive transmission. Thus, activation of nociceptive pathways may induce feedback modification of subsequent nociceptive transmission.

ENDOGENOUS CONTROL OF PAIN

The search for endogenous mechanisms that can alter the transmission of nociceptive information was stimulated by the recognition of morphine's analgesic properties and reports of stress-induced analgesia on the battlefield. The synapse between first-order and second-order neurons in the nociceptive pathway is at the center of this endogenous control system. Both segmental input from non-nociceptive afferent fibers and descending input from the brain stem affect transmission through this synapse. The mechanism for this inhibition is not entirely understood but may involve both presynaptic and postsynaptic effects.

The gate theory of pain control was put forward by Melzack and Wall[26] in 1965 to explain the inhibitory effect of large-diameter afferents on nociceptive transmission. Large-diameter (Aβ) afferent fibers conduct innocuous sensory information into the spinal cord and ascend in the ipsilateral dorsal column. Branches of these large-diameter afferents terminate on neurons in the dorsal horn of the spinal cord. Stimulation of low-threshold mechanoreceptors activates Aβ afferents and can diminish or abolish the sensation of pain from nearby areas. This effect is observed when someone achieves pain relief by rubbing the area next to an injury. The gate theory postulates that collaterals of Aβ fibers activate interneurons in the substantia gelatinosa, which inhibit lamina V cells and close the gate to nociceptive transmission. Collaterals of Aδ and C fibers inhibit the substantia gelatinosa interneurons and open the gate. Although there are anatomic correlates that support the gate theory, there is little physiologic evidence to support this model. However, no other model has been proposed to explain the inhibitory effects of large-diameter afferents on nociceptive transmission.

In addition to segmental input onto dorsal horn nociceptive cells, there is also evidence for descending input from higher centers in the brain. Electrical stimulation of the periaqueductal gray area of the mesencephalon produces analgesia, which is abolished by transection of the dorsolateral funiculus of the spinal cord.[25] Basbaum and Fields[25] proposed the following model for the descending control system. Neurons in the periaqueductal gray descend to the rostral medulla, where they terminate on and activate serotonergic neurons in the nucleus raphe magnus. The serotonergic neurons descend in the dorsolateral funiculus and terminate in the dorsal horn of the spinal cord. Activation of this descending pathway inhibits nociceptive neurons in laminae I and V of the dorsal horn either directly or via inhibitory interneurons. There is evidence in the cat and rat that other rostral medullary nuclei contribute fibers to the dorsolateral funiculus and participate in controlling nociception.[25] Details of the interactions within the periaqueductal gray, rostral medulla, and dorsal horn remain unknown at this time, so it is likely that the descending control of nociception is more involved than the scheme outlined previously.

The analgesic effects of morphine and the identification of receptors that bind morphine led to the discovery of endogenous opiates. These morphinelike compounds are normally present in the body and include met-enkephalin, leu-enkephalin, β-endorphin, and dynorphin.[27] The endogenous opiates are found throughout the nervous system, but the distribution of each opiate differs from the distribution of the others. There is also a family of opiate receptors, including μ, κ, and δ. Each receptor subtype expresses a different pattern of binding affinities for the various opiates.[28] It is likely that all three kinds of receptors participate in antinociception to some extent,[28] but their specific roles cannot be distinguished at this time. Binding of opiates to these receptors also elicits other effects such as respiratory depression, inhibition of gastrointestinal motility, and changes in emotional state.

Opiate receptors and opiatergic neurons have been found at several locations within the proposed endogenous nociceptive control pathway. Opiate receptors are present on the terminals of Aδ and C fibers in the substantia gelatinosa, and enkephalins inhibit the release of substance P by these fibers.[25] Thus, enkephalins could mediate the presynaptic inhibition of nociceptive transmission in the dorsal horn. However, enkephalinergic synapses on Aδ and C fiber terminals have not been demonstrated. The periaqueductal gray contains enkephalin and dynorphin and a high density of opiate receptors.[25] Injection of opiates into the periaqueductal gray induces analgesia.[29]

The mechanisms by which the endogenous pain control pathway is activated remain speculative. The presence of branches from ascending nociceptive pathways onto the periaqueductal gray and medulla oblongata provides an anatomic pathway by which the descending pain control system can be activated by nociceptive input. The periaqueductal gray receives descending input from cortical, limbic, and hypothalamic regions,[30, 31] which suggests that higher centers could provide some control over the pathway. Some stressful situations induce analgesia that is sensitive to naloxone (an opiate antagonist) and thus apparently use the endogenous opiate pain-control pathway.[32] However, not all forms of stress-induced analgesia are naloxone sensitive. Therefore, it is likely that nonopiate systems also participate in endogenous pain control.[32] The pathways and neurotransmitters involved in the nonopiate pathways remain unclear. Injection of vasoactive intestinal polypeptide into the periaqueductal gray produces analgesia that is not sensitive to naloxone,[33] so this may be one of the nonopiate neurotransmitters mediating endogenous control of nociceptive transmission.

References

1. Krueger L, Perl ER, and Sedivec MJ: Fine structures of myelinated mechanical nociceptor endings in cat hairy skin. J Comp Neurol 198:137–154, 1981.
2. Ganong WF: Review of Medical Physiology. San Mateo, CA, Appleton & Lange, 1991, pp 124–135.
3. Besson J-M and Chaouch A: Peripheral and spinal mechanisms of nociception. Physiol Rev 67:67–186, 1987.
4. Mountcastle VB: Medical Physiology. St. Louis, CV Mosby, 1974, pp 348–381.
5. Perl ER: Sensitization of nociceptors and its relation to sensation. Adv Pain Res Ther 1:17–28, 1976.
6. Taiwo YO and Levine JD: Effects of cyclooxygenase products of arachidonic acid metabolism on cutaneous nociceptive threshold in the rat. Brain Res 537:372–374, 1990.
7. Mizuno K, Yamamoto S, and Lands W: Effects of non-steroidal anti-inflammatory drugs on fatty acid cyclooxygenase and prostaglandin hydroperoxidase activities. Prostaglandins 23:743–757, 1982.
8. McMahon SB, and Koltzenburg M: Novel classes of nociceptors: Beyond Sherrington. Trends Neurosci 13:199–201, 1990.
9. Roberts WJ: A hypothesis on the physiological basis for causalgia and related pains. Pain 24:297–311, 1986.
10. Sato J and Perl ER: Adrenergic excitation of cutaneous pain receptors induced by peripheral nerve injury. Science 251:1608–1610, 1991.
11. Otsuka M and Yanagisawa M: Pain and neurotransmitters. Cell Mol Neurobiol 10:293–302, 1990.
12. Kuraishi Y, Hirota N, Sato Y, et al: Evidence that substance P and somatostatin transmit separate information related to pain in the spinal dorsal horn. Brain Res 325:294–298, 1985.
13. Yaksh TL, Jessell TM, Gamse R, et al: Intrathecal morphine inhibits substance P release from mammalian spinal cord in vivo. Nature 286:155–157, 1980.
14. Foreman JC: Peptides and neurogenic inflammation. Br Med Bull 43:386–400, 1987.
15. Lisney SJW and Bharali LAM: The axon reflex: An outdated idea or a valid hypothesis? News Physiol Sci 4:45–48, 1989.
16. Levine JD, Collier DH, Basbaum AI, et al: Hypothesis: The nervous system may contribute to the pathophysiology of rheumatoid arthritis. J Rheumatol 12:406–411, 1985.
17. Kelly DD: Central representations of pain and analgesia. In Kandel ER and Schwartz JH (eds): Principles of Neural Science. New York, Elsevier, 1985, pp 331–343.
18. Woolf CJ: Central and peripheral components of the hyperalgesia that follows peripheral tissue injury. In Rowe M and Willis WD (eds): Development, Organization and Processing in Somatosensory Pathways. New York, Alan R. Liss, 1985, pp 317–323.
19. Ruch TC: Visceral sensation and referred pain. In Fulton JF (ed): Howell's Textbook of Physiology. Philadelphia, WB Saunders, 1947, pp 360–374.
20. Berne RM and Levy MN: Physiology. St. Louis, CV Mosby, 1988, pp 135–157.
21. Livingston RB: Touch, pain and temperature. In West JB (ed): Physiological Basis of Medical Practice. Baltimore, Williams & Wilkins, 1991, pp 1012–1031.
22. Dennis SG and Melzack R: Pain signalling systems in the dorsal and ventral cord. Pain 4:97–132, 1977.
23. Hammond DL: New insights regarding organization of spinal cord pain pathways. News Physiol Sci 4:98–101, 1989.
24. Talbot JD, Marrett S, Evans AC, et al: Multiple representations of pain in human cerebral cortex. Science 251:1355–1358, 1991.
25. Basbaum AI and Fields HL: Endogenous pain control systems: Brainstem spinal pathways and endorphin circuitry. Ann Rev Neurosci 7:309–338, 1984.
26. Melzack R and Wall PD: Pain mechanisms: A new theory. Science 150:971–979, 1965.
27. Costa E, Mocchetti I, Supattapone S, et al: Opioid peptide biosynthesis: Enzymatic selectivity and regulatory mechanisms. FASEB J 1:16–21, 1987.
28. Dixon WR, Viveros, OH, Unsworth CD, et al: Multiple opiate receptors: Functional implications. Fed Proc 44:2851–2862, 1985.
29. Murfin R, Bennett J, and Mayer DJ: The effect of dorsolateral spinal cord (DLF) lesions on analgesia from morphine microinjected into the periaqueductal gray matter (PAG) of the rat. Neurosci Abstr 2:946, 1976.
30. Beitz AJ: The organization of afferent projections to the midbrain periaqueductal gray of the rat. Neuroscience 7:133–159, 1982.
31. Mantyh PW: Forebrain projections to the periaqueductal grey in the monkey with observations in the cat and rat. J Comp Neurol 204:349–363, 1982.
32. Watkins LR and Mayer DJ: Organization of endogenous opiate and nonopiate pain control systems. Science 216:1185–1192, 1982.
33. Sullivan TL and Pert A: Analgesic activity of non-opiate neuropeptides following injections into the rat periaqueductal grey matter. Neurosci Abstr 7:504, 1981.

CHAPTER 42

Medical Management of Chronic Pain

Bernard R. Wilcosky, Jr., M.D.

According to the International Association for the Study of Pain (IASP), pain is defined as "an unpleasant sensory and emotional experience associated with actual or potential tissue damage and described in terms of such damage." The existence of pain and suffering has been acknowledged in art and literature from the beginning of recorded history. The rudimentary arts of primitive cultures are replete with depictions of agony. Virtually no language is without one or more words for the entity we generically refer to as pain. Certainly, our individual experiences include some common threads, and failure to identify instantly with terms such as burning, aching, stinging, and throbbing is rare.

Despite this treasure of informal data, it was not until 1978 that an international body of clinical authority, under the auspices of the IASP, derived an operational definition of pain. What led to such incongruity? This seeming inability to define pain in an acceptable way results from long-standing failure to distinguish acute pain from chronic pain. There have been countless trite axioms that attempt to deal with pain. Expressions such as "a certain amount is useful," "pain is the body's message," and so on have become a part of medical folklore and, although lacking in science, may serve to describe the pain response such as that experienced after acute injury or in the immediate postoperative period. It is widely held that pain in these circumstances is a byproduct of injury and healing and serves to facilitate avoidance of further injury. In these acute circumstances, the response is relatively finite and short lived and treated adequately with common approaches to analgesia and graduated rehabilitation. These traditional views, however, fail to recognize the more pressing clinical problem of chronic pain, which may exist long after the "appropriate" healing period and may exist in the absence of definitive or demonstrable defects.

Current thought supports the notion that chronic pain is a separate clinical entity accompanied not only by subjective and objective indications of suffering but most often by psychological, social, and economic dysfunction as well.[1] There can be no doubt that chronic pain and acute pain are by no means interchangeable in presentation, implications, or consequences. For this reason, a crisp definition of the broad entity known as pain has eluded clinical scholars until recently. Even now, that definition leaves much to be desired and should be considered evolutionary. The growth of multidisciplinary interests in chronic pain has been exponential

in the last two to three decades, and these efforts will undoubtedly improve our understanding and treatment methodology in the future. It is to the recognition of chronic pain (either blatant or incipient) by the busy primary care practitioner that this chapter is dedicated. This chapter is written from the perspective of one involved in the fledgling subspecialty of pain management and with the purpose of equipping the busy practitioner with the ability to recognize chronic pain syndrome and to foster familiarity with the basic treatment options.

It should be stated from the outset that, in the context of chronic pain, to declare oneself an expert is a misnomer. Indeed, the world's experience suggests that success in this complex entity is realized best through a multidisciplinary approach. Well-organized facilities require the simultaneous services of anesthesiologists, psychologists, physiatrists, neurologists, neurosurgeons, and physical and occupational therapists. Other specialists such as speech therapists, pharmacists, dietitians, and internists are used frequently as well. Each specialist applies his or her own particular skills. Despite the diverse requirements of a particular patient, efficient coordination of this effort is essential to success.[2] Currently, most treatment facilities are directed by anesthesiologists. The extensive knowledge of pharmacology and nerve blockade renders this specialty particularly suited to this function, and many consider the treatment of chronic pain a logical extension of the basic functions of the anesthesiologist in the operating room.

As the multidisciplinary concept evolves, however, other specialties such as neurology have also stepped into the directorship or coordination role. Outside of one's individual field of expertise, the real requirement for this position is a broad appreciation of available modalities and the judicious use of appropriate consultants.

DIAGNOSIS OF CHRONIC PAIN SYNDROME

As previously stated, chronic pain may develop in the aftermath of more or less appropriate acute pain that results from injury, disease, or surgery. The evolution of chronic pain is observable in this setting because most patients are involved in a continuum of primary care. There have been attempts to delineate a specific temporal relationship between acute and chronic pain. Durations as long as 6 months and as brief as 3 months have been popularized by various authors as signaling the transition from the acute to the chronic pain state. These relationships must, by definition, remain arbitrary and artificial owing to wide interpatient variability.[1] In this specific scenario, a useful clinical guideline is to call on one's range of clinical experience regarding similar cases and generally appropriate periods of healing and rehabilitation. If these parameters are exceeded, the probability of developing chronic pain syndrome (CPS) increases, and the practitioner must be alerted to the concomitant problems that accompany the physical complaints. The history of deterioration along several axes should be actively sought. Specifically, several factors should be explored: Depression, by far, is the most common disorder that accompanies and, in fact, may in large measure define the CPS. It is my belief that, in the vast majority of patients, the depression is reactive and results from deterioration in other areas of function as well as the stress of intractable pain. The vegetative signs of depression, such as early morning awakening, loss of appetite, agitation, or withdrawal should be monitored. On occasion, patients will harbor baseline endogenous depression or even bipolar disorders that are unmasked or worsened by the superimposition of CPS. A history of suicidal ideation should also be sought. Social dysfunction may be manifested both in and outside of the home, and sexual dysfunction is not uncommon. The inability to maintain economic productivity is a major stressor in CPS. Even activities of daily living can be compromised to the extent that feeding, dressing, and bathing, as well as other elements of self-care, present major obstacles for the patient.

Medical dependency is an issue of some controversy today that is addressed in some detail. Suffice it to say that, in a broad sense, basic value systems of many patients are challenged through the necessary use of strong analgesics. Conflict and guilt are the result. It is easy to appreciate from the foregoing how the cyclic nature of CPS may become established. The patient is perpetually occupied in the examination of self-worth, which must subjectively deteriorate in this complex disorder. Once this cycle has become well established, even elimination of the pathophysiologic disorder may not completely restore function.

The recognition of demonstrable disease, past or present, may theoretically facilitate the diagnosis of CPS. At the very least, although a total understanding of ongoing symptoms may be elusive, complaints may be easier to validate.

Unfortunately, in far too many patients, the complaints arise insidiously; even costly extensive evaluations fail to reveal a physical cause, and the patient's credibility is tenuous. Physical signs are extremely helpful in this regard but may not be consistently present. The history may reveal illness or trauma so minor as to have been completely overlooked by the patient. I have attended to several such patients who were later demonstrated to have either sympathetic or somatic pain with appropriate therapeutic responses. The tragedy of this subset of patients lies in the fact that they will all too often percolate in the medical system for months or years, leaving in their wake a considerable list of frustrated and bewildered practitioners of various disciplines. This typical time-consuming sequence of events is characterized by the migration of the patient from one consultant to another, each of whom may exhaust his or her repertoire. Surgery is often performed along the way, based on ordinarily scant

indications, out of desperation. A true distinction between palliative and curative efforts is not universally understood by patients in spite of good intentions, and if procedures are unsuccessful, further uncertainty and confusion result as patients begin to direct blame inwardly for unfavorable responses. The cycle of CPS is once again perpetuated.

Most patients will fall somewhere along the continuum of extremes just depicted, and they will also vary widely with regard to overt expressions of suffering. In fact, worse outcomes are often forthcoming in patients who manifest very little outward expression of distress and may "suffer in silence." Perpetual smiles in the face of consistent complaints may mask spiraling deterioration, even to the point of suicidal ideation. In such patients, an extremely detailed history must be combined with specific inquiries to family, friends, or employers to complete the picture. As the spectrum of the problem is outlined, completeness dictates a brief discussion of yet another distinct subset of patients who suffer from recurrent episodic acute pain. Chronic conditions such as the various arthropathies are specific examples in which exacerbations and remissions are common. Good and often exceptional functional adjustments are the general rule in this population, but, again, developing features of CPS should be periodically monitored. There are some risks of contradiction in the previous statement made regarding the element of time. To clarify, it can be stated that the passage of 3 or even 6 months is not essential to the diagnosis of CPS, because many patients do have florid manifestations in much shorter times. Clinical observations are far more important. Paradoxically, once CPS is recognized, it can be considered a tenet of chronic pain management that outcome is largely dependent on timeliness of intervention. This is generally true regardless of clinical entity, from chronic discogenic back pain to other neuropathic pain states, such as reflex sympathetic dystrophy. The most common pain syndromes seen in the pain treatment setting that involve the foot and ankle occur postoperatively, such as recurrent neuroma and reflex sympathetic dystrophy, and after trauma, such as reflex sympathetic dystrophy and degenerative joint disease.

TREATMENT OF CHRONIC PAIN SYNDROMES

There are some overlaps in modalities used to treat acute and chronic pain. In general, acute pain requires fewer modalities. A useful construct is to view the treatment modalities in several broad categories: (1) cognitive-behavioral, (2) pharmacologic, (3) physical/rehabilitation, (4) neural blockade, (5) surgical/ablative, and (6) palliative technology. It should also be mentioned that, before the initiation of therapy, it is highly advisable that the patient be subjected to a multidisciplinary evaluation. The protocol at my institution (Sequoia Hospital Pain Clinic) presently requires that such an evaluation be performed by the appropriate practitioners after an initial evaluation is done by the primary pain physician, who is usually one of the attending anesthesiologists. Once the data from the evaluations are collected, the individual patient's case is discussed at a patient treatment conference, which is attended by all the respective specialties. At this time, basic conclusions can be drawn, authoritative communication can be made with the referring sources, and an individualized plan can be derived. This plan is then presented to the patient, and the interactive aspects are emphasized, and passive participation is de-emphasized.

Cognitive/Behavioral

Most CPS patients become preoccupied with their pain to the extent that it becomes the central focus of their lives. This seems to be part of the progression in CPS but must be considered maladaptive in that emphasis is placed entirely on negative developments, and reaction to positive developments (e.g., measurable increase in capacity) is absent or attenuated. The patient must be made aware of the destructive nature of this thought process; once this is accomplished, an attempt is made to modify behavior in an effort to shift emphasis to more positive aspects of life.

Coping strategies are often assessed and reinforced if necessary, and energy devoted to self-blame and guilt is redirected. The patient is taught to become an active instrument of self-recovery or improvement rather than a passive recipient of therapeutic efforts. Helplessness is de-emphasized. Family members are often recruited, shifting their role from codependent to therapeutic agent.[3] In susceptible patients, adjuncts to a pure cognitive-behavioral approach include biofeedback, guided imagery, self-hypnosis, and other relaxation techniques. As patients progress through their pain treatment programs, maintenance of cognitive-behavioral skills often becomes the principal mode of therapy.

Pharmacologic Therapy

It is rare to treat a chronic pain patient who is not now or has not in the past been availed of multiple-pharmacologic agents. Analgesics, both narcotic and non-narcotic, constitute the most common form of pain treatment. When placed into context with other modalities and not relied on solely, they continue to occupy a key berth in the chronic pain armamentarium. Useful drugs can be functionally divided into (1) narcotic, (2) non-narcotic, (3) anticonvulsants, (4) psychotropic, and (5) antidepressants.

Non-Narcotic Analgesics. Acetaminophen and its metabolites (e.g., phenacetin) are perhaps the most widely used non-narcotic analgesics in this country. Acetaminophen is considered to be as effective an analgesic as aspirin for mild to moderate pain. Although general agreement on a peripheral mechanism of analgesia is widely held, traditional thought ascribes an antipyretic but not an antiinflammatory role to the compound. Some recent studies in dental surgery have challenged this belief, and efficacy at reduction of postoperative edema was equal to that of nonsteroidal antiinflammatory drugs (NSAIDs). It has advantages over NSAIDs in that no inherent gastrointestinal irritation is observed. There is also no effect on platelet function. Hepatic toxicity is possible owing to its metabolism, but few cases have been recorded. It appears that for doses within the recommended clinical range of 650 to 1000 mg every 4 to 6 hours, toxicity is unlikely. However, patients with a compromise in hepatic function should be treated with a reduced dosage or the drug avoided altogether if a therapeutic effect is not forthcoming at smaller doses. Conversely, it is ideally suited for patients who cannot tolerate the gastrointestinal effects of NSAIDs or for patients with thrombocytopenia or other coagulopathies.

NSAIDs. Another useful and widely prescribed class of non-narcotic analgesics is the NSAIDs. Although acting peripherally, the mechanism of action is more fully understood than that of acetaminophen. These drugs inhibit the synthetic pathway of prostaglandins, which are essential to both the inflammatory response and the chemical mediation of peripheral nociception. It is an extremely important point in that a decrease in inflammation may result in analgesia. However, analgesia can be achieved in the absence of frank inflammation. Owing to the importance of prostaglandins to coagulation, gastrointestinal integrity, and renal function, the major side effects are now described. Bone marrow suppression is rare but also reported. Patient selection and careful monitoring can minimize the clinical consequences of these side effects. Generally, the elderly are at greater risk for all side effects, and thoughtful application is essential in this population.

The development of gastrointestinal symptoms does not inevitably lead to catastrophic outcomes, and these effects can be controlled in many cases through the use of particulate antacids, H_2 blockers such as cimetidine, and several recently introduced agents that act directly to reinforce the integrity of the gastric mucosa, such as sucralfate, misoprostol, or omeprazole. The basic principle of the use of these drugs to treat side effects is a clinical decision based on the individual risk-to-benefit scenario.

Aspirin is the prototype of NSAIDs. However, the list of available drugs in this category grows yearly, and all with claims of advantages in either efficacy, side effects, or both. Aspirin differs from other NSAIDs in that effects on platelet function are irreversible for the life of affected platelets, whereas other NSAIDs have transient effects. The pharmacokinetics of aspirin will allow a 4- to 6-hour dosing interval, depending on dosage; a longer interval requires a higher dose. A ceiling effect for analgesia is reported, but the absolute dose is disputed. A dose range of 650 to 1000 mg every 4 to 6 hours, with a maximum dose of 4 gr per day, should provide analgesia in patients who respond with an acceptable side effect profile. Two side effects peculiar to aspirin deserve particular mention. Salicylism is characterized by tinnitus, hearing loss, headache, dizziness, confusion, and nausea, alone or in combination. Aspirin-sensitive asthma is also reported; therefore, caution is indicated in asthmatic patients.

A complete treatise on all the other NSAIDs is well beyond the scope of this chapter, so only practical guidelines are emphasized. Common oversights, in my opinion, include a failure to ensure around-the-clock dosing compliance and abandoning the entire class of drugs based on an unsuccessful trial with a single agent. If tolerated from a standpoint of side effects, a trial should continue for at least 2 weeks. The search for a drug with efficacy and acceptable side effects may require several alternate trials. Although NSAIDs are alike in mechanism of action, several distinct chemical families are represented, and it seems reasonable to alternate chemical families rather than change to a drug with a similar chemical make-up. Salicylates include, in addition to aspirin, diflunisal, disalcid, and choline magnesium trisalicylate (Trilisate). The last has the unique property of minimal gastrointestinal irritation and no appreciable effect on platelet function as measured by bleeding time. It is, therefore, extremely useful with the elderly and patients with platelet dysfunction. The proprionic acid derivatives are represented by ibuprofen, naproxen, and their relatives. This group should be avoided in patients taking anticonvulsants or warfarin derivatives, because their metabolism is inhibited, and excessive levels may result.

Indole derivatives include sulindac and indomethacin. Sulindac has a lower incidence of renal dysfunction among the NSAIDs and may be preferred in the elderly for that reason alone. Also, the indoles do not inhibit warfarin metabolism.

The oxicam family is represented by piroxicam. The primary advantage is a long plasma half-life, which allows a single dose per day and, thus, better potential compliance.

The phenylacetic acid diclofenac has been used extensively in Europe for several years with an impressive record of efficacy in the various arthropathies. Although it has only recently been introduced in the United States, it is gaining favor in similar patient populations.

The injectable NSAID ketorolac represents a revolutionary development with analgesic efficacy that compares favorably with morphine or meperidine for postoperative pain with greater duration of action. It is also available in oral form, but advantages over other NSAIDs have not been convincingly demonstrated, and prolonged usage is prohibitive because of gastrointestinal side effects.

The use of NSAIDs for chronic pain cannot be supported by well-controlled studies at this time; however, because analgesic efficacy in patients is comparable to that of narcotics, their trial application in difficult chronic pain patients makes good empiric sense.[4–6]

Narcotics. The opiates, by far, are the oldest group of analgesic agents, and their use has been documented since the beginning of recorded history. The discovery of specific opiate receptors and the existence of endogenous opiate-like substances in the last 30 years has shed much light on their mechanism of action. These opiate-specific receptors have been identified in the brain and spinal cord, and, although evidence is inconclusive, receptors may also be present in peripheral nerves. Additionally, several subpopulations of opiate receptors have been identified, each of which has a unique profile of physiologic effects in the presence of a specific agonist. The μ receptor is believed to be the primary site of action of most opiates in clinical use today. Classic effects, in addition to analgesia, include euphoria, meiosis, respiratory depression, sedation, and so on. The precise relative magnitude of effects will vary with the neural anatomic location of the receptors; the broadest range of effects is mediated by μ receptors in the brain stem. The presence of receptors in the spinal cord makes possible specific targeting for segmental analgesia with a lesser side effect profile.

The role of the opiates in the treatment of acute pain (e.g., postoperative) is undisputed, although current data indicate that these agents are underused to the detriment of patients. Their role in the treatment of chronic pain is now a hotly debated issue, because therapeutic nihilists opine against more liberal and pragmatic forces. Evidence is rapidly gathering that refutes traditional ideas, especially regarding the touted high risks of addiction. These risks appear to be minimal in a fairly broad chronic pain population. Great strides have been made in the malignant pain population; consequently, fewer cancer patients die in pain. Exactly how rapidly clinical practice will change based on these new data remains to be seen. There appears, however, to be a very select chronic pain population who have failed all other reasonable means of pain control and for whom the chronic use of narcotics, under strictly controlled circumstances, results in a greater level of function and better quality of life. It

seems most reasonable, however, that if chronic narcotic therapy is chosen, every effort should be made to use drugs such as methadone or a slow-release morphine formulation so that plasma levels remain relatively constant and episodes of uncontrolled breakthrough pain are minimized. Some patients may not have acceptable side effects with this strategy, and shorter-acting agents may be required. However, in my opinion, regular dosing schedules with a long-acting agent should be the goal. In this regard, several states, including California, have enacted legislation to permit the compassionate use of opiates without strict limitations to the terminally ill. These measures may remove some of the obstacles to practical application of these valuable drugs on the basis of physician fears of prosecution. Some of the time-honored medical folklore embracing the issues of toxicity and addiction will be slow to fade, however.

The criteria used at my institution include but are not limited to the failure of all other reasonable and suitable therapies in a multidisciplinary environment, a written, contractual agreement wherein the patient agrees to the program structure, the ability to establish a stable dosage regimen, and, in most cases, a clear demonstration that function and quality of life are enhanced by the therapy. It can be readily appreciated that this is a highly selective therapeutic modality.

Although the prescription of narcotics for the treatment of chronic pain should be in the armamentarium of most primary care physicians, it is probably not advised for the consulting subspecialist primarily because of the relatively frequent follow-up and monitoring that are required for success.

Constipation is, by far, the most common side effect of narcotic therapy and can usually be managed by prophylactic and concurrent use of bulk-forming laxatives. Nausea may resolve with time or be managed by addition of antiemetics. Urinary retention may also be treated with cholinergics. Clearly, if multiple side effects require a polypharmaceutical offset, the propriety of continued narcotic therapy should be re-examined on the basis of a critical risk-to-benefit analysis.[6–10]

Anticonvulsants. The benefits of electrochemical stabilizing effects of the anticonvulsants have been extrapolated over the years to various pain states. Neuropathic pain is, by far, the most responsive. The classic example is the treatment of trigeminal neuralgia with carbamazepine. This drug, along with the alternative hydantoin, constitutes primary treatment for the painful neuropathic disorders, supplanting more invasive and often unsuccessful procedures commonly performed in the past. Characteristics of neuropathic pain that respond to anticonvulsants include shocklike dysesthesias and, to a lesser extent, burning hyperesthesia. The former may represent the peripheral analogue of seizure activity. Overall, hydantoin appears to be the best tolerated, but carbamazepine seems to be the most effective, although with more prominent side effects such as bone marrow suppression and hepatic dysfunction. Consequently, periodic monitoring is required. Valproic acid and clonazepam have also been used, especially when intolerance to the others is demonstrated. Suffice it to say that, under appropriate circumstances, these drugs are extremely beneficial and are often used in combination with other drugs, such as NSAID, antidepressant, or narcotic, in an attempt to address various components of the pain syndrome separately.[11–13]

Antidepressants. There is a great volume of literature to support the use of antidepressants in chronic pain patients. Many are clinically depressed, and therapeutic application is straightforward. However, it has been recognized that low-dose administration of the tricyclic antidepressants (TCAs) seems to benefit nondepressed chronic pain patients as well. Antidepressants regulate the levels of biogenic amines (norepinephrine, dopamine, serotonin, L-dopa) in the limbic system. These substances play a key role in pain modulation and emotional perception. This results in the so-called descending inhibition. Specifically, the TCAs increase the levels of serotonin in the limbic systems, thereby reducing pain perception, increasing the pain threshold, and improving sleep. Amitriptyline is, by far, the most studied of the TCAs. Of all the TCAs, amitriptyline has a relatively greater differential effect on serotonin, and it is attractive to conclude that this facet of drug action alone is responsible for analgesia. However, other tricyclics such as nortriptyline, doxepin, and desipramine are often effective as well, whereas their effects on serotonin are relatively weaker. Further, newer non-TCAs such as fluoxetine are selective for serotonin, yet their efficacy as analgesics has not been convincingly demonstrated. Given these observations, it is probable that if an analgesic effect can be attributed to antidepressants, it must reflect the fact that other biogenic amines are also involved.

The relative effect of this class of drugs on central neural transmitters is also responsible for considerable side effects. Relative cholinergic inhibition mediates dry mouth, blurred vision, urinary retention, constipation, and arrhythmias, and, at common analgesic dosages, these are the most troublesome and will often prompt therapy to be discontinued. It is also believed to be prudent, in this event to use an alternate drug. This rationale is similar to the one outlined for the NSAIDs. The burning hypersensitivity of neuropathic pain syndrome seems to respond best to antidepressants. It should be mentioned that analgesic dosage is usually less than that for depression, and typically, amitriptyline at 100 mg or less as a single nighttime dose is effective compared with 200 mg or more for the usual treatment of depression.[13] Many neuropathic pain syndromes such as traumatic peripheral nerve injuries, postherpetic neuralgia, and several metabolic neuropathies have been shown to respond to combinations of TCAs and either anticonvulsants or phenothiazines.

Psychotropics. This class of drugs is mentioned only briefly, because their usage in chronic pain treatment is not widespread. When used alone, there is not apparent analgesia. However, in combination with TCAs or narcotics, a synergism can often be appreciated. Antiemetic effects are often useful as well and may determine the practicality of these other agents in a given patient. Fluphenazine and promethazine are most often used. Mechanism of action probably involves blockade of norepinephrine. Theoretically, it appears rational to combine a phenothiazine for norepinephrine blockage and a TCA, which raises serotonin levels. In fact, it is observed that this combination is particularly effective regarding neuropathic pain. Side effects limit their use in many patients.[11, 12]

Benzodiazepines. This classification is mentioned only to discourage their use in chronic pain patients. Drug-induced depression is common, as is true psychological dependency. Occasionally, a patient will respond well to anticonvulsants but will tolerate only clonazepam. The dosages should be carefully titrated and single nighttime dosage is possible.[11, 12]

Physical/Rehabilitative

As stated, a decrement in function often accompanies CPS. In the eyes of colleagues and family members, patient suffering is often overshadowed by the obvious lack of function, because the latter is tangible and measurable and has the most direct impact on the lives of others. Central to physical dysfunction is generalized deconditioning and progressive weight gain. After long periods of inactivity because of pain, efforts to increase activity, even with good pain control, are met with lack of stamina, stiffness, soreness, and possible microinjury to selected muscle groups. Even in the absence of improvements in pain control, a good progressive and challenging physical therapy program will foster functional improvement. For this reason, physical therapy must be part of a contemporary pain treatment program. Energy spent to provide analgesia may be supporting only vegetation unless physical demands are also increased. These basic concepts must be understood by the patient and frequently reinforced by the pain treatment team because a hypokinetic profile is common.

Therapy must be well supervised and modalities de-emphasized and used only as rewards after efforts are demonstrated by the patient. Duration of therapy is important and may range from 2 to 6 months or longer to demonstrate good conditioning effect.

Occupational therapists can be used to great advantage, through the critique of patient activities and even the work place, with an eye toward modification in techniques and facilities. Often simple devices such as shower seats or reach-extension appliances can make a difference in both independent function and self-esteem.

Therapeutic massage in various forms, acupuncture, and chiropractic manipulation all have been used with varying success rates in chronic pain management. These respective effects appear transient, and mechanisms are not delineated. It is my considered opinion that the use of these modalities should satisfy the patient's need to try them; in this regard, an open mind is essential. Strict time limits should be set, however, beyond which continuance should be discouraged if results are not forthcoming.

Both the Greeks and the Romans observed that placement of electrical fish to painful areas resulted in analgesia. The modern extension involves the use of transcutaneous electrical nerve stimulation (TENS) devices. Efficacy has been demonstrated in various chronic pain states, postoperative pain, and obstetric pain. Electrodes must often be placed astride the painful areas and variations in rate, amplitude, and pulse width must be frequently made before the technique can be fully evaluated. Sensitivity to electrode pads should prompt a trial of alternate adhesives. The proposed mechanisms of action include local sympatholysis with improved microcirculation, manipulation of nociception at the spinal cord level, and, finally, augmented release of endogenous opiates. The latter appears least likely because the analgesia is not uniformly antagonized by naloxone. Because TENS is noninvasive, reversible, and involves no drugs, it should be tried early on in most chronic pain patients.[14]

Neural Blockade

Blockade of peripheral nerves or the central neural axis constitutes one of the oldest forms of pain management. In modern practice, neural blockade is diagnostic, therapeutic, or neurolytic.

Diagnostic nerve blocks help to delineate the mechanism of pain. In sympathetically maintained pain syndromes such as reflex sympathetic dystrophy, selective blockade of sympathetic outflow aids in the diagnosis, helps to form therapeutic decisions, and may, in and of itself, result in long-term therapeutic effect. When the pain mechanism is a clinical enigma, a differential block can be used via the spinal or epidural route. A catheter is commonly placed, and serial injections are made to include placebo and various concentrations of local anesthetics and, often today, narcotics. Sympathetic pain responds characteristically to low concentrations of local anesthetics, usually below that which results in frank sensory block. On the opposite end of the spectrum, frank sensory blockade should eliminate the peripheral sources of pain to include those emanating from the spinal cord. If profound sensory and motor blockade fails to relieve pain in the desired distribution, a central mechanism of pain is suggested and, more importantly, further extensive efforts directed at peripheral ablation will likely fail. If a peripheral or sympathetic mechanism is demonstrated, serial or continuous blockade is commonly used. Frequent interruption of the pain will often result in marked improvement when the blocks are discontinued.

Epidural or peripheral nerve blocks with corticosteroids and local anesthetics are frequently used to provide intermediate-term relief of pain, during which rehabilitation efforts can be intensified. Finally, neurolytic nerve blocks with phenol or alcohol can be accomplished. However, relief is seldom permanent, and postneurolytic pain may be more intense than the original symptoms. For this reason, neurolytic nerve blocks are usually reserved for terminally ill patients in whom intermediate duration is more appropriate to life expectancy.

Surgical Therapy

Surgical techniques in chronic pain treatment are also directed at lysis or attenuation of nerve supplies. Surgical sympathectomy is appropriate when positive responses to sympathetic blockade with local anesthetic are consistently demonstrated. Overall, frank causalgia, which involves major peripheral nerve injury, responds with good long-term results after surgical sympathectomy. Other sympathetically maintained pain syndromes respond less consistently, and symptom recurrence is observed. It is attractive to implicate regeneration as the culprit, but recent evidence for bilateral innervation or some crossover innervation seems more plausible.

As with chemical neurolysis, surgical neurolysis is fraught with potential complications such as neuroma formation, denervation hypersensitivity, causalgia, and postprocedure neuralgia. These may be late in developing. Thus, as tempting as it may seem to just kill the nerve, it is clearly not that simple and should be reserved for only the most refractory cases. Intracranial neurolytic procedures such as cingulotomy are possible but are reserved only for the terminally ill.

Newer Palliative Technology

In recent years, practitioners devoted to chronic pain treatment have increasingly recognized that, despite the most sophisticated diagnostic and therapeutic efforts, the source of pain is often not amenable to definitive therapy. Such patients were formerly doomed to lives of unremitting suffering and dysfunction. The last two decades have witnessed the development of two technologies—spinal cord stimulation and spinal opiates—that have furthered palliative efforts.

Spinal Cord Stimulation. Spinal cord stimulation involves the placement of a linear electrode array into the epidural space to produce mild electrical stimulation superimposed on the patient's pain distribution. It is experienced as a gentle paresthesia and is described by most patients as pleasant. The procedure is usually accomplished in two stages. Initially, a trial is conducted wherein an electrode is placed under fluoroscopic guidance with local anesthesia and mild sedation. When stimulation in the proper distribution is ascertained, the electrode is secured, and temporary percutaneous wires are attached. The trial is usually conducted over several days during which manipulation of electrode activation, amplitude, pulse width, and rates are made. The goal is 50% or greater relief of pain, and if this is achieved, a permanent implant is recommended. Depending on the particular patient requirements, the battery/transmitter may be totally implanted, or a receiver may be implanted and an external antenna and transmitter used. Considerations for success include technical ability to superimpose stimulation in the pain distribution, whether stimulation is tolerable to the patient, and whether stimulation results in pain relief. The mechanism is probably descending inhibition of peripheral pain impulses at the spinal cord "gate." A sympathetic mechanism is also suggested by the near-uniform increase in blood flow and temperature in the stimulation distribution. The primary indications are peripheral vascular disease, neuropathic pain syndromes such as postherpetic neuralgia, sympathetically maintained pain, adhesive arachnoiditis, and diabetic and other neuropathies. With careful patient screening in a multidisciplinary setting, success rates are greater than 70%. Although neurosystems are very stable after implant, some activity limitations are necessary. Practically speaking, most candidates are so markedly dysfunctional at baseline that resultant activity levels are vast improvements. Unilateral extremity pain is most responsive with bilateral pain less so. When percutaneous access to the epidural space is prohibited (e.g., prior surgery), surgical placement via laminotomy is possible. Deep brain stimulation is a possible variation but has obvious greater clinical implications.[15]

Spinal Opiates. The injection of opiates epidurally or intrathecally has become common practice today on the basis of the discovery of specific opiate receptor families in the spinal cord. The analgesia produced is therefore segmental. The primary advantage over oral or parenteral opiate therapy is a most intense analgesia, at $\frac{1}{10}$ to $\frac{1}{100}$ of the standard doses by more conventional routes. Most side effects are similar to standard routes but are markedly less with lipid-soluble agents such as fentanyl and sufentanil. Spinal opiates are most commonly used for postoperative pain. These techniques are becoming increasingly used for the treatment of refractory pain in terminally ill cancer patients. More recently, spinal opiates have been applied to the chronic benign pain syndromes, such as postlaminectomy syndrome and sympathetically maintained pain syndromes. For short- or intermediate-term use, from days to approximately 3 months, the epidural route is preferred with either a direct percutaneous or implanted catheter with subcutaneous port. Continuous infusion is most efficient, but periodic injection can be used. It is generally agreed by most practitioners that, for long-term use, the intrathecal route is preferred, and because of the risk of infection, a fully implanted pump reservoir is also preferred. Depending on the individual requirements, the pump may be fully programmable, and refills may be required every 3 to 5 weeks. Morphine is the most commonly used opiate, but most others have been used as well.[16]

Both spinal opiates and spinal cord stimulation are costly techniques. With proper patient selection, including a favorable psychological profile and good patient acceptance, the cost effectiveness of spinal opiates and spinal cord stimulation, when compared with long-term repeated acute pain management (e.g., hospital admission, emergency room visits), can be demonstrated. Several series now show continued effectiveness beyond 5 years. Once the decision is made to proceed with these palliative technologies, most practitioners recommend a trial of spinal cord stimulation, if possible, before considering spinal opiates, because the former has few associated side effects and potential complications.

References

1. Bonica JJ: The Management of Pain. New York, Lea & Febiger, 1990.
2. Aronoff GM: Evaluation and Management of Chronic Pain. Baltimore, Williams & Wilkins, 1992.
3. Spinhoven P and Linsen CJ: Behavioral treatment of chronic low back pain: #1 relation of coping strategy use to outcome. Pain 45:29–34, 1991.
4. Dewson DD and Mather IE: Non-steroidal anti-inflammatory agents. *In* Rajj PP (ed): Practical Management of Pain. Chicago, Year Book Medical Publishers, 1986, pp 523–524.
5. Flower RJ, Moncada S, and Vane JR: Analgesic antipyretic and anti-inflammatory agents: Drugs employed in the treatment of gout. *In* Gilman AG and Goodman LS (eds): The Pharmacological Basis of Therapeutics, 6th ed. New York, Macmillan, 1980.
6. Halpern LM: Analgesic and anti-inflammatory medications. *In* Tolison DC (ed): Handbook of Chronic Pain Management. Baltimore, Williams & Wilkins, 1989, pp 54–68.
7. Portenoy RK: Chronic opioid therapy in non-malignant pain. J Pain Symptom Management 4(Suppl):46–61, 1990.
8. Portenoy RK: Chronic opioid therapy for persistent non-cancer pain: Can we get past the bias? APS Bull 1(2):1,4–5, 1991.
9. Portenoy RK: Chronic opioid therapy in non-malignant pain. J Pain Symptom Management 5(Suppl):S46–S62, 1991.
10. Portenoy RK and Foley KM: Chronic use of opioid analgesics in non-malignant pain: Report of 38 cases. Pain 25:179–186, 1986.
11. Oxman T and Denson DD: Antidepressants and adjunctive psychotropic drugs. *In* Raj PP (ed): Practical Management of Pain. Chicago, Year Book Medical Publishers, 1988, pp 528–538.
12. Atkinson JH: Psychopharmologic agents in the treatment of pain syndromes. *In* Tollison DC (ed): Handbook of Chronic Pain Management, Baltimore, Williams & Wilkins, 1989, pp 69–103.
13. Aronoff GM and Evans WO: Pharmological management of chronic pain: A review. *In* Aronoff GM (ed): Evaluation and Treatment of Chronic Pain. Baltimore, Williams & Wilkins, 1987, pp 358–368.
14. Roesch R and Ulrich DE: Physical therapy management in the treatment of chronic pain. Phys Ther 1:53–57, 1980.
15. Kumar K and Wyant GM: Epidural spinal cord stimulation for relief of chronic pain. Pain Clin 12:91–99, 1986.
16. Penn RD and Paice JA: Chronic intrathecal morphine for intractable pain. J Neurosurg 67:182–186, 1987.

CHAPTER 43

Surgical Treatment of Peripheral Nerve Entrapment Syndromes

Michael S. Downey, D.P.M.

Nerve entrapments in the lower extremity are common. Although frequently overlooked and misdiagnosed, these entrapment neuropathies can be painful, unrelenting, and mentally and physically disabling for the patient. Similarly, the literature shows that medicine only recently has begun to identify the prevalence and nature of these lower extremity neuropathies. As Joplin stated more than 20 years ago when discussing nerve problems:

> A rare opportunity awaits the young surgeon who is interested in foot problems, because in this special field, which remains almost unexplored, he has a chance to exert his ingenuity as in no other branch of surgery that I know of today. There are patients everywhere waiting to be treated, and twice as many feet as there are people.[1]

This chapter explores the current status of the most common peripheral nerve entrapments of the lower extremity, including my currently preferred surgical approaches for their treatment.

CLINICAL PRESENTATION AND DIAGNOSIS

Subjective Findings

Kopell and Thompson[2] concisely described classic entrapment neuropathy as "a region of localized injury and inflammation in a peripheral nerve that is caused by mechanical inflammation from some impinging anatomic neighbor." Because accurate diagnosis is the first step in proper management of this clinical quagmire, a thorough history, including the nature, location, duration, onset, course, aggravating factors, and previous treatment of the patient's condition, should be investigated in detail.

Generally, sensory abnormalities predominate over motor dysfunction. A patient with an entrapment neuropathy typically complains of paresthesias, including sharp, shooting, or burning types of pain. Patients verbalize this discomfort in their own terms, often referring to the pain as "electric shocks," "a hot poker," "lightning bolts," or other similar depiction. This can usually be differentiated from dull or throbbing pain, as is typically associated with motor problems, mechanical problems, arthralgias, or other non-neuritic inflammatory processes. Only later in the course of an entrapment neuropathy will the discomfort become more dull or muscular in nature.

In most instances, the pain is localized to the anatomic distribution of the specific injured nerve or nerves (Fig. 43–1). The onset and duration of the pain may provide clues to the diagnosis, especially if a history of prior trauma or surgery is elicited. The resolution or progression of the pain varies widely but in many instances is described as "unrelenting" or "constant." Frequently, the pain is present or even increased with inactivity or rest and is worse at night. Temperature extremes may also exacerbate the symptoms. The clinician may quantitate the patient's perceived level of pain by asking him or her to grade it. This may be done on a simple scale of 1 to 10 (10 being the worst). Such subjective grading can be repeated later to assess the patient's envisioned improvement.

Further, evaluation of previous treatment can be enlightening. Often, the patient will have seen a multitude of physicians of varying specialties and will have had a similarly sizable list of diagnoses and treatments, with minimal to no improvement or relief. Occasionally, the patient will have been told that there is no organic cause for the pain and will have been left with the impression from previous physicians, and many times from his or her own family, that "the pain is all in my head." The patient may further express his or her mental distress and frustration by making broad, irrational statements such as "I have tried everything to relieve the pain," or "Please, just cut the foot off." The astute clinician must avoid the pitfall of joining the "bandwagon" of previous diagnoses and, in a reassuring manner, reassess the patient carefully.

Objective Findings

Objectively, the properly performed neurologic examination provides the best chance for a specific diagnostic answer. The key to the diagnosis of entrapment neuropathy is the isolation of the neuropathy to a specific nerve or nerves. In entrapment neuropathy, the stimulus intensity required to elicit a response from a specific nerve is altered. In early entrapment syndromes, a hyperesthetic or hypersensitive response is usually present. Later in the course of the nerve compression, the threshold may increase so that a greater

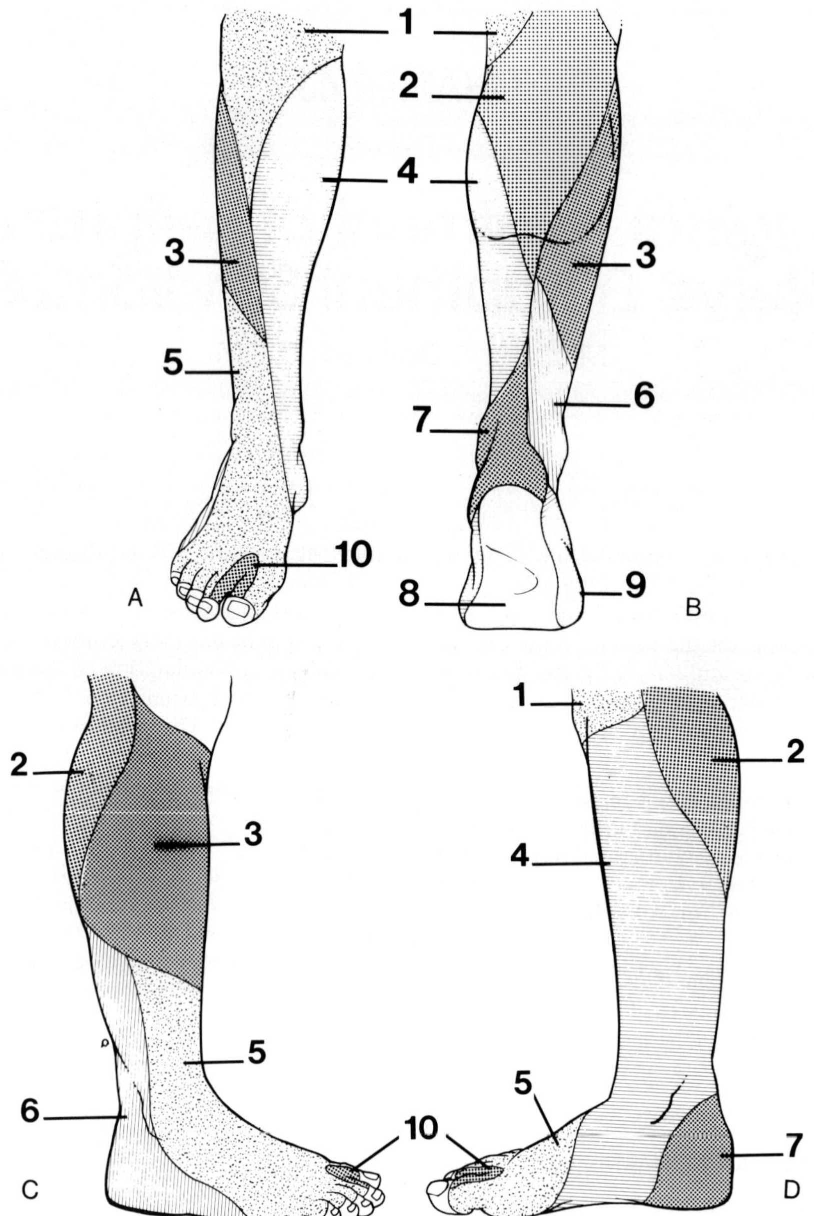

FIGURE 43–1. Anatomic sensory distribution of peripheral nerves. *A,* Anterior. *B,* Posterior. *C,* Lateral. *D,* Medial.

stimulus intensity is necessary to create the same response, resulting in hypoesthesia. Further, autonomic or trophic changes may be seen anytime, and motor changes may be seen later in the course of entrapment disorders. The clinical examination should include evaluation of the central, autonomic, and peripheral sensorimotor nervous systems. The peripheral portion of the examination should include observation, palpation, sensibility testing, reflex examination, and skeletal motor testing. Occasionally, diagnostic nerve blocks, electrodiagnosis, or advanced imaging techniques are indicated to help support or confirm the diagnosis.

Observation. The examination should begin with an inspection for any muscle atrophy, surgical cicatrices, or trophic changes. Muscle atrophy may signify damage or en-

trapment of a motor nerve or may be secondary to disuse. Surgical scars may belie an underlying nerve entrapment. Trophic changes, including ulceration, vasospasm, cyanosis, xerosis, hyperhidrosis or hypohidrosis, and increased or decreased hair or nail growth may signal autonomic nervous system dysfunction as a component of the entrapment neuropathy.

Palpation. Before external nerve manipulation, one may ask the patient to sketch or map his or her area of dysesthesia. In the office, a skin marker may be given to the patient to outline the area involved (Fig. 43–2). This may provide clues as to the specific nerve(s) involved.

Because identification of the specific nerve or nerves entrapped is the key to the diagnosis, palpation or percussion

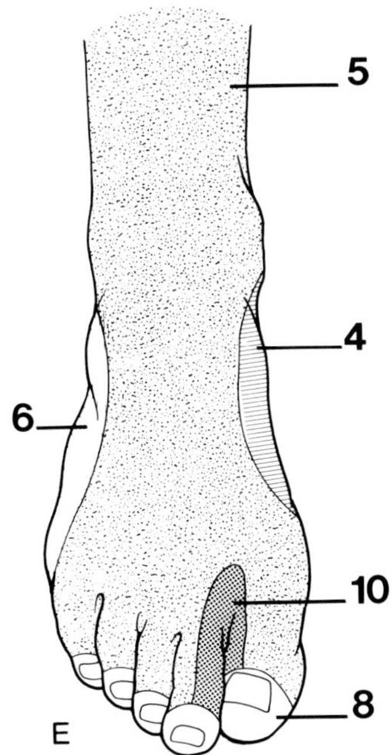
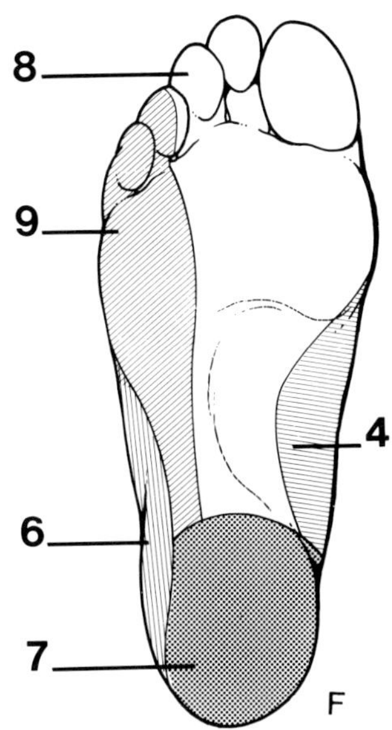

FIGURE 43–1 *Continued E,* Dorsal. *F,* Plantar. 1, Medial and intermediate femoral cutaneous nerves (L2, 3). 2, Posterior femoral cutaneous nerve (S1, 2, 3). 3, Lateral sural cutaneous nerve (L5; S1, 2). 4, Saphenous nerve (L3, 4). 5, Superficial peroneal nerve (L4, 5; S1). 6, Sural nerve (L5; S1, 2). 7, Medial calcaneal nerve branch (S1, 2). 8, Medial plantar nerve (L4, 5). 9, Lateral plantar nerve (S1, 2). 10, Deep peroneal nerve (L4, 5).

of the nerve at the suspected point of entrapment is an important diagnostic maneuver. With percussion of an injured or recovering nerve, distal tingling or paresthesias over the sensory distribution of the nerve and its terminal branches may result (see Fig. 43–1). This is Tinel's sign and is usually present except in the earliest and latest stages of a localized acquired neuropathy.

Valleix's points, or points of tenderness to pressure, may be noted along the entire course of an injured nerve. Some authors have described Valleix's sign, or phenomenon, to mean a proximal radiation of pain and paresthesias along a nerve's distribution with direct percussion at the site of suspected entrapment.[3]

Sensibility Testing. The distribution and degree of sensory aberration can be subjectively quantitated or qualitated, or both, with sensibility testing. Sensibility testing can help differentiate a peripheral nerve entrapment from lumbosacral radiculopathy. If the distribution of sensibility alteration corresponds with specific dermatomes, a spinal root impingement is suggested. The distribution of altered sensation in a local, acquired neuropathy should parallel specific peripheral nerves.[4] Whenever sensibility testing is performed, comparison should be done to the corresponding area of the contralateral, uninjured extremity when possible. The typical peripheral sensory nerve comprises three major subpopulations of fibers: type A-β, type A-δ, and type C. These fiber groups mediate different sensory stimuli.

Type A-β fibers are large, myelinated, conduct rapidly, and are sensitive to light touch and pressure. Light touch and pressure can be evaluated but are hard to quantitate. In 1922, von Frey made the first attempt to standardize the subjective sense of light touch. He accomplished this by using horse

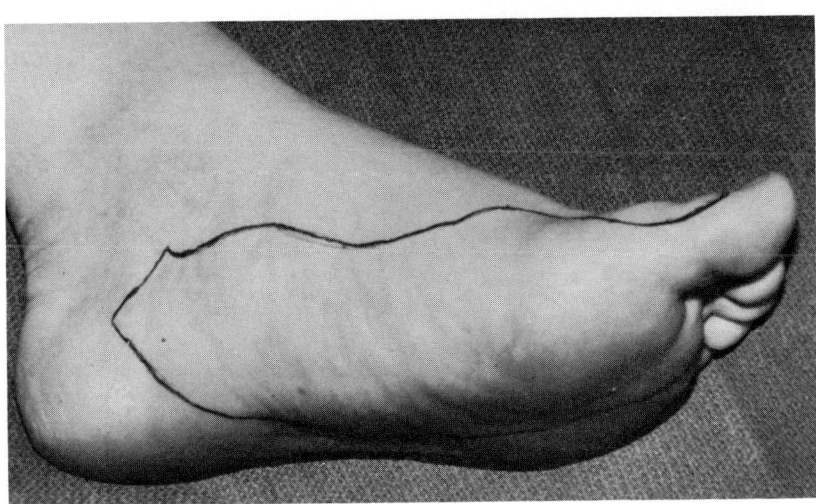

FIGURE 43–2. Area of dysesthesia as outlined by the patient with a skin marker. Note that the patient has unknowingly outlined the sensory distribution of the medial plantar nerve. This nerve was found to be compressed by a large plantar tumor.

hairs of varying stiffness and thickness. More recently, Weinstein and Semmes developed a similar evaluation tool consisting of monofilament nylon fibers of varying thickness mounted in individual lucite rods. The Weinstein-Semmes esthesiometer can be used to quantitatively measure peripheral nerve degeneration and regeneration thresholds of the slowly adapting nerve fiber system (Fig. 43–3).[5]

Type A-δ fibers are also myelinated but are smaller, slower conducting, and are sensitive to vibration. An increased sensitivity to vibration can be an early sign of nerve degeneration. However, with time, the sensitivity to vibratory stimulation decreases. A set of tuning forks with various frequencies (i.e., cycles per second) allows testing of different end organs.[5] Alternatively, if available, a vibrometer may be used to quantitate vibratory sensation.[6] Vibration perception quantitatively measures the cutaneous threshold of the quickly adapting nerve fiber system.

Type C fibers are unmyelinated, very small, very slow conducting, and are sensitive to pain and temperature. Sharp-dull or pain distinction can be easily assessed with a simple pin, sharp on one end and dull on the other. Diminished ability to differentiate between sharp and dull stimuli can indicate a nerve entrapment.[5] Hot-cold sensation can also be tested. However, many patients demonstrate hypersensitivity and intolerance to these temperature extremes. Further, appropriate equipment with calibrated thermometers is required, and this is cumbersome.

More recently, devices that allow current perception threshold testing (CPT), such as the Neurometer CPT (Neurotron, Inc., Baltimore, MD), have become available. By varying the frequency of electrical stimulation, these devices allow quantitative measurement of the three nerve fiber subgroups. Thus, the devices can evaluate and quantify both early and late entrapment neuropathy. The primary disadvantages of these devices are their cost and the time required to perform a complete lower extremity sensory examination.

With more prolonged nerve entrapment or compression, and eventual loss of nerve fibers due to wallerian degeneration, a diminished number of fibers innervate the nerve's sensory distribution. This decreased innervation density can be quantitatively measured by two-point discrimination testing. The classic Weber static two-point discrimination test is useful for assessing the innervation density of the slowly adapting fiber system and the Dellon moving two-point discrimination test for the quickly adapting nerve fiber system.[7] The instrument for two-point discrimination can be a Boley gauge, two pins, an ordinary paper clip, or an instrument specifically designed for the test (Fig. 43–4). At the knee, two-point discrimination is diminished if lost at a distance of 50 to 80 mm.[8] In the hallux, normal two-point discrimination is 5 to 8 mm.[9]

Local changes in the sympathetic nervous system also can be present. These may include (1) vasomotor changes (abnormal skin color, generally purplish or mottled); (2) pilomotor changes (loss of the piloerection response); (3) trophic changes (variations in skin texture and turgor, delayed dermal healing, slow hair and nail growth, and atrophy or tapering of the digits); and (4) sudomotor changes (altered sweat production, either increased or decreased). Many of these changes can be evaluated objectively, and unlike the other sensibility tests, the responses are involuntary.[5]

Early nerve entrapment or compression is best assessed by the tests for cutaneous pressure threshold (Weinstein-Semmes monofilaments) and cutaneous vibratory threshold (tuning fork or vibrometer). Static and moving two-point discrimination more accurately evaluate a moderate to late entrapment neuropathy (Table 43–1).

Reflex Examination and Skeletal Motor Testing. Deep tendon reflexes and cutaneous reflexes, such as the Babinski reflex, should be evaluated in every patient with a suspected neurologic problem. The patellar tendon reflex corresponds to spinal levels L2, L3, and L4, whereas the Achilles tendon reflex corresponds to spinal levels S1 and S2. If there is an upper motor neuron lesion, or if the spinal cord is severed

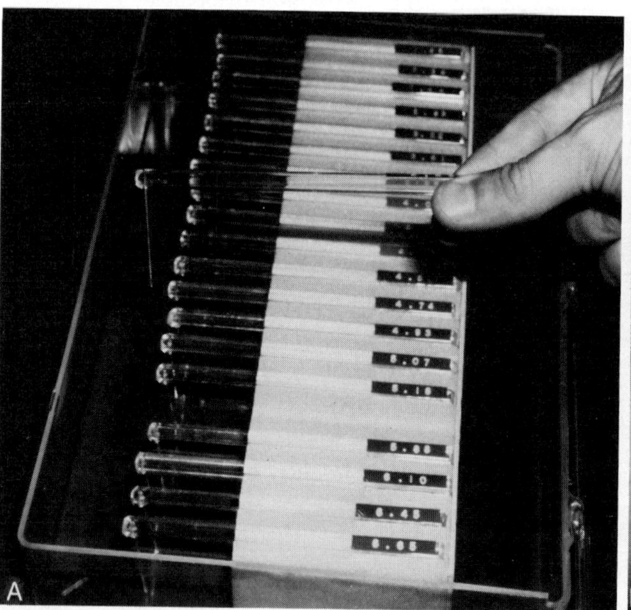
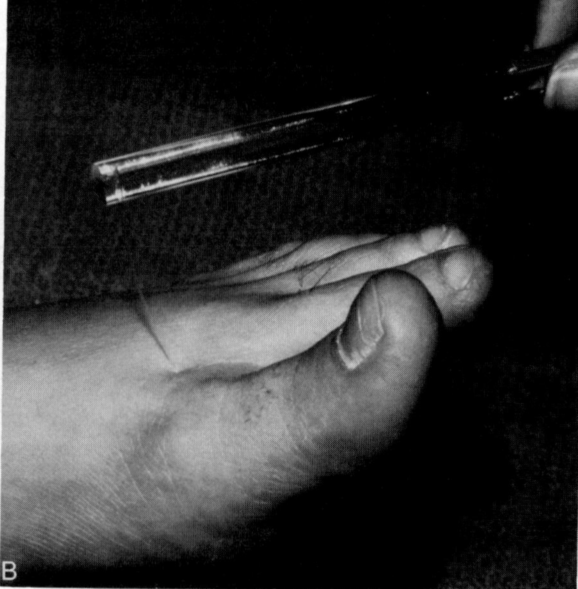

FIGURE 43–3. *A*, Weinstein-Semmes esthesiometer with multiple lucite rods with monofilament fibers of varying thickness mounted in them. *B*, Demonstration of use of one rod in the Weinstein-Semmes esthesiometer. Note the slight bend of the monofilament fiber.

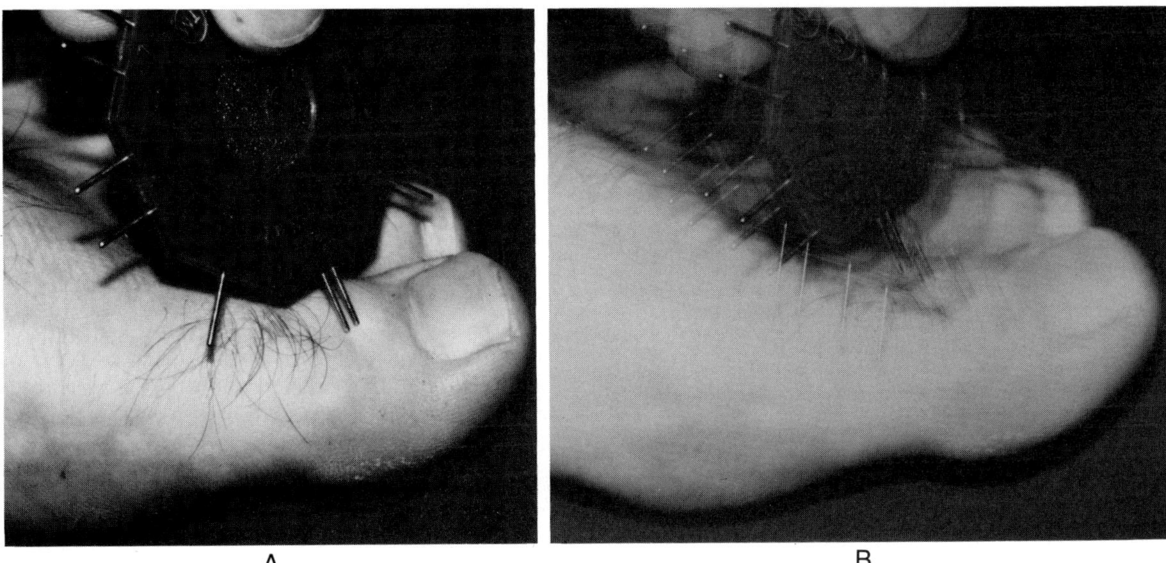

A   B

FIGURE 43–4. Use of a Mackinnon-Dellon Disk-Criminator for evaluating two-point discrimination. *A,* Static two-point discrimination. *B,* Moving two-point discrimination.

above the level of the reflex arc, a hyper-reflexia with possible associated clonus will be identified with the respective deep tendon reflex testing. Similarly, a positive Babinski test (in anyone older than 2 years of age) indicates an upper motor neuron lesion.

With advanced nerve entrapment, motor changes may be observed. Deep muscle pain, weakness, and atrophy are signs of diminished innervation to a muscle. The extrinsic muscles of the lower extremity should be assessed individually and compared with those of the contralateral extremity. Each muscle should be evaluated for mass, tone, and strength. Evaluation of individual muscles in this fashion may help differentiate lumbosacral radiculopathy from a local nerve entrapment.

Diagnostic Nerve Blocks. In most patients with suspected peripheral nerve entrapments, diagnostic nerve blocks are an integral part of the evaluation. These blocks help support or confirm the diagnosis. Once a suspected nerve entrapment is identified, a small amount of local anesthetic is infiltrated into the area of the entrapped nerve trunk. If the pain at the site of the suspected entrapment is diffuse, the block may be done to the nerve trunk proximal to the entrapment to ensure that only pain caused by the anesthetized nerve is eliminated. In this fashion, the neural pathways conducting the noxious

impulses can be defined, and both the patient and physician can judge the probable result of permanent neurectomy.

Further, local anesthetic blocks help differentiate a local, acquired entrapment neuropathy or causalgia from a sympathetically maintained pain syndrome or reflex sympathetic dystrophy syndrome (RSDS). Complete symptomatic relief with a local anesthetic block of a single peripheral nerve is not possible in RSDS because the hyperalgesia associated with RSDS is outside the distribution of any single peripheral nerve.

In an occasional patient, it will become apparent that local nerve blocks will not be tolerated. In these patients, an elaborate emotional response occurs during the injection with increased pain after the block. Generally, patients who react in this fashion are not good surgical candidates.[10]

Electrodiagnosis. The value of electrodiagnosis in the assessment and management of peripheral nerve injuries is limited. Unfortunately, the inexperienced clinician uses electrodiagnosis as a substitute or ''crutch'' in lieu of a thorough neurologic examination. To the physician experienced in peripheral nerve injuries, the appropriate use of electrodiagnostic testing is founded in an understanding of its neurophysiologic basis, and its limitations with respect to individual nerves and their anatomic anomalies. Electrodiagnosis is

TABLE 43–1

SENSORY TESTS AND NEUROPHYSIOLOGIC CORRELATIONS

Sensory Test	Pressure (Constant Touch)		Movement (Moving Touch)	
	Pressure Perception	*Static Two-Point Discrimination*	*Vibration Perception*	*Moving Two-Point Discrimination*
Test instrument	Weinstein-Semmes monofilaments	Paper clip, Boley gauge, pins, Disk-Criminator	Tuning fork Vibrometer	Paper clip, Boley gauge, pins, Disk-Criminator
Neurophysiologic correlate	Threshold	Innervation density	Threshold	Innervation density
Nerve fiber system	Slowly adapting	Slowly adapting	Quickly adapting	Quickly adapting

helpful when the subjective and objective examinations are equivocal, or it may help confirm a suspected diagnosis. However, many of the individual nerves in the foot and ankle are too small or too deep to be accurately and reproducibly evaluated via electrodiagnosis.

Diagnostic Imaging. In rare instances, diagnostic imaging may provide information related to a peripheral nerve entrapment. Magnetic resonance imaging (MRI) may allow direct imaging of an individual nerve or may provide clues to the cause of a particular entrapment neuropathy. Generally, the posterior tibial nerve, the medial and lateral plantar nerves, and large neuromas are most amenable to MRI study (Fig. 43–5).[11] Recently, MRI has been found to be helpful in the diagnosis of tarsal tunnel syndrome (Fig. 43–6).[12]

In summary, a specific nerve entrapment or compression syndrome may be not only diagnosed but also staged. With a thorough examination, the entrapment neuropathy may be classified as mild, moderate, or severe. In an early or mild entrapment neuropathy, the patient usually has symptoms related to the sensory component of that nerve. Tinel's sign is negative, and the only physical examination findings may be a hypersensitive response to tuning fork stimulation and sharp-dull testing. The Weinstein-Semmes esthesiometer may demonstrate changes as well. The symptoms in early entrapment are not persistent, there is no muscle wasting, and there is no abnormal static or moving two-point discrimination. With a moderate degree of nerve compression, the patient's symptoms are generally not persistent but are more troublesome throughout the day. Tinel's sign is usually positive, and numerous Valleix's points may be present. Tuning fork and vibration perception now become diminished. There is still minimal to no muscle wasting, and the two-point discrimination tests remain normal. In severe nerve entrapment, the patient has one or more of the following symptoms or signs: persistent sensory changes, muscle wasting, and abnormal static or moving two-point discrimination.[10]

TREATMENT

Localized, peripheral entrapment neuropathy can become a disabling condition. The more chronic and severe the entrapment, the worse the prognosis. Thus, early diagnosis remains vital to appropriate and timely treatment. Once identified, the successful treatment of nerve entrapment depends on several factors, including patient age and activity level, severity and location of the entrapment, cause of the entrapment, and condition of the local nerve trunk. Initially, in most instances, conservative measures should be promptly instituted. These conservative approaches may include medical, biomechanical, and rehabilitative management. If conservative treatment fails to relieve the pain, or if the patient is rapidly deteriorating both mentally and physically, surgical intervention is indicated. Prolonged conservative treatment should not be a substitute for surgery when surgery is indicated, because irreversible intraneural and end organ damage may occur.

Surgical management of an entrapment neuropathy usually consists of neurolysis, either external or internal, or neurectomy.

Neurolysis

Neurolysis involves the freeing of a nerve trunk or fasciculi from scar tissue and inflammatory adhesions that are preventing normal physiologic nerve conduction, inhibiting the anatomic regeneration of axons, or obstructing the nerve's blood supply. Neurolysis may be either external or internal.[5]

External Neurolysis. External neurolysis involves the surgical liberation of the entire nerve trunk from surrounding scar tissue or other mechanical irritations. External neurolysis is performed through an incision that allows the least traumatic exposure of the entrapped nerve while it minimizes the likelihood of a problematic postoperative scar. This balance

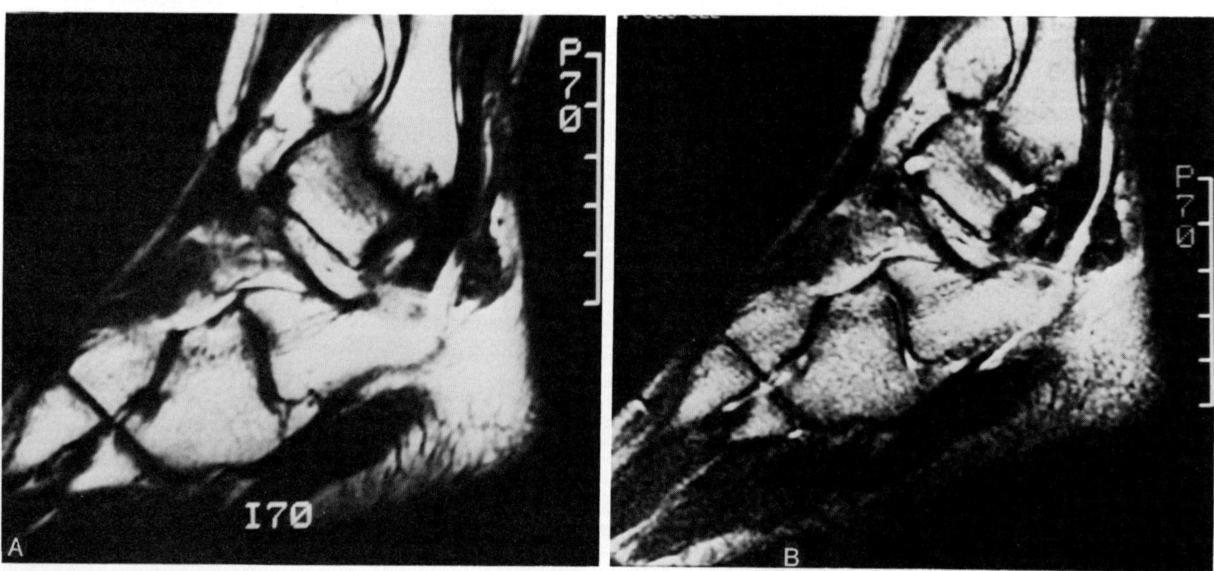

FIGURE 43–5. T_1-weighted *(A)* and T_2-weighted *(B)*, sagittal (longitudinal) plane, magnetic resonance images of a large sural neuroma. The nerve is of intermediate signal intensity, whereas the T_2-weighted image *(B)* demonstrates significant extraneural edema (high signal intensity), making the neuroma quite apparent.

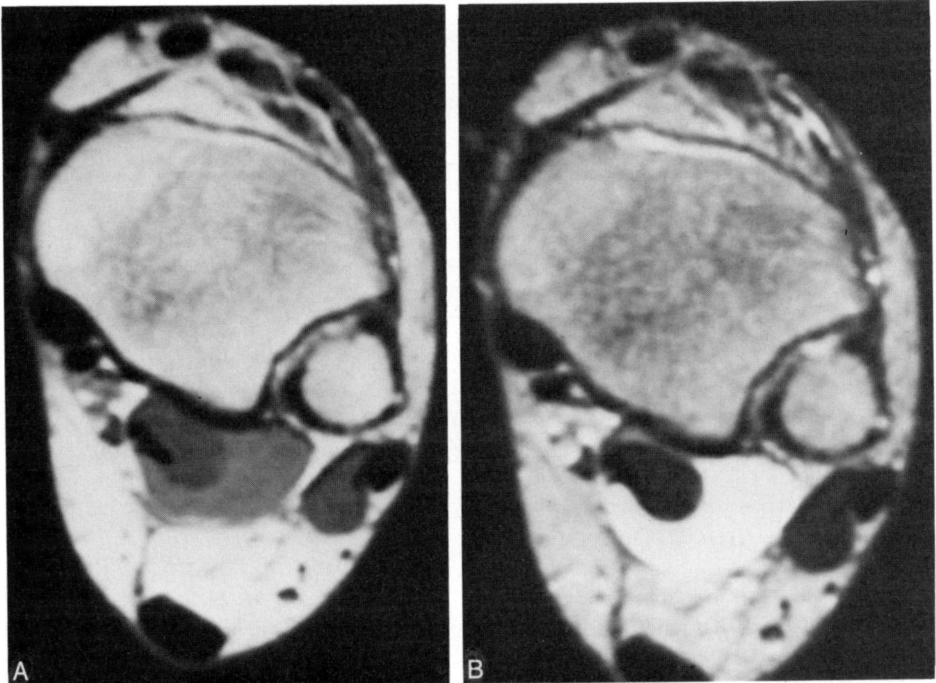

FIGURE 43–6. T_1-weighted *(A)* and T_2-weighted *(B)*, transverse (axial) plane, magnetic resonance images (MRIs) demonstrating a large ganglion of the flexor hallucis longus tendon. This patient presented with severe tarsal tunnel syndrome, and the MRI provided the first evidence of a space-occupying lesion as the probable cause.

can often be tenuous, and the surgeon should avoid the temptation to ''always get the most direct exposure'' if the resultant scar might potentially create significant mechanical sequelae. This is especially true of incisions made in weight-bearing areas or over osseous prominences. In certain instances, it is preferable to approach the area of nerve entrapment from a contiguous area of normal structure. If an old surgical scar or other scar tissue is present, the new surgical incision can be lengthened to incorporate an undamaged area. Normal tissue planes can be established in this area and continued either proximally or distally into the entrapment site. In this fashion, with careful anatomic dissection, uninvolved portions of the nerve can be identified proximal or distal to the entrapped area. The nerve trunk can then be carefully freed from any adherent scar tissue. Loupes or a surgical microscope are generally preferred to aid in this meticulous dissection process. The nerve trunk should be mobilized without damaging its outer adventitia. If the nerve is to be mobilized over a significant distance, additional care must be taken to avoid excessive damage to the nerve's segmental external blood supply.

Once freed, the nerve should be assessed for any internal damage. Visual inspection and palpation of the nerve provides some information as to probable nerve function. A neuroma in-continuity may feel more firm and appear swollen compared with the proximal and distal normal segments of the same nerve. Occasionally, intraoperative direct nerve stimulation may be necessary to determine the degree of nerve fiber function for lesions in-continuity. Direct nerve stimulation is useful for mixed nerves with a motor component (e.g., the posterior tibial nerve). Active contracture of distal musculature innervated by the stimulated nerve indicates satisfactory function of the motor nerve fibers. In most

instances, when this function is present, external neurolysis alone or combined with nerve transposition should provide adequate facilitation for additional nerve recovery.

If distal contraction is absent, intraoperative evoked nerve action potentials (NAPs) may be measured across the portion of the nerve where intraneural damage is suspected. The presence of intraoperative NAPs usually indicates that some function of the nerve remains or that regeneration is occurring and that only external neurolysis is needed. An abnormal appearance or palpatory texture of the nerve, or the absence of intraoperative NAPs, suggests the need for internal neurolysis, neurectomy, or resection of the nonconductive segment of nerve with primary neurorrhaphy or grafting. When intraoperative nerve stimulation is performed, it must be remembered that the use of a proximal tourniquet may cause temporary ischemia to the nerve, which may inhibit impulse conduction. Further, excessive manipulation of the nerve prior to conduction testing may cause a temporary neurapraxia, also inhibiting nerve conduction.

If nerve transposition is to be combined with external neurolysis, the nerve should be relocated as small a distance as possible and preferably to a protected, well-vascularized soft tissue or muscle bed (Fig. 43–7). Entubulation, or ensheathment, of the area of nerve entrapment with silicone sheets or venous grafts has been described as an alternative to transposition. Theoretically, such enswathing is designed to protect a freed portion of the nerve trunk from surrounding noxious stimuli and incarcerating scar tissue. However, by surrounding the nerve with these or other similar materials, the external vascular supply to the nerve is reduced or eliminated, and the nerve is likely to undergo ischemic changes, degeneration, and fibrosis.[13] Malay and McGlamry[3] reported two cases of silicone nerve ensheathment of the posterior

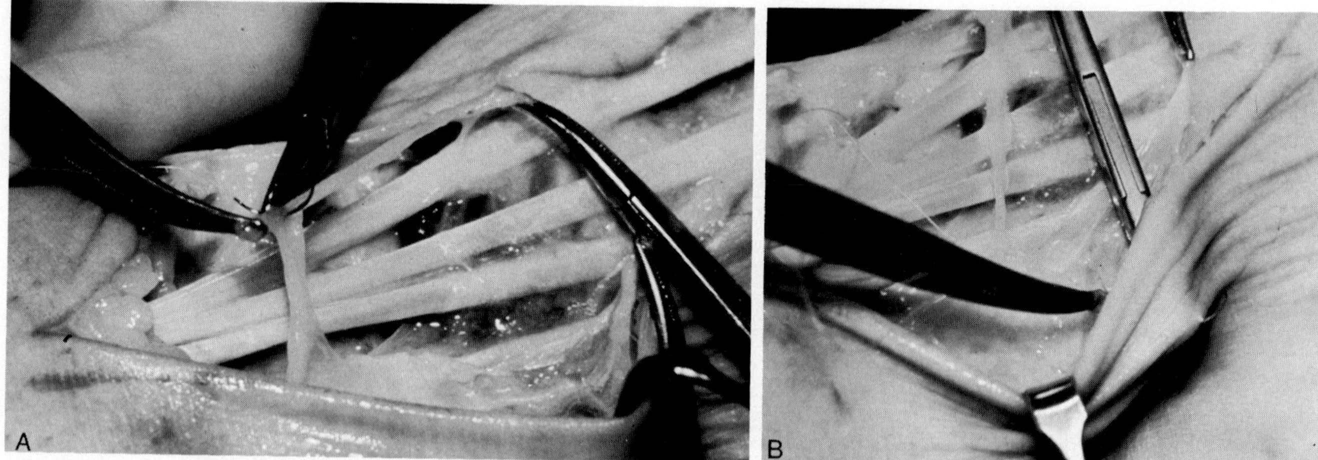

FIGURE 43–7. Transposition of intermediate dorsal cutaneous nerve. *A,* Identification of the nerve and placement of suture in the epineurium. *B,* Transposition and suture of the nerve into a more lateral position away from the skin incision and in a better soft tissue bed.

tibial nerve, with 0.02- or 0.01-in.-thick silicone elastomer sheets, in patients with recalcitrant tarsal tunnel syndrome. In these two patients, intraneural edema and dysvascularity created a recurrence of pain and the eventual need for neurectomy. While performing revisional tarsal tunnel decompression, I have similarly performed silicone ensheathment of the posterior tibial nerve with 0.007-in.-thick silicone sheeting on three occasions, with two failures requiring revisional neurectomy and with one case of partial symptomatic improvement (Fig. 43–8). Thus, it remains to be seen whether synthetic or biologic materials placed around a previously entrapped nerve will significantly enhance postneurolysis recovery.

Following external neurolysis, the nerve bed should be evaluated. In certain compression or entrapment syndromes, it may be preferable to deflate the tourniquet, if one has been used. Scrupulous hemostasis should be obtained, and a surgical drain used if necessary. Before wound closure, a small amount of soluble steroid (e.g., dexamethasone phosphate) may be dispersed over the mobilized portion of the nerve trunk to diminish postoperative edema and scar tissue formation. Wound closure is then performed in anatomic layers. The deep fascia may be left open if there is a likelihood that it might impinge or contribute to recurrent entrapment of the healing nerve segment. The subcutaneous tissue and skin closure should be supported with surgical strips, so that dehiscence may be avoided and early motion of the extremity begun in the postoperative phase.

Postoperatively, the wound is typically immobilized in a compression dressing, with or without a cast or splint, for the first 7 to 10 days. After that time, the patient is allowed to begin passive and active movement of the area and joints surrounding the nerve entrapment. However, in certain instances (e.g., following tarsal tunnel decompression), the patient will still be kept non-weightbearing. The early motion is believed to be essential in preventing the nerve from becoming readherent to its bed and the wound itself. If weightbearing has not been allowed, it is commenced after 3 to 4 weeks. Scar massage, ultrasonography, and other rehabilitative modalities may be instituted once the incision is healed.

Internal Neurolysis. As external neurolysis extirpates a peripheral nerve from its scarred bed or its surroundings, internal neurolysis involves attempts to remove or release scar tissue from within the nerve. Internal neurolysis, or endoneurolysis, should be contemplated only when the preoperative and intraoperative findings suggest intraneural fibrosis. Preoperatively, findings consistent with a severe entrapment syndrome (i.e., persistent sensory discomfort, muscle wasting, or abnormal two-point discrimination) suggest intraneural damage. Intraoperatively, damage detected on palpation (i.e., firm and indurated area within the nerve) and absent operative NAPs after external neurolysis suggest intraneural scar formation.

The operative technique for internal neurolysis is founded on the concept that injury to a peripheral nerve produces fibrosis within the connective tissue components of the nerve (Fig. 43–9). For the epineurium, this translates into a thickening in both the extrafascicular and interfascicular epineuria. The perineurium is similarly thickened, and there is also endoneurial fibrosis, but this is not released. The perineurium forms a sheath that contains the fasciculi, maintains intrafascicular pressure, and therefore preserves a vital internal milieu for the individual nerve fibers. Thus, internal neurolysis involves removal of extrafascicular epineural fibrosis and the separation of the fascicles from interfascicular epineural fibrosis. Care is taken to avoid breaching or injuring the perineurium, because this may result in ischemia and further scar tissue formation. In this fashion, internal neurolysis consists of extrafascicular and interfascicular neurolysis but does not involve intrafascicular dissection or scar release. Internal neurolysis is ideally continued until each fascicle is free from constriction, and a good fascicular pattern is obtained with observable perineurial markings.

Internal neurolysis is performed only after complete external neurolysis. Microsurgical technique and instrumentation are always used for an internal neurolysis. Loupes of at least 3.5× magnification, or preferably an operating microscope, are mandatory for satisfactory visualization. Tourniquet hemostasis is desirable so that the intraneural topographic anatomy may be easily seen. Once external neurolysis has been completed, the nerve is gently palpated and manipulated with vessel loops or Penrose drains to identify the intraneural

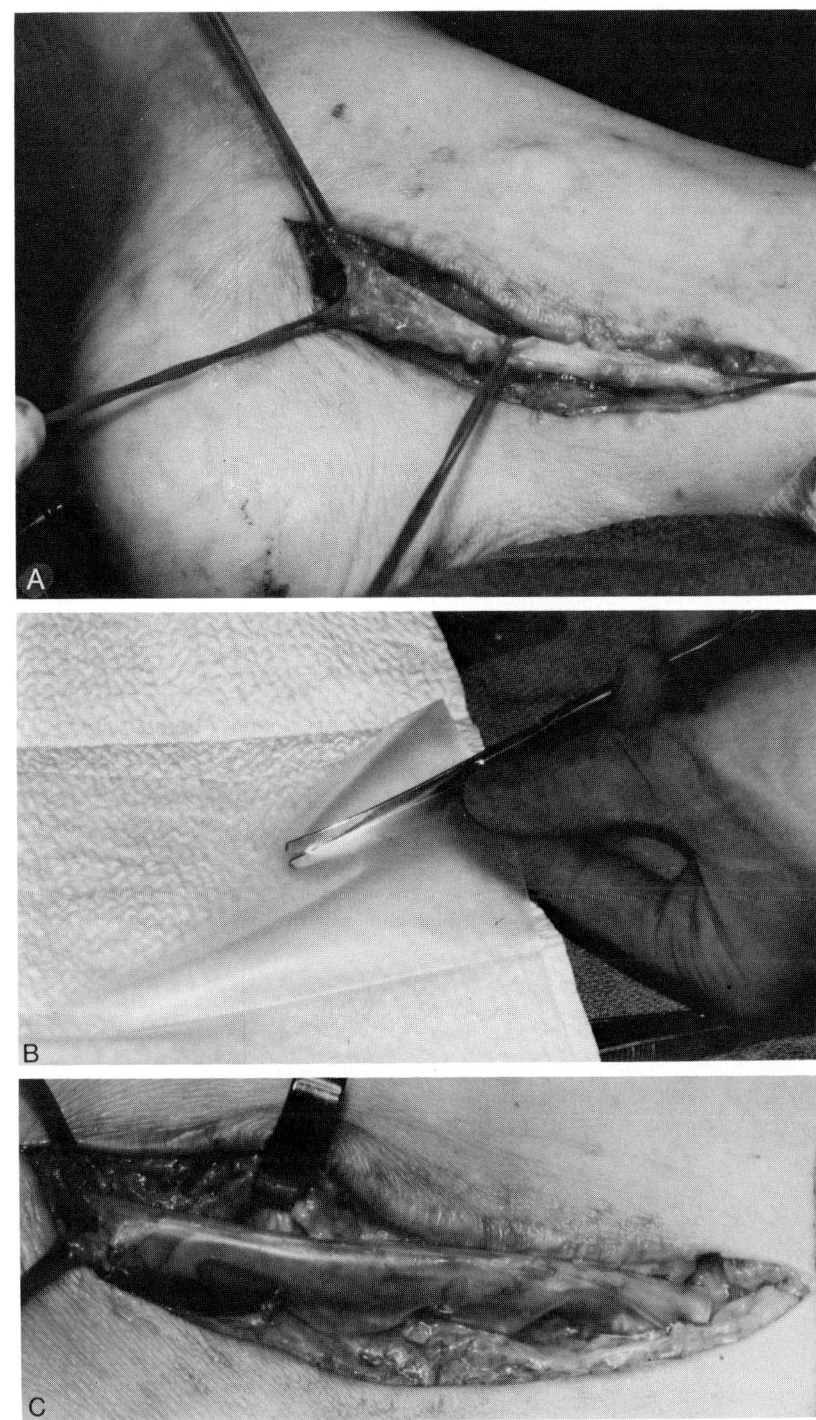

FIGURE 43–8. Entubulation of the posterior tibial nerve with silicone sheet. *A,* External neurolysis of posterior tibial nerve. *B,* Preparation of 0.007-in.-thick silicone sheeting. *C,* Sheeting placed around the nerve and sutured to maintain its approximation.

lesion or fibrosis. Using microscissors or a scalpel, the epineurium is opened over the length of the anatomic site of concern. Occasionally, this epineurotomy is facilitated by the injection of a small amount of normal saline (without preservatives) under the epineurial sheath to allow differentiation between normal intraneural architecture and scarred fasciculi that are adhered to the epineurial sheath. The saline distends the extrafascicular epineurium, allowing the epineurotomy to be performed with less risk of damage to intraneural structures. Care must be taken to avoid accidental injection of saline into the perineurial sheath because this could cause

damage to the intrafascicular nerve fibers.[5] The injection of saline does not itself accomplish interfascicular neurolysis and will not accomplish internal neurolysis alone.[14] Once the extrafascicular epineurium is incised, the incision is carried deep until the first fascicle is apparent. If good perineurial markings are noted (i.e., Fontana's bands are present, and the fascicles are soft and clearly distinct from one another), no further surgery is performed. If good perineurial markings are not noted, the epineurial sheath is gently retracted by placing of 6–0 or 7–0 sutures into the epineurium on either side of the area opened, temporarily tagging these edges to

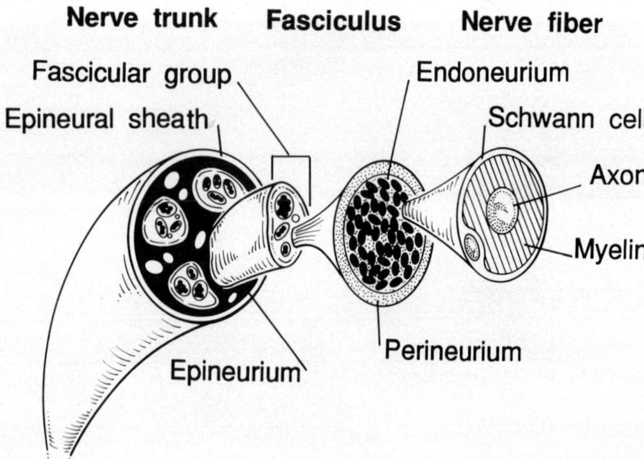

FIGURE 43–9. Functional and structural anatomy of the peripheral nerve trunk.

the surrounding nerve bed. This maneuver provides greater stability to the area, facilitating the interfascicular release. The microscissors is then placed between the two most superficial fascicles and gently slid down between them. Care must be taken to avoid damage to any interchange of nerve fibers between the adjacent fascicles. In this fashion, the individual fascicles are gently teased apart. On each fascicle, longitudinal vessels are visible in the perineurium, and these are not injured. The microdissection continues until all the fascicles have been freed and the return of good perineurial markings are noted. If a fascicle has been damaged enough to preclude satisfactory recovery, it may be resected or reconstructed with a nerve graft or nerve tube.[10]

Before closure, a small amount of soluble steroid may be placed around the nerve. The extrafascicular epineurium is not closed and may be excised if desired. As with external neurolysis, transposition of the nerve trunk should be performed if a more favorable soft tissue bed can be found.[5] If a tourniquet has been used, it may be deflated, and meticulous hemostasis obtained. Wound closure and postoperative care are the same as with an external neurolysis alone.

Neurectomy

Neurectomy involves the excision of a segment of nerve. In most instances, neurectomy should be reserved as a "last resort" surgical approach when external or internal neurolysis has failed or is not practical. At times, especially when the nerve provides critical sensation and the distal nerve and sensory receptors are available, neurectomy combined with nerve reconstruction may be the most viable approach. If function of the entrapped nerve is not critical, or if previous attempts at neurolysis or nerve reconstruction have failed, resection of the nerve with or without transposition of the remaining nerve stump is indicated.

Neurectomy is performed by isolating the entrapped portion of nerve, neuroma in-continuity, or stump neuroma. Dissection is carried proximally until normal nerve is identified. Once the normal nerve trunk is delineated, sharp sectioning of the nerve is performed as far distally as possible through this normal nerve tissue. The entrapment or neuroma site may then be excised. Once the entrapped portion of nerve has been resected, numerous operative techniques to inhibit axonal regrowth and transposition away from painful stimuli

have been described (Table 43–2). Each of these methods attempts to diminish stump neuroma formation or to transpose the nerve to an area subject to the least possible amount of mechanical stimulation.

Inhibition of axonal regrowth or stump neuroma formation has been attempted via physical, synthetic, and physiologic

TABLE 43–2
SURGICAL TREATMENT POSTNEURECTOMY

Inhibition of Axonal Regrowth
Physical containment
  Chemical treatment
    Alcohol
    Phenol
    Formaldehyde
    Nitrogen mustard
    Pepsin
    Hydrochloric acid
    Iodine
    Gentian violet
    Steroids
  Cautery
    Electrocoagulation
    Laser
    Radiofrequency current
    Cryosurgery
  Ligation
Synthetic containment
  Silicone caps
  Rubber
  Plastic
  Lucite
  Polyethylene
  Collodium
  Cellophane
  Metallic foil
  Tantalum
  Glass
  Nerve glue
Physiologic containment
  Epineurorrhaphy
  Nerve grafting

Translocation away from Painful Stimuli
Excision and retraction
Implantation into muscle
Implantation into bone
En bloc translocation

Adapted from Downey MS: Management of neurologic trauma. *In* Scurran BL (ed): Foot and Ankle Trauma. Churchill Livingstone, New York, 1989, p 245.

containment. Physical containment includes the use of alcohol, phenol, formaldehyde, nitrogen mustard, pepsin, hydrochloric acid, iodine, gentian violet, or insoluble steroids after neurectomy to attempt chemical cautery or inhibition of further neuroma formation. Further, neurectomy with electrocoagulation, laser cautery, radiofrequency current, and cryosurgery attempt thermal cautery of the nerve stump. Synthetic containment includes the use of inert materials such as silicone caps, rubber, plastic, lucite, polyethylene, collodion, cellophane, silver and gold foil, tantalum, glass, and nerve glues to attempt containment.[15–17] Physiologic containment with epineurorrhaphy has been used alone or in conjunction with physical or synthetic containment.[18, 19] Although long-term clinical studies with these varying methods are scarce, these approaches have had minimal reported success at diminishing recurrent stump neuroma formation, and some have been associated with foreign body reactions.

Transposition of a resected nerve end away from potential irritation appears to be preferable to in situ containment. Excising a neuroma and allowing the nerve end to retract proximally may be of benefit, because it allows the nerve ending to rest in a proximal site away from the surgical incision and original site of entrapment. However, if the nerve end comes to rest in a poor soft tissue bed or continues to be irritated, this approach will be doomed to failure. Resection of the classic Morton's neuroma is an example of excision of a portion of nerve with proximal retraction of the nerve stump. Alternatively, the resected end of the nerve may be transplanted into bone or muscle. The structure used should be in close proximity to the nerve ending and subject the nerve to the least possible amount of mechanical irritation. Whenever possible, I generally prefer implantation of the nerve ending into innervated, well-vascularized muscle away from denervated skin and scar tissue. Mackinnon and Dellon[10] coined the term *neurotrop(h)ism* to suggest influences that facilitate both nerve fiber maturation and appropriate direction of regeneration. Recent research suggests that cut nerve endings implanted into innervated muscle are least likely to demonstrate significant neurotrop(h)ism, thus the nerve is least likely to attempt regeneration in innervated muscle tissue.[20, 21] Implantation into muscle is accomplished by suturing the epineurium into the belly of the muscle. If the surgeon prefers or if an appropriate muscle belly is not available, bone may be used.[22, 23] A small trephine hole is made into the bone and the epineurium is sutured into the opening created, thus burying the cut end of the nerve into bone.

Finally, en bloc transfer of an intact neuroma or neuroma resection with primary neurorrhaphy or grafting may be considered. Herndon and associates[24] reported 72% minimally painful or tender results following en bloc transfer of intact neuromas with their fibrous scar tissue encapsulation to an adjacent area that was more protective and free from scar tissue. Although these results are promising, en bloc transfer would not appear to offer any advantage over implantation of a freshly cut nerve ending into bone or muscle. Hattrup and Wood[25] reported 77% (10 of 13) of their patients had diminished symptomatology following neurectomy with interfascicular grafting. However, nerve reconstruction is generally reserved for nerves with a major motor component, and when considering the foot and ankle, would be limited to recalcitrant lesions of the posterior tibial nerve.

Following neurectomy, the soft tissues should be closed in anatomic fashion. A compression dressing should be applied, and a closed suction drain used if necessary. Protected weightbearing or non-weightbearing should be considered for the first 2 to 4 weeks. Range-of-motion exercises and rehabilitative modalities should be instituted after 7 to 10 days and accelerated after wound healing.

Complications

Although it is often rewarding, peripheral nerve surgery can also be frustrating for both the surgeon and the patient. Even with an accurate preoperative diagnosis, good intraoperative technique, and proper postoperative management, uniform results are not ensured. Therefore, the preoperative development of a good patient-physician rapport with a thorough informed discussion of the procedure, alternatives, potential risks and complications, and postoperative course is critical to the success of the procedure. Aside from the complications inherent to any surgery in the lower extremity, peripheral nerve surgery has a unique set of potential complications that include recurrent entrapment and neuroma formation, sensorimotor alterations as the sensory and motor components of the nerve are altered, and reflex sympathetic dystrophy as the sympathetic component of the nerve is irritated. In any particular patient, each of these complications has the potential to cause pain greater than that experienced before surgery.

One of the primary goals of any peripheral nerve surgery is to eliminate scar tissue intraoperatively and minimize its formation postoperatively. A fine balance exists between complete nerve recovery and recurrent nerve entrapment. For example, external neurolysis can result in recurrent entrapment of the nerve to its soft tissue bed, internal neurolysis can result in recurrent intraneural fibrosis and a neuroma incontinuity, and neurectomy can result in an amputation neuroma or chronic neuritis of the transected nerve ending.

Second, sensorimotor alterations can occur following any peripheral nerve surgery. A transient period of paresthesias and hyperesthesia is to be expected in the immediate postoperative period. However, continued nerve irritation or reentrapment can cause these symptoms to continue. With time, hypoesthesia or motor changes with resultant atrophy may occur. When neurectomies are performed, altered sensation may occur by collateral sprouting as the cut nerve attempts to regenerate. Also, in my experience, nerves providing sensation in areas surrounding a transected nerve may become hyperesthetic as they attempt to provide "compensatory sensation" for the denervated area. In such instances, the patient will point to the distributional area of the previously unaffected nerve and relate pain, hyperesthesia, or paresthesias.

Third, the sympathetic fibers of any particular nerve can be irritated from any peripheral nerve surgery. If this irritation becomes severe, a true causalgia may develop. This potentially will present with burning pain, swelling, skin temperature, texture, color, and hair and nail growth changes and must be differentiated from a sympathetic-maintained pain syndrome or RSDS. Causalgia occurs from a specific peripheral nerve injury, and the resultant hyperalgesia, vasomotor, sudomotor, and trophic changes occur in the distribution of that nerve. In RSDS, the signs and symptoms occur outside the distribution of any single peripheral nerve in a more diffuse pattern. Causalgia can often be differentiated from a sympathetic-maintained pain syndrome by sensibility testing and a local anesthetic block of the potentially injured nerve. The symptoms of causalgia associated with a local nerve entrapment will be relieved by a local block, whereas the symptoms of a sympathetic-maintained pain syndrome will not. In some instances, causalgia and RSDS may occur together, in which case the local block will not provide relief. Treatment for both of these conditions should be immediate and aggressive.[26–29]

Finally, certain patients with suspected peripheral nerve pathology simply will not respond to attempted treatment. Lusskin[30] divided these types of patients into two groups: (1) those in whom the physical cause of pain seems to defy treatment; and (2) those whose complaints do not correlate well with the physical findings. Hopefully, these patients will be identified preoperatively through appropriate diagnostic and psychological evaluation. However, when the surgeon is faced with such a patient postoperatively, he or she must avoid the temptation to employ available therapeutic measures and medications, especially narcotics, in a ''shotgun'' or ''trial and error'' fashion. Even more hazardous are further surgical attempts for this ill-defined pain when there is little or no obvious gain expected. The inexperienced surgeon often applies such misguided efforts in an attempt to placate the patient, avoid litigation, and prevent their colleagues— often quite enthusiastic in their criticism—from observing their treatment failure. Invariably though, when such haphazard approaches are attempted, the pain recurs or continues, and both the patient and the physician become further dis-

illusioned. Instead, careful re-evaluation of the patient's condition, with appropriate consultation when necessary, should be performed before the initiation of any further treatment. If a nonorganic pain pattern is identified, the patient should be referred for psychological evaluation.

SPECIFIC LOWER EXTREMITY NERVE ENTRAPMENTS

Saphenous Nerve

Etiology and Specific Findings (Fig. 43–10A). Entrapment neuropathy of the saphenous nerve due to direct trauma is rather uncommon except in certain contact sports such as football.[31] Occasionally, chronic compression may occur with genu valgum and medial tibial positioning (frequently compensatory knee changes secondary to faulty foot biomechanics). However, the most frequently encountered compression neuropathy occurs as the nerve passes anteriorly over the medial malleolus and medially over the first metatarsal base. Chronic pressure from shoegear occasionally associated with a first metatarsocuneiform exostosis is often the cause of this compression. Further, postsurgical entrapment of the saphenous nerve can occur following surgical procedures for the medial column of the foot or the medial malleolus. The key diagnostic finding of saphenous nerve entrapment is pain on palpation, with the pain following a linear pattern along the course of the saphenous nerve. This pain must be anatomically differentiated from the more common symptom complex in the tarsal tunnel region. Local diagnostic blocks are particularly helpful in confirming this diagnosis.

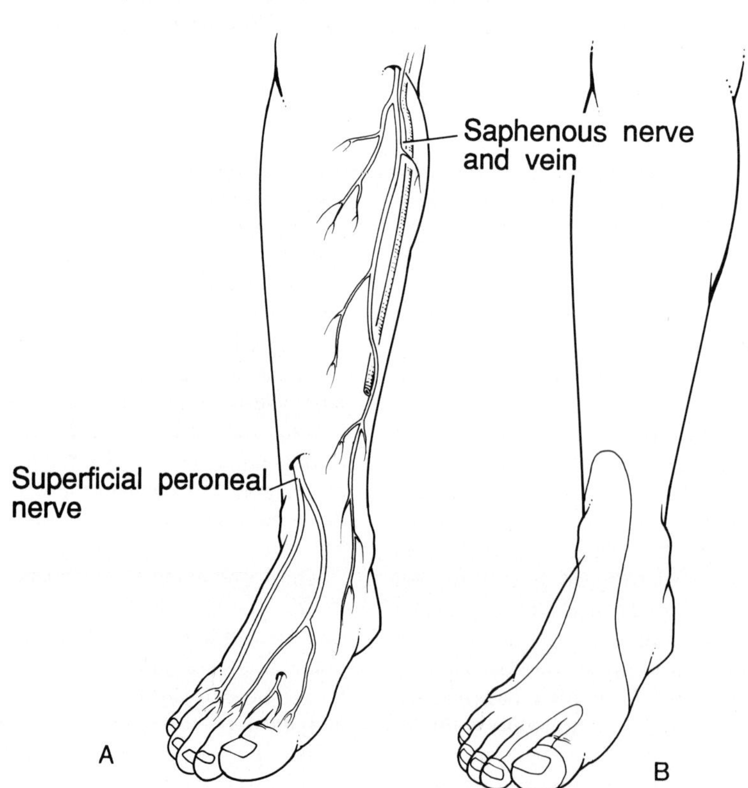

FIGURE 43–10. *A,* Courses of the superficial peroneal and saphenous nerves. *B,* Sensory distribution of the superficial peroneal nerve and its terminal branches, the medial and intermediate dorsal cutaneous nerves.

Surgical Technique. Surgical management of a local saphenous nerve entrapment most commonly involves external neurolysis with transposition of the saphenous nerve to a more favorable soft tissue bed (Fig. 43–11). If a neuroma in-continuity is identified, internal neurolysis may be necessary. However, because the terminal branches of the nerve are primarily sensory, neurectomy is preferred when severe nerve entrapment is found. Neurectomy of the saphenous nerve at the level of the foot or ankle results in loss of sensation but is usually of minimal concern to the patient previously in pain.

Superficial Peroneal Nerve

Etiology and Specific Findings (see Fig. 43–10). The superficial peroneal nerve originates from the common peroneal nerve and terminates distally by bifurcating into the medial and intermediate dorsal cutaneous nerves (MDCN

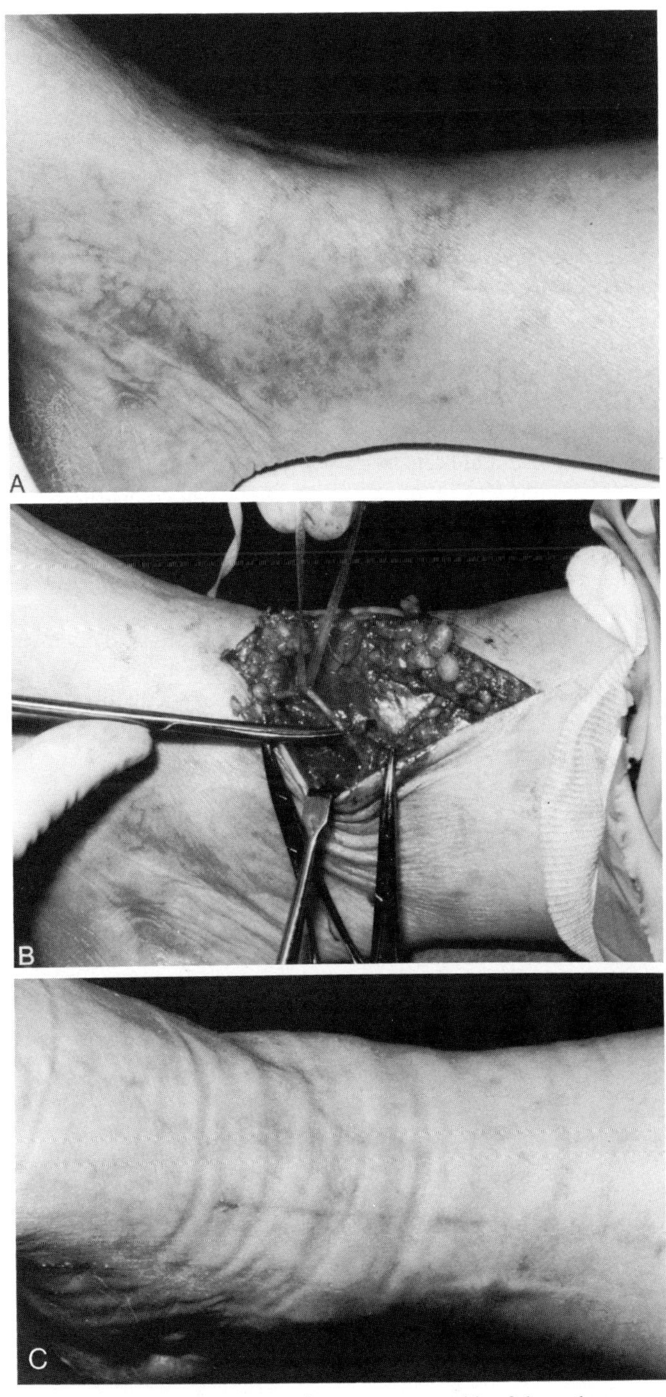

FIGURE 43–11. *A,* Preoperative appearance of patient with post-traumatic entrapment neuritis of the saphenous nerve. Note the previous laceration of the medial ankle. *B,* Isolation and external neurolysis of the saphenous nerve. The nerve was transposed away from the scar to a more favorable soft tissue bed. *C,* Four months after surgery, the patient is asymptomatic.

and IDCN, respectively). This bifurcation occurs near the junction of the middle and distal third of the leg where the nerve penetrates the deep fascia. The bifurcation may occur after the superficial peroneal nerve emerges through the deep fascia, but it occurs more often deep to the fascia. It is at the point of emergence through the deep fascia that the nerve or its branches most commonly become entrapped. Herniation of muscle through the fascial opening may cause or compound the nerve entrapment and symptom complex. Compression syndromes involving the superficial peroneal nerve may result from compartment syndromes in the anterior crural compartment. Contusions to the front of the leg (commonly seen in soccer players), fibular fractures, and tibial pilon fractures are but a few of the reported traumatic causes of anterior compartment syndrome. Any athlete may also develop shin splints secondary to faulty biomechanics, and this exertional compartment syndrome is a common cause of superficial peroneal nerve entrapment.[32] Severe involvement may disrupt motor function to the peroneus brevis and longus muscles. Traction injuries to the superficial peroneal nerve and one of its terminal branches, the IDCN, can occur with plantarflexion-inversion sprains or injuries to the foot and ankle.[33]

Symptoms of superficial peroneal nerve compression usually consist of sharp, burning pain along the nerve's distribution. Diminished sensation and altered sensibility are noted over the superficial peroneal nerve and its terminal branches. If the deep peroneal nerve and sural nerve are not involved, sensation will be normal over the contiguous surfaces of the hallux and second toe and along the lateral border of the fifth digit. Frequently, proximal and distal radiation of pain and paresthesias may be elicited on percussion of the nerve as it pierces the deep fascia about 10 to 12 cm proximal to the lateral malleolus. Forceful inversion of the foot and ankle may exacerbate any pain present, because the superficial peroneal nerve is stretched and tented over its deep fascial exit with this maneuver. Further, a muscle herniation through the deep fascial opening may be visible and palpable. This muscle bulge may become more obvious with resistive motor testing of the anterolateral crural musculature.

The suspected diagnosis of superficial peroneal nerve entrapment may be supported by electrodiagnostic studies demonstrating a change in the sensory latency of the nerve or by a diagnostic nerve block of the nerve at its point of entrapment or maximal tenderness. Finally, measurement of compartment pressures or an MRI to assess potential muscle herniation may be helpful when the diagnosis cannot be confirmed by other means.

Surgical Treatment. When conservative treatment has failed, surgical treatment most commonly involves external neurolysis (Fig. 43–12). A 5- to 8-cm longitudinal or lazy-S incision is centered over the point where the superficial peroneal nerve emerges from the deep fascia. The nerve is identified, and the fascia incised 2 cm proximal and 2 cm distal to the nerve's point of exit. If significant muscle herniation exists, the fascial incision may have to be extended and the nerve transposed. If intraneural fibrosis is identified, internal neurolysis may be necessary. Finally, if external neurolysis with or without internal neurolysis fails, neurectomy may be necessary to alleviate the patient's pain.

Medial Dorsal Cutaneous Nerve, Intermediate Dorsal Cutaneous Nerve, and Dorsal Digital Nerves

Etiology and Specific Findings (Fig. 43–13). Like the saphenous nerve, the MDCN is most frequently entrapped as it passes over the first metatarsocuneiform joint. In 20 cadaver dissections, Tobin and coworkers[34] found the proper digital branch of the MDCN to consistently cross over the first metatarsocuneiform joint. Shoegear can cause compression of the nerve at the anterior aspect of the ankle, but more frequently the MDCN is compressed where it passes dorsally

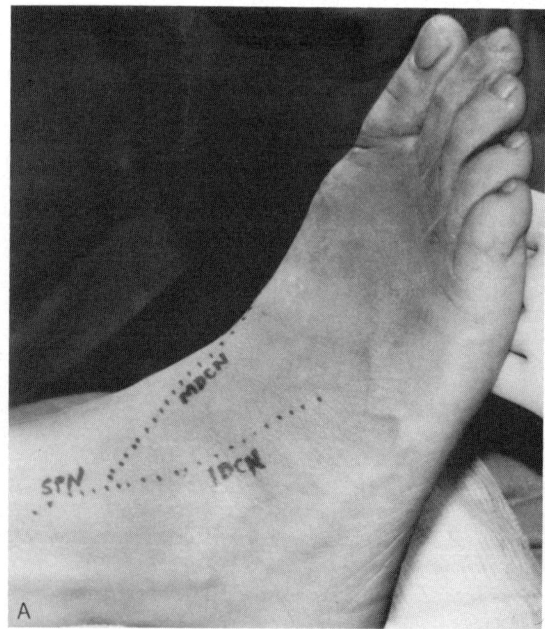

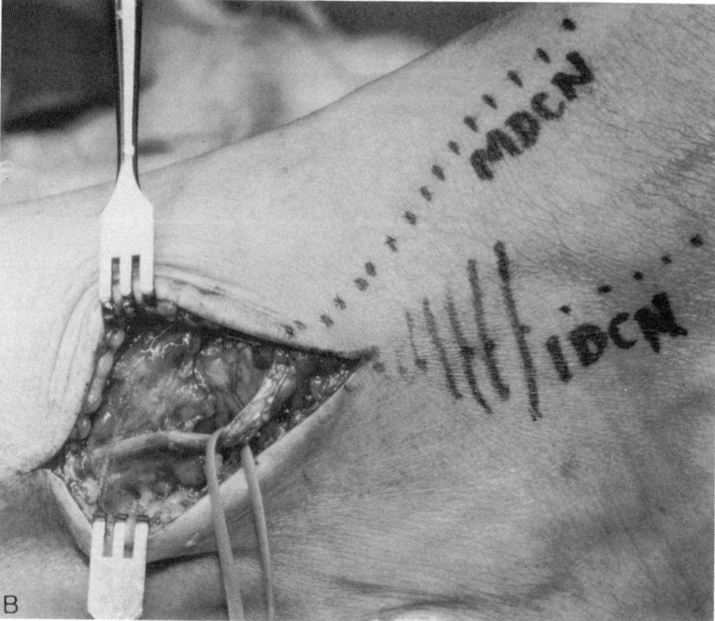

FIGURE 43–12. *A,* Preoperative marking of superficial peroneal nerve course and penetration from deep fascia. *B,* Isolation and external neurolysis of superficial peroneal nerve at point of deep fascial emergence. The deep fascial opening was also enlarged.

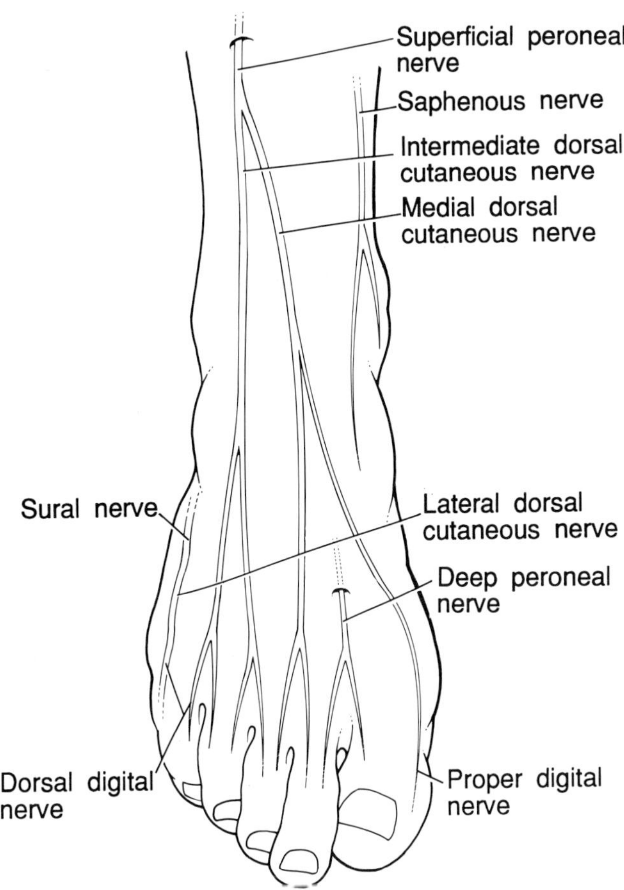

FIGURE 43–13. Typical nerve distribution of the dorsum of the foot. Numerous anastomoses and communicating branches (not pictured) may occur between these nerves.

over the first metatarsocuneiform joint. This creates a symptom complex traditionally referred to as *vamp pain*. If excessive hypermobility of the first ray has resulted in dorsal first metatarsocuneiform spurring, the symptom complex is initiated much more quickly.

The IDCN is rarely involved in primary compression neuropathologic changes. Occasionally, shoegear causes compression over the anterior aspect of the ankle or over the dorsum of Lisfranc's joint.

However, the MDCN and IDCN commonly are secondarily entrapped following surgical procedures to the dorsum of the midfoot. The MDCN, IDCN, and lateral dorsal cutaneous nerve (i.e., sural nerve) form a somewhat predictable but individually varying network over the dorsum of the midfoot. Dorsal surgical approaches to the deeper structures of the midfoot should be performed only through carefully planned incisions with significant dissection time and attention paid to avoid these dorsal cutaneous nerves. For example, excision of a simple ganglion can become a postoperative nightmare if entrapment neuropathy occurs (Fig. 43–14). Owing to the high incidence of postincisional nerve entrapment in the dorsum of the foot, Kenzora[35] labeled the medial two thirds of the dorsum of the midfoot the *neuromatous* or *N zone*.

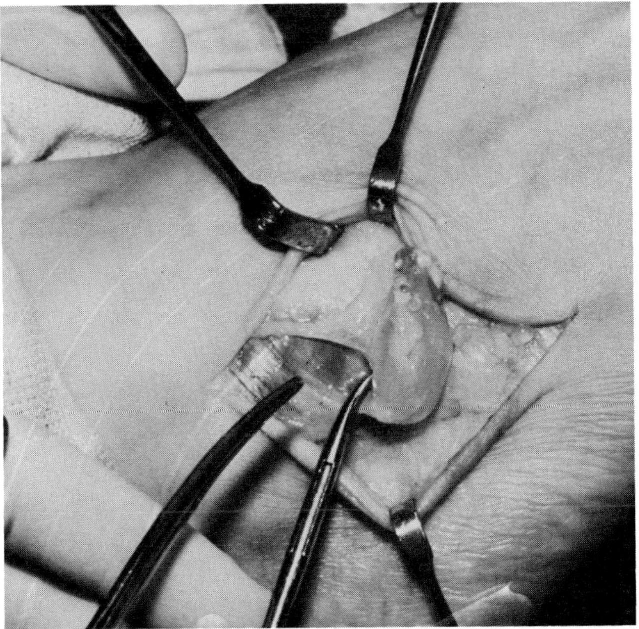

FIGURE 43–14. Excision of a ganglion from the dorsolateral aspect of the foot. Note that the intermediate dorsal cutaneous nerve is clearly impinged on by the ganglion.

The terminal digital branches of the MDCN and IDCN may become entrapped following trauma, infections, or surgery in the digits, or they may become compressed with certain digital deformities or tumors. The proper digital branch of the MDCN may be chronically traumatized dorsomedially over the first metatarsal head, especially in a patient with a bunion deformity.[36]

Confirmation of suspected MDCN and IDCN entrapment is usually based on the sensibility examination along with diagnostic nerve blocks.

Surgical Technique. Virtually all noniatrogenic MDCN and IDCN entrapments are treated by addressing the cause of the compression, thus indirectly decompressing the nerves. External and internal neurolysis are typically adjunctive but can be primary procedures if the entrapment is secondary to a prior surgical incision. When proximal neurectomy of the MDCN or IDCN is necessary, I prefer to resect the superficial peroneal nerve where it exits the deep fascia. I have found that attempts to excise portions of the MDCN and IDCN leave the resultant nerve stump in a poor soft tissue bed and in an area subject to further mechanical irritation. Attempts at burying the nerve into the extensor digitorum brevis muscle belly or the osseous structures of the midfoot leave the nerve stump susceptible to irritation from shoegear. By excising the superficial peroneal nerve where it exits the deep fascia, one essentially performs a neurectomy on both the MDCN and IDCN (Fig. 43–15). The more proximal neurectomy allows the resultant superficial peroneal nerve stump to lie in a good soft tissue bed in an area subjected to minimal mechanical irritation.

Entrapment of the terminal digital branches of these nerves is most frequently treated with decompression and external neurolysis, if the nerve is being compressed by a bony prominence, tumor, or other offending projection. Alternatively, if

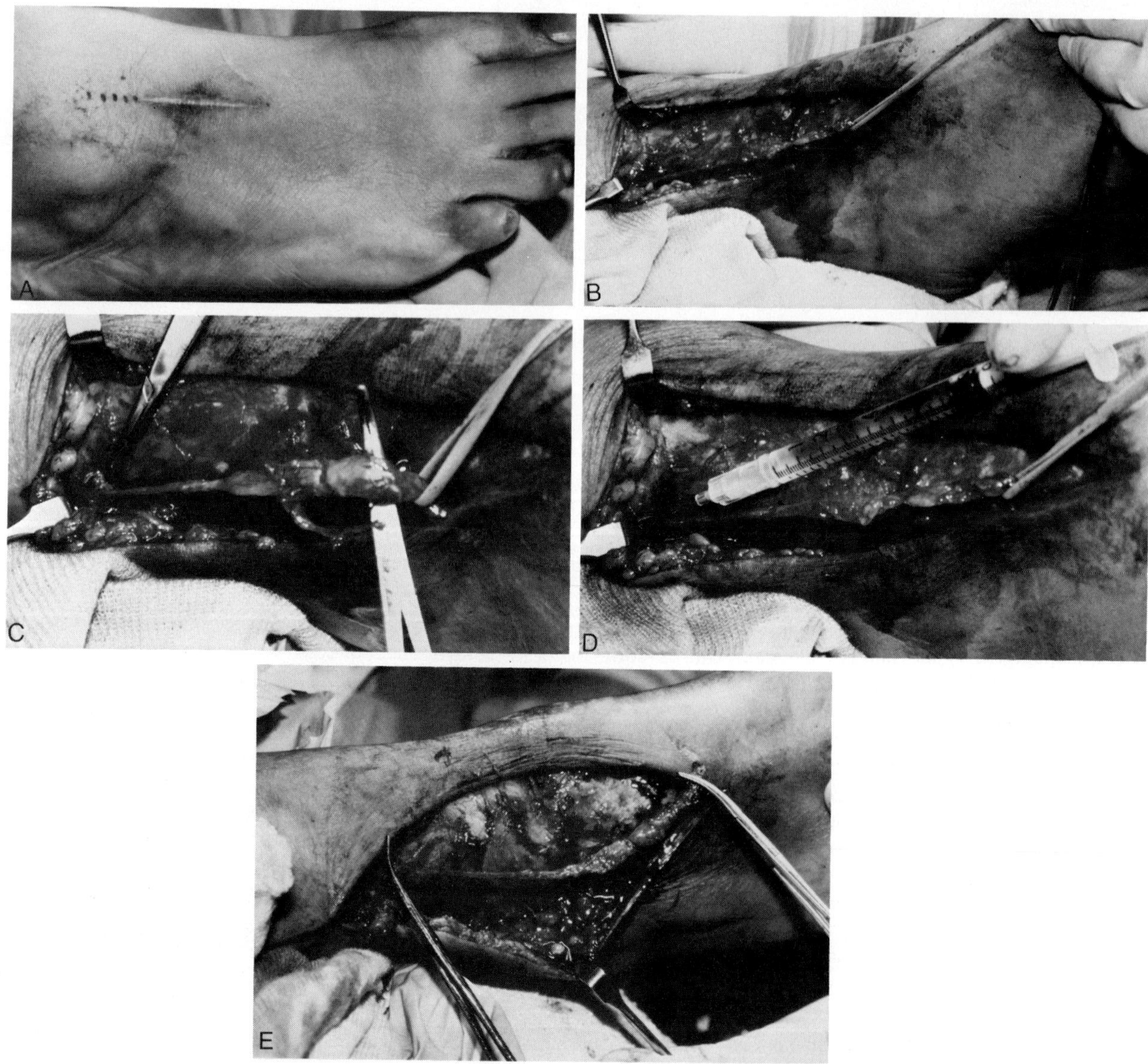

FIGURE 43–15. *A,* Preoperative photograph of a patient with postincisional entrapment neuropathy of the medial and intermediate dorsal cutaneous nerves following excision of a dorsal ganglion. *B* and *C,* Isolation of the superficial peroneal nerve. Note the extensive distal thickening and fibrosis of the nerve. *D,* Intraneural injection of the proximal nerve trunk with dexamethasone phosphate, prior to nerve resection. *E,* Resection of the superficial peroneal nerve trunk. The injected proximal nerve end is allowed to retract under the deep fascia. In this position, mechanical irritation can be minimized, and the nerve will be embedded in a good soft tissue environment.

the nerve is entrapped in scar tissue or primarily damaged itself, neurectomy generally is the treatment of choice.

Deep Peroneal Nerve

Etiology and Specific Findings (Fig. 43–16). The deep peroneal nerve, also known as the *anterior tibial nerve*, originates from the common peroneal nerve. The nerve, like the superficial peroneal nerve, can be compressed with anterior compartment syndromes. More commonly, however, the nerve is compressed at the ankle or just distal to the ankle. The nerve passes deep to the superior and inferior extensor retinacula at this level, and the resultant symptom complex has been termed the *anterior tarsal tunnel syndrome.*[37–39] Acute injuries in the form of direct trauma or severe ankle supination are clearly the most common cause of this entrapment. Biomechanically induced, chronic microtrauma in the cavus foot aggravated by tight shoegear is another frequent cause. Compression of the nerve near its origin, like compression of the common peroneal nerve itself, can result in paralysis of the anterior crural musculature with subsequent drop foot. In the leg, the deep peroneal nerve supplies muscular branches to the tibialis anterior, extensor hallucis longus, extensor digitorum longus, and peroneus tertius. Further prolonged entrapment of the nerve can affect the extensor digitorum brevis, extensor hallucis brevis, and the first and second dorsal interosseous muscles supplied by the nerve. Dellon[40] described 20 cases of compression of the deep peroneal nerve over the first and second metatarsocuneiform joints, where the nerve is bound down by the deep fascia and is crossed by the extensor hallucis brevis tendon. This symptom complex may be accentuated by talonavicular exostoses, dorsal first and second metatarsocuneiform exostoses, or post-traumatic degenerative changes in the area caused by prior Lisfranc's joint injury or dislocation. The terminal aspect of the nerve can become entrapped following a fibular sesamoid fracture or recalcitrant sesamoiditis. Finally, the nerve can become entrapped following surgery over the dorsum of the midfoot or deep in the first intermetatarsal space.

Diagnosis of an isolated deep peroneal nerve entrapment requires the identification of sensory and motor changes specific to the nerve without additional sensory and motor changes in other surrounding nerves. Typical complaints include aching and burning pain over the dorsum of the midfoot extending from the first intermetatarsal space proximally. These symptoms may be aggravated by tight shoegear and activity. Forced plantar flexion and inversion of the foot place traction on the nerve and may re-create or aggravate the symptoms. With distal entrapment, a Tinel's sign is commonly elicited with percussion of the nerve where it passes over the first and second metatarsocuneiform joints. A local diagnostic nerve block in this area helps confirm the diagnosis in these cases. Further, electromyography and nerve conduction studies may be helpful in localizing the suspected level of entrapment.

Surgical Technique. Surgery for proximal deep peroneal nerve entrapment most commonly involves external or combined external-internal neurolysis. An incision is placed over the suspected site of entrapment. Any offending osseous prominences are usually resected.

If the nerve is entrapped under the extensor retinaculum, the incision will cross the ankle joint, and a lazy S- or Z-

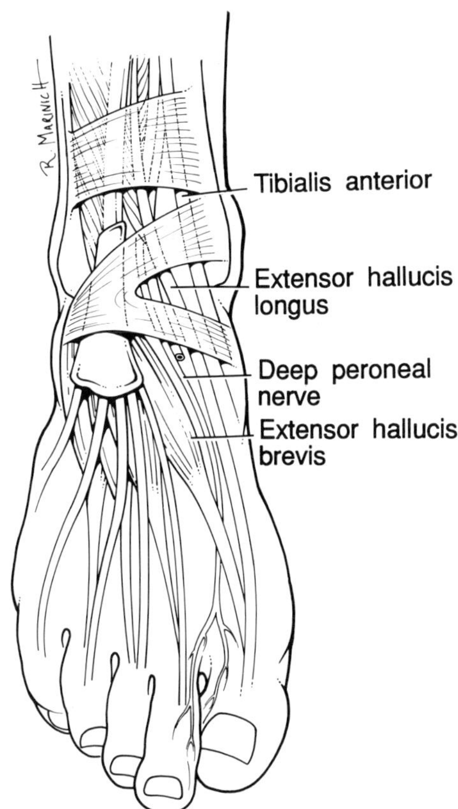

FIGURE 43–16. Course of the deep peroneal nerve. Note that the extensor hallucis brevis tendon crosses over the nerve at the first and second metatarsocuneiform joint level.

shaped approach should be used. The incision is then deepened in blunt fashion, with care paid to avoid the branches of the superficial peroneal nerve. Identification of the nerve either proximal or distal to the involved retinaculum aids in guiding the incision through the retinaculum. The retinaculum is then incised and the deep peroneal nerve isolated. External neurolysis is accomplished by mobilizing the nerve over the area of entrapment. Internal neurolysis is then performed if intraneural damage is suspected. At the surgeon's discretion, a small amount of soluble steroid may be sprinkled on the nerve. The retinaculum is left open, and the subcutaneous tissue and skin are reapproximated in anatomic fashion.

If the site of entrapment is over the proximal first intermetatarsal space and cuneiforms, the incision is carried deep in blunt fashion, with care taken to avoid damage to the MDCN as it courses distally and medially through the subcutaneous tissue. The deep fascia is then incised by tenting the fascia and opening it with a small scissors. At this level, the extensor hallucis brevis is found crossing the deep peroneal nerve and dorsalis pedis artery. This tendon may be retracted or excised as recommended by Dellon.[40] The deep peroneal nerve and dorsalis pedis artery are then found tightly adherent to the underlying osseous structures by further bands of deep fascia. This fascia is carefully opened throughout the area of entrapment and the artery retracted. Magnifying loupes are particularly helpful at this stage. The nerve is mobilized 1 to 2 cm proximal and distal to the site of entrapment. If clinically indicated, an internal neurolysis

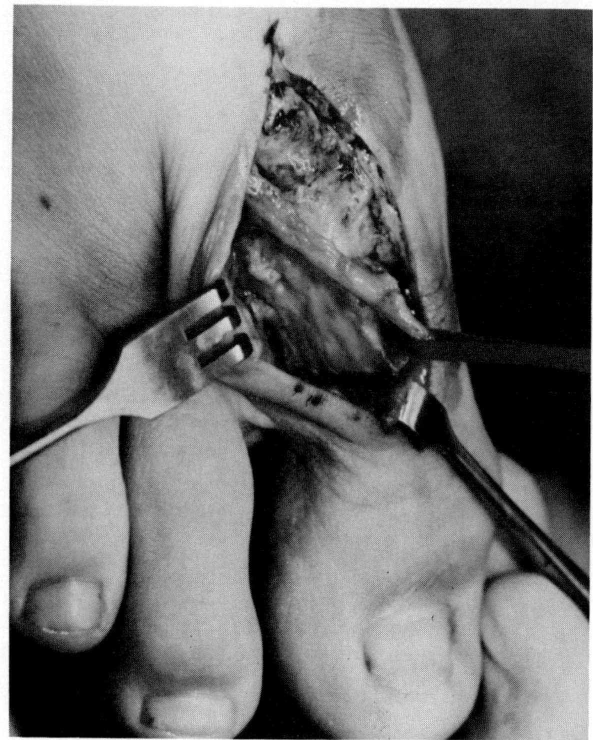

FIGURE 43–17. External neurolysis of the deep peroneal nerve in the distal first intermetatarsal space. The nerve had become entrapped following a previous fibular sesamoidectomy.

may be performed at this time. The deep fascia is then left open, and the subcutaneous tissue and skin are closed with appropriate suture. A small amount of soluble steroid may be infiltrated about the nerve prior to closure if desired. Dellon[40] reported 60% excellent results, 20% good results, and 20% poor results in 20 similar operations in 18 patients followed for an average of 25.9 months.

If the entrapment site is distal in the first intermetatarsal space, a dorsal approach is still preferred. The incision is placed over the first intermetatarsal space and carried deep. The nerve is mobilized, and external neurolysis or combined external and internal neurolysis is performed (Fig. 43–17).

Finally, in rare instances, neurectomy of a portion of the deep peroneal nerve may be necessary. In such instances, it is advisable to avoid leaving the cut end of the nerve over the dorsum of the midfoot. If the nerve must be resected over the dorsal midfoot area, the resection should be done proximal to the superior extensor retinaculum. In this fashion, the nerve stump may be buried deep in the musculature of the anterior lower leg.[41] If the nerve is to be resected in the distal first intermetatarsal space, the stump may be buried in the proximal interspace musculature.

Sural Nerve and Lateral Dorsal Cutaneous Nerve

Etiology and Specific Findings (Fig. 43–18; see also Fig. 43–13). A specific anatomic site of sural nerve compression has not been described, but sural nerve entrapment owing to direct trauma may occur anywhere along the course of the nerve. Displaced fifth metatarsal fractures can tent the nerve

or cause extraneural compression from the resultant hematoma formation. Rupture of the Achilles tendon or fracture of the ankle or hindfoot can also cause extraneural compression secondary to local edematous changes. Biomechanical irritation and compression can result from excessive pronation, excessive supination, or chronic Achilles tendinitis. Degenerative or inflammatory changes within the sural nerve, peroneal tendon sheath, and calcaneocuboid joint, with or without ganglion formation, have also been reported as causes of sural nerve entrapment.[42–46] Fracture of an os peroneum has also been reported as a cause of sural neuritis.[47] Unfortunately, sural nerve entrapment may also occur following surgical procedures on the triceps surae and Achilles tendon, the posterolateral heel, the fibular malleolus, or the lateral column of the foot, including the fifth metatarsal head and base.

Signs and symptoms of sural nerve entrapment are typically sensory and localized to the distribution of the nerve. Commonly, the sural nerve sends a communicating branch to the intermediate dorsal cutaneous nerve over the area of the sinus tarsi and the anterior calcaneal beak. Entrapment of this communicating branch may occur following fractures of the anterior calcaneus or problems around the sinus tarsi. I have seen several cases of entrapment of this communicating branch misdiagnosed and treated as sinus tarsi syndrome. Sensibility testing and diagnostic nerve blocks remain the standards for confirmation of a suspected sural nerve entrapment.

Surgical Technique. Biopsies of a portion of the sural nerve are often performed for diagnostic purposes in patients with suspected unusual neuropathies, with the assumption that the sural nerve reflects what is going on in the entire peripheral nervous system. The sural nerve is also often harvested as a donor nerve for nerve grafting. Because the sural nerve is primarily sensory, it has long been the selected nerve for such biopsies or grafts. Published reports do not describe

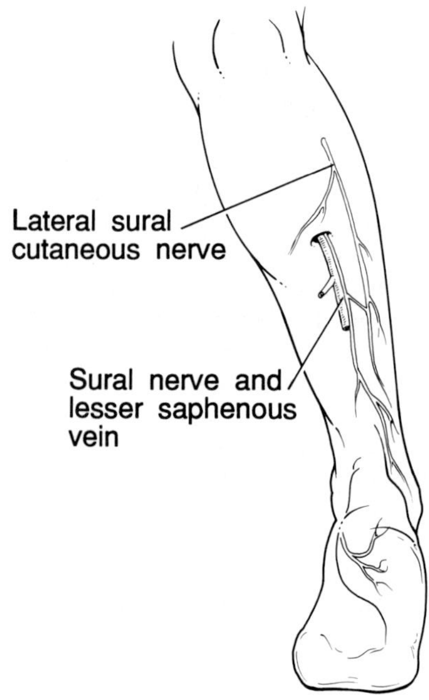

FIGURE 43–18. Courses of the lateral sural cutaneous and sural nerves.

significant sequelae or recurrent stump problems following these planned surgical neurectomies.[48] Therefore, although external neurolysis is still preferred, initial treatment for a sural nerve entrapment may be via neurectomy.

External neurolysis is performed through an incision centered over the suspected entrapment site (Fig. 43–19). The nerve is mobilized from the entrapment site. If necessary, internal neurolysis is performed. Once neurolysis is completed, the soft tissue bed is assessed, because the success of this approach appears to be directly related to the quality of the postoperative nerve environment. If the tissue bed is of poor quality, transposition may be considered. If no good soft tissue bed is available for transposition, progression to immediate neurectomy is often the best surgical option. Once the nerve is freed and a good soft tissue bed is found, closure of the subcutaneous tissue and skin is performed. As with other nerve entrapments, a small amount of soluble steroid may be dispersed over the nerve prior to closure.

If neurectomy is to be performed, the nerve should be resected proximal to the site of entrapment. In all cases, the stump of the nerve should be placed in a good soft tissue environment away from future mechanical irritation. The nerve may be transected and allowed to retract proximally, or it may be implanted into the fibula or peroneal musculature (Fig. 43–20).

Posterior Tibial Nerve, Medial and Lateral Plantar Nerves, and Medial Calcaneal Nerve

Etiology and Specific Findings (Fig. 43–21). Most frequently, the posterior tibial nerve is compressed in the fibro-osseous tarsal tunnel where the nerve runs deep to the flexor retinaculum (i.e., the laciniate ligament). Compression neuropathy in this region produces a symptom complex commonly referred to as the *tarsal tunnel syndrome* or *medial tarsal tunnel syndrome*.[49] The roof of the tarsal tunnel is the flexor retinaculum, which is a specialized, thickened band of the deep fascia that radiates in a fanlike manner from the medial malleolus to the calcaneus. Fibrous septa extend from the deep surface of the flexor retinaculum to form four compartments or channels. From anteromedial to posterolateral, the first, second, and fourth channels, respectively, contain the tibialis posterior tendon, the flexor digitorum longus ten-

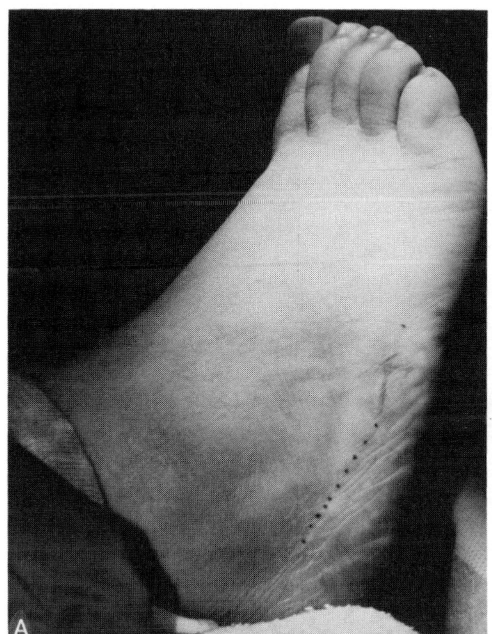
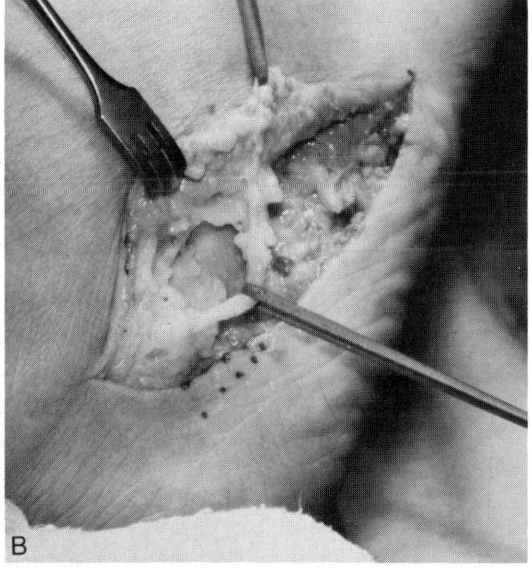
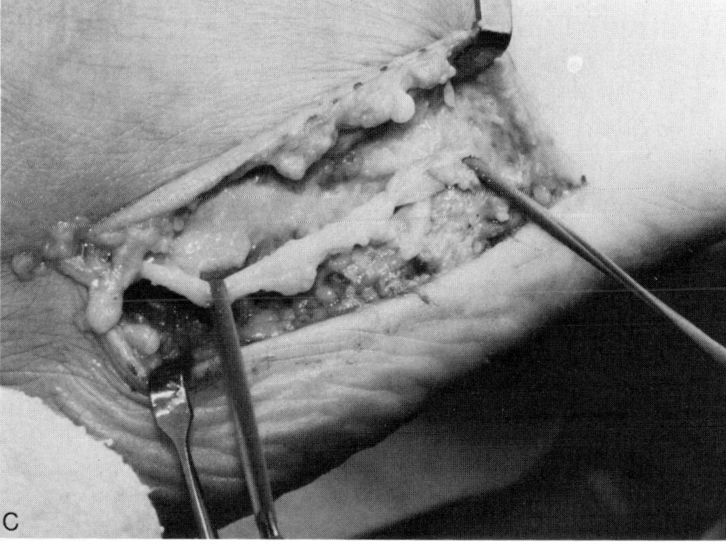

FIGURE 43–19. *A,* Preoperative appearance of a patient with sural nerve (i.e., lateral dorsal cutaneous nerve) entrapment following excision of a benign soft tissue tumor. *B* and *C,* Isolation and external neurolysis of the nerve. Note the use of vessel loops for nerve manipulation.

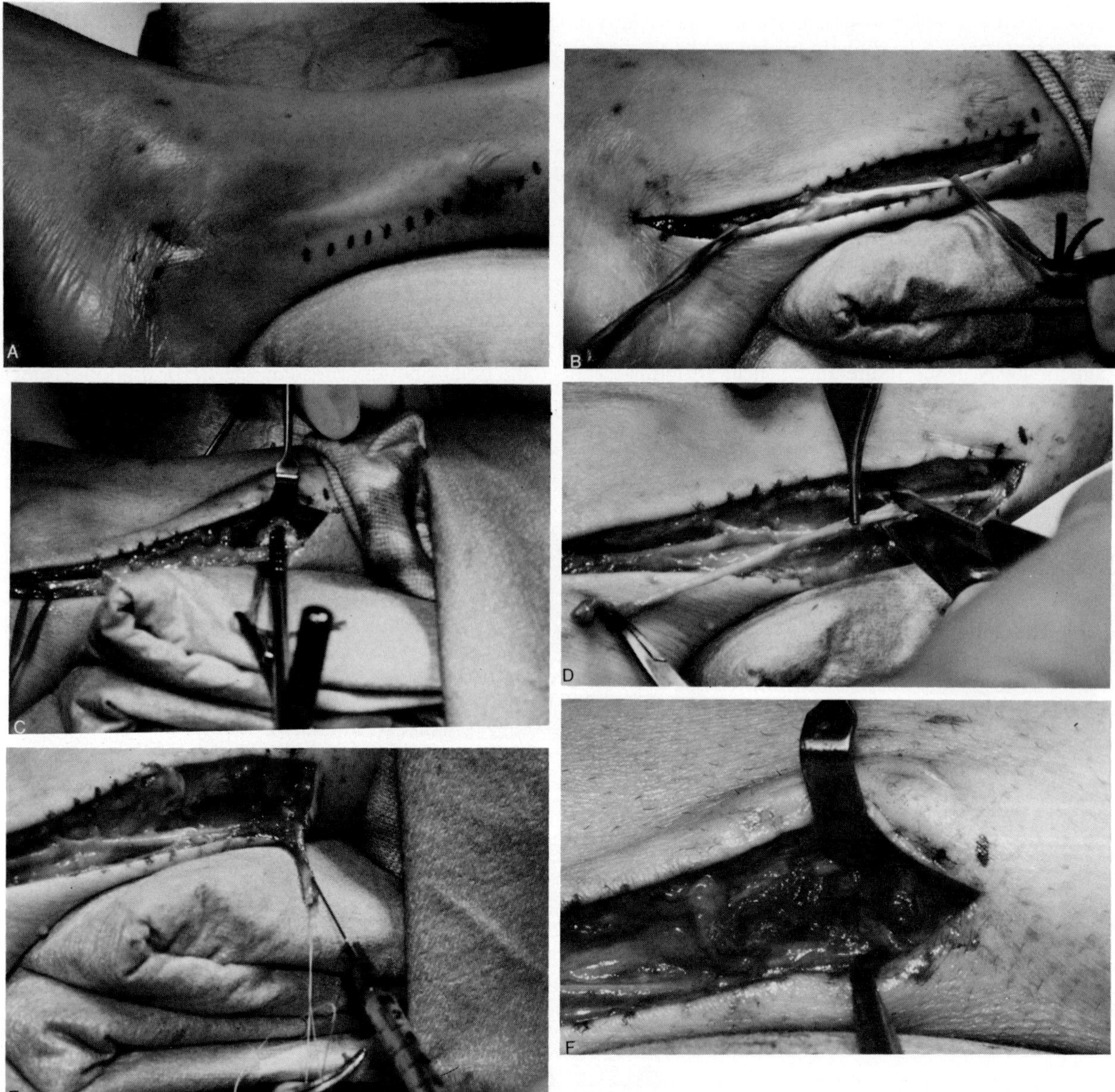

FIGURE 43–20. *A,* Preoperative appearance of patient with severe sural nerve entrapment following lateral ankle trauma and ulceration (now healed). *B,* Isolation of the sural nerve throughout the entrapment site. *C,* Use of trephine to create a small hole, or channel, in the fibula. *D,* Severance of the sural nerve proximally. *E,* Placement of an epineural suture and intraneural injection of resected nerve end with absolute alcohol. *F,* Resected sural nerve end sutured into a hole in the fibula, completing intraosseous implantation.

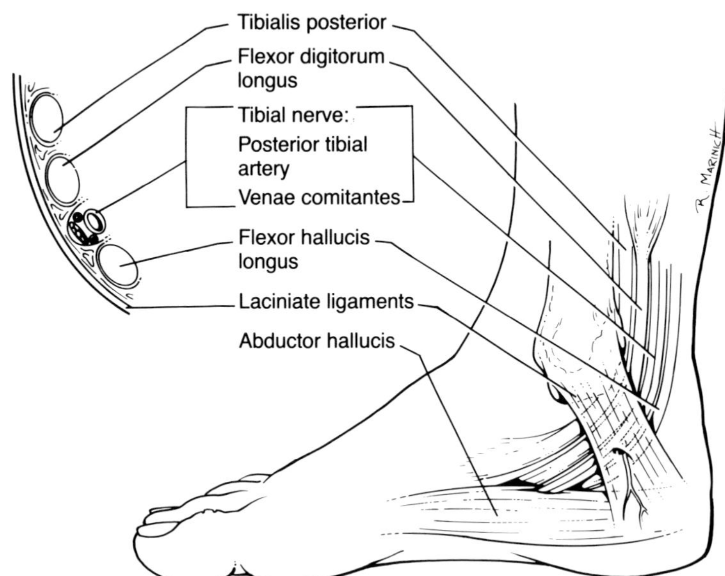

FIGURE 43–21. Course of the posterior tibial nerve beneath the flexor retinaculum (also known as the laciniate ligament). Note the medial calcaneal branch piercing the flexor retinaculum. From anteromedial to posterolateral, the contents of the tarsal tunnel are the tibialis posterior tendon; the flexor digitorum longus tendon; the posterior tibial nerve, artery, and venae comitantes; and the flexor hallucis longus tendon.

don, and the flexor hallucis longus tendon (Fig. 43–22). The posterior tibial nerve and its branches, along with the posterior tibial artery and its venae comitantes, occupy the third channel of the tunnel. The popular mnemonic, *Tom* (*TP*), *Dick* (*FDL*), *and Nervous* (*Artery/Nerve*) *Harry* (*FHL*), can be used to remember these anatomic relationships. The tunnel is narrowest at its proximal margin but is generally considered to be most constricting at its distal margin.

Studies have shown that the posterior tibial nerve divides into its terminal branches, the medial and lateral plantar nerves, either proximal to the retinaculum or, more commonly, underneath the retinaculum. Havel and colleagues[50] performed 68 cadaver dissections and found that the bifurcation occurred within the tarsal tunnel in 93% and proximal in 7%. Dellon and Mackinnon[51] made similar conclusions in 31 cadaveric foot dissections. In both studies, there were no bifurcations noted distal to the flexor retinaculum.

The origin and course of the medial calcaneal nerve branch are much more variable. Havel and coworkers[50] found the nerve to consist of a single branch in 79% of the feet they examined and multiple branches in 21%. This finding agreed with the earlier Dellon and Mackinnon study that found 75% single branches and 25% multiple branches.[51] The nerve arises either within the tarsal tunnel or proximal to the tarsal tunnel from the posterior tibial nerve or the lateral plantar nerve. Both Havel and associates[50] and Mackinnon and Dellon[10] each reported only one case of the medial calcaneal nerve arising from the medial plantar nerve, so this condition must be considered rare. When the nerve arises proximal to the tarsal tunnel, it usually remains outside the tarsal tunnel. When it arises within the tarsal tunnel, it typically pierces the flexor retinaculum to course plantarward to the heel.

Just distal to the flexor retinaculum, the medial and lateral plantar nerves continue toward the plantar aspect of the foot. As they enter the foot, these nerves each enter their own anatomic tunnels. The fibrous origins of the plantar aponeurosis form the roof over the lateral plantar nerve, and the abductor hallucis muscle forms the roof over the medial plantar nerve. A fibrous septum separates the nerves from one another. The nerves may be compressed as they abruptly change direction and enter their individual channels in the plantar vault. Compression of the medial and lateral plantar nerves in this location is intimately related to tarsal tunnel syndrome.

Tarsal tunnel syndrome most frequently occurs in adults. However, when it does present in children, it usually occurs in girls.[52]

Tarsal tunnel syndrome is most commonly caused by direct or indirect trauma to the hindfoot and ankle region with subsequent post-traumatic fibrosis.[53, 54] Etiologic factors for tarsal tunnel syndrome include biomechanical disorders (especially excessive subtalar joint pronation); an accessory or hypertrophic abductor hallucis muscle belly; tenosynovitis or ganglion formation affecting the nerve itself or tendons in the tarsal tunnel (tibialis posterior, flexor digitorum longus, and flexor hallucis longus); varices or venous incompetency of the posterior tibial venae comitantes; and post-traumatic fibrosis and scarring following calcaneal, talar, and ankle fractures.[53–58] Various tumors of the hindfoot and ankle, es-

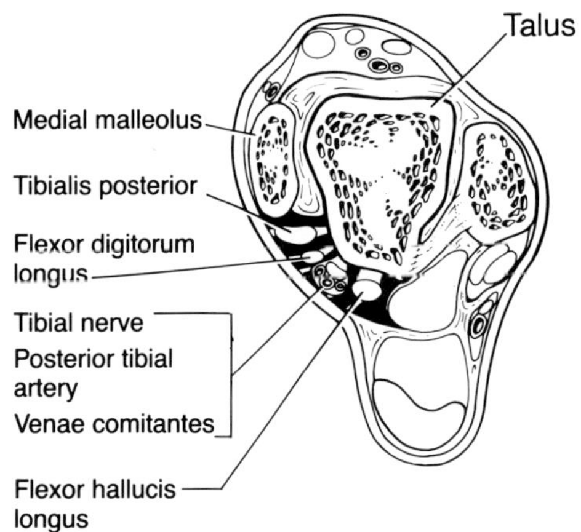

FIGURE 43–22. Transverse (axial) cross-section of the tarsal tunnel. Note that from anteromedial to posterolateral, the contents of the tarsal tunnel are the tibialis posterior tendon; the flexor digitorum longus tendon, the posterior tibial nerve, artery, and venae comitantes; and the flexor hallucis longus tendon.

pecially neurilemomas, have been reported as causes of tarsal tunnel syndrome.[59–66] Tarsal tunnel syndrome may also be associated with hyperlipidemia,[67] rheumatoid arthritis,[68, 69] regional migratory osteoporosis,[70] and lower back pain.[71] Further, tarsal tunnel syndrome is often associated with additional nerve entrapments in the same limb.[72]

Similarly, abnormal biomechanical influences, including excessive pronation of the subtalar joint, can create chronic compression of the medial and lateral plantar nerves. Direct trauma affecting the plantar aspect of the foot, local myotenositis of the intrinsic musculature, plantar fasciitis, and osseous prominences can cause extraneural compression.

The medial calcaneal branch of the tibial nerve is frequently subjected to direct trauma, especially in long-distance runners, with frequent neurilemoma formation. Post-incisional entrapment of the medial calcaneal nerve also can occur following plantar-medial surgical approaches for plantar heel spur and plantar fascial releases. "Heel neuromas" may result from direct injury or chronic compression of the medial calcaneal nerve.[73–76]

Several authors have suggested entrapment neuropathy of the muscle branch of the lateral plantar nerve that goes to the abductor digiti quinti muscle as a cause of plantar heel pain.[77, 78] The nerve branch traverses in close proximity to the medial calcaneal tuberosity and may be compressed in this area.

The diagnosis of tarsal tunnel syndrome is based on a thorough historical interview and physical findings. The distribution of sensorimotor alteration is the key to an accurate diagnosis. Symptomatology usually centers around a "pins and needles" sensation, burning pain, or numbness affecting the plantar aspect of the foot. Pain and paresthesias are aggravated by a variety of activities, and the symptoms are often worse at night. On examination, Tinel's sign can often be elicited with percussion of the flexor retinaculum. Numerous Valleix's points may be noted. Occasionally, edema may be noted posterior to the medial malleolus in the area of the tarsal tunnel. Diminished vibratory perception and abnormal two-point discrimination may be present over the plantar aspect of the foot or in the toes. Patients often state that relief is obtained with massage, foot and ankle motion, and elevation. Intrinsic muscular atrophy and associated hammertoes are late findings. Nerve conduction velocities and electromyography may be helpful in confirming the diagnosis as well as in monitoring the therapeutic regimen.[79, 80] Further, MRI may be helpful in evaluating the tarsal tunnel for a space-occupying lesion, scar tissue, varicosities, and other compressive and traction-producing lesions (see Fig. 43–6). Further, the information provided by MRI may aid in planning surgical intervention by showing the extent of the pathologic changes, their relationship to the neurovascular structures, and the extent of decompression required.[12, 81, 82] However, the clinical diagnosis of tarsal tunnel syndrome should not be reversed because of negative electrodiagnostic or MRI findings.

Neuritic heel pain may accompany tarsal tunnel complaints or may be independent of it. Entrapment of the medial calcaneal nerve branch or the muscular branch of the abductor digiti quinti from the lateral plantar nerve must be considered in any differential diagnosis of heel pain. Sharp, burning, or shooting pain in the plantar heel radiating from the tarsal tunnel area, which may be associated with paresthesias,

is characteristic of nerve entrapment of one of these branches. A positive Tinel's sign may be noted with percussion of the medial calcaneal nerve branch where it courses over the medial aspect of the heel, inferior to the tarsal tunnel. Conversely, percussion of the plantar heel may cause proximal radiation to the tarsal tunnel area. In severe cases, a neuroma of the medial calcaneal nerve branch may be palpated.

Surgical Technique. Tarsal tunnel decompression is performed with or without the use of a mid-thigh pneumatic tourniquet. If a tourniquet is used, several factors must be remembered: (1) the tourniquet creates an ischemic state, possibly making the posterior tibial nerve unresponsive to an intraoperative nerve stimulator; (2) the pulse of the posterior tibial artery will not be palpable, making entrance to the third compartment slightly more hazardous; and (3) the tourniquet should be deflated before wound closure so that absolute hemostasis is ensured.

The approach is by a 5- to 8-cm, retromalleolar, curvilinear incision extending from approximately 2 cm superior to the flexor retinaculum, gently curving distally to the proximal margin of the abductor hallucis muscle (Fig. 43–23A). The incision is deepened through the subcutaneous layer with meticulous hemostasis obtained. This dissection is typically done bluntly to avoid inadvertent damage to the medial calcaneal nerve branch. When the flexor retinaculum is reached, the subcutaneous layer is bluntly reflected.

Once the flexor retinaculum is exposed, care is taken to identify the third canal of the tarsal tunnel. The pulse of the tibialis posterior artery is palpated if there is no tourniquet to identify the third canal. If a tourniquet is used, the tibialis posterior, flexor digitorum longus, and flexor hallucis longus tendons will be palpated with the third canal lying between the flexor longus tendons. Passive manipulation of the foot, lesser digits, and hallux aids in the identification of these tendinous structures. Alternatively, the venae comitantes can usually be visualized through the flexor retinaculum. Occasionally, a perforating vein that pierces the flexor retinaculum can be used to identify the third canal because it is presumed to communicate with the venae comitantes of the posterior tibial artery (Fig. 43–23B). If the surgeon cannot locate the third canal by these methods, as often occurs in revisional tarsal tunnel surgery, the posterior tibial nerve may be identified proximal to the tarsal tunnel and followed distally. Once the third canal of the flexor retinaculum has been identified, the roof is incised in its entirety from proximal to distal, allowing access to its contents (Fig. 43–23C).

The posterior tibial nerve is isolated and freed of any constricting connective tissue or scarring. A vessel loop or Penrose drain is placed around the nerve trunk to aid in operative retraction and manipulation (Fig. 43–23D). Once the posterior tibial nerve is isolated, the dissection is carried distally until all the branches have been isolated (Fig. 43–23E). The medial calcaneal branch generally comes first, followed by the medial plantar and lateral plantar branches. Vessel loops or Penrose drains are similarly placed around the branches to aid in their operative retraction and manipulation (Fig. 43–23F). An intraoperative nerve stimulator may be used to aid in the identification of the nerve or its branches and to assess their function.

The dissection is then carried distally to the abductor canal where the plantar nerves enter the plantar vault. Dilation of

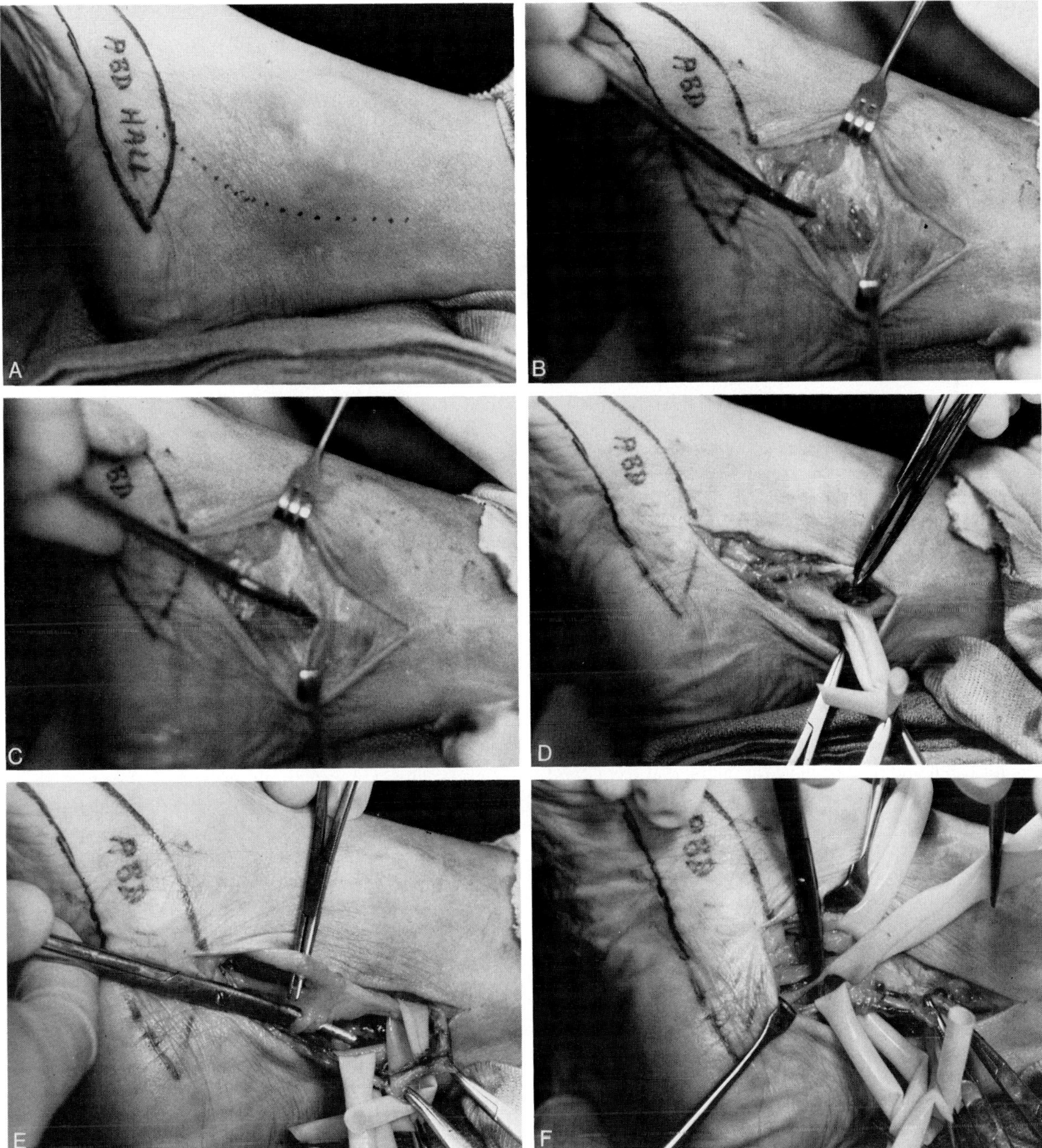

FIGURE 43–23. *A,* Incision placement for tarsal tunnel decompression. *B,* Identification of the third canal of the tarsal tunnel. Note the varicosities that can be visualized through the flexor retinaculum. *C,* Elevation and incision of the flexor retinaculum. *D,* Identification and retraction of the posterior tibial nerve with a small Penrose drain. *E,* Isolation of the branches of the posterior tibial nerve. From dorsal to plantar, they are the medial plantar nerve, the lateral plantar nerve, and the medial calcaneal nerve. Note that the posterior tibial nerve's division, in this patient, occurs under the flexor retinaculum and that the medial calcaneal nerve originates from the lateral plantar nerve. *F,* Use of Penrose drains to facilitate nerve manipulation and external neurolysis.

Illustration continued on following page

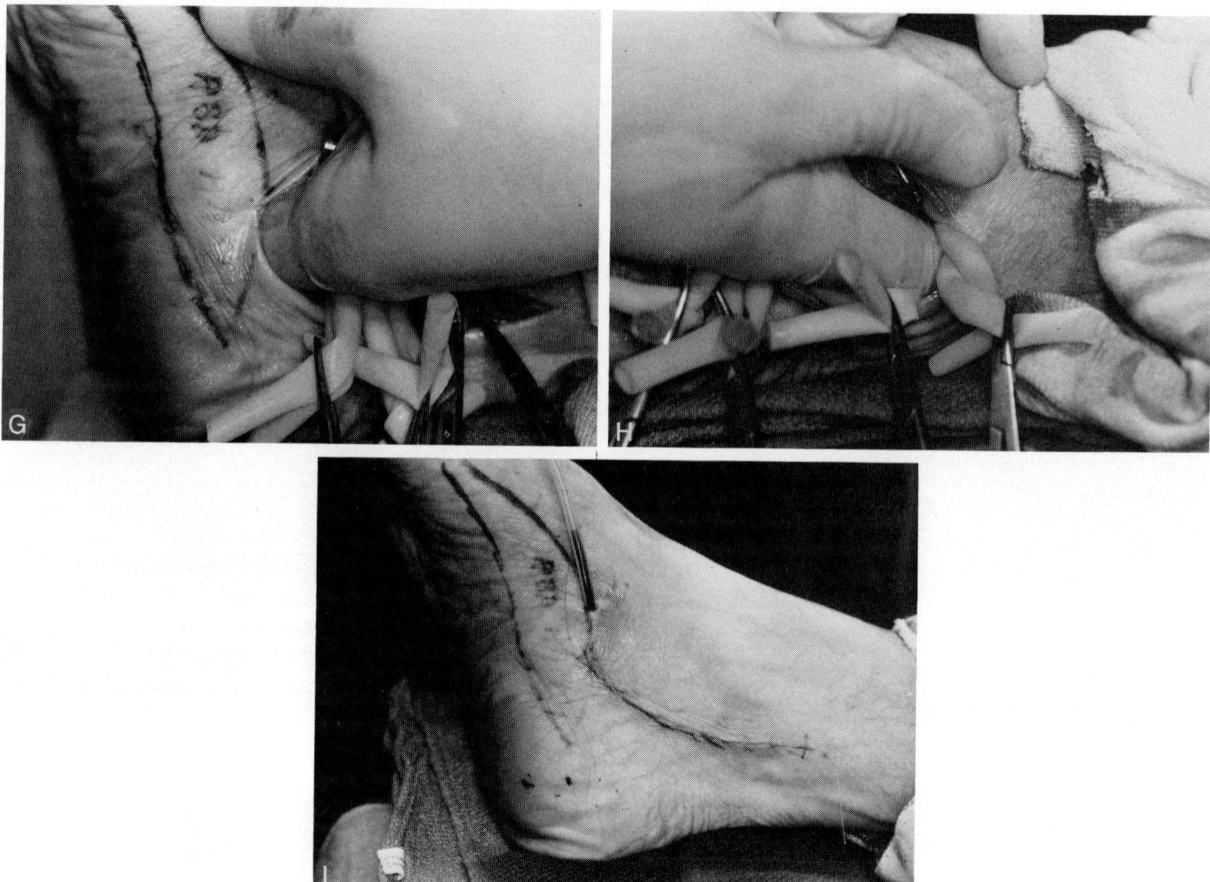

FIGURE 43–23 *Continued G,* Dilation of the abductor hiatus bluntly with the surgeon's finger. *H,* Proximal dilation of the tarsal tunnel, again bluntly with the surgeon's finger. *I,* Closure of subcutaneous tissue and skin. Note the use of a closed-suction drain in this case.

the abductor canal and the channels for the medial and lateral plantar nerves is then performed. This may be accomplished bluntly with the surgeon's finger or sharply by excising the septum between the plantar nerves (Fig. 43–23*G*).

If a local neoplasm, bony prominence, or other compressive problem is observed, it is excised. Sectioning and ligation of varicosities of the venae comitantes can be performed when these contribute to the neural compression. If an aneurysmal defect of the posterior tibial artery is identified, it may be repaired, but this should be done only by a surgeon well oriented in this vascular technique. Attention is then returned to the proximal end of the tarsal tunnel, where blunt dilation is again performed with the surgeon's finger or similar instrumentation (Fig. 43–23*H*).

Following complete external neurolysis, the nerve is assessed. If necessary, internal neurolysis is then performed. The wound is then flushed with copious amounts of sterile isotonic saline. Following complete release, the flexor retinaculum is left open to decrease the chances of postoperative fibrosis and re-entrapment. If a tourniquet has been used, it is usually deflated and hemostasis completed. A closed suction drain (e.g., TLS drain) may be used if desired. A small amount of short-acting phosphate-type steroid may be infiltrated if desired. The subcutaneous layer is then reapproximated using 3–0 and 4–0 absorbable suture (e.g., Dexon or

Vicryl). The skin is then closed with 5–0 or 6–0 absorbable (e.g., Dexon or Vicryl), or 4–0 or 5–0 nonabsorbable (e.g., Prolene or Dermalon) suture (Fig. 43–23*I*). Saline-moistened sponges and a dry sterile dressing are then applied followed by a below-knee Jones compression dressing.

A dressing change is usually performed during the first postoperative week, and a below-knee synthetic cast is applied. The patient is kept non-weightbearing with the cast intact for the first 10 to 21 days. At the second visit, the cast is bivalved down the sides and active dorsiflexion-plantarflexion exercises are begun to encourage free movement between the nerve and the related tissues in which it is embedded. Prolonged immobilization has been found to allow a greater chance of reincarceration of the nerve. At 4 weeks the patient is allowed to begin partial weightbearing, with full ambulation allowed after about 8 weeks. Scar massage, ultrasonography, and other rehabilitative modalities are begun as soon as possible.

If properly performed, tarsal tunnel decompression has predictably good results in the accurately diagnosed patient. In a review of the literature, Cimino[83] tabulated the results of 24 reports and found that 111 of 122 patients (91%) had good (i.e., resolution of symptoms) or improved (i.e., mild residual symptoms) results. In a recent study of 15 tarsal tunnel decompressions in 13 patients, Stern and Joyce[84] reported 8 (53%) with complete relief of symptoms, 3 (20%) with only mild residual symptoms, and 4 (27%) with moderate symptoms or no relief. In my experience, the most common long-term complication involves re-entrapment of the nerve. This is especially true if the procedure is the second or third decompression attempt. A traumatic episode may initiate late recurrence of tarsal tunnel syndrome following surgical decompression.[85] However, careful attention to meticulous hemostasis (often with the additional use of a closed suction drain), atraumatic technique, complete release of the flexor retinaculum with dilation of the tunnel proximally and distally, not closing the flexor retinaculum, the instillation of a short-acting steroid, and early postoperative activity have decreased the incidence of reincarceration.

Occasionally, isolated compression syndromes of the plantar nerves or medial calcaneal nerve are identified. Local neurolysis or neurectomy can be performed for the medial calcaneal heel neuroma or entrapment of the nerve (Fig. 43–24). The nerve is approached through a plantar-medial incision over the suspected site of entrapment. The deep fascia covering the abductor hallucis muscle is released. If necessary, the nerve is then followed and freed along its course distal and deep to the medial tuberosity as it approaches the abductor digiti quinti muscle.[86] Extensive entrapment of the medial and lateral plantar nerves is usually approached through a plantar Z-shaped incision over the plantar aspect of the foot (Fig. 43–25).

Plantar Digital Nerves

Etiology and Specific Findings (Fig. 43–26). The differential diagnosis for pain in the forefoot or metatarsalgia is quite substantial and certainly must include entrapment neuropathies of the plantar digital branches. These plantar digital nerves are the terminal branches of the medial and lateral plantar nerves. Distally, the nerves may be entrapped by various soft tissue masses; may be damaged directly by osseous prominences, trauma, or surgery; or may become entrapped in post-traumatic or postoperative scar tissue.[87–92] Surgical procedures involving the plantar aspects of the digits or the sesamoid apparatus may entrap the common or proper plantar digital nerves. Biomechanical derangement may also directly compress or place traction on a plantar digital nerve. Joplin's neuroma is an example of such a compression syndrome, as the proper digital nerve becomes compressed or entrapped over the medial aspect of the first metatarsal and the hallux.[1, 93, 94] More proximally, at the level of the deep transverse intermetatarsal ligament (DTIL), the nerves may become entrapped between the metatarsals and related structures where they pass deep to the DTIL. The classic Morton's

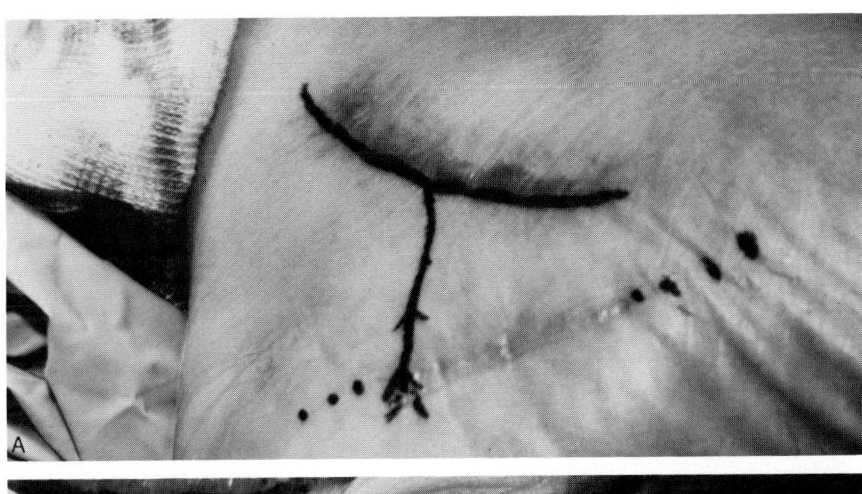
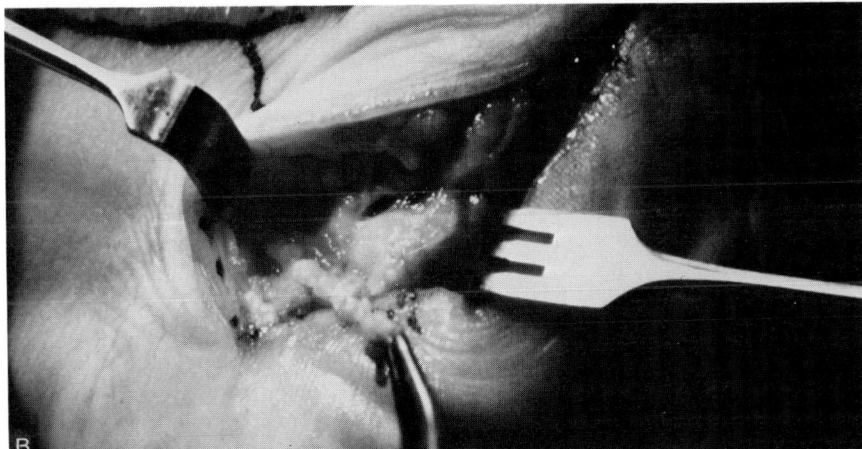

FIGURE 43–24. *A,* Preoperative photograph of patient with medial calcaneal nerve entrapment following plantar heel spur surgery. Note that the nerve is palpated and drawn preoperatively, if possible. *B,* Isolation and neurectomy of the entrapped medial calcaneal nerve branch.

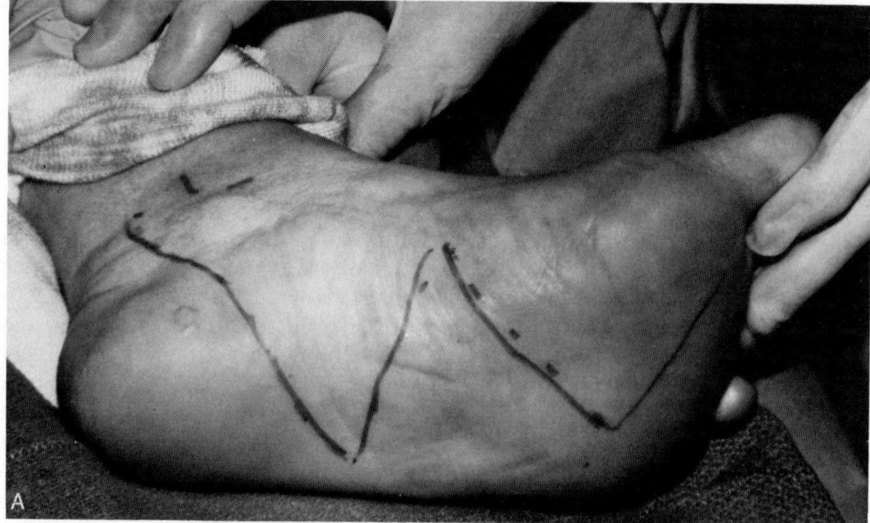

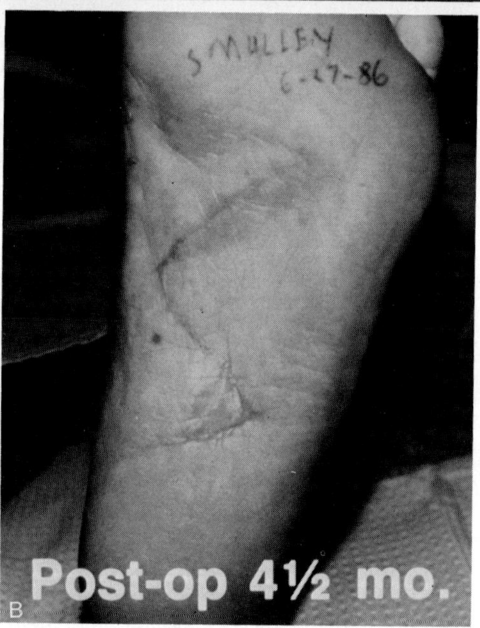

FIGURE 43–25. *A,* Use of plantar Z-shaped or zig-zag incision to release a medial plantar nerve entrapment. *B,* Healed incision 4.5 months after surgery.

neuroma is an example of such a compression syndrome. Again, post-traumatic fibrosis, tumors, infectious processes, or biomechanical abnormalities may cause compression syndromes of the nerves in this area.[95–97]

Complaints of paroxysmal or constant sharp, burning, or throbbing pain are characteristic of plantar digital nerve entrapment, such as Morton's neuritis. Numbness and paresthesias at the site of nerve entrapment are common. Patients may express their symptoms as a lancing sensation "like an electric shock" or "having a hot poker thrust into their foot." With intermetatarsal neuromas, the patient may feel a "lump," "fullness," or sensation of a "bunched up sock" on the bottom of the foot or between the toes. On rare occasions, the patient may find that the pressure from bedsheets is intolerable. The pain may radiate distally to the pulp of the involved toes or may radiate proximally up the sole of the foot. The pain may increase with weightbearing, movement of the toes, or in tight shoegear, but it is not unusual for a patient to have continued or even increased pain at rest or at night. A characteristic finding is the almost uniform desire by the patient to remove shoes and massage the feet or toes. This is especially common in patients with Morton's neuritis.[86, 98]

Much has been written regarding Morton's neuroma. This compression syndrome was first described by Durlacher[99] in 1845, but was named after Thomas G. Morton[100] who, in 1876, called it "a peculiar and painful affection of the fourth metatarsophalangeal articulation." The use of the term *neuroma* is a misnomer, because the entity is not a "true" neoplasm of cells of the nervous system. Rather, the classic Morton's neuroma is an irregular swelling with associated perineural thickening of the third common plantar digital nerve. Although the third intermetatarsal space is most commonly affected, followed by the second intermetatarsal space, these "neuromas" may occur in any of the intermetatarsal spaces.[86, 101–103] Two or more neuromas in one foot is unusual but not unreported.[103, 104] The condition most frequently affects adults between 18 and 60 years of age and is

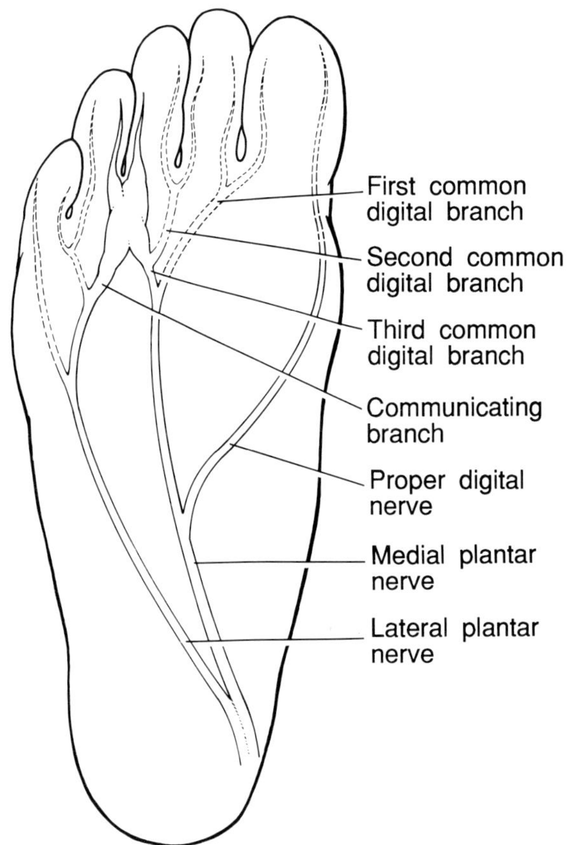

FIGURE 43–26. Typical nerve distribution on the sole of the foot. Note the neuroma depicted on the third common digital branch.

usually unilateral. Women are more often affected than men, perhaps because of the types of shoes they wear.[105] Obesity has also been described as an etiologic factor.[106] Besides the aforementioned clinical characteristics, several authors have described tests to clinically diagnose an intermetatarsal neuroma. Dorsoplantar palpation of the suspected interspace with simultaneous side-to-side compression of the forefoot has been referred to as the *lateral squeeze test* and can reproduce the symptomatology by directly trapping the neuroma between the metatarsals. Similarly, Mulder[107] described a finding which he considers pathognomonic. Mulder's test also involves transverse compression of the forefoot, combined with dorsal and plantar pressure of the intermetatarsal space, so that the suspected neuroma might be caught between the adjacent metatarsal heads. The test is positive when a palpable, often painful, click is elicited. Gauthier[108] described an increase in pain with forced extension or dorsiflexion of the metatarsophalangeal joints and relief with joint plantarflexion. If the neuroma is particularly large, it may be perceived as swelling in the intermetatarsal space or may cause divergence of the adjacent toes.[98]

As with other compression syndromes, sensibility testing remains the mainstay for the clinical diagnosis of most plantar digital nerve entrapments. With Morton's neuritis, there may or may not be a detectable sensory change in the web space between the toes adjacent to the intermetatarsal space of the suspected neuroma. Local diagnostic nerve blocks

should temporarily alleviate the patient's symptoms and help confirm the diagnosis.

Other diagnostic tests that have been suggested for plantar digital nerve entrapments, including Morton's neuromas, include electrodiagnostic tests, computed tomography (CT), high-resolution ultrasonography, and MRI. Sensory nerve conduction tests are not highly accurate, primarily because of the difficulty inherent in isolating a single plantar digital nerve with an electrode to measure sensory conduction velocity.[109] However, at least one study[110] suggested that electrodiagnostic testing may be useful, so it appears that with increased examiner interest and machine sensitivity, there may eventually be more widespread use of these techniques. CT scans have limited usefulness in evaluating soft tissues compared with high-resolution ultrasonography and MRI, and in one study, identified a neuroma in suspected cases less than 50% of the time.[111] Both high-resolution ultrasonography and MRI provide noninvasive methods for the evaluation and identification of plantar digital nerve entrapments or neuromas.[11, 112–115] However, owing to limited resolution, false-negative results may occur, and these modalities are more cost effective and better used for suspicious masses, larger neuromas, or extensive nerve entrapments.

Surgical Technique. Four different surgical approaches have been described for the resection of a Morton's neuroma. Betts[116] and others[107, 117–120] advocated a longitudinal plantar incision between the third and fourth metatarsal heads. This approach is thought to be the most direct approach to the plantar nerves. However, this approach may lead to an irritating scar on the weightbearing surface of the foot, especially if careful attention to placement of the incision between the metatarsal heads is not observed. Nissen,[121] Kaplan,[122] and more recently, Burns and Stewart[123] encouraged the use of a transverse plantar incision at the level of the distal fat pad. This was thought to be useful for exploring neighboring intermetatarsal spaces and, like the longitudinal plantar approach, preserved the DTIL. However, the transverse incision must be placed distal to the plantar fat pad to avoid the weightbearing surface, and this makes surgical exposure and exploration tedious. McElvenny[124] and Joplin[125] were the first to describe a dorsal web-splitting approach. The advocates of the dorsal web-splitting approach believed that the avoidance of a plantar weightbearing scar was advantageous. However, the retraction in the interspace is difficult, and, postoperatively, the web space is more prone to maceration, wound dehiscence, and infection. McKeever[126] first described, and Kitting and McGlamry[127] clearly illustrated, the removal of a Morton's neuroma through a longitudinal dorsal incision. The dorsal approach offers the advantage of early weightbearing and the avoidance of a plantar scar. However, it does necessitate additional dissection, including severance of the DTIL, to expose and excise the neuroma.

Regardless of which surgical approach is selected, Miller[86, 98, 128] correctly outlined several principles that must be observed to minimize complications. These include (1) gentle handling of tissues at all times; (2) meticulous hemostasis (a tourniquet is unnecessary); (3) identification of the digital branches before completing the resection; (4) removal of the neuroma without damaging the intermetatarsal artery or tendons from the lumbricales; (5) clean transection of the nerve proximally to prevent irritation or adhesions to the stump;

(6) closure of dead space as necessary, and if this is not possible, insertion of a closed suction drain; and (7) use of a firm, even, compression dressing to prevent postoperative hematoma formation.

The longitudinal dorsal incision has been my preferred approach. Generally, a tourniquet is used, and local anesthesia is infiltrated in proximal field block fashion anesthetizing the involved intermetatarsal space and the contiguous intermetatarsal spaces. A 3- to 5-cm longitudinal dorsal incision is made over the involved intermetatarsal space extending from the digital web proximally (Fig. 43–27A). The incision may be extended onto an adjacent toe to provide additional exposure. Blunt dissection is then used to traverse the subcutaneous layer, and punctilious hemostasis is obtained. A self-retaining Weitlaner retractor or Senn retractors may then be inserted to afford wound retraction (Fig. 43–27B). A large Kelly hemostat, Schink metatarsal retractor, baby Inge lamina spreader, or other similar instrument is then inserted between the metatarsals proximal to the DTIL. The DTIL is then identified and incised sharply (Fig. 43–27C and D).

Close observation of the wound generally reveals the body of the neuromatous mass. If the neuroma is not visualized, blunt probing may be performed until such visualization is achieved. A curved mosquito hemostat may then be inserted at the distal bifurcation of the nerve into digital branches. The distal digital branches are then isolated as far distally as possible, clamped, pulled proximally, and severed sharply as far distally as possible. The neuroma is then freed as far proximally as possible (Fig. 43–27E). Careful attention is paid to avoid compromise of the intermetatarsal vessels by keeping the scalpel blade coaxial to the neuroma while isolating it. A large Kelly hemostat or similar instrument may again be inserted between the metatarsals and opened to aid in separation of the metatarsals and proximal nerve trunk visualization. A small amount of soluble steroid or absolute alcohol is then infiltrated into the nerve trunk as far proximal as possible (Fig. 43–27F). The proximal nerve trunk is then placed under distal traction and severed sharply. The neuromatous mass is removed and sent for pathologic evaluation (Fig. 43–27G). The remaining nerve stump is allowed to retract proximally, hopefully to become buried in surrounding vascular, fatty, or muscular tissue away from potential mechanical irritation.

The wound is then flushed with copious amounts of sterile isotonic saline. An additional small amount of short-acting steroid may then be infiltrated if desired. A small closed suction drain (e.g., TLS drain) may be used if necessary. The DTIL may then be reapproximated if desired. However, this is not necessary, and I prefer to diminish the intermetatarsal dead space by loosely tagging the adjacent metatarsophalangeal joint capsules to one another with 3–0 absorbable suture (e.g., Dexon or Vicryl). The subcutaneous layer (4–0 absorbable [Dexon or Vicryl] sutures) and skin (5–0 absorbable [Dexon or Vicryl] or 5–0 nonabsorbable [Prolene or Dermalon] sutures) are then closed (Fig. 43–27H). A saline-moistened sponge and dry sterile dressing are then applied followed by a compressive bandage. I prefer a uniquely fashioned saline-moistened sponge to minimize edema and potential wound maceration (Fig. 43–28).

Additional longitudinal dorsal incisions may also be used to address multiple neuromas in the same foot. Care should be paid to avoid neurovascular compromise to the skin island created between incisions over adjacent intermetatarsal spaces. Alternatively, a single longitudinal dorsal incision may be placed over the intermediate metatarsal of the neighboring intermetatarsal spaces, allowing exposure to both. However, in this instance, care must be paid not to cross the involved metatarsophalangeal joint because dorsal scar contracture may result.

Postoperatively, the patient is allowed to ambulate with a surgical shoe on the first postoperative day. However, the patient is encouraged to limit activities for the first 10 to 14 days. A dressing change is performed on the third to fifth postoperative day. The dressings are removed after 14 to 17 days, and the patient is gradually returned to normal shoegear over a 4- to 6-week period.

Overall, in larger studies, satisfactory results from surgical excision of intermetatarsal neuromas have been reported to range from 76% to 97%.[101, 102, 119, 129–133] The most common postoperative complication of neuroma surgery is hematoma formation and resultant fibrosis contributing to painful plantar scar tissue or recurrent stump neuroma formation. The aforementioned principles, including the attainment of meticulous hemostasis, cannot be overstressed. Further, the use of a closed suction drain can aid in the prevention of hematoma formation. Equally important is severance of the nerve trunk as far proximal as possible and while under traction. This allows the transected nerve ending to retract proximally into the plantar vault of the foot well away from potential incarcerating scar tissue and mechanical irritation. In my experience, failure to transect the nerve trunk far enough proximal is the most common contributing cause to recurrent stump neuroma pain.

Recurrent stump neuroma pain, or neuritis of the transected nerve ending, can be a distressing problem for both the patient and the surgeon. In most instances, the symptoms become apparent between 3 and 12 weeks after the initial surgery, as the patient's postoperative pain continues and again becomes primarily neuritic in nature. In a small percentage of patients, a late or delayed return of symptoms occurs. Exquisite tenderness is typically present at the site of the nerve stump. The patient's symptoms may be similar to or different from those experienced before surgery, and frequently the patient continues or begins to complain of a painful plantar ''lump'' or sensation of ''a wrinkled stocking.'' Sensibility testing usually reveals objective hypoesthesia of the plantar aspects of the toes adjacent to the intermetatarsal space of the resected neuroma. Careful examination should be performed to ensure that the continued pain is from the plantar digital nerve stump and not from postincisional entrapment of dorsal digital nerves (i.e., if a dorsal incisional approach was used initially), adjacent intermetatarsal space neuritis or neuroma, or other causes of local peripheral neuropathy. When stump neuritis is suspected, aggressive conservative treatment, similar to that used for a primary Morton's neuroma, should be initiated immediately with corticosteroid injections, padding, and physical therapy, including ultrasound or phonophoresis. If conservative measures fail, revisional exploration of the intermetatarsal space should be considered. In most instances, recurrent stump neuritis is due to fibrous adhesions of the nerve to the plantar joint capsule of a metatarsal head.[133–135] In such instances,

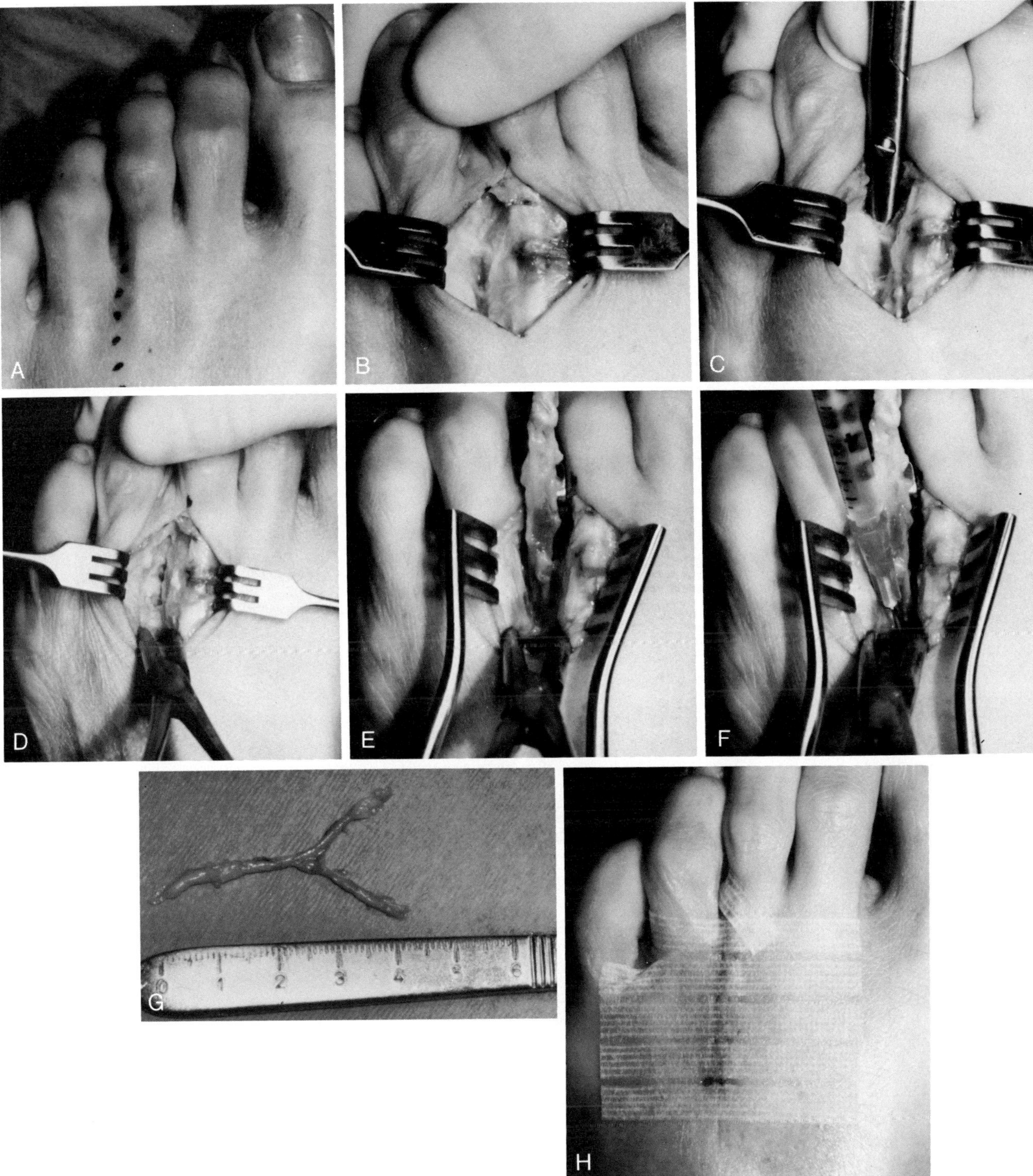

FIGURE 43–27. *A,* Dorsal incisional approach for resection of a Morton's neuroma. Note that the incision is carried distally onto the third toe to aid in exposure of the digital branches. *B,* Blunt dissection is carried deep to the extensor expansion and deep transverse intermetatarsal ligament (DTIL). *C,* The DTIL is sharply incised. *D,* A Kelly hemostat is inserted to separate the metatarsals. Plantar pressure then forces the neuroma into the wound. *E,* The neuroma is identified, and the digital branches are isolated and transected. *F,* The nerve trunk is then injected, as far proximal as possible, with soluble steroid. Distal traction is then placed on the nerve, and it is transected proximally. *G,* The resected nerve with the perineural fibrosis dissected away. *H,* Wound closure and the application of adhesive surgical strips.

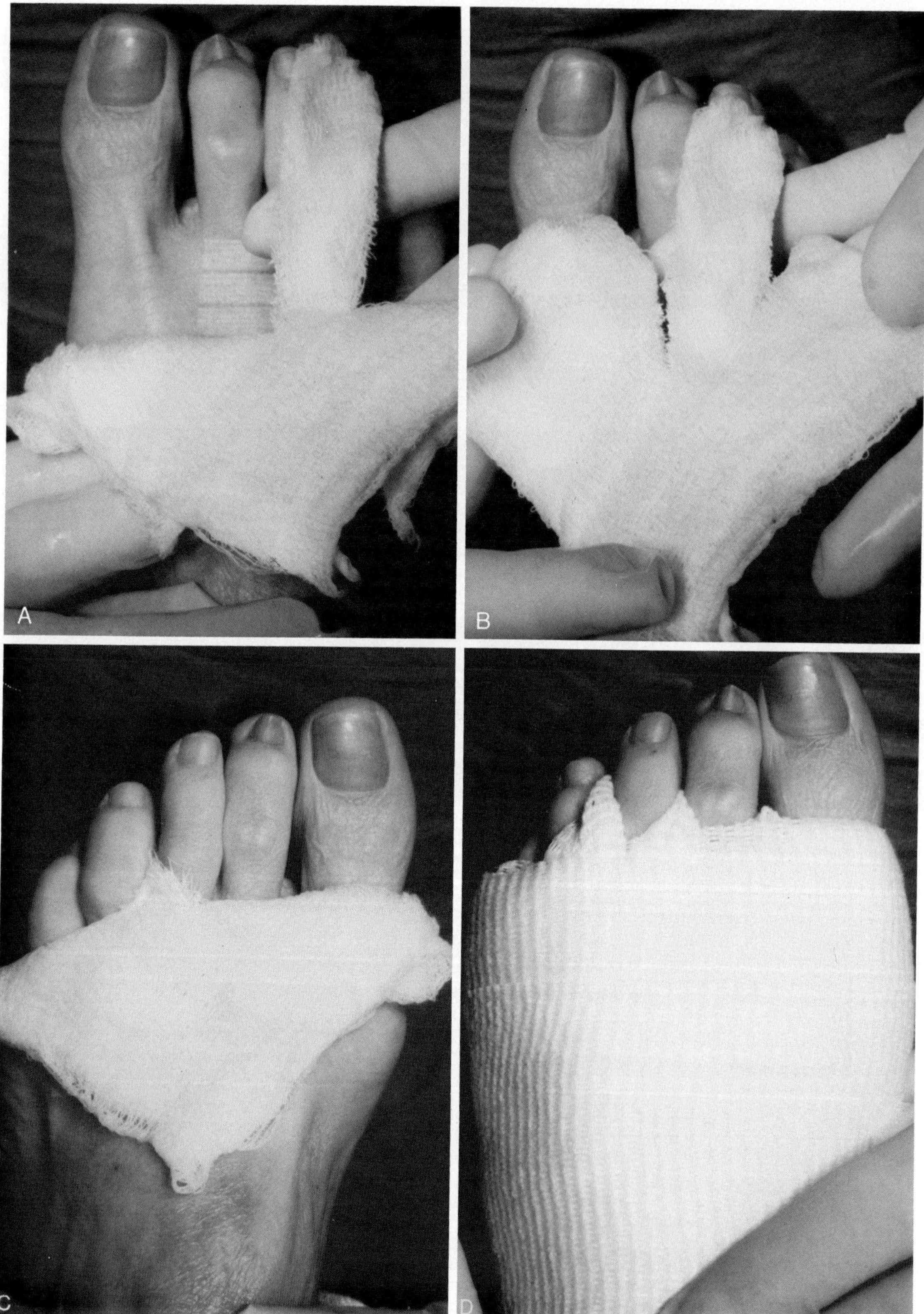

FIGURE 43–28. The author's preferred postoperative dressing following distal intermetatarsal surgery. *A,* Saline-moistened sponge is cut twice at one corner. *B,* The edges are folded back, leaving the corner protruding. *C,* The sponge is placed over the distal forefoot with the protruding corner placed into the interdigital space. *D,* The sterile gauntlet compression dressing is then completed in standard fashion.

more proximal resection of the nerve trunk is indicated. Another cause of persistent pain may be accessory plantar nerve branches that were not identified or resected at the time of the initial surgery.[133, 136–138]

When reoperation is to be performed, the approach may again be either dorsal or plantar. Most recent reports advocate either a longitudinal plantar[98, 120,131, 134, 138] or transverse plantar approach proximal to the metatarsal heads.[139] If a dorsal approach was used initially, the plantar approach avoids the tedious dissection through scar tissue and allows better proximal-plantar exposure. Other authors have espoused reoperation through a dorsal approach, employing the original dorsal incision.[119, 124] With either approach, in addition to the principles outlined earlier for a primary neuroma, the goals of revisional surgery are to (1) resect any recurrent stump neuroma and scar tissue; (2) transect the nerve trunk more proximally, allowing the nerve ending to retract into a more vascular soft tissue bed, away from potential mechanical irritation; (3) explore and resect any accessory nerve branches; and (4) minimize postoperative hematoma formation and recurrent scar tissue formation. If desired, the nerve ending may be implanted into a lumbrical muscle,[120] the adductor hallucis muscle,[10] or an adjacent metatarsal bone.[135] One would anticipate the success from revisional neuroma surgery to be less than for primary neuroma surgery. Bradley and associates[129] reported four failures in five revisional cases, but otherwise the reported success rates are surprisingly good. Beskin and Baxter[139] reported better than 50% improvement in 86.8% of their series (33 of 38), Mann and Reynolds[133] reported improvement in 9 of 11 (82%) reoperations, and Johnson and associates[138] reported subjective satisfaction in 30 of 39 (77%) reoperations. However, in these series, complete relief of pain was not typically achieved, and most patients, although improved, continued to have some pain with certain shoes and activities.

Recognizing the potential drawbacks of nerve resection, in 1979 Gauthier[108] described external neurolysis and epineurotomy of the involved plantar digital nerve with division of the DTIL. He reported stable improvement with an average follow-up time of 21 months in 252 of 304 (83%) procedures. Dellon,[140] Diebold and Delagoutte,[141] Price and Miller,[142] and Vito[143] reported similarly gratifying results with combined external and internal neurolysis in smaller series. Approaching the classic Morton's neuroma surgically with external and internal neurolysis, as opposed to neurectomy, may ultimately become the treatment of choice. However, neurectomy continues to be the more popular and commonly performed surgical approach at this time.

Other plantar digital nerve entrapments, like Morton's neuromas, can be treated with either neurectomy or neurolysis. The postoperative course is similar to that for a Morton's neuroma.

References

1. Joplin RJ: The proper digital nerve, vitallium stem arthroplasty, and some thoughts about foot surgery in general. Clin Orthop 76:199–212, 1971.
2. Kopell HP and Thompson WAL: Peripheral Entrapment Neuropathies, 2nd ed. Malabar, FL, Robert E. Krieger, 1976, pp 1–88.
3. Malay DS and McGlamry ED: Acquired neuropathies of the lower extremities. *In* McGlamry ED, Banks AS, and Downey MS: Comprehensive Textbook of Foot Surgery, 2nd ed. Baltimore, Williams & Wilkins, 1992, pp 1095–1123.
4. Merrill TJ: Peripheral nerve entrapment syndromes of the lower extremity. *In* Marcinko DE (ed): Medical and Surgical Therapeutics of the Foot and Ankle. Baltimore, Williams & Wilkins, 1992, pp 239–252.
5. Downey MS: Management of neurologic trauma. *In* Scurran BL (ed): Foot and Ankle Trauma. New York, Churchill Livingstone, 1989, pp 219–246.
6. Dellon AL: The vibrometer. Plast Reconstr Surg 71:427–431, 1983.
7. Dellon AL, Mackinnon SE, and Crosby PM: Reliability of two-point discrimination measurements. J Hand Surg 12A:693–696, 1987.
8. Omer GE Jr: Sensibility testing. *In* Omer GE Jr and Spinner M (eds): Management of Peripheral Nerve Problems. Philadelphia, WB Saunders, 1980, pp 3–15.
9. Dellon AL: Sensory recovery in replanted digits and transplanted toes: A review. J Reconstr Microsurg 2:123–129, 1986.
10. Mackinnon SE and Dellon AL: Surgery of the Peripheral Nerve. New York, Thieme Medical, 1988.
11. Hoskins CL, Sartoris DJ, and Resnick D: Magnetic resonance imaging of foot neuromas. J Foot Surg 31:10–16, 1992.
12. Downey MS: MRI of tarsal tunnel pathology. *In* Ruch JA and Vickers NS (eds): Reconstructive Surgery of the Foot and Leg: Update '92. Tucker, GA, Podiatry Institute, 1992, pp 104–110.
13. Merle M, Dellon AL, Campbell JN, and Chang PS: Complications from siliconpolymer intubulation of nerves. Microsurgery 10:130–133, 1989.
14. Brown BA: Internal neurolysis in traumatic peripheral nerve lesions in continuity. Surg Clin North Am 52:1167–1175, 1972.
15. Martini A and Fromm B: A new operation for the prevention and treatment of amputation neuromas. J Bone Joint Surg 71B:379–382, 1989.
16. Midenberg ML and Kirschenbaum SE: Utilization of Silastic nerve caps for the treatment of amputation neuromas. J Foot Surg 25:489–494, 1986.
17. Vito GR and Camasta CA: Introduction to tissue adhesives and fibrin glue. *In* Ruch JA and Vickers NS (eds): Reconstructive Surgery of the Foot and Leg: Update '92. Tucker, GA, Podiatry Institute, 1992, pp 96–99.
18. Muehleman C and Rahimi F: Effectiveness of an epineurial barrier in reducing axonal regeneration and neuroma formation in the rat. J Foot Surg 29:260–264, 1990.
19. Rahimi F and Muehleman C: Epineural capping via Surgitron and the reduction of stump neuromas in the rat. J Foot Surg 31:124–128, 1992.
20. Dellon AL and Mackinnon SE: Treatment of the painful neuroma by neuroma resection and muscle implantation. Plast Reconstr Surg 77:427–436, 1986.
21. Mackinnon SE, Dellon AL, Hudson AR, and Hunter DA: Alteration of neuroma formation by manipulation of its microenvironment. Plast Reconstr Surg 76:345–352, 1985.
22. Boldrey E: Amputation neuroma in nerves implanted in bone. Ann Surg 118:1052–1057, 1943.
23. Goldstein SA and Sturim IIS: Intraosseous nerve transposition for treatment of painful neuromas. J Hand Surg 10A:270–274, 1985.
24. Herndon JH, Eaton RG, and Littler JW: Management of painful neuromas in the hand. J Bone Joint Surg 58A:369–373, 1976.
25. Hattrup SJ and Wood MB: Delayed neural reconstruction in the lower extremity: Results of interfascicular nerve grafting. Foot Ankle 7:105, 1986.
26. Carlson T and Jacobs AM: Reflex sympathetic dystrophy syndrome. J Foot Surg 25:149–153, 1986.
27. Purdy CA and Miller SJ: Reflex sympathetic dystrophy syndrome. *In* McGlamry ED, Banks AS, and Downey MS: Comprehensive Textbook of Foot Surgery, 2nd ed. Baltimore, Williams & Wilkins, 1992, pp 1124–1135.
28. Turf RM and Bacardi BE: Causalgia: Clarifications in terminology and a case presentation. J Foot Surg 25:284–295, 1986.
29. Van Wyngarden TM and Bleyaert AL: Reflex sympathetic dystrophy involving the foot. J Foot Surg 31:75–78, 1992.
30. Lusskin R: Orthopaedic aspects of chronic pain. Foot Ankle 7:138–141, 1986.
31. Kopell HP and Thompson WAL: Knee pain due to saphenous nerve entrapment. New Engl J Med 263:351–353, 1960.
32. Garfin S, Mubarak SJ, and Owen CA: Exertional anterolateral compartment syndrome: Case report with fascial defect, muscle herniation, and superficial peroneal nerve entrapment. J Bone Joint Surg 59A:404–405, 1977.
33. Lerman BI, Gornish LA and Bellin HJ: Injury of the superficial peroneal nerve. J Foot Surg 23:334–339, 1984.
34. Tobin R, Krych S, and Harkless LB: First metatarsal-cuneiform dorsal exostosis: Its anatomical relation with the medial dorsal cutaneous nerve. J Foot Surg 28:442–444, 1989.
35. Kenzora JE: Symptomatic incisional neuromas on the dorsum of the foot. Foot Ankle 5:2–15, 1984.
36. Rosen JS and Grady JF: Neuritic bunion syndrome. J Am Podiatr Med Assoc 76:641–644, 1986.
37. Adelman KA, Wilson G, and Wolf JA: Anterior tarsal tunnel syndrome. J Foot Surg 27:299–302, 1988.
38. Cangialosi CP and Schnall SJ: The biomechanical aspects of anterior tarsal tunnel syndrome. J Am Podiatr Assoc 70:291–292, 1980.
39. Marinacci AA: Neurological syndromes of the tarsal tunnels. Bull Los Angeles Neurol Soc 33:90–100, 1968.
40. Dellon AL: Deep peroneal nerve entrapment on the dorsum of the foot. Foot Ankle 11:73–80, 1990.
41. Kenzora JE: Sensory nerve neuromas—leading to failed foot surgery. Foot Ankle 7:110–117, 1986.
42. Acciarri N, Giuliani G, Poppi M, et al: Sural neuropathy produced by intraneural ganglion. J Foot Surg 29:231–232, 1990.
43. Herrin E, Lepow GM and Bruyn JM: Mucinous cyst of the sural nerve. J Foot Surg 25:14–18, 1986.

44. Pasternack WA and Lipp RM: Idiopathic sural neuroma: A case report. J Am Podiatr Med Assoc 82:424–427, 1992.

45. Pringle RM, Protheroe K, and Mukherjee SK: Entrapment neuropathy of the sural nerve. J Bone Joint Surg 56B:465–468, 1974.

46. Raynor KJ, Raczka EK, Stone PA, et al: Entrapment of the sural nerve: Two case reports. J Am Podiatr Med Assoc 76:401–403, 1986.

47. Perlman MD: Os peroneum fracture with sural nerve entrapment neuritis. J Foot Surg 29:119–121, 1990.

48. Ortiguela ME, Wood MD, and Cahill DR: Anatomy of the sural nerve complex. J Hand Surg 12A:1119–1123, 1987.

49. Keck C: The tarsal-tunnel syndrome. J Bone Joint Surg 44A:180–182, 1962.

50. Havel PE, Ebraheim NA, Clark SE, et al: Tibial nerve branching in the tarsal tunnel. Foot Ankle 9:117–119, 1988.

51. Dellon AL and Mackinnon SE: Tibial nerve branching in the tarsal tunnel. Arch Neurol 41:645–646, 1984.

52. Albrektsson B, Rydholm A, and Rydholm U: The tarsal tunnel syndrome in children. J Bone Joint Surg 64B:215–217, 1982.

53. Grumbine NA, Radovic PA, Parsons R, and Scheinin GS: Tarsal tunnel syndrome: Comprehensive review of 87 cases. J Am Podiatr Med Assoc 80:457–461, 1990.

54. Merrill TJ and Corey SV: Tarsal tunnel syndrome: A review of 30 cases. In DiNapoli (ed): Reconstructive Surgery of the Foot and Leg: Update '90. Tucker, GA, Podiatry Institute, 1990, pp 217–220.

55. Evans C and Prior J: Iatrogenic posterior tibial neurothlipsis: A tarsal tunnel syndrome. J Foot Surg 25:194–196, 1986.

56. Gould N and Alvarez R: Bilateral tarsal tunnel syndrome caused by varicosities. Foot Ankle 3:290–292, 1983.

57. Havens RT, Kaloogian H, Thul JR, and Hoffman S: A correlation between os trigonum syndrome and tarsal tunnel syndrome. J Am Podiatr Med Assoc 76:450–454, 1986.

58. Puleo DC, Knudsen HA, and Sharon SM: Talar exostosis as a cause of tarsal tunnel syndrome. J Am Podiatr Med Assoc 77:147–149, 1987.

59. Aydin AT, Karaveli S, and Tuzuner S: Tarsal tunnel syndrome secondary to neurilemoma of the medial plantar nerve. J Foot Surg 30:114–116, 1991.

60. Brietstein RJ: Compression neuropathy secondary to neurilemoma. J Am Podiatr Assoc 75:160–161, 1985.

61. Dowling GL and Skaggs RE: Neurilemoma (schwannoma) as a cause of tarsal tunnel syndrome: A case report and review. J Am Podiatr Assoc 72:45–48, 1982.

62. Grossman MR, Mandracchia VJ, Urbas WM, and Mandracchia DM: Neurilemoma of the posterior tibial nerve with an uncommon case presentation. J Foot Surg 31:219–224, 1992.

63. Kenzora JE, Lenet MD, and Sherman M: Synovial cyst of the ankle joint as a cause of tarsal tunnel syndrome. Foot Ankle 63:181–183, 1982.

64. Levin AS, Titchenal WO, and Clark J: Tarsal tunnel syndrome secondary to neurilemoma: A case report. J Am Podiatr Assoc 67:429–431, 1977.

65. Menon J, Dorfman HD, Renbaum J, and Friedler S: Tarsal tunnel syndrome secondary to neurilemoma of the medial plantar nerve: A case report and review of the literature. J Bone Joint Surg 62A:301–303, 1980.

66. Southerland CC Jr and Spinner SM: Synovial sarcoma presenting as tarsal tunnel syndrome. J Am Podiatr Med Assoc 77:70–72, 1987.

67. Ruderman MI, Palmer RH, Olarte MR, et al: Tarsal tunnel syndrome caused by hyperlipidemia: Reversal after plasmapheresis. Arch Neurol 40:124–125, 1983.

68. Grabois M, Puentes J, and Lidsky M: Tarsal tunnel syndrome in rheumatoid arthritis. Arch Phys Med Rehabil 62:401–403, 1981.

69. Lloyd K and Agarwal A: Tarsal tunnel syndrome—a presenting feature of rheumatoid arthritis. Br Med J 3:32, 1970.

70. Byrd JW, Ricciardi JM, and Jung BI: Regional migratory osteoporosis and tarsal tunnel syndrome. Clin Orthop 157:164–169, 1981.

71. Romansky NM, Fried LC, and Frugh A: Relief of low back pain from treatment of tarsal tunnel syndrome. J Foot Surg 25:327–329, 1986.

72. Sammarco GJ, Chalk DE, and Feibel JH: Tarsal tunnel syndrome and additional nerve lesions in the same limb. Foot Ankle 14:71–77, 1993.

73. Altman MI and Hinkes MP: Heel neuroma: A case history. J Am Podiatr Assoc 72:517–519, 1982.

74. Cohen SJ: Another consideration for the diagnosis of heel pain—neuroma of the medial calcaneal nerve. J Foot Surg 13:128–130, 1974.

75. Davidson MR: Heel neuroma: Identification and removal. J Am Podiatr Assoc 67:431–435, 1977.

76. Davidson MR, Liston H, Jacoby RP, et al: Heel neuroma. J Am Podiatr Assoc 67:589–594, 1977.

77. Baxter DE and Thigpen CM: Heel pain: Operative results. Foot Ankle 5:16–25, 1984.

78. Przylucki H and Jones CL: Entrapment neuropathy of muscle branch of lateral plantar nerve: A cause of heel pain. J Am Podiatr Assoc 71:119–124, 1981.

79. DiGiacomo MA, Bernstein AL, Scurran BL, and Karlin JM: Electrodiagnosis of the tarsal tunnel syndrome. J Am Podiatr Assoc 70:94–96, 1980.

80. Goodgold J, Kopell HP, and Spielholz NI: Tarsal tunnel syndrome: Objective diagnostic criteria. N Engl J Med 273:742–745, 1965.

81. Erickson SJ, Quinn SF, Kneeland JB, et al: MR imaging of the tarsal tunnel and related spaces: Normal and abnormal findings with anatomic correlation. Am J Radiol 155:323–328, 1990.

82. Kerr R and Frey C: MR imaging in tarsal tunnel syndrome. J Comput Assist Tomogr 15:280–286, 1991.

83. Cimino WR: Tarsal tunnel syndrome: Review of the literature. Foot Ankle 11:47–52, 1990.

84. Stern DS and Joyce MT: Tarsal tunnel syndrome: A review of 15 surgical procedures. J Foot Surg 28:290–294, 1989.

85. Zahari DT and Ly P: Recurrent tarsal tunnel syndrome. J Foot Surg 31:385–387, 1992.

86. Miller SJ: Intermetatarsal neuromas and associated nerve problems. In Butterworth R and Dockery GL (eds): A Colour Atlas and Text of Forefoot Surgery. London, Wolfe Publishing, 1992, pp 159–182.

87. Berlin SJ, Donick II, Block LD, and Costa AJ: Nerve tumors of the foot: Diagnosis and treatment. J Am Podiatr Assoc 65:157–166, 1975.

88. Bratkowski B: Differential diagnosis of plantar neuromas: A preliminary report. J Foot Surg 17:99–102, 1978.

89. Chioros PG, Frankel SL, and Sidlow CJ: Sesamoid pain secondary to a plantar neuroma. J Foot Surg 26:296–300, 1987.

90. Fabrikant J and Califano PJ: Atypical neuroma of the lateral fifth metatarsal head. J Foot Surg 20:35–37, 1981.

91. Kravette MA: Peripheral nerve entrapment syndromes in the foot. J Am Podiatr Assoc 61:457–472, 1971.

92. Thul JR and Hoffman SJ: Neuromas associated with tailor's bunion. J Foot Surg 24:342–344, 1985.

93. Ames PA, Lenet MD, and Sherman M: Joplin's neuroma. J Am Podiatr Assoc 70:99–101, 1980.

94. Merritt GN and Subotnick SI: Medial plantar digital proper nerve syndrome (Joplin's neuroma)—typical presentation. J Foot Surg 21:166–169, 1982.

95. Higgins KR, Burnett OE, Krych SM, and Harkless LB: Seronegative rheumatoid arthritis and Morton's neuroma. J Foot Surg 27:404–407, 1988.

96. Miller HG, Abadesco L, and Heaney JP: Morton's neuroma symptoms from a rheumatoid nodule: A case report. J Am Podiatr Assoc 73:311–312, 1983.

97. Zivot ML, Pitzer S, Pantig-Felix L, and Nathan LE Jr: Malignant schwannoma of the medial plantar branch of the posterior tibial nerve. J Foot Surg 29:130–134, 1990.

98. Miller SJ: Morton's neuroma: A syndrome. In McGlamry ED, Banks AS, and Downey MS (eds): Comprehensive Textbook of Foot Surgery, 2nd ed. Baltimore, Williams & Wilkins, 1992, pp 304–320.

99. Durlacher L: A Treatise on Corns, Bunions, the Diseases of Nails, and the General Management of the Feet. Philadelphia, Lea & Blanchard, 1845, pp 49–50.

100. Morton TG: A peculiar and painful affection of the fourth metatarsophalangeal articulation. Am J Med Sci 71:37–45, 1876.

101. Addante JB, Peicott PS, Wong KY, and Brooks DL: Interdigital neuromas: Results of surgical excision of 152 neuromas. J Am Podiatr Med Assoc 76:493–495, 1986.

102. Gudas CJ and Mattana GM: Retrospective analysis of intermetatarsal neuroma excision with preservation of the transverse metatarsal ligament. J Foot Surg 25:459–463, 1986.

103. Silverman IJ: Three neuromas of one foot. J Am Podiatr Med Assoc 77:353–354, 1987.

104. Thompson FM and Deland JT: Occurrence of two interdigital neuromas in one foot. Foot Ankle 14:15–17, 1993.

105. Viladot A Sr: The metatarsals. In Jahss MH (ed): Disorders of the Foot and Ankle: Medical and Surgical Management, 2nd ed. Philadelphia, WB Saunders, 1991, pp 1229–1268.

106. Bartolomei FJ and Wertheimer SJ: Intermetatarsal neuromas: Distribution and etiologic factors. J Foot Surg 22:279–282, 1983.

107. Mulder JD: The causative mechanism in Morton's metatarsalgia. J Bone Joint Surg 33B:94–95, 1951.

108. Gauthier G: Thomas Morton's disease: A nerve entrapment syndrome. Clin Orthop 142:90–92, 1979.

109. Guiloff RJ, Scadding JW and Klenerman L: Morton's metatarsalgia: Clinical, electrophysiological and histological observations. J Bone Joint Surg 66B:586–591, 1984.

110. Oh SJ, Kim HS, and Ahmad BK: Electrophysiological diagnosis of interdigital neuropathy of the foot. Muscle Nerve 7:218–225, 1984.

111. Turan I, Lindgren U, and Sahlstedt T: Computed tomography for diagnosis of Morton's neuroma. J Foot Surg 30:244–245, 1991.

112. Pollak RA, Bellacosa RA, Dornbluth NC, et al: Sonographic analysis of Morton's neuroma. J Foot Surg 31:534–537, 1992.

113. Redd RA, Peters VJ, Emery SF, et al: Morton neuroma: Sonographic evaluation. Radiology 171:415–417, 1989.

114. Sartoris DJ, Brozinsky S, and Resnick D: Magnetic resonance images. J Foot Surg 28:78–82, 1989.

115. Unger HR, Mattoso PQ, Drusen MJ, and Neumann CH: Gadopentetate-enhanced magnetic resonance imaging with fat saturation in the evaluation of Morton's neuroma. J Foot Surg 31:244–246, 1992.

116. Betts LO: Morton's metatarsalgia: Neuritis of the fourth digital nerve. Med J Aust 1:514–515, 1940.

117. Bickel WH and Dockerty MB: Plantar neuromas: Morton's toe. Surg Gynecol Obstet 84:111–116, 1947.

118. Carrel JM, Sokoloff HM, Davidson DM, and Goldstein KT: Nerve surgery. In Carrel JM and Sokoloff HM (eds): American College of Foot Surgeons—Complications in Foot and Ankle Surgery: Prevention and Management, 3rd ed. Baltimore, Williams & Wilkins, 1992, pp 67–78.

119. Hoadley AE: Six cases of metatarsalgia. Chicago Med Record 5:32–37, 1893.

120. Karges DE: Plantar excision of primary interdigital neuromas. Foot Ankle 9:120–124, 1988.

121. Nissen KI: Plantar digital neuritis: Morton's metatarsalgia. J Bone Joint Surg 30B:84–94, 1948.

122. Kaplan EB: Surgical approach to the plantar digital nerves. Bull Hosp Joint Dis 11:96–97, 1950.
123. Burns AE and Stewart WP: Morton's neuroma: Preliminary report on neurectomy via transverse plantar incision. J Am Podiatr Assoc 72:135–141, 1982.
124. McElvenny RT: The etiology and surgical treatment of intractable pain about the fourth metatarsophalangeal joint (Morton's toe). J Bone Joint Surg 25:675–679, 1943.
125. Joplin RJ: Some common foot disorders amenable to surgery. Am Acad Osteopath Soc Instructional Course Lectures 15:144–158, 1958.
126. McKeever DC: Surgical approach for neuroma of plantar digital nerve (Morton's metatarsalgia). J Bone Joint Surg 34A:490, 1952.
127. Kitting RW, McGlamry ED: Removal of an intermetatarsal neuroma. J Am Podiatr Assoc 63:274–276, 1973.
128. Miller SJ: Surgical technique for resection of Morton's neuroma. J Am Podiatr Assoc 71:181–188, 1981.
129. Bradley N, Miller WA, and Evans JP: Plantar neuroma: Analysis of results following surgical excision in 145 patients. South Med J 69:853–854, 1976.
130. Gaynor R, Hake D, Spinner SM, and Tomczak RL: A comparative analysis of conservative versus surgical treatment of Morton's neuroma. J Am Podiatr Med Assoc 79:27–30, 1989.
131. Johnson KA: Interdigital neuroma. *In* Johnson KA: Surgery of the Foot and Ankle. New York, Raven Press, 1989, pp 69–82.
132. Keh RA, Ballew KK, Higgins KR, et al: Long-term follow-up of Morton's neuroma. J Foot Surg 31:93–95, 1992.
133. Mann RA and Reynolds JC: Interdigital neuroma—a critical clinical analysis. Foot Ankle 3:238–243, 1983.
134. Malay DS: Recurrent intermetatarsal neuroma. *In* McGlamry ED (ed): Reconstructive Surgery of the Foot and Leg: Update '89. Tucker, GA, Podiatry Institute, 1989, pp 321–324.
135. Nelms BA, Bishop JO, and Tullos HS: Surgical treatment of recurrent Morton's neuroma. Orthopedics 7:1708–1711, 1984.
136. Alexander IJ, Johnson KA, and Parr JW: Morton's neuroma: A review of recent concepts. Orthopedics 10:103–106, 1987.
137. Amis JA, Siverhus SW, and Liwnicz BH: Anatomic basis for recurrence after Morton's neuroma excision. Foot Ankle 13:153–156, 1992.
138. Johnson JE, Johnson KA, and Unni KK: Persistent pain after excision of an interdigital neuroma. J Bone Joint Surg 70A:651–657, 1988.
139. Beskin JL and Baxter DE: Recurrent pain following interdigital neurectomy—a plantar approach. Foot Ankle 9:34–39, 1988.
140. Dellon AL: Treatment of Morton's neuroma as a nerve compression: The role of neurolysis. J Am Podiatr Med Assoc 82:399–402, 1992.
141. Diebold PF and Delagoutte JP: True neurolysis in the treatment of Morton's neuroma. Acta Orthop Belg 55:467–471, 1989.
142. Price BA and Miller G: Internal neurolysis. J Foot Surg 31:250–259, 1992.
143. Vito GR: Decompression technique for Morton's neuroma. *In* Ruch JA and Vickers NS (eds): Reconstructive Surgery of the Foot and Leg: Update '92. Tucker, GA, Podiatry Institute, 1992, pp 111–113.

CHAPTER 44

Post-Traumatic Painful Ankle

Steven J. Palladino, D.P.M.

Chronic post-traumatic ankle pain can be frustratingly bothersome to the patient and perplexing to the treating physician. Typically, the patient presents months to years after an ''ankle'' injury, complaining of persisting or recurrent pain. Because of the number and proximity of key anatomic structures in the ankle/rearfoot region, deciphering which structure or structures are the source of the chronic pain can be prohibitively difficult if one is not well versed in the sequelae of injuries to this anatomic location.

It is hoped that the knowledgeable caregiver can offer more insight into the diagnosis and treatment of patients presenting with chronic post-traumatic ankle pain than merely to respond that the pain is ''probably arthritis'' and that treatment options are limited to living with it, using an ankle brace and taking nonsteroidal antiinflammatory drugs (NSAIDs), or having an ankle fusion. To this end, this chapter focuses on the detailed evaluation and management of chronic post-traumatic ankle pain. The potential causes of chronic post-traumatic ankle pain are presented. An initial approach directed at narrowing the list of etiologic possibilities is advocated. Further diagnostic work-up of the patient is discussed. Management alternatives for specific intra-articular entities are highlighted. In summary, this chapter attempts to expand the reader's ability to manage the patient with chronic post-traumatic ankle pain effectively and comprehensively.

COINCIDENTAL VERSUS POST-TRAUMATIC CAUSES

When evaluating a patient with chronic post-traumatic ankle pain, one must keep in mind that, although the patient relates the pain to a traumatic incident months or years before, the problem may be nothing more than chronologically coincidental with the traumatic episode. Albeit rare, it is possible for entities that are pathogenically unrelated to trauma to arise in an ankle before or after a traumatic episode. The symptoms of the unrelated condition either can be exacerbated by the trauma or can naturally progress undisturbed by the trauma. Nevertheless, as symptoms persist beyond the expected period of recovery for the given trauma, the patient mistakenly may attribute the persisting or growing symptoms to the traumatic episode and present this history when they finally seek care for the problem.

Therefore, an awareness of the variety of pathologic enti-

ties that may present with ankle pain of nontraumatic origin must also be at the command of the evaluating physician. Some of these entities are listed in Table 44–1. An exhaustive list is precluded here, as is a thorough discussion of the evaluation and management of each listed entity. However, more detailed discussions of a number of these entities can be found elsewhere in this textbook.

Nevertheless, it is apparent that in the evaluation of a patient presenting with chronic post-traumatic ankle pain, the physician's task is to decipher not only the diagnosis from among the various traumatically induced conditions (which can be further broken into extra-articular and intra-articular groups) but also the various pathologic entities that can arise independent of trauma.

EXTRA-ARTICULAR CAUSES

Although consideration must be given to coincidental, nontraumatic causes for the differential diagnosis of a patient's presenting complaint, focus must be primarily placed on the potential traumatic causes. In this endeavor, it is of great assistance diagnostically to divide the potential causes of chronic post-traumatic ankle pain into extra-articular and intra-articular sources.

As one begins to evaluate for potential extra-articular sources, it is additionally helpful to consider the potential causes by anatomic group. Specifically, the extra-articular causes of chronic post-traumatic ankle pain can be grouped into tenosynovial, neurologic, osseous, or other joint cate-

TABLE 44–1

POTENTIAL COINCIDENTAL ANKLE DISEASE WITH ORIGINS UNRELATED TO TRAUMA

Osseous Tumors	**Arthritic Diathesis**
Osteoid osteoma	Inflammatory
Osteochondroma	Seropositive
Osteoblastoma	Seronegative
Chondroblastoma	Crystalline
	Septic
Synovial Disease	Pyogenic
Pigmented villonodular synovitis	Tuberculous
Synovial chondromatosis	Fungal
	Gonococcal
Tarsal Coalition	Reactive
Talocalcaneal	
Calcaneonavicular	

TABLE 44–2

EXTRA-ARTICULAR CAUSES FOR CHRONIC POST-TRAUMATIC ANKLE PAIN

Tenosynovial
Stenosing peroneal tenosynovitis
Longitudinal peroneal tendon disruption
Subluxing peroneal tendons
Flexor hallucis longus tenosynovitis (with or without trigger toe)
Posterior tibial tenosynovitis (with or without tendon dysfunction)
Achilles tendinopathy
  Peritendinitis
  Tendinosis
  Rupture
  Enthesopathy

Neurologic
Post-traumatic focal neuropathy
  Sural nerve
  Superficial peroneal nerve
  Deep peroneal nerve
  Tarsal tunnel syndrome
Reflex sympathetic dystrophy

Osseous
Undiagnosed, nonunited, or malunited fractures
  Calcaneal stress fracture
  Calcaneal anterosuperior process fracture
  Calcaneal sustentacular fracture
  Calcaneal intra-articular (subtalar) fracture
  Calcaneal avulsion fracture of the extensor retinaculum
  Talar neck fracture (with or without avascular necrosis)
  Talar posterior lateral process fracture
  Navicular tuberosity fracture
  Navicular body fracture
  Navicular stress fracture
  Nonunion of malleolar fracture
  Tibial or fibular stress fracture
  Fractured talocalcaneal or calcaneonavicular coalition

Other Joints
Subtalar joint
  Sinus tarsi syndrome
  Subtalar joint traumatic arthritis

---

gories (Table 44–2). Thinking of the potential extra-articular sources in this manner greatly assists in the clinical examination and subsequent evaluation of the patient with chronic post-traumatic ankle pain.

Although the major emphasis of this chapter is on intra-articular sources of chronic post-traumatic ankle pain, and selected components of the extra-articular causes (nerve entrapment syndromes and tendon dysfunction) are detailed in other chapters in this text, the extra-articular causes are nevertheless briefly discussed in the context of the evaluation process of chronic post-traumatic ankle pain. The treatment of extra-articular causes of chronic post-traumatic ankle pain is not discussed in this chapter.

INTRA-ARTICULAR CAUSES

The differential diagnosis of internal derangement of the ankle joint is too frequently limited to processes that are observable on routine radiographic examination, such as transchondral talar dome fractures and post-traumatic degenerative joint disease. However, with the utilization of advanced imaging techniques, including arthroscopy, it is now known that a great variety of pathologic conditions can arise within the ankle joint as a result of single or recurrent trau-

matic episodes[1–20] (Table 44–3). Many of the causes of chronic post-traumatic ankle pain that arise from within the ankle joint cannot be imaged with standard ankle radiographs. Furthermore, it is not unusual to observe concurrent intra-articular abnormalities within the same joint. Thus, full awareness of the scope of diagnostic possibilities and careful, systematic evaluation cannot be overemphasized.

Hypertrophic Synovitis. Synovium maintains two primary functions: (1) production of synovial fluid with hyaluronic acid and (2) phagocytosis and clearing the joint of debris and wear particles. It is in the latter function that hypertrophic synovitis and chronic joint pain can develop. The mechanism for pathologic changes starts with the liberation of debris into the joint. This may occur through acute injury of the capsuloligamentous and synovial structures, acute osteochondral injury, or chronic erosion of the chondral surface. Regardless of source, the synovium must clear the debris. It is possible for the synovium's capacity to clear the joint and phagocytize debris to be exceeded. This, in turn, creates inflammatory changes within the synovium and causes it to thicken, hypertrophy, and appear more villous and opaque. The inflammatory changes as well as the mechanical irritation of the thickened synovium on the subsynovial nerves create pain. Beside pain, other secondary manifestations of chronic hypertrophic synovitis may occur, including transient effusions, fibrous synovial exudate, and fibrous bands.

Clinically, the patient presents with nonspecific joint pain or achiness, which is worse with increased activity and improves with rest. However, pain may persist at rest. Examination will reveal either generalized or focal joint line or gutter tenderness. Effusions and bogginess are rare findings. Joint motion should not be limited, unless another defect is present. Examination or imaging evidence of chondral or osteochondral defect does not preclude the possibility of hypertrophic synovitis. To the contrary, hypertrophic synovitis is often found overlaying areas of chondral or osteochondral pathology.

Synovial Impingement Syndrome. As focal areas of hypertrophic synovitis become increasingly enlarged and bulky, it is possible for those areas to become impinged between the capsule and joint surfaces. Particularly during movement, when the capsule becomes taught (anteriorly with plantarflexion and posteriorly with dorsiflexion), there is forced

---

TABLE 44–3

INTRA-ARTICULAR CAUSES FOR CHRONIC POST-TRAUMATIC ANKLE PAIN

Hypertrophic synovitis
Synovial impingement syndrome
Meniscoid body
Fibrous bands
Adhesive capsulitis
Anteroinferior tibiofibular ligament impingement
Chondromalacia
Post-traumatic degenerative joint disease
Talar dome fracture
Medial transchondral tibial impingement lesion
Loose body
Avulsion fracture
Tibial lip fracture
Anterior impingement exostosis
Fracture of the lateral process of the talus

compression of the focal areas of synovitis against the joint surface and retropressure back onto the subsynovial nerves. Furthermore, it is remotely possible for the lysozymal enzyme milieu that may exist in the impinged hypertrophic synovium to cause injury to the adjacent chondral surface, which may or may not have had prior abnormality. In any case, a vicious cycle of sorts is established.

Areas particularly predisposed to the development of synovial impingement syndrome include the anterosuperior lateral articular region, the anterior talofibular gutter region, the anterosuperior medial articular region, the anterior tibiotalar gutter region, and the posterosuperior lateral articular region. Of these, the anterosuperior lateral articular region appears to be the most common. The occurrence of synovial impingement syndromes at these particular sites may be determined by their relative predisposition to injury with ankle trauma or the relative space restriction that is created in these areas with joint movement.

Clinically, patients present with nonspecific pain ranging from achiness with activity to sharp pains that are position dependent. Physical examination may reveal generalized joint tenderness, but palpation may reveal more focal symptoms in one or more of the aforementioned sites. Motion is generally not restricted, unless another defect is present. However, selected movements may recreate the pain. Like hypertrophic synovitis, examination or imaging findings suggestive of focal chondral or osteochondral defects do not preclude the diagnosis of a synovial impingement syndrome.

Meniscoid Body. With well-established hypertrophic synovitis and synovial impingement syndrome, it is possible for the synovium to intrude between the articular surfaces of the talus and tibia or the talus and fibula. Between the surfaces, the synovium will become compressed and, over time, become a thickened, fibrous, almost hyalinized structure appearing like a meniscus or plica. Hence, the term *meniscoid body* is applied to the pathologic structure formed by this process in the ankle joint.

An alternative explanation for the development of meniscoid bodies in the lateral gutter is that, with acute collateral ligament injuries, it is possible for the torn anterior talofibular ligament to become entrapped between the fibula and the talus. In either case, it becomes possible, with joint motion, for these structures to become irritated and occasionally entrapped or pulled on, creating pain.

Meniscoid bodies are most commonly found in the anterior superior lateral triarticular region and the lateral gutter region. Clinically, patients will report intermittent and occasionally more constant pain in one of these locations, unless there is concurrent defect elsewhere in the joint. Locking and a feeling that the ankle is about to give out (which may be misconstrued as ligamentous insufficiency) may occasionally be reported. Examination may reveal pain on palpation of the specific site, especially as the joint is dorsiflexed and plantarflexed. Joint motion generally will not be limited. Once again, documentation of chondral or osteochondral abnormality in the area does not preclude the diagnosis of this soft tissue entity.

Fibrous Bands. Fibrous bands can develop within the ankle joint because of either one of two possible mechanisms. First, they may develop as a result of intra-articular scar formation after acute trauma or surgery, especially if combined with immobilization. Second, they may develop as a result of the fibrous exudative process sometimes associated with chronic hypertrophic synovitis.

The bands may connect two articular surfaces or the capsulosynovial structure with an articular surface. If substantial in size or number, the bands may restrict joint motion or cause pain. There does not appear to be any one area of the joint more predisposed than another.

Thus, clinically, patients complain of pain primarily with movement. Occasionally, locking or a feeling that the ankle is about to give out may also be present. On examination, joint motion may or may not be limited, depending on the size, number, and location of bands. Palpation of the joint will only reveal nonspecific findings.

Adhesive Capsulitis. Adhesive capsulitis is a generalized aberrant capsulosynovial response to joint injury. The inciting injury is not necessarily limited by severity. The response, however, can result in severe limitation of function. The response includes capsular thickening, extensive hypertrophic synovitis, and sometimes extensive adhesion bands, all of which contribute to a significantly reduced intra-articular volume.

Clinically, patients will complain of pain with activity and at rest. The pain can be low grade or may be disabling. Stiffness will generally be reported, and limited motion will be confirmed on examination of the affected ankle versus the unaffected side. Palpation will reveal nonspecific joint line tenderness. Examination or imaging data that suggest chondral or osteochondral abnormalities do not preclude this diagnosis.

Anteroinferior Tibiofibular Ligament Impingement. The size, extent, and structure of the anteroinferior tibiofibular ligament is known to be variable. In some individuals, the inferior aspect of this ligament is juxtaposed to the dorsolateral shoulder of the talar dome. Because the ligament is intra-articular, it is covered with synovium. With injury to this ligament or its insertions, or with any injury in the region that would create a hypertrophic synovitis around the ligament, an impingement syndrome can be created in those predisposed individuals in whom the ligament or its enveloping hypertrophic synovitis creates pressure against the moving talus. The pressure of the talus on the synovium and ligament creates pain. The direct pressure of the ligament or the lysozymal enzyme milieu of the hypertrophic synovitis can, in turn, create a chondral defect on the talus.

Clinically, the symptoms and findings of anteroinferior tibiofibular ligament impingement are virtually indistinguishable from those found in anterosuperior lateral synovial impingement syndrome. Not surprisingly, the two conditions may be observed concurrently.

Chondromalacia. Through injury, abnormal force application (wear), or other mechanisms, articular cartilage may undergo pathologic changes. Perhaps early in the pathologic sequence, these are metabolic changes within the articular cartilage, with corresponding changes in glycosaminoglycan, collagen, or cellular organization or function.

Later, clinical stages of development can be identified. Stage 1 chondromalacia demonstrates a softening of the cartilage. Stage 2 reveals fibrillation of the articular surface along with the aforementioned softening. In stage 3, the cartilage becomes more disorganized and demonstrates a deeper, shaggy, degenerative appearance. Stage 4 is represented by full-thickness loss of cartilage substance.

In the ankle, the process may be initiated by a number of

mechanisms. Direct injury to the cartilage, such as with talar dome fractures, may initiate surrounding focal chondromalacia. Chronic, repetitive, abnormal wear may also initiate a focal chondromalacia, such as that seen with various impingement syndromes. More generalized chondromalacia may be affiliated with the generalized abnormal wear created by articular malalignment either from congenital, traumatic, or iatrogenic origin.

Regardless, it is important to understand that chondromalacia, as it advances, becomes a source of increasingly abundant wear particles (or cartilage snow) within the joint. This, in turn, eventually may tax the synovium's capacity to clear the joint. Hypertrophic synovitis may ensue, resulting in pain. Articular cartilage is devoid of neural elements. Thus, the pain associated with chondromalacia is, more often than not, synovial in origin.

Clinically, the symptoms and findings of chondromalacia in the ankle joint are virtually indistinguishable from those associated with hypertrophic synovitis. As with the various forms of synovial malady, symptoms and findings may be focal or more diffuse. Crepitation with joint motion is not a frequent finding but, if present, suggests the possibility of chondromalacia, among other diseases.

Post-Traumatic Degenerative Joint Disease. Similar to chondromalacia in many ways, yet different in others, post-traumatic degenerative joint disease is among the more well-documented disorders causing chronic post-traumatic ankle pain. It arises from either direct injury to the osteochondral surface or from chronic abnormal wear associated with congenital, traumatic, or iatrogenic malalignment of the osteochondral surfaces.

Degeneration of the cartilage surface is progressive and similar to that seen in chondromalacia. However, subchondral and periarticular osseous changes are also associated, including subchondral bony sclerosis, subchondral cyst formation, and marginal osteophyte formation.

Pain may originate from the synovial response to cartilage degeneration as with chondromalacia. However, fracture of marginal osteophytes, fracture/collapse of subchondral cysts, and subchondral/periarticular intraosseous hypertension may also be sources of pain.

Clinically, patients complain of pain with activity, which may be relieved by rest in early cases but may persist in more advanced cases. The pain ranges from low grade in most cases to disabling in some. Examination by palpation may reveal joint line tenderness, which is nonspecific. Motion may or may not be limited. Crepitation may be felt with more advanced cases. Symptoms and findings of post-traumatic degenerative joint disease do not preclude the possibility of concurrent disease within the ankle joint, especially the aforementioned soft tissue pathologic components.

Talar Dome Fracture. Another well-documented source of chronic post-traumatic ankle pain is the talar dome fracture or transchondral talar dome injury. The pain from this injury initially arises from disruption of the neural elements in the injured subchondral bone. Subsequently, an additional source of pain may be developed in the form of hypertrophic synovitis and its sequelae. The synovial response is due to the debris created by the initial injury or the development of chondromalacia wear debris around the injury site.

The injuries have been classically grouped into four stages of severity. In stage 1, a compression injury to the subchondral bone is present, but the cartilage surface remains intact.

Stage 2 involves a more discernible fracture cleavage of the subchondral bone. The cartilage surface demonstrates an incomplete fissure line. In stage 3, a complete fracture fragment with cartilaginous cap is noted. The fragment is found to sit in anatomic position with a complete circumferential fissure through the cartilage surface. In stage 4, the fragment becomes displaced from its anatomic position, occasionally floating free as a loose body.

The location of the injury on the talar dome is somewhat dependent on the relative position of the joint in dorsiflexion and plantarflexion while being subjected to a deleterious inversion ankle injury. Those injuries found on the lateral shoulder of the talar dome are usually more anteriorly placed and occur with the ankle more dorsiflexed while the inversion injury takes place. Medial shoulder injuries of the talar dome are generally more posteriorly located than lateral shoulder injuries. The ankle is therefore usually more plantarflexed during the inversion episode that creates the medial shoulder injury.

Lateral shoulder fragments are generally more flake-like and are caused by a shearing component as the talus abuts the fibula during the inversion episode. In contrast, the medial shoulder fragments are deeper and cup-like, presumably from greater direct impaction forces between the talus and tibia. In either case, lateral collateral ligament disruption is generally thought to occur as a precursor to the development of the talar injury.

Clinically, it is not unusual for acute injuries to escape diagnosis, instead being labeled as ankle sprains. Patients may continue to have symptoms on a chronic basis. The pain is generally aching but may occasionally be sharp. Activities exacerbate the pain, and rest generally allows it to subside. Patients may report position-dependent pain, particularly with climbing or descending stairs. Locking or a feeling of the ankle about to give way may present on occasion. Palpation may reveal focal pain in the specific injury area but is usually nonspecific. Motion is usually not impaired. Clinically positive inversion stress or anterior drawer may be an associated finding.

Medial Transchondral Tibial Impingement Lesion. In addition to the talar dome, transchondral impaction injuries may also be found on the tibia. The injury occurs at the anterior aspect of the medial bend of the tibia (malleolar-plafond junction) as the talus impacts the area during an inversion injury. It is not known whether the injury occurs as a result of either a single traumatic episode or recurrent inversion injuries. Regardless, resultant chondromalacia and subchondral bone degeneration develop in the area of the anteromedial bend, occupying a conical area with a 6- to 8-mm base anteriorly and tapering back posteriorly as much as 8 mm. Pain may be mediated by disruption of neural elements in the subchondral bone as well as by the reactive hypertrophic synovitis that generally is juxtaposed to the lesion.

Clinically, the patient complains of a focal, activity-related pain, unless other disease is superimposed. Examination by palpation reveals focal tenderness at the anteromedial joint line. Joint motion is preserved. Clinical inversion stress or anterior drawer testing may suggest lateral collateral ligament insufficiency. Examination or imaging that suggests the occasionally associated findings of medial shoulder talar dome fracture or anterior impingement exostosis does not necessarily preclude the diagnosis of medial tibial impingement lesion with or without associated hypertrophic synovitis.

Loose Body. It must be kept in mind that the majority of bodies referred to as loose in the ankle joint actually are not. Quite frequently, they retain a capsuloligamentous attachment or are deeply embedded in and engulfed by hypertrophic synovitis, which is trying to clear the joint. Bodies may be fibrocartilaginous, cartilaginous, osteocartilaginous or osseous. Thus, radiographic detection varies with size, location, and composition.

The origin of loose bodies in the ankle may be from talar dome fractures, tibial lip injuries, or malleolar avulsion fractures. Usually, loose bodies are found in patients with a long history of recurrent ankle injuries. However, it must be kept in mind that synovial chondromatosis may present with the appearance of loose bodies in the ankle joint.

Clinically, patients may complain of vague ankle pain, occasionally focalized, especially if the body is associated with a reactive hypertrophic synovitis. If the body is indeed loose or immediately adjacent to the joint surfaces, locking or a feeling that the ankle is about to give way may be reported. Examination by palpation may reveal focal tenderness, but motion and other maneuvers will generally yield nonspecific findings, if any.

Avulsion Fractures. The types of avulsion fractures that become components of the chronic post-traumatic painful ankle are not the larger malleolar fractures. Those types are generally not missed at initial diagnosis and accordingly are usually well managed. The types usually associated with chronic ankle pain are small osseous avulsion fragments off of the malleolus. These injuries at initial diagnosis are either deemed insignificant, and thus not treatable, or are missed entirely. Regardless, these injuries do have the potential for chronic pain, although not always. The pain can arise from the development of a painful nonunion between the fragment and the malleolus or reactive synovitis associated with the fragment.

The Lauge-Hansen classification of ankle injuries suggests that fibular avulsion fragments are associated with the anterior talofibular or the calcaneofibular ligament and produced by an inversion mechanism. Tibial avulsion injuries involving the deltoid ligament can potentially be produced by three mechanisms, although two are more likely culprits in most avulsion injuries associated with chronic post-traumatic ankle pain. The abduction and the external rotation mechanisms while the foot is pronated are the more likely candidates. The external rotation mechanism while the foot is supinated is less likely to result in an untreated or incorrectly managed tibial avulsion fracture.

Clinically, in patients with chronic post-traumatic ankle pain caused by an avulsion fracture, focal pain with activity is the primary complaint unless other disease is superimposed. Palpation of the affected gutter may reproduce the pain, particularly with concurrent manipulation of the ankle. Motion is usually preserved. Although clinical stress testing may be abnormal, findings are usually equivocal or normal.

Tibial Lip Fracture. Most practitioners are well acquainted with fractures of the posterior tibial lip or posterior malleolus. The fractures are generally associated with external rotation mechanism ankle fractures, with the foot in either supination (smaller fragments) or pronation (larger fragments). Because of familiarity, these fractures are rarely missed or inappropriately treated. Therefore, these injuries

rarely result in chronic post-traumatic ankle pain. Generally, the ones that are associated with chronic pain are the larger fragments that are allowed to heal in less than anatomic reduction, leading to degenerative changes within the joint.

Probably more pertinent to the discussion of chronic post-traumatic ankle pain are the anterior tibial lip fractures that can arise from a dorsiflexion trauma. These fracture fragments can be small enough to escape initial diagnosis. The fragments are found either detached from or partially attached to the anterior tibial plafond region just medial to the insertion of the anteroinferior tibiofibular ligament.

Clinically, patients complain of generalized ankle pain, which is usually exacerbated with maximal ankle joint dorsiflexion. Locking is rare. On examination, anterior joint line tenderness may be reproduced by palpation or with maximal dorsiflexion. Overall, the joint motion is usually not restricted.

Anterior Impingement Exostosis. With recurrent abutment of the talus on the tibia in maximal dorsiflexion, an osteogenic response is created that can lead to the development of exostoses (or osteophytoses) at the anterior edge of the tibial plafond and, more prominently, the dorsal aspect of talus just within the capsular confines of the ankle joint. Although it is possible to see these processes develop as a sequela of degenerative joint disease, it is quite common to see them in the absence of substantial degenerative joint disease. In these latter cases, the individuals afflicted with chronic pain are usually actively involved in sports that create or demand repetitive maximal ankle joint dorsiflexion. Furthermore, additional mechanical factors involved with ankle joint dorsiflexion may play a role in the development of anterior impingement exostoses.

The talar exostosis is usually more prominent than the tibial exostosis (if it is present). The location of the talar exostosis is more medial than lateral at the anterior edge of the articular surface. Pain may result from direct bone-to-bone impaction injury, fracture of the exostosis, or adjacent reactive hypertrophic synovitis.

Clinically, the pain is activity related and exacerbated by activities that require maximal dorsiflexion. Palpation of the medial aspect of the anterior articular surface of the talus will generally allow the examiner to appreciate the exostosis and reproduce pain. Ankle joint dorsiflexion will generally be limited. Imaging of the exostosis does not preclude the diagnosis of other intra-articular diseases, including hypertrophic synovitis and medial transchondral tibial impingement lesions.

Fracture of the Lateral Process of the Talus. Another intra-articular fracture of the talus, albeit rare, is the fracture of the lateral process of the talus. Perhaps because of its location or because of its infrequent occurrence, the fracture is often missed, leading to the chronic post-traumatic ankle pain presentation.

The fracture is caused by an inversion mechanism while the ankle is dorsiflexed. The resultant fracture involves all or part of the lateral talar process. Because of its size and location, it is difficult to image with standard ankle radiographs.

Clinically, patients generally will complain of lateral ankle pain that is worse with movement and may persist with rest. On examination, swelling may be present laterally, along with gutter tenderness on palpation. Joint motion is usually not limited, except by pain. Stress testing will re-create the pain, but guarding will generally prevent luxation.

INITIAL DIAGNOSTIC APPROACH

From the foregoing discussion, the goals of the initial diagnostic approach are implied. Surely, the examiner must ascertain that the pain is truly post-traumatic rather than coincidental. Most importantly, however, the examiner must determine whether the pain is intra-articular or extra-articular in origin, or both. Once this is accomplished, the search for the exact cause of the chronic post-traumatic ankle pain can be pursued more aggressively.

A history of the complaint should start with the traumatic episode. How long ago did it occur? What was the initial and subsequent treatment? Were there episodes of trauma before or since the main episode? Were there symptoms before the trauma? What were the initial symptoms? How have the symptoms changed? Are any other joints painful? These and other questions can be asked to explore the relationship of the patient's complaint to a traumatic versus coincidental cause. The mechanism of injury, if recalled, may be of help in sorting out possible causes.

The history of the complaint should also explore the current symptoms. What type of pain is present? Neuritic pain can often be distinguished from pain of musculoskeletal origin. Where is the pain felt? Sometimes localization of the pain helps to rule out a number of potential causes. Exacerbating and ameliorating factors may be of some benefit in diagnosis but often not much. The severity of the pain, although important to document for evaluation of therapy, is usually of little help diagnostically. A history of locking may suggest an intra-articular cause but beyond that is somewhat nonspecific.

The medical history should be explored. An arthritic history should be investigated to rule out the possibility of coincidental disease. A history of allergy to radiographic contrast material should be obtained because these materials may be used in the future.

A physical examination should be conducted to evaluate both extra-articular as well as intra-articular disease. All the while, the examiner should be attuned to the signs of coincidental disease by observing other joints as well as the contralateral foot and ankle.

The pertinent tendon sheaths should be palpated for tenderness, bogginess, and effusion. Tendon/muscle strength should be ascertained. The pertinent nerves should be palpated and percussed at the level of the ankle. The sensory status of suspected nerves should be evaluated distal to the ankle. Signs of reflex sympathetic dystrophy should be noted. The subtalar joint should be evaluated for range of motion and quality of motion. The sinus tarsi should be carefully palpated. With a knowledge of the various extra-articular osseous causes of chronic post-traumatic ankle pain (see Table 44–2), high-risk sites can be carefully palpated.

The ankle joint itself should be systematically palpated for tenderness, bogginess, and effusion. The examiner might start from the lateral gutter and then move to the anterolateral triarticular area, across the joint line, to the anteromedial bend–shoulder region, to the medial gutter, and finally to the medial aspect of the anterior articular surface of the talus. Points of pain may correlate with intra-articular disease and a diagnosis might be suggested. The range and quality of motion should be evaluated. Restricted motion or crepitance, if found, may suggest intra-articular disease. The ankle can also be evaluated through clinical stress testing. Abnormal laxity not only suggests disease of the collateral ligaments but may be associated with additional intra-articular disease.

The initial radiographic examination should consist of weightbearing anteroposterior, mortise, and lateral ankle views and an oblique view of the foot. The radiographs should be carefully and systematically evaluated for evidence of coincidental causes (see Table 44–1) as well as extra-articular causes (see Table 44–2). On the other hand, the ankle joint itself may reveal radiographic evidence of post-traumatic degenerative joint disease, talar dome fracture, loose body, avulsion fracture, tibial lip fracture, anterior impingement exostosis, or fracture of the lateral process of the talus. On the other hand, the films may be entirely negative, yet disease may still exist.

At the completion of the screening process described so far, certain diagnoses may be excluded, whereas others may be strongly suggested. However, the screening process is not complete. The examiner should verify whether the pain is originating from within the ankle joint or external to it. Thus, it is suggested that the ankle joint be infiltrated with local anesthetic as part of the initial screening process. This will additionally serve to focus the diagnostic effort.

Either the anteromedial or anterolateral approach may be used, whichever is farthest from the area of greatest symptoms. The skin is appropriately prepared using sterile technique. At least 10 cc of 2% lidocaine or other short-onset anesthetic should be directly infiltrated into the ankle joint. No anesthetic should be injected subcutaneously because this may anesthetize extra-articular structures. After 10 to 15 minutes, the patient should be re-examined. The disappearance of symptoms suggests that the cause is intra-articular. The extra-articular structures previously mentioned should again be examined without the confusion of background joint pain. Perhaps there is also an extra-articular cause.

Variations on this protocol are possible. If the joint is effused, joint fluid can be aspirated before anesthetic infiltration and sent for synovial fluid analysis. If the joint does not accept a full 10 cc of anesthetic, and back pressure is felt earlier (at less than 5 cc), then a diagnosis of adhesive capsulitis is suggested. Some practitioners may elect to use a phosphated corticosteroid (acetated corticosteroids may initiate a crystalline arthropathy) along with the initial local anesthetic infiltration for therapeutic reasons. This should be done only when the examiner feels confident that there is no infectious component to the ankle pain. Finally, some might be concerned about the possibility of an anatomic communication between the ankle joint and an adjacent tendon sheath or the subtalar joint. If this is a concern, radiographic contrast material may be included in the local anesthetic infiltrate and a radiograph taken to verify the location of the fluid.

Combining the information of the clinical history, the examination before and after intra-articular local anesthetic infiltration, and the routine radiographic examination, the examiner should be able to narrow the potential causes to a relative few at the completion of this screening process. Most important to the follow-up evaluation process, the examiner should know whether the problem is primarily intra-articular or extra-articular.

FOLLOW-UP EVALUATION

The follow-up evaluation of chronic post-traumatic ankle pain is directed at confirming a suspected diagnosis. Thus, the test or tests used will depend largely on the circumstances of the case, namely, the possible diagnoses suggested by the initial evaluation. Cost and availability may also have a bearing on selected tests.

Of all of the tests, magnetic resonance imaging (MRI) may be one of the most versatile and, therefore, most helpful in the follow-up evaluation. Advances in MRI of the ankle region have contributed to its usefulness in the evaluation of chronic post-traumatic ankle pain. However, for the examination to be of maximal benefit, at least the following guidelines should be followed: An extremity coil should be used, T_1 and T_2 images (or reasonable substitutes) should be obtained, and the smallest slice thickness possible (less than 2 mm) should be used.

MRI may help to identify some types of coincidental disease (see Table 44–1), such as tumors, pigmented villonodular synovitis, synovial chondromatosis, and tarsal coalitions. Extra-articularly, MRI may help to identify or diagnose tenosynovial disease, subtalar joint disease, and sometimes osseous and neurologic disease (see Table 44–2). Intra-articularly, MRI may identify hypertrophic synovitis, fibrous bands, post-traumatic degenerative joint disease, talar dome fractures, medial transchondral tibial impingement lesions, loose bodies, avulsion fractures, tibial lip fractures, anterior impingement exostoses, and fractures of the lateral process of the talus.

MRI is not always specific (especially in regard to cortical bone pathology) and is costly, and its sensitivity is highly operator and technique dependent. MRI should be delayed at least 2 weeks after intra-articular injection; otherwise, false-positive synovial abnormality may be demonstrated. Although not perfect, MRI nevertheless serves as a valuable evaluation tool in chronic post-traumatic ankle pain. This statement is particularly true when both intra-articular and extra-articular causes may be concurrently present.

Many other diagnostic tests may be used, given the circumstances. Prior radiographs should be obtained, if available. Contralateral ankle radiographs may also be used for comparison purposes in the detection of subtle osseous abnormalities. If a posterior medial talar dome fracture is suspected, a mortise radiographic view while the ankle is plantarflexed may demonstrate the injury. Stress views may be used to document ligamentous insufficiency.

If arthritic diatheses cannot be ruled out, laboratory evaluation through hematology and serology may be used. Furthermore, an arthrocentesis may yield enough fluid for synovial analysis.

Tenosynovial disease can be further evaluated via intratendon sheath diagnostic local anesthetic blocks, tenosynoviography, or diagnostic ultrasonography.

Neurologic disease may be further evaluated with diagnostic local anesthetic nerve blocks or electrodiagnostic testing.

Suspected subtalar joint disease can be evaluated with diagnostic local anesthetic infiltration or arthrography.

Computed tomographic (CT) evaluation may be substituted for MRI when small osseous abnormalities in or around the ankle joint are suspected. However, the examiner would be sacrificing the diagnostic yield for soft tissue disease when utilizing CT over MRI. Furthermore, the two best planes for ankle joint evaluation are the coronal (frontal) and the sagittal. MRI offers direct imaging of both planes, whereas CT offers only a computer reconstruction of the sagittal plane. Because of MRI's advantages, plus the availability of smaller slice thicknesses and improved utility of MRI to image bone disease (particularly cancellous bone, which predominates in the ankle region), CT is being supplanted as an evaluation tool in this diagnostic exercise.

Ankle arthrography may still offer some benefits. Two-phase arthrography may be used to image talar dome fractures. However, the utility of arthrography lies primarily in its ability to detect filling defects with single-phase studies. Hypertrophic synovitis, synovial impingement syndromes, and occasionally loose bodies may be detected with this modality. Finally, adhesive capsulitis can be definitively diagnosed with single-phase arthrography. Lateral and mortise arthrograms of the ankle in adhesive capsulitis will reveal significantly restricted or absent anterior and posterior ankle joint capsular pouches and absence of filling of the distal tibiofibular recess.

On rare occasions, a three-phase technetium bone scan may be used. An absence of activity on the delayed image may effectively rule out bone and some joint disease. The examiner then can turn to soft tissue causes as possible explanations for a patient's pain. If the delayed image has focal activity, other work-up of the bone or joint disease is warranted, perhaps using CT imaging. The bone scan may be of particular assistance in cases of suspected malingering.

Finally, arthroscopic evaluation may be an important tool in the evaluation (and management) of pain that has been confirmed to be originating from within the ankle joint. It is entirely possible for some of the intra-articular causes of chronic post-traumatic ankle pain to escape diagnosis, even with tools as sophisticated as MRI. It is not unusual for causes such as hypertrophic synovitis, synovial impingement syndrome, meniscoid body, fibrous bands, anteroinferior tibiofibular ligament impingement, chondromalacia, medial transchondral tibial impingement lesion, and tibial lip fracture to be initially diagnosed during arthroscopic evaluation. However, compared with MRI, diagnostic arthroscopy is invasive, more expensive, and also highly dependent on the proficiency of the arthroscopist. Nevertheless, the advantages over MRI are that arthroscopy is usually more specific diagnostically, is occasionally more sensitive, and offers the capacity for simultaneous therapeutic intervention.

In summary, the follow-up evaluation of chronic post-traumatic ankle pain is dependent on the identification of an intra-articular versus an extra-articular source of pain. In the absence of suspected coincidental disease, intra-articular disease is often evaluated further with MRI or occasionally via arthroscopy. However, other modalities may be used and have been identified. The follow-up of extra-articular disease is structure dependent, as discussed. In the event of concurrent intra-articular and extra-articular disease, then MRI is advised.

MANAGEMENT OF INTRA-ARTICULAR DISEASE

The management of intra-articular causes of chronic post-traumatic ankle pain is by no means standardized. The management protocol must be tailored to the individual patient using age, type of work, activities, aspirations, apprehensions, previous treatments, and other factors as guides. Treatment protocols may range from nonspecific symptomatic intervention to disease-specific therapeutic programs.

NSAIDs may be used alone or in conjunction with other therapeutic modalities to reduce synovial inflammation and pain.

Physical therapy modalities such as ice and interferential current may also be used as adjunctive methods to reduce synovial inflammation and pain.

Intra-articular injections may be used therapeutically in two ways. First, phosphated corticosteroid may be used to reduce synovial inflammation. However, multiple injections should be avoided because of the possibility of potentiating degenerative joint disease. Furthermore, corticosteroids should be avoided in the presence of healing fractures of the talar dome, tibial lip, and lateral talar process. Second, local anesthetic (with or without corticosteroid) may be injected into the joint under pressure as a fluid distention adhesiotomy treatment for adhesive capsulitis or adhesive bands.

Orthoses and braces may be used to redistribute forces within the joint or reduce joint motion, which, in turn, reduces pain. These modalities are best applied in cases of post-traumatic degenerative joint disease as a substitute for fusion.

Rocker-soled shoes can similarly reduce the need for ankle motion and thus reduce pain. Again, these additions are usually substitutes for fusion of a degenerated ankle.

Cast immobilization may be attempted to symptomatically quiet an ankle that is afflicted with soft tissue sources of pain or degenerative joint disease. The exception is adhesive capsulitis, in which case the ankle should be mobilized. More important, cast immobilization should be considered as a treatment option of chronic presentations of stages 1 and 2 talar dome fractures and lateral talar process fractures. However, the chronicity of these fractures may suggest surgical options.

The length and extent of conservative care in chronic post-traumatic ankle pain cases are ill-defined. Factors that determine the length and extent of conservative care include those listed at the outset of this discussion. Additional factors include the relative lack of conservative disease-specific treatments and the existence of surgical disease-specific treatments. Regardless, this issue must be decided on an individual basis.

Open surgery may be used for virtually every intra-articular cause of chronic post-traumatic ankle pain. However, arthroscopic surgery generally has proven to be an equally effective treatment approach but with less morbidity and faster recovery. An experienced ankle arthroscopist is capable of addressing intra-articular disease as follows: hypertrophic synovitis, synovectomy; synovial impingement syndrome, synovectomy; meniscoid body, resection and synovectomy; fibrous bands, resection; adhesive capsulitis, adhesiotomy and synovectomy; anteroinferior tibiofibular ligament impingement, partial resection and synovectomy;

chondromalacia, shaving; post-traumatic degenerative joint disease, shaving and therapeutic lavage or arthroscopic ankle fusion; talar dome fracture, excision and curettage; medial transchondral tibial impingement lesion, curettage; loose body, excision; avulsion fractures, excision with or without syndesmorraphy; tibial lip fracture, excision; anterior impingement exostosis, resection; fracture of the lateral process of the talus, resection or percutaneous fixation. Nevertheless, open surgery may be required for fixation or excision of lateral talar process fractures, posterior medial talar dome fracture excision, resection of large anterior impingement exostoses, and ankle fusion. Clearly, though, arthroscopic surgery has become the more common method of surgical therapy in cases of chronic post-traumatic ankle pain.

Finally, in cases in which symptoms have been resolved, it is important to consider rehabilitation of the patient's extremity. The chronicity of these cases occasionally contributes to loss of mobility and strength. These areas should be addressed in physical rehabilitation programs as symptoms subside.

References

1. Bassett FH, Gaits HS, Billys JB, et al: Talar impingement by anteroinferior tibiofibular ligament. J Bone Joint Surg 72A:55, 1990.
2. Chen Y-C: Arthroscopy of the ankle joint. *In* Watanabe M (ed): Arthroscopy of Small Joints. Tokyo, Igaku-Shoin, 1985, pp 104–127.
3. Fallat LM: Accuracy of diagnostic arthroscopy of the ankle joint. J Foot Surg 26:26, 1987.
4. Ferkel RD, Karzel RP, DelPizzo W, et al: Arthroscopic treatment of anterolateral impingement of the ankle. Am J Sports Med 19:440, 1991.
5. Flick AB and Gould NC: Osteochondritis dissecans of the talus (transchondral fractures of the talus): Review of the literature and new surgical approach for medial dome lesions. Foot Ankle 5:165, 1985.
6. Guhl JF: Ankle Arthroscopy: Pathology and Surgical Techniques. Thorofare, NJ, Slack Publishing, 1988.
7. Hawkins RB: Arthroscopic treatment of sports-related anterior osteophytes in the ankle. Foot Ankle 9:87, 1988.
8. Lundeen RO: Medial impingement lesion of the tibial plafond. J Foot Surg 26:37, 1987.
9. Lundeen RO: Arthroscopic evaluation of traumatic injuries to the ankle and foot. Part II: Chronic posttraumatic pain. J Foot Surg 29:59, 1990.
10. Lundeen RO: Manual of Ankle and Foot Arthroscopy. New York, Churchill Livingstone, 1992.
11. Lundeen RO and Hawkins RB: Arthroscopic lateral ankle stabilization. J Am Podiatr Med Assoc 75:372, 1985.
12. Lundeen RO and Stienstra JJ: Arthroscopic treatment of transchondral lesions of the talar dome. J Am Podiatr Med Assoc 77:456, 1987.
13. Martin DF, Curl WW, and Baker CL: Arthroscopic treatment of chronic synovitis of the ankle. Arthroscopy 5:110, 1989.
14. McCarroll JR, Schrader JW, Shelbourne KD, et al: Meniscoid lesions of the ankle in soccer players. Am J Sports Med 15:255, 1987.
15. Myerson MS and Allon SM: Arthroscopic ankle arthrodesis. Contemp Orthop 19:21, 1991.
16. Palladino SJ and Chan R: Adhesive capsulitis of the ankle. J Foot Surg 26:484, 1987.
17. Ray RG and Kriz BM: Anterior inferior tibiofibular ligament. Variations and relationship to the talus. J Am Podiatr Med Assoc 81:479, 1991.
18. Schonholz GJ: Arthroscopic Surgery of the Shoulder, Elbow, and Ankle. Springfield, IL, Charles C Thomas, 1987.
19. Wolin I, Glasman F, and Sideman S: Internal derangement of the talofibular component of the ankle. Surg Gynecol Obstet 91:193, 1950.
20. Yu GV, Boberg JS, Cavaliere R, and Mahan KT: The acute ankle: Differential diagnosis. *In* Scurran BL (ed): Foot and Ankle Trauma. New York, Churchill Livingstone, 1989, pp 511–566.

CHAPTER 45

Compartment Syndromes

Paul D. Dayton, D.P.M., and Richard T. Bouché, D.P.M.

The devastating result of an untreated compartment syndrome was first recognized by von Volkmann in the late 19th century. Although at that time details of the pathophysiology were not known, an important connection was established linking this "ischemic contracture" to extremity trauma. By the mid-1900s, the compartment syndrome that von Volkmann described in the forearm was well known in the compartments of the lower leg. It was not until the works of contemporary investigators that compartment syndrome was recognized as a distinct clinical entity and direct correlation made to closed-compartment pressure.

Failure to diagnose and treat compartment syndrome on an emergent basis will lead to permanent extremity disability, including selective neuromuscular dysfunction, drop foot and claw foot. Compartment syndrome is a true emergency because resultant dysfunction, sepsis, or chronic disabling pain may make amputation necessary. The pioneering works defined the anatomic and clinical basis for compartment syndrome and provided clinical descriptions as well as objective pressure studies that serve as the foundation of our current understanding of compartment syndrome. Recently, these basic ideas have been expanded to include descriptions of acute compartment syndrome in the arm, lower leg, and foot, and have led to a better understanding of chronic exercise-induced compartment syndrome.

Early theories related the cause of compartment syndrome to pressure from external bandages, direct arterial injury or thrombosis, nerve injury, and venous obstruction. Although these are represented in the spectrum of compartment syndrome and crush injury, none alone explains the clinical and pathologic findings of compartment syndrome in total. The current literature proposes a model based on the effects of increased closed-compartment pressure on local vasculature, leading to a decrease in local circulation and compartment ischemia. Circulatory compromise may result from the following:

1. Lowering of the transmural pressure gradient in small arterioles to the so-called critical closing pressure at which active vessel closure takes place, as described by Burton.[1]
2. Capillary collapse is effected directly from the increased local tissue pressure.[2]
3. Arterial spasm caused by increased tissue pressure action on local receptors.[3, 4]
4. Impaired venous drainage secondary to venous collapse

and increased venous pressure, which leads to capillary congestion and decreased perfusion.[2, 5]

The result is ischemia of neurologic and muscular components in the compartment. A self-perpetuating cycle is established as ischemia induces increased vascular permeability and intravascular fluid escape, adding to the mounting compartment pressure.

Many factors can effect increased tissue pressure and act as the first link in the pressure cycle of compartment syndrome. Certainly, any event that increases compartment content such as bleeding, inappropriate infusion of fluids, muscle edema, or vascular exudation can start the cycle. Similarly, any decrease in the compartment size that can be caused by tight bandages, compression stockings, tourniquets, medical antishock trousers,[6, 7] or closure of fascial defects must be considered as a potential cause. Simply stated, compartment syndrome results when interstitial pressure is increased in a compartment possessing nonyielding osseous or fascial boundaries to a point at which the local tissue perfusion pressure is overcome. Failure to recognize or a delay in reestablishing local circulation on an emergent basis will cause neuromuscular ischemic necrosis and extremity disability.

ACUTE COMPARTMENT SYNDROME

Although acute traumatic incidents commonly associated with fracture have made up the largest group of compartment syndromes, isolated soft tissue injury, crush injury, abnormal bleeding, burn injury, postrevascularization edema, venous obstruction, arterial occlusion or embolus, exercise, and iatrogenic infusion injury are potentially causative. Ischemic damage is a common factor in all instances. The diagnostic and therapeutic goals, however, will differ with each cause. There are basic tenets of care followed in all instances. Compartment syndrome is best assessed initially with a detailed history and physical examination; objective clinical testing is used as an adjunct, and therapy must be instituted emergently (Table 45–1).

The clinical signs of compartment syndrome are well known and include one or more of the following:

1. Pain out of proportion to the injury (i.e., pain not relieved by fracture reduction, immobilization, and appropriate pain medication) is a good indicator. Pain is usually poorly localized and subjectively may be noted

TABLE 45–1

DIFFERENTIAL DIAGNOSIS OF COMPARTMENT SYNDROME CAUSES

Soft tissue contusion
Crush
Bleeding disorder
Postrevascularization edema
Venous obstruction
Arterial occlusion
Burn
Iatrogenic infusion of fluid
Prolonged compression after drug overdose
Medical antishock trousers
Exercise

as a deep burning or a sensation of a constricting band or covering. Pain, however, is not absolute. Descriptions have been given of painless compartment syndrome.[8]

2. Pain with movement of the joints distal to the ischemic compartment is a very reliable sign. Stretch of the ischemic muscular components causes increased pain.
3. Paresthesia and subsequent sensory loss will be noted along the course of the nerves within the compartment.
4. The skin over the compartment may be tense and waxy in appearance.
5. Absence of pulse distal to the compartment is an unreliable sign of compartment syndrome because pressures need not be suprasystolic to produce compartment syndrome. This is more characteristic of arterial occlusion.
6. In some cases, elevation of the extremity may produce increased pain, and dependency may relieve it. This is due to a relative change in intravascular pressure and therefore perfusion pressure with elevation or dependency.[9]
7. Muscle weakness may be evident.
8. Advanced signs such as muscle paralysis and complete anesthesia are indicative of prolonged ischemia and are related to a poor prognosis for total recovery.[10]

These signs are variable in number and magnitude and can be confusing in the face of skeletal or soft tissue trauma. A high index of clinical suspicion is needed to separate findings that are a direct result of trauma and those related to compartment syndrome (Table 45–2).

When considering the effects of ischemia on the neurologic and muscular structures, duration of ischemia and absolute pressure are critical factors. Partial ischemia, like total ischemia, will lead to damage if given sufficient time. Skeletal muscle contractability has been shown to remain intact for up to 3 hours under total ischemia, whereas nerve tissue conductivity is lost after just 70 to 75 minutes.[11] This is clinically evident to those who have used tourniquet hemostasis for extremity procedures. Signs of paresthesia and hypoesthesia occur after a very short application. Clinical muscle function remains intact, and complete return of neuromuscular function is evident shortly after deflation.

Histologically, muscle damage does not become apparent until approximately 2 days after the ischemic episode and subsequent revascularization.[12] In the hours directly after ischemia, reactive edema and inflammatory changes become evident. Again, the magnitude of this change is dependent on the duration of ischemia. Later, as the inflammatory and regenerative processes are activated, muscle necrosis and microscopic signs of degeneration become evident. Animal studies[11] have shown that after 4 hours of ischemia, there is no permanent damage histologically or clinically, whereas periods of 6 to 8 hours caused extensive damage evidenced by cell death and clinical dysfunction. This correlates with clinical findings of ischemic damage and compartment syndrome.

Pressure Recording

Compartment pressure monitoring has become an important tool in the diagnosis and management of compartment syndromes. Although clinical recognition through basic physical examination and clinical judgment is the cornerstone of diagnosis, objective data obtained through compartment pressure monitoring can clarify equivocal situations and aid in the decision and timing of fasciotomy. Not all compartment syndromes will have the classic presentation (e.g., some will lack the most important sign of pain out of proportion and exhibit only early neurologic change). To allow these cases to progress to the point at which advanced sensory loss or muscle weakness is evident before instituting therapy will certainly decrease chances for total functional recovery. Conversely, clinically obvious cases may not require compartment pressure monitoring. With knowledge of proper measurement technique and guidelines for normal and abnormal pressures at hand, the decision as to when to institute therapy will be clear-cut.

Normal compartment pressures have been established and guidelines given for pressures capable of effecting circulatory interrruption and therefore producing acute compartment syndrome. Mubarak, Hargens, and Owen[13] measured resting pressure in the leg of 4 mm Hg $\pm$ 4 mm Hg using a wick catheter. Similar pressures have been obtained by other in-

TABLE 45–2

CLINICAL SIGNS OF COMPARTMENT SYNDROME

Compartment	Hypoesthesia	Pain	Weakness	Tenseness
Anterior	First interspace	Ankle plantarflexion, toe flexion	Ankle dorsiflexion, toe extension	Anterior leg
Lateral	Dorsal foot	Ankle plantarflexion, foot inversion	Ankle dorsiflexion, foot eversion	Lateral leg
Deep posterior	Plantar foot	Ankle dorsiflexion, foot eversion, toe extension	Ankle plantarflexion, foot inversion, toe flexion	Medial leg
Superficial posterior	Dorsolateral foot	Ankle dorsiflexion	Ankle plantarflexion	Calf

vestigators.[14] Normal pressures in the foot have been shown to be 5 mm Hg ± 3 mm Hg with a range of 1 to 12 mm Hg.[15] Values may vary with the type of instrumentation used. Wick[13] and slit[16] catheters have been touted to be more accurate than the plain-needle technique, having less standard deviation between values and better long-term monitoring capabilities. The plain-needle technique was noted in one investigation[16] to give false high values at absolute pressures of less than 50 mm Hg and false low values between 50 and 100 mm Hg. Recently, a side-ported 18-gauge needle was used to make 94 separate compartment pressure measurements with a standard deviation of less than 3 mm Hg and obtained normal values consistent with those previously published.[15]

Regardless of the method used to measure compartment pressure, several points of technique need to be stressed:

1. Saline injection must be kept to a minimum to avoid inducing local edema, which will introduce error. In my experience, 0.1 to 0.2 cc of saline have not presented a problem when used to clear the portal.
2. Patient positioning and instrument calibration are vital for accurate measurement. Patients are positioned supine with the extremities at heart level. Positioning of the instrumentation should be consistent.
3. Experience with measurement adds to the reliability.
4. All compartments in the involved extremity should be checked.

Guidelines for compartment pressure threshold requiring fasciotomy have been determined by several authors and generally follow similar recommendations. Whitesides and colleagues[17] advocated that compartment pressure of 20 to 30 mm Hg be closely monitored with repeat measurements at 1- to 2-hour intervals. Fasciotomy would be carried out when the pressures approach to within 10 to 30 mm Hg that of diastolic blood pressure. Variations in diastolic pressure that can occur with pain and shock are accounted for with this method. Hargens and associates[18] recommended that fasciotomy be performed when pressures are >30 mm Hg past 8 hours from the traumatic event and clinical signs are present to suggest compartment syndrome.

As noted previously, compartment pressures need not be suprasystolic or even supradiastolic to impede compartment circulation and produce compartment syndrome. In fact, cessation of local circulation was shown to occur at pressures of 40 to 55 mm Hg applied by an external compression sleeve.[2] Matsen and Krugmire[5] noted the variability of subjects' tolerance to increased compartment pressure and indicated that there is a threshold beyond which permanent injury is likely. They found that when the compartment pressure was less than 45 mm Hg and fasciotomy was not performed, long-term follow-up showed no functional deficits. Clinical signs of ischemia were variable. When pressures in excess of 55 mm Hg were encountered, clinical signs of neuromuscular dysfunction were marked, and fasciotomy was suggested because damage was believed to be certain.

Clinical correlation should be made between absolute compartment pressure and the patient's history, symptoms, and clinical signs. Keeping these factors in mind, several guidelines are suggested. Compartment pressures of 0 to 20 mm Hg are normal. Pressures of 20 to 30 mm Hg are borderline, the patient should be closely monitored, and repeat or continuous pressure measurements should be taken. Pressures of 30 to 45 mm Hg should be carefully correlated, and if clinical signs are sufficient, fasciotomy is performed. Also, if these pressures persist for longer than 6 hours, fasciotomy should be considered. A resting pressure of greater than 45 mm Hg is diagnostic of compartment syndrome, and fasciotomy is mandatory. It must be remembered that there is a ±4 to 5 mm Hg error in measurement and that two separate measurement techniques may not produce the same value. It is best to stay with only one technique so that the absolute values have more reliability. Because advanced signs such as muscle weakness and anesthesia along a nerve branch may not be evident until permanent damage is well under way, pressure monitoring should be started early in the course, even when only subtle signs are present. Admission for observation and pressure monitoring is a reasonable course of action when compartment syndrome is suspected but not confirmed. Pressure survey of all compartments of either the foot or leg should be made because compartment syndrome is not necessarily isolated to one compartment. Pressure monitoring is continued until pressures normalize, clinical signs resolve, and symptoms subside.

Whitesides and associates[19] popularized the needle manometer technique of tissue pressure measurement in which an 18-gauge needle was connected to an extension tube and filled on its distal half with saline and proximally with air. A meniscus is seen at the interface. An air-filled syringe with a three-way stopcock is hooked to a mercury manometer and to the proximal end of the tube with the needle. When the stopcock is open and the needle is placed in the compartment, depression of the syringe will produce pressure in the system. At the point at which the system pressure just surpasses the tissue pressure, the meniscus in the tubing will begin to move. A reading that should closely approximate the tissue pressure can be read from the manometer (Fig. 45–1).

Variations on this method using alternate probes and pressure-recording devices can also be used.[13–16] Most commonly, we have used a system with an 18-gauge side-ported needle and a standard arterial monitor/tubing and transducer setup. This method is both simple and accurate. If dynamic measurements or prolonged monitoring is necessary, a flexible intravenous catheter can be used as the probe. Self-contained

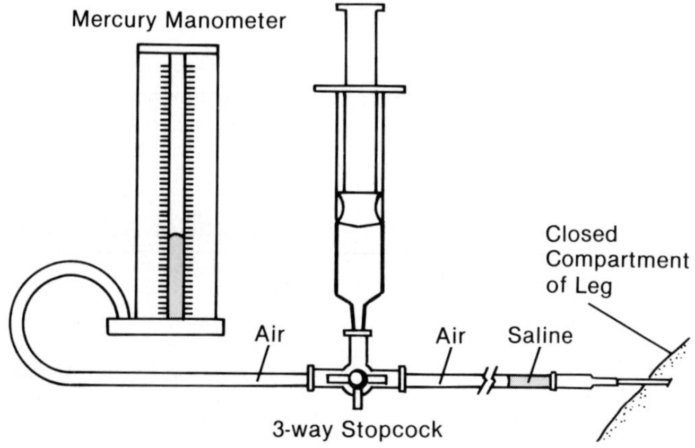

FIGURE 45–1. Needle manometer method of compartment pressure measurement. (From Bouché RT: Chronic compartment syndrome of the leg. J Am Podiatr Med Assoc 80:638, 1990.)

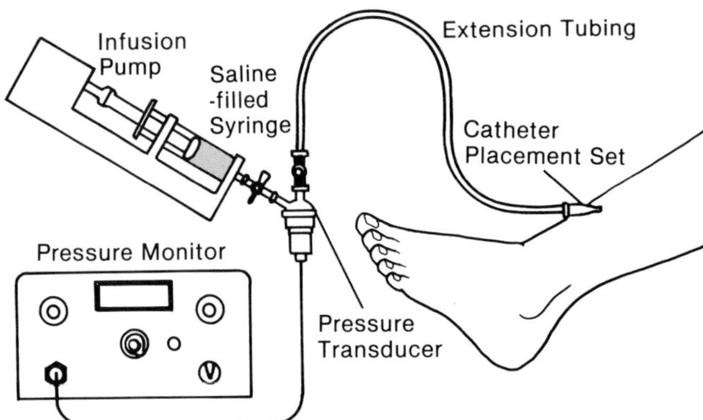

FIGURE 45–2. Infusion technique of pressure measurement. (From Bouché RT: Chronic compartment syndrome of the leg. J Am Podiatr Med Assoc 80:639, 1990.)

pressure monitoring devices are also available and are useful in acute and chronic measurements (Figs. 45–2 and 45–3).

Management

Failure to recognize and treat compartment syndromes on an emergent basis consistently leads to poor functional results and dramatically increases the potential for complications. Immediately, there is risk of massive necrosis, setting the stage for local or systemic sepsis. Myoglobinuria and renal failure can occur, and cardiac arrhythmias and death are possible. Late complications include extremity disability, contracture, and chronic pain.

The devastating results of delayed treatment are illustrated in a review of 46 extremities with compartment syndrome.[20] Normal functional results were shown in 68% of the patients when fasciotomy was performed within 12 hours of the initial symptoms and signs. The complication rate was 4.5%. Conversely, when fasciotomy was delayed beyond 12 hours, 92% of patients had permanent functional deficits and 54% had perioperative complications. Significant among the complications was a near 50% infection rate when fasciotomy was delayed. In one half of these cases, amputation was the eventual outcome. Systemic sepsis and myoglobinuric renal failure was also encountered in the delayed group.

Jepson[21] was the first to demonstrate experimentally the utility of fasciotomy in relieving compartment pressure and re-establishing compartment circulation. Currently, fasciot-omy is universally recommended as the only predictable treatment, with variations only in the technique with which the compartment is opened.

When clinical signs of compartment syndrome are first noted, all bandages, casts, and splints are widely opened or removed. The extremity is placed at heart level to avoid both dependent edema and increased compartment ischemia secondary to decreased perfusion pressure. Pulses are carefully evaluated, and if evidence of arterial injury or occlusion is present, arteriography or exploration is performed. Similarly, deep venous thrombosis, cellulitis, and nerve injury should be ruled out. The extremity is closely monitored both clinically and with compartment pressure evaluation. If clinical evidence is overwhelming or threshold compartment pressures are reached, emergency fasciotomy is performed. As stated previously, time is the critical factor when dealing with the ischemic tissue damage associated with compartment syndrome. A maximum 6-hour grace period from the earliest signs of ischemia to fasciotomy is acceptable. Many times, this grace period has passed when initial evaluation is made. Further delays should be avoided, and the diagnosis should be confirmed and treatment rendered immediately.

The technique of fasciotomy varies with the compartment in question. There are, however, universal guidelines that relate to all compartment syndromes:

1. Tourniquets are not used so that ischemia is not prolonged and muscle viability and vascular integrity can be assessed.
2. Subcutaneous fasciotomy alone is inadequate and should not be performed. The wound is left widely open because skin alone can act as the limiting envelope.[22]
3. Muscle debridement is kept to a minimum at the initial operation. This is because muscle, even if noncontractile or exhibiting a dull or cyanotic appearance, may have potential for regeneration.[12, 23] If necessary, necrotic muscle is debrided at a subsequent operation.
4. Postischemic rebound swelling is expected after fasciotomy. For this reason, all bandages and splints must be carefully applied so as not to impede circulation further.
5. The wound must be carefully monitored for signs of sepsis at regular intervals. If necrotic tissue, hematoma, or abscess is noted, subsequent debridement is performed.

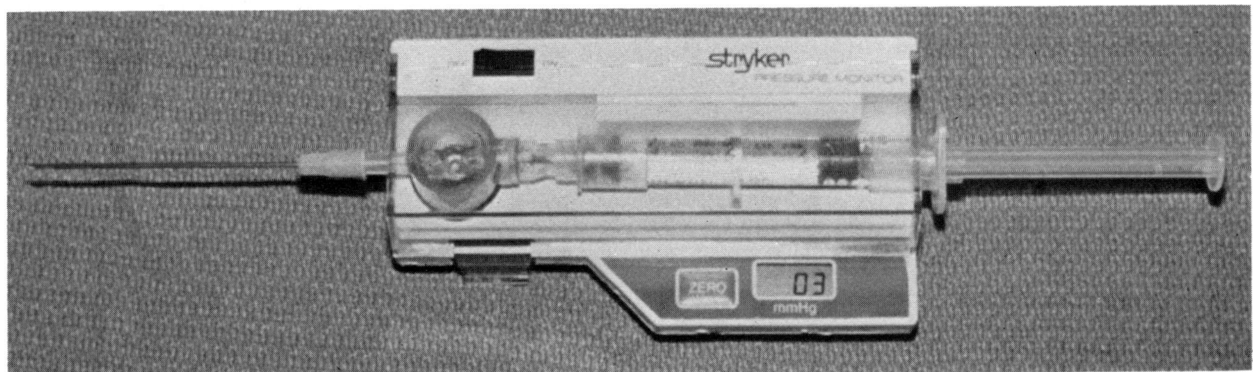

FIGURE 45–3. Self-contained pressure measurement device. (Courtesy of the Stryker Corporation, Kalamazoo, MI.)

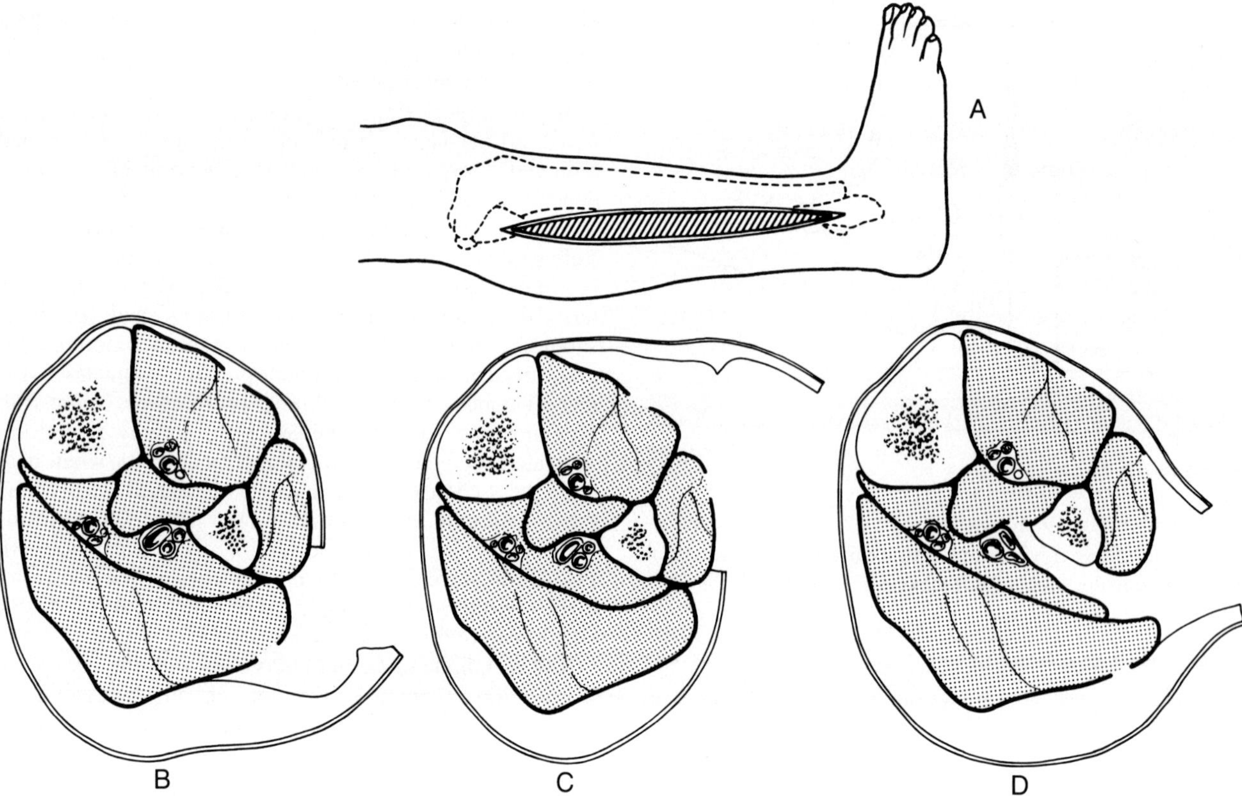

FIGURE 45–4. Single-incision parafibular approach to a lower leg fasciotomy. (From Davey JR, Rorabeck CH, and Fowler PJ: The tibialis posterior muscle compartment. Am J Sports Med 12:391, 1984.)

6. Antibiotic prophylaxis may be elected and is usually directed at the *Staphylococcus* species.
7. Fractures in need of rigid fixation techniques are addressed at the time of initial fasciotomy to provide improved stability for soft tissue and vascular healing.
8. The patient should be monitored for cardiac arrhythmias and myoglobinuria as well as sepsis.
9. Hypothermic therapy[24] and sympathetic blocks[8, 25, 26] have not been proven effective in treating compartment syndrome and should not be used in place of fasciotomy or to prolong the time until it is performed.

Lower Leg

Fasciotomy of the leg can be performed using several methods. In all cases, Matsen and colleagues[27] advised that all compartments of the leg be opened even if only one shows classic signs of compartment syndrome. Abnormal pressures have been noted in all compartments even when only one is clinically diagnosed, and postfasciotomy ischemic contracture has been noted when those compartments are left intact. Significant overlap and confusion of symptoms prevent the clinician from conclusively ruling out an individual compartment.

A one- or two-incision approach may be used to expose the four compartments of the leg. The parafibular[27] approach uses a single incision from the neck of the fibula to the lateral malleolus on the lateral aspect of the leg. The anterior and lateral compartment fascia is directly visualized and opened along its entire extent. Care is taken to preserve the superficial peroneal nerve branches as they pierce the fascia. The posterior skin flap is elevated, and the superficial posterior

compartment fascia is opened. At this point, the lateral compartment musculature is retracted anteriorly. The exposed fibular attachment of the soleus is elevated and fasciotomy of the deep posterior compartment performed. Alternatively, a second incision on the medial aspect of the leg can be substituted to expose the superficial posterior compartment.[28] Elevation of the medial soleus attachment exposes the deep posterior compartment. A transfibular technique has been described in which the fibula is removed from the lateral incision approach, leaving the distal 3 inches intact.[29] This can lead to valgus deformity in the ankle, especially when used on children. The success of the parafibular approach makes this a less desirable choice. When fasciotomy is completed, the skin is left open and postoperative wound care is instituted (Fig. 45–4).

Wound closure can be considered when postischemic edema has subsided, usually from 3 to 7 days. In some cases, the wound edges can be mobilized and delayed primary closure performed. It has been helpful in other cases to use serially applied tape strips or elastic bands at the wound edges to bring them into apposition in several days' time. In the remaining cases, meshed skin graphs are necessary.

Foot

Pedal compartment syndrome exhibits the same general clinical and objective findings already discussed with several exceptions. These exceptions are related to the compact anatomic nature of the foot and the small mass of muscle therein. In some cases, the symptomatology of foot compartment syndrome is less dramatic than that in the arm and the leg. A relatively smaller muscle mass produces less ischemic pain and blunting of clinical signs and symptoms. In addition, the layered nature of the neurologic, muscular, and osseous anatomy makes for overlap and confusion of symptoms directly related to fracture, contusion, and nerve compression with those of early compartment syndrome. Ambiguity of the clinical signs in pedal compartment syndrome may be responsible for its low incidence of reports. Additionally, these factors make the objective findings from compartment pressure monitoring much more important in the foot, and monitoring should be considered at a lower threshold. Some groups now recommend tissue pressure measurement in all major foot injuries.[30] They have reported neuromuscular dysfunction and joint contracture after calcaneal fracture in 7 of 17 patients, which led to plantar muscular scarring and claw-toe deformities. Calcaneal fracture and crush injury with or without fracture are at high risk for compartment syndrome and need to be closely monitored.

When fasciotomy of the plantar foot is necessary, all fascial spaces must be opened. Generally, the plantar aspect of the foot is divided into the following compartments with their muscular contents:

1. *Medial*: abductor hallucis, flexor hallucis brevis
2. *Central*: flexor digitorum brevis, lumbricals, adductor hallucis (transverse and oblique heads)
3. *Lateral*: abductor digiti minimi, flexor digiti minimi brevis
4. *Interosseous*: dorsal and plantar interossei
5. Recent experimental evidence suggests that there is an additional compartment with distinct fascial boundaries and containing only the quadratus plantar muscle[31]: The *calcaneal compartment* has been shown to communicate with the deep posterior compartment of the leg and has no connection to the adjacent foot compartments. Occult isolated compartment syndrome in the calcaneal compartment has been theorized to explain claw-toe deformity sometimes seen after calcaneal fracture (Fig. 45–5).

Foot fasciotomy is generally performed through a medial longitudinal incision that is a modification[32] of the approach used by Grodinsky[33] and Loeffler and Ballard[34] to treat plantar space abscess. The incision parallels the plantar aspect of the first metatarsal from the plantar calcaneal tubercle to the first metatarsal head. The medial compartment is approached directly through the overlying fascia. The central compartment fascia is then exposed by plantar retraction of the adductor hallucis muscle belly. Blunt dissection is used to separate the muscular layers of the central compartment and to open the interosseous, adductor, and calcaneal compartments. Care is taken to protect the plantar neurovascular structures running through the area. The medial fascial boundary of the lateral compartment is then opened. All hematomas are evacuated, and the wound is left widely open. Protective wound interface and compressive dressings are carefully applied. Postoperative care follows the same courses as described for the leg. Fractures can be addressed through the same incision or through additional dorsal incisions. A lateral approach for calcaneal fractures is not contraindicated after fasciotomy (Fig. 45–6).

A second technique has been described[35] using two dorsal incisions centered over the second and fourth metatarsals. All plantar compartments are approached blindly through the

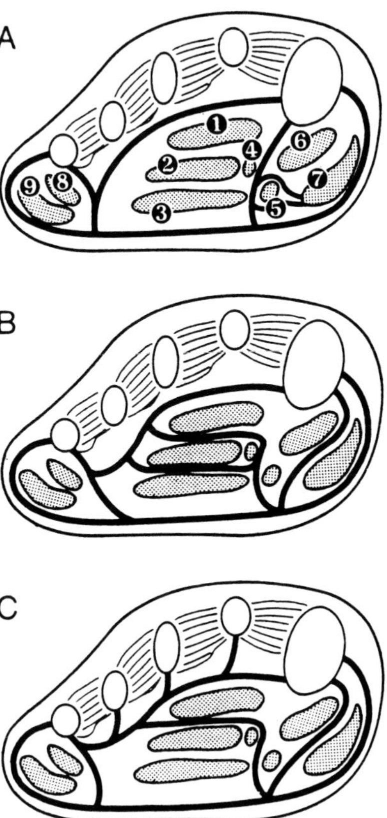

FIGURE 45–5. Alternate descriptions of the fascial boundaries of the plantar space of the foot. (From Goldman FD: Deep space infections in the diabetic patient. J Am Podiatr Med Assoc 77:431, 1987.)

intermetatarsal spaces. The advantage of this technique is that fractures in the forefoot and midfoot can be directly addressed. In an experimental trial[32] comparing decompression by the dorsal approach with that of the medial, both approaches were found to be effective within the experimental design. There was a difference noted in the time for pressure equalization; the dorsal approach took 11 minutes and the medial approach 1 minute.

Because injection of saline was used to simulate the pressure of compartment syndrome, one must question whether fasciotomy was producing decompression that would be applicable to clinical compartment syndrome or merely draining the compartment. Similarly, one questions whether this technique would be completely effective clinically, especially because it provides no expansion route for the edematous muscle mass within a compartment. Certainly, hematoma could be drained, and if this were the sole cause of the pressure-induced ischemia, this would likely be effective. In our experience, medial longitudinal fasciotomy in pedal compartment syndrome allows explosive expansion of swollen muscle into the wound. Closure of the skin over this mass is impossible without significant tension and increased pressure. In this situation, we are not confident in the ability of the dorsal approach producing decompression (Fig. 45–7).

CHRONIC COMPARTMENT SYNDROME

Compartment pressure can increase to a critical level after strenuous exercise, resulting in ischemic extremity pain.[36, 37]

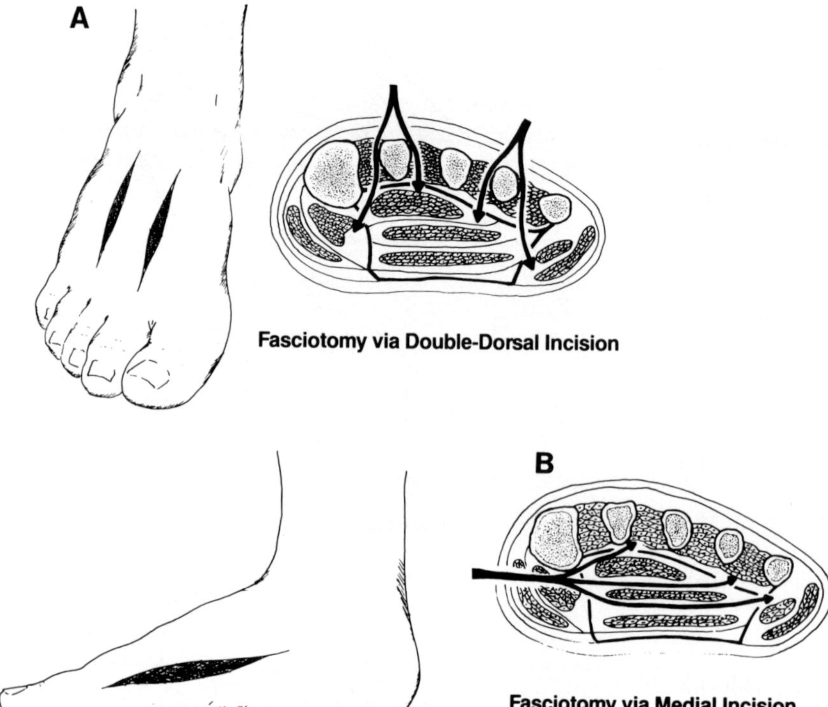

FIGURE 45–6. *A,* Dorsal approach to foot fasciotomy. *B,* Medial approach to foot fasciotomy. (From Myerson M: Acute compartment syndromes of the foot. Bull Hosp J Dis Orthop Inst 47:251, 1987.)

Symptoms will resolve with rest and recur on resumption of the offending activity once the critical pressure is realized. Although other names have been used to describe this phenomenon of transient exercise-induced ischemia, chronic compartment syndrome is the most descriptive. Chronic compartment syndrome must be separated from acute exercise-induced compartment syndrome in which pressure increase and ischemia are sustained. Chronic compartment syndrome is marked by transient clinical signs of ischemia resolving usually with the cessation of exercise or shortly thereafter. Although it is not an emergency, chronic compartment syndrome is an important cause of leg pain that can result in considerable disability in the athlete or active individual.

Increased tissue pressure may result from increased muscle mass seen with exercise, impairing local circulation. Exercise has been shown to raise muscle weight by 20%.[38] Postexercise muscle edema is influenced by increased blood flow[38] and fluid retention.[39] Hypertrophy of muscle cells from repeated exercise may also increase compartment pressure.[37] Decreased compartment volume from tight or thickened fascia and external pressure from casts, braces, and taping may increase pressure.

The existence of chronic compartment syndrome was first noted in the literature in 1956.[40] Chronic compartment syndrome is commonly encountered in endurance activities, but any activity requiring sustained extremity exertion may cause it. More importantly, it must be remembered that an *acute* compartment syndrome may also develop after strenuous exercise. In today's society, in which exercise for health is emphasized and many older and previously sedentary individuals are taking up athletic endeavors, compartment syndromes, both chronic and acute, will certainly become more prevalent. This is supported by the increase in literature reports of compartment syndromes.

Chronic compartment syndrome predominantly affects the

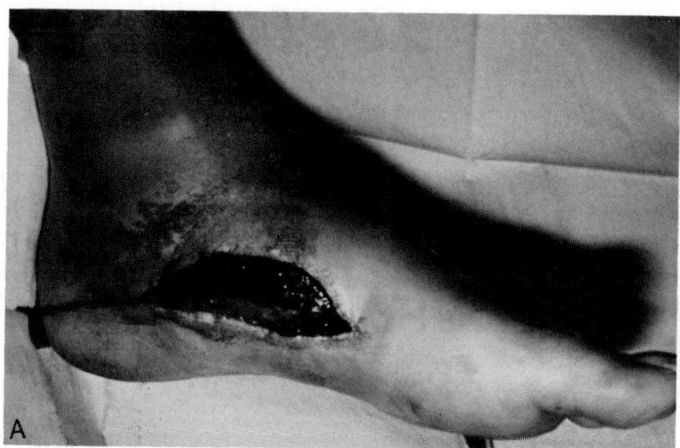

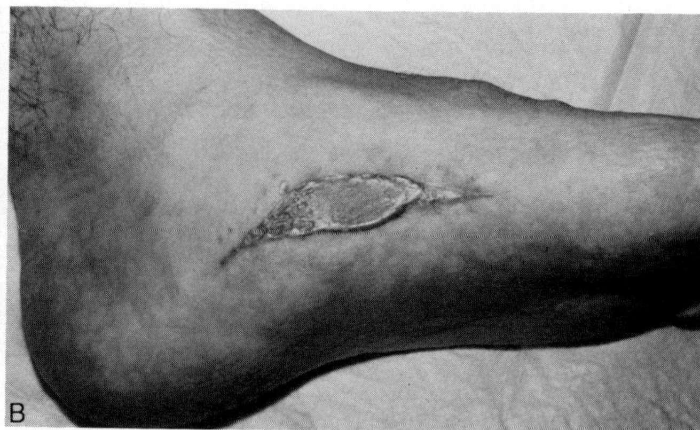

FIGURE 45–7. *A,* Immediately after a medial fasciotomy. *B,* Three months after closure with a split-thickness skin graft.

lower leg,[36, 37] but involvement of the posterior thigh[41] and most recently the foot[42] has been described. Isolated or combined anterior, lateral, deep posterior, and superficial posterior compartment syndromes have been described,[36, 37, 43–45] although their absolute frequency is not known.

Diagnosis

Diagnosis of chronic compartment syndrome, like that for acute compartment syndrome, relies heavily on clinical history. Chronic pain in the involved compartment arises usually after a consistent duration of activity and prevents further activity. Pain is variable in nature, ranging from vague, diffuse pain to well-localized, sharp pain. Rest provides relief from the pain, although pain relief is not immediate. Other complaints may include paresthesia or numbness of the distal nerve distributions, temporary footdrop,[45] a feeling of weakness or imbalance, pain with passive stretch of involved muscles, and muscle herniation.

Physical examination is directed at accurate localization of the pain and determination of the distribution of the neuromuscular deficits. At rest, there is no obvious physical findings, although muscle herniations may be present (Fig. 45–8). In fact, these are present in greater than 40% of cases of chronic compartment syndrome compared with less than 15% of normal extremities.[43, 44] Exercise until symptoms occur is necessary before accurate examination can be performed. Reproducing the activity in which symptoms are

encountered is important rather than using standardized clinical maneuvers that may not reproduce symptoms and therefore may give an inaccurate clinical assessment. Muscle herniations become more prominent after exercise. Palpation of the involved compartment reveals local tenseness and pain. Passive stretch of the compartment musculature increases the pain. A marked strength deficit is usually noted with manual muscle testing. Pedal pulses and distal capillary fill remain normal. After exercise is completed, these clinical findings usually resolve in minutes to hours, depending on the duration of exercise and the severity of the problem.

Differential diagnosis should include stress fracture, stress reaction, tendinitis, muscle strain, tibial stress syndrome (shin splints), and recurrent muscle cramps. Less common problems to consider are nerve lesions, claudication, and superficial/deep vein thrombophlebitis.

Pressure Measurements

Compartment pressure measurements have been used in the diagnosis of chronic compartment syndrome as in acute compartment syndrome and are used to confirm the diagnosis or to clarify equivocal situations. Normal ranges for compartment pressure stated earlier are the basis for comparison. Abnormal pressures are evaluated in the relaxation phase of muscle contraction. Compromise of local circulation is, therefore, related to increased relaxation pressures. Peak pressures, which can easily reach the 50 to 100 mm Hg range with muscle contraction, are not diagnostic. Furthermore, sustained increases in compartment pressure after cessation of activity are an important sign of compartment syndrome. Pedowitz and coworkers[43] gave the following parameters for the diagnosis of chronic compartment syndrome: resting pressure >15 mm Hg, with a 1-minute postexercise pressure of >30 mm Hg or a 5-minute postexercise pressure of >20 mm Hg. Other authors gave similar recommendations.[45, 46]

Management

Initial treatment of chronic compartment syndrome consists of activity modification and rest. Unfortunately, conservative therapy including retraining and physical therapy have not been effective, and usually a full return to previous activity level is not possible.[37, 44, 47] When permanent activity modification is not acceptable, compartment fasciotomy may be elected. High success rates have been reported with surgical treatment.[36, 37, 45, 47]

Fasciotomy for chronic leg compartment syndrome can be performed through limited skin incisions, provided the underlying fascia is completely opened. This is typically done through a small vertical or transverse incision at the midportion of the leg overlying the lateral crural septum on the lateral side and just posterior to the tibia on the medial side. A long-handled surgical scissors with the jaws blocked open 2 to 3 mm can be used carefully in a small incision and run distally then proximally to open the extent of the compartment. If fasciotomy cannot be completed by feel, accessory incisions must be made at several intervals to ensure complete fasciotomy. Care must also be taken to avoid the superficial peroneal nerve in the distal third of the leg. When fascial defects are present, the skin incision is placed over the herniation and the fasciotomy is initiated at that point.

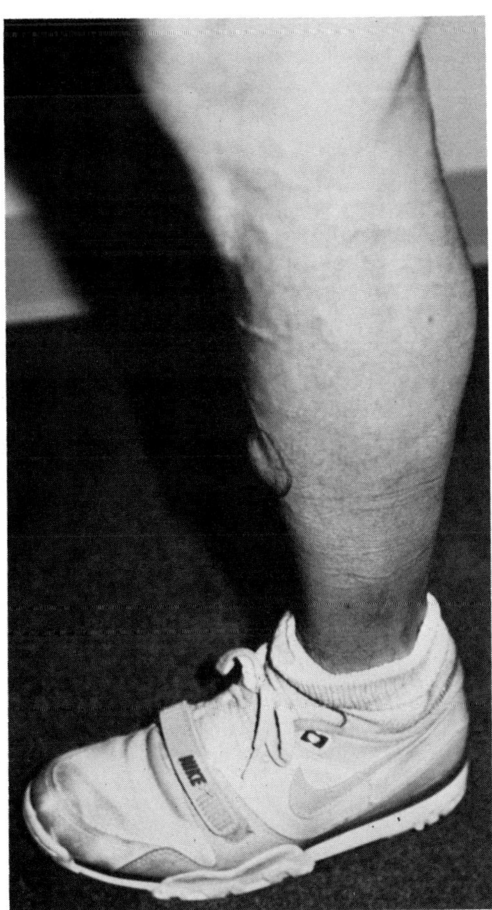

FIGURE 45–8. Fascial herniation of the anterior compartment.

Fascial defects are never repaired because this can induce an acute compartment syndrome.[37] Postoperatively, the extremity is placed in a compressive bandage and is non-weightbearing for 1 week. Progression to full weightbearing is made when the incisions are healed, and athletic activity may be resumed at approximately 6 weeks.

Technique for fasciotomy of the foot in the treatment of chronic pedal compartment syndrome has not been described. Release of fascial envelopes of the foot has been described in the discussions on acute compartment syndrome. Although one report of the diagnosis and treatment by fasciotomy of chronic pedal compartment syndrome exists,[42] further experimental studies are needed to document the existence of this disorder and determine appropriate diagnostic parameters and treatment.

ESTABLISHED VOLKMANN'S CONTRACTURE

An extremity can be rendered functionally useless by the sequelae of an improperly managed compartment syndrome. Ischemic necrosis of the muscular and neural components gives way to replacement with noncontractile and afunctional scar tissue. Joints are in fixed contracture devoid of voluntary and passive function. Sensation is impaired or absent. The extremity appears atrophic with tight contracture of the overlying skin. Acute skin ulceration may occur, or decreased friction resistance may lead to chronic skin breakdown over prominences. Bone and articular cartilage can be affected by ischemia, leading to impaired fracture healing and altered bone development in children.[48] Chronic, indolent pain may be evident weeks to months after the ischemic event.

Ischemia produces functional impairment through several mechanisms. Fibrotic replacement of involved muscle groups directly produces weakness. Fixed contracture at the involved joints becomes evident as the scar contracts. Seddon[49] described the scar formation in the arm to be a fusiform mass, with the central portion more dense than the periphery on the basis of the vascular distribution of the compartment and the usual proximal arterial trunk involvement in elbow fractures. In the lower extremity compartments, generalized compartment swelling and ischemia seem to give rise to scar replacement that begins at the periphery and moves inward.[50] Nerve damage, initially from direct ischemic damage and later through compression or traction from the surrounding scar, leads to further weakness and sensory disruption. Neurologically mediated weakness may also result in progressive contractures. Typically, however, the contractures after compartment syndrome are coincident with the ischemic episode, unlike contractures after direct nerve trauma, which produce contracture through muscle imbalance over weeks, months, or years.

Differential diagnosis includes isolated nerve or vessel damage, infection, tenodesis after injury and immobilization, malunion, and reflex sympathetic dystrophy.

Clinical Presentation and Evaluation

The clinical presentation of Volkmann's ischemic contracture depends on the compartment involved. Deep posterior compartment involvement of the leg leads to equinovarus hindfoot contracture, ankle joint contracture, flexion contracture of the toes, plantar anesthesia, and intrinsic foot muscle

paralysis. Foot ulceration may be a prominent component because of altered sensation. Anterior compartment ischemia leads to footdrop initially and later to extension contracture at the ankle and toes. Anesthesia in the first toe web and paralysis of the short extensor to the toes are evident because of involvement of the deep peroneal nerve. Lateral compartment involvement leads to impaired eversion and superficial peroneal distribution anesthesia. Superficial posterior compartment involvement leads to flexion contracture across the ankle as well as varus hindfoot deformity.

In the foot, plantar intrinsic muscle contracture leads to fixed claw-toe formation. Loss of intrinsic muscle function leads to long flexor contracture of the toes and extension contracture at the metatarsophalangeal joints. Hypoesthesia or anesthesia along the medial and lateral plantar nerve distributions is noted. Scar tissue replacement of the plantar muscle groups and atrophy of the plantar fat pad and skin lead to pain with ambulation and the possibility of ulceration. The foot becomes stiff, and shock absorption and adaptive function are lost.

Clinical evaluation of the ischemically damaged extremity begins with a recount of the timing of injury, onset of symptoms, appearance of deformities, and any treatments undertaken to date. After a complete history is elicited, detailed clinical examination is necessary to determine the exact involvement of muscle groups, nerve branches, and associated musculoskeletal components. In the case of severe contracture, it may be difficult to assess the degree of damage accurately. Muscles with retained contraction must be identified and may be candidates for tendon transfers. Those with no function but retained vascularity may regenerate. Nerve branches with partial remaining function may respond to neurolysis. Major arterial damage needs to be assessed and proper steps for reconstruction taken.

If the pattern of weakness, anesthesia, vascular compromise, atrophy, and contracture cannot be clearly delineated, clinical studies should be undertaken. An arteriogram should be performed to identify arterial interruption. Electromyography may be an asset in quantifying muscle damage and muscle recovery. This may not always be reliable, especially when necrosis and scarring are spotty.[51] If focal scarring produces localized nerve entrapment, this may be identifiable by nerve conduction studies. When scarring is widespread, it is difficult to determine accurately, either clinically or electronically, the extent of damage, and a clear picture may only be obtained on exploration. Computed tomography (CT) and magnetic resonance imaging (MRI) may be useful in determining the extent of ischemic muscle damage. Landi and coauthors[52] showed the utility of CT in differentiating replacement fibrosis secondary to ischemia (true Volkmann's ischemia) from contracture produced by tenodesis after immobilization for fracture healing (pseudo-Volkmann's contracture). Hypodensity of the involved muscle groups correlated precisely to fibrotic replacement of muscle seen at surgical exploration in eight patients in their study. MRI is likely to produce an even more accurate assessment.

Conservative Management

Initial treatment of established Volkmann's ischemic contracture is always conservative. In the early stages before contractures become fixed, the extremity is splinted to attempt contracture prevention. Daily passive joint range-of-motion exercises are important in reducing or preventing contracture. Conservative treatments are started as early as practical or when pain and the need to splint local fracture or vascular injuries allow. This assumes that ischemic contracture is diagnosed in its early stages because response will be poor when contracture is established. Rehabilitation should include strengthening and proprioceptive programs. Bracing and accommodative shoe insoles may be necessary to gait or to reduce friction and ulceration.

Surgical Management

Recommendations for timing of operative reconstruction after ischemia vary depending on variable reports of spontaneous recovery. It is generally held that spontaneous recovery will occur to varying degrees in the first 3 to 18 months after ischemia[48, 51, 53] and, therefore, only conservative treatments should be chosen during this time. When spontaneous recovery and conservative efforts reach a plateau, operative intervention is necessary if function has not been restored to an acceptable level or if deformity or pain prevent ambulation. Initially, operation is for exploration and survey of the extent of damage. Concomitantly or subsequently, operation can provide several benefits:

1. Joint contractures can be freed by tendon release, joint capsule release, infarct excision, and muscle slides. These improve position and restore some function. This operation is carried out late to provide opportunity for spontaneous recovery.
2. Release of nerve branches entrapped in scar tissue can provide sensory and motor function restoration and relieve pain. In the case of clinically obvious focal nerve entrapment, early exploration may prevent progressive damage.
3. Tendon transfer can be used to improve function. This, again, is a delayed procedure and is usually performed after exploration and infarct excision.
4. Stabilization procedures such as ankle arthrodesis or subtalar arthrodesis may be needed to restore and maintain functional extremity position.
5. Muscle transplantation has been used to restore function but requires adequate local vascularization and innervation.[54]

The leg compartments are explored through a wide incision similar to that used for fasciotomy, as described earlier in this chapter. In the foot, a medial approach is used to expose the intrinsic muscle origins, the porta pedis, and the tarsal tunnel. Exposure of all components of the compartment is necessary. The exact degree of damage can sometimes be appreciated only at this stage. All frankly necrotic and homogeneously fibrotic tissue is excised. If a particular muscle group is partially involved, a slide is performed by detaching the entire origin of the muscle and all surrounding adhesions. Fibrosis enveloping joint capsules and tendon sheaths is released and excised as necessary to provide mobilization. Tendon lengthenings are generally not done because of rapid postoperative recontracture. All neurovascular components are explored and released if entrapped. Tendon transfers may be carried out at this time or after rehabilitation is attempted. The extremity is splinted in corrected position, and passive

mobilization is begun at approximately 2 weeks or when the incisions are stable. Physical therapy progresses to active exercise and re-education. Weightbearing is delayed until 6 to 8 weeks postoperatively. Subsequent operations may be performed to address digital contractures and joint instability or to improve function further with tendon transfer or muscle transplantation. Night-brace therapy is used for several months after reconstruction to prevent recontracture. In those cases in which pain is intractable or deformity is severe or in which chronic skin breakdown and infection predominate, amputation may be needed.

References

1. Burton AC: On the physical equilibrium of small blood vessels. Am J Physiol 164:319–329, 1951.
2. Ashton H: The effect of increased tissue pressure on blood flow. Clin Orthop 113:15–26, 1975.
3. Eaton RG, Green WT, and Stark HA: Volkmann's ischemic contracture in children. J Bone Joint Surg 47A:1289, 1965.
4. Eaton RG and Green WT: Epimysiotomy and fasciotomy in treatment of ischemic contracture. Orthop Clin North Am 3:175–186, 1972.
5. Matsen FA and Krugmire RB: Compartmental syndromes. Surg Gynecol Obstet 147:943–949, 1978.
6. Teeny SM and Wiss DA: Compartment syndrome: A complication of use of the MAST suit. J Orthop Trauma 1:236–239, 1987.
7. Aprahamian C, Gessert G, Bandyk DF, et al: MAST-associated compartment syndrome (MACS): A review. J Trauma 5:549–555, 1989.
8. Eaton RG and Green WT: Volkmann's ischemia: A volar compartment syndrome of the forearm. Clin Orthop 113:58–64, 1975.
9. Matsen FA, Mayo KA, Krugmire RB, et al: A model of compartment syndrome in man with particular reference to the quantification of nerve function. J Bone Joint Surg 59A:648–653, 1977.
10. Rorabeck CH and Macnab I: The pathophysiology of anterior tibial compartmental syndrome. Clin Orthop 113:52–57, 1975.
11. Whitesides TE, Harada H, and Morimoto K: The response of skeletal muscle to temporary ischemia: An experimental study. J Bone Joint Surg 53A:1027, 1971.
12. Sanderson RA, Foley RK, McIvor GW, et al: Histological response on skeletal muscle to ischemia. Clin Orthop 113:27–35, 1975.
13. Mubarak SJ, Hargens AR, and Owen CA: The wick catheter technique for measurement of intramuscular pressure. J Bone Joint Surg 58A:1016–1020, 1976.
14. Nkele C, Aindow J, and Grant L: Study of pressure of the normal anterior tibial compartment in different age groups using the slit-catheter method. J Bone Joint Surg 70A:98–101, 1988.
15. Dayton P, Goldman FD, and Barton E: Compartment pressure in the foot: Analysis of normal values and measurement technique. J Am Podiatr Med Assoc 80:521–525, 1990.
16. Rorabeck CH, Castle GS, and Hardie R: Compartmental pressure measurements: An experimental investigation using the slit catheter. J Trauma 21:446–449, 1981.
17. Whitesides TE, Haney TC, Morimoto K, et al: Tissue pressure measurements as determinant for the need of fasciotomy. Clin Orthop 113:43–51, 1975.
18. Hargens AR, Akeson WH, Mubarak SJ, et al: Tissue fluid pressures: From basic research tools to clinical applications. J Orthop Res 7:902–909, 1989.
19. Whitesides TE, Harada H, and Morimoto K: Compartment syndromes and the role of fasciotomy: Its parameters and techniques. Instr Course Lect 26:179–196, 1977.
20. Sheridan GW and Matsen FA: Fasciotomy in the treatment of acute compartment syndrome. J Bone Joint Surg 58A:112–114, 1976.
21. Jepson PN: Ischemic contracture: Experimental study. Ann Surg 84:785–795, 1926.
22. Gaspard DJ and Kohl RD: Compartmental syndromes in which the skin is the limiting boundary. Clin Orthop 113:65–68, 1975.
23. Clark L: An experimental study of the regeneration of mammalian striped muscle. J Anat 80:20, 1947.
24. Matsen FA, Questad K, and Matsen AL: The effect of local cooling on post fracture swelling: A controlled study. Clin Orthop 109:201, 1975.
25. Holden CE: Compartmental syndromes following trauma. Clin Orthop 113:95–102, 1975.
26. Sarokhan AJ and Eaton RG: Volkmann's ischemia. J Hand Surg 8:806–809, 1983.
27. Matsen FA, Winquist RA, and Krugmire RB: Diagnosis and management of compartmental syndromes. J Bone Joint Surg 62A:286–291, 1980.
28. Mubarak SJ and Owen CA: Double-incision fasciotomy of the leg for decompression of compartment syndromes. J Bone Joint Surg 59A:184–187, 1977.
29. Kelly RP and Whitesides TE: Transfibular route for fasciotomy of the leg. J Bone Joint Surg 49A:1022, 1967.
30. Mittlmeier T, Machler G, and Lob G: Compartment syndrome of the foot after intraarticular calcaneal fracture. Clin Orthop 269:241–248, 1991.
31. Manoli A and Weber TG: Fasciotomy of the foot: An anatomical study with special reference to release of the calcaneal compartment. Foot Ankle 10:267–275, 1990.
32. Myerson MS: Experimental decompression of the fascial compartments of the

foot—The basis for fasciotomy in acute compartment syndromes. Foot Ankle 8:308–314, 1988.

33. Grodinsky M: A study of the fascial spaces of the foot and their bearing on infections. Surg Gynecol Obstet 49:737–751, 1929.

34. Loeffler RD and Ballard A: Plantar fascial spaces of the foot and a proposed surgical approach. Foot Ankle 1:11–14, 1980.

35. Mubarak SJ and Hargens AR: Compartment Syndromes and Volkmann's Contracture. Philadelphia, WB Saunders, 1981.

36. Styf JR and Korner LM: Chronic anterior-compartment syndrome of the leg: Results of treatment by fasciotomy. J Bone Joint Surg 68A:1338–1347, 1986.

37. Fronek J, Mubarak SJ, Hargens AR, et al: Management of chronic exertional anterior compartment syndrome of the lower extremity. Clin Orthop 220:217–227, 1987.

38. Barcroft H and Dornhorst AC: The blood flow through the human calf during rhythmic exercise. J Physiol 109:402, 1949.

39. Jacobsson S and Kjellmer I: Accumulation of fluid in exercising skeletal muscle. Acta Physiol Scand 60:286, 1964.

40. Mavor GE: The anterior tibial syndrome. J Bone Joint Surg 38B:513–517, 1956.

41. Raether PM and Lutter LD: Recurrent compartment syndrome in the posterior thigh. Report of a case. Am J Sports Med 10:40, 1988.

42. Bouche RT: Chronic compartment syndrome of the leg. J Am Podiatr Med Assoc 80:633–647, 1990.

43. Pedowitz RA, Hargens AR, Mubarak SJ, et al: Modified criteria for the objective diagnosis of chronic compartment syndrome of the leg. Am J Sports Med 18:35–40, 1990.

44. Reneman RS: The anterior and the lateral compartmental syndrome of the leg due to intensive use of muscles. Clin Orthop 113:69–79, 1975.

45. Mannarino F and Sexson S: The significance of intracompartmental pressures in the diagnosis of chronic exertional compartment syndrome. Orthopedics 12:1415–1418, 1988.

46. Rorabak CH, Bourne RB, Fowler PJ, et al: The role of tissue pressure measurement in diagnosing chronic anterior compartment syndrome. Am J Sports Med 16:143–146, 1988.

47. Martens MA and Moeyersoons JP: Acute and recurrent effort-related compartment syndrome in sports. Sports Med 9:62–68, 1990.

48. Bajpai J, Sinha BN, and Srivastava AN: Clinical study of Volkmann's ischemic contracture of the upper limb. Int Surg 60:162–164, 1975.

49. Seddon HJ: Volkmann's contracture: Treatment by excision of the infarct. J Bone Joint Surg 38B:152–174, 1956.

50. Griffiths DL: Volkmann's ischemic contracture. Br J Surg 28:239–260, 1940.

51. Gershuni DH: Volkmann's contracture of the lower extremity: Pathology and reconstruction. *In* Mubarak SJ (ed): Compartment Syndrome and Volkmann's Contracture. Philadelphia, WB Saunders, 1981.

52. Landi A, De Santis G, Torricelli P, et al: CT in established Volkmann's contracture in forearm muscles. J Hand Surg 14B:49–52, 1989.

53. Kikuchi S, Hasue M, and Watanabe M: Ischemic contracture in the lower limb. Clin Orthop 134:185–191, 1978.

54. Zuker R: Volkmann's ischemic contracture. Clin Plast Surg 16:537–545, 1989.

Index

Note: Page numbers in *italics* refer to illustrations; page numbers followed by t refer to tables.

Aβ fibers, in entrapment syndromes, 687–688, *688*

Aδ fibers, 675
 in entrapment syndromes, 688

Abductor hallucis muscle, strain of, athletic injuries and, 254

Abrasion chondroplasty, in hallux limitus/ rigidus, 539–540, *540*

Abrasive wear, 94

Abscess(es), osteomyelitis and, 343, *344*
 soft tissue, imaging in, 393, *393*
  magnetic resonance imaging in, 357

Absorbable fixation, implants and, 99–100

Absorptive powders, wound healing and, 60

Accessory ligaments, of synovial joints, 5

Acetaminophen, in chronic pain syndrome, 680

Acetazolamide, anesthesia and, 475–476

Acetylsalicylic acid. See *Aspirin.*

Achilles tendon, advancement of, anterior, 606–608
  complications of, 607–608
  indications for, 606
  postoperative care and, 607
  technique for, 606–607, *607*
 in equinus, 294, *294, 295*
 contracture of, in paralytic disorders, 286
 rupture of, 246–247
  following glucocorticoid injection therapy, 448
 tendinitis of, in seronegative spondyloarthropathies, 134
 tenosynovitis of, rheumatoid arthritis and, 121

Acquired immunodeficiency syndrome (AIDS). See *Human immunodeficiency virus (HIV) infection.*

Acrodermatitis continua of Hallopeau, 194

Acrokeratosis paraneoplastica, 189

Acrolentiginous melanoma, 196

Activated oxygen, inflammation and, 41, 46

Acumed Great Toe System, *523,* 523–524

Acyclovir, in herpes simplex virus infections, 305

Adenosine triphosphate (ATP), muscle activity and, 68

Adhesive capsulitis, of ankle, 616
 post-traumatic ankle pain and, 720

Adhesive wear, 94, *95*

Adipose synovial membrane, 6

Adrenocortical insufficiency, signs and symptoms of, 440, 440t

Adrenocorticotrophic hormone (ACTH), anesthesia and, 472
 in gout, 148, 432

Afferent neurons, 674–675

Age. See also *Children; Elderly patients.*
 musculoskeletal tumors and, radiographic appearance of, 324
 nonunions and, 26–27

Airway management, anesthesia and, 478–480

Akin-type procedure, in hallux limitus/rigidus, 537

Albright's sign, in basal cell nevus syndrome, 196

Alcohol, avascular necrosis of bone and, 639–640
 gout and, 142–143

Aldosterone, anesthesia and, 472t

Allergic dermatitis, implants and, 95

Allergic reactions. See *Hypersensitivity reactions.*

Allogeneic, autolyzed, antigen-extracted (AAA) bone, chemosterilized, 25–26

Allogenic tissue. See *Allografts.*

Allografts, 23, 25–26
 arthrodesis and, in rheumatoid arthritis, 563

Alloimplants, 23, 25–26
 chemosterilized, allogenic, autolyzed, antigen-extracted bone for, 25–26
 demineralized bone matrix for, 26

Allopurinol, 411t, 426t, 426–427
 anesthesia and, 474
 in gout, chronic gouty arthritis and, 149

Amino amides, as local anesthetics, 476

Amino esters, as local anesthetics, 476

Aminoglycosides, drug interactions of, 407
 in septic arthritis, 215t

Amitriptyline, in chronic pain syndrome, 682

Amoxicillin, in septic arthritis, 215t

Amoxicillin/clavulanic acid, in septic arthritis, 215t

Amphiarthroses, 1, 2

Amphotericin B, in septic arthritis, 215t

Ampicillin, in septic arthritis, 215t

ANA test, 225, *225,* 225t

Anaerobic infections, septic arthritis and, 209

Analgesics, in osteoarthritis, 131
 non-narcotic, in chronic pain syndrome, 680

Anaphylactoid reactions, nonsteroidal anti-inflammatory drugs and, 402–403
 to salicylates, 407

Anemia, anesthesia and, 465–466
 in rheumatoid arthritis, 108, 110, 460

Anesthesia, 464–480
 airway management and, 478–480
 drug therapy and, 468–476
  antimalarials and, 471–472
  antimetabolites and, 471
  gold salts and, 470
  gout medications and, 474–476
  immunosuppressives and, 470–471

Anesthesia *(Continued)*
  nonsteroidal anti-inflammatory drugs and, 469–470
  D-penicillamine and, 471
  salicylates and, 468–469
  steroids and, 472t, 472–474
 in healthy patients, 464, 465t
 in systemic disease, 464–468
  anemia and, 465–466
  blood transfusions and, 466
  cardiac, 464–465
  diabetes mellitus and, 466–468, 467t, 468t
  of peripheral nervous system, 466
  pulmonary, 464
  renal, 466
  vasculitis and vasospasm and, 465
 local, agents for, 476t, 476–478
  for glucocorticoid injection therapy, 446
 regional, 479

Aneurysmal bone cyst, radiographic appearance of, 330, *331*

Angiitis. See *Vasculitis.*

Angiolipomas, 630, *631*

Angiomatosis, bacillary, in HIV infection, 305

Angiotensin (ANG), nonsteroidal anti-inflammatory drugs and, 399

Ankle, anatomy of, 612–613
 capsule and, 612
 cartilage and, 612
 subchondral bone and, 612
 synovial fluid and, 613
 synovium and, 613
 arthritic process in, 613–616
  chondral lesions and, *613,* 613–614, *615*
  osteochondral lesions and, 614
  synovial and related soft tissue disorders and, 614, 616, *616*
 arthrodesis of, in rheumatoid arthritis, 570–575, *571, 572, 574*
 arthrography of, 367, *368*
  normal arthrographic anatomy and, *366,* 366–367, *367*
 arthroscopy of. See *Arthroscopy, of ankle.*
 biomechanics of, gait and, 72, 72–73
  in joint diseases, 80
  pathologic gait and, 78–80, *79, 80*
 fractures of, arthroscopy and, 619–621, *621*
  imaging in, 386, *387*
  post-traumatic ankle pain and, 722
 impingement of, posterior, 243
 instability of, arthroscopy and, 621
 limited dorsiflexion of. See *Equinus deformity.*
 muscle action on, 73, *73*
 post-traumatic pain in, 718–725
  coincidental causes versus, 718, 718t

Ankle *(Continued)*
extra-articular causes of, 718–719, 719t
follow-up evaluation of, 724
initial diagnostic approach to, 723
intra-articular causes of, 719t, 719–723
management of intra-articular disease and, 724–725
rheumatoid arthritis and, 122
septic arthritis in, treatment outcome in, 216t
sprains of, 243–245, *244*
sequelae of, 245t, 245–246
Ankylosing spondylitis (AS). See also *Seronegative spondyloarthropathies.*
clinical features of, 132
differential diagnosis of, 135, 136
exercises for, 454t
HLA measurement in, 226–227
preoperative and postoperative considerations in, 462
spine involvement in, 135–136
Ankylosis, of foot, bony, in rheumatoid arthritis, imaging and, 310, *312*
imaging and, 319
Antacids, anesthesia and, 468
drug interactions of, 404t, 405
gastrointestinal function and, 401
Antalgic gait, 76, *76*
Anterolateral system, pain and, 676
Anthranilic acids, 410t, 416. See also specific drugs.
Antibacterial agents, wound healing and, 60
Antibiotics. See also specific drugs.
in rheumatoid arthritis, 430
in septic arthritis, 214, 214t, 215t
prophylactic, in seronegative spondyloarthropathies, 137
Anticardiolipin syndrome, livedo vasculitis in, 173–174
Anticonvulsants, drug interactions of, 405t, 407
in chronic pain syndrome, 681
local anesthesia and, 477
Antidepressants, in chronic pain syndrome, 681–682
Antidiuretic hormone, nonsteroidal anti-inflammatory drugs and, 399
Antihypertensive agents, drug interactions of, 406–407
Antimalarial agents, 410t, 418–419. See also specific drugs.
anesthesia and, 471–472
Antimetabolites, 411t
anesthesia and, 471
Antinuclear antibodies (ANAs), measurement of, 224t, 224–225
Antiseptic agents, wound healing and, 60
Aortic arch arteritis. See *Takayasu's arteritis.*
Aortic arch syndrome. See *Takayasu's arteritis.*
Apophysitis, calcaneal, 241–242
Apropulsive gait, 78
Arachidonic acid cascade, inflammation and, 34–36
cyclooxygenase pathway and, 35, *35*
lipoxygenase pathway and, 35–36
Arch, collapse of, rheumatoid arthritis and, 120
transverse, loss of, rheumatoid arthritis and, 120
Areolar synovial membrane, 6
Arginine vasopressin (AVP), nonsteroidal anti-inflammatory drugs and, 399
Arterial insufficiency, correction of, nonhealing wounds and, 59
Arterial supply, of joints, 13
Arteriography, *375*, 375–376, *376*
Arterioles, of bone, 18
Arteritis, 162. See also *Polyarteritis; Vasculitis.*
giant cell, rheumatoid arthritis versus, 114

Arteritis *(Continued)*
Takayasu's. See *Takayasu's arteritis.*
temporal, 163–164
Arthralgia, in HIV infection, 304
in polyarteritis nodosa, 163
in systemic lupus erythematosus, 154
Arthritis, gouty. See under *Gout.*
in ankle. See under *Ankle.*
in systemic lupus erythematosus, 154
polyarticular, imaging in, 385
post-traumatic, of ankle, arthroscopy in, 619–621, *621*
proliferative, of ankle, arthroscopy in, 622–624
psoriatic. See *Psoriatic arthritis (PA).*
rehabilitation in. See *Rehabilitation.*
rheumatoid. See *Rheumatoid arthritis (RA).*
septic. See *Septic arthritis.*
Arthritis mutilans, 133
Arthrocentesis. See *Joint aspiration.*
Arthrodesis, for calcaneal deformity, 289
in poliomyelitis, 285
in rheumatoid arthritis, 559–576, *560*
bone grafting and, 563
general principles for, 560–562, *561*
in children, *575*, 575–576
indications for, 559–560
of ankle, 570–575, *571*, *572*, *574*
of first metatarsophalangeal joint, 564–565, *566*
of hallux interphalangeal joint, 563–564, *564*, *565*
of subtalar joint, 568–570, *569*, *570*
of talonavicular joint, 567–568, *567–569*
of tarsometatarsal junction, 565–566, *566*
pantalar, 575
postoperative immobilization and, 575
surgical considerations in, 562, *563*
triple, 570
in valgus deformity, *297*, 297–298, 298t
of metatarsophalangeal joints, first, 512, 545–557
contraindications to, 546
fixation and, 552–553, *554–556*
in rheumatoid arthritis, 564–565, *566*
indications for, 546
joint resection techniques and, 547–548, *548–553*, *550–552*
position of fusion and, 546–547, 547t
rationale for, 545–546
results with, 553, 556–557
in hallux limitus, 535–536
subtalar, in calcaneovalgus deformity, 656
surgical anatomy and, 656, *657*
in rheumatoid arthritis, 568–570, *569*, *570*
Arthrography, 366t, 366–370
double-contrast, 367
in post-traumatic ankle pain, 724
normal ankle anatomy and, *366*, 366–367, *367*
single-contrast, 367
technique for, 367–370
ankle and, 367, *368*
calcaneocuboid joint and, 368, *369*
posterior subtalar joint and, 368, *368*, *369*
small joints of foot and, 368–370, *370*
Arthroplasty, failed, as indication for arthrodesis, in rheumatoid arthritis, 559–560
infection following, imaging in, 359
joint sepsis following, 218
of ankle, 572, *572*
of forefoot, 496–515, *497*
dorsal approach for, 506–508, *509*, 510–511
dorsal transverse approach for, 511

Arthroplasty *(Continued)*
first metatarsophalangeal joint and, 511–512
hallux interphalangeal joint and, 512–513
historical background of, 496, 498–499, *498–502*, 501
implant. See *Implant arthroplasty, of forefoot.*
lesser metatarsophalangeal joints and, 512
perioperative medical considerations for, 503
plantar transverse approach for, 511
postoperative care and, 513
procedural decision-making for, 503, *504–506*, 506
resection, 511–512
results with, 513–514
of metatarsophalangeal joints, 492, *492*
implant arthroplasty and, 492
resection, of metatarsophalangeal joints, 545
Arthroscopy, in septic arthritis, 217, *217*
of ankle, 616–625
in ankle arthritis secondary to instability, 621
in inflammatory arthritis, 622–624
crystalline, 624
rheumatoid, 622–624
in osteoarthritis, 618–619
in post-traumatic ankle pain, 724
in post-traumatic arthritis, 619–621, *621*
in septic arthritis, 624–625
neuropathic joint and, 621–622
Arthrosis, of central metatarsophalangeal joint, 481–495
adjunctive osseous procedures for, 494, 494t
adjunctive soft tissue procedures for, 492, *493*, 494, *494*
clinical evaluation and, 487–489, *488*, 489t, *490*
functional forefoot anatomy and, *482–486*, 482–487
pathophysiology and, 481–482, 482t
postoperative management and, 494–495
primary surgical procedures for, 491–492
severity level classification and, 489
Arthrotomy, in septic arthritis, 216–217
Articular cartilage, 28–29, *29*, *30*
alterations in loading conditions and, 66
biochemical alterations in, 66, *66*
collagen fibers of, 28–29
components of, biomechanics of, 65–66, *66*
extracellular matrix of, 29, *30*
fluid phase of, 66
glycosaminoglycans of, 29
lubrication of, 9
nonsteroidal anti-inflammatory drugs and, 403
of synovial joints, 2, *2–4*, *3–5*
septic arthritis and, 211
stress-strain state of, 66
superficial layer of, 28
tangential layer of, 28
tidemark of, 28
water content of, 29
zones of, 28
Ascending pathways, pain and, 675–676
Aseptic necrosis, of bone, following glucocorticoid injection therapy, 445
Aspirin, 407. See also *Salicylates.*
drug interactions of, 404t, 405, 406, 407, 408
enteric-coated, 409t
gastrointestinal function and, 400
hepatic function and, 402
in chronic pain syndrome, 680
Assistive devices, 455
Ataxia, in cerebral palsy, 292

Atherosclerosis, in diabetes mellitus, 56
 xanthomas and, 183t
Athletic injuries, 234–257
 Achilles rupture and, 246–247
 ankle impingement and, 243
 ankle sprains and, 243–245, *244*
  sequelae of, 245t, *245*–246
 calcaneal apophysitis and, 241–242
 friction blister and, 234–235
 heel disorders and, *242,* 242–243
 iliotibial band syndrome and, *252,* 252–253
 Jones fracture and, *238,* 238–239
 metatarsalgia and, 236
 metatarsophalangeal joint sprain and, *237,*
  237–238
 midfoot sprain and, 239–240, *240*
 muscle strain and, 253–255
 neuroma and, 235, *235*
 os navicularis syndrome and, 239, *239*
 patellofemoral pain syndrome and, 249–252,
  250t, *251*
 plantar fasciitis and, *240,* 240–241
 plantar forefoot neuritis and, 235–236
 sesamoiditis and, 236–237
 stress fracture and, *255,* 255–257, *256*
 superficial peroneal nerve neuropraxia and,
  247, 247–248
 tibial stress syndrome (shin splints) and, 85,
  248, 248–249, *249*
Atrophic nonunions, 27
Atrophy, of muscle, following glucocorticoid
  injection therapy, 445
 imaging in, 391
Auranofin, 410t, 419
Aurothioglucose (ATG), 410t, 419
Austin osteotomy, in hallux limitus/rigidus, 537,
 538
 Youngswick modification of, 538
Autogeneic tissue. See *Autografts.*
Autogenous tissue. See *Autografts.*
Autogenous weld, 22
Autografts, 23
 arthrodesis and, in rheumatoid arthritis, 563
 in brachymetatarsia, 671
 nonvascularized, 24–25
 vascularized, 24
  free, 24
  pedicled, 24
Autoimmune disorders, diabetes mellitus and,
 280
 exocrinopathy and. See *Sjögren's syndrome.*
Autoimmunity, rheumatoid arthritis and, 103
Autologous tissue. See *Autografts.*
Avascular necrosis, of bone, 639–649
  diagnosis of, 640–641
  etiology of, 639t, 639–640
  idiopathic, 649
  osteochondritis dissecans and, 644–646,
   645, 646
  osteochondroses and, 641–644, 642t
  postoperative, 646–648, *647*
  trauma and, 648–649, *649*
Avulsion fractures, of ankle, arthroscopy and,
 619
 of extensor digitorum brevis, following ankle
  sprains, 246
 post-traumatic ankle pain and, 722
Azapropazone, 425
 drug interactions of, 407
Azathioprine, 411t, 422–423
 anesthesia and, 470–471
 in rheumatoid arthritis, 429–430
Aztreonam, in septic arthritis, 215t

B lymphocytes, inflammation and, 46–47
Bacillary angiomatosis, in HIV infection, 305
Back pain, leg-length inequality and, *87,* 87–88
 orthotics in, 89
Bacterial cell wall antigens, in synovial fluid, in
  septic arthritis, 213
Bacterial fatty acids, in synovial fluid, in septic
  arthritis, 213
Bacterial infections. See also specific organisms.
 cutaneous, in HIV infection, 188
 of skin, in HIV infection, 305
 septic arthritis and, 208
Bacteroides fragilis infections, septic arthritis
  and, 209, 215t
Baker's cysts, in knee, rheumatoid arthritis and,
 123
Balanitis, circinate, in Reiter's syndrome, 133
Basal cell carcinoma, in basal cell nevus
  syndrome, 195, *195*
Basal cell nevus syndrome, *195,* 195–196
Basophils, inflammation and, 47
Bazex's syndrome, 189
Beau's lines, *198,* 198–199, *199,* 199t
Bebax shoe, in calcaneovalgus deformity, 654,
  654t
 in metatarsus adductus, 660, *661*
Behçet's syndrome, 164–165, *165*
 arthritis related to, rheumatoid arthritis ver-
  sus, 114
 HLA measurement in, 226t
Benoxaprofen, 415
 platelet function and hematologic system and,
  402
Benzbromarone, 427
Benzodiazepines, in chronic pain syndrome, 682
Beta-blocking agents, drug interactions of, 406–
 407
Betamethasone, anesthesia and, 472t
 for injection therapy, 443t
  dosage of, 444t
Betamethasone phosphate-acetate mixture, in
  neuroma, 235
Bicitra, preanesthetic, in gout, 475
Bio-Action Great Toe Implant, 522–523, *523*
Biocompatibility, of implants, 91, 93t
Biointegration, implant fixation using, 98
Biomaterials. See *Implant(s); Implant
  arthroplasty.*
Biomechanics, 65–89
 of ankle joint, 80
 of articular cartilage components, 65–66, *66*
 of bone, 65
 of gait. See *Gait, biomechanics of.*
 of midtarsal joint, 82
 of skeletal muscle, 66, *67, 68, 68*
 of subtalar joint, 80–82, *81*
Biomet Total Toe System, 522, *522*
Biopsy, musculoskeletal tumors versus, 324
 of soft tissue tumors, indications for, 630
Blastomyces dermatitidis infections, septic
  arthritis and, 210
Blastomycosis, septic arthritis and, 210
Bleeding. See *Hemorrhages.*
Blister, friction, 234–235
Blood dyscrasias, nonsteroidal anti-
  inflammatory drugs and, 402
Blood supply, of forefoot, 380–381
 of hindfoot, 377
 of long bones, 18, *19*
  afferent supply, 18, *19*
 of midfoot, 379
 of synovial membrane, 13
 of tendons, 577, 579
Blood transfusions, anesthesia and, 466
Blue toe syndrome, 184, *184*
Bone(s), 15–28

Bone(s) *(Continued)*
 avascular necrosis of. See *Avascular necrosis,
  of bone.*
 biomechanics of, 65
 blood supply of, 18, *19*
 cancellous. See *Cancellous bone.*
 composition and structure of, 17–18
 cortical. See *Cortical bone.*
 development of, 15
 electrical properties of, 19
 fractures of. See *Fracture(s).*
 immature (fibrous; woven), 17
 lamellar, 17
 lyophilized. See *Alloimplants.*
 mass lesions in, radiographic appearance of,
  324
 mature (lamellar), 17
 of forefoot, 380, *380, 381*
 of hindfoot, 377, *377, 378*
 of midfoot, 378, *379*
 ossification of, endochondral, 15–16, *16*
  membranous, 16–17
 spongy. See *Cancellous bone.*
 trabecular. See *Cancellous bone.*
 woven, 17
Bone blocking procedures, for calcaneal
  deformity, 289–290, *290*
Bone cyst, aneurysmal, radiographic appearance
  of, 330, *331*
 unicameral, radiographic appearance of, 337,
  337
Bone grafts, 23–28
 allografts and alloimplants as, 25–26
 arthrodesis and, in rheumatoid arthritis, 563
 in brachymetatarsia, 671
 mechanisms of repair of, 23–24
 nonvascularized, 24–25
 vascularized, 24
Bone healing, primary, 16–17
 secondary, 16, *16*
Bone marrow, necrosis of, 648
 tumors of, radiographic appearance of, 330–
  332
Bone marrow injection, percutaneous, 25
Bone mineral content (BMC), osteopenia and, in
  diabetic foot, 269–270
Bone repair, endochondral, 16, *16*
Bony erosions, in inflammatory disease, 308
Borrelia burgdorferi infections, septic arthritis
  and, 210
Boutonnière deformity, in rheumatoid arthritis,
  115, *115*
Brachial arteritis. See *Takayasu's arteritis.*
Brachymetatarsia, *671,* 671–672
 surgical treatment of, 671–672
Bracing, in calcaneovalgus deformity, 655
 in metatarsus adductus, Wheaton brace and,
  660–661
 in post-traumatic ankle pain, 725
 in rheumatoid arthritis, 127–128
Bradykinin, inflammation and, 40, 41, *44*
Breslow thickness, 196
Bridging external callus, fracture healing and,
 22
Brucella infections, arthritis related to,
  rheumatoid arthritis versus, 113
Bruise, "stone," 241
Buccal ulceration, in Behçet's syndrome, *165*
Bullae, hemorrhagic, in cutaneous vasculitis,
  202, *202*
 in erythema multiforme, 190, *190*
Bullosis diabeticorum, 178
Bunion(s), dorsal, in paralytic disorders, 290,
  291
 treatment of, 290
 rheumatoid arthritis and, 119, *119*

Bunion(s) *(Continued)*
  tailor's, in diabetes mellitus, 278, *278*
Bunionectomy, Keller. See *Keller bunionectomy.*
Bupivacaine, 476, 476t, 477
Bursae, 10–11
Bursitis, retrocalcaneal, in rheumatoid arthritis, imaging and, 310, *312*
Bursography, 375
Butterfly rash, in systemic lupus erythematosus, 153, *154*, 154, 171, *171*
Buttonhole deformity, in rheumatoid arthritis, 115, *115*

C fibers, 675
  in entrapment syndromes, 688
Cachectin. See *Tumor necrosis factor (TNF).*
Caisson disease, avascular necrosis of bone and, 640
Calcaneal apophysitis, 241–242
  avascular necrosis of bone in, 643, *644*
Calcaneal brace, in calcaneovalgus deformity, 655
Calcaneal deformities, in paralytic disorders. See *Paralytic disorders, calcaneal deformities in.*
  in rheumatoid arthritis, of foot, imaging and, 310
Calcaneal nerve entrapment, 706–709
  etiology of, 705
  surgical treatment of, 706, *707–710*, 708–709
Calcaneal osteotomy, of Evans. See *Evan's calcaneal osteotomy.*
Calcaneocuboid joint, arthrography of, 368, *369*
Calcaneofibular ligament (CFL), sprain of, 243–245, *244*
Calcaneovalgus deformity, 652–657
  clinical signs in, 652, *652*
  etiology of, 652–653, *653*
  radiologic evaluation of, 653, *653*
  treatment of, 653–657
    conservative, 653–656
    surgical, 656–657
Calcaneus, fractures of, imaging in, 385–386
Calcaneus gait, following Achilles tendon advancement, 607–608
Calcification, of musculoskeletal tumors, 323, *323*
Calcified zone, of synovial joints, 4
Calcinosis, in dermatomyositis, *160*, 160–161
Calcinosis cutis, 170, *170*
Calcium hydroxyapatite crystal deposition disease, 150
  imaging and, 315
Calcium pyrophosphate dihydrate deposition disease (CPPD), 149. See also *Chondrocalcinosis; Pseudogout.*
  chronic arthropathy in, 150
  in diabetic foot, 280
  of foot, imaging and, 315
Calcium pyrophosphate dihydrate deposition disease (CPPD) *(Continued)*
  rheumatoid arthritis versus, 113–114
Calcium salt crystals, in articular cartilage, of synovial joints, 5
Calf pump failure, in chronic venous insufficiency, 57
Callotasis, in brachymetatarsia, *671*, 672
Callus, distraction of, in brachymetatarsia, *671*, 672
  hard, fracture healing and, 22
  ''horse hoof,'' 26
  soft, fracture healing and, 22
Calor, 34

Campylobacter infections, in Reiter's syndrome, 132
Cancellous bone, 17, 18, *18*
  grafts and, 24–25
Candida albicans, in HIV infection, 305
Candida infections, cutaneous, in HIV infection, 188
  in diabetes mellitus, 179
  septic arthritis and, 210
Capacitive coupling, for nonunions, 27
Capillary hemangiomas, 634
Caplan's syndrome, in rheumatoid arthritis, 108
Capsular ligaments, of synovial joints, 5
Capsulitis, adhesive, of ankle, 616
  post-traumatic ankle pain and, 720
Caput ulnae syndrome, rheumatoid arthritis and, 116, *117*
Carbamazepine, in chronic pain syndrome, 681
Carbon fiber–reinforced plastic (CFRP), implant fixation using, 98
Carbonic anhydrase inhibitors, drug interactions of, 405t
Carcinoma, basal cell, in basal cell nevus syndrome, 195, *195*
Cardiopulmonary system, in systemic lupus erythematosus, 155t
Cardiovascular system, nonsteroidal anti-inflammatory drugs and, 402
Cartilage, 28–31
  articular. See *Articular cartilage.*
  calcification of, musculoskeletal tumors and, 323, *323*
  chondrocytes in, 28
  in rheumatoid arthritis, 104
Cartilage rearrangement, in hallux limitus/rigidus, 538–539, *540*
Cartilage repair, 30–31
  depth of injury and, 30–31
  techniques for, 31
Cartilaginous joints, 1–2
Casting, in calcaneovalgus deformity, 653–654, *654*
  in medial tibial torsion, *664*, 664–665
  in metatarsus adductus, 659–661
  in neuroarthropathy, of diabetic foot, 267
  in post-traumatic ankle pain, 725
Catabolin, septic arthritis and, 211
Causalgia, 674
Cavernous hemangiomas, 633–634
Cavity, of synovial joints, 2, *2*
Cavus deformity, 668–671
  area of, 668–669
  degree of, 669
  tendon transfers in, Hibbs tenosuspension procedure and, 600
  treatment of, 669–671
    conservative, 669–670
    surgical, 670–671
      in forefoot, 670–671
      in hindfoot, 670, *670*
Cefazolin, in septic arthritis, 215t
Cefixime, in septic arthritis, 215t
Ceftazidime, in septic arthritis, 215t
Ceftriaxone, in septic arthritis, 215t
Cefuroxime, in septic arthritis, 215t
Cefuroxime axetil, in septic arthritis, 215t
Cellular factors, inflammation and, 41, 46–48
Cellular zone, of articular cartilage, 28
Cellulitis, imaging in, 393, *393*
  in diabetes mellitus, 179
Central nervous system. See also *Spinal cord.*
  in systemic lupus erythematosus, 155t
  nonsteroidal anti-inflammatory drugs and, 403
  pain perception and, 676
Cephalexin, in septic arthritis, 215t

Cephalosporins, third-generation, in septic arthritis, 215t
Ceramic implants, 92t, 97, 99
Cerebral cortex, pain perception and, 676
Cerebral palsy (CP), 290–298
  clinical types of, 290–292
  equinus deformity in, 292–294
    nonoperative treatment of, 292
    postoperative care and, 294
    spastic, surgical treatment of. See also *Achilles tendon, advancement of, anterior.*
    surgical treatment of, 292, *293–295*, 294
  spastic activity of tibialis posterior tendon in, split tibialis posterior tendon transfer and, 605
  treatment of, 292–298
  valgus deformity in, 297–298
    treatment of, *297*, 297–298, 298t
  varus deformity in, 294–297, *296*
    treatment of, 296–297
Cerebrotendinous xanthomatosis, 182–183
Cervical spine, arthritis of, airway management and, 478
  in rheumatoid arthritis, 105t, 105–106, 116–117, 460
Charcot-Marie-Tooth (CMT) disease, peroneal muscle weakness in, 78–79
Charcot's arthropathy, 204–205, *205*
  treatment of, 206
Charcot's changes, 58
Charcot's joints. See *Neuroarthropathy.*
Cheilectomy, in hallux limitus/rigidus, 536–537, *537*
Chemical nociceptors, 674
Chemokinesis, 36
Chevron-type procedure, in hallux limitus/rigidus, 537
Children, congenital deformities in, 652–672. See also specific deformities.
  nonsteroidal anti-inflammatory drugs in, 403
  rheumatoid arthritis in. See *Juvenile rheumatoid arthritis (JRA).*
  septic arthritis in, 207
Chlamydia infections, in Reiter's syndrome, 132
Chloroprocaine, 476, 476t
Chloroquine, anesthesia and, 471–472
Chlortenoxicam, 417
Cholestyramine, drug interactions of, 404t
Choline magnesium trisalicylate, 409t
  in chronic pain syndrome, 680
Chondral lesions, in ankle, *613*, 613–614, *615*
Chondroblastoma, radiographic appearance of, 329, *329*
Chondrocalcinosis, asymptomatic, 149–150
Chondrocalcinosis articularis. See *Calcium pyrophosphate dihydrate deposition disease (CPPD).*
Chondrocytes, in articular cartilage, of synovial joints, 3, *4*, 4
Chondroma, periosteal, radiographic appearance of, 329, *329*
Chondromalacia, 83
  post-traumatic ankle pain and, 720–721
Chondromyxoid fibroma, radiographic appearance of, 329
Chondroplasty, abrasion, in hallux limitus/rigidus, 539–540, *540*
Chondrosarcoma, radiographic appearance of, 327–328, *328*
Chopart's joint, arthrography of, 369
Chronic pain syndrome (CPS), diagnosis of, 678–679
  medical dependency and, 679
  treatment of, 678–684
    cognitive/behavioral therapy in, 680

Chronic pain syndrome (CPS) *(Continued)*
neural blockade in, 682–683
pharmacologic, 680–682, 683–684
physical/rehabilitative modalities in, 682
spinal cord stimulation and, 683
surgical, 683
Chrysotherapy. See *Gold salts.*
Cigarette smoking, limited joint mobility and, 272
Cimetidine, anesthesia and, 468
drug interactions of, 404t, 405–406
Ciprofloxacin, in septic arthritis, 215t
Circinate balanitis, in Reiter's syndrome, 133
Circulus articularis vasculosus, 13
Citrobacter infections, septic arthritis and, 215t
Clark's test, in patellofemoral stress syndrome, 251
Claudication, in rheumatoid arthritis, 107
Clearance, of nonsteroidal anti-inflammatory drugs, 398–399
Clindamycin, in septic arthritis, 215t
Clonazepam, in chronic pain syndrome, 682
Closing base wedge osteotomy, in metatarsus adductus, 661
Clotting system, inflammation and, 41, *45*
Clubbing, of digits, *198*, 198–199
Coarctation, reverse. See *Takayasu's arteritis.*
Coccidioidomycosis, imaging in, 359
septic arthritis and, 210
Cock-up hallux deformity, Jones tenosuspension and, 608
Cognitive/behavioral therapy, in chronic pain syndrome, 680
Colchicine, 411t, 412t, 424–425
anesthesia and, 475
in gout, 432
acute gouty arthritis and, 147–148
intercritical, 148
Cold therapy, 451
Collagen, breakdown of, wound healing and, 56
glutaraldehyde cross-linked, implant fixation and, 99
in articular cartilage, 28–29, 66
of synovial joints, 3, 4–5
in hyaline cartilage, of ankle, 612
in tendons, age-related changes in, 11
synthesis of, wound healing and, 55, 56
Collagenases, in rheumatoid arthritis, 104
Colloidal bismuth subcitrate, gastrointestinal function and, 401
Compartment syndromes, 726–735
acute, 726–731, 727t
pressure recording in, 727–729, *728, 729*
surgical management of, 729–731
in foot, 730–731, *731, 732*
in lower leg, 730, *730*
chronic, 731–734
diagnosis of, 733, *733*
management of, 733–734
surgical, 733–734
pressure measurements in, 733
clinical signs of, 727t
Complement, measurement of, 223, 223t, 224t
Complement fixation, vasculitis and, 201
Complement system, inflammation and, 40, *42–44*
Complete blood cell count, in gout, 147
with hematocrit, nonsteroidal anti-inflammatory drugs and, 407
Compression force, 65
Computed tomography (CT), 322, 381–382
in avascular necrosis of bone, 641
in neoplasms and related disorders, 383
in osteomyelitis, 345–346
in post-traumatic ankle pain, 724
in tendinitis, 580–581

Computed tomography (CT) *(Continued)*
in tendon dysfunction, 583
three-dimensional reconstruction and, 381–382, *382*
Concentric contraction, 66
Congenital deformities, 652–672. See also specific deformities.
Connective tissue diseases (CTDs), 152–167. See also *Dermatomyositis/polymyositis (DM/PM); Rheumatoid arthritis (RA); Scleroderma; Sjögren's syndrome; Systemic lupus erythematosus (SLE); Vasculitis.*
mixed, *165*, 165–167
clinical features of, 165t, 166–167
pathology of, 166
preoperative and postoperative considerations in, 461–462
treatment and prognosis of, 167
of foot, imaging and, 315, *317*
radiography in, 308t
overlap syndromes and, 165–166, 166t, 167, 167t
preoperative and postoperative considerations in, 460–462
preoperative evaluation and, 459t
Continuous passive motion (CPM), in septic arthritis, 218
Contraction time, 66
Contrast baths, 451
Contrast radiography, 365–376. See also specific modality.
contrast agents and, 365–366
adverse reactions to, 365–366
Conventional radiography. See *Plain radiography.*
Corrosion products, released by metal implants, 95
Corrosive wear, 94
Corrugated pattern, in peroneal tendons, 371, *371*
Cortical bone, 17–18, *18*
grafts and, 24–25
Corticocancellous grafts, 25
Corticosteroids. See also specific corticosteroids.
anesthesia and, 472t, 472–474
drug interactions of, 404t, 405
in gout, 432
acute gouty arthritis and, 148
local therapy using, avascular necrosis of bone and, 640
in gout, 475
in post-traumatic ankle pain, 725
Corticosterone, *438*
anesthesia and, 472t
Corticotropin. See *Adrenocorticotrophic hormone (ACTH).*
Cortisol. See *Hydrocortisone.*
Cortisone, *438*
anesthesia and, 472t
Corynebacterium minutissimum infections, in diabetes mellitus, 179–180, *180*
Coumarin, drug interactions of, 406
Counter Rotational System (CRS), in calcaneovalgus deformity, 654–655, *655*
Coxsackie virus infections, cutaneous manifestations of, 184–185, *185*
"Crab meat" appearance, of synovium, 614, *616*
Cracchiolo procedure, 499–501, *500*
Cranial arteritis, 163–164
C-reactive protein (CRP), 221
Creep, of implants, 93
Crepitation, in patellofemoral stress syndrome, 251

Crescentic osteotomy, in metatarsus adductus, *662*, 662–663
CREST syndrome, 156, 170, *170*
Cricoarytenoid arthritis, airway management and, 478–479
Crithidia luciliae test, for antinuclear antibody measurement, 225
Crohn's disease. See *Inflammatory bowel disease (IBD).*
Cross-sectional imaging, 377–394
computed tomography in, 381–382
three-dimensional reconstruction and, 381–382, *382*
foreign bodies and, 385
in arthritis, 385
in neoplasms and related disorders, 383–385
imaging methods and, 383–385
in osteomyelitis, 392–394
in postoperative assessment, 394
in tarsal coalition and normal variants, 391, *391*
in trauma, 385–391
magnetic resonance imaging and, 382–383
ultrasound imaging and, 383
Crutches, following arthrodesis, 562
Cryoglobulinemia, cutaneous manifestations of, 176, *176*
Cryotherapy, 451
Cryptococcus infections, septic arthritis and, 210
Crystal(s), examination for, in septic arthritis, 212
in synovial fluid, 231, *231*
Crystal chemotactic factor, 432
Crystalline deposition disease. See also *Calcium hydroxyapatite crystal deposition disease; Calcium pyrophosphate dihydrate deposition disease (CPPD); Gout.*
drug therapy in, 424–427
exercises for, 454t
preoperative evaluation in, 459t
Cuneiforms, first, open wedge osteotomy of, in metatarsus adductus, 663
Current perception threshold testing (CPT), in entrapment syndromes, 688
Cushioning, 86, *86*
in osteoarthritis of knee, 88–89
Cutaneous. See also under *Nail(s); Skin.*
Cutaneous arteriospasm, Raynaud's phenomenon and, 203–204
Cutaneous atrophy, in systemic lupus erythematosus, 171, *171*
Cutaneous leiomyomas, 634
Cutaneous nerve entrapment, dorsal. See *Dorsal cutaneous nerve entrapment.*
Cutis marmorata, 173
Cutting cones, 22
Cyanosis, Raynaud's phenomenon and, 203–204
Cyclophosphamide, 411t, 423
anesthesia and, 470–471
Cyclosporin A, 411t, 423
Cyclosporine, anesthesia and, 471
in psoriasis, 195
Cyst(s), benign, magnetic resonance imaging and, 628, *628*
epidermoid, radiographic appearance of, 333
of bone. See *Bone cyst.*
synovial, in knee, rheumatoid arthritis and, 123
Cytokines. See also specific cytokines.
inflammation and, *36*, 36–39
Cytomegalovirus infections, imaging in, 362
Cytoprotective agents, drug interactions of, 405–406
Cytotoxic agents, 421–422. See also specific drugs.

Dactylitis, in HIV infection, 304
de Quervain's tenosynovitis, 116
Débridement, arthroscopy and, 620–621
  in septic arthritis, 216
  of muscles, fasciotomy and, 729
  of necrotic tissue, nonhealing wounds and, 59
Débriding agents, wound healing and, 60
Deep bursae, 11
Deep peroneal nerve entrapment, 701–702
  etiology and specific findings in, 701, *701*
  surgical technique for, 701–702, *702*
Deep transverse intermetatarsal ligament
    (DTIL), plantar digital nerve entrapment
    and, 709
Deep zone, of synovial joints, 3
Deformity. See also specific deformities.
  as indication for arthrodesis, 559
Degenerative disease. See *Osteoarthritis (OA).*
Degranulation, wound healing and, 52
11-Dehydrocorticosterone, *438*
Delayed union, of ankle fractures, arthroscopy
    and, 620
Demineralized bone matrix (DBM), 26
Denis Browne bar, in calcaneovalgus deformity,
    655
11-Deoxycortisol, *438*
Dermatitis, allergic, implants and, 95
Dermatomyositis/polymyositis (DM/PM), 159–
    161, 160t
  clinical features of, *160*, 160–161
  cutaneous manifestations of, 171–172, *172*,
    173
  functional scale for, 451t
  of skin and nails, in HIV infection, 305
  pathology of, 159–160, 160t
  treatment of, 161
Dermopathy, diabetic, 178–179, *179*
Desipramine, in chronic pain syndrome, 682
Desmoid tumors, 633, *635*
  extra-abdominal, magnetic resonance imaging
    and, 629–630
11-Desoxycorticosterone, anesthesia and, 472t
Dexamethasone, anesthesia and, 472t
  for injection therapy, 443t
    dosage of, 444t
Dextranomer powder (Debrisan), wound healing
    and, 60
Diabetes mellitus, anesthesia and, 466–468,
    467t, 468t
  avascular necrosis of bone and, 640
  cutaneous manifestations of, 177–180, *178–
    180*
  dermopathy in, 178–179, *179*
  foot in. See *Diabetic foot.*
  nonhealing wounds in, 56
Diabetic foot, 178, 261–280
  autoimmune-related disorders and, 280
  bunions and, 278, *278*
  chondrocalcinosis and, 280
  diffuse idiopathic skeletal hyperostosis of,
    270–271
    evaluation of, 270
    pathogenesis of, 270
    treatment of, 270–271
  drop foot and, 276–277
  equinus and, 277–278
  fascial disorders of, 273–275, *274*
    evaluation of, 274–275
    pathogenesis of, 274
    treatment of, 275
  gait disturbances and, 277
  gout and, 279, *280*
  hallux limitus and, 278–279, *279*
  hallux valgus and, 278
  imaging of, 319, *319*, 359, *360*, 394
  infections of, *179*, 179–180, *180*

Diabetic foot *(Continued)*
  intrinsic minus foot and, 275–276, *276*
  limited joint mobility in, 271–273
    evaluation of, 272–273, *273*
    pathogenesis of, 271–272
    treatment of, 273
  neuroarthropathy of, 56, 204, *205*, 261–268,
    262–264
    classification of, 265, 266t
    evaluation of, 265–266
    pathogenesis of, 262, *264*, 264–265
    treatment of, 266–268
  osteoarthritis of, 279
  osteolysis of, *268*, 268–269
    evaluation of, 268–269
    pathogenesis of, 268
    treatment of, 269
  osteopenia of, generalized, 269–270
  pseudogout and, 280
  tendon xanthomas of, 275
Diabetic neuropathy, 56
Diaphyses, 15
  of mature long bones, 17–18
Diatrizoates, 365
Diazepam, local anesthesia and, 477
Diclofenac, 410t, 416
  drug interactions of, 406, 407
  in chronic pain syndrome, 681
Dicloxacillin, in septic arthritis, 215t
Didanosine (ddI), in HIV infection, 302
Dideoxycytidine (ddC), in HIV infection, 302
Diet, in rheumatoid arthritis, 430
Differentiation clusters (CD), in HIV infection,
    300–301, *301*
  inflammation and, 46
Diffuse idiopathic skeletal hyperostosis (DISH),
    135
  in diabetic foot. See *Diabetic foot, diffuse
    idiopathic skeletal hyperostosis of.*
Diffuse plane xanthomas, 183, *184*, 184
Diflunisal, 409t
  drug interactions of, 406
Digit(s), clubbing of, *198*, 198–199
  deformities of, rheumatoid arthritis and, 119–
    120, *120*
  implant arthroplasty and, 525, 525–526, *526*
  mallet toes and, following Hibbs tenosuspen-
    sion procedure, 602
  sausage, in seronegative spondyloarthropa-
    thies, 134
Digital implants, 525, 525–526, *526*
Digital subtraction arteriography (DSA), 376,
    376
Digitorum longus tendon, anatomy of, 372–373
Digoxin, drug interactions of, 405t, 407
Dimethylcysteine. See D-*Penicillamine.*
Direct coupling, 452
Discoid lupus erythematosus, overlapping
    pathologic and clinical manifestations of,
    166t
  overlapping serologic manifestations of, 167t
Discs, of synovial joints, 9–10
  blood supply of, 13
  functions of, 10
Disease-modifying agents and remissive drugs
    (DMARDs), 397, 398t, 410t, 418–422. See
    also specific drugs.
  in rheumatoid arthritis, 125
  in seronegative spondyloarthropathies, 136
Distal interphalangeal (DIP) joints, rheumatoid
    arthritis and, 115
Dorsal cutaneous nerve entrapment, 702–703
  etiology and specific findings in, 702, *702*
  medial, 698–701, *699–700*
  surgical technique for, 702–703, *703*
Double-support phase of stance, 69

Doxepin, in chronic pain syndrome, 682
Dressings, wound healing and, 60
Drop foot, 79, *79*
  in diabetes mellitus, 276–277
  tendon transfers in, of tibialis posterior ten-
    don, 602
Drug therapy, 397–432. See also specific drugs
    and drug types.
  gout induced by, 142–143
  in bacillary angiomatosis, in HIV infection,
    305
  in candidal paronychia, 179
  in chronic pain syndrome, 680–682
  in dermatomyositis, 161
  in erythema nodosum, 191
  in gout. See *Gout, treatment of.*
  in herpes simplex virus infections, in HIV in-
    fection, 305
  in HIV infection, 302
  in metatarsalgia, 236
  in metatarsophalangeal joint sprain, 238
  in mixed connective tissue disease, 167
  in necrobiosis lipoidica diabeticorum, 178
  in polymyositis, 161
  in post-traumatic ankle pain, 725
  in pseudogout, 150
  in psoriasis, 195
  in pyoderma gangrenosum, 193
  in Raynaud's phenomenon, 206
  in rheumatoid arthritis, 124–125, 427–430
    injection therapy and, 125
    oral medications in, 124–125
    surgery and, 460–461
  in sarcoidosis, 192
  in scleroderma, 159
  in septic arthritis, 214, 214t, 215t
    treatment outcome with, 216t
  in seronegative spondyloarthropathies, 432
  in Sjögren's syndrome, 162
  in systemic lupus erythematosus, 155
  in tendinitis, 581
  in vasculitis, 205
  on osteoarthritis, 430–431
Dupuytren's disease of palmar fascia (DDPF),
    in diabetic foot. See *Diabetic foot, fascial
    disorders of.*
DuVries-Dickson procedure, 499
Dynamic stabilizing insole system, in
    calcaneovalgus deformity, 655–656, *656*,
    657
Dysbaric osteonecrosis, 640
Dysbetalipoproteinemia, type III, xanthomas
    and, 183t
Dyskinesia, in cerebral palsy, 291
Dyslipoproteinemias, 182
Dystonia, in cerebral palsy, 291
Dystrophic nonunions, 27

Eicosanoids, inflammation and, 34
Elastic element, 93
Elasticity, modulus of, 91
Elbow, rheumatoid arthritis and, 116
  septic arthritis in, treatment outcome in, 216t
Elderly patients, nonsteroidal anti-inflammatory
    drugs in, 403–404
  salicylates in, 124
  septic arthritis in, 207–208
Electrical potentials, of bone, 19
Electrical stimulation, 453. See also
    *Transcutaneous electrical nerve stimulation
    (TENS).*
  for nonunions, 27–28
  wound healing and, 61

Electrodiagnostic testing, in entrapment
syndromes, 689–690
in plantar digital nerve entrapment, 711
Electrokinetics, of bone, 19
''Elephant foot,'' 26
Elephantiasis, cutaneous manifestations of, *187*,
187–188
ELISA double-binding test, for rheumatoid
factor, 222–223
Enchondroma, radiographic appearance of, 328–
329
Endochondral bone repair, 16, *16*
Endochondral ossification, 15–16, *16*
bone healing and, 20
Endogenous opiates, 676–677
Endosteum, 18
Endotendineum, 11
Endothelial cells, inflammation and, 47–48
Endotracheal intubation, anesthesia and, 479
Enflurane, epinephrine for, 477
Enterobacter infections, septic arthritis and,
215t
Enterococcus infections, septic arthritis and,
215t
Entheseal arthropathies, 309
Entheses, 11, *11*
in ankylosing spondylitis, 132
Enthesopathy, in HIV infection, 304
Entrapment syndrome. See *Nerve entrapment
syndromes.*
Environmental factors, gout and, 142–143
Enzyme-linked immunosorbent assay (ELISA),
for HIV infection detection, 301
for rheumatoid factor, 222, 222–223
Eosinophil(s), inflammation and, 47
Eosinophilia, in rheumatoid arthritis, 110
Eosinophilic granuloma, radiographic
appearance of, 337–338, *338*
Epidermal regeneration, wound healing and, 54
Epidermoid cyst, radiographic appearance of,
333
Epimyothelial islands, in Sjögren's syndrome,
161
Epinephrine, local anesthesia and, 477–478
Epiphyseal arteries, 18
Epiphysis, 15
Epitendineum, 11
Equino-adducto-varus foot, gait pattern in, 79–
80, *80*
Equinovarus deformity, tendon transfers in, of
tibialis posterior tendon, 602, *603*
Equinus deformity, *665*, 665–667
clinical diagnosis of, 666
gait pattern in, 78, *79*, 81
in cerebral palsy. See *Cerebral palsy (CP),
equinus deformity in.*
in diabetes mellitus, 277–278
in paralytic disorders, 286, *287*
osseous, 80
spastic, 667–668
in cerebral palsy, Achilles tendon transfer
in. See *Achilles tendon, advancement
of, anterior.*
peroneal, 81
treatment of, 667–668
conservative, 667–668, *668*
surgical, 668
tendon transfers in, Hibbs tenosuspension
procedure and, 600
treatment of, 297, *297*
conservative, 666
surgical, 666–667
Erosive osteoarthritis, of foot, 315
Eruptive xanthomas, 183, *184*
Erysipelas, in diabetes mellitus, 179

Erythema, periungual, in systemic lupus
erythematosus, 154, *156*
Raynaud's phenomenon and, 203–204
Erythema multiforme (EM), 189–190, *189–191*
major, 189–190, *190*
Erythema nodosum, 190–191, *191*
Erythema nodosum leprosum, 191
Erythrasma, in diabetes mellitus, 179–180, *180*
Erythrocyte sedimentation rate (ESR), 220–221
in rheumatoid arthritis, 110
in seronegative spondyloarthropathies, 134
Erythromycin, in bacillary angiomatosis, in HIV
infection, 305
Escherichia coli infections, septic arthritis and,
209, 215t
Ethambutol, in septic arthritis, 215t
Ethyl chloride, for glucocorticoid injection
therapy, 446
Etodolac, 410t, 413
Evan's calcaneal osteotomy, in calcaneovalgus
deformity, 656–657
indications for, 656, *657*
procedure for, 656–657, *658*
Ewing's sarcoma, radiographic appearance of,
331–332, *333*
Exercise(s), 453–455, 454t
following hallux limitus/rigidus repair, 543,
543
isokinetic, 455
isometric, 454–455
mobilization and, 455
range-of-motion, 455
strengthening, 454–455
stretching, 68
Exocrinopathy, autoimmune. See *Sjögren's
syndrome.*
Extensor digitorum brevis, avulsion fracture of,
following ankle sprains, 246
Extensor digitorum longus (EDL) tendon, 485–
486
Extensor hallucis longus tendon, anatomy of,
372–373
Extensor subluxation, gait and, 80
Extracapsular accessory ligaments, of synovial
joints, 5
Extracellular matrix, of articular cartilage, 29,
30
Extractable nuclear antigen, 224
Exudative stage of cartilage repair, 30
Eye(s), in rheumatoid arthritis, 108
in Sjögren's syndrome, 161, *162*

Factor XII, inflammation and, 40
Factor XIIA, inflammation and, 40
Familial Mediterranean fever, arthritis related
to, rheumatoid arthritis versus, 113
Famotidine, anesthesia and, 468
Farr method, for antinuclear antibody
measurement, 225
Fascia, of forefoot, 381
of hindfoot, 377–378
of midfoot, 379, *379*
Fasciitis, nodular, 631, *634*
plantar, *240*, 240–241
Fasciotomy, in compartment syndromes, acute,
729
of lower leg, 730, *730*
chronic, 733–734
Fat pads, of synovial joints, 10
Fatigue fracture. See *Stress fractures.*
Fatigue testing, of implants, 93–94, *94*
Fatty acids, bacterial, in synovial fluid, in septic
arthritis, 213
fish oil, 424

Felty's syndrome, in rheumatoid arthritis, 108
Femur, fracture of neck of, avascular necrosis
and, 648
Fenbufen, drug interactions of, 407
Fenoprofen, 414–415
anesthesia and, 470
Fenoprofen calcium, 410t
in gout, acute gouty arthritis and, 148t
Fibrin, inflammation and, 41
Fibrinopeptides, inflammation and, 41
Fibroblasts, 18
inflammation and, 48
wound healing and, 53
Fibrocortical defect, radiographic appearance of,
332–333
Fibromas, chondromyxoid, radiographic
appearance of, 329
magnetic resonance imaging and, 629, *629*
nonossifying, radiographic appearance of,
332–333
ossifying, radiographic appearance of, 327,
328
Fibromatosis, plantar, 631–632, *633*, *634*
in diabetic foot, 274
radiographic appearance of, 334, *335*
Fibronectin, inflammation and, chronic, 49
would healing and, 55
Fibronexus, 55
Fibrosarcomas, 636
of nerve sheath. See *Schwannomas, malig-
nant.*
Fibrositis, functional scale for, 451t
Fibrous bands, post-traumatic ankle pain and,
720
Fibrous bone, 17
Fibrous dysplasia, imaging in, 385
radiographic appearance of, 333, *334*
Fibrous joints, 1
Fibrous synovial membrane, 6
Fibula, stress fracture of, 256
Fillauer bar, in calcaneovalgus deformity, 655
Finger, Hippocratic, 198
Fish oil, fatty acid supplementation, 424
Fistulas, osteomyelitis and, 342
rheumatoid arthritis and, 122
Fixation. See also *specific types of fixation.*
arthrodesis and, of ankle, 573–575, *574*
of hallux interphalangeal joint, 564
of metatarsophalangeal joint, 552–553,
554–556, 557
of subtalar joint, 569–570, *570*
of talonavicular joint, 568, *569*
of implants. See *Implant(s), fixation of.*
Flatfoot. See *Equinus deformity.*
Flexible fixation, implants and, 98–99
Flexor digitorum brevis (FDB) tendon, 486
Flexor digitorum longus (FDL) tendon, 486
anatomy of, 372, *372*, *373*
Flexor hallucis longus tendon, anatomy of, 372,
372, *373*
Flexor tenosynovitis, rheumatoid arthritis and,
115
Fluconazole, in septic arthritis, 215t
Fluidotherapy, 453
Fluoxetine, in chronic pain syndrome, 682
Fluphenazine, in chronic pain syndrome, 682
Flurbiprofen, 410t, 415
anesthesia and, 470
drug interactions of, 406–407
Folliculitis, in diabetes mellitus, 179
Foot. See also *Digit(s); Forefoot; Heel;
Hindfoot; Midfoot.*
arch of. See *Arch.*
compartment syndrome in, 730–731, *731*, *732*
diabetic. See *Diabetic foot.*
drop. See *Drop foot.*

Foot *(Continued)*
dysfunction of, tendinitis and, 578–579
"elephant," 26
equino-adducto-varus, gait pattern in, 79–80, *80*
imaging of, 307t, 307–321
general principles in, 307–308, 308t, *309*
in connective tissue disease, 308t , 315, *317*
in crystal deposition diseases, 315, *316*, *317*
in gout, 308t
in infections and neuroarthropathy, 308t, 315, 317, *318–320*, 319–320
in osteoarthritis, 308t, *314*, 314–315
in psoriatic arthritis, 308t
in Reiter's syndrome, 308t
in rheumatoid arthritis, 308t, 309–310, *309–313*
in seronegative spondyloarthropathies, 310, *313*, 313–314, *314*
in sesamoid bone disorders, 320–321
intrinsic minus, in diabetes mellitus, 275–276, *276*
phalanges of, avascular necrosis in, 649
rheumatoid arthritis of, 117–122
arch collapse and, 120
bunion and, 119, *119*
digital deformities and, 119–120, *120*
extra-articular involvement and, 121–122
forefoot splaying and, 120
hallux valgus and, 119, *119*
plantar fasciitis and, 120
progressive joint deformity and, 120–121
signs and symptoms in, 118
talonavicular joint involvement and, 118–119, *119*
tenosynovitis and, 121
transverse arch and, 120
types of feet and, 126–127
serpentine, 658–659
splay, in diabetes mellitus, 278
surgery of, anesthesia for, 473
in seronegative spondyloarthropathies, 136–140
ulcers of, 128, *128*
Footwear. See *Shoes.*
Forces, bending, 65
compression, 65
gait biomechanics and, 69, *69*
production of, by muscles, 68
torsional, 65
Forefoot, anatomic structures of, 380–381
arthroplasty of. See *Arthroplasty, of forefoot; Implant arthroplasty, of forefoot.*
functional anatomy of, *482–486*, 482–487
reconstruction of, 129
rheumatoid arthritis of, imaging and, *309*, 309–310, *310*
splaying of, 120
surgery of, in cavus deformity, 670–671
Forefoot adductus, 659
Forefoot neuritis, plantar, 235–236
Foreign antigens, rheumatoid arthritis and, 427
Foreign bodies, imaging and, 385
Foreign-body reaction, implant arthroplasty and, 527
Fowler-Philip angle, 242, *242*
Fracture(s). See also *specific anatomic sites and types of fractures.*
avascular necrosis and, 648–649, *649*
Jones, *238*, 238–239
nonunion of. See *Nonunions.*
plating of, 23
Fracture healing, 19–23
primary, 22–23

Fracture healing *(Continued)*
rigid fixation and, 23
secondary, 19–20
stages of, *20*, 20–22
Freeze-dried allograft. See *Alloimplants.*
Freiberg's disease, 644, *644*, 644t, *645*
Fretting corrosion, 94
Friction blister, 234–235
Functional assessment, 450, 451t
Fungal infections, cutaneous, in HIV infection, 188
septic arthritis and, 210, 215t
Furlong casting procedure, modified, 660, *660*
Furunculosis, in diabetes mellitus, 179
Fusobacterium necrophorum infections, septic arthritis and, 209

Gait, biomechanics of, 69–76
ankle joint and, *72*, 72–73
forces and lever arms and, 69, *69*
hip joint and, 70–71, *71*
knee joint and, 71–72, *72*
midtarsal joint and, 74–76, *75*, *76*
normal gait cycle and, 69, *70*
pathologic gait and. See *Pathologic gait.*
phases of gait and, 69–70
subtalar joint and, 73–74, *74*
calcaneus, following Achilles tendon advancement, 607–608
disturbances of, in diabetes mellitus, 277
pathologic. See *Pathologic gait.*
pendulum, 80
waddling, 80
Gait cycle, biomechanics of, normal, 69, *70*
stance phase of, 69–70, *70*
swing phase of, 68, *70*
GAIT implant, 520, *520*
surgical technique for, 521
Gallium-67 citrate (^{67}Ga citrate), 351, *354*, 355, *356*
"Gamekeeper's thumb," 116
Gangliography, 373, *373*, 375
Ganglion, 632, *634*
Gangrene, dry, in diabetes mellitus, 179, *179*
in polyarteritis nodosa, 163, *163*
Ganley splint, in calcaneovalgus deformity, 654, *655*
in metatarsus adductus, 660
Garré's sclerosing osteomyelitis, 342
Gastrocnemius muscle, lengthening of, in equinus deformity, 666–667, *667*
strain of, athletic injuries and, 254
Gastrointestinal system, in Sjögren's syndrome, 162
in systemic lupus erythematosus, 155t
infections of, arthritis related to, rheumatoid arthritis versus, 114
nonsteroidal anti-inflammatory drugs and, 400–401
Gate theory, of pain control, 676
Gaucher's disease, avascular necrosis of bone and, 640
General anesthesia. See also *Anesthesia.*
intubation and, 479
Genetic disorders. See also *specific disorders.*
nonhealing wounds in, 57
Genu valgum, 78, *78*
"Geographic tongue," in Reiter's syndrome, 133
Geriatric patients. See *Elderly patients.*
German measles, imaging in, 359, *362*
Germinal zone, of growth plate, 16, *16*
Giant cell arteritis, 163–164
rheumatoid arthritis versus, 114

Giant cell tumors, of bone, radiographic appearance of, 329–330, *330*
of tendon sheath, magnetic resonance imaging and, 628
reparative granulomas and, radiographic appearance of, 330, *330*
Gliding zone, of synovial joints, 3
Glomus tumor, radiographic appearance of, 332
Glucocorticoids, 437–448, *438*. See also *specific glucocorticoids.*
anesthesia and, 473–474, *474*
in rheumatoid arthritis, 125
surgery and, 461
insufficiency of, signs and symptoms of, 440, 440t
local therapy using, 442–448
agents available for, 443t, 443–444, 444t
allergic reactions to, 445
aseptic necrosis of bone following, 445
choice of agent and dose for, 445–446
contraindications to, 442
in rheumatoid arthritis, 125
in seronegative spondyloarthropathies, 136
injection techniques for, 446–448
muscle atrophy following, 445
neuropathic arthropathy following, 445
postinjection flares and, 444–445
septic arthritis following, 445
relative anti-inflammatory potency of, 441, 441t, 443–444
systemic therapy using, 437–441, 439t–441t
guidelines for, 441, 441t
prolonged, effects of, 438–440, 439t
Glucose, blood levels of, anesthesia and, 467t, 467–468, 468t
in synovial fluid, 231
in septic arthritis, 213
Gluteus medius limp, 77
Glycoproteins, HIV infection and, 300, *300*
Glycosaminoglycans (GAGs), nonsteroidal anti-inflammatory drugs and, 403
of articular cartilage, 29
Gold salts, 410t, 419–420
anesthesia and, 470
in rheumatoid arthritis, 125, 430
surgery and, 461
in seronegative spondyloarthropathies, 136
Gold sodium thiomalate (GST), 410t, 419
Gomphoses, 1
Gonococcal arthritis-dermatitis syndrome, 186–187, *187*
Gonorrhea, arthritis related to, rheumatoid arthritis versus, 113
cutaneous manifestations of, 186
septic arthritis and, 208–209
Gottron's papules, in dermatomyositis, 160
in dermatomyositis/polymyositis, 171, 172, *172*
Gout, 141–149
acute, pathogenesis of, 143
synovial analysis in, 229t
treatment of, 431–432
asymptomatic hyperuricemia and, clinical manifestations of, 143–144
treatment of, 149
causes of, 142t
chronic tophaceous, clinical manifestations of, 144–145
cutaneous manifestations of, *181*, 181–182, *182*
classification of, 141, 142t
clinical evaluation of, 145–147
laboratory studies, 146t, 146–147
radiographic findings in, 145–146
clinical manifestations of, 143–145

Gout (*Continued*)
cutaneous manifestations of, *181*, 181–182, *182*
diagnosis of, criteria for, 146t
differential diagnosis of, 147
disease association with, 143
functional scale for, 451t
gouty arthritis and, 34
acute, clinical manifestations of, 144
chronic, treatment of, 148–149
idiopathic, 431
in diabetic foot, 279, *280*
intercritical, clinical manifestations of, 144
treatment of, 148
of ankle, arthroscopy in, 624
of foot, imaging and, 315, *316*, *317*
radiography in, 308t
pathophysiology of, 141–143, 142t
preoperative and postoperative considerations in, 462–463
prevalence and incidence of, 141
primary, 141, 431
pathophysiology of, 142t
rheumatoid arthritis versus, 113–114
secondary, 141, 431
pathophysiology of, 142t, 142–143
synovial fluid analysis in, 231, *231*
treatment of, 147–149, 148t
pharmacologic, 431–432
in chronic tophaceous gout, 182
Gram's stain, in septic arthritis, 212
Granulocyte colony-stimulating factor (G-CSF), inflammation and, 39
Granulocyte macrophage colony-stimulating factor (GM-CSF), inflammation and, 38–39
Granulomas, eosinophilic, radiographic appearance of, 337–338, *338*
reparative, radiographic appearance of, 330, *330*
Granulomatosis, Wegener's, 163
Granulomatous infections, imaging in, 359
"Grasshopper" deformity, rheumatoid arthritis and, 115
Ground substance, in articular cartilage, of synovial joints, 5
Growth factor therapy, wound healing and, 61
Growth plate, 15–16
zones of, 16, *16*
Guaiac stool tests, nonsteroidal anti-inflammatory drugs and, 407–408
Guttate psoriasis, 194

Haemophilus influenzae infections, septic arthritis and, 209
Hageman factor. See *Factor XII.*
Haglund's deformity, 242
Hallucal interphalangeal joint, arthrodesis of, in rheumatoid arthritis, 563–564, *564*, *565*
arthroplasty of, 512–513
Hallux, scar contracture of, following Jones tenosuspension, 608, *609*
Hallux limitus. See also *Hallux limitus/rigidus.*
in diabetes mellitus, 278–279, *279*
nonsurgical treatment of, 535
surgical treatment of, joint-destructive procedures for, 535–536, *536*
Hallux limitus/rigidus, classification of, 532–533, *533*, *534*, 535
clinical findings and evaluation in, *531*, 531–532, *532*
etiology of, 530–531
first metatarsophalangeal joint motion and, anatomy and mechanics of, 529–530, *529*, *530*

Hallux limitus/rigidus (*Continued*)
measurement of, 530, *530*
imaging in, 532, *533*
primary, 530, 531
secondary, 530
surgical treatment of, 535–544
abrasion chondroplasty and, 539–540, *540*
cartilage rearrangement and, 538–539, *540*
cheilectomy and, 536–537, *537*
combination procedures and, 540–541, *541*, *542*, 543
complications of, 544
metatarsophalangeal joint arthrodesis in, 546, 546t
plantar-flexion procedures and, 537–538, *539*
postoperative care and, 543, *543*
reconstructive techniques for, 536
shortening procedures and, 537, *538*
Hallux rigidus. See also *Hallux limitus/rigidus.*
imaging and, 314–315
Hallux valgus, in diabetes mellitus, 278
rheumatoid arthritis and, 119, *119*
Halothane, epinephrine for, 477
Hand, rheumatoid arthritis and, 115–116, *115–117*
Hand-foot-mouth disease, cutaneous manifestations of, 184–185, *185*
Hardness testing, of implants, 94–95, *95*
Healing. See also *Fracture healing; Wound healing.*
of tendons, 577–578
Heart, in rheumatoid arthritis, 107–108
Heart disease, anesthesia and, 464–465
Heat, inflammation and, 34
Heat therapy, 451–453, 452t
Heel, lover's, in Reiter's syndrome, 133, *133*
neuritic pain in, 706
posterior disorders of, athletic injuries and, 242, 242–243
Heel lifts, in leg-length inequality, 88
Heel wedging, in osteoarthritis of knee, 88
Heliotrope rash, in dermatomyositis/polymyositis, 171–172, *172*
Hemangiography, 375
Hemangiomas, 633–634
radiographic appearance of, 332
Hematocrit, nonsteroidal anti-inflammatory drugs and, 407
Hematogenous osteomyelitis, 340
Hematogenous spread, septic arthritis and, 210
Hematologic disorders, nonhealing wounds and, 57–58
Hematologic studies, 220–232, 228t. See also specific studies.
Hematologic system, in systemic lupus erythematosus, 155t
nonsteroidal anti-inflammatory drugs and, 401–402
Hematomas, of muscle, imaging in, 390–391
Hemi-implants, for forefoot implant arthroplasty, 517–518, *518*
Hemodynamic studies, in avascular necrosis of bone, 640–641
Hemorrhages, salicylates and, 124
splinter, 199, *199*, 199t
Hemorrhagic bullae, in cutaneous vasculitis, 202, *202*
Hemorrhagic papules, in cutaneous vasculitis, 202, *202*
Hemostasis, wound healing and, 52
Henoch-Schönlein purpura, 174, *175*
Heppenstall's classification of fracture repair, 20–22
Herpes simplex virus infections, in HIV infection, 305

Herpetic whitlow, in HIV infection, 305
Heyman-Herndon tarsometatarsal capsulotomy, in metatarsus adductus, 663
Hibbs tenosuspension procedure, 600–602
complications of, 602
indications for, 600–601, *601*
technique for, *601*, 601–602, *602*
High-voltage direct-current stimulators (HVDCSs), 453
Hindfoot, anatomic structures of, 377–378
rheumatoid arthritis of, imaging and, 310, *311*, *312*
surgery of, in cavus deformity, 670, *670*
Hip, biomechanics of, gait and, 70–71, *71*
pathologic gait and, 76–77, *77*
in seronegative spondyloarthropathies, 134
pain in, leg-length inequality and, 88, *88*
orthotics in, 89
rheumatoid arthritis and, 122, 123
septic arthritis in, treatment outcome of, 216t
Hippocratic finger, 198
Histamine, inflammation and, 40
HIV. See *Human immunodeficiency virus (HIV) infection.*
Hoffmann-Clayton type procedure, 499, *499*
variations of, 501
Hole saw, for metatarsophalangeal joint arthrodesis, 552
Homogenous tissue. See *Allografts.*
Homografts. See *Allografts.*
Hormones, rheumatoid arthritis and, 427
"Horse hoof" callus, 26
Howel-Evans syndrome, 188
H_2-receptor antagonists, gastrointestinal function and, 401
Human immunodeficiency virus (HIV) infection, 300–306
clinical presentation of, 302–305, *303*, 303t
dermatologic manifestations and, 304–305
musculoskeletal manifestations and, 304
neurologic manifestations and, 303–304
vascular manifestations and, 305
cutaneous manifestations of, 188
pathogenesis of, *300*, 300–301, *301*
staging of, 301–302, 302t
testing for, 301
treatment of, 302
Human leukocyte antigens (HLA), diabetes mellitus and, 280
in ankylosing spondylitis, 132
in inflammatory bowel disease, 134
in seronegative spondyloarthropathies, 134–135
measurement of, 226t, 226–227, 227t
rheumatoid arthritis and, 427–428
Humoral factors, inflammation and. See *Inflammatory reaction, humoral factor(s) in.*
Hutchinson's freckle, 196
Hyaline cartilage, of ankle, 612
Hyaluronic acid, nonsteroidal anti-inflammatory drugs and, 403
of mucin, 9
Hydantoin, in chronic pain syndrome, 681
Hydrocolloid dressings, wound healing and, 60
Hydrocortisone, *438*
anesthesia and, 472, 472t, 473
for injection therapy, 443t
dosage of, 444t
Hydrocortisone sodium succinate, 440
Hydrogel dressings, wound healing and, 60
5-Hydroperoxyeicosatetraenoic acid (5-HPETE), inflammation and, 35
12-Hydroperoxyeicosatetraenoic acid (12-HPETE), inflammation and, 36

15-Hydroperoxyeicosatetraenoic acid (15-HPETE), inflammation and, 36
Hydrotherapy, 452–453
Hydroxyapatite, implant fixation and, 99
Hydroxychloroquine, anesthesia and, 471–472
  in rheumatoid arthritis, 125
    surgery and, 461
Hydroxychloroquine sulfate (HCS), 410t, 418–419
  in rheumatoid arthritis, 429–430
5-Hydroxyeicosatetraenoic acid (5-HETE), inflammation and, 35
12-Hydroxyeicosatetraenoic acid (12-HPETE), inflammation and, 36
15-Hydroxyeicosatetraenoic acid (15-HPETE), inflammation and, 36
5-Hydroxytryptamine (5-HT), inflammation and, 40
Hygiene, in rheumatoid arthritis, 128
Hyperbaric oxygen (HBO), wound healing and, 60–61
Hypercholesterolemia, xanthomas and, 183t
Hyperlipoproteinemia, xanthomas and, 183t
Hypersensitivity reactions, glucocorticoid injection therapy and, 445
  nonsteroidal anti-inflammatory drugs and, 402–403
  to contrast agents, 365–366
  to salicylates, 407
Hypersensitivity vasculitis, 164
Hyperthyroidism, cutaneous manifestations of, 181
Hypertrophic osteoarthropathy, 198, *198*
Hypertrophic synovitis, post-traumatic ankle pain and, 719
Hyperuricemia, 142, 142t. See also *Gout.*
Hypoglycemic agents, drug interactions of, 405t, 406
Hypothyroidism, cutaneous manifestations of, *180*, 180–181
Hypoxanthine guanine phosphoribosyl transferase (HGPRT) deficiency, gout and, 142–143

Ibuprofen, 410t, 414
  anesthesia and, 469–470
  drug interactions of, 406, 407
  in chronic pain syndrome, 680–681
  in gout, acute gouty arthritis and, 148t
  in osteoarthritis, 431
Ice, cold therapy using, 451
Ichthyosis, 193, *193*
IL. See *Interleukin* entries.
Iliotibial band (ITB) syndrome, *84*, 84–85, *85*
  athletic injuries and, 252, 252–253
Imaging. See also specific modalities.
  cross-sectional. See *Cross-sectional imaging.*
  in ankle sprains, 244
  in avascular necrosis of bone, 641
  in calcaneovalgus deformity, 653, *653*
  in diabetic osteolysis, 269
  in entrapment syndromes, 690, *690, 691*
  in gout, 145–146
  in hallux limitus/rigidus, 532, *533*
  in metatarsus adductus, 658–659, *659*
  in neuroarthropathy, of diabetic foot, 265–266
  in post-traumatic ankle pain, 724
  in rheumatoid arthritis, 109
  in septic arthritis, 213
  in seronegative spondyloarthropathies, 135
  in tendinitis, *580*, 580–581
  in tendon dysfunction, 583
  of bone and joint infections. See *Osteomyelitis, imaging in.*

Imaging *(Continued)*
  of foot. See *Foot, imaging of.*
  of musculoskeletal tumors. See *Tumor(s), imaging of.*
Imipenem, in septic arthritis, 215t
Immature bone, 17
Immobilization, following arthrodesis, in rheumatoid arthritis, 575
  for nonunions, 27
  in neuroarthropathy, of diabetic foot, 267
  in post-traumatic ankle pain, 725
  in tendinitis, 581
  postoperative, in septic arthritis, 217–218
Immune complexes, in synovial fluid, 231
Immunoglobulins, IgD, 110
  IgE, 110
  IgG, 110
  IgM, 109–110, *110*
  in rheumatoid arthritis, 109–110, *110*
Immunology, of vasculitis, 201
Immunosuppressive agents, 411t, 422–423. See also specific drugs.
  anesthesia and, 470–471
  septic arthritis and, 207
Impact stage, of fracture healing, 20
Impetigo, in diabetes mellitus, 179
Impingement exostosis, anterior, 722
Implant(s), 91–101, 92t, 97t. See also *Implant arthroplasty.*
  biocompatibility of, 91, 93t
  biologic reaction to, *95*, 95–96, *96*
  failure of, 100–101, 101t
    biologic, 100, 101t
    mechanical, 100–101, 101t
    structural, 101, 101t
  fixation of, 97–100
    absorbable, 99–100
    biologic, 97–98, *98*
    collagen for, 100
    flexible or less rigid, 98–99
    hydroxyapatite for, 100
  fracture or deformation of, *526*, 526–527
  mechanical properties of, 91, 93–95
    fatigue testing and, 93–94, *94*
    hardness testing and, 94–95, *95*
    tensile testing and, 91, 93, *93, 94*, 94t
  osteomyelitis and, 343, *349*
  septic arthritis and, 210
Implant arthroplasty, implant complications and, *526*, 526–527, *527*
  in hallux limitus, 535, *536*
  lesser metatarsophalangeal joints and, *524*, 524–525
  of forefoot, 516–527
    biomaterials for, 516–517
    digital implants and, *525*, 525–526, *526*
    first metatarsophalangeal joint and, 512
      hemi-implants and, 517–518, *518*
      surgical technique for, 520–522, *521*
      total hinged implants and, 518–522, *519, 520*
      two-component implants and, 522–524, *522–524*
Indirect coupling, 452
Indium-111–labeled white blood cells (¹¹¹In-WBCs), 355, *357*
Indole(s), hepatic function and, 402
  in chronic pain syndrome, 681
Indole carboxamides, 418
Indoleacetic acids, 409t, 412–413. See also specific drugs.
Indomethacin, 409t, 412, 413
  anesthesia and, 469
  drug interactions of, 406–407, 408
  in chronic pain syndrome, 681
  in gout, acute gouty arthritis and, 147, 148t

Indomethacin *(Continued)*
  in osteoarthritis, 431
Induction stage, of fracture healing, 20–21
Inductive coupling, for nonunions, 27
Infants, septic arthritis in, 207
Infarcts, in cutaneous vasculitis, 203
Infections. See also specific sites and infections.
  arthritis related to, rheumatoid arthritis versus, 113
  bacterial. See *Bacterial infections.*
  cutaneous manifestations of, 184–188, *185–188*
  fungal. See *Fungal infections.*
  in Reiter's syndrome, 132
  metatarsophalangeal joint arthrodesis and, 546
  of foot, radiography in, 308t
  of skin, in diabetes mellitus, 179
  postoperative, imaging in, 359
    in rheumatoid arthritis, 460
  preoperative and postoperative considerations in, 462
  preoperative evaluation in, 459t
  viral. See *Viral infections.*
Infective osteitis, 340
Infiltrative fasciitis, 631, *634*
Inflammation, in rheumatoid arthritis, 106t, 106–108, *107*
Inflammation stage, of fracture healing, 21–22
Inflammatory arthropathies, degenerative disease versus, 308
  metatarsophalangeal joint arthrodesis in, 546
  of ankle, arthroscopy in, 622–624
  of foot, imaging and, 308–314
Inflammatory bowel disease (IBD). See also *Seronegative spondyloarthropathies.*
  arthritis related to, rheumatoid arthritis versus, 114
  clinical features of, 133–134
  differential diagnosis of, 136
Inflammatory cells, septic arthritis and, 211
Inflammatory osteoarthritis, of foot, 315
Inflammatory phase, of bone healing, 20, 20–22
  of wound healing, 52–53
Inflammatory reaction, 34–49
  acute, 34, 48–49, *49*
  cellular factors in, 41, 46–48
    basophils as, 47
    endothelial cells as, 47–48
    eosinophils as, 47
    fibroblasts as, 48
    mast cells as, 47
    monocytes and macrophages as, 41, 46
    natural killer cells as, 48
    neutrophils as, 41
    platelets as, 47
    synovial cells as, 48
    T and B lymphocytes as, 46–47
  chronic, 34, 49
  humoral factor(s) in, 34–41
    activated oxygen as, 41, *46*
    arachidonic acid cascade as, 34–36
    clotting system as, 41, *45*
    complement system as, 40, *42–44*
    cytokines as, *36*, 36–39
    kinin system as, 40–41, *44*
    platelet-activating factor as, *39*, 39–40
    vasoactive amines as, 40
  implants and, 96
  in seronegative spondyloarthropathies, 134
Inflammatory stage, of cartilage repair, 30
Infracalcaneal bursa, glucocorticoid injection therapy in, 448
Infrared equipment, 453
Injection therapy. See *Glucocorticoids, local therapy using.*

Insoles, in rheumatoid arthritis, 126–127
Insulin, anesthesia and, 468
Interferon, inflammation and, 38
Interleukin-1 (IL-1), 36–37
  wound healing and, 53
Interleukin-2 (IL-2), 37
Interleukin-3 (IL-3), 37
Interleukin-4 (IL-4), 37
Interleukin-5 (IL-5), 37
Interleukin-6 (IL-6), 37–38
Interleukin-7 (IL-7), 38
Interleukin-10 (IL-10), 38
Intermediate dorsal cutaneous nerve (IDCN)
    entrapment, 698–701
  etiology and specific findings in, *699*, 699–
    700
  surgical technique for, *700*, 700–701
Intermediate zone, of synovial joints, 3
Interphalangeal joints. See *Distal
    interphalangeal (DIP) joints*; *Proximal
    interphalangeal (PIP) joints.*
Intertarsal joints, glucocorticoid injection
    therapy in, 447
Interzonal mesenchyme, 2
Intestinal lipodystrophy, arthritis related to,
    rheumatoid arthritis versus, 114
Intima, synovial, 6, *6*
Intoe, in children. See *Tibia, medial torsion of.*
Intra-articular folds, of synovial joints, 10
Intracapsular accessory ligaments, of synovial
    joints, 5
Intravenous drug abuse, septic arthritis and, 208
Intrinsic minus foot, in diabetes mellitus, 275–
    276, *276*
Inverse psoriasis, 194
Iothalamates, 365
Iselln's apophysis, *661*, *661*
Isoflurane, epinephrine for, 477
Isogeneic tissue, 23
Isografts, 23
Isokinetic contraction, 68
Isokinetic exercise, 455
Isometric contraction, 66, 68
Isometric exercise, 454–455
Isoniazid, in septic arthritis, 215t
Isotonic contraction, 68
Isotope studies. See *Radionuclide imaging.*

Jaccoud's arthritis, rheumatoid arthritis versus,
    113
Joint(s). See also specific joints.
  blood supply of, 13
  cartilaginous, 1–2
  embryology of, 2–3
  fibrous, 1
  fluid in. See *Synovial fluid.*
  in systemic lupus erythematosus, 154, 155
  infections of, rheumatoid arthritis and, 122
  neuropathic. See *Neuroarthropathy.*
  peripheral, in seronegative spondyloarthropa-
    thies, 135
  synovial. See *Synovial joints.*
Joint aspiration, 228
  glucocorticoid injection therapy and, 446–447
  in gout, 146
    acute gouty arthritis and, 148
  in septic arthritis, 212
Joint capsule, in rheumatoid arthritis, 104
  of ankle, 612
  of synovial joints, 2, *2*, 5
Joint mobility, limited, in diabetic foot. See
    Diabetic foot, limited joint mobility in.
Joint space narrowing, radiography and, 308
Jones fracture, *238*, 238–239

Jones tenosuspension, 608–609
  complications of, 608–609, *609*
  indications for, 608, *608*
  postoperative care and, 608
  technique for, 608
Joplin's neuroma, 709
Juvenile rheumatoid arthritis (JRA), 136
  arthrodesis in, *575*, 575–576
  preoperative and postoperative considerations
    in, 461

Kallikrein, inflammation and, 41
Kaposi's sarcoma, in HIV infection, 188, *188*,
    304–305
Kawasaki disease, 164
Kayger's triangle, in Achilles rupture, 246
Keller bunionectomy, 496, 529, 535, 564
  modified, in seronegative spondyloarthropa-
    thies, 138–140
  procedure for, *139*, 139–140
Kelokian push-up test, 488, *488*, 489, 494
Keratinocytes, wound healing and, 53, 54
Keratoconjunctivitis sicca. See *Sjögren's
    syndrome.*
Keratoderma(s), 188t, 188–189
Keratoderma blenorrhagicum (KB), in Reiter's
    syndrome, 132–133, 177, *177*
Keratoderma climactericum, 189
Ketoconazole, in septic arthritis, 215t
Ketoprofen, 410t, 415
  anesthesia and, 470
  drug interactions of, 406, 407
  in gout, acute gouty arthritis and, 148t
  in osteoarthritis, 431
Ketorolac, anesthesia and, 470
  in chronic pain syndrome, 681
Kidneys. See *Renal* entries.
Kinin system, inflammation and, 40–41, *44*
Kininogen, high-molecular-weight,
    inflammation and, 40–41
Kirschner wires, for arthrodesis, in rheumatoid
    arthritis, 562, *563*
  of hallux interphalangeal joint, 564
  of metatarsophalangeal joints, 552
Knee, anatomy of, *2*
  avascular necrosis in, 649
  biomechanics of, gait and, 71–72, *72*
    pathologic gait and, *77*, 77–78, *78*
  iliotibial band and, *84*, 84–85, *85*
  osteoarthritis of, 88–89
    pedal considerations in, 88–89, *89*
  patellofemoral pain and, *83*, 83–84
    orthotics in, 84
  rheumatoid arthritis of, 122–123
  septic arthritis of, treatment outcome in, 216t
Koebnerization, foot surgery and, in
    seronegative spondyloarthropathies, 137
Köhler's disease, 643, *643*

La Porta implant, *519*, 519–520
  surgical technique for, 521, *521*
Laboratory studies, 220–232. See also specific
    studies and types of studies.
  preoperative, 459t, 459–460
    anesthesia and, 465t
Labra, of synovial joints, 10
Lacelike pattern, in gout, 315
Lachman test, modified, 488
Lactate, wound healing and, 55
Lactate dehydrogenase, in synovial fluid, in
    septic arthritis, 213
Lamellae, in bone, 17

Lamellar bone, 17
Lamina splendens, of synovial joints, 5
Langerhans' cell disease, radiographic
    appearance of, 337–338, *338*
Laryngoscopy, flexible fiber-optic, anesthesia
    and, 479
Lawrence total implant, 520, *520*
  surgical technique for, 521
LE prep, 225–226, *226*
Leg(s), fasciotomy of, 730, *730*
  unequal length of. See *Leg-length inequality
    (LLI).*
Legg-Calvé-Perthes disease, avascular necrosis
    of bone in, *642*, 642–643
Leg-length inequality (LLI), 86–88
  back pain and, *87*, 87–88
  hip pain and, 88, *88*
  in poliomyelitis, 285–286
Leiomyomas, 634, 636
Leiomyosarcomas, 637
Lentigo maligna, 196
Lesch-Nyhan syndrome, 142
Less rigid implantation, implants and, 98–99
Lesser Metacarpal Cap, *524*, 524–525
Leukocytes. See also specific leukocytes.
  wound healing and, 52–53
Leukocytoclastic angiitis, 164
Leukocytoclastic vasculitis, 174, *174*, *175*
Leukotrienes, inflammation and, 35–36
Levamisole, 424
Lever arms, gait biomechanics and, 69, *69*
Lidocaine, 476, 476t, 477
Ligaments, 12
  injuries of, imaging in, 389–390, *390*
  of forefoot, 380
  of hindfoot, 377
  of midfoot, 378
  rupture of, following glucocorticoid injection
    therapy, 445
  weak, in calcaneovalgus deformity, 653, *653*
Light therapy, wound healing and, 61
Limited joint mobility (LJM), in diabetic foot.
    See *Diabetic foot, limited joint mobility in.*
Limp, gluteus medius, 77
Lining cell layer, of synovial membrane, 6, *7*, 8,
    8
Lipids, in articular cartilage, of synovial joints,
    5
Lipodermatosclerosis, 56
Lipodystrophy, intestinal, arthritis related to,
    rheumatoid arthritis versus, 114
Lipomas, 630–631, *631–633*
  magnetic resonance imaging and, 628, *628*
  radiographic appearance of, 333–334, *334*
Lipoprotein lipase deficiency, xanthomas and,
    183t
Liposarcomas, 636
  radiographic appearance of, 334, *335*
Lipoxin A (LxA), 36
Lipoxin B (LxB), 36
Lisfranc fractures, 386
Lithium, drug interactions of, 405t, 407
Livedo reticularis, 173–174, *174*
  in cutaneous vasculitis, 202–203, *203*
Livedo vasculitis, 173–174
Liver, nonsteroidal anti-inflammatory drugs and,
    402, 408
Liver enzyme–inducing agents, drug interactions
    of, 406
Liver function tests, nonsteroidal anti-
    inflammatory drugs and, 407
Load, velocity and, 68
Local anesthetics, 476t, 476–478
  for glucocorticoid injection therapy, 446
Löfgren's syndrome, 192

Loose bodies, post-traumatic ankle pain and, 722

Lornoxicam, 417

Lover's heel, in Reiter's syndrome, 133, *133*

Low back pain (LBP), leg-length inequality and, 87, 87–88

Lubricin, in synovial fluid, 9

Lupus erythematosus (LE), 170–171. See also *Discoid lupus erythematosus; Systemic lupus erythematosus (SLE).*

Lupus erythematosus (LE) cell test, 225–226, *226*

Lupus foot, 315, *317*

Lupus pernio, 191–192

Lyme disease, septic arthritis and, 210

Lymphangiomas, radiographic appearance of, 332

Lymphatic system, of synovial membranes, 13

Lymphatic vessels, of forefoot, 381
 of hindfoot, 378
 of midfoot, 380
 of synovial subintima, 8

Lymphedema. See also *Elephantiasis.*
 nonhealing wounds and, 58

Lymphocytes, inflammation and, 26–27
 chronic, 49
 wound healing and, 52

Lymphokines, wound healing and, 53

Lymphomas, radiographic appearance of, 332

Lyophilized bone. See *Alloimplants.*

Lysosomal enzymes, in rheumatoid arthritis, 104

Lytic regions, of musculoskeletal tumors, 323, *323*, 326, *326*
 radiographic appearance of, 330, *330*, *331*

McCune-Albright syndrome, 333

Macrophage colony-stimulating factor (M-CSF), 39

Macrophages. See *Monocytes/macrophages.*

Magnesium salicylate, 409t

Magnetic resonance imaging (MRI), 322, 382–383
 contraindications to, 382–383
 in avascular necrosis of bone, 641
 in entrapment syndromes, 690, *690*, *691*
 in fibrosarcomas, 636
 in leiomyosarcomas, 637
 in lipomas, staging of, 630, *632*, *633*
 in liposarcomas, 636
 in malignant schwannoma, 637
 in neoplasms and related disorders, 383–385, *384*
 in osteomyelitis, 355, 357–359, *358*
 in plantar fibromatosis, 634
 in post-traumatic ankle pain, 724
 in seronegative spondyloarthropathies, 135
 in soft tissue tumors, 627t, 627–630, *628*, *629*
 in tendinitis, 581
 in tendon dysfunction, 583

Major histocompatibility complex (MHC), 46

Malignancies. See also specific malignancies.
 nonhealing wounds and. See specific disorders.
 radiographic appearance of, in bone-forming tumors, 325–326
  in cartilage-forming tumors and, 327–328
 staging of, in soft tissue tumors, 626–627

Malignant fibrous histiocytoma, radiographic appearance of, 335, *336*

Mallet toes, following Hibbs tenosuspension procedure, 602

Malunion, of ankle fractures, arthroscopy and, 620

Manual muscle testing, 450

Marrow necrosis, 648

Marrow tumors, radiographic appearance of, 330–332

Martel's sign, in gout, 145

Massage, in chronic pain syndrome, 682

Mast cells, inflammation and, 47
 chronic, 49

Matrix, in tendons, age-related changes in, 11
 ossification of, of musculoskeletal tumors, 323

Matrix flow, 31

Maturation stage, of cartilage repair, 30

Mature bone, 17

Mechanical nociceptors, 673

Meclofenamate, in gout, acute gouty arthritis and, 148t

Meclofenamate sodium, 410t, 416

Medial dorsal cutaneous nerve (MDCN) entrapment, 698–701
 etiology and specific findings in, 698–699, *699*, 700
 surgical technique for, *700*, 700–701

Medullary callus, late, fracture healing and, 22

Mees' lines, 197, *197*, 198t

Mefenamic acid, 416

Megakaryocytes, inflammation and, 47

Melanoma(s), 196–197
 acrolentiginous, 196
 nodular, 196
 subungual, *196*, 196–197, *197*
 superficial spreading, 196, *196*

Membranous ossification, 16–17

Menisci, of synovial joints, 9–10
 blood supply of, 13
 functions of, 10

Meniscoid body, in ankle, 614, *616*
 post-traumatic ankle pain and, 720

Meniscoid folds, 10

Mepivacaine, 476, 476t, 477

Mesenchyme, 2

Mesotendon, 12

Metacarpophalangeal (MCP) joints, rheumatoid arthritis and, 115–116

Metal implants, 92t, 99
 alloys for, 96, 97t
 corrosion products released by, 95
 passivation of, 94–95

Metalloproteinases, wound healing and, 54–55

Metaphyseal arteries, 18

Metaphyses, 15
 of mature long bones, 18, *18*

Metatarsal bones, 482
 avascular necrosis of heads of, 649
 fifth, avulsion of, following ankle sprains, 246
 internal, stress fracture of, 256–257
 short, congenital, *671*, 671–672
  surgical treatment of, 671–672

Metatarsal length pattern formulas, 482

Metatarsalgia, 236

Metatarsophalangeal (MTP) joint(s), arthrodesis of. See *Arthrodesis, of metatarsophalangeal joints, first.*
 arthroplasty of. See *Arthroplasty, of forefoot.*
 central, arthrosis of. See *Arthrosis, of central metatarsophalangeal joint.*
 first, arthrodesis of, in rheumatoid arthritis, 564–565, *566*
  arthroplasty of, 511–512
  aspiration of, 228, *229*
  functional anatomy of, 483
  imaging of, 315
  limited dorsiflexion of. See *Hallux limitus.*
  measurement of motion of, 530, *530*

Metatarsophalangeal (MTP) joint(s) *(Continued)*
 normal motion of, anatomy and mechanics of, *529*, 529–530, *530*
  osteoarthritis of, imaging and, 314–315
  sprain of, *237*, 237–238
 fusion of. See *Arthrodesis, of metatarsophalangeal joints.*
 glucocorticoid injection therapy in, 447
 hallux limitus/rigidus and. See *Hallux limitus; Hallux limitus/rigidus; Hallux rigidus.*
 implant arthroplasty of. See under *Implant arthroplasty.*
 in gout, 145–146
 instability of, 488, *488*
 joints, arthrography of, 369–370, *370*
 Keller procedure and. See *Keller bunionectomy.*
 lesser, arthroplasty of, 512
 metatarsalgia and, 236
 release of, 492, *493*, 494, *494*
 rheumatoid arthritis and, 118, 119–120, *120*

Metatarsophalangeal (MTP) joint luxation test, 488

Metatarsus adductus, 657–663
 atavistic form of, 658
 radiologic evaluation of, 658–659, *659*
 serpentine, 658–659
 total, 658
 treatment of, 659–663
  conservative, 659–661
  surgical, 661–663

Metatarsus primus adductus, 658

Metatarsus primus elevatus, in paralytic disorders, 290, *291*
 treatment of, 290

Methicillin-resistant *Staphylococcus aureus* (MRSA), septic arthritis and, 208

Methotrexate (MTX), 411t, 421–422
 anesthesia and, 471
 drug interactions of, 405t, 407, 408
 in psoriasis, 195
 in rheumatoid arthritis, 429–430
 in seronegative spondyloarthropathies, 136

Methoxyflurane, contraindication to, in gout, 476

Methylprednisolone, anesthesia and, 472t, 473
 for injection therapy, 443t
  dosage of, 444t

Metoclopramide, anesthesia and, 468–469

Metronidazole, in septic arthritis, 215t

Microangiopathy, in diabetes mellitus, 179, *179*

Midazolam, local anesthesia and, 477

Midfoot, anatomic structures of, 378–380
 rheumatoid arthritis of, imaging and, 310, *311*, *312*
 sprain of, 239–240, *240*

Midtarsal joint, biomechanics of, gait and, 74–76, *75*, *76*
 in joint diseases, 82

Mineralocorticoids, anesthesia and, 474

Minocycline, in rheumatoid arthritis, 430
 in septic arthritis, 215t

Mixed connective tissue disease. See *Connective tissue diseases (CTDs), mixed.*

Mobilization, 455

Modified Lachman test, 488

Modulus of elasticity, 91

Moist heat packs, 453

Molecular mimicry hypothesis, of rheumatoid arthritis, 427–428

Molluscum contagiosum, in HIV infection, 305

Monocytes/macrophages, inflammation and, 41, 46
 chronic, 49
 wound healing and, 52, 53, 54

Monokines, wound healing and, 53

Morganella infections, septic arthritis and, 215t
Morphea, 170
Morton's neuromas, 235, *235*, 709–711, *711*
    imaging in, 385
    surgical technique for, 711–712, *713*, *714*,
        715
Moth-eaten pattern, of musculoskeletal tumors,
    323, *323*
Mucin, in synovial fluid, 9
Mucin clot test, in seronegative
    spondyloarthropathies, 135
Mucocutaneous lymph node syndrome, 164
Mueller-Weiss syndrome, 649
Mulder's click sign, 235
Mulder's test, 711
Multiple myelomas, radiographic appearance of,
    330–331, *332*
Murphy procedure. See *Achilles tendon,*
    advancement of, anterior.
Muscle(s), action of, on ankle, 73, *73*
    biomechanics of, 66, *67*, 68, *68*
    contraction of, 66, 68
    débridement of, fasciotomy and, 729
    imbalance of, in calcaneovalgus deformity,
        652–653
    in systemic lupus erythematosus, 154
    injuries of, imaging in, 390–391
    of forefoot, 380, *380*, *381*
    of hindfoot, 377, *377*, *378*
    of midfoot, 378–379, *379*
    restoration of balance of, in poliomyelitis,
        284–285, 285t
    strain of, athletic injuries and, 253–255
    testing of, in rheumatoid arthritis, 127
    treatment of, in rheumatoid arthritis, 127
Muscle fibers, 66
Muscle pain, in rheumatoid arthritis, 107
Muscle strength, assessment of, 450
Muscle tension, 66, 68, *68*
Musculoskeletal system, disorders of. See also
        specific disorders.
    in HIV infection, 304
    in scleroderma, 158–159
    in systemic lupus erythematosus, 154, 155t
"Mushrooming," in gout, 146
Myalgia, in polyarteritis nodosa, 163
Mycobacterium avium-intracellulare, 209
Mycobacterium infections, 209
    nontubercular, septic arthritis and, 215t
Mycobacterium kansii, 209
Mycobacterium leprae, 209
Mycobacterium marianum, 209
Mycobacterium tuberculosis, 209, 215t
Myelomas, multiple (plasma cell), radiographic
    appearance of, 330–331, *332*
Myelomeningoceles, avascular necrosis of bone
    and, 640
Myositis, exercises for, 454t
Myxedema, cutaneous manifestations of, 180,
    180

N zone, 699
Nabumetone, 410t, 417–418
Nafcillin, in septic arthritis, 215t
Nail(s), 197–199
    Beau's lines and, *198*, 198–199, *199*, 199t
    disorders of. See specific disorders.
    in psoriasis, 194–195, *195*
    periungual erythema and, in systemic lupus
        erythematosus, 154, *156*
    transverse white bands of, 197, *197*, 198t
Nail folds, in dermatomyositis/polymyositis,
    172, *173*
Nail pits, in psoriasis, 194–195

Naphthylalkanones, 410t, 417–418. See also
        specific drugs.
Naproxen, 410t, 414
    anesthesia and, 469–470
    drug interactions of, 406, 407
    in chronic pain syndrome, 680–681
    in gout, acute gouty arthritis and, 148t
Narcotics. See *Opiates.*
Natural killer (NK) cells, inflammation and, 48
Navicular bone, avascular necrosis of, 643, *643*,
    649
Necrobiosis lipoidica diabeticorum (NLD), 178,
    178
Necrosis, aseptic, of bone, following
        glucocorticoid injection therapy, 445
    avascular. See *Avascular necrosis.*
Necrotic nonunions, 27
Necrotic ulceration, in rheumatoid arthritis, 173,
    173
Needle aspiration, in septic arthritis, 214, 216
Needle biopsy, percutaneous, of synovium, 232,
    232
Neisseria infections. See also *Gonorrhea.*
    arthritis related to, rheumatoid arthritis ver-
        sus, 113
Neoangiogenesis, wound healing and, 54
Neoplasia. See *Tumor(s); specific tumors.*
Nerve blocks. See *Neural blocks.*
Nerve entrapment syndromes, 685–715. See
        also specific nerves.
    clinical presentation and diagnosis of, 685–
        690
        objective findings and, 685–690
        subjective findings and, 685, *686–687*
    recurrent, postoperative, 695
    treatment of, 690–696
        surgical, 690–696
Nerve sheath, fibrosarcoma of. See
        Schwannomas, malignant.
Nerve supply, of forefoot, 381
    of hindfoot, 377
    of joints, 13–14
    of midfoot, 379
    of synovial subintima, 8
Neural blocks, diagnostic, in entrapment
        syndromes, 689
    in chronic pain syndrome, 682–683
    sciatic-femoral, agents for, 477
Neurapraxia, of superficial peroneal nerve, *247*,
    247–248
Neurectomy, 694t, 694–695
    complications of, 695–696
Neurilemomas, 636
    radiographic appearance of, 334–335, *336*
    tarsal tunnel syndrome and, 706
Neurinomas, radiographic appearance of, 334–
    335, *336*
Neuritis, forefoot, plantar, 235–236
Neuroarthropathy, following glucocorticoid
        injection therapy, 445
    hypertrophic, 198, *198*
    of diabetic foot. See *Diabetic foot, neuroar-*
        thropathy of.
    of foot, radiography in, 308t
    preoperative and postoperative considerations
        in, 463
    preoperative evaluation and, 459t
Neurofibromas, 636
    radiographic appearance of, 335
Neurofibrosarcomas. See *Schwannomas,*
        malignant.
Neurologic disorders. See also specific disorders
        and nerves.
    in HIV infection, 303–304
Neurolysis, 690–694
    external, 690–692, *692*, *693*

Neurolysis *(Continued)*
    internal, 692–694, *694*
        complications of, 695–696
Neuromas, athletic injuries and, 235, *235*
    glucocorticoid injection therapy and, 448
    Joplin's, 709
    Morton's. See *Morton's neuromas.*
    recurrent stump neuroma pain and, 712, 715
Neuromatous zone, 699
Neurometer CPT, in entrapment syndromes, 688
Neuropathic joint. See *Neuroarthropathy.*
Neuropathy, arthroscopy and, 621–622
    diabetic, 56
    entrapment. See *Nerve entrapment syn-*
        dromes; specific entrapment syndromes.
    in rheumatoid arthritis, 107
    peripheral. See *Peripheral neuropathy.*
    sensorimotor, in rheumatoid arthritis, 107
    sensory, in HIV infection, 303–304
Neurosarcomas. See *Schwannomas, malignant.*
Neurotropism, 695
Neurovascular disorders, rheumatoid arthritis
        and, 122
Neutrophils, inflammation and, 41
    acute, 48–49, *49*
    wound healing and, 52–53
Nifedipine, in Raynaud's phenomenon, 206
Nizatidine, anesthesia and, 468
Nociceptors, 673–674
Nodular fasciitis, 631, *634*
Nodular melanoma, 196
Nodules, in cutaneous vasculitis, 203
    rheumatoid, in rheumatoid arthritis, 106, 173,
        173
    subcutaneous, in erythema nodosum, 190,
        191
Nonossifying fibromas, radiographic appearance
    of, 332–333
Nonsteroidal anti-inflammatory drugs
        (NSAIDs), 397–418, 425. See also specific
        drugs.
    allergic reactions to, 402–403
    anesthesia and, 469–470
    articular cartilage and, 403
    bronchopulmonary system and, 402
    cardiovascular system and, 402
    central nervous system and, 403
    clinical pharmacology of, 398–399
    drug interactions of, 404t, 404–407, 405t, 408
    gastrointestinal function and, 400–401
    in children, 403
    in chronic pain syndrome, 680–681
    in elderly patients, 403–404
    in gout, acute gouty arthritis and, 147, 148t
        intercritical, 148
    in metatarsalgia, 236
    in metatarsophalangeal joint sprain, 238
    in osteoarthritis, 431
    in post-traumatic ankle pain, 725
    in rheumatoid arthritis, 124–125, 429
        surgery and, 460–461
    in seronegative spondyloarthropathies, 136
    laboratory and clinical monitoring and, 407–
        408
    liver and, 402
    platelet function and hematologic system and,
        401–402
    renal function and, 399–400
    side effects of, 124–125
    skin and, 402
    specific agents, 408, 409t–412t, 412–418
    volume of distribution of, 399
Nonunions, 26–27
    atrophic, 27
    biologic failures and, 26–27
        rationale for treatment of, 28

Nonunions *(Continued)*
  defect type of, 27
  dystrophic, 27
  necrotic, 27
  of ankle fractures, arthroscopy and, 620
  rationale for treatment of, 27–28
  technical failures and, 26
    rationale for treatment of, 27–28
Nortriptyline, in chronic pain syndrome, 682
Nutrient arteries, of long bones, 18

Observation, in entrapment syndromes, 868
Occlusive dressings, wound healing and, 60
Occupational therapy, in chronic pain syndrome, 682
Oil spots, in psoriasis, 195
Oligoarthritis, in HIV infection, 304
Olive oil supplementation, 424
Omeprazole, anesthesia and, 468
  gastrointestinal function and, 401
Onychodystrophy, in psoriasis, 195
Onychomycosis, white, proximal, in HIV infection, 305
Open wedge osteotomy, of first cuneiform, in metatarsus adductus, 663
Opiates, endogenous, 676–677
  in chronic pain syndrome, 681
  spinal, in chronic pain syndrome, 683–684
Oral contraceptives, drug interactions of, 404t
Oral lesions, in hand-foot-mouth disease, 185, *185*
  in Reiter's syndrome, 133
Orthotics. See also *specific orthotics.*
  in calcaneovalgus deformity, 655
  in cavus deformity, 669
  in equinus deformity, 666
  in metatarsus adductus, 661, *661, 662*
  in patellofemoral pain, 84
  in post-traumatic ankle pain, 725
  in rheumatoid arthritis, 126–127
Os navicularis syndrome, 239, *239*
Osgood-Schlatter disease, avascular necrosis of bone in, 643
Osseous equinus, 80
Ossification, endochondral, 15–16, *16*
  bone healing and, 20
  membranous, 16–17
  of matrix, of musculoskeletal tumors, 323
Ossifying fibromas, radiographic appearance of, 327, *328*
Osteitis, infective, 340
Osteoarthritis (OA), exercises for, 454t
  functional scale for, 451t
  imaging in, 385
  in diabetic foot, 279
  inflammatory (erosive), of foot, 315
  inflammatory disease versus, 308
  injection therapy in, 442–443
  of ankle, arthroscopy in, 618–619
  of foot, imaging and, *314*, 314–315
    radiography in, 308t
  of knee, pedal considerations in, 88–89, *89*
  post-traumatic ankle pain and, 721
  preoperative and postoperative considerations in, 462
  preoperative evaluation in, 459t
  rehabilitation in. See *Rehabilitation.*
  rheumatoid arthritis versus, 113
  septic arthritis and, 208
  synovial analysis in, 229t
  tendinitis and, 579
  treatment of, pharmacologic, 430–431
Osteoarthropathy. See *Neuroarthropathy.*

Osteoblastomas, radiographic appearance of, 326
Osteoblasts, 17
  bone repair and, 27
Osteochondral lesions, fractures and, imaging in, 390, *391*
  in ankle, 614
Osteochondritis dissecans, avascular necrosis of bone in, 644–646, *645, 646*
  staging of, 646, *646*
  synovial analysis in, 229t
Osteochondromas, radiographic appearance of, 326–327, *327*
Osteochondroses. See also *specific disorders.*
  avascular necrosis of bone in, 641–644, 642t
Osteoclasts, 17
Osteoconduction, bone grafts and, 23–24
  implant fixation using, 97, 98
Osteocytes, 17
Osteogenesis, bone grafts and, 23
Osteoid, 17
Osteoid osteomas, radiographic appearance of, 326, *326*
Osteoinduction, bone grafts and, 23
Osteointegration, implant fixation using, 97–98, *98*
Osteolysis, diabetic. See *Diabetic foot, osteolysis of.*
Osteomyelitis, classification of, 342–343
  hematogenous spread and, 342, *342, 343*
    spread from contiguous focus of infection and, 342–343, *344*
  hematogenous, 340
  imaging in, 340–359, 392–394 , *392*
    algorithm for, 362, *362*
    cellulitis and, 393, *393*
    computed tomography and, 345–346
    healing and, 393
    magnetic resonance imaging and, 355, 357–359, *358*
    plain film screen radiography and, 343, 345, *345–350*
    practical applications of, 359–362
    radionuclide imaging and, 351, *352–354,* 355, *356, 357*
    septic arthritis and, 393–394
  of foot, imaging and, 315, 317, 319, 320, *320*
  pathophysiology of, 340, *341*
  sclerosing, Garré's, 342
  septic arthritis and, 218
  tuberculous, imaging in, 359, *361*
Osteonecrosis. See also *Avascular necrosis, of bone.*
  dysbaric, 640
Osteopathy, diabetic. See *Diabetic foot, osteolysis of.*
Osteophytosis, in degenerative disease, 308
Osteoporosis, following glucocorticoid injection therapy, 445
  in rheumatoid arthritis, 460
  of hallux interphalangeal joint, arthrodesis and, 564
Osteoprogenitor cells, 18
Osteosarcomas, radiographic appearance of, *325,* 325–326, *326*
Osteotomy, Austin, in hallux limitus/rigidus, 537, *538*
  Youngswick modification of, in hallux limitus/rigidus, 538
  calcaneal, of Evans. See *Evan's calcaneal osteotomy.*
  closing base wedge, in metatarsus adductus, 661
  crescentic, in metatarsus adductus, *662,* 662–663
  for calcaneal deformity, 289, *289*

Osteotomy *(Continued)*
  in cavus deformity, 670, *670*
  open wedge, of first cuneiform, in metatarsus adductus, 663
  plantar-flexory base, in hallux limitus/rigidus, 540–541, *542*
  Watermann-type, in hallux limitus/rigidus, 538–539, *540*
''Overhanging edge'' appearance, in gout, 315
Oxicams, 410t, 416–417. See also *specific drugs.*
  in chronic pain syndrome, 681
Oxygen, activated, inflammation and, 41, 46
  muscle activity and, 68
Oxygen therapy, wound healing and, 60–61
Oxyphenbutazone, platelet function and hematologic system and, 402

Pachydermoperiostosis, 198–199
Paget osteosarcomas, radiographic appearance of, 325, *325*
Paget's disease, imaging in, 385
Pain. See also *Chronic pain syndrome.*
  as indication for arthrodesis, in rheumatoid arthritis, 559
  assessment of, 450
  control of, endogenous, 676–677
    gate theory of, 676
    transcutaneous electrical nerve stimulation and, 453
  following ankle sprains, 246
  inflammation and, 34
  physiology of, 673–677
    ascending pathways and, 675–676
    endogenous pain control and, 676–677
    peripheral afferents and, 674–675
    receptors and, 673–674
    spinal cord interactions and, 675
  recurrent stump neuroma pain and, 712, 715
  referred, 675
Pallor, Raynaud's phenomenon and, 203–204
Palmoplantar pits, in basal cell nevus syndrome, 195, *195*
  in general population, 196
Palmoplantar psoriasis, 194, *194*
Palmoplantar xanthomas, 183–184, *184*
Palpable purpura, in cutaneous vasculitis, 174, *174, 175,* 202, *202*
Palpation, in entrapment syndromes, 686–687, *687*
Panmetatarsal head resection, in seronegative spondyloarthropathies, 137–138
  procedure considerations for, 138, *138, 139*
Panmetatarsectomy, forefoot arthroplasty and, 506–508, *509,* 510–511
Pannus, septic arthritis and, 211
Pantalar arthrodesis, in rheumatoid arthritis, 575
Papillon-Lefèvre syndrome, 188–189
Papules, hemorrhagic, in cutaneous vasculitis, 202, *202*
Paraffin wax, heat therapy using, 453
Paralytic disorders. See also *Cerebral palsy (CP); Poliomyelitis.*
  calcaneal deformities in, 287–290, *289*
    arthrodesis for, 289
    bone blocking procedures for, 289–290, *290*
    osteotomies for, 289, *289*
    tendon transfers for, 288–289
  equinus deformity in, 286, *287*
  midtarsus primus elevatus (dorsal bunion) in, 290, *291*
    treatment of, 290

Paralytic disorders *(Continued)*
  valgus deformities in, tendon transfer for, 286–287
  varus deformities in, tendon transfer for, 286, *288*
Parasitic infections, septic arthritis and, 210
Paratenonitis, 578
Parkinson's disease, rheumatoid arthritis versus, 115
Paronychia, candidal, in diabetes mellitus, 179, *179*
Parotid gland, in Sjögren's syndrome, 161
Passivation, of metal implants, 94–95
Patellofemoral pain, *83*, 83–84
Patellofemoral pain syndrome (PPS), athletic injuries and, 249–252, 250t, *251*
Pathologic gait, antalgic, 76, *76*
  apropulsive, 78
  biomechanics of, *76*, 76–80
    ankle joint and, 78–80, *79*, *80*
    hip joint and, 76–77, *77*
    knee joint and, *77*, 77–78, *78*
  drop foot and, 79, *79*
  extensor subluxation and, 80
  in equino-adducto-varus foot, 79–80, *80*
  in equinus, 78, *79*, 81
  pendulumlike (waddling), 80
  short-lever push-off, 80–81, *81*
  short-limb, 76
  steppage, 77, *77*
  Trendelenburg, 76–77, *77*
Pediatric patients. See *Children*; specific pediatric disorders.
Peg-and-hole interlock, for metatarsophalangeal joint arthrodesis, 550–551, *551*, 552, *552*, 557
Pendulum-like gait, 80
Penicillamine, 410t
  in rheumatoid arthritis, 430
    surgery and, 461
D-Penicillamine, 410t, 420–421
  anesthesia and, 471
Penicillin, in septic arthritis, 215t
  penicillin V, in septic arthritis, 215t
Peptococcus anaerobius infections, 209
Percutaneous needle biopsy, of synovium, 232, *232*
Periarteritis nodosa. See *Polyarteritis nodosa (PAN)*.
Pericarditis, in rheumatoid arthritis, 107–108
Perichondrium grafting, for cartilage repair, 31
Periosteal chondroma, radiographic appearance of, *329*, *329*
Periosteal reaction, musculoskeletal tumors and, 323–324, *324*
Periosteum, 18, *18*
Peripheral afferents, 674–675
Peripheral neuropathy, anesthesia and, 466
  in HIV infection, 303–304
  in polyarteritis nodosa, 163
  in Sjögren's syndrome, 162
  in systemic lupus erythematosus, 153–154
Peritendinitis crepitans, 579
Periungual erythema, in systemic lupus erythematosus, 154, *156*
Peroneal(s), subluxating, following ankle sprains, 245
Peroneal brevis tendon, 371, *371*
  transfer of, 609–610
Peroneal longus tendon, 371, *371*
  tenosynovitis of, 121
  transfer of, 609
Peroneal muscle, weakness of, in Charcot-Marie-Tooth disease, 78–79
Peroneal nerve, superficial, neurapraxia and, 247–248, *247*

Peroneal nerve entrapment, 697–698
  etiology of, 697–698
  surgical treatment of, 698, *698*
Peroneal spastic flatfoot. 81
  complications of, 610
  indications for, 609
  postoperative care and, 610
  technique for, *609*, 609–610, *610*
Pes planus deformity, in rheumatoid arthritis, 107
  imaging and, 310
Pes valgus. See *Valgus deformity*.
Phagocytes, inflammation and, 41, 46
Phalanges, avascular necrosis in, 649
  erosions of, in scleroderma, 158, *159*
Phenobarbital, drug interactions of, 406
Phenylacetic acid, 410t, 416. See also specific drugs.
  in chronic pain syndrome, 681
Phenylbutazone, 409t
  drug interactions of, 407
  hepatic function and, 402
  in gout, 147, 148t
  platelet function and hematologic system and, 402
Phenylephrine, local anesthesia and, 478
Phenytoin, drug interactions of, 406, 407
Photosensitivity, in systemic lupus erythematosus, 155
Physical modalities, in chronic pain syndrome, 682
Physical therapy, in post-traumatic ankle pain, 725
Physis. See *Growth plate*.
"Piano key" sign, 116, *117*
Piezoelectricity, of bone, 19
"Pig skin" appearance, in myxedema, 180, *180*
Pigmented villonodular synovitis (PVNS), 632–633, *635*
  radiographic appearance of, *338*, 338–339
Pirenzepine, gastrointestinal function and, 401
Piroxicam, 410t, 416–417
  in chronic pain syndrome, 681
  in gout, 148t
Pirprofen, drug interactions of, 406
Plain radiography, 322
  in neoplasms and related disorders, 383
  in osteomyelitis, 343, 345, *345–350*
  in tendon dysfunction, 583
Plantar digital nerve entrapment, 709–715
  etiology and specific findings in, 709–711, *711*
  surgical technique for, 711–712, *713*, *714*, 715
Plantar fascia, athletic injuries and, 254–255
  insertion of, glucocorticoid injection therapy in, 448
  sectioning of, in seronegative spondyloarthropathies, 137, *137*
Plantar fasciitis, *240*, 240–241
  rheumatoid arthritis and, 120
Plantar fibromatosis, 631–632, *633*, *634*
  in diabetic foot, 274
Plantar forefoot neuritis, 235–236
Plantar interdigital ligaments, 483, *484*
Plantar nerve entrapment, 706–709
  etiology of, 705
  surgical treatment of, 706, *707–710*, 708–709
Plantar xanthomas, 183–184, *184*
Plantar-flexion procedures, in hallux limitus/rigidus, 537–538, *539*
  plantar-flexory base osteotomy and, in hallux limitus/rigidus, 540–541, *542*
Plasma cell myeloma, radiographic appearance of, 330–331, *332*

Plasmacytomas, radiographic appearance of, 330–331, *332*
Plasminogen-activating factor, inflammation and, 41
Plate fixation, metatarsophalangeal joint arthrodesis and, 553, *556*
Platelet(s), inflammation and, 47
  nonsteroidal anti-inflammatory drugs and, 401–402
  salicylates and, 469
Platelet-activating factor (PAF), inflammation and, *39*, 39–40
Platelet-derived growth factor (PDGF), wound healing and, 53
Platelet-derived wound-healing factors (PDWHFs), 61
Pleuritis, in rheumatoid arthritis, 107–108
Podagra. See *Gout*.
Poliomyelitis, 284–286
  etiology of, 284
  fixed deformities in, 285
  leg-length discrepancies in, 285–286
  restoration of muscle balance in, 284–285, 285t
Polyarteritis, overlapping pathologic and clinical manifestations of, 166t
  overlapping serologic manifestations of, 167t
Polyarteritis nodosa (PAN), 163, *163*
  cutaneous manifestations of, 176, *176*
Polydioxanone (ORTHOSORB), implant fixation and, 99
Polyethylene implants, ultra-high molecular weight, 97
Polyglactin 910, implant fixation and, 99
Polyglycolic acid, implant fixation and, 99, 100
Poly-L-lactic acid, implant fixation and, 99, 100
Polymer implants, 92t, 96–97
  biodegradable, self-reinforced, 99
Polymerase chain reaction (PCR) test, for HIV infection, 301
Polymethylmethacrylate implants, 97
Polymyalgia rheumatica, rheumatoid arthritis versus, 114
Polymyositis, 159–161, 160t. See also *Dermatomyositis/polymyositis (DM/PM)*.
  clinical features of, *160*, 160–161
  exercises for, 454t
  overlapping pathologic and clinical manifestations of, 166t
  overlapping serologic manifestations of, 167t
  pathology of, 159–160, 160t
  treatment of, 161
Polyol metabolic pathway, in limited joint mobility, of diabetic foot, 272
Potassium salicylate, 409t
Prednisolone, anesthesia and, 472t
  for injection therapy, 443t
    dosage of, 444t
Prednisone, 439–440, 441
  anesthesia and, 472t
  in gout, 432
  in rheumatoid arthritis, 428–429
Prekallikrein activator, 40
Preoperative evaluation, 457–460, 458t
  history in, 457, 458t
  laboratory studies in, 459t, 459–460
  physical examination in, 457–459, 459t
Pressure measurement, in compartment syndromes, acute, 727–729, *728*, *729*
  chronic, 733
Prilocaine, 476, 476t
Primary bone healing, 16–17, 22–23
Probenecid, 411t, 425
  anesthesia and, 474
  drug interactions of, 404t, 406, 408
  in gout, chronic gouty arthritis and, 148–149

Procaine, 476, 476t
Prodrugs, gastrointestinal function and, 400
Progressive systemic sclerosis. See
　Scleroderma.
Proliferative arthritis, of ankle, arthroscopy in,
　622–624
Proliferative fasciitis, 631, *634*
Proliferative phase, of bone healing, 20, *20*
　of wound healing, 53–55
Proliferative stage, of cartilage repair, 30
Promethazine, in chronic pain syndrome, 682
Pronation, of subtalar joint, 74
Properdin pathway, 40
Properdin system, inflammation and, 40
Propionic acid, 410t, 414–416. See also specific
　drugs.
　anesthesia and, 469–470
　hepatic function and, 402
　in chronic pain syndrome, 680–681
Prostaglandins, 398
　gastrointestinal function and, 401
　nonsteroidal anti-inflammatory drugs and, 398
Prostheses. See *Implant(s)*.
Protein, in synovial fluid, 231
Proteoglycans, in articular cartilage, 65–66
　wound healing and, 55
Proteus mirabilis infections, septic arthritis and,
　215t
Proteus vulgaris infections, septic arthritis and,
　215t
Prothrombin, inflammation and, 41
Proximal interphalangeal (PIP) joints,
　rheumatoid arthritis and, 115, *115*
Proximal white onychomycosis, in HIV
　infection, 305
Pseudogout. See also *Calcium pyrophosphate
　dihydrate deposition disease (CPPD)*.
　acute, 150
　in diabetic foot, 280
　of ankle, arthroscopy in, 624
　preoperative and postoperative considerations
　　in, 463
　synovial analysis in, 229t
Pseudomonas infections, cutaneous, in HIV
　infection, 188
　Pseudomonas aeruginosa, imaging in, 359
　　septic arthritis and, 215t
　Pseudomonas cepacia, septic arthritis and,
　　215t
　septic arthritis and, 208
Pseudosarcomatous fibromatosis (fasciitis), 631,
　634
Psoriasis, 193–195, *194*, *195*
　guttate, 194
　in HIV infection, 305
　inverse, 194
　palmoplantar, 194, *194*
　pustular, generalized (von Zumbusch's pso-
　　riasis), 194, *194*
　localized, 194
Psoriasis vulgaris, 194, *194*
Psoriatic arthritis (PA). See also *Seronegative
　spondyloarthropathies*.
　clinical features of, 133
　differential diagnosis of, 136
　HLA measurement in, 226t
　in HIV infection, 304
　of foot, imaging and, 313–314, *314*
　radiography in, 308t
Psychotropic drugs, in chronic pain syndrome,
　682
Pulmonary disease, anesthesia and, 464
　in rheumatoid arthritis, 460
　interstitial fibrosis and, 108
Pulsed electromagnetic field (PEMF), for
　nonunions, 27

Pulseless disease. See *Takayasu's arteritis*.
Puncture wounds, imaging in, 359
Purified protein derivative (PPD) test, 209
Purpura, Henoch-Schönlein, 174, *175*
　palpable, in cutaneous vasculitis, 174, *174*,
　　175, 202, *202*
Pustular psoriasis, generalized (von Zumbusch's
　psoriasis), 194, *194*
　localized, 194
Pyoderma, in diabetes mellitus, 179
Pyoderma gangrenosum (PG), *192*, 192–193
Pyrazoles, 409t, 412. See also specific drugs.
　drug interactions of, 406
　hepatic function and, 402
　platelet function and hematologic system and,
　　402
Pyrrolacetic acid, 409t, 413–414. See also
　specific drugs.

Q angle, 83, *83f*
Quinolone, in septic arthritis, 215t

Radial zone, of synovial joints, 3
Radioimmunoassay (RIA), for rheumatoid
　factor, 222, *222*
Radionuclide imaging, 322
　in avascular necrosis of bone, 641
　in osteomyelitis, 351, *352–354*, 353, *356*, *357*
　in post-traumatic ankle pain, 724
Range of motion, assessment of, 450
Range-of-motion exercise, 455
Ranitidine, drug interactions of, 406
Rash, butterfly, in systemic lupus
　erythematosus, 153, *154*, 154, 171, *171*
　heliotrope, in dermatomyositis/polymyositis,
　　171–172, *172*
　in dermatomyositis, 160
"Rat bite" erosions, in gout, 145
Raynaud's disease, 169
Raynaud's phenomenon, 169, 170t, *203*, 203–
　204
　cutaneous arteriospasm and, 203–204
　in scleroderma, 157
　sympathetic versus local control and, 204
　treatment of, 205–206
Raynaud's syndrome, cutaneous manifestations
　of, 169–170, *170*, 170t
Reactive oxygen species, inflammation and, 41
Reamer systems, for metatarsophalangeal joint
　arthrodesis, 550–552, *551*, *552*
Redness, inflammation and, 34
Referred pain, 675
Reflexes, in entrapment syndromes, 688–689
Regional anesthesia, 479
Rehabilitation, 449–455
　assistive devices in, 455
　following hallux limitus/rigidus repair, 543,
　　543
　functional assessment and, 450, 451t
　in chronic pain syndrome, 682
　pain assessment and, 450
　physical examination and, 449–450
　physical modalities in, 450–453
　range-of-motion assessment and, 450
　strength assessment and, 450
　therapeutic exercise in, 453–455, 454t
Reiter's cells, in seronegative
　spondyloarthropathies, 135
Reiter's disease. See *Reiter's syndrome (RS)*.
Reiter's syndrome (RS). See also *Seronegative
　spondyloarthropathies*.

Reiter's syndrome (RS) *(Continued)*
　arthritis related to, rheumatoid arthritis ver-
　　sus, 113
　clinical features of, 132–133, *133*
　cutaneous manifestations of, 176–177, *177*,
　　189
　differential diagnosis of, 136
　of foot, imaging and, 313–314, *314*
　radiography in, 308t
Relaxation time, 66
Remissions, in rheumatoid arthritis, 109
Remodeling phase, of bone healing, 20
　of wound healing, 56
Remodeling stage, of cartilage repair, 30
　of fracture healing, 22
Renal disease, anesthesia and, 466
Renal function tests, nonsteroidal anti-
　inflammatory drugs and, 407
Renal system, in rheumatoid arthritis, 108
　in systemic lupus erythematosus, 155t
　nonsteroidal anti-inflammatory drugs and,
　　399–400
Reparative granuloma, radiographic appearance
　of, 330, *330*
Reparative phase of bone healing, 20, *20*
Resistance arm, 69
Resting zone, of growth plate, 16, *16*
Retinacula, 12
Retrocalcaneal bursitis, in rheumatoid arthritis,
　imaging and, 310, *312*
　in seronegative spondyloarthropathies, imag-
　　ing and, 314
Reverse coarctation. See *Takayasu's arteritis*.
Revision surgery, metatarsophalangeal joint
　arthrodesis for, 546
Rheumatic fever, acute, synovial analysis in,
　229t
　arthritis related to, rheumatoid arthritis ver-
　　sus, 113
Rheumatic vasculitis, 174, *174*, *175*
Rheumatoid arthritis (RA), 34, 103–129. See
　also *Sjögren's syndrome*.
　antinuclear antibodies in, 224t, 224–225
　arthrodesis in. See *Arthrodesis, in rheumatoid
　　arthritis*.
　causes of, 427–428
　clinical findings with, 115–123
　　in cervical spine, 116–117
　　in lower extremities, 117–123
　　in upper extremities, 115–116
　cutaneous manifestations of, 172–173, *173*
　diagnosis of, 111t, 111–112, 112t
　differential diagnosis of, 112t, 112–115
　　arthritis associated with infections and, 113
　　CPPD and, 113–114
　　degenerative or traumatic arthritis and, 113
　　diffuse connective tissue disease and, 114
　　enteric disease–related arthritis and, 114
　　giant cell arteritis and, 114
　　gout and, 113–114
　　Parkinson's disease and, 115
　　polymyalgia rheumatica and, 114
　　spondyloarthropathies and, 114
　erythrocyte sedimentation rate in, 221
　etiology and incidence of, 103–104
　exercises for, 454t
　functional scale for, 451t
　HLA measurement in, 227, 227t
　immunoglobulins in, 109–110, *110*
　juvenile. See *Juvenile rheumatoid arthritis
　　(JRA)*.
　laboratory studies in, 110–111, 228t
　management of, 123–129
　　conservative, 125–128
　　general considerations in, 123–124, 124t
　　pharmacologic, 124–125

Rheumatoid arthritis (RA) *(Continued)*
  surgical, 128–129
  of ankle, arthroscopy in, 622–624
  of foot, imaging and, 309–310, *309–313*
    radiography in, 308t
  overlapping pathologic and clinical manifestations of, 166t
  overlapping serologic manifestations of, 167t
  pathogenesis of, 9, 104–105
  pathology of, 105–108
    inflammation and vasculitis and, 106t, 106–108, *107*
    rheumatoid nodules and, 106
    spinal involvement and, 105t, 105–106
  patterns of onset and disease course in, 108–109
  preoperative and postoperative considerations in, 460–461
  radiographic findings in, 109
  rheumatoid factor in, 110
  septic arthritis and, 208
  stages of, drug therapy and, 428–430, *429*
  synovial analysis in, 229t
  tendinitis and, 579
  treatment of, pharmacologic, 427–430, 460–461
    step-down bridge approach to, 428–429, *429*
Rheumatoid factor (RF), in rheumatoid arthritis, 110, 173, 428
  in seronegative spondyloarthropathies, 135
  in Sjögren's syndrome, 161
  measurement of, 221–223, *222*, 222t, *223*
Rheumatoid nodules, in rheumatoid arthritis, 106, 173, *173*
Rheumatoid variants, 309
Richner-Hannert syndrome, 189
Rickettsia rickettsii infections, cutaneous manifestations of, 185, *185*
Rifampicin, drug interactions of, 406
Rifampin, in septic arthritis, 215t
Rigid fixation, debate on, 23
  implants and, 97–98, *98*
Rigidity, in cerebral palsy, 291
Roberts plate, in calcaneovalgus deformity, 655
  in equinus deformity, spastic, 667
Rocker-soled shoes, in post-traumatic ankle pain, 725
Rocky Mountain spotted fever, cutaneous manifestations of, 185, *185*
Rose-Waaler test, 222, 222t
Rubella infections, imaging in, 359, *362*
Rubor, 34
Runners, leg-length inequality in, 87

Salicylates, 408, 409t. See also specific drugs.
  anesthesia and, 468–469
  hepatic function and, 402
  high-dose, 425
  in chronic pain syndrome, 680
  in gout, chronic gouty arthritis and, 149
  in rheumatoid arthritis, 124
  side effects of, 124
Salicylic acid, gastrointestinal function and, 400
Salicylsalicylic acid, 407
Salivary glands, in Sjögren's syndrome, 161
Salmonella infections, arthritis related to, rheumatoid arthritis versus, 113
  in Reiter's syndrome, 132
  septic arthritis and, 209, 215t
Salsalate, 407, 409t
Saphenous nerve entrapment, 696–697
  etiology and specific findings in, 696, *696*
  surgical technique for, 697, *697*

Sarcoidosis, cutaneous manifestations of, 191–192, *192*
Sarcolemma, 66
Sarcomas. See also specific types of sarcomas.
  high-grade, 627
  low-grade, 626–627
  synovial, 636–637
    radiographic appearance of, 335, 337, *337*
Sausage digit, in seronegative spondyloarthropathies, 134
Scarring, in systemic lupus erythematosus, 171, *171*
Schleichender ersatz, 23–24
Schober test, in seronegative spondyloarthropathies, 134
Schwannomas, 636
  benign, radiographic appearance of, 334–335, *336*
  malignant, 637
    radiographic appearance of, 335
Sciatica, in seronegative spondyloarthropathies, 134
Sciatic-femoral nerve block, agents for, 477
Scintigraphy. See *Radionuclide imaging.*
Scleroderma, 155–159, 157t
  classification of, 157t
  clinical features of, 157–159, 158t
  cutaneous manifestations of, 170, *170*
  exercises for, 454t
  functional scale for, 451t
  overlapping pathologic and clinical manifestations of, 166t
  overlapping serologic manifestations of, 167t
  pathology of, 157
  preoperative and postoperative considerations in, 461
  treatment of, 159
Screw fixation, metatarsophalangeal joint arthrodesis and, 553, *554–556*, 557
Secondary bone healing, 16, *16*, 19–20
Sensibility testing, in entrapment syndromes, 687–688, *688*, *689*, 689t
  in plantar digital nerve entrapment, 711
Sensorimotor alterations, following surgery in nerve entrapment syndromes, 695
Sensorimotor neuropathy, in rheumatoid arthritis, 107
Sensory neuropathy, in HIV infection, 303–304
Sensory receptors, 673–674
Sensory tests, in entrapment syndromes, 689t
Septic arthritis, 207–218
  acute, synovial analysis in, 229t
  classification of, by source, 210–211
  clinical presentation of, 207
  diagnosis of, 212–213
    aspiration in, 212, 212t
    laboratory studies in, 212–213
    radiography in, 213
  following glucocorticoid injection therapy, 445
  fungal, 210
  gonococcal, 208–209
  imaging in, 357, *358*, 359, 393–394
  in HIV infection, 304
  mycobacterial, 210
  nongonococcal, 209
  of ankle, arthroscopy in, 624–625
  of foot, imaging and, 315, 317, *318*, 319
  osteomyelitis and, 218
  parasitic, 210
  pathophysiology of, 211–212
  predisposing factors for, 207–208
  spirochetal, 210
  treatment of, 213t, 213–218
    aftercare and, 217–218
    antibiotics in, 214, 214t, 215t

Septic arthritis *(Continued)*
    drainage in, 214, 216t, 216–217
    variables affecting, 214, 216t
  tuberculous, 209
  viral, 210
Seronegative spondyloarthropathies, 132–140.
    See also *Ankylosing spondylitis (AS); Inflammatory bowel disease (IBD); Psoriatic arthritis (PA); Reiter's syndrome (RS).*
  clinical features of, 132–134
  differential diagnosis of, 135–136
  functional scale for, 451t
  HLA measurement in, 226t, 226–227
  imaging in, 135, 309
  laboratory studies in, 134–135
  of foot, imaging and, 310, *313*, 313–314, *314*
  physical findings in, 143
  preoperative and postoperative considerations in, 462
  preoperative evaluation in, 459t
  treatment of, 136
    foot surgery in, 136–140
    pharmacologic, 432
Serotonin, 40
Serpentine, S-shaped foot, 658–659
Serratia infections, septic arthritis and, 208, 215t
Sesamoid bones, 12
  imaging and, 320–321
  stress fracture of, 257
Sesamoiditis, 236–237
Sever's disease. See *Calcaneal apophysitis.*
Sgarlato implant, 524, *524*
Sharpey's fibers, 11
Sheep cell agglutination test, 222, 222t
Shigella infections, arthritis related to, rheumatoid arthritis versus, 113
  in Reiter's syndrome, 132
Shin splints, 85, *248*, 248–249, *249*
Shoes, Bebax, in calcaneovalgus deformity, 654, 654t
  in metatarsus adductus, 660, *661*
  cushioning of, 86, *86*
    in back pain, 89
    in hip pain, 89
    in osteoarthritis of knee, 88–89
  in metatarsus adductus, 661
    Bebax, 660, *661*
  in rheumatoid arthritis, 126–127, *127*
  rocker-soled, in post-traumatic ankle pain, 725
Short leg syndrome, 87
Shortening procedures, in hallux limitus/rigidus, 537, *538*
Short-lever push-off gait, 80–81, *81*
Short-limb gait, 76
Shoulder, in seronegative spondyloarthropathies, 134
  rheumatoid arthritis and, 116
  septic arthritis in, treatment outcome in, 216t
Sicca syndrome. See *Sjögren's syndrome.*
Silicone rubber implants, 96–97
Sinography, *374*, 375
  technique for, 375
Sinus tarsi syndrome, following ankle sprains, 245
Sjögren's sicca complex. See *Sjögren's syndrome.*
Sjögren's syndrome, 161–162
  clinical features of, 161–162, *162*
  cutaneous manifestations of, 177
  HLA measurement in, 227t
  in rheumatoid arthritis, 108
  overlapping pathologic and clinical manifestations of, 166t

Sjögren's syndrome *(Continued)*
overlapping serologic manifestations of, 167t
pathology of, 161
preoperative and postoperative considerations in, 462
treatment of, 162
Skeletal motor testing, in entrapment syndromes, 689
Skin, 169–197. See also specific disorders.
in HIV infection, 304–305
in limited joint mobility, of diabetic foot, 272
in polyarteritis nodosa, 163, *163*
in scleroderma, 156, 157–158, *158*, *159*
in systemic lupus erythematosus, 153, *154*, 154, 155t, 171, *171*
infections of, rheumatoid arthritis and, 122
nonsteroidal anti-inflammatory drugs and, 402
of lower extremity, examination of, 169
rashes and. See *Rash.*
Skin care, in rheumatoid arthritis, 128
Slow-acting antirheumatic drugs (SAARDs), 397
Slow-reacting substance of anaphylaxis (SRS-A), inflammation and, 36
Smoking, limited joint mobility and, of diabetic foot, 272
Sodium bicarbonate, preanesthetic, in gout, 475
Sodium citrate, preanesthetic, in gout, 475
Sodium salicylate, 409t
in rheumatoid arthritis, 124
Sodium urate crystal deposition disease. See *Gout.*
Soft callus stage of fracture healing, 22
Soft tissue disorders, in seronegative spondyloarthropathies, 135
of ankle, 614, 616
radiographic appearance of, 324
Soleus, accessory, imaging of, 391, *391*
Soudre autogene, 22
Spastic flatfoot, peroneal, 81
Spasticity, in cerebral palsy, 291
Spinal cord, interactions within, physiology of pain and, 675
stimulation of, in chronic pain syndrome, 683
Spine, cervical. See *Cervical spine.*
in Reiter's syndrome, 133
Spinothalamic tract, pain and, 675–676
Splay foot, in diabetes mellitus, 278
Splinter hemorrhages, 199, *199*, 199t
Splinting, Ganley, in calcaneovalgus deformity, 654, *655*
in metatarsus adductus, 660
Spondyloarthropathies, rheumatoid arthritis versus, 114
seronegative. See *Ankylosing spondylitis (AS); Inflammatory bowel disease (IBD); Psoriatic arthritis (PA); Reiter's syndrome (RS); Seronegative spondyloarthropathies.*
Spongy bone. See *Cancellous bone.*
Sporothrix infections, septic arthritis and, 210
Sprains, midfoot, 239–240, *240*
of ankle, 243–245, *244*
sequelae of, 245t, 245–246
of metatarsophalangeal joints, first, *237*, 237–238
Squeeze test, lateral, in plantar nerve entrapment, 711
S-shaped foot, 658–659
Stainless steel implants, 96
Stance phase of gait, biomechanics of, 69–70, *70*
double-support phase of, 69
Staphylococcus aureus, in septic arthritis, 215t
osteomyelitis and, 342
septic arthritis and, 208, 209

Staphylococcus epidermidis, cutaneous, in HIV infection, 188
septic arthritis and, 209
Staphylococcus infections, coagulase-negative, in septic arthritis, 215t
groups A and B, in septic arthritis, 215t
septic arthritis and, 218
Steady-state potentials, of bone, 19
Steinmann pins, 552, 562, *563*
Stenosing tenosynovitis (STS), 579–580
etiology of, 582–583
of thumb, 116
treatment of, 581, *582*
Step-down bridge approach, in rheumatoid arthritis, 428–429, *429*
Steppage gait, 77, *77*
Steroid(s). See also specific steroids and types of steroids.
avascular necrosis of bone and, 640
Steroid myopathy, exercises for, 454t
Stevens-Johnson syndrome, 189–190, *190*
''Stone bruise,'' 241
Strains, implants and, 91
muscular, athletic injuries and, 253–255
Streptococcus aureus, in diabetes mellitus, 179
Streptococcus infections, septic arthritis and, 218
Streptomycin, in septic arthritis, 215t
Stress, glucocorticoids and, 440
implants and, 91
Stress fractures, 85–86
athletic injuries and, *255*, 255–257, *256*
imaging in, 386–388, *388*
Stress testing, in ankle sprains, 244
Stress-generated electrical potentials, of bone, 19
Stress-strain curve, 91, 93, *93*, *94*
Stretching exercises, 68
Subchondral bone, anatomy of, 612
Subcutaneous nodules, in erythema nodosum, 190, *191*
Subintima, synovial, 6, *6*, 8
Substance P, peripheral afferents and, 674–675
Substrate phase of wound healing, 52–53
Subtalar joint, arthrodesis of, in calcaneovalgus deformity, 656
surgical anatomy and, 656, *657*
in rheumatoid arthritis, 568–570, *569*, *570*
biomechanics of, gait and, 73–74, *74*
in joint diseases, 80–82, *81*
glucocorticoid injection therapy in, 447–448
posterior, arthrography of, 368, *368–369*
supination of, 74
Subungual melanoma, *196*, 196–197, *197*
Sucralfate, drug interactions of, 404t, 405
gastrointestinal function and, 401
Sulfasalazine, 411t, 423–424
in rheumatoid arthritis, 125, 429–430
in seronegative spondyloarthropathies, 136
Sulfidopeptide leukotrienes, inflammation and, 36
Sulfinpyrazone, 411t, 425
drug interactions of, 408
in gout, 149
Sulfonylureas, drug interactions of, 406
Sulindac, 409t, 412, 413
hepatic function and, 402
in chronic pain syndrome, 681
in gout, acute gouty arthritis and, 148t
Sullivan's sign, in neuroma, 235
Superoxide ions, inflammation and, 36
Supination, of subtalar joint, 74
Suprofen, 415
Sural nerve entrapment, 702–703
etiology and specific findings in, 702, *702*
surgical technique for, 702–703, *703*, *704*

Surgery. See also specific types of surgery and specific procedures.
anesthesia for. See *Anesthesia.*
avascular necrosis of bone following, 646–648, *647*
glucocorticoid therapy and, 441
in Achilles rupture, 246–247
in ankle sprains, 245
in arthropathy, 206
in calcaneovalgus deformity, 656–657
in chronic pain syndrome, 683
in equinus deformity, 666–667
in cerebral palsy, 292, *293*, 294
spastic, 668
in gout, chronic gouty arthritis and, 149
in metatarsus adductus, 661–663
indications for, 661
in neuroarthropathy, of diabetic foot, 267–268
in nonunions, 28
in post-traumatic ankle pain, 725
in rheumatoid arthritis, 128–129
in septic arthritis, treatment outcome with, 216t
in systemic lupus erythematosus, 155
in tendinitis, 581–582, *582*
in tendon dysfunction, 584–586, *585*, *586*
in valgus deformity, 297, 297–298, 298t
perioperative considerations and, 457–463. See also under specific procedures.
in connective tissue disease, 460–462
in crystal-induced arthropathies, 462–463
in infectious arthropathies, 462
in neuroarthropathy, 463
in osteoarthritis, 462
in spondyloarthropathies, 462
in vasculitis, 462
preoperative evaluation and. See *Preoperative evaluation.*
postoperative imaging and, 394
preoperative evaluation and. See *Preoperative evaluation.*
risk of, 457, 458t
septic arthritis induced by, 210
soft tissue tumors and, 630
Surgical drainage, in septic arthritis, 214, 216t, 216–217
Sutures, 1
''Swan-neck'' deformity, rheumatoid arthritis and, 115–116
Swanson double-stemmed hinge implant, 524, *524*
Swanson flexible toe implant, 518–519, *519*
surgical technique for, 521–522
Swelling, inflammation and, 34
Swing phase of gait, 69, *70*
Sympathetic nervous system, Charcot's arthropathy and, 204
Raynaud's phenomenon and, 204
Symphyses, 1, 2
Symptom-modifying antirheumatic drugs (SMARDs), 397, 398t
Synchondroses, 1–2
Syndesmophytes, in seronegative spondyloarthropathies, 135
Syndesmoses, 1
Syngeneic tissue, 23
Syngrafts, 23
Synostoses, 1, 81
Synovectomy, arthroscopy and, of ankle, 617
central metatarsophalangeal joint arthrosis and, 491
Synovial biopsy, 231–232, *232*, 232t
in septic arthritis, 216
Synovial cells, inflammation and, 48
Synovial cysts, in knee, rheumatoid arthritis and, 123

Synovial fluid, 2, *2*, 9
  aspiration of, glucocorticoid injection therapy and, 446–447
  characteristics of, 229t
  differential diagnosis of, by groups, 230t
  functions of, 9
  normal, 231
  of ankle, 613
Synovial fluid analysis, 228–229, 229t, 230t, 231, *231*
  in septic arthritis, 212–213
Synovial impingement syndrome, post-traumatic ankle pain and, 719–720
Synovial joints, 2, *2*, 3–10
  articular cartilage of, 2, *2–4*, 3–5
  discs of, 9–10
  fat pads of, 10
  fluid in. See *Synovial fluid* entries.
  intra-articular folds of, 10
  joint capsule of, 2, *2*, 5
  labra of, 10
  menisci of, 9–10
  superficial zone of, 3
  synovial membrane of, 2, *2*, 5–6, *6–8*, 8–9
  tangential zone of, 3
Synovial membrane, blood supply of, 13
  functions of, 8
  hypertrophy of, septic arthritis and, 211
  of ankle, anatomy of, 613
    disorders of, 614, 616, *616*
  of synovial joints, 2, *2*, 5–6, *6–8*, 8–9
Synovial sarcomas, 636–637
  radiographic appearance of, 335, 337, *337*
Synovial tissues, in rheumatoid arthritis, 104
Synovitis. See also *Tenosynovitis*.
  hypertrophic, post-traumatic ankle pain and, 719
  of ankle, following ankle sprains, 245
    rheumatoid arthritis and, 122
  of metatarsophalangeal joints, pathophysiology of, 481–482
    rheumatoid arthritis and, 120
  villonodular, pigmented, 632–633, *635*
    radiographic appearance of, *338*, 338–339
Syphilis, congenital, imaging in, 359, *361*
  cutaneous manifestations of, 185–186, *186*
  in HIV infection, 305
  septic arthritis and, 210
Systemic lupus erythematosus (SLE), 152–155, *153*, 153t
  antinuclear antibodies in, 224
  clinical features of, 153–154, *154*, 155t, *156*
  cutaneous manifestations of, 170–171, *171*, *172*
  exercises for, 454t
  functional scale for, 451t
  HLA measurement in, 227t
  overlapping pathologic and clinical manifestations of, 166t
  overlapping serologic manifestations of, 167t
  pathology of, 152–153
  preoperative and postoperative considerations in, 461
  synovial analysis in, 229t
  treatment of, 154–155
Systemic sclerosis. See *Scleroderma*.

T lymphocytes, inflammation and, 46–47
Tabes dorsalis, 186
Tailor's bunions, in diabetes mellitus, 278, *278*
Takayasu's arteritis, 164
  HLA measurement in, 227t
Talar dome fractures, post-traumatic ankle pain and, 721

Talar dome lesions, following ankle sprains, 246
Talocalcaneal articulation. See *Subtalar joint*.
Talofibular ligament, sprain of, 243
Talonavicular (TN) joints, arthrodesis of, in rheumatoid arthritis, 567–568, *567–569*
  rheumatoid arthritis and, 118–119, *119*, 120–121
  imaging and, 310, *311*
Talus, fractures of, imaging in, 386
  of lateral process, post-traumatic ankle pain and, 722–723
  of talar neck, avascular necrosis and, 648, *649*
Tarsal coalition, imaging in, 391, *391*
Tarsal navicular stress fractures, 257
Tarsal tunnel syndrome, anterior. See *Peroneal nerve entrapment*.
  medial. See *Tibial nerve entrapment*.
  rheumatoid arthritis and, 121
Tarsometatarsal capsulotomy, Heyman-Herndon, in metatarsus adductus, 663
Tarsometatarsal joint, glucocorticoid injection therapy in, 447
Tarsometatarsal junction, arthrodesis of, in rheumatoid arthritis, 565–566, *566*
Tarsonavicular bone, avascular necrosis of, 649
Technetium-99m methylene diphosphonate (^{99m}Tc-MDP), 351, *352*, *353*
Telos test, in ankle sprains, 244, *244*
Temperature, muscle activity and, 68
Temporal arteritis, 163–164
Temporomandibular joint, airway management and, 479
Tendinitis, 578–582
  classification of, 579–580
  diagnosis of, *580*, 580–581
  etiology of, 578–579
  treatment of, 581–582, *582*
Tendinous xanthomas, 182–183, *183*
Tendon(s), 11, *11*, 577–586
  advancement of, in tendon dysfunction, *585*, 585–586, *586*
  anatomy of, 370–373, *371–373*
  blood supply of, 577, 579
  excision of degenerated portions of, in tendon dysfunction, 585
  healing of, 577–578
  injuries of, imaging in, 388–389, *389*, *390*
  motion of, 577
  of forefoot, 380, *380*, *381*
  of hindfoot, 377, *377*, *378*
  of midfoot, 378–379, *379*
  rupture of, following glucocorticoid injection therapy, 445, 448
    spontaneous, 582
  sesamoid bones in, 12
  structure and function of, 577–578
  xanthomas of, in diabetic foot, 275
Tendon dysfunction, 582–586
  diagnosis of, 583, *584*
  etiology of, 582–583
  treatment of, 583–586, 584t, *585*, *586*
Tendon sheaths, 11–12, *12*
  anatomy of, 370–373, *371–373*
  giant cell tumors of, magnetic resonance imaging and, 628
Tendon transfers, 588–610
  conditions amenable to, 593–596
  for calcaneal deformity, 288–289
  general principles for, 588–591
    muscle and joint mechanics and, 590, *590*
    phasic conversion and, 590–591
  Hibbs tenosuspension procedure and. See *Hibbs tenosuspension procedure*.
  in valgus deformities, 286–287, 297
  in varus deformities, 286, *288*, 296

Tendon transfers *(Continued)*
  Jones tenosuspension. See *Jones tenosuspension*.
  of flexor tendons, central metatarsophalangeal joint arthrosis and, *491*, 491–492
  preoperative evaluation and, 591–593
    electrodiagnostic testing in, 592
    history in, 591, *591*
    physical examination in, 591–592
    radiographic, 592–593, *593*
  surgical techniques for, *596*, 596–597, *598*, *599*
Tenidap sodium, 418
Tenography, 370–373, 371t
  in tendinitis, 580, *580*
  in tendon dysfunction, 583
  technique for, 373
  tendon and tendon sheath anatomy and, 370–373, *371–373*
Tenosynovitis, 578. See also *Tendinitis*.
  chronic, 579
  de Quervain's, 116
  flexor, rheumatoid arthritis and, 115
  of flexor tendons, 372, *373*
  rheumatoid arthritis and, 121
  stenosing, 579–580
    of thumb, 116
Tenoxicam, 417
  drug interactions of, 406
Tensile testing, of implants, 91, 93, *93*, *94*, 94t
Tetany, 66
Tetracaine, 476t
Tetrahydroindoles, 410t
Therapeutic exercises. See *Exercise(s)*.
Thermal nociceptors, 673
Thompson/Doherty test, in Achilles rupture, 246
Thrombin, inflammation and, 41
Thrombocytosis, in rheumatoid arthritis, 110
Thrombophlebitis, in Behçet's syndrome, 164–165
Thrombosis, in rheumatoid arthritis, 106–107, *107*
Thromboxane A$_2$ (TXA$_2$), nonsteroidal anti-inflammatory drugs and, 399, 401
Thumb, "gamekeeper's," 116
  stenosing tenosynovitis of, 116
Thyroid disease, cutaneous manifestations of, *180*, 180–181
Tiaprofenic acid, 415–416
  drug interactions of, 407
Tibia, medial tibial stress syndrome and, 85
  medial torsion of, 663–665
    diagnosis of, 663–664
    treatment of, *664*, 664–665
  stress fracture of, 256
Tibial lip fractures, post-traumatic ankle pain and, 722
Tibial muscle, strain of, 254
Tibial nerve entrapment, 705–706
  etiology of, 703, 705–706, *705*
  surgical treatment of, 706, *707–710*, 708–709
Tibial stress syndrome (TSS), 248, 248–249, *249*
  medial, 85
Tibialis anterior tendon, anatomy of, 372–373
Tibialis anterior tendon transfer, in varus deformity, 296
  split, 597, 599–600
    complications of, 600
    in varus deformity, 296
    indications for, 597
    postoperative care and, 599–600
    technique for, 597, 599–600, *599*
Tibialis posterior tendon, anatomy of, 371–372, *372–373*
  lengthening of, in varus deformity, 296–297

Tibialis posterior tendon *(Continued)*
  tenosynovitis of, rheumatoid arthritis and, 121
Tibialis posterior tendon dysfunction (TPTD),
    582
  etiology of, 582, 583
  stages of, changes associated with, 584, 584t
  treatment of, 583–586, 584t, *585, 586*
Tibialis posterior tendon transfer, 602–605
  complications of, 605, *605*
  indications for, 603
  postoperative care and, 605
  split, 605–606
    in varus deformity, 296
    indications for, 605
    postoperative care and, 606
    technique for, 605–606
  technique for, 603–605, *604*
Tibiofibular joint, proximal, glucocorticoid
    injection therapy in, 448
Tibiofibular ligament impingement,
    anteroinferior, 720
Ticarcillin/clavulanic acid, in septic arthritis,
    215t
Tidemark, of articular cartilage, 28
  of synovial joints, 4, 5
Tinea infections, in diabetes mellitus, 179
Tinel's sign, in entrapment syndromes, 690
Tinnitus, salicylates and, 408, 469
Toes. See *Digit(s).*
Tolmetin, 409t, 413–414
  drug interactions of, 406
  in gout, acute gouty arthritis and, 148t
Tophi, *181,* 181–182, *182,* 431
  gouty, 144–145
Torsional force, 65
Total hinged implants, for forefoot implant
    arthroplasty, 518–522, *519, 520*
Tourniquets, fasciotomy and, 729
Toxic epidermal necrolysis (TEN), 189, 190,
    191
Toygar's angle, in Achilles rupture, 246
Trabecular bone. See *Cancellous bone.*
Tracheostomy, anesthesia and, 479
Transchondral fractures, of ankle, arthroscopy
    and, 619–620
Transchondral tibial impingement, medial, 721–
    722
Transcutaneous electrical nerve stimulation
    (TENS), in chronic pain syndrome, 682
  pain modulation using, 453
Transfusion therapy, anesthesia and, 466
Transitional zone, of growth plate, 16, *16*
  of musculoskeletal tumors, 323, *323*
  of synovial joints, 3
Transverse white bands, 197, *197,* 198t
Trauma. See also *Athletic injuries; Fracture(s);*
    specific injuries.
  arthritis of ankle following, arthroscopy in,
    619–621, *621*
  avascular necrosis of bone following, 648–
    649, *649*
  tendinitis and, 578
Tremor, in cerebral palsy, 291–292
Trendelenburg gait, 76–77, *77*
Treponema pallidum infections. See *Syphilis.*
Triamcinolone, anesthesia and, 472t
  for injection therapy, 443t
    dosage of, 444t
Trichophyton rubrum infections, in HIV
    infection, 305
Tricyclic antidepressants (TCAs), in chronic
    pain syndrome, 682
Trimethoprim-sulfamethoxazole, in septic
    arthritis, 215t
Tuberculous arthritis, 209
Tuberous xanthomas, 183, *183*

Tumor(s). See also specific tumors.
  imaging of, 322–339
    bone marrow, 330–332
    bone-forming, benign, 326–327
      malignant, 325–326
    cartilage-forming, benign, 328–329
      malignant, 327–328
    classification in, 324–325
    eosinophilic granulomas and, 337–338, *338*
    epidermoid cysts and, 333
    fibrocortical defect and, 332–333
    fibromatosis and, 334, *335*
    fibrous dysplasia and, 333, *334*
    general features in, 322–324
      previous biopsy or treatment and, 324
      staging and, 324
    giant cell, 329–330
    lipomas and, 333–334, *334*
    liposarcomas and, 334, *335*
    malignant fibrous histiocytomas and, 335,
      336
    modalities used in, 322
    neurilemomas and, 334–335
    neurofibroma and, 335, *336*
    nonossifying fibroma and, 332–333
    pigmented villonodular synovitis and, *338,*
      338–339
    schwannomas and, 335
    synovial sarcomas and, 335, 337, *337*
    unicameral bone cysts and, 337, *337*
    vascular, 332
  soft tissue, 626–637. See also specific tumors.
    intracapsular excision of, 630
    morphologic features of, magnetic reso-
      nance imaging and, 627t, 627–630,
      629, 728
    staging of, 626–627, 627t
    surgical considerations for, 630
Tumor necrosis factor (TNF), inflammation and,
    38
  wound healing and, 53
Turf toe, *237,* 237–238
Twenty-four-hour urinary uric acid
    measurement, in gout, 147
Twitch, 66
Two-component implants, for forefoot
    arthroplasty, 522–524, *522–524*
Two-point discrimination testing, in entrapment
    syndromes, 688, *689*
Tylosis, 188t, 188–189
Type A lining cells, of synovial membrane, 6, *7,*
    8–9
Type B lining cells, of synovial membrane, 6, 8,
    8

Ulcer(s), buccal, in Behçet's syndrome, *165*
  necrotic, in rheumatoid arthritis, 173, *173*
  of foot, in rheumatoid arthritis, 128, *128*
  oral, in hand-foot-mouth disease, 185, *185*
Ulcerative colitis. See *Inflammatory bowel
    disease (IBD).*
Ultra-high molecular weight polyethylene
    implants, 97
Ultrasonography, 383
  heat therapy using, 452
  in neoplasms and related disorders, 383
  in tendinitis, 580
  in tendon dysfunction, 583
  indications for, 383
  wound healing and, 61
Unicameral bone cyst, radiographic appearance
    of, 337, *337*

University of California Biomechanics
    Laboratory (UCBL) device, in tendon
    dysfunction, 584
  in valgus deformity, 297
Unna's boot dressings, wound healing and, 60
Urethritis, nongonococcal, in Reiter's syndrome,
    132
Uric acid, gout pathophysiology and, 141–143,
    142t
  serum level of, 227
    in gout, 146–147
  24-hour urinary uric acid measurement and,
      in gout, 147
Uricosuric agents, 411t, 425, 427. See also
    specific drugs.
Urinalysis, nonsteroidal anti-inflammatory drugs
    and, 407
Urticarial vasculitis, 174

Valgus deformity, in cerebral palsy, 297–298
    treatment of, *297,* 297–298, 298t
  in paralytic disorders, tendon transfer for,
      286–287
Valleix's points, in entrapment syndromes, 690
Valproic acid, drug interactions of, 407
Vancomycin, in septic arthritis, 215t
Varus deformity, in cerebral palsy, 294–297,
    296
  surgical treatment of, 296–297
  in paralytic disorders, tendon transfer for,
      286, *288*
Vascular disorders, 201–206. See also specific
    disorders.
  in diabetes mellitus, 179, *179*
  in HIV infection, 305
Vascular tumors, leiomyomas and, 634, 636
  radiographic appearance of, 332
Vasculitis, *162,* 162–165, 201–203. See also
    *Behçet's syndrome; Mucocutaneous lymph
    node syndrome; Polyarteritis nodosa;
    Takayasu's arteritis; Temporal arteritis;
    Wegener's granulomatosis.*
  anesthesia and, 465
  clinical features of, 163–165
  cutaneous, in systemic lupus erythematosus,
      154
  hypersensitivity, 164
  immunologic factors in, 201
  in rheumatoid arthritis, 106t, 106–108, *107*
  leukocytoclastic, 164, 174, *174, 175*
  livedo, 173–174
  pathology of, 163
  preoperative and postoperative considerations
      in, 462
  preoperative evaluation in, 459t
  rheumatoid arthritis and, 122
  skin lesions associated with, 202–203
  treatment of, 205
  urticarial, 174
Vasoactive amines, inflammation and, 40
Vasospasm, anesthesia and, 465
Veins, of joints, 13
Velocity, load and, 68
Venography, 375, *375*
Venous insufficiency, chronic, nonhealing
    wounds in, 56–57
Venous ulceration, treatment of, nonhealing
    wounds and, 59–60
Verrucae, in HIV infection, 305
Vincula, 12
Viral infections. See also specific infections.
  imaging in, 359, 362
  of skin, in HIV infection, 305
  septic arthritis and, 210

Viscoelasticity, of implants, 93
Viscous element, 93
Volkmann's contracture, 734–735
    clinical presentation and evaluation of, 734
    management of, conservative, 734–735
        surgical, 735
von Zumbusch's psoriasis, 194, *194*

Waddling gait, 80
Warfarin, drug interactions of, 406
Water content, of articular cartilage, 29
Watermann-Green technique, in hallux limitus/
    rigidus, 539
Watermann-type osteotomy, in hallux limitus/
    rigidus, 538–539, *540*
Wear products, of implants, 95
Weber static two-point discrimination testing, in
    entrapment syndromes, 688, *689*
Wegener's granulomatosis, 163
Weight reduction, in gout, intercritical, 148
Weil design hammertoe implant, 525, *525*
Weinstein-Semmes esthesiometer, in entrapment
    syndromes, 690
Westergren method, for erythrocyte
    sedimentation rate measurement, 220
Wet-to-dry dressing, wound healing and, 60
Wheaton brace, in metatarsus adductus, 660–
    661
Whipple's disease, arthritis related to,
    rheumatoid arthritis versus, 114
    HLA measurement in, 226t

"Whiskering," in seronegative
    spondyloarthropathies, 310, *313*
White blood cell count, in seronegative
    spondyloarthropathies, 135
    in synovial fluid, 231
        septic arthritis and, 212
    indium-111 labeled, 355, *357*
White blood cell trapping theory, 57
White procedure, in equinus deformity, 292,
    293, 294
Whitman plate, in equinus deformity, 667
Wintrobe method, of erythrocyte sedimentation
    rate measurement, 220
Woodruff screw, 553, *554–556*
Wound(s), nonhealing, treatment of, 58–61
        direct care in, 60–61
        evaluation in, 58–59, *59*
        specific, 59–60
Wound contraction, 55
Wound healing, 52–61
    disease states and, 56–58
    in seronegative spondyloarthropathies, 136–
        137
    normal, 52–56
        proliferative phase of, 53–55
        remodeling phase of, 56
        substrate phase of, 52–53
Woven bone, 17
Wright's stain, 135
Wrist, rheumatoid arthritis of, 116, *117*
    septic arthritis of, treatment outcome in, 216t

Xanthelasmas, 183, *184*

Xanthine oxidase inhibitors, 411t, 425–427,
    426, 426t. See also specific drugs.
    in gout, chronic gouty arthritis and, 149
Xanthoma striatum palmare, 183, *184*, 184
Xanthomas, 182–184
    eruptive, 183, *184*
    in diabetic foot, 275
    palmoplantar, 183–184, *184*
    syndromes associated with, 182, 183t
    tendinous, 182–183, *183*
    tuberous, 183, *183*
Xanthomonas maltophilia infections, septic
    arthritis and, 215t
Xenogeneic tissue, 23
Xenografts, 23
Xerostomia. See *Sjögren's syndrome.*

Yellow nail syndrome, 199, *199*
Yersinia infections, arthritis related to,
    rheumatoid arthritis versus, 113
    in Reiter's syndrome, 132
    Yersinia enterocolitica, arthritis related to,
        rheumatoid arthritis versus, 114

Zero-order release acetylsalicylic acid, 409t
Zidovudine (AZT), in HIV infection, 302
Zomepirac, anaphylaxis induced by, 402–403
Zomepirac acid, 413
Zone of hypertrophy, of growth plate, 16, *16*
Zone of proliferating cells, of growth plate, 16,
    16

ISBN 0-7216-3716-7

1039877

GWUMC
P16MGZ